Manic-Depressive Illness

Collaborators

S. Nassir Ghaemi, M.D., M.P.H.
Associate Professor of Psychiatry and Public Health
Emory University

Constance Hammen, Ph.D.
Professor of Psychology and Psychiatry
University of California, Los Angeles

Terence A. Ketter, M.D.
Professor of Psychiatry
Stanford University School of Medicine

Husseini K. Manji, M.D., FRCPC
Director, Mood and Anxiety Disorders Program
National Institute of Mental Health

Francis M. Mondimore, M.D.
Assistant Professor of Psychiatry
The Johns Hopkins University School of Medicine

James B. Potash, M.D., M.P.H.
Associate Professor of Psychiatry
The Johns Hopkins University School of Medicine

Harold A. Sackeim, Ph.D.
Professor of Psychiatry and Radiology
College of Physicians and Surgeons of Columbia University

Myrna M. Weissman, Ph.D.
Professor of Epidemiology in Psychiatry
College of Physicians and Surgeons of Columbia University

AND

Hagop S. Akiskal, M.D.
Professor of Psychiatry
University of California, San Diego

Gabrielle A. Carlson, M.D.
Professor of Psychiatry and Pediatrics
Stony Brook University School of Medicine

Miriam Davis, Ph.D.
Adjunct Assistant Professor of Epidemiology
  and Biostatistics (as of 2006)
The George Washington University School of Public Health
  and Health Services

J. Raymond DePaulo, Jr., M.D.
Professor of Psychiatry
The Johns Hopkins University School of Medicine

Jan Fawcett, M.D.
Professor of Psychiatry
University of New Mexico School of Medicine

Daniel Z. Lieberman, M.D.
Associate Professor of Psychiatry
The George Washington University Medical Center

Teodor T. Postolache, M.D.
Associate Professor of Psychiatry
University of Maryland School of Medicine

SECOND EDITION

MANIC-DEPRESSIVE ILLNESS
Bipolar Disorders and Recurrent Depression

FREDERICK K. GOODWIN, M.D.
Professor of Psychiatry
The George Washington University Medical Center

KAY REDFIELD JAMISON, PH.D.
Professor of Psychiatry
The Johns Hopkins University School of Medicine

OXFORD
UNIVERSITY PRESS

2007

OXFORD
UNIVERSITY PRESS

Oxford University Press, Inc., publishes works that further
Oxford University's objective of excellence
in research, scholarship, and education.

Oxford   New York
Auckland   Cape Town   Dar es Salaam   Hong Kong   Karachi
Kuala Lumpur   Madrid   Melbourne   Mexico City   Nairobi
New Delhi   Shanghai   Taipei   Toronto

With offices in
Argentina   Austria   Brazil   Chile   Czech Republic   France   Greece
Guatemala   Hungary   Italy   Japan   Poland   Portugal   Singapore
South Korea   Switzerland   Thailand   Turkey   Ukraine   Vietnam

Published by Oxford University Press, Inc.
198 Madison Avenue, New York, New York 10016

www.oup.com

Oxford is a registered trademark of Oxford University Press

Library of Congress Cataloging-in-Publication Data
Goodwin, Frederick K., 1936–
Manic-depressive illness : bipolar disorders and recurrent depression / Frederick
K. Goodwin, Kay Redfield Jamison ; with Nassir Ghaemi . . . [et al.]. —
2nd ed.
p. ; cm.
Includes bibliographical references and index.
ISBN-13: 978-0-19-513579-4
1. Manic-depressive illness.   I. Jamison, Kay R.   II. Ghaemi, S.
Nassir.   III. Title.
[DNLM: 1. Bipolar Disorder.   WM 207 G656m 2007]
RC516.G66 2007
616.89'5—dc22   2006026791

Please visit this volume's companion Web site at
www.oup.com/us/manicdepressiveillness2e

Citation to this volume should be given in the following way: Goodwin, F. K., and Jamison,
K.R. (2007). *Manic-Depressive Illness: Bipolar Disorders and Recurrent Depression,*
2nd edition. New York: Oxford University Press.

9 8 7 6 5 4 3 2

Printed in the United States of America
on acid-free paper

The original version of this book, published in 1990, was a unique contribution to the literature on manic-depressive illness. For a long time, certainly since Bleuler and Schneider developed broad criteria for schizophrenia, manic-depressive illness had been neglected both as a clinical diagnosis and as a topic for research. The influence of psychoanalysis and Meyer's psychobiology exacerbated this neglect. Meaningful attention to the illness began to increase with the discovery of lithium as a surprisingly effective treatment for mania (this book is very appropriately dedicated to John Cade and Mogens Schou). But it was Goodwin and Jamison's work, coming at a time when manic-depressive illness remained curiously marginalized in the scientific literature, that gave the subject the treatment it deserved. Remarkably, their text was lengthy enough to allow detailed accounts and comprehensive summaries of all the available literature while at the same time being accessible in style and presentation, with an authentic continuity in the voice of its two authors.

Kay Jamison and Fred Goodwin are, of course, giants in this field, and their contribution seemed even then a remarkable one: Jamison for her profound clinical and psychological understanding, and Goodwin for his immense pharmacological and biological knowledge. To attempt a repeat of their efforts in a new edition was an enormous challenge, especially since the rapid expansion of scientific and clinical information that has occurred in the last 20 years has made the single- or dual-author textbook an increasingly endangered species. The authors' solution for this new edition of *Manic-Depressive Illness* is an innovative one that works exceedingly well: by enlisting the help of close colleagues with various specialized interests and producing an interpretive synthesis of those views through the filter of their own unparalleled expertise, they have avoided creating a compilation of chapters written by individual authors and preserved the unity and structure of the original work.

The book is divided into five parts covering the diagnosis, clinical characteristics, psychology, pathophysiology, and treatment of manic-depressive illness. It is an exceptional record of the current state of the art, and we are confident that it will satisfy the most discriminating readers, from those who simply want to acquaint themselves with a single aspect of the illness and its many manifestations to those who wish to use this text as the basis for a comprehensive understanding of the subject.

A number of key differences between this and the first edition of the book deserve to be highlighted. The discussion of the spectrum diagnoses has been greatly expanded and informed by an increase in empirical work on the topic: diagnoses such as bipolar-II were not as commonly accepted prior to the publication of the *Diagnostic and Statistical Manual*, 4th edition (DSM-IV) in 1994, and the previously underappreciated topic of mixed states, especially depressive mixed states, is now properly included. Phenomenological studies of manic-depressive illness in children, women, and the elderly are now examined. The chapter on course of illness incorporates some major new outcome studies that began in the 1990s and have since expanded. The treatment chapters are, inevitably, greatly expanded to review the literature on benchmark therapies such as electroconvulsive therapy and lithium, as well as to accommodate the new literature on atypical antipsychotics, novel anticonvulsants, antidepressants, and structured psychosocial interventions. These chapters are also preceded by a discussion of the research methods now needed to evaluate increasingly complex clinical trials. Studies of molecular genetics, second messenger and intracellular mechanisms, and functional imaging were just starting two decades ago, but are quite central now. Even the historical assessment of how the illness was understood in previous eras is being revised on the basis of new evidence discussed in this edition.

The title of the second edition remains *Manic-Depressive Illness*, with the addition of a subtitle, *Bipolar Disorders and Recurrent Depression*. As in the first edition, the main emphasis is on the inclusive Kraepelinian concept of manic-depressive illness, a perspective too easily lost within the post–DSM-III nosology of mood disorders. This second edition underlines how Kraepelin's "central insight—that all of the recurrent major mood disorders (in today's terms) belonged together under the rubric of *manic-depressive illness*—still provides the best model for what we know to date, as well as for understanding emerging clinical, pharmacological, and genetic data."

We have no doubt that this second edition of *Manic-Depressive Illness*, like the first, will have an immense impact on the field; it will be a great resource for research, and it will help improve diagnosis and treatment of those who suffer from the illness. While the volume of new work it describes is encouraging, however, manic-depressive illness remains a much lower public health priority than schizophrenia and depression, not to mention many physical conditions, as evidenced by the relative paucity of research funds devoted to its study. Hence this second edition

can help us all in an important additional task: to promote awareness and investment of both time and money in this major illness by the best and brightest around the world. As Kraepelin said, "What goal could be more sacred than that of caring for a brother in distress, especially when the affliction stems from his very humanity . . . and when it cannot be halted by reason, rank or riches?"[1]

GUY GOODWIN, M.D.
Oxford

ATHANASIOS KOUKOPOULOS, M.D.
Rome

---

[1] Emil Kraepelin, quoting Anton Mueller, in *Hundert Jahre Psychiatrie* (Berlin: Verlag von Julius Springer, 1918), p. 112.

ACKNOWLEDGMENTS

Without the sustained commitment and clinical and scientific expertise of our collaborators, whose names appear opposite the title page, there would be no second edition of *Manic-Depressive Illness*. We are immensely indebted to them for their time and scholarship. The collaborators' individual contributions ranged from a slight to substantial updating of a first-edition chapter (retaining the original organization and most of the original material) to, in a few instances, the drafting of an entirely new chapter; most contributions fell somewhere in between. They followed general guidelines formulated by us, including our specifications about the conceptualization and usage of the terms *manic-depressive illness* and *bipolar disorder*, the critical need for rigorous and impartial review, and the shared goal of contributing to a book that would maintain the unified authorship voice of the first edition. There was extensive interaction between us and our collaborators throughout, with many drafts of each chapter going back and forth.

In each case the last draft provided to us by a collaborator was revised and updated, usually extensively, by one or both of us. When our judgment about a specific clinical or scientific point differed from that of a collaborator, which was not infrequently the case, we carefully considered the collaborator's point of view before making a final decision. In the end, the two authors take responsibility for the contents of the book.

The collaborators would like to acknowledge the contributions of Po Wang and John Brooks (Dr. Ketter); Susan Bachus, Lisa Catapano, Guang Chen, Jing Du, Holly A. Giesen, Fatemi Hosein, Libby Jolkovsky, Celia Knobelsdorf, Phillip Kronstein, Rodrigo Machado-Vieira, Andrew Newberg, Jennifer Payne, Jorge Quiroz, Giacomo Salvadore, Peter J. Schmidt, Jaskaran Singh, and Carlos A. Zarate, Jr. (Dr. Manji); Al Lewy, Joseph Soriano, John Stiller, Leonardo Tonelli, and Thomas Wehr (Dr. Postolache); Gregory Fuller (Dr. Potash); Rice Fuller (Dr. Sackeim); and Helena Verdeli (Dr. Weissman). Drs. Goodwin and Jamison would like to acknowledge additional colleagues who reviewed chapters or otherwise provided input: Jules Angst, Ross Baldessarini, Robert Belmaker, Charles Bowden, Joseph Calabrese, Kiki Chang, Guy Goodwin, Heinz Grunze, Dean Jamison, Athanasios Koukopoulos, Andreas Marneros, Roger Meyer, Gary Sachs, Mauricio Tohen, Eduardo Vieta, Jeremy Waletzky, and Peter Whybrow.

Dr. Goodwin's two research assistants, Mark Goldstein and Jaclyn Saggese Fleming, worked full time on this book and were essential to its production, Mr. Goldstein during the critical first two years of the project and Mrs. Fleming during the final three. Not only were they responsible for many of the literature searches and the preparation of tables and figures, they also often went beyond that, preparing summaries of critical areas of research. During the final two years in particular, Mrs. Fleming was the indispensable hub of the whole operation, coordinating the work of both the authors, the input from all of our collaborators, the work of our chief medical editor, and the editorial and production staff at Oxford University Press. She did this with a rare combination of intelligence, care and thoroughness, organization, blinding speed, and good humor. The ability of Mr. Goldstein and Mrs. Fleming to perform at such a high level is consistent with their career trajectories—Mr. Goldstein is already in medical school and Mrs. Fleming is in a post-baccalaureate biology program.

Dr. Goodwin is further indebted to his executive assistant, Joanne Davis, for facilitating his work on this book by skillfully keeping other aspects of his professional life on track. Dr. Goodwin would also like to acknowledge his first mentor, William E. Bunney, Jr., M.D., and his long-term colleague Dennis Murphy, M.D., who together contributed so much to the emergence of manic-depressive illness as a major focus of research at the National Institute of Mental Health. He would also like to thank the George Washington University Medical Center's Department of Psychiatry and Behavioral Sciences and its chairman, Jeffrey Akman, M.D., for support. Finally, the unceasing encouragement and support of Rosemary Goodwin, M.S.W., has been, as always, a mainstay.

Dr. Jamison would like to acknowledge the invaluable contributions of Silas Jones, William Collins, and Ioline Henter. It has been a delight to work with them and it would have been impossible to complete this book without their help. She would also like to acknowledge the support of her colleagues in the Department of Psychiatry at the Johns Hopkins School of Medicine. Adam Kaplin, M.D., Ph.D., has been particularly helpful and generous with his time. Most deeply she would like to extend her heartfelt appreciation to her psychiatrist, Daniel Auerbach, M.D., who not only taught her how to live with manic-depressive illness but also encouraged her to study and write about it. His profound clinical understanding of the medical and psychological aspects of bipolar disorder were life saving; they have also strongly influenced her research, clinical practice, and writing. She owes a deep debt as well to her late husband, Richard Wyatt, M.D. He too encouraged her to write about manic-depressive illness, from both a clinical and personal perspective, and provided the kind of love and support that made it possible. He was a wonderful husband, colleague, and friend.

It is impossible to overstate the contribution of our medical editor, Rona Briere. Her consummate editing abilities, coupled with an extraordinary level of professionalism and intellectual integrity, made working with her both an education and a pleasure. Alisa Decatur meticulously prepared the manuscript of each chapter, tracked and reconciled the text citations and reference lists, edited the references, and performed numerous additional tasks that were invaluable in finalizing the book. Deb Uffelman and Gerald Briere assisted with proofreading and preparation of the reference lists. We are also grateful to Marion Osmun, Nancy Wolitzer, and Sarah Harrington at Oxford University Press for their dedication, skill, and

impressive ability to implement and meet near-impossible deadlines.

During the time that this book was in preparation, Dr. Goodwin received research support from George Washington University Medical Center, the Foundation for Education and Research on Mental Illness, the Dalio Family Foundation, GlaxoSmithKline, Pfizer, Eli Lilly, and Solvay. He has received honoraria from GlaxoSmithKline, Pfizer, Solvay, and Eli Lilly and unrestricted educational grants to support the production of this book from Abbott, AstraZeneca, Bristol Meyers Squibb, Forest, GlaxoSmithKline, Janssen, Eli Lilly, Pfizer, and Sanofi. Dr. Goodwin has been a consultant and/or advisor for Eli Lilly, GlaxoSmithKline, Pfizer, Janssen, Novartis, and Solvay. He is not a shareholder in any pharmaceutical or biotechnology company. He is a partner in Best Practice Project Management, Inc.

Dr. Jamison, as a MacArthur fellow, received generous financial support from the John D. and Catherine T. MacArthur Foundation, as well as funding from the Dana Foundation. She has received occasional lecture honoraria from AstraZeneca, GlaxoSmithKline, and Eli Lilly. She has received no research support from any pharmaceutical or biotechnology company, nor is she a consultant to, or shareholder in, any pharmaceutical or biotechnology company. As with the first edition of this text, all of her royalties go directly to a not-for-profit foundation that supports public education about manic-depressive illness.

F.K.G. AND K.R.J.

Contents

Melancholia is the beginning and a part of mania . . . . The development of a mania is really a worsening of the disease (melancholia) rather than a change into another disease.

—Aretaeus of Cappadocia, ca. 100 AD[1]

It has been 17 years since the publication of the first edition of this text; they have been the most explosively productive years in the history of medical science. In every field relevant to our understanding of manic-depressive illness—genetics, neurobiology, psychology and neuropsychology, neuroanatomy, diagnosis, and treatment—we have gained a staggering amount of knowledge. Scientists and clinicians have gone an impressive distance toward fulfilling the hopes articulated by Emil Kraepelin in the introduction to his 1899 textbook on psychiatry. Those who treat and study mental illness, he wrote, must first, from bedside observation, delineate the clinical forms of illness; they must define and predict its course, determine its causes, and discover how best to treat and then ultimately prevent insanity. Psychiatry, he argued, was a "young, still developing science," and it must, "against sharp opposition, gradually achieve the position it deserves according to its scientific and practical importance. There is no doubt that it will achieve the position—for it has at its disposal the same weapons which have served the other branches of medicine so well: clinical observation, the microscope and experimentation."[2] Kraepelin was right, as usual. And he was remarkably astute in his observations and predictions about the immensely complex group of disorders collectively known as manic-depressive illness.

Manic-depressive illness magnifies common human experiences to larger-than-life proportions. Among its symptoms are exaggerations of normal sadness and joy, profoundly altered thinking, irritability and rage, psychosis and violence, and deeply disrupted patterns of energy and sleep. In its diverse forms, manic-depressive illness afflicts a large number of people—the exact number depending on how the illness is defined and how accurately it is ascertained. First described thousands of years ago, found in widely diverse cultures, manic-depressive illness always has fascinated medical observers, even as it has baffled and frightened most others. To those afflicted, it can be so painful that suicide seems the only means of escape; indeed, manic-depressive illness is the most common cause of suicide.

We view manic-depressive illness as a medical condition, an illness to be diagnosed, treated, studied, and understood within a medical context. This position is the prevailing one now, as it has been throughout history. Less universal is our diagnostic conception of manic-depressive illness, which evolved as we were writing both editions of this book. Derived from the work of Kraepelin, the "great classifier," our conception encompasses roughly the same group of disorders as the term *manic–depressive illness* in European usage. It differs, however, from contemporary concepts of bipolar disorder. Kraepelin built his observations on the work of a small group of nineteenth-century European psychiatrists who, in their passion for ever finer distinctions, had cataloged abnormal human behavior into hundreds of classes of disorder. More than any other single individual, Kraepelin brought order and sense to this categorical profusion. He constructed a nosology based on careful description, reducing the categories of psychoses to two: manic-depressive illness and dementia praecox, later renamed *schizophrenia*.

It is to Kraepelin, born in the same year as Freud, that we owe much of our conceptualization of manic-depressive illness. It is to him that we owe our emphasis on documenting the longitudinal course of the illness and the careful delineation of mixed states and the stages of mania, as well as the observations that cycle length shortens with succeeding episodes; that poor clinical outcome is associated with rapid cycles, mixed states, and coexisting substance abuse; that genetics is central to the pathophysiology of the disease; and that manic-depressive illness is a spectrum of conditions and related temperaments.

Kraepelin's model consolidated most of the major affective disorders into one category because of their similarity in core symptoms; presence of a family history of illness; and, especially, the pattern of recurrence over the course of the patient's lifetime, with periods of remission and exacerbation and a comparatively benign outcome without significant deterioration. Kraepelin viewed mania as one manifestation of the illness, not as the distinguishing sign of a separate bipolar disorder as it is regarded in today's American (and increasingly worldwide) diagnostic practice.

The European and American concepts of manic-depressive illness began to diverge almost immediately after Kraepelin's ideas became widespread in the early years of the twentieth century. Europeans, adhering to a traditional medical disease model, emphasized the longitudinal course of the illness in both research and clinical work. Ever pragmatic, Americans wanted to treat the illness with the techniques at hand, which at that time were derived from the "moral treatment" movement in mental hospitals and the emerging dynamic therapies based on psychoanalytic theory. Research and clinical efforts in the United States thus slighted clinical description and genetics and turned instead to the psychological and social contexts in which the symptoms of the illness occurred.

Exploration of the linkages between clinical typology and family history led to the formulation of the bipolar–unipolar distinction, by which manic-depressive patients were grouped according to the presence or absence of a prior history of mania or hypomania. First proposed by a German, Karl Leonhard, the distinction was elaborated by other Europeans, such as Jules Angst and Carlo Perris, and by the Washington University group in St. Louis, Missouri, the neo-Kraepelinians who gave impetus to the new concern for an etiology-free, description-based diagnostic system in the United States.

The bipolar–unipolar distinction represented a logical refinement of the already well-defined Kraepelinian model, with its emphasis on recurrence and endogeneity. As useful as the distinction is in both research and clinical contexts, it proved to be problematic when applied to the much broader American conception of affective disorders. The bipolar subgroup was clearly defined, but the other component of Kraepelinian manic-depressive illness—endogenous, recurrent unipolar depression—was obscured by its confusion with other affective disorders. In American usage, *unipolar* disorder came to mean any mood disorder that was not bipolar, regardless of its severity or course. Although the third edition of the *Diagnostic and Statistical Manual* (DSM-III) clarified the situation somewhat by requiring that criteria for major affective disorder be met before the bipolar–unipolar distinction is drawn, a diagnosis of unipolar disorder was still broader than the Kraepelinian concept since it did not require a prior course of illness. Even the DSM-III/IV category of

recurrent depression is overly broad, requiring only two episodes in a lifetime.

Our own struggle to confine and limit the focus of the first edition of this text followed a course similar to the larger historical one. We started with a framework of Kraepelinian manic-depressive illness, that is, recurrent major affective illness with and without mania. Later, we focused more exclusively on bipolar disorder as a way of imposing workable boundaries on the scope of our efforts. Once thoroughly immersed in the subject, however, we became increasingly convinced that isolating bipolar disorder from other major depressive disorders and unduly emphasizing polarity over cyclicity (as do DSM-III and DSM-IV) prejudges the relationships between bipolar and unipolar illness and diminishes appreciation of the fundamental importance of recurrence. By the end, we had returned to a position close to where we began, convinced of the value of the original unified concept of manic-depressive illness, albeit with a special emphasis on the bipolar form. Scientific and clinical advances of the past two decades have only added to the strength of our belief that, as important as polarity is, cyclicity or recurrence is fundamental to understanding manic-depressive illness. This conviction is made clear in the second edition's new title: *Manic Depressive Illness: Bipolar Disorders and Recurrent Depression*. Genetic findings will have the ultimate etiologic and diagnostic say, of course, but in the interim we think a broader rather than narrower concept of the illness is warranted by the data; we also think it is heuristically most valuable.

DIMENSIONS OF THE ILLNESS

It bears repeating that the presence or absence of mania in addition to depression is but one critical aspect of manic-depressive illness. The other is cyclicity, which may ultimately prove to be as useful as polarity in differentiating forms of affective illness. The classic European focus on longitudinal studies has provided an ample database for redirecting the emphasis of pathophysiology to mechanisms of cyclicity— that is, the biology of recurrence. To conduct such research, an investigator must analyze each patient's biological functioning over time and relate it to the natural course of illness. The priority that American clinicians are beginning to assign to recurrence is a tribute to the persuasiveness of our European colleagues' meticulous longitudinal clinical observations. Kraepelin's descriptions have been enduring: again and again during our study of the contemporary literature, we returned to his original writings to rediscover modern ideas. To a remarkable degree, his work anticipated, explicitly and implicitly, contemporary theoretical developments. One example is the spectrum concept—the continuity of manic-depressive symptoms with normal fluctuations in mood, energy patterns, and behavior—a concept whose database has greatly expanded since the publication of the first edition.

The longitudinal view provided by Kraepelin and many others both before and since persuaded us to survey the literature on recurrent unipolar illness along with that on bipolar illness, our primary focus. If we had confined ourselves to the bipolar literature, we would have excluded many potentially relevant data and insights. This recognition of the essential unity of major recurrent affective illness is evident throughout the book. When discussing lithium prophylaxis in Chapter 20, for example, we point out that similarities between recurrent unipolar and bipolar illness constitute firm ground for speculating about common neurobiological substrates.

The issue of cyclicity opens up many new areas of inquiry. Manic and depressive episodes can be predicted to revert to normal at some finite time, either spontaneously or in response to effective treatment. The opportunity to compare biological measures during the illness with the same measures in the recovered state is essential in psychobiological research, since it permits longitudinal studies that can circumvent the problem of variability among individuals. The recurrent pattern of the illness—that of recovery to normal or change to an opposite state—makes it an unsurpassed paradigm for separating state and trait variables in mental illness. The regularity of recurrence in some patients permits the clinical investigator to anticipate the onset of an episode and thus to schedule data collection at critical points. The frequent rapidity of the switch from one state to another, especially the switch into mania, allows for intensive efforts to understand the relationships between stress and biological changes in the onset of illness by looking at the temporal sequence of events—one approach to the ultimate question of causality.

The bipolar form of the illness also is an interesting study in the coexistence of opposites or, more precisely, deviations from normal in opposite directions. Even lay observers may recognize that bipolar disorder is at times accompanied by periods of euphoric mood, productivity, and high energy, but at other times by despair and profound lassitude. Clinicians see a more subtle manifestation of this Janus-like illness in lithium's effects in preventing its apparently opposite expressions. Lithium's dual action, perhaps diminishing some of the silver lining along with the cloud, challenges the clinician's psychotherapeutic skills in managing the issue of treatment acceptance, especially medication adherence.

THE SCIENCE OF THE ILLNESS

Over the past six decades, research has yielded effective treatments that have radically altered clinical work in manic-depressive illness. Principally, it was the discovery of lithium that galvanized the treatment community, instilling new hope among clinicians, their patients, and the public. Also important, the emergence of lithium, the antidepressants, the antipsychotics, and the anticonvulsants gave birth to whole new fields of scientific investigation. Studies of the illness have dominated biological psychiatry, which itself has begun to lead the profession. Manic-depressive illness has been an increasingly important focus of work in other disciplines as well. Insights gained from the study of an illness that is biological in origin yet psychological in expression have underscored the urgency and inevitability of paradigms of mental illness that give balanced attention to biology, psychology, and the environment. Methodologies developed expressly for studies of manic-depressive illness have been incorporated as standard tools of clinical investigation in other areas of biomedical and behavioral research in psychopathology. Because symptoms of the illness shade over into normal human experience, it provides a model for the study of normal states as well.

Nearly 60 years have passed since the initial clinical observation of lithium's effectiveness in treating manic-depressive illness and 50 years since early clinical trials—most important, those completed by Mogens Schou, Poul Christian Baastrup, G. P. Hartigan, and Alec Coppen—were conducted so that lithium could be approved for general clinical use throughout the world. More recently, research on manic-depressive illness has played a central role in efforts to apply new and emerging techniques, such as molecular genetics, to the study of psychiatric conditions. The application of these techniques depends on the use of sensitive and reliable epidemiological and diagnostic case-finding methodologies to identify family pedigrees with a high incidence of the illness. Preliminary results suggest that several genotypes underlie different forms of manic-depressive illness. It is also possible that, as with the multiple genetic forms of diabetes, several genotypes are expressed in clinical phenomena commonly associated with the illness.

Research on manic-depressive illness also has contributed new, empirically based theories about the pathophysiology of psychiatric disorders, including the influence of the physical environment—light and temperature in particular—on their course and expression. Of equal interest are efforts to describe mechanisms by which the psychosocial environment interacts with the individual's biology to produce symptoms. One of the most promising lines of inquiry grew out of longitudinal observations: external stress appeared to activate or precipitate some initial episodes of illness, but eventually the illness seemed to take on a life of its own, since later episodes began without obvious precipitating stress.

OVERVIEW OF THIS TEXT

In a text of this size and scope, a certain amount of redundancy is inevitable. Issues pertaining to the dimensional aspects of manic-depressive illness, such as severity, polarity, and cyclicity, are introduced in the first two chapters and then discussed further throughout the book. Where an issue could logically be discussed in more than one chapter, our decisions on placement occasionally were somewhat arbitrary.

Clinical Description and Diagnosis

The text is divided into five parts, the first of which focuses on clinical phenomenology and diagnosis. Chapter 1 traces the evolution of the concept of the illness, which has remained remarkably consistent since the time of Hippocrates, and describes the spectrum of the illness in detail. We highlight the fact that diagnostic and subgroup boundaries represent somewhat arbitrary distinctions, with individual patients often falling in a gray area. Also emphasized is the spectrum of manic states, which, unlike the well-described depressive spectrum, is often overlooked. We stress that while the spectrum concept has validity and utility, there are risks in subclassifying the bipolar forms of the illness to such an extent that they are confusing, on occasion to the detriment of both clinical and research purposes.

We begin the chapter on clinical description (Chapter 2) with classic descriptions of the illness by early clinical observers who worked in the era before effective medications altered the natural expression of the illness; these are followed by patients' descriptions of their experiences of the illness. We also review data-based studies of mania, mixed states, and bipolar depression, with a particular emphasis on new research findings pertaining to mixed states and bipolar depression.

Chapter 3 guides the clinician through the problems of diagnosis. Most important is the differential diagnosis of bipolar disorder and unipolar depression, schizophrenia, organic brain disorders, substance abuse, and borderline personality disorders. The shortcomings of our current diagnostic systems, including their emphasis on polarity rather than cyclicity, the absence of a category for highly recurrent depression, the underrecognition of bipolar-II disorder, and the inadequacy of the diagnostic criteria for mixed states, are discussed in detail.

Clinical Studies

The second part covers various clinical aspects of manic-depressive illness. Appropriately, we begin in Chapter 4 with a discussion of course and outcome, fundamental characteristics of the illness that provide the basis for differentiating it from schizophrenia. In addition to its obvious importance for clinicians who are assessing prognosis and planning treatment, natural course is important to scientists since it offers many useful clues as to pathological processes. We consider historical observations on course and outcome together with data gathered from the large-scale studies conducted since the first edition of this text.

Chapter 5, on epidemiology, argues that manic-depressive illness, especially its bipolar form, is more common than is usually thought. Among the most important recent observations are the early age at onset documented in careful community surveys; determinations of the rates of bipolar-II and bipolar spectrum disorders; and the results of several important international studies, including those of death and disability, that document the high toll exacted by manic-depressive illness worldwide.

The next three chapters highlight special clinical aspects of manic-depressive illness. Chapter 6 addresses aspects of the illness in children and adolescents. Because there are essentially no data on highly recurrent depression in these populations, the chapter focuses exclusively on bipolar disorder, which all too often goes unrecognized in youth. Although relatively rare in prepubertal children, classic bipolar disorder often begins in adolescence; indeed, well over one-third of all cases begin before the age of 20. Were the kindling hypothesis substantiated, early recognition and immediate, vigorous treatment would be expected to reduce subsequent pathology. Early treatment would reduce the psychological scarring caused by untreated illness, as well as the high mortality rate from suicide, which is disproportionately likely to occur early in the course of bipolar disorder. All too typical is the individual, initially treated in his or her mid- to late twenties, who has already lived with the disorder for more than a decade, a period critical for life's major beginnings in relationships, education, and career. The research findings on childhood bipolar disorder published since the first edition of this text have been prodigious, but continue to be marked by confusion and controversy. Even so, many more young children with severe mood lability and behavioral dyscontrol are now being identified and treated with mood stabilizers, antipsychotics, and antidepressants.

A focus on the young highlights the frequent coexistence of drug and alcohol abuse among young manic-depressive patients. Growing recognition of the frequent coexistence of the illness with substance abuse prompted us to devote an entire chapter (Chapter 7) to describing these problems and another (Chapter 24) to reviewing their treatment. In these two chapters, we also discuss other important comorbid conditions, such as anxiety disorders, eating disorders, cardiovascular disease, thyroid dysfunction, overweight and obesity, and migraine, as well as their treatment. The presence of a depressive or anxiety disorder can double the chances of subsequent substance abuse. Conversely, illicit drugs and alcohol can adversely affect the course and treatment of manic-depressive illness by altering the same brain mechanisms that regulate mood, including the potential for kindling.

As with substance abuse and other comorbid conditions, the importance of suicide in manic-depressive illness is reflected in our devoting two chapters to the subject—one describing rates, putative causes, and clinical correlates (Chapter 8), and another detailing preventive measures (Chapter 25). The high mortality associated with this illness cannot be overemphasized. Fortunately, considerable progress has been made in understanding the causes of suicide in manic-depressive patients, in addition to the accumulating evidence that lithium exerts a strong protective influence.

The reader may note that there is no chapter on gender differences in manic-depressive illness, reflecting the relative scarcity of literature on this subject. However, reports of male–female differences are noted throughout the book; here we summarize those for which there is general agreement: the first episode is more likely to be mania in males and depression in females, while women have more mixed episodes (consistent with a predominance of depression) and are overrepresented among rapid cyclers; consistent with the general population, men are more likely to have comorbid substance abuse and histories of pathological gambling and conduct disorder, while women are more likely to have comorbid eating disorders as well as changes in appetite and weight during depressive episodes; and, in contrast to the general population, the completed suicide rate for bipolar women is higher than that for bipolar men. It may be that the risk of suicide associated with manic-depressive illness is so powerful that it overrides the usual male–female patterns. Bipolar women generally are more likely than their male counterparts to seek treatment, but there is as yet no consensus regarding gender differences in response to mood stabilizers.[3]

Psychological Studies

Manic-depressive illness has been a rich source of theory and data for investigators interested in psychological mechanisms. The third part of the book considers these developments. Manic-depressive illness has contributed to the general study of psychology by serving as a paradigm for explorations of state and trait differences. It also has been a model for the general psychological assessment of cognition and for the more specific differentiation of cognition in manic and depressive states from that in schizophrenia. We begin with a survey of what is known about neuropsychological deficits in mood disorders, including recent research documenting significant impairments in intellec-

tual functioning, attention, learning and memory, and executive functioning (Chapter 9).

The psychological manifestations of manic-depressive illness, observable in personality and behavior as well as cognitive patterns, can result in profound discord in family life and other social relationships; this is especially true for those with the bipolar form of the illness. In Chapter 10 we review studies of personality functioning in manic and depressed states and how it compares with that in normal states in patients themselves and in the general population. We also discuss personality disorders that commonly coexist with manic-depressive illness, as well as the effects of medication on personality. The chapter then addresses interpersonal aspects of the illness, with emphasis on the bipolar subgroup.

Chapter 11 is devoted to the wide array of methods that now exists for assessing manic, mixed, and depressive states; these assessment measures add the perspective of formal psychological evaluation to the discussion of differential diagnosis in Chapter 3.

Widespread interest in creativity, the subject of Chapter 12, has lent visibility to this aspect of the study of manic-depressive illness. The age-old link between "madness" and creativity has been studied with increasingly sophisticated methods in recent years. Research has demonstrated that it is not schizophrenia but manic-depressive illness, especially its bipolar forms, that is more often associated with creative accomplishment. Among the most interesting developments in this field is the hypothesis that the genetic predisposition for manic-depressive illness also confers a creative edge on affected individuals and their close relatives. Explorations of the characteristics that help make some individuals more creative than others should have implications for the general population. Among the positive features of the bipolar form of the illness being examined in relation to creativity are the heightened energy level and speed of cognition of hypomania, linked to a global, inclusive associative process, and certain temperamental factors; positive (and painful) experiences derived from having affective illness are salient as well. In addition to raising important psychological, social, and ethical issues, these and related positive features of the bipolar form of the illness can play a key role in reducing the burden of stigma borne by patients. Understanding these features is, of course, necessary in dealing with one of the most sensitive and difficult issues in treatment—medication adherence.

Pathophysiology

The size of the fourth part of the book, the largest, testifies to the wealth of biological knowledge that has accrued through research on manic-depressive illness. The illness has come to represent an extraordinarily rich source of information about the interrelationships between behavioral and biological phenomena; certainly it has stimulated fascinating and productive theories about brain–behavior relationships.

We begin with a survey of the salient literature on genetics (Chapter 13). In this chapter we review genetic epidemiology, results of studies using the linkage method, alternative phenotypic definition, association methods, gene expression and pathogenesis, pharmacogenetics, and genetic counseling. We then look at the future of the field, including new technologies and what we can expect to learn from each.

Chapter 14, on neurobiology, provides the conceptual base necessary for an appreciation of the biochemical and pharmacological studies whose review follows. Much of modern neurobiology and neuropharmacology has been driven by efforts to understand the effects of mood-altering drugs. Indeed, attempts to understand why certain drugs affect mood have inspired major hypotheses about the neurobiology of behavior. The chapter also describes animal models designed to simulate affective illness and reviews the formidable literature on the major neurotransmitter, neuroendocrine, and neuropeptide systems involved in manic-depressive illness, along with extensive new findings related to postsynaptic signal transduction networks and gene expression.

With the emergence of highly sophisticated brain-imaging technologies, it has become important to review the anatomical correlates of mania and depression critically, if only to help guide the application of imaging approaches; we do so in Chapter 15. Functional neuroimaging work has advanced rapidly in recent years. We review research findings on cerebral activity in normal, depressed, and manic states, as well as summarize what is known about baseline cerebral activity markers of treatment response.

Chapter 16 covers sleep and biological rhythms, reflecting our judgment that these two fields, which developed independently of one another, have found a natural point of convergence in the pathophysiology of manic-depressive illness. It is increasingly clear that sleep physiology is important to circadian physiology and that sleep disturbances seen in affective illness reflect disturbances in circadian rhythms. This area of study has, in our estimation, yielded some of the most interesting developments in understanding manic-depressive illness. The identification of seasonal affective disorder, for example, represents a systematic, quantitative rediscovery of ancient observations of seasonality in mood disorders and suicide. The speed with which the initial observation of seasonal mood disorder was incorporated into the DSM nosology testifies to the responsiveness of our current diagnostic system. Research

on biological rhythms has spawned the development of three novel physiological but nonpharmacological treatments for mood disorders—sleep deprivation, phase advance, and high-intensity light—that are described in Chapter 19 on the treatment of acute depression, especially in bipolar patients. At a more general level, the contemporary focus on biological rhythms has given rise to environmental psychiatry, and thus the discussion of the subject in Chapter 16 emphasizes the subtle environmental influences on manic-depressive illness and offers relevant clinical suggestions.

Treatment

The final part of the book covers all aspects of the treatment of manic-depressive illness. It is traditional in its organization, separating acute from prophylactic treatment and medical from psychological treatment. Despite this division, we wish to emphasize the profound importance of integrating medical and psychological approaches. Although the structure of this part of the book is traditional, the organization of each chapter is not. Each begins with practical recommendations for clinical management and then reviews the treatment literature, highlighting areas inadequately explored in existing reviews, including the efficacy of lithium in treating depression as well as mania and the quality of the prophylactic response. We discuss treatment controversies such as antidepressant-induced mania, mixed states, and rapid cycling; the use of adjunctive treatments for breakthrough episodes during prophylactic treatment with mood stabilizers; the important but often overlooked distinction between prevention of relapse and prevention of recurrence (new episodes); the relative efficacy and side-effect profiles of the mood stabilizers and the antipsychotics; and the use of alternative or adjunctive approaches for patients who do not respond to initial treatment. It has been of great, often life-saving clinical importance to now have anticonvulsant and antipsychotic medications that provide an alternative for those patients who do not respond to or will not take lithium. We make clear our belief that lithium remains the gold standard of treatment, however, despite an increasing tendency to use less-proven medications.

The two chapters on adherence and psychotherapy (Chapters 21 and 22, respectively) should be read together. Our purpose here is not to provide a general psychotherapy primer but to focus on issues of special importance to the psychotherapy of manic-depressive illness, especially the bipolar form. These issues include fears of recurrence, the psychological scars left by the illness, and concerns about genetic vulnerability. The central issue in the psychological management of bipolar patients is medication adherence. Recent studies suggest that outcomes of medical treatment are substantially enhanced by adjunctive psychotherapy, no doubt reflecting the contribution of improved adherence. In our discussion of adherence, we return to the core issue of the paradox of drugs that are often very effective, yet can have an impact on some aspects of the illness that may be valued by the patient. Given clinicians' all-too-common tendency to be unaware of subtle adherence problems, we believe this issue warrants a separate chapter.

Chapter 23 is devoted to the special issues that arise in treating children and adolescents with bipolar illness. Chapter 24 deals with the treatment of comorbid conditions such as anxiety disorders, substance abuse, and medical conditions that frequently accompany manic-depressive illness.

The fact that manic-depressive illness is often lethal bears repeated mention. We have underscored this fact by summarizing what is known about rates and clinical correlates of suicide in Chapter 8; in Chapter 25, we emphasize clinical methods we believe to be most useful in reducing the risk of suicide among acutely ill patients. We emphasize again the fundamental premise that the best approach to the prevention of suicide is the effective and aggressive treatment of the underlying illness.

THE DEVELOPMENT OF THIS BOOK

The overwhelming size of the literature on manic-depressive illness makes it all but impossible for clinicians and researchers to keep pace with the latest findings and to see the broader clinical, human, and scientific picture. The National Library of Medicine's Medline file on bipolar disorder alone has grown from 16 citations in 1950; to approximately 600 citations in 1990, the year the first edition of this book was published; to more than 1,100 citations in 2006. We were aware of the problem before we began writing the first edition of this book. As we struggled through the scientific literature that had grown exponentially since 1990, we once again were concerned that the very magnitude of the new, scattered evidence threatens the ability to form a coherent overall view of the illness. In recent decades, research on manic-depressive illness has contributed to an extraordinary expansion of the knowledge base in increasingly specialized fields. The productivity of the research enterprise has generated diverse points of focus, which are often appreciated only by individuals in a given subfield. An unfortunate outgrowth of such specialization is that the wealth of new information typically has been made available only in the form of individual research reports or reviews of selected areas; at best, these occasionally are published in edited volumes.

Working during this period of extraordinary productivity and ferment in the study of manic-depressive illness, we saw the need for a comprehensive book that would attempt to impose order on a rich but vast and disparate literature. We were convinced that this goal could be accomplished only by seeing the subject through from beginning to end—in other words, by writing a book rather than editing a collection. We were able to accomplish this by jointly authoring the first edition. As indicated in our acknowledgments and in the list of collaborators for this edition, however, we found it imperative to seek the help of colleagues; we could not have completed this book without them. Our intent was to go beyond a review of the literature—to assess the nodal points in knowledge of the illness, to integrate them in a way that would enhance the quality of clinical care available, and to suggest opportunities for future research. In the early twenty-first century, manic-depressive illness continues to present new challenges and questions that extend from the realm of basic neurobiological science to those of clinical practice and social ethics. The skill the field brings to identifying these questions will determine the strategies formulated to answer them, and in turn will bear directly on future advances in treatment and prevention.

Throughout the writing of this edition of the book, as during the first, we have been impressed time and again by the excellent science, imaginative clinical research, and profoundly important treatment advances generated by our colleagues. We are delighted to acknowledge our debt to them, both for their science and for the lives they have saved. As before, our debt to our students and patients is immeasurable.

NOTES

1. Cited in Marneros, A., and Angst, J. Bipolar disorders: Roots and evolution (p. 6). Translated from the Greek by A. Marneros. In Marneros, A., and Angst, J. (2000). *Bipolar Disorders: 100 Years After Manic-Depressive Insanity.* Dordrecht, The Netherlands: Kluwer.
2. Kraepelin, E. (1990). *Psychiatry: A Textbook for Students and Physicians*, Sixth Edition. Translated by Helga Metoui. Canton, MA: Science History Publications, p. 8. Originally published as *Psychiatrie. Ein Lehrbuch fur Studierende und Arzte.* Leipzig: Johann Ambrosius Barth, 1899.
3. For reviews of gender differences in bipolar disorder, see Taylor and Abrams, 1981; Leibenluft, 1996; Blehar et al., 1998; Robb et al., 1998; Hendrick et al., 2000; and Kawa et al., 2005.

REFERENCES

Blehar, M.C., and Oren, D.A. (1997). Gender differences in depression. *Medscape Womens Health*, 2(2), 3.

Blehar, M.C., and Rudorfer, M.V. (1998). Women's mental health research—what is the need? *Psychopharmacol Bull*, 34(3), 237–238.

Blehar, M.C., DePaulo, J.R., Gershon, E.S., Reich, T., Simpson, S.G., and Nurnberger, J.I. (1998). Women with bipolar disorder: Findings from the NIMH Genetics Initiative sample. *Psychopharmacol Bull,* 34(3), 239–243.

Dorr, D.A., Rice, J.P., Armstrong, C., Reich, T., and Blehar, M. (1997). A meta-analysis of chromosome 18 linkage data for bipolar illness. *Genet Epidemiol,* 14(6), 617–622.

Hendrick, V., Altshuler, L.L., Gitlin, M.J., Delrahim, S., and Hammen, C. (2000). Gender and bipolar illness. *J Clin Psychiatry,* 61(5), 393–396, quiz 397.

Kawa, I., Carter, J.D., Joyce, P.R., Doughty, C.J., Frampton, C.M., Wells, J.E., Walsh, A.E., and Olds, R.J. 2005. Gender differences in bipolar disorder: Age of onset, course, comorbidity, and symptom presentation. *Bipolar Disord,* 7(2), 119–125.

Leibenluft, E. (1996). Women with bipolar illness: Clinical and research issues. *Am J Psychiatry,* 153(2), 163–173.

Robb, J.C., Young, L.T., Cooke, R.G., and Joffe, R.T. (1998). Gender differences in patients with bipolar disorder influence outcome in the medical outcomes survey (SF-20) subscale scores. *J Affect Disord,* 49(3), 189–193.

Stuart, S., O'Hara, M.W., and Blehar, M.C. (1998). Mental disorders associated with childbearing: Report of the Biennial Meeting of the Marce Society. *Psychopharmacol Bull,* 34(3), 333–338.

Taylor, M.A., and Abrams, R. (1981). Gender differences in bipolar affective disorder. *J Affect Disord,* 3(3), 261–271.

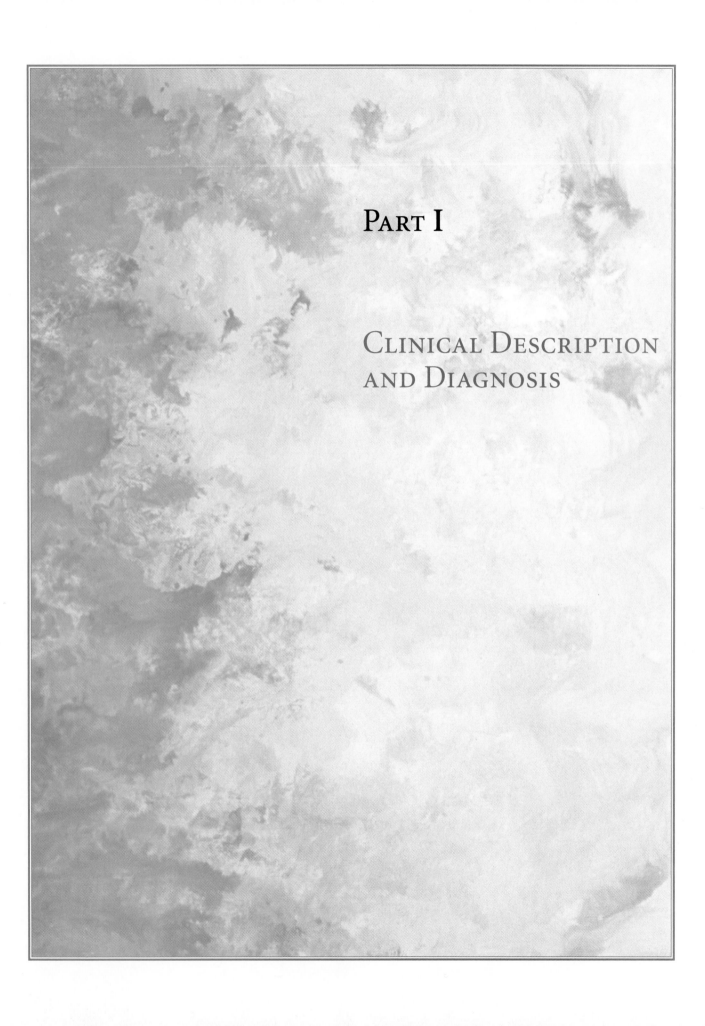

Part I

Clinical Description and Diagnosis

1
Conceptualizing Manic-Depressive Illness: The Bipolar–Unipolar Distinction and the Development of the Manic-Depressive Spectrum

Manic-depressive insanity . . . includes on the one hand the whole domain of the so-called periodic and circular insanity, on the other hand simple mania, the greater part of the morbid states termed melancholia and also a not inconsiderable number of cases of amentia [confusional insanity].

—Emil Kraepelin[1] (1921, p. 1)

It was the work of Angst and Perris that helped spread my theory that unipolar and bipolar diseases . . . have different clinical pictures. The bipolar form displays a considerably more colorful appearance; it varies not only between the two poles, but in each phase offers different pictures. The unipolar forms . . . return, in a periodic course, with the same symptomatology.

—Karl Leonhard (1979, pp. 3–4)

Medical conceptions of mania and depression are as old as medicine itself. From ancient times to the present, an extraordinary consistency characterizes descriptions of these conditions. Few maladies have been represented with such unvarying language. Yet while the essential features are recognizable in the medical literature through the centuries, the boundaries that define mania and depression and the relationship between them have changed during that time. In this chapter, we begin by reviewing the historical roots of our current concepts. We then discuss the two different but overlapping conceptualizations of manic-depressive illness: the bipolar–unipolar distinction and the manic-depressive spectrum.

HISTORICAL ROOTS

Pre–Nineteenth-Century Ideas

The medical writers of ancient Greece conceived of mental disorders in terms that sound remarkably modern.[2] They believed that melancholia was a psychological manifestation of an underlying biological disturbance, specifically, a perturbation in brain function. In documents dating back to the fifth and fourth centuries BC, Hippocrates and his school[3] described melancholia as a condition "associated with 'aversion to food, despondency, sleeplessness, irritability, restlessness,' and they stated that fear or depression that is prolonged means melancholia" (Jackson, 1986, p. 30). Early conceptions of melancholia and mania were, however, broader than those of today. The two terms, together with phrenitis, which corresponds roughly to an acute organic delirium, made up all mental illness throughout

most of the ancient period. As Jackson (1986, p. 249) pointed out, "disorders similar to our mania and our melancholia constituted significant portions of the larger groupings of mental disorders that were subsumed under those rubrics in ancient times."

As they did with other illnesses, the Hippocratic writers argued forcefully that mental disorders were not due to supernatural or magical forces, beliefs that characterized most primitive societies and that have resurfaced from time to time throughout history. In Greece, "Hippocrates did not encounter excessive resistance in the magical sphere because these diseases had long been interpreted as phenomena deriving from an underlying humoural disturbance" (Roccatagliata, 1986, p. 170). This essentially biological explanation for the cause of melancholia, which survived until the Renaissance, was part of the prevailing understanding of all health as an equilibrium of the four humors—blood, yellow bile, black bile, and phlegm—and all illness as a disturbance of this equilibrium. First fully developed in the Hippocratic work *Nature of Man* (ca. 400 BC), the humoral theory linked the humors with the seasons and with relative moistness. An excess of black bile was seen as the cause of melancholia, a term that literally means "black bile." Mania, by contrast, was usually attributed to an excess of yellow bile.

Aristotle, who differed with the Hippocratic writers by seeing the heart rather than the brain as the dysfunctional organ in melancholy, introduced the notion of a "predisposition" to melancholy. The "marker" of that predisposition was a relative excess of black bile, which he thought was common in small amounts in all people. As Whitwell[4] (1936, p. 59) pointed out, Aristotle thought those with the excess had melancholic temperaments that were associated with being gifted:

> Aristotle appears to have been the first to draw attention to the problem of the frequent occurrence of melancholia, or at least a degree of mental depression in the case of philosophers, statesmen, artists and poets, and he gives as examples Plato, Socrates and Empedocles. This is a question which is constantly recurring in later literature, the explanation of which is attempted by Marsilius Ficinus.[5]

Deliberations on the relationship between melancholia and mania date back at least to the first century BC, as noted by Soranus of Ephesus: "The followers of Themison, as well as many others, considered melancholy a form of the disease of mania" (Jackson, 1986, p. 250). Soranus himself (fl. 100 AD) believed that melancholia and mania were two distinct diseases, but with similar prodromal symptoms and requiring similar treatments (Jackson, 1986, p. 250):

> For Soranus, mania involved an impairment of reason with delusions; fluctuating states of anger and merriment, although sometimes of sadness and futility and sometimes "an overpowering fear of things which are quite harmless"; "continual wakefulness, the veins are distended, cheeks flushed, and body hard and abnormally strong"; and a tendency for there to be "attacks alternating with periods of remission." Melancholia involved being "downcast and prone to anger and . . . practically never cheerful and relaxed"; "signs . . . as follows: mental anguish and distress, dejection, silence, animosity toward members of the household, sometimes a desire to live and at other times a longing for death, suspicion . . . that a plot is being hatched against him, weeping without reason, meaningless muttering, and again, occasional joviality"; and various somatic symptoms, many of them gastrointestinal.

Aretaeus of Cappadocia, who lived in the second century AD, appears to have been the first (whose work has survived to modern times) to bring together the syndromes described in Greek medicine and propose that mania was an end stage of melancholia, a view that was to prevail for centuries to come. Roccatagliata (1986, p. 229), who referred to Aretaeus as "the clinician of mania," noted that he "isolated . . . a form of mental disease presenting phases of depression alternating with phases of mania," and reported Aretaeus's characterization of the illness:

> "Some patients after being melancholic have fits of mania . . . so that mania is like a variety of being

melancholy." He described a kind of cyclothymia which presented only intermittent stages of mania: "It arises in subjects whose personality is characterised by gayness, activity, superficiality and childishness." The mania was expressed in "furor, excitement and cheerfulness." Other types of mania, he said, had delirious manifestations of an expansive type, so that the patient "has deliriums, he studies astronomy, philosophy . . . he feels great and inspired." So he identified a bipolar cyclothymia, a monopolar one consisting only of manic phases, and a paranoid psychosis which he considered akin to schizophrenic mania.

Although Aretaeus included syndromes that today might be classified as psychoses beyond mania, his clear descriptions of the variety of manic conditions influenced medicine for many centuries, and have a modern ring to them (Roccatagliata, 1986, pp. 230–231):

> According to Aretaeus, the classical form of mania was the type that was associated with melancholia: the patient who previously was gay, euphoric, and hyperactive suddenly "has a tendency to melancholy; he becomes, at the end of the attack, languid, sad, taciturn, he complains that he is worried about his future, he feels ashamed." When the depressive phase is over, such patients go back to being gay, they laugh, they joke, they sing, "they show off in public with crowned heads as if they were returning victorious from the games; sometimes they laugh and dance all day and all night." In serious forms of mania, called furor, the patient "sometimes kills and slaughters the servants"; in less severe forms, he often exalts himself: "without being cultivated he says he is a philosopher . . . and the incompetent [say they are] good artisans . . . others yet are suspicious and they feel that they are being persecuted, for which reasons they are irascible."

Aretaeus believed that mania was a brain dysfunction that "deprived its imaginative functions" (Roccatagliata, 1986, p. 229). Melancholy, similarly, had an endogenous etiology; melancholic delirium arose (Roccatagliata, 1986, p. 231):

> "without motive, like the loss of reason, insomnia, and despair." The vital tone was subject to typical circadian variations, which in melancholy were inverted with respect to the normal person, so that the patients "wake up suddenly and are seized by a great tiredness."

The next important medical writer, Galen of Pergamon (131–201 AD), firmly established melancholia as a chronic and recurrent condition. His few comments on mania included the observation that it can be either a primary disease of the brain or secondary to other diseases. Galen's "contribution" was, in the opinion of most medical historians, his brilliant, all-encompassing elaboration of the humoral theory, a system so compelling that it dominated—and stifled—medical thought for more than a millennium.

Medical observations in succeeding centuries continued to reflect these conceptions of depression and mania laid down in classical Greece and Rome. As Jackson (1986) observed, most authors wrote of the two conditions as separate illnesses, but usually in adjoining chapters and ascribing them to humoral causes that suggested a close connection between them. Yet where mania and depression are considered in the historical medical literature, a link is almost always made, as can be seen in the time line in Box 1–1.

As we have seen, from classical Greece until the Middle Ages, mental and physical afflictions were primarily the concern of medical doctors. As illness gradually became the responsibility of the priests, the above early insights were submerged. The period that followed was, in retrospect, a dark age, when mental illness was generally attributed to either magic or sin or possession by the devil.

By the late Middle Ages, empirical science had attracted interest and the beginnings of acceptance, engendered by the ascendancy of Baconian philosophy. At that point, however, in the clinical realm now encompassed by psychiatry, scientific interpretations were limited to anatomical, physiological, and pathological studies of the brain.

Empirical clinical observations without religious overtones did not reappear until the beginning of the seventeenth century. A key figure in this descriptive renaissance was Felix Platter, who in 1602 published his systematic observations and classifications of mental disorders. Although his descriptions of mania and melancholia were extensive and methodical, there was little to suggest the longitudinal or recurrent nature of the illness, or the distinctions between manic-depressive illness[6] and what is now known as schizophrenia.

A unique eighteenth-century discussion of manic-depressive illness can be found in a 1759 monograph by Andres Piquer ("the Spanish Hippocrates"), physician to King Ferdinand VI of Spain ("Discurso sobre la Enfermedad del Rey nuestro Senor Fernando VI"), recently republished with an introduction by Eduard Vieta and Demetrio Barcia. Piquer diagnosed the king with "melancholic-manic affect" (p. 17), clearly anticipating later French and German authors in viewing this condition as a single illness: "Melancholy and mania, although treated in many medical books separately, are one and the same illness, and only differ according to the various grades of activity and diversity of affective states that occur in both." (pp. 57–58; translated

segments by Nassir Ghaemi) Piquer went on to quote Hippocrates and Arateus in support of his view.

As noted previously, the subsequent literature of the seventeenth and eighteenth centuries is replete with clinical observations of manic and depressive symptomatology. As pointed out by Pichot (1995), the disciples of Esquirol played a critical role as they paved the way for recognition of the mental disease that ultimately came to be known as manic-depressive insanity through the work of Kraepelin (1899). For instance, Jules Baillarger[7] wrote in 1854:

> There exists a special type of insanity characterized by two regular periods, the one of depression and the other of excitement. . . . This type of insanity presents itself in the form of isolated attacks; or, it recurs in an intermittent manner; or, the attacks might follow one another without interruption.

This theme is echoed in subsequent French psychiatric writing:

> By circular insanity, or *folie à double forme*, we understand a special form of mental derangement, the attacks of which are characterised by a regular sequence of two periods—one of depression, and another of excitement, or inversely. (Ritti, 1892)[8]

There are literally thousands of such observations, for the most part disconnected from one another. Many are accompanied by hastily erected classification systems and etiological speculations, which sometimes anticipate contemporary theory to a striking extent. As Jelliffe (1931) wrote, the "epidemic of classification" was further spread by the powerful influence of Linnaeus's work on the classification of plants. Even more new empirical observations were added when the advent of autopsies opened the door for neuropathologic observations and their attendant speculations. This evidence was gathering in a conceptual climate still dominated by the traditional separation of the mind ("soul") from the body. The era was not yet ready for a new synthesis or unifying insights, despite its increasing need of them.

Nineteenth-Century Ideas

The explicit conception of manic-depressive illness as a single disease entity dates from the mid-nineteenth century. As noted above, the French "alienists," Falret and Baillarger, independently and almost simultaneously formulated the idea that mania[9] and depression could represent different manifestations of a single illness. Students of Esquirol and, therefore, intellectual descendants of Pinel, they had been strongly influenced by Pinel's sharp disdain for the "classification epidemic," as well as by contemporary arguments for a unitary concept of general paresis.

ca. 400 BC   An excess of black bile was seen as the cause of melancholia, a term that literally means "black bile." Mania, by contrast was usually attributed to yellow bile. (Hippocrates)

ca. 150 AD   "Some patients after being melancholic have fits of mania . . . so that mania is like a variety of being melancholy." (Aretaeus of Cappadocia[b])

ca. 575   "Those affected with such a condition are not suffering from melancholia only, for they tend to become maniacal periodically and in a cycle. Mania is nothing else but melancholia in a more intense form." (Alexander of Tralles[c])

ca. 1000   "Undoubtedly the material which is the effective producer of mania is of the same nature as that which produces melancholia." (Avicenna[d])

ca. 1300   "Mania and melancholia are different forms of the same thing." (Joh. Gaddesden[e])

ca. 1500   "[Melancholia] manifestly differs from what is properly called mania; there is no doubt, however, that at some time or other, authorities agree that it replaces melancholia." (Joh. Manardus[f])

ca. 1549   "Perturbation of the spirit of the brain when mixed with and kindled by other matter can produce melancholia, or if more ardent, mania." (Felix Platter[g])

ca. 1672   "[Manics and melancholics] are so much akin, that these Distempers often change, and pass from one into the other; for the Melancholick disposition growing worse, brings on Fury; and Fury or Madness [mania] growing less hot, oftentimes ends in a Melancholick disposition. These two, like smoke and flame, mutually receive and give place to one another." (Thomas Willis[h])

ca. 1735   "If Melancholy increases so far, that from the great Motion of the Liquid of the Brain, the Patient be thrown into a wild Fury, it is call'd Madness [mania]. Which differs only in Degree from the sorrowful kind of Melancholy, is its Offspring, produced from the same Causes, and cured almost by the same Remedies." (Herman Boerhaave[i])

ca. 1759   "Melancholy and mania, although treated in many medical books separately, are one and the same illness, and only differ according to the various grades of activity and diversity of affective states that occur in both."—Andres, Piquer (quoted in "El trastorno bipolar en el siglo XVIII," by Eduard Vieta and Demetrio Barcia, 2000, Burdeos, Spain: Mra ediciones, pp. 57–58, segment translated by Nassir Ghaemi).

ca. 1806   "[Mania is] often no other than a higher degree of melancholia. . . . [I]t does not appear to me any wise difficult to suppose, that the same state of the brain may in a moderate degree give melancholia; and in a higher, that mania which melancholia so often passes into." (William Cullen[j])

ca. 1845   "Several distinguished masters, Alexander de Tralles, and Boerhaave himself, were of the opinion, that melancholy . . . was only the first degree of mania. This is in some cases true. There are in fact, some persons who, before becoming maniacs, are sad, morose, uneasy, diffident and suspicious." (Jean-Etienne-Dominique Esquirol[k])

---

[a]Although the idea for this time line was ours, locating the quotations would have been next to impossible without the excellent historical sources cited for each. We are especially indebted to Whitwell (1936), Jackson (1986), and Roccatagliata (1986). The quotations, particularly those from the Middle Ages, do not always represent prevailing thought, but they do illustrate the thread of this theme throughout history. Also, when the conditions we would characterize as manic-depressive illness were interpreted as medical rather than philosophical or religious problems, a relationship between mania and depression was almost always suggested, explicitly or implicitly.

[b]Cited by Whitwell (1936, pp. 163–164). From *De acut, et diut, morborum, causis, signis, et curatione* (Paris), 1554. Transl. R. Moffatt.

[c]Quoted by Whitwell (1936, p. 175), who gave Trallianus's birth and death dates as 525–605, from Trallianus Alexander: *Medici libri duodecim*, interpret, Guintherius (Basil), 1556.

[d]Quoted by Whitwell (1936, p. 181), who gave Avicenna's birth and death dates as 980–1037. Whitwell cited as a source Opera, ed.: *Alpagus et Benedictus* (Venet.), 1582, and *Morb. Ment.* (Paris) 1659. Italics in original.

[e]Quoted by Whitwell (1936, p. 196), who gave Gaddesden's birth and death dates as 1280–1361. Source cited is Gaddesden Joh.: *Practica Johanni Anglica—Rosa medicina nuncupata* (Papiae), 1492. Transl. Wolffe.

[f]Cited by Whitwell (1936, p. 205), who gave Manardus's birth and death dates as 1462–1536. Citation given is Manardus Joh: *Epist. Med.* (Venet.), 1542. Italics in original.

[g]Quoted by Whitwell (1936, p. 98), who gave Platter's birth and death dates as 1536–1614. Although it is not clear which of Platter's works is the source of this quotation, Whitwell later quoted from *Praxeos medicae Tomi tres* (Basil), 1656, and *Histories and Observations* (London: Culpeper and Cole), 1664.

[h]Quoted by Jackson (1986, p. 255) from Willis, T.: *Two Discourses Concerning the Soul of Brutes*. Transl. S. Pordage (London: Thomas Dring), Ch. Harper and John Leigh,^ 1683, pp. 201, 205.

[i]Quoted by Jackson (1986, p. 256) from Boerhaave, H.: *Boerhaave's Aphorisms: Concerning the Nature and Cure of Diseases, Which Is That of a Vital and Sensitive Man. The First Is Physiological Shewing the Nature, Parts, Powers, and Affections of the Same. The Other Is Pathological, Which Unfolds the Diseases Which Affect It and Its Primary Seat; to Wit, the Brain and Nervous Stock, and Treats of Their Cures: with Copper Cuts* (London: W and J Innys), 1735, pp. 323–324.

[j]Quoted by Jackson (1986, p. 259) from Cullen, W.: *First Lines of the Practice of Physic*. 2 vols., in 1. ed. J. Rotheram (New York: E. Duyckinck), 1806, p. 497.

[k]Quoted by Jackson (1986, p. 262) from Esquirol, E.: *Mental Maladies: A Treatise on Insanity*. Transl. E. K. Hunt (Philadelphia: Lea and Blanchard), 1845, pp. 381–382.

In 1854, Falret described a circular disorder (*la folie circulaire*), which for the first time expressly defined an illness in which "this succession of mania and melancholia manifests itself with continuity and in a manner almost regular" (perhaps a foreshadowing of the modern concept of rapid cycling). In the same year, Baillarger (1854) described "double insanity" (*la folie à double forme*), emphasizing that the manic and depressive episodes were not two different attacks but rather two different stages of the same attack. Thus, cyclicity with or without clear-cut remission was already being described in these pioneering French contributions. Although clearly anticipating Kraepelin's later synthesis, these descriptions nonetheless focused on chronic illness with poor prognosis; the relationship of these "forms" to other varieties of mania or melancholia was not delineated. Other valuable contributions were made by Griesinger (1867), who provided rich clinical descriptions of melancholia and mania, although he described primarily chronic states with poor prognosis. As Aretaeus had centuries before, Griesinger conceived of mania as an end stage of a gradually worsening melancholia and of both as different stages of a single, unitary disease (Jackson, 1986).

Although mild cases of mania had been described by the ancients, as well as by Falret, Esquirol, and other observers, Mendel (1881) was the first to define *hypo*mania as "that form of mania which typically shows itself only in the mild stages abortively, so to speak." Kahlbaum (1882) described circular disorders (cyclothymia), which were characterized by episodes of both depression and excitement but did not end in dementia, as chronic mania or melancholia could. Despite these contributions, most clinical observers continued to regard mania and melancholia as separate entities, chronic in nature, and following a deteriorating course. Nonetheless, some German authors during this period, such as Hecker (see the translation by Koukopoulos, 2003), reserved cyclothymia for the milder, nondeteriorating, forms observed in private clinical practice. Hecker's work is actually quite consistent with what today we have come to recognize as bipolar-II disorder:

> Virtually all of the [patients with cyclothymia] presented with a depressive state. The state of excitation—and I should like to emphasize this—had escaped the attention, in the majority of milder cases, of the patient's doctor, his family and friends, and the patient himself. The patients only became aware of it when I described the characteristics of this state to them. Even more often, however, it was the patients themselves who, having up until that moment considered them as their 'healthiest' periods, were forced to recognize that they were ill in these periods also.

The Kraepelinian Synthesis

It was left to Kraepelin to segregate the two major psychotic illnesses—manic-depressive insanity and dementia praecox—from one another and clearly draw the perimeter around manic-depressive illness. The early editions of his textbook of psychiatry contained the seeds of his later synthesis, particularly his special emphasis on careful diagnosis based on both longitudinal history and the pattern of current symptoms. Nevertheless, these early editions still reflected a struggle with the then-traditional categories of melancholia and circular psychosis. In the sixth edition, published in 1899, the term *manic-depressive* encompassed the circular psychoses and simple manias. Kraepelin expressed doubt that melancholia and the circular psychoses (a category that includes today's bipolar and schizoaffective disorders) were really separate illnesses, but he was still reluctant to take a definite stand.

By 1913, in the eighth edition of Kraepelin's text, virtually all of the major clinical forms of melancholia had been subsumed under "manic-depressive illness." Under his unitary concept, much of what had once been considered involutional melancholia was reclassified as mixed states,[10] based on a follow-up study by his pupil, Dreyfus.[11] Kraepelin placed special emphasis on the features of the illness that differentiated it most clearly from dementia praecox (schizophrenia): the periodic or episodic course, the more benign prognosis, and a family history of manic-depressive illness.

Within a relatively short time, Kraepelin's views were widely accepted, thus bringing some unity to European psychiatry. His was the first fully developed disease model in psychiatry to be backed by extensive and carefully organized observations and descriptions. This model did not exclude psychological or social factors, and in fact, Kraepelin was one of the first to point out that psychological stresses could precipitate individual episodes. By including "slight colourings of mood," which "pass over without sharp boundary into the domain of personal predisposition," he also provided the basis for the development of spectrum concepts, described later in this chapter.

Wide acceptance of Kraepelin's broad divisions led to further exploration of the boundaries between manic-depressive illness and dementia praecox, the delineation of similarities across the two, and the possibility that subgroups could be identified within each. Kraepelin's extraordinary synthesis is important not because it drew the ultimately "correct" picture of nature, but because it built a solid and empirically anchored base for future work. This was his major accomplishment. Indeed, as we will see later, his central insight—that all of the recurrent major mood disorders (using current nomenclature) belonged together under the rubric of *manic-depressive illness*—still provides the best model for what we know to date, as well as for understanding emerging clinical, pharmacological, and genetic data.

Post-Kraepelinian Developments

After Kraepelin, the evolution of the concept of manic-depressive illness proceeded differently in Europe and the United States (Pichot, 1988). Europeans continued to place primary emphasis on the traditional medical disease model of mental illness, whereas psychiatrists in the United States were profoundly influenced by the new perspectives of psychoanalysis and other theories emphasizing psychological and social factors. During the first half of the twentieth century, the views of Meyer (1866–1950) gradually assumed a dominant position in American psychiatry, a position maintained for several decades. Meyer believed that psychopathology emerged from interactions between an individual's biological and psychological characteristics and his social environment.[12]

The disease model, by contrast, is based on the premise that clinical phenomena in a given patient are understandable (and therefore potentially predictable) in terms of a given disease with a specific natural history and pathophysiology. European psychiatry in the nineteenth and early twentieth centuries had successfully employed this traditional medical disease model in the definition and treatment of general paresis secondary to syphilis of the central nervous system and organic syndromes associated with vitamin deficiencies (especially pellagra).[13] Failure to identify mechanisms of pathophysiology in the major so-called functional psychoses, including manic-depressive illness, stimulated doubts about the continued usefulness of the model, particularly since the prevailing biological hypotheses emphasized infectious agents and neuropathological lesions. Consistent with this pessimism was the failure of the biologically based treatments of the time. In this climate, it is not surprising that American psychiatrists, manifesting the national penchant for pragmatism, were drawn to treatment approaches that emphasized psychological and social factors. When the Meyerian focus, considerably influenced by psychoanalysis, turned to manic-depressive illness, the individual and his environment were the natural focus, and clinical descriptions of symptoms and the longitudinal course of the illness were given less emphasis.[14]

Until the latter part of the twentieth century, the American nosological systems for affective disorders reflected these competing sets of etiological assumptions. Depression was divided into several dichotomies: reactive–endogenous, neurotic–psychotic, and, more recently,

primary[15]–secondary. Forgotten in these conceptions is the fact that a single parameter cannot differentiate aspects of illness that are at least partially independent of one another: severity, "neurotic features," thought disorder, precipitating events, physiological symptoms, and genetic vulnerability. Dichotomous systems thus foundered on their a priori assumptions about etiology. Even the primary–secondary distinction, although free of assumptions about severity, quality of symptoms, and precipitating events, is based on another supposition: it assumes that depression or mania associated with other illnesses is relatively free of genetic influence, an assumption that has not been supported by the data (Andreasen et al., 1988).[16]

In Europe, the post-Kraepelinian evolution of the concept of manic-depressive illness took a different turn. The European psychosocial and psychoanalytical traditions continued to develop in relative isolation from the mainstream of psychiatry, which largely retained its medical or disease orientation; psychoanalytic thinking per se did not have as important an influence on the European concept of manic-depressive illness as it did on the American concept. Although Kraepelin's fundamental distinction between manic-depressive illness and dementia praecox endured (Mayer-Gross et al., 1955), nosological disputes soon arose. *└ study of diseases*

In his classic contributions to descriptive psychiatry, Bleuler (1924) departed from Kraepelin by conceptualizing the relationship between manic-depressive (affective) illness and dementia praecox (schizophrenia) as a continuum without a sharp line of demarcation.[17] *boundary* Bleuler believed that a patient's location on the spectrum depended on the number of schizophrenic features he demonstrated. In that sense, Bleuler considered the affective symptoms to be nonspecific. These issues are explored more fully in Chapter 3.

Bleuler also broadened Kraepelin's concept of manic-depressive illness by designating several subcategories and using the term *affective illness*. The influence of his modifications of Kraepelin's taxonomy could be seen in the *International Classification of Diseases* (ICD) (8th and 9th editions) and the closely related early versions of the *Diagnostic and Statistical Manual*, the first and second editions (DSM-I and -II). Bleuler's subcategories of affective illness anticipated the principal contemporary subdivision of the classic manic-depressive diagnostic group—the bipolar–unipolar distinction.

THE BIPOLAR–UNIPOLAR DISTINCTION

From its inception, Kraepelin's unitary concept of manic-depressive illness was criticized for being too inclusive, but it was not until 1957 that Leonhard proposed a classification system that went beyond clinical description alone. Leonhard observed that, within the broad category of manic-depressive illness (i.e., recurrent affective illness), some patients had histories of both depression and mania, whereas others had depressions only. He then noted that patients with a history of mania (whom he termed *bipolar*) had a higher incidence of mania in their families as compared with those with recurrent depressions only (whom he termed *monopolar*). In 1966, Angst and Perris independently provided the first systematic family history data to support Leonhard's distinction, validating it by an independent criterion—family history. As discussed in Chapter 13, some of the subsequent family history studies are consistent with a model in which bipolar and the more highly recurrent forms of unipolar depression are variants of the same fundamental disorder (Kraepelin's manic-depressive illness), with bipolar illness representing the more severe end of the spectrum.

The bipolar–unipolar distinction was formally incorporated into the American diagnostic system, DSM, the third edition (DSM-III), in 1980; was subsequently carried forward into DSM, the fourth edition (DSM-IV); and became explicit in the international classification system in ICD-10. Unfortunately the structure of DSM-IV (see Fig. 3–1 in Chapter 3), which breaks out bipolar disorder as a separate illness distinct from all other mood disorders (i.e., from the depressive disorders) obscures the fact that originally, the bipolar–unipolar distinction was conceived of as a way to distinguish two forms of a *recurrent* illness. In other words, the DSM structure gives precedence to polarity over cyclicity, obscuring the reality that one rather common variant of unipolar illness is as recurrent or cyclic as bipolar illness. Further, DSM-IV really has no language for the unipolar patient with frequent recurrences, since its "recurrent" category is so broad as to include patients with only two depressions in a lifetime (see Chapter 3 for a more extensive discussion of this point).

Before the mid-1970s, the scientific literature on manic-depressive illness typically did not include information on the number of patients with or without a history of mania. During the past three decades, however, the bipolar–unipolar distinction has been examined in numerous studies encompassing family history, natural course, clinical symptoms, personality factors, biological measures, and response to various pharmacological treatments. The question of bipolar–unipolar differences in clinical features of depression is reviewed in this chapter; these as well as other reported bipolar–unipolar differences (e.g., biological, pharmacological, psychological) are summarized in Table 1–1 and further detailed in the relevant chapters (including this one—see also Table 1–3 on clinical differences later in the chapter). Our purpose in outlining these reported differences here is to introduce a framework helpful in understanding them.

An Overview of Differentiating Features

The criteria that distinguish bipolar from unipolar illness have changed over the years, at least among American investigators. As noted above, in the original descriptions of Leonhard and the subsequent studies of Angst and colleagues (1998), Perris and colleagues (1971), and Winokur and colleagues (1981), both *bipolar*[18] and *unipolar* were used to describe patients with a phasic or cyclic course of recurrent episodes, characterized by autonomous "endogenous" features and clear functional impairment. It is worth repeating that in DSM-III and -IV, *unipolar* has come to mean all depressed patients without a history of hypomania or mania (i.e., to mean simply nonbipolar)—a heterogeneous population that includes both highly recurrent and nonrecurrent depressions, not to mention patients who might have been classified as "neurotic," "reactive," "characterological," or "atypical" in other diagnostic systems. As Roth (1983, pp. 47–48) observed about DSM-III:

> The significant point in this context is that Leonhard intended that bipolar–unipolar dichotomy for endogenous states alone. . . . When the endogenous syndrome is discarded, unipolar disorders become a large and compendious bag to be commingled with a wide variety of disorders of affect, including neuroses of different kinds.

The critical issue of recurrence is further obscured by DSM-IV, which does not include an item concerning prior history or course, despite evidence suggesting a clear distinction between family history and course in different illness subtypes (Winokur, 1979).[19] We believe that the next revision of the DSM and ICD systems should include a category (and operational definition) for the more recurrent forms of unipolar depression, which might be designated as "highly recurrent," or "cyclic." A related contributor to unipolar heterogeneity is the subgroup of unipolar patients with certain bipolar-like characteristics, as discussed below.

Bipolar groups are also heterogeneous. Most studies, particularly those first to use the distinction, did not specify criteria for bipolar beyond indicating a "history of mania." In many studies, bipolar included only those patients with a history of frank mania requiring hospitalization; in others, the bipolar group included patients with milder symptoms (hypomania). Then, Goodwin and colleagues at the National Institute of Mental Health (NIMH) suggested that bipolar patients could be classified more meaningfully as either bipolar-I or bipolar-II (Dunner et al., 1976b). They based this recommendation on their studies of hospitalized depressed patients who met criteria for primary

TABLE 1–1. Overview of Reported Differences between Bipolar and Unipolar Depression

Phenomenology of Depression	Bipolar (I and/or II)	Unipolar
Depressive Symptoms	See Table 1–3	See Table 1–3
Natural Course		
Age at onset	Younger	Older
	Narrower range	Broader range
Number of episodes	More	Fewer
Length of depressive episode[a]	Shorter	Longer
Cycle length	Shorter	Longer
Precipitants of episodes	More important at illness onset than for later episodes	Relation to illness onset not clear
Interepisode mood shifts	More	Fewer
Marital Status	Single status not a risk factor for episodes	Single status a risk factor
Epidemiology		
Lifetime risk	1.2–1.5%	5–10%
Proportion of major affective illness	20–50%	50–80%
Gender ratio	F=M	F>M
Substance abuse	More frequent	Less frequent
Suicide	Unclear	Unclear
Personality		
Depression/introversion	Less	More
Impulse control	Less	More
Stimulus seeking	More	Less
Personality profile	More normal	Less normal
Hyperthymic temperament	More	Less
Cyclothymia	More	Less
Family History/Genetics		
Monozygotic twin concordance rates	Higher	Lower
Mania among first-degree relatives	More	Less
Biological/Physiological		
Monoaminergic function (metabolites, receptors, neuroendocrine response, electrolytes, etc.)	Some studies report UP–BP differences (see Chapter 15)	
Pain sensitivity	Less	More
Hemispheric function dysfunction	More nondominant	?
Brain imaging parameters	? (see Chapter 15)	?

(continued)

TABLE 1–1. **Overview of Reported Differences between Bipolar and Unipolar Depression** *(continued)*

Phenomenology of Depression	Bipolar (I and/or II)	Unipolar
Sleep/Rhythms		
Sleep duration	Longer	Shorter
Phase advance	Less frequent (?)	More frequent (?)
Seasonal patterns	Fall/winter depression	Spring depression (?)
	Spring/summer mania	
Pharmacological Response		
Response to antidepressants	Less (?)	More (?)
Speed of response to antidepressants	More rapid (?)	Less rapid (?)
Tolerance to antidepressants	More frequent	Less frequent
Antidepressant response to mood stabilizers	More frequent	Less frequent
Manic/hypomanic response to antidepressants	More frequent	Less frequent
Prophylactic response to lithium	Equivalent when bipolar and unipolar cycle length are comparable	
Prophylactic response to antidepressants	Poor	Good

[a]Studies demonstrating longer duration of episodes with unipolar versus bipolar depression are generally not corrected for number of episodes. See text.

Note: See individual chapters for details. Some of the bipolar–unipolar comparisons included both bipolar-I and -II, while others focused on either one or the other, an obvious source of heterogeneity. Not all of the reported differences have been replicated uniformly, which is not surprising given the heterogeneity of both the bipolar and "unipolar" groups (for example, early-onset, highly recurrent unipolar depression will be closer to bipolar depression in clinical characteristics). The sequence of the table follows that of the chapters in this volume.

F = female; M = male; UP–BP = unipolar–bipolar.

major affective disorders; that is, they had no prior history of another psychiatric diagnosis. Bipolar-I patients were defined as those with a history of mania severe enough to have resulted in treatment, usually hospitalization. Such full-blown mania was often accompanied by psychotic features. Bipolar-II patients, by contrast, had, in addition to major depression requiring hospitalization, a history of hypomania—that is, specific symptoms of sufficient magnitude to be designated as abnormal by the patient or the family and to result in interference with normal role functioning, but not severe enough to result in hospitalization.

This original distinction between bipolar-I and -II is different from that made in subsequent studies that also employed the bipolar-II terminology.[20] Whereas the work of Dunner and colleagues (1976b) and the NIMH Collaborative Program on the Psychobiology of Depression-Clinical Studies, as well as that of Angst and colleagues (2005) in their long-term follow-up study, emerged from observations of hospitalized depressed patients without other psychiatric diagnoses, many of the more recent studies were conducted in patients in whom neither the depressed nor the hypomanic phase was severe enough to require hospitalization and in whom concomitant diagnoses (principally borderline personality disorder and substance abuse disorder) were not uncommon (Coryell et al., 1985, 1995; Endicott et al., 1985). Such definitional broadening is not universally accepted (Ghaemi et al., 2002). Thus, Baldessarini (2000) pointed out that mood fluctuations can be found in many if not most psychiatric disorders and expressed concern that the continued broadening of the bipolar diagnosis risks weakening the core concept of bipolar disorder. Similar concerns were expressed by van Praag (1993), and we agree.

Angst (1978), having earlier recognized the problem of the range of meanings that could confuse application of the bipolar-II category, proposed a nomenclature that would account for milder forms of both depression and mania. He divided bipolar patients into Md and mD, with *M* and *D* indicating episodes of mania and depression requiring hospitalization, and *m* and *d* episodes clearly different from normal but not of sufficient severity to necessitate hospitalization. Although Angst's mD group is analogous to the original definition of bipolar-II of Dunner and colleagues (1976b), other systems have no subcategory analogous to his Md group. This is unfortunate, since Angst reported interesting differences among these subgroups. For instance, the ratio of females to males is substantially higher in the predominantly depressed subgroups (unipolar and Dm), whereas males are a higher proportion of the predominantly manic subgroups (MD and Md); these data are consistent with the higher female-to-male ratio in bipolar-II compared with bipolar-I disorder (Weissman et al., 1996; Cassano et al., 1999). More recently, Angst completed a long-term follow-up study of his original 1959–1963 cohort. He concluded that the Md group, compared with their MD counterparts, have a more favorable course and are less likely to require long-term maintenance medication, while their first-degree relatives have a lower affective morbidity risk (Angst et al., 2004).

The extent of overlap between Angst's dm category and the bipolar-II outpatients in subsequent studies (by Akiskal, Benazzi, and others) cannot be assessed because Angst's system defines d episodes by an absence of hospitalization for depression, whereas a bipolar-II diagnosis is based on meeting DSM-IV criteria for major depression. Angst's dm grouping is inherently broader than bipolar-II and includes patients who would be classified as cyclothymic in DSM-III and -IV (see Chapter 3). Whatever the level of depressive severity,[21] however, bipolar-II patients represent a very important group. Moreover, as discussed below, both family history and pharmacological response data indicate that, while in some respects bipolar-II should be considered an intermediate form between bipolar-I and unipolar,[22] some of the data are consistent with its being a distinct subgroup.

As noted in the first edition of this text, one problem complicating research on bipolar-II disorder has been the poor reliability of the diagnosis, which results principally from the difficulty of establishing a history of hypomania (Andreasen et al., 1981; Dunner and Tay, 1993). Depressed patients are especially poor at recalling prior episodes of hypomania. Fortunately, family members generally do better. Moreover, the sensitivity to hypomania can be increased by multiple interviews over time (Rice et al., 1986). And current data indicate excellent reliability when clinicians trained in recognizing bipolar-II make the diagnosis (Dunner and Tay, 1993; Simpson et al., 2002). Other issues

involved in making a DSM diagnosis of hypomania include the not-always-warranted primacy accorded to elated mood over dysphoric mood and the durational requirement of 4 or more consecutive days, both of which have been widely criticized by clinical researchers (see the discussion in Chapter 3).

Most significant, contemporary data necessitate revision of the more traditional view of bipolar as substantially less common than unipolar illness. In Egeland and Hotstetter's (1983) study, using sensitive methods of ascertainment and considering cyclothymia, bipolar-II, and bipolar-I together, the incidence of bipolar disorder was approximately equal to that of unipolar illness—that is, it accounted for 50 percent of major affective illness.[23] Angst and colleagues (1978) also found that the ratio of bipolar to unipolar illness was about 1:1 in patients followed for up to 16 years, a ratio very close to that noted in the subsequent follow-up of that cohort, in which only 46 percent of the patients were still unipolar (Angst et al., 2002, 2004). Other recent studies using this broader definition of bipolar have found a similarly high bipolar/unipolar ratio.[24]

Unfortunately, many studies of recurrent affective illness employ relatively insensitive methods of ascertainment and correspondingly rigid criteria for an episode. Although such inflexible criteria are useful for certain research purposes, they exclude many patients from consideration. Egeland and Hotstetter (1983) referred to the bipolar illness typically cited in the literature (i.e., bipolar-I) as the "tip of the iceberg" of bipolarity. Current data indicate that manic-depressive spectrum conditions (see below), many of them below the threshold of mania, may be found in 5–8 percent of the population (Angst, 1978) (see Chapter 5). However, the validity of the diagnoses in most of these surveys (obtained by trained lay interviewers) has been questioned, primarily because estimates based on diagnoses by experienced clinicians tend to be substantially lower (see Chapters 4 and 5).

A broad range of bipolar–unipolar differences have been reported (see Table 1–1). They include four separate spheres of data—genetic, clinical, biological, and pharmacological. Considerable caution is warranted in interpreting these differences, however, given the heterogeneity in both groups. While most of these studies have focused on bipolar-I patients (reducing heterogeneity on that side),[25] the unipolar groups have been highly heterogeneous with respect to the critical variable of recurrence or cycle length; clearly the unipolar groups represented in Table 1–1 have generally not been selected for frequent recurrences (Cassano et al., 1992; Winokur et al., 1993, 1994, 1995; Judd et al., 2003a). Indeed, to our knowledge, there have been no studies comparing bipolar and unipolar illness in which the groups have actually been matched for episode frequency. This is a serious limitation in light of the increasing evidence that more highly recurrent unipolar patients appear to be quite similar to bipolar patients in some important respects (e.g., early age at onset, family history of mania, "atypical" features, and prophylactic response to lithium).

Implicit in the foregoing discussion of bipolar–unipolar distinctions is the need for a more explicit focus on the relationship between cyclicity and polarity. To what extent do differences in cyclicity contribute to or obscure reported bipolar–unipolar differences? In other words, how are we to know whether a given bipolar–unipolar difference is a function of the presence or absence of a history of mania/hypomania, or occurs because the bipolar group is more cyclic or recurrent than the unipolar group? These important questions are discussed later in the chapter. The relationship between polarity per se and other dimensions of affective illness—family history, age at onset, severity, psychotic features, response to treatment, and biological markers—generally has been studied one dimension at a time. A more comprehensive understanding of these interrelationships awaits studies that employ simultaneous weighing of multiple dimensions.

Unipolar Mania

The classic studies of Leonhard (1957), Perris (1966), Angst (1966), and Winokur and colleagues (1969) noted the relatively rare occurrence of manic patients with no apparent history of depression. In Leonhard's series, "pure mania" represented 9 percent of the bipolar group, whereas in the other studies it made up less than 5 percent. Although Leonhard initially considered patients with pure mania a separate group, subsequent studies indicated that they could not be distinguished from bipolar patients by either family history, course, treatment, or clinical features of mania. Thus, pure mania has generally been considered a variant of bipolar illness. Present knowledge suggests the likelihood that patients so identified either have had unreported depressions or have not been followed long enough to rule out future depressions. For some unipolar manic patients, depressive episodes are subsyndromal: they fail to be diagnosed because they lack a prominent or reported mood component; that is, the depressions manifest themselves primarily as episodes of increased sleep, decreased energy, and slowed thinking.

Abrams and colleagues[26] (Abrams and Taylor, 1974; Abrams et al., 1979) prompted a reevaluation of this question by reporting a 28 percent and an 18 percent incidence of unipolar mania among two relatively large independent samples of manic patients (N=127 for the two samples). Among the problems with these two studies, however, is the method used to ascertain a history of depression.[27] Like previous authors, Abrams and Taylor found that their "unipolar manics" did not differ fundamentally from the bipolar patients in demographic characteristics, family history variables, symptoms, or response to "doctor's choice" treatment.

Nurnberger and colleagues (1979) surveyed 241 bipolar-I patients in a lithium clinic and found that 16 percent had not been medically treated for depression, although most of them did show depressive features on a systematic interview. These authors, like other investigators, concluded from their review of phenomenological and family history data that unipolar mania is a variant of bipolar illness, not a separate entity. The NIMH Collaborative Program on the Psychobiology of Depression-Clinical Studies followed 27 patients (from a pool of 163 bipolar-I patients) initially admitted with a diagnosis of unipolar mania (Solomon et al., 2003) and found that 7 of them suffered no episodes of major depression during the 15- to 20-year follow-up; that is, unipolar mania represented 4 percent of the total bipolar sample. Yazici and colleagues (2002), by contrast, found that unipolar mania accounted for 16 percent of patients in their lithium clinic in Turkey, the higher rate perhaps reflecting cultural differences; that study also revealed a significantly higher rate of psychotic features associated with unipolar mania. Shulman and Tohen (1994) found the rate of unipolar mania to be 12 percent in a group of 50 elderly manic patients.

Perugi and colleagues (1998a) reported that hyperthymic temperament was the baseline in many unipolar manic patients, whose course appeared to be more chronic than that of the typical bipolar patient. Unlike the work of Angst and colleagues (2004), who reported a relatively favorable course among their pure M and Md patients, the findings of the two aforementioned studies suggest that unipolar mania represents a prognostically unfavorable variant of bipolar-I disorder. Yet this discrepancy may reflect differences in the populations designated as unipolar manics. For example, a late-onset bipolar disorder with predominantly manic course has been described, and is associated with evidence of organic contributions and negative family history for bipolarity (Shulman and Post, 1980; Moorhead and Young, 2003). The condition of these patients is best considered a phenocopy of mania, and should probably be excluded from the manic-depressive spectrum.

Future studies attempting to evaluate the validity of the concept of unipolar mania will have to employ careful diagnostic criteria, sensitive methods of ascertainment (especially family informants), and extensive follow-up periods. As the evidence now stands, we would agree with most authorities in the field that the existence of true unipolar mania as a separate entity is questionable. In our discussions here, it is included in the bipolar group.

False Unipolar Patients

As reviewed in the first edition of this volume, patients classified as unipolar who subsequently experience a manic or hypomanic episode—so-called *false unipolars*—confound studies of bipolar–unipolar differences (unipolar patients with some bipolar characteristics—sometimes called *pseudounipolar*—represent a different issue and are discussed below). Obviously, substantial numbers of false unipolar patients in a sample could distort or conceal bipolar–unipolar differences.

Table 1–2 presents data from three longitudinal studies (Perris, 1968; Angst et al., 1978; Grof, unpublished). The number of false unipolar patients is expressed as a percentage of the total unipolar group and as a function of numbers of depressive episodes without a mania. One might have expected the percentage of false unipolar patients to decrease as the group was "purified" by requiring more episodes of depression, that is, allowing more and more opportunity for latent bipolarity to express itself. In fact, however, the denominator (i.e., the number of true unipolar patients) also decreases as patients with more episodes are selected, since the unipolar patients who have only one, two, or three episodes are dropped. Thus, the actual percentage of false unipolar patients in the apparent unipolar population is relatively stable beyond the second episode, so that the convention of requiring more than two episodes of depression before diagnosing unipolar illness is ineffective in reducing the percentage of false unipolar patients. However, this convention does reduce the heterogeneity among unipolar groups

with respect to recurrence, increasing the chances that bipolar–unipolar comparisons will really be about polarity, as noted above. Perris's (1966) bipolar–unipolar studies come closest to this in that his unipolar patients had all experienced at least three depressions. But the median number of episodes experienced by his unipolar patients was still substantially below that of his bipolar group.

A number of important studies of the unipolar-to-bipolar conversion conducted since 1990 are not included in Table 1–2 because they do not provide this type of analysis. They generally found rates of conversion from an initial unipolar to a subsequent bipolar diagnosis that range up to 50 percent;[28] the highest rate was found in the study of the Angst group, which had the longest follow-up period. Generally, the younger the age at onset of depression, the higher was the rate of subsequent conversion to bipolar (see, for example, Rao et al., 1995; Geller et al., 2001). These issues are detailed in Chapter 4.

We have already noted that some unipolar patients have bipolar-like courses—namely early age at onset and frequent recurrences. Akiskal and Mallya (1987) pursued this observation by examining unipolar patients for depressive symptoms that might be considered analogous to mania/hypomania. Koukopoulos and Koukopoulos (1999) described these agitated depressions as "depressive mixed states," a concept that overlaps considerably with "agitated depression" (see Chapter 2). Depressive mixed states were studied more systematically in the Ravenna–San Diego Collaborative Study.[29] In that research, only three "manic-hypomanic" symptoms were required, the most frequent being psychomotor agitation (which was not goal directed), distractibility, and racing–crowded (predominantly

TABLE 1–2. **Estimates of Percent False Unipolar Using Different Cutoff Points for "Unipolar Depression"**

Required Number of Depressive Episodes	FALSE UNIPOLAR %		
	Grof (Unpublished)	Perris (1968)	Angst et al.[a] (1978)
1	18.5	—	28.4
2	15.3	13.1	26.2
3	11.9	11.4	22.5
4	13.2	12.5	22.9
5	7.8	10.7	25.0

[a]The larger percentages from the Angst et al. data may reflect a sampling bias toward more recurrent forms of the illness.

negative) thoughts, all symptoms traditionally associated with agitated depression.

The examination of depressive "mixed states" has accelerated since the first edition of this text was produced. For example, Benazzi (2001) found that 49 percent of his bipolar-II patients had three or more concurrent manic-like symptoms, versus only 3 percent of his unipolar patients. Likewise, Sato and colleagues (2003) found significantly more manic-like symptoms in their bipolar depressed patients—especially irritability, racing thoughts, and distractibility—than in their unipolar patients. In their study of 441 bipolar patients, Bauer and colleagues (2005) found that 70 percent had "clinically significant" manic-like symptoms while in a depressive episode. Maj and colleagues (2003) compared bipolar-I patients who became agitated when depressed with those who did not and found that one in four of the former had other manic-like symptoms, such as racing thoughts and pressured speech. In a more recent study of major depressive disorder, Maj and colleagues (2006) compared agitated patients with the same number of nonagitated patients, and found more bipolar relatives among the former. Serretti and Olgiati (2005) analyzed the patterns of "manic" symptoms in 372 patients diagnosed with major depressive disorder and identified agitated activity as the most frequent (18 percent), followed by irritable mood (7 percent), distractibility (3 percent), reduced need for sleep (2 percent), and reckless activity (2 percent). Note that in these studies, the most frequent "manic" symptom identified was psychomotor agitation, which recalls our speculation in the first edition of this text that agitation in unipolar depression may be analogous to mania in bipolar illness. However, we noted that manic hyperactivity and depressive agitation generally connote different phenomena, the former being more variable and goal directed, and the latter more repetitive, stereotyped, and purposeless.

The contention that these conditions should be called "mixed states" (and therefore bipolar) rather than "agitated depression" can complicate the interpretation of bipolar–unipolar differences because it broadens the concept of bipolarity to include patients *without* a history of mania or hypomania. While the finding of an elevated risk for bipolarity in first-degree relatives of agitated unipolar patients reinforces the conclusion that activation/agitation in a subgroup of unipolar patients may be a marker of a bipolar diathesis, it falls short of being an adequate basis for designating such unipolar patients as bipolar per se (Goodwin and Ghaemi, 2000). The contemporary delineation of depressive mixed states harkens back to Kraepelin (1899), who cited the existence of certain manic-like signs and symptoms during recurrent depression in some patients as he developed his argument for the essential unity of the recurrent affective disorders as manic-depressive

illness. Clearly this is a critical issue and one that is central to the discussion of mood disorders. The centrality of mixed affective states, along with the belief that recurrence/cyclicity is as or more defining a feature than polarity per se, underscores our use of the more inclusive diagnostic term manic-depressive illness. Future research on depressive mixed states and their relationship to bipolar disorder will in time clarify which characteristics of depression and mania are most important to differentiating among and understanding the affective illnesses.

The Primacy of Mania

Koukopoulos (2006) has made a novel suggestion about the relationship between mania and depression that may explain the occurrence and frequency of mixed states, as well as the connection between manic and depressive episodes in the course of this illness. According to his hypothesis, mania is primary, with depression being the consequence of a preceding mania. Thus according to this perspective, the recurrent unipolar subgroup of manic-depressive illness does not really exist since all depressive presentations are preceded by a manic presentation. Obviously, this hypothesis would require a much broader notion of mania than occurs in DSM-IV, one corresponding to concepts used 100 years ago and into ancient times. In this model, mania represents any kind of "excitement" or agitation. Thus in mania's most severe forms, we have type I bipolar disorder, while in its less severe forms, hypomania or hyperthymic personality precedes depressive episodes. Even with respect to nonrecurrent major depression, other manifestations of excitation (e.g., stress-induced anxiety conditions) could be seen as precursors of a later major depressive episode. As with any bold hypothesis, numerous objections can be made to the thesis of Koukopoulos; however, it is testable, and considering it in examining the spectrum of mood conditions may be heuristically useful.

Clinical Differences between Bipolar and Unipolar Depression

In his early observations, Leonhard noted that his bipolar patients (proportion of bipolar-I versus -II not specified) showed more symptomatic variability from episode to episode than did his recurrent unipolar patients, whose depressive symptoms he characterized as "stereotyped" (Leonhard, 1957). This differential brings to mind more recent comparisons in which bipolar-II depressed patients have been noted to have less stability and uniformity of symptoms across episodes than unipolar patients (Hantouche and Akiskal, 2005). Many studies over several decades, the results of which are summarized in Table 1–3, have found unipolar and bipolar-I differences over a wide

TABLE 1–3. Clinical Differences between Bipolar (Primarily Bipolar-I) and Unipolar Depressions

Symptom	Clinical Comparisons	Studies
Anxiety	UP > BP	Greenhouse and Geisser, 1959; Beigel and Murphy, 1971a; Brockington et al., 1982; Mitchell et al., 2001; Sato et al., 2005; Vahip et al., 2005
Tension/fearfulness	BP > UP	Perlis et al., 2006
Somatic complaints	UP > BP	Greenhouse and Geisser, 1959; Beigel and Murphy, 1971a; Vahip et al., 2002
Psychomotor retardation	BP > UP	Beigel and Murphy, 1971a; Himmelhoch et al., 1972; Kotin and Goodwin, 1972; Dunner et al., 1976a; Katz et al., 1982; Mitchell et al., 2001
	UP > BP	Popescu et al., 1991; Mitchell et al., 1992
Psychomotor agitation	UP > BP	Greenhouse and Geisser, 1959; Beigel and Murphy, 1971a; Katz et al., 1982; Kupfer et al., 1974
Atypical features	BP-II > UP	Ebert et al., 1993; Perugi et al., 1998c; Agosti and Stewart, 2001; Benazzi and Akiskal, 2001; Mitchell et al., 2001; Angst et al., 2002; Ghaemi et al., 2004; Akiskal and Benazzi, 2005; Hantouche and Akiskal, 2005
	BP-II = UP	Horwath et al., 1992; Robertson et al., 1995; Posternak and Zimmerman, 2002; Sullivan et al., 2002
Appetite loss	UP > BP	Papadimitriou et al., 2002
Depressive mixed states	BP > UP	Benazzi, 2001; Perugi et al., 2001; Maj et al., 2003; Sato et al., 2003; Akiskal and Benazzi, 2005; Bauer et al., 2005
Symptomatic variability across episodes	BP-I/-II > UP	Leonhard, 1957; Hantouche and Akiskal, 2005
Mood lability within episode	BP > UP	Brockington et al., 1982a; Hantouche and Akiskal, 2005
Irritability	BP-II > UP	Fava and Rosenbaum, 1999; Deckersbach et al., 2004; Perlis et al., 2004; Perugi et al., 2004; Benazzi and Akiskal, 2005
Insomnia (initial)	UP > BP	Mitchell et al., 2001; Hantouche and Akiskal, 2005
Insomnia (late)	BP > UP	Vahip et al., 2002
Hypersomnia	BP > UP	Mitchell et al., 2001
Postpartum episodes	BP > UP	Reich and Winokur, 1970; Kadrmas et al., 1979
Pain sensitivity	UP > BP	Davis and Buchsbaum, 1981
Fragmented REM sleep	BP > UP	Duncan et al., 1979; Mendelson et al., 1987; Rao et al., 2002

(continued)

TABLE 1–3. **Clinical Differences between Bipolar (Primarily Bipolar-I) and Unipolar Depressions** *(continued)*

Symptoms	Clinical Comparisons	Studies
Weight loss	UP >BP	Abrams and Taylor, 1980
Psychotic features	BP >UP	Guze et al., 1975; Akiskal, 1983c ; Coryell et al., 1985; Endicott et al., 1985; Parker et al., 2000; Mitchell et al., 2001
Comorbid substance abuse	BP >UP	Regier et al., 1990; Judd et al., 2003a; Marneros and Goodwin, 2006

BP = bipolar; UP = unipolar.

range of clinical features. We have already noted the heterogeneity in both the bipolar and unipolar groups (especially the latter), which makes any generalizations difficult to say the least. In addition to the unknown variability in extent of recurrence (cycle lengths), most of these studies did not control for differences in severity of depression or age at onset.[30]

It is worth noting that the comparisons in Table 1–3 are predominantly between unipolar and bipolar-I patients (although several of the studies refer only to "bipolar" without specifying subtype). Indeed, it has been suggested that bipolar–unipolar differences become clearer when the bipolar-II group is excluded. The most widely replicated studies point to a picture of the bipolar-I depressed patient as having more mood lability, psychotic features, psychomotor retardation, and comorbid substance abuse. In contrast, the typical unipolar patient in these studies had more anxiety, agitation, insomnia, physical complaints, anorexia, and weight loss. As noted in the table, there are a number of other features for which there is only one study or conflicting studies; certainly some of the apparent disagreement may be related simply to inadequate description of the bipolar or unipolar samples.

There is a much smaller body of data on unipolar–bipolar-II comparisons, and most of these data focus on depressive "mixed states" (more frequent in bipolar-II, as discussed above and in Chapter 2) and on so-called atypical features. Atypical depression was originally described in unipolar patients on the basis of a group of symptoms including hypersomnia, increased weight and appetite, leaden paralysis, interpersonal rejection sensitivity, and preferential response to monoamine oxidase inhibitors (MAOIs) (reviewed by Raskin and Crook, 1976). Given the suggestion of earlier studies that MAOIs are preferentially effective in bipolar depression (Himmelhoch et al., 1991), an interest in the relationship between atypical features and bipolar illness has developed. Following up on studies of atypical features reviewed in the first edition, a number of more recent

studies have reported more atypical symptoms in bipolar-II than in unipolar depressed patients.[31] On the other hand, not all investigators have found such differences.[32,33] Some of these latter studies, however, did not systematically assess bipolar-II as recommended by Dunner and Tay (1993) and Ghaemi and colleagues (2002), among others. As noted above, heterogeneity among samples of unipolar patients is another potential source of divergent findings. For example, Benazzi (2003) found that some bipolar–unipolar differences depended on the age at onset in the unipolar sample: only those unipolar patients with later age at onset were significantly different from the bipolar-II group with respect to bipolar family history, atypical features, number of episodes, and depressive mixed states.

Another approach to examining the relationship between atypical depression and bipolar disorder was pursued by Akiskal and Benazzi (2005). They examined 602 consecutively evaluated outpatients with DSM-IV major depression (58 percent were bipolar-II,[34] 42 percent unipolar), 43 percent of whom met DSM-IV criteria for atypical features, in agreement with the data of Perugi and colleagues (1998a) and Angst and colleagues (2002). They found a robust association between atypical features (especially leaden paralysis and hypersomnia) and a bipolar family history.[35] In a recent analysis of this same cohort, Akiskal and Benazzi (2006) found that hypomania scores (using The Hypomania Interview Guide) were distributed normally, not bimodally and there was a "dose response" relationship between these scores and the extent of bipolar family history, both findings suggesting that highly recurrent unipolar and bipolar II are on the same spectrum rather than representing seperate categories. On this basis, Akiskal and Benazzi suggested that atypical depression may represent a bridge between unipolar and bipolar-II disorder.

Heun and Maier (1993) interviewed 80 bipolar and 108 unipolar patients and 80 controls, along with their first-degree relatives, and found that while the morbid risk for bipolar-I was equivalent in relatives of the bipolar-I and -II groups (and was higher for both than for the unipolar group), the morbid risk for bipolar-II distinguished the relatives of this group (6.1 percent) from those of the bipolar-I group (1.8 percent). Like the findings of earlier studies (Dunner et al., 1976b; Gershon et al., 1982), these data suggest that bipolar-II may be genetically heterogeneous, some evidence being consistent with categorical integrity (Simpson et al., 1993) and some with a bipolar-I–bipolar-II spectrum. (These genetic issues are discussed more thoroughly in Chapter 13.)

Clinical Differences between Bipolar-I and -II Depressions

In the first edition, we reported on a series of NIMH clinical, genetic, pharmacological, and biological studies of bipolar–unipolar differences in which bipolar-I and -II patients were analyzed separately (Dunner et al., 1976a; Dunner, 1980). On some measures (for example, a family history of mania), the bipolar-I and -II groups were similar to one another and dissimilar to the unipolar patients. On other measures (for example, age at onset), the bipolar-II group appeared to be intermediate between the bipolar-I and unipolar groups. Finally, on some measures (for example, "atypical" features of depression), the bipolar-II patients were more similar to the unipolar than to the bipolar-I patients. One problem limiting interpretation of this interesting series of studies is the fact that the initial diagnosis of depressive illness was made prior to the availability of formal diagnostic criteria; thus, even though all of the patients had depressions severe enough to require hospitalization, the unipolar groups were undoubtedly heterogeneous.

Endicott and colleagues (1985) advanced the field by applying the formal Research Diagnostic Criteria (RDC) to 122 bipolar-I, 66 bipolar-II, and 104 recurrent unipolar depressed patients (two or more episodes of major depressive disorder). In the earlier study of Dunner and colleagues (1976) of patients hospitalized for depression, the age at onset of the bipolar-II group was intermediate (consistent with a spectrum based on severity of mania), whereas in the study of Endicott and colleagues (1985), the age at onset of the two bipolar groups was similar and different (younger) from that of the unipolar group. On the other hand, bipolar-II and unipolar patients were similar (and different from bipolar-I patients) in that both had higher proportions of time spent depressed, a finding that was confirmed and extended by the longitudinal NIMH Collaborative Program on the Psychobiology of Depression-Clinical Studies (Judd et al., 2003c) (see Chapter 4). Bipolar-II females had higher rates of alcoholism than unipolar or bipolar-I females, consistent with the earlier findings of Dunner and colleagues (1979), and they

were more likely to suffer from premenstrual dysphoria. Most important, Coryell and colleagues (1984) and Endicott and colleagues (1985) found that bipolar-I and -II patients tended to breed true. That is, bipolar-I patients tended to have bipolar-I relatives and bipolar-II patients to have bipolar-II relatives, a finding that is in agreement with the data of Fieve and colleagues (1984)[36] and Simpson and colleagues (1993) and partly with those of Gershon and colleagues (1982).

Table 1–4 updates those findings with studies published since the first edition. One important question is how these reported bipolar-I–bipolar-II differences may affect our understanding of the relationship between unipolar and bipolar depression and the concept of the manic-depressive spectrum. Focusing on the most replicated findings, a picture emerges of the bipolar-II patient as more likely to be female, with less severe but more frequent and more chronic depressions, shorter interepisode intervals, and more comorbid anxiety and alcohol abuse (the latter among females). By contrast, the bipolar-I patient has more severe and prolonged depressions with more psychosis and hospitalizations. With regard to age at onset, agitation, irritability, and frequency of rapid cycling, there is no consensus on bipolar-I–bipolar-II differences.

Examining Tables 1–3 and 1–4 together, one notes that bipolar-II is closer to unipolar in some respects (e.g., percent female and time spent depressed), but closer to bipolar-I in others (e.g., number of episodes and substance abuse).

As noted earlier, the DSM-IV construct of bipolar-II requires a threshold of 4 or more days. However, findings of more recent studies suggest that 2 days may be a more appropriate threshold (judged on the basis of external validating strategies, such as age at onset, depressive recurrence, and familial bipolarity). These are mainly cross-sectional studies from different clinics in the United States (Akiskal and Mallya, 1987; Manning et al., 1997) and Italy (Cassano et al., 1992; Benazzi, 2001). Epidemiologic data reveal that most hypomanias are of 1–3 days' duration (Wicki and Angst, 1991). It is interesting to note that if one takes a dimensional view of hypomania in manic-depressive illness (symptoms rather than syndrome), bipolar–recurrent unipolar differences are attenuated (Cassano et al., 2004);[37] these clinical observations require independent validation by external markers, such as family history and prospective course.

Few long-term studies have been conducted with lower thresholds for hypomania. The two exceptions are derived from the prospective NIMH Collaborative Program on the Psychobiology of Depression-Clinical Studies, which showed, first, longitudinal stability of bipolar-II over time (Coryell et al., 1995) and, second, no significant differences in clinical and course parameters when either 2- or 7-day

TABLE 1–4. **Clinical Differences between Bipolar-I and Bipolar-II**

Symptom	Clinical Comparisons	Studies
Anxiety	BP-II > BP-I	Dunner et al., 1976b; Hantouche et al., 1998; Judd et al., 2003c
Time spent in depression (major and minor)	BP-II > BP-I	Endicott et al., 1985; Vieta et al., 1997; Judd et al., 2003
Interepisode intervals	BP-II < BP-I	Judd et al., 2003b
Number of episodes	BP-II > BP-I	Vieta et al., 1997; Judd et al., 2003c; Akiskal and Benazzi, 2005
Rapid cycling	BP-II > BP-I	Coryell et al., 1992; Maj et al., 1999; Baldessarini et al., 2000
	BP-II = BP-I	Vieta et al., 1997; Coryell et al., 2003
Psychotic features	BP-I > BP-II	Vieta et al., 1997; Mitchell et al., 2001
Suicide/suicide attempt	BP-II > BP-I	Dunner et al., 1976; Goldring and Fieve, 1984; Arato et al., 1988; Rihmer and Pestality, 1999
	BP-I = BP-II	Coryell et al., 1989; Vieta et al., 1997
Premenstrual dysphoria	BP-II > BP-I	Endicott et al., 1985
Hospitalizations	BP-I > BP-II	Vieta et al., 1997
Agitation; irritability	BP-I > BP-II	Dunner et al., 1976b; Hantouche et al., 1998; Serretti and Olgiati, 2005
Alcohol abuse (females)	BP-II > BP-I	Dunner et al. 1976b; Endicott et al., 1985; Ferrier et al., 2001
Percent female	BP-II > BP-I	Weissman et al., 1996; Cassano et al., 1999
Severity of depressive episodes	BP-I > BP-II	Coryell et al., 1985; Vieta et al., 1997; Benazzi, 1999
Length of depressive episode	BP-I > BP-II	Coryell et al., 1985
Percent medicated	BP-I > BP-II	Coryell et al., 1985

BP = bipolar.

thresholds were applied to RDC-defined bipolar-II patients (Judd et al., 2003b). Akiskal and Pinto (1999) suggested that those with the shortest duration of hypomania are more unstable and have a highly recurrent course, typically arising from a cyclothymic temperamental base, which they designate bipolar-II ½.[38] It remains to be seen whether such continued splitting of diagnostic groups is productive or is simply confusing to the field. This is an empirical question, one that will be resolved ultimately by genetic studies. It is noteworthy that Angst and Gamma (2002), in defining subthreshold bipolarity, set no thresholds for the duration of hypomania as long as the hypomania is recurrent.

EMERGENCE OF THE MANIC-DEPRESSIVE SPECTRUM

The concept of a spectrum is used in two different ways in the description of affective disorders, both clearly delineated by Kraepelin. On the one hand, spectrum conceptualizes a continuum between bipolar and unipolar illness—historically, this is the manic-depressive spectrum. On the other hand, a spectrum is a way to conceptualize the relationship between full-blown affective illness, either bipolar or unipolar, and milder states or characteristics that might be construed as temperament. When we refer to the manic-depressive spectrum here, we are using it in this latter way.

Kraepelin (1921, p. 1) was the first to formally posit a continuum between the psychotic and less severe of affective disorders, merging imperceptibly with normality (although this concept was implicit among many of the ancient physicians):

Manic-depressive insanity . . . [includes] certain slight and slightest colourings of mood, some of them periodic, some of them continuously morbid, which on the one hand are to be regarded as the rudiment of more severe disorders, on the other hand pass without sharp boundary into the domain of personal predisposition. In the course of the years I have become more and more convinced that all the above-mentioned states only represent manifestations of a single morbid process.

As we noted in the first edition, the classic descriptions cited in Chapter 2, systematic observations reported in the literature, and our own research and clinical experience and that of our colleagues all convince us that the cardinal features of manic-depressive illness are dimensional, that is, distributed along a spectrum. Indeed, to give emphasis to the spectrum concept in the first edition, we devoted a separate chapter to it. Our 1990 conclusion was echoed by an international panel of experts that summarized the increasingly rich and sophisticated database supporting such a spectrum (Akiskal et al., 2000). More recently, Ghaemi and colleagues (2004) proposed a definition of bipolar spectrum disorder (or as we would prefer for clarity, the manic-depressive spectrum), which is outlined in Box 1–2.

We further explore the spectrum model here because it introduces concepts that shaped the formal diagnostic systems reviewed in Chapter 3, and it clarifies our own conceptions of manic-depressive illness, implicit in discussions throughout this volume.

Although diagnosis is central to all of medicine, the assumptions underlying its various meanings are seldom examined. The most common medical classification model—the categorical approach—posits discrete diagnostic entities or discrete subtypes within a larger diagnostic group. Dimensional approaches, the most common competing model, characterize the individual patient according to where he or she falls on a number of separate dimensions. In this model, each individual represents the point of intersection of multiple parameters. Both models have gained support from studies using discriminate function analysis and other statistical techniques. Clearly, the categorical approaches tend to prevail, not because they are supported more compellingly by the empirical evidence, but because they are much easier to grasp conceptually and to deal with statistically. Indeed, multidimensional approaches, however eloquently descriptive of an individual patient, will remain essentially unhelpful if they cannot test generalizations—that is, be applied to prediction.

Contrary to the common assumption, the categorical approach does not preclude the concept of a continuum (Grayson, 1987; Kraemer et al., 2004). A diagnostic category need not have absolutely discrete and discontinuous boundaries. Let us suppose for the moment that individuals with depressive disorders are distributed more or less evenly along a continuum with self-limiting grief reactions on one end and severe, disabling major depressive illness on the other (Kendell, 1968; Goodwin, 1977). Even if discontinuity (i.e., clustering at discrete points along the spectrum) is not

---

BOX **1–2.**   **A Proposed Definition of Bipolar Spectrum Disorder**

A. At least one major depressive episode
B. No spontaneous hypomanic or manic episodes
C. Either one of the following, plus at least two items from criterion D, or both of the following plus one item from criterion D:
    1. A family history of bipolar disorder in a first-degree relative
    2. Antidepressant-induced mania or hypomania
D. If no items from criterion C are present, six of the following nine criteria are needed:
    1. Hyperthymic personality (at baseline, nondepressed state)
    2. Recurrent major depressive episode (>3)
    3. Brief major depressive episodes (on average, <3 months)
    4. Atypical depressive features (increased sleep or appetite)
    5. Psychotic major depressive episode
    6. Early age at onset of major depressive episode (before age 25)
    7. Postpartum depression
    8. Antidepressant tolerance ("wear-off," acute but not prophylactic response)
    9. Lack of response to >3 antidepressant treatment trials

Source: Ghaemi et al., 2004.

---

demonstrable, a useful category can still be defined by establishing a minimum (or maximum) threshold of symptoms for inclusion in the category; consider, for example, hypertension and hypothyroidism. And the pattern of illness characteristics—symptoms, course, family history, and treatment response, for example—reflects a convergence of several dimensional variables. Such a model should be acceptable to those who are comfortable with large, internally variable categories—the "lumpers"—as well as to those who want to create a new category for every variant—the "splitters." This conception is simply for the sake of narrative convenience, not to reflect a conviction that any particular group has discrete, discontinuous boundaries. On the contrary, and as we emphasized in the first edition of this book, we are impressed with the subtlety of the shadings.[39] How these issues bear on diagnosis is discussed in Chapter 3.

Exploration of spectrum models is important for several reasons. The reliable characterization and validation of subsyndromal states similar to bipolar illness would enhance research on genetic markers and modes of genetic transmission, as discussed in Chapter 13, as well as provide an approach for identifying individuals at risk for the development of full-blown bipolar illness (Alda, 2004). Additionally, a spectrum model would permit the evaluation of treatments for attenuated variants, including the question of whether early intervention could lessen the chance of progression to bipolar illness. Existing prospective and retrospective data indicate that approximately one-third of individuals with subthreshold conditions phenomenologically related to bipolar illness (i.e., cyclothymia) will go on to develop the full bipolar syndrome (Akiskal et al., 1979a, 1995; Depue et al., 1981, 1989; Cassano et al., 2002, 2004). The possibility that this progression may be hastened by treatment with antidepressant drugs (see Chapter 19) lends further urgency to identifying subsyndromal precursors of bipolar disorder. Indeed, the term *bipolar spectrum*, which conveys the continuum of cyclothymia with bipolar-II and with hypomanias associated with antidepressants, is a logical extension of concepts laid out long ago by Kraepelin and his predecessors.

The concepts of secondary depression and secondary mania have received considerable attention because they are important to differential diagnosis (see Chapter 3) and because they may shed light on the pathophysiology of mood states (see Chapter 14). Reexamined in light of spectrum models, secondary mania and depression, like their primary counterparts, also appear to be expressions of an underlying diathesis, but a weaker one, which therefore requires a greater perturbation to be expressed clinically. This possibility is most credible in the case of pharmacologically induced hypomanias.

Bearing on the concept of a manic-depressive spectrum (i.e., the relationship between unipolar and bipolar illness), recent data from the French national EPIDEP (Epidemiology of Depression) study (Akiskal et al., 2003a) suggest a familial vulnerability for hypomania associated with antidepressant pharmacotherapy, which is similar to that for spontaneous bipolar-II disorder (see Table 1–1), but one that is probably less severe than that associated with spontaneous hypomanic episodes. For this reason, Akiskal and colleagues (2003a) have suggested the term *bipolar-III* for this group of patients. A prospective study by Kovacs and colleagues (1994) showed that many dysthymic children followed up beyond puberty do switch to hypomania and/or mania even without pharmacological treatment. These data suggest a threshold of vulnerability among subjects with early-onset dysthymia that may not routinely require external triggers, such as antidepressants.

Along the same lines, Akiskal and colleagues (1979b) reported that familial affective "loading" (defined as more than three affected members in a pedigree) predicted those "neurotic depressives" who progressed to hypomania and/or mania during prospective follow-up. In another study, Akiskal and colleagues (1978) followed 100 outpatients with mild depressive states—variously referred to as "neurotic," "reactive," or "situational"—for 3 to 4 years. They found that 40 percent developed a major affective disorder, and nearly half of these were bipolar.

The terminology applied to the "soft bipolar spectrum" includes overlapping conditions in the less-than-manic range. The soft spectrum includes Dunner and colleagues' (1980) "bipolar, not otherwise specified," as well as conditions described by Akiskal and Akiskal (1988) as depressions arising from cyclothymic and hyperthymic temperament. In addition, it includes hypomanic reactions occurring during antidepressant and other somatotherapies for depression.

An elevated risk for familial bipolarity (Cassano et al., 1992; Akiskal, 2001) represents the main external validation of the bipolar nature of these "soft" phenotypes. Akiskal and colleagues (2003a) and Hantouche and colleagues (2003a) have suggested that within the broadly conceived cyclothymic temperamental domain there are "dark" and "sunny" types. Although family history for bipolar disorder is equally high in both groups, in clinical practice bipolar-II associated with the darker core cyclothymic temperament is more likely to be diagnosed as a personality disorder. There is little justification for this practice, because as in the case of full-blown bipolar patients, those with spectrum diagnoses in the broad cyclothymic–bipolar-II realm are equally likely to engage in dramatic and socially inappropriate behaviors (Akiskal, 1994; Deltito et al., 2001). In the end, it may not be easy to distinguish among clinical, subclinical, subthreshold, and personality expressions of bipolarity (Akiskal et al., 1979a; Sass et al., 1993; Akiskal, 2001). Again, it is important to stress that although the spectrum concept is essential, there must be concern that the spectrum of bipolarity can become so far extended that it becomes theoretically and clinically meaningless (if not actually damaging, as would be the case with a diagnostic overinclusiveness resulting in the inappropriate diagnosis and treatment of individuals with intense normal variants of temperament).

The Akiskal and Pinto (1999) formulation acknowledging more subtle intermediary forms, a formulation indebted to the observations of many earlier clinicians and investigators, captures the dilemmas of the clinician and the researcher working within a spectrum model of bipolar illness from the most severe (mood-incongruent mania) to the least severe (hyperthymic temperament). Similar dilemmas are encountered when exploring the manic-depressive spectrum between bipolar disorder and unipolar depression.

Using both clinical and nonclinical populations of college students, Depue and colleagues developed a systematic approach to the evaluation of subsyndromal affective states, focusing particularly on bipolar forms. The touchstone of this series of studies was the development of the General Behavioral Inventory (GBI), a self-report measure of traits that can assess the pattern of cyclothymia over time (Depue et al., 1981; Depue and Klein, 1988). Each of its

73 items, drawn from clinical descriptions of hypomania and depression and focused on lability, incorporates the dimensions of intensity, duration, and frequency. (The GBI is described in more detail in Chapter 11.) GBI scores for depression are distributed across normal, cyclothymic, and bipolar-II populations; each group merges imperceptibly into the other, consistent with the concept of a spectrum.[40] These studies imply that the concept of a depressive spectrum applies equally to bipolar and unipolar depression, challenging the conventional wisdom that neurotic depression should be subsumed entirely in the unipolar spectrum.

Unfortunately, the cyclothymic scale introduced by Depue and colleagues did not command sufficient interest in the literature, conceivably because its system for assessing mood lability, intensity, and cyclicity was quite elaborate. A new instrument was subsequently developed to measure the broader temperamental domain of bipolarity (Akiskal et al., 1998b): the temperament scale of Memphis, Pisa, Paris, and San Diego (TEMPS), which, while lacking the psychometric sophistication and strong validating research base of the GBI, appears to be somewhat less unwieldy from a psychometric standpoint and represents the dominant tendency for each of the cyclothymic, hyperthymic, irritable, and depressive types.[41]

As noted earlier, and as elaborated in Chapter 2 on clinical description, Kraepelin described a "manic temperament," which he originally termed "constitutional excitement." The antithesis of the "depressive temperament," the manic temperament, at its most severe, was defined as a handicapping condition marked by desultory, incoherent, and aimless thought; hasty and shallow judgment; restlessness; and exalted, careless, and confident mood. Kraepelin viewed the manic temperament as a "link in the long chain of manic-depressive dispositions," which in its least severe form could still be considered normal.

Akiskal and colleagues (1979a) characterized—and psychometrically validated (Akiskal et al., 1998b)—the most discriminatory features of what they termed the "hyperthymic temperament," representing the softest expression of Kraepelin's manic type. Like cyclothymia, hyperthymia represents a trait and possibly a lifelong disposition, with a familial excess of bipolar disorder as compared with depressive states without bipolar temperaments (Cassano et al., 1992; Akiskal, 2001; Akiskal et al., 2005). Unlike the studies of Kagan and colleagues (see Chapter 10), however, these studies of temperament have not been carried out across the lifetime or in a prospective context, which limits our understanding of the relationship among measured "hyperthymia," subsyndromal illness, and actual illness.

In his discussion of the manic spectrum based on cross-sectional observations, Klerman (1981) described a continuum from normal happiness or joy through cyclothymic personality, nonpsychotic hypomania, and psychotic mania. It is clear, however, that this string of states does not reflect a spectrum of ever-increasing happiness and joy, since these pleasant emotions are replaced by qualitatively very different moods and sensations as one crosses the line from hypomania into mania. Klerman's recommendation that the term "elations" be used to encompass the spectrum of mania emphasizes mood over other important features, such as energy level, activity, behavior, and cognition. As noted earlier, the terminology can be confusing. In Klerman's spectrum, cyclothymic personality falls between normal happiness and hypomania. In DSM-IV, a diagnosis of cyclothymia requires hypomanic episodes. In this diagnostic system, cyclothymia is differentiated from bipolar-II major affective disorder on the basis of its less severe depressions, which do not meet criteria for major depressive disorder. Using elation as the criterion for the manic spectrum also is reminiscent of older formulations in which depression and mania were at opposite ends of a continuum, with normal in the middle. Such a continuum is quite limited as a model, primarily because it cannot account for mixed states, which, as discussed in Chapter 2, are quite common. Some believe it preferable to consider the depressive and manic spectra as independent and capable of interacting in a variety of combinations and permutations.[42] It is interesting that in both the Endicott (1989) and the Angst and Gamma (2002) schema, the manic-depressive spectrum is dominated by depressive recurrences, with very mild and short hypomanias. This conception is in line with our view that recurrence and cyclicity are more fundamental than polarity, which in turn accords with Kraepelin's nosologic position. We remain concerned, however, that relatively little research has been conducted on the continuum of manic states (Jamison, 2004), a concern we expressed in the first edition of this text.

As reviewed in Chapter 2, severe psychotic features, including mood incongruence, are extensively documented for bipolar patients in both the classical and the recent literature. The boundary between severe mania and schizobipolar disorder is not clear (see Chapter 3). Suffice it to say that new data appear to be consistent with the view that schizobipolar patients lie on a continuum with severe mania, whether one examines family history (Van Eerdewegh et al., 1987; Toni et al., 2001) or course (Cutting, 1990).

If we integrate the depressive and manic spectra, we can construct an overall spectrum of bipolar illness. At one end is cyclothymic personality; then cyclothymic disorder (bipolar, other in Dunner's terms or md in Angst's terms[43]); followed by bipolar-II disorder (mD or bipolar disorder, not otherwise specified, in DSM-IV); then Md (often misdiagnosed as unipolar mania); and finally MD (i.e., bipolar-I), which is the core critical bipolar disorder.[44] Figure 1–1 illustrates this spectrum by displaying the mood variation characteristic of each subgroup. Note that in this spectrum, we implicitly consider mania to be more severe than depression, since the Md form is closer than mD (bipolar-II) to the severe end of the spectrum. Current international data indicate that much of the bipolar spectrum is in the midrealm (type II) and beyond.[45]

As presented here, the spectra are only descriptive. They do not necessarily imply a progression, nor do they require that all these states share some unitary relationship. Individuals fitting the description of cyclothymic personality, for example, may have a family history or response to treatment unrelated to bipolar-I disorder. The data reviewed in this chapter suggest, however, that a large percentage of individuals with soft or subsyndromal states apparently analogous to bipolar disorder do indeed belong in the bipolar spectrum by virtue of their positive family history and their tendency to progress to full clinical disorder. While those on the soft end of the spectrum may not be bipolar in the formal sense of having a history of diagnosable mania or hypomania, many of them no doubt have a bipolar diathesis.

Once we move beyond the temperaments into cyclothymic disorder (described more fully in Chapter 2), the evidence argues compellingly for the inclusion of cyclothymic disorder in the bipolar spectrum. Cycles of mood and energy can continue indefinitely, constituting a mild form of bipolar illness, or they can progress to a more severe expression of the disorder, sometimes after years.

As noted in Chapter 2, Kraepelin assumed that cyclothymia is part of the bipolar spectrum, and modern investigators[46] have argued persuasively for its inclusion on the basis of (1) family history data linking cyclothymia with the more severe forms of bipolar illness, (2) overlap and similarity of symptom patterns between cyclothymia and bipolar disorder, (3) comparability of rates for pharmacologically induced hypomania, and (4) the subsequent development of full syndromal illness in many patients initially diagnosed as cyclothymic. In some instances, cyclothymia can be regarded as a milder expression of bipolar illness and in others as a precursor to the full syndrome.

Some bipolar-II patients show considerable erratic "character" pathology (often referred to as "cluster B" or borderline—see Chapters 2 and 10), interepisode lability, and related problems of substance abuse. Conventional wisdom (e.g., DSM-IV) would suggest that an intrinsic association of these features with bipolar disorder is less convincing, on the assumption that such features are simply a consequence of the fact that bipolar-II patients often lead chaotic lives, have poor or unpredictable social support systems, and fail to adhere to medications.[47] Nonetheless, new findings from the French EPIDEP study, as described in Chapter 2, suggest that from a familial standpoint, these patients may be as bipolar as those with bipolar-II. Perugi and colleagues (1999, 2003) have proposed a common link among these cyclothymic traits, borderline personality, and atypical depression.

Criticism notwithstanding, the concept of a manic-depressive spectrum appears to be shaping a new paradigm, much of it extending into the domain of traditional depressive disorders. Indeed, whether one examines bipolar pedigrees (Gershon et al., 1982; Tsuang et al., 1985), offspring of bipolars (Akiskal et al., 1985), epidemiologic samples (Angst et al., 2003), or the microstructure of the course of bipolar-I and -II disorders (Judd et al., 2002, 2003b), bipolar illness is

Figure 1–1. Range of total mood variation by subgroup.

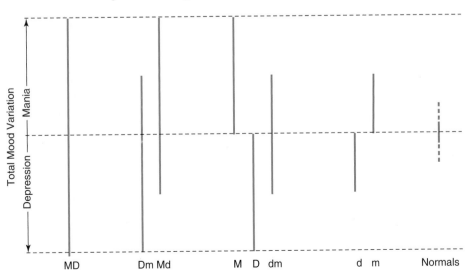

dominated by depressive symptomotology.[48] In this respect, bipolar-I and -II appear to be quite similar (Judd et al., 2003a). This is where a great deal of the disability associated with the illness appears to reside—in the subdepressive symptomotology between episodes (Altshuler et al., 2002). Given that the depressive dominance is found in epidemiologic samples and in pedigree and family studies, one cannot criticize the foregoing clinical studies on the basis of tertiary referral bias, by which the more depression-prone bipolar patients are retained in follow-up studies. As detailed in Chapter 2, the depressive phase of bipolar disorder and depressive presentations in clinical practice represent a highly important aspect of bipolarity.

The spectrum concept is not just a recent peculiarity of the clinical and research focus on soft bipolarity. As reviewed here and in Chapter 2, these concepts are ancient. Indeed, it has been suggested that all major mental disorders can perhaps best be characterized in spectrum models (Maser and Akiskal, 2002). As noted earlier, Baldessarini (2000) criticized the concept of a broad bipolar spectrum on methodological grounds, arguing that it risks diluting the concept of bipolar disorder, thereby reducing the rigor of contemporary research. We agree. It is true that most authors cited by Baldessarini as having made major contributions to the field (from Aretaeus on) endorsed a broad conceptualization of manic-depressive illness; as we noted earlier, however, "manic-depressive spectrum" denotes something different from "bipolar spectrum."

While the more recently proposed soft forms of bipolarity make some clinical and intuitive sense to us, they still require considerably more research from a wider range of independent research groups focused on external validators, especially family history, treatment response, and long-term outcome. For the clinician dealing with individuals, deciding whether one is encountering one end of a normal range of behavior, a personality disorder, or manic-depressive illness requiring treatment remains a challenge.

CONCLUSIONS

The existence of the "softer" phenotypes on the fringes of classic or "hard" bipolar phenotypes that encroach into the territory of unipolar depression indicates the need for at least a partial return to the unitary Kraepelinian concept of manic-depressive illness. While some view the bipolar spectrum as the modern heir of this classic broader position, subsuming all conditions under the rubric of "bipolar" is a less than totally satisfactory way to emphasize the close relationship between bipolar illness and highly recurrent unipolar depression (many patients with the latter condition, after all, remain nonbipolar in the usual sense).

If our diagnostic systems were to return to the Kraepelinian position of taking recurrence as the first principle for organizing the affective disorders (as we propose in Chapter 3), one would not have to posit that all early-onset recurrent depressions are part of the bipolar spectrum. On the other hand, contemporary studies[49] of "depressive mixed states" appear to provide some empirical support for Kraepelin's descriptions of "excited depression" and "depression with flight of ideas," apparently representing those highly recurrent unipolar patients who, despite not having a history of manic or hypomanic episodes, may have enough manic-like features when depressed, as well as sufficient bipolarity in their family histories, to be considered part of the bipolar spectrum in the sense of having some bipolar diathesis. For conceptualizing the relationship between bipolar disorder per se and recurrent depressive disorders, however, we still prefer the Kraepelinian concept of manic-depressive illness because it is unitary; all recurrent affective illness is encompassed, although Kraepelin anticipated the later bipolar–unipolar subdivision. Indeed, while much future research needs to be conducted to fully validate the concept of a manic-depressive spectrum, the pendulum appears to have shifted distinctly in favor of the Kraepelinian position, which includes much of the domain of frequently recurrent depression under the broad manic-depressive rubric.

Finally, we should reiterate why the exploration of spectrum models of manic-depressive illness is so important. First, for the bipolar subgroup, validation of subsyndromal states will enhance research on genetic markers and modes of genetic transmission. Second, it will allow the identification of individuals potentially at risk for the development of full bipolar illness, opening up the possibility of trials of early interventions that could reduce the likelihood of progression. Lastly, the model of a manic-depressive spectrum increases clinicians' awareness of the close relationship between bipolar illness and some forms of unipolar depression (an understanding that has been undermined by the structure of DSM-IV). It is only this awareness that can help the clinician avoid the all-too-common misdiagnosis of bipolar patients as unipolar, a mistake that can lead to the almost always ill-advised treatment decision, discussed in Chapter 19, of administering an antidepressant in the absence of a mood stabilizer.

NOTES

1. The authors acknowledge a deep intellectual debt to the great German psychiatrist Emil Kraepelin. Kraepelin, the son of an actor, was born in 1856 in Neustrelitz, near the Baltic Sea. His older brother Karl, a biology teacher, influenced Emil's decision to become a doctor and an academician. Interested in

psychiatry while still at the Würzburg Medical School, Kraepelin, upon graduation in 1878, studied with the neuroanatomists Bernard von Gudden and P. E. Flechsig. He then turned to experimental psychophysiological research, under the tutelage of Wilhelm Wundt. He held psychiatric hospital appointments in Munich, Leubus, and Dresden. In 1886, he became professor of psychiatry in Dorpat, then moved to the same position in Heidelberg in 1890 and to Munich in 1904 [or 1903?]. In 1922, he retired from teaching and became head of the Research Institute of Psychiatry in Munich.

According to Alexander and Selesnick (1966), Kraepelin's training, personality, and dedication were well suited to the task of classifying and generalizing the myriad clinical observations made during the nineteenth century: "He learned early to respect authority, order, and organization. . . . "Imperial German psychiatry" was said to have gained its prominence under the "chancellorship" of Kraepelin, one of Bismarck's admirers" (pp. 162–163). As Bismarck unified Germany, Kraepelin brought order to the balkanized psychiatry of the turn of the century. The first edition of his textbook, which he continued to revise throughout his life, was published in 1883. In succeeding editions, he refined and expanded the textbook from the brief outline of the first edition to the 2,425 pages of the ninth edition, published in 1927, a year after his death. The textbook was notable for its division of major psychiatric illness into two categories and for its emphasis on prognosis. The third and fourth parts of the eighth edition, covering manic-depressive "insanity" and paranoia, were published separately in 1921, and it is that monograph that is cited throughout this book.

Zilboorg (1941), from his psychoanalytical perspective, summarized the personal observations of Kraepelin from those who knew him personally:

[They] tell of his rather pleasant, responsive personality, of his tactful ability in bringing people together to work as an organized group, and of his great gifts as a teacher; yet it is curious that his scientific personality was so very detached, almost distant from the inner life of the patient. To Kraepelin a mentally sick person seems to have been a collection of symptoms. He was a true son of the great, energetic, and creative age that was interested greatly in humanity but comparatively little in man. Perhaps this trait in Kraepelin as a psychiatrist, which today would be considered a defect, was the very characteristic which helped rather than hindered him in the creation of his great system and school. He was able to collect and to study thousands of case histories, covering not only the story of each illness, but the history of each patient's life before the illness and a follow-up history of his life after he left the hospital. Dealing with such large masses of data, Kraepelin was able to sort out everything these many individuals had in common, leaving out of consideration the purely individual data. He thus arrived at an excellent general picture, at a unique perspective of a mental illness as a whole. But he seems to have been almost unaware that in his careful study he lost the individual. (p. 452)

Berrios and Hauser (1988) took issue with this assessment, noting the "great depth and beauty" of Kraepelin's late conceptual writing. They quoted from a 1920 work: "If these observations approximate the truth we will have to look for the key to the understanding of the clinical picture primarily in characteristics of the individual patient . . . his expectations play a decisive role."

2. For the material in this section we are indebted to the historians in our field, especially to Jackson (1986) and Roccatagliata (1986) for their extensive scholarship. Whitwell (1936), in his modestly titled *Historical Notes on Psychiatry*, provided translations of ancient manuscripts and insights into the apparent manic-depressive symptoms of literary and historical figures, such as Orestes, Saul, and Herod the Great. Although not as sharply focused on affective illness, other sources have proved valuable in understanding the historical context in general medicine and psychiatry; they include Ackerknecht (1959, 1982), Zilboorg (1941), Alexander and Selesnick (1966), and Wightman (1971).

3. Medical historians believe that the works attributed to Hippocrates probably represent the work of his school. According to Ackerknecht (1982, p. 55), for example:

From fifty to seventy books were later attributed to Hippocrates, and in the third century B.C. they were collected in Alexandria into the Corpus Hippocraticum. It is not known which of these books, if any, were actually written by the great physician. As a matter of fact, none of them contains the ideas attributed to him in the writings of Plato and Menon.

4. Quoted by Whitwell (1936, p. 212) from Pratensis Jason: *De cerebri morbis* (Basil), 1549.

5. According to Jackson (1986, p. 100), Marsilius Ficinus (Marsilio Ficino) was a fifteenth-century philosopher, physician, and priest who revitalized Aristotle's views "with far-reaching effects on his own and later times."

6. Despite the presence of schizophrenic-like symptoms during the manic episodes, the diagnosis of manic-depressive illness was confirmed on follow-up. Demographic data suggested that the patients in this study were like manic-depressive patients in other studies in relapse frequency, duration of illness, and other features.

7. Quoted by Jackson (1986, p. 263) from Baillarger, 1854, p. 352.

8. Quoted by Jackson (1986, p. 268) from Ritti, A.: "Circular insanity." In *A Dictionary of Psychological Medicine Giving the Definition, Etymology and Synonyms of Terms Used in Medical Psychology, with the Symptoms, Treatment and Pathology of Insanity and the Law of Lunacy in Great Britain and Ireland*, edited by D. Hack Tuke, 2 vols. (Philadelphia: P. Blakiston), 1892, p. 214.

9. Some psychoanalytic writers implied that different phases of manic-depressive illness were linked through some underlying mechanism. Prominent here is the conception of mania as a defense against depression (see Chapter 11). This analytical formulation, reminiscent of the earliest observations that mania grew out of melancholia, could be said to have anticipated the current continuum model.

10. Some investigators (e.g., Koukopoulos et al., 1983; Akiskal and Akiskal, 1988; Cassano et al., 1988) focused on the opposite temperaments—depressive and hyperthymic—and proposed that a fundamental characteristic of bipolarity is the shift from one temperamental state into the opposite

extreme in the form of an episode. Thus, depressive temperaments are vulnerable to a swing into hypomania or mania, whereas those with hyperthymic temperaments are likely to swing into depressions. According to Akiskal and colleagues (1998b), such propensities may serve as the basis for mixed states (see Chapter 2).

11. The very existence of depressive mixed states (isolated intradepressive "manic" symptoms) argued for a continuum, which is consistent with the contemporary work of Benazzi and Akiskal (2001) and Sato and colleagues (2003).

12. Although not incompatible with Kraepelin's descriptions of manic-depressive illness, Meyer's approach implied a different conceptual framework. The Meyerians, although allowing for the operation of biological and genetic factors, understood them as part of an individual's vulnerability to specific psychological and social influences. This perspective was symbolized by the rubric "manic-depressive reaction" in the first official diagnostic manual of the American Psychiatric Association, published in 1952.

13. This would apply most clearly to German and British psychiatry, perhaps less so to French psychiatry (Leff, 1977).

14. This emphasis on presenting episode rather than course was somewhat ironic, because Meyer's own writings emphasized a longitudinal perspective.

15. *Primary* is defined as depression in the absence of any preexisting or antecedent psychiatric or medical disorder.

16. At any rate, from a clinical and epidemiologic standpoint, current data indicate that the foregoing depressive dichotomies are best regarded as part of a depressive spectrum (Judd and Akiskal, 2000).

17. To Bleuler, a patient was predominantly schizophrenic or predominantly manic-depressive. Patients were distributed all along this spectrum, and an individual patient could be at different points on the spectrum at different times.

18. Compared with unipolar patients, bipolar depressed patients were reported to have lower ratings of anxiety, anger, and physical complaints (Beigel and Murphy, 1971b); more psychomotor retardation (Beigel and Murphy, 1971b; Himmelhoch et al., 1972; Kotin and Goodwin, 1972; Dunner et al., 1976a; Katz et al., 1982); lower levels of measured physical activity (Kupfer et al., 1974); and more total sleep time (Hartmann, 1968; Kupfer et al., 1972; Duncan et al., 1979).

19. Winokur divided his primary unipolar patients (none of whom had a family history of mania) into familial pure depressive disease (FPDD), sporadic pure depressive disease (SPDD), and depression spectrum disease (DSD). (*Primary* was defined as depression in the absence of any preexisting or antecedent psychiatric or medical disorder.) The two pure types had no other preceding psychiatric diagnoses and no alcoholism among first-degree relatives. The distinction between them was that FPDD patients had a first-degree relative with primary depression, whereas SPDD patients did not. DSD patients were those with alcoholism or antisocial personality among first-degree (male) relatives; they were predominantly female patients with early onset. Winokur (1980) suggested that genetically, the FPDD subtype was closely related to bipolar illness.

20. Akiskal, 1981, 1983a, 1998; Benazzi, 1997, 2001, 2003; Akiskal and Pinto, 1999; Angst and Marneros, 2001; Benazzi and Akiskal, 2001, 2003; Marneros, 2001; Hantouche et al., 2003b.

21. Some of the differences among individual manic-depressive patients reflect differences in the illness per se, whereas others reflect the interaction of the illness with individual characteristics, some of which certainly involve genetic differences unrelated to manic-depressive illness. The reactive–endogenous and neurotic–psychotic dichotomies (or spectra) should not be taken simply as a reflection of differential severity, that is, from mild to severe in consequences for the patient. As observed by Lewis (1936, p. 998):

> It may be said, simply, that severe emotional upsets ordinarily tend to subside, but that mild emotional states, when often provoked or long maintained, tend to persist, as it were, autonomously. Hence the paradox that a gross blatant psychosis may do less damage in the long run than some meager neurotic incubus: a dramatic attack of mania or melancholia, with delusions, wasting, hallucinations, wild excitement and other alarms, may have far less effect on the course of a man's life than some deceptively mild affective illness which goes on so long that it becomes inveterate. The former comes as a catastrophe, and when it has passed the patient takes up his life again, active, cheerful, normal in every way, while with the latter he may never get rid of his burden.

22. Akiskal et al., 1977, 1979a; Depue et al., 1981; Egeland and Hotstetter, 1983; Akiskal and Pinto, 1999; Angst and Marneros, 2001; Marneros, 2001; Ghaemi et al., 2002.

23. It is possible that the high bipolar/unipolar ratio in Egeland's Amish data reflects special genetic factors limited to that population. As noted below, however, Angst's (1978) group also found a 1:1 ratio of bipolar to unipolar illness when the sample was followed for many years and hypomania was ascertained.

24. Ghaemi et al., 1999; Goldberg et al., 2001; Dilsaver and Akiskal, 2005; Hantouche and Akiskal, 2005; Rybakowski et al., 2005; Sharma et al., 2005; Smith et al., 2005.

25. Some bipolar–unipolar differences become more clear when bipolar-II is deleted from the comparison.

26. In their second study, however, Abrams and Taylor (1979) found a higher morbid risk for unipolar depression in unipolar manic patients compared with bipolar patients.

27. The method relied on reports of the manic patients themselves at or near admission, presumably while they were still ill. Davenport and colleagues (1979) at NIMH showed (as common sense would suggest) that manic patients report substantially fewer past depressive episodes than their families remember.

28. Akiskal et al., 1995, 2005; Coryell et al., 1995; Goldberg et al., 2001; Angst et al., 2005.

29. Benazzi and Akiskal, 2001; Maj et al., 2003; Akiskal and Benazzi, 2004; Biondi et al., 2005; Sato et al., 2005; Serretti and Olgiati, 2005.

30. Even in the study by Katz and colleagues (1982), which employed prior screening by the Research Diagnostic Criteria (RDC) (see Chapter 3), greater heterogeneity in the unipolar group is plausible since the research criteria allowed for sleep and appetite changes in either direction. In fact, Kupfer and colleagues (1975), examining unipolar depressed patients with a variety of clinical and personality measures, described a subgroup with symptoms similar to those of

bipolar depression. Like bipolar patients, these unipolar depressed patients were more retarded, had lower levels of anxiety, and ate and slept more. They, like the bipolar patients, had been hospitalized more often in the past than the unipolar patients, although the incidence of past depressive episodes, suicide attempts, and substance abuse was similar for all the patients. Kupfer suggested that this subgroup of unipolar patients may share some common biological and pharmacological response characteristics with bipolar patients. Overlapping with this grouping are the unipolar patients described by Winokur and Clayton (1967) as having familial pure depressive disease and by Mendels (1976) as "pseudounipolar." In a similar vein, Benazzi (2003) described a group of early-onset unipolar patients who, unlike later-onset patients, were very similar to his bipolar-II group.

31. Ebert et al., 1993; Perugi et al., 1998a; Serretti et al., 1998; Akiskal et al., 2000; Agosti and Stewart, 2001; Mitchell et al., 2001; Angst et al., 2002; Benazzi, 2003; Ghaemi et al., 2004; Akiskal and Benazzi, 2005; Hantouche and Akiskal, 2005.

32. Horwath et al., 1992; Robertson et al., 1996; Levitan 1997; Posternak and Zimmerman, 2002; Sullivan et al., 2002.

33. The negative studies generally involved small and/or unbalanced samples.

34. The DSM IV criteria were modified to require only 2 days for hypomania.

35. Other features that have been reported to differentiate unipolar from bipolar-II patients are irritability and agitation, symptoms that overlap with the concept of depressive "mixed states."

36. Unpublished data cited by Dunner (1987).

37. In the Cassano et al. study (2004), recurrent unipolar patients endorsed a substantial number of manic/hypomanic symptoms over their lifetimes.

38. Hantouche and colleagues (2003b) and Akiskal and colleagues (2003b) have argued for the existence of such a bipolar-II variant on the basis of clinical, psychometric, and temperamental characteristics; further, the bipolar nature of the more unstable bipolar-II ½ patients is suggested by the observation that the rates of familial bipolarity in bipolar-II and bipolar-II ½ groups are highly similar.

39. Even within categories, variation always occurs. Cantor and Genero (1986, p. 236) pointed out that the "natural" categories into which human beings organize their perceptual experiences do not have "obvious necessary and sufficient criterial properties, so that boundaries between closely related categories are ill-defined." People find it extraordinarily difficult or impossible to specify criteria for common object categories, such as furniture, birds, fruit, or clothing. Instead, they identify correlated features that imply a continuum of category membership, ranging from a prototype (an apple is a very typical fruit, for example) to a more atypical member (a tomato is a fruit often thought to be a vegetable). Assigning such atypical members to one category or another can be difficult, and the overlap of characteristic features from one category to another also "runs counter to the intuitive notion of well-defined, orthogonal categories with clearly demarcated boundaries."

40. With appropriate cut-off scores, the GBI can be used for case identification in either nonclinical or clinical populations. It may be particularly useful in family studies. For example, evaluated against clinically determined DSM-III diagnoses, the GBI was found to have a sensitivity of 90 percent and a specificity of 98 percent when used with adolescent offspring of bipolar-I parents and parents with nonaffective major psychiatric diagnoses (Klein et al., 1986b). Originally structured to identify only bipolar affective states, the GBI has been broadened to apply to the separation of bipolar from unipolar subjects with considerable success (Depue et al., 1989).

41. TEMPS exists in an interview format (TEMPS-I) (Akiskal et al., 1998a; Placidi et al., 1998) and a self-rated autoquestionnaire version (TEMPS-A) (Akiskal and Akiskal, 2005). The cutoffs, determined by extreme distributions based on z-scores (corresponding to +2 standard deviations), represent individuals at putative risk for clinical bipolar disorder. Akiskal (1995) actually proposes that temperaments can both provoke and react to life events, thereby leading to complex life situations, emotional arousal, and, eventually, affective episodes. This viewpoint is supported by data on juvenile subjects indicating that cyclothymic reactivity is associated with stress, anxiety, and behavioral disturbances (Signoretta et al., 2005). Only new research will reveal the extent to which the promise of TEMPS-A will be justified. Such research is in progress.

42. Joffe et al., 1999; Angst and Marneros, 2001; Angst et al., 2003.

43. The DSM-III-R category bipolar disorder–not otherwise specified, was originally meant to apply to bipolar-II patients; however, many such patients meet DSM-III-R criteria for bipolar major affective disorder, given that the criteria for major depression are broad enough to encompass a wide range of severity. On the other hand, cyclothymia in DSM-III-R reflects a milder state, referred to by Dunner as "cyclothymic personality," that is also milder than the cyclothymia described by Akiskal.

44. More recently, using nonclinical community samples, Angst (1991) identified recurrent brief depression (RBD) or recurrent brief hypomania (RBM), each with a minimum of 12 episodes a year. He suggested that these are part of the bipolar spectrum.

45. Akiskal and Mallya, 1987; Cassano et al., 1992; Simpson et al., 1993; Benazzi, 1997; Manning et al., 1997; Hantouche et al., 1998; Angst and Gamma, 2002; Mainia et al., 2002.

46. Akiskal et al., 1977, 1978, 1979a, 1983: Depue et al., 1978; Waters, 1979; Akiskal, 1981, 1983a,b.

47. As detailed in Chapter 21, nonadherence is a major problem for both bipolar-I and bipolar-II patients, although the factors that contribute to it may be different in each group.

48. This predominance of depression in bipolar disorder might be reconciled with the proposal of Koukopoulos and others that mania represents the underlying state in bipolar disorder by noting that many depressions in the bipolar spectrum involve activation and other manic-like symptoms.

49. The widespread use of effective pharmacological treatments, along with earlier recognition, probably accounts for the fact that contemporary studies of manic-depressive illness are more dependent on outpatient samples, whereas earlier studies were predominantly of inpatients.

2 Clinical Description

[N]otwithstanding manifold external differences certain *common fundamental features* yet recur in all the morbid states mentioned. Along with changing symptoms, which may appear temporarily or may be completely absent, we meet in all forms of manic-depressive insanity a quite definite, narrow group of disorders, though certainly of very varied character and composition. Without any one of them being absolutely characteristic of the malady, still in association they impress a uniform stamp on all the multiform clinical states.

—*Emil Kraepelin (1921, p. 2)*

To understand manic-depressive illness—to diagnose it accurately and to treat it effectively—requires close familiarity with what Kraepelin calls "the common fundamental features" of the disease. This chapter gives a general clinical description of hypomania and mania, bipolar depression and recurrent unipolar depression, and mixed states, as well as the cyclothymic and other temperamental traits that often underlie these states. Clinical description is approached from three perspectives: that of uniquely experienced classic clinical observers, such as Kraepelin; that of manic-depressive patients themselves (especially the bipolar subgroup); and that of contemporary investigators who have conducted data-based clinical studies. By combining these perspectives (at the unavoidable cost of some redundancy), we hope to capitalize on the descriptive and heuristic strengths of each while avoiding the limitations of any one alone.

We have chosen to cite extensively the classic clinical literature, most of which predates the modern treatment era. We have done this for several reasons. First, descriptions found in these sources are powerful and have not been surpassed; Kraepelin, particularly, remains without peer. Second, the lack of effective treatments and the provision of residential care for patients over many years, often lifetimes, allowed prepharmacotherapy clinicians to observe the natural course of the illness in all its severity. Third, modern diagnostic systems, although vital in advancing treatment and research, have resulted in less emphasis on clinical description and proportionately more emphasis on quantifications susceptible to stastistical analysis, employing symptom checklists, rating scales, and diagnostic algorithms. Regrettably, few psychiatric residents, graduate students, scientists, and clinicians now read Kraepelin and Bleuler. Fewer still have read Aretaeus,

Griesinger, Weygandt, Falret, Jaspers, Baillarger, Campbell, or Henderson and Gillespie. We believe the clinical writings of these classic authors provide both historical perspective and a singular understanding of the nature of manic-depressive illness.

The accounts of manic-depressive (predominantly bipolar) patients presented in this chapter provide the personal dimension missing from clinicians' and researchers' reports, however astute their observations. These descriptions, which vary widely, reflect both the nature of the illness and the nature of the people suffering from it. In the scientific literature, relatively scant attention is paid to firsthand accounts of manic-depressive illness; rather, the emphasis is on the use of objective observer ratings as a basis for studying and describing major affective disorders, including their psychotic variants. One reason for this virtual exclusion of experiential information is that firsthand accounts are subjective and necessarily biased. Thus, patients may remember with clarity some aspects of their disorder and forget or ignore others; they may verbalize what is easiest to describe and say little about aspects less readily articulated. They may relate only those experiences most novel to them, thus giving disproportionate weight to out-of-the-ordinary events, or they may describe what they think the observer wishes to hear. In addition, moods can radically alter memory and perception, resulting in state-dependent distortions. Finally, those individuals most capable of discussing their experiences in an articulate manner may belong, by virtue of this fact, to a more introspective and less representative group.

These are legitimate concerns for anyone desiring systematic, clear-cut, and reducible data. Clinicians have long been aware, however, that experiential accounts are vital to an understanding of individuals and their illnesses.

Likewise, the heuristic value of hypotheses generated from patients' descriptions of their feelings, thoughts, and behaviors is well established. Good clinical management of manic-depressive illness, both pharmacological and psychotherapeutic, depends upon recognizing the concerns of patients and the consequences (both negative and positive) the illness has for them. Descriptive information gathered from patients also has been important in clinical research, such as that describing the switch process (Bunney et al., 1972a,b,c), unraveling the paradoxical effects of lithium as both antidepressant and antimanic agent (Goodwin et al., 1969), and elucidating the occasional positive qualities of manic states (Jamison, 1993, 2004; Jamison et al., 1980), as well as the clinically related difficulties some patients have in adhering to a treatment regimen (see Chapter 21).

There are strong limitations on the effective use of language to describe unusual events, such as extreme moods, gross cognitive and perceptual distortions, and both subtle and profound changes in sensory experience. Despite the shortcomings of language and the highly personalized vocabulary often used by patients in describing their manic-depressive illness, certain words, phrases, and metaphors are chosen time and again, forming a common matrix of experiences. Often these images center on nature, weather, the day–night cycle, and the seasons; often, too, they convey unpredictability, periodicity, violence, tempestuousness, or a bleak dearth of feelings. Religious themes and mystical experiences pervade the language, conveying an extraordinary degree and type of experience—beyond control, comprehension, or adequate description.

At a narrower conceptual level, certain individual words and phrases are heard repeatedly by clinicians treating patients with manic-depressive illness. Depression is associated with common language fragments. The patient is "slowed down," "in a fog," or "exhausted" and describes life as having "lost its color," "dull, flat, and dreary." Everything is "hopeless," "heavy," "too much of an effort," "drab, colorless, pointless." Life is a "burden"; there is no point to living; all is meaningless. Hypomania and mania elicit descriptions of a more vivacious and energetic kind. Life is "effortless," "charged with intensity," and filled with special meaning. The patient is "upbeat," "racing," "full of energy," "speeded up," "wired," "hyper," "high as a kite," "moving in the fast lane," "ecstatic," "flying." Other people are described as "too slow" and unable to "keep up."

Clinical descriptions derived from data-based studies compensate, in part, for the selective attention of both clinicians and patients. They provide a more objective view of the frequency and character of symptoms in manic-depressive illness. In selecting such studies for review in this chapter, we have to some extent emphasized manic states, partly because differential diagnosis can be problematic in mania (see Chapter 3), and partly because more systematic studies of symptoms and their syndromic profiles have been carried out on mania than on bipolar depression, recurrent unipolar depression, mixed states, or cyclothymia. Moreover, we agree with Koukopoulos (2005) and those before him (Pinel, 1801; Heinroth, 1818; Griesinger, 1845) that mania is the fundamental clinical state in bipolar disorder.

In the first edition of this volume, we noted the relative scarcity of data-based studies of bipolar depression and mixed states as a cause for both surprise and concern. This was in contrast to an exceedingly large general literature on depression, one that seldom differentiated bipolar depression from the many nonbipolar forms. Fortunately, there has been a proliferation of studies of both bipolar depression and mixed states in recent years, and their inclusion here is an important addition to the first edition. Older data-based clinical studies, although using standardized diagnostic criteria and making the necessary distinctions between bipolar and unipolar depression, tended not to focus on clinical patterns of bipolar depression but on such issues as psychotic versus nonpsychotic status. Typically, bipolar patients were excluded from these samples. There is next to no research on the nature of depressions in unipolar patients with highly recurrent illness, which were included in Kraepelin's concept of manic-depressive illness, and how they may differ from that of depressions in patients with the less recurrent unipolar forms.

The same caveats about methodology that apply to earlier research findings on manic-depressive illness in general, particularly the bipolar form, apply as well to the older studies discussed in this chapter. First, diagnostic criteria, especially for mixed states, varied greatly across studies. Second, investigators often failed to specify the stage, severity, or duration of the affective state. Third, measurement techniques lacked sophistication; there was a tendency, for example, to measure only the presence or absence of a symptom rather than its intensity, constancy, and duration. Other methodological problems were widespread. The pioneering clinical study of mania, bipolar depression, and mixed states conducted by Winokur and colleagues (1969), for example, although an invaluable contribution to the literature, involved the analysis of data based on multiple episodes (e.g., 100 episodes of mania in 61 patients). To the extent that a given individual showed a similar symptom pattern from one affective episode to another, a contaminating element was introduced. Early clinical studies, while often methodologically flawed, were nonetheless important for the questions they raised and the patients they studied, individuals whose illnesses were generally uncomplicated by changes in clinical presentation due to treatment, especially antidepressant use. We have included the findings of many of these pre-1990 studies because of their historical as well as clinical and scientific interest.

With greater attention to clinical research on bipolar disorder since 1990, the limitations of the older literature have to some extent been addressed. For instance, the twin French collaborative studies of the clinical epidemiology of mania (EPIMAN) and bipolar depression (EPIDEP) have focused on carefully measured clinical nuances of manic, mixed, and bipolar-II disorders, as well as their temperamental foundations (e.g., Hantouche et al., 1998). *Bipolarity beyond Classic Mania*, an extensive examination of soft bipolar variants (Akiskal, 1999), and a European monograph entitled *Bipolar Disorder One Hundred Years after Manic Depressive Illness* (Marneros and Angst, 2000) were published to pay tribute to—and extend—Kraepelin's clinical vision and methodology. Another trans-Atlantic monograph, *Bipolar Disorders*, focuses on mixed, atypical, and rapid-cycling bipolar disorder (Marneros and Goodwin, 2003). Finally, an entire issue of the *Journal of Affective Disorders* devoted to "soft" and "hard" phenotypes within the bipolar spectrum was published in 2003. The data-based contributions of this monograph came from the United States, France, Italy, Switzerland, and Germany, countries where clinical research is currently being conducted on the phenomenology of the broadly conceived manic-depressive spectrum.

In this chapter we address only those aspects of symptom presentation relevant to clinical description. These include the observable patterns of mood, energy, sleep, thought, and behavior typically used in clinical diagnosis. (Detailed discussion of related topics is found in Chapters 1, 3, 9, 10, and 15.) Before proceeding, we emphasize that while many generalizations can be drawn from clinical descriptions of manic-depressive illness, individuals are bound to differ widely with regard to an illness that is at once genetically based, environmentally influenced, and psychologically expressed. Kraepelin (1921), although committed to the idea and practice of classification, also was sensitive to the infinite capacity for individual expression in the illness. Referring to the subclassifications proposed by earlier writers, he concluded (p. 139): "I am convinced that that kind of effort . . . must of necessity wreck on the irregularity of the disease." The clinical differences seen across individuals can be striking (as are, more often, the similarities), but it remains unclear to what extent one episode resembles another in a given individual. Anecdotal accounts, along with several studies discussed later, support some constancy of clinical presentation, including the presence or absence of melancholic and psychotic features, in the same patient across time.[1]

Finally, although much of the clinical description presented here emphasizes differences among clinical states, we stress from the outset that the coexistence of affective states is fundamental to bipolar disorder and that oscillation into, out of, and within the various forms and states of manic-depressive illness is, in its own right, a hallmark of the disease. As we shall see, "pure" affective states are rare: mania is often complicated by depressive symptoms, and conversely, depression, especially the bipolar form, usually is accompanied by at least one or more symptoms of mania. Bauer and colleagues (2005), for example, found in their study of 441 bipolar patients that clinically significant depressive symptoms occurred in 94 percent of those with mania or hypomania, while 70 percent of patients in a depressive episode had clinically significant manic symptomatology. Thus, far from being a "bipolar" disorder, with the assumption of clinically opposite states, the illness is characterized by co-occurrence of manic and depressive symptoms more often than not. Bauer and colleagues (2005) also found that depressive and manic symptoms were positively, not inversely, correlated, suggesting that "a dimensional conceptualization of mood state in this disorder is more valid than the categorical conceptualization presumed by both the DSM [*Diagnostic and Statistical Manual*] and ICD [International Classification of Diseases]" (p. 88).

Patterns of manic and depressive symptoms clearly have a cyclic quality, but their overlapping, transitional, and fluctuating aspects are enormously important in describing and understanding the illness overall. Thus, Kraepelin (1921, p. 54) wrote:

> The delimitation of the individual clinical forms of the malady is in many respects wholly artificial and arbitrary. Observation not only reveals the occurrence of gradual transitions between all the various states, but it also shows that within the shortest space of time the same morbid case may pass through most manifold transformations.

Campbell (1953, pp. 112–113) emphasized this fundamentally dynamic nature of bipolar illness by comparing the illness to a film:

> The fluidity, change, and movement of the emotions, as they occur in the ever-changing cyclothymic process, may be compared to the pictures of a cinema, as contrasted with a "still" photograph. Indeed, the psychiatrist, observing a manic-depressive patient for the first time, or as he undergoes one of the many undulations in mood, from melancholia to euphoria or from hypomania to a depression, is reminded of the experience of entering a movie during the middle of the story. No matter where one takes up the plot, the story tends to swing around again to the

point where it started. The examiner may observe the manic-depressive patient first in a manic reaction, later in a depression, but eventually, if followed long enough, in another manic reaction. Like the movie, which is a continuous but constantly changing process, the cyclothymic process is also continuous even though for the moment the observer is attracted by the immediate cross-section view. This conception of change, or constant undulation of the emotions, is much more accurate than a static appraisal.

In the following sections, we address in turn manic, depressive, and mixed states and cyclothymia. For each we present clinical description in three general areas of functioning: mood, cognition and perception, and activity and behavior.

MANIC STATES

Classic Clinical Descriptions

Manic states are typically characterized by heightened mood, more and faster speech, quicker thought, brisker physical and mental activity levels, greater energy (with a corresponding decreased need for sleep), irritability, perceptual acuity, paranoia, heightened sexuality, and impulsivity. The degree, type, and chronicity of these cognitive, perceptual, and behavioral changes determine the major subclassification of mania, namely hypomania or mania. In hypomania, the above changes are generally moderate and may or may not result in serious problems for the individual experiencing them. In more intense episodes, however, they profoundly disrupt the lives of patients, their families, and society.

Mood

Mood in hypomania is usually ebullient, self-confident, and exalted, but with an irritable underpinning. Most early clinical descriptions emphasized the elevated, volatile, and fluctuating nature of hypomanic mood. Campbell (1953, pp. 151, 153) described its euphoric aspect:

> Associated with the euphoria there is a genuine feeling of well-being, mentally and physically, a feeling of happiness and exhilaration which transports the individual into a new world of unlimited ideas and possibilities. . . . When a 19-year-old [hypo]manic was advised that he was indeed ill, he replied, "if I'm ill, this is the most wonderful illness I ever had."

Kraepelin (1921, p. 56) likewise described the euphoric aspect of hypomanic mood, but also emphasized the integral quick changes, irritability, and extreme volatility:

Mood is predominantly exalted and cheerful, influenced by the feeling of heightened capacity for work. The patient is in imperturbable good temper, sure of success, "courageous," feels happy and merry, not rarely overflowingly so. . . . On the other hand there often exists a great emotional irritability. The patient is dissatisfied, intolerant, fault-finding . . . he becomes pretentious, positive, regardless, impertinent and even rough, when he comes up against opposition to his wishes and inclinations; trifling external occasions may bring about extremely violent outbursts of rage.

Mood in acute mania is not well described by the classic writers, perhaps because extreme changes in cognition and behavior are more clearly observable than subjective mood states. Two thousand years ago, however, Aretaeus of Cappadocia noted that those who are manic are gay, active, and expansive. They are naturally joyous; they laugh and they joke: "they show off in public with crowned heads as if they were returning victorious from the games; sometimes they laugh and dance all day and all night" (quoted in Roccatagliata, 1986, pp. 230–231). Kraepelin (1921, p. 63), writing centuries later, agreed, but stressed the instability of the manic mood:

> Mood is unrestrained, merry, exultant, occasionally visionary or pompous, but always subject to frequent variation, easily changing to irritability and irascibility or even to lamentation and weeping.

Jaspers (1997, p. 596; first published in 1913) emphasized the essential liveliness of mood and behavior in *pure mania*, making the distinction, as Kraepelin had, between pure and mixed manic states:

> The feeling of delight in life is accompanied by an increase in instinctual activities: increased sexuality, increased desire to move about; pressure of talk and pressure of activity which will mount from mere vividness of gesture to states of agitated excitement. The psychic activity characterized by flight of ideas lends an initial liveliness to everything undertaken but it lacks staying-power and is changeable. All intruding stimuli and any new possibility will distract the patient's attention. The massive associations at his disposal come spontaneously and uncalled for. They make him witty and sparkling; they also make it impossible for him to maintain any determining tendency and render him at the same time superficial and confused.

Cognition and Perception

Cognition and perception, especially the former, are strongly altered in hypomania. Falret (1854, cited in Sedler, 1983) wrote that "profusion of ideas [in manic states] is prodigious," and most early clinicians emphasized that, to a point, associational fluency is furthered by mild hypomania. Bleuler (1924, pp. 466, 468), for example, commented that thought remains relatively intact in the less severe forms of mania:

> The *thinking* of the manic is flighty. He jumps by by-paths from one subject to another, and cannot adhere to anything. With this the ideas run along very easily and involuntarily, even so freely that it may be felt as unpleasant by the patient. . . . Because of the more rapid flow of ideas, and especially because of the falling off of inhibitions, artistic activities are facilitated even though something worth while is produced only in very mild cases and when the patient is otherwise talented in this direction. The heightened sensibilities naturally have the effect of furthering this.

Tuke (1892, p. 765), in his *Dictionary of Psychological Medicine*, described the quickened senses so many manic patients appear to have:

> Increased acuity in the perception of sense impressions certainly exists. Attention is lively and sharp though entirely unstable. The acute maniac appears to see and hear better than a sane person because every impression tells upon him. . . . Everything attracts his notice.
> The filling of the mind with an enormous number of sense impressions, the blurring as it were of the mental canvas by the superposition of a crowd of details . . . account in a great degree for the confusion of memory which is one of the ordinary phenomena of mania. . . . Objects seen appear to serve chiefly as the starting-point of trains of ideas which change rapidly with slight changes in the visual surroundings.

Thinking becomes fragmented and often psychotic in acute mania. Coherence gives way to incoherence; rapid thinking proceeds to racing and disjointed thinking; distractibility becomes all-pervasive. Paranoid and grandiose delusions are common, as are illusions and hallucinations. In Kraepelin's (1921, p. 62) description, patients

> show themselves sensible and approximately oriented, but extraordinarily distractible in perception and train of thought. Sometimes it is quite impossible to get into communication with them; as a rule, however, they understand emphatic speech, and even give isolated suitable replies, but they are influenced by every new impression; they digress, they go into endless details.

Kraepelin (pp. 68–69) went on to describe the progressively worsening clinical state of *delusional mania*:

> The Delusions and Hallucinations, which in the morbid states hitherto described are fugitive or merely indicated, acquire in a series of cases an elaboration which calls to

mind paranoid attacks. His surroundings appear to the patient to be changed; he sees St. Augustine, Joseph with the shepherd's crook, the angel Gabriel, apostles, the Kaiser, spirits, God, the Virgin Mary.[2] . . . The delusions, which forthwith emerge, move very frequently on religious territory. . . . He preaches in the name of the holy God, will reveal great things to the world, gives commands according to the divine will.

Benjamin Rush (1812, pp. 244–245), author of the first major psychiatric treatise published in the United States, gave a particularly graphic account of the grandiose and "disjointed or debilitated faculties of the mind" in an acutely delusional manic patient:

> The following short extract, taken down by Mr. Coats, from the constant conversation of a young man of a good education, and respectable connections, now deranged in the Pennsylvania Hospital, will exhibit an affecting specimen of this disjointed state of the mind, and of the incoherence of its operations. "No man can serve two masters. I am king Philip of Macedonia, lawful son of Mary queen of Scots, born in Philadelphia. I have been happy enough ever since I have seen general Washington with a silk handkerchief in High-street. Money commands sublunary things, and makes the mare go; it will buy salt mackerel, made of tenpenny nails. Enjoyment is the happiness of virtue. Yesterday cannot be recalled. I can only walk in the night-time, when I can eat pudding enough. I shall be eight years old tomorrow. They say R. W. is in partnership with J. W. I believe they are about as good as people in common—not better, only on certain occasions, when, for instance, a man wants to buy chincopins, and to import salt to feed pigs. Tanned leather was imported first by layers. Morality with virtue is like vice not corrected. L. B. came into your house and stole a coffee-pot in the twenty-fourth year of his majesty's reign. Plumb-pudding and Irish potatoes make a very good dinner. Nothing in man is comprehensible to it. Born in Philadelphia. Our forefathers were better to us than our children, because they were chosen for their honesty, truth, virtue and innocence. The queen's broad R originated from a British forty-two pounder, which makes two [*sic*] large a report for me. I have no more to say. I am thankful I am no worse this season, and that I am sound in mind and memory, and could steer a ship to sea, but am afraid of the thriller. ****** ****** son of Mary queen of Scots. Born in Philadelphia. Born in Philadelphia. King of Macedonia."

Activity and Behavior

Activity and behavior are greatly increased and diversified in mania. Patients appear to be indefatigable; they are rash, virulently opinionated, and interpersonally aggressive. Additionally, as Campbell (1953, pp. 152, 154–155) wrote:

> The manic patient may expend a considerable amount of his energy and pressure of ideas in writing. His writing is demonstrative, flashy, rhetorical and bombastic. He insists that the physician must read every word, even though the content is biased, full of repetition, rambling and circumstantial. Capital letters are used unnecessarily, sentences are underscored and flight of ideas and distractibility destroy the coherence of the theme. The subject of the manic's writing often pertains to the correction of wrongs, religious tangents, gaining his freedom, institution of lawsuits. . . . One patient made three visits to Washington to obtain a patent on a cotton-chopping machine; another attempted to speak to the President by long-distance telephone to warn him that the Russians might land on the coast of Florida. Urged on by the pressure of ideas as well as an excess of physical energy the manic patient has an inner drive which will not allow him to rest.

For many patients, excessive energy translates directly into pressured writing and an inordinate production of written declarations, poetry, and artwork. Kraepelin (1921, pp. 34–36) gave a concise description of this phenomenon, along with a specimen of handwriting produced during mania (see Fig. 2–1):

Figure 2–1. Specimen of handwriting produced during mania. (*Source*: Kraepelin, 1921, p. 35. Reproduced with permission.)

The handwriting of the patients may at first be quite regular and correct. In consequence of the excitability, however, it usually becomes gradually always larger, more pretentious and more irregular. There is no more consideration for the reader; the letters run through one another, are scribbled; more words are underlined; there are more marks of exclamation; the flourishes become bolder. . . . The number of documents produced by manic patients is sometimes astonishing, though certainly they themselves do not count on their being read; the pleasure of writing itself is the only motive.

The progression from hypomania to acute mania is usually accompanied not only by instability of mood and a sense of impending doom or premonitions of madness, but also by increasingly erratic behavior. Rush (1812, p. 142) made this clear in his monograph *Medical Inquiries and Observations upon the Diseases of the Mind*:

Its premonitory signs are, watchfulness, high or low spirits, great rapidity of thought, and eccentricity in conversation, and conduct; sometimes pathetic expressions of horror, excited by the apprehension of approaching madness; terrifying or distressing dreams; great irritability of temper; jealousy, instability in all pursuits; unusual acts of extravagance, manifested by the purchases of houses, and certain expensive and unnecessary articles of furniture, and hostility to relations and friends.

Sexual or erotic excitement is common in mania. Aretaeus of Cappadocia (150 AD) (quoted in Jelliffe, 1931, p. 20), for example, wrote that "a period of lewdness and shamelessness" exists in mania. Likewise, Kraepelin (1921, p. 22) noted that sexual excitability "is increased and leads to hasty engagements, marriages by the newspaper, improper love-adventures, conspicuous behaviour, fondness for dress, on the other hand to jealousy and matrimonial discord." Tuke (1892, pp. 764–765) described this as well:

A very common symptom in maniacal conditions is erotic excitement. This varies from a mere coquetry, a somewhat extended application of the command "love one another," an undue attention to the opposite sex, and so forth, up to the extreme of salacity, when the mind is wholly occupied by the urgent sexual appetite, and all restraint is abandoned.

Particularly dramatic and extreme among the clinical features of acute mania are the frenetic, seemingly aimless, and occasionally violent activities of manic patients. Bizarre, driven, paranoid, impulsive, and grossly inappropriate behavior patterns are typical. Kraepelin (1921, pp. 64–65) provided a graphic overview of these behaviors:

The patient cannot sit or lie still for long, jumps out of bed, runs about, hops, dances, mounts on tables and benches, takes down pictures. He forces his way out, takes off his clothes, teases his fellow patients, dives, splashes, spits, chirps and clicks. . . . [There are] discharges of inner restlessness, shaking of the upper part of the body, waltzing about, waving and flourishing the arms, distorting the limbs, rubbing the head, bouncing up and down, stroking, wiping, twitching, clapping and drumming. . . . [Death may be caused] by simple exhaustion with heart failure (collapse) in long continuing, violent excitement with disturbance of sleep and insufficient nourishment, by injuries with subsequent blood-poisoning.

Delirious mania, or Bell's mania, is a relatively rare, grave form of mania characterized by severe clouding of consciousness. When Bell (1849) described the syndrome in the mid-nineteenth century, he noted its sudden onset and symptoms of severe insomnia, loss of appetite, disorientation, paranoia, and extremely bizarre hallucinations and delusions.[3] Kraepelin (1921, pp. 70, 71) also remarked upon the syndrome's acute onset and noted that patients were "stupefied, confused, bewildered," in addition to being completely disoriented as to time and place. At the core of the illness he found a "dreamy and profound clouding of consciousness, and extraordinary and confused hallucinations and delusions." Griesinger (1867) also emphasized the acute onset of the syndrome and observed that the primary emotion experienced by patients is anxiety. Bond (1980) noted that acute delirious mania can be distinguished by its precipitous onset, with or without premonitory signs of irritability, insomnia, or emotional withdrawal; the presence of the hypomanic or manic syndrome at some point during the illness; development of the signs and symptoms of delirium; a personal and/or family history of either mania or depression; and responsiveness to standard treatments for mania. (Patients with delirious mania often respond to electroconvulsive therapy, despite the delirium [Mann et al., 1986; Fink 1999].)

Mayer-Gross and colleagues (1960, pp. 213–214) gave a general overview of extreme manic confusion, emphasizing the medical gravity of the untreated clinical situation:

These states are seriously debilitating and may endanger life. *Sleep* is severely disturbed in these graver psychoses, but it is also shortened in the milder forms. Another bodily symptom is the exhaustion which supervenes on months of hyper-activity and reduced sleep. The intake of food may be seriously interfered with, for the manic may never take an uninterrupted meal, being constantly diverted to something else. *Body-weight*, which increases in the milder stages, rapidly drops, and very careful nursing is required. . . . The possibility that the atypical features in manic confusion or delirium are due to nutritional deficiencies of the same kind as those sometimes causing delirium in infective illness, cannot be excluded.

Mood during delirious mania may shift rapidly between extreme melancholia and mania, suggesting a clinical link to mixed states. In Kraepelin's (1921, p. 71) words, mood is "very changing, sometimes anxiously despairing ('thoughts of death'), timid and lachrymose, distracted, sometimes unrestrainedly merry, erotic or ecstatic, sometimes irritable or unsympathetic and indifferent." The extreme cognitive and perceptual changes during delirious mania are manifested primarily through clouding of consciousness, hallucinations, and delusions. The profoundly disturbed and psychotic behavior of delirious mania underscores the origin of the phrase "raving maniac." Kraepelin (1921, pp. 71–72) graphically described this behavior:

> At the beginning the patients frequently display the signs of senseless raving mania, dance about, perform peculiar movements, shake their head, throw the bedclothes pellmell, are destructive, pass their motions under them, smear everything, make impulsive attempts at suicide, take off their clothes. A patient was found completely naked in a public park. Another ran half-clothed into the corridor and then into the street, in one hand a revolver in the other a crucifix. . . . Their linguistic utterances alternate between inarticulate sounds, praying, abusing, entreating, stammering, disconnected talk, in which clang-associations, senseless rhyming, diversion by external impressions, persistence of individual phrases, are recognised. . . . Waxy flexibility, echolalia, or echopraxis can be demonstrated frequently.

More recently, Fink (1999, pp. 57–58) described a series of modern cases of delirious mania:

> Patients with delirious mania are excited, restless, fearful, paranoid, and delusional. They sleep poorly, are often confused and disoriented, and they confabulate. The onset develops within a few hours or a few days. Fever, rapid heart rate, tachycardia, hypertension, and rapid breathing are common. Patients hide in small spaces, close the doors and blinds on the windows, remove their clothes, and run nude from their home. Garrulous, incoherent, and rambling speech alternates with mutism. Negativism, stereotypy, grimacing, posturing, echolalia, and echopraxia occur. When examined, they are poorly oriented for place, date and time, are unable to recall their recent experiences, or numbers given them.

Fink argued that we do not know the true incidence of delirious mania, nor do we have adequate diagnostic criteria to distinguish it reliably from malignant catatonia, excited catatonia, rapid-cycling mania, or mania with psychotic features.

Chronic mania was observed and described by many early clinicians, including Pinel (1801), Esquirol (1838), Griesinger (1865), Schott (1904), Kraepelin (1921), and Wertham (1929). According to Schott, only the lack of recovery distinguished the chronic from the acute form of the illness (see also Chapter 4). A first manic episode after the age of 40 was thought to put the patient at much higher risk for chronicity than one occurring earlier (Henderson and Gillespie, 1956), an observation consistent with the results of subsequent research (see Chapter 4). Wertham (1929) outlined the central features of chronic mania: reduced intellectual productivity and general activity levels, increased behavioral stereotypy, and an overall intellectual weakening. Hare (1981), in an excellent historical review of the concept of mania, discussed the declining interest in the subject of chronic mania after the nineteenth century. He attributed this in part to the decreasing morbidity of manic illness, and maintained that improvements in general health and hygiene had resulted in significant changes in the manifestation, severity, and consequences of mania. He acknowledged, however, that there still existed "the ghost as it were, of a process of mental enfeeblement which can occur in affective psychosis and which generally *did* occur, to a more severe degree, until towards the end of the nineteenth century" (p. 97).

Kraepelin (1921, pp. 161–162) provided an overview of the intellectual and emotional blunting in chronic mania; he also drew a distinction between chronic mania and extreme, continuous, rapid cycling and discussed possible contributory factors:

> Here manic features dominate the picture. The patients are in general sensible and reasonable, and perceive fairly well; memory and retention are also fairly well preserved. On the other hand there exist increased distractibility, wandering and desultoriness of thought, a tendency to silly plays on words, poverty of thought. The patients have no understanding of their state, consider themselves perfectly well and capable of work.
>
> Mood is exalted, but no longer exultant, enjoying activity, but silly and boastful; occasionally it comes to flaring up without strength or durability. The finer emotions are considerably injured. . . . Only the coarser enjoyments, eating, drinking, smoking, snuffing, still arouse in them vivid feelings, further the satisfaction of their personal wishes and wants; everything else has become to them more or less indifferent. . . .
>
> At this point we have to mention in a few words another group of cases, in which the psychic decline

reveals itself in continual, abrupt fluctuation between lachrymose anxiety, irritability, and childish merriment. States of this kind sometimes appear to be developed from a continuous accumulation of short circular attacks.

Subjective Experiences of Patients

Mood

In his memoir *Wisdom, Madness, and Folly: The Philosophy of a Lunatic*, John Custance (1952, p. 30), a writer and former Royal Navy intelligence officer who suffered from bipolar illness, described the sense of well-being at the beginning of his manic episodes:

> First and foremost comes a general sense of intense well-being. I know of course that this sense is illusory and transient. . . . Although, however, the restrictions of confinement are apt at times to produce extreme irritation and even paroxysms of anger, the general sense of well-being, the pleasurable and sometimes ecstatic feeling-tone, remains as a sort of permanent background of all experience during the manic period.

As it progresses, this feeling of well-being often is accompanied by a sense of benevolence and communion with nature; frequently it is associated with what Henderson and Gillespie (1956) and others have called a "heightened sense of reality." These feelings, analogous to the beatific and mystical experiences of saints and other religious leaders, share certain features with contemporary experiences of "universal communion" induced by mescaline, LSD, and other hallucinogenic substances. The interaction among emotional, cognitive, and sensory–perceptual changes is complex, as we see in the following passages by Custance (1952, pp. 37, 40):

> It is actually a sense of communion, in the first place with God, and in the second place with all mankind, indeed with all creation. It is obviously related to the mystic sense of unity with the All. . . .
> A feeling of intimate personal relationship with God is perhaps its paramount feature. . . .
> The sense of communion extends to all fellow-creatures with whom I come into contact; it is not merely ideal or imaginative but has a practical effect on my conduct. Thus when in the manic state I have no objection to being more or less herded together—as is inevitable in public Mental Hospitals—with men of all classes and conditions. Class barriers cease to have any existence or meaning.

Likewise, poet Theodore Roethke (quoted in Seager, 1991, p. 101) captured the mystical merging of identity in his description of the early, euphoric stage of one of his manic episodes:

> For no reason I started to feel very good. Suddenly I knew how to enter into the life of everything around me. I knew how it felt to be a tree, a blade of grass, even a rabbit. I didn't sleep much. I just walked around with this wonderful feeling. One day I was passing a diner and all of a sudden I knew what it felt like to be a lion. I went into the diner and said to the counter-man, "Bring me a steak. Don't cook it. Just bring it." . . . I went to the Dean [at the university where Roethke taught] and said, "I feel too good. Get me down off this." So they put me into the tubs.

Cognition and Perception

During hypomanic and manic states, thinking becomes very fluid and productive—to the point of loosening of normal patterns of association, as well as racing thoughts and flight of ideas. The dendritic, branching-out quality of manic thinking was described by nineteenth-century art critic and writer John Ruskin (quoted in Rosenberg, 1986, p. 151):

> I roll on like a ball, with this exception, that contrary to the usual laws of motion I have no friction to contend with in my mind. . . . I am almost sick and giddy with the quantity of things in my head—trains of thought beginning and branching to infinity, crossing each other, and all tempting and wanting to be worked out.

Perhaps most pathognomonic of hypomanic and manic cognitive patterns are flight of ideas and the subjective experience of racing thoughts. The overwhelming and often terrfying nature of racing thoughts is expressed below in one patient's account of manic illness. Grandiosity of delusional proportions and a compelling sense of moral and social awareness also are described (Reiss, 1910):

> The condition of my mind for many months is beyond all description. My thoughts ran with lightning-like rapidity from one subject to another. I had an exaggerated feeling of self importance. All the problems of the universe came crowding into my mind, demanding instant discussion and solution—mental telepathy, hypnotism, wireless telegraphy, Christian science, women's rights, and all the problems of medical science, religion and politics. I even devised means of discovering the weight of a human soul, and had an apparatus constructed in my room for the purpose of weighing my own soul the minute it departed from my body. . . .
> Thoughts chased one another through my mind with lightning rapidity. I felt like a person driving a wild horse with a weak rein, who dares not use force, but lets him run his course, following the line of least resistance. Mad

impulses would rush through my brain, carrying me first in one direction then in another. To destroy myself or to escape often occurred to me, but my mind could not hold on to one subject long enough to formulate any definite plan. My reasoning was weak and fallacious, and I knew it.

Russian poet Velimir Khlebnikov (quoted in Markov, 1975, pp. 362–363), hospitalized for his erratic behavior and wild mood swings, described a euphoric grandiosity that ratcheted upwards into a delusional system of cosmic proportions. He was convinced that he possessed equations "for the stars, equations for voices, equations for thoughts, equations of birth and death." The artist of numbers, he believed, could draw the universe:

Working with number as his charcoal, he unites all previous human knowledge in his art. A single one of his lines provides an immediate lightninglike connection between a red corpuscle and Earth, a second precipitates into helium, a third shatters upon the unbending heavens and discovers the satellites of Jupiter. Velocity is infused with a new speed, the speed of thought, while the boundaries that separate different areas of knowledge will disappear before the procession of liberated numbers cast like orders into print throughout the whole of Planet Earth.

Here they are then, these ways of looking at the new form of creativity, which we think is perfectly workable.

The surface of Planet Earth is 510,051,300 square kilometers; the surface of a red corpuscle—that citizen and star of man's Milky Way—0.000, 128 square millimeters. These citizens of the sky and the body have concluded a treaty, whose provision is this: the surface of the star Earth divided by the surface of the tiny corpuscular star equals 365 times 10 to the tenth power (365×10^{10}). A beautiful concordance of two worlds, one that establishes man's right to first place on Earth. This is the first article of the treaty between the government of blood cells and the government of heavenly bodies. A living walking Milky Way and his tiny star have concluded a 365-point agreement with the Milky Way in the sky and its great Earth Star. The dead Milky Way and the living one have affixed their signatures to it as two equal and legal entities.

The perceptual and somatic changes that almost always accompany hypomania and mania reflect the close and subtle links among elevated mood, a physical sense of well-being, expansive and grandiose thoughts, and heightened perceptual awareness. Custance (1952, p. 16) described the temporal ordering of somatic, mood, and cognitive symptoms during the initial phases of his manic episodes:

Thus at the onset of phases of manic excitement I have sometimes noticed the typical symptoms, the pleasurable tingling of the spinal chord [sic] and warm sense of well-being in the solar plexus, long before any reaction in the mental sphere occurred. The same thing happens with the sinking feeling of fear and horror which accompanies extreme depression.

Clearly, as with virtually all signs and symptoms of bipolar illness, perceptual and somatic changes vary in degree and kind—from mild increases in awareness of objects and events actually present in the individual's environment to total chaotic disarray of the senses, resulting in visual, auditory, and olfactory experiences unrelated to existing physical phenomena. At the milder end of perceptual change, one patient described the relationship of heightened awareness, strongly charged but normal emotional reactions, and psychotic perceptions (Coate, 1964, p. 1):

In normal life at times of strong emotion, and especially at moments of great fear, we find that we are more keenly aware than usual of the external details of our world. The sunshine on wet roofs across the way, the faded edge to the blue window curtain, a scent of pipe tobacco in the room, the way the man in the armchair clasps and unclasps his hands—all is more clearly etched in consciousness because of the feeling aroused by the nearness of enemy bombers, or the gravity of an operation taking place next door, or the tenseness of waiting until an expected person, acutely loved or deeply hated, will walk in. In psychotic states, where the fate of the whole universe may be at stake, awareness of material objects and of trivial events can be heightened to an extent that is outside the range of sane experience.

Custance wrote of his sensory experiences while in the preliminary stage of a manic episode (1952, pp. 31–32):

The first thing I note is the peculiar appearances of the lights—the ordinary electric lights in the ward. They are not exactly brighter, but deeper, more intense, perhaps a trifle more ruddy than usual. Moreover, if I relax the focusing of my eyes, which I can do very much more easily than in normal circumstances, a bright star-like phenomenon emanates from the lights, ultimately forming a maze of iridescent patterns of all colours of the rainbow, which remind me vaguely of the Aurora Borealis. . . . Connected with these vivid impressions is a rather curious feeling behind the eyeballs, rather as though a vast electric motor were pulsing away there.

All my other senses seem more acute than usual. Certainly my sense of touch is heightened; my fingers are much more sensitive and neat. . . .

My hearing appears to be more sensitive, and I am able to take in without disturbance or distraction many different sound-impressions at the same time.

Custance (1952, p. 59) also described specific physical sensations he experienced during his manic episodes. His perceived imperviousness to pain and cold, as well as his delusional beliefs about electrical and other influences, occur in many manic patients:

> Metabolism is rapid. I can stand cold without difficulty or discomfort; an inner warmth seems to pervade me. I can, for example, walk about naked out of doors on quite cold nights—to throw off my clothes is incidentally a strong impulse and presumably symbolises the freedom from restraint which is a feature of the whole condition. My skin seems peculiarly resistant; I have walked barefooted on stony and thorny ground, squeezed myself naked through furze fences and so on without suffering discomfort. Perhaps this is akin to the strange feats of fire walkers or dancing Dervishes. It certainly seems to show the influence of mind over matter. I fear nothing—freedom from fear is another notable symptom—so nothing seems to hurt me.

Activity and Behavior

Behavioral changes during mania include increases in psychomotor activity and in the pressure and rate of speech; heightened irritability and aggressive behaviors; increases in spending and other impulsive behaviors; hypersexuality; and frenzied, bizarre, often aimless activity. Detailed clinical descriptions of these behavioral changes—especially those by Kraepelin—were given earlier in this chapter, and specific discussions of hypomanic and manic behavior can be found elsewhere in the volume. We present here first-person accounts of only a few common or especially interesting behavioral changes in manic states. Two passages describe increased enthusiasm for and involvement in a wide variety of creative interests and activities. The first, from Coate (1964, pp. 84–85), reflects the clear influence of mood and grandiosity on thinking and behavior. The sense of time urgency and the special significance of events and objects also are evident:

> I must record everything and later I would write a book on mental hospitals. I would write books on psychiatric theory too, and on theology. I would write novels. I had the libretto of an opera in mind. Nothing was beyond me. My creative impulse had found full outlet and I had enough now to write to last me for the rest of my life.
>
> I made notes of everything that happened, day and night. I made symbolic scrap-books whose meaning only I could decipher. I wrote a fairy tale; I wrote the diary of a white witch; and again I noted down cryptically all that was said or done around me at the time, with special reference to relevant news bulletins and to jokes which were broadcast in radio programmes. The time, correct to the nearest minute, was recorded in the margin. It was all vitally important. The major work which would be based on this material would be accurate, original, provocative, and of profound significance. All that had ever happened to me was now worthwhile.

Because her thinking was not yet psychotically fragmented or delusional, Coate was able to concentrate intensely and to keep in order a broad diversity of ideas and sensations. This ability is not uncommon in hypomania, although many bipolar patients who experience scattered thinking early in their episodes never go through this hyperalert but concentrated phase. Those who do and who also possess creative ability find this stage can be an exceptionally productive one (see Chapter 12). For Custance (1952, pp. 244–245), both creativity and learning were heightened:

> In some forms of insanity, including especially mania, this ripening of the instinct, this eager readiness to absorb and learn new things, to become interested in fresh games, sports and forms of work, seems to recur. It certainly does in my own case. I have, in actual fact, learnt more while confined in Mental Hospitals than anywhere else, including my School and University. I have learnt drawing, shorthand, some languages, studied philosophy and psychology as deeply as I was able, collected and systematically written down and filed innumerable scraps of information on all sorts of subjects, and, above all, read in the book of human nature, which is as it were exposed in the raw. I know the history, background and medical diagnosis of many of the patients in the wards I have been in. Finally I have written this book.

A common aspect of the manic state is impulsive and irrational financial behavior. The psychological and interpersonal consequences, as well as the economic ones, can be devastating. The return of postmanic reason and subsequent awareness of financial extravagances and other painfully embarrassing actions often occur in the harsh context of severe postmanic depression. The humorous aspects of many manic purchases often obscure the acute shame and dire financial consequences experienced by patients with bipolar illness:

> When I am high I couldn't worry about money if I tried. So I don't. The money will come from somewhere; I am entitled; God will provide. Credit cards are disastrous, personal checks worse. Unfortunately, for manics anyway, mania is a natural extension of the economy. What with credit cards and bank accounts there is little beyond reach. So I bought twelve snake bite kits, with a sense of urgency and importance. I bought precious stones, elegant and unnecessary furniture, three watches within an hour of one another (in the Rolex rather than Timex

class: champagne tastes bubble to the surface, are the surface, in mania), and totally inappropriate siren-like clothes. During one spree in London I spent several hundred pounds on books having titles or covers that somehow caught my fancy: books on the natural history of the mole, twenty sundry Penguin books because I thought it could be nice if the penguins could form a colony, five Puffin books for a similar reason, on and on and on it went. Once, I think, I shoplifted a blouse because I could not wait a minute longer for the woman-with-molasses feet in front of me in line. Or maybe I just thought about shoplifting, I don't remember, I was totally confused. I imagine I must have spent far more than $30,000 during my two major manic episodes, and God only knows how much more during my frequent milder manias.

But then back on lithium and rotating on the planet at the same pace as everyone else, you find your credit is decimated, your mortification complete: mania is not a luxury one can easily afford. It is devastating to have the illness and aggravating to have to pay for medications, blood tests, and psychotherapy. They, at least, are partially [tax] deductible. But money spent while manic doesn't fit into the Internal Revenue Service concept of medical expense or business loss. So, after mania, when most depressed, you're given excellent reason to be even more so. (Jamison, 1995, pp. 74–75)

Clinical Studies

Mania is a complex, volatile, and fluctuating cauldron of symptoms. "The form and ways which mania manifests are manifold," said Aretaeus (translated by Jelliffe, 1931, p. 20) nearly 2000 years ago. "Some are cheerful and like to play . . . others passionate and of destructive type, who seek to kill others as well as themselves." Although classically described as a state of extraordinary energy and activity, mania can also present clinically as manic stupor and "catatonia." Manic mood, frequently characterized as elated and grandiose, as often as not is riddled with depression, panic, and extreme irritability; mania without significant mixed features is what is known as "classic" mania. For years, mania was differentiated mistakenly from schizophrenia because it reputedly lacked a thought disorder. It now is recognized as an often floridly psychotic condition, as we shall see below.

Manic episodes differ from person to person and in the same individual from time to time, although Falret (1854, cited in Sedler, 1983) and Kraepelin (1921) noted a tendency for constancy in symptom patterns across episodes in the same individual. While few systematic data are available on this latter point, Wellner and Marstal (1964, p. 176), reporting on a study of 279 manic episodes in 221 patients, concluded that "atypical attacks are followed by atypical, and typical by typical significantly more often than not

($p = 0.002$), indicating the patients' inclination to reproduce the type of their psychoses." Beigel and Murphy (1971a) found that patients with multiple manic attacks tended to exhibit similar behavior and mood patterns during subsequent episodes. Two more recent studies (Cassidy et al., 2001a; Woods et al., 2001) demonstrated that manic and mixed episodes show diagnostic stability over time; the interepisode stability of depressive mixed states, while significant, is considerably less pronounced than is the case for manic states (Sato et al., 2004). Francis and colleagues (1997) found that the symptom profile of catatonia is highly consistent across episodes, while Cassidy and colleagues (2002), who evaluated 77 bipolar patients during two distinct manic episodes separated, on average, by 2 years, concluded that manic symptomatology remains generally consistent from episode to episode. Specifically, they found that severity of mania, dysphoria, hedonic activation, psychosis, and irritable aggression tends to correlate across episodes; psychomotor symptoms do not.

Regardless of the degree of constancy of the clinical picture across attacks, it is clear that symptoms vary widely during any given manic episode as it progresses through various stages. These stages, characterized by Carlson and Goodwin (1973) and discussed more fully below, begin with elation or irritability, evolve into a more severe form as arousal and hyperactivity escalate, and culminate in floridly psychotic disorganization.

Mood

Research on mood symptoms in mania, summarized in Table 2–1, demonstrates that most patients, on average, are depressed (46 percent) or labile (49 percent) nearly as often as they are euphoric (63 percent) or expansive (60 percent); they are irritable (71 percent) even more often. The depression, irritability, and mood lability are generally seen less often in early stages of an episode, although few studies have specified the stage, level, or severity of mania at the time of observation.

Winokur and colleagues (1969) observed depressed mood in 68 percent of their manic patients, as well as more severe depressive symptoms (including depressive delusions and psychomotor retardation) in a significant subgroup. They found that "short depressive contaminations in the manic episode" were significantly more common in women (79 percent) than in men (49 percent) (p. 64). Like many investigators, they were particularly impressed by the volatility of mood during manic episodes:

In our series of patients, the degree of mood elevation varied from patient to patient and from time to time during the same episode. The changes in mood were capricious, responding to internal as well as external stimuli

TABLE 2–1. **Mood Symptoms during Mania: Percent Displaying Symptoms**

Study	Patients (N)	Irritability (%)	Euphoria (%)	Depression (%)	Lability (%)	Expansiveness (%)
Clayton et al., 1965	31		97			
Winokur et al., 1969	100[a]	85	98	68[b]	95	
Beigel and Murphy, 1971a	12		67	92		
Kotin and Goodwin, 1972	20			100		
Carlson and Goodwin, 1973	20	100	90	55	90	
Taylor and Abrams, 1973	52	81	31			66
Murphy and Beigel, 1974	30			90		
Winokur and Tsuang, 1975	94	70	92[c]			
Abrams and Taylor, 1976	78	76	44		59	
Leff et al., 1976	63		97			
Loudon et al., 1977	16	75	81[d]	63[e]	56	44
Taylor and Abrams, 1977	119	81	39		52	60
Carlson and Strober, 1979	9[f]	100	89			
Prien et al., 1988	103			67[g]		
Cassidy et al., 1998[h]	316	51	59	29[i]	42	
Serretti and Olgiati, 2005	158	91				
Total n[j]	1121					
Weighted Mean[j]		71	63	46	49	60

[a]100 episodes, 61 patients.
[b]Depressive delusions in 24%, suicidal ideation in 7%.
[c]Irritable only (8%), euphoric only (30%), irritable and euphoric (62%).
[d]Hypomanic affect.
[e]Suicidal ideation in 25%.
[f]Adolescents.
[g]Mild depression (45%), moderate to severe depression (22%).
[h]High threshold value used for signs and symptoms.
[i]Dysphoria.
[j]Winokur et al. not included in calculation because units are in episodes, not in patients.

and so very changeable that they defied measurement. . . . In only 5% was the mood unchanging over a period of hours or days. (p. 62)

As noted earlier, Carlson and Goodwin (1973) described progressive stages of mania, from mild hypomania to delirious psychotic mania. The principal features of the three stages are outlined in Table 2–2; the relationship of these stages to daily behavioral ratings is illustrated in Figure 2–2. The stages were inferred from a study of 20 hospitalized, unmedicated bipolar patients who had experienced a manic episode at some time during their hospitalization.

TABLE 2–2. Clinical Features of the Stages of Mania

	Stage I	Stage II	Stage III
Mood	Lability of affect; euphoria predominates; irritability if demands not satisfied	Increased dysphoria and depression; open hostility and anger	Clearly dysphoric; panic-stricken; hopeless
Cognition	Expansivity, grandiosity, overconfidence; thoughts coherent but occasionally tangential; sexual and religious preoccupation; racing thoughts	Flight of ideas; disorganization of cognitive state; delusions	Incoherent, definite loosening of associations; bizarre and idiosyncratic delusions; hallucinations in one-third of patients; disorientation as to time and place; occasional ideas of reference
Behavior	Increased psychomotor activity; increased initiation and rate of speech; increased spending, smoking, telephone use	Continued increased psychomotor acceleration; increased pressured speech; occasional assaultive behavior	Frenzied and frequently bizarre psychomotor activity

Source: Adapted from Carlson and Goodwin, 1973.

Figure 2–2. Relationship between states of a manic episode and daily behavior ratings. (*Source*: Carlson and Goodwin, 1973.)

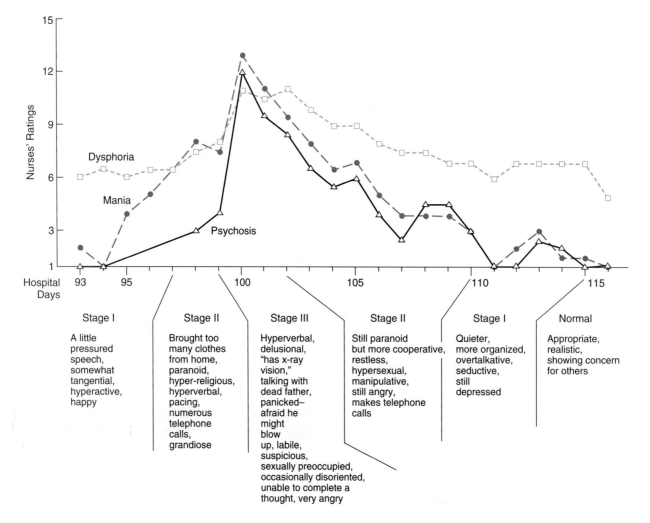

Manic episodes were identified by means of global mania ratings determined twice a day by consensus of the nursing research team, and were corroborated by the psychiatrists' and nurses' written descriptions of patients' affect, psychomotor activity, and cognitive state. The sequence of mood, cognitive, and behavioral symptoms over the course of the episode was recorded. Based on analysis of this information, the patients' longitudinal course was divided into three stages, with predominant mood as the primary criterion—from the euphoria of stage I, to the anger and irritability of stage II, to the severe panic of stage III. In some of the patients, the onset of mania (the switch) was gradual, clearly unfolding in a sequence until the full syndrome had developed. In others, the onset was sudden and dramatic; even in these cases, however, the earlier stages were present, if transient.

As Carlson and Goodwin elaborated, the initial phase of mania (stage I) typically is characterized by increased activity; by a labile mood that can be euphoric, irritable, or both; and by expansive, grandiose, and overconfident thoughts. Thinking remains coherent but is often tangential. Patients describe this change as "going high" and frequently report racing thoughts. In some instances, the "high" does not go beyond stage I, which corresponds to hypomania.

Many episodes progress to the next stage, however. Psychomotor activity increases—evident in the even more rapid speech—and the mood state becomes more labile, characterized by a mix of euphoria and dysphoria. Irritability turns into open hostility and anger, and the accompanying behavior often is explosive and assaultive. As racing thoughts progress to a definite flight of ideas, cognition becomes increasingly disorganized. Preoccupations intensify, with grandiose and paranoid trends that are apparent as frank delusions. This level, which corresponds to acute mania, is designated as stage II.

In some patients, the manic episode progresses further to an undifferentiated psychotic state (stage III), experienced by the patient as clearly dysphoric, usually terrifying, and accompanied by frenzied movement. Thought processes that earlier had been only difficult to follow become incoherent, and definite loosening of associations often is seen. Delusions commonly are bizarre and idiosyncratic, and some patients experience ideas of reference, disorientation, and a delirium-like state. This phase of the syndrome is difficult to distinguish from other acute psychoses, at least superficially. In general, as the manic episode unfolds, stage I is dominated by elation (or irritability) and grandiosity, stage II by increasing hyperactivity and arousal, and stage III by florid psychotic disorganization.

In the Carlson and Goodwin study, many of the rated items showed graded continuous distributions, whereas others evidenced definite thresholds involving apparently qualitative shifts. The level of psychomotor activity escalated continuously through all three stages, and ratings for manic mood increased in like manner through stages I and II. Ratings of psychosis, by contrast, were not clearly distributed along a continuum. This point is illustrated by the case example presented in Figure 2–2. As can be seen, stage III mania was characterized by the relatively abrupt and initial appearance of hallucinations, formal thought disorder in the Schneiderian sense, and organic delirium.

In their study of mania, Kotin and Goodwin (1972) found depressive affect to be pervasive. Indeed, in 10 of their 20 manic patients the mean depression rating was significantly higher during the manic episode than during nonmanic, depressed periods in the hospital. The authors noted that mania and depression ratings were correlated positively in a majority of patients both during manic periods and for the entire hospital stay. These findings, observed the authors, "are contrary to the common view that a patient is either manic or depressed" (p. 683). Recent studies of mania, discussed later, bear out its mixed nature.

Cognition and Perception

Nonpsychotic cognitive symptoms are common during mania. Grandiosity and flight of ideas—experienced subjectively as racing thoughts—were observed in approximately three-quarters of the manic patients described in the clinical studies summarized in Table 2–3. Less clearly and more variably defined were distractibility, poor concentration, and confusion, a fact that may account in part for the broader range of results on these variables—16 to 100 percent for distractibility, for example, and 8 to 58 percent for confusion. Definitions were especially wide-ranging for confusion—from "somewhat confused and unable to follow the gist of a conversation" to the more severe clinical usage of the term to denote disorientation and serious memory disturbance.

Thought Disorder.   There is no single or comprehensive definition of formal thought disorder. Instead, thought disorder has been used as a general phrase to describe problems with the ability to attend to, abstract, conceptualize, express, or continue coherent thought. Deficits in thought and language were at one time described in general terms; today these deficits are defined by specific measures (e.g., the Thought Disorder Index or the Scale for the Assessment of Thought, Language and Communication). This increased specificity makes it possible to disentangle, at least in part, disorders of thought from those of language or speech (accordingly, we discuss the

TABLE 2–3. **Cognitive Symptoms during Mania (Excluding Psychotic Features)**

Study	Patients (N)	Grandiosity (%)	Flight of Ideas/ Racing Thoughts (%)	Distractibility/ Poor Concentration (%)	Confusion[a] (%)
Lundquist, 1945	95				23
Clayton et al., 1965	31	79	100	97	58
Winokur et al., 1969	100[b]	86	93	100	8
Carlson and Goodwin, 1973	20	100	75	70	35
Taylor and Abrams, 1973	52		77		33
Abrams and Taylor, 1976	78	71	41		26
Leff et al., 1976	63		49	16	
Loudon et al., 1977	16	50	58[c]	75	
Taylor and Abrams, 1977	119				27
Carlson and Strober, 1979	9	67	56	67	
Braden and Ho, 1981	11		91[d]	55	
Cassidy et al., 1998	316	72	78		
Serretti and Olgiati, 2005	158		95	97	
Total n[e]	968				
Weighted mean[e]		73	76	75	29

[a]Disorientation and memory lapses; unclear criteria in some studies.
[b]100 episodes, 61 patients.
[c]Flight of ideas=25%.
[d]Persistent=55%.
[e]Winokur et al. not included in calculation because units are in episodes, not in patients.

latter separately below). Although difficult, this distinction is important, since it is possible to have either disorder without the other (Holzman et al., 1985). Much of thought is nonverbal, and individuals often say one thing while thinking another. Here we use as a working definition of thought disorder one provided by Solovay and colleagues (1987, p. 13): thought disorder "is not intended to denote a unitary dimension or process; rather, it refers to any disruption, deficit, or slippage in various aspects of thinking, such as concentration, attention, reasoning, or abstraction."

Certain psychotic features of mania and bipolar depression—delusions and hallucinations—are relevant but not central to the concept of thought disorder. The specificity of thought disorder to the major psychoses—mania and schizophrenia—represents an important conceptual issue and is a major focus here. Results of recent genetic studies indicate that psychosis may be an overlapping feature of bipolar illness and schizophrenia (see Chapter 13); therefore, studies that address the similarities and dissimilarities in the psychotic presentation of the two illnesses are of particular interest. Holzman and colleagues (1985, p. 228) asked: "Is thought disorder a nonspecific accompaniment of psychotic behavior, whatever the etiology of that psychosis, just as fever is nonspecific for a variety of systemic conditions; or is there a set of specific disorders of thinking that accompanies specific psychotic conditions?"

Several methods have evolved for studying thought and communication disorders in schizophrenia and affective illness. These methods were categorized by Harvey (1983) as (1) clinical (the examination of speech patterns on the basis of clinical interactions, e.g., in the manner of Kraepelin and Bleuler); (2) laboratory (the study of underlying cognitive processes that result in or contribute to disordered speech); and (3) natural-language (the examination of speech samples from a variety of sources in an attempt to "identify the discourse processes that lead to the problems listeners have in understanding the speech of psychotics" [p. 368]). Several specific measures have been developed, three of which, summarized below, form the basis for most of the research relevant to the study of thought disorder in bipolar illness. Taken together, these three measures can provide a reasonably comprehensive assessment of formal thought disorder.

Holzman and colleagues (1985) developed the Thought Disorder Index using verbal protocols (most typically verbatim responses to the Rorschach test). Based on earlier indices (Watkins and Stauffacher, 1952; Rapaport et al., 1968), the Thought Disorder Index comprises 23 categories of thinking disturbances evaluated at four levels of severity (Johnston and Holzman, 1979; Shenton et al., 1987; Solovay et al., 1987). The least severe level includes vagueness and peculiar verbalizations; the most severe includes thought contamination and neologisms.

Andreasen (1979a,b) characterized different language behaviors that she considered to be subtypes of thought disorder and developed them into another measure, the Scale for the Assessment of Thought, Language and Communication. Some subtypes occur frequently in psychotic speech (e.g., poverty of content of speech, pressure of speech, tangentiality, derailment, loss of goal, and perseveration), whereas others are relatively uncommon and, correspondingly, less useful (e.g., clanging, blocking, echolalia, neologisms, and word approximations).

Finally, Harrow and colleagues[4] have used a battery of measures taken from the Wechsler Adult Intelligence Scale (WAIS) (Social Comprehension Subtest), the Goldstein-Scheerer Object-Sorting Test, and the Gorham Proverbs Test to assess bizarre and idiosyncratic thinking and behavior, as well as conceptual style. Detailed discussions of the development, reliability, and validity of their test battery are provided elsewhere.[5]

Virtually all studies of formal thought disorder in mania and schizophrenia, the results of which are summarized in Table 2–4, have found comparably high levels in both diagnostic groups.[6] In fact, although Resnick and Oltmanns (1984) observed more thought disorder in schizophrenic patients, Harrow and colleagues (1982) found a trend toward greater levels in manic patients.[7] There is,

therefore, no indication that thought disorder per se is in any way specific to schizophrenia. This observation is consistent with the evidence for the strong presence in mania, as well as in schizophrenia, of psychotic features, such as hallucinations and delusions. (See Chapter 13 for discussion of potential genetic factors underlying psychosis in both bipolar disorder and schizophrenia.) Findings of qualitative comparisons of manic and schizophrenic thought disorder are less consistent, although increased pressure of speech appears to be more characteristic of mania,[8] as are increased derailment, loss of goal, and tangentiality (Andreasen, 1984; Simpson and Davis, 1985). Poverty of speech and other negative symptoms were reported by Andreasen (1984) to be more characteristic of schizophrenic thought, although Ragin and Oltmanns (1987), using the same scale, did not confirm this finding. More recent studies have found greater poverty of thought, less complexity of speech, and less overall quantity of speech in schizophrenic than in manic patients.[9]

Studies of differences between manic and schizophrenic patients on measures of idiosyncratic and/or bizarre thinking have yielded mixed results, with some authors finding higher levels in manic patients (Andreasen and Powers, 1975; Harrow et al., 1982) and others higher levels in schizophrenic patients (Simpson and Davis, 1985; Shenton et al., 1987; Docherty et al., 1996). In general, investigators have found that those with mania have more complex speech than those with schizophrenia (Thomas et al., 1996; Lott et al., 2002). Simpson and Davis (1985) made the useful distinction that manic patients appear to be more disordered in *thought structure*, whereas schizophrenic patients appear to be more disordered in *thought content*. Jampala and colleagues (1989, p. 462) argued that manic patients with formal thought disorder may "have a more severe rather than a different condition than manic patients without formal thought disorder. The fact that more manic patients with formal thought disorder had a first-degree relative with affective illness supports this interpretation."

Qualitative differences in thought disorder between mania and schizophrenia are more distinct in the use of combinatory thinking, the "tendency to merge percepts, ideas, or images in an incongruous fashion" (Shenton et al., 1987, p. 23). In a study of 20 manic patients, 43 schizophrenic patients, and 22 normal subjects, Solovay and colleagues (1987), using the Thought Disorder Index, found no significant difference in the quantity of thought disorder in manic and schizophrenic patients, but did note that manic thought disorder was "extravagantly combinatory, usually with humor, flippancy, and playfulness." Schizophrenic thought disorder, by contrast, was "disorganized, confused, and idealistically fluid, with many peculiar words and

TABLE 2–4. Thought Pathology in Mania and Schizophrenia: Similarities and Differences

Study	Thought Disorder Measure	Similarities	Differences
Breakey and Goodell, 1972	Bannister Grid Text	Same frequency of thought disorder	
Andreasen and Powers, 1975	Goldstein–Scheerer Object Sorting Test		**Manic patients:** ↑ behavioral overinclusion; ↑ conceptual overinclusion, ↑ idiosyncratic thinking **Schizophrenic patients:** ↑ underinclusiveness
Grossman et al., 1981	Gorham Proverbs Test Goldstein–Scheerer Object Sorting Test Wechsler Adult Intelligence Scale (WAIS), Social Comprehension Subtest	Similar in overall level of severity, course of disturbance, and loose association of ideas; intermingling of inappropriate personal ideas or concerns into responses to neutral stimuli; gaps in communication of ideas, odd outlooks, and other manifestations of bizarre thinking	**Manic patients:** ↑ behavioral activity and responsiveness, ↓ response time on word association test, ↓ deficits in behavioral activity or impoverished activity, ↑ grandiose ideas
Harrow et al., 1982	Gorham Proverbs Test Goldstein–Scheerer Object Sorting Test WAIS, Social Comprehension Subtest		**Manic patients:** may be more thought disordered than schizophrenics, "although the results are not conclusive"; ↑ bizarre–idiosyncratic thinking
Andreasen, 1984	Scale for the Assessment of Thought, Language and Communication	Similar in number of abnormalities	**Manic patients:** more positive thought disorder; ↑ tangentiality, ↑ derailment, ↑ incoherence, ↑ illogicality, ↑ pressure of speech **Schizophrenic patients:** more negative thought disorder, ↑ poverty of speech, ↑ poverty of content **Schizoaffective patients:** thought disorder is midway between that of manic and schizophrenic patients
Resnick and Oltmanns, 1984	Global ratings of thought disorder		**Manic patients:** less overall thought disorder; ↑ pressure of speech

Reference	Measure	Findings
Simpson and Davis, 1985	Scale for the Assessment of Thought, Language and Communication; Brief Psychiatric Rating Scale	**Manic patients:** more disordered thought structure; ↑loss of goal, ↑tangentiality, ↑derailment, ↑circumstantiality, ↑illogicality, ↑pressure of speech, ↑incoherence **Schizophrenic patients:** more disordered thought content; ↑hallucinatory statements, ↑hallucinatory behavior, ↑unusual thought content
Ragin and Oltmanns, 1987	Scale for the Assessment of Thought, Language and Communication	**Manic patients:** ↑ pressure of speech Similar levels of poverty of speech, derailment, loss of goal
Shenton et al., 1987	Thought Disorder Index	**Manic patients:** ↑ combinatory thinking High level of thought disorder in both manic and schizophrenic patients **Schizophrenic patients:** overall higher level of thought disorder; ↑idiosyncratic and autistic thinking, ↑absurdity, ↑confusion **Schizoaffective patients:** thinking disorders more similar to those of schizophrenic patients than to those of manic patients
Solovay et al., 1987	Thought Disorder Index	**Manic patients:** Thought disorder "extravagantly combinative, usually with humor, flippancy and playfulness" Equal amount of thought disorder **Schizophrenic patients:** "disorganized, confused, and ideationally fluid, with many peculiar words and phrases"
Jampala et al., 1989	Authors' measures of thought disorder	**Manic patients:** ↑flight of ideas **Schizophrenic patients:** ↑non sequiturs, ↑tangentiality, ↑driveling, ↑neologisms, ↑private use of words, ↑paraphasias

(continued)

47

TABLE 2–4. Thought Pathology in Mania and Schizophrenia: Similarities and Differences *(continued)*

Study	Thought Disorder Measure	Similarities	Differences
Docherty et al., 1996	Communication Disturbance Index	Structural unclarities; confused, wrong words and vague references	**Manic patients:** ↑ amount of speech; ↑ ambiguous word meanings **Schizophrenic patients:** ↑ references to information unknown to listener
Thomas et al., 1996	Brief Syntactic Analysis		**Schizophrenic patients:** ↓ complexity of speech
Lott et al., 2002	Authors' measures of thought, language, and communication	Most measures of deviant speech	**Manic patients:** ↑ complexity of speech **Schizophrenic patients:** ↑ poverty of speech

phrases." The authors elaborated further on these differences (pp. 19–20):

> [M]anic thought disorder manifests itself as ideas loosely strung together and extravagantly combined and elaborated . . . appearance of irrelevant intrusions into social discourse that may at times appear inappropriately flippant and playful. . . . Schizophrenic thought disorder, on the other hand, seems devoid of the playful, compulsively elaborative, and ideationally loose constructions of the manic patients. Characteristic of the schizophrenic patients in this study were fluid thinking, interpenetrations of one idea by another, unstable verbal referents, and fragmented and elliptical communications.

These differences are portrayed in Figure 2–3, which shows standardized Thought Disorder Index scores (on factors derived from a principal components analysis) for 12 schizoaffective (manic) and 10 schizoaffective (depressed) patients, as well as for the manic, schizophrenic, and normal subjects discussed earlier (Shenton et al., 1987). Of note, on the one "manic" factor (combinatory thinking), schizoaffective manic patients were most similar to the manic group, but on the five "schizophrenic" factors (idiosyncratic thinking, autistic thinking, fluid thinking, absurdity, and confusion), they performed more like the schizophrenic patients. The schizoaffective depressed patients more strongly resembled the normal subjects. Andreasen (1984) found that her schizoaffective patients were midway in thought disorder between the manic and schizophrenic patients. Jampala and colleagues (1989) observed a greatly increased rate of flight of ideas in their manic patients (72 percent) compared with schizophrenic patients (10 percent).

In summary, although the overall amount of thought disorder does not differentiate manic from schizophrenic patients, qualitative differences do exist. Manic patients are more likely than schizophrenics to exhibit more pressured and complex speech; grandiosity; flight of ideas; combinatory and overinclusive thinking; and a strong affective component to thought that is characterized by humor, playfulness, and flippancy. The causal relationships among affect, psychomotor acceleration, and the often strikingly different manifestations of the underlying thought disorders in mania and schizophrenia remain unclear.

A few studies have followed the course of manic thought disorder over time. Andreasen (1984) observed that most manic patients, unlike schizophrenic patients, demonstrated a reversible thought disorder. Other than a continuing pressure of speech, they showed nearly complete recovery over time. Schizoaffective patients, to a lesser

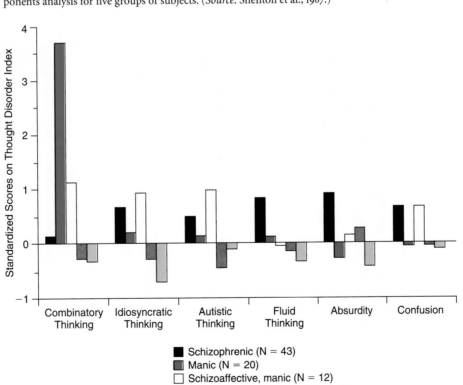

Figure 2–3. Standardized Thought Disorder Index scores on factors derived from principal components analysis for five groups of subjects. (*Source*: Shenton et al., 1987.)

extent than the manic patients, also recovered. Ragin and Oltmanns (1987), on the other hand, found that manic patients displayed moderate levels of derailment and loss of goal at initial testing and, unlike other thought-disordered subjects, did not show significant decreases in either of these features at follow-up. The most extensive longitudinal studies of manic thought disorder were conducted by Harrow and colleagues (Harrow et al., 1982, 1986; Grossman et al., 1986). Using a battery of cognitive tests designed to assess bizarre–idiosyncratic thinking (Goldstein-Scheerer Object Sorting Test, Gorham Proverbs Test, and WAIS Social Comprehension Subtest), the investigators tested manic thought disorder in the acute phase (Harrow et al., 1982), 1 year after hospitalization (Harrow et al., 1986), and 2 to 4 years after hospitalization (Grossman et al., 1986). Initial levels of manic thought pathology and changes over time were compared with those obtained for schizophrenic and nonpsychotic psychiatric patients and normal subjects. The results of these comparisons are summarized in Figure 2–4 and presented in further detail below.

In the acute phase, manic patients were extremely thought disordered; 94 percent showed some definite evidence of abnormal thinking, and 73 percent of hospitalized manic patients demonstrated severe levels of bizarre–idiosyncratic thinking. There were no significant differences

in levels of thought disorder between medicated and unmedicated manic patients. Manic patients were at least as thought disordered as, if not more so than, schizophrenic patients (Harrow et al., 1986).

In the short-term follow-up phase (7 weeks), manic thought disorder in medicated patients improved, although some patients continued to show severe thought disorder. Manic patients did not show a more rapid reduction in thought pathology relative to the schizophrenic patients (Harrow et al., 1982).

One year after hospital discharge, a "surprisingly large number" of manic patients showed relatively severe bizarre–idiosyncratic thinking or positive thought disorder (Fig. 2–4). There was also a significant reduction in severity of thought pathology for both manic and schizophrenic patients at follow-up. Manic patients showed a greater reduction in pathology (from 73 to 27 percent rated as severe or very severe) relative to the schizophrenic patients (from 50 to 27 percent) (Harrow et al., 1986).

Two- to 4-year follow-up data revealed that of the manic patients, 30 percent had severe or very severe thought disorder, and another 30 percent had definite signs of abnormal thinking. Of the 14 formerly hospitalized manic patients who showed severe or very severe thought disorder, only 4 were rehospitalized at the time of the follow-up assessment.

Figure 2–4. Composite level of thought disorder during and after hospitalization in manic, schizophrenic, and nonpsychotic psychiatric patients and normal subjects. (*Source*: Grossman et al., 1986; Harrow et al., 1982, 1986.)

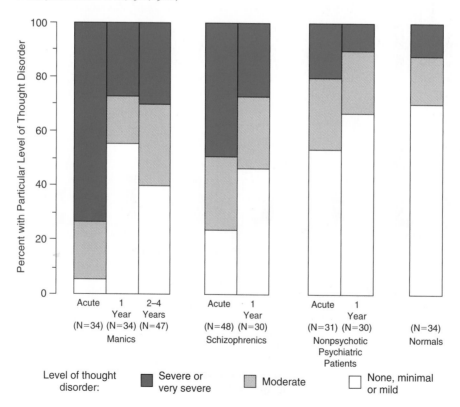

TABLE 2–5. Relationship of Manic Behavior and Psychosis to Thought Disorder in 47 Formerly Hospitalized Manic Patients at 2- to 4-Year Follow-Up

	No or Mild Thought Disorder (%) (n = 19)	Signs of Abnormal Thought Disorder (%) (n = 14)	Severe or Very Severe Thought Disorder (%) (n = 14)
Ratings of Manic Behavior			
None	58	71	29
Equivocal	42	7	36
Definite	0	21	36
Ratings of Psychosis			
None	74	29	43
Equivocal	26	36	29
Definite	0	36	29

Source: Grossman et al., 1986. Reprinted with permission from the *American Journal of Psychiatry*, Copyright 1986, American Psychiatric Association.

Positive thought disorder was associated with manic behavior; that is, those patients who showed more manic behaviors had more severe thought disorder (see Table 2–5). There was a significant correlation between thought disorder and psychosis, but psychotic symptoms alone did not account for all of the variance associated with thought disorder at follow-up. Manic patients with more than one previous hospitalization or with a more chronic manic course had significantly more thought disorder than patients with only one or no previous hospitalizations (Grossman et al., 1986).

These findings of Harrow's group are indicative of the fact that manic thought disorder can prevail long past an acute episode, a point suggesting the need for caution in accepting assumptions of a relatively benign course of illness or of a return to normality for all patients with bipolar illness (see Chapter 4 for further discussion of the problematic course of bipolar disorder). The findings must be tempered, however, by certain methodological constraints, especially one relevant to recent investigations. In the current era, manic-depressive patients seen and treated in university teaching hospitals represent a disproportionately ill and treatment-refractory group. Bipolar patients with a more typical (i.e., salutary) course are now treated, for the most part, by the general psychiatric community. Those patients less responsive to standard medical interventions are more frequently referred to research centers for evaluation and treatment. Further confounding interpretation of the above findings are issues of patient nonadherence to medication regimens (see Chapter 21), medication side effects, and seasonal biases (e.g., annual assessments, if completed 1, 2, or 4 years after an acute episode, may increase the likelihood of testing during a periodic recurrence rather than a remission). The continuance of significant thought pathology in many manic patients is of both clinical and theoretical relevance and is an important area for further research (see Perugi et al., 1998a, for a discussion of cognitive decline in chronic mania).

Linguistic and Communication Patterns. Investigators have found differences in linguistic patterns between manic and schizophrenic patients (Kagan and Oltmanns, 1981; Harvey, 1983; Ragin and Oltmanns, 1987). Hoffman and colleagues (1986) found that total speech deviance and utterance length were greater in manic than in schizophrenic patients. The authors concluded that "manic speech difficulties were due to shifts from one discourse structure to another, while schizophrenic speech difficulties reflected a basic deficiency in elaborating any discourse structure" (p. 836). In a related study, Fraser and colleagues (1986) found that schizophrenic patients had less syntactically complex speech than manic patients. This finding is consistent with those of the more recent work of Thomas and colleagues

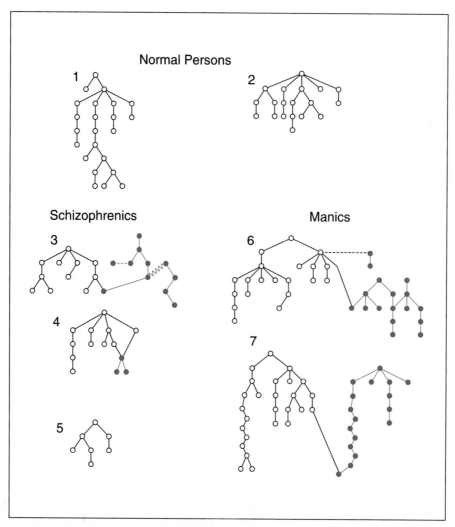

Figure 2–5. Sample of discourse structures taken from three groups. Note: Nodes correspond to statements generated by text. Linkages are formed from dependency relations. Substructures identified by open circles correspond to largest subtree embedded in segment. Jagged line indicates nontransitive dependency; broken lines represent nondependent associations. Upward branching nodes can be seen to receive more than one chain of superordinate statements. Two manic patients have larger subtrees compared with three schizophrenic patients. 1, 2, and 5 are well-formed trees. (*Source*: Hoffman et al., 1986.)

(1996) and Lott and colleagues (2002), who also found that manic speech was more complex. The structural differences in language are schematized in Figure 2–5. Hoffman and colleagues (1986) speculated that the shift from one discourse structure to another is related to the manic patient's increased distractibility and general level of overactivation, each of which involves both verbal and nonverbal behavior. Distractibility in bipolar illness, which is pervasive and often severe, is discussed in detail in Chapter 9.

Predictability of verbal communication has been studied through close analysis, a measure of the ability of normal subjects to guess words deleted from transcripts of speech samples. Using this technique, Ragin and Oltmanns (1983) found that depressed speech was the most predictable,

schizophrenic the least, and manic somewhere in between. Andreasen and Pfohl (1976) analyzed the frequency of syntactical elements in speech samples taken from 16 manic and 15 depressed patients. Their results are summarized in Table 2–6 and as follows by the authors (p. 1366):

The analysis of syntactical elements was particularly useful in distinguishing between the two groups . . . [D]epressive speech tends to be more vague, qualified, and personalized, while manic speech is more colorful and concrete . . . [D]epressed patients tend to qualify more, to talk more in terms of a "state of being," and to talk more both about themselves and other people. Manics, on the other hand, tend to talk more about things

TABLE 2–6. Frequency of Syntactical Elements in Manic and Depressed Patients

Manic = Depressed	Manic > Depressed	Depressed > Manic
• Lexical diversity (number of words, number of different words) • Syntactical complexity	• Colorfulness • Action verbs • Adjectives • Concreteness • Words reflecting power and achievement	• Vagueness • Qualifying adverbs • First-person pronouns • Overstatement

Note: Sample = 16 manic patients, 15 depressed patients.
Source: Adapted from data in Andreasen and Pfohl, 1976.

than about people, to discuss them in terms of action, and to use more adjectives to describe them.

Delusions and Hallucinations. Problems in the assessment of delusions and hallucinations are many and troublesome. Orvaschel and colleagues (1982) found that family reports of affective delusions identified only 18 percent of probands who admitted such symptoms on direct interview with the Schedule for Affective Disorders-Lifetime (SADS-L). In a study of psychosis in 89 bipolar patients, Rosen and colleagues (1983a) found that 49 (55 percent) emerged as psychotic on the basis of interviews (SADS) alone. After a review of all interviews and prior records, however, 63 were identified as psychotic. Price and colleagues (1984), like Orvaschel and colleagues (1982), found a lack of reliability in reports from family members. Yet as Pope and Lipinski (1978) observed in their early review of the literature, the general findings of all these studies, despite wide differences in time, setting, and sample selection, are reasonably consistent.

Table 2–7 summarizes findings from 33 studies of psychotic features in mania. Approximately two-thirds of the bipolar patients in these studies were found to have a lifetime history of at least one psychotic symptom (phase of illness usually unspecified, but when specified, more often manic). The range of rates was 47 to 90 percent. These results are consistent with Carlson and Goodwin's (1973) finding that 30 percent of their bipolar-I patients (i.e., those with a history of mania) did not progress to stage III mania. Rosenthal and colleagues (1979) also observed that 33 percent of their bipolar-I patients never became formally psychotic during mania. The high prevalence of psychotic features in these studies is consistent with the presence of a psychosis factor in most factorial studies of mania and with Koukopoulos's (2005) assertion that the manic syndrome is basically a psychotic condition.

Some evidence suggests that early age at onset of bipolar illness is likely to be associated with an increased rate of psychotic symptoms. Carlson and Strober (1979) found that bipolar illness first appearing during adolescence was characterized by especially florid psychotic symptoms. Rosenthal and colleagues (1980) observed that those bipolar-I patients who also met Research Diagnostic Criteria (RDC) for schizoaffective illness had a younger age at onset and more non-Schneiderian delusions and hallucinations. Rosen and colleagues (1983b) found a negative correlation of 0.4 between age at onset and psychotic symptom score. The authors also suggested that their findings raise the possibility that RDC schizoaffective disorders are really a form of bipolar-I disorder. More recent, larger studies have not found a significant correlation between early age at onset and psychotic symptoms, however (Perugi et al., 2000; Toni et al., 2001; Baethge et al., 2005). Age-specific issues relevant to delusions and hallucinations are discussed more fully in Chapter 6.

Akiskal and colleagues (1983) reported that in patients who switched from depression to mania during a prospective observation period of 3–4 years, the index depressive episode was often psychotic. Findings of a new study (Othmer et al., in press) based on more than 1,000 outpatients confirm the strong association between early-onset psychotic depression and eventual manic switch.

Some evidence relates the presence of psychotic symptoms to severity of illness. Abrams and Taylor (1981) found "only a trend" toward an association between severity of manic syndrome and "schizophrenic features," including delusions and hallucinations. Carlson and Goodwin (1973), however, reported covariance between ratings of psychosis and ratings of manic severity. Likewise, Young and colleagues (1983) found a positive relationship between total score on the Mania Rating Scale and the presence of psychotic symptoms. More recently, Baethge and colleagues (2005) found that hospitalizations for bipolar patients who had hallucinations averaged 17 percent longer than those for bipolar patients who did not.

TABLE 2–7. Psychotic Symptoms during Mania

Study	Patients N	DELUSIONS				HALLUCINATIONS				Presence or History of Psychotic Symptoms[a] (%)	Thought Disorder (%)	First-Rank Schneiderian Symptoms (%)
		Any (%)	Grandiose (%)	Persecutory/ Paranoid (%)	Passivity (%)	Any (%)	Auditory (%)	Visual (%)	Olfactory (%)			
Lange, 1922	700						7				8	
Bowman and Raymond, 1931–1932a,b	1009			20			17	9				
Rennie, 1942	66	24				22						
Lundquist, 1945	95					13						
Astrup et al., 1959	96			18	9		24					9
Clayton et al., 1965	31	73			47							
Winokur et al., 1969	100[b]	48		19	22		21	9				
Beigel and Murphy, 1971a	12			33								
Carlson and Goodwin, 1973	20	75		65	20	40						
Carpenter et al., 1973	66											23
Taylor and Abrams, 1973b	52		60	42			48	27	15			12
Murphy and Beigel, 1974	30			23								
Guze et al., 1975	19									53[b]		
Abrams and Taylor, 1976	78			55			44					
Leff et al., 1976	63	67										
Loudon et al., 1977	16		43	25								

54

Study	n									
Taylor and Abrams, 1977	119	52	65		47				84	11
Carlson and Strober, 1979	9	56			33				44	
Rosenthal et al., 1979	66	35[c]	35[c]		30[c]	21[c]		67[c]		
Brockington et al., 1980[a]	32		53		34				9	34
Rosenthal et al., 1980	71	41	30		30	25		74[c]		34
Rosen et al., 1983a	89							55 (71)[e,f]		
Rosen et al., 1983b	71							75[c]		
Winokur, 1984	122	54	4		14	9		64[c]		
Endicott et al., 1986	298[d]							47[c]		
Black and Nasrallah, 1989	467	44		14	13	6				
Vieta et al., 1997	34[g]							90		
Cassidy et al., 1998	316							78–90[h]		
Coryell et al., 2001	139							65		
Suppes et al., 2001	214[g]							67		
Serretti et al., 2002	863[g]	61		31				50		
Keck et al., 2003	352[c]	17	34	25	25	22		68		
Baethge et al., 2005	196(48)[i]			11 (23)[i]						
Total n	5973									
Weighted means (individual episode data[a])		53	31	39	18	14	15	61	19	17

(continued)

TABLE 2–7. **Psychotic Symptoms during Mania** (continued)

Study	Patients N	DELUSIONS				HALLUCINATIONS				Presence or History of Psychotic Symptoms[a] (%)	Thought Disorder (%)	First-Rank Schneiderian Symptoms %
		Any (%)	Grandiose (%)	Persecutory/ Paranoid (%)	Passivity (%)	Any (%)	Auditory (%)	Visual (%)	Olfactory (%)			
Weighted means[j] lifetime data[a]	—	35	22	—	18	10	—			60	9	34
Weighted means[j] (all)	53	31	29	12	23	18	12	15		61	19	18

[a]Lifetime or course of illness.
[b]100 episodes, 61 patients.
[c]Phase of illness not specified.
[d]Bipolar fraction unclear.
[e]38 reported psychotic symptoms during manic phase only, 6 during both manic and depressed phases, and 5 during depressed phase only.
[f](71) refers to total % psychotic (only 55% were considered psychotic on the basis of interview alone).
[g]Bipolar I patients only.
[h]Low and high symptom threshold values.
[i]Mixed mania figures are in parentheses.
[j]Winokur et al. not included in calculation because units are in episodes, not in patients.

The relationship between the presence or a history of psychotic features and the long-term course of illness is unclear. While several studies have not found a correlation between psychosis and poorer outcome,[10] many more have.[11] There is even more agreement that mood-incongruent psychotic features predict a less positive course.[12] Only one early investigation (Abrams and Taylor, 1983) and a single recent study (Keck et al., 2003) found otherwise. Keck and colleagues hypothesized that their findings, which are at variance with most others, may reflect the high morbidity and poor functional outcome in the great majority of the patients they studied. There does not appear to be a significant correlation between psychosis and an increased likelihood of attempting suicide (Grunebaum et al., 2001; Black et al., 2003; Keck et al., 2003; see Chapter 8).

Young and colleagues (1983) examined the relationship between psychotic features and other manic symptoms. They found no association of psychotic features with insight, disruptive–aggressive behavior, appearance, and rate and amount of speech, or with demographic variables, such as age, gender, and race. They did find, however, that psychotic patients were significantly more likely than nonpsychotic patients to have grandiose and expansive mood, increased psychomotor activity and energy, and increased sexual interest, and were also more likely to report sleep-disturbance symptoms. Baethge and colleagues (2005), who studied hospitalized bipolar patients, found that those who reported hallucinations were less well educated and had higher anxiety scores, longer hospitalizations, and less insight into their illness. Comparisons of bipolar-I and -II patients have found, as one would expect, a greatly elevated rate (nearly three-fold) of psychotic symptoms in those with bipolar-I (Vieta et al., 1997; Suppes et al., 2001; Serretti et al., 2002).

Finally, Endicott and colleagues (1986) studied 1,084 first-degree relatives of 298 probands with schizoaffective, psychotic, and nonpsychotic unipolar and bipolar major depressive disorders. They found that over the course of a lifetime, bipolar disorder and psychosis were positively associated in both probands and relatives. Bipolar illness in a proband did not predict psychosis in relatives, however, whereas psychosis in a proband was related to increased risk of psychosis (but not to bipolarity) in relatives. According to Endicott and colleagues, these findings suggest that, although bipolarity and psychosis often occur in the same individuals, they may not reflect the same genetic influence. The authors speculated that "the risk for the 'expression' of psychotic symptoms is increased in individuals who also have had a bipolar disorder" (p. 11). Interestingly, Winokur and colleagues (1986; Winokur and Kadrmas, 1989) showed that the risk for psychosis, as well as polyepisodic course in bipolar patients, is predicted by a history of mania and polyepisodic course in the family.

Delusions, like thought disorder, vary widely in severity, fixedness, content, and effect on overt behavior (Jaspers, 1913; Kraepelin, 1921; Garety, 1985). The degree to which they are contingent upon fluctuating affect also varies.

Manic delusions are usually grandiose and expansive in nature, often religious, and not infrequently paranoid. They generally can be differentiated from schizophrenic delusions by their tendency to be wish-fulfilling in nature and oriented more toward communion than segregation (Lerner, 1980). Winokur and colleagues (1969, p. 70) distinguished the presentations of delusions in the two illnesses as follows:

> The delusions that are seen in schizophrenia usually last for months or years and are often primary; that is, they do not explain a real or disordered perception. They fulfill the definition of a delusion as a fixed, false belief. In mania the delusions are quite different. They are often evanescent, appearing or disappearing during the course of a day, or even during an interview. They also vary with the patient's total state, being more frequent when he is more active; and his flights of ideas become more pronounced and fading as he becomes more quiet. Frequently they are extensions of the patient's grandiosity.
>
> At times the patient can be talked out of his delusion, and at other times he gives the impression that he is only being playful rather than really being deluded. In our group the delusions were often secondary to the patient's exalted affect. This was especially true of those patients who felt their mood could be described only as a religious experience.
>
> The most subtle and earliest distortions of reality are manifest in the frequent extravagance and grandiose self-image expressed by the patients.

Kraepelin (1921, pp. 68–69) also emphasized the changing nature of manic delusions (especially when contrasted with those expressed during the depressive phase, which he thought were for the most part "uniformly adhered to"): manic delusions "change frequently, emerge as creations of the moment and again disappear"; they "move very frequently on religious territory," tending to be grandiose; and "patients often narrate all sorts of journeys and adventures, secret experiences." He also reported that the same delusional ideas often appeared again in subsequent attacks. Winokur and colleagues (1969, p. 72), like Kraepelin, suggested that delusions of mania are "not well systematized and, apart from grandiose optimism, tend not to be acted upon." They attributed the fact that manic patients seldom act on their delusions (a point perhaps worth disputing) to the brief duration of the delusions and the patient's "inability to make any sort of concerted action." They noted further that both manic and depressive delusions, which occur primarily in the most disturbed patients, tend to be appropriate to the patient's mood and not to be systematized. The same investigators found that religious themes were the most common manic delusions in both men (27.0 percent) and women (30.1 percent). Political themes were more common in men (18.9 percent) than in women (3.2 percent), and sexual and financial themes were about equally common (13.5 and 9.5 percent, respectively, in men; 5.4 and 7.9 percent, respectively, in women).

Hallucinations, or perceptions of sensory impressions without the existence of external physical stimuli, represent a fascinating, not uncommon, and yet relatively unstudied part of the clinical phenomenology of affective illness. They occupy a portion of the continuum of dream-state–illusory–hallucinatory phenomena, which ranges from distortions and misperceptions on the one hand to the total conjuring of fully developed images on the other. Hallucinations can vary in a wide range of aspects, such as their extent (frequency and duration), location, constancy, intensity, effect on overt behavior, affect produced, content, and causal attributions (Lowe, 1973). Yet despite these complexities, hallucinations are most commonly presented in the psychiatric research literature as simply present or absent in a given sensory modality (e.g., auditory or visual).

Hallucinations generally occur less frequently than delusions in both the manic and depressed phases of bipolar illness, although Carlson and Strober (1979) reported a significantly higher rate of hallucinations in bipolar depression. Baethge and colleagues (2005) found comparable rates of hallucinations in mania and depression, but twice as high a rate in bipolar mixed patients (see Table 2–8). The lifetime history data presented earlier in Table 2-7 suggest that at least half of all patients report a history of delusions, but only about a fifth report the experience of hallucinating while depressed or manic. Auditory hallucinations, averaged across the data-based studies, are more common than visual ones.

Kraepelin (1921, pp. 5–6) found that in mania, the perception of external impressions was "invariably encroached upon" and that defective perceptions often were related to "extraordinary distractibility of attention." He described not only the blurring of illusions, hypnagogic phenomena, and hallucinations, but also their overlap with mood and thinking in the bipolar form of manic-depressive illness (pp. 8, 11):

Isolated hallucinations are observed frequently and in the most different states, although they do not very often

appear conspicuously in the foreground. It is generally a case of illusionary occurrences, the appearance of which is favoured by the incompleteness and slightness of perception, but especially by the lively emotions peculiar to the disease. The substance of the illusions therefore is invariably in close connection with the trains of thought and the moods of the patients. . . .

Auditory hallucinations frequently appear only in the night-time, or at least much more then. They seem, as a rule, not to possess complete sensory distinctness. They are voices "as in a dream". . . . Their origin is relatively seldom referred to the external world. . . . Much more frequently the hallucinations have their seat in the patient's own body.

In an early study, Bowman and Raymond (1931–1932b) compared hallucinations in 1,009 patients with manic-depressive psychoses, 1,408 with schizophrenia, and 496 with general paresis. They found an overall tendency for more women than men to have a history of hallucinations (especially of a visual nature), and observed that women with "seclusive personalities" were at particularly high risk for auditory and visual hallucinations. A recent study of hallucinations in bipolar patients also found that women were more likely than men to report hallucinations (Baethge et al., 2005). Bowman and Raymond found no significant relationship between the presence of hallucinations and religion, age at admission, or level of intelligence. They did observe a close relationship between the clinical nature of the hallucinations in bipolar illness and those present in patients with general paresis. This latter finding is consistent with Lowe's (1973) conclusion that bipolar hallucinations resemble more those of the organic psychoses than those of schizophrenia or paranoia. (This similarity to organic psychosis [toxic versus defect] is also discussed in Chapters 3, 9, and 15.)

Winokur and colleagues (1969) found that manic hallucinations tended to be brief, grandiose, often part of a delusional idea, usually religious ("the face of God," "Heaven in all its glory"), and frequently in the form of a command from God. Manic and depressive hallucinations shared a fragmented and fleeting quality and usually occurred in the most severely disturbed patients. The authors stressed the theoretical importance of a severity profile in bipolar illness, after noting that hallucinations—the least common of symptoms—were also the first symptoms to disappear during recovery from a manic episode, followed in turn by delusions, flight of ideas, push of speech, and distractibility (a general pattern later confirmed by Carlson and Goodwin, 1973).

Although finding hallucinations of generally limited use in differential diagnosis, D.W. Goodwin and colleagues

TABLE 2–8. **Comparison of Psychotic Features during Mania and Bipolar Depression**

Category of Symptoms	PERCENTAGE OF PATIENTS					
	Winokur et al., 1969[a]	Carlson and Strober, 1979	Rosenthal et al., 1980	Black and Nasrallah, 1989	Mantere et al., 2004	Baethge et al., 2005
Delusions						
Mania	48	56	96[c]	44		
Depression	33	66	28	12		
Hallucinations						
Mania	21[b]	33	66	14		11 (23[d])
Depression	6[b]	50	24	8		11
Psychotic Symptoms[e]						
Mania					44	
Depression					9	
Mixed					40	

[a]100 episodes, 61 patients.
[b]Episodes of auditory hallucinations only.
[c]Includes delusions during euthymic states.
[d]Mixed state.
[e]Delusions or hallucinations not specified. Bipolar-I patients.

(1971), in one of the few (albeit small) phenomenological studies, were able to draw several conclusions about the nature of hallucinations in their 28 patients (7 bipolar) with affective illness: (1) the modality of hallucinations (e.g., auditory or visual) was not consistent from one affective episode to another; (2) patients with affective illness were far more likely than those with schizophrenia to hallucinate only when no other person was there; (3) color was usually normal; (4) the people who appeared in the hallucination were usually of normal size and appearance; (5) the hallucinations were intermittent; (6) they were often in several sensory modalities; and (7) accusatory voices were not specific to affective illness—indeed, they were more common in schizophrenia.

Lowe (1973) studied 22 bipolar patients in a particularly intensive and interesting investigation of hallucinations. In comparing these patients with others who had organic, paranoid, or schizophrenic psychoses, he found that they reported mainly auditory and visual hallucinations when manic; that these hallucinations were less frequent and briefer than those occurring in other neuropsychiatric conditions; that in retrospect, the hallucinations were believed by patients to be "less real" but were also perceived to be less controllable; that women were more likely to report rarer types of hallucinations; and finally, that the patients always believed the hallucinations to be experienced only by themselves. Consistent with other investigators, Lowe concluded that manic hallucinations were more similar in nature to those reported by patients with organic psychoses than to those reported by patients with schizophrenia or paranoia.

Lerner (1980), who also investigated qualitative differences between the psychotic experiences of mania and schizophrenia, concluded that mania was more characterized by enhanced sensory awareness and ecstatic or beatific experiences. Manic hallucinations tended to be more of the visual type; strikingly vivid and associated with bright, colorful sensations; and often coupled with intensely pleasurable or ecstatic feelings (similar to psychedelic experiences). Silberman and colleagues (1985) compared histories of transient sensory phenomena akin to hallucinations in 44 euthymic affective patients (34 bipolar), 37 patients with a history of complex partial seizures, and 30 hypertensive controls. Affective and epileptic patients were similar in their reports of sensory changes, including visual and auditory hallucinations and altered perceptual intensities. Epileptic patients, however, were far more likely to have experienced epigastric, vestibular, and gustatory hallucinations.

In summary, hallucinations occur less frequently than delusions in both the manic and depressed phases of bipolar illness. Hallucinatory phenomena appear to represent the extreme end of the symptomatic picture, being nonexistent in milder forms of depression and mania and most pronounced in the gravest, most delirious states. Hallucinations during mania are frequently ecstatic and religious in nature, brief and fleeting in duration, and inconstant in their modality of expression. They appear qualitatively, at least in the few studies in which they have been addressed, to be more similar to organic than to schizophrenic psychoses. Gender differences in the experience of hallucinatory phenomena are unclear, although there is some evidence that women are more likely to report having had hallucinations.

Activity and Behavior

The results of studies of activity and behavior during manic states, summarized in Table 2–9, show that disturbed sleep and speech, as well as hyperactivity, are common in mania. About 80 percent of manic patients have either insomnia or a decreased need for sleep. Virtually all, 80–90 percent, exhibit hyperverbosity and rapid or pressured speech. An overwhelming majority are hyperactive, more than half are hypersexual, and one in four exhibits catatonia. There are few studies of gender differences in manic activity and behavior, although a recent New Zealand investigation of 90 bipolar males and 121 bipolar females found that men were significantly more likely to report the presence of "problem behaviors" (the nature of which was not specified) and "excitement or inability to hold a conversation" (Kawa et al., 2005, p. 122). Gender differences in manic sexual behavior are discussed in Chapter 10.

Factorial Studies of Mania

Although a great deal of research has been done on the factorial structure of nonbipolar depressive disorders, the literature on the structure of bipolar depressive states is relatively sparse (reviewed in Azorin, 2000). Until recently, this was also the case for mania. Initially, Beigel and colleagues (1971) concluded, on the basis of a relatively small National Institute of Mental Health (NIMH) sample, that pure manic and dysphoric subtypes could be delineated. Subsequently, new data derived from large clinical samples have confirmed this conclusion, but also painted a much more complex clinical portrait of mania.[13] The French EPIMAN study (Akiskal et al., 2003a) is multicentered, with patient information being collected by means of a standardized protocol in at least four regions of France. The main findings of this study are generally consistent with those of earlier research in indicating that further phenomenological understanding of mania requires a multidimensional perspective. The authors of this study went beyond the euphoric–dysphoric dichotomy and proposed the existence of independent euphoric, depressive, hostile, psychotic, and deficit factors, each of which was correlated with a core activation (disinhibition–instability) factor of mania.

Like Bauer and colleagues (1994), Akiskal and colleagues (2001) concluded that, rather than euphoria/irritability, the central definitional focus of mania should be psychomotor activation. This conclusion is consistent with the emphasis of Heinroth (1818) and Koukopoulos (2005), which posits that excitement is the fundamental state of the bipolar subgroup of manic-depressive illness. By incorporating new features of mania derived from the EPIMAN study (e.g., pathological gregariousness and overfamiliarity) and using clinical expertise, different groups of investigators have developed a factorial structure of mania that incorporates psychomotor activation as the major criterion, along with mood disturbance, other signs and symptoms, and a lack of insight and judgment; this work, in conjunction with that of other investigators, has led to proposed changes in the DSM-IV criteria for mania. Ghaemi and colleagues (1995) also underscored the cognitive dysfunction in the areas of insight and judgment in mania; similar findings were reported by Dell'Osso and colleagues (2000). Interestingly, insight appears to be less impaired during mixed mania (Cassidy et al., 2001a; see Chapters 21 and 22).

Table 2–10 summarizes the findings of factorial studies of the structure of mania. It is clear that current diagnostic systems fail to reflect the actual complexity of the state. Nor do most diagnostic formulations adequately capture the essential relationship, indeed the often total overlap, between major subtypes of mania and mixed states. Virtually all investigations of the structure of mania have noted common underlying dimensions: a mood component, characterized by either predominantly euphoric or dysphoric qualities; psychomotor activation; psychotic features; and irritability and/or aggression.

There are fewer data on the structure of hypomania, but as with mania, cardinal manifestations are irritability, coupled with heightened activation and behavioral excess. Serretti and Olgiati (2005) compared patterns of manic symptoms in 158 bipolar-I and 122 bipolar-II patients (see Table 2–11). The bipolar-I patients had a higher prevalence of reckless activity, distractibility, psychomotor agitation, irritable mood, and increased self-esteem. Juruena and colleagues (2006) compared 27 bipolar-I patients with

TABLE 2–9. Activity and Behavior Symptoms during Mania

Study	Patients (N)	Hyper-activity (%)	Decreased Sleep[a] (%)	Violent/ Assaultive Behavior (%)	Rapid/ Pressured Speech (%)	Hyper-verbosity (%)	Nudity/ Sexual Exposure (%)	Hyper-sexuality (%)	Extrav-agance (%)	Religiosity (%)	Head Decoration (%)	Regression (Pronounced) (%)	Catatonia (%)	Fecal Inconti-nence/ Smearing (%)
Lange, 1922	700											27		
Allison and Wilson, 1960	24							70						
Clayton et al., 1965	31		94		100			74						
Winokur et al., 1969	100[b]	76	90		99			65	69					
Carlson and Goodwin, 1973	20	100		75	100	100		80		50		45		
Taylor and Abrams, 1973	52	100		48	100		23				33		14	19
Abrams and Taylor, 1976	78	100		46	100		33				38			14
Leff et al., 1976	63	81	63			86		27	32					
Loudon et al., 1977	16	56	69		75			25		25				
Taylor and Abrams, 1977[c]	123			46			29				32		28	10
Carlson and Strober, 1979	9	100	78			89		78				56		

(continued)

TABLE 2–9. Activity and Behavior Symptoms during Mania (continued)

Study	Patients (N)	Hyper-activity (%)	Decreased Sleep[a] (%)	Violent/ Assaultive Behavior (%)	Rapid/ Pressured Speech (%)	Hyper-verbosity (%)	Nudity/ Sexual Exposure (%)	Hyper-sexuality (%)	Extrav-agance (%)	Religiosity (%)	Head Decoration (%)	Regression (Pronounced) (%)	Catatonia (%)	Fecal Inconti-nence/ Smearing (%)
Abrams and Taylor, 1981	111												19	
Bräunig et al., 1998	61												31	
Cassidy et al., 1998	316[d]	85	79	46	80									
Krüger et al., 2003	99												27[c]	
Serretti and Olgiati, 2005	158	98	99		93									
Total n[f]	1857													
Weighted mean[f]		90	83	47	88	89	29	51	32	39	34	28	24	13

[a]Includes decreased need for sleep and insomnia.
[b]100 episodes, 61 patients.
[c]Calculations based on a sample of 119 patients (except for catatonia rating).
[d]Based on high-threshold scores.
[e]Of mixed manic patients, 62% displayed catatonia; of pure manic patients, only 5%.
[f]Winokur et al. not included in calculation because units are in episodes, not in patients.

TABLE 2–10. Findings of Factorial Studies of the Structure of Mania

Study	Sample Size	Assessment Tool	Primary Factors	Core Dimensions/ Clusters
Murphy and Beigel, 1974	30	MSRS		I. Euphoria–grandiosity II. Paranoia–destructiveness
Double, 1991	81	RDC MRS CPRS	10 nondelineated factors	I. (Mild) excitation II. Elation–pressured speech–flight of ideas III. Psychosis–severity IV. Psychomotor activation–aggressive overactivity
Cassidy et al., 1998	237	DSM-III-R MSRS Clinical assessment	1. Dysphoric mood 2. Psychomotor pressure 3. Psychosis 4. Euphoric mood 5. Irritability, aggression	
Dilsaver et al., 1999	105	RDC DSM-III-R	1. Manic activation 2. Depressed state 3. Sleep disturbance 4. Irritability/paranoia	I. Mania with depressed mood II. Mania without depressed mood
Cassidy et al., 2001a	327	DSM-III-R SMS	1. Hypomania; low psychosis; mild, classic mania 2. Severe, classic "pure" mania; devoid of dysphoric features 3. Grandiosity and psychosis, but without marked psychomotor pressure, sleep disturbance, hypersexuality, humor, and irritable paranoia 4. Dysphoria; complete absence of euphoric mood or humor; little grandiosity or hypersexuality 5. Dysphoria, but less than factor 4. Higher levels of grandiosity, humor, psychomotor activation, hypersexuality	Hypomania Acute mania Delusional mania Depressive or anxious mania Mixed state

(continued)

TABLE 2–10. **Findings of Factorial Studies of the Structure of Mania** (continued)

Study	Sample Size	Assessment Tool	Primary Factors	Core Dimensions/ Clusters
Swann et al., 2001	162	DSM-III-R SADS ADRS	1. Impulsivity 2. Hyperactivity 3. Anxious pessimism 4. Distressed appearance 5. Hostility 6. Psychosis	I. Depressive II. Delusional III. Classic IV. Irritable
Sato et al., 2002	576	DSM-IV GAF AMDPS	1. Depressive mood 2. Irritable aggression 3. Insomnia 4. Depressive inhibition 5. Pure mania 6. Emotional liability/agitation 7. Psychosis	I. Pure mania II. Aggressive mania III. Psychotic mania IV. Depressive (mixed) mania
Akiskal et al., 2003a	104	DSM-IV MSRS GAF HDRS	1. Disinhibition 2. Hostility 3. Deficit 4. Psychosis 5. Elation 6. Depression 7. Sexuality	
González-Pinto et al., 2003	103	DSM-IV MRS HDRS	1. Depression 2. Dysphoria 3. Hedonism 4. Psychosis 5. Activation	I. Hedonism II. Dysphoria III. Activation

ADRS = Affective Disorders Rating Scale; AMDPS = Association for Methodology in Psychiatry System; CPRS = Comprehensive Psychopathology Rating Scale; DSM-III-R = *Diagnostic and Statistical Manual*, 3rd edition, revised; DSM-IV = *Diagnostic and Statistical Manual*, 4th edition; GAF = Global Assessment of Functioning; HDRS = Hamilton Depression Rating Scale; MRS = Mania Rating Scale (Young); MSRS = Manic State Rating Scale; MVAS-BP = Multiple Visual Analogue Scales of Bipolarity; RDC = Research Diagnostic Criteria; SADS = Schedule for Affective Disorders; SMS = Scale for Manic States.

25 bipolar-II patients. Those with bipolar-I reported a higher frequency of racing thoughts, grandiosity, impaired judgment, and decreased total sleep time. Patients with bipolar-II disorder experienced 3.5 times more depressive episodes and four times the rate of lifetime substance abuse disorders. Benazzi (2005) emphasized that there are no clear boundaries between mania and hypomania and that overactive behavior during hypomania is at least as important as hypomanic mood. To date, fewer factors have been derived for hypomania: energy–activity; irritability–racing thoughts, which, as noted earlier, is putatively a

dysphoric expression of hypomania (Benazzi and Akiskal, 2003); and, more recently, an "elevated mood" factor that includes elevated mood and increased self-esteem (Benazzi, 2006). Hantouche and colleagues (2003) also found a dual structure of hypomania, although the factors were slightly different: one factor was defined by positive (driven–euphoric) features, and the other by greater irritability and risk taking.

The factorial structure of mania and hypomania is a relatively new area of clinical investigation, and future studies are needed to follow up on this preliminary work.

TABLE 2–11. **Occurrence of Manic Symptoms in Bipolar-I and -II**

Symptom	BP-I (n = 158) (%)	BP-II (n = 122) (%)	Probability	Risk Ratio	95% Confidence Interval
Excessive activity	98.1	96.7	0.47	1.32	0.56–3.13
Reckless activity	72.1	41.8	<0.01	1.81	1.40–2.33
Distractibility	96.8	79.5	<0.01	3.67	1.64–8.22
Reduced need for sleep	98.7	96.7	0.41	1.71	0.55–5.32
Agitated activity	87.9	52.4	<0.01	3.13	2.08–4.71
Pressured speech	93.0	86.0	0.07	1.48	0.93–2.38
Racing thoughts	94.9	89.3	0.11	1.52	0.87–2.67
Elevated mood	90.5	94.2	0.27	0.82	0.60–1.10
Irritable mood	91.1	68.8	<0.01	2.34	1.48–3.71
Increased self-esteem	86.7	63.9	<0.01	1.97	1.37–2.84

Source: Adapted from Serretti and Olgiati, 2005.

In particular, little is known about the longitudinal stability of these factors, although the findings of one short-term follow-up study suggest such a possibility for the manic and mixed subtypes (Cassidy et al., 2002).

DEPRESSIVE STATES

Classic Clinical Descriptions

The bipolar depressive states, in sharp contrast to the manias, are usually characterized by a slowing or decrease in almost all aspects of emotion and behavior: rate of thought and speech, energy, sexuality, and the ability to experience pleasure. As with the manic states, severity varies widely. Symptoms can range from mild physical and mental slowing, with very little distortion in cognition and perception, to profound depressive stupors, delusions, hallucinations, and clouding of consciousness. Of the three major symptomatic groups we have been examining—mood, cognition and perception, and activity and behavior—mood is perhaps the least variable across the continuum of depressive states, although, as we shall see, irritability and anger often accompany the more usual melancholic picture. Cognition and perception, on the other hand, change profoundly, as do activity and behavior. We begin with extensive classic descriptions of depressive mood, then discuss changes in cognition and perception and activity and behavior in various depressive states (i.e., nonpsychotic, psychotic, and stuporous depressions). Cognition and perception are treated most extensively in the discussion of psychotic depression, whereas activity and behavior figure more prominently in the discussion of stuperous depression. First, however, we present an ancient description of melancholia from Aretaeus (*Extant Works*, pp. 299–300):

The patients are dull or stern, dejected or unreasonably torpid, without any manifest cause: such is the commencement of melancholy. And they also become peevish, dispirited, sleepless, and start up from a disturbed sleep.

Unreasonable fear also seizes them, if the disease tend to increase, when their dreams are true, terrifying, and clear: for whatever, when awake, they have an aversion to, as being an evil, rushes upon their visions in sleep. They are prone to change their mind readily; to become base, mean-spirited, illiberal, and in a little time, perhaps, simple, extravagant, munificent, not from any virtue of the soul, but from the changeableness of the disease. But if the illness become more urgent, hatred, avoidance of the haunts of men, vain lamentations; they complain of life, and desire to die. In many, the understanding so leads to insensibility and fatuousness, that they become ignorant of all things, or forgetful of themselves, and live the life of the inferior animals. . . . They are voracious, indeed, yet emaciated; for in them sleep does not brace their limbs either by what they have eaten or drunk, but watchfulness diffuses and determines them outwardly.

Mood

Mood in all of the depressive states is bleak, pessimistic, and despairing. A deep sense of futility is often accompanied, if not preceded, by the belief that the ability to experience pleasure is permanently gone. The physical and mental worlds are experienced as monochromatic, as shades of gray and black. Heightened irritability, anger, paranoia, emotional turbulence, and anxiety are common. The frightening lack of color and the inability to experience meaningful emotional responses were described by Campbell (1953, p. 106):

> General impairment in emotional feeling is another symptom often described by the manic-depressive patient in a depressive episode. In addition to distortions in sensing impressions, such as a queer, odd or unreal feeling, the patient may complain of a universal dulling of the emotional tone. This symptom, like the feeling of unreality, frightens the patient because it tends to alienate him from his environment. Indeed, it is an important constituent of the patient's fear of insanity. It is bad enough not to speak the same language as other people—it is worse not to feel the same emotions.

Mayer-Gross and colleagues (1960, p. 209) emphasized the negative cognitive and affective tone of depressed patients:

> There is a diminished capacity for normal affective response to sad as well as happy events, a phenomenon which is merely one aspect of a *generalized insufficiency of all mental activities*. . . . Whatever is experienced seems to be painful. Even enjoyable experiences have this effect, partly by making the patient more acutely aware of his incapacity for normal appreciation, partly because he is at once sensible of any unfortunate aspect they may have; he may in fact show considerable ingenuity in seeing the bad side of everything. Past, present, and future are alike seen through the same dark and gloomy veil; the whole of life seems miserable and agonizing. The depth of the affect cannot easily be measured from its *outward expression*. The silent shedding of tears may be seen in an otherwise expressionless face; another patient will mock at himself and at his complaints with a grim and sardonic but surprising humour or call himself a fraud or a fool: in another a sudden smile or expression of gaiety will deceive the physician about the severity of the underlying emotion.

Cognition and Perception

Most mental activity is markedly slowed during depression. By definition, patients with nonpsychotic depression do not manifest clouding of consciousness, nor do they experience delusions or hallucinations. Suicidal thinking, however, is often of dangerous proportions, and morbidly ruminative and hypochondriacal thinking is common. The profoundly slowed but nonpsychotic nature of this type of depressive thought and its indecisive and ruminative quality are portrayed in the following passage from Kraepelin (1921, p. 75)[14]:

> Thinking is difficult to the patient, a disorder, which he describes in the most varied phrases. He cannot collect his thoughts or pull himself together; his thoughts are as if paralyzed, they are immobile. . . . He is no longer able to perceive, or to follow the train of thought of a book or a conversation, he feels weary, enervated, inattentive, inwardly empty; he has no memory, he has no longer command of knowledge formerly familiar to him, he must consider a long time about simple things, he calculates wrongly, makes contradictory statements, does not find words, cannot construct sentences correctly.

Jaspers (1997, p. 597; first published in 1913) described the profound impairment of will, pervasive gloom, and dearth of ideas in depression. The central core of pure depression, he wrote, is formed from

> an equally unmotivated and profound sadness to which is added a retardation of psychic events, which is as subjectively painful as it is objectively visible. All instinctual activities are subjected to it. The patient does not want to do anything. The reduced impulse to move and do things turns into complete immobility. No decision can be made and no activity begun. Associations are not available. Patients have no ideas. They complain of a complete disruption of memory. They feel their poverty of performance and complain of their inefficiency, lack of emotion and emptiness. They feel profound gloom as a sensation in the chest or body as if it could be laid hold of there. The depth of their melancholy makes them see the world as grim and grey. They look for the unfavourable and unhappy elements in everything. They accuse themselves of much past guilt (self-accusations, notions of having sinned). The present has nothing for them (notions of worthlessness) and the future lies horrifyingly before them (notions of poverty, etc.).

Activity and Behavior

Like thought and verbal expression, activity and behavior are slowed in bipolar depression. Fatigue, lack of activity, withdrawal from the company of others, impairment in the volition of will, and profoundly altered sleep and eating patterns are hallmarks of this type of depression (see Chapter 16 for detailed discussion of altered sleep and activity patterns). Campbell (1953, p. 85) described the fatigued, psychomotorically retarded appearance of depressed patients:

> Depressed mood is often suggested by the bearing, gait or general appearance of the patient. The depressed individual usually walks slowly and reacts sluggishly. He appears to push himself along, as if he were being held back, rather than propelling himself with normal agility. There are no unnecessary movements with the hands or feet, the patient sitting in a languorous but not restful posture. The shoulders sag, the head is lowered and the entire body seems to droop; loosely hanging clothes sometimes suggest the weight loss often present in the melancholic individual. Everyone is acquainted with the tendency of the angles of the mouth to turn down in the saddened person; a smile, when it occurs, must be forced, and even then there is something sickly or distorted in its expression. The facial musculature of the depressed individual lacks tone, giving the face an inert, myasthenic appearance. The upper eyelids also manifest this careworn expression. . . .
>
> The eyes, which normally portray the spark, vitality and curiosity of the personality, are dull and lustreless. In some individuals the eyes have a faraway, unnatural stare, which even the layman recognizes as a mark of extreme pre-occupation or mental illness.

Disturbances in both the quality and quantity of sleep during depression can be profound but variable. Jaspers (1997, p. 234) noted that depressive sleep is

> sometimes abnormally deep, so that patients sometimes feel as if they had been dead. It may however be abnormally light and the patients never feel refreshed, but have vivid, restless and anxious dreams, and feel as if only half of their being had been asleep, the other half had stayed awake and watched. *Duration of Sleep* may be very lengthy . . . in some depressed states. The patients are always wanting to sleep and sometimes sleep twelve hours uninterruptedly. On the other hand we find sleep abnormally curtailed. The patients go to sleep but are awake again soon after and then lie awake all night long. Or they only manage to get off to sleep towards morning.

Suicide is an all-too-frequent outcome of bipolar depression (see Chapter 8). In the words of Kraepelin (1921, pp. 25, 87–88):

> The torment of the states of depression, which is nearly unbearable, according to the perpetually recurring state-

ments by the patients, engenders almost in all, at least from time to time, weariness of life, only too frequently also a great desire to put an end to life at any price. . . .
>
> The extraordinarily strong tendency to suicide is of the greatest practical significance. Sometimes it continually accompanies the whole course of the disease, without coming to a serious attempt owing to the incapacity of the patients to arrive at a decision. . . . Sometimes the impulse to suicide emerges very suddenly without the patients being able to explain the motives to themselves. . . .
>
> Occasionally after indefinite prodromata the first distinct morbid symptom is a suicidal attempt. Only too often the patients know how to conceal their suicidal intentions behind an apparently cheerful behaviour, and then carefully prepare for the execution of their intention at a suitable moment.

Psychotic depression (Kraepelin's *melancholia gravis*) is characterized by the same signs and symptoms as those present in nonpsychotic depression, usually in worsened form, with the addition of delusions and/or hallucinations. The following is Bleuler's (1924, pp. 475–476) description of the nature and extent of depressive delusions, hallucinations, and paranoia, as well as their primary content areas of expression (somatic, religious, and financial):

> In the severer cases delusions are invariably present and may stand in the foreground. At the same time the hallucinations usually but not always increase. . . . The devil appears at the window, makes faces at the patients. They hear themselves condemned, they hear the scaffold erected on which they are to be executed, and their relatives crying who must suffer on their account, or starve or otherwise perish miserably.
>
> But the *delusions* especially are never absent in a pronounced case and always as delusions of economic, bodily, and spiritual ruin. The patients think that they became poor, and it does no good to show them their valuables or their balance in the bank; that has no significance for them. Debts are there anyway, or demands are to be expected that will wipe out everything.

A more severe form of psychotic depression, although still less severe than delirious depression, was termed by Kraepelin *fantastic melancholia* (equivalent to Griesinger's *melancholia with delusions,* or what other clinicians have called *depressive insanity*). Delusions and hallucinations are more pronounced, some clouding of consciousness usually occurs, and violent excitement can alternate with mild stuporous states. As described by Kraepelin (1921, pp. 89–95):

> [a] further, fairly comprehensive group of cases is distinguished by a still greater development of *delusions*. We

may perhaps call it "fantastic melancholia." Abundant *hallucinations* appear. . . . [T]here are also multifarious delusional interpretations of real perceptions. The patient hears murderers come; some one is slinking about the bed; a man is lying under the bed with a loaded gun; an electro-magnet crackles. . . . The trees in the forest, the rocks, appear unnatural, as if they were artificial, as if they had been built up specially for the patient, in fact, even the sun, the moon, the weather, are not as they used to be. . . .

Hypochondriacal delusions usually reach a considerable development; they often completely resemble those of the paralytic. . . .

Consciousness is in this form frequently somewhat clouded. The patients perceive badly, do not understand what goes on, are not able to form clear ideas. They complain that they cannot lay hold of any proper thought, that they are beastly "stupid," confused in their head, do not find their way, also perhaps that they have so many thoughts in their head, that everything goes pell-mell. . . .

The Volitional Disorders are also not quite uniform. The activity of the patients is frequently dominated by volitional inhibition; they are taciturn, even mute, cataleptic; they lie with vacant or strained expression of countenance in bed. . . .

At times more violent states of excitement may be interpolated. The patients scream, throw themselves on the floor, force their way senselessly out, beat their heads, hide away under the bed, make desperate attacks on the surroundings. . . . Serious attempts at suicide are in these states extremely frequent.

Delirious melancholia represents the most severe stage of cognitive and perceptual distortion and disorientation. Delusional thought becomes progressively unclear and fragmented, and hallucinations are particularly vivid, bizarre, and frightening. It is a depressive state characterized predominantly by clouding of consciousness. Kraepelin (1921, pp. 95–97) wrote more than anyone since about the mental and physical aspects of this stage of depression:

Gradual transitions lead to a last, delirious group of states of depression, which is characterized by *profound visionary clouding of conscience*. Here also numerous, terrifying hallucinations, changing variously, and confused delusions are developed. . . .

During these changing visionary experiences the patients are outwardly for the most part strongly inhibited; they are scarcely capable of saying a word. They feel confused and perplexed; they cannot collect their thoughts, know absolutely nothing any longer, give contradictory, incomprehensible, unconnected answers, weave in words which they have heard into their detached,

slow utterances which they produce as though astonished. . . . For the most part the patients lie in bed taking no interest in anything.

Depressive stupor, the most severe form of psychomotor retardation, often constitutes an acute medical emergency. Although it is rarely seen today, it is an important clinical presentation and one that provides insight into the severity of the illness prior to the modern treatment era. The state was described by Henderson and Gillespie (1956, p. 258):

This condition may be defined as a state of intense psychic inhibition during which regression may occur to an infantile, if not more primitive level. The patient, usually, is confined to bed, is mute, inactive and unco-operative. His bodily needs require attention in every way; he has to be fed, washed and bathed. Precautions have to be taken to prevent the retention of faeces, urine and saliva. In some cases all attempts at movement are strongly resisted. In other cases the muscles are more flaccid, and the body and limbs can be moulded into any position. On the surface it may seem as if there was a total absence of feeling or emotion, but that is often more apparent than real, for, after recovery, many patients give a vivid account of the distress which they have experienced. The idea of death is believed by some to be almost universal in stupor reactions, and may be regarded as a form of expiation for the wickedness for which they hold themselves responsible. Some patients may have a clear appreciation of their position and surroundings throughout the whole period of the stupor, but in the majority a considerable dulling of consciousness occurs.

During all these stages of depression the *physical health* suffers greatly. The patient becomes weak, loses weight, has a poor appetite, a coated tongue, and constipation. The circulation is enfeebled, and there is cyanosis, especially of the extremities.

Subjective Experiences of Patients

Mood

Mood in bipolar depression tends to be dominated by a dull, flat, and colorless sense of experience; by despair, hopelessness, and pessimism, often fueled by marked physical and mental lethargy; and by a sharp decrease in the pleasure obtained from ordinarily gratifying events, interests, and people.

Depression is paralyzing and suffocating to those in its grasp. Five years before she killed herself, Sylvia Plath (1982, p. 240) wrote of this in her journal: "I have been and am battling depression. I am now flooded with despair, almost hysteria, as if I were smothering. As if a great muscular owl were sitting on my chest, its talons clenching and constricting my heart." British writer Alan Garner (1997, pp. 208–209) portrayed the deadening and the horror of the beginning of his manic-depressive breakdown:

> The next thing I remember is that I was standing in the kitchen, the sunlit kitchen, looking over a green valley with brook and trees; and the light was going out. I could see, but as if through a dark filter. And my solar plexus was numb.
>
> Some contraption, a piece of mechanical junk left by one of the children, told me to pick it up. It was cylindrical and spiky, and had a small crank handle. I turned the handle. It was the guts of a cheap musical box, and it tinkled its few notes over and over and over again, and I could not stop. With each turn, the light dimmed and the feelings in my solar plexus spread through my body. When it reached my head, I began to cry with terror at the blankness of me, and the blankness of the world.
>
> A scene from Eisenstein's "Alexander Nevsky" swamped my brain: the dreadful passage in which Nevsky dupes the Teutonic Knights onto the frozen lake, and the ice breaks, and their faceless armour takes them under. The cloaks float on the water before being pulled down, and the hands clutch at the ice floes, which flip over and seal in the knights.
>
> All that helplessness, cold and horror comprised me. I was alone in the house, and throughout the afternoon I turned the tinkle tinkle tinkle of the broken toy, which became the sound of the ice. My body was as heavy as the armour and the waterlogged cloaks as I slid beneath the ice.
>
> When the family came home, I was lying on the kitchen settle, in a foetal position, without moving or speaking, until I went to bed at midnight. Sleep was unconsciousness without rest. . . .
>
> I was incapable of emotion except that of being incapable of emotion. I had no worth. I poisoned the planet.

Composer Hugo Wolf's account of his depression (quoted in Walker, 1968, p. 322) focused, as have many descriptions written by depressed or formerly depressed individuals, on the painful contrast between the subjective experience of an arid, sterile reality and a perception of the external world as an unobtainable, visible but not habitable world of light, warmth, and creation:

> What I suffer from this continuous idleness I am quite unable to describe. I would like most to hang myself on the nearest branch of the cherry trees standing now in full bloom. This wonderful spring with its secret life and movement troubles me unspeakably. These eternal blue skies, lasting for weeks, this continuous sprouting and budding in nature, these coaxing breezes impregnated

with spring sunlight and fragrance of flowers . . . make me frantic. Everywhere this bewildering urge for life, fruitfulness, creation—and only I, although like the humblest grass of the fields one of God's creatures, may not take part in this festival of resurrection, at any rate not except as a spectator with grief and envy.

The sense of lost energy is of singular importance in understanding the subjective experience of depression. The ebb and flow of life's force or vitality and its painful absence in depression were described by F. Scott Fitzgerald in *The Crack-Up* (1956, p. 74; first published in 1936), a harrowing account of his nervous breakdowns:

> [O]f all natural forces, vitality is the incommunicable one. In days when juice came into one as an article without duty, one tried to distribute it—but always without success; to further mix metaphors, vitality never "takes." You have it or you haven't it, like health or brown eyes or honor or a baritone voice. "*Ye are the salt of the earth. But if the salt hath lost its savour, wherewith shall it be salted?*"—Matthew 5:13[15]

Cognition and Perception

Cognitive changes during depression can be subtle or profound and often are a combination of both. Depressed patients frequently complain that their process of thinking has slowed down. They are confused and ruminative, cannot concentrate, and feel inadequate and useless. John Custance (1952, p. 62) wrote:

> I seem to be in perpetual fog and darkness. I cannot get my mind to work; instead of associations "clicking into place" everything is inextricable jumble; instead of seeming to grasp a whole, it seems to remain tied to the actual consciousness of the moment. The whole world of my thought is hopelessly divided into incomprehensible watertight compartments. I could not feel more ignorant, undecided, or inefficient. It is appallingly difficult to concentrate, and writing is pain and grief to me.

Irrational fears, which can range from fear and panic to obsession and delusion, are common in depression. Fitzgerald (1956, p. 75) summed up the experience as "the dark night of the soul":

> Now the standard cure for one who is sunk is to consider those in actual destitution or physical suffering—this is an all-weather beatitude for gloom in general and fairly salutary day-time advice for everyone. But at three o'clock in the morning, a forgotten package has the same tragic importance as a death sentence, and the cure doesn't work—and in a real dark night of the soul it is always three o'clock in the morning, day after day.

Robert Schumann (quoted in Niecks, 1925, p. 142) was even more explicit about his terror:

> I was little more than a statue, neither cold nor warm; by dint of forced work life returned gradually. But I am still so timid and fearful that I cannot sleep alone. . . . Do you believe that I have not courage to travel alone to Zwickan for fear that something might befall me? Violent rushes of blood, unspeakable fear, breathlessness, momentary unconsciousness, alternate quickly.

Preoccupation with sin and perceived religious transgressions are not uncommon in severe depression, and many deeply depressed patients would empathize with Cowper's "strong sense of God's wrath, and a deep despair of escaping it." William James wrote definitively of this preoccupation, as well as of religious ecstasies, in *The Varieties of Religious Experience* (1902).

Finally, as noted above, thoughts of suicide often accompany the despair, apathy, guilt, and feelings of inadequacy associated with depression. Extensive discussion of suicidal thoughts and behaviors is given in Chapter 8; here we present one woman's description of the depression leading up to a nearly lethal suicide attempt (Jamison, 1995; pp. 110–111, 113):

> A floridly psychotic mania was followed, inevitably, by a long and lacerating, black, suicidal depression; it lasted more than a year and a half. From the time I woke up in the morning until the time I went to bed at night, I was unbearably miserable and seemingly incapable of any kind of joy or enthusiasm. Everything—every thought, word, movement—was an effort. Everything that once was sparkling now was flat. I seemed to myself to be dull, boring, inadequate, thick brained, unlit, unresponsive, chill skinned, bloodless, and sparrow drab. I doubted, completely, my ability to do anything well. It seemed as though my mind had slowed down and burned out to the point of being virtually useless. The wretched, convoluted, and pathetically confused mass of gray worked only well enough to torment me with a dreary litany of my inadequacies and shortcomings in character, and to taunt me with the total, the desperate, hopelessness of it all. What is the point in going on like this? I would ask myself. Others would say to me, "It is only temporary, it will pass, you will get over it," but of course they had no idea how I felt, although they were certain that they did. Over and over and over I would say to myself, If I can't feel, if I can't move, if I can't think, and I can't care, then what conceivable point is there in living?
>
> The morbidity of my mind was astonishing: Death and its kin were constant companions. I saw death everywhere, and I saw winding sheets and toe tags and body bags in my mind's eye. Everything was a reminder that everything ended at the charnel house. My memory always took the black line of the mind's underground system; thoughts would go from one tormented moment of my past to the next. Each stop along the way was worse than the preceding one. . . .
>
> At the time, nothing seemed to be working, despite excellent medical care, and I simply wanted to die and be done with it. I resolved to kill myself. I was cold-bloodedly determined not to give any indication of my plans or the state of my mind; I was successful.

Activity and Behavior

Although social isolation, psychomotor retardation or agitation, and other behavioral changes accompany depression, changes in sleep patterns are among the most pervasive, quantifiable, and pathognomonic symptoms. They are also highly distressing for patients. (Research on sleep disturbances is discussed in detail in Chapter 16.) Sylvia Plath—probably bipolar, certainly hospitalized and treated for severe depression—described her experience thus in her autobiographical novel *The Bell Jar* (1971, pp. 142–143):

> I hadn't washed my hair for three weeks. . . .
>
> I hadn't slept for seven nights.
>
> My mother told me I must have slept, it was impossible not to sleep in all that time, but if I slept, it was with my eyes wide open, for I had followed the green, luminous course of the second hand and the minute hand and the hour hand of the bedside clock through their circles and semicircles, every night for seven nights, without missing a second, or a minute, or an hour.
>
> The reason I hadn't washed my clothes or my hair was because it seemed so silly.
>
> I saw the days of the year stretching ahead like a series of bright, white boxes, and separating one box from another was sleep, like a black shade. Only for me, the long perspective of shades that set off one box from the next had suddenly snapped up, and I could see day after day after day glaring ahead of me like a white, broad, infinitely desolate avenue.
>
> It seemed silly to wash one day when I would only have to wash again the next.
>
> It made me tired just to think of it.
>
> I wanted to do everything once and for all and be through with it.

Likewise for Scott Fitzgerald (1956, pp. 72–73; first published in 1936), sleep and hating to face the night became sources of terror:

> [E]very act of life from the morning toothbrush to the friend at dinner had become an effort . . . hating the night

when I couldn't sleep and hating the day because it went towards night. I slept on the heart side now because I knew that the sooner I could tire that out, even a little, the sooner would come that blessed hour of nightmare which, like a catharsis, would enable me to better meet the new day.

Clinical Studies

There has been much less quantitative study of the clinical features of bipolar depression than is the case for either mania or nonbipolar depression. In fact, the substantial literature on depression seldom differentiates bipolar from unipolar depression,[16] and until recently, bipolar depression was usually excluded from study and discussion. Further complicating matters, bipolar depression has frequently been misdiagnosed as unipolar depression, or not discussed in the context of its often mixed forms. For our data-based clinical description of bipolar depression, we have relied primarily upon the early monograph of Winokur and colleagues (1969), Benazzi's series of outpatient studies,[17] and the work of several other researchers (Perugi et al., 1998a; Koukopoulos and Koukopoulos, 1999; Mitchell et al., 2001). Specific comparisons of bipolar and unipolar depression are presented in Chapter 1.[18] In this section we present the findings of data-based studies with regard to symptom presentation in bipolar depression, psychotic features, depressive mixed states, and bipolar–unipolar differences in depressive symptomatology.

Mood

Winokur and colleagues (1969) studied the symptomatology and clinical course of 21 treated bipolar depressed patients (5 men and 16 women, with a combined total of 33 separate depressive episodes). They described the onset of depression as abrupt in 5 episodes (15 percent) and gradual in 28 (85 percent). Mood was observed to be melancholic or tearful in virtually all patients (100 and 94 percent, respectfully), with approximately half (52 percent) displaying hopelessness. Fully three-fourths of bipolar depressed patients were described as irritable, almost as high a percentage (85) as was found by the same authors in manic patients (see Table 2–1). Irritability, which is pervasive during bipolar depression (Deckersbach et al., 2004; Benazzi and Akiskal, 2005), is considered more extensively later in this section, as well as in the subsequent discussion of mixed depressive states.

Cognition and Perception

Winokur and colleagues (1969) found widespread cognitive and perceptual changes during bipolar depression. Self-deprecatory and self-accusatory thoughts were present in almost all patients (97 and 91 percent, respectively).

With few exceptions, patients also reported substantially impaired cognitive ability: 91 percent reported poor concentration, diminished clarity of thought, and/or diminished speed of thought. Half complained of poor memory. Suicidal thoughts were common (82 percent), a figure in close agreement with the rate (83 percent) found in a later study of bipolar depressed adolescents (Carlson and Strober, 1979).

Frequencies of thought disorder in manic, depressed, and normal subjects (as measured by the Scale for the Assessment of Thought, Language and Communication) were analyzed in three early studies (Ianzito et al., 1974; Andreasen 1979a, 1984). Manic patients were more likely than depressive patients to exhibit pressured speech, distractibility, derailment, illogicality, loss of goal, perseveration, and a higher overall global rating of thought disorder. Depressed patients, by contrast, were more likely than manic patients to demonstrate poverty of speech. There were no differences between manic and depressed patients in ratings of poverty of content of speech, tangentiality, clanging, neologisms, word approximations, circumstantiality, echolalia, blocking, or stilted speech. When compared with normal subjects, depressed patients displayed greater poverty of content of speech, as well as increased tangentiality, circumstantiality, and self-reference. Normal subjects were more likely than depressed patients to exhibit derailment. Andreasen (1979a,b, 1984) found less evidence of thought disorder in her depressed patients than in schizophrenic patients, perhaps reflecting either true differences or differences in illness severity, assessment techniques, and diagnostic criteria (bipolar–unipolar differences were not specified).

Delusions and hallucinations often occur in severe bipolar depression, but they are less frequent than psychotic symptomatology in mania. Depressive delusions tend to focus on fixed ideas of guilt and sinfulness, poverty, hypochondriacal and somatic concerns, and feelings of persecution.[19] As shown in Table 2–8 (presented earlier), delusions were present in 12 to 66 percent of bipolar depressive episodes versus 44 to 96 percent of manic episodes. Hallucinations, less common in both mania and depression, were relatively more frequent in manic episodes. Several investigators have found a constancy in the presence or absence of psychotic symptoms across major depressive episodes,[20] although generalizability from unipolar to bipolar depression has not been demonstrated. Charney and Nelson (1981) found that 95 percent of their delusional patients but only 8 percent of their nondelusional patients had experienced prior delusional episodes. Among patients whose index admission was psychotic, 89 percent of all previous episodes had been psychotic as well. Helms and Smith (1983) reported that 92 percent of their psychotic depressive patients with recurrent illness had experienced another admission for psychotic depression, while Lykouras and colleagues (1985) found that 92 percent of their delusional depressive patients had experienced previous episodes with delusional ideation, compared with 36 percent of their nonpsychotic depressive patients. Nelson and colleagues (1984, p. 298) observed:

> It would appear that the presence of delusions during an index episode of depression may be not merely an indicator of severity of that episode, but additionally a distinct stable trait which would be expressed in the biologically vulnerable individual during prior and subsequent episodes.

Aronson and colleagues (1988), studying bipolar as well as unipolar delusional depressive patients, also found a consistency of psychotic expression across episodes, as well as an association with a marked rate of relapse. They noted that psychoticism may be an independent variable that can present in either bipolar or nonbipolar depression. The question of whether psychoticism is to some extent independent of polarity and diagnosis (for example, schizophrenia and bipolar illness) is discussed in Chapter 13, as are family-history studies of bipolar and unipolar delusional depression; additional reviews of clinical correlates of unipolar delusional depression are presented elsewhere.[21] A recent large-scale analysis (N = 4,274) of three family studies found that the diagnosis of bipolar-I was far more predictive of psychotic symptoms during depression than was the diagnosis of recurrent major depression (odds ratio [OR] = 5.13) (Goes et al., in press).

Bipolar patients who experience psychotic depressions tend to have a more severe and more chronic course than those who do not. They also have fewer atypical features and less Axis I comorbidity (Benazzi, 1999c).

Activity and Behavior

Activity, behavior, and somatic symptoms during bipolar depression as noted by Winokur and colleagues (1969) are summarized in Table 2–12; comparison figures from Carlson and Strober (1979) and Casper and colleagues (1985) also are given. Sleep difficulties are pronounced and pervasive. Fatigue and psychomotor retardation are seen in approximately three-fourths of bipolar depressed patients; loss of appetite and sexual drive are common as well. Women are more likely than men to report weight and appetite changes during periods of bipolar depression (Benazzi, 1999; Kawa et al., 2005). Most patients have somatic complaints, and the majority report a diurnal mood variation (most feel worse in the morning and better in the evening).

MIXED STATES

Mixed states, in which symptoms of depression and mania combine, represent a complex and often confusing aspect of the clinical presentation of bipolar illness. They can be conceived of as transitional states from one phase of illness to another or as independent clinical states combining various mixes of mood, thought, and activity components. To a considerable extent, mixed states are even more vulnerable to the inadequacies of modern diagnostic systems than other types or stages of affective illness. Indeed, systematic diagnostic criteria, impressively standardized for most other types and phases of affective disorders, are least validated for mixed states. Differential diagnosis—especially among mixed states, agitated depressions, and borderline pathologies—can be a difficult clinical problem (see Chapter 3).

Mixed states are broadly defined as the simultaneous presence of depressive and manic symptoms. Yet we know, for example, as noted earlier, that mania frequently is accompanied by moderate to severe depression. Should depression during mania be conceptualized as a mixed state, a typical mania, an atypical mania, or a severe (stage-related) form of mania? Should a mixed depressive episode be defined by the presence of four manic symptoms or only two? Are the diagnostic criteria of DSM-IV prohibitively strict, as most researchers think? (According to DSM-IV, a diagnosis of mixed states requires that all of the criteria, except duration, for both a manic and a depressive episode be met "nearly every day" during at least a 1-week period, and that the symptoms be severe enough to cause "marked impairment" or necessitate hospitalization, or that there be psychotic features.) Until more systematic and discriminating definitions and criteria are developed, the pragmatism of the immediate clinical or research issue will determine the answers to such questions.

Classic Clinical Descriptions

Mixed states are important for both theoretical and clinical reasons. (Their implications for pathophysiology are discussed in Chapter 17 and for treatment in Chapters 18 and 19.) Despite the diagnostic difficulties noted above, their existence has been recognized for centuries. A seventeenth-century physician (Brouchier, 1679; cited in Dewhurst, 1962, p. 122) described the alternating and combining qualities of mania and melancholy in one of his patients, a Lady Grenville. Characterizing the illness as "her Ladyship's annual raving," he wrote to her husband:

> For there are twin symptoms, which are her constant companions, Mania and Melancholy, and they succeed each other in a double and alternate act; or take each other's place like the smoke and flame of a fire; so that the

TABLE 2–12. **Activity, Behavior, and Somatic Symptoms in Bipolar Depression**

	PERCENTAGE OF PATIENTS		
Category of Symptoms	Winokur et al., 1969[a]	Carlson and Strober, 1979	Casper et al., 1985
Sleep Disorder			
Insomnia	100		
Global sleep disturbance			85
Difficulty falling asleep	58		
Early-morning awakening	27		77
Hypersomnia	23		
Activity			
Fatigue	76		
Psychomotor retardation	76	83	
Social withdrawal	100		
Weight and Appetite			
Loss of appetite	97	50	45
Increase in appetite			23
Loss of weight			26
Libido			
Loss of sexual interest	73		77
Somatic Complaints	67		
Diurnal Mood Variation	64		72

[a]100 episodes, 61 patients.

noble patient is first melancholy, while her animal spirits are unable to disentangle themselves from the dense cloud of fumes which surround them; and then maniacal, when the saline and sulphureous atoms of the blood are stirred up and loosened by the immoderate heat of their surroundings.

Heinroth (1818) delineated, in detail, mixed states of exaltation and depression (see Marneros, 2001). Later in the mid-nineteenth century, Falret (cited in Sedler, 1983) noted the strong depressive quality often observed before, during, and after manic episodes, as well as *melancolie anxieuse.* The latter state, he wrote, is "characterized by constant pacing and inner turmoil, which incapacitates these patients

so they cannot concentrate, and this state sometimes ends up as manic agitation." Kraepelin (1921, pp. 4, 191–192) described mixed states and their similarities and dissimilarities to manic and depressive states as follows:

> We observe also clinical "*mixed forms,*" in which the phenomena of mania and melancholia are combined with each other, so that states arise, which indeed are composed of the same morbid symptoms as these, but cannot without coercion be classified either with the one or with the other. . . . The mixed states frequently fall outside the limits of the ordinary states in a very conspicuous way. . . . Our customary grouping into manic and melancholic attacks does not fit the facts, but requires substantial

enlargement, if it is to reproduce nature. At the same time it turned out that this enlargement ran out in the direction not of the fitting in of fresh morbid symptoms, but only of the different combination of morbid symptoms known for long. Further, it was seen that the mixed states, even when they appeared not as interpolations but as independent attacks, behaved with regard to their course and issue quite similarly to the usual forms, and lastly, that they might in the same morbid course simply take the place of the other attacks especially after a somewhat long duration of the malady.

Kraepelin conceptualized mixed states as primarily transitional phenomena, but recognized their existence as individual attacks that frequently occur in later stages of the illness, often associated with poor outcome. Table 2–13 summarizes Kraepelin's classification and description of mixed states, which he conceptualized as different combinations of the manic and depressive symptoms of mood, activity, and thought. Below is Kraepelin's (1921, pp. 103–104) description of two of the most important kinds of these mixed states, *depressive* or *anxious mania* and *excited depression*:

Depressive or Anxious Mania—If in the picture depression takes the place of cheerful mood, a morbid state arises, which is composed of flight of ideas, excitement, and anxiety. The patients are distractible, absent-minded, enter into whatever goes on round them, take themselves up with everything, catch up words and continue spinning out the ideas stirred up by these; they do not acquire a clear picture of their position, because they are incapable of systematic observation, and their attention is claimed by every new impression. They complain that they must think so much, their thoughts come of themselves, they have a great need of communicating their thoughts, but easily lose the thread, they can be brought out of the connection by every interpolated question, suddenly break off and pass to quite other trains of thought. Many patients display a veritable passion for writing, and scrawl over sheets and sheets of paper with disorderly effusions. At the same time ideas of sin and persecution are usually present, frequently also hypochondriacal delusions, as we have formerly described them.

Mood is anxiously despairing; it gives itself vent in great restlessness, which partly assumes the form of movements of expression and practical activity, but partly also passes over into a wholly senseless pressure of activity. The patients run about, hide away, force their way out, make movements of defense or attack; they lament, scream, screech, wring or fold their hands, beat them together above their head, tear out their hair, cross themselves, slide about kneeling on the floor. With these are associated rhythmical, rubbing, flourishing, snatching,

turning, twitching movements, snapping with the jaw, blowing, barking, growling. If one will, one might here speak of a "depressive" or "anxious" mania.

Excited Depression—If in the state described the flight of ideas is replaced by inhibition of thought, there arises the picture of excited depression. It is here a case of patients who display, on the one hand, extraordinary poverty of thought but, on the other hand, great restlessness. They are communicative, need the doctor, have a great store of words, but are extraordinarily monotonous in their utterances. To questions they give short answers to the point, and then immediately return to their complaints again, which are brought forth in endless repetition, mostly in the same phrases. About their position in general they are clear; they perceive fairly well, understand what goes on, apart from delusional interpretation. Nevertheless they trouble themselves little about their surroundings, they are only occupied with themselves.

Mood is anxious, despondent, lachrymose, irritable, occasionally mixed with a certain self-irony. Sometimes one hears from the patients witty or snappish remarks. Delusions are frequently present, but they are usually scantier and less extraordinarily spun out than in the form just described. The excitement of the patients also is usually not so stormy or protean. They run hither and thither, up and down, wring their hands, pluck at things, speak loud out straight in front of them, give utterance to rhythmic cries and torment themselves as well as their surroundings often to the uttermost by continuous, monotonous lamenting.

Jaspers, while noting occasional ambiguity in Kraepelin's nosology of mixed states, acknowledged its clinical utility. The many possible combinations of components—euphoria, flight of ideas, and pressure of movement on the one hand, and sadness and retardation of thought and of movement on the other—made possible a better understanding of the wide variety of affective states seen in clinical practice. Thus, Jaspers (1997, p. 598; first published in 1913) described a mixed melancholia, one that he suggested might be characterized as a "querulant mania" or "nagging depression" in some, and as a "wailing melancholia" in others:

In this state the over-valued or compulsive depressive ideas become delusionlike. They are fantastically elaborated (the patients are the cause of all the misfortune in the world; they are thought to be beheaded by the devil, etc.). The ideas are believed even though the patient seems relatively sensible. Underlying the experiences there are a host of *body sensations* (which soon lead to hypochondriacal delusions: the patients are filled up to the neck with excreta; the food falls through the empty body right to the bottom); then there are the most severe

TABLE 2–13. Kraepelin's Classification of Mixed States

	I. Depressive or Anxious Mania	II. Excited or Agitated Depression	III. Mania with Poverty of Thought
Mood	*Anxiety*	*Anxiety*	*Elation*
	Anxiously despairing.	Anxious, despondent, lachrymose, irritable, occasional self-irony.	Cheerful, pleased, unrestrained; somewhat irritated, repellent, or afterwards breaking into a merry laugh.
Activity	*Overactivity*	*Overactivity*	*Overactivity*
	Great restlessness; wholly senseless pressure of activity.	They run hither and thither, wring their hands, pluck at things; loud rhythmic cries; monotonous lamenting.	Excitement is often limited to making faces, dancing about, throwing things, changes in dress; many conduct themselves so quietly and methodically that superficial excitement does not appear at all; incapable of regular occupation, very abrupt, short-lived, impulsive outbursts of violence.
Thought	*Flight of Ideas*	*Inhibition of Thought*	*Inhibition of Thought*
	Distractible, absent-minded; incapable of systematic observation; veritable passion for writing with disorderly effusions; thoughts come of themselves.	Delusions are frequently present; extraordinary poverty of thought; extraordinarily monotonous in utterances; perceive well, understand what goes on, apart from delusional interpretation.	Perceive slowly and inaccurately; cannot immediately call things to mind. Their conversation is monotonous, not infrequently making an impression of weak-mindedness; state is subject to great fluctuation.
Summary			
Mood	Depressed	Depressed	Manic
Activity	Manic	Manic	Manic
Thought	Manic	Depressed	Depressed

(continued)

TABLE 2–13. **Kraepelin's Classification of Mixed States** *(continued)*

	IV. Manic Stupor	V. Depression with Flight of Ideas	VI. Inhibited Mania
Mood	*Elation*	*Depression*	*Elation*
	Cheerful; smile without recognizable cause; supportive, erotic.	Cast-down and hopeless; anxiety; sad and moody.	More exultant, occasionally irritable, distractible, inclined to jokes.
Activity	*Gross Motor Retardation*	*Motor Retardation*	*Motor Retardation*
	Usually inaccessible; lie quiet in bed; decorate themselves, without sign of restlessness or excitement. Not infrequently catalepsy can be demonstrated. Unexpectedly give utterance to loud and violent abuse, throw their food, suddenly take off their clothes, and immediately sink back into inaccessibility.	They read much, show interest in, and have understanding of their surroundings, although almost mute, and rigid in their whole conduct.	In outward behaviors, conspicuously quiet; it appears, however, as if a great inward tension existed, as patients may suddenly become very violent.
Thought	*Inhibition of Thought*	*Flight of Ideas*	*Flight of Ideas*
	Occasionally isolated delusions of changing content find utterance; for the most part they prove themselves fairly sensible and well oriented.	Incited by delusions; occasionally patients who cannot give utterance in speech are capable of writing; often desultory, full of ideas of sin and delusional fears; heaping up of synonymous phrases, jumping off to side thoughts, show flight of ideas, recognizable only in writings.	They easily fall into chattering talk with flight of ideas and numerous clang associations.
Summary			
Mood	Manic	Depressed	Manic
Activity	Depressed	Depressed	Depressed
Thought	Depressed	Manic	Manic

Source: Kraepelin, 1921. Reproduced with permission.

forms of *depersonalization* and *derealisation*: the world is no more, they themselves no longer exist, but still since they seem to exist they will have to live for ever (nihilistic delusions); finally there is extreme *anxiety*: the patients seek relief from this by keeping constantly on the move and indulging in a monotonous pressure of talk which almost becomes verbigeration: 'God, God, what will come of it, all, everything is gone, everything is gone, everything is gone, what will come of it?' etc. Even when the anxiety and melancholy have lifted, the patterns of movement, the facial expression and pressure of talk seem to maintain an *ossified* state until—often after a considerable time—the phase finally abates and recovery commences.

Manic stupor, according to Kraepelin's student and colleague Weygandt (1899, translated into English in the *Harvard Review*, 2002, p. 276), is the most important of the mixed states:

> Manic stupor as a phase of manic-depressive insanity is characterized by psychomotor inhibition and manic, elevated mood, with inhibition of thought (which usually occurs in a depressive state) instead of flight-of-ideas. This condition can occur transiently during a manic or depressive episode, particularly during switching from the manic phase to the depressive, when a shift has already taken place in psychomotor activity but not in affect . . . .
>
> The psychopathological condition is usually characterized by psychomotor manifestations (specifically stupor) as the prominent feature: some patients lie [in bed] showing very severe inhibition for a long time. Their limbs are cold; they refuse food, and every attempt to feed them is vain due to their opposition; for months they are mute. Only the facial expression, which shows no trace of depression and often shows a slight smile, reveals that a case is not typical circular [manic-depressive] stupor with depressed mood. In other cases, the [psychomotor] block is less intense: such patients may answer if asked questions, but they speak in a soft voice and hesitate before replying. They prefer not to speak spontaneously at all. Furthermore, these patients want to stay in bed all the time and refuse to work. Considerable retardation in their movements can be observed immediately: the gait is heavy and leaden; they hesitate to shake hands; and their writing is clearly slowed down. In less severe cases, the [psychomotor] block is occasionally interrupted by a fast, goal-directed movement.

Campbell (1953, pp. 144, 146), with his characteristic and important emphasis on the ever-fluctuating nature of moods, reiterated the mixed nature of most of the emotional and physical states associated with bipolar illness:

> There are more mixed reactions of this disease than is generally realized. It could truly be stated that, to some extent, all manic-depressive reactions are "mixed" types, in that the symptomatology is anything but static.
>
> The mixed type of manic-depressive psychosis epitomizes the entire cyclothymic process, in that it contains the symptoms characteristic of the various phases. Whether it is a sustained reaction or represents a phase of metamorphosis between the major forms, the mixed type emphasizes the underlying similarities between the depressive and hypomanic, the fact that the manic and depressive reactions may be superimposed, and that the same individual possesses the potentialities for either form. . . . Manic-depressive is a dynamic, constantly changing process which, at times, may manifest symptoms of both phases simultaneously. It is in the mixed form that the observer graphically realizes the homogeneity of the entire process.

Subjective Experiences of Patients

The extreme mental anguish often experienced during mixed states, including the terrifying thoughts and feelings associated with racing thoughts, delusions, and auditory hallucinations, was described by one bipolar patient whose mixed state was experienced at the height of a manic episode that, prior to that point, had been purely euphoric (as had countless hypomanias). Despite the strong and prolonged preponderance of classic euphoric mania in each of her episodes, the occasional transition into a mixed state was a potent feature of her illness. The simultaneous existence of suicidal thinking and mania is clearly portrayed in this description (Jamison, 1995, pp. 82–83):

> I felt infinitely worse, more dangerously depressed, during this first manic episode than when in the midst of my worst depressions. In fact, the most dreadful I have ever felt in my entire life—one characterized by chaotic ups and downs—was the first time I was psychotically manic. I had been mildly manic many times before, but they had never been frightening experiences—ecstatic at best, confusing at worst. I had learned to accommodate quite well to them. I had developed mechanisms of self-control, to keep down the peals of singularly inappropriate laughter, and had set rigid limits on my irritability. I avoided situations that might otherwise trip or jangle my hypersensitive wiring, and I learned to pretend I was paying attention or following a logical point when my mind was off chasing rabbits in a thousand directions. My work and professional life flowed. But nowhere did this, or my upbringing, or my intellect, or my character, prepare me for insanity.
>
> Although I had been building up to it for weeks, and certainly knew something was seriously wrong, there was

a definite point when I knew I was insane. My thoughts were so fast that I couldn't remember the beginning of a sentence halfway through. Fragments of ideas, images, sentences raced around and around in my mind like the tigers in a children's story. Finally, like those tigers, they became meaningless melted pools. Nothing once familiar to me was familiar. I wanted desperately to slow down but could not. Nothing helped—not running around a parking lot for hours on end or swimming for miles. My energy level was untouched by anything I did. Sex became too intense for pleasure, and during it I would feel my mind encased by black lines of light that were terrifying to me. My delusions centered on the slow painful deaths of all the green plants in the world—vine by vine, stem by stem, leaf by leaf they died and I could do nothing to save them. Their screams were cacophonous. Increasingly, all of my images were black and decaying.

At one point I was determined that if my mind—by which I made my living and whose stability I had assumed for so many years—did not stop racing and begin working normally again, I would kill myself by jumping from a nearby twelve-story building. I gave it twenty-four hours. But, of course, I had no notion of time, and a million other thoughts—magnificent and morbid—wove in and raced by. Endless and terrifying days of endlessly terrifying drugs—Thorazine, lithium, valium, and barbiturates—finally took effect. I could feel my mind being reined in, slowed down, and put on hold. But it was a very long time until I recognized my mind again, and much longer until I trusted it.

In the nineteenth century, composer Hector Berlioz (1966, translated by Cairn, 1970, pp. 226–228), described his episodes of "spleen," or depression, one type of which he characterized as an agitated and deeply "malignant" state:

The fit fell upon me with appalling force. I suffered agonies and lay groaning on the ground, stretching out abandoned arms, convulsively tearing up handfuls of grass and wide-eyed innocent daisies, struggling against the crushing sense of absence, against a mortal isolation.

Yet such an attack is not to be compared with the tortures that I have known since then in ever-increasing measure. What can I say that will give some idea of this abomidable disease? . . .

There are . . . two kinds of spleen; one mocking, active, passionate, malignant; the other morose and wholly passive, when one's only wish is for silence and solitude and the oblivion of sleep.

George Gordon, Lord Byron (in a letter dated August 1819) described his agitated and fluctuating moods during one of his many mixed depressive episodes:

I am so bilious—that I nearly lose my head—and so nervous that I cry for nothing—at least today I burst into tears all alone by myself over a cistern of Gold fishes—which are not pathetic animals. . . . I have been excited—and agitated and exhausted mentally and bodily all this summer—till I really sometimes begin to think not only "that I shall die at top first"—but that the moment is not very remote—I have had no particular cause of grief—except the usual accompaniments of all unlawful passions.

In a letter to a friend (written in December 1793), Scottish poet Robert Burns, who was also afflicted with a vexacious melancholia on and off throughout his life, provided a particularly graphic description of the terrible agitation that can accompany depression (*The Letters of Robert Burns*, ed. G.R. Roy, 1985):

Here I sit, altogether Novemberish, a damn'd mélange of Fretfulness & melancholy; not enough of the one to rouse me to passion; nor of the other to repose me in torpor; my soul flouncing & fluttering round her tenement, like a wild Finch caught amid the horrors of winter newly thrust into a cage.

Clinical Studies

To date, the best historical discussions of mixed states are those of Weygandt (1899), Kraepelin (1921), Campbell (1953), Winokur and colleagues (1969), Himmelhoch (1979), and Koukopoulos (Koukopoulos et al., 1992; Koukopoulos and Koukopoulos, 1999). These authors described the clinical course, presentation, and correlates of mixed states, as well as hypotheses regarding their etiology and nature (including their relationship to the continuum hypothesis of affective illness, kindling and rapid cycling, and mixed-heredity hypotheses).

Reported rates of mixed states vary as a function of the inclusion criteria—that is, whether the diagnostic criteria are narrow or broad—and the nature of the rating scales employed,[22] as reflected in the wide range of rates reported by the 18 studies summarized in Table 2–14. An average of 28 percent of affectively ill patients experienced mixed states across these studies. By any standard, mixed states are not as rare as they once were reputed to be. (Kraepelin and Weygandt, of course, were fully aware of how common mixed states are. In a study of 150 manic-depressive patients at the Heidelberg Psychiatric Clinic, 36 percent were diagnosed with a form of mixed states: 15 percent with sustained mixed episodes, 8 percent with agitated depression, 7 percent with manic stupor, and 6 percent with unproductive mania [Weygandt, 1899].)

Symptomatic presentations of mixed states range from a single opposite-state symptom found in the midst of an

TABLE 2–14. **Rates of Mixed Manic States in Representative Studies**

Study	Patients (N)	%
Winokur et al., 1969	61	16
Kotin and Goodwin, 1972	20	65
Himmelhoch et al., 1976	84	31
Akiskal and Puzantian, 1979	60	25
Nunn, 1979	112	36
Prien et al., 1988	103	67
Secunda et al., 1988	18	44
Post et al., 1989	48	46
Dell'Osso et al., 1991	108	45
McElroy et al., 1995	71	40
Perugi et al., 1997	261	>50[a]
Akiskal et al., 1998a	104	37
Cassidy et al., 1998	237	14
Dilsaver et al., 1999	105	54
Cassidy et al., 2001	327	13
Sato et al., 2002	576	10
Gonzalez-Pinto et al., 2003	103	24
Krüger et al., 2003	99	39
Total no. of patients	2,497	
Weighted mean		28[b]

[a]Because of the sampling methods, the use of enriched criteria from European concepts of mixed states (Berner et al., 1992) and various thresholds for diagnosing mixed states beyond the strict DSM-IV guidelines, the rate of mixed states in this study cannot be given as a single round figure. If excluded, weighted mean becomes 26%.

[b]Assuming the minimum 50% for Perugi et al.

otherwise "pure" manic or depressive syndrome (such as depressive mood during mania or racing thoughts during depression) to more complex mixes of mood, thought, and behavior. Documentation of the frequent occurrence of depressive mood during mania was presented earlier in Table 2–1. Kotin and Goodwin (1972) systematically inves-

tigated the relationship of depression to mania in 20 hospitalized patients. Through an analysis of nurses' and physicians' behavioral ratings and notes, they found a statistically significant positive association between mania and depression in the majority of cases.

Racing thoughts during depression can be considered another type of mixed state, one observed by earlier clinicians (Kraepelin, 1921; Lewis, 1934). More recently, this state was examined by Ianzito and colleagues (1974) and Braden and Qualls (1979). Ianzito's group found a relatively low rate of racing thoughts in their 89 depressed inpatients (5 percent), but they used the Present State Exam, which emphasizes the pleasurable and exciting quality as well as the rapidity of thought. Braden and Qualls, by contrast, found that one-third to one-half of their depressed inpatients reported racing thoughts, with a definite diurnal variation (worsening in the evening, greatest severity at bedtime). They drew the following conclusion (pp. 17–18):

> In bipolar patients and cyclothymics, the racing thoughts may occur in both "high" and "low" states. The symptom may thus be related more to the underlying pathology of the affective illness than to the characteristics of either "pole."

Other authors (Akiskal and Mallya, 1987; Koukopoulos and Koukopoulos, 1999; Benazzi and Akiskal, 2001) have favored the interpretation that racing—especially "crowded"—thoughts are indicative of mixed depressive states, and have invoked a significant excess of bipolar family history as validation of the bipolar nature of the phenomenon.

The symptomatic presentation of severe mixed states has been characterized in a variety of studies as dysphoric mood alternating with elevated mood, racing thoughts, grandiosity, suicidal ideation, persecutory delusions, auditory hallucinations, severe insomnia, psychomotor agitation, and hypersexuality (Cassidy et al., 1998; Perugi et al., 2001a; Brieger et al., 2003). Kotin and Goodwin (1972, p. 60) summarized their clinical impressions of mixed states as follows:

> Mania was nevertheless clearly identifiable by pressure of speech, increased motor activity, anger, intrusiveness, grandiosity, and mood instability. Depression during mania was frequently evidenced by expressed feelings of helplessness and hopelessness and thoughts of suicide. Sleep disturbance, irritability, anorexia, and many other symptoms are common to both conditions.

In their early study, Winokur and colleagues (1969) documented the course and symptoms of mixed states; the quantitative results of their work are given in Table 2–15. They concluded that the single most striking feature of

TABLE 2–15. **Symptoms of Mixed Manic-Depressive Psychosis**

Category of Symptoms	Percentage of Patients
Mood	
Depressed	100
Euphoric	100
Irritable	100
Labile	100
Hostile	79
Cognition and Perception	
Distractibility	100
Grandiosity	57
Flight of ideas	43
Delusions (depressive)	36
Delusions (nondepressive)	21
Auditory hallucinations	14
Visual hallucinations	7
Disorientation	7
Activity and Behavior	
Increased psychomotor activity	100
Insomnia	93
Pressure of speech	93
Decreased sexual interest	63
Suicidal threats or attempts	43
Increased alcohol intake	43
Anxiety attacks	43
Extravagance	14

Note: Based on 14 episodes of mixed manic-depressive psychosis in 10 patients.
Source: Adapted from Winokur et al., 1969.

mixed states was variability and lability of mood: "It is this panoply of varying and contrasting emotions which makes these patients difficult to diagnose" (p. 81). Winokur's group observed that mixed states tended to resemble mania in push of speech, physical activity, and hyperactivity. Delusions, on the other hand, tended to be depressive in nature, as did mood and vegetative signs and symptoms. The authors found that in 79 percent of cases, mixed states were gradual; that there was prior depression of appreciable clinical proportions in 71 percent of patients; that diurnal variation occurred in 64 percent; that the average period from onset to euthymia was 24 days; and that more than half (57 percent) of mixed episodes were followed by a depression.

Women made up 60 percent of Nunn's (1979) sample of patients with mixed states, consistent with the finding of Himmelhoch and colleagues (1976a) that 55 percent of their sample were women. Winokur and colleagues (1969) found a far more striking gender difference: 9 of their 10 patients with mixed episodes were women, and 13 of the 14 episodes they analyzed were experienced by women. The degree of this discrepancy almost certainly is due to the more stringent criteria used by these authors in defining mixed states. In the most comprehensive study to date, 908 bipolar patients were followed over a period of 7 years to assess mixed and euphoric hypomanias (Suppes et al., 2005). Mixed hypomania was more common than euphoric hypomania, and women were significantly more likely to experience a mixed symptomatic picture ($p < .001$).

Himmelhoch and colleagues (1976a) found no correlation between mixed states and severity of illness or rapidity of mood swings. They did find, however, that patients with mixed states were far more likely to have a history of substance abuse, especially alcoholism. This has been confirmed in some studies (Sonne et al., 1994; McElroy et al., 1995; Goldberg et al., 1999) but not in subsequent, larger investigations (Brieger, 2000; Cassidy et al., 2001). Current data indicate that mixed mania, unlike pure mania, which peaks in the spring, is more likely to peak in the late summer (Cassidy and Carroll, 2002), and both types of episodes tend to remain consistent over a prospective course (Cassidy et al., 2001b; Woods et al., 2001; Suppes et al., 2005). A recent study (Sato et al., 2006) found significant seasonal differences between 95 bipolar depressive patients and 77 unipolar patients with depressive mixed states when compared with 786 unipolar depressive patients without mixed states. Depressive episodes peaked in the spring in those without mixed states, but in those with mixed states (whether bipolar or unipolar), there was a significant autumn peak in depressive episodes. (It is not clear why unipolar patients with mixed states were not diagnosed as bipolar by the researchers.)

Winokur and colleagues (1969) examined the nature of delusions during mixed states and found, not surprisingly, that the type of delusion fluctuated with the patient's mood. Although depressive delusions were more frequent, manic-like delusions (nondepressed, grandiose, all religious) also occurred. Himmelhoch (1979, p. 453) emphasized the importance of manic delusions in differentiating unipolar agitated depression from mixed states:

> The clue to recognizing it [a mixed state] is the presence of distinct maniacal coloration of the psychotic material in the midst of all the severe depressive symptomatology . . . [for example] . . . grandiose, radiant, beatific religious delusions . . . out of tune with the patient's misery.

Recent studies have found a significant rate of delusions (23 percent) or delusions and/or hallucinations (40 percent) in mixed states (Mantere et al., 2004; Baethge et al., 2005). As some overlap exists between depressive and manic signs and symptoms (insomnia, anorexia, psychomotor agitation), the question arises of what constitutes the depressive manifestations "uncontaminated" by mania that would be suitable for the diagnostic assessment of mixed states. On the basis of a comprehensive review of the data (McElroy et al., 1992; Bauer et al., 1994, Cassidy et al., 1998), Akiskal and colleagues (2000) proposed the following depressive symptoms to support a diagnosis of dysphoric mania: depressed and/or labile mood, irritability, anhedonia, hopelessness/helplessness, suicidal thinking or behavior, guilt, and fatigue. Nonspecific symptoms, according to these authors, include agitation, changes in weight, and insominia.

Akiskal (1992b) proposed that mixed states arise when temperament and episodes are opposite in polarity—that is, mania arising from a depressive temperament and depression arising from a hyperthymic temperament. There has now been some preliminary validation of this view in several Italian, French, and German studies (Dell'Osso et al., 1991; Perugi et al., 1997; Brieger et al., 2003), but the diverse presentation of mixed states makes any single explanation necessarily incomplete and premature. Temperament may be decisive in determining the manifestation of mixed states in some individuals but ultimately is far less important than other factors—for example, comorbidity, chronicity of illness, medication effects—in many or even most patients.

While much of the research on mixed states has been in dysphoric or depressive mania, depressive mixed states (hypomanic behavior and/or symptoms intruding into depressive episodes) have been described since Kraepelin's (1899) and Weygandt's (1899) original contributions in this area. The most common manifestations of the excitatory pole in depressive mixed states are psychomotor activation and/or agitation, irritability and mood lability, racing or crowded thoughts, and sexual arousal, as well as severe insomnia, panic attacks, and suicidal crises in severely complicated variants.[23] Indeed, increased suicidality and the risk of suicide are particularly associated with mixed states (Hantouche et al., 2003; Strakowski et al., 1996; Marneros et al., 2004; see Chapter 8). A recent study of bipolar adolescents found that mixed states contributed independently to the risk of suicidal behavior, but the increased risk was among the girls only (Dilsaver et al., 2005). In a meta-analysis of risk factors for suicide and attempted suicide, Hawton and colleagues (2005) at the University of Oxford also found mixed states to be a significant risk factor.

Consistent with Aretaeus, who had observed that melancholics could be "angry without reason," Mammen and colleagues (2004) found that 39 percent of their bipolar patients reported anger attacks during depression. Such attacks may well represent a form of depressive mixed state.

As discussed in Chapter 1, Benazzi and Akiskal (2005) compared the relationship between irritability and other clinical features in a large number of bipolar-II and unipolar major depressive subjects. Major depressive episodes with irritability were present in 60 percent of their bipolar-II patients and in 37 percent of their depressive patients. In the bipolar-II patients, those who presented with irritability had a significantly younger age at index episode, higher rates of atypical depressive features, and more significant Axis I comorbidity relative to those who did not. They also were more likely to meet the study criteria for depressive mixed states, defined by the investigators as a major depressive episode plus three or more concurrent intradepressive hypomanic symptoms (whether occurring in the bipolar-II or major depressive patients). In the unipolar patients, those who presented with irritability had a significantly younger age at onset and higher rates of atypical depression; they were also more likely to meet criteria for a depressive mixed state and to have a family history of bipolar illness. According to the authors, their data demonstrate that irritability may be a good marker of depressive mixed states, a view consistent with that of others who have found high rates of irritability and anger attacks associated with these states (e.g., Fava and Rosenbaum, 1999; Deckersbach et al., 2004; Perlis et al., 2004). The relationship between age at onset and mixed states is unclear. Some investigators have found that earlier age at onset is associated with mixed states (Nunn, 1979; Post et al., 1989; McElroy et al., 1997), but others have not (Marneros et al., 1991a,b; Strakowski et al., 1996; Perugi et al., 1997).

In their discussion of depression with manic features, Koukopoulos and Koukopoulos (1999) suggested that all types of agitated depressions should be called "mixed depression." They proposed that the following diagnostic criteria be used: (1) major depressive episode and (2) at least two of the three symptoms of motor agitation, psychic agitation or intense inner tension, and racing or crowded thoughts. Perugi and colleagues (2001) have distinguished between depressive mixed states and non-mixed bipolar depression on the basis of depressive mixed states being characterized by fewer episodes of longer duration; less cyclicity; greater likelihood of mixed state at first episode; more previous mixed episodes; less interepisode remission; more incongruent psychotic features; and more agitation, irritability, pressured speech, and flight of ideas.

CYCLOTHYMIA AND MANIC-DEPRESSIVE TEMPERAMENTS

Classic Clinical Descriptions

Cyclothymia and related temperamental types represent a significant portion of the manic-depressive spectrum. The relationship of predisposing personalities (or temperaments) and cyclothymia to the subsequent development of manic-depressive illness is a fundamental one (as discussed further below, as well as in Chapters 1, 5, 6, and 10). *Cycloid temperament*, a generic term for the spectrum of manic-depressive personality types, is generally manifested as predominantly depressive, manic or hypomanic, irritable, or cyclothymic.[24] Campbell (1953, pp. 25–26) described these personality types and their relationship to manic-depressive illness and to one another:

> The term *cycloid personality* is an overall or general appellation, indicating all forms of the prepsychotic manic-depressive personality. The cycloid personality may occur in one of three forms, with innumerable gradations and mixtures between the three. First, is the hypomanic personality, the overactive, jovial, friendly, talkative and confident individual who, if he becomes psychotic, *usually* develops the manic form of manic-depressive psychosis. . . . Second, is the depressive type, the worried, anxious, thoughtful, sorrowful, individual who, if he becomes psychotic, *usually* develops the depressive form of manic-depressive psychosis. The third form of the cycloid personality is the cyclothymic personality who may have mixed traits, or be euphoric and friendly at one time, and depressed and pessimistic at another, and who may develop either a manic or depressive reaction, or swing from one into the other. It is important to realize

that the manic reaction, melancholia, hypomanic reaction, cyclothymic personality, cycloid personality, depressive personality and periodic insanity, are all a part of the same disease process, and that any one of these may change into any other.

The generic term *cycloid personality* used by Kretschmer encompasses all types of prepsychotic personality in manic-depressive patients. Kretschmer, too, stressed the overlap among these personality types (1936; cited in Campbell, 1953, pp. 26–27):

> Men of this kind have a soft temperament which can swing to great extremes. The path over which it swings is a wide one, namely between cheerfulness and unhappiness. . . . Not only is the hypomanic disposition well known to be a peculiarly labile one, which also has leanings in the depressive direction, but many of these cheerful natures have, when we get to know them better, a permanent melancholic element somewhere in the background of their being. . . . The hypomanic and melancholic halves of the cycloid temperament relieve one another, they form layers or patterns in individual cases, arranged in the most varied combinations.

Clearly, not all cyclothymic or cycloid personalities go on to develop the full manic-depressive syndrome, and here we concern ourselves primarily with clinical descriptions of the range of cycloid temperaments and cyclothymic disorders. Kraepelin (1921, pp. 119–120) described a *depressive temperament*, which is characterized by a "permanent gloomy emotional stress in all the experience of life":

> Patients, as a rule, have to struggle with all sorts of internal obstructions, which they only overcome with effort; . . . they lack the right joy in work. . . . From youth up there exists in the patients a special susceptibility for the cares, the difficulties, the disappointments of life . . . in every occurrence feel the small disagreeables much more strongly than the elevating and satisfying aspects. . . . Frequently . . . a capricious, irritable, unfriendly, repellent behaviour is developed. The patients are occupied only with themselves, do not trouble themselves about their surroundings. . . .
>
> Every task stands in front of them like a mountain; life with its activity is a burden which they habitually bear . . . without being compensated by the pleasure of existence.

In manic temperament, Kraepelin went on to say, the patients' "understanding of life and the world remains superficial"; their "train of thought is desultory, incoherent, aimless"; and their mood is "permanently exalted, careless, confident." (Centuries earlier, Aretaeus [cited in

Roccatagliata, 1986, p. 229] had described a predominantly manic form of illness that arose in those "whose personality is characterized by gayness, activity, superficiality and childishness." The mania itself was manifest in "furor, excitement and cheerfulness") Kraepelin (1921, pp. 126–128) said that such patients are

> convinced of their *superiority* to their surroundings. . . . Towards others they are haughty, positive, irritable, impertinent, stubborn. . . . *unsteadiness and restlessness* appear before everything. They are accessible, communicative, adapt themselves readily to new conditions, but soon they again long for change and variety. Many have belletristic inclinations, compose poems, paint, go in for music. . . . Their mode of expression is clever and lively; they speak readily and much, are quick at repartee, never at a loss for an answer or an excuse. . . . With their surroundings the patients often live in constant *feud.*

Kraepelin also discussed a milder form of manic temperament within the "domain of the normal," but still a "link in the long chain of manic-depressive dispositions," a form that progresses to what he termed the *irritable temperament.* In Kraepelin's (1921, pp. 129–131) words:

> It concerns here brilliant, but unevenly gifted personalities with artistic inclinations. They charm us by their intellectual mobility, their versatility, their wealth of ideas, their ready accessibility and their delight in adventure, their artistic capability, their good nature, their cheery, sunny mood. But at the same time they put us in an uncomfortable state of surprise by a certain restlessness, talkativeness, desultoriness in conversation, excessive need for social life, capricious temper and suggestibility, lack of reliability, steadiness, and perseverance in work, a tendency to building castles in the air . . . periods of causeless depression or anxiety. . . .
>
> The *irritable temperament,* a further form of manic-depressive disposition, is perhaps best conceived as a *mixture of the fundamental states* . . . in as much as in it manic and depressive features are associated. . . . The patients display from youth up extraordinarily great fluctuations in emotional equilibrium and are greatly moved by all experiences, frequently in an unpleasant way. While on the one hand they appear sensitive and inclined to sentimentality and exuberance, they display on the other hand great irritability and sensitiveness. They are easily offended and hot-tempered; they flare up, and on the most trivial occasions fall into outbursts of boundless fury. "She had states in which she was nearly delirious," was said of one patient; "Her rage is beyond all bounds," of another. It then comes to violent scenes with abuse, screaming and a tendency to rough behaviour. . . . The patients are positive, always in a mood for a fight, endure no contradiction, and, therefore, easily fall into disputes with the people round them, which they carry on with great passion. . . . The colouring of mood is subject to frequent change. . . .
>
> Their power of imagination is usually very much influenced by moods and feelings. It, therefore, comes easily to delusional interpretations of the events of life. The patients think that they are tricked by the people round them, irritated on purpose and taken advantage of.

Cyclothymic temperament is characterized, according to Kraepelin (1921, p. 131), by "frequent, more or less regular fluctuations of the psychic state to the manic or to the depressive side." He described cyclothymic individuals as follows (p. 132):

> These are the people who constantly oscillate hither and thither between the two opposite poles of mood, sometimes "rejoicing to the skies," sometimes "sad as death." To-day lively, sparkling, beaming, full of the joy of life, the pleasure of enterprise, and pressure of activity, after some time they meet us depressed, enervated, ill-humoured, in need of rest, and again a few months later they display the old freshness and elasticity.

Kretschmer (1936, p. 132) pointed out a tendency of these individuals to drift toward either mania or depression:

> The temperament of the cycloids alternates between cheerfulness and sadness, in deep, smooth, rounded waves, only more quickly and transitorily with some, more fully and enduring with others. But the mid-point of these oscillations lies with some nearer the hypomanic, and with others nearer the depressive pole.

Slater and Roth (1969, pp. 206–207) provided a general description of the "constitutional cyclothymic," emphasizing the natural remissions and seasonal patterns often inherent in the temperament. The alternating mood states, each lasting for months at a time, are continuous in some individuals but subside, leaving periods of normality, in others. In Slater and Roth's words, the cyclothymic constitution

> is perhaps less frequent than the other two "basic states," but its existence in artists and writers has attracted some attention, especially as novelists like Björnsen and H. Hesse have given characteristic descriptions of the condition. Besides those whose swings of mood never intermit, there are others with more or less prolonged *intervals of normality.* In the hypomanic state the patient feels well, but the existence of such states accentuates his feeling of insufficiency and even illness in the depressive phases. At such times he will often seek the advice of his practitioner,

complaining of such vague symptoms as headache, insomnia, lassitude, and indigestion. . . . In typical cases such alternative cycles will last a lifetime. In cyclothymic artists, musicians, and other creative workers the rhythm of the cycles can be read from the dates of the beginning and cessation of productive work. Some cyclothymics have a *seasonal rhythm* and have learned to adapt their lives and occupations so well to it that they do not need medical attention.

According to Koukopoulos (2003, p. 202), observing a cyclothymic patient who is depressed, "one is spontaneously reminded of a machine in which the oil has run dry and the gears grind on in laborious suffering, rasping against one another until they seize up in pain." When hypomanic, on the other hand, the patient is entirely different (p. 203):

> Instead of the inhibition that was previously felt, the course of thoughts is now faster, the perception of external impressions easier and more immediate, so the patient appears to be more intelligent, full of wit and more entertaining than in the healthy days. As for the increased capacity for criticizing, which as already mentioned may present itself also in the depressive state, this may now become so strong as to be considered vexing by the patient himself. It often betokens itself by an arrogant, mocking smirk. The elevated mental capacity leads in the majority of cases to a restless, non-stop activity and dynamism which develops in the widest variety of directions. It is not only the stamina of the patient, which appears greater than that of the healthy days, but the level of skill and ability that is increased in various ways. Many, for instance, who had a rather mediocre voice and in their depressive intervals—were without much musical talent—now sing not only with great eagerness, but also with a better tone of voice and a livelier expressiveness. Others display, in manual tasks and their mode of dress, a skill and taste which they did not formerly possess. And others manifest a literary bent that was quite alien to them before.

> All these characteristics are, as I observed above, due to the expression of the expansive mood, which as a rule sweeps over the patient suddenly. All at once he sees the rosy side of life and at the same time feels a desire to have others partake in his joy, to help his fellow men and carry out activities that frequently bear fruit in the fields of charity and humanitarian interests.

Clinical Studies

Compelling evidence argues for including cyclothymia as an integral part of the spectrum of manic-depressive illness. The data presented here describe several aspects of cyclothymia: its clinical presentation; symptomatic patterns of mood, cognition, and behavior; and subsequent development of full affective episodes in cyclothymic patients.[25] (Related issues are discussed in Chapters 1, 10, and 11.)

In his early review of the literature, Waters (1979) cited widespread agreement that mood and energy swings often precede clinical illness by years. In a study of 33 patients with definite bipolar illness, he found that one-third reported bipolar mood swings or hypomania predating the actual onset of their illness. These subsyndromal mood swings were characterized by (1) onset in early adulthood; (2) occurrence most often in spring or fall; (3) occurrence on an annual or biennial basis; (4) onset unrelated to current life events (with the exception of the first episode); (5) persistence of symptoms for 3 to 10 weeks; (6) a change in energy level, rather than the experience of dysphoria; and (7) sensitivity to lithium treatment (comparable to that for manifest bipolar illness). More recently, Kochman and colleagues (2005) assessed 80 depressed children and adolescents with the Kiddie-SADS semistructured interview and a newly developed questionnaire to measure cyclothymic–hypersensitive temperament. At the end of the 2- to 4-year follow-up period, 43 percent of the sample had been diagnosed as bipolar. Of the children and adolescents who had been categorized as cyclothymic–hypersensitive, 64 percent developed bipolar disorder; of those who had not been so categorized, only 15 percent experienced a hypomanic or manic episode ($p < .001$).

In a study of the natural course or progression of cyclothymia, that is, the relationship of cyclothymic states to the subsequent development of bipolar affective episodes, approximately one-third (36 percent) of 50 cyclothymic patients, in contrast to only 4 percent of 50 nonaffective controls, developed full syndromal depression, hypomania, or mania (Akiskal et al., 1979b). Of the 25 cyclothymic patients requiring antidepressant medication for their depressive illness, 11 (44 percent) became hypomanic. This rate was comparable to the switch rate in bipolar controls (35 percent).

Akiskal and colleagues further described and quantified these "subsyndromal" mood swings. Box 2–1 presents revised operational criteria for cyclothymia based on a population study that tested the authors' clinically derived criteria (Akiskal et al., 1979a, 1998b). Their original sample of 50 cyclothymic patients was characterized by the following: a female/male ratio of 3:2; young age at onset, which is consistent with other data suggesting an onset of first symptoms between ages 12 and 14 (Akiskal et al., 1977; Depue et al., 1981); and a tendency for the first clinical presentation to be perceived as a personality rather than a mood disorder, with family members and friends describing the

BOX 2–1. Validated Criteria for Cyclothymic Temperament

Biphasic subclinical mood swings with abrupt and labile shifts, and with variability in duration, measured from hours to a few days. At least four of the following constitute the habitual long-term baseline of the subject:

- Lethargy alternating with eutonia
- Shaky self-esteem alternating between low self-confidence and overconfidence
- Decreased verbal output alternating with talkativeness
- Mental confusion alternating with sharpened and creative thinking
- Unexplained tearfulness alternating with excessive punning and jocularity
- Introverted self-absorption alternating with uninhibited people seeking

Source: Akiskal et al., 1998b. Reprinted with permission from Elsevier.

patient as "high-strung," "explosive," "moody," "hyperactive," or "sensitive."

Mood, cognitive, and behavioral patterns in 46 patients with cyclothymia were studied by Akiskal and colleagues (1977); although based on a small sample, their findings are useful in providing an overall view of cyclothymic states. As might be expected, the mood and cognitive aspects parallel, in milder form, those for mania and depression. Three-fourths of Akiskal and colleagues' patients met criteria for alternating patterns of sleep disorder, fluctuating levels in the quality and quantity of work or school productivity, and financial disinhibition. One-half of the patients reported periods of irritability or aggressiveness, patterns of frequent shifts in interests or plans, drug or alcohol abuse, or fluctuating levels of social interaction. Episodic promiscuity or extramarital affairs were reported by 40 percent of the sample, and joining new movements with zeal, followed by disillusionment, by 25 percent. Although frequencies of specific behavior patterns are of interest, replicated and comparison population figures are necessary. Thus we await more detailed studies of cognitive and perceptual changes across mood states, much larger sample sizes, and replications utilizing more standardized measures.

Cyclothymia is a common temperamental variant, occurring in 0.4 to 6.3 percent of the population (Depue et al., 1981; Placidi et al., 1998; Chiaroni et al., 2005). According to Akiskal (1998), the most frequent subtypes of cyclothymia are *pure cyclothymia* (equal proportion of depressive and hypomanic swings, alternating in an irregular fashion), *predominantly depressed cyclothymia* (depressive periods dominating the clinical picture,

interspersed with "even," "irritable," and occasional hypomanic periods), and *hyperthymia* (hypomanic traits—decreased need for sleep, expansive behavior, "wild lifestyle"—dominating, with occasional depressive and irritable episodes). Systematic qualitative data to verify this taxonomy do not exist, however.

Discriminatory criteria for the irritable temperament have remained elusive (Akiskal, 1992a; Akiskal et al., 1998b). The hyperthymic type, by contrast, is probably distinct from the cyclothymic (Akiskal, 1992a). Indeed, in a factor analytic study of temperaments in an Italian student population, the cyclothymic and hyperthymic types emerged as separate superfactors (Akiskal et al., 1998b). The hyperthymic type is best described as adaptive-trait hypomania (which distinguishes it from hypomanic episodes), consisting of the triad of high energy, overconfidence, and cheerfulness, with virtually no depressive dips (which distinguishes this type from the cyclothymic type proper). Again, while such speculations are interesting, they need greater validation and replication.

The validated criteria for the cyclothymic type summarized in Box 2–1 portray a temperament with greater instability than the hyperthymic type, and for that reason one perhaps more proximal to bipolar disorder; indeed, cyclothymia often precedes or underlies bipolar-II disorder (Hantouche et al., 1998; Perugi and Akiskal, 2002). Of the affective temperaments, cyclothymia is the most correlated with emotional and behavioral problems (Signoretta et al., 2005).

On the other hand, the hyperthymic type represents a more adaptive set of traits. The criteria for hyperthymic temperament, as validated by Akiskal and colleagues (1998a), require that four of the following traits (which constitute the habitual long-term functioning of the individual) be present: (1) warm, people seeking, or extraverted; (2) cheerful, overoptimistic, or exuberant; (3) uninhibited, stimulus seeking, or risk taking; (4) overinvolved and meddlesome; (5) vigorous, overenergetic, and full of plans; (6) self-assured, overconfident, or boastful; and (7) overtalkative or articulate. Researchers in Italy (Maremmani et al., 2005) compared responses from 1,010 students aged 14 to 26 on Cloninger's revised Tridimensional Personality Questionnaire (TPQ) (Cloninger, 1987) and on the semi-structured affective temperament interview (TEMPS-I) (Placidi et al., 1998). The TPQ constructs of gregariousness, exploratory excitability, uninhibited optimism, attachment, confidence, extravagance, independence, vigor, and impulsiveness correlated highly with the temperamental construct of hyperthymia. Jamison (2004) has discussed at length the relationship among exuberant, hyperthymic, and extraverted temperaments, as well as the relationship between such temperaments and psychological resilience (see also Chapter 10).

Psychiatric studies of temperament would benefit enormously from the addition of the perspectives and methodologies used by developmental psychologists who have studied early manifestations of temperament and the development of temperament over time, from infancy to adulthood. Particularly relevant here is the paradigm used by Jerome Kagan and colleagues in their important studies of inhibited and uninhibited temperaments.[26] At present, we lack the sophisticated developmental and genetic approaches that ultimately will provide the kind of information needed to adequately understand the manic-depressive spectrum of temperaments.

CONCLUSIONS

This chapter has presented a clinical description of manic-depressive illness (with emphasis on the bipolar form) that combines three methods of observation: descriptions of both ancient and modern clinical observers, first-person accounts from patients with manic-depressive illness, and results obtained from clinical studies. Each method is unique, invaluable, but incomplete. Good clinical description is beholden to all three perspectives.

Pathognomonic cycles of mood and activity serve as a background for ongoing fluctuations in thinking, perception, and behavior. The bipolar form of manic-depressive illness encompasses the extremes of human experience. Moods swing between euphoria and despair, irritability and panic. Cognition can range from psychosis or delirium to a pattern of fast, clear, and sometimes creative associations; it can also manifest as retardation so profound that consciousness is clouded. Behavior can be seductive, hyperactive–expansive, and dangerous; or it can be reclusive, sluggish, and suicidal.

The rapid undulations and combinations of such extremes result in an intricately textured clinical picture. It is important to note that the designation "mixed states" is often arbitrary. Indeed, manic patients are depressed and irritable at least as often as they are elated, and bipolar depressed patients are frequently agitated and may have racing thoughts.

NOTES

1. Falret, 1854 (translated by Sedler, 1983); Kraepelin, 1921; Campbell, 1953; Wellner and Marstal, 1964; Beigel and Murphy, 1971a; Cassidy et al., 2001a, 2002; Woods et al., 2001; Sato et al., 2004.

2. Kraepelin continued:

> Statues salute him by nodding; the moon falls down from the sky; the trumpets of the Day of Judgment are sounding. He hears the voice of Jesus, speaks with God and the poor souls, is called by God dear son. There are voices in his ears; the creaking of the floor, the sound of the bells take on the form of words. The patient has telepathic connection with an aristocratic fiancée, feels the electric current in the walls, feels himself hypnotized; transference of thought takes place.

3. As discussed later in this chapter, Carlson and Goodwin (1973), in their systematic study of the stages of mania, found that mania usually evolves gradually. In their hospitalized patients, the early stages of mania could be discerned in nurses' recordings of mood and behavior reviewed after the apparently sudden onset of manic episodes.

4. Harrow et al., 1972a,b, 1982, 1983, 1986; Harrow and Quinlan, 1977; Harrow and Prosen, 1978.

5. Harrow et al., 1972a,b, 1986; Himmelhoch et al., 1973; Adler and Harrow, 1974; Harrow and Quinlan, 1977; Grossman et al., 1981.

6. Breakey and Goodell, 1972; Grossman et al., 1981; Andreasen, 1984; Shenton et al., 1987; Solovay et al., 1987.

7. The discrepancy between the results of these two groups may be due in part to differences in the assessment of thought disorder. Resnick and Oltmanns (1984) used a global rating, whereas Harrow and colleagues (1982) used specific tests.

8. Andreasen, 1984; Resnick and Oltmanns, 1984; Simpson and Davis, 1985; Ragin and Oltmanns, 1987.

9. Morice and Ingram, 1983; Morice and McNicol, 1986; Docherty et al., 1996; Thomas et al., 1996; Lott et al., 2002.

10. Pease, 1912; Rosenthal et al., 1979; Harrow et al., 1990; Goldberg et al., 1995; Keck et al., 2003.

11. Beigel and Murphy, 1971b; Murphy and Beigel, 1974; Taylor and Abrams, 1975; Rosen et al., 1983b; Young et al., 1983, Winokur et al., 1985; Coryell et al., 1990, 2001; Tohen et al., 1990; Young and Klerman, 1992; Toni et al., 2001.

12. Brockington et al., 1983; Winokur, 1984; Coryell et al., 1990; Miklowitz, 1992; Tohen et al., 1992; Fennig et al., 1996; Perugi et al., 1999; Strakowski et al., 2000.

13. Double, 1990; Bauer et al., 1994; Cassidy et al., 1998; Dilsaver et al., 1999; Perugi et al., 2001b; Swann et al., 2001; Sato et al., 2002.

14. Suicidal behavior, discussed in the next section, is covered more fully in Chapter 8.

15. All quotations from this source are from F. Scott Fitzgerald, *The Crack-up*, copyright © 1945 by New Directions Publishing Corp. Reprinted by permission of New Directions Publishing Corp.

16. It is even more rare for a clinical study of unipolar depression to differentiate the highly recurrent form (part of Kraepelin's manic-depressive illness) from the nonrecurrent form.

17. Benazzi, 1999b, 2000a,b, 2001, 2003, 2004.

18. More specialized reviews of related clinical topics can be found in Chapters 1, 8, 9, 10, 11, and 16.

19. Kraepelin, 1921; Bowman and Raymond, 1931–1932a; Schneider, 1959; Beck, 1967; Winokur et al., 1969.

20. Charney and Nelson, 1981; Frangos et al., 1983; Helms and Smith, 1983; Winokur, 1984. Baethge et al., 2005.

21. Charney and Nelson, 1981; Frances et al., 1981; Glassman and Roose, 1981; Coryell and Tsuang, 1982; Nelson et al., 1984; Spiker et al., 1985; Roose and Glassman, 1988.

22. McElroy et al., 1992, 1995; Cassidy and Carroll, 1998; Cassidy et al., 1998; Sato et al., 2002.

23. Akiskal and Mallya, 1987; Koukopoulos and Koukopoulos, 1999; Benazzi, 2000b; Benazzi and Akiskal, 2001; Sato et al., 2003; Biondi et al., 2005; Benazzi, 2006; Oedegaard et al., 2006.

24. Reiss, 1910; Kraepelin, 1921; Bleuler, 1924; Kretschmer, 1936; Campbell, 1953; Slater and Roth, 1969.

25. *Cyclothymia* in the German literature refers to the temperament as well as the full range of bipolar disorders. In the English literature, it is restricted to a subthreshold disorder.

26. Kagan et al., 1988, 1992; Kagan, 1989; Kagan and Snidman, 1991; Fox et al., 2001; Schwartz et al., 2003.

3 Diagnosis

The symptom-complexes of pure mania and depression seem extraordinarily "natural" to us because of the thread of meaningful connection which runs through their individual features, but very many of these patients do not correspond at all to these "natural" complexes which are only ideal types of construct.

—*Karl Jaspers (1913, p. 597)*

The history of psychiatric diagnosis has been notable for its confusion, reflected in the myriad overlapping systems for classifying and subdividing depressive disorders. As discussed in Chapter 1, however, Kraepelin brought order to the diagnosis of depression by grouping all of the recurrent affective disorders under the rubric of manic-depressive illness, a broad category later divided into unipolar and bipolar subgroups. Although the original meaning of *unipolar* as a form of recurrent affective disorder has been obscured in our current diagnostic system, bipolar illness has remained a relatively consistent and stable diagnostic category; characterizing patients as bipolar leads to valid predictions about family history, course, prognosis, and treatment response. In this chapter, we review the formal criteria for the diagnosis of manic-depressive illness, focusing on the bipolar form. With the category thus defined, we then reexamine the boundaries it shares with other major diagnostic categories, some of which were introduced in our earlier discussion of the manic-depressive spectrum (see Chapter 1). Here the focus is on clinical decision making.

A reading of the relevant literature makes clear that reliable diagnosis of manic-depressive illness requires a longitudinal as well as a cross-sectional view of the patient.[1] This literature also charts a course for clinicians, underscoring the need to meet repeatedly with the patient and to seek out other people, particularly family members, who can help in forming an accurate picture of the patient's history, symptoms, and behavior. Such practices decrease the clinician's dependence on cross-sectional data and increase the reliability of diagnoses. Clinicians will need to remain careful and skilled diagnosticians even if future genetic and biological studies provide more clues as to the etiology of manic-depressive illness. This is so because both the bipolar and highly recurrent unipolar forms of manic-depressive illness undoubtedly involve complex interactions among genetic and environmental factors that do not allow for the kinds of direct cause-and-effect relationships seen, for example, with inborn errors of metabolism.

The first section of this chapter summarizes the development of contemporary diagnostic systems. This is followed by a review of the diagnostic criteria for those disorders salient to diagnosis of manic-depressive illness. We then examine findings of recent studies addressing the key issue of whether psychotic conditions should be classified as separate conditions or as falling along a continuous spectrum. Finally, we look at the problem of differential diagnosis of bipolar disorder and other disorders with which it shares overlapping features.

DEVELOPMENT OF CONTEMPORARY DIAGNOSTIC SYSTEMS

Successive versions of the *International Classification of Diseases* (ICD), now in its tenth revision (Sato et al., 2002), represent the official diagnostic system used by clinicians throughout most of the world. The major exception, of course, is the United States, where clinicians use the American Psychiatric Association's (APA) *Diagnostic and Statistical Manual*, the fourth edition of which (DSM-IV) was published in 1994. The different diagnostic systems are illustrated in Boxes 3–1a and 3–1b. Two European systems of classification are also important—the Present State Examination (PSE)-Catego (Wing and Nixon, 1975) and the system developed by the Association for Methodology and Documentation in Psychiatry (Guy and Ban, 1982).

diff. diag.

BOX **3–1a.**   **DSM-IV Mood Disorders**

Depressive Disorders

2.96	Major depressive disorder
	.2x single episode
	.3x recurrent
300.4	Dysthymic disorder
	—specify if: early onset/late onset
	—specify: with atypical features
311	Depressive disorder not otherwise specified

Bipolar Disorders

296	Bipolar I disorder
	.0x single manic episode
	—specify if mixed
	.40 most recent episode hypomanic
	.4x most recent episode manic
	.6x most recent episode mixed
	.5x most recent episode depressed
	.7 most recent episode unspecified
296.89	Bipolar II disorder
	—specify (current or most recent episode) hypo-manic/depressed
301.13	Cyclothymic disorder
296.8	Bipolar disorder not otherwise specified
293.83	Mood disorder due to (indicate the general medical condition)
	—specify type: with depressive/manic/mixed features
	—specify if: with onset during intoxication/withdrawal
	—see substance-related disorders for codes
	for specific drugs of abuse
	for other agents (including antidepressants)
292.84	Code as other substance–induced mood disorder
296.90	Mood disorder not otherwise specified
295.70	Schizoaffective disorder
	—specify: bipolar type/depressive type
295.40	Schizophreniform disorder
	—specify: with or without good prognostic features
298.8	Brief psychotic disorder
	—specify: with or without marked stressor, with postpartum onset
298.9	Psychotic disorder not otherwise specified

Source: Reprinted with permission from the *Diagnostic and Statistical Manual of Mental Disorders,* Fourth Edition, Text Revision (Copyright 2000). American Psychiatric Association.

BOX **3–1b.**   **ICD-10 Mood Disorders (Affective Disorder)**

F 32	Depressive episode
F 33	Recurrent depressive disorder
F 34	Persistent mood (affective) disorders
F 34.1	Dysthymia
F 34.8	Other persistent mood (affective) disorders
F 34.9	Persistent mood (affective) disorders, unspecified
F 38	Other mood (affective) disorders
F 38.0	Single mixed affective episode
F 38.1	Recurrent brief depressive episode
F 31	Bipolar affective disorder (BAD)
F 30	Manic episode
	—specify if hypomania, mania with or without psychosis
F 31.0	BAD, current episode hypomania
F 31.1, 31.2	BAD, current episode manic with or without psychosis
F 31.6	BAD, current episode mixed
F 31.3, 31.4, 31.5	BAD, current episode depressed with or without psychotic symptoms
F31.8	Other bipolar affective disorders
	—specify if bipolar-II disorder or recurrent manic episodes
F 34.0	Cyclothymia
F 31.9	BAD, unspecified
F 10-19	Mental and behavioral disorders due to psychoactive substance abuse
F 25.0	Schizoaffective disorder, manic type
F 25.1	Schizoaffective disorder, depressive type
F 25.2	Schizoaffective disorder, mixed type
F 25.9	Schizoaffective disorder, unspecified
F 23	Acute and transient psychotic disorder
F 23.2	Acute schizophrenic-like psychotic disorder

Source: From *International Classification of Diseases,* 10th edition. Reprinted with permission from WHO.

ICD-6 through ICD-9 and DSM-I and DSM-II

The first effort to establish a universal diagnostic system for psychiatric illnesses was made by the World Health Organization (WHO) in its 1948 ICD-6, formerly the International Classification of Causes of Death. The ICD was designed as a system that could be applied throughout the world; thus its developers attempted to encompass a great variety of conceptual backgrounds, which in turn resulted in overlap among many of its categories. The 16 different subtypes of affective disorder in ICD-9, grouped under eight different main headings, cannot readily be compared with the descriptive diagnostic systems that have recently evolved from systematic research on these disorders.

The APA's first diagnostic manual (DSM-I) was published in 1952. Although developed independently of the ICD, the American system likewise was not derived from systematic research. In DSM-I, manic-depressive reaction appeared along with psychotic depressive reaction as subcategories of affective reactions, which in turn formed one of four categories of psychosis.

In 1968, the eighth revision of the ICD appeared, as did the revised APA manual (DSM-II); the two generally paralleled each other. Manic-depressive reaction became manic-depressive illness and, with involutional melancholia, was classified under major affective disorders. Psychotic depressive reaction was removed from the affective disorders category and became a separate class. As was true of prior versions, the categories in ICD-9, which appeared in 1978, overlapped conceptually.

Empirically Based Systems: Research Diagnostic Criteria, DSM-III-R, and ICD-10

The transition from DSM-II to DSM-III and more recent systems has been characterized by a movement from psychiatric dogmas to greater reliance on empirical research. ICD-9 and DSM-II were fundamentally flawed, despite their greater use of descriptive material and implicit recognition of the bipolar–unipolar distinction, because they were essentially compromises constructed around isolated, mutually exclusive belief systems about etiology. In DSM-II, each school of psychiatric thought appeared to be assigned its own category, which reflected its own etiologic assumptions. For example, a presumed psychosocial etiology was the defining characteristic for depressions not associated with physiological disturbances or major functional impairment. Depressions associated with these latter features were presumed to be endogenous, that is, biological in origin. In both ICD-9 and DSM-II, manic-depressive illness stayed in the "endogenous" column. Neurotic (reactive) depression and psychotic depressive reaction (or reactive depressive psychoses) were excluded from the manic-depressive illness

category, implying that the presence of precipitating factors was incompatible with such a diagnosis.

Clearly, what was desperately needed was a nosological system that was etiologically neutral, a system that would allow independent assessment of the types and severity of symptoms, the presence of precipitating events, the extent of functional impairment, personality characteristics, and the presence of other psychiatric diagnoses. Without such a system, the long-standing debate pitting biological predispositions against psychological causes and social influences would remain an exercise in polemics. Likewise, attempts to foster understanding of manic-depressive illness by bridging these insular schools of thought would continue to flounder, as would efforts to clarify the relationship between affective illness and schizophrenia.

The evolution of psychiatric nosology toward DSM-III was propelled by the rise in influence of the "neo-Kraepelinian" school, based in the United States at Washington University at St. Louis. The shift was toward descriptive criteria, based to the extent possible on empirical evidence, with no etiologic commitments. Since diagnostic validity was and remains elusive, the framers of DSM-III sought to at least establish diagnostic reliability—agreed-upon empirically testable definitions—which is a prerequisite to validity. A precursor to DSM-III was the Research Diagnostic Criteria (RDC)[2] (Spitzer et al., 1978).

The systems as they have evolved thus far are by no means ideal. For example, as illustrated in Figure 3–1, the organization of both DSM-III and DSM-IV implies that bipolar disorder is distinct from all forms of major depression. This division discourages consideration of underlying unifying relationships between bipolar and the more highly recurrent forms of unipolar disorder, including the possibility that they fall along a continuum (Angst et al., 2003; Smith et al., 2005; see also Chapter 1). It appears that

Figure 3–1. DSM-IV classification of mood disorders. NOS = not otherwise specified.

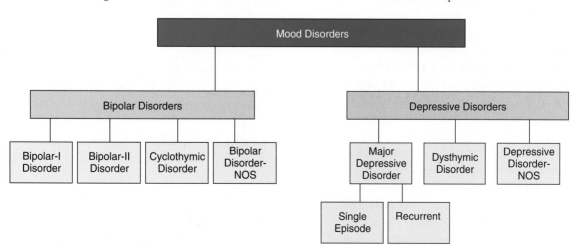

the designers of DSM-III and -IV arbitrarily chose polarity over cyclicity or recurrence as the primary principle for organizing a diagnostic system. This approach left the depressive disorder category as hopelessly heterogeneous, defined only by not being bipolar (see Chapter 1). Another drawback of DSM-III, DSM-III-R, and DSM-IV is that they lack the rich clinical descriptiveness of ICD-9.

Other criticisms can be made of the DSM-IV system in general, not just of the bipolar category. First, natural course, longitudinal patterns, and family history in recurrent affective illness are not included in the DSM-IV criteria, despite their clear importance. The lack of attention to course means that the DSM-IV schema often results in defining an episode more reliably than the disorder. For example, in longitudinal studies of patients with mixed affective and schizophrenic symptoms, numerous investigators[3] have noted a significant proportion who undergo syndrome shifts; that is, at one point in their history they can be diagnosed as schizophrenic, and at another as having an affective disorder.

Other studies of diagnostic stability—defined as the degree to which a diagnosis is confirmed at subsequent assessment points (Fennig et al., 1994)—have shown a similar propensity to diagnostic shifting, with an original diagnosis of unipolar depression later changing to one of bipolar disorder.[4] In a 20-year follow-up of 406 hospitalized depressed patients initially diagnosed as unipolar (Angst et al., 2005), the diagnoses were changed to bipolar at a rate of approximately 1.5 percent per year (1 percent to bipolar-I, 0.5 percent to bipolar-II), cumulatively 39.2 percent over the 20-year follow-up period; those with six or more depressive episodes were especially likely to be rediagnosed as bipolar. In an interesting study of the relationship of diagnostic criteria to the stability of the bipolar diagnosis, Amin and colleagues (1999) found that 91 percent of those diagnosed as bipolar according to ICD-10 maintained that diagnosis at a 3-year follow-up, compared with only 78 percent of those so diagnosed using DSM-IV (see also Chapter 3).

Another problem with DSM-IV is that since all criteria are weighted equally, a DSM-IV diagnosis cannot by itself replicate the complex process of pattern recognition by which the experienced clinician arrives at a diagnosis. The limitations of the system were emphasized by van Praag (1993, p. 97):

> One can witness a standardized interview degenerating into a question-and-answer game: answers being taken on face value, not caring for the meaning behind the words, disregarding the as-yet-unspoken and oblivious to the emotional content of the communication. . . . There is the danger of the desk researcher studying rating scale and standardized interview results rather than actual patients. These may be data collected not by himself, but by a research assistant with little psychiatric experience and training.

ICD-10 became official in 1993. Heavily influenced by the development of DSM-IV, it groups all mood disorders together by replacing manic-depressive psychosis with bipolar affective disorder and recurrent depressive disorders. ICD-10 does stay more true to the original Kraepelinian vision by linking the two recurrent forms of major affective disorder.[5] Neurotic depression, reactive depressive psychosis, and affective (cyclothymic) personality disorder are relocated to the major groups of affective disorders. The classification scheme for ICD-10 is reviewed in Box 3–1b, presented earlier.

Transition from DSM-III-R to DSM-IV

DSM-III-R was criticized for its definitions of mood disorders on a number of grounds. First, bipolar-II disorder was only a residual category and not recognized as a distinct presentation. Second, there was no operational definition of rapid cycling or mixed states. Third, there was no duration requirement for manic, mixed, or depressive episodes in bipolar disorder, leading to some confusion in distinguishing among rapid cycling, mixed episodes, and cyclothymic disorder. Fourth, certain system-level flaws from prior DSM criteria persisted, such as an absence of clinical description and no information regarding age at onset, course, or family history.

DSM-IV was introduced in 1994. Major revisions are as follows:

- Bipolar-II is designated as a diagnostic entity in its own right.
- Antidepressant-induced mood states are excluded from the diagnosis of bipolar disorder.
- Episodes are descriptive but not formally categorized with codes; instead, mood disorders are coded as either recurrent or single episode. This simple distinction between recurrent and single episode is still too broad since it includes everyone with more than one episode; more useful would be a further distinction between those with two to four (recurrent) and more than four (highly recurrent) episodes.
- Information on course, age, and gender is included. A time specification of 1 week is given for manic or mixed episodes.
- Criteria for mixed states are explicitly stated.
- A separate definition of rapid cycling is provided, based on empirical data supporting a definition of four or more episodes per year (see Chapter 4).

DSM-IV makes no change in the overall diagnostic schema for major depressive disorder.

Of the above changes, perhaps the most important clinically are the introduction of bipolar-II disorder, the definition of rapid cycling, the definition of mixed episodes, and the exclusion of antidepressant-induced mood states from the diagnosis of bipolar disorder. In general, it would appear that the DSM-IV task force attempted to balance the expansion of the bipolar diagnosis to include type II and a clearly defined rapid-cycling course with more restrictive definitions of mixed states and antidepressant-induced mania.

On the latter point, there is indeed significant evidence that antidepressant-induced mania is a predictive marker for bipolar disorder (Akiskal and Benazzi, 2003; Akiskal et al., 2003). The exclusion of this diagnostic group is not supported clinically or empirically by most of the available evidence. To quote Dunner (1998) (a member of the DSM-IV task force):

> There was a sense from the Task Force that bipolar conditions should not be overdiagnosed in the community; if they are, lithium might be too broadly applied to patients with mood disorders. . . . The criteria for bipolar II were defined in a way that is somewhat restrictive. . . . Hypomanic episodes occurring in response to treatment with antidepressant pharmacotherapy would not count toward the diagnosis of bipolar II but would instead be termed substance-induced hypomania. Frankly, this latter option makes little sense to me and is inconsistent with the natural course of bipolar disorder. . . . It is difficult to induce mania or hypomania in a true unipolar patient; there is a likelihood that patients who develop hypomania in response to treatment are actually bipolar.

Given the (probably unfortunate) reality that the majority of patients with bipolar disorder take antidepressants most of the time, it can be difficult to be sure about the identification of true spontaneous manic or hypomanic episodes.

The definition of mixed episodes (discussed further below) in DSM-IV requires that complete criteria for a major depressive episode and a manic episode be met simultaneously for 1 week. This strict definition can exclude many classic descriptions of dysphoric mania and agitated depression that have historically been referred to as mixed states and appear to share characteristics distinct from pure depression or pure mania (see Chapter 2). As discussed below, these more broadly defined mixed states may be valid categories that are, unfortunately, excluded from DSM-IV.

Finally as noted above, DSM-IV continues to leave unaddressed Kraepelin's original observation of the essential unity of the recurrent affective disorders, both bipolar and unipolar, and the possibility that these two recurrent subgroups exist along a spectrum with intermediate forms.

Thus, while DSM-IV incorporates some useful new features, it leaves considerable room for improvement. It may be hoped that this will be accomplished. The APA and the National Institute of Mental Health (NIMH) have commissioned a series of white papers on various diagnostic issues as a way to launch the process of the development of DSM-V. Also, the APA and WHO are jointly sponsoring a series of conferences to stimulate and coordinate the empirical research necessary to fill key information gaps relevant to improving current diagnostic systems; the promotion of international collaborations is a key goal of the APA–WHO effort (American Psychiatric Association, 2005). Figure 3–2 presents our proposal for the organization of mood disorders in DSM-V.

We now turn to the specific diagnostic criteria set forth in DSM-IV. For mania, depression, and mixed states, the criteria define episodes; for bipolar-II disorder, cyclothymia, and schizoaffective disorder, they include a definition of the disorder. The role of biological correlates of diagnosis is reviewed in Chapters 9, 13, 14, and 15.

DIAGNOSTIC CRITERIA

When making a diagnosis, the clinician should assess presenting signs and symptoms, and weigh them together with the patient's history and prior response to treatment, as well as the family's history. Individual symptoms—even clusters of symptoms—examined at one point in time often lack diagnostic specificity, although such cross-sectional views are sometimes the only ones available. In the following sections, we use the relevant DSM-IV categories as a framework for discussing diagnostic criteria for mania and hypomania, depression, mixed states, cyclothymia, and schizoaffective disorder. We also review problems involved in applying the DSM-IV criteria.

Mania and Hypomania

The DSM-IV definition of a manic episode is given in Box 3–2. Among the criteria for mania, perhaps the most objective is decreased need for sleep. In more subtle cases of hypomania in particular, this feature—decreased need for sleep—appears to be the most reliable single indicator of the diagnosis (Rice et al., 1992) and can alert the clinician to explore for other manic features.

As detailed in Chapter 2, the structure of mania has been examined in recent phenomenological studies using factor analytic and other methods. These studies have revealed that the most common signs of mania are motor activation, flight of ideas, pressured speech, and decreased sleep, while elated mood and increased sexuality are decidedly less common. These studies have also identified four types of mania that coincide with Kraepelin's observations:

H types of mania

BOX 3–2.   DSM-IV Definition of a Manic Episode

DSM-IV (p. 328) defines a manic episode as follows:

Criterion A: A *manic episode* is a distinct period during which there is an abnormally and persistently elevated, expansive, or irritable mood. This period of abnormal mood must last at least 1 week (or less if hospitalization is required).

Criterion B: The mood disturbance must be accompanied by at least three additional symptoms from a list that includes inflated self-esteem or grandiosity, decreased need for sleep, pressure of speech, flight of ideas, distractibility, increased involvement in goal-directed activity or psychomotor agitation, and excessive involvement in pleasurable activities with a high potential for painful consequences. If the mood is irritable (rather than elevated or expansive), at least four of the above symptoms must be present.

Criterion C: The symptoms do not meet criteria for a mixed episode.

Criterion D: The disturbance must be sufficiently severe to cause marked impairment in social or occupational functioning or to require hospitalization, or it is characterized by the presence of psychotic features.

Source: Reprinted with permission from the *Diagnostic and Statistical Manual of Mental Disorders*, Fourth Edition, Text Revision (Copyright 2000). American Psychiatric Association.

dysphoria opp. of euphoria
· depression & indifference

hypomania, acute mania, delusional mania, and depressive or anxious mania. *ie., hearing voices*

As in DSM-III-R, diagnostic criteria for manic episodes in DSM-IV include psychotic features—even the Schneiderian first-rank symptoms that some investigators have thought to be pathognomonic of schizophrenia. The framers of DSM-IV (and its DSM-III-R precursor) departed from earlier diagnostic systems because evidence had accumulated to confirm the presence of considerable thought disorder and gross psychotic content in patients clearly defined as manic by all other indicators, corresponding to Kraepelinian delusional mania. Specific exclusionary criteria are used to rule out other psychotic or secondary mental disorders, a point developed later in the section on differential diagnosis.

The diagnostic distinction between pure mania and mixed states is supported by the identification in these studies of a factor linking dysphoria in mania with depressed mood, lability, guilt, anxiety, suicidality, and the absence of elation. This finding supports the idea of frequent mixed states in manic presentations, as well as the validity of the distinction between pure mania and mixed states (see Chapter 2).

Impulsivity as a prime phenomenological feature of mania has also been underscored by the recent studies reviewed in Chapter 2. Using the Barratt Impulsiveness Scale, Swann and colleagues (2003) found that impulsivity appears to persist even outside of the acute mood state in

Figure 3–2. Mood disorders in DSM-V: a proposal. BP = bipolar; NOS = not otherwise specified.

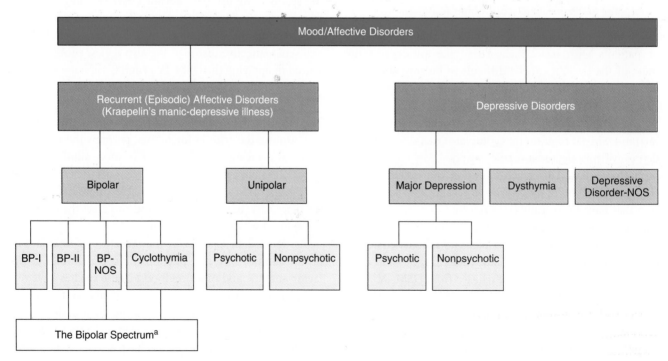

BOX 3–3.   DSM-IV Definition of a Hypomanic Episode

DSM-IV (p. 335) defines a hypomanic episode as follows:

Criterion A: *Hypomanic episode* is defined as a distinct period during which there is an abnormally and persistently elevated, expansive, or irritable mood that lasts at least 4 days.

Criterion B: Normal mood must be accompanied by at least three additional symptoms from a list that includes inflated self-esteem or grandiosity (nondelusional), decreased need for sleep, pressure of speech, flight of ideas, distractibility, increased involvement in goal-directed activities or psychomotor agitation, and excessive involvement in pleasurable activities that have a high potential for painful consequences.

Criterion C: If the mood is irritable rather than elevated or expansive, at least four additional symptoms must be present (from a list identical to that provided for a "manic episode")....Hypomanic episodes must be clearly different from the individual's usual nondepressed mood, and there must be a clear change in functioning that is not characteristic of the individual's usual functioning.

Criterion D: These changes in mood and functioning must be observable by others.

Criterion E: In contrast to a manic episode, a hypomanic episode is not severe enough to cause marked impairment in social or occupational functioning or to require hospitalization, and there are no psychotic features.

Source: Reprinted with permission from the *Diagnostic and Statistical Manual of Mental Disorders*, Fourth Edition, Text Revision (Copyright 2000). American Psychiatric Association.

---

bipolar disorder, suggesting that it may represent both a state and a trait feature of the illness.

Research on the structure of manic episodes indicates that they are stable, appearing with similar presentations if and when they recur. The symptom factors reviewed in Chapter 2 have been found to be highly correlated in separate episodes.

The inclusion of hypomanic episodes in DSM-IV was based on accumulating empirical evidence that hypomania could be diagnosed reliably by experienced clinicians using semistructured interviews (Dunner and Tay, 1993; Simpson et al., 2002; Benazzi, 2003); that it was stable; and that it could be distinguished from bipolar-I disorder or unipolar depression on the basis of symptoms, course, family history, and treatment response (Coryell et al., 1989; Dunner and Tay, 1993).[6] The diagnostic criteria for a hypomanic episode in DSM-IV, which are much more specific than those in DSM-III-R, are listed in Box 3–3.

The key differentiating feature between a manic and hypomanic episode in DSM-IV is not in the manic symptoms themselves, as they are largely the same for both diagnoses. Rather, the key difference is in the impact of those symptoms on social or occupational functioning. In a manic episode, social or occupational functioning must be characterized by "marked" impairment. In a hypomanic episode, "the episode is not severe enough to cause marked impairment in social or occupational functioning, or to necessitate hospitalization, and there are no psychotic features." In simple terms, there should be no such thing as a hypomanic hospitalized patient; if manic-like symptoms lead to hospitalization, the diagnosis must be mania, not hypomania. The same holds true if psychosis is present. With regard to functional impairment, much hinges on one's definition of the word "marked," which DSM-IV has left deliberately vague, perhaps reflecting the limited literature on the subject. Indeed, the main reason for the low reliability of a bipolar-II diagnosis in many routine clinical settings is that clinicians disagree on the limits of marked functional impairment. Hypomanic episode is one of the few if not the only major Axis I primary psychiatric diagnosis in DSM-IV in which marked impairment of social or occupational functioning is not part of the definition of the syndrome; indeed as noted, the clinician must rule out such impairment before making the diagnosis. Almost all the impairment in bipolar-II is due to the depressive phase. As Vieta and colleagues (1997, p. 100) observed:

> It is worth emphasizing that although bipolar-II disorder is milder than bipolar-I disorder in terms of manic symptoms, it is not less severe in terms of depressive morbidity. In fact, bipolar-II disorder is more severe in terms of an increased propensity for rapid-cycling and a greater number of mood episodes than bipolar-I disorder.

Another important difference between the DSM-IV definitions of mania and hypomania has to do with the duration of the syndrome, defined as 1 week for the former and a minimum of 4 days for the latter. Clinical and research experience suggests that 2 to 3 days of hypomania appears to identify a cohort of patients with a variant of bipolar illness that is milder in manic symptomatology than the classic form (Angst, 1998). Duration of 1 day or less of hypomania is more controversial, often making it difficult to distinguish the state from the rapid mood alternations of borderline personality disorder or normal variants in temperament. The following is Dunner's (1992, p. 13) account of how the 4-day minimum criterion came to be set:

> The initial definition proposed by Dunner et al. had posited a 3-day or longer duration of hypomania. This definition was based on a study of "normal" women who were being assessed for a premenstrual mood disturbance and who on interview were sometimes found to have 1–2 days

of hypomanic symptoms. Because 1–2 days of hypomania could occur in "normal" women, the proposed minimal criteria for the duration of hypomania for bipolar II patients became 3 days or more. There were no data to support the minimal duration criteria [sic] for hypomania, and the ICD-10 group had arbitrarily chosen 4 days or more as the minimal criterion. The [DSM-IV] Work Group opted for that definition in order to be consistent.[7]

Just as with mania, an exclusive focus on euphoria can miss patients in whom irritability is the primary manifestation, with hypomania, overactivity can be a more sensitive (but less specific) indicator of hypomania than euphoria (Akiskal, 2005). Angst and Cassano (2005) have argued for broadening this concept so that overactivity and/or euphoria and/or irritability are used together.

Bipolar-II disorder is defined as at least one hypomanic episode along with at least one major depressive episode. The diagnostic criteria for this condition are listed in Box 3–4. If a patient meets criteria for hypomania and has a history of depressions not severe enough to be designated as major depression, the appropriate DSM-IV diagnosis is

---

BOX **3–4.**   **DSM-IV Definition of Bipolar-II**

DSM-IV (p. 359) defines bipolar-II as follows:

Criterion A: The essential feature of bipolar-II disorder is a clinical course that is characterized by the occurrence of one or more major depressive episodes.

Criterion B: Accompanied by at least one hypomanic episode.

Criterion C: The individual experiences rapidly alternating moods (sadness, irritability, euphoria) accompanied by symptoms of a manic episode and a major depressive episode. The presence of a manic or mixed episode precludes the diagnosis of bipolar-II disorder.

Criterion D: Episodes of substance-induced mood disorder (due to the direct physiological effects of a medication, other somatic treatments for depression, drugs of abuse, or toxin exposure) or of mood disorder due to a general medical condition do not count toward a diagnosis of bipolar-II disorder. In addition, the episodes must not be better accounted for by schizoaffective disorder and are not superimposed on schizophrenia, schizophreniform disorder, delusional disorder, or psychotic disorder not otherwise specified.

Criterion E: The symptoms must cause clinically significant distress or impairment in social, occupational, or other important areas of functioning.

Source: Reprinted with permission from the *Diagnostic and Statistical Manual of Mental Disorders*, Fourth Edition, Text Revision (Copyright 2000). American Psychiatric Association.

---

cyclothymia (discussed below), which is not easily distinguishable from bipolar-not otherwise specified (NOS).

Additional discussion relevant to the bipolar-II diagnosis is included in Chapters 1 and 2. For example, Benazzi and Akiskal (2005) have offered a definition of trait mood lability and suggested that it can be used as a screening tool for bipolar-II.

Depression

DSM-IV criteria for a major depressive episode are presented in Box 3–5. As with the criteria for mania, the boundaries of major depressive disorder were considerably broadened in DSM-III-R through the incorporation of additional psychotic features, including mood-incongruent delusions, and this broadened definition carries over into DSM-IV. We return to this issue later in the section on differential diagnosis. The required minimum 2 weeks' duration is regarded as too short by many clinicians, who prefer the 1 month originally given in the criteria of Feighner and colleagues (1972).

As noted earlier in this chapter and in Chapter 1, one of the major, and in our opinion unfortunate, changes in the transition to ICD-10 and DSM-IV is that both of these nosologies, as a first principle, separate bipolar disorder from major depression (single or recurrent), thereby reinforcing the bipolar–unipolar dichotomy. Within the DSM-IV framework, there is no attempt to differentiate bipolar from unipolar depression on any grounds other than the presence or absence of a history of mania. Clinical features reported to differentiate bipolar from unipolar depression as described in Chapter 1 are not incorporated into the DSM-IV system. In contrast, ICD-9, under the rubric of manic-depressive psychoses–depressed type, properly emphasized the recurrent nature of endogenous forms of depression, implying that such depressions are closely related to bipolar illness (i.e., Kraepelin's manic-depressive illness).

Mixed States

The factor analytic studies referred to earlier (and reviewed in Chapter 2) reported two types of mixed states with marked lability of mood: one displayed depression with labile periods of pressured, irritable hostility and paranoia; the other displayed an incongruous mix of elated mood and psychosis, which would switch frequently to anxiety, depression, and irritability.

Kraepelin originally viewed mixed states as the most common form of manic-depressive illness. In fact, in the 1899 edition of his textbook, he placed a great deal of emphasis on six types of mixed states, including forms that clinicians today may label as mania (dysphoric mania) or depression (agitated depression, depression with racing

BOX 3–5.   DSM-IV Definition of a Major Depressive Episode

DSM-IV (p. 320) defines a major depressive episode as follows:

Criterion A1: The essential feature of a major depressive episode is a period of at least 2 weeks during which there is either depressed mood or the loss of interest or pleasure in nearly all activities. In children and adolescents, the mood may be irritable rather than sad. The individual must also experience at least four additional symptoms drawn from a list that includes changes in appetite or weight, sleep, and psychomotor activity; decreased energy; feelings of worthlessness or guilt; difficulty thinking, concentrating, or making decisions; or recurrent thoughts of death or suicidal ideation, plans, or attempts. To count toward a major depressive episode, a symptom must either be newly present or must have clearly worsened compared with the person's pre-episode status. The symptoms must persist for most of the day, nearly every day, for at least 2 consecutive weeks. The episode must be accompanied by clinically significant distress or impairment in social, occupational, or other important areas of functioning. For some individuals with milder episodes, functioning may appear to be normal, but requires markedly increased effort. The mood in a major depressive episode is often described by the person as depressed, sad, hopeless, discouraged, or "down in the dumps."

Criterion A2: Loss of interest or pleasure is nearly always present, at least to some degree.

Criterion A3: When appetite changes are severe (in either direction), there may be a significant loss or gain in weight, or, in children, a failure to make expected weight gains may be noted.

Criterion A4: The most common sleep disturbance associated with a major depressive episode is insomnia.

Criterion A5: Psychomotor changes include agitation (e.g., the inability to sit still, pacing, hand-wringing; or pulling or rubbing of the skin, clothing, or other objects) or retardation (e.g., slowed speech, thinking, and body movements; increased pauses before answering; speech that is decreased in volume, inflection, amount, or variety of content, or muteness).

Source: Reprinted with permission from the *Diagnostic and Statistical Manual of Mental Disorders*, Fourth Edition, Text Revision (Copyright 2000). American Psychiatric Association.

thoughts) (Marneros, 2001; Salvatore et al., 2002).[8] Recent work has confirmed that agitated depression and dysphoric mania are distinguishable syndromes—the differences lying primarily in manic-like symptoms, with depressive and anxiety features being rather similar (Swann et al., 1993). Koukopoulos (1999) considers agitated depression to be a mixed depressive state, as did Kraepelin (1921) and Waygandt (1899). This category can include cases without motor agitation but with intense psychic agitation or inner tension. To clarify the differential diagnosis between anxiety and

inner agitation, Koukopoulos has proposed certain criteria[9] (Koukopoulos et al., 2005).

A third kind of mixed state, unique to bipolar-II disorder, has also recently been proposed: the "depressive mixed state" (Benazzi, 2000b). This condition, described more fully in Chapters 1 and 2, reflects the occurrence of a major depressive episode and *at least three* hypomanic symptoms in an individual with bipolar-II disorder (past pure depressive and spontaneous "hypomanic" episodes).

Compared with DSM-III-R and ICD-10, DSM-IV provides a more definitive treatment of mixed episodes. DSM-IV still does not, however, provide separate empirically derived criteria for mixed states, but instead refers to the criteria for mania and depression. DSM-IV also avoids addressing criteria for the diagnosis of agitated depression or dysphoric mania. The main DSM-IV and ICD-10 criteria for bipolar-I disorder, most recent episode mixed, are provided in Box 3–6. DSM-IV's description is more extensive than in the past, whereas the ICD-10 definition is somewhat vague and spotty.

Despite the advance toward a clear definition of mixed episodes, the DSM-IV criteria remain unlinked to empirical

BOX 3–6.   DSM-IV and ICD-10 Definitions of a Mixed Episode

DSM-IV (p. 333) defines a mixed episode as follows:

Criterion A: A *mixed episode* is characterized by a period of time (lasting at least 1 week) in which the criteria are met both for a manic episode and for a major depressive episode nearly every day.

The individual experiences rapidly alternating moods (sadness, irritability, euphoria) accompanied by symptoms of a manic episode and a major depressive episode. The symptom presentation frequently includes agitation, insomnia, appetite dysregulation, psychotic features, and suicidal thinking.

The ICD-10 definition is as follows (p. 58)[a]:

Bipolar affective disorder, current episode mixed: The patient has had at least one authenticated hypomanic, manic, depressive, or mixed affective episode in the past, and currently exhibits either a mixture or a rapid alternation of manic and depressive symptoms.

[a]In the first edition, we also referred to the Vienna Research Criteria for Mixed States, which before DSM-IV provided the clearest definition. Unlike DSM-IV, the Vienna Research Criteria were derived more directly from empirical studies of mixed states. It appears the DSM-IV task force felt the need to provide a clear definition of mixed states in light of the burgeoning literature on the topic. Yet it chose to use the most restrictive definition possible, contrary to the empirical evidence supporting somewhat broader definition of mixed states (see discussion in the text).

Source: Reprinted with permission from the *Diagnostic and Statistical Manual of Mental Disorders*, Fourth Edition, Text Revision (Copyright 2000). American Psychiatric Association.

studies of such episodes—specifically those studies that support the validity of definitions in which criteria for mixed episodes are met by mania accompanied by as few as two or more depressive symptoms (dysphoric mania) (McElroy et al., 1992). Using this definition, for instance, one study (reviewed in Chapter 18) suggested greater treatment response with valproate than with lithium.

Some research suggests that, under the narrow DSM-IV criteria, fewer than 10 percent of episodes in patients with bipolar disorder meet criteria for a mixed episode. One study reviewed in Chapter 2 found that only 54 percent of 143 broadly defined mixed states (using Kraepelinian definitions) met DSM-III-R (or DSM-IV) criteria for a mixed episode (Perugi et al., 1997). Data suggest that using broader criteria for mixed states, incorporating the clinical concept of dysphoric mania and perhaps also agitated depression, in patients with bipolar disorder would result in more than 50 percent of episodes in bipolar disorder being diagnosable as mixed states.

Further work is needed to demonstrate empirically the appropriate boundaries for mixed states. Findings of other studies reviewed in Chapter 2 suggest that the DSM-IV criteria will need to be broadened. For instance, when dysphoric mania was defined as two or more depressive criteria plus a manic episode (McElroy et al., 1992), 36 percent of manic episodes were identified as dysphoric (Hantouche et al., 2001). In a study of the "depressive mixed state," Perugi and colleagues (1997) found that 32 patients with depressive mixed states could be distinguished from 36 patients with pure bipolar depression by the presence of increased cyclicity with greater frequency of episodes in the latter group, as opposed to longer episodes with less interepisode recovery in the depressive mixed state group (Perugi et al., 2001).

There is also some evidence, reviewed in Chapter 19, that patients with depressive "mixed states" (analogous or perhaps identical to agitated depression), unlike those with pure depression, may not respond well to antidepressants and may even worsen with their use. Thus it would appear that depressive mixed states are distinct from pure major depression in phenomenology, course, treatment response, and family history, a supposition that may justify a broadening of DSM-IV criteria for mixed episodes. It is also important to recall the point made in Chapters 1 and 2 that, while irritability often occurs in mixed states, irritability is nonspecific, occurring also in pure mania as well as in pure depression.

Cyclothymia

Consistent with our discussion of cyclothymia in Chapter 2, DSM-IV notes that the boundaries between this disorder, bipolar disorder, and bipolar-NOS are not well de-fined, and that many investigators believe cyclothymia to be simply a mild form of bipolar illness. The DSM-IV definition of cyclothymia is presented in Box 3–7.

Note that DSM-IV allows for a dual diagnosis of a major depressive, manic, or mixed episode and cyclothymia if such episodes occur after the described 2-year period. The clinical relevance of this provision is not clear. DSM-IV also allows for a dual diagnosis of borderline personality disorder, noting that the two disorders are sometimes difficult to distinguish. We find the notion of combining two diagnoses because they are difficult to differentiate questionable at best; we discuss problems involving borderline personality disorder comorbidity in Chapter 2 and in the section on differential diagnosis below.

It should be noted that the DSM-IV residual category of bipolar-NOS allows for the inclusion of many suspected

---

BOX 3–7. DSM-IV Definition of Cyclothymia

DSM-IV (p. 363) defines cyclothymia as follows:

Criterion A: *Cyclothymic disorder* is a chronic, fluctuating mood disturbance involving numerous periods of hypomanic symptoms and numerous periods of depressive symptoms.

Criterion B: The hypomanic symptoms are of insufficient number, severity, pervasiveness, or duration to meet full criteria for a manic episode, and the depressive symptoms are of insufficient number, severity, pervasiveness, or duration to meet full criteria for a major depressive episode. During the 2-year period (1 year for children or adolescents), any symptom-free intervals last no longer than 2 months.

Criterion C: The 2-year period of cyclothymic symptoms must be free of major depressive, manic, and mixed episodes.

Criterion D: After the initial 2 years of the cyclothymic disorder, manic or mixed episodes may be superimposed on the cyclothymic disorder, in which case both cyclothymic disorder and bipolar-I disorder are diagnosed. Similarly, after the initial 2 years of cyclothymic disorder, major depressive episodes may be superimposed on the cyclothymic disorder, in which case both cyclothymic disorder and bipolar-II disorder are diagnosed. The diagnosis is not made if the pattern of mood swings is better accounted for by schizoaffective disorder or is superimposed on a psychotic disorder, such as schizophrenia, schizophreniform disorder, delusional disorder, or psychotic disorder not otherwise specified.

Criterion E: The mood disturbance must also not be due to the direct physiological effects of a substance (e.g., a drug of abuse, a medication) nor a general medical condition (e.g., hyperthyroidism).

Source: Reprinted with permission from the *Diagnostic and Statistical Manual of Mental Disorders*, Fourth Edition, Text Revision (Copyright 2000). American Psychiatric Association.

cases of bipolar disorder that are excluded by the manual's rather strict definitions of hypomania and mixed episodes. Thus, bipolar-NOS

> includes disorders with bipolar features that do not meet criteria for any specific Bipolar Disorder. Examples include 1. Very rapid alternation (over days) between manic symptoms and depressive symptoms that do not meet minimal duration criteria for a Manic Episode or a Major Depressive Episode; 2. Recurrent Hypomanic Episodes without intercurrent depressive symptoms; 3. A Manic or Mixed Episode superimposed on Delusion Disorder, residual Schizophrenia, or Psychotic Disorder not otherwise specified; 4. Situations in which the clinician has concluded that a Bipolar Disorder is present but is unable to determine whether it is primary, due to a general medical condition, or substance induced. (p. 366)

In effect, most cases of bipolar spectrum illness that are more atypical than bipolar-II disorder or cyclothymia fall under the nonspecific rubric of bipolar-NOS. We should note here that, although DSM-IV does not address bipolar spectrum disorder (which is covered in Chapter 1), there is an emerging literature proposing criteria for its diagnosis.[10]

Schizoaffective Disorder

In DSM-I and -II, schizoaffective illness was included as a subtype of schizophrenia, reflecting the broad Bleulerian concept of schizophrenia as discussed later in this chapter. Subsequent research (reviewed in Chapter 2) documented the frequent occurrence of Schneiderian first-rank[11] and related schizophrenic symptoms (e.g., catatonic features, paranoia, bizarre behavior, formal thought disorder) in individuals whose family history, natural course, other symptoms, and treatment outcome clearly placed them in the manic spectrum. American psychiatry departed significantly from the Bleulerian tradition when, in DSM-III, the scope of affective illnesses was substantially broadened to include nonaffective psychotic symptoms. Schizoaffective illness was moved from schizophrenia to an intermediate category labeled "psychotic disorders not elsewhere classified." With DSM-III-R and ICD-9, schizoaffective disorder was given its own criteria. Those criteria essentially restated the acute symptoms required for a diagnosis of schizophrenia, but without continuous signs of illness for 6 months or more. The schizoaffective category was thus reserved for patients who met the acute symptomatic criteria for mania (or depression) and for schizophrenia and who had delusions or hallucinations in the absence of prominent mood symptoms for more than 2 weeks. (If the delusions or hallucinations were present for less than 2 weeks, the patient met criteria for a primary affective disorder.)

In DSM-IV, the main change is in criterion C. This criterion had previously been worded as follows: "Schizophrenia has been ruled out, [when] the duration of all episodes of a mood syndrome has not been brief relative to the total duration of the psychotic disturbance." In DSM-IV, this wording is somewhat clearer: "Symptoms that meet criteria for a mood episode are present for a substantial portion of the total duration of the active and residual periods of the illness." By still using the somewhat deliberately vague phrase "substantial portion," the DSM-IV definition seeks to increase the relevance of mood symptoms to the definition of schizoaffective disorder. In other words, one might diagnose DSM-IV schizoaffective disorder in a person with prominent mood syndromes and only a relative excess of psychotic symptoms (e.g., 2 weeks of psychosis outside of a mood syndrome). Yet one would not diagnose the disorder in a person with prominent chronic psychosis and only brief mood episodes (e.g., 2 weeks of a major depressive episode). Mood episodes must be relatively frequent and lengthy in the DSM-IV definition of schizoaffective disorder. Otherwise, the appropriate diagnosis would appear to be schizophrenia with comorbid major depressive episodes (in the case of depression). This tendency of the DSM-IV definition of schizoaffective disorder to be weighted toward the presence of mood symptoms is intended to focus this diagnosis on persons whose illness is closely related to mood disorders.

Some controversy persists over whether this newly delineated category is closer to affective illness or to schizophrenia, or whether it is a valid diagnosis in its own right. There are at least five major schools of thought on the matter, among them that schizoaffective illness represents

- A separate illness.
- An intermediate form on the continuum of psychosis.
- Comorbidity of schizophrenia and affective disorders.
- A more severe variant of bipolar disorder.
- A less severe variant of schizophrenia.

Some investigators believe that since patients with mood-incongruent symptoms are now included under mood disorders in DSM-IV, the remaining individuals with a mix of schizophrenic and affective symptoms (particularly depressive symptoms) are closer to the schizophrenic end of the schizoaffective spectrum (Kendler et al., 1986). As outlined in Chapter 13, family history studies support an association between DSM-III-R (or RDC) schizoaffective disorder and manic-depressive illness, as well as schizophrenia. Yet most studies have not found that schizoaffective disorder runs in families, as would be expected if it were a separate disease entity (Kendler et al., 1993). The genetic finding of co-occurrence of schizophrenia and bipolar disorder in at least some genealogies of schizoaffective disorder supports most strongly two of the above five models—either the continuum (described below) or co-morbidity perspective. The latter perspective, perhaps the newest, holds that schizoaffective disorder results when schizophrenia and bipolar disorder (two relatively common medical conditions) happen to occur in the same individual.

The position that schizoaffective illness will ultimately occupy on the spectrum of schizophrenia and affective illness may depend on whether one is referring to schizomanic or schizodepressive conditions. The schizomanic condition clearly appears to be associated more closely with affective illness, with a somewhat worse course than bipolar disorder (Gershon et al., 1982; Coryell et al., 1990). Schizoaffective depressed patients, by contrast, often demonstrate outcomes or neuropsychological profiles similar to those of the schizophrenic pole (Brockington et al., 1980; Tsuang and Coryell, 1993; Evans et al., 1999).[12]

An integrative perspective on these models and the associated data may be similar to that proposed by Tsuang and Simpson (1984). According to this perspective, in some individuals with predominantly manic symptoms and less pronounced psychosis, the diagnosable schizoaffective condition may represent a more severe variant of bipolar disorder. In individuals with predominantly psychotic symptoms and less pronounced mood symptoms (which are solely depressive), the diagnosable schizoaffective condition may represent a less severe variant of schizophrenia. And in others with a nearly equal mix of psychosis and mood symptoms (both mania and depression), the diagnosable schizoaffective disorder may represent a true comorbidity of schizophrenia and bipolar disorder, a condition not likely to be very common. Indeed, recent epidemiological studies have found the community prevalence of schizoaffective disorder to be a fraction of a percent, as might be expected if the comorbidity model is correct (Kendler et al., 1993, 1996). In contrast, clinical samples often show quite high diagnostic rates for schizoaffective disorder, perhaps reflecting the fact that those with more than one condition are more likely to come to clinical attention. In addition, higher rates of schizoaffective diagnosis could reflect the clinical tendency at times to overdiagnose schizoaffective disorder rather than engage in the arduous task of identifying psychotic and mood syndromes.

Problems in Applying the DSM-IV Criteria

We have discussed conceptual problems inherent in the DSM-IV system, including those engendered by the separation of bipolar disorder from depressive disorders. Here we note the practical problems that arise when applying this system in the clinical context.

As noted above, DSM-IV lists bipolar disorder first and then assigns depressive disorders to a totally separate category. This separation of categories at the outset is incompatible with the reality of clinical practice, where assessing patients with depressive symptoms is the most common diagnostic decision faced. The clinician's first task is to determine whether the patient meets criteria for major depressive disorder or dysthymia, and then to review the individual's history for evidence of bipolar or unipolar illness (if at all possible with the assistance of a family member). Compounding the problems caused by separating bipolar and depressive disorders "from the top," milder depressive states are listed only under the depressive disorders—that is, the nonbipolar disorders. A patient who is mildly or moderately depressed and also has a history of mania finds a niche in this system only by some awkward fitting. The system implies more homogeneity and separateness for the bipolar category than is justified by the data.

Clinical Summary

The nosological systems that evolved during the latter part of the 20th century are in many respects superior to those used earlier. They are, for the most part, etiologically neutral, allowing for independent assessment of the types and severity of symptoms, the presence of precipitating events, the extent of functional impairment, personality characteristics, and the presence of other psychiatric diagnoses. Problems remain in the classification of manic-depressive illness, however. For example, DSM-IV implies that bipolar disorder is a separate illness and fundamentally different from all forms of unipolar depression; this supposition goes beyond the data, especially with respect to the more recurrent forms of unipolar depression. Also troubling is the absence from all categories of affective illness of criteria concerning long-term course and family history and the failure to provide for a mild form of depression in bipolar illness. These and other features of the system are problematic for clinical as well as conceptual reasons.

THE PSYCHOSES: SEPARATE OR CONTINUOUS?

In the first edition of this volume, we emphasized the controversial and important topic of whether psychotic conditions should be classified as a few major conditions or as one continuous spectrum. The ensuing decade and a half has not resolved this debate, though overall, perhaps, the available evidence is accumulating more in support of than against the Kraepelinian dichotomy. Readers interested in the history of this topic may refer to Tables 3–1a and 3–1b.

TABLE 3–1a. The Two-Entities Tradition

Author	Schizophrenia	Manic-Depressive Illness
Kraepelin, 1896	Characterized by a steady downhill course into chronic dementia	Characterized by an episodic course with intermittent recovery.
Bleuler, 1911	Certain symptoms are specific and pathognomonic—namely, those symptoms that define splitting of thought from feeling and behavior.	Symptoms are nonspecific; diagnosis is made only after schizophrenia is excluded.
Kraepelin, 1919	Some patients appeared to recover.	Some patients followed a progressive chronic course.

TABLE 3–1b. A Schizophrenia–Affective Continuum

Study	Findings
Kasanin, 1933	Coined the term "schizoaffective psychosis" to describe a group of relatively young patients with good premorbid adjustment who in response to stress developed the rapid onset of a psychosis characterized by "marked emotional turmoil" and "false sense impressions," but without "passivity."
Langfeldt, 1937	Coined the term "schizophreniform" to describe patients who today would probably be referred to as schizoaffective.
Slater and Roth, 1969	Contended that the patient with a mix of affective and schizophrenic symptoms who is observed long enough can usually be confidently diagnosed as having either an affective illness or schizophrenia.
Brockington and Leff, 1979	Applied eight different published definitions of schizoaffective illness to a sample of patients, and found virtually no agreement among the various definitions.

The Two-Entities Tradition

Kraepelin's (1913) lucid discrimination of pattern in a mass of confusing clinical phenomena led him to propose a dichotomy of fundamentally different classes of psychotic illness. Lacking knowledge of etiology or pathophysiology, he based the distinction on family history, age at onset, course, and outcome. In his original formulation, dementia praecox was marked by a steady downhill course into chronic dementia, and manic-depressive illness followed an episodic course with intermittent recovery.

Kraepelin's original contribution was followed rapidly by the revision of Bleuler (1968), who changed the term "dementia praecox" to "schizophrenia," extended the condi-

tion's boundaries, and focused on intrapsychic symptoms. The concept of manic-depressive illness, in contrast, grew increasingly narrow with time, especially in the United States, where it attracted little interest on the part of psychoanalytic groups. A U.S.–U.K. study (Copper et al., 1972) highlighted how far American clinicians had likely gone in overdiagnosing schizophrenia and underdiagnosing manic-depressive illness. With the introduction of DSM-III, this situation gradually began shifting back to one of greater balance, though there is some evidence that bipolar disorder is still misdiagnosed as schizophrenia, particularly, perhaps, in state hospitals in the United States or in developing nations (Vieta and Salva, 1997; Ghaemi et al., 1999).

A Schizophrenia–Affective Disorder Continuum

As noted previously, the complex concept of schizoaffective disorder could be seen as a rejection of the Kraepelinian dichotomy, as suggested by Crow (1998); on the other hand, the available evidence does not support the validity of schizoaffective disorder as a unique disease entity. This view was well expressed as early as 1969, in the revision of Mayer-Gross' *Clinical Psychiatry*, in which Slater and Roth contended that the patient with a mix of affective and schizophrenic symptoms who is observed long enough can usually be confidently diagnosed as having either affective illness or schizophrenia. This assertion implies that, by and large, the schizoaffective category has reflected incomplete or imperfect diagnoses rather than a meaningful diagnostic entity.

This observation is supported in part by epidemiologic studies of schizoaffective disorder conducted since the first edition of this book was published in 1990. In both the Roscommon study (2003) and the National Comorbidity Survey, schizoaffective disorder appeared to represent a small fraction of 1 percent of the population (Kendler et al., 1993, 1996). This finding contrasts with what one might expect from the unitary psychosis model, in which schizoaffective presentations, occurring in the middle of the psychotic continuum, would be presumed to be quite frequent. The Roscommon family study in particular also appeared to provide a new explanation for schizoaffective disorder—the idea of comorbidity. It could be that if families with propensities to develop schizophrenia and bipolar disorder were to merge, some offspring would develop both types of symptoms, presenting phenotypically as schizoaffective disorder. The genetic data from that study strongly support this interpretation.

Some support for a continuum model is provided by the observation that neurobiological studies have not clearly distinguished between affective disorders and schizophrenia (Crow, 1990). This observation, if accurate in the long run, does not necessarily entail the continuum model, however. Two diseases can be different phenomenologically, as well as in their etiologies, but share many pathophysiological mechanisms. In the case of the brain, the presence of many shared "final common pathways" is a well-known feature of brain function. In any case, the neurobiological or neuropsychological findings of some studies do suggest differences between patients with schizophrenia and those with affective disorders (Keri et al., 2001), although there are enough conflicting reports to leave this question open (see Chapters 9, 14, and 15). Ketter and colleagues (2004) have proposed a mixed dimensional/categorical model that they believe allows for a more flexible approach to considering pathophysiological findings and treatment options. It is their view that a dimensional construct may be best when evaluating relationships between biological or other variables and symptoms such as psychosis in bipolar disorder or schizophrenia, while a categorical construct allows evaluation of diagnostic reliability.

Findings of a carefully conducted nosological study by Kendler and colleagues (1998) argue against the concept of a nosologic continuum. That study assessed diagnostic groupings based on family data, as well as symptom groupings. It found that most patients appeared to fall into different diagnostic categories rather than one (as suggested by Crow). Similarily, based on a factor analysis of a group of 191 psychotic patients whose diagnoses included schizophrenia and mood disorders with psychosis, Dikeos and colleagues (2006) concluded that diagnosis by itself explained the large majority of the clinical characteristics examined, although dimensional measures were more useful than diagnosis as predictors of clinical course. Others who have explored the predictive value of diagnostic versus dimensional measures in psychotic patients across both schizophrenic and affective disorder patients include van Os and colleagues (1996, 1998), Toomey and colleagues (1998), Ventura and colleagues (2000) and Serretti and colleagues (2001). Finally, another view, closer to that of Crow, is expressed by Craddock and Owen (2005, p. 364) who pointed to the emerging evidence for shared and overlapping susceptibility genes as "the beginning of the end for the Kraepelinian dichotomy," a topic that is explored in Chapter 13.

DIFFERENTIAL DIAGNOSIS

Until the 1980s, the most commonly encountered problems in making differential diagnoses of bipolar illness involved its overlapping boundaries with schizophrenia and schizoaffective illness, as well as with personality disorders, especially borderline disorders. These two major differential diagnoses remain highly important, but to them must be added the most clinically significant problem—the differential diagnosis of bipolar disorder and unipolar depression. Bipolar illness also must be distinguished from schizophreniform disorder, brief reactive psychosis, cycloid psychosis, atypical psychosis, organic brain disorders, and epilepsy. The overlap between primary affective diagnoses and substance abuse is of such importance that we address it in a separate chapter (see Chapter 7).

Schizophrenia and Schizoaffective Disorder

As discussed previously, the clinician should be able to assign the great majority of patients a diagnosis of either affective illness or schizophrenia by carefully applying the diagnostic criteria shown in Box 3–8. Schizoaffective

---

BOX 3–8.   DSM-IV Definition of Schizoaffective Disorder

DSM-IV (p. 309) defines schizoaffective disorder as follows:

Criterion A: The essential feature of schizoaffective disorder is an uninterrupted period of illness during which, at some time, there is a major depressive, manic, or mixed episode concurrent with symptoms that meet Criterion A for schizophrenia.

Criterion B: In addition, during the same period of illness, there have been delusions or hallucinations for at least 2 weeks in the absence of prominent mood symptoms.

Criterion C: Finally, the mood symptoms are present for a substantial portion of the total duration of the illness.

Source: Reprinted with permission from the *Diagnostic and Statistical Manual of Mental Disorders,* Fourth Edition, Text Revision (Copyright 2000). American Psychiatric Association.

---

disorder can sometimes be excluded by considering previous episodes; a history of either clear affective illness or clear schizophrenia cautions against diagnosing a present episode as schizoaffective.

Mania versus Schizophrenia or Schizoaffective Disorder

Differentiating mania from schizophrenia or schizoaffective illness is a diagnostic challenge often faced by clinicians. Viewed cross-sectionally, acute symptoms of irritability, anger, paranoia, thought disorder, and catatonic-like excitement cannot distinguish mania from schizophrenia. Because presenting symptoms can be similar in mania and schizophrenia, the clinician must give equal attention to the level of premorbid functioning, family history, natural course, and the character of any prior episodes. This differential diagnosis has been made more rational and straightforward by the previously discussed broadening of the criteria for mania to include a range of psychotic features.

A key DSM-IV criterion for diagnosing psychotic mania or depression in the presence of schizophrenic symptoms is the more or less continuous prominence of the affective symptoms. Thus, bizarre mood-congruent delusions or hallucinations (including Schneiderian first-rank symptoms) are not inconsistent with a diagnosis of mania as long as they have been accompanied substantially by affective symptoms most of the time (the DSM-IV criteria for mania allow for up to 2 weeks of delusions or hallucinations free of other prominent manic symptoms, whereas the RDC allow for 1 week).

If the period of quiet (i.e., affect-free) delusions or hallucinations is substantial (by criterion, exceeding 2 weeks), a diagnosis of either schizophrenia or schizoaffective illness should be considered. Schizophrenia would be diagnosed if, in addition, the patient continuously manifested overt signs of a psychotic illness for at least 6 months, and the manic symptoms were brief relative to the duration of the schizophrenic symptoms. On the other hand, schizoaffective illness, manic type, would be diagnosed if the criterion of 6 months of continuous psychotic illness were not met, but there had been more than 2 weeks of quiet delusions or hallucinations.

It is now well recognized that strict application of the Bleulerian concept of thought disorder as pathognomonic of schizophrenia can result in misdiagnosis of manic-depressive patients (see Chapters 1 and 10). More than a quarter of patients with mania have "classic" Bleulerian symptoms of schizophrenia (Pope and Lipinski, 1978).[13] See Chapter 2 for further discussion of psychosis and thought disorder in mania and schizophrenia.

Bipolar Depression versus Schizophrenia or Schizoaffective Disorder

As with mania, the DSM-IV criteria for differentiating bipolar depression from schizophrenia and schizoaffective disorder focus on the prominence of the affective symptoms, their temporal relationship to the psychotic or schizophrenic symptoms, and the length of time the patient has been continuously delusional or hallucinatory. (As for mania, the DSM-IV criteria for major depression allow for up to 2 weeks of "mood-free" delusions or hallucinations, whereas the RDC allow for 1 week.) These criteria reemphasize classic descriptions that include considerable psychosis among the affective disorders.

Studies emerging since the first edition of this book was published have emphasized other clues to psychosis in the depressive syndrome, which are especially relevant to many bipolar patients with psychotic depression (Schatzberg and Rothschild, 1992). Those clues include relatively intact insight, marked guilt, and marked psychomotor changes. Intact insight in particular can lead to an increased effort on the part of the patient to mask psychotic symptoms.

Mixed Bipolar States versus Schizophrenia or Schizoaffective Disorder

Mixed bipolar states can pose special problems of differential diagnosis because of their instability, the often confusing mix of manic and depressive symptoms, and the fact that these states occur most characteristically in association with the most severe stage of mania (stage III) (Carlson and Goodwin, 1973). Frequently associated with mixed states is the presence of alcohol or drug intoxication, which can further mask pure affective symptoms and confuse differential diagnosis.

Clinical Summary

The clinician can distinguish manic-depressive illness from schizophrenia or schizoaffective disorder in most cases by careful attention to the patient's personal and family history, premorbid functioning, age at onset, and sequence and patterning of symptoms. In manic-depressive illness, delusions or hallucinations generally follow a period of either manic or depressive symptoms, and affective symptoms are prominent almost continuously.

Unipolar Depression

As noted in Chapter 1, evidence has begun to accumulate over the last decade that the misdiagnosis of bipolar disorder as unipolar depression is a major clinical problem. There are likely five primary causes for this development: (1) patients' lack of insight with regard to manic as opposed to depressive symptoms; (2) clinicians' neglect of information available from family members or other third parties; (3) clinicians' relative focus on euphoric rather than dysphoric or irritable mood as a criterion for hypomania; (4) the structure of DSM-IV, which by separating out bipolar from all depressive disorders has obscured the close relationship between early-onset recurrent depression and bipolar disorder; and (5) widespread interest in and use of "second-generation" antidepressants.

In some clinical studies, between 40 and 60 percent of patients with bipolar disorder appear to have been misdiagnosed with unipolar depression in both inpatient and outpatient psychiatric settings (Benazzi, 1999; Ghaemi et al., 1999, 2000). Data that are not widely known because they were collected as part of a family history study (Tsuang et al., 1980) illustrate the extent of the problem. When patients who had previously been hospitalized for mania were evaluated by an extensive research diagnostic interview several years later (but without input from a family member), about 60 percent had forgotten or denied that they had ever been manic. These findings, reported in the United States, appear to hold true in other countries as well; similar results were found in Spain, for example, although the latter study also noted a high rate of misdiagnosis as schizophrenia and personality disorder (Vieta and Salva, 1997). In another study, careful evaluation of the history of 108 patients in primary care revealed that 48 (44 percent) had hypomanic symptoms, thus indicating an apparent misdiagnosis rate of about 40 percent in the primary care setting as well (Manning et al., 1997). Hence careful attention to the differential diagnosis of bipolar disorder and unipolar depression is essential.

As we note throughout this text, much of the problem of the misdiagnosis of bipolar disorder as unipolar depression has to do with the structure of DSM-IV itself (recall Fig. 3–1). Since DSM-III, the diagnostic system used in the United States has separated bipolar disorder from all depressive disorders "from the top," as does ICD-10. Major depressive episodes are always identified initially as unipolar (not bipolar), and a diagnosis of bipolar disorder relies entirely on diagnosis of a spontaneous manic or hypomanic episode. By excluding antidepressant-related mania or hypomania and by providing a very strict definition of mixed episodes, DSM-IV makes it likely that unipolar depression will be diagnosed more and bipolar disorder less frequently.

Unfortunately, in the case of the depressed patient, a diagnosis of bipolar disorder becomes entirely dependent on obtaining a history of past spontaneous mania or hypomania. A number of factors—related to both patient and clinician—mitigate against a complete and accurate diagnosis in such circumstances (see Box 3–9).

Among patient factors, lack of insight is perhaps most important. Researchers have demonstrated that about half of patients with acute mania lack insight into their symptoms (Amador et al., 1994; Ghaemi et al., 1995). Thus among depressed patients, that proportion or more would be unable to provide an accurate history of mania simply because they had never recognized having its symptoms. For example, in one study, patients reported prodromal

---

BOX 3–9. Patient, Clinician, and Illness Factors Leading to Misdiagnosis of Bipolar Disorder as Unipolar Depression

Patient Factors

- Lack of insight with regard to mania
- Impaired memory during the depressive state and/or memory selective for past depressions (state-dependent memory)
- Experiencing of hypomania as normal "good times"
- Cultural positive feedback for manic/hypomanic symptoms

Clinician Factors

- Failure to include a family member in the diagnostic evaluation
- Structure of DSM-IV, which, "from the top," separates bipolar from all depressions
- Inadequate knowledge of manic criteria
- Intuitive "prototype" approach to diagnosis
- Practical desire to make a diagnosis (e.g., unipolar depression) for which many effective treatments exist
- Lack of awareness of the high population rate of bipolar illness

Illness Factors

- First episode of illness is often depression, not mania
- Dysphoric depression is not conceptualized as a mixed state
- Depressive episodes last longer than the often fleeting hypomanic states

behavioral symptoms of mania only half as frequently as did family members (Keitner et al., 1996). These data strongly support the need to obtain family or other third-party reports (e.g., teachers, halfway-house staff, social workers, psychotherapists, friends) in assessing the bipolar diagnosis. In fact, one might reasonably say that it is virtually impossible to rule out bipolar disorder with any degree of confidence in the absence of third-party reports.

Depressed patients' self-reports are also impaired by the depressive state. As is well known, depression not only impairs memory but also makes it more likely that memories will focus on past depressions—that is, memory can be state dependent. Thus, even if patients had previously possessed some insight into their manic symptoms, they might have difficulty recalling those symptoms clearly and accurately enough for the clinician to make a definitive diagnosis. Also, patients are often in such psychic pain during a depressive episode that they may be unmotivated to search their memory carefully for times when they may have felt better (albeit pathologically). Even then the mania may be remembered simply as "good periods."

Even more challenging is the ascertainment of prior hypomania, given the ill-defined boundary between hypomania and normal good mood (Gershon et al., 1982). Indeed, patients often cannot distinguish the hypomanic state, since they may not view it as behaviorally different from their usual personality—a phenomenon recognized by DSM-IV in requiring third-party reports for the diagnosis of hypomania. Cultural factors are also relevant: in the United States, hypomanic traits are often prized and socially promoted, making it difficult for some patients, as well as some observers, to recognize them as "abnormal."

Clinician-related factors are important as well. First and foremost, clinicians are often not aware of manic symptoms. In one study, clinicians could not describe accurately more than three of the seven manic criteria when asked to write them down, as compared with their ability to describe seven of the eight major depressive criteria (Sprock, 1988). This apparent ignorance of the features of mania may be due in part to the "prototype" phenomenon (Cantor et al., 1980), which relates to diagnosis by clinical intuition alone. Clinicians often practice with prototypes of the common syndromes in mind—the "typical" patient with depression, schizophrenia, or mania. Experience over the years has taught, however, that such prototypes need to be augmented by careful attention to empirically based diagnostic criteria. Furthermore, prototypes usually represent cross-sectional symptomatic presentations (e.g., the manic patient is agitated and grandiose); we know that such observations need to be augmented with longitudinal data regarding age at onset and course, as well as family history and prior medication responses.

In the past, such intuitive diagnostic techniques tended to lead to overdiagnosis of schizophrenia and probably to underdiagnosis of major depression as well. In the last decade or so—in part as a result of major continuing medical education programs often underwritten by the pharmaceutical industry (with interests in the multitude of new antidepressants)—much greater attention has been paid to major depression, and clinicians now routinely apply DSM-IV diagnostic criteria to that disorder. The evidence suggests, in contrast, that many if not most clinicians fail to apply the diagnostic criteria for mania routinely, and instead rely on a largely intuitive approach to diagnosis of the condition. With this approach, it is likely that only patients with pure euphoric mania at the time of the evaluation will be diagnosed; mixed episodes, rapid-cycling episodes, and bipolar depressed patients will tend to be missed.

Clinicians are practitioners first and foremost. The recent tendency to diagnose bipolar disorder less frequently may relate to the relative paucity of mood-stabilizing options. The advent of new mood stabilizers appears to be generating increased interest in bipolar disorder. Unfortunately, a recent survey of the members of the National Depressive and Manic-Depressive Association (now renamed the Depression and Bipolar Support Alliance) in the United States failed to find improvement in diagnosis of bipolar disorder in 2000 (Lewis, 2001) relative to 1994 (Lish et al., 1994). About half of patients had initially been misdiagnosed with unipolar depression, and the accurate diagnosis of bipolar disorder had usually been delayed by about a decade after initial evaluations with mental health professionals. On average, more than three mental health professionals had been seen before the accurate diagnosis of bipolar disorder had been made.[14] Relatively recent clinical studies have confirmed these findings. Thus, despite increasing attention to affective disorders in recent years, follow-up of treatment experience in a U.S. advocacy group population (which admittedly is probably not representative of bipolar illness generally) revealed little improvement during the last decade in the ability of U.S. practitioners to diagnose bipolar disorder (Hirschfeld et al., 2003). In one study, the mean time to a bipolar-I diagnosis from the first visit to a mental health professional (6 years) was twice that for unipolar depression (3.3 years), and the mean time to the correct diagnosis of bipolar-II disorder was even longer (nearly 12 years) (Ghaemi et al., 2000).

Of relevance to bipolar diagnosis is a self-report questionnaire, the Mood Disorder Questionnaire (MDQ), developed as a screening instrument for bipolar disorder (Hirschfeld et al., 2000).[15] This questionnaire reflects DSM-IV criteria. Patients are asked to report whether they have experienced those symptoms, whether the symptoms occurred simultaneously, and whether they led to significant social and occupational dysfunction. The sensitivity or true positive rate (the proportion of those actually ill thus identified) and specificity or true negative rate (the proportion of those not ill thus identified) of this self-report questionnaire depend on the population it is used to evaluate. Thus, as discussed more thoroughly in Chapter 11, relatively high sensitivity was achieved among patients from a university affective disorders clinic with a high proportion of bipolar-I patients who, moreover, were likely to have been educated about their illness. By contrast, in a community-based sample (where a screening instrument is presumably most useful), sensitivity was only 28 percent; that is, the MDQ missed more than 70 percent of those diagnosed as bipolar by a clinician using the Structured Clinical Interview for DSM (SCID) (Zimmerman et al., 2004). Similarly, in an independent validation study with a clinical sample, the MDQ was found to be more diagnostically sensitive for 26 patients with bipolar-I disorder (69 percent) than for 8 patients with bipolar-II disorder (30 percent) (Miller et al., 2002). Further, patients with impaired insight would be expected to deny their symptoms on the MDQ.[16] These studies suggest that the MDQ may be more useful in a clinical than in a community setting (Hirschfeld et al., 2003). Modifications to the MDQ that might increase its utility as a screening tool in community samples have been discussed by Miller and colleagues (2004) (see Chapter 11).

Besides the issue of differential sensitivity in community versus clinical settings, the larger question is whether it is appropriate to use the MDQ as a diagnostic tool without further clinical assessment. Here the concept of predictive value is relevant (Phelps and Ghaemi, 2006). Sensitivity and specificity are characteristics of a scale; predictive values are characteristics of a sample to which the scaled is applied. If the underlying prevalence of an illness is low, then even a highly sensitive scale can have a low positive predictive value, just as a highly specific scale can have a weak negative predictive value. For instance, if the MDQ, based on its two main validation studies, is applied in a community setting where the baseline rate of bipolar illness is 10 percent, a positive predictive value of less than 45–51 percent is obtained. In other words, only about half of the MDQ-positive subjects actually have bipolar disorder. In contrast, the negative predictive value of the MDQ in such settings would be quite high, over 92–97 percent. Thus in the community setting, the MDQ can help rule out but not rule in bipolar disorder. This limitation again highlights the importance of combining the MDQ or any self-report diagnostic scale with clinician-based interview evaluations. Further, this limitation should be taken into account in some quite large research studies that assume that MDQ-positive scores are equivalent to a valid bipolar diagnosis.

In addition to clinician and patient factors, an important natural history factor can make it likely for bipolar disorder to be misdiagnosed as unipolar depression: the occurrence of depressive episodes before manic episodes in the onset of the illness (false unipolar depression). As noted in Chapters 1 and 4, this is a frequent presentation in bipolar illness, especially in females. Again, it is important to recognize that there is a relationship between false unipolar depression and age at onset. As detailed in Chapter 4, the risk of switching from false unipolar depression to bipolar disorder is highest in childhood and young adulthood, occurring at a rate of about 3 to 5 percent per year; it then decreases by the late 30s, at which point it flattens out to about 1 percent per year. Thus in any depressed child or young adult, the index of suspicion for bipolar disorder should be high, as opposed to depressed individuals in their 30s or older.

In addition to identifying past hypomanic or manic symptoms, clinicians should seek to assess clinical data in three areas that can better delineate the distinction between unipolar and bipolar depression: natural course (especially age at onset and episode frequency), family history, and treatment response.[17] (For a more detailed analysis of the distinction between unipolar and bipolar depression, see Chapter 1.)

Attention-Deficit Hyperactivity Disorder (ADHD)

In children, a major differential for the diagnosis of bipolar disorder is ADHD, a topic discussed in more detail in Chapter 6. A principal overlap in symptomatology is distractibility, which is one of the criteria for mania. Child psychiatrists report that co-occurrence of marked irritability and aggression, often with major depressive episodes, should raise suspicion of bipolar disorder, at least comorbid with ADHD (Danielson et al., 2003; Fergus et al., 2003; Scheffer and Niskala Apps, 2004; Citrome and Goldberg, 2005). Retrospective data in adults suggest that in patients with bipolar disorder, symptoms of ADHD or anxiety disorder may predominate in childhood, and mood symptoms in adolescence and early adulthood (Sachs et al., 2000). Thus in some patients, ADHD may represent an early manifestation of an overall illness that later presents as a mood disorder. Another particularly informative feature is family history of bipolar disorder, which markedly increases the likelihood of bipolar disorder as opposed to ADHD. Also, if stimulant medications are ineffective or cause worsened aggression and irritability or even manic symptoms, the likelihood of bipolar disorder increases.

Finally, further research is required to establish the validity of adult ADHD. This is especially urgent now, given that adult ADHD is becoming an increasingly common diagnosis (some of this increase in diagnosis is, no doubt, in response to a new agent being marketed with this condition as an indication).

In the National Comorbidity Survey, adult ADHD was diagnosable in about 4.4 percent of the adult population (Kessler et al., 2006). However, 86 percent of these individuals were also diagnosable with mood or anxiety disorders. The authors, and many ADHD experts view these data as simply representing comorbidity; thus the importance of diagnosing and treating adult ADHD is emphasized. An equally possible if not more logical conclusion would be that since adult ADHD is hardly diagnosable without concomitant other mood or anxiety disorder diagnoses, those other diagnoses may account for most if not all of the cognitive symptoms that are labeled ADHD. This perspective flows from an appreciation of the concept of diagnostic hierarchy, whereby mood disorders in particular can cause other kinds of symptoms (whether psychotic, anxiety, or cognitive); thus those other diagnoses should not be made in the presence of an active mood disorder (Surtees and Kendell, 1979). In other words, if those mood or anxiety disorders are adequately treated, the cognitive symptoms will improve, suggesting that no separate ADHD diagnosis is necessary. Such extensive overlap between diagnoses should raise the possibility of a single diagnosis with multiple manifestations, not simply the concept of multiple diagnoses. Further, advocates for the diagnosis of adult ADHD often point to retrospective data in adults with bipolar disorder, in which 9.5 percent of such patients are retrospectively diagnosable with ADHD in childhood (Nierenberg et al., 2005). Yet such data do not necessarily support the common presence of ADHD in adulthood, but rather are compatible with the alternative view that many children with purported ADHD develop bipolar disorder in adulthood, raising the possibility that the ADHD-like presentation in childhood may have represented an early manifestation of the bipolar illness. In other words, instead of thinking that such persons had one illness in childhood and have another in adulthood, it may be more plausible that the same illness manifested itself differently at different ages, with ADHD-like symptoms in childhood and more classic bipolar symptoms in adulthood.

In sum, given these possibilities, we would urge caution in the diagnosis and treatment of adult ADHD, always giving preference to initially diagnosing and treating mood disorders until euthymia is achieved before making the ADHD diagnosis or seeking to treat it with stimulants. Most experts would agree (given the abuse potential of stimulants) that prescribing such agents for cognitive symptoms of distractibility without first trying to treat concurrent mood or anxiety conditions is not scientifically or clinically well informed.

Brief Psychotic Disorder

Brief psychotic disorder is a DSM-IV category (see Box 3–10) reserved for individuals who experience a psychotic episode lasting from a day to a month with "eventual full return to premorbid level of functioning." The psychotic symptoms may or may not follow immediately after a major psychological or social stress, or they may occur postpartum. If the criteria for mania or major depressive episode are met, the affective diagnosis takes precedence. Often, individuals initially placed in the category of brief psychotic disorder eventually show symptoms that permit a diagnosis of either bipolar illness or schizophrenia. In particular, postpartum psychosis (often with depressive features) is highly associated with bipolar illness and may represent the first episode of the disorder (with manic episodes to follow) (Viguera and Cohen, 1998).

Cycloid Psychosis

The concept of cycloid psychosis, first described by Leonhard (1957), like that of schizoaffective disorder, a hybrid rooted in the overlapping symptoms of schizophrenia and recurrent (predominantly bipolar) affective illness, was discussed in more detail in the first edition of this volume. The condition occurs predominantly among females and

---

BOX 3–10.   DSM-IV Definition of a Brief Psychotic Episode

DSM-IV (p. 139) defines a brief psychotic episode as follows:

Criterion A: The essential feature of brief psychotic disorder is a disturbance that involves the sudden onset of at least one of the following positive psychotic symptoms: delusions, hallucinations, disorganized speech (e.g., frequent derailment or incoherence), or grossly disorganized or catatonic behavior.

Criterion B: An episode of the disturbance lasts at least 1 day but less than 1 month, and the individual eventually has a full return to the premorbid level of functioning.

Criterion C: The disturbance is not better accounted for by a mood disorder with psychotic features, by schizoaffective disorder, or by schizophrenia and is not due to the direct physiological effects of a substance (e.g., a hallucinogen) or a general medical condition (e.g., subdural hematoma).

Source: Reprinted with permission from the *Diagnostic and Statistical Manual of Mental Disorders,* Fourth Edition, Text Revision (Copyright 2000). American Psychiatric Association.

has a good prognosis. One study of 73 inpatients who met Perris's (1988) criteria for cycloid psychosis concluded that it is best regarded as an atypical variety of affective psychosis (Cutting, 1990). However, a more recent controlled family study of cycloid psychosis found a significantly lower morbidity risk for bipolar illness in first-degree relatives compared with relatives of patients with bipolar illness (Pfuhlmann et al., 2004). The authors concluded, therefore, that cycloid psychosis cannot be integrated into either the bipolar or the schizophrenic spectrum, but exists as an independent entity. Because of these conflicting results, further research is needed. Given the genetic vulnerability to psychosis that may cross the schizophrenia–affective boundary, it will be interesting to see what genetic studies of cycloid psychosis ultimately reveal.

Psychotic Disorder-Not Otherwise Specified

Classically, atypical psychosis was diagnosed in patients who had schizophrenic symptoms but showed rapid fluctuations in emotional states, an episodic course, and a generally favorable outcome. Mitsuda (1965) concluded from his study of monozygotic twins that atypical psychosis could be distinguished genetically from schizophrenia and, to a lesser extent, from manic-depressive illness. However, the relationship between this disorder and the cycloid psychosis delineated by Leonhard (1957) and Perris (1990) is not clear.

In DSM-IV, psychotic disorders-NOS is a residual category for patients with psychotic symptoms who do not meet criteria for any other DSM-IV disorder. For purposes of differential diagnosis, such patients would appear to fall in the schizoaffective spectrum.

Borderline Personality Disorder

The overlap between bipolar disorder and borderline personality disorder is quite controversial, and is discussed in more detail in Chapters 10 and 11. As a clinical rule of thumb, however, it may be good practice to use great caution in diagnosing borderline personality disorder in the midst of an active affective disorder (Parker et al., 2004). In other words, during a major depressive or hypomanic/manic episode, patients often may meet criteria for borderline personality disorder, whereas once the episode has ended, borderline features are no longer evident. Thus if possible, it is best to evaluate borderline personality disorder during periods of euthymia.

Making a differential diagnosis between bipolar depression and the depressive affect associated with borderline personality disorder involves attention to issues of lability, reactivity, and the overall symptom cluster. The depressive affect associated with borderline personality disorder is marked by considerable day-to-day or even hour-to-hour

variability, whereas the depressive mood associated with a bipolar episode is generally experienced as a discrete episode with a clear onset and termination and a relatively stable course during the episode. The mood of the borderline patient is more likely to remain reactive to the environment and, although intensely dysphoric, to change quickly with an appropriate stimulation or intervention. As noted earlier, the symptom cluster of bipolar depression generally involves pervasive changes in the regulation of sleep and appetite (usually hyperphagia and hypersomnia). These features are not associated as prominently with depressive mood in the borderline patient unless bipolar disorder also is present.

In evaluating elevated mood, duration is important as well. Given the extreme lability of mood in borderline personality disorder, mood elevation probably does not last long enough to meet the criteria for mania. On duration alone, the mood elevation in borderline personality disorder could overlap with that in hypomania or cyclothymia. The usual associated symptoms of hypomania, however, such as racing thoughts and decreased need for sleep, are generally not part of the mood lability of the borderline patient. The absence of events either precipitating or terminating the hypomanic mood would also suggest a true case of bipolar disorder, as would a positive family history of the disorder, although the latter would not be conclusive. In practical terms, emphasis on the linkage between borderline and bipolar diagnoses is important because all too often, the diagnosis of bipolar disorder is missed when borderline features are also present, especially in adolescents. As discussed in Chapter 6, bipolar disorder can be especially difficult to diagnose in this age group, since a wide range of apparently nonspecific symptoms is common. Not infrequently, moreover, individuals rediagnosed as bipolar on follow-up experienced their first manic or hypomanic episode after exposure to an antidepressant drug. The possibility of this outcome argues for considerable care in ruling out a bipolar diathesis before treating depressive syndromes in adolescents with presumed borderline features.

It is our impression that many patients who may have bipolar disorder, particularly the rapid-cycling type II variety, receive a diagnosis of borderline personality disorder because of an overreliance on the intuitive prototype approach described above. The clinical picture of the rapid-cycling bipolar patient can approximate that of borderline personality cross-sectionally. However, careful application of the criteria for mania or hypomania often distinguishes rather clearly between patients with bipolar disorder and characterological illness (Akiskal, 2005; Benazzi, 2000a).[18] In some settings, moreover, patients with borderline personality disorder may be mistakenly diagnosed as bipolar when the clinician relies overly on mood lability alone for a bipolar diagnosis, rather than assessing both the full criteria for a mood episode and the unique course features associated with bipolar disorder (Berns et al., 2003).

Organic Brain Disorders

Since manic-depressive illness has its own underlying biological foundation, differentiating it from secondary brain disorders can be semantically and diagnostically confusing. DSM-IV represents an advance over DSM-III-R in this regard. Whereas DSM-III-R applied the term "organic" to disorders in which psychological and behavioral abnormalities are "associated with transient or permanent dysfunction of the brain," DSM-IV refers to "secondary" psychiatric disorders, in which symptoms are secondary to a specific medical condition, a specific medication or other substance, or identifiable conditions such as delirium or dementia of the Alzheimer's type. With DSM-IV, the designations "functional" and "organic" were replaced by "primary," meaning no definitive established etiology, and "secondary," with reference to the specific established etiology. This terminology is more precise and accurate, and allows for the fact that many primary psychiatric disorders, such as manic-depressive illness, may have biological etiologies that are not yet identifiable. The catch-all DSM-III-R diagnoses of "organic mood syndrome" and "organic personality syndrome," which often overlapped with manic-depressive illness, do not appear in DSM-IV.

The absence of specific pathognomonic neuropsychiatric manifestations of secondary brain disorders means that differentiating these disorders from bipolar illness requires an understanding of the variety of potentially associated conditions. Some behavioral features—principally changes in cognitive function, including impairment of orientation, memory, general intellectual function, and judgment—are more prominent in most of these disorders than in bipolar illness (see Chapter 9). Of comparable importance in making a differential diagnosis is a history of bipolar illness. However, the absence of such a history does not rule out primary bipolar illness, especially when the patient is still within the age of risk for onset of the disorder; here a positive family history of bipolar disorder can be helpful.

A standard neurological examination usually does not aid in differential diagnosis, since in most organic psychiatric syndromes, the results of such an examination remain normal until the disease is far advanced. The so-called soft neurological signs often thought to mark secondary brain disease have not proven to be specific.

Neuropsychological testing can be helpful in quantifying the extent of impairment but is not particularly useful in the initial differential diagnosis. This is so because, as detailed in Chapter 9, both depression and mania can be associated with substantial disturbances in responses on a wide variety of neuropsychological tests designed to measure cognitive changes. Procedures such as magnetic resonance imaging (MRI), computed tomography (CT) scans, and electroencephalograms (EEGs) may be helpful, but unless they can identify a localized lesion, they have not yet proven reliable in differentiating secondary brain disorder from bipolar illness. Newer methods, such as functional MRI (fMRI), positron emission tomography (PET), and single photon electromagnetic transmission (SPECT), provide enhanced functional assessments of anatomic function, which can be particularly useful in assessing changes during varying mood states. However, their utility remains limited primarily to research.

The Concept of Secondary Affective Episodes

Krauthammer and Klerman (1978) made an important conceptual contribution by reviewing the literature for reports of manic syndromes occurring shortly after medical, pharmacological, or other somatic dysfunctions. As described previously, DSM-IV places a great deal of emphasis on secondary causes of mania or hypomania. Box 3–11 lists conditions that have been associated with secondary manic or hypomanic symptoms.

Studies of secondary mania are uncommon. One study found that EEG abnormalities in patients with bipolar disorder predicted better valproate than lithium response (Stoll et al., 1994). Studies of secondary depression are more common. Its occurrence is frequently related to stroke or other neurological disorders (Whyte and Mulsant, 2002).

In general, while the primary–secondary distinction in psychiatry has not been carefully validated, it appears to have clinical utility and theoretical attraction.[19] As discussed in Chapter 1, however, an alternative to dividing mania and depression into primary and secondary categories is a spectrum model reflecting varying levels of vulnerability. The greatest vulnerability would be expressed as a *primary* case, in which little or no external stress was required; lower levels of vulnerability might show up only as *secondary* cases, that is, requiring the operation of external factors for the episode to appear. (For a more complete discussion of secondary affective presentations, see Chapter 17.)

We now review three specific secondary conditions: two related but nonaffective states—delirium and dementia—and epilepsy.

Delirium

The DSM-IV diagnostic criteria for delirium are given in Box 3–12. Severe (stage III) mania (Carlson and Goodwin, 1973) can involve clouding of consciousness, occasionally rendering it difficult to differentiate from delirium

BOX 3–11. DSM-IV Features Associated with Secondary Mania or Hypomania

DSM-IV (p. 328) defines features associated with a manic episode as follows:

Individuals with a manic episode frequently do not recognize that they are ill and resist efforts to be treated. Ethical concerns may be disregarded even by those who are typically very conscientious. The person may be hostile and physically threatening to others. Some individuals, especially those with psychotic features, may become physically assaultive or suicidal. Adverse consequences of a manic episode (e.g., involuntary hospitalization, difficulties with the law, or serious financial difficulties) often result from poor judgment and hyperactivity. Some individuals describe having a much sharper sense of smell, hearing, or when catatonic symptoms (e.g., stupor, mutism, negativism, and posturing) are present, the specifier with catatonic features may be indicated (see p. 382). Mood may shift rapidly to anger or depression. Depressive symptoms may last moments, hours, or, more rarely, days. Not uncommonly, the depressive symptoms and manic symptoms occur simultaneously. No laboratory findings that are diagnostic of a manic episode have been identified. However, a variety of laboratory findings have been noted to be abnormal in groups of individuals with manic episodes compared with control subjects. Laboratory findings in manic episodes include polysomnographic abnormalities, increased cortisol secretion, and absence of dexamethasone nonsuppression. There may be abnormalities involving the norepinephrine, serotonin, acetylcholine, dopamine, or gamma-aminobutyric acid neurotransmitter systems, as demonstrated by studies of neurotransmitter metabolites, receptor functioning, pharmacological provocation, and neuroendocrine function.

DSM-IV (p. 335) defines features associated with a hypomanic episode as follows:

Associated features of a mixed episode are similar to those for manic episodes and major depressive episodes. Individuals may be disorganized in their thinking or behavior. Because individuals in mixed episodes experience more dysphoria than do those in manic episodes, they may be more likely to seek help. Laboratory findings for mixed episode are not well studied, although evidence to date suggests physiological and endocrine findings that are similar to those found in severe major depressive episodes.

Source: Reprinted with permission from the *Diagnostic and Statistical Manual of Mental Disorders*, Fourth Edition, Text Revision (Copyright 2000). American Psychiatric Association.

BOX 3–12. DSM-IV Definition of Delirium

DSM-IV (p. 127) defines delirium as follows:

Criterion A: The essential feature of a delirium is a disturbance of consciousness that is accompanied by a change in cognition that cannot be better accounted for by a preexisting or evolving dementia. The disturbance develops over a short period of time, usually hours to days, and tends to fluctuate during the course of the day. The disturbance in consciousness is manifested by a reduced clarity of awareness of the environment. The ability to focus, sustain, or shift attention is impaired.

Criterion B: There is an accompanying change in cognition (which may include memory impairment, disorientation, or language disturbance) or development of a perceptual disturbance.

Criterion C: In mild delirium, disorientation to time may be the first symptom to appear. Disorientation to self is less common. Language disturbance may be evident as dysnomia (i.e., the impaired ability to name objects) or dysgraphia (i.e., the impaired ability to write). In some cases, speech is rambling and irrelevant, in others pressured and incoherent, with unpredictable switching from subject to subject. The disturbance develops over a short period of time and tends to fluctuate during the course of the day.

Source: Reprinted with permission from the *Diagnostic and Statistical Manual of Mental Disorders*, Fourth Edition, Text Revision (Copyright 2000). American Psychiatric Association.

(see Chapter 2) (Fink, 1999). Indeed, delirious mania was well described by Kraepelin (1921) and others. The absence of the preceding stages of mania or of a history of mania is sometimes helpful in making this differential diagnosis. Perceptual disturbances usually have a more sudden onset in delirium than in stage III mania. The sustained euphoria (or irritability) characteristic of mania, by contrast, is not likely in delirium.

As with all diagnoses of organic brain disorders, indications (from the patient's history, physical examination, or laboratory data) of a specific organic etiological factor are important to the diagnosis. As noted in Chapter 7, manic episodes are commonly associated with substance abuse, particularly in young patients, and here the challenge is to differentiate a pure organic delirium from a manic episode precipitated and colored by alcohol or drugs.

Dementia

The DSM-IV criteria for dementia, given in Box 3–13, overlap somewhat with those for delirium. The considerable attention that has been paid to differentiating between true dementia and depressive pseudodementia is often justified since the pseudodementia associated with depression is highly treatable. Recent data suggest, however, that depression in the elderly can often herald dementia, making the distinction less exclusive than may earlier have been assumed (Jorm, 2000). As discussed in Chapter 9, bipolar patients in particular often experience profound deficits in

BOX 3–13.   DSM-IV Definition of Dementia

DSM-IV (p. 139) defines dementia as follows:

Criterion A1: The essential feature of a dementia is the development of multiple cognitive deficits that include memory impairment and at least one of the following cognitive disturbances: aphasia, apraxia, agnosia, or a disturbance in executive functioning. Memory impairment is required to make the diagnosis of a dementia and is a prominent early symptom.

Criterion A2a: Deterioration of language function (aphasia) may be manifested by difficulty producing the names of individuals and objects.

Criterion A2b: Individuals with dementia may exhibit apraxia (i.e., impaired ability to execute motor activities despite intact motor abilities, sensory function, and comprehension of the required task).

Criterion A2c: Individuals with dementia may exhibit agnosia (i.e., failure to recognize or identify objects despite intact sensory function).

Criterion A2d: Disturbances in executive functioning are a common manifestation of dementia and may be related especially to disorders of the frontal lobe or associated subcortical pathways.

Criterion B: The items in both Criterion A1 (memory impairment) and Criterion A2 (aphasia, apraxia, agnosia, or disturbance in executive functioning) must be severe enough to cause significant impairment in social or occupational functioning (e.g., going to school, working, shopping, dressing, bathing, handling finances, and other activities of daily living) and must represent a decline from a previous level of functioning. The nature and degree of impairment are variable and often depend on the particular social setting of the individual.

Source: Reprinted with permission from the *Diagnostic and Statistical Manual of Mental Disorders,* Fourth Edition, Text Revision (Copyright 2000). American Psychiatric Association.

cognition and memory, and consequently are sometimes misdiagnosed as having primary dementia. This misdiagnosis occurs most frequently with elderly patients, in whom clinicians tend to neglect affective symptoms and focus instead on somatic and cognitive symptoms. Although a history of manic or depressive episodes is quite helpful in making this differential diagnosis, it cannot be used absolutely: on the one hand, a small percentage of bipolar patients do not have their first episode until they are in their 50s or 60s; on the other hand, bipolar patients may independently develop dementia later in life. Since a high proportion of late-onset bipolar patients have frequent cycles (see Chapter 4), the clinical picture may convey chronicity and therefore appear to be associated with an organic etiology.

Other aspects of the depressive syndrome, such as sleep and appetite dysregulation, are not especially helpful in differentiating bipolar illness from dementia. Neuropsychiatric testing can be useful, especially if a focal lesion is involved, but it cannot be relied upon to establish a clear differential because bipolar depression can also be associated with profound cognitive impairment. As with other differential diagnostic questions, it is important to look for atypical forms of mania in the patient's history, particularly episodic irritability or agitation in the absence of euphoria. The periods of secondary affective lability sometimes associated with primary dementing illnesses do not appear as discrete episodes. Obviously, a definitive diagnosis can be made if an organic cause for the dementia can be uncovered. Box 3–14 lists diseases or conditions that have been associated with dementia.

Because of its enormous public health importance, the issue of acquired immunodeficiency syndrome (AIDS) dementia deserves special attention (Melton et al., 1997). The human immunodeficiency virus (HIV) belongs to a class of retroviruses that are neurotrophic; that is, they have a special affinity for the nervous system. By the time AIDS has reached its peak, involvement of the central nervous system is almost universal. More important to the issue of

BOX 3–14.   DSM-IV Definition of Diseases Associated with Dementia

DSM-IV (pp. 133–134) defines the physical examination findings and general medical conditions associated with dementia as follows:

The associated physical examination findings of dementia depend on the nature, location, and stage of progression of the underlying pathology. The most common cause of dementia is Alzheimer's disease, followed by vascular disease, and then by multiple etiologies. Other causes of dementia include Pick's disease, normal-pressure hydrocephalus, Parkinson's disease, Huntington's disease, traumatic brain injury, brain tumors, anoxia, infectious disorders (e.g., human immunodeficiency virus [HIV], syphilis), prion diseases (e.g., Creutzfeldt-Jakob disease), endocrine conditions (e.g., hypothyroidism, hypercalcemia, hypoglycemia), vitamin deficiencies (e.g., deficiencies of thiamine, niacin, vitamin B), immune disorders (e.g., polymyalgia rheumatica, systemic lupus erythematosus), hepatic conditions, metabolic conditions (e.g., Kufs' disease, adrenoleukodystrophy, metachromatic leukodystrophy, and other storage diseases of adulthood and childhood), and other neurological conditions (e.g., multiple sclerosis).

Source: Reprinted with permission from the *Diagnostic and Statistical Manual of Mental Disorders,* Fourth Edition, Text Revision (Copyright 2000). American Psychiatric Association.

differential diagnosis, however, is the finding that among 20–25 percent of AIDS patients, the presenting symptoms originate in the central nervous system. These early AIDS symptoms may be difficult to distinguish from depression (Price et al., 1986; Bridge et al., 1988). Mania has also been reported as an early symptom (Gabel et al., 1986; Lyketsos et al., 1997; Yang et al., 2005). As the condition progresses, memory, concentration, and rapid alternating movements are impaired. Other indications include pyramidal tract signs, ataxia, leg weakness, and tremor. AIDS dementia becomes the presumptive diagnosis when the antibody test is positive. In addition, neuropsychological tests and MRI scans may be helpful in making the differential diagnosis. Of course it must be remembered that bipolar patients may also have AIDS, perhaps at a higher rate than comparable populations, given the prominence of reckless sexual behavior during mania.

Epilepsy

Epilepsy comprises a group of disorders of the central nervous system that, like other organic disorders, must be differentiated from bipolar illness. The condition is commonly associated with psychiatric symptoms, which can be divided into those occurring during actual seizure activity and those manifested only during interictal periods.

Findings of epidemiologic surveys of large numbers of patients with epilepsy (see, e.g., Gibbs and Gibbs, 1952) indicate that psychotic symptoms are about 10 times more likely to occur in association with temporal lobe than with generalized epilepsy (reviewed by McKenna et al., 1985; Kanner, 2004). The psychoses associated with temporal lobe epilepsy were initially described at a time when the broad Bleulerian concept of schizophrenia was prevalent. It is thus not surprising that patients with these psychoses tended to be described as schizophrenic, and less frequently as affectively ill. Clinically, these psychoses are generally mixed syndromes with a prominence of visual and olfactory hallucinations, rapid fluctuations of mood, catatonic features, and dreamlike states—all of which occur in an episodic course.

In his studies of patients with temporal lobe epilepsy, Flor-Henry (1969) found that 40 percent had either manic-depressive or schizoaffective features, and 42 percent had predominantly schizophrenic symptoms. Further frustrating attempts to understand the association between psychosis and temporal lobe epilepsy is the fact that patients can at times manifest predominantly affective symptoms and at other times predominantly schizophrenic symptoms. Flor-Henry also found an association between ictal laterality and type of mood syndrome: left-side epileptic foci in temporal lobe epilepsy were associated with depressive syndromes, whereas right-side epileptic foci were associated

with manic syndromes. While intriguing, this observation has not been well replicated. Conversely, Post and Weiss (2004) at the NIMH observed a relatively high frequency of epileptic-like phenomena in bipolar patients, particularly those with rapid cycles.

The specific relationship between epilepsy per se and bipolar disorder is relatively understudied. The most recent study of the topic compared 13 patients with generalized epilepsy and interictal manic episodes and 13 patients with primary bipolar disorder (Kudo et al., 2001). In that study, patients with epilepsy and mania tended to experience somewhat less severe manic episodes than did patients with primary bipolar disorder. The epileptic patients also tended to have substance-induced episodes somewhat more frequently than the primary bipolar disorder group. The epileptic foci were frontal or temporal in location.

Clinical Summary

Given the possibility that the pathophysiology of manic-depressive illness may overlap with that of some identifiable brain disorders, differential diagnosis cannot easily be reduced to simple formulas. For practical purposes, however, a differential diagnosis is critical to making an accurate treatment selection and prognosis. Thus, the clinician's first task when presented with manic or depressive symptoms is to consider other (possibly correctable) factors that might explain the symptoms. The absence of a personal or family history of affective illness and poor response to traditional treatments for manic-depressive illness are important clues suggesting the possibility of an organic etiology (McElroy et al., 1992). Although no single medical screening test is definitive, certainly a neurological examination, formal neuropsychiatric testing, an MRI, an EEG, a CT scan, and a chemical screen for metabolic and toxic disturbances should supplement the careful taking of the patient's history. Where the evidence points to a possible commingling of manic-depressive illness and a seizure disorder diathesis, anticonvulsants with a primary effect on temporal lobe disorders (e.g., carbamazepine, valproate, or lamotrigine) should be the treatment of choice.

CONCLUSIONS

To make an accurate diagnosis of bipolar disorder, the patient's history should be reviewed carefully with the patient *and* a family member; this focus on history is at least as important as a full description of the presenting episode. Whenever possible, the onset, duration, and treatment response of all past episodes should be recorded on a life chart, along with important life events. Much of this information can be obtained before the initial appointment by having the patient and family members fill out a life chart form. The most important differential diagnostic issue in evaluating depression is determining whether the patient has a unipolar or bipolar form of the illness. Obviously, this distinction must rest on knowledge of the patient's history, especially any prior episodes of mania or hypomania. Once again we must emphasize the importance of obtaining information from the family, especially given that impairment of insight is a major problem in about half of patients with bipolar disorder. Without family input, more than half of patients with a prior history of mania will deny or forget it, and the resulting overdiagnosis of unipolar depression is even more likely when the bipolar history involves hypomania only.

If the patient has had two or more previous depressions without evidence of mania or hypomania, an age at onset above 25 or 30, and a family history negative for bipolar disorder, it is reasonably safe to assume a unipolar diagnosis, even though about 10 percent of such patients will later develop a manic episode and be reclassified as bipolar. In children and adolescents presenting with depression, the likelihood of an eventual bipolar course is much higher. As noted above, a family history of mania can provide an important clue to a possible bipolar diathesis, and may be helpful in choosing a mood stabilizer over an antidepressant for the treatment of highly recurrent depression. When manic-like symptoms characterize the presenting picture, the clinician may face difficult questions of differential diagnosis. If a patient is in the hyperactive psychotic state described as stage III mania (see Chapter 2) and a complete patient or family history is not available, the clinician must rely on an analysis of the presenting symptoms. (If there is a history of manic or depressive episodes, especially with well intervals, bipolar illness is the presumptive diagnosis, despite the atypical presenting symptoms.)

The principal alternative diagnoses that should be ruled out in diagnosing the manic phase of bipolar illness are acute schizophrenia and psychoses secondary to substance abuse or a general medical condition, although the latter can, and often do, occur in an individual with bipolar illness. The presence of delusions (including paranoid delusions), hallucinations, and thought disorder does not support a diagnosis of schizophrenia over that of mania. Schizophrenia should be suspected, however, if the delusions are organized into a formal and stable system that has continued for a considerable time in the absence of prominent mood symptoms. As a practical matter, differentiating acute stage III mania from schizoaffective illness and schizophrenia is not absolutely critical, since the initial treatment—antipsychotic medication (especially an atypical agent)—often is essentially the same for all three. If an affective component is suspected, the addition of a mood stabilizer, such as lithium or an anticonvulsant, should be considered. When the acute psychotic episode is under control, differential diagnosis often becomes clearer, even if information on the patient's personal or family history is still missing. If delusions or hallucinations persist in the absence of manic mood or hyperactivity (i.e., the patient is quietly delusional), schizophrenia or schizoaffective disorder is the more appropriate diagnosis. If the patient meets criteria for both schizophrenia and affective illness in the present episode or by history, schizoaffective illness is the appropriate diagnosis. Care should be taken to avoid overuse of the schizoaffective diagnosis simply because the patient's past history is unavailable. Distinguishing between bipolar disorder and schizophrenia can be particularly difficult in an adolescent because at that age, psychotic features are especially common in manic syndromes.

When vivid hallucinations (especially visual ones) or delusions dominate the clinical picture, particularly in a young person, a drug-induced state should be suspected, and a urine screen becomes especially important. Indeed, for most adolescent patients, it is sensible to employ a urine screen routinely. True mania may be present even if these suspicions are borne out, because it is not at all uncommon for initial manic episodes to be precipitated by drugs of abuse. In such cases, differential diagnosis can be difficult during the acute phase.

When presented with milder manic-like symptoms (or a history of such symptoms), the clinician must differentiate between clinical hypomania and normal elevated mood. Here it is important to recall the spectrum concepts outlined in Chapter 1. The threshold for a DSM-IV diagnosis of hypomanic episode is reached when (1) elation, excitement, and/or irritability cluster in discrete episodes lasting at least 4 days; (2) the symptomatic criteria outlined previously are met; (3) symptoms are out of proportion to any environmental precipitant; (4) symptoms represent a clear change in the individual's normal functioning; and/or (5) the episodes have a high potential to result in negative social, professional, and/or financial consequences. While the criteria for hypomania can be met without (4) or (5), the latter are prominent in the DSM-IV definition of a hypomanic episode. Again, we cannot overstate the importance of obtaining corroborating information from a spouse or other family member in evaluating the presence (or history) of hypomanic symptoms.

When presented with psychotic depressive symptoms, the clinician faces a somewhat different diagnostic challenge. Again, assuming that no history is available, one must rule out schizophrenia and schizoaffective illness, drug-induced states, and dementia. If delusions are present, they should be depressive in content to support an affective diagnosis. Among the depressive disorders, delusions are more likely to be associated with the bipolar form. Differentiating the bipolar form of manic-depressive illness from personality disorders or post-traumatic stress disorder (PTSD) is complex. Frequently, the conditions can co-occur. If any acute episodes meet the criteria for mania or hypomania, bipolar disorder should be diagnosed, regardless of the extent of concomitant PTSD or personality disorder features. If the course is almost completely characterized by physical or sexual trauma, along with the typical features of borderline personality (interpersonal conflict and rage, repeated self-injury, manipulative relationships), then the occurrence of mood lability *by itself* likely will not justify the bipolar diagnosis. Again, attention should be paid to family history, and more emphasis placed on course of illness rather than acute presentation.

NOTES

1. Andreasen et al., 1981; Tsuang et al., 1981; Andreasen and Grove, 1982; Keller and Baker, 1991; Blacker and Tsuang, 1992; Dunner, 1992; DeBattista et al., 1998; Goodwin and Ghaemi, 1998.

2. The RDC, together with the Schedule for Affective Disorders and Schizophrenia, proved to be reliable diagnostic instruments when used by interviewers from different centers around the country to rate past psychiatric symptoms and lifetime diagnoses in patients who were mentally ill at the time of assessment. However, the lifetime diagnoses of hypomania and recurrent unipolar depression were not as reliable as other categories (Keller et al., 1981).

3. Angst, 1980; Marneros et al., 1988, 1989, 1991, 2000; Maj et al., 1989.

4. Akiskal et al., 1995; Goldberg et al., 1995, 2001, Kessing, 2005.

5. Outside the United States, most of the rest of the world is characterized by geographically stable populations, making it easier to recognize the recurrent nature of the affective disorders.

6. Not all studies are consistent. For instance, one study found that bipolar-II disorder was much less stable (33 percent unchanged diagnostically 6 years later) than bipolar-I disorder (60 percent unchanged); it also found that decreased need for sleep was the best predictor among diagnostic criteria for bipolar-II disorder (Rice et al., 1992). Dunner also found that the reliability of the bipolar-II diagnosis was much greater when made by clinicians with expertise in mood disorders than when based solely on research diagnostic instruments such as the Structured Clinical Interview for DSM (SCID) (Dunner and Tay, 1993).

7. Testing the DSM-IV definition, Benazzi (2001) reported that almost all patients who met the DSM-IV definition of bipolar-II disorder also experienced 2 to 3 days of hypomania.

8. A recent excellent historical review demonstrated that Kraepelin's original conception of mixed states was derived largely from Weygandt, and that Kraepelin and Weygandt viewed mixed states not as uncommon, but as being the most common form of manic-depressive illness (Salvatore et al., 2002).

9. Along with major depression and inner agitation, at least three of the following symptoms must be present: (1) racing or crowded thoughts, (2) irritability or unprovoked feelings of rage, (3) absence of signs of retardation, (4) talkativeness, (5) dramatic descriptions of suffering or frequent spells of weeping, (6) mood lability and marked emotional reactivity, and (7) early insomnia (which is often associated with racing or crowded thoughts).

10. See Chapter 2; also, especially, Akiskal, 1996, 2002; Ghaemi et al., 2002.

11. The Schneiderian first-rank symptoms that overlap most commonly between schizophrenia and manic-depressive illness include thought broadcasting, thought insertion, experiences of influence, delusional perceptions, and incomplete auditory hallucinations (Schneider, 1959). Descriptive data suggest that manic patients with first-rank and/or catatonic symptoms cannot be distinguished from those without such symptoms on the basis of family history or treatment response (Jampala et al., 1989). Jampala and colleagues (1985) reported that manic patients with so-called emotional blunting—"a constricted, inappropriate, unrelated affect of diminished intensity, with indifference or unconcern for loved ones, lack of emotional responsivity, and a loss of social graces"—had family histories suggestive of schizophrenia, but with a pattern of treatment response related more closely to mania without emotional blunting.

12. Schizoaffective depressed patients do not have a history of mania; that is, they are unipolar.

13. The following case history reported by Pope (1983, pp. 326–327) illustrates the devastation that can follow the misdiagnosis of manic-depressive illness as schizophrenia:

> Ms. B, a 28-year-old woman, had been a psychiatric inpatient in a state hospital for the greater part of nine years. She had first been admitted at the age of 19 when she developed psychotic symptoms. . . . A history taken at that time by the admitting psychiatrist elaborately described her delusions and hallucinations but gave no information about whether Ms. B displayed mood change, activity change, an increase or decrease in energy level, or other affective symptomatology. No family history data were elicited. . . . Ms. B had been treated with virtually every antipsychotic drug available but had never been treated with lithium or ECT [electroconvulsive therapy]. . . . [Her] hospital records revealed that she had had periods of unusual irritability, coupled with increased activity and talkativeness . . . [and] had also displayed distractibility, grandiosity, and interpersonal intrusiveness. However, during most of her hospitalization, she was described as apathetic, with hypersomnia of 10 to 11 hours a night, lacking in energy and concentration, eating poorly, and displaying little interest in social contact. She was also markedly self-deprecating and was described as having long guilty ruminations on religious themes. She had made two suicide attempts during these periods.
>
> During Ms. B's ninth year in the hospital, her 21-year-old brother was admitted to a private psychiatric hospital. He was suffering from a relatively typical manic episode . . . [and] responded relatively well to lithium carbonate. When the brother's psychiatrist learned of Ms. B's illness, he elicited more information about the family and discovered that a maternal aunt and the

maternal grandmother had had major depressive episodes. This evidence seemed to support his theory that Ms. B was suffering from a chronic form of bipolar disorder. . . . [T]he brother's psychiatrist made further inquiries about the possibility of the sister's being given a trial of lithium carbonate. The doctors at the state hospital refused, saying that the patient was "clearly schizophrenic." . . . However, after a great deal of pressure from Ms. B's mother, [they] reluctantly agreed to start Ms. B on lithium.

Within about three weeks Ms. B became markedly less agitated, less irritable, and more cooperative with staff. Shortly thereafter she was discharged to the quarterway house. Within two months, she transferred to a halfway house setting and was able to engage in a productive job with only a modest degree of supervision. However, she then became somewhat more depressed, and shortly thereafter stopped both her lithium and her antipsychotic drugs. Within a week, she had become sleepless, hyperactive, irritable, distractible, and grandiose. She was readmitted to the state hospital where she was treated with antipsychotic drugs but not with lithium. In spite of the clear temporal association between use of lithium and clinical response, the doctors claimed that the patient's "schizophrenic" symptoms ruled out a diagnosis of manic-depressive illness, and were unwilling to resume lithium therapy. At last report Ms. B's mother was still battling with the state hospital to reinstitute lithium.

14. Although the association's samples are not likely to be representative of patients with bipolar disorder in general, the point is that in this sample, early ascertainment of bipolarity had not improved recently.

15. The MDQ is a five-part questionnaire. The first part comprises 13 brief yes-or-no statements related to manic symptoms, all of which begin with the precursor "Has there ever been a period of time when you were not your usual self and. . . ." These questions assess various bipolar symptoms, such as hypersexuality ("you were much more interested in sex than usual?") and racing thoughts ("thoughts raced through your head or you couldn't slow your mind down?"). The second part is one yes-or-no question, which asks whether those manic symptoms occurred simultaneously. The third part has the subject evaluate the problems caused by those manic behaviors along a four-point scale, ranging from "no problem" to "serious problem." The fourth and fifth parts assess bipolar disorder in the subject's relatives and previous bipolar diagnoses, respectively.

16. One study found that 93 percent of patients who joined a voluntary bipolar disorder case registry accurately reported having bipolar disorder in agreement with a research diagnostic interview (Cluss et al., 1999). However, 94 percent of these patients had previously been diagnosed by professionals with bipolar disorder. It would appear likely that they would be influenced by such professional interactions. What is of concern for a screening instrument is how well it accurately diagnoses individuals who have never been correctly diagnosed with bipolar disorder despite having the condition, and in those circumstances, impairment of insight would appear to predict low accuracy of self-report.

17. Mitchell et al., 1992; Akiskal et al., 1995; Akiskal, 1996; Benazzi, 2000b; Benazzi and Rihmer, 2000; Ghaemi et al., 2004; Akiskal and Benazzi, 2005.

18. It also has been suggested that personality inventories, such as Cloninger's Temperament Character Inventory, may be used to distinguish between bipolar disorder and borderline personality disorder (Atre-Vaidya and Hussain, 1999).

19. In their review of reported reserpine-induced depressions, Goodwin and Bunney (1971) found that the great majority of reserpine "depressions" were, in fact, pseudodepressions that did not mimic the full natural syndrome. Those with full endogenous or melancholic symptoms generally had a personal or family history of affective illness. These authors inferred that reserpine merely uncovered a vulnerability rather than inducing depression de novo (see Chapter 19).

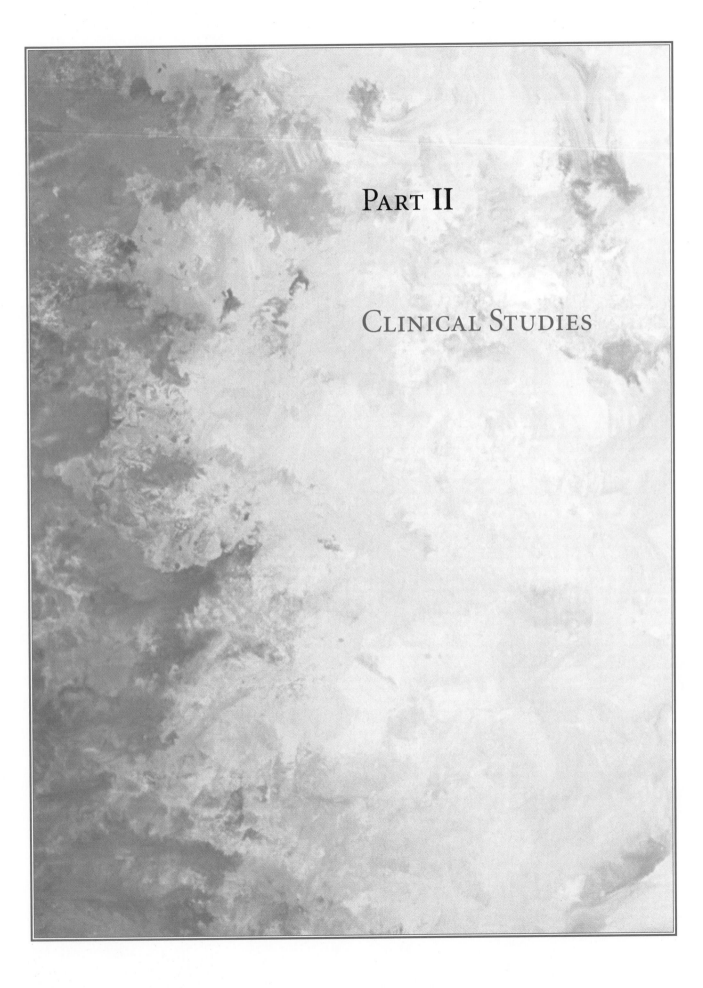

PART II

CLINICAL STUDIES

4 Course and Outcome

The universal experience is striking, that the attacks of manic-depressive insanity . . . never lead
to profound dementia, not even when they continue throughout life almost without interruption. . . . As a rule the disease runs its course in isolated attacks more or less sharply defined
from each other or from health, which are either like or unlike, or even very frequently are
[the] perfect antithesis.

—*Emil Kraepelin (1921, p. 3)*

Emil Kraepelin's central insight, one that continues as an
organizing principle in modern descriptive psychiatry, was
his division of the major psychoses into two groups based
largely on course and outcome. He observed that whereas
dementia praecox (schizophrenia) tends to be chronic and
to follow a deteriorating course, manic-depressive illness is
episodic and ultimately exacts a less devastating toll from
those affected. Today we face a paradox: whereas the discovery of the prophylactic potential of lithium and, subsequently, some of the anticonvulsants and atypical antipsychotics has revived interest in the natural course of
manic-depressive illness, widespread use of these prophylactic agents, as well as antidepressants, has substantially
altered that course. Investigators must confront the fact
that "natural" course now includes the largely unquanti-
fied effects of routine, acute, and prophylactic treatment.

In this chapter, after briefly reviewing salient methodological issues, we examine findings of the literature on the
following aspects of the course and outcome of manic-
depressive illness: premorbid functioning, age at onset,
number of episodes, frequency of episodes (cycle length),
onset and duration of episodes, polarity, pattern, precipitants of episodes, long-term outcome, mortality, the course
of bipolar-II disorder, and mechanisms of recurrence. Studies assessing the impact of prophylactic treatment are reviewed in Chapter 20, and biological correlates of natural
course are covered in Chapter 14.

METHODOLOGICAL ISSUES

As with most fields of inquiry, studies of the course and outcome of manic-depressive illness involve methodological
complexities that should be kept in mind when interpreting
the study results. Two issues are especially important.

The first relates to patient selection. The index hospitalization required in many older outcome studies can produce either underestimates or overestimates of recurrence.
Underestimates can result when, during a single hospitalization, a patient has multiple rapid cycles that are counted
as a single episode. On the other hand, overestimates can
result from basing recurrence rates on hospital admission
data, because those data exclude patients who experience a
single episode, recover without hospitalization, and never
have a recurrence. While some recent studies (virtually all
of which focused on the bipolar subgroup) have avoided
these problems by recruiting patients from the general
community, other samples (e.g., those of the Stanley Foundation Bipolar Network) have been drawn from clinics in
which sicker, treatment-resistant patients tend to be overrepresented. Indeed, clinical samples are, by definition, not
representative, because a substantial portion of the bipolar
population is not receiving treatment at any given time.

The second issue has to do with diagnosis. Many of
the classic studies of natural course do not distinguish
between the bipolar and recurrent unipolar subgroups.
Numerous interpretive problems result, particularly in
studies from the United States, where diagnostic criteria
for unipolar illness (i.e., depressions that are not bipolar)
allow for considerable heterogeneity (see the discussions of
this issue in Chapters 1 and 3). For this reason, we emphasize the literature on bipolar patients, although some conclusions may be relevant to the more recurrent forms of
unipolar illness as well. Furthermore, most classic studies
of bipolar patients have involved patients hospitalized for
mania and thus have not included the bipolar-II subgroup.
The extent to which patients with schizoaffective features
are included in the sample is another diagnostic issue (see
the later discussion).

In addition to these issues, a traditional methodological problem is the lack of a generally accepted convention for collecting data on the course of manic-depressive illness or for defining recovery and relapse. Standardized methods for charting the course of the illness, proposed for both retrospectively derived data (Post et al., 1988; Honig et al., 2001) and prospectively derived data (Keller et al., 1987; Leverich et al., 2001), have improved this situation but are still far from universally applied. These methods have clinical as well as research uses. For example, detailed description of the prior course of the illness may reveal that medications, such as lithium, given to the patient in the past were mistakenly judged ineffective when they actually led to improvement. Conversely, charting may uncover instances in which certain drugs, such as antidepressants, exacerbated the course of the illness. In addition, previously unrecognized associations of episode onsets with anniversaries, life events, or other stressors may aid in psychotherapeutic understanding and behavioral management. These standardized charting methods are all the more important in industrialized countries, where population mobility is exacerbating a situation in which there are increasingly fewer opportunities for a single clinic or clinician to follow a cohort of patients over a lifetime.

A final methodological consideration in reviewing this literature is its largely retrospective nature, a troublesome aspect given the problems inherent in recalling the past, especially for depressed patients. Future studies need to be prospective and to focus on patients in naturalistic treatment settings.

PREMORBID FUNCTIONING

The distinction between "premorbid" functioning in children and childhood manifestations of full-blown manic-depressive illness can be somewhat arbitrary, because the disorder may present a different clinical picture in childhood than in adolescence or adulthood. We discuss clinical manifestations of possible childhood variants of the illness, as well as premorbid functioning in its early-onset forms, in Chapter 6, issues of premorbid/underlying personality in Chapter 10, and issues of neurocognitive development in Chapter 9. Here we focus on other measures of premorbid functioning (e.g., social, academic) in samples that do not include childhood-onset recurrent mood disorder.

In the original Kraepelinian definition, patients with manic-depressive illness were free of any morbid symptoms before the onset of their illness. Some modern data are consistent with this impression. In an elegant prospective study, Reichenberg and colleagues (2002) examined results from an extensive array of tests designed to measure level of functioning in persons who later developed schizoaffective,

schizophrenic, or nonpsychotic bipolar disorder. Patients were matched with normal controls on age and education level. The nonpsychotic bipolar group showed no significant impairment on intellectual tests, reading/writing, or various behavioral measures.[1] Schizophrenic patients displayed premorbid impairment across most measures of intellectual and behavioral functioning, whereas schizoaffective patients showed less consistent impairment, suggesting a psychotic continuum of premorbid impairment.[2]

Some studies of premorbid functioning in psychotic bipolar patients paint a picture slightly different from the Kraepelinian model. For example, in their retrospective analysis comparing a large sample of bipolar and unipolar patients, Stephens and McHugh (1991) found significantly greater premorbid impairment on descriptive measures of social and work functioning in the bipolar group, which also had significantly higher rates of mood-congruent psychosis; however, the unipolar group was not selected for the more recurrent form. In a retrospective study using maternal interviews, Cannon and colleagues (1997) compared hospitalized schizophrenic patients with hospitalized psychotic bipolar patients and healthy controls on measures of premorbid social functioning and school performance. The psychotic bipolar group scored significantly worse than healthy controls on premorbid social adjustment measures, but significantly better than schizophrenic patients. Other studies have corroborated the finding that patients with psychotic and/or severe forms of bipolar disorder displayed significantly less premorbid impairment than did schizophrenic patients, lending weight to the notion that degree of premorbid impairment is an important distinction between bipolar disorder and schizophrenia.[3] Nevertheless, it appears that subtle premorbid dysfunction (especially cognitive dysfunction) may exist in some patients with bipolar disorder, particularly those with psychotic forms of the illness. More prospective data from epidemiologic samples, employing *Diagnostic and Statistical Manual* (DSM)-IV diagnoses and incorporating both psychotic and nonpsychotic forms of the disorder, are needed to further elucidate the premorbid phenomenology of bipolar disorder.

AGE AT ONSET

The age when manic-depressive illness most often begins (in both its bipolar and recurrent unipolar forms) is intrinsically important to genetically vulnerable individuals and their clinicians and may offer clues to future course. In this section, we examine the literature on this issue in general; Chapter 6 focuses on studies of early onset in prepuberty and adolescence, and Chapter 13 examines how differences in age at onset relate to estimates of the degree of genetic vulnerability.

We pooled data from 15 studies published after 1990 (i.e., since the first edition of this text appeared) reporting average age at onset in samples of patients with bipolar illness (summarized in Table 4–1) and derived a weighted mean of 22.2 years.[4] When gender was specified, the difference for males and females was not significant (Fogarty et al., 1994; Hendrick et al., 2000; Suppes et al., 2001). Studies reporting separate figures for bipolar-I and -II disorder showed similar averages for the two groups (McMahon et al., 1994; Judd et al., 2003).

It is interesting that the post-1990 mean is 6 years younger than the weighted mean taken from the 22 pre-1990 studies examined in the first edition, which used the same basic inclusion criteria. Because the data are not normally distributed, however, these figures may be misleading. Averages can be raised by a relatively small number of patients with late onset, for example. When median age at onset is reported, it is usually in the early twenties. Here again, these medians are several years younger than those found in the literature before 1990.

As noted earlier, some of the variance across individual studies in Table 4–1 is related to differing criteria for onset. In general, the age when symptoms first appear is younger than the age when patients meet diagnostic criteria, and the age of first clinical contact is later still. (Studies of first hospitalization are not included in Table 4–1 because this measure says very little about age at onset.) Some studies have used age at first clinical contact on the assumption that dating of initial symptoms would be too imprecise. Egeland and colleagues (1987a), however, using information gleaned from patient charts and interview records to compare six clinical indices of onset for bipolar disorder, obtained high interrater reliability ($r = .89$) using the measure of first achievement of Research Diagnostic Criteria (RDC) for a major affective disorder.[5] As might be expected, the ages obtained with this measure are significantly younger than those derived from first treatment or first hospitalization.

Indeed, the literature is consistent in finding a significant time gap between onset of the illness and first treatment. Meeks (1999) found that mean age at first symptoms in a bipolar and unipolar population was almost 6 years younger than age at first treatment. A demographic study of the first 261 patients in the Stanley Foundation Bipolar Network (which may represent patients on the more severe end of the spectrum) revealed an 8-year difference between age at first diagnosis and age at first medical treatment (22.9 and 30.4 years, respectively), whereas age at first symptoms was only 2 years before age at diagnostic onset (Suppes et al., 2001). In a Stanley Foundation recruitment survey administered by Kupfer and colleagues (2002), more than 50 percent of a large bipolar sample indicated that they had received no treatment for their first affective episode. Thus it is to be expected that age at first treatment is a poor indicator of onset. Although retrospective self-reporting has its own pitfalls—which should be controlled for whenever possible with corroborating family reports and medical/academic records—using "first episode" as an onset measure with standardized (*International Classification of Diseases* [ICD]-10 or DSM-IV) criteria appears to be the most accurate indicator.

The lower age at onset in more recent studies reflects, in part, a cohort effect that is supported in the literature. For example, Chengappa and colleagues (2003) examined two separate cohorts of patients with bipolar disorder in a large patient sample and found that the more recent cohort had a mean age at onset 3 years younger than that of the older cohort. When the investigators examined a third, still more recent cohort in a post hoc analysis, they found that onset occurred at an even younger age, with a statistically significant different mean among the three cohorts. Kupfer and colleagues (2002) made similar findings in their examination of separate birth cohorts in a patient population from the Stanley Center's Bipolar Disorder Registry: the earliest birth cohort (1900–1939) was 3.5 years older at onset than the later two cohorts.

Researchers have advanced several hypotheses to explain this reduction in age at onset. Changes in nosology and illness definition could be a partial explanation. With the exception of the retrospective studies, the data in Table 4–1 were taken largely from samples of patients diagnosed in the past three decades (Stephens and McHugh, 1991). Many of these patients might have been classified as "schizophrenic" 50 years ago. The diagnostic inclusion of more psychotically ill subgroups could lower the age at onset, particularly in light of the earlier impairment observed in these groups (as discussed earlier). Genetic anticipation could play a role in the heightened predisposition to development of the disorder with each subsequent generation (see Chapter 13). Some investigators have proposed that the increasing use of antidepressants and stimulants in adolescents and children may help induce the onset of bipolar disorder at an earlier age in those already susceptible (Goodwin and Ghaemi, 1998; Cicero et al., 2003; Reichart, 2004).[6] This phenomenon would be consistent with what we know about the effect of antidepressants on mania induction and cycle acceleration, but more research is necessary to draw a solid conclusion. Similar to the antidepressant association is the hypothesis that the increased use of recreational drugs and alcohol among young people contributes to earlier onset. Here again, sound evidence is lacking, and it is difficult to establish a unidirectional association between onset of affective symptoms and onset of drug use.[7]

To gauge more accurately the distribution of the published ages at onset in the bipolar patient population, we

TABLE 4–1. **Average Age at Onset in Studies Since 1990**

Study	Sample	Average Age at Onset (Years)	Purpose/Design	Other Findings
Stephens and McHugh, 1991	235 bipolar	26.7	Retrospective analysis of notes on patients treated and monitored at a large institution, 1913–1940	Average age at onset lower in bipolar than in unipolar patients by approximately 6 years; average of 6 years between average age at onset and age at first admission
Kessler et al., 1993; Weissman et al., 1996	116 bipolar	23.3	Data from national comorbidity survey	—
Fogarty et al., 1994	22 bipolar	20.3: 20.5 male, 20.0 female	Determined clinical characteristics of mania by survey of randomly selected households	Age at onset: 5th percentile, ~9.0; 50th percentile, ~18.5; 95th percentile, ~25.5
Benazzi, 1999	186: 45 bipolar-I, 141 bipolar-II	26.7: 28.5 bipolar-I, 26.0 bipolar-II	Determined first episode using retrospective Structured Clinical Interview for DSM (SCID)/patient interview	No significant difference in age at onset ($p=.53$) in bipolar-I vs. bipolar-II
Meeks, 1999	86 bipolar	24.9	Determined factors of functioning in late-life bipolar disorder through patient interviews conducted three times over 8 months	Early onset related to poor functioning, increase in episode number and severity
Hendrick et al., 2000	37 bipolar-II	20.5: 21.8 male, 19.6 female	Gender comparison for average age at onset and a number of other clinical variables; first episode determined by retrospective questionnaire	—
Johnson et al., 2000	190 bipolar	31.4 (range 14.0–78.0)	Examined relationship between average age at onset and family history, early life events; average age at onset = first episode as determined by retrospective questionnaire	
Bellivier et al., 2001	211 bipolar-I	25.9 (standard deviation 4.5)	Used admixture analysis (a clustering method) to determine average age-at-onset distribution patterns/first diagnosis	Three subgroups of bipolar patients based on average age-at-onset distribution with distinct clinical profiles; findings support average age-at-onset subtypes

Study	Sample	Age at onset	Method	Findings
McElroy et al., 2001	288 bipolar (I or II)	22.3: 26.0 noncomorbid diagnosis, 20.3 comorbid diagnosis	Compared attributes of bipolar patients with comorbid Axis I diagnosis and purely bipolar patients through retrospective interviews	Comorbidity related to earlier average age at onset
Suppes et al., 2001	261: 211 bipolar-I, 42 bipolar-II, 5 bipolar–not otherwise specified (NOS), 3 schizoaffective–bipolar type	22.9: 23.4 (±11.0) male, 22.5 (±10.0) female	Descriptive analysis of demographic features and course for 261 recruits in Stanley Foundation Bipolar Network; average age at onset ascertained by first full syndrome development using SCID	Early average age at onset associated with increased mood switching, worsening course of illness, history of early abuse
Carlson et al., 2002	123 bipolar	25.66 (standard deviation 9.9)	Outcome as a function of early vs. late average age at onset, first-episode SCID history, records, third-party interviews	22% <19.0, 78% >19.0. Early average age at onset an independent influence on poor functioning
Dittmann et al., 2002	152 bipolar	24.4 (standard deviation 10.9)	Follow-up of 152 patients entered in Stanley registry clinical sample, mostly hospitalized	No associations with age at onset included in this report
Judd et al., 2002, 2003	232 bipolar	22.2	Combined data reported in two studies on bipolar-I and -II patients from National Institute of Mental Health's Collaborative Depression Study. Average age at onset based on Research Diagnostic Criteria for first episode	Average age at onset did not correspond with measures of chronicity in either bipolar-I or bipolar-II group. Median age: bipolar-I = 21.0; bipolar-II = 19.0 (nonsignificant)
Kupfer et al., 2002	2,308 bipolar	19.8	Analysis of clinical and demographic characteristics of respondents to a Stanley recruitment survey; average age at onset determined by self-report using DSM-IV criteria for first manic or depressive episode	Median age = 17.5; younger cohort (1950–1959) had higher median average age at onset (22.5) than two older cohorts (1940–1949 = 19.0; 1900–1939 = 19.0); more than 50% of participants received no treatment for first episode

Note: Weighted means; 15 studies since 1990 (N = 4,494) = **22.2**; studies before 1990 (N = 4,210) = **28.1**; studies 1907–present (N = 8,704) = **25.1**.

123

pooled data from seven studies specifying the number of patients with first episodes beginning in each decade of life (a total of 2,968 patients). This finer-grained analysis resulted in a peak in the age range of 15 to 19, followed closely by the 20–24 and 10–14 ranges, which were almost equal (Fig. 4–1). Note that the age-at-onset distribution is similar for men and women. Note also that this distribution provides only a rough picture and is heavily influenced by the large cohort of bipolar survey participants recruited by the Stanley Center Bipolar Registry, in which the largest subset (approximately 26 percent) of a sample of 2,308 participants were aged 15 to 19 (Kupfer et al., 2002).[8] Still, the rising concentration of bipolar diagnosis before age 20 is a clear trend in the recent literature and is consistent with Epidemiological Catchment Area (ECA) data showing hazard rates for the development of mania to be at their highest in the 15–19 age range (Burke et al., 1990).

Some investigators have defined two primary groups by age at onset—early and late (Carlson et al., 2000; Schurhoff et al., 2000; Suppes et al., 2001; Patel et al., 2006), with bimodal cutoff points ranging from the late teens (Goldstein and Levitt, 2006) to the mid-twenties (Grigoroiu-Serbanescu et al., 2001). Others have proposed three subgroups of onset—early (child or early adolescent), intermediate or typical (late adolescent, young adult), and later life (after age 35) (Sax et al., 1997; Bellivier et al., 2001; Mick et al., 2003; Lin et al., 2006). These hypotheses can be difficult to verify because "early," "late," and varying degrees of intermediate categories have tended to be defined inconsistently and arbitrarily.[9] However, Bellivier's group (2001)

used "admixture analyses" to determine the subgrouping model of best fit in a sample of 211 patients. Their findings correspond to an early–intermediate–late model (that is, a trimodal distribution), with mean onset at ages 16.9, 26.9, and 46.2, respectively. In a subsequent study (Bellivier et al., 2003), this group tested the fitness of this model on a different patient population (N=368). The model fit within the bounds of statistical sameness, further validating the trimodel distribution of onset age. Also, Bellivier and colleagues (2001) reported that bipolar siblings of a patient in a particular subgroup were statistically more likely to be part of the same age subset (p=.0001), a finding that supports a genetic etiological component to age-at-onset subgroups. A similar familial aggregation by age at onset was recently reported by Lin and colleagues (see Chapter 13).

Very late onset (i.e., after age 60) generally has been considered rare (Carlson et al., 1974; Loranger and Levine, 1978), although some data suggest that it may be more common than previously thought (Spicer et al., 1973; Shulman and Post, 1980; Stone, 1989; Wylie et al., 1999; Almeida and Fenner, 2002; Kessing, 2006). Angst and colleagues (1978) reported a secondary peak of late onset among women in the 40–50 age range (see Fig. 4–1). Patients with very late onset are less likely to have a family history of the disorder and more likely to be organically impaired. For example, Tohen and colleagues (1994) compared two groups of elderly patients, one with late-onset mania (first episode after age 65) and one with multiple manic episodes before age 65. The former group was significantly more likely to

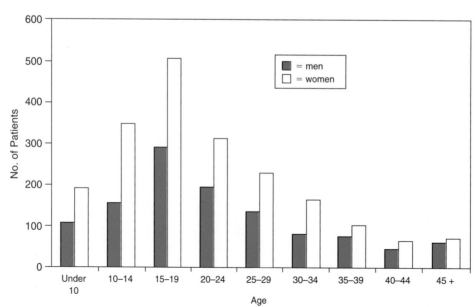

Figure 4–1. Distribution of age at onset (years) in bipolar-I and -II patients across seven studies.

experience neurological abnormalities.[10] These observations highlight the importance of differential diagnosis of primary mood disorders and mood disorders that occur secondary to specific neuropathology (see Chapter 3).

It is not yet clear to what extent grouping patients by age at onset really identifies distinct subgroups with differential phenomenology, pathophysiology, family history, outcome, and/or treatment response. Studies examining family history in early- versus late-onset groups have generally shown more genetic loading for recurrent mood disorder associated with early onset (see below).[11] But age at onset did not differ significantly in several studies comparing patients with mixed and pure mania (McElroy et al., 1995[12]; Akiskal et al., 1998; Brieger et al., 2003), and it does not appear to be a distinguishing feature of bipolar-I versus bipolar-II disorder (Benazzi, 1999). On the other hand, early onset has shown rather consistent correlations with certain clinical features, including rapid cycling, presence of comorbid anxiety disorder, suicidal behavior, psychotic features, and treatment resistance.

Carlson and colleagues (2002) reported that patients with an early onset (before age 19) had significantly worse outcomes on a variety of measures than those with later onset (after age 19).[13] Likewise, a French study of 58 early-onset (before age 18) versus 39 late-onset (after age 40) bipolar patients found that the former group experienced more psychosis (in agreement with the data of McGlashan [1988] and Schulze et al. [2002]), mixed episodes, panic disorder comorbidity, and lithium resistance and were more likely to have first-degree relatives with bipolar disorder (Schurhoff et al., 2000).[14] Among 320 bipolar-I and -II patients, those with onset younger than age 18 had more comorbid anxiety, rapid cycling, suicidality, and substance abuse compared with those with an onset above age 18 (Carter et al., 2003). An examination of a large cohort of Stanley Foundation Bipolar Network patients showed significant correlations between early onset (up to age 17) and greater incidence of learning disabilities, rapid-cycling course, and family history of bipolar disorder (Suppes et al., 2001),[15] while Ernst and Goldberg (2004) found that onset below age 19 was associated with more rapid cycling and comorbid substance abuse.[16] Engstrom and colleagues (2003) reported lower levels of treatment response and significantly greater numbers of suicide attempts in early- versus late-onset patients in a Swedish population.

Although the evidence for a connection between early onset and the complicating illness features described is compelling, one must exercise caution when using cross-sectional studies to distinguish damaging effects of the illness from so-called "clinical subtype" features. That is, worse outcomes in early-onset patients could be a factor of longer duration of illness rather than a phenotypic characteristic.

The issue of duration of illness is discussed later in this chapter.

The genetic literature is discussed in detail in Chapter 13, but it is worth noting here that newer linkage/mapping studies, coupled with older family studies, support the proposition that different age-at-onset subsets represent genetically heterogeneous groups of bipolar patients. Several studies cited in the first edition of this text reported that earlier onset was linked to higher familial bipolar morbidity and to early onset in bipolar relatives (Baron et al., 1981; Smeraldi et al., 1982–1983). Grigoroiu-Serbanescu and colleagues (2001), using segregation analysis of a large sample of 177 bipolar-I probands and 2,407 relatives, found that early-onset bipolar-I disorder was transmitted with a different pattern of heritability (non-mendelian major gene model) than late-onset bipolar-I. Recently, polymorphisms in serotonin transporter (5-HTTLPR) and a glycogen synthase kinase (GSK3-β) were associated with age at onset within bipolar populations (Bellivier et al., 2002; Benedetti et al., 2002). A recent chromosomal linkage study also confirmed the heritability of onset age, linking it to three chromosomal regions (Faraone et al., 2004). Taken as a whole, the evidence for age at onset as a possible marker for genetic subtypes of bipolar disorder is robust (see the review by Leboyer and colleagues [2005]).

The association between psychotic features and early onset among bipolar patients has considerable support in the literature. In an extensive review, Angst (1986c) cited 10 studies reporting this relationship, a conclusion supported by Blumenthal and colleagues (1987) in their study of the Amish and confirmed by subsequent research (Dell'Osso et al., 1993; Verdoux and Bourgeois, 1993; Schulze et al., 2002). Yet adolescent-onset mania is not always associated with psychotic features, as evidenced by cross-sectional comparison studies (Coryell and Norten, 1980; McElroy et al., 1997). A more recent cross-sectional study comparing early with non-early onset groups likewise failed to find a significantly higher presence of psychotic features in the former (Perlis et al., 2004). However, cross-sectional studies cannot determine subsequent development of psychosis and may easily miss prior psychotic features, especially if the investigators rely on patient recall. Taken as a whole, the evidence for a connection between psychotic features and younger age at onset is strong. Coupled with the association between premorbid impairment and level of psychosis discussed earlier, this evidence supports the hypothesis that pervasive psychotic features mark a more severe form of the disorder that sometimes entails earlier syndromal manifestation and is more often characterized by premorbid impairment. The relationship between age at onset and episode frequency is discussed later in this chapter.

NUMBER OF EPISODES

In his classic 1921 monograph, Kraepelin noted that of 459 manic-depressive patients he had studied (which included unipolar patients), only 55 percent had experienced more than one episode and only 28 percent more than three. A careful reading of Kraepelin's clinical descriptions suggests, however, that many of his ostensibly single-episode patients were in fact severely and chronically ill and had experienced multiple episodes, which at that time required continuous hospitalization (the single hospitalization being counted as single episode).

Considered together, findings of longitudinal studies of manic-depressive patients not taking prophylactic medication (Table 4–2), which included those with both bipolar and unipolar forms of the illness, indicate that most patients—particularly those studied in the past 35 years—had more than one episode.[17] Table 4–2 also indicates that most patients with major affective disorder (i.e., Kraepelinian manic-depressive illness) have a recurrent course. Many textbooks, apparently relying on older data, fail to emphasize this point sufficiently.

The near-total likelihood of recurrence is supported by recent research. In a 4-year naturalistic follow-up study of 75 bipolar patients, only 28 percent remained in remission (Tohen et al., 1990). If relapse were to continue at this rate over the long term (18 percent per year), fewer than 1 percent of patients would remain in remission at about 10 years' follow-up. In the National Institute of Mental Health's (NIMH) Collaborative Program on the Psychobiology of Depression-Clinical Studies (CDS), relapse into a new episode within 5 years was observed in 81 to 91 percent of patients, the variability in percentage being related to the polarity of the index episode (i.e., depressive, mixed, or manic states) (Keller et al., 1993).

In contrast, relapse in unipolar depression is not as frequent and is more dependent on the number of previous episodes, with a much higher risk of relapse after the third major depressive episode. In a separate analysis of the data from the NIMH Collaborative Program on the Psychobiology of Depression-Clinical Studies, the 5-year recurrence rate was 64 percent among 380 patients with unipolar depression, rising to 80 percent at 10 years and 85 percent at 15 years (Mueller et al., 1999). In a Japanese collaborative study (Kanai et al., 2003), 95 previously untreated unipolar depressed subjects (70.5 percent first episode, 29.5 percent recurrent; mean age 44.3) were followed for 6 years. In this cohort, lower rates of relapse were seen, with only 45 percent experiencing a new episode at 6 years. This lower relapse rate may reflect the fact that, unlike the CDS cohort, most of these patients had not already experienced recurrent major depressive episodes. The lower rate of episode

recurrence in unipolar compared with bipolar disorder does not address the issue of subsyndromal chronicity, however (see later discussion).

Angst (1980) subdivided his patients into three categories according to their pattern of recurrence: MD, Md, and Dm. As described in Chapter 2, MD represents the core illness, with both major manic and major depressive episodes; Md patients have full manic episodes, but their depressive episodes do not require hospitalization; and Dm patients have been hospitalized for depression, but their manic episodes are not severe enough for hospitalization (i.e., they have a history of hypomania).[18] Angst's MD patients showed a tendency toward having the most episodes. In the larger cohort described in the CDS, however, Dm (bipolar-II) patients had the most prior episodes, although this number was not significantly different from that for bipolar-I patients (Coryell et al., 1989).[19]

As noted earlier in our discussion of methodological issues, some differences among studies relate to varying definitions of what counts as an episode. Some studies underestimate recurrence because they rely solely on hospitalization as a marker of episodes.[20] Other studies may be prone to overestimate recurrence because of treatment factors, such as use of antidepressants and selection of lithium clinic patients for study.

On the question of the contribution of antidepressant drugs, it is important to note that the highest relapse rates generally are the most recent. Thus it is conceivable, as suggested in the first edition of this text and by Koukopoulos and colleagues (1980) and Wehr and Goodwin (1987), that the increased use of antidepressants may have influenced the results. Indeed, in his analysis of the incidence of manic switches in one hospital studied over six decades, Angst (1985) noted a four-fold increase when the pretreatment decades were compared with the decades after electroconvulsive therapy (ECT) and antidepressant drugs became widely used. Some more recent studies (Altshuler et al., 1995; Ghaemi et al., 1999, 2000), but not all (Altshuler et al., 2001), support the possible impact of anti-depressants. Although other explanations, such as better diagnostic detection of mania, are plausible, these explanations also are consistent with the hypothesis that effective antidepressant treatments altered the course in some manic-depressive patients (perhaps particularly those with the bipolar form) toward more frequent recurrences. The evidence for and against this hypothesis is reviewed extensively in Chapter 19.

Another possibility is that a bias toward higher relapse rates is likely when an outcome study draws all of its subjects from patients referred to a lithium maintenance clinic. The studies of Angst and of Grof cited elsewhere in this chapter, however, included all patients who came to

TABLE 4–2. **Total Number of Episodes**

Study	Sample Size	Years of Observation	TOTAL EPISODES (%)				Comments
			1	2–3	4–6	7+	
Kraepelin, 1921	459	Variable, up to a lifetime R	45	27	—	28	Many "single-episode" patients were chronically hospitalized with continuous cycling
Pollock, 1931	5,739	11 R	55	35	8	2	Excluded episodes occurring before index admission
Rennie, 1942	66	26 R	8	29	26	37	"Several" had 20 or more episodes
Lundquist, 1945	103	20% <10 R 38%, 10–20 R 42%, 20–30 R	50	25	—	25	28% were chronic and were included in the "single-episode" category; excluded episodes occurring before index admission
Stenstedt, 1952	62	1.2–20+ R	26	42	—	32	Included nonrecovered patients as single-episode
Bratfos and Haug, 1968	42	1–12 P	13	42	—	45	"Not free of symptoms for any length of time"; half of these were "chronic"
Perris, 1968	131	19.6 R	0	17	40	43	Average number of episodes: bipolar=7, unipolar=4
Carlson et al., 1974[a]	53	10 P	4	17	32	47	One third of these were rapid cyclers (4 or more episodes/year).
Angst, 1978, 1979b[a]	95	26 P, R	0	8	22	69	16% had >20 episodes. "New episode" required >4 weeks asymptomatic interval
Zis et al., 1980	105	P, R	6	13	33	48	—
Fukuda et al., 1983	96	18–28 R	15	40	20	25	Hospitalized; questionnaire and chart review; no treatment with lithium, but other drugs used
Total	**6,951**		**0–55**	**13–42**	**8–40**	**2–69**	

Note: Studies reported here included both bipolar and unipolar patients.
P = prospective; R = retrospective.
[a]These studies included some patients treated prophylactically; most of the other studies included patients treated acutely.
Source: Update of Goodwin and Jamison (1984).

the clinic for treatment of an episode without regard to previous episodes (i.e., not just those deemed eligible for maintenance treatment). Other studies appear to have focused primarily on those judged eligible for lithium maintenance (Baldessarini et al., 1999, 2000). As noted earlier, both underestimations and overestimations of true natural recurrence rates have occurred in the literature. It appears that some recent studies may be prone to overestimation of recurrence rates as a result of the uncontrolled effects of treatment and to potential selection bias, although underestimation also occurs.[21]

FREQUENCY OF EPISODES (CYCLE LENGTH)

Cycle length is defined as the time from the onset of one episode to the onset of the next. Variation in cycle length reflects primarily variation in the length of the symptom-free interval, because the duration of episodes tends to be relatively constant in a given individual. Onset is used to calculate cycle length because it is generally easier to pinpoint than termination of an episode. In addition, treatment can easily obscure an episode's natural length. Most investigators agree that cycle length tends to grow shorter with subsequent recurrences; that is, episodes become more frequent. What is not as clear is the proportion of bipolar patients whose illness accelerates. After three to five episodes, however, the extent of shortening slows considerably and approaches a leveling off, or maximum frequency of episodes.

In the first edition of this text, we speculated that episode frequency might represent a familial trait, as suggested by Gershon and colleagues (1982). Subsequently, Fisfalen and colleagues (2005), examining 86 families with at least three members with a major affective disorder, found that episode frequency (evenly distributed over a wide range) was correlated among relatives (r = 0.56, p < .004). They also noted that, compared with the lowest quartile of episode frequency, the highest quartile was significantly (and independently) associated with bipolar-II, early age at onset, psychotic features, alcoholism, and suicidal behavior.

Decrease in Well Intervals with Increasing Number of Episodes

Kraepelin was the first to report that intervals of euthymia appear to decrease in duration in manic-depressive illness with increasing numbers of affective episodes. This observation later became a central impetus for the kindling model, with its prediction that episodes become more frequent over time, and that euthymic intervals between episodes become increasingly shorter. This observation was subsequently confirmed in a number of clinical studies. Recently, however, some methodological flaws underlying those

studies have been identified, and not all of the study findings have been consistent.

Figure 4–2 illustrates the relationship between average cycle length and episode number. This graph is based on six studies involving a total of 20,660 patients. Despite substantial individual variability, the averages show a remarkably consistent pattern across the studies. For example, note the pattern in the 105 bipolar patients of Zis and colleagues (1979): the average cycle length between the first and second episodes was 36 months, diminishing to about 24 months, then to 12 months. In 46 bipolar patients studied by Roy-Byrne and colleagues (1985a), the mean cycle lengths for the first seven episodes were 53, 28, 25, 20, 12, 15, and 9 months. In 95 bipolar patients from Angst's Zurich clinic, the median first cycle length was 48 months, compared with 22 months for the second cycle, 24 for the third, 14 for the fourth, and 12 for the fifth (Angst, 1981b). The longer average cycle length in the Kraepelin data reflects the inclusion of unipolar patients, whose cycles are longer than those of bipolar patients (Angst, 1981b; Fukuda et al., 1983).

The findings of the six studies illustrated in Figure 4–2 are consistent with the retrospective data of Taschev (1974), who found the average second cycle to be as long as the first, but the fourth cycle to be half as long as the second. A prospective study of patients in the 1980s (Keller et al., 1982) also documented the increasing probability of an

Figure 4–2. Episode number versus cycle length. BP = bipolar, UP = unipolar. (*Source*: Update of Goodwin and Jamison, 1984.)

earlier relapse with each episode, a finding suggesting that some fundamental characteristics of the illness course may persist despite treatment. The methodological consideration of "Slater's fallacy"—the impact of the number of episodes on cycle length—needs to be taken into account when assessing these studies, however (see later discussion).

Recent studies have not been consistent with regard to the progressive shortening of cycle length. In a reanalysis of his Zurich cohort (identified 1959–1963, followed to 1997; N = 220 bipolar patients), Angst and Selloro (2000) found shortening of cycle length in the first few but not in later episodes. In the studies of Winokur and colleagues (1993) and Turvey and colleagues (1999), who analyzed data from the same large NIMH cohort, bipolar patients did not appear to have more frequent and shorter episodes with time, nor was there a correlation between poor outcome and such a course. Rather, poor outcome was associated with "polyphasic" mood episodes; that is, immediate switching from mania to depression to mania without intervening euthymia.

Findings of other contemporary studies suggest that at least a subgroup of patients with bipolar disorder do experience a progressive shortening of cycle length. For instance, Goldberg and Harrow (1994) reported that 50 percent of 20 bipolar patients with two or more previous hospitalizations had experienced intervals between episodes of less than 1 year (defined as "kindlers"), whereas 19 other patients with fewer than two hospitalizations had experienced intervals between episodes of more than 1 year ("nonkindlers"). At 4.5-year follow-up, the kindlers were more likely to have had a recurrence than the nonkindlers. In a hospital-based case register study, Kessing and colleagues (1998a) found that 40 percent of a large sample (N = 1,712) had shortening between first and second intervals, and 25 percent of this sample showed progressive shortening across two consecutive intervals.

The considerable individual variability in patterns of relapse was pointed out by Kraepelin (1921, p. 149):

> If we give no more examples that is not because those already given represent adequately the multiplicity of the courses taken by manic-depressive insanity; it is absolutely inexhaustible.

The complexity of this topic increases when we pay attention to the above-noted methodological problem first raised by Eliot Slater in 1938 but ignored by most researchers until recently. Slater's fallacy, as revived by Oepen and colleagues (2004), posits that patients with more episodes tend also to have shorter cycle lengths, and those with fewer episodes to have longer cycle lengths.[23] Thus if the two groups are pooled, as in Kraepelin's original data, it will ap-

pear as if cycle length decreases with more episodes in the sample as a whole, whereas this apparent effect may be an artifact of pooling the two distinct subgroups of patients, those with few and those with many episodes. To truly demonstrate shortening of cycle length, then, one would need to correct for number of episodes.

Because this important methodological point went underrecognized for decades, we reanalyzed the studies described in the first edition of this text with regard to cycle length, as well as newer studies conducted since 1990. We found that the majority of studies either did not correct for number of episodes or did not address the subject. A number of investigators, however, without directly referring to Slater's finding, appear to have been cognizant of this issue.[23] In two of these studies (Bratfos and Haug, 1968; Angst et al., 1973), correction for number of episodes led to results similar to those reported by Slater; that is, no consistent evidence of progressive shortening of well intervals. In two other studies (Roy-Byrne et al., 1985a; Goldberg and Harrow, 1994), however, a "sensitization" or "kindling" pattern was identified in about half of patients with refractory bipolar disorder and not in the others (see Fig. 4–2). In a large Norwegian community-based study of hospitalized bipolar patients, half of those with three or fewer episodes also appeared to have progressive shortening of intervals of wellness, but a similar pattern was seen in only 25 percent of patients with four or more episodes (Kessing et al., 1998a). Slater's fallacy was also avoided in a contemporary Italian study of 426 hospitalized research patients with mood disorders (182 unipolar, 244 bipolar) (Cusin et al., 2000). In that study, in which all patients had experienced periods of euthymic recovery (continuous and rapid-cycling courses were excluded), progressive shortening of cycle length was observed (based on retrospective evaluation) after correction for total number of episodes, up to a plateau of about one episode per year. In a recent 40-year follow-up of Angst's Zurich cohort (N = 406, 186 with recurrent unipolar depression, 220 with bipolar disorder), Kessing and colleagues (2004) specifically conducted their analysis to control for Slater's fallacy by using a Cox regression model in which one of the variables was episode number, thus adjusting the overall hazard ratio for number of previous episodes. They found an increased likelihood (hazard ratio) of more episodes with increasing number of episodes (e.g., the hazard ratio for 1 episode was 1.0 as the reference point, while for 4 episodes it was 1.52 and for 10 episodes 2.19).

In these studies, then, correction for episode frequency revealed decreasing length of well intervals mainly in the first three episodes, with unchanging well intervals of about one per year for further episodes, which in fact was what the Goodwin group found earlier (Zis et al., 1980). These findings suggest that studies of well intervals that fail to capture the first three episodes of illness are unlikely to observe any kindling-like effect. This point may be relevant to some studies that fail to find this effect, such as that of Turvey and colleagues (1999), in which the first episode was captured in only 15 percent of subjects recovered from the index episode. On the other hand, the recent data from the McLean-Harvard First-Episode Mania Study do not show evidence of shortened intervals of wellness, although the period of follow-up was brief (2 to 4 years) (Tohen et al., 2003).[24]

As alluded to earlier, if the finding of shortening of well intervals cannot be applied to an entire sample of patients with manic-depressive illness, the question arises of whether it may be a subgroup effect. It is important to note that Post and colleagues (Post et al., 1986a; Post, 1990) proposed the kindling hypothesis as relevant to only a subset of patients with bipolar illness, particularly those who are unresponsive to lithium, more responsive to anticonvulsants, and with other "nonclassical" features of the illness. Granting Slater's critique, such a proposal would not be inconsistent with the available literature.

Clearly, the kindling model does not depend solely on the prediction of shortening of euthymic intervals of wellness. As discussed previously, the model makes other predictions as well, such as increasing frequency of episodes, increasing episode duration with time, decreasing importance of psychosocial triggers with time, and increasing treatment resistance with greater numbers of episodes (or differential efficacy in early versus later phases of illness). An important issue bearing on the generalizability of the kindling model is the proportion of patients with bipolar disorder whose course is consistent with these predictions.

Research on psychosocial triggers of episodes has revealed interesting data regarding this issue. Kendler and Karkowski-Shuman (1997) analyzed their sample of patients with recurrent unipolar depression so as to account for "within-person analyses." They reported on a sample of 2,395 female twin pairs followed for 9 years, in whom later mood episodes were associated less and less frequently with psychosocial triggers, as predicted by the kindling model.[25] They concluded (p. 542):

> These results indicate the observed decline in the association between stressful life events and depressive onsets with increasing numbers of previous depressive episodes is a true within-individual phenomenon and cannot be explained by systematic differences between the kind of individuals who have a low versus high number of previous depressive episodes.

Is there any evidence that episodes increase in frequency over time? Kessing and Andersen (1999) reported that such was the case for both unipolar depression (15 percent increased risk of recurrence with each episode)

and bipolar disorder (9 percent) in a case register study of all hospitalized admissions in Denmark (7,925 unipolar, 2,011 bipolar; 1971–1993 time frame). A similar conclusion was reached by Bockting and colleagues (2006) on the basis of a study of 172 patients meeting DSM-IV criteria for recurrent unipolar depression.

Increasing treatment resistance with number of episodes has been reported in some studies (e.g., Koukopoulos et al., 2000) but not in others (e.g., Baldessarini et al., 1999). Kessing and colleagues (1998b) failed to find other evidence of worsened outcome, such as increased mortality, associated with a sensitization pattern of progressive shortening of cycle length, although there was an interesting association between that kindling-like pattern and an increased risk of dementia.[26]

Recall that the kindling model predicts that outcome will be worse after more episodes. The outcome of both untreated and treated courses could be expected to reflect this pattern. This prediction is supported by some but not all studies. For instance, Gitlin and colleagues (1995) found that more previous episodes predicted earlier relapse at 4.3-year follow-up (2.2 versus 3.5 years; $p = .007$), a finding similar to that of Goldberg and Harrow (1994) noted earlier. On the other hand, in a 4.6-year study of outcome among 360 bipolar-I ($n = 220$) and bipolar-II ($n = 140$) patients on lithium maintenance therapy, Baldessarini and colleagues (1999) did not confirm the kindling-based prediction of worsening outcome with each successive episode. These investigators assessed delay in beginning lithium treatment after onset of bipolar illness and compared response to lithium treatment in subgroups of patients with few (0 to 4), some (4 to 9), or many (more than 10) mood episodes before treatment began. They reported no difference in lithium treatment response among these conditions; that is, lithium response was neither better nor worse if patients had experienced few or many previous mood episodes, or if they had begun lithium treatment soon after the onset of their illness as opposed to later. It is worth noting that lithium treatment had not been started until an average of 8 years after the onset of illness in this sample, which suggests that a significant delay occurred in most patients. Also, because this study was naturalistic, information about previous episodes and onset of illness was retrospective and subject to recall bias. It is notable that the average age at onset of bipolar illness in this sample (29.6 years)[27] was much older than the age in most other studies, a fact that may suggest the effects of recall bias or a difference in patient selection. It is also relevant that the kindling model may not be pertinent to the long-term outcome of lithium treatment. In the early work of Post and colleagues (Post and Weiss, 1989; Post, 1990), kindling was invoked to explain the treatment-refractory course of illness in those patients who failed to respond to lithium and who appeared to respond to anticonvulsant agents.

Taken as a whole, the findings reviewed here, although not decisively confirming the validity or generalizability of the kindling model, appear to suggest its relevance to at least some patients with manic-depressive illness, including both bipolar and recurrent unipolar forms.[28]

Other Cycle-Length Patterns

The relationship between frequency of episodes and age at onset remains somewhat unclear. Several older studies[29] found an increasing frequency of relapse with increased age at onset, but two studies failed to show this association (Dunner et al., 1980; Roy-Byrne et al., 1985a), and two found the opposite (Okuma and Shimoyama, 1972; Winokur and Kadrmas, 1989).[30] A multiple-regression analysis of the 105 bipolar patients studied by Grof and colleagues (1995) showed that the patient's age and age at onset each contributed independently to the prediction of relapse (Zis et al., 1979). Onset in the 20s was associated with a 20 percent probability of recurrence within 24 months, onset in the 30s with a 50 percent probability, and late onset (age 50 years or older) with a very high (80 percent) probability. Only the first cycle length (the time between the first and second episodes) was related to age at onset, however.[31]

A final question about the pattern of cycles in bipolar illness is whether burnout occurs. Kraepelin observed that the illness tends to decline after the fourth decade, although he did not elaborate on his observation. In a prospective follow-up study of 215 bipolar patients (150 bipolar-I, 65 bipolar-II) over a period of 17 to 21 years, Angst (1986d) found no age-related decrease in frequency of episodes; 26 percent of the bipolar patients (versus 42 percent of the unipolar patients) were free of relapses over 5 or more years, although most patients were still actively ill through their 60s, when the follow-up usually ended. Likewise, findings of recent studies do not generally support the concept of burnout (Goldberg and Harrow, 1999), although long-term follow-up from adulthood into the elderly years is rare.

Rapid Cycling

The inclusion of rapid cycling in DSM-IV was based to a large extent on a study by Bauer and colleagues (1994), who compared 120 patients with rapid-cycling bipolar disorder and 119 non–rapid-cycling patients. They found that 45 percent of the rapid cyclers had bipolar-II disorder, compared with 38 percent of the non–rapid cyclers, a difference that did not achieve statistical significance. Those with rapid cycling, not surprisingly, had more episodes in a 12-month prospective follow-up period; there were also more females in the rapid-cycling group. Based on these differences in course and demographics, the investigators supported the differentiation of rapid-cycling bipolar disorder as a valid course specifier for inclusion in DSM-IV. They also supported the cutoff definition of four episodes per year, because of an increase in the number of patients who experienced four to eight episodes per year, versus two to three episodes, during the prospective follow-up (although this was observed only among the females). It is notable that this was an observational study, in which adjustments were not made for potential confounding variables or effect modifiers. Therefore, similarities or differences between the two groups in this study may or may not be related to rapid cycling per se. This limitation holds for most of the research on rapid cycling.

Rapid cycling is thought to be equally common in type I and type II bipolar illness, but there is no firm consensus on this point.[32] Indeed, rapid-cycling unipolar depression (although uncommon) has been reported. It has generally been thought that rapid cycling develops later in the course of the illness and may reflect underlying pathophysiological mechanisms, such as the progressive kindling, or sensitization, discussed earlier (Fig. 4–3.). Late rapid cycling may also reflect the impact of certain treatments, especially antidepressants, in accelerating the natural course of the illness (see Chapter 19). The concept of rapid cycling as a later manifestation of bipolar illness has been proposed but is not supported by all investigators (see the later discussion) (Coryell et al., 1992). There may also be a predominance of rapid cycling in females (Koukopoulos et al., 1980; Coryell et al., 1992; Bauer et al., 1994), although Kupka and colleagues (2005) examined 539 outpatients in the Stanley Network and found that female preponderance was limited to those with eight or more episodes per year.

Box 4–1 highlights what is known about the relationship between rapid-cycling and non-rapid-cycling bipolar disorder. A study of the frequency distribution of cycle lengths could answer the question of whether rapid cycling represents a distinct subgroup or is simply one end of a continuum. Cycle-length data presented by Coryell and colleagues (1992) do not support a separate short-cycle-length group. The existing family history data also are more consistent with the continuum notion, in that the families of rapid-cycling patients have the same frequency of non-rapid-cycling affective disorders as families of non-rapid-cycling patients (Nurnberger et al., 1988b; Wehr et al., 1988; Coryell et al., 1992). The largest single prospective study of rapid cycling (Coryell et al., 1992) found that it is transient and not associated with the end stage of severe bipolar illness. The data in this study are based on the CDS, conducted in five tertiary-care academic health centers, in which 243 bipolar and 674 unipolar patients were

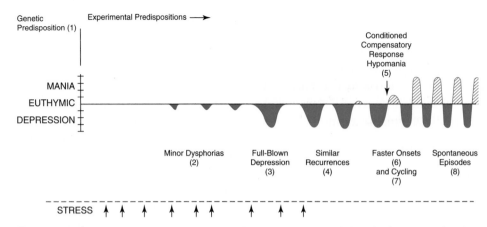

Figure 4–3. Behavioral sensitization paradigm of progressive course of illness leading to rapid cycles. (*Source:* Post et al., 1986a.)

- Data are insufficient to determine whether cycle length is distributed normally.
- In general, rapid-cycling patients appear to be related genetically and phenotypically to non-rapid-cycling patients (Nurnberger et al., 1988b; Wehr et al., 1988; Coryell et al., 1992).
- Illness in rapid-cycling patients can include a non-rapid-cycling course.
- Rapid cycling may be viewed as an extreme development of tendencies inherent in a non-rapid-cycling course:
  — Increasing frequency of episodes[*] (Grof et al., 1974)
  — Switches into new episodes with no normal interval between[*] (Winokur et al., 1969)
  — Circularity of episodes (Koukopoulos and Reginaldi, 1973)
- Rapid cycling may exhibit a somewhat different pharmacological response profile.
- Relative frequency in bipolar-I versus -II is unsettled.

*Potentiated by antidepressants, which are also capable of inducing rapid cycling (Wehr and Goodwin, 1979, 1987).

---

followed for 1 to 5 years, with interviews conducted every 6 months. The investigators found that 45 patients, all but one of them bipolar, developed a rapid-cycling course in the first year of follow-up; however, this group did not experience a lower rate of recovery at 5-year follow-up. Only 1 of the 39 rapid cyclers followed for the full 5 years continued to have four or more episodes in each year. In years 3 to 5, rapid cyclers did not differ from non–rapid cyclers in recovery from their index episode at the beginning of the study. However, there was a statistical trend for rapid cyclers to be less likely to experience a final follow-up year with no affective symptoms (only 10 percent of rapid cyclers, versus 49.5 percent of non–rapid cyclers; $p = .09$).

Although the CDS has the major advantage of being the kind of careful prospective, naturalistic study needed by the field, it is limited by those same study methods. Patients who remained in the study after having been recruited into one of the five tertiary-care centers in which it was conducted may not have been representative of the larger population of patients with rapid-cycling bipolar disorder—individuals whose chaotic lives often do not allow for long-term prospective follow-up in a systematic research study. Nonetheless, one cannot ignore the findings of this study, especially given the fact that, in a separate cohort, Maj and colleagues (1994) also found that only 18.9 percent of 37 individuals with rapid cycling continued to experience four or more episodes per year during 5-year follow-up. Future prospective research on more community-based samples may clarify these questions that are so important to the estimation of prognosis in individual patients.

Rapid cycling appears to represent a generally treatment-refractory state compared with non–rapid cycling. Most of the studies on this issue have involved lithium, which has led to the common belief that rapid-cycling patients do not respond well to lithium and respond better to anticonvulsants. In fact, as discussed in Chapters 18, 19, and 20, it appears that most rapid-cycling patients do not respond particularly well to any medication—lithium or anticonvulsants. Alternatively, as suggested by a number of investigators (Koukopoulos et al., 1983; Wehr et al., 1988; Baldessarini et al., 2000), the responsiveness of rapid-cycling patients to mood stabilizers may be greatly enhanced when concomitant antidepressant use is avoided.

Recent genetic studies on rapid cycling have yielded instructive, if inconclusive, results. Associations have been reported with the serotonin transporter gene polymorphism (Rousseva et al., 2003) and with a low-activity allele for the catechol-O-methyltransferase (COMT) gene (Kirov et al., 1998; Papolos et al., 1998), although the COMT allele association was not seen in a study of 52 children (mean age 10.9 years) (Geller and Cook, 2000). A family history study in 165 patients with rapid-cycling bipolar disorder did not identify major differences in familial mental illness compared with non-rapid-cycling bipolar disorder, with the exception of a suggestion of more substance abuse among relatives of rapid-cycling bipolar probands (Lish et al., 1993).

Taken together, the data tend to favor the concept that rapid cycling represents one extreme of a bipolar spectrum of cyclicity, but it is generally not a stable characteristic in an individual patient.

ONSET AND DURATION OF EPISODES

Often, the onset of manic episodes is abrupt, developing over a few days. Depressive episodes develop more gradually, over weeks, although bipolar depressive episodes are more abrupt in onset than unipolar depressive episodes (Winokur, 1976; Molnar et al., 1988; Keitner et al., 1996).

As we noted in the first edition, some patients experience a "hypomanic alert" (Jacobsen, 1965), a period of days or even weeks of hypomanic symptoms before the switch into mania. The most common prodrome is sleep disturbance, which had a prevalence of 77 percent in one study (Jackson et al., 2003). Family members are twice as likely as patients to observe early behavioral symptoms of mania (Keitner et al., 1996) (see Chapter 22).

Older estimates of the average duration of episodes in manic-depressive illness were derived from studies conducted before medications were available. In the CDS 5-year follow-up of a largely treated sample, the mean time to recovery was 6 weeks with pure mania, 11 weeks with pure depression, and 17 weeks with mixed states (Coryell et al., 1990). In a follow-up study conducted by Angst and Preisig (1995), the mean episode length was 4.3 months. Pure manic and pure depressive episodes lasted the same amount of time—approximately 3 months. Mixed episodes also lasted about 3 months, but "cyclic" episodes were longer (mean 4.2 months). The Baltimore site of the ECA community-based study of psychiatric disorders found that episodes lasted a median of 8 to 12 weeks (Eaton et al., 1997), with depressions lasting longer than manias. Maj and colleagues (2003) found longer duration of agitated depressive episodes compared with nonagitated depression in bipolar-I disorder (mean time to 50 percent recovery, 12 versus 9 weeks; N = 120) (Maj et al., 2003).

POLARITY

Estimates of the proportion of bipolar patients who begin the illness with a manic episode range from 34 to 79 percent, averaging just over 50 percent. It is important to recognize that the other half of patients with the bipolar form of manic-depressive illness will go undiagnosed as bipolar at the onset of their condition, because they initially experience only major depressive episodes[33]; this condition is sometimes called "false" unipolar depression. This dilemma arises from the current DSM nosology (see Chapters 1 and 3), which places primary emphasis on polarity at the expense of cyclicity or recurrence. This approach guarantees an initial misdiagnosis in many patients who have bipolar disorder but have not yet experienced their first manic episode. The problem was less acute with the classic construct of manic-depressive illness, which took into account other course factors, such as recurrence of episodes, as well as family history.

One study of false unipolar depression examined 17,447 patients with mood disorders who were hospitalized in Denmark over a 22-year period (1971–1993) (Kessing, 1999). Among those whose first episodes were depressive, if a manic episode was to develop, it usually did so within 5 years. Patients with false unipolar depression experienced more recurrent depressive episodes than did patients with true unipolar depression.[34]

It is also important to recognize that there is a relationship between false unipolar depression and age at onset (see Chapter 1). An often-cited figure is that 1 to 2 percent of patients with depression may experience a hypomanic/manic episode in every year of follow-up. This figure is based on the CDS cohort (Coryell et al., 1995), in which 10.2 percent of a depressed subgroup (mean age 36.8 years) had a manic or hypomanic episode during 10 years of follow-up. A younger age at onset within this cohort was associated with increased risk of manic/hypomanic switch, however. Other younger cohorts have confirmed higher natural switch rates to mania (see Chapter 6). For example, in a group of 72 depressed children (mean age 10.3 years), Geller and colleagues (2001) found that 49 percent had experienced a manic or hypomanic episode at 10-year follow-up. In a group of 74 depressed young adults (mean age 23.0 years), Goldberg and colleagues (2001) observed that 46 percent had experienced a manic or hypomanic episode at 15-year follow-up. Thus the risk of switching from false unipolar depression to bipolar disorder is highest in childhood and young adulthood, occurring at a rate of about 3 to 5 percent per year; it then decreases by the late 30s, at which point it flattens out to about 1 percent per year.

Studies showing the highest estimates of manic onset utilize first hospitalization as the onset criterion. It is possible that these high estimates result from underestimation of depressive onsets, because many depressions do not require hospitalization. On the other hand, hypomanic onsets are probably underestimated compared with depressive onsets, because patients are more likely to experience (and report) depressive symptoms as illness. Angst (1978) reported manic onset of illness in the majority of his bipolar sample (N = 95), where onset was defined as the first occurrence of symptoms requiring treatment. On the other hand, Roy-Byrne and colleagues (1985a), who defined onset as the first symptoms meeting the RDC for an affective episode, found that 60 percent of 71 bipolar patients had a depressive first episode.

Onset may influence the later pattern of illness. Perris and d'Elia (1966) reported that among patients with a manic first episode, 62 percent went on to have a predominantly manic course, and only 25 percent a predominantly depressive course. It is interesting that a predominantly manic course may herald a better outcome. In a hospital chart review study based on the premedication treatment era, Stephens and McHugh (1991) reported on outcomes in 297 bipolar and 945 unipolar patients admitted to the Johns Hopkins Hospital from 1913 to 1940. Only 2 percent of all patients with mood disorder experienced unipolar manic episodes, and their outcome was best (75 percent recovered or improved), followed by that of those with unipolar depression (69 percent) and bipolar disorder (57 percent) (Stephens and McHugh, 1991). This report is supported by another study of 320 patients with bipolar-I disorder (Perugi et al., 2000), in whom depressive episode onset was associated with higher levels of later rapid-cycling course, as well as suicide attempts. Later psychotic features were more likely to be associated with manic onset, however. In light of these findings of a relationship between polarity at onset and subsequent course, a recent report that the polarity of onset appears to be familial (Kassen et al., 2006) is especially interesting.

It has generally been observed that women tend to be more likely to have a predominantly depressive pattern to their bipolar illness, and men a predominantly manic pattern.[35] More recent data have not uniformly supported these findings, however. In one chart review of 131 patients (63 women and 68 men) (Hendrick et al., 2000), there were no statistically significant gender differences in age at onset, number of depressive or manic episodes, and number of hospitalizations for depression. However, women had been hospitalized for mania significantly more often than men, whereas substance abuse, although high in both groups, was more prevalent among men. Also, in a cross-sectional analysis of 500 subjects in the NIMH Systematic Treatment Enhancement Program for Bipolar Disorder (STEP-BD) study cohort, there were no gender differences in number of past depressive versus manic episodes (87.4 percent of women and 86.8 percent of men had experienced three or more manic episodes; 92.1 percent of women and 92.3 percent of men had experienced three or more depressive episodes) (Baldassano et al., 2002).[36] As noted earlier in relation to age at onset of depression and false unipolar depression, polarity distinctions are not stable until approximately age 40.[37] Before that age, depressed individuals remain at a relatively elevated risk of eventual occurrence of manic or hypomanic episodes.

Some investigators have noted that polyphasic polarity patterns are associated with poor outcomes (Turvey et al., 1999; Maj et al., 2002). For instance, Maj and colleagues (2002) compared 10-year outcome in 97 patients with bipolar disorder whose index episode included switching from one mood phase to another and 97 patients whose index episode was monophasic. Overall, they found that a subgroup of those who switched had experienced multiple polarity switches (n = 23) and had worse outcomes (ill 56 percent of the time during the follow-up period), compared with those who had one polarity switch (ill 26 percent of the time; n = 74) or those with a monophasic index episode (ill 20 percent of the time; n = 97).

A related question (discussed further in Chapter 19) is whether depression that occurs alone (preceded and followed by euthymia) is different in duration or risk of an antidepressant-related manic switch from depression that occurs immediately following mania. This pattern of differential risk was noted in a post hoc analysis of a small randomized clinical trial comparing the addition of paroxetine to a mood stabilizer (lithium or valproate) with a combination of the two mood stabilizers (Goldberg, 2001). Another study (Gitlin et al., 2003) examined 72 prospectively observed depressive episodes in 28 patients with bipolar-I disorder. It was found that 65 percent of depressive episodes were monophasic, and 35 percent were postmanic. Duration of episodes was somewhat longer in the monophasic group (82 ± 65 days) than in the postmanic group (62 ± 48 days). Antidepressant-induced manic switching was also higher in the postmanic group (36 percent, 4 of 11 patients) than in the monophasic group (26 percent, 9 of 34 patients). Although the authors interpreted these differences as unimportant because of a lack of statistical significance, there is a large risk of type II false-negative error due to the small sample size. Whether future research will confirm this suggestion of higher susceptibility to antidepressant-induced mania and perhaps an increased cycling rate in those with polyphasic as compared to monophasic depressive episodes remains an open question.

The features of a manic episode may also be related to the course of illness. In a retrospective assessment, Swann and colleagues (2001) found that mania with depressive features (mixed states) was associated with an earlier onset of illness and more prior episodes than mania with irritable features (but no concomitant depressive affect).

PATTERN

The topic of episode pattern is of historical importance. Early investigators demonstrated that three basic patterns were apparent: mania followed by depression and then a well interval (MDI), depression followed by mania and then a well interval (DMI), and continuous cycling (MDMD).[38] There is some evidence from these studies that the MDI pattern may have the best outcome (Koukopoulos et al., 1980) and the MDMD pattern the worst. As we suggested in the first edition, the DMI pattern appears to be associated with mania occurring after treatment of the depressive phase with antidepressants (Maj et al., 1989).

Contemporary studies of episode pattern are not entirely consistent with this older literature. In a study of all hospitalized cases of bipolar and unipolar disorders in Denmark over a 22-year period (1971–1993; N = 17,447), the DMI and MDI courses were associated with a similar number of recurrences (Kessing, 1999). On the other hand, in a recent reanalysis of data from the CDS in which 165 bipolar-I patients were followed for 15 years, Turvey and colleagues (1999) reported that mood episodes beginning with depression (depression only or depression followed by mania) were associated with worse 15-year outcomes than those beginning with mania. Also, polarity sequences tended to remain stable over time: 75 to 80 percent of individuals whose first observed mood episode began with mania continued to have mood episodes beginning with mania, and 55 to 60 percent of those whose mood episodes began with depression also maintained that pattern. This study is the longest outcome study assessing polarity. Its findings suggest that patterns of mood episodes are sustained over time and that the poorer prognosis of depressive as opposed to manic episodes persists in the long run.

Finally, it should be noted that some confusion regarding the patterning of episodes has been introduced by recent treatment guidelines asserting that the polarity of the index episode predicts the polarity of a relapse following the episode. As discussed in detail in Chapters 17 and 20, this conclusion should apply only to those relapses that occur shortly after remission is achieved, and these generally occur as a result of an effective treatment's being withdrawn before the continuation phase of treatment is completed. In an analysis of the course of patients on placebo participating in an 18-month study of maintenance treat-ment with lithium or lamotrigine when the time frame beyond the continuation phase of treatment was examined the next new episode was almost always (85 percent of the time) of opposite polarity confirming classic observations (F. Goodwin and Calebrese [in preparation]).

PRECIPITANTS OF EPISODES

Findings of most studies of diagnostically heterogeneous groups of depressed patients suggest that stressful life events, such as losing a loved one, changing jobs, or moving, are more frequent during the 3 to 12 months preceding the onset of a depressive episode. Although the literature on events precipitating depression is extensive, that pertaining specifically to bipolar patients is more modest. It comprises primarily interesting but ultimately inconclusive case reports (reviewed by Ellicott, 1988), an intriguing report on increased relapses among bipolar patients after a hurricane,[39] and 14 systematic studies, all but 3 of which were retrospective. These studies are outlined in Table 4–3; their conclusions are summarized in Box 4–2. Taken together, they provide considerable support for the importance of stressful events in the onset of episodes in bipolar patients.

Although some theories assign primary causal importance to psychosocial environmental forces, it is now generally accepted that environmental conditions—psychosocial or physical—contribute more to the timing of an episode than to underlying vulnerability, which is largely genetic (see Chapter 13). Thus modern biological theory reaffirms the classic position of Kraepelin (1921, pp. 180–181):

> We must regard all alleged injuries as possibly sparks for the discharge of individual attacks, but that the real cause of the malady must be sought in permanent internal changes, which at least very often, perhaps always, are innate. . . . Unfortunately, the powerlessness of our efforts to cure must only too often convince us that the attacks of manic-depressive insanity may be to an astonishing degree independent of external influences.

Early precipitating events, rather than merely influencing the timing of an episode, may actually activate the preexisting vulnerability, thereby making the individual more vulnerable to subsequent episodes, as recently demonstrated by Dienes and colleagues (2006). The theoretical significance of this possibility, proposed by Post and colleagues (1986a), is elaborated in Chapters 14 and 17.

More recent evidence supports the conclusion that the influence of life events in triggering mood episodes is more prominent in earlier than in later phases of bipolar disorder. The studies summarized in Table 4–3 (total of 688 patients) generally support this observation.

TABLE 4–3. Life Events, Kindling, and Mood Episodes in Bipolar Disorder

Study	Sample Size	Life Event (LE) Method	Findings	Supports Kindling	Comments
Ambelas, 1979	67	Paykel LE scale	First-episode patients were overrepresented in LE-associated mania.	Yes	Retrospective only; hospitalized manic episodes assessed
Dunner et al., 1979b	79	Own LE questionnaire	52% reported LEs before first episode, compared with 15% before subsequent episodes.	Yes	Retrospective study of outpatients; not limited to hospitalized episodes
Glassner and Haldipur, 1983	53	Own interview with patients and families	23% of early-onset bipolar patients (age <20) had LEs before episodes, compared with 63% of late-onset bipolar patients (age >20). However, early-onset patients had the same percentage LEs before first and subsequent episodes (23%), as did late-onset patients (64% and 61%, respectively).	Indeterminate	Retrospective; included inpatients and outpatients
Perris et al., 1984	149	Own LE interview	More patients with later episodes than first episode of depression reported no preceding negative LEs (50% vs. 38%; $p < .02$) or conflict events (81% vs. 57%; $p < .001$).	Yes	Prospective; combined bipolar and recurrent unipolar disorders in sample
Bidzinska, 1984	36	Puzynski LE questionnaire	LEs preceded more of first three episodes (2.6) than fourth through sixth episodes (1.9; $p < .05$).	Yes	Retrospective; compared findings with those of studies of unipolar patients, in which results did not support kindling; criteria for episodes unclear

136

Study	N	Measure	Finding	Kindling supported?	Comments
Swann et al., 1990	66	Two Schedule for Affective Disorders and Schizophrenia (SADS) scale items asking clinicians and patients to give impressions of stressful LEs and current episode	Perceived roles of stressful LEs (combined clinician and patient scores) were greater in patients with fewer previous episodes (3.7) than in those with more previous episodes (13.4; $p < 0.05$).	Yes	Retrospective; careful rating scale and diagnostic assessments; data for bipolar and unipolar patients not separate
Winokur et al., 1993	148	None	Patients with one or more previous episodes were more likely than first-episode patients to have a recurrence in 2-year follow-up (0.64 episodes vs. 0.46; $p = .18$), but not statistically significant.	Indeterminate	Prospective; episodes based on Research Diagnostic Criteria and not just hospitalization, up to 5-year follow-up
Palao et al., 1997	26	Scale of Assessment of LE and Social Support of the California Department of Mental Health	Fewer LEs were found before the first episode of bipolar disorder compared with the following two episodes ($p < .02$).	No	Outpatients; complete data not available, presented as abstract; method for assessing episodes not clear (apparently retrospective)
Hlastala et al., 2000	64	SADS-Lifetime (SADS-L) or Structured Clinical Interview for DSM (SCID)	Number of episodes experienced did not appear to have a significant effect on reactivity of bipolar-I patients to external stressors.	No	Prospective

Note: Total sample = 688 (limited to patients identified as having bipolar disorder, with exception of Perris et al., 1984).

BOX 4–2. Precipitants of Episodes in Bipolar Illness: Conclusions

- All studies found significantly more stress prior to manic episodes, compared with various control groups.
- Only one study (Kennedy et al., 1983) involved a within-patient comparison (i.e., controlling for inherent stress vulnerability). It found significantly more stressful events preceding a manic episode.
- The onset of initial (or early) episodes is more likely to be associated with stress than is that of later episodes (five of six studies), which is consistent with the kindling hypothesis.
- Although bipolar–unipolar differences have been observed in some studies, there is no consistent pattern.
- Work-related events may be particularly important precipitating factors for manic or hypomanic relapses.
- Cyclothymia is associated with an increased response to stress, consistent with its being part of the bipolar spectrum (Depue et al., 1981).
- Manic patients frequently create stressful life events.
- Stressful events often lead to sleep loss, which in turn can precipitate mania.
- Stress can lead to increased alcohol and drug use, both of which can result in sleep loss and/or mania.

Recently, Kendler and colleagues (2000) conducted a large twin study involving 2,395 individuals with unipolar depression, interviewed four times over a period of 9 years, and found that stressful life events were increasingly less associated with triggering a major depressive episode over time. This pattern held for the first nine episodes, then tapered off. Although this study investigated unipolar disorder, its findings on precipitation of episodes appear to be highly relevant to mood disorders in general. A major strength of this study is that it employed a twin research paradigm and therefore could control for the effects of the environment, as opposed to genetics, in a way that clinical studies cannot. Employing this paradigm and mathematical models that can be used to predict genetic versus environmental causation, the investigators were able to suggest that the relationship between life events and major depressive episodes was causal and not simply correlational. Similar findings have reported from non-twin studies of recurrent unipolar depression (Brown et al., 1994; Hammen et al., 2000; Bockting et al., 2006.)

The older literature on an association between life events and relapse is supported by a study of 62 patients with bipolar disorder (Hunt et al., 1992), in which a more frequent rate of severe life events (19 percent) was found in the month before relapse, compared with the background monthly rate of such events (5 percent), during the 2-year follow-up period. In another study, recovery from mood episodes in 67 hospitalized patients with bipolar-I disorder was delayed three-fold in the presence of a precipitating negative life event (Johnson and Miller, 1997).

Because external life events have been established as associated with mood episodes, recent research has focused on other aspects of the psychosocial circumstances of individuals with bipolar disorder. For instance, Staner and colleagues (1997) reported that, among 27 patients with bipolar disorder in remission for 1 year, social support, self-esteem, and attributional styles were not associated with increased risk of subsequent episodes of bipolar illness, but social maladjustment was.

Specific life events that deserve separate mention are pregnancy and childbirth. The earlier literature suggested a significant risk of postpartum (puerperal) depression or mania.[40] More recent data indicate a high risk of depression during pregnancy or the postpartum period in bipolar women (30 to 50 percent), as well as some risk of mood instability during pregnancy itself.[41,42] The treatment implications of pregnancy and the postpartum period of treatment are discussed in Chapter 20.

Comorbidity of personality disorders may be another factor that interacts with psychosocial stressors in increasing the risk of relapse in bipolar disorder (see Chapter 10). In one study of 52 euthymic U.S. military veterans with bipolar disorder, 38 percent met DSM-III-R criteria for personality disorder, which, in an unadjusted analysis, was associated with lower employment status and increased substance abuse (Kay et al., 2002). In another study, 72 bipolar-I patients were assessed dimensionally for the presence of hyperthymic versus depressive temperaments. Adjusted for age, sex, and occupational level in a multiple-regression analysis, higher depressive temperament trait scores were associated with greater number of mood episodes, especially of depressive polarity, and more suicide attempts (Henry et al., 1999). The interaction between personality and psychosocial stressors is an important clinical and research topic for further evaluation.

Drugs and physical illness, unlike life events, are sometimes not recognized as significant precipitating factors for manic or depressive episodes, but they should be (Table 4–4). Both drugs and alcohol can, in their own right, precipitate manic episodes, and they also can impair both the quantity and quality of sleep, thereby increasing the probability of mania. The special situation of mania precipitated by antidepressant treatment is discussed in detail in Chapter 19; we review some of that literature here as it relates to precipitation of mood episodes.

In his cohort study, Angst (1981a) found no association between long-term administration of antidepressants and recurrence, although he did not report the raw data. Turvey

TABLE 4–4. Conditions and Drugs Reported to Precipitate Manic Episodes

General Category	Specific Factor	Study
Endocrine States or Substances	Cushings (increased steroids)	Glaser, 1953; Goolker and Schein, 1953
	Hyperthyroidism	Corn and Checkley, 1983
	Androgens	Freinhar and Alvarez, 1985b
	Steroid and steroid withdrawal	Goldstein and Preskom, 1989; Pope and Katz, 1988; Venkatarangam et al., 1988; Viswanathan and Glickman, 1989
Drugs	Isoniazid[a]	Chaturvedi and Upadhyaya, 1988; Jackson, 1957; Kane and Taylor, 1963
	Procarbazine	Mann and Hutchinson, 1967
	Levodopa	O'Brien et al., 1971; Ryback and Schwab, 1971; Van Woert et al., 1971; Chase et al., 1973
	Methyldopa withdrawal	Labbate and Holzgang, 1989
	Hallucinogens (e.g., LSD, PCP and mescaline)	
	Cocaine[b]	
	Alcohol[b]	
	Bromide	Sayed, 1976
	Sympathomimetic amines	Waters and Lapierre, 1981
	Cimetidine; amantadine	Hubain et al., 1982; Lazare, 1979; Rego and Giller, 1989
	Tolmetin	Sotsky and Tossell, 1984
	Iproniazid	Crane, 1956
	Methylphenidate	Koehler-Troy et al., 1986
	Triazolam	Weilburg et al., 1987
	Zidovudine[c]	Maxwell et al., 1988; O'Dowd and McKegney, 1988; Schaerf et al., 1988;
	Busipirone	Wright et al., 1989; Liegghio and Yeragani, 1988; Price and Bielefeld, 1989
	Alprazolam	France and Krishnan, 1984
	Lorazepam	Rigby et al., 1989
	Guanfacine[d]	Horrigan and Barnhill, 1999
	Lisinopril[d]	Skop and Masterson, 1995
Metabolic Conditions	Postoperative state	Muncie, 1934
	Hemodialysis	Cooper, 1967
Infections	Influenza	Maurizi, 1985; Steinberg et al., 1972
	Q Fever	Schwartz, 1974
	Post–St. Louis type A encephalitis	Weisert and Hendrie, 1977
	Cryptococcal meningitis	Johnson and Naraqi, 1993
Central Nervous System (CNS) Pathology Neoplasms[a]	Suprasellar diencephalic tumor	Guttman and Hermann, 1932; Greenberg and Brown, 1985
	Head trauma	Stern and Dancey, 1942; McKeown and Jani, 1987; Jorge et al., 1993

(continued)

TABLE 4–4. **Conditions and Drugs Reported to Precipitate Manic Episodes** *(continued)*

General Category	Specific Factor	Study
	Parasagittal meningioma	Oppler, 1950
	Benign pheno-occipital tumor	Bourgeois and Campagne, 1967
	AIDS	Dauncey, 1988; Gabel et al., 1986; Kermani et al., 1985; Mijch et al., 1999
	Creutzfeld-Jakob Disease	Lendvai et al., 1999
	Syndenham's chorea	Black and Perlmutter, 1997
	Multiple sclerosis	Casanova et al., 1996; Heila et al., 1995
	Chondroma	Salazar-Calderon et al., 1993
Vascular Lesions[e]	Aneurysm	Jampala and Abrams, 1983
	Infarction	Cummings and Mendez, 1984; Fujikawa et al., 1995; Kulisevsky et al., 1993; Vuilleumier et al., 1998
Other	Epilepsy—right temporal focus	Rosenbaum and Barry, 1975
	Vitamin B_{12} deficiency	Goggans, 1984
	L-glutamine	Mebane, 1984
	Aspartame	Walton, 1986
	Metrizamide as a contrast agent in myelography	Kwentus et al., 1984

Note: This table is based on the definition of secondary mania provided by Krauthammer and Klerman (1978); the data have been updated by our own review and those of Lazare (1979), Yassa and colleagues (1988a), and Sultzer and Cummings (1989).

[a]Mania induced by antidepressants (tricyclic monoamine oxidase inhibitors [MAOIs] and selective serotonin reuptake inhibitors [SSRIs]) is thoroughly discussed in Chapter 20. Reports of antipsychotic-induced mania are discussed in Chapter 18.

[b]The impact of alcohol and illicit drug abuse on manic-depressive illness is detailed in Chapters 7 and 21.

[c]Used for treatment of acquired immunodeficiency syndrome (AIDS).

[d]Antihypertensive medications.

[e]A comprehensive review of secondary mania in association with central nervous system (CNS) pathology can be found in Chapter 17.

and colleagues (1999), analyzing the CDS data, reported that polyphasic as opposed to monophasic mood episodes were not associated with antidepressant use. Although polyphasic mood episodes were associated with poor outcome and initial depression was correlated with polyphasic mood episodes, antidepressant use could not be shown to be a factor in the poor outcome later observed. This study was a longer-term reanalysis of the same sample previously discussed (with similar findings) by Coryell and colleagues (1992). Because treatments were not randomized, one cannot know what influenced clinicians to use or not use antidepressants.

Other investigators, using other samples, have reported different results. As detailed earlier, Altshuler and colleagues (1995) found that about 25 percent of bipolar patients appeared to show an association between antidepressant use and rapid cycling. This figure was confirmed by Ghaemi and colleagues (2000), who reported that 24 percent of individuals treated in a university-affiliated health maintenance organization demonstrated such an association. Although these latter reports are retrospective, rather than prospective like the CDS, the inability to replicate the findings of the CDS in other samples raises questions about the generalizability of the CDS sample.

Wehr and colleagues (1987a) proposed that sleep reduction may be the common denominator of several disparate events and stressors that reportedly precipitate mania. Indeed, this suggestion is well supported by our clinical experience. Sleep loss is common to reports of manic episodes following (1) various stressful events, such as bereavement (e.g., Krishnan et al., 1984); (2) the postpartum state; and (3) jet lag associated with flying across time zones. Selective serotonin reuptake inhibitor (SSRI) antidepressants are capable of destabilizing sleep patterns. Because of the importance of this issue, we outline in Chapter 19 specific approaches designed to minimize sleep loss in bipolar patients.

Another important potential trigger for mood episodes is the season of the year. Issues regarding light and seasonality were addressed extensively in the first edition and are further discussed in Chapter 16 of this volume. In the context of course of illness, patients with bipolar and recurrent unipolar conditions often experience seasonal patterns. In one study published since the first edition of this text, 49 percent of 146 patients who met DSM-III-R criteria for seasonal affective disorder (Faedda et al., 1993) were diagnosable with bipolar disorder, mainly type I (30 percent of the total sample; 19 percent were type II), meaning that these patients tended to experience full manic episodes in spring or summer. While winter depression is often the focus in the diagnosis and treatment of seasonal affective disorder, the high likelihood of summer mania should also be noted.[43]

LONG-TERM OUTCOME

The literature on long-term outcome in bipolar disorder can be quite confusing. We have already noted some problems that can contribute to this confusion, such as effects of treatment in studies done in the modern era, selection bias in studies from academic health centers, and lack of adjustment through appropriate statistical techniques (e.g., multivariate regression) for other potential predictors of outcome (such as socioeconomic status and antidepressant use). Another problem is multiple publications over time based on the same dataset, which can appear to readers to represent different datasets. For this reason, we have grouped studies of long-term outcome by their initial recruitment location, rather than by specific publications.

The literature from the 1970s and 1980s on long-term outcome in bipolar illness tended to find somewhat better outcomes than have more recent studies. For instance, in a report on a 35-year follow-up of the original 100 patients admitted for mania in the Iowa 500 study, Tsuang and colleagues (1979) found that when marital, residential, occupational, and psychiatric (symptomatic) status were combined, outcome was good in approximately 64 percent of patients, fair in 14 percent, and poor (i.e., chronic) in 22 percent. This study, while more than 25 years old, still encompasses the modern era in which pharmacological treatments were available.

Modern Prospective Cohort Studies

Since 1990, there have been reports on 11 prospective cohort studies of natural history in manic-depressive illness, all but one of which were limited to bipolar disorder (Table 4–5).[48] The two largest and most carefully examined are the CDS and McLean-Harvard first-episode cohorts, which are discussed at the end of this section. Two more recent cohorts are those of the Stanley Foundation Bipolar Network and STEP-BD. Longitudinal outcome data are beginning to become available from both of these studies.

The Zurich cohort consisted of 406 patients, 186 with unipolar depression and 220 with bipolar disorder, initially recruited on admission to a psychiatric hospital during 1959–1963 and then reinterviewed at 5-year intervals. In a follow-up period that lasted up to 20 years, Angst and colleagues (2005) reported that only 24 percent of the bipolar sample and only 30 percent of the unipolar sample had fully remitted (that is, had experienced no further episodes). Many patients, however, had experienced periods free of illness, comprising on average about 80 percent of the time; chronically ill outcomes were seen in only 16 percent of the bipolar and 13 percent of the unipolar sample. In a recent reanalysis involving a follow-up period of more than 40 years, only 16 percent of the total sample had fully recovered by age 68 (Global Assessment Scale score above 60, with no episodes in the past 5 years), and 52 percent still had recurrent episodes. A subgroup (16 percent) remained chronically ill, and 7.8 percent had committed suicide (Angst and Preisig, 1995).

The Chicago cohort consisted of 139 hospitalized patients, 73 with mania and 66 with unipolar depression, recruited from area hospitals in the late 1980s. Outcome was assessed with a scale that incorporated both symptomatic and functional assessments. In a follow-up period that lasted on average 1.7 years, 25 percent of unipolar and 19 percent of bipolar subjects had a good outcome, while 14 percent of unipolar versus 25 percent of bipolar subjects had a consistently poor outcome (Harrow et al., 1990). In a follow-up that extended up to 5 years (mean 4.5 years), outcomes looked somewhat better, with 41 percent of unipolar and bipolar subjects demonstrating a good outcome, versus 14 percent of unipolar and 22 percent of bipolar subjects having a consistently poor outcome (Goldberg et al., 1995).

The University of California-Los Angeles (UCLA) cohort consisted of 82 bipolar patients recruited to the university outpatient clinic from 1984 to 1990, followed for a minimum of 2 years (which led to the exclusion of 78 patients initially recruited) and then for up to 5 years (mean 4.3 years) (Gitlin et al., 1995). Among this sample, 37 percent had relapsed at 1-year follow-up and 73 percent at 5 years, with only 17 percent consistently euthymic. Most relapses (70 percent) involved multiple episodes.

The Cincinnati cohort consisted of two groups. The first comprised 134 hospitalized patients with DSM-III-R bipolar disorder recruited from their academic psychiatric units during 1992–1995. At 1-year follow-up (Keck et al., 1998), 48 percent had experienced syndromal recovery; 26 percent symptomatic recovery (full remission); and 24 percent functional recovery (defined as regaining premorbid occupational and residential status), which was associated with higher initial socioeconomic status and paralleled

TABLE 4–5. **Prospective Cohort Natural-History Studies in Manic-Depressive Illness Since 1990**

Study	Sample Size	Follow-up Period	Findings
Chicago cohort (Harrow et al., 1990; Goldberg et al., 1995)	139	Up to 4 years	22% poor overall outcome, 41% good overall outcome in bipolar subgroup
McLean/Harvard cohort I (Tohen et al., 1990)	75	Up to 4 years	Multiepisode cohort; 100% follow-up obtained. 28% poor functional outcome; only 28% episode-free
National Institute of Mental Health (NIMH) Collaborative Program on the Psychobiology of Depression-Clinical Studies cohort (Coryell et al., 1993, 1994, 1995; Akiskal et al., 1995, 1998; Judd et al., 1998; Turvey et al., 1999; Judd et al., 2002, 2003)	428	Up to 20 years	Mood symptoms presented in about one half of the follow-up period, primarily those associated with chronic subsyndromal depression
University of California-Los Angeles (UCLA) cohort (Gitlin et al., 1995)	82	Up to 5 years	Only 17% "consistently euthymic"
Cincinnati cohort I (Keck et al., 1998)	134	Up to 1 year	48% syndromal recovery; 28% symptomatic recovery; 24% functional recovery
Cincinnati cohort II (Strakowski et al., 1998)	50	Up to 1 year	First-episode mania cohort. 30% not improved; 30% with continued subsyndromal symptoms
McLean/Harvard cohort II (Tohen et al., 2000, 2003)	173	Up to 4 years	First-episode cohort; classic Kraepelinian features; almost complete syndromal recovery (98%), but less symptomatic (72%) and functional (43%) recovery
Stanley Foundation Bipolar Network cohort (Post et al., 2001, 2003; Suppes et al., 2001; Keck et al., 2003)	648	Up to 1 year	33% were substantially well, 67% mostly ill; 63% had a prospective rapid cycling course; cohort was depressed for 33% of the follow-up period and manic for 11%
Systematic Treatment Enhancement Program for Bipolar Disorder (STEP-BD) cohort (Kogan et al., 2004)	1000	Up to 5 years	Prospective data pending
Jorvi Bipolar Study cohort (Mantere et al., 2004)	191	N/A	A polyphasic episode was current in 51.3%, rapid cycling in 32.5%, and psychotic symptoms in 16.2%; mixed episodes occurred in 16.7% of bipolar-I and depressive mixed states in 25.7% of bipolar-II patients
Zurich cohort (Angst and Preiseg, 1995)	406	Up to 40 years	Only 16% fully recovered; only 16% had chronic outcome

symptomatic recovery. Incidentally, only 47 percent of patients were fully adherent to treatment at follow-up, which is consistent with the literature reviewed in Chapter 21. A second Cincinnati cohort project, initiated in 1996, recruited bipolar patients hospitalized with their first manic episode. The initial 50 subjects enrolled between 1996 and 1998 were characterized at about 6.8 months of follow-up (Strakowski et al., 2000). On average, the subjects remained in a full syndromal mood episode for about 30 percent of the follow-up period, spending an additional

30 percent of the time in subsyndromal mood states. Initial mood-incongruent psychosis predicted worse outcome than initial mood-congruent psychosis (after adjusting for some clinical factors with analysis of covariance).

The CDS and McLean-Harvard cohorts can be seen as complementary, because they represent different types of patients. Data on the CDS cohort were collected at five U.S. academic health centers. The cohort consisted of patients in their 30s and 40s initially, whose illness usually had begun a decade or more earlier with depression as its primary presenting feature (for which the patients had been treated primarily with antidepressants), and who tended to have comorbid diagnoses. This represents a "modern" manic-depressive illness cohort, with nonclassical features of illness. The McLean-Harvard cohort consisted completely of hospitalized bipolar patients, most of whom were psychotic and experiencing their first manic episode. Most were insured, of middle to high socioeconomic status, and with few psychiatric comorbidities. This cohort is close to a modern analogue of the classic patients of the pretreatment era, similar to those Kraepelin described from among psychotic patients hospitalized at the Munich asylum. As Grof and colleagues (1995) suggested, it could be that the natural history of the bipolar variant of classic Kraepelinian manic-depressive illness is quite different from that of the bipolar disorder identified in many cohorts today. At any rate, differences in findings among contemporary cohorts need to be assessed in light of the different samples they represent. Each cohort is discussed below in turn.[45]

The CDS has produced the most published data in recent years on the course of manic-depressive illness. The sample in that study consisted of roughly one-third outpatients and two-thirds inpatients initially recruited during the years 1978–1981 at five U.S. academic health centers. This cohort has now been followed for up to 25 years, with a retention rate in follow-up of more than 80 percent. As of 2003, about 80 percent of this cohort was reportedly in continued treatment with pharmacotherapy (R. Keller, personal communication, 2003). At 5-year follow-up, more previous episodes predicted more relapses but also quicker recovery (recovery at 6 months was 55 percent for a first episode, 73 percent for one or two previous episodes, and 90 percent for more than three previous episodes). Psychosis predicted only 37 percent recovery at 6 months, versus 65 percent in nonpsychotic patients. At 5-year follow-up, all of the patients initially treated for pure mania had recovered, compared with 89 percent of those with pure depression and 83 percent of those with mixed states. Despite ongoing "high-intensity somatotherapy" in the majority of subjects (75 percent), early relapse rates were relatively high: at 6 months, 20 percent of patients with pure mania had relapsed, compared with 33 percent of those with pure depression and 36 percent of those with mixed states. By 1 year, 48 percent of patients initially with pure mania had had a relapse, versus 57 percent of those with mixed states; at 5 years, these rates were up to 81 and 91 percent, respectively. Relapse rates among those initially treated for depression were similar to those among patients with mixed episodes (Keller and Boland, 1998). The question of antidepressant-induced worsening of the long-term course of bipolar illness also raises the possibility that these poor outcomes may have occurred in part because of (rather than despite) the high-intensity somatotherapy received by patients (although adherence to treatment was not reported).

Despite sustained syndromal recovery for 2 years, most of the sample of 148 bipolar and 240 unipolar patients experienced severe impairment of psychosocial functioning (Coryell et al., 1993). In the index episode, the co-occurrence of psychotic features with mixed states (depressive symptoms during acute mania) was associated with more long-term psychosis than was the co-occurrence of index psychotic features with pure mania (Coryell et al., 2001).

Other analyses of the CDS data were reviewed earlier in the discussion of kindling. More recent results from the CDS are presented later in the discussion of subsyndromal outcomes.

The McLean-Harvard First-Episode Mania Study consisted of two cohorts. The first (Tohen et al., 1990) included 75 bipolar patients who were recruited over a 1-year period (1983–1984) from the psychiatric units of McLean Hospital after admission for acute mania and followed for up to 4 years (100 percent of subjects were followed for the entire outcome period). This was primarily a multiple-episode cohort (68 percent). The second cohort (Tohen et al., 2000, 2003) started with bipolar patients in their first hospitalized episode; 173 such patients were recruited from 1989 to 1996 at the same hospital and followed for up to 4 years. The characteristics of this second cohort were as follows: 84.9 percent were Caucasian, with gender about equally distributed; 88.6 percent were psychotic; 75.3 percent were in a pure manic (not mixed) episode; only 18.7 percent had substance abuse comorbidity; and only 8.4 percent had another psychiatric comorbidity. As noted earlier, this second cohort can be viewed as representing close to the classic Kraepelinian description of what would now be referred to as the bipolar subgroup of manic-depressive illness.

In the first, multiple-episode cohort (Tohen et al., 1990), 28 percent were unable to work or study at 4-year follow-up, and 19 percent were unable to live independently. Only 28 percent were episode-free, and 28 percent had experienced three or more relapses, with a predominance of manic polarity. Poor occupational and residential status was correlated with subsyndromal interepisode illness (r=.42 to .46). After Cox proportional hazard regression to predict time to relapse, adjusted for 13 risk factors, the statistically significant main predictors were, in order of magnitude, past alcoholism (hazard ratio [HR]=3.9), index psychosis (HR=2.2), and index depressive symptoms during the manic episode (HR=2.0). A reanalysis assessing psychotic features found that mood-incongruent psychosis in particular predicted a quicker relapse (adjusted HR=2.6) (Tohen et al., 1992).

In the second McLean-Harvard cohort (patients initially hospitalized for mania/mixed states), those with past substance abuse were less likely than nonabusers to be recovered at 2-year follow-up (86 versus 98.5 percent). Among patients with initial mixed episodes, only 33 percent were living independently at 2 years, compared with 82 percent of those who had been admitted for pure mania. Further, although almost all patients had recovered syndromally at 2 years (98 percent), fewer (72 percent) had achieved full remission, and only 43 percent had recovered functionally (defined as regaining premorbid occupational and residential status). New episodes had been experienced by 59 percent of patients—20 percent mania, 20 percent depression, and 19 percent polyphasic switches (Tohen et al., 2000, 2003). These data suggest that functional recovery lags behind episode recovery and, further, that complete symptomatic remission does not ensure functional recovery, even in a classic Kraepelinian group of patients with relatively good prognosis. Predictors of earlier syndromal recovery (using Cox regression to adjust for other clinical factors) were as follows: short initial hospitalization (HR=1.99; 95 percent confidence interval [CI]=1.36 to 2.93), female gender (HR=1.72; 95 percent CI=1.16 to 2.56), and fewer index depressive symptoms (HR=1.65; 95 percent CI=1.14 to 2.39). For functional recovery (using multiple logistic regression), predictors were older than age 30 at index episode (odds ratio [OR]=3.28; 95 percent CI=1.58 to 6.82) and shorter initial hospitalization (OR=2.82; 95 percent CI=1.36 to 5.88). Further analyses suggest that initial pure mania and mood-congruent psychosis predicted manic relapse, whereas initial mixed episode predicted depressive relapse. Further, there appeared to be more manic relapse among those with lower baseline occupational status and more depressive relapse among those with higher status.

In the Stanley Foundation Bipolar Network cohort (N=258) (Nolen et al., 2004), poor prognostic factors at 1 year of prospective follow-up (in an adjusted multivariate regression model) were comorbid substance abuse, more than 10 prior manic or depressive episodes, family history of substance abuse, past rapid-cycling course, and poor occupational functioning at study entry. In a German subgroup of this cohort (n=152), predictors of poor outcome at 2.5 years of follow-up were bipolar-I disorder, comorbid Axis I disorders, and past rapid cycling (Dittmann et al., 2002).

In the first 1,000 subjects analyzed in the STEP-BD cohort, early age at onset (Perlis et al., 2004), past substance abuse (Weiss et al., 2005), and past comorbid attention-deficit disorder (Nierenberg et al., 2005) were associated with poor outcome (age-at-onset data only, based on an adjusted multivariate regression model).

Other Features of Long-Term Outcome

Another feature of long-term outcome that may be related to poor occupational functioning is cognitive impairment.[46] Findings of a number of studies indicate that cognitive impairment and neuroanatomical changes may be associated with the long-term effects of multiple mood episodes and/or duration of illness and/or treatment in both recurrent unipolar and bipolar patients (see Chapters 9 and 14). In one study using magnetic resonance imaging (MRI), lateral ventricles were larger in multiple-episode patients with bipolar disorder compared with 17 first-episode patients and 32 healthy subjects (Strakowski et al., 2002). In another study, duration of bipolar disorder (N=43) was associated with impaired performance on general memory tasks (Donaldson et al., 2003). In neither of these studies, however, was the potential impact of pharmacological treatment evaluated. Neuropsychological test abnormalities were confirmed in another study of 26 euthymic patients with recurrent unipolar or bipolar illness, with an association being found between degree of neuropsychological impairment and number of past hospitalized episodes (Tham et al., 1997). This finding was confirmed in another study of 25 euthymic patients with bipolar disorder compared with 22 age-matched normal controls (van Gorp et al., 1998).

It has been suggested that neuropsychological dysfunction may be a consequence of increased activity of the hypothalamic–pituitary–adrenal axis during mood episodes, which has been shown to lead to excitotoxic damage to sensitive brain regions, particularly the hippocampus (Lee et al., 2002). Hippocampal atrophy is more likely to occur in patients with greater numbers of mood episodes than in those with fewer mood episodes or in normal controls (Altshuler et al., 1991), and pilot data (detailed in Chapter 14) suggest that patients taking lithium, compared with similar patients not taking lithium, do not suffer such atrophy (Moore et al., 2000).

It should be noted that studies in this area focus primarily on symptomatic outcome, although some recent studies have begun to focus on functional outcome. As previously noted, these two kinds of outcome are correlated, but not completely. In other words, while episode recurrence and subsyndromal chronicity are, not surprisingly, both associated with worse functional outcomes, about 40 percent of euthymic patients with minimal detectable symptoms still appear to be functionally impaired. Long-term state-independent cognitive impairment is one likely explanation for this asymptomatic functional impairment, but this link remains to be established.

Beyond functional recovery, moreover, the question of quality of life remains. Even if patients are working and living in normal circumstances, the quality of their work and level of satisfaction with life remain largely unexamined by standard functional outcome measures. In a study of 50 euthymic persons with bipolar disorder, Sierra and colleagues (2005) found that quality of life was lower than in normal controls, and Yatham and colleagues (2004) found that some aspects of quality of life may be worse in bipolar compared with unipolar depression. Findings of another study from Europe were more optimistic, noting some improvement in recent years in bipolar patients' reports of their quality of life as they learned more about the nature of their disorder and the need for treatment (Morselli et al., 2004). With regard to pharmacological treatment, our review of the quality-of-life literature revealed that, although mood-stabilizing treatments clearly improve symptomatic outcomes in the majority of patients with bipolar disorder, their effect on quality of life remains to be established (Revicki et al., 2005).

Finally, with regard to subsyndromal morbidity and interepisode symptoms, the most recent reanalysis of the CDS data (Judd et al., 2002) found chronic subsyndromal depression to be the main outcome of treated bipolar-I disorder. In a follow-up period ranging up to 20 years (mean 12.8 years; N=146), patients were symptomatic 47 percent of the time. During these symptomatic periods, patients were predominantly depressed (67 percent of symptomatic period, 32 percent of total follow-up period), rather than manic or hypomanic (19 and 9 percent, respectively) or in mixed states (13 and 6 percent, respectively). Depressive periods were almost three times more likely to be spent in subsyndromal states (25 percent of total period) than in major depressive states (9 percent of total follow-up period). In sum, these data reflect primarily subsyndromal or interepisode periods of chronicity. The fact that depressive rather than manic symptoms are responsible for the bulk of the morbidity and functional impairment associated with bipolar disorder has also been noted in a community survey using self-reports (Calabrese et al., 2004).

It should be noted that similar rates of subsyndromal chronicity were reported in the CDS cohort for patients with unipolar depression (N=431) (Judd, 1998). This cohort consisted of a first-episode group (28 percent; n=122), a recurrent-depression group (48 percent; n=205), and a "double-depression" group meeting criteria for recurrent episodes and dysthymia (24 percent; n=104). In a follow-up of up to 20 years (mean 8.7 years), patients were symptomatic 59 percent of the time. During these symptomatic periods, depressive symptoms were again almost three times more likely to be associated with subsyndromal states (43 percent of total follow-up period) than with major depressive states (15 percent of total period).

As a result of these studies, Judd and colleagues (2002) and others (Kupka et al., 2005) have urged a shift in long-term studies to focus on chronicity and subsyndromal morbidity. One example of such work is a study that found subsyndromal depressive morbidity in bipolar disorder (N=25) to be associated with increased functional impairment (Altshuler et al., 2002).

It is also notable that subsyndromal manic morbidity was found to be most prominent in a 4-year follow up of children (N=86; mean age at baseline 10.8 years) (Geller et al., 2004). In this cohort, patients spent 57 percent of the follow-up time in manic or hypomanic states, versus 47 percent in depressive states and 37 percent in mixed states. (The total exceeds 100 percent because mixed states were included in all three categories.) These findings suggest that the chronic subsyndromal depressive course is a feature of adult bipolar disorder, whereas in children a more chronic manic/mixed course predominates (see Chapter 6).

A number of considerations arise in interpreting the results of outcome studies. The first is the extent to which these outcomes reflect natural history as opposed to being either attenuated or exacerbated by treatment effects. Most of the investigators cited earlier noted that their patients were treated primarily according to current standards, although information on specific treatments was not provided. When treatment effects were addressed, it was generally in the context of the assumption that continuing morbidity had to be occurring despite these effective treatments. Another possibility exists, however: that in some cases, treatment is only minimally beneficial or neutral, but capable of exacerbating the course of bipolar illness. As noted earlier and discussed in detail in Chapter 19, this possibility is especially salient for antidepressants, which may lead to subsyndromal cycling states that could in turn account for the outcomes described by Geller and colleagues (2004). The issue of how to treat subsyndromal chronic bipolar depression is a vexing problem for clinicians and an important unanswered question for researchers. If antidepressants are related to cycling, one option would be to decrease their use. On the other hand, if antidepressants were not being used, their possible benefits in some patients would be missed. The use of cognitive-behavioral and other psychotherapies would appear to be appropriate in this situation (see Chapter 22), although this approach has not been well studied. Other behavioral interventions, such as enhancement of sleep hygiene, have also been suggested (Morris, 2002; see also Chapter 16).

MORTALITY

Suicide is a frequent outcome of manic-depressive illness; in bipolar patients, it occurs more frequently early in the course of the illness (see Chapter 8). Although suicide is the single most important factor contributing to increased mortality in manic-depressive patients,[47] other causes, such as the increased risk of cardiovascular disease, contribute as well. Indirect consequences of psychotic behavior during untreated episodes—including malnutrition, exposure, and exhaustion—all compromise general health and presumably contribute to a higher mortality rate. So, too, do smoking and alcohol and drug abuse. As reviewed in Chapters 14 and 15, some of the biological dysfunction noted in manic-depressive patients involves systems other than the brain. These dysfunctions could also contribute to higher-than-normal mortality rates.

Recent studies of mortality in bipolar disorder are listed in Table 4–6, along with the weighted mean standardized mortality ratio (SMR) from studies reviewed in the first edition of this text.[47] Early studies of mortality rates in manic-depressive illness, which did not separate bipolar from unipolar forms, claimed substantially increased mortality—up to six times the rate expected for the same age group in a normal population. More recent studies have found a less striking but still considerable increase in mortality, averaging approximately 2.3 times the expected rate in the general population. This difference in results probably reflects improvements in psychiatric care, particularly the availability of specific treatments for the depressive and manic phases. Thus in Derby's (1933) study, 22 percent of hospitalized manic patients died, and 40 percent of these deaths were from "exhaustion," whereas in the Iowa 500 follow-up, Tsuang and colleagues (1980) found a significant increase only in "circulatory" deaths and only among women. Corroborating the earlier Iowa findings in a follow-up of 1,593 affective patients, Black and colleagues (1987a) noted that non-suicide-related deaths were excessive only among those patients with a concurrent medical disorder.

The largest recent prospective study of mortality in bipolar disorder involved up to 38 years of follow-up of depressed hospitalized patients in Zurich. Angst and colleagues (1999) reported that, overall, these patients demonstrated increased mortality compared with the general population, with a 61 percent higher risk of death (SMR = 1.6). The greatest risk was associated with suicide (SMR = 18), but statistically significant risks were also associated

with cardiovascular disease (SMR = 1.6) and accidents (SMR = 1.9). Those with bipolar depression were somewhat less likely to commit suicide than those with unipolar depression (SMR = 12.3 versus 26.7) but somewhat more likely to die from cardiovascular disease (SMR = 1.8 versus 1.4). Treated patients had lower suicide risks than untreated persons with bipolar disorder (SMR = 6.4 versus 29.2), but confounding factors were not controlled statistically in this observational study. It is also noteworthy that since cardiovascular disease is much more common than suicide, the absolute amount of improvement in mortality associated with suicide was the result primarily of decreased cardiovascular-related mortality. In concluding this discussion of mortality it is important to note that, with adequate lithium treatment, the mortality associated with bipolar illness can be reduced to a level indistinguishable from that of the general population, an effect no doubt related, at least in part, to the antisuicide effect of lithium (Muller-Oerlinghausen et al., 1996; Tondo et al., 2001). This point is discussed in greater detail in Chapters 8 and 25.

BIPOLAR-II DISORDER

The course of bipolar-II disorder has not been as well studied as that of bipolar-I illness; moreover, one of the issues in research on bipolar-II disorder is the relative lack of reliability for this diagnosis (see Chapter 3). The CDS in particular, however, has begun to shed light on the course of this condition. In 5-year follow-up, while bipolar-II subjects were less likely than bipolar-I subjects to be hospitalized, no other clinical differences in outcome (cycle length, number of mood episodes, suicide attempts) were found (Coryell et al., 1989b). Depressive episodes and symptom severity did not differ between the two groups, nor did frequency or duration of hypomanic versus manic episodes (in the bipolar-I group). Differences in psychosocial outcome between the two groups also were not evident. Manic episodes, by definition, occurred exclusively in the bipolar-I group. In a follow-up period of up to 10 years, only 7.5 percent (N = 64) of individuals with bipolar-II illness switched to type I. However, if one includes dropouts from follow-up in that study, which may reflect the disinclination of more severely ill patients to continue to participate in the biennial interviews, rates of switch from type II to type I approach 15 percent. In a follow-up of up to 20 years, the primary morbidity over time was chronic subsyndromal depression, and the prominence of depression was even more pronounced than in the bipolar-I cohort (Judd et al., 2003). During the follow-up period (mean 13.4 years; N = 86), patients were symptomatic 54 percent of the time. During these symptomatic periods, patients were predominantly depressed (93 percent of symptomatic period,

TABLE 4–6. Contemporary Studies of Mortality in Bipolar Disorder

Study	Sample Size	Duration of Observation (Years)	Deceased (%)	Standard Mortality Ratio[a]	Suicide % of all Deaths	Cardiovascular Disease % of all Deaths	Comments
Sharma and Markar, 1994	472	12–17	12.1	—	15.7	42.1	Population included psychiatric patients who had at least one episode of mania; SMR for CVD=3.0; and for suicide=23.4
Ahrens et al., 1995	473 F 354 M	6.75 (avg.)	4.9 5.9	1.23 1.07	21.7 9.5	30.4 33.3	Patient sample included BP, UP, and SZA patients attending outpatient lithium clinic; suicide mortality greater than expected, but overall mortality and CVD-caused mortality not different from general population
Broderson et al., 2000	133	16	30.1	2.50	27.5	17.5	All patients admitted to psychiatric hospital and given lithium prophylaxis; Dx=BP, UP, atypical affective disorders; SMR for CVD=1.23 and for suicide=20.5
Hoyer et al., 2000	34,465 F 19,638 M	1–20	26.8 32.4	1.8 2.2	17.9 23.1	26.5 28.5	Main analysis included hospitalized BP and UP patients; SMR for CVD=1.5, $p<.0001$ and SMR for suicide=17.12, $p<.0001$
Kallner et al., 2000	299 F 198 M	1–30	15.1 18.7	1.3	25.6	20.7	424 BP, 97 UP; all started on prophylactic lithium; SMR for suicide=14.0 ($p<.001$)
Ösby et al., 2001	8808 F 6578 M	11.5 (mean) 10.5 (mean)	19.8 26.1	27 2.5	18.7 20.1	29.9 32.1	Included only BP patients; all causes of death and diagnoses obtained from Swedish national registers; SMR for CVD=2.6 (F), 1.9 (M) and for suicide=22.4 (F), 22.9 (M)

(continued)

TABLE 4–6. Contemporary Studies of Mortality in Bipolar Disorder *(continued)*

Study	Sample Size	Duration of Observation (Years)	Deceased (%)	Standard Mortality Ratio[a]	Suicide % of all Deaths	Cardiovascular Disease % of all Deaths	Comments
Angst et al., 2002	291 F	34–38	72.2	1.59	13.8	35.2	186 UP and 220 BP; BP patients had SMR for CVD=1.84 vs. UP SMR for CVD=1.36; treated BP patients had lower SMR for CVD than untreated (1.68 vs. 2.23)
	115 M		82.6	1.64	15.8	26.3	
Weighted mean pre-1990s[b]				2.28			

BP = bipolar; CVD = cardiovascular disease; Dx = diagnosis; UP = unipolar; SMR = standard mortality ratio; SZA = schizoaffective.

[a]Ratio of observed mortality to expected mortality based on a normal demographically matched comparison population.

[b]Based on a total of 7,584 subjects from 11 pre-1990 studies in which excess mortality was determined.

50 percent of total follow-up period), and minimally hypomanic (2.4 and 1.3 percent, respectively) or mixed (4.3 and 2.3 percent, respectively). Depressive symptoms were almost three times more likely to be subsyndromal (37 percent of total follow-up period) compared with major depression (13 percent); again, then, these data reflect primarily subsyndromal or interepisode chronicity.

Vieta and colleagues (1997) reported that bipolar-II (n = 22) compared with bipolar-I patients (n = 38), had more past depressive episodes (5.6 versus 2.6), more hypomanic episodes (7.0 versus 3.2), and, of course, more total lifetime episodes (12.6 versus 6.3). Again, bipolar-I disorder was associated with more hospitalizations (3.0 versus 1.0).

The phenomenon of double-depression refers to the persistence of milder depressive states (dysthymia) following recovery from an episode of major depression (Keller et al., 1983). Klein and colleagues (1988) noted that, compared with other unipolar patients, those with double-depression had a higher incidence of hypomanic episodes during follow-up.

MECHANISMS OF RECURRENCE

Considering that recurrence is a major characteristic of manic-depressive illness, particularly in the bipolar form, it is surprising how little attention has been paid to its underlying mechanisms. None of the dominant neurotransmitter theories attempts to account for repeated episodes.

As noted earlier, the most widely cited explanation of the recurrent course of bipolar disorder is kindling, proposed by Post (1990) on the basis of experimental work on rodents (Weiss et al., 1990). The neurobiology of kindling is discussed extensively in Chapter 14, and earlier in this chapter we reviewed those aspects of the course of the illness that are relevant to evaluating this model. Those points bear repeating here.

Epileptic seizures are known to be generated by repeated subthreshold stimulation. The kindling model assumes that repeated stress and trauma can induce a similar progressive process in bipolar patients. Numerous studies have found fewer precipitants with increasing number of episodes in bipolar illness. Kindling may also be applicable in some cases to atypical DSM-IV bipolar disorder, with patients often reporting childhood traumas in retrospect. Unfortunately, none of the other predictions suggested by the kindling model appears to apply to classic bipolar disorder. For example, the kindling model would predict that patients treated later, after "a latency" and after more episodes, would have worse outcomes, but this hypothesis is not supported by the data (Baldessarini et al., 1999; Baethge et al., 2005). The kindling model would also predict that cycle length would shorten with more episodes,

but this is not a characteristic feature of later episodes of bipolar illness. Although regression analysis of cycles would create such an impression (Angst et al., 1970), progressive shortening is demonstrable only in a subgroup of patients, the MD type—patients who experience both major depressions and full manias (Angst, 1986c). Furthermore, 7 to 8 percent of patients actually show a gradual lengthening of cycle (Lat, 1973). Similarly, the kindling model might predict that patients fully stabilized after long-term lithium treatment would experience fewer episodes after gradual discontinuation than before the treatment, and this certainly is not the case.

Other proposed explanations of recurrence include those derived from biological rhythm models (see Chapter 16), especially catastrophe theory, based on a nonphysiological intersection of several endogenous rhythms. Other investigators have concluded that, in some cases, recurrent patterns of deterministic chaos may underlie the course of bipolar disorder (Bauer and Whybrow, 1988; Post et al., 1995).

CONCLUSIONS

The natural course and outcome of manic-depressive illness contribute to its definition and its differentiation from schizophrenia. For the clinician, understanding natural course can help answer a patient's questions about the most important estimate of all, the prognosis: Will it return, and when? Here we summarize the key points of this chapter that can help answer these questions.

Despite substantial methodological problems of both earlier and recent studies and limited data from prospective follow-up studies, the literature on the course and outcome of manic-depressive illness supports the following conclusions:

- The bipolar subtype has the earliest age at onset, followed by the more recurrent forms of unipolar depression, followed by the less recurrent forms. For the bipolar subgroup, the representative value varies with the definition of onset, ranging from the appearance of first symptoms (such as mood lability) before age 20 to the first hospitalization (in the 25–30 age range).
- Almost all bipolar patients experience relapse, given adequate observation time. Results of contemporary studies indicate higher relapse rates than those found in earlier studies; extended use of antidepressants may have contributed to this increase. Highly recurrent unipolar depression is a risk factor for developing bipolar illness.
- Cycle length does not change predictably with time, although it may shorten progressively in the initial stages of illness in a subgroup of individuals.

- An appreciable proportion of bipolar patients develop rapid cycling. Rapid cycling may represent one extreme of the bipolar spectrum rather than a completely autonomous group. The nosological status of rapid cycling remains unclear, however.

- The literature shows rather consistently that manic episodes are briefer than depressive or mixed episodes. The average episode duration remains stable throughout the illness.

- About 1–2% per year of unipolar patients experience a first manic or hypomanic episode, suggesting that over a long period of follow-up, a large minority of previously diagnosed unipolar patients will switch to diagnosable bipolar disorder. The pattern of initial depression followed later by mania is associated with poor long-term outcome. Antidepressants may have a role in hastening poor long-term outcome.

- Psychosocial and physical stresses continue to appear to be robust predictors of the timing of relapse, although these severe life events most likely interact with a patient's underlying vulnerability in a complex manner. Life events appear to be associated with relapse more in earlier than in later phases of bipolar illness.

- Long-term data suggest that up to one third of bipolar patients achieve complete remission, and a similar number achieve complete functional recovery. Although syndromal recovery is two or more times more frequent, fewer patients go on to recover premorbid levels of function. Chronic persistence of symptoms can be expected in about 20% of cases, and social incapacity in about 30%. Poor outcome in recent studies may be influenced by selection bias toward the inclusion of more severely ill patients in tertiary care centers. In the community setting, outcomes could be better than those cited here. Early age at onset, depression, mixed episodes, psychosis, substance abuse, medication noncompliance, and probably the long-term use of antidepressants are all associated with poor outcome. Mortality and suicide rates are increased in bipolar illness but can be substantially reduced by adequate lithium treatment.

- There are several interesting theories of the mechanisms of recurrence, including chronobiological explanations and kindling theory. Kindling may represent a subgroup effect, being relevant to a more severe or atypical subgroup of individuals with bipolar disorder.

NOTES

1. Behavioral, intellectual, and language tests were part of the standard examination battery administered by the Israeli Draft Board Registry. Anyone previously diagnosed with the aforementioned disorders by the time of the draft examinations or directly thereafter was excluded from the study. The experimental group was culled from those who developed the disorders at least 1 year after examination. To control for instability of diagnosis, the authors included only patients whose diagnosis after a 4-year follow-up was the same as the entry diagnosis.

2. Psychotic bipolar patients were excluded from this study because part of the cohort had been assessed using *International Classification of Diseases* (ICD)-9 criteria, before the bipolar definition had been broadened to include more psychotic features.

3. van Os et al., 1995; Bromet et al., 1996; Vocisano et al., 1996; McClellan et al., 2003.

4. While some of these data were taken from subanalyses of large epidemiological samples, most were gathered from clinical populations. We discuss age-at-onset results from epidemiological samples in Chapter 6. Although it is impossible to eliminate selection bias completely, we took care here to select only those patient samples that appeared to represent the general bipolar population.

5. Reliability measures were based on age-at-onset assessments made by two independent physician raters. Reliability coefficients for first treatment and first hospitalization were 0.94 and 0.97, respectively.

6. One must also consider the possible contributions of changes in maternal behavior (smoking and drinking during pregnancy), as well as changes in dietary factors, such as decreased intake of omega-3 fatty acids (since World War II) due to changes in infant formulas (see Chapter 5).

7. It is likely that the lower age at onset seen in more recent birth cohorts results from a confluence of these multiple factors.

8. Additional information about this survey was obtained from the study authors for the present review. Although subject to recall bias and not administered by a trained clinician, the survey used to determine age at onset did adhere to DSM-IV episodic criteria. Furthermore, to control for underreporting of later ages at onset, the authors did not include the youngest cohort of participants (born after 1959) in their analyses.

9. For example, Mick and colleagues (2003) compared measures of cognitive and global functioning, comorbidity, and clinical features across three groups arbitrarily designated as childhood, adolescent, and adult onset. They found significantly more comorbid anxiety disorders in the child and adolescent groups compared with the adult group, but no difference among groups in cognitive or global functioning. However, there was a trend for more rapid cycling and mixed episodes in the earlier-onset group, although the sample size lacked the power to permit evaluation of statistical significance for some of these measures.

10. Neurological abnormalities were descriptive and based on medical records. Among 14 patients in the elderly-onset mania group, 10 had neurological problems such as seizures, gait disturbance, recurrent cerebral contusions, and cerebral infarcts.

11. Winokur and colleagues (1993) found no association between a family history of bipolar disorder and age at onset. Lish (1994) and colleagues, however, found a significant correlation between childhood/adolescent onset and a family history of the disorder. This finding was replicated by Engstrom and colleagues (2003). Johnson and colleagues (2000) reported that patients with a family history of bipolar disorder had a significantly lower age at onset than those with no such family history.

12. However, a recent study from this group did find that mixed episodes were more common in a bipolar group with an early age at first hospitalization (younger than 18) compared with those first hospitalized in their twenties (Patel et al., 2006).

13. Although this study included patients with adolescent onset (minimum age = 15), the authors confirmed the diagnosis at intake and at follow-up with clinician-administered Structured Clinical Interview for DSM (SCID) results and corroborating evidence from family reports, as well as school and medical records.

14. Here again, both early- and late-onset groups were adults at the time of assessment (mean age 33.6 and 60.2, respectively). Diagnosis was verified with DSM-IV criteria and corroborating medical records, as well as family interviews.

15. At the time of assessment, the sample included all adults (mean age 43.1) diagnosed with DSM-IV bipolar disorder. Age at onset was determined by clinician-administered questionnaire, medical records, and family interviews in some cases. Confirming other reports, Suppes and colleagues (2001) also found a highly significant relationship between incidence of childhood sexual abuse and early onset (p ≤ .001), a possible triggering phenomenon discussed in Chapter 7.

16. As in most studies of this kind, Ernst and Goldberg ascertained age at onset retrospectively, in this instance using life charts.

17. Perris (1968) found 83 percent with four or more episodes and 43 percent with seven or more. In a 1978 paper, Angst (1978) updated a careful longitudinal study of 95 bipolar patients who at that time had been followed for an average of 26 years (standard deviation ±11.9). The study included both retrospective and prospective phases, the latter involving direct patient and family contact at least every 5 years. Patients by and large did not receive prophylactic treatment, although most had individual episodes treated with medications. The number of episodes ranged from 2 to 54, with a median of 9; 84 percent had 5 or more episodes, 69 percent had 7 or more, and 42 percent had 11 or more. A naturalistic study of 51 bipolar patients who received unsystematic acute and prophylactic treatment showed that all but 2 of the patients had experienced 3 or more episodes, with a median of 15 (Roy-Byrne et al., 1985a). Although this finding is consistent with earlier data, it is important to remember that the patient groups are not comparable, because the research setting of the Roy-Byrne study tended to select treatment-resistant patients. In a chart review study of 236 bipolar patients from the prepharmacotherapy era (between 1920 and 1950), Winokur and Kadrmas (1989) found that, during a follow-up period averaging 2.4 years, 28 percent had 1 episode, 22 percent had 2, 14 percent had 3, 11 percent had 4, 4 percent had 5, 2 percent had 6, 0.8 percent had 7, 0.4 percent had 8, and 11 percent had 9 or more.

18. Angst's Dm group is roughly analogous to the bipolar-II subgroup in DSM-III-R, although hospitalization is not necessary for the diagnosis of either major depression or mania in DSM-III-R.

19. Today, given modern treatment, relatively few patients would actually meet this criterion (i.e., hospitalization).

20. In their 1979 review of the literature on the natural course of manic-depressive illness (both unipolar and bipolar, with the index episode usually a hospitalization), Zis and Goodwin (1979) divided studies that showed low rates of relapse from those that showed high rates. They found that those with low relapse rates were marred by methodological limitations, including short duration of observation, focus on episodes involving hospitalization, exclusion of episodes preceding index admission, inclusion of nonrecovered patients, combined episodes treated as single episodes, and high unipolar/bipolar patient ratio. For example, studies with low relapse rates tended to include only episodes requiring hospitalization, introducing a bias toward patients with longer and more severe episodes. Thus in Perris's 1968 study, only 40 percent of patients had had four or more episodes involving hospitalization, but when all episodes were included, more than 80 percent had had four or more. Obviously, excluding episodes preceding the index hospital admission also leads to underestimation. When, for instance, Bratfos and Haug (1968) included preadmission episodes, the proportion of patients with single episodes dropped to 13 percent.

As noted previously, early studies often found a high proportion of single-episode patients because they included in that single-episode count the many chronic patients who in fact had had multiple (but uncounted) episodes while hospitalized. Cutler and Post (1982a) traced the long-term course of illness in a group of bipolar patients who were chronically hospitalized in a state institution. Their detailed analysis indicated that each of these patients displayed a pattern similar to what Kraepelin had observed more than half a century earlier: multiple, discrete episodes embedded in a single long-term hospitalization. Estimates of relapse rates probably were lower than justified in the older studies, even when based on patients who were not chronically hospitalized. In those cases, combined episodes (e.g., a mania followed by a depression, perhaps interspersed with a brief well interval) may have been counted as a single episode. The presence of a continuously circular course (Koukopoulos et al., 1980) or rapid cycles (Dunner et al., 1976b) makes it more likely that multiple episodes will be counted as one.

21. It may also be that recurrence is related to other features of bipolar illness, such as age at onset and genetic risk. This interesting possibility has not been adequately explored since the time of a chart review conducted during the prepharmacology era (Winokur and Kadrmas, 1989), which suggested that certain clinical features may be associated with the illness's natural tendency to recur. Winokur and Kadrmas found that, compared with patients who had only one or two episodes during a follow-up period averaging 2.4 years, patients with a polyepisodic course (more than three episodes) were more likely to have had an early age at onset, a finding that replicates an earlier report by Okuma and Shimoyama (1972). Winokur and Kadrmas also found that a polyepisodic course was associated with a more insidious onset of the index episode and a greater frequency of bipolar illness in first-degree relatives. They speculated that this last finding could indicate that cyclicity more than polarity is genetically transmitted: the more total episodes, the greater the likelihood of manic episodes.

22. In 1938, Eliot Slater of the Maudsley Hospital in London published a paper ("On the Periodicity of Manic Depressive Insanity") (Slater, 1938a) in which he reexamined cases of patients who had been the source for Kraepelin's data regarding the shortening of cycle length. Unfortunately perhaps for later generations, Slater's paper, published in a German psychiatric

journal that was prominent before World War II, lapsed into obscurity in succeeding decades, especially in the non-German-speaking world. (This lack of attention in the Anglo-American setting is particularly ironic given that Slater was an Englishman.) In our review, we found the initial peer review and the most extensive discussion of "Slater's fallacy" in English in a 1996 paper by Haghighat (1996), who also noted earlier citations in book chapters by Angst (1988). In 2000, Angst and Sellaro (2000) again referred to Slater's report in English, and we recently obtained an English translation of the original paper.

In that study, Slater reviewed 116 charts of patients diagnosed by Kraepelin in Munich with manic-depressive illness. Among the features he assessed, Slater highlighted his reexamination of Kraepelin's report of decreasing intervals of wellness with an increase in the number of episodes, which became a central feature of what would later be called the kindling model. Slater confirmed that the duration of mood episodes appeared to increase to a small degree over time. However, his key finding was that the apparent decrease in euthymic intervals between episodes was a statistical artifact. Slater pointed out that "people who have longer intervals between episodes will not fall ill as often as those in whom the intervals are shorter." In other words, if all patients are included in the analysis, some will experience only two episodes and others six, for example. It may be that those with six episodes have short periods of wellness between episodes, whereas those with two episodes experience long periods of wellness. If those two types of patients are added together, as was done by Kraepelin, there will appear to be a progressive decrease in euthymic intervals. The actual state of affairs will not necessarily be so. One would have to demonstrate that intervals of wellness shortened over time *in the same patients*, whether they had two episodes or six. In sum, interepisode intervals of wellness need to be corrected for the number of episodes. When Slater made this correction, Kraepelin's finding vanished (except to a small degree for earlier episodes). In a recent outcome study of first-episode manic patients at McLean Hospital, Baldessarini and colleagues (2000) found the same effect. Taken as a group, the sample appeared to demonstrate progressive shortening of intervals of wellness, but when the data were corrected for number of episodes, there was no apparent shortening of well intervals.

We would like to acknowledge and thank Dr. Ross Baldessarini for bringing this long-neglected paper to our attention. We would also like to acknowledge and thank our colleague, Dr. Godehard Oepen, for assistance in translating and interpreting Slater's study.

23. Bratfos, 1968; Bratfos and Haug., 1968; Angst et al., 1973; Roy-Byrne et al., 1985a; Goldberg, 1993; Goldberg and Harrow, 1994; Kessing, 1998; Kessing et al., 1998a; Cusin et al., 2000.

24. Another study found that number of episodes did not predict recurrence at 1-year prospective follow-up (Staner et al., 1997). Such short-term studies are less useful in refuting kindling hypotheses, however, because the kindling model is a long-term model. The studies of the groups led by Coryell and colleagues (2001) and Baldessarini and colleagues (1999) were longer-term (up to 10 years).

25. Kendler and Karkowski-Shuman (1997) also assessed this finding within individuals by stratifying their dataset by individual and assuming a separate hazard function for their Cox proportional hazards model for each person in the study.

26. In a study with the methodological limitation of including only hospitalized patients, there was no evidence of a difference in episode severity in individuals experiencing their first manic episode as opposed to one of multiple episodes (Keck et al., 1995). However, because all patients were hospitalized, differential severity may have been difficult to detect.

27. The sample was from the Mediterranean island of Sardinia.

28. Independent confirmation or refutation of the kindling model based on other lines of evidence may gradually develop. For instance, Huber and colleagues (2001) presented a mathematical nonlinear model of sensitization. This model has two components: a positive feedback loop (more episodes lead to more episodes) and a long time interval. The authors showed that this mathematical model can support autonomous disease progression as well as irregular rapid cycling as an end stage of disease, as predicted by the kindling hypothesis.

29. Swift, 1907; MacDonald, 1918; Pollock, 1931; Angst and Weis, 1967; Zis et al., 1979.

30. The 1989 study of Winokur and Kadrmas (1989), although limited by its chart review methodology, is nevertheless of interest because it is based on the prepharmacology era. The authors reported that patients with a polyepisodic course (more than three episodes per average follow-up of 2.4 years) were significantly more likely to have an early age at onset (before age 20) than those with one or two episodes.

31. Another question is whether episodes come in bursts or clusters, as originally described by Kraepelin in his studies of predominantly chronic patients with frequent relapses. As discussed in Chapter 20, this issue is important in assessing prophylactic treatment, and indeed in making treatment decisions. If episodes of manic-depressive illness characteristically occur in clusters, it may be difficult to interpret prophylactic trials in individual patients. The evidence on this issue is somewhat conflicting. Saran (1970) compared episode frequencies in six untreated bipolar patients for 2 years before and 3 years after an arbitrary point in time. Even in such a small number of patients, there was some suggestion of episode clustering. In a 2- to 20-year follow-up (mean 5.6 years) of patients admitted for manic episodes, Winokur (1975) found that 91 percent of first-episode patients had experienced another episode during follow-up, compared with only 53 percent of those with a history of previous episodes—a result interpreted as evidence of episode clustering. Angst and colleagues (1970) did not find different relapse rates before and after lithium treatment. It is also worth noting that there may be some methodological issues with extrapolating from such group findings to clustering in individual patients.

32. For example, Kupka and colleagues (2005) found more bipolar-I than bipolar-II patients among 539 outpatients in the Stanley Network.

33. In a study of 320 hospitalized patients with bipolar-I disorder, the polarity of the first episode was determined to be major depressive in 52 percent, mixed in 26 percent, and pure manic in 22 percent. Patients whose illness began with depression were more likely to develop a rapid-cycling course and experienced more suicide attempts but less psychosis than the other groups. The mixed group tended to be more

chronic and made frequent suicide attempts but generally did not experience a rapid-cycling course (Perugi et al., 2000).

34. In this study, the incidence of false unipolar (pseudounipolar) depression was strikingly low (4.4 percent) and out of line with the rest of the psychiatric literature. This observation may suggest that studies based on hospitalization will overreport the incidence of manic as opposed to depressive episodes, because the latter lead less frequently to hospitalization than the former.

35. Taschev, 1974; Angst, 1978; Koukopoulos et al., 1980; Roy-Byrne, 1985a; Coryell et al., 1989b.

36. The literature is inconsistent in the relationships reported between predominantly manic or predominantly depressive episodes and age at onset or family history of affective disorder. Three studies (Mendlewicz et al., 1972a; Taylor and Abrams, 1973a; Stone, 1989) found a positive family history of affective disorder to be associated with an earlier age at onset, but this finding was not replicated by Winokur (1975). An association between earlier age at onset and a higher proportion of manic episodes in the course of illness was reported by Mendlewicz and colleagues (1972a) and by Angst (1978), but not by others (Taylor and Abrams, 1973a; Carlson et al., 1977; Roy-Byrne et al., 1985a).

37. Other studies have tended to confirm the general observation of stability of polarity in the course of illness, but most have not addressed or corrected for age (Cassidy, Cassidy, Perugi, Woods). The one study (Perugi et al., 2000) with data on age at onset in the 20s found consistent polarity for manic and mixed episodes in the course of illness. Among those patients whose illness began with a depressive episode, however, future episodes were equally likely to be manic/mixed versus depressed.

38. Winokur et al., 1969; Angst, 1978; Koukopoulos et al., 1980; Roy-Byrne and colleagues, 1985a.

39. Sleep deprivation would appear to be a likely explanation for hurricane-induced manias; this recalls the earlier suggestion of Wehr and colleagues (1987a) that sleep loss is the final common pathway by which various stressors can trigger mania (Aronson and Shukla, 1987).

40. Bratfos and Haug, 1968; Reich and Winokur, 1970; Kendell et al., 1976, 1987; Kadrmas, 1979.

41. Viguera and Cohen, 1998; Viguera et al., 2002; Akdeniz et al., 2003.

42. The occurrence of sexual abuse as a precipitant or predictor of mood episodes has also been studied. In one study, the rate of self-reported childhood sexual abuse was high in 142 persons with DSM-III-R bipolar disorder (18 percent of women and 4 percent of men) and was similar to the rates found in a unipolar comparison group of 191 persons (16 percent in women, 3 percent in men) (Hyun, 2000).

43. An interesting suggestion has been made that part of the mechanism for seasonal instability in psychiatric conditions may be attributable not only to increased sunlight, but also to increased ambient light due to the cycles of the moon (Raison, 1998; also see Chapter 16).

44. Here we are excluding lithium prophylaxis studies (O'Connell et al., 1991; Maj et al., 1995), which are discussed in Chapter 22. We are also excluding retrospective cohort studies, of which there have been a number, including a Cologne cohort (Marneros et al., 1990; Deister and Marneros, 1993), a Johns Hopkins cohort (Stephens and McHugh, 1991), an Indian cohort (Khanna et al., 1992), a Danish cohort (Kessing, 1998, 1999), an Italian cohort (Cusin, 2000), and a Taiwanese cohort (Tsai, 2001).

The Cologne cohort consisted of 106 patients with DSM-III mood disorders, a subgroup of a total cohort of 402 patients (the rest with psychotic disorders). With a mean of 27.9 years of outcome data, 64 percent of the mood disorder sample was fully remitted (Marneros et al., 1990). Subclassification of bipolar and unipolar conditions was not performed. In multivariate analysis, male gender was a major predictor of poor functional outcome (Diester et al., 1993). Other apparent predictors were an "asthenic low self-confident" premorbid personality and a higher number of mood episodes.

The Johns Hopkins cohort, also mentioned in this chapter in the discussion of polarity, consisted of patients hospitalized between 1913 and 1940, and therefore represents a true pretreatment natural-history sample. The study group consisted of 914 patients with at least 5 years of medical record follow-up data. With a mean follow-up of 13.5 years, only 11 percent of the bipolar group (n=297) and 22 percent of the unipolar group (n=945) did not experience future mood episodes. About one third of the total sample had a chronic outcome, somewhat worse in the bipolar subgroup (43 percent), and 13 percent committed suicide.

The Indian cohort consisted of 95 patients with bipolar disorder hospitalized in an academic psychiatric hospital over a period of 3 months in 1989. Medical records were assessed for course of illness. The main findings were more manic than depressive episodes and worse outcomes in those with initial manic episodes (unadjusted for other clinical factors statistically). The sample was predominantly male (84 percent) and predominantly manic (83 percent of first episodes reported). Interestingly, not a single case of a rapid-cycling course or of polyphasic episodes was documented, a finding that one might speculate is related to lack of antidepressant exposure in a setting in which many patients remain untreated.

The Denmark cohort is described further in this chapter in the discussion of kindling.

The Italian cohort consisted of 244 patients with bipolar disorder with 14-year outcome data. The main finding was that an initial manic as opposed to depressive episode predicted a higher frequency of episodes in the outcome period.

In the Taiwanese cohort, 101 patients with bipolar disorder were identified by hospital records and agreed to follow-up after 15 years. The main predictor of poor psychosocial outcome was medication nonadherence, which was observed in 33 percent of the sample.

45. Although the second McLean-Harvard cohort is a proxy for a first-episode study, it is notable that 24.7 percent had experienced previous nonhospitalized major depressive episodes. Therefore, this subgroup did not really consist of first-episode bipolar subjects.

46. In Chapter 9, we review the evidence that some neurocognitive impairment may exist even prior to the onset of the illness.

47. In a postmortem study of 122 bipolar patients, for example, Taschev (1974) found that 27 percent had died by suicide. Among manic patients from the Iowa 500 series, Winokur and Tsuang (1975b) found that 8.5 percent of the deaths were

suicides. Perris and d'Elia (1966) found that 11 percent of the deaths in their patients had resulted from suicide, exactly the same proportion as in Tsuang's (1978) 40-year follow-up. Reviewing the literature, Guze and Robins (1970) noted that about 15 percent of all deaths among patients with major affective disorders can be traced to suicide. See Chapter 9 for a more comprehensive review.

48. The large epidemiologic study on the association between depression and its treatment and cardiovascular disease (known as the SAD HEARTS study) was not included. While it provides an invaluable amount of information on the relationship between depression and heart disease, the study focused exclusively on unipolar patients, and the majority were nonrecurrent, having fewer than two episodes.

5 Epidemiology

Seek the points of contact which may reveal the underlying law. Some things can be learned
only by statistical comparison.

—Sir William Osler (in Thayer, 1920, p. 52)

Epidemiology, which has been called the basic science of public health, is the study of the distribution of disorders in human populations, the variation in rates that may provide clues to their cause, and the risk factors associated with their onset and course. Epidemiology focuses on populations rather than individuals. An observation that a disorder is considerably higher in one group than another can be used to identify an epidemic or determine protective factors. Studying the variation in rates by specific characteristics (risk factors) yields clues as to how altering those characteristics may interrupt the process that leads to a disorder. This information also provides a scientific basis for assessing the overall health status of a population and identifying who is or is not receiving treatment.

Epidemiologic methods are common to studies of all chronic noninfectious diseases, including psychiatric disorders. These methods fall into three categories (see the review by Rothman and Greenland, 1998): *descriptive* methods, used to study the rates of disorder in a population; *analytic* methods, used to explore variations among different groups in order to identify risk factors; and *experimental* methods, used to test the association between a risk factor and a disorder by controlling the risk factor to see whether a reduction in onset or reoccurrence results. In this chapter, we focus primarily on results of descriptive studies. We begin by reviewing the application of epidemiologic methods in studies of psychiatric disorders, and then examine the key methodological issues that arise in such studies. Next we summarize the methods and results of epidemiologic studies of manic-depressive illness, with an emphasis on the bipolar subgroup. (The term *manic-depressive illness* in the pre–*Diagnostic and Statistical Manual* [DSM]-III literature sometimes referred to patients

that would be called bipolar in today's nosology, while in other contexts, the term referred to all recurrent mood disorders.) The studies we review are of the bipolar subgroup and involve community surveys of adults and of children and adolescents, as well as studies conducted by the World Health Organization (WHO). Finally, we review what is known about correlates, or features associated with bipolar disorder.

APPLICATION OF EPIDEMIOLOGIC METHODS IN STUDIES OF PSYCHIATRIC DISORDERS

Population samples are utilized to understand the full magnitude of a disorder, as well as its spectrum, including mild and untreated forms. WHO's international projections of the disability associated with mood disorders in both developing and developed countries (discussed later in this chapter) have garnered the attention of mental health planners and have made international epidemiologic data on mood disorders the focus of considerable interest.[1] Yet epidemiologic methods utilizing large-scale studies of populations have been applied to psychiatric disorders relatively recently. The first large-scale epidemiologic studies of psychiatric disorders were reported in the 1980s. Since then, there has been a rapid increase in the number of such studies. Moreover, their quality has improved significantly.

Over the past decade, much more reliable data on the rates of psychiatric disorders have become available as concern regarding biases, inconsistencies, and inadequacies in the psychiatric epidemiology literature has led investigators to become increasingly more systematic and sophisticated in their methodologies. Yet although the newer epidemiologic data on bipolar disorder are the product of considerable advances in methodology, they are not without difficulties:

- The findings almost always are based on structured interviews conducted by nonclinicians; studies comparing such data with diagnoses by experienced clinicians tend to show only modest correspondence.
- The relatively low prevalence of bipolar disorder requires large population samples for accurate estimates.
- There is an absence of community-based data on highly recurrent major depression, which falls within the spectrum of bipolar disorder (see Chapter 1).
- The boundary between normal mood and mild hypomania that may also be part of the spectrum, or an early sign of the illness, is ambiguous.
- Controversy exists about the nature of the disorder's clinical presentation in children and adolescents, which may complicate the ascertainment of true age at onset.
- One of the most important risk factors for bipolar disorder, family history, has not been included in epidemiologic surveys.

These problems do not in general apply to the same extent for major depression, which has a considerably higher prevalence than bipolar disorder and for which there is a more extensive body of research on first presentation in children and adolescents, although, as noted above, there is virtually no information on the more recurrent forms of depression in these age groups.

In the late 1970s, the National Institute of Mental Health (NIMH) sponsored the development of a diagnostic instrument, the Diagnostic Interview Schedule (DIS), suitable for use in large-scale epidemiologic studies of psychiatric disorders (Robins et al., 1981). In 1980, the Epidemiologic Catchment Area (ECA) study was initiated (Robins and Regier, 1991). This study included more than 18,000 adults aged 18 and older living in five U.S. communities (New Haven, Connecticut; Baltimore, Maryland; Piedmont County, North Carolina; St. Louis, Missouri; and Los Angeles, California). Using the DIS as the diagnostic instrument, lay interviewers generated DSM-III diagnoses (American Psychiatric Association [APA], 1980). The study was longitudinal, with a 1-year follow-up to determine incidence (i.e., first onset). Oversampling of African Americans, the elderly, Hispanic Americans, and the rural poor ensured that accurate rates of disorders and treatment needs among these groups could be ascertained.

The ECA demonstrated that the use of comparable and reliable methods allows rates of psychiatric illness to be compared across geographic regions. Over the course of the 1980s, comparable epidemiologic studies were undertaken in Edmonton, Canada (Orn et al., 1988); Puerto Rico (Canino et al., 1987); the former Republic of West Germany

(Wittchen et al., 1992); Florence, Italy (Faravelli et al., 1990); Paris, France (Lépine et al., 1989); Beirut, Lebanon (Karam, 1992); Christchurch, New Zealand (Wells et al., 1989); Taiwan (Hwu et al., 1989); and Korea (Lee et al., 1990a,b). A collaboration among the lead investigators—called the Cross-National Collaborative Group—was undertaken to conduct joint analyses (Weissman et al., 1996).

In the 1990s, the National Comorbidity Study (NCS) was initiated in the United States (Kessler et al., 1994). This study was unique in that it was a national probability sample, and it used a new diagnostic method, the Composite International Diagnostic Interview (CIDI) (WHO, 1990), which had the capacity to generate both *International Classification of Diseases* (ICD) (WHO, 1991) and DSM-III diagnoses (see Chapter 11). Thus, it was possible to use variable diagnostic criteria to make direct comparisons with cross-national studies.

The ECA, the Cross-National Collaborative Group, and the NCS, as well as other epidemiologic surveys in different parts of the world, demonstrated that the majority of psychiatric illnesses had their onset in childhood and adolescence.[2] The pressing need for a direct epidemiologic study of children became apparent, but such studies of children present even more methodological problems than those of adults. Many questions arise: Should the diagnostic criteria used with adults also be used with children (a question discussed below under methodological issues)? Who is the best informant? Should parents, children, or both be interviewed? What risk factors should be included? What is the youngest age at which psychiatric disorders can be meaningfully assessed? These questions have not yet been fully resolved. Nonetheless, the National Institute of Mental Health's (NIMH) Methods for the Epidemiology of Child and Adolescent Mental Disorder (MECA) study was initiated in the 1990s in New Haven, Connecticut; Westchester County, New York; Atlanta, Georgia; and Puerto Rico. Its purpose is to develop and test methods for a large national epidemiologic study (Lahey et al., 1996). Other studies of children are also under way, as described later.

Because of the relative lack of information on the epidemiology of childhood psychiatric disorders, NIMH has begun to capitalize on ongoing national physical health surveys of children by adding questions about mental health. These surveys include the National Health and Nutrition Examination Survey (U.S. Department of Health and Human Services [US DHHS], 1998) for children aged 8 to 18, the National Health Interview Survey (US DHHS, 1996) for those aged 4 to 17, and the National Household Survey on Drug Abuse (US DHHS, 1999) for those aged 12 to 17. The first two surveys are investigating the comorbidity of psychiatric with physical problems, and the third is examining comorbidity with drug abuse. The inclusion of questions on mental health in ongoing national surveys of physical health among young people in the United States provides much-needed monitoring data on both psychiatric disorders in children and the relationship of these disorders to physical health. It is not clear whether bipolar disorder will be examined separately from other mood disorders.

By 1995, the availability of epidemiologic information from community surveys had made possible the first textbook on psychiatric epidemiology (Tsuang et al., 1995). At the close of the twentieth century, WHO, in collaboration with The World Bank and Harvard University (Murray et al., 1994), turned to developing methods for assessing the global burden of disease. Given changing disease patterns, including a decrease in communicable diseases, as well as increasing longevity, investigators sought measures other than the traditional mortality used in international projections. They found that four psychiatric disorders, including bipolar disorder, appeared among the top 10 disabling illnesses in both developed and developing countries. This information drew worldwide attention and laid the groundwork for the future generation of epidemiologic studies, which are global in scope.

METHODOLOGICAL ISSUES

The chapter on epidemiology in the first edition of this text focused on methodological problems because at the time there were more problems than data. Although these problems cannot be ignored in interpreting the growing body of data now emerging, we need not dwell on them because they have been addressed in many of the more recent studies. Therefore, this section reviews only those methodological issues that are particularly relevant to current understanding of the epidemiology of bipolar disorder.

Variable Diagnostic Criteria

During the past decade, methods for obtaining diagnostic data have improved significantly. Reliability across interviewers has improved, and many new approaches to diagnostic interviews are available. Yet despite these improvements, different diagnostic interview formats yield different rates of psychiatric disorders. Even when the same methods are used, comparing published rates across studies can be difficult because of differences in data presentation. Some investigators confine the data to cases that show an episodic pattern of mania and major depression (bipolar-I), whereas others include cases with a pattern of hypomania and major depression (bipolar-II). Still others combine bipolar-I and -II rates or include cyclothymia. For major depression, most investigators do not separate out the more recurrent forms (which are part of the manic-depressive spectrum) from the less recurrent forms, and some older studies reporting rates of manic-depressive illness do not separate the bipolar from the recurrent unipolar groups. The Cross-National Collaborative Group, mentioned earlier, was formed to address these differences in the reported data by standardizing methods for analysis and data presentation. The results of the group's efforts are presented in Table 5–1.

As detailed in Chapter 3, DSM-III, DSM-III-R, and DSM-IV improved specification of the diagnostic criteria for bipolar disorder; however, slight changes in the criteria over time have made comparisons of studies conducted even less than a decade apart problematic. In DSM-III, hypomania was classified as a disturbance similar to but not as severe as a manic episode, but no specific criteria were given (APA, 1980, p. 209) (see Chapter 3). Hypomania first appeared as a specific diagnostic entity in DSM-III-R, where it was defined as a distinct period of elevated mood but not severe enough to warrant the diagnosis of mania (APA, 1986, p. 218). In the 1990s, DSM-IV operationalized the criteria for hypomania,

TABLE 5–1. One-Year Disorder Prevalence (Percent Standard Error), Before and After Applying Clinical Significance Criteria

Disorder	Survey	Before CS	After CS
Unipolar major depression	Epidemiologic Catchment Area	4.9 (0.3)	4.0 (0.3)
	National Comorbidity Study	8.9 (0.6)	5.4 (0.5)
Bipolar-I disorder	Epidemiologic Catchment Area	0.9 (0.1)	0.5 (0.1)
	National Comorbidity Study	1.3 (0.2)	1.3 (0.2)

Note: Encompasses ages 18–54 years.
CS = clinical significance.
Source: Narrow et al., 2002.

requiring a persistently elevated, expansive, or irritable mood for at least 4 days (APA, 1994, p. 338); these criteria are consistent with those of ICD-10.

Even when diagnostic criteria are clear, mild forms of mania (such as hypomania) can fail to be detected. Most hypomanic episodes go undiagnosed even by psychiatrists, who when asking about episodes of depression may not elicit information about periods of unusual activity before and after an episode. As we emphasized in the first edition of this book, unless the patient and a family member are both carefully questioned about past hypomania, the bipolar nature of a depression may be missed (Simpson et al., 1993; Angst and Gamma, 2002). Indeed, hypomania is not well defined in research instruments. In community surveys, as the data presented later in this chapter suggest, it is exceedingly difficult to distinguish mild states of euphoria due to positive changes in a subject's life from the abnormal highs of hypomania; many patients initially diagnosed as having agitated depressions subsequently turn out to have had dysphoric hypomanias. In short, misdiagnosing and overlooking hypomanic states often leads to an underestimate of the true rate of bipolar disorder.[3] (See Chapters 1 and 3 for a detailed discussion of these issues.) Higher incidence rates are obtained when a broader range of cases belonging to the presumed spectrum of bipolar disorder, such as cyclothymia or atypical bipolar illness, are included in the survey.

In the absence of a clear understanding of the pathophysiology involved, the distinctions among bipolar disorders, highly recurrent unipolar disorder, other mood disorders, and psychotic disorders remain unclear (see Chapters 1 and 3). These distinctions are especially difficult to make in community studies that include greater numbers of mild and untreated cases. At the psychotic end of the spectrum, a large number of patients have illnesses with features of both schizophrenia and bipolar disorder, termed schizoaffective disorder. The line between hypomania and mania is also difficult to draw, and DSM-IV offers differential diagnoses depending on the severity of symptoms and impairment. Patients with bipolar-II disorder are unlikely to present for treatment for hypomania, and even more unlikely to report it as pathology in community surveys (Akiskal, 1995, 1996; Coryell et al., 1995). Therefore, as shown later, the rates of bipolar-II are low in community surveys and are likely to be underestimated. (The reliability of diagnosis of bipolar-I and bipolar-II in community surveys is discussed further in the presentation of results of U.S. surveys.) Thus the distinction between bipolar-I and bipolar-II disorder is usually based on retrospective accounts, limiting reliability (Dunner and Tay, 1993). Moreover, applying criteria related to the clinical significance of a disorder based on impairment and the need for treatment

can markedly alter rates (Narrow et al., 2002) (see the later discussion).

Age-Specific Issues

The criteria for diagnosing bipolar disorder in children are even less clear than those used for adults (for example, see the discussion of problems in defining age at onset in children and adolescents later in this chapter and in Chapter 6). Indeed, since 1980 (DSM-III, DSM-III-R, and DSM-IV), adult criteria have been applied to diagnose mania and depression in children without taking into account differences in age and developmental stage (Sanchez et al., 1999). Bipolar disorder in young people may therefore be misdiagnosed or underdiagnosed. Moreover, although mania in youth can be a severe illness frequently associated with mixed features, psychosis, rapid cycling, and comorbid disruptive disorders, there is often a clinical bias against making a diagnosis of mania in children. And the relationship between bipolar disorder and other, more prevalent childhood psychiatric illnesses, such as attention-deficit hyperactivity disorder (ADHD), is problematic (see the later discussion of surveys of children and adolescents). Estimates of the age at onset of bipolar disorder must take into account this lack of clarity regarding first presentation of the disorder in youth. Eventually, longitudinal studies of children from families with a high risk of bipolar disorder may clarify issues of first presentation (see Chapter 6).

The effects of duration and severity on prevalence must also be considered when reviewing the literature on prevalence of childhood bipolar disorder (Sanchez et al., 1999). DSM-III-R removed the 7-day minimum duration criterion for mania required by DSM-III. Consequently, reports based on DSM-III-R criteria may overdiagnose mania, especially in childhood. In DSM-IV, the duration criterion was reinstated, and the severity requirement was added.

In April 2000, NIMH convened a group of experts for a Bipolar Child Roundtable to discuss possible approaches for addressing outstanding issues related to research on prepubertal bipolar disorder. The major issues of relevance to epidemiology addressed at the roundtable were the earliest age at which bipolar disorder can be diagnosed and the predictive value of the early manifestations of bipolar illness in children and adolescents. The experts generally agreed that a diagnosis of bipolar disorder using DSM criteria is possible in prepubertal children.

Discussion among the expert group resulted in agreement on two basic definitions: (1) a narrow phenotype that adheres strictly to bipolar-I and bipolar-II criteria, and (2) a broader phenotype that encompasses more heterogeneity—basically bipolar-not otherwise specified (NOS)—and includes children who do not quite meet the criteria (especially the durational criterion) for an episode but still are severely impaired by symptoms of mood instability. Consensus on the former phenotype was that it can be diagnosed with available psychiatric assessment instruments, such as the semistructured Kiddie Schedule for Affective Disorders and Schizophrenia (KSADS) (Chambers et al., 1985). For clear communication, however, the importance of establishing thresholds for the boundaries between bipolar disorder subtypes (bipolar-I, bipolar-II, and cyclothymia) was emphasized because homogeneity is essential for biological, genetic, and epidemiologic research.

Currently, children with severely impairing mood disturbance who do not meet full DSM-IV criteria for bipolar-I or -II are not included in research studies and are difficult to assess in epidemiologic studies because of the perceived uncertainty of diagnosis. The expert group agreed that bipolar-NOS could be used as a working diagnosis to advance research on this broader phenotype, as long as the children were well described (with particular attention to symptoms of ADHD). Because available diagnostic instruments may not generate a reliable and replicable diagnosis of bipolar-NOS, it was recommended that careful assessment include all of the behaviors that are impairing, giving consideration when relevant to the frequency with which they occur, as well as their severity. Examples of the behaviors to be included are aggressiveness, agitation, explosiveness, irritability, mood lability (fluctuation independent of input), thought disorder (paranoia, misinterpretation of social cues), communication disorder (pragmatic language disorder that can look like flight of ideas, receptive and expressive language disorder that can interfere with the accurate performance and interpretation of structured interviews), and cognitive ability/cognitive impairment (significantly low intelligence quotient [IQ], reading disabilities).

Once agreement has been reached on exclusion criteria (certain comorbidities, such as pervasive developmental disorder and/or physical disease) as well as inclusion criteria for the broader phenotype, it should be possible to address questions about relationships among the disorders—for example, whether bipolar-NOS or its subtypes are precursors of bipolar-I and/or bipolar-II or have a different course. The expert group noted, for instance, that whereas the course of classic bipolar illness includes well periods, these children tend not to have such periods. Moreover, it should be possible to identify and fully characterize children who have bipolar symptoms and are severely impaired and to follow them prospectively, with attention to developmental stages and transitions, in order to resolve whether they have a childhood-onset variant of bipolar disorder (see Chapter 6 for a more complete discussion).

Validation studies also need to take developmental manifestations into account. The expert group suggested that studies could encompass children as young as 4 years of age. Reconstruction of the history of adults with early-onset bipolar illness may be useful as well. For example, in studies of the offspring of bipolar parents, which should include all of their children, parents should be asked about their own age at onset. The group deemed it important also that children with possible bipolar disorder, as well as their parents, be interviewed with developmentally appropriate measures.

Information about instruments currently employed in NIMH-funded studies of childhood-onset bipolar disorder was assembled for use at the roundtable. The most commonly used diagnostic instrument is KSADS—in most cases, the Washington University (St. Louis) version (WASH-U-KSADS) or KSADS with the WASH-U-KSADS sections on mood disorders and rapid cycling added. Ancillary instruments being used include the Child Behavior Checklist (CBCL) (Achenbach, 1991a,b).

Efforts that might be undertaken to resolve the diagnostic issues raised above include the following: describing the course of bipolar-I, bipolar-II, cyclothymia, and bipolar-NOS, with attention to the impact of development on changing patterns of symptoms; establishing the predictive validity of bipolar disorder in prepubertal children; defining thresholds for and boundaries between bipolar-I, bipolar-II, and cyclothymia in prepubertal children; and identifying occasions on which combining versus separating bipolar-I and -II would be appropriate (in treatment studies of mania, for example, where severity is an issue, combining manic with hypomanic patients may be inappropriate). Although future epidemiologic studies will need to incorporate the clinical findings of studies conducted to date, the unresolved issues of diagnosis in children described here make the accuracy of estimates of rates of childhood bipolar disorder and determinants of age at onset uncertain. See Chapter 6 for a comprehensive discussion of these issues.

Epidemiologic findings for the elderly are also ambiguous. In geriatric inpatient units, the prevalence of treated bipolar disorder has been described as reaching 10 percent (Yassa et al., 1988). Yet there is a disparity between the prevalence of bipolar disorder among elderly patients in hospitals and elderly individuals living in the community. Moreover, the rates of bipolar disorder are dramatically lower among community-dwelling elderly people than among younger persons (Shulman and Hermann, 1999). One reason for this is the increased early mortality from medical causes, such as cardiovascular disease and suicide among those with the disorder (Snowdon, 1991).

Diagnostic Methods

Over the years, we have seen the development of a number of structured interview instruments that have improved the precision with which psychiatric disorders can be identified and their rates estimated (see Chapters 3 and 11). Yet different diagnostic criteria or revised versions of the same criteria can affect rates and their comparisons. Thus differences among diagnostic instruments used in community studies may explain some of the variation in the rates obtained.

The DIS (Robins et al., 1981a), mentioned earlier, is a highly structured interview designed for large-scale epidemiologic studies. It generates DSM-IV diagnoses in computer algorithm form for the major psychiatric disorders. The CIDI (WHO, 1990; Wittchen et al., 1998a), also noted previously, consists of state-of-the-art structured diagnostic interviews based on the DIS and generates DSM-IV and ICD diagnoses. Trained lay interviewers administer both the DIS and the CIDI. The two instruments differ in that the DIS includes impairment criteria when generating diagnoses, whereas the CIDI does not. Moreover, after an initial round of questions about symptoms, the CIDI returns to reassess those symptoms, while the DIS asks about symptoms only once. A modification of the CIDI made by the University of Michigan Institute for Social Research (UM-CIDI) (Kessler, 1995) simplified that instrument's complex questions. Qualifiers such as "a lot" (as in the question, "Did the symptom interfere with your life and activities a lot?") were clarified (as in the question, "How much did the symptom interfere with your life or activities—a lot, some, a little, not at all?").

Another semistructured interview instrument is the Schedule for Affective Disorders and Schizophrenia (SADS) (Endicott and Spitzer, 1978), which is tied to the Research Diagnostic Criteria (RDC) (Spitzer et al., 1978) and the DSM. This instrument has been used less often than the DIS or the CIDI in community surveys because it must be administered by trained mental health professionals.

The Structured Psychopathological Interview and Rating of the Social Consequences of Psychiatric Disturbances for Epidemiology (SPIKE for the original German) (Angst et al., 1984) is yet another semistructured clinical interview. It allows the assessment of 29 separate syndromes, including hypomania, in terms of symptoms, their length, their frequency of occurrence, subjective suffering, social consequences, treatment, and family history, and generates DSM-III diagnoses.

The Structured Clinical Interview for DSM (SCID) is a semistructured clinical interview used for making a major Axis I DSM-III-R or DSM-IV diagnosis. Through a decision-tree approach, the SCID guides the clinician in testing diagnostic hypotheses as the interview is conducted (see Chapter 11 for a discussion of issues involved in using decision trees). The output of the SCID is a record of the presence or absence of each of the disorders being considered for current episodes (past month) and for lifetime occurrence.

The Diagnostic Interview for Genetic Studies (DIGS) (Nurnberger et al., 1994) yields DSM-IV and RDC diagnoses and requires trained clinical interviewers. Questions on mania/hypomania in the mood disorder module are designed to assess current and most severe disorder, presence of psychotic features, impairment, organic factors, and treatment seeking. Mixed affective states and cycling are also assessed. The DIGS was designed for large-scale genetic studies and has not been used in community-based epidemiologic studies (see Chapter 13).

Finally, with few exceptions (Italy, Israel, Switzerland), the larger epidemiologic community surveys use trained nonclinical interviewers because it is costly and usually infeasible to send doctoral-level clinicians to conduct in-home interviews with thousands of subjects. Results of testing the congruence between findings obtained by nonclinical and clinical interviewers are described later in the presentation of the ECA findings.

Nonresponse or Refusal to Participate in the Survey

Another bias in community surveys that may affect the rates of bipolar disorder obtained is the failure of some subjects to participate, which may occur in the early phase of sample designation and again at measurement and interviewing. Because one cannot assume that nonresponse is randomly distributed across the intended sample, it can be a major source of bias. Nonresponse bias that occurs during the process of selecting and contacting the sample includes sample mortality, sample loss, and missing data (Badawi et al., 1999); also significant is refusal to respond in the middle stages of data collection.

The predictors of nonresponse bias were investigated in a 15-year follow-up of individuals in a probability sample from the household population of the Baltimore, Maryland, ECA. Mania was found to be associated with increased mortality, some of which may be related to the high rates of suicide, alcohol and drug abuse, and cardiovascular disease among this population (Badawi et al., 1999).

In the NCS, a special effort was made to estimate the rate of disorders among people who initially refused to participate in the survey. The results indicated that these individuals had higher rates of mental disorders, including bipolar disorder, than those who agreed to participate. Such data might be used to adjust prevalence estimates.

Other Issues

Sample Size

The relatively short duration of many manic and depressive episodes and the presence of mixed states cause difficulties in assessment. Short episodes are counted in some studies but overlooked in others that use diagnostic instruments with long-duration criteria. Short episodes also are responsible for large differences in rates of point and annual prevalence. Gagrat and Spiro (1980) explained this difficulty and underscored the problems created by studying a phenomenon with a low baseline rate. As they noted, point prevalence studies for a short-duration disorder with a yearly prevalence of 0.7 percent would require the screening of very large numbers of people. Even allowing for a mean duration of manic episodes of 2 months (a mean duration of 2 months assumes that many of the manic episodes in the community are shortened by treatment), the point prevalence rate would be on the order of 0.2 percent if the annual prevalence in the population at large were 1.0 percent. This means it would be necessary to screen 1,000 people to find 2 active cases. Epidemiologic studies of several hundred thousand people at a time would be required to determine the point prevalence in the population at large. Moreover, it is questionable whether current epidemiologic research instruments would be reliable in such studies.

Except for demographic characteristics such as age and gender, the relatively low prevalence of bipolar disorder makes estimates of variations in rates by risk factor difficult even in reasonably sized epidemiologic surveys. For example, in a sample of 5,000, which would be considered a reasonably sized community survey, a lifetime prevalence of 2 percent for a disorder would yield at most 100 cases. Few epidemiologic studies have 5,000 subjects. When the population is segmented by age, gender, and race, moreover, the sample size in each group dwindles rapidly. Finally, as discussed later, time constraints prevent any one study from including all the relevant risk factors, and multiple instruments are required.

Incidence and Prevalence Rates

Population measures of disease frequency include incidence and prevalence rates, the latter divided by different points in time (period prevalence). *Incidence* is defined as the number of new cases of disease in a *population at risk* for that disease per unit time. Incidence rates are used to determine differences in risk factors and are always difficult to obtain because they require a longitudinal study to identify new cases. Determining the incidence of bipolar disorder is yet more difficult because of the problems of determining subtle changes in mood and of knowing

when a case of major depression converts to bipolar. The lack of clarity of presentation in children and the need for large samples, as discussed previously, can further compound the problem. Indeed, few of the epidemiologic studies published since the first edition of this text have provided incidence data. The 13-year follow-up of the Baltimore ECA (described later) excluded incidence data for bipolar disorder because of an insufficient sample size (Badawi et al., 1999). Likewise, a 40-year follow-up of the Stirling County study in Nova Scotia assessing the incidence of depression did not include bipolar disorder (Murphy et al., 2000).

Prevalence is defined as the number of existing cases of disease in a *total population* per period of time. Prevalence rates can help identify unmet need. The studies reviewed in this chapter provide data on period prevalence, usually annual and lifetime. The lifetime prevalence is the proportion of the population that has had a disease at some point during a lifetime (Kramer et al., 1980). It is the rate obtained in response to the question, "Have you ever had . . . ?" Lifetime prevalence as a measure has been criticized for numerous reasons, including problems of recall. However, it is still applied widely as one of the imperfect but useful tools available for counting cases.

Functional Impairment

The assessments used in recent epidemiologic studies require some evidence of functional impairment to determine the clinical significance of the case. Questions about impairment of major roles or treatment seeking are designed to elicit this information. Variations in these questions can seriously alter rates among studies, as revealed by the comparison of the rates in the ECA and the NCS, described later.

Age at Onset

Different methods may be used for computing the age at onset of bipolar disorder. One method is to use two measures of central tendency: the mean or average age at onset and the median, or the age that corresponds to the 50th percentile of the distribution. An advantage of using this method is that age at onset can be summarized as one estimate. The disadvantage is that both the mean and the median can be biased by extreme values at either the lower or higher end of the distribution of ages.

Another method for analyzing age at onset is to compute the incidence (or hazard) rate of bipolar disorder for each age of life. This is done by taking the number of new cases that appear at each age and dividing it by the population at risk for that age. The major advantage of this method is that trends in incidence rates can be compared across all ages, although the population at risk becomes smaller as age increases, inflating the incidence rate for older ages.

COMMUNITY SURVEYS AMONG ADULTS

In this section we review the methods and results of two surveys conducted among adults in the United States in the late 1970s, the two major epidemiologic studies conducted during the 1980s and 1990s, and comparable cross-national studies conducted throughout the world since the 1980s. Recent epidemiologic studies conducted among children and adolescents are discussed in the next section. Studies were included if they used standardized diagnostic assessments and defined sampling methods. When raw data were available, we undertook data analysis. In some cases, we used published results, so there is no standard presentation across sites; for example, bipolar-I and -II were sometimes combined in published results, and sometimes only annual, not lifetime, prevalence rates were given. The data presented are primarily annual and lifetime prevalence rates and incidence rates, where available.

New Haven Survey

The first community survey to use standardized diagnostic assessments and criteria was the New Haven survey, which was conducted in 1975 using the SADS-Lifetime (SADS-L) diagnostic instrument, based on the RDC (Weissman and Myers, 1978). This survey, considered a pilot study because it was a follow-up of a cohort identified 10 years earlier, included only 511 adults. A lifetime rate of 0.6 percent for bipolar-I was reported. The addition of bipolar-II raised the rate to 1.2 percent. Bipolar disorder was represented equally in males and females. These findings are comparable to those of subsequent large-scale community surveys.

The Amish Study

The Amish study of Egeland and colleagues (1983) is unusual in its assessment of the prevalence of affective disorders in a population that is culturally and genetically homogeneous. This subculture, a highly conservative Protestant religious sect in Pennsylvania, offered an "unheralded opportunity to study multigenerational pedigrees with large sibships" (Egeland and Hostetter, 1983, p. 70). Variables that confounded past research are not present in this population; for example, alcohol and drug abuse are virtually nonexistent, and criminal acts and violence are rare. Other obstacles had to be overcome, however. In applying specific diagnostic criteria to this group, the RDC definitions for mania and depression needed to be considered within the context of Amish culture. For example, manic behaviors to the Amish include racing one's horse

and carriage too fast, buying or using machinery or worldly items, using the public telephone excessively, and planning vacations during the wrong season (Egeland et al., 1983).

The Old Order Amish, 12,500 people who live primarily in Lancaster County, Pennsylvania, keep extensive genealogical and medical records of ancestors going back 30 generations (Egeland and Hostetter, 1983). The Amish study, which spanned the 5-year period from 1976 to 1980, attempted to identify all individuals who were actively ill, thus yielding incidence and period prevalence rates. As the authors noted, the close interactions among the Amish prevented even mild cases of emotional disturbance from being overlooked. Once an active case had been identified, medical records were abstracted and sent to a psychiatric board, which made a consensus diagnosis based on the RDC. If medical records did not exist, patients were interviewed directly using the SADS-L.

Reliability estimates were made based on the agreement between board consensus and a separate psychiatrist's diagnosis (Hostetter et al., 1983). Kappa statistics for reliability generally were high and consistent for any major affective disorder, for unipolar depression, and for bipolar-I disorder (0.87, 0.95, and 0.86, respectively). Only with bipolar-II disorder was the kappa coefficient much lower (0.68), suggesting a possible misrepresentation of this diagnosis among the Amish and less reliability in the diagnostic category. Indeed, the problem of unreliability in estimates of bipolar-II in community samples was found in subsequent studies described later.

During the survey period, 112 cases of mental illness were reported, 80 percent of which were affective disorders (71 percent major affective disorders), involving 1 percent of the Amish population (Egeland and Hostetter, 1983). A further breakdown of these rates revealed that 34 percent of the psychiatric cases were either bipolar-I or bipolar-II disorder, and 37 percent were unipolar depression. The remaining 9 percent comprised minor depression and hypomania (8 and 1 percent, respectively). As the authors pointed out, both the rate of major affective disorders and the rate of mental illness in general appeared to be below the general population average.

The most interesting finding is the apparent equivalence in rates of bipolar and unipolar illness. Other studies have shown a lopsided ratio. Weissman and Klerman (1978) and many subsequent investigators have found an almost 4:1 unipolar:bipolar diagnosis ratio across the United States, and some studies have shown a 10:1 ratio. In an attempt to explain these discrepant findings, Egeland and Hostetter (1983) noted that their sample of bipolar patients would have been greatly reduced had not community reports of behaviors suggestive of a "high" led to early SADS-L interviewing. In fact, the Amish data may more accurately reflect the actual bipolar:unipolar ratio. Recent clinical research indicates that many cases diagnosed as unipolar illness may be variants of bipolar disorder (see Chapters 1, 2, 13, and 19). Another explanation for the discrepancy is the finding of Egeland and colleagues (1983) that 79 percent of their bipolar-I patients had previously been diagnosed as schizophrenic. Cultural factors may be partly responsible for this incidence of misdiagnosis: earlier clinicians, unfamiliar with the customs of the Amish, may have viewed thought disorder, paranoia, and grandiosity as symptoms of schizophrenia rather than mania (Egeland and Hostetter, 1983; Egeland et al., 1983). Of particular note are grandiose symptoms with marked religious overtones, because religion is central to the Amish. If other manic symptoms are not noted or are overlooked (as is apparent in early medical records), these symptoms may easily be seen as schizophrenic. Likewise, it is probable that Amish individuals who are the most ill stay within the community, whereas the less ill may emigrate.

Among both bipolar and unipolar patients in the Amish study, gender was equally distributed. Although this finding is consistent with others for bipolar illness, the majority of subsequent studies have found a 2:1 female:male ratio for unipolar depression. The most obvious explanation for this discrepancy, according to Egeland and Hostetter (1983), is that alcoholism and sociopathy do not mask depression in Amish males as they do in males in the general population.

Although the findings of this study have been debated, they provide a view of major affective disorders relatively untainted by violence, alcohol and drug abuse, and other variables that might otherwise mask such a disorder's presence.

Epidemiologic Catchment Area Study

The ECA study, conducted during 1980–1984, was the first comprehensive epidemiologic study of mental illness in the United States. It was designed to obtain accurate and uniform epidemiologic data on mental disorders in the United States that would be comparable across sites, as well as to assess the adequacy of services to the mentally ill (Regier et al., 1984). The design required representative sampling of populations from both community and institutional settings at two different time points 1 year apart (waves 1 and 2). In wave 1, prevalence data were gathered for lifetime, annual, 6-month, 1-month, and 2-week periods. Wave 2 was a follow-up to ascertain rates of relapse and remission, as well as to determine incidence rates (Eaton et al., 1989).

More than 18,000 people were interviewed by lay interviewers, who used the DIS, together with criteria from the DSM-III, RDC, and Feighner diagnostic systems. (The latter two sets of diagnostic criteria are now used infrequently.) Subjects were first asked whether they had ever experienced a symptom at any time during their lives and whether they had experienced impairment in life activities from that symptom. For each symptom, the interviewer ascertained whether alcohol, drugs, medication, or physical illness was the underlying cause. Subjects were then asked whether they had experienced the symptom during the last 2 weeks, the last month, the last 6 months, and the last year, and this information was used to generate a diagnosis for period prevalence. The DIS determined the severity of a disorder in addition to its presence and duration.

The DIS appears to have relatively high reliability for diagnosing major depression but considerably less reliability for manic episodes. In comparing the agreement between the DIS administered to the same subjects by a lay interviewer and a physician, the kappa statistic for major depression was found to be 0.50 and for mania 0.21 (Helzer et al., 1985). Some questions remain about the continued use of the DIS and interpretation of the data it yields (see, e.g., Anthony et al., 1985). The accuracy of lifetime recall has been questioned, as has the lack of comparability of diagnoses made by lay interviewers and by experienced clinicians, whose pattern recognition and access to family history are likely to produce a more accurate diagnosis. Robbins and colleagues (1982) compared 1-month prevalence rates of depression and mania at two ECA sites (St. Louis and Baltimore) based on diagnoses by lay interviewers and psychiatrists using the DIS. Although the rates were not significantly different in Baltimore, both disorders were diagnosed three times more often by psychiatrists than by lay interviewers in St. Louis. A recent study of 41,838 individuals in the Swedish Twin Registry underscores the considerable problem in interpreting findings obtained by lay interviewers (Soldani et al., 2005). Telephone screening for mania, when compared with actual hospitalization and other medical records, resulted in spuriously high false-positive rates for mania in particular and for bipolar disorder in general. The investigators concluded that instead of the reported rate of 1.6 percent, a more accurate estimate would be 0.9 percent. These discrepancies suggest that some caution should be applied in interpreting ECA data, although the study is methodologically superior overall to past attempts at estimating the prevalence and incidence of bipolar illness.

The lifetime and annual prevalence and annual incidence for bipolar-I disorder for the total noninstitutionalized ECA sample and each of the five sites are presented in Table 5–2. The total sample size was 18,571 respondents aged 18 and older, 59 percent of whom were female. The overall response rate was 76 percent. The lifetime

TABLE 5–2. **Lifetime and Annual Prevalence/100 (Standard Error) and Incidence Rate/100 of Bipolar-I Disorder in Five Epidemiologic Catchment Area Sites**

Parameter	New Haven, CT	Baltimore, MD	St. Louis, MO	Durham, NC	Los Angeles, CA
Number in sample	5,034	3,481	3,004	3,921	3,131
Response rate (%)	77	78	79	79	68
% Female	59	62	60	60	53
Lifetime prevalence/100					
Total	1.2 (0.21)	0.6 (0.20)	1.0 (0.20)	0.3 (0.14)	0.6 (0.16)
Males	1.0 (0.27)	0.7 (0.22)	1.1 (0.30)	0.1 (0.11)	0.6 (0.23)
Females	1.3 (0.30)	0.5 (0.24)	1.0 (0.27)	0.6 (0.25)	0.5 (0.21)
M/F Ratio	0.8	1.4	1.1	0.2	1.2
Annual prevalence/100					
Total	1.0 (0.16)	0.5 (0.14)	1.0 (0.20)	0.2 (0.08)	0.4 (0.13)
Males	0.9 (0.22)	0.5 (0.21)	1.0 (0.30)	0.0	0.3 (0.15)
Females	1.1 (0.23)	0.5 (0.18)	1.0 (0.27)	0.4 (0.16)	0.5 (0.20)
M/F Ratio	0.8	1.0	1.0	0.0	0.1
Annual Incidence/100					
Total	0.6 (0.12)	0.2 (0.09)	0.1 (0.07)	0.3 (0.10)	0.5 (0.15)
Males	0.4 (0.15)	0.0	0.0	0.1 (0.09)	0.5 (0.21)
Females	0.7 (0.19)	0.4 (1.6)	0.2 (0.13)	0.5 (0.18)	0.5 (0.20)

Note: Encompasses ages 18 years and older.

prevalence of bipolar-I disorder was 0.8/100, ranging from 0.3/100 at Durham to 1.2/100 at New Haven. In general, the lifetime prevalence was the same for males and females, with slightly higher rates for males at Baltimore (M/F ratio = 1.4) and higher rates for females at Durham (M/F ratio = 0.2). The overall annual prevalence was 0.6/100, and the incidence was 0.4 per 100 cases per year. There was a tendency for females to have a higher incidence rate of bipolar-I than males, but this varied by site. The mean age at onset of bipolar-I disorder ranged from 14.6 years at St. Louis to 22.3 years at Baltimore (overall at the five sites, 18.6 years; overall median age, 18 years). (See the later discussion of the Cross-National

Collaborative Group for results and a discussion of rates for bipolar-II.)

The ECA also examined the use of mental health services by patients with bipolar disorder (Narrow et al., 1993; Regier et al., 1993). Overall, 61 percent of all individuals with bipolar disorder had been treated in the service sector within the past year—46 percent by specialty mental health providers and 29 percent by general medical providers. This was the highest rate of use of mental health services in the affective disorder group. It translates, on a population level, to approximately 1.1 million people with bipolar disorder making 16 million visits to outpatient mental health care facilities in the year before their wave 1 interview (Narrow et al., 1993).

One-third (33.4 percent) of bipolar patients receiving inpatient care did so at a general hospital facility, 19.5 percent at a private mental hospital, and 34.4 percent at a Veterans Affairs (VA) psychiatric hospital unit. The rest were treated at state and county facilities, community mental health centers, alcohol/drug units, or nursing home facilities.

National Comorbidity Survey

The NCS, administered by the staff of the Survey Research Center at the University of Michigan in Ann Arbor, was conducted between 1990 and 1992, or 10 years after the ECA. It was based on a probability sample of 8,098 individuals aged 15 to 54 from the noninstitutionalized populations of the 48 conterminous states; the response rate was 84 percent. Subjects were interviewed using the UM-CIDI, which made DSM-III-R diagnoses (Kessler et al., 1994). Unlike the ECA, which was based on five geographic sites, the NCS included a representative national sample from across the United States. Diagnoses known to have a low prevalence in population-based surveys (e.g., somatization disorder) or poor interrater reliability in the ECA (e.g., obsessive-compulsive disorder) were excluded. Respondents as young as age 15 were included because there was an interest in the comorbidity of substance abuse and other psychiatric disorders, and because the ECA had shown that the rates of psychiatric disorders were higher in younger than in older persons. Ten years after the NCS was completed, Kessler and colleagues (2005) conducted a replication (the NCS-R) of their initial study. Face-to-face diagnostic interviews were carried out on 9,282 English-speaking subjects by professional interviewers from the Institute for Social Research at the University of Michigan. DSM-IV diagnoses were generated based on the World Mental Health Survey initiative version of the CIDI (WMH-CIDI).

Table 5–3 shows the rates obtained for bipolar-I disorder in the NCS and NCS-R. Data on rates for bipolar-II were not reported in the NCS because of the unreliability of diagnosis of this disorder (see the later discussion); these rates were, however, ascertained in the replication study. The NCS and NCS-R rates shown in the table were adjusted for nonresponse and weighted to the sociodemographic characteristics of the target population from the 1989 U.S. National Interview Survey (US DHHS, 1992) and from the 2000 U.S. Census, respectively. In the NCS, the lifetime prevalence of bipolar-I disorder was 1.7 percent, with equal rates in males and females. The annual prevalence was 1.3 percent, also with equal rates by gender. The rates of bipolar-I were about twice as high in the NCS as in the ECA. The mean age at onset for bipolar-I disorder was 23.3 years (median 21 years). This onset age is about 3 years later than that found in the ECA.

The lifetime prevalence of bipolar-I disorder in the NCS-R was slightly lower, 1.0, than that reported in the NCS. The NCS-R found a lifetime prevalence of 1.1 in females and 0.8 in males. The annual prevalence for the total sample was 0.6. The mean age at onset for bipolar-I was 21.4 (median 19 years). For bipolar-II in the NCS-R, the lifetime prevalence was 1.1 (males, 0.9; females, 1.3); the annual prevalence was 0.8 (males, 0.7; females, 0.9); and the mean age at onset was 25.2 years (median 20 years).

There has been some debate about the reasons for the discrepancies in findings between the ECA and the NCS, and several attempts have been made to understand how differences between the two instruments (Table 5–4) might explain these discrepancies (Kessler et al., 1997; Regier et al., 1998; Narrow et al., 2002). The most obvious difference is the sampling frame. The ECA encompassed five selected sites, compared with a probability sample of all 48 conterminous states in the NCS. The ECA included persons living in institutions (prisons, boarding houses, nursing homes, and hospitals), while the NCS did not. The age structure of the two samples was also different, as mentioned earlier. Even when comparable age groups (18 to 54 years) are considered, however, the lifetime rate of bipolar disorder in the NCS remains at 1.7.

The controversy over which results are closer to the actual prevalence has not been resolved. However, there is agreement that any differences in rates are not true differences, but likely due to differences in sampling and methods between the studies (see note 2 for details). Moreover, although the rates of bipolar disorder are disparate between the ECA and NCS, the actual range of rates is not that large, and the demographic risk factors (discussed later) do not vary greatly between the two studies.

Table 5–5 compares the rates of bipolar-I disorder by demographic characteristics using an identical age group (18 to 54 years) to see whether the patterns of variation are similar. There are no significant differences in the rates of bipolar-I disorder by gender, educational level, or rural/urban domicile in either the ECA or the NCS. There is no difference in the rates by family income in the ECA. In the NCS, however, there is an inverse relationship between the rates of bipolar disorder and family income: the lower the income, the higher the rates ($p = .04$). Persons who are separated or divorced have higher rates in both the ECA ($p = .02$) and the NCS ($p = .002$). The age at onset is 5 years younger in the ECA compared with the NCS ($p = .001$).

Cross-National Collaborative Group

The success of the ECA in the United States led to the conduct of similar studies using the DIS in various parts of the world. Data from some countries began to appear in the late 1980s. However, it was difficult to make cross-national

TABLE 5–3. Lifetime and Annual Prevalence of Bipolar-I Disorder
in the U.S. National Comorbidity Survey (NCS)
and in the U.S. National Comorbidity
Survey Replication (NCS-R)

Parameter	NCS (1994)	NCS-R (2005)
Number in sample	8,098	9,282
Response rate (%)	84	71
Interview measure	UM-CIDI	CIDI
Diagnostic outcome	DSM-III-R	DSM-IV
Interviewers	Lay	Lay
% Female	52	52
Lifetime prevalence/100 (Standard Error)		
Total	1.7 (0.20)	1.0 (0.1)
Males	1.6 (0.28)	0.8 (0.1)
Females	1.7 (0.28)	1.1 (0.2)
Annual prevalence/100 (Standard Error)		
Total	1.3 (0.18)	0.6 (0.1)
Males	1.4 (0.25)	0.6 (0.1)
Females	1.3 (0.24)	0.7 (0.1)
Age at Onset (years)		
Mean	23.3 (0.9)	21.4 (1.2)
Median	21.0	19.0

CIDI = Composite International Diagnostic Interview; DSM = *Diagnostic and Statistical Manual*; UM-CIDI = University of Michigan Institute for Social Research's modification of the CIDI.
Sources: Kessler et al., 1994; National Comorbidity Study Replication (2005).

comparisons, even with studies using the same diagnostic assessment methods, because of variability in the data presentation. As noted earlier, the Cross-National Collaborative Group was formed in the 1990s to directly compare rates and risks for psychiatric disorders and to help overcome this problem of disparate presentation of data by standardizing analysis across sites. The hope was that real differences in rates by country, not due to differing analytic methods, might thereby emerge. Ten countries, including the United States, that had used Version III of the DIS and DSM-III formed the collaboration. Only 7 of these 10 provided data

on bipolar disorder; nonetheless, these 7 countries represent diverse geographic, political, and cultural areas in North America, the Caribbean, Europe, Asia, and the Pacific Rim. The investigators in each country translated the DIS; details on the translation and the methodology employed are included in the references for each study. In addition to the ECA, data were obtained from the following sources:

• The Edmonton Survey of Psychiatric Disorders (Orn et al., 1988) was conducted in the city of Edmonton, Alberta, Canada.

TABLE 5–4. Comparison of the Epidemiologic Catchment Area Study (ECA) and the National Comorbidity Survey (NCS)

Parameter	ECA	NCS
Date conducted	1980–1984	1990–1992
Sample size	18,571	8,089
Site	5 U.S. sites	48 U.S. states
Age range (years)	18–65	15–54
Instrument	DIS	CIDI
Diagnosis	DSM-III	DSM-III-R
Interviewers	Lay	Lay

CIDI = Composite International Diagnostic Interview; DIS = Diagnostic Interview Schedule; DSM = *Diagnostic and Statistical Manual.*

- The Puerto Rico Study of Psychiatric Disorders (Canino et al., 1987) included persons living in households throughout Puerto Rico, in addition to household members temporarily away and those in institutions.
- The Munich Follow-up Study (Wittchen et al., 1992) was a 7-year follow-up investigation of a stratified random general population sample drawn from the former West Germany.
- The Taiwan Psychiatric Epidemiology Project (Hwu et al., 1989) sampled three population areas representing metropolitan Taipei and township and rural areas.
- The Korean Epidemiologic Study of Mental Disorders (Lee et al., 1990a,b) sampled persons in urban Seoul and in scattered rural regions across South Korea.
- The Christchurch Psychiatric Epidemiology Study (Wells et al., 1989) included adults living in Christchurch on the South Island of New Zealand.

Table 5–6 shows the target population and sample size, response rate, and gender and age distributions for each study that collected data on bipolar disorder. Statistical analyses of these data standardized the rates at each site to the age and gender distribution of the ECA. Because of different age distributions at each site, analysis was restricted to the 18- to 64-year age group (26 to 64 years in West Germany). The standardization was performed according to methods described by Breslow and Day (1987). Weighted prevalence rates yielded estimates that would be derived if each site had the same age and gender distribution as the ECA. The ECA, Edmonton, Puerto Rico, Munich, Taiwan,

Korea, and Christchurch surveys collected data on both bipolar-I and bipolar-II disorder, which are the basis for the rates presented here; the NCS data are shown for comparison purposes. Note that both the ECA and NCS rates presented in the following tables may vary slightly from the rates presented earlier in Tables 5–2 and 5–3 because of the differing age ranges included.

The lifetime prevalence for bipolar-I range from 0.3 percent in Taiwan to 1.7 percent in the United States (NCS) (Weissman et al., 1996) (Table 5–7). The rates are moderately consistent cross-nationally. The male/female ratio is almost equal for the United States and Taiwan. Men have slightly higher rates than women in the Edmonton, Puerto Rico, and New Zealand surveys, and much higher rates in the Korea survey. Mean age at onset is on average 6 years younger for bipolar-I than for major depression, ranging from 17 in Edmonton to 27 in Puerto Rico (median 18 to 25). The West German rates are not stable because of the small sample size. The data on mean age at onset for bipolar-I may represent underestimates, because some of those surveyed had not yet passed through the age of risk, and no one older than age 64 was included.

The lifetime rates for bipolar-II are lower than those for bipolar-I, a result that probably reflects the difficulty of distinguishing mild highs from normal mood fluctuations in a community sample, as discussed previously. The rates are relatively consistent across sites (range 0.1 to 0.9 percent). There is no consistent gender ratio, although the rate of bipolar-II disorder is more often higher among females than males, a result suggested by clinical studies (Leibenluft, 1996). These rates, too, are probably underestimates. The lower rates of bipolar-II compared with bipolar-I reflect the uncertainty associated with diagnosis of bipolar-II in a nonpatient sample—a conclusion discussed previously and also reached by Kessler and colleagues (1997) in their validity study of the NCS.

Table 5–8 shows the very high rates of suicide attempts among persons with versus those without bipolar-I disorder in the United States and five other countries in the 1980s and 1990s (see Chapters 8 and 25). These figures were adjusted for age and gender at each site. Regardless of the variation in rates of bipolar disorder across countries, the association with suicide attempts is consistent and strong: the difference in prevalence of suicide attempts among those with and without bipolar disorder (odds ratio) ranges from 5.5 to 25.7/100.

Table 5–9 shows the significant association between panic disorder and bipolar disorder (see Chapter 7). Although the actual numbers of persons with this comorbidity were quite small in Puerto Rico, Taiwan, Korea, and Christchurch, the association is statistically significant across all sites. The association between the two disorders

TABLE 5–5. Lifetime Prevalence/100 (Standard Error) of Bipolar-I Disorder by Demographic Characteristics in the United States

Characteristic	ECA (1980)	NCS (1990)
Gender		
Male	1.0 (0.16)	1.6 (0.29)
Female	1.1 (0.17)	1.8 (0.30)
p Value	.43	.77
Mean age at onset, years	18.7 (6.1)	24.0 (7.5)
Median	18	22
Educational level		
Less than high school	1.3 (0.25)	2.2 (0.61)
High school graduate	1.1 (0.21)	2.0 (0.36)
College or higher	0.9 (0.16)	1.2 (0.27)
p Value	.33	.12
Total Family Income		
$0–$19,999	1.2 (0.22)	2.7 (0.53)
$20,000–$34,999	0.7 (0.21)	1.4 (0.38)
$35,000–$69,999	1.2 (0.33)	1.6 (0.34)
$70,000+	N/A	0.8 (0.39)
p Value	.34	.04
Marital status		
Married	0.8 (0.13)	1.3 (0.22)
Separated/divorced	1.6 (0.40)	3.8 (0.93)
Never married	1.3 (0.23)	1.8 (0.48)
p Value	.02	.002
Domicile		
Rural	0.9 (0.26)	1.3 (0.39)
Urban	1.1 (0.13)	1.8 (0.24)
p Value	.63	.31

Note: Encompasses ages 18–54 years.
ECA = Epidemiologic Catchment Area study; NCS = National Comorbidity Study.

TABLE 5–6. **Target Population, Sample Size, Response Rate, and Gender and Age Distributions for the Cross-National Sites**

Characteristic	ECA[a]	NCS[b]	Alberta, Edmonton	Puerto Rico	West Germany	Taiwan	Korea	New Zealand
Size of target population	1,198,000[c]	247,005,000[d]	397,965[e]	1,792,127[c]	29,240,900[f]	1,681,118[c]	13,520,908[c]	181,000[g]
Total number in study, age 18+ years	18,571	8,098	3,258	1,513	481	11,004	5,100	1,498
Response rate (%)	76	84	72	91	76	90	83	70
% Female	59	52	59	57	52	48	52	66
% Age at Interview (years)								
18–25	14	19	22	22	N/A	25	20	20
26–45	33	59	46	50	55	43	49	55
46–64	21	16	21	28	45	24	30	24
65+	31	N/A	11	N/A	N/A	7	0.5	N/A

Note: Figures shown are in raw percentages; percentages may not add to exactly 100 at certain sites because of missing values
N/A = not assessed.
[a]U.S. Epidemiologic Catchment Area Study, 1980.
[b]U.S. National Comorbidity Survey, 1990.
[c]Population figures according to 1980 census.
[d]Population figures drawn from 1990 U.S. Census of 48 conterminous states.
[e]Population figures according to 1981 census.
[f]Population figures according to 1974 census of West Germany, former Federal Republic of Germany.
[g]Population figures according to 1986 census.

TABLE 5–7. Lifetime Prevalence/100 (Standard Error) of Bipolar-I Disorder in Samples of the Cross-National Collaborative Group Study

Survey Site	Overall	Males	Females	M/F Ratio	Age at Onset (years)	Median Age at Onset (years)
United States						
ECA, 1980	0.9 (0.10)	0.8 (0.14)	1.0 (0.15)	0.7	18.1 (0.68)	18
NCS, 1990[a]	1.7 (0.21)	1.6 (0.29)	1.8 (0.30)	0.9	24.0 (0.92)	23
Edmonton	0.6 (0.16)	0.7 (0.25)	0.5 (0.21)	1.4	17.1 (1.12)	22
Puerto Rico	0.6 (0.23)	0.8 (0.38)	0.5 (0.27)	1.6	27.2 (3.40)	18
Munich[b]	0.5 (0.37)	N/A	1.0 (0.71)	N/A	29.0	25
Taiwan	0.3 (0.06)	0.3 (0.09)	0.3 (0.07)	1.0	22.5 (1.90)	22
Korea	0.4 (0.09)	0.6 (0.16)	0.2 (0.09)	3.0	23.0 (2.54)	18
Christchurch	1.5 (0.36)	1.7 (0.56)	1.2 (0.45)	1.4	18.2 (5.90)	N/A

Note: Encompasses ages 18–64 years unless otherwise noted.
N/A = not assessed.
[a]Ages 18–54 years.
[b]Ages 26–64 years. Only one case of bipolar disorder was reported.

TABLE 5–8. Lifetime Prevalence/100 (Standard Error)[a] of Suicide Attempts in Persons with and without Bipolar-I Disorder

Survey Site	Persons with Bipolar Disorder	Persons without Bipolar Disorder	Odds Ratio (95% CI)[b]	p Value
United States				
ECA, 1980	23.9 (4.70)	2.9 (0.18)	9.6 (5.6–16.6)	.0001
NCS, 1990[c,d]	40.5 (6.08)	4.2 (0.33)	15.8 (9.3–26.9)	.0001
Edmonton	44.5 (12.72)	3.6 (0.38)	25.7 (8.6–76.6)	.0001
Puerto Rico	24.5 (25.50)[e]	5.8 (0.67)	5.6 (1.0–29.8)	.04
Taiwan	11.8 (5.84)[e]	0.7 (0.08)	18.1 (5.8–57.0)	.0001
Korea	15.1 (8.40)[e]	3.1 (0.25)	5.5 (1.5–20.2)	.01
Christchurch	32.7 (11.69)	4.0 (0.59)	13.1 (4.2–41.1)	.0001

Note: Encompasses ages 18–64 years unless otherwise noted.
CI = confidence interval.
[a]Standardized to U.S. 1980 Census.
[b]Odds ratio adjusted by age and gender at each site.
[c]Ages 18–54 years.
[d]Weighted to 1989 National Health Interview Survey.
[e]Indicates cells with a frequency of 5 or less.

TABLE 5–9. Lifetime Prevalence/100 (Standard Error)[a] of Panic Disorder in Persons with and without Bipolar-I Disorder

Survey Site	Persons with Bipolar Disorder	Persons without Bipolar Disorder	Odds Ratio (95% CI)[b]	p Value
United States				
ECA, 1980	16.2 (4.09)	1.5 (0.13)	12.8 (6.8–24.1)	.0001
NCS, 1990[c,d]	27.0 (5.49)	3.1 (0.28)	12.5 (6.9–22.6)	.0001
Edmonton	16.7 (9.55)	1.3 (0.68)	16.5 (4.0–67.6)	.0001
Puerto Rico	49.6 (18.00)[e]	1.3 (0.33)	79.2 (17.3–323)	.0001
Taiwan	14.5 (6.36)[e]	0.3 (0.06)	53.5 (17.9–160)	.0001
Korea	9.0 (6.70)[e]	1.7 (0.19)	14.1 (2.6–77.3)	.002
Christchurch	20.6 (10.09)[e]	1.8 (0.40)	17.2 (4.3–69.1)	.0001

Note: Encompasses ages 18–64 years unless otherwise noted.
CI = confidence interval.
[a]Standardized to U.S. 1980 Census.
[b]Odds ratio adjusted by age and gender at each site.
[c]Ages 18–54 years.
[d]Weighted to 1989 National Health Interview Survey.
[e]Indicates cells with a frequency of 5 or less.

has also been noted in genetic studies showing an increased familial aggregation of panic disorder in probands with bipolar disorder (MacKinnon et al., 1998). The meaning of these results and whether they represent a specific genetic subtype are unclear (see Chapter 13).

Table 5–10 shows the significant association between substance abuse or dependence and bipolar disorder in all countries except Puerto Rico and New Zealand. These results suggest that cultural differences in substance abuse may explain some of the association (see Chapter 7).

Other International Studies

The data reported in the preceding section are from seven countries that used the DIS in their surveys and provided raw data for analyses. The NCS used the CIDI, not the DIS, but the raw data were available so that direct comparisons, with standardization for age and gender, could be made, thus reducing methodological differences as a source of variance in rates. Other well-designed epidemiologic studies have been conducted cross-nationally and published in the last decade; these studies have limitations for present purposes, however, in that they group all affective disorders together and do not present rates for bipolar disorder separately. Results of studies that do report on bipolar-I or bipolar-II disorder are presented separately from the results of the Cross-National Collaborative Group study in Table 5–11, even if the former studies used the same diagnostic measures, as they employed somewhat different methods for either data collection or analysis that could explain differences in the results. Because the raw data were not available, standardization for age and gender differences could not be performed. Therefore, only published rates are presented. A uniform presentation across sites as shown in Tables 5–7 through 5–10 is not possible.

Iceland

The Icelandic study was drawn from a case register and represented a birth cohort born in 1931 and residing in Iceland on December 1, 1986; 2,396 persons met these criteria. Among 1,195 persons randomly selected, 862 interviews (79 percent) were completed. DSM-III diagnoses were derived from DIS interviews administered by trained lay interviewers. The lifetime prevalence rates for bipolar-I (0.2 percent) and bipolar-II (0.5 percent) were low, with equal gender ratios (Stefansson et al., 1991). The sample of bipolar subjects was too small to permit interpretation of associations with marital status. The lower rates obtained in this study could be explained by the age of the cohort (about 56) at the time of the interview.

TABLE 5–10. Lifetime Prevalence/100 (Standard Error)[a] of Any Substance Abuse or Dependence (Alcohol or Drug) in Persons with and without Bipolar-I Disorder

Survey Site	Persons with Bipolar Disorder	Persons without Bipolar Disorder	Odds Ratio (95% CI)[b]	p Value
United States				
ECA, 1980	57.2 (5.51)	17.5 (0.41)	7.6 (4.7–12.1)	.0001
NCS, 1990[c,d]	58.2 (6.11)	23.4 (0.69)	5.0 (3.0–8.4)	.0001
Edmonton	60.0 (12.53)	20.1 (0.82)	6.4 (2.1–19.5)	.001
Puerto Rico	0.0	12.8 (1.00)	—	—
Taiwan	19.3 (7.13)	6.7 (0.25)	3.3 (1.2–9.0)	.02
Korea	54.8 (11.68)	22.8 (0.61)	4.6 (1.3–12.5)	.02
Christchurch	23.7 (10.60)	20.9 (1.23)	0.8 (0.9–2.8)	.77

Note: Encompasses ages 18–64 years unless otherwise noted.
CI = confidence interval.
[a]Standardized to U.S. 1980 Census.
[b]Odds ratio adjusted by age and gender at each site.
[c]Ages 18–54 years.
[d]Weighted to 1989 National Health Interview Survey.

Shantin (Hong Kong)

A large-scale community survey was conducted in Shantin using the DIS and DSM-III (Chen et al., 1993). A two-phase design yielded 7,229 respondents. A flagged sample was given the Self-Reporting Questionnaire (SRQ) as a screen and the full DIS. The DIS was administered only to respondents among an unflagged sample who were positive on one of the screens of the SRQ. With this design, the lifetime prevalence of bipolar disorder was very low, and similar for males (0.15 percent) and females (0.16 percent). These rates are slightly lower than those reported for the two Asian countries (Taiwan and Korea) in the Cross-National Collaborative Group study (see Table 5–7). Chen and colleagues (1993) suggested that the difference could be due to the location of their study; because Shantin was a new town attracting healthy workers, people with serious mental illnesses would not have relocated there.

Hungary

A national community study was conducted in Hungary to estimate the prevalence of affective disorders in the adult population aged 18 to 64, sampled from the registries of 15 general practitioners in five different geographic areas

(Szadoczky et al., 1998). In this study, 2,953 respondents were interviewed using the DIS. The lifetime prevalence for bipolar-I was 1.5/100, similar to the U.S. rate; for bipolar-II, the lifetime rate was 2.0/100. There were few differences in the rates by gender. The first symptoms were reported slightly earlier for females (at 17.9 years) than for males (at 22 years), and the highest risk for first onset of bipolar-I was at ages 15 to 19. Persons with bipolar disorder had a higher level of education, a higher rate of unemployment in males, and a higher rate of marital disruption or never being married compared with those without the disorder.

Florence, Italy

This study included a community sample of 1,000 people in Florence, Italy, drawn from the registries of general physicians (Faravelli et al., 1990). In contrast to the majority of the other epidemiological surveys, the interviews were carried out by qualified psychiatrists or third-year trainees. The annual prevalence for bipolar-I was 1.9/100 for females and 0.6/100 for males, for an overall prevalence of 1.3/100. These rates are again in the same range as the U.S. rates, except for higher rates in females. For bipolar-II disorder, the overall prevalence was 0.2/100. The high annual rates of bipolar disorder are similar to lifetime rates

TABLE 5–11. Prevalence/100 of Bipolar Disorder from Other Cross-National Community Surveys

Study	Country/Year	Sample Size	Age Range (Years)	Diagnostic Method	Diagnosis	Time Period	Prevalence/100
Angst et al., 1984	Zurich, Switzerland, 1978–1982	4,547	19–20	SPIKE	BP-I	Annual	0.7
Faravelli et al., 1990	Florence, Italy, 1987	1,000	15–89	DIS	BP-I BP-II	Annual Annual	1.3 0.2
Stefansson et al., 1991	Iceland, 1987	862	Cohort born in 1931	DIS	BP-I BP-II	Lifetime Lifetime	0.2 0.5
Chen et al., 1993	Shantin, Hong Kong, 1984–1986	7,229	18–64	DIS	BP I or II	Lifetime	Males, 0.15; females, 0.16
Levav et al., 1993	Israel, 1987	2,741	24–33	SADS	BP-I BP-II	6 months	0.7 0.9
Brewin et al., 1997	Nottingham, England, 1992–1994	397,048[a]	16–64	SCAN, SANS	BP	2-year incidence	0.005
Szadoczky et al., 1998	Hungary, 1998	2,953	18–64	DIS	BP-I BP-II	Lifetime Lifetime	1.5 2.0
Scully et al., 2000	Ireland, 1995–2000	29,542	Not stated	SCID-III-R	BP	Annual incidence	0.0022: males, 0.00037; females, 0.00060
Kringlen et al., 2001	Oslo, Norway, 1994–1997	2,066	18–65	CIDI	BP	Lifetime Annual	1.6 0.9
Andrade et al., 2002	São Paulo, Brazil, 1994–1996	1,464	18+	CIDI	BP	Lifetime Annual Annual incidence	1.0 0.5 0.3
Regeer et al., 2002	Netherlands, 1996–1999	7,067	18–64	CIDI	BP-I BP-NOS	Lifetime	2.0
Mitchell et al., 2004	Australia	10,641	18+	CIDI	BP[b]	Annual	0.5
Negash et al., 2005	Butajira, Ethiopia	68,378	15–49	CIDI	BP-I	Lifetime	0.5: males, 0.6; females, 0.3
Vicente et al., 2006	Chile	2,978	15+	CIDI	BP-I	Lifetime	1.9: males, 1.5; females, 2.2

BP = bipolar; BP-NOS = bipolar disorder–not otherwise specified; CIDI = Composite International Diagnostic Interview; DIS = Diagnostic Interview Schedule; SANS = Schedule for Assessment of Negative Symptoms; SCAN = Schedules for Clinical Assessment in Neuropsychiatry; SCID = Structured Clinical Interview for DSM; SPIKE = Structured Psychopathological Interview and Rating of the Social Consequences of Psychiatric Disturbances for Epidemiology.

[a] Population at risk from 1991 Nottingham population census.
[b] Euphoric type.

reported in other studies, a result that may be attributable to having the interviews conducted by psychiatrists, who were better able to probe for symptoms of mania. Also, this study assessed only mood disorders; therefore, the results may include other disorders with mood disturbance. The low rate of bipolar-II disorder found in this study again suggests the difficulty of discriminating between mild mood disorders and normal mood in a community survey. This was also the only epidemiologic study to report rates of recurrent depression (annual prevalence 2.6 percent).

Israel

In an epidemiologic study of mental disorders among young adults in Israel, a 10-year birth cohort (1949–1958) was interviewed by psychiatrists using the Israeli version of SADS, based on RDC criteria. A two-stage screening process was used. Subjects scoring positive on the screen (about a fifth of the sample) received the full diagnostic interview by a psychiatrist. The screened positive sample included 2,741 Israeli-born offspring of Jewish immigrants. The 6-month prevalence was 0.7 percent for bipolar-I disorder and 0.9 percent for bipolar-II disorder. Annual or lifetime prevalence rates were not reported. The rates did not vary significantly by gender. The 6-month prevalence of *definite* bipolar-I disorder was higher among Israelis of European ethnicity (0.61) compared with Israelis of North African ethnicity (0.15, $p < .05$) (Levav et al., 1993). There were no significant differences by education.

Zurich, Switzerland

Subjects for the Zurich Cohort Study were drawn from the total population of the canton of Zurich. The sample was the result of a two-stage design that selected subjects at high risk for psychiatric disorders and applied random controls for 4,547 subjects at the ages of about 19 (males) and 20 (females). Reassessments were conducted when the subjects were about 22, 27, 29, and 34 years of age. Screening took place in 1978, the first and second interviews were conducted in 1979 and 1981, and the last (fifth) interview was conducted in 1993. Each interview covered the previous 12 months. Symptomatology was assessed using SPIKE (Angst et al., 1984), administered by trained clinical psychologists in the subjects' homes. SPIKE is a semistructured clinical interview, which, as noted earlier, allows the assessment of 29 separate syndromes, including hypomania, in terms of symptoms, their length, their frequency of occurrence, subjective suffering, social consequence, treatment, and family history.

The 1-year prevalence of bipolar-I disorder was 0.7 percent (Angst et al., 1984). The study identified brief hypomania (recurrent and sporadic), a condition characterized by short episodes of 1 to 3 days' duration and high recurrence, as a new diagnostic group with a 1-year prevalence rate (cumulative) of 2.8 percent (see later discussion).

The lifetime prevalence of bipolar spectrum disorder, which included a full range of manic symptoms (see the later discussion of bipolar spectrum) was 5.5 percent (Angst, 1995). Overall, the study demonstrated the high prevalence rates of DSM-IV hypomania and brief hypomania among the general population and the clinical and social relevance of these diagnoses. Because this was a prospective study with five waves of interviews focusing on rates from the previous year, it may have been more successful than other studies at identifying fluctuating hypomanic episodes. There have been no other epidemiologic studies of comparable design.

Ireland

A prospective study in rural Ireland of 29,542 subjects from 39 electoral districts was initiated in 1995–2000 to assess all *first episodes* of bipolar disorder. The SCID-III-R (Spitzer et al., 1992) and DSM-III-R were used. As of 2002, the annual incidence of bipolar-I for women was 0.0006 and for men was 0.00037; the overall incidence was 0.0022.[5]

Nottingham, England

This study estimated the incidence rate of ICD manic psychosis in first referrals to general adult psychiatric clinics over the 2-year period 1992–1994. It differs from the others reviewed here in that it was not community based. Therefore, patients who did not present for treatment—most likely milder cases—were not included (Brewin et al., 1997). New patients were evaluated with the Schedule for Clinical Assessment in Neuropsychiatry (SCAN) (WHO, 1994) and the Schedule for Assessment of Negative Symptoms (SANS) (Andreasen, 1982). Using the 1991 Nottingham population census as the population at risk (denominator) and new referrals meeting the ICD criteria for manic psychosis as the case (numerator), the incidence rate was 0.005, with a slightly higher rate among females (Brewin et al., 1997).

Norway

A sample of 2,066 subjects aged 18 to 65, randomly selected from the Norwegian National Population Registry, was interviewed with the CIDI between 1994 and 1997 (Kringlen et al., 2001). The overall annual prevalence of bipolar disorder was 0.9 percent (0.8 percent for males and 1.0 percent for females). The overall lifetime prevalence for bipolar disorder was 1.6 percent, with little difference by gender (1.7 percent for males and 1.4 percent for females). These rates are close to those found in the NCS, which also used the CIDI.

The Netherlands

A prospective survey of 7,067 subjects aged 18 to 64 years from the Dutch general population was conducted at three points in time between 1996 and 1999, using the CIDI (de Graaf et al., 2002; Regeer et al., 2002). Summing of the responses at the three points yielded a lifetime prevalence for bipolar-I or bipolar-NOS of 2.4 percent. A clinical reappraisal, blind to the original diagnosis, was conducted by trained clinicians using the SCID. The results led to a reduction of the rate to 2.0 percent. The annual incidence was 0.3 and was higher in females than in males, but these rates are based on small numbers (Bijl et al., 2002).

São Paulo, Brazil

A community survey of a sample of 1,464 adults living in one catchment area of a large hospital complex in São Paulo was conducted using the CIDI (Andrade et al., 2002). The lifetime and annual rates of bipolar disorder were 1.0 and 0.5, respectively. The rates among men and women were similar. Data on the association with other demographic characteristics were not presented for bipolar disorder separately from other mood disorders.

Chile

The CIDI was administered to a stratified random sample of 2,978 individuals from four provinces representative of Chile's population aged 15 and above (Vicente et al., 2006). The lifetime and annual rates of manic disorder were 1.9 and 1.4, respectively. Lifetime rates were higher in women (2.2) than in men (1.5).

Bipolar Spectrum

The rates of bipolar disorder reported above may be underestimates because many subjects who have brief recurrent hypomanic episodes may not be captured in surveys (see Chapters 2 and 3). Moreover, there is controversy about what symptoms should be included in the full spectrum of bipolar disorder. Some epidemiologic data on the spectrum that include hypomanic episodes are now available.

The relatively low reported rates of hypomania noted in previous surveys may be due to the fact that hypomania is frequently unrecognized by subjects themselves as a pathological condition. However, there may be a wide bipolar spectrum in clinical samples (Angst, 1998). The bipolar spectrum includes mania, hypomania, recurrent brief hypomania, sporadic brief hypomania, and cyclothymia. Modern concepts of bipolar disorder are still developing and can include bipolar-I and -II, hypomania, cyclothymia, mania with depression, and depression with hypomania, as well as highly recurrently major depression.[6] Six subtypes of bipolar disorder were described by Klerman (1981): (1) mania, (2) hypomania, (3) hypomania or mania precipitated by drugs, (4) cyclothymic personality, (5) depression with a familial history of bipolar disorder, and (6) mania without depression. The concept of "soft" bipolar spectrum (Akiskal, 1996) includes Klerman's subtypes 3 through 6, as well as recurrent depression without spontaneous hypomania but with hyperthymic temperament (Angst, 1998). Epidemiologic studies have found lifetime prevalence rates for certain segments of the bipolar spectrum that range from 3.0 to 8.3 percent (Table 5–12). The further the spectrum is extended, however, the lower is the diagnostic reliability.

In this context, longitudinal epidemiologic studies of young adults to determine instances of subtle onset of symptoms could provide data for use in testing the hypothesis of a bipolar spectrum. However, almost all epidemiologic studies are cross-sectional. One attempt to study the spectrum was the longitudinal study of Angst (1998), discussed previously. In that study, the cumulative prevalence (based on four interviews over 12 years) for DSM-IV hypomania/mania was 5.5 percent. Brief (recurrent or sporadic) hypomania had a prevalence of 2.8 percent. Therefore, the inclusion of brief hypomania raised the Zurich rate for bipolar spectrum to 8.3 percent (Akiskal 2000). All of the subgroups in this study—those that met the DSM-IV criteria for hypomania and those with sporadic or brief recurrent hypomania—had similar symptom profiles and a family history of depression (Angst, 1998). Angst recommended that the bipolar spectrum be broadened to include brief hypomania in light of its high prevalence and clinical relevance.

The largest study of bipolar spectrum disorder included more than 85,000 adults in the United States and used the Mood Disorder Questionnaire (MDQ), a screening instrument of uncertain reliability. This study found a rate of bipolar spectrum of 3.7 percent. The relationship between data on bipolar spectrum obtained from a screening questionnaire and from a full diagnostic interview is unclear, however (Hirschfeld et al., 2001, 2003a,b; see Chapter 11).

The recent NCS-R found a lifetime prevalence of bipolar spectrum of 4.4 percent: 1.4 percent for bipolar-I, 1.6 percent for bipolar-II, and 1.4 percent for bipolar subthreshold (defined as those individuals who have euphoria or irritability plus two other symptoms for 4 days or longer with at least mild impairment and a history of major depression). Males were more likely to be diagnosed with subthreshold bipolar disorder than were females (1.7 and 1.0 percent, respectively) (Kessler et al., 2006).

Bipolar spectrum is an ambiguous classification and includes subtypes that are subtle and difficult to diagnose. There is general agreement, however, that bipolar disorder encompasses a broad spectrum and that clinically

TABLE 5–12. Lifetime Prevalence/100 of Bipolar Spectrum Disorder

Study	Country	Age Range (Years)	Diagnostic Method	Time Period	Prevalence/100
Oliver and Simmons, 1985	United States	15+	DIS	Lifetime	3.3
Faravelli and Incerpi, 1985	Italy	15–89	DIS	Annual	3.4
Szadoczky et al., 1998	Hungary	18–64	CIDI	Lifetime	5.1
Weissman and Meyers, 1978	United States	18–64	SADS-L	Lifetime	3.0
Heun and Maier, 1993	Germany	20–60	SADS-L	Lifetime	6.5
Levav et al., 1993	Israel	24–33	SADS-L	6-month	2.6
Angst, 1998	Switzerland	19–35	SPIKE	Lifetime	5.5[a]
Hirschfeld et al., 2002	United States	18+	MDQ	Lifetime	3.7
Judd and Akiskal, 2003	United States	18+	DIS	Lifetime	6.4
Moreno and Andrade, 2005	Brazil	18+	CIDI	Lifetime	8.3
Kessler et al., 2006	United States	18+	CIDI	Lifetime	4.4
Faravelli et al., 2006	Italy	14+	MINI	Lifetime	5.5

CIDI = Composite International Diagnostic Interview; DIS = Diagnostic Interview Schedule; MDQ = Mood Disorder Questionnaire; MINI = Mini International Neuropsychiatric Interview; SADS-L = Schedule for Affective Disorders and Schizophrenia-Lifetime; SPIKE = Structured Psychopathological Interview and Rating of the Social Consequences of Psychiatric Disturbances for Epidemiology.

[a]8.3 if brief hypomania is included.

significant cases within that spectrum are not captured in epidemiologic or even clinical studies.

COMMUNITY SURVEYS WITH CHILDREN AND ADOLESCENTS

As discussed earlier, the onset and clinical presentation of bipolar disorder in children and adolescents are less clear than in adults (see also Chapter 6). Moreover, there is considerable controversy about clinical presentation in children (Geller et al., 2002; Lewinsohn et al., 2003; Biederman et al., 2004). In particular, there is controversy as to whether hyperactive, inattentive children with emotional lability represent early presentations of mania or ADHD. Biederman (1995), Farone and colleagues (1997), Geller and colleagues (1998), and Wozniak and colleagues (1995) examined ADHD uncomplicated by any other psychiatric disorder in an effort to understand the possible symptomatology of childhood mania. Biederman and colleagues (1995) found that 96 percent of children referred with symptoms of mania fulfilled criteria for a diagnosis of ADHD; however, only 16 percent of the children referred with symptoms of ADHD met the criteria for mania. The diagnosis of bipolar disorder in pediatric populations is complicated by insufficient information on the clinical development of childhood symptomatology into adulthood; a clinical bias against a diagnosis of mania in childhood (Carlson, 1996), similar to the bias seen 20 years ago against the diagnosis of depression in children (Angold, 1988); and overlap of symptomatology between bipolar

disorder and other, more prevalent childhood psychiatric illnesses (ADHD and conduct disorder) (see Chapter 6).

Compared with the gender distribution in adulthood, reports of mania in childhood based on clinical and epidemiologic studies suggest that prepubertal onset of mania may be more frequent in boys than in girls (Varanka et al., 1988; Geller et al., 1998). The incidence of mania appears to increase after the onset of puberty, and the prevalence of mania during late adolescence is estimated to approximate that in adulthood.[7]

Table 5–13 presents the prevalence rates of bipolar disorder from community-based epidemiologic studies of adolescents. Only the MECA study included children; all of the other studies included only adolescent samples. The table demonstrates the paucity of data in this area. Note that the considerable variation in age ranges included in the different studies affects the rates derived and accounts for discrepancies shown in the table.

Results of both the NCS and the MECA study are on public-use tapes, making it possible to undertake the analyses presented here. The NCS, as described previously, included subjects aged 15 to 54. In that study, the lifetime rate for bipolar-I was 1.3/100 among 468 adolescents aged 15 to 17.

The MECA study was conducted among a population-based sample of children and adolescents (see Table 5–13). As noted, this is the only published epidemiologic study to include children; however, the sample was too small to be divided by age, and pubertal status was not obtained. Probability household samples of 1,285 youths aged 9 to 17 were selected at four sites (Atlanta, Georgia; New Haven,

TABLE 5–13. Prevalence/100 of Bipolar Disorder from Studies in Adolescents

Study	Country (Year)	Sample Size	Age Range (Years)	Diagnostic Method	Diagnosis	Time Period	Prevalence/100
NCS, unpublished	United States (1992)	468	15–17	CIDI	BP-I	Lifetime	1.4
MECA, unpublished	United States (1992)	1,285	9–17	DISC	Mania	6-month	1.2
					Hypomania	6-month	0.6
Lewinsohn et al., 1995	Western Oregon (1987)	1,709	14–18	KSADS/LIFE	BP	Lifetime	1.0
Wittchen et al., 1998	Bavaria, Germany (1988)	3,021	14–24	CIDI	BP-I	Annual	1.4
						Lifetime	0.4
					BP-II	Annual	0.4
						Lifetime	0.4
Aalto-Setälä et al., 2001	Helsinki, Finland (2000)	647	Follow-up of high school students, 20–24	SCAN	BP-I	1-month	0.2
					BP-II	1-month	0.5
					BP-NOS	1-month	0.2

Note: Only the MECA study included children.

BP = bipolar; BP-NOS = bipolar disorder–not otherwise specified; CIDI = Composite International Diagnostic Interview; DISC = Diagnostic Interview Schedule for Children; KSADS = Kiddie Schedule for Affective Disorders and Schizophrenia; LIFE = Longitudinal Interval Follow-up Evaluation; MECA = Methods for the Epidemiology of Child and Adolescent Mental Disorder; NCS = National Comorbidity Study; SCAN = Schedules for Clinical Assessment in Neuropsychiatry.

Connecticut; Westchester County, New York; and Puerto Rico). Lay interviewers administered a computer-assisted version of the NIMH Diagnostic Interview Schedule for Children (DISC) 2.3 and structured interviews to assess demographic variables, functional impairment, risk factors, service utilization, and barriers to service utilization (Lahey et al., 1996). Data were collected from both children and their parents. A clinician interviewer, again using DISC 2.3, reassessed 247 of these parent–child pairs 1 to 3 weeks later. The test-retest reliability of the interviews with the parents was generally good for most diagnoses but less satisfactory for the interviews with the children. The current (6-month) prevalence for mania was 1.2/100 and for hypomania was 0.6/100 (unpublished data). Annual rates were not available.

Gould and colleagues (1998) examined the relationships among suicidal ideation, suicide attempts, and mania in the MECA study. They found that 4.5 percent of youths having had suicidal ideation and 7.1 percent of those having made a suicide attempt had experienced manic symptoms, compared with 0.9 percent of those who had neither had suicidal ideation nor made an attempt. The comparison of these two groups was statistically significant. There were 16 children with mania—3 with suicidal ideation (18.7 percent), 3 who had made a suicide attempt (18.7 percent), and 10 who had neither had suicidal ideation nor

made an attempt (62.5 percent; $p < .005$ ideation versus none; $p < .001$ attempt versus none).

A community sample of 1,709 adolescents (aged 14 to 18 years) was randomly selected from nine senior high schools representative of urban and rural districts in western Oregon (Lewinsohn et al., 1995). The adolescents were interviewed initially between 1987 and 1989 using KSADS (with combined features of the epidemiologic and present state versions). Parents were not interviewed. At approximately 1 year, a follow-up interview (the Longitudinal Interval Follow-up Evaluation [LIFE]; Keller et al., 1987) and KSADS were administered to determine the presence of psychiatric disorders since the initial interview. The lifetime prevalence of bipolar disorder (primarily bipolar-II and cyclothymia) was approximately 1.0 percent. An additional 5.7 percent of the sample (termed "core positive subjects") reported experiencing a distinct period of abnormally elevated, expansive, and/or irritable mood, although they never met the criteria for bipolar disorder per se. Both bipolar and "core positive" patients exhibited significant functional impairment and high rates of comorbidity (anxiety and disruptive behavior), suicide attempts, and use of mental health services. The prevalence, age at onset, phenomenology, and course of bipolar disorder in adolescents were similar for both males and females.

To examine the course of adolescent depression, a follow-up was conducted to compare the rates of mood and other mental disorders between ages 19 and 24 for adolescents with a history of depression and those with adolescent adjustment disorder with depressed mood, those with nonaffective disorders, and those with no disorder. The study participants were followed-up again when they reached age 24. The follow-up sample (739 subjects) had low rates of dysthymia and bipolar disorder (less than 1 percent). In accord with other results, a small percentage (0.9 percent) of children and adolescents with major depression had experienced manic/hypomanic episodes.[8]

The same community sample in Oregon was used to compare the incidence and prevalence of bipolar disorder among adolescents and young adults, to explore the stability and consequences of adolescent bipolar disorder in young adulthood, to determine the rate of transition from depression to bipolar disorder, and to evaluate the significance of subsyndromal bipolar disorder (SUB) (Lewinsohn et al., 1995). The results show a lifetime prevalence of bipolar disorder of approximately 1.0 percent during adolescence and 2.0 percent during young adulthood. Lifetime prevalence of SUB was approximately 5.0 percent. Fewer than 1.0 percent of adolescents with depression had converted to bipolar disorder by age 24 (Lewinsohn et al., 2000). The bipolar disorder and SUB subgroups both had elevated rates of antisocial and other personality disorder symptoms. Both showed significant impairment in psychosocial functioning and had made greater use of mental health services. In general, adolescents with bipolar disorder showed significant continuity across developmental periods and had adverse outcomes during young adulthood. Adolescent SUB was also associated with adverse outcomes in adulthood, but not with increased incidence of bipolar disorder, a finding that questions the validity of the SUB diagnoses.

A study conducted in Bavaria, Germany, among a sample of 3,021 adolescents and young adults aged 14 to 24 using the CIDI and DSM-IV revealed a lifetime prevalence of 1.4/100 for bipolar-I and 0.4/100 for bipolar-II (Wittchen et al., 1998a). The annual rates were 1.3/100 and 0.4/100, respectively. The version of the CIDI used in this study also included questions about disabilities and impairment, operationalized as the assessment of economic, social, and leisure impairment during the worst episode and 1 month before the interview. Among those youths with any bipolar disorder, 94 percent considered themselves very impaired.

A 5-year follow-up of 647 high school students aged 20 to 24 in Helsinki, Finland, found 1-month prevalence rates of 0.2 percent for bipolar-I, 0.5 percent for bipolar-II, and 0.2 percent for bipolar-NOS, with a total rate of bipolar disorder of 0.9 percent (Aalto-Setälä et al., 2001). Given

that these rates are monthly, they do not diverge greatly from the annual rates reported in Germany among a similar age group.

GLOBAL BURDEN OF DISEASE STUDIES

In recent decades the patterns of disease and mortality in developing countries have grown to resemble those of high-income countries, with a preponderance of burden resulting from chronic diseases. To quantify these changes the World Bank, in collaboration with WHO, undertook a systematic assessment of the global burden of disease (GBD) in 1990 (World Bank, 1993b; Murray et al., 1994; Murray and Lopez, 1996). The burden of disease was measured in disability-adjusted life years (DALYs), which are the sum of life years lost to premature mortality (YLL) and life years lost to disability (YLD). The 1990 GBD assessment confirmed a major epidemiological transition resulting from both decreasing birth rates and decreasing rates of death from communicable diseases. As the birth rate of a population drops, the number of adults increases relative to the number of children, and a greater proportion of health care resources is accordingly focused on adults. Then, as fatalities from acute diseases become increasingly preventable, and public health and medicine achieve growing success in controlling and stabilizing the effects of such chronic diseases as cancer, cardiovascular conditions, and AIDS, people live longer with the disabling effects of their illness. The disability from disease results in the inability to work or carry out daily activities of living.

A major assessment of the global burden of disease and risk factors, updated to 2001, has recently been published (Lopez et al., 2006). Self-inflicted injuries, overwhelmingly attributable to psychiatric illnesses—especially unipolar and bipolar disorders—are the sixth leading cause of death in adults 15–59 in low and middle-income countries and the second in high-income countries (Table 5–14). Unipolar depression ranks first in disability in both low and middle-income and high-income countries (Table 5–15).

Questions have been raised about the severity weights for mental disorders used in the GBD study and whether the weights for depression and substance abuse may have been overestimated (Andrews et al., 1998; Vos and Mathers, 2000). In a study from the Netherlands in which the burden of disease in 1994 in terms of DALYs was estimated by using data from Dutch vital statistics, registries, and surveys with Dutch disability weights, depression ranked eighth, accounting for 112,800 DALYs in that year. This figure represented 4.4 percent of the DALYs for all diseases, compared with a figure of 3.7 percent in established market economy populations from the GBD study (Melse et al., 2000).

TABLE 5–14. **The 10 Leading Causes of Death in Adults Ages 15–59, by Broad Income Group, 2001**

	LOW- AND MIDDLE-INCOME COUNTRIES				HIGH-INCOME COUNTRIES		
	Cause	Deaths (millions)	Percentage of total deaths		Cause	Deaths (millions)	Percentage of total deaths
1	HIV/AIDS	2.05	14.1	1	Ischemic heart disease	0.13	10.8
2	Ischemic heart disease	1.18	8.1	2	Self-inflicted injuries	0.09	7.2
3	Tuberculosis	1.03	7.1	3	Road traffic accidents	0.08	6.9
4	Road traffic accidents	0.73	5.0	4	Trachea, bronchus, and lung cancers	0.08	6.8
5	Cerebrovascular disease	0.71	4.9	5	Cerebrovascular disease	0.05	4.4
6	Self-inflicted injuries	0.58	4.0	6	Cirrhosis of the liver	0.05	4.4
7	Violence	0.45	3.1	7	Breast cancer	0.05	4.0
8	Lower respiratory infections	0.33	2.3	8	Colon and rectal cancers	0.04	3.1
9	Cirrhosis of the liver	0.32	2.2	9	Diabetes mellitus	0.03	2.1
10	Chronic obstructive pulmonary disease	0.32	2.2	10	Stomach cancer	0.02	2.0

Source: Mathers et al., 2006.

TABLE 5–15. **The 10 Leading Causes of Disability (Years Lived with Disability) by Broad Income Group, 2001**

LOW- AND MIDDLE-INCOME COUNTRIES			HIGH-INCOME COUNTRIES		
Cause	YLD (millions of years)	Percentage of total YLD	Cause	YLD (millions of years)	Percentage of total YLD
1 Unipolar depressive disorders	43.22	9.1	1 Unipolar depressive disorders	8.39	11.8
2 Cataracts	28.15	5.9	2 Alzheimer's and other dementias	6.33	8.9
3 Hearing loss, adult onset	24.61	5.2	3 Hearing loss, adult onset	5.39	7.6
4 Vision disorders, age-related	15.36	3.2	4 Alcohol use disorders	3.77	5.3
5 Osteoarthritis	13.65	2.9	5 Osteoarthritis	3.77	5.3
6 Perinatal conditions	13.52	2.8	6 Cerebrovascular disease	3.46	4.9
7 Cerebrovascular disease	11.10	2.3	7 Chronic obstructive pulmonary disease	2.86	4.0
8 Schizophrenia	10.15	2.1	8 Diabetes mellitus	2.25	3.2
9 Alcohol use disorders	9.81	2.1	9 Endocrine disorders	1.68	2.4
10 Protein-energy malnutrition	9.34	2.0	10 Vision disorders, age-related	1.53	2.1

Source: Mathers et al., 2006.

In a study from Victoria, Australia, rates of bipolar disorder were estimated from published studies by applying the Dutch disability weights (Vos and Mathers, 2000). The DALYs rates for depression were 7.7 for females and 5.3 for males, and those for bipolar disorder were 1.3 for females and 1.4 for males. These rates were lower than those for the established market economies in the WHO study—for depression, 10.7 for females and 6.0 for males, and for bipolar disorder, 2.1 for females and 2.2 for males. The burden of major depression was found to be higher for females than for males, but that of bipolar disorder did not differ by gender (Vos and Mathers, 2000), as determined from the gender ratios in the tables presented earlier.

Psychiatric disorders are expected to represent a greater global share of the disability burden than cardiovascular disease by 2020 (Murray and Lopez, 2000). Indeed, the results of the World Bank Development Study and the Murray and Lopez report caught the attention of the administration of WHO and helped spur the initiation of the World Mental Health Study, 2000, which is described next.

World Mental Health Study, 2000

The beginning of a new generation of cross-national studies of mental disorders was marked by a study in 2000 by the WHO International Consortium of Psychiatric Epidemiology (ICPE), which encompassed countries and geographic areas not included in previous cross-national studies.[9] The first prevalence rates, based on use of the CIDI to generate DSM–IV diagnoses, were from a sample of 29,644 persons participating in population surveys in North America (Canada and the United States [the NCS]), Latin America (Brazil and Mexico), and Europe (Germany, the Netherlands, and Turkey). Although the rates for bipolar disorder were not presented separately, the lifetime rates of any mood disorder (depression, dysthymia, and/or mania) are as follows: Turkey, 7.3 percent; Mexico, 9.2 percent; Canada, 10.2 percent; Brazil, 15.5 percent; Germany, 17.1 percent; the Netherlands, 18.9 percent; and the United States (the NCS), 19.4 percent. These, the first estimates from the consortium, show that mood disorders are highly prevalent throughout the world.

Additional surveys are to be conducted by the consortium in Mexico, Colombia, France, Italy, Belgium, the Ukraine, South Africa, Indonesia, China, and New Zealand and may include an adolescent sample. Data from the ICPE on individual mood disorders, including mania and disorder subtypes, are forthcoming (R.C. Kessler, Department of Health Care Policy, Harvard Medical School, personal communication, 2002). These data will encompass bipolar disorder and bipolar spectrum, as well as impairment, course, and current symptoms. Reappraisals of clinical data are also under way.

ASSOCIATED FEATURES

In this section, we summarize what is known about the correlates of bipolar disorder. These variables are often called "risk factors," but to avoid possible causal implications, we use instead the term "associated features." Some of this information has been presented earlier (e.g., in our review of cross-national studies or variation in rates by marital status or age), and some is discussed in detail in other chapters. Here we summarize that material, along with other information available from analytical epidemiologic studies. Analysis of data on associated features from community surveys is problematic except for such broad factors as age and gender because large samples are necessary for a disorder of relatively low prevalence. Therefore, few community-based epidemiologic studies of bipolar disorder are able to examine associated features beyond age, age at onset, and gender.

Temporal Variations

Gershon and colleagues (1987) observed birth cohort changes in mania among relatives of bipolar and schizoaffective patients. Using life table analysis, they found higher rates of bipolar disorder among those cohorts born after the 1940s, suggesting that the cumulative hazard for the disorder in a given age group is greater in those born after that decade. Gershon and colleagues (1987) concluded that cohorts with the highest rates of affective illness appear to have been born in the decades after World War II (these findings are the same for bipolar and major depressive disorders).

Somewhat similar findings were derived independently in the ECA (Lasch et al., 1990). Respondents were divided into eight birth cohorts, each spanning a 10-year interval. Actuarial life table analysis showed variations in the risk of mania by birth cohort, with the greatest risk seen among the post-1935 cohorts.

Various explanations have been proposed to account for these results (Klerman and Weissman, 1989). The temporal variations noted could be due to differential mortality and institutionalization, which could have removed older persons and earlier birth cohorts from the source populations, while changes in diagnostic criteria and the inclusion of persons with milder forms of bipolar disorder could have increased the rates in cohorts born after 1935. The onset of the "antidepressant era" in the early 1960s and the subsequent 10-fold increase in the use of this class of drugs, beginning with the appearance of "second-generation" antidepressants in the 1990s, may well have played a significant role. Dietary changes (including lower (compared with breast milk) concentrations of omega-3 fatty acids in infant formulas, discussed later, and younger age at first alcohol or drug use) and increased smoking in women must also be considered. It may be noted that there is some consensus that higher rates of bipolar disorder in the 1990 NCS compared with the 1980 ECA are due to methodological differences, as discussed earlier, rather than to temporal variations. Recall, memory, and a general reporting bias may also have contributed to the observed temporal variations in mania—specifically, a decline in the memory of lifetime events among the elderly or a conscious effort not to report them.

Gender

Mood disorders as a group are consistently more prevalent among women than men, but the difference is due to the higher prevalence of unipolar major depression in women. When only subjects with bipolar disorder are considered, nearly equal gender ratios have been found across most but not all national and cross-national studies, as reported earlier. Variations in one direction or another are likely due to the instability of small samples.

Social Class

In the first edition of this text, we reviewed more than 30 early studies of the association between social class and manic-depressive illness published between 1913 and 1989. We discussed in detail the considerable methodological problems involved in virtually every one of the studies but were impressed, nonetheless, by the overall association between bipolar illness and one or more measures reflecting upper social class.[10] The complexities are many, of course. We discuss in Chapter 12 the possible links among creativity, educational and occupational achievement, and certain behavioral, temperamental, cognitive, and behavioral characteristics associated with bipolar illness. Education and occupational achievement are, of course, associated with higher social class. It is also possible that characteristics associated with mild manic states, such as increased energy, risk-taking sexual drive, productivity, and social outgoingness, make some individuals more attractive and therefore, on occasion, more likely to marry into a higher social class.

More recent epidemiologic data show an equal distribution of the disorder among all social classes and educational levels. While bipolar illness in a small minority of patients may facilitate achievement and may aid the creative process (see Chapter 12), it is likely that most of the earlier association between bipolar disorder and higher social class had to do with diagnostic practices and inaccuracies in the concept. Upper- and middle-class people were more likely to be diagnosed as bipolar, whereas lower-class individuals, especially the urban poor, were (and still are) more likely to be diagnosed as schizophrenic (often mistakenly so) and consequently treated as such. Criteria for social class also varied widely across studies. Nonetheless, these investigations remain interesting for their span over many decades, their historical significance, and their great range across countries and cultures.

Most newer studies have failed to find a significantly lower than expected rate of bipolar disorder associated with indices of upper social class (educational status, occupation, economic status, or parental social class). In both the ECA and the NCS, lower educational level was not found to be associated with an increased risk of bipolar disorder. The NCS found an association between rates of bipolar illness and lower family income; it is unclear, however, whether the latter is a direct consequence of the illness or a trigger for its onset. Abood and colleagues (2002) examined 90 patients with bipolar-I disorder from a publicly financed service in Dublin to assess the association of the disorder with social advantage. Although not a representative sample, when compared with other psychiatric patients, excluding those with schizophrenia, the bipolar patients had similar demographic and socioeconomic characteristics (including more frequent residential moves).

On the other hand, a sample of 130 patients meeting DSM-III-R criteria for bipolar disorder and depression were compared on their and their relatives' occupational levels (Verdoux and Bourgeois, 1995). Occupational level did not differ significantly between unipolar and bipolar probands, although higher levels predominated among bipolar probands' brothers and children. A comparison of entire groups including probands and all their relatives revealed a social advantage for the relatives of bipolar patients. These results are consistent with the downward-drift hypothesis of bipolar disorder, which suggests that if there is any social advantage among bipolar patients, it may be reflected in the higher social class of their relatives. The devastation of the illness may erase these advantages and result in the association between the disorder and lower income seen in the NCS or the increased rates among the homeless discussed later. Consistent with this hypothesis is a recent study (Tsuchiya et al., 2004) finding that higher

parental educational level and greater parental wealth were associated with an elevated risk for bipolar disorder, but that the patients themselves were more likely to be unemployed and less well educated. The authors concluded that socioeconomic status may deteriorate as a result of the negative consequences of the disease (as described in Chapter 4). It may also be that milder forms of the illness on occasion lead to high achievement, but that the illness expressed in offspring of successful individuals is of a more severe nature (see Chapter 13, in particular the discussion of the phenomenon of anticipation).

Race/Ethnicity and Cultural Differences

A number of studies have examined racial similarities and differences in the prevalence and incidence of bipolar illness. Many factors apart from the previously discussed sources of variance cloud the accurate determination of these rates, including inadequate sampling from different socioeconomic groups, cultural differences and consequent problems regarding presentation, the misdiagnosis of schizophrenia noted earlier, and possible racial insensitivity among early researchers. These factors must be accounted for in such analyses.

Lewis and Hubbard (1931), Faris and Dunham (1939), Helzer (1975), and Weissman and Myers (1978) found equal rates of diagnosis of bipolar illness among African Americans and Caucasians. Likewise, the ECA revealed no significant difference in the prevalence or incidence of bipolar disorder among races (Robins and Regier, 1991). The NCS, on the other hand, indicated that African Americans had significantly lower rates of mania than Caucasians (Kessler et al., 1994). There is also some evidence that African Caribbean and African individuals are less likely to have experienced a depressive episode before the onset of first mania, and more likely to have more severe psychotic symptoms during their first mania, relative to Caucasian Europeans (Kennedy et al., 2004). In the study of the Cross-National Collaborative Group, the rates among the two Asian samples (Taiwan and Korea) and the Hispanic sample (Puerto Rico) were compared with those among the primarily Caucasian samples from Edmonton, Canada; West Germany; and Christchurch, New Zealand. The Asian samples clearly showed the lowest rates of bipolar disorder, but these rates were still within the same general range as those of the other sites. Moreover, the Asian sites (Taiwan, Korea, Hong Kong) generally showed the lowest rates for all psychiatric disorders.

In general, the newer epidemiologic data are consistent with the results of earlier studies in indicating no strong association between race/ethnicity and bipolar illness, with the possible exception of the unexplained lower rates of many psychiatric disorders in Asian countries. Too few Asians were included in the ECA and NCS to study the consistency of this finding among Asians living in the United States. Such data could aid in understanding whether low rates of bipolar disorder are intrinsic to Asian people or affected by environmental factors. Selective migration could also be at play in that families or persons with bipolar disorder may be more likely to emigrate. Future studies and the new worldwide epidemiologic study of the ICPE, described previously, may clarify this issue.

Marital Status

Epidemiologic studies investigating marital status among bipolar patients have revealed that the disorder is slightly more common among single and divorced persons. The ECA revealed that individuals who are separated or divorced are more likely to suffer from bipolar disorder as compared with married or never-married individuals (see Table 5–7). In a Hungarian national survey (Szadoczky et al., 1998), bipolar disorder was found to be more frequent among those who were separated and divorced. The rate among those never married was high as well. Early onset of the illness may contribute to the latter phenomenon, negatively influencing personality development and thus causing difficulties in establishing and maintaining interpersonal connections.

As Krauthammer and Klerman (1979) pointed out, marital status may change as a result of the disorder, rather than leading to its onset. On the other hand, it is plausible that being single or divorced constitutes a risk for bipolar illness in some populations; it is also plausible, indeed likely, that stressful marriages may precipitate affective episodes and, conversely, that supportive marriages may have a protective effect.

While persons with bipolar disorder are more likely than those in the general population to be single, divorced, or in a disrupted marriage, we know of no evidence to support a causal relationship between the disorder and marital status. The establishment of such a link is hampered by small sample sizes and a lack of clarity as to the direction of causality in studies addressing the question. Therefore, although it is likely that symptoms of untreated mania are disruptive to forming or sustaining intimate relationships, this hypothesis is not supported empirically. (See Chapter 10 for further discussion of the effect of bipolar disorder on interpersonal relationships.)

Urban/Rural Comparisons

No urban/rural differences in rates of bipolar disorder were found in the ECA or the NCS. In Taiwan, the lifetime prevalence was higher in metropolitan Taipei (1.6 percent) than in small towns (0.7 percent) and rural villages (1.0

percent) (Hwu et al., 1989). In Korea, the lifetime prevalence of mania was similar in metropolitan Seoul (0.4 percent) and in rural regions (0.4 percent) (Lee et al., 1990b). Urban/rural differences in prevalence rates of affective disorders, when they exist, may relate to the interplay among such factors as place of residence, migration patterns, socioeconomic status, diet, and environment, rather than just one variable.

The Homeless and the Institutionalized

Homelessness and mental illness among the homeless population have become a special interest of many mental health professionals. The homeless population itself is difficult to define, and ascertaining the prevalence of mental disorders within this community is even more problematic. In 1990, the lifetime and 5-year prevalence of all types of homelessness in the United States was estimated at 14.0 percent (26 million people) and 4.6 percent (8.5 million people), respectively. Lifetime "literal homelessness" (sleeping in shelters, abandoned buildings, bus and train stations, and the like) was 7.4 percent (13.5 million people). Among those who had ever been literally homeless, the 5-year (1985–1990) prevalence of self-reported homelessness was 3.1 percent (5.7 million people) (Link et al., 1994). More recent follow-up studies of the homeless, however, indicate that these figures overestimate the persistence of the problem and the number of homeless with psychiatric problems (Phelan and Link, 1999).

Among the mental disorders that exist within this population, schizophrenia, substance abuse, personality disorders, and affective disorders are the most prevalent (Arce and Vergare, 1984). Affective disorders make up 5 to 30 percent of mental disorders found among the homeless. The most comprehensive and standardized of the studies addressing this issue (Koegel et al., 1988) used the DIS to diagnose mental disorders among the mentally ill homeless in Los Angeles. Over the course of their lifetimes, these homeless individuals were 3.4 times more likely to have had any affective disorder, 17.7 times more likely to have had a manic episode, and 2.9 times more likely to have had a major depressive episode relative to people in the general population. Similarly, over a period of 6 months, the risk ratios for a mental disorder were many times greater among the homeless than in the general population (6.1, 37.5, and 5.0, respectively).

One must keep in mind when examining these data that these are prevalence rates within the mentally ill homeless population, and not within the general homeless population. Still, when these data are converted to rates within the general homeless population, the resulting proportions are higher than those among the general population. One other note regarding prevalence rates within this population is that substance abuse can easily coexist with or mask other underlying mental disorders, especially affective disorders. Therefore, these already high rates of bipolar disorder may be underestimates.

A more recent study of 1,022 homeless men living in shelters or on the street in Munich, Germany, using the SCID, also revealed high rates of mood disorders (lifetime prevalence of 32.8 percent for any mood disorder and of 5.2 percent for bipolar disorder). The highest rate was found for substance abuse (79.6 percent), particularly alcohol dependence (72.7 percent) (Fichter et al., 2001). A lifetime rate of bipolar disorder (3.6 percent), based on the CIDI, was found among 838 homeless men and women in a study conducted in Paris in 1996 (Kovess and Lazarus, 1999). Comparable studies in other European countries did not report bipolar disorder separately from other mood disorders (Vázquez et al., 1997; Muñoz et al., 1998; Babidge et al., 2002).

Some studies have oversampled the incarcerated (Buhrich et al., 2000) and the institutionalized (Robins and Regier, 1991). These groups were found to have higher rates of bipolar disorder than the general population. For example, Blazer (1985) found a lifetime prevalence of 5.4 percent for those living in prisons and 9.7 percent for those living in nursing homes. Yet the studies showed that the inclusion of these populations added only a small fraction (1.0 percent) to the estimated percentage of the general population having a mental disorder. Therefore, their inclusion or exclusion has little effect on community rates.

Pregnancy and Menopause

Childbearing represents a special risk for the onset of bipolar-I disorder in women. As shown by both epidemiologic and clinical studies, the first onset of bipolar disorder is almost always in the childbearing years (Blehar et al., 1998). As noted in Chapter 20, almost one-half of bipolar-I women who had been pregnant reported having experienced severe emotional disturbances in relationship to childbearing, with almost one-third citing episodes during pregnancy. Nair and colleagues (2000) hypothesized that subsets of women with a history of repeated reproductive-related mood disorders may be especially vulnerable to mood disturbances during perimenopause and menopause. In their study, two-thirds of perimenopausal bipolar-I women reported frequent mood disturbances, and almost 20 percent of postmenopausal bipolar-I women had experienced severe emotional disturbances during the menopausal transition.

Smoking

Bipolar disorder is associated with increased risk of smoking. A case-control study carried out in Alava, Spain, including patients with a DSM-III-R diagnosis of bipolar-I disorder found that smoking was more prevalent among bipolar patients than among the general population. Most patients had begun to smoke before the onset of bipolar disorder; thus vulnerability to bipolar illness (not the illness itself) may make subjects more likely to become smokers (Gonzalez-Pinto et al., 1998).

The NCS included questions on smoking. About 69 percent of respondents with bipolar-I were current smokers, and 82 percent had ever smoked. These rates were quite different from those among respondents without mental illness or with other psychiatric disorders (Lasser et al., 2000). For example, the 82 percent of bipolar respondents who had ever smoked is a significantly higher proportion than the 59 percent of subjects with major depression and the 72 percent of drug abusers who had ever done so. Analysis of the 2001–2002 National Epidemiologic Survey on Alcohol and Related Conditions found that nicotine dependence occurred in 40 percent of all cases (Grant et al., 2005). Moreover, studies that have addressed smoking in bipolar patients have noted their difficulty in quitting (Glassman, 1993).

Comorbid psychiatric and medical conditions are discussed in Chapter 7.

Omega-3 Fatty Acids

Essential fatty acids are crucial components of synaptic cell membranes (see Chapter 14). The essential long-chain polyunsaturated fatty acids, omega-3 and omega-6, cannot be formed in the human body, so dietary intake is their only source. Sources of omega-3 fatty acids include fish and seafood, particularly oily fish (cod, salmon, tuna, haddock, and scallops).

Hibbeln (1998) found that greater seafood consumption was related to lower lifetime prevalence rates of major depression across nine countries ($r = .84$, $p < .005$). Frequent fish consumption (at least twice a week) was revealed to be an independent factor for a reduced risk of depressive symptoms (odds ratio = 0.63) and suicidal thinking (odds ratio = 0.57) in a restricted geographic region within a single country. The use of omega-3 supplements in the treatment of depression and bipolar disorder is discussed in Chapters 19 and 20.

Relating data on fish consumption in a country to independently collected epidemiologic data on rates of a disorder requires many assumptions about the quality, time, and sample structure of both datasets and yields at best a rough estimate of correlations. However, the data are consistent with a growing body of literature. Tanskanen and colleagues (2001) reported lower rates of suicidal ideation among frequent consumers of lake fish in Finland and a decrease in suicide risk among daily fish consumers in

Japan followed over 17 years. Nonetheless, well-controlled studies in bipolar and unipolar patients are needed before definitive conclusions can be reached about the role of omega-3 fatty acids.

Family History

There is strong agreement that bipolar disorder is heritable. While family studies cannot determine heritability, one of the strongest predictors of first onset of bipolar illness is a family history of the disorder. Unfortunately, family history is excluded from epidemiologic studies, mainly because collecting accurate information on family history is time-consuming.

As detailed in Chapter 13, the morbid risk for bipolar disorder among first-degree relatives of bipolar probands is elevated substantially over the risk in the general population. Furthermore, adoption studies have shown that the monozygotic-to-dizygotic concordance ratio is higher for bipolar disorder than for unipolar depression, indicating greater genetic involvement in the former condition. A number of genetic linkage and association studies are under way to determine the genes involved.

CONCLUSIONS

In its calculations of rates of disability, WHO has ranked bipolar disorder among the top 10 disabling disorders in both developed and developing countries. It is not easy to summarize the results of epidemiologic studies of bipolar disorder from around the world, especially in light of a number of methodological problems. Nonetheless, it is possible to derive reasonable estimates of the prevalence and incidence of the disorder.

Findings of recent studies generally indicate an overall lifetime prevalence of bipolar-I disorder of about 1 percent. The range of rates is not great, even from diverse countries. In the United States, Europe, Scandinavia, the South Pacific, South America, and the United Kingdom, the lifetime prevalence of bipolar-I disorder ranges from 0.2 percent (Iceland) to 2.0 percent (the Netherlands and Hungary). Most rates are around 1 to 1.5 percent. The exceptions are Iceland (0.2 percent) and three Asian countries with lifetime rates of 0.015 to 0.3 percent. The reasons for the markedly low Asian rates, which are also low for a number of other mental disorders, are unclear. Studies of Asians living outside the continent are needed to determine whether these low rates are related to genetic differences, to living in Asian countries, or to ascertainment factors.

Studies that include a broad bipolar spectrum produce much higher lifetime prevalence rates of 3.0 to 8.3 percent. While there have been efforts to determine the rates of bipolar-II and milder forms of bipolar disorder

in community surveys, it is difficult to distinguish between normal moods and mild hypomania in nonpatient populations, making the validity of these findings questionable. Moreover, all of these rates for bipolar spectrum may be underestimates because they do not include patients with highly recurrent major depression, some of whom may fall within the bipolar spectrum (see Chapter 1).[11]

Several features associated with bipolar disorder have been studied. Most studies with large sample sizes have not shown strong differences in rates of bipolar disorder by gender. Persons who are separated or divorced have higher rates of the disorder than their married counterparts. Differences by social class and racial group have been less well studied. Smoking is more prevalent among those with bipolar disorder than among the general population. And pregnancy and menopause represent vulnerable periods for women in the development of manic episodes.

A family history of bipolar disorder in first-degree relatives remains the strongest predictor of risk of onset of bipolar disorder. However, it is also a risk factor not usually included in epidemiologic surveys.

NOTES

1. Cowley and Wyatt, 1993; World Bank, 1993a,b; Murray and Lopez, 1996.
2. In the ECA and the NCS, the diagnostic interviews (the DIS and the UM-CIDI, respectively) contained questions designed to determine the clinical significance of each symptom involved in the disorder (Narrow et al., 2002). Questions in the two surveys were similar, and information was obtained as to whether the symptom was severe enough to require telling a doctor or any professional about it, to take medicine for it, and/or to interfere with usual activities. Symptoms failing to meet any of these criteria were not identified as clinically significant and did not count toward making the diagnosis. The ECA used this approach for most disorders. However, neither the ECA nor the NCS applied these criteria at the symptom level for major depression or bipolar disorder. In both cases, questions about clinical significance were asked only after all symptoms had been obtained and diagnostic criteria met. Applying clinical significance criteria at the symptom level and not at the end of the diagnostic stage reduced the overall rates of mental disorders in both surveys. The impact was greater in the NCS, and the disparity in rates between the ECA and the NCS was reduced, with an estimated 18.5 percent annual rate of any disorder.

   Applying the clinical significance criteria in the ECA reduced the annual rate of unipolar depression by about 18 percent and that of bipolar disorder by 44 percent (see Table 5–1) (Narrow et al., 2002). The rate of unipolar major depression was reduced to 4.0 percent, compared with 4.9 percent without the clinical significance criteria. The clinical significance criteria had a greater effect on major depression prevalence rates in the NCS than on those in the ECA, drawing the two rates closer together. The annual prevalence estimate for unipolar major depression in the NCS fell from 8.9 to 5.4 percent. The annual prevalence of bipolar-I disorder did not change in the NCS and remained at 1.3 percent, but dropped to 0.5 percent in the ECA. Thus, the gap between the ECA and NCS widened. There is controversy about the manipulation of rates based on treatment need (Narrow et al., 2002). Wakefield and Spitzer (2002) noted that basing disorders on stringent impairment criteria, which led to reduced rates in the NCS, helped resolve discrepancies between the 1980 and 1990 surveys. However, they suggested that these revised prevalence rates are not necessarily a valid redefinition of the disorders, but may reflect an inadequate measure of treatment need. Use of the impairment or treatment criteria, they noted, means that disorders that are real but do not interfere significantly with life are ignored.

Another way of examining diagnostic validity, used in the NCS, is through a clinical reappraisal of potential mania cases. Kessler and colleagues (1997) concluded that validity was satisfactory on bipolar-I, as judged by the reappraisal, only for cases of mania with elevated mood or increased activity, decreased need for sleep, and elevated self-esteem or grandiosity. Requiring these symptoms reduced the prevalence of mania to 0.3 percent. However, the authors cautioned that, because of a significant number of CIDI false-negative findings in the clinical reappraisals, these clinically confirmed CIDI cases may underestimate by half the actual rate of mania in the community. If this statement holds true, the extrapolated estimate of 0.6 percent for bipolar-I disorder is closer to the ECA rate. The authors were unable to document an algorithm with acceptable concordance with clinical diagnosis for bipolar-II, and they concluded that bipolar-II prevalence was not valid in their sample.

Another analysis of factors that may have contributed to the differences between ECA and NCS rates was conducted by Regier and colleagues (1998). Their analysis produced rates of psychiatric disorder from each survey by controlling for demographic variables; standardizing the weights in both surveys to the age, sex, and racial distributions of the 1990 census; formulating diagnoses according to DSM-III; and restricting the age range to 18 to 54 years. Using this method, the lifetime rate of any DSM-III disorder for the first wave of interviews was 36 percent. Adding the cases from the second wave produced a rate of 47 percent, consistent with the rate of 48 percent from the single-wave NCS. Annual rates of mania produced in this way were almost identical to those in the

ECA and the NCS. The annual rate of bipolar-I for the first wave of the ECA using these conventions was 0.9 percent; adding cases from the second wave produced a rate of 1.0 percent. The annual rate in the NCS was 1.1 percent with these conventions.

That such modifications can reduce or increase disparate rates concerns health policy planners and insurers, who base the direct costs of service delivery for a disorder on its prevalence rate. The WHO initiative to revise the CIDI by including impairment criteria for each disorder is addressing this issue (Regier and Burke, 2000). However, there is still no fully satisfactory method of calculating the actual rates.

3. Simpson et al., 1993; Benazzi, 1997; Koukopoulos and Koukopoulos, 1999; Dilsaver and Akiskal, 2005; Rybakowski et al, 2005; Sharma et al., 2005.

4. Dilling and Weyerer, 1984; Henderson et al., 2000; Murphy et al., 2000; World Health Organization International Consortium of Psychiatric Epidemiology, 2000.

5. Scully et al., 2000, 2002a,b; Baldwin et al., 2002.

6. Angst, 1978; Dunner et al., 1982; Akiskal et al., 2000; Cassano et al., 2000; Angst et al., 2002.

7. Research on minors often makes a distinction by pubertal status. Puberty has been shown to differentiate the onset and clinical course of mood disorders in longitudinal and epidemiologic studies (Angold et al., 1998, 1999; Weissman et al., 1999a,b). The rates and gender ratios of depression change dramatically at puberty, with a marked increase occurring in overall rates, especially among females. Some studies separate prepubertal children from adolescents, others focus on one or the other, and still others merge the two. Most studies use chronological age to designate pubertal status; a few use Tanner staging (see Angold et al., 1998, 1999). We recognize the importance of these age distinctions and make them where the necessary data are available. In the absence of such data or the need to make an age-specific point, however, we use the term *children* to describe minors.

8. Strober et al., 1993; Lewinsohn et al., 1995; Rao et al., 1995; Geller et al., 1998.

9. More information on the ICPE can be obtained from http://www.hcp.med.harvard.edu/icpe/.

10. For example, Hollingshead and Redlich, 1958; Parker et al., 1959; Rao, 1966; Hare, 1968; Rowitz and Levy, 1968; Bagley, 1973; Gershon and Liebowitz, 1975; Petterson, 1977; Coryell et al., 1989.

11. Indeed, Kraepelin's "manic-depressive illness" included both bipolar and highly recurrent unipolar subgroups.

6 Children and Adolescents

In rare cases the first beginnings can be traced back even to before the tenth year. . . . The greatest frequency of first attacks falls, however, in the *period of development* with its increased emotional excitability between the fifteenth and the twentieth year.

—Emil Kraepelin (1921, p. 167)

Bipolar disorder commonly manifests itself in adolescence or young adulthood, but classic descriptions and numerous case studies also demonstrate the existence of the disorder in children. In recent years, identification of these earliest forms of the disorder has been the subject of an explosion of interest among clinicians, scientists, the public, and the media.[1] This interest has been driven in part by the emerging hypothesis of bipolar disorder as a progressive neurobiological process that may worsen with succeeding episodes, so that early identification and treatment may have important implications for attenuating the course of illness. Increasingly, moreover, parents are seeking answers and help for their children who display bewildering or overwhelmingly severe symptoms and are at increased risk for serious behavioral and educational problems, as well as suicide (see Hellander and Burke, 1999; Lewinsohn et al., 2003). Aside from treatment considerations, childhood-onset bipolar disorder also raises important conceptual and etiological questions: Are there different subtypes with differing causes and courses? What are the defining distinctions between pediatric bipolar illness and other psychiatric disorders of childhood, such as attention-deficit hyperactivity disorder (ADHD)? Is the rate of childhood bipolar disorder increasing, and if so, why? Is the course of the disorder different for early versus adult onset? Although this book is about manic-depressive illness, which includes both bipolar and recurrent unipolar forms, the pediatric literature rarely distinguishes recurrent from nonrecurrent forms of unipolar depression; this chapter limits its focus to the bipolar subgroup.

We begin with a review of research on childhood- and adolescent-onset bipolar disorder. We then examine the epidemiology and implications of bipolar disorder in these populations. Finally, we present the findings of studies of high-risk subjects that have attempted to identify characteristics of children of bipolar parents, with particular emphasis on early markers of potential bipolar illness. Unfortunately, many unresolved issues remain. The interest in manifestations of bipolar disorder among children and young adolescents is far greater than the yield from research addressing the key questions involved.

Throughout the discussion, we attempt to identify problems with the methods used in existing studies, as well as research needed to address important issues. One of the most pervasive difficulties stems from the failure of many studies to distinguish between childhood- and adolescent-onset bipolar disorder; this occurs, for example, when vague terms such as "juvenile-onset bipolar disorder" and "pediatric bipolar disorder" are used or when child and adolescent samples are combined in the same study. This is a widespread problem in the study of adolescent bipolar disorder, where distinctions are seldom made between childhood and adolescent *onset*. Some studies of adolescents with bipolar disorder include patients whose symptoms actually first occurred before age 12 or before puberty. As detailed in chapter 4, age at onset is also defined differently in various studies—for example, as age at first diagnosable symptoms of mania or at first symptoms of any affective disorder, or as age at first actual diagnosis of mania or depression by a mental health professional. Studies have employed different diagnostic criteria as well, and many have included clinical populations with a mix of bipolar-I and other bipolar spectrum disorders, despite the fact that there is very little information specifically on bipolar-II disorder in children or adolescents (see Chapter 3). Finally, one of the greatest methodological gaps is the paucity of longitudinal studies of either childhood or adolescent bipolar disorder. Such studies are essential to clarify diagnostic controversies and to map the course of the disorder and the implications of its early onset.

CHILDHOOD-ONSET BIPOLAR DISORDER

Although occurrences of mania and depression in adolescence are well established, the frequency of early-childhood onset of bipolar disorder remains controversial. Kraepelin (1921) found that 0.4 percent of his patients had displayed manic features before age 10. Despite historical records of case studies documenting apparent bipolar illness in children, however, theorists believed for an extended period in the mid-twentieth century that bipolar disorder in children before puberty was not possible (reviewed in Faedda et al., 1995). For instance, Anthony and Scott (1960) examined the psychiatric literature from 1884 to 1954 and uncovered only 28 cases of alleged manic episodes in young children. After applying systematic diagnostic criteria to these clinical reports, they dismissed all of the cases as misdiagnosed and concluded that a classic clinical presentation of manic-depressive illness in childhood had yet to be demonstrated.

Recent years have seen a growing acceptance that prepubertal forms of mania can be identified. Opinions range from certainty that characteristic patterns of symptoms signal childhood bipolar disorder in substantial numbers, even if in a form that may not precisely follow that of classic forms of the disorder, to more cautious views that prepubertal mania exists, but that many such complex cases may be misinterpreted as bipolar disorder. Difficulty in applying the adult criteria for bipolar disorder in the *Diagnostic and Statistical Manual*, 4th edition (DSM-IV) to children is at the heart of the controversy. In the following sections, we present research on characteristics of bipolar disorder in children and discuss the controversies related to its diagnosis.

Symptoms and Clinical Presentation

Manic Features

The appearance and diagnosis of mania is considered a distinctive indicator of bipolar disorder in children. However, the diagnosis of mania in children is controversial and fraught with pitfalls, as reviewed below.

Even as young as preschool age, some children appear to present relatively classic manic symptoms, including DSM-IV–defined mania or hypomania with elated mood and/or grandiosity; flight of ideas or racing thoughts; poor judgment, such as excessive silliness, uninhibited people-seeking, hypersexuality, or daredevil acts; talking fast; and distractibility, with increased energy, activity, and agitation (e.g., Geller et al., 2000a, 2002c). In their study of 93 children

with prepubertal and early-adolescent onset of bipolar disorder (mean age at onset 7.3 years), Geller and colleagues (1998b, 2002c) found that five mania-specific symptoms were especially likely to discriminate bipolar children from children with ADHD or normal comparison groups: elation, grandiosity, flight of ideas/racing thoughts, decreased need for sleep, and hypersexuality. Table 6–1 presents examples of manic symptoms in children compared with normal characteristics of youngsters of similar age (Geller et al., 2002b).

Geller and colleagues (2002c) also found that 60 percent of their sample had symptoms of psychosis, including 50 percent who had grandiose delusions. In a later follow-up study, they found that psychosis predicted more weeks ill with mania or hypomania (Geller et al., 2004). In their review of psychotic symptoms in pediatric bipolar disorder, Pavuluri and colleagues (2004) found that the prevalence of psychotic features ranged from 16 to 88 percent; most common were mood-congruent delusions, especially of the grandiose type. Biederman and colleagues (2004c) found that nearly 1 in 4 of the 298 bipolar patients they studied were psychotic or had a history of psychosis. Likewise, in their study of 263 bipolar children and adolescents, Birmaher and colleagues (2005b) found that one-third (33.1 percent) of their subjects had a history of psychosis.

Geller and colleagues required elation and/or grandiosity for the diagnosis of mania in children, as did Leibenluft and colleagues (2003a). This is an important, if still preliminary, consensus of clinical researchers, although, as Carlson (2005) pointed out, uncertainty remains about what actually constitutes these two symptoms. Methods of assessment vary widely, as do cultural expectations and developmental factors, and all are likely to influence the ascertainment of both euphoria and grandiosity (Breslau, 1987; Shaffer, 2002; Harrington and Myatt, 2003). Some studies have defined mania by the presence of highly labile moods with intense irritability, rage, explosiveness, and destructiveness; extreme agitation; and behavioral dysregulation (e.g., Biederman et al., 2000a). Irritability, and indeed rage, are noted as prominent features in many bipolar children (e.g., Faraone et al., 1997b; Carlson and Kelly, 1998; Geller et al., 2002c). The children are often aggressive and frequently are described by their parents as "out of control." Not surprisingly, they are often seen in hospital settings, and overall their functioning is marked by severe impairment in social and academic as well as family roles (Geller et al., 2000a). Box 6–1 presents a mother's diary of the behaviors of her 9-year-old bipolar son, conveying a sense of the severe but characteristic features of the disorder. Suicidal thoughts and behaviors are not uncommon.

TABLE 6–1. Examples of Core Symptoms of Mania among Children

Normal Child	Child with Mania
	Elated Mood
Child was extremely happy on days family went to Disneyland, on Christmas morning, during grandparents' visits (joy appropriate to context, not impairing).	7-year-old boy repeatedly taken to principal for clowning and giggling in class; had to leave church for similar behaviors. 9-year-old girl continually danced around at home, stating, "I'm high, over the mountain high" after suspension from school.
	Grandiosity
After school hours, 7-year-old boy played at being a firefighter, directing other firefighters and rescuing victims. Child did not call fire station and tell firefighters what to do.	7-year-old boy stole go-cart because he wanted to have it; knew stealing was wrong, but did not believe it was wrong for *him* to steal. 8-year-old girl, failing in school, spent evenings practicing for when she would be the first female President. She was also planning how to train her husband to be the First Gentleman.
	Decreased Need for Sleep
Normal children sleep approximately 8 to 10 hours a night and are tired the next day if they sleep fewer hours than usual.	8-year-old boy chronically stayed up until 2 AM rearranging the furniture or playing games. He then awoke at 6 AM for school and was energetic throughout the day without evident fatigue.
	Poor Judgment: Hypersexuality
7-year-old child played doctor with a friend of the same age. 12-year-old boy looked at his father's pornographic magazines.	7-year-old girl touched the teacher's breasts and propositioned boys in class. 10-year-old boy used explicit sexual language in restaurants and public places. Girl faxed a note to the local police station asking police to___her.
	Racing Thoughts
Normal children do not report racing thoughts.	Children tend to give concrete answers to describe racing thoughts: A girl pointed to the middle of her forehead and stated, "I need a stoplight up there." Others: "It's like an energizer bunny in my head." "My thoughts broke the speed limit." "I don't know what to think first."

Source: Adapted from Geller et al., 2002a. Reprinted with permission from Mary Ann Liebert, Inc.

BOX 6–1.   Twelve Days in May: Diary of a Mother of a Nine-Year-Old Bipolar Child

5/11   Hypomanic, bizarre evening. "I hate me; kill me; Why am I like this?" Very rough with younger brother.

5/12   Good morning, dropped off well at school. Pretty good mood coming off bus, but more defiance in the afternoon. Uneventful evening. Went to bed well.

5/13   Up early, dressed well, good mood but problems on the bus. Kids teasing him. Teacher called and reported very bizarre behavior at school. She also reported a lot of ADHD symptoms—very fidgety, unable to remain seated in the afternoon, cruises around classroom, ran out of classroom, pestering other kids, unable to follow directions, not remaining on task or completing work.

5/14   Teacher reported a great day in school. Good mood after school.

5/15   Good A.M.—off to school well. Very defiant after school. Angered by new doctor. Got very angry in car—punching me, destructive to car, scribbling on dashboard, dumping over trash. Had to be restrained in office—punching, kicking, swearing—settled down at end of meeting and apologized.

5/16   Happy mood in A.M., but doing goofy, impulsive things—squirted water on dad's work shirt, squirted water on table and floor. Very aggressive after school—threatening me, hitting, increase in defiance. Aggressive toward other students.

5/17   Had a good time with grandparents. Crying a lot in the afternoon.

5/18   "Mixed," very irritable to hypomanic—increase in goal-directed activities, very easily frustrated and angered.

5/19   Good and uneventful day.

5/20   Very irritable in A.M.—threatened father—said: "I'm going to kill you someday." Manic after school—very goal-directed—taking all the tools out of the basement to use up in his room (hammer, sander, drill, staple gun). Very angry when I intervened—very loud, shouting, laughing, singing, dancing, "I don't feel good today. I want to kill myself. When I grow up, I am going to kill myself because being bipolar is bad." Hallucinating in afternoon—auditory and visual; goblin, clown, queen. "I hear the devil, I hear penises in your brain, Mom." Very hyperactive, and not rational. Gave him Risperdal and he went to sleep.

5/21   Hypomanic, happy in the afternoon.

5/22   Woke up laughing—found some needlepoint yarn and needles under the bed. "I'm giving myself a lab test"—trying to stick needles into his arm. Giddy, shouting "hubba, hubba, hubba, howdy, howdy" over and over again, very wound up. Settled down and watched some TV. Pleasant and more normal, but talkative in the afternoon. Easier to please. More irritable after dinner. Fascinated with knives, demonstrated how he would stab a wolf. Very quiet in my lap. He said: "I love you, Mom. You don't love me, you want me to die. I will if you want me to."

Source: Papolos and Papolos, 2002, pp. 22–23. © 2002 by Demitri Papolos and Janice Papolos. Used with permission of Broadway Books, a division of Random House, Inc.

Depressive Features

For many individuals, bipolar disorder first emerges in the form of depressive episodes in childhood (e.g., Geller et al., 1994; Lish et al., 1994). Although depression in children may be readily diagnosed using adult criteria, the majority of such cases probably go undetected and untreated. Even if they are detected, however, there is presently no certain way of knowing the extent to which early-onset depression presages childhood-onset bipolar disorder; the issue is an important question not only clinically but for research as well.

As noted previously, studies of bipolar illness have often combined childhood- and adolescent-onset populations, and longitudinal studies of the outcomes of depression in children have been rare. Given that unipolar depression in children is substantially more prevalent than mania and is characterized by marked clinical and etiological heterogeneity, it is difficult to identify predictors specific to eventual bipolarity. Wozniak and colleagues (2004) compared 109 children with unipolar depression and 43 children with bipolar depression (all had been diagnosed with ADHD as well) and found that the bipolar children were more severely depressed and anhedonic, were more often suicidal, expressed greater hopelessness, and were more likely to need medication and hospitalization. They also had higher rates of comorbidity with conduct disorder, oppositional defiant disorder, agoraphobia, obsessive-compulsive disorder, and alcohol abuse (see Chapter 7 for a detailed discussion of comorbidity in bipolar disorder). A family history of bipolar disorder was more than twice as likely in the bipolar group as in the unipolar children (20 versus 8 percent).

Most follow-up studies of depressed children have yielded little information on predictors of bipolarity because of the limited size of samples that have converted to a bipolar course. Recently, Luby and Mrakotsky (2003) attempted to identify differences in symptoms among depressed preschoolers with and without a family history of bipolar disorder. Only one symptom (restlessness/"moves around a lot") distinguished the groups, but its association with the emergence of bipolarity remains to be seen. Geller and colleagues (1994) found that among a sample of 79 severely depressed children (ages 6 to 12), 32 percent switched to bipolar-I or bipolar-II during a 2- to 5-year follow-up. When the same subjects were recontacted in young adulthood (mean age 21), 49 percent were found to have switched to bipolar disorder, including 33 percent with bipolar-I (Geller et al., 2001b). The authors found that parental and grandparental mania was a significant predictor of bipolar switching.

Unfortunately, this information has sometimes been misstated. Although Geller and colleagues (2001b) did indeed find a 33 percent rate of switching to bipolar-I disorder among their severely depressed sample of children, their sample may be atypical and perhaps biased by high rates of referral for suspected bipolar disorder. The rate of switching is likely to be substantially lower in more typical outpatient samples. For instance, Weissman and colleagues (1999b) followed up on outpatient children with prepubertal depression an average of 11 years later, and found that only 6 percent had developed bipolar disorder, although this rate was much higher than that among comparison groups. Lewinsohn and colleagues (2000) found that fewer than 1 percent of adolescents with depression in a community sample switched to bipolar disorder. Differences in rates among these studies are likely due to differing diagnostic and exclusion criteria in the samples. Most clinical samples are small and can be greatly affected by variations in level of severity; family history of bipolar disorder; use of alcohol, stimulants, antidepressants, or other drugs; and other unspecified or unknown factors. Clearly, further research is needed on the predictors of switching among depressed children so as not to exaggerate, or even mislabel, bipolarity in children, yet provide accurate information to enable early treatment of those who truly have or are likely to develop the illness.

Diagnostic Controversies

Despite general agreement that bipolar disorder can emerge in childhood, several problems make it difficult to validate some of the assertions made about diagnosis of bipolar children. Three related issues are discussed here: comorbidity and indistinct diagnostic boundaries, the validity and meaning of a diagnosis of mania, and the lack of developmental guidelines.

Comorbidity and Indistinct Diagnostic Boundaries

As noted earlier, the great majority of cases of childhood-onset bipolar disorder also meet criteria for other disorders, including ADHD, conduct disorder, and oppositional defiant disorder.[2] Findings of the major studies of comorbidity in childhood-onset bipolar disorder are presented in Table 6–2. As can be seen in the table, many clinical investigations have documented a high rate of comorbid anxiety disorders as well.[3] (There is some indication that bipolar-II children and adolescents, like adults, are more likely to have comorbid anxiety disorders than those with bipolar-I disorder [Axelson et al., 2006].) Perhaps nothing has fueled the controversy as much as the potentially confusing overlap of symptoms between mania and disruptive behavioral disorders.

Many studies have shown that children with a bipolar diagnosis have a high probability of being diagnosed with ADHD. Geller and colleagues (2000a), for example, found this to be the case in 98 percent of their sample (see also Biederman et al., 2000a; Sachs et al., 2000; Spencer et al., 2001). Considerably lower rates have been found by other researchers, however (Masi et al., 2003; Faedda et al., 2004; Jaideep et al., 2006). Some investigators have argued that many children diagnosed with ADHD also have bipolar disorder. Biederman and colleagues (1996) identified psychiatrically referred children with ADHD, who were then assessed for the presence of mania at baseline and at 1 and 4 years later. Bipolar disorder was diagnosed in 11 percent of the ADHD children at baseline and in an additional 12 percent at the 4-year follow-up. Arguing that a substantial number of children diagnosed with ADHD may actually have unrecognized bipolar disorder, Biederman fueled a controversy that is still active (Wozniak et al., 1995; Faraone et al., 1997b; Biederman, 1998). Many investigators have also observed high rates of conduct disorder and oppositional defiant disorder (e.g., Biederman et al., 2000a; Geller et al., 2000b; Wozniak et al., 2001), as well as substance abuse and anxiety disorders (e.g., Birmaher et al., 2002), among bipolar children (see also reviews in Biederman et al., 2000a, and Papolos, 2003).

What is the meaning of the overlap between mania and ADHD (or other disruptive behavior disorders)? There are several different perspectives on this question. One general argument is that the comorbidity is simply an artifact of overlapping symptomatology. Three more specific arguments are that the ADHD–mania overlap is (1) true comorbidity (coexistence of separate disorders), potentially marking a genetically mediated subtype; (2) artifactual, reflecting severe psychopathology that is not specifically bipolar; and (3) artifactual, possibly reflecting a developmental manifestation of bipolar disorder in children.

The general argument that bipolar comorbidity may be a result of overlap of symptoms suggests that diagnostic inaccuracies are caused by indistinct symptom boundaries, clinician bias, or biased diagnostic expectations due to ascertainment source. Biederman and his colleagues at

TABLE 6–2. Comorbidities in Samples of Bipolar Children

Characteristic	Faraone et al., 1997a (child outpatient)	Carlson and Kelly, 1998 (child inpatient)	Tillman et al., 2003 (child outpatient)
Sample size	68	60	93
Source of sample	Outpatient psychopharmacology clinic	Children's inpatient unit	Research study, outpatient
Assessment used	KSADS	KSADS	WASH-U KSADS
Mean age (yrs)	7.9	8.7	10.9
% Male	78	91	61
Comorbidities			
% ADHD	93	66	87
% ODD/CD	91/38	75/54	79
% OCD	10		
Anxiety disorders	56	14	23 syndromal
% substance abuse disorders	—	None	Not stated
% psychosis	31	10	Not stated
% no comorbidity	Not stated	0	Not stated
% With >1 diagnosis	Probably high	Average: 3 diagnoses	98 (≥4 diagnoses: 20.4)

ADHD = attention-deficit hyperactivity disorder; KSADS = Kiddie Schedule for Affective Disorders and Schizophrenia; OCD = obsessive-compulsive disorder; ODD/CD = oppositional defiant disorder/conduct disorder; WASH-U KSADS = Washington University at St. Louis modification of KSADS.

Source: Updated from Geller et al., 1999. Reprinted with permission.

Massachusetts General Hospital studied large numbers of children with comorbid ADHD and bipolar disorder. They argued, through the use of various diagnostic algorithms, that the presence of the two separate diagnoses was valid and was not a result of overlapping symptoms such as talkativeness, hyperactivity–psychomotor agitation, or distractibility (e.g., Milberger et al., 1995; reviewed in Spencer et al., 2001). Moreover, Biederman and colleagues (1998) found that children with comorbid diagnoses of mania and ADHD ascertained from ADHD clinics and from a study of mania differed minimally in symptoms of either mania or ADHD.

Additionally, Biederman and colleagues (2004c) hypothesized that the comorbid combination of the two disorders may mark an etiological subtype. In family–genetic studies, Faraone and colleagues (1997b) found that first-degree relatives of children with bipolar disorder and ADHD had both disorders at rates greater than would be expected by chance alone. On the basis of these and other family patterns observed across several studies, they posited that the combination of ADHD and bipolar disorder is familially distinct and may be a marker of a subtype of very early–onset bipolarity.

Geller and colleagues (1998a, 2002b) also found high rates of comorbid ADHD and bipolar disorder. ADHD occurred among 97 percent of prepubertal bipolar children and 74 percent of bipolar adolescents. Even with ADHD, the bipolar children were distinctly different from ADHD-only children in symptoms of mania, as illustrated in Figure 6–1 (Geller et al., 1998b). As noted earlier, in a study comparing 93 participants with childhood- and early-adolescent–onset mania, 81 with ADHD and no mania, and 94 community controls, Geller and colleagues (2002b) found that, despite the high rate of ADHD–bipolar comorbidity, five symptoms distinguished most clearly between bipolar and ADHD samples: elation, grandiosity, flight of ideas/racing thoughts, decreased need for sleep, and hypersexuality. These findings appear to argue against the possibility that ADHD comorbidity is an artifact of overlapping symptoms—provided, as noted later, that children otherwise meet the full criteria for mania in DSM-IV.

Whereas Biederman and colleagues (1996) argued that the combination of ADHD and bipolar disorder in children marks a subtype of bipolar disorder, Geller and colleagues (1998a) suggested that ADHD in child bipolar samples may be a "phenocopy" ADHD, driven by developmentally prevalent high energy in children. That is, high energy combined with emerging bipolar symptoms promotes the hyperactivity, impulsivity, and attentional problems that are viewed as ADHD. Geller predicted that the

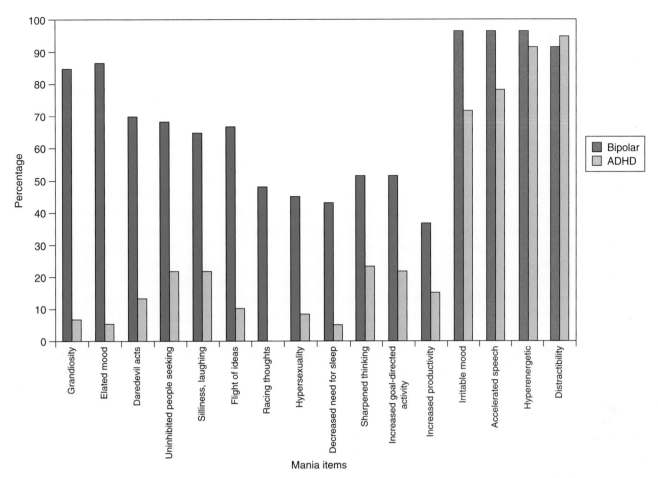

Figure 6–1. Baseline percentage of mania items in bipolar versus ADHD groups. (*Source:* Geller et al., 1998a. Reprinted with permission from Elsevier.)

ADHD will "decrease" to population levels by adulthood (e.g., Geller and Luby, 1997). Thus, ADHD may be a prodrome or developmentally expressed version of bipolarity in some children, rather than a separate disorder. Obviously, prospective longitudinal follow-up of samples of young bipolar patients would help resolve such diagnostic issues through clarification of clinical course and outcome (see reviews by Kim and Miklowitz, 2002; Kent and Craddock, 2003).

While it is doubtless likely that comorbid conditions can obscure the recognition of an underlying bipolar illness, the complex symptomatology involved may also have the opposite effect: clinicians are urged to consider bipolar disorder as an explanation for diffuse and difficult symptoms. A widely visible Web site for bipolar disorder in children, for example, listed the following as possible symptoms, among others more specific to typical mania: explosive, lengthy, and often destructive rages; separation anxiety; defiance of authority; hyperactivity, agitation, and distractibility; bed-wetting and night terrors; strong and frequent cravings; and daredevil behaviors.[4] Obviously,

although such symptoms may occur in children with bipolar disorder, each is also nonspecific. Precise diagnostic definitions that can help separate truly bipolar manifestations from overlapping conditions are needed to avoid misdiagnosis, as well as to facilitate recognition of bipolar illness.

Questions about the Validity of the Diagnosis of Mania in Children

Is severe behavioral dysregulation "mania," and does "mania" always mean bipolar disorder? Multiple, intense, and severe symptoms may be caused by brain injury, other forms of organic disorder (e.g., Carlson and Kelly, 1998), or severe disinhibition related to adverse medication responses (Carlson and Mick, 2003) (see also Chapter 3). Carlson (1998) noted that, in the child psychiatry literature, several nonspecific terms—such as "multidimensionally impaired" and "multiple complex developmental disorder"—are used to describe children with numerous, severe, disruptive behaviors that do not fit any typical diagnostic picture, as well as children suffering from some forms of head injury, pervasive developmental disorder, or other medical conditions. In the past, some of these children were labeled as "minimally brain damaged" or "hyperkinetic." Many of these historical syndromes have been described in terms that bear a marked resemblance to contemporary descriptions of childhood mania.

A related issue raised by Carlson and others is the possibility that mania or manic-like symptoms may occur as a dimension of disorder or serve as a marker of severe psychopathology without necessarily indicating the presence of a bipolar syndrome. Carlson and colleagues (1998) recruited a sample of boys aged 6 to 10 who had heterogeneous disruptive and/or depressive symptoms. The boys' mothers were asked about the presence of manic symptoms, and their responses led the researchers to distinguish three groups: those boys with at least two manic symptoms, and two matched comparison groups—those seen immediately next in the series of interviews but without manic symptoms, and those matched on the first group's comorbid disruptive symptoms (conduct disorder, ADHD, or oppositional defiant disorder) but without manic symptoms. The authors found that although the boys with symptoms of mania differed significantly from the nonmanic "next" control group, most of those differences disappeared in a comparison with the group with comorbid conditions. The presence of manic symptoms uniquely predicted significant emotionality and generally predicted more severe psychopathology (Carlson and Youngstrom, 2003). The investigators are continuing to study these children over time, attempting to determine whether some are truly bipolar, while in others the manic-like symptoms may serve mainly as markers for "behavioral and emotional multimorbidity." Similarly, Hazell and colleagues (2003) followed up boys aged 9 to 13 who met criteria for ADHD plus mania. When the boys were reevaluated after 6 years, there were no clear cases of bipolar disorder among those with prior manic symptoms; however, the boys with earlier manic symptoms had lower overall global functioning.

Geller and colleagues (2002) have reoperationalized several of the DSM criteria (most notably euphoria and grandiosity) to make them what the authors believe to be developmentally appropriate for children. Not everyone agrees with this reformulation, however (Harrington and Myatt, 2003). In a recent cross-national (United States and United Kingdom) study of five cases of children with mood symptoms in whom bipolar disorder might have been a diagnostic consideration, disagreement on diagnosis occurred in three of the five cases. The reason for this appears to be differing interpretations of specific symptoms. DSM's reliance on symptom counts (used in the United States) may result in a conceptualization that dif-

fers from the gestalt of bipolar disorder as described in the International Classification of Diseases (ICD)-10, used in the United Kingdom. Specifically, in a preadolescent patient with classic mania, agreement was close (96.4 percent of United States and 88.9 percent of United Kingdom physicians made a manic diagnosis). In the prepubertal child with both ADHD and manic-like symptoms, however, 86.2 percent of U.S. child psychiatrists diagnosed mania, in contrast to only 31.1 percent of their U.K. colleagues (Dubicka et al., 2005).

It may be noted that among adolescent samples in community populations, Lewinsohn and colleagues (1995) and Klein and colleagues (1996) observed manic-like symptoms or hypomania associated with impairment and various forms of psychopathology. Upon follow-up at age 24, those diagnosed earlier with bipolar disorder (mostly bipolar-II or cyclothymia) continued to show recurrent or chronic bipolar symptoms, but few of those with adolescent "subclinical" bipolar symptoms of mania/hypomania had developed full-blown bipolar disorder (Lewinsohn et al., 2000). Overall, studies of manic symptoms in children and adolescents may indicate true bipolar disorder in some cases, but in other cases these symptoms may be mainly markers for severe emotionality and disruptive behaviors.

Finally, a significant issue in the diagnosis of mania concerns the duration of affective cycles. Many children labeled "bipolar" may have numerous mood shifts within a day and have chronic symptoms and impairments not consistent with the adult concept of "episodes." As noted by Leibenluft and colleagues (2003a), in the absence of validated criteria for the duration of an episode in children, some investigators have defined episodes to be as brief as a few hours. Leibenluft and colleagues (2003b) suggested that within such brief periods, it is quite difficult to determine whether episodes are accompanied by the required DSM-IV criterion B changes in behavior. Thus, investigators' and parents' subjective impressions may be used to make diagnoses, contributing to the diagnostic confusion and heterogeneity in research samples. Tillman and Geller (2003) have proposed specific definitions of rapid, ultrarapid, and ultradian cycling, as well as distinctions between episodes and cycles. If used systematically in research, such definitions might help characterize the course of illness in bipolar children and contribute to diagnostic validity.

Lack of Data and Insufficient Knowledge of Developmental Issues

A further challenge to diagnosing bipolar disorder in children is the limited utility of applying to this population features of adult bipolar symptoms and course. Diagnostic confusion about how to interpret specific symptoms (e.g., hyperactivity, irritability) arises in part from developmental considerations for which little information is presently available. As Carlson (1998) noted, many of the other features of bipolar syndrome, such as grandiosity and elation, have not been systematically defined in developmentally appropriate and precise ways or evaluated in context. Simply hearing a child utter the words "I can fly," for instance, without considering the child's developmental stage and environmental context, could lead clinicians to misinterpret the statement as indicating grandiosity when it means nothing of the kind. Geller and colleagues (2002b) would argue that such states can be distinguished from normal childhood experiences; however, the issue must not hinge only on the experience and skill of a researcher or clinician, but rather on developmentally informed and validated criteria.

An intriguing suggestion that symptoms of bipolar disorder may have a developmental progression has been made by Post and colleagues (2002). These investigators studied three volunteer samples of parents: those with children who had been diagnosed with bipolar disorder or with psychiatric (nonbipolar) disorders, and those who were not ill. The parents were asked to identify their children's symptoms retrospectively during each year of life. Ages at which children displayed empirically derived clusters of symptoms were compared for the three groups. It appeared that among the bipolar children, an irritability–dyscontrol factor (e.g., impulsivity, tantrums, aggression, hyperactivity), emerging at age 1 to 3 years, was the first feature to distinguish among the groups. A depression factor began to differentiate the bipolar children from others by age 8 to 12. A mania factor (e.g., racing thoughts, grandiosity, mood elevations, bizarre behavior) did not begin to differentiate the bipolar children until ages 7 to 12, whereas a distinguishing psychosis–suicidality factor emerged at ages 9 to 12. Despite significant methodological limitations (including a lack of confirmatory diagnosis of the bipolar children, a mixed-disorder comparison group, and parental retrospective accounts), this study highlights the need for further investigation of the possible developmental progression of manifestations of bipolar symptoms.

Researchers have also urged further study of child-appropriate definitions of mania, as well as attention to traits and behaviors that may represent prodromal or subsyndromal forms of bipolar disorder (Shaffer, 2002; Coyle et al., 2003; Carlson, 2005). As we argue later, studies of children of bipolar parents may be an especially fruitful way to help identify some of the early indicators of mania and progression of symptoms in children known to be at risk for bipolar disorder.

Finally, it may be noted that boys tend to predominate in research samples of bipolar children (e.g., Faraone et al.,

1997b; Geller et al., 1998b). Indeed, this is true for most forms of childhood disorder, particularly disruptive disorders (ADHD, oppositional defiant disorder, conduct disorder), but also anxiety and depression prior to adolescence. Thus, gender differences may not be remarkable in young samples. In a study of 298 bipolar patients under the age of 18, Biederman and colleagues (2004a) found few significant differences in clinical features between males and females, although males were more likely to have ADHD as well as bipolar disorder; they were also less likely to have a chronic course. On the other hand, it is possible that this gender distribution in research samples signals under-recognition of mania in girls, inasmuch as they tend to be less aggressive and therefore may not attract as much attention as boys exhibiting destructive and risk-taking behaviors. Also, girls' initial mood disorder may more often be depression rather than mania. Therefore, developmental studies of bipolar disorder and manic symptoms need to address gender-relevant manifestations.

Current Suggestions for Assessment and Diagnosis of Bipolar Disorder in Children

In view of the varied opinions and relative paucity of data on assessment and diagnosis of bipolar disorder in children—and mindful of the high stakes involved in terms of accurate detection and early treatment—the National Institute of Mental Health (NIMH) convened the Bipolar Child Research Roundtable in 2000 (NIMH Research Roundtable on Prepubertal Bipolar Disorder, 2001) to share information and make recommendations. The roundtable members recommended that children who clearly meet current DSM-IV criteria for symptoms of bipolar-I or bipolar-II disorder—including core symptoms of grandiosity and/or elation (e.g., Geller et al., 2000a)—be distinguished from those with heterogeneous presentations who do not meet the full criteria but suffer from mood and behavior disturbances (prototypically, irritability or rage episodes) and severe impairment and *may* have bipolar disorder (e.g., Carlson et al., 1998; Biederman et al., 2000b). It was recommended that the latter be diagnosed as bipolar–not otherwise specified (NOS). The roundtable members noted that both of these groups are likely to have mixed states, chronic symptomatology, or long episodes with ultradian or continuous cycling. They speculated that many if not most suspected cases of bipolar disorder in children would be diagnosed bipolar-NOS, with a minority representing classic bipolar-I disorder. They also recommended that children be evaluated by clinicians who are well trained in mood disorders in youth, although there is a scarcity of such training (e.g., Coyle et al., 2003). The *Treatment Guidelines for Children and Adolescents with Bipolar Disorder,* published by the Child Psychiatric Workgroup on Bipolar Disorder, additionally stresses the importance of interviewing at least one parent, and ideally both; obtaining comprehensive school and medical histories; and encouraging family members to keep daily logs of the child's mood, energy, sleep, and unusual behaviors in the 2 weeks before the first visit to the clinician (Kowatch et al., 2005).

Leibenluft and colleagues (2003b) have suggested even further distinctions to improve the validation of diagnostic criteria for childhood bipolar disorder, proposing a phenotypic system of four categories ranging from narrow- to broadband subtypes. Their narrow phenotype includes the classic hallmark symptoms (e.g., elevated mood, grandiosity) and full-duration episodes. This phenotype is distinct from ADHD, despite overlapping symptoms, because ADHD is not episodic, and the associated symptoms occur only during hypomanic or manic episodes. At the broadest end of the spectrum, the system includes many children who are currently labeled as bipolar but do not meet criteria for the authors' narrower definitions. These children have severe mood and behavioral dysregulation, chronic hyperarousal, and negative reactivity to emotional stimuli, including severe rages, with no intervening periods of normal mood or adaptive functioning. Between these narrow and broad extremes lie two intermediate phenotypes: (hypo)mania-NOS, including hallmark symptoms but short episodes (although lasting at least 1 to 3 days), and irritable (hypo)mania, lacking elevated or expansive mood but with distinct episodes that meet DSM-IV duration criteria. Thus far, however, there are limited data to support these distinctions. Whether the proposal of Leibenluft and colleagues proves useful or not, it clearly addresses the crucial need for more homogeneous research samples that can help clarify and validate the construct of bipolar disorder in children.

Course of Disorder

Children diagnosed with bipolar disorder typically do not display course features commonly associated with classic bipolar disorder in adults, such as distinct mood episodes that endure for days or weeks (often clearly manic or depressive) separated by periods of being relatively well. Instead, bipolar children frequently display mixed mood states, extremely rapid cycling, and chronic psychopathology. The controversy over diagnostic criteria, including duration of episodes in children with purported bipolar disorder, is discussed further below.

Faraone and colleagues (1997b) found mixed states in 59 percent of children diagnosed with bipolar disorder, while Geller and colleagues (2002a) reported a rate of 55 percent. Geller's group (2002b) found that 87 percent of their sample had ultradian cycles (variation within a 24-hour period). Moreover, these children were chronically ill and

had been mood-disordered for an average of more than 3 years before entering the study. Craney and Geller (2003) concluded that typical youngsters with childhood-onset bipolar disorder in their sample were more severely ill than typical individuals with young adult–onset mania, and much more likely to display mixed mania, ultradian cycling, psychosis, and treatment resistance. Biederman and colleagues (2004a) found that the course of pediatric bipolar disorder was severe and chronic and was frequently characterized by severely impaired psychosocial functioning; they also observed chronic symptomatology in their bipolar–ADHD sample (Biederman et al., 1998). A prospective follow-up study of pediatric bipolar disorder in 22 boys with comorbid ADHD found that although 50 percent had remitted from the full syndrome of bipolar disorder at follow-up, 80 percent had failed to attain functional remission or euthymia over a course of 10 years (Biederman et al., 2004a). The course of the disorder, the investigators concluded, was "chronic, protracted, and dysfunctional" (p. 521). Many other investigators also have found that early onset of bipolar illness is associated with a poorer course (Carlson et al., 2002; Schneck et al., 2004; Birmaher et al., 2006). Some have argued that there may be periods of exacerbation of manic symptoms despite interepisode persistence of less severe mania, as is the case for many adult bipolar patients (Staton and Lysne, 1999).

Longitudinal research on the course of the disorder among carefully diagnosed bipolar children is sparse and greatly needed. Geller and colleagues (2000a) found 1-year mania recovery rates of 37 percent in their combined sample of youngsters with childhood- and early-adolescent–onset bipolar disorder, and substantial relapse rates within the year among those who recovered. At 2-year follow-up, the recovery rate was 65 percent, but 55 percent of those who had recovered relapsed (Geller et al., 2002a; Craney and Geller, 2003).

Thus the few outcome studies of childhood bipolar illness that exist indicate a highly pernicious course with substantial chronicity. Findling and colleagues (2001), for example, found that none of the 56 bipolar-I children they studied had interepisode recovery (defined as a 2-month period of remission of affective symptoms). Further longitudinal research is needed, however, to learn more about long-term course and outcome in children and their predictors, as well as to resolve some of the perplexing diagnostic issues in childhood bipolar disorder discussed above.

ADOLESCENT-ONSET BIPOLAR DISORDER

The onset and first diagnosis of bipolar disorder frequently occur in adolescence. For the most part, adolescent-onset bipolar disorder is clinically similar to adult bipolar disorder. Until recently, however, relatively little research had been conducted in adolescent populations.

Despite current awareness, adolescent bipolarity often was not recognized as such in the past. Diagnostic errors were common, reflecting biases of the time. These biases included the above-noted reluctance to accept the existence of youthful onset of bipolar disorder and a common tendency to assume that psychotic symptoms such as thought disorder, grandiosity, and bizarre delusional and hallucinatory phenomena are pathognomonic of schizophrenia (Carlson and Goodwin, 1973). Additionally, morbid preoccupations, frenzied behavior, moodiness or rapid mood swings, irritability, defiance, and a host of other disturbances were often regarded as exaggerations, if not typical manifestations, of adolescence. As discussed earlier, moreover, even when recognized as clearly pathological, disturbed behaviors in youths have been difficult to distinguish from alcohol and drug abuse disorders, conduct and other disruptive behavior disorders, and personality disorders. These diagnostic challenges remain today.

In recent years, however, several factors have contributed to the increased recognition and accurate diagnosis of adolescent bipolar disorder. These factors include greater awareness of the existence of severe mood pathology in adolescents, improved diagnostic criteria and interview methods for identifying depression and mania in younger populations, and increased availability of effective pharmacological and psychotherapeutic treatments for mood disorders. Increasingly, adult diagnostic criteria are being applied reliably and effectively to the diagnosis of bipolar disorder in adolescents. There is a general consensus that adolescent-onset bipolar disorder is a relatively common presentation and that, as noted, it essentially resembles the disorder in adults.

Symptoms and Clinical Presentation

Diagnosis

Adolescent onset of bipolar-I disorder may first present with major depression, mania, or a mixed state. The diagnosis is typically defined by DSM-IV criteria or by equivalent criteria used for adults (see Chapter 3; see also McClellan and Werry, 1997; Lewinsohn et al., 2003). Manic episodes, of course, provide the most unambiguous indicator of bipolar disorder. Symptoms such as elated mood, grandiosity, excessive activity, decreased need for sleep, hypersexuality, and racing thoughts are similar in both adolescents and adults, with differences only in developmental presentation. Geller and Luby (1997), for example, described grandiose beliefs in adolescents who, despite a lack of talent, believe they can become a rock star; whose excessive

activity takes the form of making curtains, illustrating a book, rearranging furniture, and making multiple phone calls all within a relatively brief period; or whose reduced need for sleep may take the form of sneaking out and partying all night. Engagement in high-risk pleasurable activities may involve a heightened interest in sex and risky sexual experiences, excessive spending through the use of parents' credit cards, taking dares, or driving more recklessly than their peers.

The assessment of bipolar illness in adolescents can be complicated. Tillman and colleagues (2004) found poor concordance between the symptom descriptions given by parents and offspring. Children and adolescents, for example, report the presence of racing thoughts and decreased need for sleep significantly more than do their parents, perhaps reflecting the reality that external and disruptive behaviors are more likely to be noted by parents. Other investigators have found high rates of bipolar spectrum in young people with recurrent depression (Smith et al., 2005), findings consistent with those of studies showing that adults with bipolar disorder tend to underreport hypomanic symptoms and impairment (Angst et al., 2003; Judd and Akiskal, 2003; Youngstrom et al., 2004). Supplemental assessment measures, such as the General Behavior Inventory and the Young Mania Rating Scale, add to diagnostic validity (Youngstrom et al., 2001, 2003; Findling et al., 2002). (See Chapter 11 for a more detailed discussion.)

Manic Features

Although the phenomenology of adolescent-onset mania has been studied incompletely, existing research clearly indicates a heterogeneity that may reflect different subgroups. Pooled data from several investigations of mania in adolescents have revealed pressured speech, euphoria, and hyperactivity to be the most common symptoms, similar to what has been found for adults (Faedda et al., 1995). Lewinsohn and colleagues (1995) noted a much higher frequency of elevated–expansive mood than irritability in their community sample (which, however, consisted primarily of those with bipolar spectrum rather than bipolar-I disorder). Faraone and colleagues (1997b), on the other hand, found relatively high rates of irritability and low rates of euphoria in their clinical sample of young manic patients. Both the Lewinsohn and Faraone subjects reported high rates of increased activity, grandiosity, and distractibility.

In an analysis of the symptoms of mania in 115 adolescents with manic or subsyndromal manic episodes, Lewinsohn and colleagues (1995) identified two factors: (1) behavioral disorganization, consisting of decreased need for sleep, flight of ideas, distractibility, and poor judgment; and (2) inflated self-esteem and increased activity. The former factor was correlated more highly than the latter with functional impairment (school, family, and social), and the authors speculated that individuals scoring high on this factor might be more likely to experience psychotic symptoms during severe manic episodes. Even in adolescents with only subthreshold bipolar disorder, Lewinsohn and colleagues (2003) noted substantial impairment, comorbidity, and increased risk of suicide attempts (18 percent, compared with 3 percent in never mentally ill controls).

Mania in adolescents often includes psychotic features (see Chapter 2). Several studies have found that between one third and one half of adolescent bipolar patients have prominent psychotic symptoms.[5] Kafantaris and colleagues (1998) found that half of the bipolar youths in their study who presented with psychotic mania had no prior psychiatric history and appeared to have experienced an acute onset after having functioned relatively well to that point. The authors suggested that this sudden-onset, psychotic subgroup may represent "classic" bipolar disorder. A recent study of 43 bipolar adolescents found that, in most, the prodromal onset was either slow with gradual deterioration (47 percent) or slow with quick worsening (39 percent). Rapid onset of illness was relatively uncommon (14 percent) (Correll et al., 2005). There is suggestive evidence that there are ethnic differences in psychotic features expressed during mania. A recent study compared clinical features in 17 bipolar African American adolescents and 61 bipolar Caucasian adolescents. Fully 90 percent of the African Americans had psychotic symptoms, as compared with only 30 percent of the Caucasian adolescents (p < .001) (Patel et al., 2006). These results are consistent with differences found between Caucasian and African American adult bipolar patients (Strakowski et al., 1996; Kirovetal, 1999).

Mixed mania and rapid-cycling mania are also common in those adolescents with bipolar disorder. Kutcher and colleagues (1998) studied a small, carefully ascertained clinical sample of 28 bipolar-I youths and found that the majority had mixed mania (74 percent), rapid cycling (76 percent), or both during their first (retrospectively assessed) episode. Fewer than 10 percent of the sample demonstrated a classic euphoric mania during their initial manic episode. Mixed episodes were reported by Faraone and colleagues (1997b) in 71 percent of a sample of 17 patients with adolescent onset of mania. McElroy and colleagues (1997) found that adolescents with bipolar disorder had a higher frequency of mixed episodes than was the case among comparison adult bipolar patients, but the investigators did not distinguish between childhood and adolescent onset in their adolescent sample. Findling and colleagues (2001) compared 56 children and 34 adolescents with bipolar-I disorder and found that 56 percent of the adolescents had rapid cycling and 21 percent mixed states; proportions among children with bipolar-I disorder were similar. However, many of the adolescents with bipolar disorder in that study appeared to have had childhood onset. Finally, Strober and colleagues (1995) reported that the index episode in their inpatient sample (which was the first episode in 56 percent of the cases studied) was mixed in 19 percent and rapid cycling in 19 percent, with the other cases being "pure" depression or mania. An unresolved issue is whether rapid cycling or mixed states are particularly associated with bipolar adolescents with childhood onset, a typical developmental manifestation of bipolar illness in young people, or a subtype of bipolar-I disorder marking a course that may differ from more "classic" cycling episodes.

Depressive Features

For a substantial number if not the majority of individuals with adolescent-onset bipolar disorder, the illness starts with depression, thereby delaying recognition and diagnosis of the bipolar course. Kutcher and colleagues (1998) found that depressions were the first affective episodes in 75 percent of their sample of adolescents with bipolar-I disorder. Likewise, a community sample of adolescents with bipolar spectrum disorders revealed that 61 percent had experienced an initial depressive episode before mania or hypomania occurred (Lewinsohn et al., 1995). And among those who responded to a volunteer survey of members of the National Depressive and Manic-Depressive Association (now called the Depression and Bipolar Support Alliance), both early age at onset (childhood or adolescence) and female gender were associated with higher rates of initial depressive symptoms or both depressive and manic symptoms (Lish et al., 1994). The studies of Kutcher and colleagues (1998) and Lewinsohn and colleagues (1995) did not evaluate initial symptom presentation by gender status.

The switch rate of adolescent major depression to eventual mania or hypomania is quite variable across studies. Interpretation of this variation is complicated by the above-noted common practice of mixing children and adolescents in the same study samples. For instance, in a review of seven studies of more than 250 depressed children and adolescents followed for 2 to 4 years, Faedda and colleagues (1995) found a mean rate of switch from depression to eventual mania of about 25 percent. A review by Kovacs (1996) yielded a switch range of 8 to 37 percent; her own longitudinal study of 92 depressed children followed for 5 to 10 years yielded a rate of 21 percent. More recently, Birmaher and colleagues (2006) conducted a 2-year prospective study of 263 children and adolescents (mean age 13 years) with bipolar-I (n=152), bipolar-II (n=19), and BP-NOS (n=92). Of the bipolar-II subjects, 21 percent converted to bipolar-I; 20 percent of the bipolar-NOS subjects converted to bipolar I, and 10 percent converted to bipolar-II. Females were more likely to convert than males (odds ratio, 3.2; 95 percent confidence interval [CI] 1.33–7.50). The findings are of considerable interest but somewhat difficult to interpret because of the mixed age range of the sample. Such variations in rates of switching among studies may depend on the mean age and age ranges of the sample, the diagnostic criteria used, the ascertainment source (that is, whether the study involved community, outpatient, or inpatient populations), and the extent to which the initial depressive episode was treated with antidepressants (see Chapter 23). In contrast to the high switch rate in Kovacs' childhood sample, for instance, Weissman and colleagues (1999a) revisited 10 to 15 years later an outpatient sample that had been diagnosed with major depression during adolescence, and found that only 4.1 percent had developed bipolar-I disorder and 1.4 percent bipolar-II disorder. As discussed earlier, severe depression during childhood (rather than adolescence) may portend higher rates of eventual bipolarity (e.g., Geller et al., 1994).

Further studies are needed not just on adolescent depression switch rates, but also on characteristics that link adolescent and childhood depression to eventual bipolar disorder (e.g., State et al., 2002). Strober and Carlson (1982) studied 60 inpatient depressed adolescents and identified several features predictive of eventual bipolarity: rapid onset of the depressive episode, psychomotor retardation, psychotic features, family history of mood disorders (especially bipolar), and antidepressant-related onset of mania or hypomania. It should be noted, however, that a recent study of switching during a 2-year period among adults with first-onset psychotic depression showed no association of switching with medication use, earlier age at onset, or family history of bipolar disorder (DelBello et al., 2003). A 15-year follow-up study of 74 young adults hospitalized for major depression (average age 23) found that 27 percent of the study group had experienced at least one episode of hypomania and another 19 percent an episode of mania (Goldberg et al., 2001). Psychosis during the depressive episode was significantly correlated with a switch into manic states (see Chapter 19). Predicting bipolar switching in cases of adolescent depression is an important area for further study because of speculation that treatment with antidepressant medications in the absence of knowledge of underlying bipolarity precipitates switches from depression to mania or hypomania and predicts a more adverse course of bipolar disorder with rapid cycling (see Chapter 19).

Depressive symptoms in adolescents with bipolar disorder tend to be quite similar to those seen in adults, although psychotic features are more common in the younger age group (Carlson and Strober, 1979; Chambers et al., 1982; Friedman et al., 1983). Preoccupation with death and thoughts of suicide are common, and suicide attempts are frequent (see Box 6–2 for one 15-year-old bipolar girl's account of her experience during a suicidal depression). Lewinsohn and colleagues (2003), for example, found that 44 percent of the bipolar adolescents in their sample had attempted suicide; in comparison, 22 percent of the adolescents with major depression had attempted suicide, as had 18 percent of those with subsyndromal bipolar disorder syndrome (defined by the investigators as abnormally and persistently elevated, expansive, or irritable mood plus one other DSM-III-R manic symptom, but never having met criteria for full bipolar disorder).

Course of Disorder

Longitudinal studies of youths with bipolar-I disorder are rare; therefore, most data on the course of the illness come from retrospective accounts or short-term treatment outcome studies (e.g., Kafantaris et al., 1998; Kutcher et al., 1998). The latter studies certainly document the likelihood of further episodes and hospitalizations, but more information is needed to clarify the predictors of relatively better or worse outcomes and responsiveness to treatment in patients with adolescent onset.

Strober and colleagues (1995) conducted one of the few longitudinal studies, a 5-year naturalistic follow-up of 54 adolescents (mean age 16.0) who had been inpatients diagnosed with bipolar-I disorder (although age at first diagnosable episode was not reported). The rate of recovery from the index episode was high (96 percent), with only 2 of the patients failing to achieve recovery during the 5-year period. However, time to recovery was affected by the polarity of the index episode: median time to recovery was significantly longer for those who had pure depressive episodes (26 weeks) compared with those who had pure manic (9 weeks) or mixed (11 weeks) episodes. The majority (56 percent) of those who recovered remained free of major relapses during the follow-up period, and the probability of relapse did not vary by polarity of the index episode (although among those who had multiple relapses, most had mixed or cycling index episodes). Suicide attempts sufficient to require medical attention occurred in 20 percent of the adolescents during the 5-year follow-up (Strober et al., 1995). None of the clinical or demographic factors that were evaluated in the study significantly predicted relapse, and all participants were treated aggressively. Thus it is important to note that the information on course derived from this study cannot be generalized to untreated bipolar disorder in adolescents.

BOX **6–2.**   **Drowning in My Personal Hell**

I'm being plunged into dark and murky waters
Someone or something is holding me there
I can't see—everything is black
I try to swim, to get away, back to the top, but the force
    is holding me too tight
Reluctantly I give up
I feel myself slipping down
Down, down, I am slipping down
My head aches with the pressure, but I keep sinking
With each inch, I grow colder
With each second, my lungs grow tighter
I pray to God to save me
There is no answer
I am deep now, buried under the layers of the sea
The water seems to be eating me
I wonder if I have entered Hell
All I want is to die
I want to relieve the pressure, the cold, the dark
I've already lost myself
My self is looking at me from above
She is miles from me
She is happy—she was me, but no more
It doesn't matter anymore
I'm not mad, not sad or scared
I am no one; I am nothing
I feel myself slipping down to the sea floor
And I watch shadows of the sun laugh at me as I die

—Katrina Skefos, 15-year-old girl with bipolar disorder. Reprinted with permission.

A 2-year prospective study of adolescent-onset psychotic disorders by McClellan and colleagues (1999) included a comparison of a small group of bipolar youths with patients who had schizophrenia. The results indicated that 50 percent of the bipolar youths had an episodic course, and 40 percent were chronically impaired (but fared significantly better than the schizophrenic youths). Rajeev and colleagues (2003) observed adolescent-onset patients with bipolar mania for 6 months; like Strober and colleagues (1995), but unlike McClellan and colleagues (1999), they found 96 percent recovery and very little chronicity. Recently, researchers at the University of Pittsburgh, Brown University, and the University of California-Los Angeles conducted a longitudinal study of 263 bipolar children and adolescents (13.0 ±3.1 years old); they interviewed their subjects on average every 35 weeks for 94.8 ±51.5 weeks using the Longitudinal Interval Follow-up Evaluation. Although two thirds of the subjects recovered

from the index episode, 50 percent had at least one syndromal recurrence (Birmaher et al., 2005b). Subjects were symptomatic for the majority (60 percent) of the follow-up period; almost one quarter (22 percent) of the time was spent in full syndromal episodes.

Additional research is needed on predictors of treatment responsiveness in bipolar adolescents (see Chapter 23). Moreover, given the potential for misdiagnosis of bipolar disorder in youths, further studies of the potentially adverse effects of antidepressant medications and stimulants used to treat ADHD are warranted (e.g., Soutullo et al., 2002).

Pre- and Postmorbid Adjustment and Functioning

Premorbid adjustment would appear to be an important clue to the possible presence of subclinical symptoms in childhood prior to the onset or diagnosis of bipolar disorder (see also Chapter 4). However, relatively few studies have reported information on prior adjustment. In the study by Kutcher and colleagues (1998), 90 percent of bipolar-I patients with adolescent onset had excellent or average peer relationships, and more than 60 percent had good to excellent academic achievement, before their diagnosis. Such findings suggest that many youths with adolescent-onset bipolar disorder have relatively good functioning before being diagnosed. In the study by McClellan and colleagues (1999), better premorbid functioning predicted higher levels of functioning over 2 years and was a more significant predictor than diagnosis in a sample of schizophrenic and bipolar adolescents.

Once initiated, however, the course of bipolar disorder in adolescents is associated with considerable impairment. Kutcher (2000) found that a bipolar-I adolescent-onset sample followed for a mean of 4.6 years after their initial manic episode had lower rates of high school graduation and lower full-scale IQ scores than those of unipolar and non-ill controls (see also Quackenbush et al., 1996). They also had significantly worse problems with peers and greater dissatisfaction with peer relationships than the comparison groups. Likewise, in a cross-sectional study that included adolescents with mania and distinguished between childhood and adolescent onset, Faraone and colleagues (1997a) found significantly worse functioning on most social, peer, recreational, and family variables, as well as school performance, among bipolar youths compared with normal controls. Few differences in functioning were observed between childhood- and adolescent-onset bipolar youths, except that manic adolescents generally had worse relationships with parents than did manic children. A recent comparison of 18 bipolar adolescents and 18 normal control subjects found that adolescents with bipolar

BOX 6–3.   One Adolescent's Experience with Bipolar Illness

The following is a first-person account of a hypomanic episode followed by severe depression in a 17-year-old girl. She went on to experience several further depressive and hypomanic episodes before becoming floridly manic in her 20s. This passage depicts the resilient recovery described by Carlson and Strober (1979), but it also underscores the disconcerting ability of some adolescents to continue the illusion of normal functioning even though seriously ill. It also illustrates many of the obscuring issues of adolescence and the effects of intense peer loyalties.

I was a senior in high school when I had my first attack of manic-depressive illness; once the siege began, I lost my mind rather rapidly. At first, everything seemed so easy. I raced about like a crazed weasel, bubbling with plans and enthusiasms, immersed in sports, and staying up all night, night after night, out with friends, reading everything that wasn't nailed down, filling manuscript books with poems and fragments of plays, and making expansive, completely unrealistic, plans for my future. The world was filled with pleasure and promise; I felt great. Not just great, I felt *really* great. I felt I could do anything, that no task was too difficult. My mind seemed clear, fabulously focused, and able to make intuitive mathematical leaps that had up to that point entirely eluded me. Indeed, they elude me still. At the time, however, not only did everything make perfect sense, but it all began to fit into a marvelous kind of cosmic relatedness. . . .

Unlike the very severe manic episodes that came a few years later and escalated wildly and psychotically out of control, this first sustained wave of mild mania was a light, lovely tincture of true mania; like hundreds of subsequent periods of high enthusiasms it was short-lived and quickly burned itself out; tiresome to my friends, perhaps; exhausting and exhilarating to me, definitely; but not disturbingly over the top. Then the bottom began to fall out of my life and mind. My thinking, far from being clearer than a crystal, was tortuous. I would read the same passage over and over again only to realize that I had no memory at all for

what I just had read. Each book or poem I picked up was the same way. Incomprehensible. Nothing made sense. I could not begin to follow the material presented in my classes, and I would find myself staring out the window with no idea of what was going on around me. It was very frightening. . . .

Each day I awoke deeply tired, a feeling as foreign to my natural self as being bored or indifferent to life. Those were next. Then a gray, bleak preoccupation with death, dying, decaying, that everything was born but to die, best to die now and save the pain while waiting. I dragged exhausted mind and body around a local cemetery, ruminating about how long each of its inhabitants had lived before the final moment. I sat on the graves writing long, dreary, morbid poems, convinced that my brain and body were rotting, that everyone knew and no one would say. Laced into the exhaustion were periods of frenetic and horrible restlessness; no amount of running brought relief. For several weeks, I drank vodka in my orange juice before setting off for school in the mornings, and I thought obsessively about killing myself. It was a tribute to my ability to present an image so at variance with what I felt that few noticed I was in any way different. Certainly no one in my family did. Two friends were concerned, but I swore them to secrecy when they asked to talk with my parents. One teacher noticed, and the parent of a friend called me aside to ask if something was wrong. I lied readily: I'm fine, but thank you for asking.

I have no idea how I managed to pass as normal in school, except that other people are generally caught up in their own lives and seldom notice despair in others if those despairing make an effort to disguise the pain. I made not just an effort, but an enormous effort not to be noticed. I knew something was dreadfully wrong, but I had no idea what, and I had been brought up to believe that you kept your problems to yourself. Given that, it turned out to be unnervingly easy to keep my friends and family at psychological bay.

Source: Jamison, 1995, pp. 36–39. Reprinted with permission.

disorder displayed significantly more deficits in social skills performance; however, no significant differences emerged between the groups in social skills knowledge (Goldstein et al., 2006).

Thus whereas some individuals with adolescent-onset bipolar disorder—especially those with severe childhood psychopathology—may have a relatively poor course of illness and adjustment, many cases of more "classic" bipolar disorder emerge in adolescence. Such individuals may have relatively favorable outcomes in the long run and adequate if not excellent adjustment in the short run (Carlson and Strober, 1979). Box 6–3 presents a first-person account of a posthypomanic depressive episode in an adolescent who, although she subsequently developed full-blown psychotic manias, went on to have good academic and social functioning.

Comorbidity

Comorbidity complicates the diagnostic and clinical picture of adolescent-onset bipolar disorder, as it does for childhood-onset illness. Tables 6–3 and 6–4, respectively, display the results of the major studies of comorbidity among adolescent-onset and combined samples of adolescent- and child-onset bipolar subjects. Nowhere is the question of the meaning of comorbidity more complex than with adolescent-onset bipolar disorder, because the co-occurrence of psychiatric syndromes can be due to several factors. There are, for example, indistinct diagnostic boundaries and overlapping symptoms. Irritability, impulsivity, and excessive activity, for instance, are symptoms shared by bipolar and other syndromes. Moreover, there is a causal relationship between bipolar illness and other disorders, in that symptoms of mania or depression may lead to substance or alcohol abuse. (Likewise, substance abuse can precipitate mood disorders.) Too, there are shared genetic or other risk factors, such as parental assortative mating, and similar or related genes may be implicated in both ADHD and bipolar disorder. Considerable research, including carefully designed longitudinal studies, is needed to help clarify the meaning of comorbid conditions in those with childhood- and adolescent-onset bipolar disorder.

Comorbid conditions that commonly complicate differential diagnosis include drug or alcohol abuse, conduct disorder, and ADHD, all of which may involve manic-like symptoms of irritability, disruptiveness, hostility, impulsiveness, distractibility, antisocial behaviors, and the like. Psychotic symptoms may be mistaken for schizophrenia, and drug and alcohol abuse may obscure and complicate the diagnosis of mania, depression, or mixed states.

Comorbidity with personality disorders may also complicate the diagnosis of bipolar disorder in adolescents. Although relatively few studies of Axis II disorders in bipolar youths have been conducted, this important topic should be pursued because personality pathology not only makes differential diagnosis potentially difficult; it also affects the interpretation of studies of course and treatment outcome. A small study by Kutcher and colleagues (1990), for example, revealed a rate of 15 percent for borderline personality disorder among euthymic bipolar adolescents, and the presence of that disorder predicted worse responsiveness to lithium. Mood instability, impulsiveness, an inclination to suicide, irritability, and other characteristics of borderline personality disorder represent a conceptual challenge in determining the boundary between severe mood disorder and personality pathology. Such issues are pursued in greater detail in Chapter 10. It

TABLE 6–3. Comorbidities in Samples of Bipolar Adolescents

Characteristic	Faraone et al., 1997 (teen outpatient)	Kafantaris et al., 1998 (teen inpatient)
Sample size	17	28
Source of sample	Outpatient psychopharmacology clinic	Adolescent inpatient treatment
Assessment used	KSADS	KSADS
Mean age (yrs)	15.8	15.8
% male	65	44
Comorbidities		
% ADHD	59	21
% ODD/CD	71/35	
% OCD	38	
% anxiety disorders	59	33
% substance abuse disorders	35	Specifically excluded
% psychosis	35	48
% no comorbidity	Not stated	31
% With >1 diagnosis	Probably high	Not stated

ADHD = attention-deficit hyperactivity disorder; KSADS = Kiddie Schedule for Affective Disorders and Schizophrenia; OCD = obsessive-compulsive disorder; ODD/CD = oppositional defiant disorder/conduct disorder.

Source: Updated from Geller et al., 1999. Reprinted with permission.

TABLE 6–4. Comorbidities in Combined Samples of Bipolar Children and Adolescents

Characteristic	Kowatch et al., 2000 (child and teen outpatient)	Frazier et al., 2001 (child and teen outpatient)
Sample size	42	23
Source of sample	Outpatient treatment study	Outpatient olanzapine trial
Assessment used	KSADS	KSADS
Mean age (yrs)	11	10.2
% Male	62	57
Comorbidities		
% ADHD	71	78
% ODD/CD	38/7	100/35
% OCD	Not stated	35
% anxiety disorders	17	57
% substance abuse disorders	2	Not stated
% psychosis	Not stated	44
% no comorbidity	Not stated	Not stated

ADHD = attention-deficit hyperactivity disorder; KSADS = Kiddie Schedule for Affective Disorders and Schizophrenia; OCD = obsessive-compulsive disorder; ODD/CD = oppositional defiant disorder/conduct disorder.

is likely that mood instability and cognitive and behavioral dysfunction due to bipolar disorder in childhood and adolescence contribute to the development of personality pathology.

Studies vary in the rates of comorbid diagnosis reported among individuals with adolescent-onset bipolar disorder. Lewinsohn and colleagues (1995, 2003) found high rates of comorbid anxiety disorders (33 percent), substance abuse, and disruptive behavior disorders (22 percent each), as well as ADHD (11 percent), in their community sample of youths with bipolar spectrum disorders. Kutcher and colleagues (1998) found that 61 percent of their adolescent-onset sample had no psychiatric diagnoses other than mood disorders; among those who did, generalized anxiety disorder (21 percent), ADHD (11 percent), and conduct disorder (11 percent) were observed most frequently. Findling and colleagues (2001) also observed high levels of comorbidity (76 percent overall, including 62 percent with ADHD) among adolescents with bipolar-I disorder (many of whom, however, probably had had childhood onset). ADHD as a comorbid condition is of particular interest, as discussed earlier, because of the problem of differential diagnosis, markedly different treatment strategies, and the possibility that comorbid ADHD may identify a genetic subtype and predict a worse course and poorer response to lithium (e.g., Strober et al., 1998).

A recent European study of 98 consecutively referred bipolar children and adolescents found that 38 percent were comorbid for ADHD (Masi et al., 2006). The mean age at onset for bipolar disorder was 10.0 ±3.2 years and for ADHD was 3.7 ±1.1 years. The bipolar patients with comorbid ADHD were predominantly male (73 percent) and younger, had an earlier age at onset of their bipolar illness (8.1 ±2.8 years versus 11.1 ±2.9 years, p <.000), were more likely to exhibit a chronic rather than episodic course (67 versus 33 percent), were more likely to have irritable rather than elated mood (62 versus 36 percent), and were likely to have overall greater psychiatric impairment. As the authors of the study pointed out, these differences are important:

> An identification of ADHD may help to identify a specific subgroup of patients, with a more homogeneous course, outcome, and response to treatments. From a neurobiological standpoint, the identification of common biological pathways may help to more deeply define the links in the pathophysiology of both disorders, which are still under question. (p. 380) (see also Geller et al., 2006)

Neurodevelopmental Aspects of Adolescent Bipolar Disorder and the Issue of Puberty

Many studies use the term "prepubertal" or "pubertal" onset, but the vast majority have neither verified the pubertal status of research participants nor articulated a model of early-onset bipolar disorder in which "puberty" plays a role in pathophysiology. The issue is important, however, given the frequent onset of bipolar disorder in adolescence, apparently after pubertal changes.

A neurodevelopmental emphasis has emerged in the field of schizophrenia (e.g., Lenzenweger and Dworkin, 1998), helping to identify early markers of neurocognitive impairment that are predictive of eventual schizophrenia, as well as to generate etiological models pertinent to abnormal brain development. Benes (1999) and others have noted the significance of puberty for the development of neural circuits that are relevant to mental disorders. Walker (2002), for example, explored the role played by hormones in neuromaturation, speculating that vulnerability to mental disorders such as schizophrenia, severe depression, and bipolar illness is mediated in part by the effects of hormones on gene expression. Further research on the development of the brain and on the role of pubertal changes in neurodevelopmental processes might help clarify whether pubertal effects are indeed significant in triggering underlying vulnerabilities to bipolar disorder.

A small body of research has begun to emerge on the neurocognitive, neuroanatomic, and neurochemical correlates of bipolar disorder in adolescents (e.g., Davanzo et al., 2003; DelBello et al., 2004; see also Chapters 9, 14, and 15). Sigurdsson and colleagues (1999), for example, reviewed chart notes for a sample of bipolar adolescents and found significantly greater evidence of delays in linguistic, social, and motor development among bipolar youths compared with those with early-onset unipolar depression, and especially among those who developed psychotic symptoms. Although the neurodevelopmental differences were relatively general and nonspecific, these findings are compatible with the hypothesis that such impairments are indicators of neurocognitive vulnerability factors for bipolar disorder. A growing literature suggests that bipolar youths are more likely than controls to demonstrate impairment on a wide variety of neuropsychological measures, including executive functioning, sustained attention, and working memory (Dickstein et al., 2004; Meyer et al., 2004; Doyle et al., 2005). These deficits, in turn, contribute to substantial academic difficulties (Pavuluri et al., 2006). There is accumulating evidence that comorbid ADHD significantly contributes to the cognitive deficits (McClure et al., 2005; Rucklidge, 2006).

In related work, Friedman and colleagues (1999) conducted a magnetic resonance imaging (MRI) study of adolescent bipolar and schizophrenic patients compared with non-ill youths. They found few differences among the patient groups, but the schizophrenic and bipolar youths differed significantly from normal controls on various measures, including reduced intracranial volume and increased frontal sulcal prominence, among others. These results are consistent with neurodevelopmental abnormalities and

raise many intriguing questions for further study (see also Botteron et al., 1995, and the review by Todd and Botteron, 2002). It should be noted, however, that such studies need to verify age at onset and clarify whether state or trait markers of disorder are being identified. Recent studies by Blumberg and colleagues (2003a, 2003b) found that adolescents with bipolar illness show decreased volumes of medial temporal lobe structures (with greater effect sizes in the amygdala than in the hippocampus) and signal increases in the subcortical portions of the frontal striatal circuits. Additional discussion on the need to pursue potential markers of neurodevelopmental vulnerability for bipolar disorder is presented in our later review of the offspring of bipolar parents (see also Chapters 13, 14, and 15).

EPIDEMIOLOGY OF BIPOLAR DISORDER IN CHILDREN AND ADOLESCENTS

Three problems limit understanding of the prevalence of bipolar disorder in young populations: epidemiologic surveys encompassing children and adolescents have been rare (see Chapter 5); few have included bipolar disorder as an object of inquiry; and in most of the studies that are available, data have not been presented separately for children and adolescents or specified age at onset.

Chapter 5 (see especially Table 5–13) presents the results of community-based epidemiologic studies that have included children and adolescents, and those findings are not duplicated here. The sparse data available from representative community and psychiatric samples illustrate several patterns that are generally accepted and confirmed by clinical studies. First, childhood bipolar-I disorder is rare in community samples (although, of course, more prevalent in clinical samples). Second, bipolar disorder occurs among adolescents at about the same rate as in the general adult population. Third, subsyndromal forms of bipolar disorder can be identified in child and adolescent samples, and can reflect prodromal or stable dimensional traits of the bipolar spectrum that may be associated with impairment of functioning.

Some have asserted that the frequency of bipolar disorder in youngsters is increasing. There has been some evidence that rates of childhood- or adolescent-onset bipolar disorder have increased in more recent cohorts (e.g., Rice et al., 1987; Chengappa et al., 2003; Kessler et al., 2005) and that this increase is not due to increased ascertainment alone. It is difficult to determine the validity and generalizability of this conclusion, however, given the lack of epidemiologic surveys with comparable data over time, as well as the lack of consistent diagnostic criteria. Moreover, increasing rates of apparent mania in clinical samples of children and adolescents may reflect methodological matters, such as age-related changes in awareness and memory, temporal changes in morbidity and sample availability, and diagnostic practices (see Chapter 5).

At the same time, it has been argued that changes in health practices and environmental factors may induce earlier expression of bipolar disorder—or actual increased rates of bipolarity. Such factors may include widespread and increased use of stimulant and antidepressant medications (e.g., Zito et al., 2002) that could trigger bipolar rapid-cycling patterns in susceptible children or decrease the age at onset (DelBello et al., 2001); alcohol and drug use at younger ages, possibly inducing earlier onset of bipolar symptomatology; earlier onset of puberty; and exposure to maternal health risks during pregnancy (e.g., smoking, drug and alcohol intake, dietary reductions in omega-3 fatty acids, social stressors). Also, as noted in Chapter 13, genetic anticipation effects may promote earlier onset. These issues are clearly important, with critical implications for etiology and treatment, and require further study.

IMPLICATIONS OF CHILDHOOD AND ADOLESCENT ONSET OF BIPOLAR DISORDER

Other chapters in this volume address some of the implications of the onset of bipolar disorder in childhood and early adolescence, including effects of age at onset on course (Chapter 4), epidemiology and the possibility of cohort changes in age at onset (Chapter 5), genetic implications of early onset (Chapter 13), and treatment considerations (Chapter 23). A few important issues merit emphasis here, however, including the implications of childhood and adolescent onset for treatment and prevention.

Clinical Implications

Even apart from the goal of validating the diagnostic features of childhood bipolar disorder, it is important to study whether the outcomes and features of childhood-onset cases of the disorder differ from those of adolescent- and adult-onset cases. If, as discussed earlier, childhood onset reflects a particularly virulent form of the disorder, then relatively chronic symptomatology, mixed-state episodes, and rapid cycling might be expected to continue. It is possible, however, that such atypical features reflect developmental manifestations of nonspecific severe dysregulation, with maturity revealing a more recognizable episodic course with relatively better interepisode functioning. To answer this question, relevant longitudinal studies would need to separate out the effects on course and functioning that are due to comorbid childhood psychopathology—and indeed, to determine whether such

clinical conditions reflect true cases of multiple disorders or diffuse, severe bipolar symptomatology.

Preliminary studies suggest that early onset may indeed portend a worse course. Unfortunately, these studies do not always differentiate childhood from adolescent onset. Carlson and colleagues (2000) found that early-onset psychotic manic patients (onset before 21 years of age) had significantly poorer recovery between episodes, more manic episodes, and more time in the hospital during 2-year follow-up as compared with later-onset psychotic manic patients. Early-onset patients also were more likely than later-onset patients to have mixed episodes. The early-onset patients were significantly more likely to be male, high school dropouts, and never married. In a subsequent study of the same sample, Carlson and colleagues (2002) performed a separate analysis for the effects of "early onset" of bipolar disorder and comorbid childhood psychopathology. They determined that the two factors had somewhat independent effects in predicting outcome, with childhood disorders being more likely to predict poor functional outcome and early age at bipolar onset being related to continuing symptoms.

Similarly, Schurhoff and colleagues (2000) found that a group of bipolar patients with early onset (before age 18) was significantly more impaired, had more psychotic features, and had poorer response to lithium prophylaxis than a group with late onset (after age 40). Also, the early-onset group had more first-degree relatives with bipolar disorder. These findings are consistent with those of the above-noted retrospective self-report volunteer survey of members of the National Depressive and Manic-Depressive Association (Lish et al., 1994). Those who reported early (childhood/adolescent) onset (60 percent) were compared with adult-onset respondents on various indicators of functioning. Onset in childhood and adolescence was associated with significantly greater likelihood of social morbidity, as indicated by dropping out of school, financial difficulties, marital problems, being unmarried, alcohol and drug abuse, injury to self or others, and minor crime. Those with early onset also reported significantly more recurrent bipolar illness. Statistical analyses indicated that the effects on social morbidity were due to independent contributions by frequency of recurrences and early onset. Those with early-onset bipolar disorder reported that their initial symptoms were more likely to be depressive than manic and that their recurrences were predominantly depressive as well.

Neither the study of Schurhoff and colleagues (2000) nor the National Depressive and Manic-Depressive Association survey evaluated effects of childhood comorbid disruptive disorders. However, this is an important consideration in interpreting the effects of early age at onset, because those conditions may confound the results of such analysis, with outcomes perhaps being attributed inaccurately to bipolar disorder. A further consideration is that childhood or early-adolescent onset of bipolar disorder may cause later comorbid conditions (see the earlier discussion of comorbidity). For instance, Tohen and colleagues (1998) found that early age at onset, male gender, and the presence of mixed states predicted the development of substance abuse in bipolar patients (see Chapter 7).

Other methodological issues also need to be considered in studies of the effects of age at onset. As noted, few longitudinal studies exist; most data are therefore based on retrospective reports or short-term follow-up. Moreover, many studies have had small sample sizes. In addition, studies may differ as to whether they assess separately for psychotic features, effects of prior depressive histories and comorbid childhood disorders, and clinical presentation (such as mixed or cycling episodes)—all of which may affect prognosis. Despite these limitations, it appears that childhood and adolescent onset may portend greater functional impairment, and possibly a more difficult clinical course.

Implications for Treatment and Prevention

As noted elsewhere in this volume, two treatment issues are salient in considering the implications of childhood and early-adolescent onset of bipolar disorder (see Chapter 23). One is that misdiagnosis may worsen the course of bipolar illness. For instance, antidepressant-induced rapid cycling in adults may have a counterpart in children who have been erroneously diagnosed as having nonbipolar depression. It has been speculated that some cases of rapid or ultra-rapid cycling in children may stem from antidepressant treatment for depression—although the role of such treatments in this age group has not been thoroughly investigated. It has also been theorized that stimulants used to treat ADHD may worsen the course of bipolar disorder in children. Some have suggested that the widespread use of antidepressant and stimulant medications in U.S. children may have led to more cases of childhood onset of bipolar disorder in the United States than in European and other nations, where such medications are used less frequently in children (e.g., Reichart et al., 2000). These hypotheses require empirical validation, and in fact one review of the findings of preliminary studies casts doubt on notions of the negative impact of antidepressants and stimulants (e.g., Meyer et al., 2004). Further studies are vital to provide guidelines for maximally effective interventions for children with probable mood disorders.

The second treatment issue is the widely cited hypothesis that bipolar disorder is a progressive illness with neurobiological "kindling"—that is, episodes beget episodes (see, for example, Post, 2006, and Chapter 4). If this were in fact the case, vigorous early intervention with mood-stabilizing drugs to prevent episodes would have critical and positive implications for long-term outcome. The successful use of such interventions would then depend on research aimed at identifying the earliest valid markers of bipolar disorder. At the very least, early recognition and diagnosis of established cases could have important consequences for treatment and eventual course. These are not easy tasks, however. Underrecognition of childhood disorders and underutilization of treatment are rampant problems in public health, not limited to mood disorders.

STUDIES OF CHILDREN AT HIGH RISK

Children at risk for bipolar disorder as a result of parental bipolar illness represent an ideal sample for the study of potential antecedents (see Chapter 13 for a full discussion of the genetics of bipolar disorder). The high-risk methodology in psychopathological research—that is, the study of children of psychiatrically ill parents—has been employed productively for more than 25 years to accomplish several interrelated goals. First, examination of early signs of a disorder in offspring helps clarify the course of the illness from its initial expression to its unfolding over the course of development. Identification of early signs of bipolar disorder in a prospectively followed high-risk sample is an especially useful approach to validation of the developmental manifestations of symptomatology and establishment of diagnostic certainty. Second, assessment of putative markers of a disorder can help flag those who will eventually develop it, and thereby identify possible targets for early intervention (a potentially important accomplishment for children with bipolar disorder, as discussed earlier). Third, study of such markers and other environmental and contextual factors that influence children's development can help clarify the psychological processes by which possible genetic predispositions are, or are not, manifested as disorders.

Despite their usefulness, however, offspring studies of bipolar disorder have limitations. For one thing, these high-risk children represent a unique sample not necessarily generalizable to the entire population of bipolar probands. By definition, youngsters in families with a bipolar parent experience both the genetic risk (perhaps a uniquely strong one) and the environmental impact of living with such a parent. The challenge to researchers is to disentangle these interrelated factors. Eventually, more precise knowledge of genetic factors will yield a greater understanding of the contributions of psychological and environmental factors to bipolar outcomes among those at risk. At the same time, while the majority of current offspring studies, as designed, do not clarify genetic contributions as such, they do shed light on early signs of bipolar disorder in children and young adolescents.

There are numerous methodological obstacles to be overcome in studies of high-risk children, including issues of diagnosis (how broad a spectrum of bipolarity to include, how comorbid conditions should be conceptualized and analyzed), evaluation of outcomes, and assessment of the many factors in families with bipolar illness that contribute to children's adjustment. Too, because the age range for the onset of bipolar disorder extends over decades, a cross-sectional evaluation of children is likely to be misleading (some children diagnosed with major depression or ADHD, for example, may later convert to bipolarity). Moreover, sample sizes in many high-risk studies have been small, and interviewers have not been blind to parental diagnosis. Finally, the majority of high-risk studies of children having a parent with bipolar disorder were not specifically designed to assess early signs of bipolarity and thus may not have realized their full potential. Research on children at risk for bipolar disorder is less well advanced than is the case for other major disorders, such as schizophrenia or unipolar depression. The latter fields have produced intriguing insights into the neurodevelopmental and neurocognitive markers of schizophrenia and of family and psychosocial risk factors in depression. Studies of families at high risk for bipolar disorder, by contrast, have been less common and less methodologically sophisticated. However, this situation is changing rapidly with improved diagnostic methods, theoretical developments to guide the search for potential markers and risk factors and mechanisms of action, and increased interest among researchers and affected families alike in learning more about options for early intervention.

Recent and Direct-Interview Studies of Children of Bipolar Parents

Early offspring studies were unsystematic or methodologically limited but still contributed important evidence regarding the risk to children of bipolar parents. Information from these early studies is presented in Box 6–4. In the following sections, we summarize the results of more methodologically sophisticated work. Before proceeding, however, we must make clear that the term "children" of bipolar parents refers generally to both preadolescent and adolescent offspring; as with the early-onset literature generally, the results of the great majority of studies have not been separated out by age.

Clinical Outcomes in Controlled Studies

Table 6–5 summarizes numerous high-risk studies that we selected because they had comparison groups and used adequate measures for assessing children's clinical status.

Specifically, both the child and a parent were interviewed, using well-established structured or semistructured interview methods to assign diagnoses. Many of the studies were attentive to matching bipolar and comparison families on demographic factors, and several also included diagnostic information on the nonproband parent. These studies represent the current state of the art of research on the offspring of bipolar parents.

The studies are relatively consistent in reporting higher rates of lifetime diagnosis among children of bipolar parents compared with those of non-ill controls. The diagnoses include the full range of childhood mood, anxiety, and behavioral disorders. Most of the studies found that children of bipolar parents were particularly likely to display mood disorders—chiefly depression, but also forms of bipolar disorder. A recent study (Klimas-Dougan et al., 2006) found slightly increased rates of major depressive disorder in children of mothers who had bipolar disorder (12 percent) or major depression (17 percent) as compared with children of mothers who were psychiatrically well (8 percent). Much more striking, however, the children of bipolar mothers showed far more neurocognitive deficits—in executive functioning, perceptual memory, and sustained attention—than the children of either the unipolar or psychiatrically well mothers. There were no differences in verbal memory between the high-risk and control children.

Only a few investigators looked for sampled subclinical manifestations of bipolar illness. Decina and colleagues (1983) observed the presence of subclinical symptoms—including expansiveness, excitability, need for constant attention and admiration, need for reassurance, and other traits potentially suggestive of hyperthymic or depressive personality—in half of nondiagnosed offspring. Depressive traits were observed in a substantial proportion of children of bipolar parents by Grigoroiu-Serbanescu and colleagues (1991). Reichard and colleagues (2005) administered the General Behavior Inventory (GBI) and the Kiddie Schedule for Affective Disorders and Schizophrenia (KSADS) to 129 adolescents and young adult offspring of bipolar parents at initial assessment and 14 months later. At 5-year follow-up, both the GBI and the Structured Clinical Interview for DSM (SCID) were administered. The scores on the Depression scale of the GBI for the offspring who later developed bipolar disorder were significantly higher than those for the offspring who did not. For the offspring with unipolar depression at the first assessment, the scores on the Depression scale were significantly higher for those who converted to bipolar disorder than for those who did not. Carlson and Weintraub (1993) found that young-adult offspring of bipolar parents scored significantly higher on a scale rating of subsyndromal bipolarity than

BOX **6–4.** Early Studies of Children of Bipolar Parents

The earliest studies of the impact on children of having a bipolar parent either were uncontrolled observations with no systematic comparison groups or consisted of psychiatric comparisons in studies of children of schizophrenic patients. Typically, the clinical studies had very small samples, and the assessment of the children was conducted by investigators who were not blinded to the parents' diagnosis. Early methods of assessing children typically relied on unsystematic observations or parent reports, which may be biased. In addition, the initial studies were generally guided by the assumption that risk was due exclusively to genetic factors, so that family (and spousal) characteristics were largely unreported. Despite these limitations, however, intriguing patterns began to emerge.

The earliest high-risk studies were conducted on schizophrenic patients and often included a comparison group of parents with affective disorders or psychotic mood disorders. As a result of the use of earlier diagnostic frameworks, such as DSM-I or DSM-II, the affective disorder groups contained a mix of unipolar and bipolar families, and some of those diagnosed as schizophrenic may have been bipolar. The St. Louis High-Risk Study (e.g., Worland et al., 1979) and the Stony Brook High-Risk Project (Weintraub and Neale, 1984) included hospitalized depressed comparison subjects, both unipolar and bipolar. The Stony Brook sample represents what is probably the largest comparative high-risk study, involving 113 children of unipolar parents, 73 of bipolar parents, 57 of schizophrenic parents, and 297 of normal parents.

Other studies were well designed in terms of careful diagnostic evaluations and comparisons with at least one other normal or psychopathological group but were limited in their assessment of the children (e.g., parent report only, nondiagnostic methods) or had small samples. These included studies by Conners and colleagues (1979) comparing children of 16 bipolar and 43 "other psychopathology" (primarily unipolar depressed) groups, and those by Greenhill and colleagues (1980) reporting on offspring of 7 bipolar and 2 unipolar parents. Other studies did not include a comparison group: Kuyler and colleagues (1980) studied 49 children of 27 parents, and Waters and colleagues (1983) sampled adult offspring of 17 bipolar parents. Investigations by McKnew and colleagues (1979) and Cytryn and colleagues (1982) were forerunners of later well-designed work by Gershon and colleagues (1985), which is listed in Table 6–2 as an example of a good case-control study with direct diagnostic evaluations of children. A study by LaRoche and colleagues (1987) that included 37 offspring of 21 bipolar families is unique because it reported 3 to 7 years of follow-up data on the children.

Virtually all of these studies found high rates of psychiatric disorders among children of bipolar parents—higher than in normal comparisons or than would be expected in the general population. Most of the studies specifically indicated higher levels of affective disorders in offspring. Among the adult offspring studied by Waters and colleagues (1983), 9 (17 percent) of 53 had been diagnosed as bipolar by young adulthood. The LaRoche and colleagues (1987) follow-up, including offspring up to age 25, found that 24 percent had been diagnosed, mainly in the affective disorder spectrum. Two studies compared offspring of bipolar and unipolar parents. Conners and colleagues (1979) found higher rates of symptoms and disorders among the children of unipolar depressed parents, whereas offspring of unipolar and bipolar parents in the Stony Brook sample did not differ from each other but were significantly more symptomatic than children of non-ill controls (Weintraub, 1987).

Two additional studies from the 1980s are informative. Zahn-Waxler and colleagues (1988) compared 7 children of bipolar parents with 12 control children. The unique features of this investigation were the inclusion of infants studied up to age 5 or 6 years and the intensive study of family relationships and children's psychosocial development. The offspring of the bipolar parents displayed a range of behavioral and adjustment difficulties that persisted at follow-up. This study was eventually expanded as the Radke-Yarrow and colleagues (1992) investigation, which is reported in the text, along with the data yielded on toddler development and parent–child relations.

An investigation by Akiskal and colleagues (1985) focused on affective symptoms in referred children who were known to be offspring or siblings of adult bipolar patients. Although not a traditional high-risk study, the work was aimed at identifying possible signs and symptoms of bipolarity in youngsters at risk. Using the investigators' Mood Clinic Data Questionnaire, which included diagnostic criteria as well as subclinical symptoms, the study revealed several features characteristic of the sample. Onset of systems before puberty was rare, and all bipolar diagnoses occurred after puberty. Acute depressive episodes and dysthymic-cyclothymic disorders were the most common symptom patterns. By the end of 3 years of follow-up, bipolar outcomes were prominent: 19 (28 percent) of 68 children were bipolar-I, and 12 (18 percent) were bipolar-II; 2 were rapid cyclers, and 6 were cyclothymic. There were no signs of bipolarity in 43 percent of the children; the authors argued, however, that 7 of these children were "pseudo-unipolar" and potentially at risk for bipolarity, as suggested by pharmacological hypomania.

TABLE 6–5. High-Risk Studies with Comparison Groups and Direct Assessment of Children: Clinical Findings

	HIGH RISK		COMPARISON		ASSESSMENT	
Study	Parents	Children	Parents	Children	Method	Findings
Decina et al., 1983	11 BP-I, 7 BP-II (7 fathers, 11 mothers)	14 M, 17 F (ages 7–14)	14 with no disorder	10 M, 8 F (ages 7–14)	Direct interview of child and parent; semistructured interview with some KSADS items.	Significantly higher rates of mood disorders in bipolar offspring than in offspring of non-ill parents; 50% of bipolar offspring had some psychiatric diagnosis. Presence of subclinical affective symptoms suggestive of depressive or hyperthymic personality.
Klein et al., 1985	24 BP (11 fathers, 13 mothers)	19 M, 18 F (ages 15–21)	14 with psychiatric disorders (outpatient) (10 fathers, 4 mothers)	13 M, 9 F (ages 15–21)	Direct interview of child; structured interview (KSADS) modified to include cyclothymia.	Significantly higher rates of mood disorders (38%) in offspring sample compared with psychiatric sample (5%). High rate of cyclothymia (9 of 16 youths). Higher risk of mood disorders if mother bipolar.
Gershon et al., 1985	19 BP-I (sex unspecified) and spouses; (12 had unspecified diagnoses)	12 M, 17 F (ages 6–17)	22 with no disorder (sex unspecified)	16 M, 21 F (ages 6–17)	Direct interview of child and parent; structured interview (KSADS-E); used "NIMH criteria," similar to RDC.	3 (10%) of 29 offspring of bipolar parents had mania/hypomania vs. none for controls. Overall, 66% of offspring of bipolar parents vs. 43% of controls had some diagnosis. No significant effect of two ill parents.

(continued)

TABLE 6–5. High-Risk Studies with Comparison Groups and Direct Assessment of Children: Clinical Findings *(continued)*

| Study | HIGH RISK | | COMPARISON | | ASSESSMENT | |
	Parents	Children	Parents	Children	Method	Findings
Nurnberger et al., 1988	(1) 23 BP or schizoaffective (sex unspecified; one parent ill); (2) 9 families with two ill parents (both BP or schizoaffective, or one ill and the other with "loaded" family history of disorder; sex unspecified)	(1) 15 M, 23 F (ages 15–25); (2) 9 M, 6 F (ages 15–25)	39 with no disorder (sex unspecified)	18 M, 21 F (ages 15–25)	Direct interview of child; structured interview (SADS-L adapted for children).	67–74% of offspring of one or two ill parents had disorders vs. 31% of normal controls. Over 1- or 2-year follow-up, increased rates of disorder were found in offspring of bipolar parents, including major affective illness and affective spectrum disorders.
Grigoroiu-Serbanescu et al., 1989	28 BP-I mothers, 19 BP-I fathers; spouses (34 no disorder, 13 other disorder)	34 M, 38 F (ages 10–17)	61 couples with no disorder	34 M, 38 F (ages 10–17)	Direct interview of child and parent; structured interview (KSADS-E); reported point prevalence.	7 (10%) of 72 offspring had affective disorder (1 bipolar); there were also significantly higher rates of anxiety disorders, ADHD, and personality disorders than in control offspring. Severity of illness in offspring was related to severity of illness in parent and psychopathology in spouse of bipolar parent.
Hammen et al., 1990	14 BP mothers[a] and spouses (7 fathers with no disorder, others with varied disorders)	8 M, 10 F (ages 8–16)	(1) 16 unipolar mothers and spouses (5 fathers no disorder, others with varied disorder); (2) 14 medically ill	(1) 10 M, 12 F; (2) 9 M, 9 F; (3) 19 M, 19 F (all groups ages 8–16)	Direct interview of child and parent; structured interview (KSADS-E).	Rates of current and past affective and disruptive behavior disorders were significantly higher in unipolar and bipolar groups. Cumulative probability of major depression was .67 in

Study	Sample	Measures	Results
	mothers and spouses (5 fathers no disorder, others varied disorders); (3) 24 non-ill mothers and spouses (15 fathers with no disorder, others varied disorders)		unipolar, .33 in bipolar, .45 in medical, and .12 in non-ill groups through 3-year follow-up. By age 19, the cumulative probability of any significant diagnosis in bipolar offspring was .75 (.85 in unipolar group). Bipolar offspring had later age at onset.
Radke-Yarrow et al., 1992	22 BP mothers[b] (5 BP-I, 17 BP-II) and spouses (14 unipolar fathers, 8 fathers with no disorder) (1) 41 unipolar mothers[d] and spouses (22 fathers with depression or anxiety disorder, 19 fathers with no disorder); (2) 37 mothers with no disorder and spouses (37 fathers with no disorder)[c] Sibling pairs: 22 ages 1½–3½[c], 22 ages 5–8[b] (gender not specified, stated as "approximately equal" in each group) (1) Sibling pairs: 41 ages 1½–3½[c], 41 ages 5–8[c]; (2) sibling pairs: 37 ages 1½–3½[c], 37 ages 5–8[c]	Age <4 yr: psychiatric evaluation based on observation of standardized play sessions, mothers' reports on CBCL; age >4 yr: CBCL, structured interview of child (Child Assessment Scale), DSM-III criteria	Outcomes varied by children's age and maternal group, mother or psychiatrist report. Generally, children of bipolar and unipolar mothers were more likely than control children to have disruptive and depressive disorders. Offspring of bipolar mothers had later onset than those of unipolar mothers. No differences between groups with one and two ill parents.
Carlson and Weintraub, 1993 (follow-up of Weintraub and Neale, 1984)	134 children of BP parents originally studied at ages 7–16; follow-up of 125 after age 18 211 of 240 in original group of children of parents with unipolar depression, schizophrenia, substance abuse; 98 of 108 in original group of children of normal controls	Results reported on adult follow-up based on SCID interviews, DSM-III criteria.	4.8% of offspring of bipolar parents had definite bipolar disorder, 53% had some diagnosis overall. In childhood, 28% had behavior problems, 30% had attention problems (all significantly higher than normal controls but not "other" controls). Such problems predicted mood disorders in adulthood.

(continued)

TABLE 6–5. High-Risk Studies with Comparison Groups and Direct Assessment of Children: Clinical Findings (*continued*)

Study	HIGH RISK		COMPARISON		ASSESSMENT	
	Parents	Children	Parents	Children	Method	Findings
Todd et al., 1996	30 families selected because adult bipolar proband or proband's adult sibling was in bipolar pedigree study (NIMH Genetic Initiative Study); 12 parents affected: 8 BP-I, 1 BP-II, 3 unipolar depressed	Total sample across 30 families: 24 M, 26 F (ages 6–17); 23 offspring of affected families	18 sets of parents with no disorder	27 offspring of nonaffected families	Direct interview of child and parent, structured interview (Diagnostic Interview for Children and Adolescents–Revised) with revised mania sections.	9 offspring of 23 affected parents had affective disorder (including 5 bipolar), compared with 3 of 27 with unaffected parents.
Birmaher et al., 2005	132 BP: 56% BP-I, 36% BP-II, 8% BP-NOS or cyclothymia (79% mothers)	210: 49% F (average age = 12.0 yr)	79: 29% MDD, 9% dysthymia (90% mothers)	138: 57% F (average age = 11.5 yr)	Parental interview. Children assessed by KSADS-PL, K-MRS, KSADS-P. Family history obtained via FHRDC, DSM-IV diagnosis.	Offspring of BP parents showed 7.7-fold higher risk for any BP disorder, 4.0-fold risk for any mood disorder, and 2.2-fold risk for anxiety disorders.
Jones et al., 2006	19 BP-I, 1 BP-II (5 fathers, 15 mothers)	6 M, 19 F (ages 13–19)	19 with no disorder	6 M, 16 F (ages 13–19)	SADS-L, Self-report measures, actigraph, Social Rhythm Metric, diaries	Significantly higher rates of mood disorders in children of bipolar parents (CBP) (14/19) than in offspring of non-ill parents (CC) (2/19), p<.001. CBP had stronger ruminative coping styles and significantly greater self-esteem variation, but did not differ in positive affect. CBP exhibited shorter and less variable sleep latency.

212

Study	High-risk sample	Comparison sample	Measures	Findings
Klimas-Dougan et al, 2006	25 BP mothers[b] 37 MDD mothers[d] 43: 61% F (average age = 15.1 yr) 72: 64% F (average age = 16.0 yr)	26 psychiatrically well mothers 50: 48% females (average age = 15.3 yr)	Administered a battery of neuropsychological tests, including Wisconsin Card Sorting Test, Trail Making Test, California Verbal Learning Task, Continuous Performance Task, and WISC-R/WAIS	Lifetime MDD diagnosis: children of bipolar mother, 12%; MDD mother, 17%; well mother, 8%. Children of BP mothers exhibited deficits in executive functioning, perceptual memory, and sustained attention, but not in verbal memory. These deficits were not found in children of MDD mothers or in healthy control mothers.

[a] 3-year follow-up data reported here, with reduced sample numbers due to attrition (see Hammen et al., 1987, for initial results). Father data based on mothers' FHRDC reports; high rates of divorce in unipolar and bipolar families.

[b] n = 26 BP mothers reported later in study (Radke-Yarrow, 1998).

[c] 3-year follow-up also.

[d] n = 42 unipolar mothers reported later in study (Radke-Yarrow, 1998).

ADHD = attention-deficit hyperactivity disorder; BP = bipolar; BP-NOS = bipolar-not otherwise specified; CBCL = Child Behavior Checklist (Achenbach, 1991); F = female; FHRDC = Family History Research Diagnostic Criteria; K-MRS = Kiddie Mania Rating Scale; KSADS = Kiddie Schedule for Affective Disorders and Schizophrenia for School-Age Children; KSADS-E = KSADS-Epidemiological Version; KSADS-P = KSADS-Present State; KSADS-PL = KSADS-Present and Lifetime version; M = male; MDD = major depressive disorder; NIMH = National Institute of Mental Health; RDC = Research Diagnostic Criteria; SADS = Schedule for Affective Disorders and Schizophrenia; SADS-L = SADS-Lifetime; SCID = Structured Clinical Interview for DSM. WAIS = Wechsler Adult Intelligence Scale; WISC-R = Wechsler Intelligence Scale for Children-Revised.

Source: Updated from Geller et al, 1998a.

did the offspring of both normal and "other" parents. A study by Klein and colleagues (1985) is noteworthy for the development and testing of a scale specifically for cyclothymic symptoms; it was found that more than half of the offspring of bipolar parents who had a diagnosis of affective disorder met criteria for cyclothymia.

Hirshfeld-Becker and colleagues (2006) compared 34 offspring of bipolar parents with 244 offspring of parents without bipolar disorder. Children (ages 2–6) had been classified in laboratory assessments as behaviorally inhibited, disinhibited, or neither. Offspring of bipolar parents had significantly higher rates of disinhibition than offspring of parents without bipolar disorder (53 versus 34 percent; odds ratio = 2.62, 95 percent CI = 1.22 − 5.62). The association between parental bipolar disorder was even stronger among the offspring of parents with bipolar-I illness (67 versus 34 percent; odds ratio = 5.01, 95 percent CI = 1.84 − 13.62). There was no difference in the rate of inhibition between the offspring of parents with and without bipolar disorder.

In one of the rare follow-up designs, Hammen and colleagues (1990) found that, despite relatively high rates of diagnosis over time, children of bipolar mothers were generally less chronically and severely impaired than those of unipolar mothers. The largest follow-up study, conducted by Carlson and Weintraub (1993) with 125 young-adult offspring of bipolar parents, found a rate of definite bipolar disorder of nearly 5 percent, as well as higher rates of diagnosis overall relative to normal comparison groups; generally, however, the bipolar offspring did not differ in symptoms and functioning from offspring of parents with other disorders (e.g., unipolar depression, schizophrenia, substance abuse).

A recent 5-year prospective study of adolescent offspring of parents with bipolar disorder found that the lifetime prevalence rate of bipolar disorder in the offspring increased from 3 to 10 percent at follow-up. The lifetime prevalence of overall mood disorders increased to 40 percent and of overall psychopathology to 59 percent (Hillegers et al., 2005). With the exception of one individual, all of the adolescent subjects subsequently diagnosed with bipolar illness first presented with a unipolar expression; this initial diagnosis occurred an average of 4.9 years (standard deviation = 3.4 years) before the first hypomanic or manic expression.

In their longitudinal study of young children of unipolar and bipolar mothers, Radke-Yarrow and colleagues (1992) initially found worse functioning in offspring of unipolar mothers, but in later analyses (Radke-Yarrow, 1998), the differences between unipolar and bipolar groups were negligible. This work is unique in that the sample was recruited to include mothers with sibling pairs—one of

toddler age (1½–3½) and the other of early school age (5–8); the families were studied at three points in time over a 10-year period. The young children of bipolar mothers, who suffered mainly from depression (bipolar-II), tended to have depressive and disruptive disorders; offspring in early adolescence had a diagnosis rate of 58 percent, especially for depressive and anxiety disorders, but they also had higher rates of disruptive disorders than children of well mothers. At younger ages, the offspring of unipolar mothers tended to have slightly more diagnoses than those of bipolar mothers, but both groups were substantially more likely to have disorders than the children of well mothers. By early adolescence, however, the children of bipolar mothers had similar rates of disruptive and anxiety disorders and higher rates of depression than children of unipolar depressed women. Of interest, it appeared that those offspring in all groups with early signs of disruptive disorders (20 percent) were more likely than those without such signs (2 percent)[1] to develop bipolar disorder by adulthood. The combination of a bipolar mother and an early history of chronic disruptive disorder was highly predictive of eventual bipolar disorder by adulthood—although the actual number of cases was small (Meyer et al., 2001).

A recent University of Pittsburgh study (Birmaher et al., 2005a) evaluated the lifetime prevalence of psychiatric disorders in 210 offspring of 132 parents with bipolar disorder. Rates of illness in these high-risk children were compared with those in 138 offspring of 79 community controls who were healthy or had nonbipolar psychiatric illnesses and who were matched by age, sex, and neighborhood. The offspring of parents with bipolar illness showed a 7.7-fold higher risk for bipolar disorder and a 4-fold increased risk for any mood disorder. The median age at onset for bipolar illness in the offspring was 9, but the rates of mood disorders rose steeply during adolescence. There were no differences in the rates of ADHD between the offspring of bipolar parents and those of controls.

The studies listed in Table 6–5 generally indicate few gender differences overall, although there may be gender-typical patterns of disorders, such as more disruptive behavior disorders in boys and more depressive disorders in girls. Moreover, although a few studies compared outcomes for children with one versus two ill parents, no definite conclusions could be drawn. There appears to be an increased likelihood that a bipolar adult will marry a person who also has a diagnosable disorder (nonrandom mating), thereby making it more likely that the couple's children will acquire a mix of genetic predispositions, in addition to being raised in a potentially disruptive family environment as a result of parental impairment or marital distress. There is a need for further evaluation of the impact of the marital relationship, as well as the gender and mental health of the spouse, as psychosocial contributors to outcomes among offspring (see Chapter 10).

The results of these case-control studies, along with those of other designs that did not include comparison groups but did report children's diagnoses, were summarized in a meta-analysis by Lapalme and colleagues (1997). They concluded that 52 percent of the offspring of bipolar parents met criteria for a diagnosis of at least one psychiatric disorder, compared with 29 percent of children of parents with no disorders—a highly statistically significant difference. (Note that these figures should be viewed as approximations because some of the samples overlapped, potentially causing cases to be counted more than once.) Aggregating across various samples makes it easier to see the specific concentration of mood disorders in the offspring. In total, 26.5 percent of the offspring of bipolar parents had an affective disorder (including major, minor, and intermittent depression and dysthymia, as well as mania, hypomania, cyclothymia, and hyperthymic states), compared with 8.3 percent of children of non-ill parents. Bipolar disorder occurred in 5.4 percent of the offspring of bipolar parents but in none of the children of non-ill parents. Obviously, this figure cannot be taken as a final estimate of risk for bipolarity because most of the children had not passed—or even entered—the age of risk. However, the figure does suggest that the majority of offspring of a bipolar parent fail to manifest diagnosable bipolar disorder at an early age.

Despite the overall consistency of the findings of these studies, there remain significant gaps in our knowledge of children's risk. Few of the studies included young children, while most included both older children and adolescents. The developmental manifestations of bipolar disorder, therefore, have not been fully tested in adequately large samples. The general lack of longitudinal studies means that the continuity or changes in symptom expression over time remain obscure. Although several studies attempted to evaluate subsyndromal symptoms of mood disorders or personality characteristics,[6] there is currently little consensus on the best and most valid instruments for this purpose. Additionally, future researchers will need to articulate theoretical models with specific variables—including both neurobiological and psychological factors—that might be measured as markers or mechanisms of risk. To date, little information exists about the predictive value of the bipolar parent's clinical history—including not only course subtypes, but also the role of the history of manic and depressive features of the illness, age at onset, and response to treatment. Moreover, virtually no studies have considered the potential impact on children of parental comorbidity, such as substance abuse or ADHD.

Most of the early studies and the case-control investigations discussed previously reported clinical diagnostic outcomes but did not include measures of children's personality, adaptive behaviors, and functioning in typical roles. Such variables are important to characterize potential markers of bipolar disorder—unique attributes that define both positive aspects of bipolar heritage and predictors of later adjustment, including coping capabilities that may affect mental health status. A brief review of relevant findings is presented in Box 6–5.

Recent Offspring Studies with Novel Designs

Several more recent studies have provided useful information about future directions for research on risk factors and mechanisms in bipolar families. Duffy and colleagues (1998) reported on a pilot study comparing adolescent children of bipolar parents who were characterized as responsive or nonresponsive to lithium monotherapy. Children of lithium-responsive parents had fewer psychiatric disorders and good premorbid adjustment, and their disorders tended to be mood related, compared with the children of lithium-nonresponsive parents, who had a broad range of psychopathology and more frequent comorbidity. Of interest, over follow-up of up to 5 years, all of the affectively ill children of lithium-responsive parents had remitting episodes and/or episodic courses, whereas the affectively ill children of lithium-nonresponsive parents had chronic mood disorders and continuing comorbidity (Duffy et al., 2002).

Todd and colleagues (1996) used a unique offspring design to examine psychiatric disorders in children with extended bipolar pedigrees (see Table 6–5). They evaluated children and adolescents from 14 extended families with at least two adult bipolar members. The sample included children in 12 families in which a parent was a bipolar proband or an affectively ill sibling of a bipolar proband, and 18 families in which neither parent had an affective disorder. As expected, offspring who had a parent with a mood disorder had a five-fold higher risk for developing an affective disorder than children of healthy parents. Degree of risk was associated with genetic relatedness to the affected members of the pedigree. Children of ill parents were also at apparent risk for anxiety disorders, but not for disruptive behavior disorders. The use of within-pedigree comparisons helps control for environmental factors that might contribute to disorder, and the results of such comparisons further support the hypothesis of genetic factors as a mechanism of risk.

Chang and colleagues (2000) documented initial results of a study of 60 offspring of 37 families (no comparison group). The mean age of the children was 11.1 years (standard deviation = 3.5 years), and the youngsters were evaluated by both parent and child interviews. Overall, 51 percent

In addition to the subclinical affective traits and related characteristics noted in the text, several early studies identified personality traits associated with children at high risk for bipolar disorder; these included aggressiveness (e.g., Worland et al., 1979; Kron et al., 1982), extraversion, introversion, and impulsiveness (Kron et al., 1982).

Data collected on participants in the Gershon and colleagues (1985) study and reported by Pellegrini and colleagues (1986) documented personal and social resources of the children of bipolar parents. There were no overall differences between offspring of bipolar versus control parents on such variables as IQ, social problem-solving ability, self-esteem, and perceived competence. LaRoche and colleagues (1987) also found no significant overall differences in self-esteem. However, Pellegrini and colleagues (1986), reported that those offspring of bipolar parents who did not have psychiatric disorders scored significantly in the more positive direction on the measures, relative to all the other groups, whereas those with psychiatric disorders had significantly less positive scores. Also, nondisordered offspring of bipolar parents reported significantly more supportive relationships and resources available to them than did the disordered youths. Although the direction of causality cannot be determined, superior competence and self-esteem may serve as resilience factors for children at risk and help protect them from the development of psychological disorders.

The findings of Pelligrini and colleagues (1986) are consistent with those of a Stanford study of 53 children and adolescent offspring of bipolar parents that found "super-normal" temperamental characteristics in the offspring who were diagnosis-free. That is, unaffected children and adolescents were more likely to approach new situations, things, and people; to have regular sleeping patterns; and to have lower energy and activity levels (Chang et al., 2003). The authors posited that these "exceptional" temperaments may protect against, or reflect an inherent brain chemistry that is resistant to, psychiatric disorders. Because there were no follow-up data on these offspring, however, it may be that the "exceptional" temperament only postpones onset, although that in its own right would be beneficial. It is possible that some of these well "super-normal" offspring may have inherited very mild subsyndromal variations of a hypomanic temperament; this may in turn provide a protective resilience and energy.

Nurnberger and colleagues (1988) included in their study measures of subsyndromal affective symptoms, as well as the personality trait of sensation seeking. On this measure, they found that children of bipolar parents displayed personality patterns suggestive of disinhibition, and they speculated that such offspring may be prone to respond to dysphoria with disinhibitory behaviors such as drug and alcohol abuse and high-risk behaviors.

Although based on only 7 boys of bipolar parents and 20 controls, a study by Zahn-Waxler and colleagues (1984a, 1984b) is unique in the intensity of its observations and in the young age (2–3yr) of the children involved. In laboratory observations of numerous real-life situations, the investigators found that the toddlers of bipolar parents displayed notable interpersonal difficulties and emotionality. For instance, they showed difficulties in peer interactions (e.g., sharing) and maladaptive aggression, as well as heightened distress and preoccupation in response to simulated conflict and suffering, among others. Although the children of bipolar parents did not display cognitive deficits, they did show more insecure attachment and deficits in taking another's perspective (Zahn-Waxler et al., 1984c). Radke-Yarrow's (1998) report on the expanded study also indicated significantly higher rates of insecure attachment among the children of bipolar mothers, compared with both the well and the unipolar groups. Nevertheless, these toddlers were seen as being relatively socially skilled. As they grew older, however, more disruptive and emotional disorders emerged that were associated with impaired functioning. For instance, peer relationships were rated as poor for 42 percent of the offspring of bipolar women, and 23 percent were doing poorly academically. The investigators found that, overall, 27 percent of the younger and 30 percent of the older siblings showed significant functioning problems in multiple areas (compared with very few of the children of well mothers). The findings of these studies suggest the value of intensive observation of high-risk children in stressful and challenging situations as a way of identifying potential deficits in emotional and behavioral regulation that may portend bipolar disorder.

Anderson and Hammen (1993) compared offspring in the University of California-Los Angeles (UCLA) high-risk study on social competence and academic functioning measures. They discovered that, although the offspring of unipolar mothers were the most impaired of all of the groups, the children of bipolar mothers were actually comparable to the children of non-ill mothers. The investigators predicted that, despite the symptomatology of the bipolar group and the likely increasing risk as they grew older, they were somewhat protected by positive social skills and successful academic achievement, compared with children in the unipolar group. Carlson and Weintraub (1993) evaluated young-adult functioning in their follow-up study of children of bipolar parents compared with a mixed group of offspring of parents with "other" psychopathology and with offspring of non-ill parents. They found that the Global Adjustment Scale scores of the young-adult offspring of bipolar parents were significantly lower than those of children from normal families but did not differ from the scores of offspring of parents with "other" psychopathology. Osher and colleagues (2000) compared the Rorschach responses of a small sample of offspring of manic-depressive parents and controls. They found indicators of thought disorder and unconventional perceptions, suggesting that these might be markers for manic-depressive illness.

The differing results across studies of offspring characteristics reflect a lack of standard batteries of measures (or theoretically driven explorations). The varying methods employed reveal an array of both positive and problematic attributes of children at risk for bipolar disorder. Future studies will be needed to determine whether there are consistent patterns of traits and characteristics that can inform predictions of eventual outcomes.

of the children had a definite diagnosis—chiefly ADHD, depressive disorders, and bipolar disorder (15 percent). Predictors of (childhood) bipolar disorder in the offspring were early onset of parental bipolar disorder and parental childhood ADHD. Children who had two parents with a mood disorder (bipolar or unipolar) tended to show somewhat different symptoms than those with only one ill parent, including increased severity of depressed mood and irritability and rejection sensitivity.

Egeland and colleagues (2003) reported on possible prodromal signs of bipolar disorder in 100 Amish children with a bipolar-I parent and matched controls. Annual evaluations of the children for 7 years, up to age 19 (mean age 14), were retrospectively reviewed and rated blindly by clinicians according to level of possible risk for future development of bipolar-I disorder. On the basis of their symptoms, 38 percent of the children of a bipolar parent were rated as being "at risk," compared with 17 percent of controls. The authors found many depression-related symptoms, as well as anxiety/fearfulness, hyperalertness, and anger dyscontrol, among others. In contrast to the findings of some other studies, however, they found little evidence of disruptive disorders, ADHD, or conduct problems in the Amish sample, and the symptoms observed had an episodic rather than a continuous and chronic course. Further follow-up of the offspring will be useful to determine whether the "risk" symptoms identified by these investigators do indeed portend bipolar-I disorder.

Relatively unremarkable rates of disorder among adolescent offspring were observed in a Dutch volunteer sample (largely from a manic-depressive association; see Wals et al., 2001). A 27 percent lifetime rate of mood disorders was found—not dissimilar to Dutch national norms—although there was no directly studied comparison group. The investigators speculated that the sample may have included relatively healthier bipolar parents than those ascertained primarily from treatment sources.

Mechanisms of Risk to Children of Bipolar Parents

Perhaps with the exception of the study of Todd and colleagues (1996), which linked children's psychopathology to the degree of genetic relatedness in a bipolar pedigree study, the high-risk offspring studies reviewed here cannot serve to confirm a genetic mode of transmission of risk for psychopathology. Rather, most of the studies were designed on the assumption of genetic transmission. Nonetheless, it is recognized that children in such families not only inherit whatever genes predispose to bipolar illness, but also "inherit" parents who are potentially impaired in the parental role at least periodically, and whose environments may be stressful because of instability in marital, occupational, and financial circumstances associated with the effects of

the illness. Moreover, a diathesis–stress perspective shared by most forms of psychopathology would lead to the expectation that even in the presence of genetic diatheses, information on additional variables, such as neurocognitive and biological factors, may be needed to determine whether—or when and how—an at-risk person develops a disorder. And because bipolar disorder manifests very different courses among affected individuals, it is important to link course and outcome features of the illness in parents to children's risk for disorder; also of interest are certain parental demographic features. Additional analyses are therefore needed to advance understanding of the varied outcomes of high-risk offspring of bipolar parents, and perhaps to shed light more generally on factors that affect the nature and timing of the course of the illness.

Family Life and Environment

Few bipolar high-risk studies have examined the association of children's psychiatric outcomes with characteristics of family life and environment. Marital conflict and disturbances of family climate and parent–child communication almost certainly have significant negative effects on children's adjustment. Obviously, the quality of relationships in families with bipolar parents is likely to play an important role in children's risk or resilience in the face of genetic predisposition (see Chapter 10 for further discussion of parenting characteristics in bipolar families).

A few bipolar high-risk studies have examined the role of such factors. LaRoche and colleagues (1987) found that among families with a bipolar mother, the father's report of marital dissatisfaction was the strongest predictor of the presence of a diagnosis in the offspring; in slightly different analyses, the mother's report of marital distress was also a significant predictor. The offspring who had disorders reported more negative quality of their relationship with both parents, compared with youngsters who did not have a diagnosis. Hammen (1991) also assessed marital functioning and other forms of stress in high-risk families. Both unipolar and bipolar mothers had high rates of divorce and current relationship stress compared with controls. In all groups, mothers' chronic stress and negative life events contributed to the prediction of worse outcomes in their children. Grigoroiu-Serbanescu and colleagues (1989) performed descriptive evaluations of "familial atmosphere" and determined that the greatest severity of psychopathology in offspring was associated with the highest levels of physical and verbal conflict within the family. Geller and colleagues (2002a) found that bipolar youths who lived in intact biological families were significantly more likely to recover than those in other living situations (Fig. 6–2).

A National Institute of Mental Health study found that bipolar women had higher levels of marital stress than

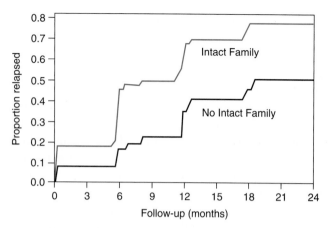

Figure 6–2. Two-year rate of recovery by living situation in subjects with a prepubertal and early adolescent bipolar disorder phenotype. Fifty-eight of the 89 subjects had recovered by 24 months. There was a significant difference between the 39 recovered subjects who lived with their intact biological families and the 19 who resided in other living situations (Cox model $\chi^2 = 7.40$, degrees of freedom [df] = 1, $p = .007$). The Kiddie Mania (K-M) estimate for recovery in intact families was 76.5% (95% confidence interval [CI] = 64.8–88.1), and for recovery in other living situations it was 50.0% (95% CI = 34.1–65.9). (*Source:* Geller et al., 2002. Reprinted with permission from the *American Journal of Psychiatry,* Copyright 2002, American Psychiatric Association.)

unipolar or well women; marital stress tended to be associated with other forms of family stress and maladaptive functioning as well, however, which made the effects difficult to disentangle (Radke-Yarrow, 1998). The combination of low maternal scores on global functioning and high indices of family stress (including marital conflict) was a strong predictor of depression in offspring, especially older children. In a more recent analysis, Meyer and colleagues (2004) reported that frequent maternal expressions of anger and irritability (perhaps themselves manifestations of mixed mania and therefore of genetic importance) during children's early years were associated with the development of mania in adulthood, even after controlling for maternal psychiatric features. Although based on a small sample, the results of this study hint that highly stressful family environments may contribute to the timing—or even the expression—of bipolar features in those at genetic risk (see also Miklowitz et al., 1988). In a 4-year prospective study of 86 prepubertal and early-adolescent bipolar patients, Geller and colleagues (2004) found that low maternal warmth predicted faster relapse after recovery from mania. In an earlier study, the same investigators had found that patients with prepubertal and early-onset adolescent bipolar disorder who were exposed to low levels of maternal warmth were four times more likely to relapse after recovery than those exposed to high levels of maternal warmth (Geller et al., 2002b). This effect

is clearly shown in Figure 6–3. It is not clear to what extent maternal warmth reflects an additional underlying vulnerability factor or if maternal warmth is decreased or adversely affected by the demands of caring for a child with bipolar illness.

One particularly dramatic example of family and environmental dysfunction concerns physical and sexual abuse. Analysis of data collected by the Stanley Foundation Bipolar Network showed that early traumatic abuse experiences were associated with a worse course of illness, including earlier onset, suicidality, and more rapid cycling (Leverich et al., 2002). Other investigators found elevated rates of childhood sexual abuse—significantly higher for males—among bipolar adults compared with those with unipolar depression (Hyun et al., 2000). There is also a highly significant association between those reporting childhood sexual abuse and auditory hallucinations (Hammersley et al., 2003). The findings of these studies suggest that among those with a predisposition to develop bipolar disorder, childhood trauma may play a role in the course of the illness; that parents who abuse children have a more severe or comorbid form that is genetically transmitted (as well as psychologically traumatic); or that children with early onset and impaired functioning may experience more severe abuse. It may be noted that self-reports

Figure 6–3. Two-year rate of relapse after recovery by high versus low levels of maternal–child warmth in subjects with a prepubertal and early-adolescent bipolar disorder phenotype. Thirty-two of the 58 recovered patients relapsed after recovery. There was a significant difference between the 21 relapsers with low maternal–child warmth and the 11 with high maternal warmth (Cox model $\chi^2 = 9.84$, degrees of freedom [df] = 1, $p = .002$). The Kiddie Mania (K-M) estimate for relapse by low maternal–child warmth was 100.0% (95% confidence interval [CI] = not applicable when K-M = 100.0%) and by high maternal–child warmth was 42.2% (95% CI = 23.2–61.2). (*Source:* Geller et al., 2002a. Reprinted with permission from the *American Journal of Psychiatry,* Copyright 2002, American Psychiatric Association.)

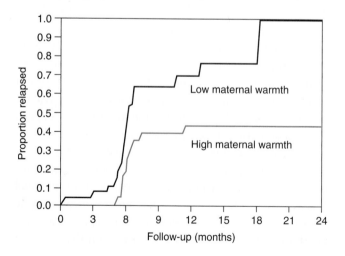

of trauma may overestimate its actual incidence, although this possibility has not been sufficiently investigated in bipolar illness.

A recent Dutch study of 132 offspring (mean age 16) of bipolar parents found that the relationship between stressful life events and the onset or recurrence of a DSM-IV mood disorder was almost entirely accounted for by the offspring's prior symptoms of depression and anxiety. The researchers concluded that the frequently hypothesized association between stressful life events and the precipitation of mood disorders may be a spurious one (Wals et al., 2005). The association between stressful life events and the onset or recurrence of a mood disorder was also independent of gender and familial loading. See Chapters 4 and 10 for a more complete discussion of life events and bipolar illness.

Neurocognitive and Biological Studies of High-Risk Youth

To date, few studies have included evaluation of potential neurocognitive and structural and functional brain markers of bipolar disorder. (See Chapters 9 and 15 for a detailed discussion of neurocognitive features of bipolar illness in general.) Because this approach has proven to be extremely fruitful in high-risk studies of schizophrenia, it is likely that such research on bipolar disorder will proliferate. Preliminary studies are beginning to emerge. For example, small samples of children at risk because of parental bipolar disorder or children/adolescents diagnosed with bipolar disorder have shown significant differences from normal controls on neurochemical abnormalities (Cecil et al., 2003), neuroanatomical features (DelBello et al., 2004), and neuropsychological performance (Dickstein et al., 2004). One study of neurocognitive effects in at-risk youth is especially interesting. Meyer and colleagues (2004) examined the outcomes after 23 years of offspring of bipolar, unipolar, and control women in the NIMH's longitudinal study of young children of women with affective disorders (Radke-Yarrow et al., 1992). They found that the majority of the offspring of bipolar mothers who later developed bipolar disorder had shown impairment on a neurocognitive test of executive functioning when they were adolescents.

In their analysis, Meyer and colleagues (2004) found that offspring in families with maternal bipolar disorder were substantially more likely to show impairment in neurocognitive functioning when tested in adolescence if they were also exposed to high levels of maternal anger and irritability during childhood. The investigators hypothesized that the maternal behavior was a potent stressor interacting with their offspring's genetic liability for bipolar disorder, potentially affecting brain development

and increasing their risk for eventual development of the disorder. Direct causality has not been established, however, and it should be kept in mind that severely ill children have an impact on the degree of maternal irritability that is expressed. One study of 140 offspring of parents with bipolar disorder found lower birth weight in offspring to be significantly correlated with greater psychopathology (Wals et al., 2003); the authors suggested that this observed relationship might be due to a shared environmental or genetic factor that influences both. Other investigators have reported a more general association among birth weight, cognitive functioning, and psychopathology (Eaton et al., 2001).

Potential mechanisms underlying bipolar disorder were suggested by Leibenluft and colleagues (2003a), who specifically indicated possible applications to childhood-onset mania (and presumably, by extension, to children at risk because of parental bipolar disorder). Drawing on the work of various investigators, they suggested paradigms for physiological assessment, along with functional neuroimaging measures, of latency, magnitude, and recovery of emotional reactions to affective stimuli—as well as the relationships between attentional and emotional regulation processes in possibly bipolar children. Research aimed at clarifying underlying maladaptive processes in bipolar disorder that can be identified in at-risk samples of children holds promise for advancing understanding, and possibly detection, of bipolar disorder in the young.

Parents' Clinical and Demographic Features and Children's Outcomes

Findings thus far have been mixed on the extent to which there is increased risk to children if both parents are bipolar or if psychiatric disorder occurs in the first-degree relatives of a parent with bipolar disorder.[7] These mixed findings are likely attributable to design and sampling variations.

Few studies have examined features of parental bipolar course and their influence on children's disorders. An exception is Duffy and colleagues (1998), whose earlier-cited work suggests that parental responsiveness to lithium, which in turn is related to the presence of more "classic" bipolar illness, may be an important predictor. The most comprehensive analyses of clinical features as predictors of children's outcomes were reported by Grigoroiu-Serbanescu and colleagues (1989), who determined that severity of children's psychiatric disorders was significantly related to severity of the illness in the bipolar parent, number of manic and mixed (but not depressive) episodes, younger age at onset in the parent, and presence of psychopathology in the coparent. LaRoche and colleagues (1987) found that duration of parental illness was related to children's risk for disorder, but the nature of the episodes and the age at onset were not specified. Radke-Yarrow (1992) and Radke-Yarrow and colleagues (1998) reported a significant correlation between mothers' time in affective episodes and low levels of functioning (as assessed by the Global Assessment of Functioning) on the one hand and several measures of children's symptoms on the other, but did not distinguish between maternal manic and depressive symptoms.

Of interest, the study of Radke-Yarrow and colleagues (1992) included an evaluation of maternal Axis II disorders. It was found that two thirds of the bipolar mothers had at least one personality disorder, and personality disorder pathology measured dimensionally was significantly related to the extent of children's symptoms and disorders. Likewise, Hodgins and colleagues (2002) speculated that bipolar parents' high levels of trait neuroticism may expose their children to relatively stressful environments and models of poor coping, as well as to the genetic transmission of neuroticism that influences susceptibility to stress reactivity. Their proposal, similar to models of intergenerational transmission proposed by Hammen (1991), is that family discord and stress factors contribute to the risk of development of disorders in children.

It may be noted that there is a lack of information on the similarity of parent and child bipolar symptoms in cases of early-onset bipolar disorder. Follow-up studies are needed as well to evaluate possible similarities in course and treatment responsiveness.

Demographic factors have likewise not been fully explored, although they have been addressed in a modest number of studies. Grigoroiu-Serbanescu and colleagues (1989) found that gender of the bipolar parent did not make a difference in children's outcomes. On the other hand, Klein and colleagues (1985) found that bipolar mothers, compared with bipolar fathers, were more likely to have children with affective symptomatology. Several studies have included or controlled for socioeconomic status of bipolar parents. Grigoroiu-Serbanescu and colleagues (1989), for example, reported that lower socioeconomic status in their Romanian sample was associated with greater psychopathology in children.

Clearly, more research is needed to shed light on both clinical and demographic factors associated with bipolar parents that may moderate the effects of their disorder on outcomes among their offspring.

CONCLUSIONS

Increasing interest in mood disorders of children and adolescents has stimulated research and careful clinical observations aimed at identifying the clinical features, precursors, and course of bipolar disorder in these populations. However, numerous gaps in knowledge remain. For many years, unclear diagnostic criteria led to frequent misdiagnosis of bipolar disorder in children and adolescents. Today, pediatric bipolar disorders are increasingly being diagnosed and treated. Nonetheless, additional studies are needed to refine the predictive utility of age at onset of first symptoms, and to determine the correlates of illness course and level of functioning. Although "classic" bipolar features, including distinct affective episodes and good interepisode functioning, appear to be rare in children, some children display severe and chronic signs of emotional instability, behavioral dysregulation, and cognitive changes that are consistent with mania, and that appear to resemble bipolar mixed states and ultrarapid cycling. Whether such patterns mark developmentally consistent manifestations of bipolarity or reflect other traits or disorders not yet understood remains uncertain, however.

Diagnostic problems are compounded by the considerable overlap between presumed mania and ADHD, as well as other comorbid disorders, such as substance abuse, anxiety, and disruptive behavior disorders. Clearly, longitudinal studies are needed to determine the unique developmental manifestations of manic symptoms and whether possible manic syndrome or symptoms in children portend bipolar disorder in adolescence or later. Moreover, the significance of manic symptoms in children remains to be clarified, in particular whether they represent an especially severe and disabling form of the illness or a nonspecific indicator of psychopathology. Some have proposed that early-onset mania presenting with comorbid ADHD may represent an etiological subtype marked by familial concentrations of bipolar disorder and ADHD. Presently, it is recommended that a diagnosis of bipolar disorder be reserved for children who meet DSM-IV criteria for mania, and that bipolar-NOS be used for those with severe emotional and behavioral dysregulation when boundaries with disruptive behavior disorders are unclear.

Parental bipolar disorder in families of children with manic symptoms would appear to be a potentially validating criterion, but further research is needed to identify early markers (endophenotypes) of childhood bipolar disorder. The stakes are high for such severely ill children, because early valid diagnosis and empirically supported treatment could greatly improve their lives and future functioning. Studies of children of bipolar parents employing the high-risk methodology (that is, the study of children of psychiatrically ill parents) represent a design uniquely suited to refining the assessment and diagnosis of precursor forms of bipolar disorder. Moreover, such studies may prove crucial in identifying markers of risk processes that interact with genetic diatheses, although few studies to date have examined the neurobiological or developmental abnormalities that may signal onset of or vulnerability to bipolar disorder. The studies of high-risk children conducted thus far have clearly indicated that the offspring of bipolar parents have elevated rates of psychopathology, developing in childhood and adolescence. A significant proportion develop bipolar disorder—and the rate is likely to grow still higher as these offspring pass through the age of risk in late adolescence and adulthood. Longitudinal research on such samples is needed to help clarify the developmental progression of the disorder; its earliest symptoms; and predictors of its course, including adverse family and environmental experiences.

NOTES

1. See excellent reviews by Faedda et al., 1995; Geller and Luby, 1997; Coyle et al., 2003; Carlson, 2005.
2. See Biederman et al., 2000a, 2004c; Geller et al., 2000b; Masai et al., 2003.
3. Masi et al., 2001; Wozniak, 2002; Faedda et al., 2004; Harpold et al., 2005.
4. This statement appeared on the Web site of the Child and Adolescent Bipolar Foundation, http://www.bpkids.org (accessed August 31, 2006).
5. See Strober et al., 1995; Faraone et al., 1997a; McElroy et al., 1997; Kafantaris et al., 1998.
6. Decina et al., 1982; Gershon et al., 1985; Klein et al., 1985; Nurnberger et al., 1988; Grigoroiu-Serbanescu et al., 1989, 1991; Birmaher et al., 2005a,b.
7. See Gershon et al., 1985; LaRoche et al., 1987; Grigoroiu-Serbanescu et al., 1989; Radke-Yarrow et al., 1992; Todd et al., 1996.

7 Comorbidity

The patient who has for years before his illness shown morbid traits, who has been anxious, or quarrelsome, or suspicious, or odd, or solitary, or obsessional, or in some other way has shown that he is constantly at odds with himself, as well as with his surroundings—such a patient is not going to be cured of his maladjustment by having an affective flare-up. A sortie does not end a siege.

—*Sir Aubrey Lewis (1936, p. 997)*

Comorbidity in manic-depressive illness, in which the mood disorder is complicated by the presence of one or more additional disorders, is the rule rather than the exception, especially for the bipolar subgroup. Data from the Stanley Foundation Bipolar Network, a consortium of bipolar specialty clinics in academic health centers around the world, indicate that 65 percent of patients with bipolar disorder have a comorbid condition. Of these patients, almost a quarter have three or more diagnoses (Fig. 7–1) (McElroy et al., 2001).

Unfortunately, disorders that can accompany affective illness tend to be underrecognized and undertreated (Simon et al., 2004a). Poor recognition of comorbid conditions may be related to the way in which clinicians diagnose their patients. Psychiatric evaluation is often directed toward identifying a single diagnosis that will account for all or most of a patient's symptoms, rather than identifying multiple conditions. This expectation can lead to important disorders being overlooked, and the partially diagnosed and incompletely treated patient may be left with considerable symptomatology and disability, even after the primary disorder has been effectively treated. In the case of bipolar disorder, which can be destabilized by certain classes of medication, the clinician must also be wary of worsening one illness while treating another. For example, treating panic disorder with a selective serotonin reuptake inhibitor (SSRI) may trigger a switch to a manic or mixed episode. (The difficulties involved in the treatment of comorbid conditions are addressed in Chapter 24.) Proper attention to management of comorbidities can reduce their impact on a patient's functioning and general health. Unfortunately, even with the best treatment, the presence of one or more comorbid disorders tends to lead to a poorer outcome compared with uncomplicated manic-depressive illness.

Some investigators have evaluated the total burden of comorbidity by surveying multiple diagnostic categories, while others have focused in more detail on specific conditions. Studies taking a comprehensive approach to the presence of comorbidity have found that, especially for the bipolar subgroup, an uncomplicated recurrent mood disorder is unusual. The National Comorbidity Survey (NCS) of more than 58,000 individuals found that, among bipolar patients with "classic" features such as euphoria, grandiosity, and the ability to maintain energy without sleep, all met the *Diagnostic and Statistical Manual* (DSM)-III-R criteria for at least one other mental disorder. Fully 95 percent met the criteria for three or more disorders (Kessler et al., 1997). This, for reasons discussed below, is almost certainly a considerable overestimate. Another study, involving 3,258 randomly selected household residents of Edmonton, Alberta, found similarly high rates of comorbidity. Based on surveys performed by trained lay interviewers using the Diagnostic Interview Schedule (DIS), comorbidity with other disorders occurred in 92 percent of subjects who had experienced a manic episode. The generalizability of this particular study may be limited, however. The lifetime prevalence of mania identified by the lay interviewers was lower than in most other studies—only 0.6 percent. Consequently, the interviewers may have been identifying only a subset of patients with bipolar disorder who had more severe psychopathology. Also, as discussed later, there are significant discrepancies between the high rates of comorbidity identified by nonclinician versus clinician interviewers. For example, experienced clinicians in the Stanley Network identified social anxiety disorder in only 16 percent of their bipolar patients, compared with nearly 50 percent identified by nonclinicians in the NCS study.

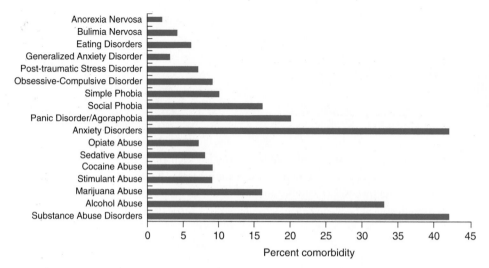

Figure 7–1. Axis I psychiatric comorbidities. Percent comorbidity in bipolar patients enrolled in the Stanley Bipolar Treatment Network. (*Source*: Adapted from McElroy et al., 2001. Reprinted with permission from the *American Journal of Psychiatry*, Copyright 2001. American Psychiatric Association.)

Guo and colleagues (2005) used a claims database to evaluate rates of bipolar comorbidity. They analyzed a large managed-care population of 123,292 patients who had been given an *International Classification of Diseases 9* (ICD-9) diagnostic code for bipolar disorder by their treating clinician. The prevalence of comorbid anxiety disorders was 36.7 percent, but the rate of comorbid substance disorders was only 12.0 percent. The low level of comorbid substance abuse/dependence in this population may have been due to the fact that individuals with commercial health insurance were more likely to be employed, whereas substance-related disorders often lead to the loss of a job or chronic unemployment (Leino-Arjas et al., 1999).

Data obtained from structured clinician interviews also reveal high levels of comorbidity in bipolar patients. Bauer and colleagues (2005) evaluated intake assessment data, obtained by clinicians using the Structured Clinical Interview for DSM (SCID), on subjects recruited as part of the Veterans Affairs (VA) Cooperative Study No. 430. In this sample of hospitalized bipolar veterans, 57 percent had at least one current comorbid disorder. More than one comorbid disorder was found in 30 percent of the patients, and 9 percent had three or more comorbidities. As in the preceding studies, the two most common comorbidities were anxiety and substance abuse disorders. At least one anxiety disorder was currently present in 38 percent of the sample; the lifetime rate was 43 percent. The similarity between current and lifetime rates suggests a high degree of chronicity. Post-traumatic stress disorder (PTSD) was present in 25 percent, panic disorder in 17 percent, and obsessive-compulsive disorder (OCD) in 8 percent. Current substance abuse disorders were present in 34 percent; alcohol (26 percent), marijuana (7 percent), and cocaine

(7 percent) were the most commonly abused substances. The lifetime rate for substance abuse disorders was considerably higher, 72 percent.

The VA investigators also evaluated correlates of anxiety and substance-related disorders and found them to be distinct. Compared with bipolar patients with no comorbidity, those with comorbid substance abuse/dependence had more marital problems and a higher probability of presenting with depression; they also had more medical conditions during the index hospitalization and were less able to work. Comorbid anxiety disorders were associated with earlier age at onset of bipolar disorder, rapid cycling, a greater likelihood of presenting with depression, a higher rate of suicide attempts, and a greater number of manic and depressive episodes in the year preceding hospitalization. Vieta and colleagues (2001), in their Barcelona Stanley Foundation Study of 129 bipolar-I outpatients in remission, found that comorbid bipolar patients had a higher number of mixed features, depressive episodes, and suicide attempts. The different patterns of correlates led Bauer and colleagues (2005) to speculate that distinct genetic subtypes of bipolar disorder were represented by patients who had comorbid anxiety disorders compared with those with comorbid substance abuse disorders. The association of discrete subtypes of bipolar disorder with specific comorbid presentations is discussed in further detail later.

Patients in the Bauer and colleagues (2005) VA study were all hospitalized and had either bipolar-I or bipolar-II disorder. However, it is not only the most severely ill patients who experience comorbid conditions. Patients with soft-spectrum bipolarity—those who, although they do not meet the full DSM criteria for bipolar disorder, nonetheless experience significant symptoms of depressed and elevated moods—also have high rates of comorbidity (Maremnani et al., 2006). For example, in the Zurich cohort study (Angst, 1998), a 15-year prospective study of 4,547 young adults, 78 percent of patients with brief hypomanic episodes had a lifetime prevalence of at least one anxiety disorder. Panic disorder was the most common anxiety disorder, affecting 12 percent of all patients; 32 percent experienced panic attacks without meeting the full criteria for panic disorder. Binge eating (13 percent) and alcohol abuse disorders (23 percent) were also common in this cohort. Patients with major depressive disorder have more anxiety and substance abuse disorders than the general population, but significantly fewer than patients with bipolar disorder (Chen and Dilsaver, 1995b).

Although comorbid conditions tend to be underdiagnosed, they can also be overdiagnosed. Manic-depressive illness, as we have emphasized, is highly variable in its presentation. Patients with completely different clinical presentations and courses are given the same DSM-IV diagnosis. Diagnostic criteria for mood disorders include symptoms of anxiety; conduct disturbance; cognitive impairment; and changes in eating, energy levels, sleeping, and sexual functioning. Comorbid diagnoses can be inflated by the confounding of symptoms with diagnoses. Nonclinician interviewers in particular, who estimate the presence of psychiatric disorders using a symptom checklist, are at greater risk for overestimating comorbidity than are experienced clinicians, who use pattern recognition to make diagnoses. Thus before one can properly interpret studies of comorbidity, the method used to establish diagnoses must be explicit.

In the remainder of this chapter, we review the findings of the literature on the major comorbid conditions in manic-depressive illness, with an emphasis on the bipolar subgroup. There is little published information on the more recurrent forms of unipolar depression per se. We address in turn alcohol and drug abuse/dependence disorders, anxiety disorders, other psychiatric illnesses, and medical illnesses.

ALCOHOL AND DRUG ABUSE/DEPENDENCE DISORDERS

Several general methodological issues arise in the study of alcohol and drug abuse/dependence in manic-depressive patients. We begin by considering these, and then turn to specific diagnostic issues. First, it is often difficult to obtain accurate histories of alcohol and drug abuse from patients; compounding the problem, clinicians tend to skirt this general line of inquiry. Second, patients vary tremendously in the development and expression of both manic-depressive illness and substance abuse/dependence disorders. Third,

many studies do not adequately differentiate substance abuse from the more serious and persistent disorder of true alcohol or drug dependence.

Inconsistency and unreliability of diagnostic criteria are particular problems when investigators attempt to diagnose and study more than one disorder and then to determine which is primary and which secondary. Schuckit (1986) summarized several major sources of diagnostic confusion related to alcohol and mood disorders: (1) alcohol can cause depressive symptoms; (2) signs of temporary serious depression can follow prolonged drinking; (3) drinking can escalate during affective episodes in some patients, especially during mania; (4) depressive symptoms and alcohol problems occur in other psychiatric disorders; and (5) a subset of manic-depressive patients have independent alcohol abuse disorder. Differentiating symptoms caused by a primary psychiatric disorder from those secondary to substance abuse can be difficult. Affective, cognitive, and psychotic symptoms can result from alcohol and from a wide variety of classes of drugs, such as amphetamines, cocaine, and hallucinogens. Likewise, alcohol and other drugs can both mask and precipitate affective symptoms. Indeed, Kraepelin (1921) observed many years ago that manic attacks occasionally begin with delirium tremens. More recently, manic attacks induced by lysergic acid diethylamide (LSD) and phenylcyclidine (PCP) have been observed in biologically vulnerable individuals. These issues are discussed in more detail later in this chapter. Obtaining a detailed chronology of the onset of symptoms (i.e., whether difficulties with substance abuse predated affective symptoms or vice versa), ascertaining the severity of presenting symptoms, and taking a thorough family history can aid in making a correct differential diagnosis (Hesselbrock et al., 1985; Schuckit, 1986). Correct diagnosis, in turn, is essential to good medical and psychological care (see Chapter 24). In a 5-year prospective study of 27 bipolar-I patients in whom the onset of alcohol abuse disorder preceded the onset of bipolar disorder, and 33 patients in whom that order was reversed, Strakowski and colleagues (2005) found that those who abused alcohol first were more likely to recover and recovered more quickly. Those whose illness preceded their alcohol abuse spent more time affectively ill and experienced more symptoms of alcohol abuse.

Alcohol Abuse/Dependence

In a letter to a friend, the poet Edgar Allan Poe wrote about alcohol and mental illness from a deeply personal perspective:

> I became insane, with long periods of horrible sanity. During these fits of absolute unconsciousness I drank, God only knows how much or how long. As a matter of

course, my enemies referred the insanity to the drink, rather than the drink to the insanity.

Separating the insanity from the drink remains a difficult problem in the differential diagnosis and treatment of affective illness and substance abuse disorders. A relationship between alcohol and mood disorders has been observed for more than 2,000 years. Plato (cited in Ackerknecht, 1959) referred to alcoholism as a demonstrable cause of mania. Soranus (c. 100 AD, cited in Zilboorg, 1941) echoed the sentiment that excessive use of alcohol frequently caused mania and criticized those who prescribed it as a treatment. Aretaeus (c. 90 AD, cited in Whitwell, 1936) suggested that symptoms of mania may be produced by an excess of wine or opiates but concluded that the resulting states cannot properly be termed mania, just temporary deliria. Early in the twentieth century, Kraepelin (1921, p. 178) summarized his findings on alcohol dependence in manic-depressive illness as follows:

> Alcoholism occurs among male patients in about a quarter of the cases, but is to be regarded as the consequence of debaucheries committed in excitement, not as a cause.

Differing views about whether alcohol abuse disorder precedes or follows the onset of manic-depressive illness persist today, and there is a growing appreciation of the importance of recognizing this comorbidity (dual diagnosis).

Rates of Mood Disorders among Patients with Alcohol Abuse/Dependence

The lack of consistency in diagnostic criteria has led to widely disparate estimates of the rates of mood disorders in patients with alcohol abuse disorder. These estimates have ranged from 3 to 98 percent, depending on whether clinical scales or more formal diagnostic criteria were used (Keeler et al., 1979; Himmelhoch et al., 1983). Estimates of the prevalence of mood disorders in those with alcohol dependence range from 12 to 57 percent when mood disorders are defined by formal diagnostic criteria, but are as high as 98 percent when rating scales are used (Bernadt and Murray, 1986).

Rates of Alcohol Abuse/Dependence among Patients with Mood Disorders

The Epidemiological Catchment Area (ECA) data for alcohol abuse/dependence in patients with affective illness show a high lifetime prevalence rate (Table 7–1) of 17 percent in unipolar depressed patients (the proportion with recurrent depressions was not specified) and a strikingly higher rate, 46 percent, in bipolar-I patients (Regier et al., 1990). Three other studies (Freed, 1969; Morrison, 1974; Estroff et al., 1985) found that when bipolar patients in clinical settings were systematically queried, they reported rates of alcohol abuse/dependence of about 60 to 75 percent. Compared with patients with other psychiatric diagnoses, those with bipolar disorder were at particularly high risk of developing an alcohol problem during their lifetime. This can be seen in Figure 7–2, which shows the lifetime prevalence of alcohol abuse disorder in individuals with selected psychiatric diagnoses and in the general population.

Most studies have found alcohol abuse disorder comorbidity is more frequent in bipolar patients than in those with any other mood disorder. The ECA study of alcohol abuse/dependence and psychiatric comorbidity (Helzer and Pryzbeck, 1988) found that mania was strongly associated with alcohol abuse/dependence (odds ratio = 6.2) but

TABLE 7–1. **Lifetime Prevalence Rates for Alcohol and Drug Abuse/Dependence in Persons with Mood Disorders and in the General Population**

Type of Abuse/Dependence	Bipolar-I (%)	Bipolar-II (%)	Major Depression (%)	General Population (%)
Alcohol	46	39	17	13.5
Abuse only	15	18	5	
Dependence	31	21	12	
Drug	41	21	18	6.2
Abuse only	13	9	7	
Dependence	28	12	11	

Note: Data are from the Epidemiological Catchment Area (ECA) study and are based on DSM-III diagnosis.
ECA = Epidemiological Catchment Area.
Source: Regier et al., 1990.

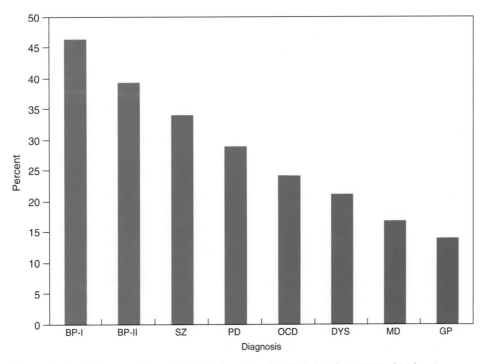

Figure 7–2. Lifetime prevalence of alcohol abuse disorder. BP-I=bipolar-I; BP-II=bipolar-II; DYS=dysthymia; GP=general population; MD=major depression; OCD=obsessive-compulsive disorder; PD=panic disorder; SZ=schizophrenia. (*Source:* Regier et al., 1990.)

that major depression was not (odds ratio=1.7); more highly recurrent or cyclic depressions were not analyzed separately. Bipolar-I was associated with a higher lifetime rate of alcohol abuse/dependence than bipolar-II (46 versus 39 percent) or unipolar depression (17 percent) (Regier et al., 1990).

A study of 267 patients enrolled in the Stanley Foundation Bipolar Network found that, as in the general population, more men (49 percent) than women (29 percent) with bipolar disorder met the criteria for lifetime alcohol abuse. Likewise, a recent study of 211 bipolar patients found that men had significantly higher rates of comorbid alcohol abuse/dependence (Kawa et al., 2005). However, having bipolar disorder raised a woman's risk of having an alcohol-related disorder to a much greater degree than it did for a man. Compared with nonbipolar patients, the odds ratio of having an alcohol-related disorder among those with bipolar disorder was 7.35 for women and 2.77 for men (Frye et al., 2003). Men and women with bipolar disorder also have different risk factors for comorbid alcohol-related diagnoses. In men, the risk appears to be more associated with a genetic predisposition. Specifically, men with bipolar disorder and comorbid alcohol abuse/dependence have a more extensive family history of both disorders compared with men with noncomorbid bipolar disorder. Women with bipolar disorder and alcohol-related disorders, on the other hand, do not have as great a family loading. Comorbid alcohol abuse/dependence in women is associated more with a greater familial burden of depressive episodes and anxiety disorders (Frye et al., 2003).

Elderly bipolar patients are also at increased risk for alcohol abuse. A community survey compared 84 elderly (ages ≥65 years) bipolar respondents with 8,121 elderly respondents without bipolar disorder; those with bipolar illness had a significantly higher lifetime and 12-month prevalence of alcohol disorders (p <.001) (Goldstein et al., 2006).

In summary, many studies, using a wide variety of diagnostic criteria and patient populations and conducted over a period of more than 50 years, have been quite consistent in finding significantly elevated rates of alcohol abuse/dependence in manic depressive illness, particularly the bipolar form. Conversely, they have found a significantly increased proportion of patients with manic-depressive illness within populations of alcohol abusers.

Drug Abuse/Dependence

The data on rates of comorbid bipolar illness and drug abuse/dependence are much less extensive and consistent than those on comorbid alcohol-related disorders, in no small part because of the illegal nature of drug-related disorders. The ECA data for drug abuse/dependence in patients with mood disorders show strikingly high lifetime prevalence rates of 18 percent in unipolar depressed patients and 41 percent in bipolar-I patients (Regier et al., 1990), nearly identical to the rates for alcohol-related disorders (see Table 7–1). In the general population, drug abuse/dependence is significantly less common than alcohol-related disorders (see also Table 7–2).

Determining the sequence of comorbid mood disorders and drug abuse/dependence presents the same methodological problems as those encountered in the case of alcohol-related diagnoses. The ECA data show that the affective disorder is 1.3 times more likely to occur before the drug abuse disorder (see the later discussion).

Cocaine

An interview study of patients voluntarily enrolled in a bipolar disorder case registry found that 3.4 percent met the diagnostic criteria for cocaine abuse, and 6.7 percent met the criteria for cocaine dependence (Chengappa et al., 2000). Consistent with other findings on drug abuse problems, more patients with bipolar-I than with bipolar-II abused cocaine.

Data of this sort cannot address the nature of the relationship between the mood and drug disorders. Clearly there are features of bipolar illness that can increase the likelihood of cocaine abuse, such as a desire to relieve the psychomotor retardation of bipolar depression and a desire to reinduce, prolong, or accelerate elevated mood and energy states. Weiss and Mirin (1986), for example, found that the majority of their bipolar patients reported using cocaine more often when manic than when depressed. This finding is consistent with that of Estroff and colleagues (1985), who observed that 58 percent of their manic bipolar patients abused cocaine, compared with 30 percent of their depressed bipolar patients.[1]

Opiates and Central Nervous System Depressants

In a study of 533 opiate and depressant abusers, 24 percent of the total subjects were diagnosed with major depressive disorder, and 5.4 percent were either bipolar-I or bipolar-II (Kosten and Rounsaville, 1986). Mirin and colleagues (1984) found a similar rate of unipolar depression among opiate addicts, but twice the rate of bipolar illness among abusers of these central nervous system (CNS) depressants. They also found that nearly three times more female than male opiate addicts were diagnosed as bipolar (10.8 versus 3.7 percent). These rates of bipolar illness are substantially higher than those found in the general population. Estroff and colleagues (1985) examined drug abuse in bipolar patients in their drug treatment clinic and reported that 25 percent of their manic patients abused heroin, compared with 20 percent of their depressed bipolar patients. The small sample size of this study limits its generalizability, however. Miller and colleagues (1989), studying a larger sample, found that only 5 percent of their manic patients abused opiates.

TABLE 7–2. **Rates of Drug Abuse/Dependence in the General Population**

Study	Total Population (%)	Male (%)	Female (%)	Prevalence
Regier et al., 1988 (ECA)				
Drug abuse/dependence	5.9			Lifetime
	2.0			6-month
Kessler et al., 1994 (NCS)				
Drug abuse	4.4	5.4	3.5	Lifetime
	0.8	1.3	0.3	12-month
Drug dependence	7.5	9.4	5.9	Lifetime
	2.8	3.8	1.9	12-month
Narrow et al., 2002 (ECA and NCS)	1.3	1.8	0.7	1-month
Drug abuse disorder using "clinical significance" criteria	1.7			12-month

ECA = Epidemiological Catchment Area; NCS = National Comorbidity Survey.

Overall, the rates of bipolar illness in opiate abusers, although not as dramatically high as in cocaine abusers, are greater than those found in the general population, but not as high as the rates of unipolar depression among those with opiate dependence.

Marijuana

Marijuana (cannabis) is the most widely abused illicit drug in the United States. According to the 2000 National Household Survey on Drug Abuse, 6.3 percent of Americans aged 12 or older were current abusers; approximately 59 percent of them abused only marijuana, and another 17 percent abused another illicit drug as well (Office of Applied Studies, 2001). Marijuana abuse is more prevalent among patients with bipolar disorder than in the general population. A study of 3,536 patients from 14 European countries, for example, found that 12 percent of patients being treated for mania were current abusers of marijuana (Reed et al., 2005). Other studies have found a wide range of rates of marijuana abuse in bipolar disorder—from 15 to 65 percent—but all rates have been high.[2] Marijuana, which has both sedative and psychedelic properties, can cause a variety of mood-related effects. Acute intoxication is associated with euphoria, anxiety, agitation, and grandiosity. Chronic abuse can lead to low-grade lethargy and depression, sometimes accompanied by anxiety, paranoia, and memory loss. A recent study of 52 bipolar alcohol-dependent patients found that 48 percent reported marijuana abuse; those that did had significantly more psychiatric comorbidity, in addition to more severe alcohol and other drug abuse (Salloum et al., 2005).

Hypotheses about the Relationship between Bipolar Illness and Alcohol and Drug Abuse

Relationship of Alcohol and Drug Abuse to Phase of Illness

Although it is perhaps more intuitive to link increased alcohol consumption with the depressed phase of bipolar illness, evidence suggests that the link is as or more common with hypomania, mania, and mixed or transitional states. Indeed, bipolar patients who increase their alcohol consumption generally do so during the manic phase (Zisook and Schuckit, 1987). Table 7–3 summarizes six studies of the relationship between alcohol intake and phase of illness. Alcohol, to a point, does appear to provide some relief for the irritability, restlessness, and agitation associated with mania. In this sense, although its use is damaging overall, it is not surprising that alcohol consumption increases during mania.

There is some evidence that bipolar patients (38 percent) are more likely than unipolar patients (15 percent) to increase their drinking when in a depressive episode (Bernadt and Murray, 1986). The tendency for bipolar patients to drink more heavily when depressed may reflect the increased agitation and perturbation associated with coexisting transitional or mixed states. In an early study, Winokur and colleagues (1969) found that the percentage of bipolar patients increasing their alcohol consumption was higher during mixed and manic states (43 and 42 percent, respectively) than during bipolar depression (27 percent). Himmelhoch and colleagues (1976a) noted that the major differ-

TABLE 7–3. Relationship between Alcohol Consumption and Phase of Bipolar Illness

Study	DEPRESSED PHASE (%)			MANIC PHASE (%)		
	Increase	Decrease	No Change	Increase	Decrease	No change
Minski, 1938	100	0	0	29	0	71
Mayfield and Coleman, 1968	26	43	31	83	0	17
Winokur et al., 1969	27	0	73	42	0	47
Reich et al., 1974[a]	3	0	97[a]	50	0	50[a]
Hensel et al., 1979[b]	21	22	57	14	7	79
Bernadt and Murray, 1986	38	25	36	20	23	57

[a]No information given as to decrease or no change.
[b]Depressed phase approximated, excluding unipolar patients.

entiating feature between patients in mixed and nonmixed states was their rate of alcohol and drug abuse; the former patients were twice as likely to abuse these substances.

As noted earlier, findings of clinical research suggest that bipolar patients abuse cocaine when depressed, but are even more likely to do so while hypomanic or manic. Patients increased their cocaine abuse during the latter states not only to alleviate associated dysphoria, but also to bring about, sustain, or heighten the high-energy, euphoric state. These mood-altering uses of cocaine have been discussed by several investigators. The use of cocaine in hypomanic states was described by Khantzian (1985, p. 1263) as a means "to augment a hyperactive, restless lifestyle." Gawin and Kleber (1986, pp. 110–111) discussed the use of cocaine by cyclothymic individuals:

> Cocaine use did not precipitate manic episodes, and it was initially well controlled. . . . Cocaine use early on reestablished hypomanic functioning during dysthymic cycles. However, cocaine use eventually was extended to continuously regulate mood state. When these subjects began to perceive that cocaine use was harmful, they successfully refrained from cocaine during dysthymic phases. Paradoxically, 80% described that when mood state improved toward hypomania, judgment of the seriousness of cocaine-related problems deteriorated, and cocaine use recurred.

The use of cocaine for control of both depressed and elated phases of bipolar illness was described by Weiss and Mirin (1984, pp. 49–50):

> We were impressed by the perceived utility of [cocaine] in the regulation of both dysphoric and elated mood. Typically, depressed patients reported symptom relief at moderate doses but also noted the need to gradually increase the dose or the frequency of drug administration. . . . Bipolar and cyclothymic patients hospitalized for chronic cocaine use reported that they used the drug most frequently to enhance endogenously elevated mood in the manic phases of their illness.

Self-Medication Hypothesis

The hypothesis that alcohol and drug abuse/dependence occurs in an effort to self-medicate mood disorders has been suggested in various ways for more than a thousand years. In 1884, Freud recognized that cocaine, with its mood-elevating properties, could be used as a potent antidepressant. Later, Milkman and Frosch (1973; quoted in Khantzian, 1985, p. 1260) wrote:

> [H]eroin addicts preferred the calming and dampening effects of opiates and seemed to use them to shore up tenuous defenses and reinforce a tendency toward withdrawal

and isolation, while amphetamine addicts used the stimulating action of amphetamines to support an inflated sense of self-worth and a defensive style involving active confrontation with their environment.

As we have seen, however, contrary to theories positing the use of stimulants to counter depressive states, most patients report using cocaine primarily when hypomanic or manic to enhance or induce euphoric moods associated with those states. Weiss and colleagues (1988), for example, found that the majority of their bipolar and cyclothymic patients abusing cocaine claimed that they were not self-medicating depression but lengthening and intensifying the euphoric effects of hypomania. These same authors had noted earlier (Weiss and Mirin, 1984, p. 50) that the manic phase of bipolar and cyclothymic cocaine abusers was characterized by euphoria, whereas "substance abusers who experienced dysphoria during mania or hypomania seemed to prefer to 'self-treat' their symptoms with opiates or other central nervous system depressants (including alcohol)."

This notion of using opiates to self-treat dysphoric feelings echoes similar results from Rounsaville and colleagues (1982) and Castaneda and colleagues (1989) and, in part, those of Khantzian (1974) and of Wurmser (1974, p. 358), who suggested that the abuse of opiates was a mechanism for combating the "psychologically disorganizing effects of overwhelming rage" (Weiss and Mirin, 1987). Evidence suggests, however, that alcohol and such drugs as heroin and PCP also may produce increased symptoms of dysphoria, irritability, and anxiety.

Why, then, do bipolar patients continue to abuse cocaine, even after they have alleviated the painful state from which they were trying to escape? Weiss and colleagues (1986) hypothesized that low to moderate doses of cocaine may make affectively ill patients feel better (as Post and colleagues, 1974b, found in depressed patients) by relieving anxious, agitated feelings, and that this effect promotes further drug use. Other factors then assume importance in maintaining drug-abusing behavior, and a chronic dependence often results (Castaneda et al., 1989). This may be true as well for opiate and alcohol abuse in manic and depressed patients who continue to drink or abuse drugs despite realizing the substances' adverse effects on mood (Weiss and Mirin, 1987).

Self-medication of affective illness by alcohol has been postulated, but it is less well supported by the evidence than such use of cocaine and opiates. Reich and colleagues (1974), like many other clinicians, observed that increased alcohol consumption appeared to be a type of self-medication, an attempt to slow down, relax, and take the edge off the dysphoria. They hypothesized that excessive alcohol use is a sign of more severe mania and represents an attempt to control manic symptoms, especially sleep disturbance and hyperactivity. Noting that patients with mixed states are twice as likely as other patients to abuse drugs and alcohol, Himmelhoch and colleagues (1976a) suggested that the switch phase could be dysphoric and uncomfortable, and substance abuse could be used to self-medicate this dysphoria. Weiss and Mirin (1987) posited that, in addition to self-medication, the increased use of drugs and alcohol during manic episodes could be attributed to impulsiveness, recklessness, and poor judgment. Liskow and colleagues (1982) suggested that "drinking may simply be another manifestation of mania—manics tend to do more of everything" (p. 145) and noted that "the self-medication hypothesis relating alcoholism to affective disorder appears to be simplistic if not entirely erroneous" (p. 146).

The self-medication hypothesis in substance abuse among affectively ill patients is likely to be debated for some time before being resolved. The ECA data discussed earlier show a greatly increased rate of major depression preceding substance abuse, rather than substance abuse preceding depression. Recently, a study of 45 patients with bipolar disorder and substance dependence found that nearly all patients said they had initiated substance abuse because of symptoms of bipolar disorder; of these, most (78 percent) cited depression, followed by racing thoughts (58 percent). Two thirds (67 percent) of the patients reported improvement in at least one symptom as a result of the substance abuse (Weiss et al., 2004).

In summary, not all studies have supported the validity of the self-medication hypothesis. It is probable that a subgroup of bipolar patients abuses alcohol and other drugs to intensify elevated mood and energy states, while another subgroup abuses the same substances to ameliorate or self-medicate their manic, depressive, or mixed symptoms. Some do both.

Precipitation of Illness

An underlying bipolar illness may be precipitated by alcohol or drug abuse. For example, the first manic episode in a biologically vulnerable individual may be triggered by hallucinogen or stimulant abuse. Interactions among predisposed individuals, their substance abuse patterns, and the onset of abnormal mood episodes have been observed by many clinicians and investigators.

The most demonstrable drug-induced psychoses in manic-depressive patients are those resulting from hallucinogenic drugs such as LSD and PCP. The psychotic symptoms associated with the abuse of these drugs have been well documented by several authors (e.g., El-Guebaly, 1975; Bowers, 1977; Erard et al., 1980). Amphetamine abuse was noted by Ellinwood and Petrie (1979) to be a precipitant of psychosis. Many of the presenting symptoms (e.g., delusions of persecution and grandeur and visual and auditory hallucinations) are present in manic psychoses. Evidence from animal studies shows that cocaine is a potent inducer of a process analogous to kindling in the CNS (sensitization) (Post et al., 1984). The role of kindling–sensitization processes in the pathophysiology of manic-depressive illness is discussed in Chapter 14.

There may be important differences between patients who develop substance abuse after the emergence of manic-depressive illness and those who develop substance abuse first. Since the literature on the sequential relationships between major depression and substance abuse typically does not differentiate more recurrent from less recurrent forms of depression, our focus once again is on the bipolar subgroup. In a retrospective study of 188 patients, those with bipolar disorder who later developed a substance abuse disorder had a younger age at onset of mood symptoms (13.5) compared with bipolar patients who never developed such a disorder (22.7) (Feinman and Dunner, 1996). As noted earlier, Strakowski and colleagues (2005), in a 5-year follow-up study of 144 bipolar-I patients, found that those whose alcohol abuse disorder preceded the onset of bipolar disorder were older and tended to recover more quickly than those whose bipolar illness proceeded their alcohol abuse disorder. This later age at onset in the alcohol-first group was found in the 2001–2002 National Epidemiologic Survey on Alcohol and Related Conditions as well (Goldstein and Levitt, 2006). This may mean that an early onset predisposes bipolar patients to future substance abuse, or there may be a subpopulation at risk for both an early onset of bipolar disorder and substance abuse. Of particular note in the Feinman and Dunner study, patients whose drug abuse came first had a later onset of mood symptoms than those with primary bipolar disorder, and later even than that of patients with uncomplicated bipolar disorder (i.e., no substance abuse at all). One might speculate that these patients had a less active form of bipolar disorder, perhaps one that required triggering by substance abuse before symptoms of abnormal mood could emerge.

Differences between primary and secondary substance abuse disorders were examined in a 5-year prospective follow-up study of 70 patients with alcohol abuse and bipolar disorder (Winokur et al., 1995). In this study, as in that conducted by Feinman and Dunner (1996), bipolar disorder that developed after exposure to alcohol abuse appeared to be less severe than that which developed spontaneously. Patients with primary alcohol abuse had fewer episodes of abnormal mood during the 5-year follow-up period.

The concept of activation of a latent bipolar vulnerability by the abuse of mood-altering substances illustrates the challenges involved in studying comorbid populations. As the two studies just discussed suggest, substance abuse may unmask a less severe form of bipolar disorder that might never have been expressed had the patient not been exposed to alcohol or drugs. Because these patients have an inherently less severe form of mood disorder, their inclusion in studies can lead to the occasional finding that comorbid patients have a more benign clinical course compared with non-drug-abusing patients with bipolar disorder. Alternatively, the indiscriminate blending of patients with secondary and primary bipolar disorder can lead to a washing out of potential differences between comorbid and noncomorbid groups. It appears to make a difference whether the substance abuse is a cause or a result of bipolar mood fluctuations. This methodological and diagnostic issue is one of many that complicate the study of the two illnesses.

From a clinical standpoint, if substance abuse is able to unmask a latent bipolar disorder, bipolar parents who pass along a genetic vulnerability to their children should be counseled on the importance of helping their children avoid substance abuse. Abuse of illicit drugs can cause significant morbidity and mortality in any child, but those who have a genetic predisposition toward development of a mood disorder are at particularly high risk of harm.

Modification of Course

Alcohol and drug abuse may modify the course and expression of manic-depressive illness. Substance abuse problems can lead to more severe psychopathology and less favorable outcomes in a number of ways, including higher rates of mixed states, rapid cycling, impulsivity, aggression, and destabilization of sleep patterns. They may also slow the time to recovery, increase the probability of treatment nonadherence, and decrease the effectiveness of prescribed medications. As reviewed in Chapter 8, the mortality associated with substance abuse and depressive disorders is cause for particular concern. More than 90 percent of suicides are associated with a psychiatric disorder (Institute of Medicine, 2002), but the association is stronger for some conditions than others. Two of the highest-risk conditions are bipolar disorder and substance abuse, and there appears to be an often dangerous interaction between the two. Harris and Barraclough (1997) examined the effect of comorbid substance abuse on suicide rates in 7,819 patients with bipolar disorder, unipolar depression, or schizophrenia. Substance abuse problems increased the lifetime risk of suicide in all of the patients, but the increase was greatest among those with bipolar disorder (recurrent unipolar patients were not identified separately).

Rapid-cycling bipolar disorder, defined by four or more mood episodes per year, tends to have a more treatment-resistant course, and a link between the risk of rapid cycling

and substance abuse has long been considered likely. In the Systematic Treatment Enhancement Program for Bipolar Disorder (STEP-BD), a multicenter project designed to evaluate the longitudinal outcome of patients with bipolar disorder, the first 500 patients were evaluated for clinical characteristics associated with rapid cycling (Schneck et al., 2004). The investigators found a correlation between substance abuse and rapid cycling but concluded that the direction of causality was unknown; that is, it was not clear whether the substance abuse destabilized the bipolar disorder and led to rapid cycling, or the more severe psychopathology associated with rapid cycling predisposed to substance abuse. The authors did find that among rapid cyclers, those with bipolar-I were more likely than those with bipolar-II to abuse substances.

Mixed states, like rapid cycling, are characterized by greater psychopathology and associated with less favorable treatment outcomes than bipolar illness uncomplicated by these states (see Chapter 1). The observation that alcohol and drug abuse is significantly higher in patients with mixed mania has been reported by several authors (Winokur et al., 1969; Himmelhoch et al., 1976a; Himmelhoch and Garfinkel, 1986). Other investigators, however, have not found a higher frequency of substance abuse disorders in patients with mixed states (Cassidy et al., 2001; Brieger, 2005). Himmelhoch and colleagues (1976a, p. 1065) noted that "drug abuse (particularly alcohol and sedatives) alters the clinical presentation of manic-depressive swings, and the impact of oversedation or withdrawal or both on a 'pure' affective state is to make it dysphoric and mixed." More recently, Goldberg and colleagues (1999) studied the long-term effects of substance abuse on the course of bipolar-I disorder. They found that in a sample of hospitalized patients, substance abuse was more common among those who had mixed states. Remission during hospitalization was less likely among those with mixed mania, current substance abuse, or even a past history of substance abuse in the absence of current substance abuse. This finding raises the possibility that early or nonchronic substance abuse can have long-term negative effects on the course of bipolar disorder.

Although substantial data support the contention that alcohol abuse has a deleterious effect on mood disorders, less is known about the impact of moderate alcohol use. For healthy males, moderate alcohol use can have health benefits through a reduction in mortality from cardiovascular disease (Gaziano et al., 2000), but for patients with mood disorders, the negative effects on mood may outweigh the benefits. A study of 84 adult outpatients with bipolar-I or -II disorder who did not have active substance abuse disorders examined the relationship of moderate alcohol use to symptoms of mania and depression. On average, these patients consumed only 2.2 alcoholic beverages per week. Overall, beer consumption was not associated with mood symptoms; the consumption of distilled spirits, however, was associated with a lifetime number of manic episodes (Goldstein et al., 2005).

Comorbid substance abuse is reported to increase a bipolar patient's risk of experiencing a switch to mania when treated with an antidepressant (see Chapter 19). A recent controversial meta-analysis failed to find an increased risk of manic switch when the combination of a mood stabilizer[3] and an antidepressant was used to treat bipolar depression; however, all of the trials reviewed excluded patients with substance abuse disorder (Gijsman et al., 2004), and were therefore not representative of patients seen in clinical practice.

A smaller, retrospective investigation that did include substance abusers studied 53 DSM-IV bipolar patients. Fully 60 percent of those with comorbid substance abuse had a history of antidepressant-induced mania or hypomania, compared with 18 percent of patients with no substance abuse history. None of the patients without a substance abuse history switched into mania if they were taking a concomitant mood stabilizer during periods of antidepressant treatment. In the subgroup with comorbid substance abuse, however, 29 percent of the patients taking both an antidepressant and a mood stabilizer experienced antidepressant-induced mania or hypomania (Goldberg and Whiteside, 2002).

The effect of marijuana on mood changes was examined in a group of 50 patients with new-onset bipolar disorder. (Strakowski et al., 2000). Patients were followed for a period that ranged from 16 to 104 weeks. During this period, on average, patients met the full criteria for marijuana dependence or abuse 13 percent of the time. Patients who experienced a longer duration of marijuana abuse/dependence also had longer periods of mania. It is not clear whether the drug contributed to the maintenance of the manic state, or manic patients were more likely to abuse it as a result of symptoms associated with their elevated mood. A recent study carried out in the Netherlands, however, found that while use of marijuana at baseline increased the risk for manic symptoms during follow-up, manic symptoms at baseline did not predict the onset of marijuana use during follow-up (Henquet et al., 2006).

Evidence generally points to a destabilizing effect of marijuana. Its effect on mood was evaluated in participants in the 1980 ECA study, who were then questioned in a follow-up investigation conducted between 1994 and 1996 (Bovasso, 2001). Marijuana abuse was associated with subsequent depressive symptoms in individuals who had had no depression at the beginning of the study. Specifically, participants with no baseline depressive symptoms who had a diagnosis of marijuana abuse were four times more likely than those with no marijuana abuse to have depressive symptoms at the follow-up assessment. Suicidal ideation and anhedonia were both associated with abuse of the drug. Shedding light on causality, depressive symptoms at baseline did not predict later development of marijuana abuse, supporting the theory that the abuse of the drug led to the depression, rather than the reverse. An Australian study of 81 patients with recent-onset psychosis (bipolar disorder, schizophrenia, delusional disorder, substance-induced psychosis) found that a higher frequency of marijuana use was predictive of psychotic relapse, after controlling for medication adherence, other substance abuse, and duration of untreated psychosis (Hides et al., 2006). An increase in psychotic symptoms was also predictive of relapse to marijuana use.

Treatment nonadherence may be a mediator of poorer outcome among manic-depressive patients with substance abuse. Personality factors, attitudes toward medication, and the experience of side effects have all been associated with nonadherence (see Chapter 21); it is only more recently that attention has been given to the role of comorbid substance abuse (Haywood et al., 1995; Swartz et al., 1998; Perlick et al., 2004). Patients with substance abuse are likely to have poor insight into both their substance abuse and their mood disorder, and the denial of the need for medication is a common reason for nonadherence in this population, especially in the bipolar subgroup (Keck et al., 1997). Calabrese and Delucchi (1990) found that poor medication adherence associated with comorbid alcohol, marijuana, or cocaine abuse led to poor outcomes in rapid-cycling patients being treated with lithium or valproate. The efficacy of these medications was not affected by comorbid substance abuse in medication-adherent patients.

The disorganized lifestyle that accompanies substance abuse, difficulties in personal relationships and employment, and the experience of more adverse effects due to the interaction between medications and alcohol and drugs (e.g., fatigue, headache, irritability, destabilized sleep, neurocognitive side effects) also contribute to the poorer clinical outcomes seen in bipolar patients with substance abuse problems. (See Chapter 4 for further details on the relationship between substance abuse and the clinical course of bipolar disorder.)

ANXIETY DISORDERS

While comorbidity implies the presence of two separate disorders, individual symptoms of anxiety—agitation, accelerated thought processes, restlessness, social anxiety, irritability, and dysphoric mood—are common features of depression, mixed states, and mania (Young et al., 1993; Gibb et al., 2005). In one study, 39 percent of a group of inpatients with bipolar disorder had symptoms of anxiety that were an integral part of their mood episodes (Cassidy et al., 1998). Thus it is not surprising that epidemiologic studies have found full-syndrome anxiety disorders to be common in bipolar populations. McElroy and colleagues (2001) observed a 42 percent rate of anxiety disorders in a group of 288 outpatients with bipolar-I or -II disorder, nearly the same rate noted earlier for anxiety *symptoms*. This rate was identical to the rate of substance abuse in the same clinical sample. The presence of at least one Axis I anxiety diagnosis was associated with a history of development of both cycle acceleration and more severe episodes over time. Table 7–4 summarizes the rates of comorbid anxiety disorders in this sample of bipolar patients.

In contrast to substance abuse, which is more common in bipolar-I than bipolar-II patients, comorbidity of anxiety disorders may be more common in patients with bipolar-II disorder (Judd et al., 2003a). In a recent Finnish study (Mantere et al., 2006), for example, rates of comorbid anxiety were similar in bipolar-II disorder and major depression (56.5 percent and 52.5 percent, respectively), but lower in bipolar-I patients (35.6 percent). This association may be related to the fact that bipolar-II patients have a more chronic course, more major and minor depressive episodes, and shorter well intervals between episodes.

Panic disorder and OCD are particularly common comorbidities in patients with bipolar disorder. In the ECA study, 21.0 percent of patients with either bipolar-I or bipolar-II disorder met criteria for lifetime panic disorder, and 21.0 percent met criteria for lifetime OCD, compared with 0.8 and 2.6 percent, respectively, in the general population (Robins and Regier, 1991). Table 7–5 provides an overview of studies of the comorbidity of bipolar and anxiety disorders.

Sociodemographic risk factors associated with bipolar–anxiety comorbidity were derived from the Netherlands Mental Health Survey and Incidence Study, a prospective epidemiological study of 7,076 adults aged 18 to 64 years. Comorbid mood and anxiety disorders, but not pure mood disorders (depression, bipolar disorder, and dysthymia), were associated with female gender, younger age, lower educational level, and unemployment (de Graaf et al., 2002).

There appears to be an interaction between mood and anxiety disorders in that each illness can be triggered or worsened by the other. Bipolar patients with high anxiety scores are more likely than those with low anxiety to have made suicide attempts, to abuse alcohol, and to respond less favorably to lithium treatment (Young et al., 1993). An analysis of a cross-sectional sample from the STEP-BD project found that the presence of a comorbid anxiety disorder was associated with younger age at onset of bipolar disorder, decreased likelihood of recovery, poorer role functioning, and lower quality of life (Otto et al., 2006). Comorbid anxiety and bipolar disorders were also associated with substance abuse and a greater risk of suicide attempts in the STEP-BD data.

TABLE 7–4. **Percent of 288 Bipolar Patients Who Also Met Criteria for Various Anxiety Disorders**

Disorder	Lifetime %	Current %
Anxiety disorders	42	30
Panic disorder/agoraphobia	20	9
Social phobia	16	13
Simple phobia	10	8
Obsessive-compulsive disorder	9	8
Post-traumatic stress disorder	7	4
Generalized anxiety disorder	3	3
Other anxiety disorders	3	2

Source: Sasson et al., 2003. Adapted from McElroy et al., 2001.

TABLE 7–5. Overview of Studies of Comorbidity of Bipolar and Anxiety Disorders

Study	Population	Sample Size	Comorbidity Findings
Savino et al., 1993	Patients with PD	108	Total comorbidity with BP was 13.5%; 2.1% had BP-I; 5% had BP-II; 6.4% had cyclothymia
Young et al., 1993	Patients with BP-I and -II	81	32% met criteria for PD and/or GAD
Bowen et al., 1994	Patients with PD	108	23.1% had comorbid BP
Kessler et al., 1994, 1997	NCS; noninstitutionalized civilian population, subgroup with BP-I	130	33.1% had comorbid PD; 47.2% had comorbid social phobia
Chen and Dilsaver, 1995b	ECA database, subgroup with BP	168	20.8% had comorbid PD; 21.0% had comorbid OCD
Keck et al., 1995	Patients with BP	71	10% had OCD; 17% had PTSD; 16% had "any" anxiety disorder (including PD, agoraphobia, social phobia, simple phobia)
Krüger et al., 1995	Patients with BP	37	35% had comorbid OCD
Lensi et al., 1996	Patients with OCD	263	1.5% had BP-I; 13.0% had hypomania (most after treatment with antidepressant)
Dilsaver et al., 1997	Patients with BP	129	Comorbidity with PD varied with episode: BP depression, 62.3%; pure mania, 2.3%
Perugi et al., 1997	Patients with OCD	315	15.7% had comorbid BP; 13.6% had BP-II; 2.0% had BP-I
Pini et al., 1997	Patients with BP depression	24	36.8% had PD; 21.1% had OCD; 31.6 % had GAD; none had social phobia
Szadoczky et al., 1998	Hungarian National Epidemiologic Survey, subgroup with BP	149	10.6% had comorbid PD; 3.2% had comorbid OCD; 7.8% had comorbid social phobia; 12.9% had specific phobia; 14.4% had GAD

(continued)

TABLE 7–5. **Overview of Studies of Comorbidity of Bipolar and Anxiety Disorders** *(continued)*

Study	Population	Sample Size	Comorbidity Findings
McElroy et al., 2001	Patients with BP	288	42% had a comorbid Axis I anxiety disorder; 20% had PD with agoraphobia; 16% had social phobia; 10% had simple phobia; 6% had GAD; 7% had PTSD; 9% had OCD

BP = Bipolar disorder; ECA = Epidemiologic Catchment Area; GAD = generalized anxiety disorder; NCS = National Comorbidity Survey; OCD = obsessive-compulsive disorder; PD = panic disorder; PTSD = post-traumatic stress disorder.
Source: Adapted from Freeman et al., 2002.

Not all studies of comorbid anxiety and bipolar disorders have found a less favorable outcome. In a French study that evaluated 318 consecutively hospitalized bipolar patients, comorbidity with anxiety disorders was not correlated with severity of bipolar illness, as defined by number of previous hospitalizations, psychotic features, abuse of alcohol and drugs, and violent and nonviolent suicide attempts (Henry et al., 2003). This study also differed from other investigations in finding that comorbid patients, compared with bipolar patients without anxiety, responded less well to anticonvulsants but equally well to lithium; other studies have found anticonvulsants to be more effective than lithium in this population (see Chapter 24). The authors noted that only 21 percent of the patients in the study had a history of substance abuse. This relatively low rate of substance abuse may explain why the comorbid anxiety disorders had less of a negative impact on the clinical course of the bipolar disorder and its treatment than has been found in other studies.

Determining the prevalence of comorbid anxiety disorders and elucidating the nature of their interaction with bipolar disorder is scientifically important as well as clinically useful. Some investigators have suggested that genetic heterogeneity of bipolar illnesses may be responsible for the comorbidity with anxiety disorders (MacKinnon et al., 2003). That is, different forms or subphenotypes of bipolar disorder appear to aggregate in families and may be associated with different combinations of susceptibility genes and comorbid presentations (see Chapter 13). Ultimately, genetic research will provide a more fundamental understanding of comorbidity.

Panic Disorder

Panic disorder is one of the most common comorbid anxiety disorders seen in bipolar patients (McElroy et al., 2001). Data from the ECA study found that the lifetime prevalence of panic disorder among individuals with bipolar disorder was 21 percent, compared with 10 percent among those with unipolar depression and 0.8 percent of the general population (Chen and Dilsaver, 1995b). Conversely, patients with panic disorder have high rates of bipolar disorder, ranging from 6 to 23 percent (Savino et al., 1993; Bowen et al., 1994; Perugi et al., 1999).

Comorbid panic disorder can negatively affect the course of bipolar disorder. In a sample of 66 patients with bipolar-I disorder, comorbid panic symptoms were associated with more prior depressive episodes, higher levels of depressive symptoms, and greater suicidal ideation during the acute treatment phase. Patients who reported high lifetime scores on the panic–agoraphobia spectrum took 27 weeks longer for their depressive episodes to remit than those who reported low scores (44 versus 17 weeks) (Frank et al., 2002).

Not only is the bipolar disorder more severe in comorbid patients, but so, too, is the anxiety disorder. The NCS found that the co-occurrence of bipolar disorder and panic attacks was associated with earlier onset of panic attacks (age 17.1 versus 22.0 years) and, not surprisingly, with significantly greater panic symptomatology (Goodwin and Hoven, 2002). Comorbid substance dependence, specific phobia, and generalized anxiety disorder were each independent correlates of the co-occurrence of bipolar disorder and panic attacks.

Evidence suggests that panic disorder may be genetically related to bipolar disorder. The National Institute of Mental Health's (NIMH) Bipolar Genetics Initiative, which focused on family members of probands with bipolar disorder, found that panic disorder occurred in 17 percent of relatives who had a recurrent major affective disorder, compared with only 3 percent of those who did not (MacKinnon et al., 2002). Conversely, 90 percent of first-degree relatives with panic disorder also had a major affective disorder (MacKinnon et al., 1997).

It has been observed that some forms of rapid cycling and panic disorder are phenomenologically linked by sudden shifts in affect. Consequently, a logistic regression analysis of rapid mood switching as a function of familial risk for panic disorder was performed on data gathered from subjects in the NIMH Bipolar Genetics Initiative (MacKinnon et al., 2003). The analysis found that familial panic disorder increased the odds of rapid mood switching, suggesting that this comorbid presentation may stem from a genetically distinct subtype of bipolar disorder. Similarly, family clusters or specific susceptibility genes have been identified for bipolar disorder with psychotic features (Potash et al., 2001) and for suicidality in the context of alcohol abuse/dependence and bipolar disorder (Potash et al., 2001). A study of bipolar patients that focused on siblings found that those who did not suffer from a mood disorder had a low rate of panic disorder (3 percent) compared with those who had bipolar disorder (32 percent) (Doughty et al., 2004).

The pathophysiology underlying the close relationship between the two disorders is not fully understood. Dysregulation of the serotonin system probably plays a role in the overlap of mood and anxiety disorders, and the fact that SSRIs are first-line agents in the treatment of panic disorder suggests a role for serotonin in the pathophysiology of that disorder. SSRIs and postsynaptic serotonin receptor antagonists are also commonly used to treat mood disorders, but the role of serotonin in bipolar disorder is complex. As detailed in Chapter 14, some studies have found abnormalities in levels of 5-hydroxyindolacetic acid (5-HIAA) in patients with bipolar disorder (Young et al., 1994); however, this finding is not consistent across all studies (Berrettini et al., 1985). Patients with both bipolar disorder and panic disorder have been found to have noradrenergic hyperactivity. Increased plasma levels of the main norepinephrine metabolite, 3-methoxy-4-hydroxyphenylglycol (MHPG), have been found in patients with mania and depression (Swann et al., 1983). Several lines of evidence suggest that catecholamines, especially norepinephrine, are also implicated in the etiology and symptomatology of panic disorder. Significantly higher baseline levels of norepinephrine excretion are seen in patients with panic disorder compared with healthy controls (Bandelow et al., 1997).

As reviewed in Chapter 24, SSRIs and serotonin/norepinephrine reuptake inhibitors (SNRIs) may be used to treat comorbid anxiety in bipolar disorder. However, they carry the risk of inducing manic and mixed episodes, as well as longer-term cycle acceleration.

The efficacy of benzodiazepines in panic disorder suggests that dysregulation of the gamma-aminobutyric acid (GABA) system may also contribute to the etiology of this illness. Evidence for GABA abnormalities in bipolar disorder, however, is uneven and conflicting. For example, effective mood stabilizers such as valproate have putative effects on the GABA system. Valproate increases functional levels of GABA in the brain, apparently by activating the biosynthetic enzyme glutamic acid decarboxylase and inhibiting the degradative enzyme GABA-transaminase. Other mood-stabilizing anticonvulsants also modulate the GABA system. However, the relevance of this neurotransmitter to unstable mood in bipolar disorder remains unknown. (See Chapter 14 for more information on the role of specific neurotransmitters in manic-depressive illness.)

Social Anxiety Disorder and Social Phobia

In the NCS, an epidemiologic study based on nonclinician assessments, nearly one-half of patients with bipolar disorder met criteria for a lifetime comorbid social anxiety disorder, compared with 13.3 percent of the general population (Kessler et al., 1994). However, data from the Stanley Foundation Bipolar Network, obtained by clinicians using structured diagnostic interviews with a clinical population, reveal social anxiety disorder in only 16 percent of bipolar patients (McElroy et al., 2001). As with panic disorder, there appears to be a mutual-risk interaction, such that patients with social anxiety disorder also have high rates of bipolar disorder. Symptoms of social anxiety tend to disappear during hypomanic episodes, when excessive social inhibition is replaced by disinhibition. There may be an underlying social behavior dysregulation connecting the two disorders (Perugi et al., 2001). A recent study of 57 patients with social anxiety disorder found that a subgroup improved while taking antidepressants, and indeed presented with clear hypomania. Without antidepressant therapy, the symptoms of social anxiety returned (Valengaet et al., 2005).

Although social anxiety disorder is a serious illness and is strongly associated with functional impairment, feelings of social isolation, and suicidal ideation (Olfson et al., 2000), it tends to go unrecognized and untreated (Weiller et al., 1996). Clinicians who treat patients with bipolar disorder should be particularly wary of failing to identify this potentially disabling disorder. However, just as with panic disorder, treatment decisions can be complex. For example, in a study of 32 patients with social anxiety disorder, 14 (78 percent) of 18 patients who responded to a monoamine oxidase inhibitor (MAOI) became hypomanic (Himmelhoch, 1998) (see Chapter 24).

Obsessive-Compulsive Disorder

Analysis of data from the ECA study showed a lifetime prevalence of OCD of 21.0 percent in patients with bipolar disorder; this was significantly higher than the rates of 12.2 percent in unipolar depression and 2.5 percent in the general population (Chen and Dilsaver, 1995a). As with anxiety disorders in general, bipolar-II is more common than bipolar-I among patients with OCD (Perugi et al., 1997, 2002). Among patients with bipolar-I disorder, those with episodes of mixed mania may be more likely to have comorbid OCD than those with pure euphoric mania (McElroy et al., 1995). The presence of comorbid OCD leads to greater bipolar morbidity and possibly to greater mortality due to suicide (Krüger et al., 2000). Compared with bipolar patients without OCD, those with OCD have more severe symptomatology, including more lifetime suicidal ideation, suicide attempts, and comorbid panic disorder.

The phenomenology of comorbid OCD is somewhat different from that of "pure" OCD. The onset of the illness is more gradual, and the course tends to be episodic rather than continuous. There are higher rates of sexual and religious obsessions and a lower rate of checking rituals (Perugi et al., 1997, 2002). The episodic nature of OCD in bipolar patients may be related to the course of the mood disorder. In one study (Strakowski et al., 1998), the symptoms of both OCD and bipolar disorder cycled together in 7 of 16 patients. There were no cases of OCD that persisted in the absence of an affective syndrome. These data showing such a tight correlation between the symptom emergence of the two illnesses suggest the possibility that the two represent variability in the expression of a single underlying CNS dysfunction.

Post-Traumatic Stress Disorder

Although PTSD is a less common comorbidity than some of the other anxiety disorders, it is substantially more common in bipolar patients than in the general population. A meta-analysis of eight studies representing a total of 1,214 bipolar patients found that the mean lifetime prevalence of PTSD in those patients was 16.0 percent, a rate roughly double that of the general population (Otto et al., 2004). Table 7–6 summarizes the seven studies.

Little is known about why there is a relatively high rate of comorbidity of the two disorders, but there are some characteristics of bipolar disorder that place a patient at risk for the development and exacerbation of PTSD and vice versa. Pretrauma psychiatric illness, including some symptoms of depression and hypomania, increase a patient's vulnerability to developing PTSD after trauma (Schnurr et al., 1993). Abnormal mood at the time of the trauma can reduce resilience. For example, unrealistic and exaggerated negative attitudes common in depression can aggravate a patient's response to stressful events.

The impulsivity and poor judgment associated with elevated mood states place patients at risk for the occurrence of traumatic events such as assault and motor vehicle accidents. In one study of the general population, 51 percent of women and 61 percent of men reported a history of exposure to trauma (Kessler et al., 1995), and while some studies have found no difference among bipolar patients (Neria et al., 2002), others have found rates as high as 98 percent (Mueser et al., 1998). The experience of psychosis, which may occur in the context of a manic or depressive episode, is often a highly traumatic event in itself. Psychosis fundamentally disrupts an individual's notion of self and expectations of the future. Psychosis as part of an abnormal mood episode occurs in the setting of a highly volatile

TABLE 7–6. **Prevalence of Post-Traumatic Stress Disorder (PTSD) in Samples of Patients with Bipolar Disorder**

Study	Sample Characteristics	Sample Size	Rate of PTSD (%)
Keck et al., 1995	BP patients admitted for mania or mixed mania	71	17
Kessler et al., 1997	National general population survey; respondents with BP-I characterized by euphoria, grandiosity, and excessive energy	29	39
Mueser et al., 1998	Inpatients and outpatients with BP	50	40
Strakowski et al., 1998	BP patients, manic or mixed; first admission for psychosis	77	21
McElroy et al., 2001	BP-I and BP-II outpatients recruited from the community	288	7
Neria et al., 2002	BP patients; first admission for psychosis	102	11
Simon et al., 2003	BP-I and BP-II, treatment-seeking outpatients	122	19

BP = bipolar disorder.
Source: Otto et al., 2004. Reprinted with permission from Blackwell Publishing.

emotional state that further diminishes a patient's capacity to adaptively tolerate this type of stress.

On the other hand, for some patients or situations, euphoria or an underlying hyperthymic temperament associated with bipolar disorder may increase resilience in the face of trauma. That is, some patients with bipolar disorder have temperamental features that protect them at least partially from the adverse psychological consequences of severe stress. Persistent optimism and self-confidence can enable an individual to avoid some of the emotional injury that occurs in the face of trauma and continue to function in an adaptive way in situations in which others would experience high levels of distress and functional impairment (Jamison, 2004). The tendency to shift focus rapidly, not always a positive attribute of a hyperthymic temperament, may be protective during periods of intense stress by allowing the individual to avoid ruminating and fixating on traumatic experiences. The hyperthymic individual is also future oriented, a trait that decreases the deleterious influence of past events.

Symptoms of PTSD can aggravate the course of bipolar disorder. Stress of any kind places bipolar patients at risk for the emergence of a mood episode. PTSD is commonly associated with chronic overarousal that occurs in addition to the acute overarousal experienced in response to environmental cues. One of the consequences of overarousal is sleep disturbance, which can have a direct impact on the course of bipolar disorder (see Chapter 16). Chronic symptoms of avoidance seen in patients with PTSD can lead to social isolation, which is associated with more depression and longer recovery times in bipolar patients (Johnson et al., 1999).

Like panic disorder and bipolar illness, PTSD has been associated with chronic noradrenergic hyperactivity (Kosten et al., 1987). One consequence of this abnormality is a decrease in the number and sensitivity of alpha-2-adrenergic receptors (Maes et al., 1999). The serotonin system is almost certainly involved as well. Large placebo-controlled trials have demonstrated the efficacy of SSRIs in the treatment of PTSD (see Chapter 24), supporting the view that pathology associated with the serotonin system plays an important role in the development and maintenance of the disorder.

The presence of comorbid PTSD increases the morbidity, mortality, and functional impairment associated with bipolar disorder. Data from the STEP-BD project reveal that patients with comorbid PTSD have a lower likelihood of being in remission from bipolar disorder, are more likely to abuse substances, have higher rates of suicide, and have lower role attainment and quality of life compared with bipolar patients without PTSD (Simon et al., 2004b).

OTHER PSYCHIATRIC ILLNESSES

Attention-Deficit Hyperactivity Disorder

The overlap of symptoms seen in bipolar disorder with those seen in attention-deficit hyperactivity disorder (ADHD) can make it difficult to separate the two illnesses. This is especially true in children, in whom mood disorders manifest somewhat differently than in adults, and who may have difficulty in accurately describing their internal affective states. Distractibility, physical hyperactivity, and pressured speech can be symptoms of either bipolar disorder or ADHD. See Chapter 6 for an extensive review of the comorbidity of ADHD and other disorders in children and adolescents. See also Chapter 9 for an in-depth discussion of the pervasive attentional deficits associated with bipolar illness, even when the illness is in remission.

The rate of comorbidity for ADHD is much lower in bipolar adults than in children. Most children aged 12 and younger with bipolar disorder meet the criteria for ADHD (Findling et al., 2001), whereas comorbid ADHD was found in just 9 percent of the first 1,000 adult patients enrolled in the STEP-BD project (aged 15 and older) (Kogan et al., 2004). Among adult patients with early-onset bipolar disorder (before age 13), the rate rose to 20 percent (Perlis et al., 2004). ADHD affects approximately 4 percent of adults in the general population (Kessler, 2004).

Data from a large claims database revealed that adults diagnosed with ADHD were significantly more likely to have a comorbid diagnosis of bipolar disorder or major depressive disorder than non-ADHD patients (Secnik et al., 2005). Adults diagnosed with ADHD had significantly higher outpatient, inpatient, and prescription drug costs than noncomorbid patients with a mood disorder. A study based on structured psychiatric interviews found that 88 percent of adults with comorbid ADHD and bipolar disorder had the bipolar-II subtype (Wilens et al., 2003). This is another example of a comorbidity that is chronic in nature, being associated with the more chronic form of bipolar disorder. Compared with patients with pure ADHD, those with both bipolar disorder and ADHD had more DSM-IV symptoms of ADHD (14.8 versus 11.4 percent), poorer global functioning, and more additional comorbid psychiatric disorders (3.7 versus 2.0 percent). Based on the outcome of their analysis, the authors concluded that the observed symptomatology in the comorbid group supported the construct of two separate disorders that were distinguishable clinically.

Eating Disorders

Only a few studies have assessed the co-occurrence of bipolar disorder and eating disorders in community samples. One study of 3,258 Canadian adults found no overlap between 22 individuals diagnosed with lifetime bipolar disorder and 4 individuals diagnosed with anorexia nervosa; other eating disorders were not assessed (Fogarty et al., 1994). More recent studies, which differed somewhat by including subthreshold hypomania and binge eating, did find associations. Among 891 randomly selected schoolgirls, approximately one-quarter of those with an eating disorder had subthreshold bipolar disorder, compared with 3.8 percent of those with no eating disorder (Lewinsohn et al., 2000). However, the rate of full-syndrome bipolar disorder was similar among the girls with and without an eating disorder. Binge eating has been found to be specifically associated with hypomania. A comparison of patients with a history of hypomania, patients with a history of depression, and a control group with no abnormal mood episodes found that the rate of binge eating was highest in the group with a history of hypomania (Angst, 1998).

Studies of clinical populations have also found connections between bipolar disorder and eating disorders. Data gathered from clinical populations may differ from community data, however, because subjects currently in treatment typically have higher levels of distress and comorbidity than do community samples.[4] Consistent with this pattern, bipolar-II disorder was found to be common among hospitalized patients with eating disorders. An evaluation of a group of 15 bulimics and 7 anorexics found that 19 of the 22 had a major mood disorder; 1 had bipolar-I disorder, and 13 had bipolar-II (Simpson et al., 1992). In a larger sample, patients with bipolar disorder were found to have a lifetime prevalence of bulimia of 4 percent (bipolar-I, 3 percent and bipolar-II, 6 percent) and a lifetime prevalence of anorexia nervosa of 2 percent (bipolar-I, 2 percent and bipolar-II, 4 percent) (McElroy et al., 2001). Analysis of the first 500 patients in the STEP-BD investigation found that the rate of bulimia in bipolar women was relatively high (12 percent), as was true for the rate in bipolar men (2 percent) (Baldassano et al., 2005). In the only study assessing binge eating and bipolar disorder (Krüger et al., 1996), the rate found in the bipolar patient sample (13 percent) was significantly higher than that reported for the general population (5 percent) (Spitzer et al., 1993). In a comprehensive review of comorbid bipolar and eating disorders, McElroy and colleagues (2005) found a particularly strong association between bulimia nervosa and bipolar-II disorder. Their summary of eating disorders in patients with bipolar disorder is given in Table 7–7.

Axis II Disorders

Affective instability is a common feature of certain personality disorders, especially those found in cluster B. Because of the frequency with which these disorders are seen in

bipolar patients and the effect they have on clinical course, Chapter 10 focuses specifically on this topic.

MEDICAL ILLNESSES

In addition to psychiatric disorders, bipolar patients experience certain general medical conditions at a higher rate than the general public. Some of this excess morbidity is associated with adverse effects of medications used to treat bipolar disorder and some with lifestyle. In other cases, the etiology of the comorbidity is not fully understood. Because many patients with serious mental illnesses have difficulty obtaining adequate medical care, the treating psychiatrist may be the only physician caring for these patients on a regular basis, and therefore should screen them for common medical problems.

Cardiovascular Disease

Cardiovascular disease accounts for the majority of the mortality seen with metabolic syndrome (discussed later). Obesity, glucose dysregulation, and dyslipidemia are all risk factors for cardiovascular disease, and consequently patients with bipolar disorder experience cardiovascular mortality at elevated rates compared with the general population (Weeke, 1979; Sharma and Markar, 1994). The mortality ratio of bipolar patients versus the general population for cardiovascular disease is 3.0. Additionally, when all the symptoms of the metabolic syndrome are controlled for, bipolar disorder continues to be an independent risk factor for cardiovascular mortality (Norton and Whalley, 1984). Before the modern era of psychopharmacology, death from manic exhaustion was not uncommon; many such deaths were attributable to cardiac events (Derby, 1933; Cade, 1979). In a long-term study that followed a group of 406 patients for more than 30 years, mortality due to circulatory disorders was second only to suicide as a cause of death among patients with bipolar disorder (Angst et al., 2002). A large study of 15,386 patients hospitalized in Sweden for bipolar disorder between 1973 and 1995 found that the most frequent cause of death was cardiovascular disease, followed by suicide and cancer. The observed number of cardiovascular deaths among male patients was 1.9 times the expected number. Among females, the mortality rate was 2.6 times the expected number (Osby, 2001).

Increased platelet aggregation and low-grade systemic inflammation seen in depressed patients may be mechanisms by which a mood disorder is a significant and independent risk factor for ischemic heart disease (Musselman et al., 1996). Patients with bipolar disorder also are more likely to smoke and to have a history of hypertension (Yates and Wallace, 1987; Johannessen et al., 2006).

TABLE 7–7. **Studies of Eating Disorders in Patients with Bipolar Disorder**

Study	Study Population	Assessment Instrument; Diagnostic Criteria	Eating Disorder Findings
Strakowski et al., 1992	41 inpatients with BP and first-episode mania (25 women)	SCID; DSM-III-R	7.3% had BN: 12.0% of women and no men had BN
Strakowski et al., 1993	60 inpatients with BP-I and first-episode mania	SCID; DSM-III-R	6.6% had BN
McElroy et al., 1995	71 inpatients with BP-I and acute mania (39 women)	SCID; DSM-III-R	8.5% had AN or BN
Krüger et al., 1996	61 euthymic outpatients with BP-I ($n=43$) or BP-II ($n=18$) (38 women)	Semistructured Clinical Interview; DSM-IV	13.1% had BED; 37.7% had recurrent binge eating episodes
Schuckit et al., 1996	14 women with BP and 1,176 with other psychiatric disorder[a]	SAGA; DSM-III-R	Of women with BD, none had AN and 7.1% had BN, compared with 0.3% and 0.6%, respectively, of controls ($p<.01$ for BN)
Cassano et al., 1998	47 inpatients with BP-I with psychotic features	SCID; DSM-III-R	6.4% had AN or BN
Edmonds et al., 1998	64 persons with BP-I ($n=44$) or BP-II ($n=11$) from a BP registry	DIGS; DSM-IV	7.3% had a DSM-IV ED
Pini et al., 1999	125 patients with BP-I with psychotic features (69 women)	SCID; DSM-III-R	4.0% had BN and 2.4% had AN
McElroy et al., 2001	288 outpatients with BP-I or BP-II (162 women)	SCID; DSM-IV	5.9% had AN or BN
Vieta et al., 2001	129 outpatients with BP-I (76 women)	SCID; DSM-IV	2.3% had BN
MacQueen et al., 2003	139 outpatients with BP-I or BP-II (94 women)	SCID; DSM-IV	15% had an ED

AN = anorexia nervosa; BED = binge eating disorder; BN = bulimia nervosa; BP = bipolar disorder; DIGS = Diagnostic Interview for Genetic Studies; ED = eating disorder; SAGA = Semi-Structured Assessment for the Genetics of Alcoholism; SCID = Structured Clinical Interview for DSM.

[a]Subjects were participants in the Collaborative Study of the Genetics of Alcoholism.

Source: Reprinted from McElroy et al., 2005 with permission from Elsevier.

Thyroid Dysfunction

Thyroid dysfunction associated with bipolar disorder is a significant problem. In addition to the medical morbidity associated with thyroid problems, mood states and affective stability are intimately connected to proper functioning of the hypothalamic–pituitary–thyroid axis (see Chapter 14). Patients with thyroid disease have higher rates of panic disorder, simple phobia, OCD, major depressive disorder, bipolar disorder, and cyclothymia than the general population (Placidi et al., 1998). Bipolar women have higher rates of comorbid thyroid disease than men; analysis of the first 500 STEP-BD participants, for example, found rates of 26.9 percent in females and 5.7 percent in males (Baldassano et al., 2005). Hypothyroidism is the most frequent manifestation of thyroid dysfunction. The most common psychiatric symptoms related to hypothyroidism are depression and cognitive dysfunction. Fatigue, weight gain, dry skin, hair loss, intolerance to cold, and irritability are also seen. Abnormally elevated levels of thyroid hormone can cause dysphoria, anxiety, restlessness, and emotional lability (Trzepacz et al., 1988).

Problems with the hypothalamic–pituitary–thyroid axis are more prevalent in patients with mood disorders than in the general population; however, many studies have included large numbers of patients taking lithium or carbamazepine, which may account for some of the high prevalence found. (The association between mood stabilizers and thyroid function is discussed in Chapter 20.) Nevertheless, the effects of lithium and carbamazepine do not fully explain the association between bipolar disorder and thyroid dysfunction. In a sample of bipolar patients who had never been treated with either lithium or carbamazepine, the rate of thyroid hypofunction was 9 percent (Valle et al., 1999). Hypofunction was determined on the basis of serum levels for total thyroxine (T_4), total triiodothyronine (T_3), and thyroid-stimulating hormone (TSH) levels. Bipolar-II patients showed significantly lower levels of thyroid functioning than those with bipolar-I disorder, as measured by higher TSH levels. Primary hypothyroidism was diagnosed in 3 percent of a general population sample (Flynn et al., 2004).

The relationship between thyroid hypofunctioning and rapid cycling is unclear. In the sample just described, no difference in thyroid parameters was observed between rapid-cycling and non-rapid-cycling bipolar patients. Other studies, however, have found hypothyroidism to be a risk factor for rapid cycling. For example, in a sample of 30 patients with rapid-cycling bipolar disorder, 60 percent also had hypothyroidism (Bauer et al., 1990). Subclinical hypothyroidism, in which thyroid hormone levels are low compared with controls but still fall within the broad normal range, has been found to be associated with rapid cycling (Kusalic, 1992), although more recently, doubt has been cast on this association (Post et al., 1997). Identifying subclinical hypothyroidism in bipolar patients may be almost as important as identifying overt dysfunction. In 1974, Wenzel and colleagues introduced a system for grading hypothyroidism. In this classification, grade 1 represents overt hypothyroidism, as defined by decreased serum T_4. Grades 2 and 3 define subclinical hypothyroidism. Grade 2 is characterized by increased TSH with normal T_4, and grade 3 by the presence of an isolated exaggeration of the TSH response to stimulation by thyroid-releasing hormone (TRH) (Wenzel et al., 1974).

Subclinical hypothyroidism can influence the outcome of mood disorders even in samples of patients with otherwise normal thyroid indices. Frye and colleagues (1999) assessed thyroid function prospectively in 52 outpatients with bipolar disorder. Even though their free thyroxine index (FTI) values were within the normal range, patients with lower mean FTI values had more affective episodes and more severe depressive symptoms. Cole and colleagues (2002) found less favorable treatment response in bipolar patients with low-normal FTI and high-normal TSH. Others have found subclinical hypothyroidism to be associated with an elevated lifetime prevalence of depression (Haggerty et al., 1993). The rate of subclinical hypothyroidism is particularly high (30 percent) in patients with refractory, treatment-resistant depression (Howland, 1993). The relationship between subclinical hypothyroidism and treatment response is discussed further in Chapter 19.

Hyperthyroidism has also been linked to depressive disorders in some studies (Kathol et al., 1986; Placidi et al., 1998), but not all (Fava et al., 1995; Engum et al., 2002; Thomsen and Kessing, 2005); it has also been linked to mania in a case series (Brownlie et al., 2000), but this finding was not confirmed in a controlled study (Cassidy et al., 2002). In a recent large historical cohort study of 133,570 patients with a clinical diagnosis of osteoarthritis, depressive disorder, or bipolar disorder (610 of whom had hyperthyroidism), patients with bipolar disorder had a hazard ratio for hyperthyroidism of 1.59 ($p < .052$) compared with the arthritis controls, and 1.86 ($p < .014$) compared with those with depression (Thomsen and Kessing, 2005).

Although the evidence for a link between mood disorders and decreased thyroid function is more consistent than that for a link to increased thyroid function, the hypothesis that some mood disorders may be linked to dysregulation of thyroid function is consistent with most of the data. Clearly, all patients with a mood disorder should be tested routinely for thyroid abnormalities, including abnormal levels of TSH and free T_4. Even in the context of normal T_4, elevated TSH should prompt a further workup and consideration of thyroid supplementation. The absence of abnormal TSH should not rule out hypothyroidism in a patient with clinical manifestations of the disease because many patients with both major depression and bipolar disorder fail to mount a TSH response to a TRH challenge (Gold et al., 1977). Evaluation of thyroid abnormalities is particularly appropriate in rapid-cycling and treatment-resistant patients.

Overweight and Obesity

Obesity is a leading cause of preventable death in the United States, and the prevalence of overweight and obesity is increasing. A survey of 4,115 adult men and women conducted in 1999 and 2000 as part of the National Health and Nutrition Examination Survey found that 64.5 percent of the U.S. population is overweight (body mass index [BMI] ≥25), and 30.5 percent is obese (BMI ≥30) (Flegal et al., 2002). A separate, smaller study of 50 bipolar patients, which used the same BMI standard, found an obesity rate that was only slightly higher (32 percent). The number of previous depressive episodes was correlated with the likelihood of being overweight or obese. Most of the weight gain occurred during acute rather than maintenance treatment, and the increase in BMI was related to the severity of the depressive episode, as measured by the patient's score on the Hamilton Rating Scale for Depression (Fagiolini et al., 2002). Although several studies have found significant obesity in bipolar patients (Elmslie et al., 2000, 2001; Fagiolini et al., 2002; McElroy et al., 2002), it is difficult to ascertain the degree to which the obesity is secondary to medications used to treat bipolar disorder or to the illness per se (see review by Toalson et al., 2004).

Longitudinal studies of children and adolescents have found a positive association of major depressive disorder with adult BMI. This association persisted even after controlling for age, gender, substance abuse, social class, pregnancy, and medication exposure (Pine et al., 2001). An important implication of the last of these factors (medication exposure) is that there is a baseline risk for elevated BMI that is independent of the weight gain associated with psychotropic medication. Yet despite the multiple etiologic factors that link mood disorders with obesity, of greatest concern to the clinician is the fact that mood-stabilizing medications frequently cause weight gain (see Chapter 20). Evidence for this conclusion comes from the Stanley Foundation Bipolar Network. Both current weight and the BMI of patients in this study were correlated with the number of weight gain–associated psychotropics to which patients had been exposed (McElroy et al., 2002). Atypical antipsychotic medications are associated specifically with central obesity, which occurs when the main deposits of body fat are localized around the abdomen. Accumulating evidence suggests that central deposition of body fat is a risk factor independent of overall obesity for mortality due to cardiovascular disease, hypertension, and type II diabetes (Donahue et al., 1987).

Other medications used to treat bipolar disorder, including lithium, valproate, and some antidepressants, have also been associated with weight gain. Thus far, there has been less concern regarding the development of metabolic syndrome with these drugs than with the atypical antipsychotics.

Beyond weight gain caused by medications, symptoms of bipolar disorder itself can lead to obesity. Depressed mood leads to lower levels of activity. Atypical features such as hyperphagia, hypersomnia, "leaden paralysis," and carbohydrate craving are seen more commonly in bipolar depression than in major depressive disorder and are more liable to lead to weight gain. It should be noted that manic syndromes are associated with loss of appetite, hypophagia, hyperactivity, and weight loss. In the majority of bipolar patients, however, depressive symptoms are far more frequent than manic symptoms (Judd et al., 2003b). Depression is often accompanied by hypercortisolemia, which is also associated with central obesity. Even in the context of normal body weight, hypercortisolemia has been associated with excess visceral fat deposition as measured by computed tomography (CT) scan (Weber-Hamann et al., 2002).

Overweight and obesity, in addition to being a result of bipolar disorder, can worsen the disorder by exacerbating depression. The Western emphasis on being thin as a desirable physical trait can lead to negative body-image problems among overweight individuals. Overweight and obese individuals may also be targets of discrimination. The socioeconomic effects of excess weight were studied in a group of 10,039 randomly selected young people, who were evaluated for weight and BMI and then followed-up 7 years later. Women who had been overweight had completed fewer years of school, were less likely to be married, and had lower household incomes than those who had not been overweight; these findings were independent of baseline socioeconomic status. Men who had been overweight also were less likely to be married. In contrast, people with other chronic health conditions did not differ in these ways from the nonoverweight subjects (Gortmaker et al., 1993).

Among individuals seeking weight loss treatments, rates of mood disorders have ranged from a low of 8 percent (Wise and Fernandez, 1979) to a high of 60 percent (Hudson et al., 1988). Although there can be an overrepresentation of psychopathology among treatment-seeking patients, studies using community samples have yielded similar results. A national survey of 40,086 adults examined the relationship between body weight and clinical depression, suicidal ideation, and suicide attempts. Among women, increased body weight was associated with major depression and suicidal ideation; in men, there was also an association with suicide attempts (Carpenter et al., 2000).

Diabetes

Because overweight and obesity are associated with diabetes, many of the risk factors that have been linked to weight gain apply also to the development of diabetes. The prevalence of reported diabetes mellitus was found to be approximately three times higher in a sample of 345 hospitalized bipolar patients (9.9 percent) than in the general population (3.4 percent) (Cassidy et al., 1999). Patients in this sample also had a more severe course of their mood disorder and significantly more lifetime psychiatric hospitalizations than the nondiabetic subjects. Age at first hospitalization and duration of psychiatric disorder were similar in the two groups. Patients with bipolar disorder and comorbid diabetes have also been reported to be more likely to experience rapid cycling and to have a chronic rather than an episodic course of illness (Ruzickova et al., 2003). A comparison of 26 diabetic and 196 nondiabetic subjects from a community-based project carried out in Canada found that the disability rates for bipolar disorder were significantly different (Ruzickova et al., 2003); 81 percent of comorbid patients were receiving disability compensation payments for bipolar disorder, compared with only 30 percent of bipolar patients without diabetes.

When patients with diabetes are being treated, lithium should be used with care. Patients with juvenile-onset insulin-dependent diabetes are susceptible to diabetic nephropathy, and the risk is increased by the presence of hypertension. On the other hand, there is evidence that when lithium is combined with an oral hypoglycemic medication or insulin, it has an assisting hypoglycemic effect in diabetic patients (Hu et al., 1997). Fasting blood glucose levels were found to be decreased in patients taking lithium combined with other therapy, but not in those being treated with a hypoglycemic agent alone. A possible explanation for this finding is that lithium increases the sensitivity of glucose transport to insulin in skeletal muscle and adipocytes (Tabata et al., 1994). The authors of this study noted that the effects of lithium on glucose transport and metabolism in skeletal muscle were strikingly similar to the effects of exercise.

Dysregulation of the hypothalamic–pituitary–adrenocortical axis occurs frequently in patients with mood disorders. Hypercortisolemia, associated with depressive states, can lead to insulin resistance. Conversely, diabetic vascular CNS lesions may contribute to mania. Weber-Hamann and colleagues (2002) found that postmenopausal women who had depression also had significantly higher levels of free cortisol than age-matched controls. Elevated levels of cortisol can lead to decreased insulin receptor sensitivity through currently unknown mechanisms (Perry et al., 2003).

A more hypothetical link between bipolar disorder and diabetes relates to intracellular signal transduction involving the enzyme glycogen synthase kinase-3-β (GSK-3β). Alterations in GSK-3β functioning play a role in insulin resistance. Insulin inhibits GSK-3β, which results in enhanced glucose transport into skeletal muscle. Insulin-mediated inhibition of GSK-3β leads as well to increased glucose utilization and the production of glycogen (Orena et al., 2000). GSK-3β is also one of the targets for lithium action. Lithium significantly inhibits brain GSK-3β at concentrations relevant for the treatment of bipolar disorder (Gould et al., 2004). In addition to its role in glucose regulation, active GSK-3β facilitates apoptosis in neurons, while inhibition of GSK-3β attenuates cellular apoptosis, resulting in a neuroprotective effect (Hetman et al., 2000). Disturbances in the GSK-3β signal transduction pathway associated with diabetes may affect the viability of neurons that play a role in mood stabilization. Diminished insulin-mediated inhibition of GSK-3β may have an effect opposite to that of lithium and may ultimately lead to an accentuation of psychiatric symptoms related to bipolar disorder. For a more detailed discussion of the neuroprotective role of lithium and its putative significance for lithium's mood-stabilizing effects, see Chapter 14.

Migraine Headaches

The lifetime prevalence of migraine is markedly higher among individuals with mood disorders (Swartz et al., 2000; Fasmer, 2001; Odegaard and Fasmer, 2005) than in the general population. Bipolar women especially are more likely to suffer from migraines (Blehar et al., 1998; Calabrese et al., 2002). The Canadian Community Health Survey (N = 36,984) found that individuals with bipolar disorder had a higher prevalence of migraine than the general population (24.8 versus 10.3 percent; $p < .05$); the sex-specific prevalence of comorbid migraine in bipolar disorder was 14.9 percent for males and 34.7 percent for females. Bipolar males with comorbid migraine reported an earlier age at onset of bipolar illness ($p < .05$) and a higher lifetime prevalence of comorbid anxiety disorders ($p < .05$) than bipolar males without migraine. Bipolar females with comorbid migraine had more additional comorbid medical disorders ($p < .05$) than bipolar females who did not have migraines (McIntyre et al., 2006). Most strikingly, bipolar-II patients are far more likely to suffer from migraines than bipolar-I patients (77 and 14 percent, respectively), leading Fasmer (2001, p. 894) to suggest that bipolar-I and bipolar-II are "biologically separate disorders [which points] to the possibility of using the association of bipolar II disorder with migraine to study both the pathophysiology and the genetics of this affective disorder."

The comorbidity of migraine in women with bipolar-I disorder may be mediated by shared hormonal mechanisms that influence the timing of recurrence or complicate treatment. Both clinical and community studies using standardized diagnostic criteria have provided evidence of this comorbidity, independently of which illness caused the patient to seek treatment (Angst and Merikangas, 1992). In another study (Merikangas and Angst, 1992), bipolar-II disorder in probands was associated with an increased risk of migraine in relatives.

CONCLUSIONS

The scientific principle of parsimony holds that one should not increase, beyond what is necessary, the number of entities required to explain an observed phenomenon. In many cases, attributing all of a patient's symptoms to a single diagnostic entity is an appealing strategy. Symptoms that might be caused by a comorbid illness—such as excessive worry (generalized anxiety disorder), social avoidance (social anxiety disorder), distractibility (ADHD), and low energy and fatigue (diabetes)—are consistent with a diagnosis of affective disorder. Nevertheless, a large body of evidence derived from rigorously conducted studies unambiguously supports the presence of extensive comorbidity in bipolar illness, although with what frequency and which diagnosis subtype is open to debate (while substance abuse is more common in bipolar-I than in bipolar-II patients, the opposite is true for anxiety and eating disorders). It is probably appropriate, therefore, to begin by assuming that symptoms such as those cited above are not part of the core bipolar or unipolar presentation, and then to evaluate the patient systematically for the presence or absence of suspected comorbid illnesses. At the very least, all bipolar patients should be screened routinely for both psychiatric and medical comorbidities.

This type of comprehensive evaluation is time-consuming. Complicating the clinician's task, one of the most common comorbidities—substance abuse—is likely to be actively concealed by a patient during psychiatric consultation. Self-report screening questionnaires are useful when well-validated instruments are available. If the patient fills out such a questionnaire before seeing the clinician, less time need be devoted to ruling out comorbid diagnoses. Additionally, as a clinician works with a patient over time, a deeper understanding of the patient's symptoms and level of functioning develops, increasing the likelihood of uncovering additional disorders or problems.

As with other psychiatric illnesses, patients with recurrent affective disorders often fail to experience a complete remission of symptoms and a return to premorbid levels of functioning. The widespread prevalence of comorbidities, often missed by the diagnosing clinician, offers an opportunity to improve outcomes substantially by identifying and treating such problems as substance abuse, thyroid dysfunction, and anxiety. Patients who fail to respond adequately to multiple trials of medication should not be considered treatment resistant until a comprehensive assessment for untreated comorbidities has been undertaken. (See Chapter 24 for a discussion of the treatment of comorbid conditions.)

NOTES

1. These percentages are substantially higher than noted in the bipolar case registry (Chengappa et al., 2000), because in the Estroff et al. (1985) study, cocaine abuse was observed during an active episode of either mania or depression.

2. Estroff et al., 1985; Winokur et al., 1998; Goldberg et al., 1999; Cassidy et al., 2001.

3. Nearly 70 percent of all of the patients included in the analysis were participants in a study in which the concomitant mood stabilizer was olanzapine, which was considered placebo for purposes of the analysis. A smaller, well-designed study of lithium with antidepressants versus placebo did find a higher switch rate in the antidepressant plus lithium group, but in the meta-analysis this study was overwhelmed by the huge olanzapine study. See Chapter 19 for additional discussion of this study.

4. As noted in the introduction to this chapter, however, there are biases that operate in the other direction, namely the tendency of nonclinician interviewers to overdiagnose when using symptom checklists.

8 Suicide

The patients . . . often try to starve themselves, to hang themselves, to cut their arteries; they
beg that they may be burned, buried alive, driven out into the woods and there allowed to
die . . . . One of my patients struck his neck so often on the edge of a chisel fixed on the ground
that all the soft parts were cut through to the vertebrae.

—*Emil Kraepelin (1921, p. 25)*

Patients with depressive and manic-depressive illness are far more likely to commit suicide than those with other psychiatric or medical illnesses. An analysis of nearly 250 studies, reported over a 30-year period, found that mood disorders carry the highest risk of suicide (Fig. 8–1; see also Juurlink et al., 2004). Yet despite this high risk, the lethality of manic-depressive illness is often underemphasized. We believe suicide is far too common in untreated, inadequately treated, or treatment-resistant manic-depressive illness. Suicide is often preventable if a correct diagnosis is made, if acute and chronic suicide risk factors are recognized and acted upon, and if appropriate treatment is provided (see Chapter 25).

We begin the chapter with a look at diagnostic and methodological issues related to the study of suicide in bipolar and unipolar depressed patients. Next, we present findings on suicide rates. We then address causes of suicide, including the contributions of genetic, family, biological, and psychosocial factors. Finally, we review psychiatric and medical comorbidities and other clinical correlates of suicidal states.

DIAGNOSTIC AND METHODOLOGICAL ISSUES

It has long been recognized that suicidal thinking and behavior are associated with both bipolar and unipolar major depressive disorders (see Chapter 2). More recently, the *Diagnostic and Statistical Manual*, 4th edition (DSM-IV) incorporated into its diagnostic criteria for major depression a specific criterion for suicidal potential: "Recurrent thoughts of death (not just fear of dying), recurrent suicidal ideation without a specific plan, or a suicide attempt or a specific plan for committing suicide" (p. 327).

Studies of suicide have used several outcome measures—ideation, suicide attempts, and completed suicide. Over the years, researchers have recognized that these end points reflect a wide range of thoughts and behaviors. Today, the focus is on the use of more nuanced measures, such as the type (e.g., violent versus nonviolent) and the severity (e.g., Beck Scale of Suicidal Ideation, Schedule for Affective Disorders and Schizophrenia [SADS] suicide subscale) of the attempt. Suicidal ideation without particular information about plans or means is common in manic-depressive illness. Yet it is neither a sensitive nor a specific predictor of suicide, at least over the long term (see Chapter 25), and scales for rating suicidal ideation and intent therefore lead to high false-positive and false-negative rates (Jacobs et al., 2003). This chapter thus places greater emphasis on actual suicide attempts, especially those of high lethality (although, unfortunately, most studies of suicide attempts do not rate lethality), and completed suicide.

The approaches taken in research on suicide have generally ignored the presence of two distinct populations. The first comprises those individuals who commit suicide who have never been diagnosed with a psychiatric disorder. This group accounts for approximately 50 percent of all suicides, even though retrospective studies have found that a psychiatric diagnosis could be established in more than 90 percent of such cases (Henriksson et al., 1993; Cheng et al., 2000). This finding was the basis for *The Surgeon General's Call to Action to Prevent Suicide* (U.S. Public Health Service, 1999), which cited stigma, lack of public education about psychiatric disorders, and insufficient financial resources as barriers to diagnosis and treatment for those at risk of committing suicide. It also addressed the need to train physicians to recognize and treat conditions, such as depression or bipolar disorder, that can lead to increased suicide risk.

The other group of concern encompasses the remaining 50 percent of individuals who commit suicide despite

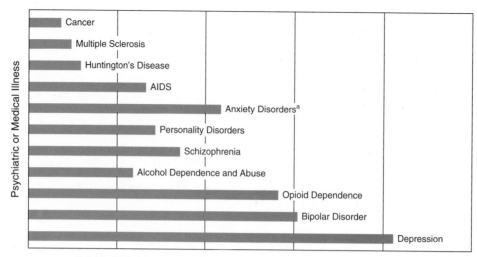

Figure 8–1. Suicide risk in psychiatric or medical illness: number of times the expected rate in the general population. [a]Obsessive-compulsive disorder and panic disorder. (*Source:* Adapted from Harris and Barraclough, 1997. Reprinted with permission from the *American Journal of Psychiatry*, copyright 2001, American Psychiatric Association.)

having been in recent contact with a clinician or diagnosed with or treated for a psychiatric disorder. Robins (1981) reported that 50 percent of his sample of suicides had seen a physician within 1 month of committing the act. Likewise, Barraclough (1970) found that 70 percent of those who had committed suicide had been in touch with a physician within 1 month, and nearly 50 percent within 1 week, of their death. And upon reviewing 40 published studies over the next decade, Luoma and colleagues (2002) concluded that 45 percent of those who had committed suicide had had contact with their primary care physician within 1 month of their death; 20 percent had been in contact with mental health services. Moreover, it has been reported that 6 to 10 percent of suicides occur in hospitals each year (Robins, 1981). Thus, despite ongoing treatment or health care contact, a significant number of patients are not being identified as being at acute risk for suicide. Others do not receive adequate treatment or fail to adhere to clinical recommendations (see Chapter 21). Many deaths could be prevented if physicians in both primary and specialty care settings became more alert to acute risk factors for suicide (see Chapter 25).

Other methodological problems limit interpretation of the findings of suicide studies. Diagnostic criteria often are unclear, and bipolar and unipolar distinctions only recently became standard in the literature. It is important to keep in mind that the definition of manic-depressive illness changed with the adoption of DSM-III in 1980 (see Chapter 3). The DSM-III nomenclature replaced the diagnosis manic-depressive disorder with that of bipolar disorder. Prior to this, a diagnosis of manic-depressive disorder had required a history or presence of recurrent depression *or* an episode of mania, thus encompassing the broader group of patients that is the focus of this volume (see Chapter 1). The narrower bipolar diagnosis required the presence or history of an episode of mania or hypomania; patients with recurrent depression were subsumed under the unipolar depression diagnosis, and recurrent unipolar was broadened to include anyone with more than one episode. This shift in diagnostic practice has made it more difficult to interpret secular trends. In this chapter, we employ the diagnostic terms relevant to particular studies, but otherwise (as throughout the volume) use "manic-depressive illness" to refer to the broader concept of recurrent major affective disorder; we use "bipolar disorder" to refer to the bipolar spectrum.

Particularly critical is the enormous range across studies in the length of follow-up periods; this broad range necessarily results in variable periods of risk for suicide. Moreover, when studies include only patients who have been hospitalized, suicide rates are likely to be higher, reflecting a greater severity of illness. Most early studies of suicide in manic-depressive illness were of hospitalized patients; many more recent studies are of outpatients or combinations of outpatients and inpatients. Because suicide risk is one of the most decisive criteria for admission to a psychiatric hospital, studies of hospitalized patients are necessarily skewed toward a greater likelihood of suicide.

SUICIDE RATES

In this section, we begin by reviewing suicide rates among the general population and among bipolar and unipolar depressed patients. We then present specific rates according to diagnosis (bipolar versus unipolar; bipolar-I versus bipolar-II), gender, and seasonality.

Rates in the General Population

In the United States in 2002, there were 31,655 deaths recorded as suicide.[1] This figure represents an overall suicide rate of 10.99 per 100,000 population (National Center for Injury Prevention and Control [NCIPC], 2005). Worldwide, an estimated 900,000 suicide deaths occur each year (World Health Organization [WHO], 2001); a figure of 1.5 million is projected for 2020 (Bertolote and Fleischmann, 2002). The estimated global suicide rate is 17.7 per 100,000 for males and 10.7 per 100,000 for females (Mathers et al., 2006). Many cultural factors, including religion and the adequacy of public health reporting systems, result in a wide range in the reporting and occurrence of suicide—from a low in Islamic countries to a high in Eastern Europe (the rates of suicide per 100,000 population are, for example, 33.1 in Hungary, 35.5 in the Russian Federation, and 41.9 in Lithuania [World Health Organization, 2001]).

Rates in Manic-Depressive Illness

Early studies documented a strikingly high lifetime rate of suicide, 15 percent, among patients with manic-depressive illness. The estimated rate today has dropped by about one half, except for patients early in the course of illness. The higher rates in most early studies (published before the mid-1980s) almost certainly reflect poorer clinical outcomes before the widespread use of lithium and other mood stabilizers, tricyclic antidepressants, and selective serotonin reuptake inhibitors (SSRIs). The figure of 15 percent lifetime risk also reflects suicide risk in clinical populations with severe, untreated manic-depressive illness.

Guze and Robins (1970) were the first to document systematically the extent of suicide risk in manic-depressive illness. They reviewed 14 follow-up studies, 2 population surveys, and 1 family study and found that at least 12 percent of all deaths among manic-depressive patients had been the result of suicide (in these early studies, patients with recurrent depressions were diagnosed as manic-depressive). In 9 of the studies, 12 to 19 percent of deaths had been due to suicide, and in the other 8 studies, the suicide rate ranged from 35 to 60 percent. The authors concluded that by the time all the patients in these studies had died, about 15 percent would have committed suicide, a rate at least 30 times that found in the general population.

Subsequent analyses buttressed these early findings. Our own review of 30 studies of completed suicide (1937–1988), presented in the first edition of this text, found a mean lifetime rate of 19 percent in patients with severe manic-depressive illness (range 9 to 60 percent). In 13 of the 30 studies, the figure was in the 10 to 30 percent range. In one fifth of the studies, at least half of the manic-depressive patients had died because of suicide. Similarly, a study of nearly 500 bipolar patients (mostly untreated or inadequately treated) over a 17-year period (1970–1987) found a suicide rate of 15 percent (Sharma and Markar, 1994).

The high suicide rate in manic-depressive illness is also documented by comparison with suicide rates in the general population. Harris and Barraclough (1997) calculated standardized mortality ratios (SMRs) in a meta-analysis of 14 studies reported from 1945 to 1992 ($N = 3,700$ bipolar patients). They found that the SMR for suicide in bipolar disorder was about 15 times higher than expected (see Fig. 8–1). Increased risk was associated with recent hospital discharge, a suicide attempt within the previous 5 years, and current alcohol abuse. The authors found a somewhat higher SMR, 20.4, for suicide in patients with major depression.

More recent studies, however, have found significantly lower rates of suicide (in the range of 5 percent lifetime risk) among never-hospitalized patients with bipolar disorder of moderate severity (see Tondo et al., 2003, for a review). But these lower suicide rates do not apply early in the course of illness. A study from the United Kingdom found a lifetime suicide rate of 6 percent for patients with affective disorders (depression and bipolar disorder), but the rate increased to 23 to 26 percent early in the course of bipolar illness (Inskip et al., 1998) (see later discussion).

There are several possible explanations for this marked decrease over time in reported suicide rates in bipolar disorder. A major reason, alluded to earlier, is most likely the increased use of lithium and other medications in the treatment of manic-depressive illness since 1980 (see Chapter 25). Other reasons for the decline are probably methodological. The findings of newer studies, which often have focused on outpatient populations or mixed inpatient and outpatient populations, reflect suicide rates in less severely ill patients. In their review, Tondo and colleagues (2003) suggested that reported rates are lower because most of the patients among whom the rates were ascertained were never hospitalized. They also pointed out that more recent studies, by reflecting the milder range of illness severity, underestimate the risk in more severely ill patients. They noted as well that, compared with a general population of patients, there is a lower ratio of attempts to fatalities in patients with major mood disorders. In their view, this finding suggests a high lethality and intent in affectively ill patients. The SMR for bipolar patients, based on a review of 28 studies from 1945 to 2000, was 22.1. Rates of suicide averaged about 0.376 percent per year.

Bostwick and Pankratz (2000) directly calculated the rates of suicide in hospitalized affectively ill patients versus other groups. In their meta-analysis, they reanalyzed both the Guze and Robins (1970) study and our own analysis of 30 studies (cited earlier), in addition to more recent studies (up to 1998). Using a different metric (case-fatality prevalence) they found lifetime suicide rates of 8.6 percent for patients hospitalized for suicide risk, 4.0 percent for those not hospitalized, and 2.2 percent for mixed inpatient/outpatient populations; the rate was less than 0.5 percent for the non–affectively ill population. The authors did not separate the risk for bipolar and unipolar disorders.

Bipolar–Unipolar Differences

Most studies have tended to find somewhat higher suicide rates in unipolar depression than in bipolar disorder (e.g., Harris and Barraclough, 1997; Osby et al., 2001; Angst et al., 2002). Others, however, have found either no bipolar–unipolar difference[2] or higher rates among patients with bipolar disorder (e.g., Rihmer and Pestality, 1999; Bottlender et al., 2000). The reason for these disparate findings, in our view, lies largely in the heterogeneity of the unipolar population and the underdiagnosis of mixed states and other forms of bipolarity.

The broad definition of unipolar depression in today's nomenclature simply means that the diagnosis is not bipolar; that is, a unipolar diagnosis encompasses patients with all degrees of recurrence, ranging from single-episode depression to highly recurrent or cyclic depression (see Chapter 2). Yet the research literature rarely has distinguished among unipolar patients on the basis of differences in their patterns of recurrence, which may in turn reflect different suicide risks depending on comorbidities, course of illness, and other clinical factors noted throughout this chapter. We believe that patients with recurrent unipolar depression may be likely to have suicide rates as high as or higher than those with bipolar disorder, whereas patients with less recurrent forms of unipolar depression are likely to have lower rates. Because the majority of unipolar patients have at least some recurrence, their inclusion could be expected to skew the unipolar category to higher rates. This might explain why Harris and Barraclough's meta-analysis (see Fig. 8–1) and other studies have found somewhat higher rates in unipolar depression than in bipolar disorder. A compounding problem is that, as we have seen (see Chapter 19), a substantial percentage of patients with major depression eventually convert to bipolar

illness. Finnish researchers have found that these patients form a subgroup that is particularly prone to suicide (Sokero et al., 2005).

What also may contribute to the apparently higher suicide rates in unipolar illness is the tendency to misdiagnose bipolar-II disorder as unipolar depression. Rihmer and Kiss (2002) argued that patients with bipolar-II disorder are often misdiagnosed and then included as unipolar patients. The unipolar category would thereby be erroneously elevated because the suicide rate in bipolar-II is higher than that in unipolar depression (Rihmer and Kiss, 2002) (Table 8–1). A final problem is that some patients diagnosed as having "agitated depression" may in fact have mixed states associated with bipolar disorder. This, too, would falsely raise the suicide rate in unipolar depression, particularly because mixed states carry a relatively higher suicide risk (see later discussion). If suicide occurs early in the course of affective illness, it may well be that patients who otherwise might have gone on to have a recurrent or bipolar course will have been diagnosed as having had a single episode of depression, again spuriously elevating the rate in unipolar illness.

The search for bipolar–unipolar differences, while important, may obscure the more significant point that all studies show greatly elevated suicide rates in both unipolar and bipolar groups in comparison with other medical and psychiatric populations (Sharma and Markar, 1994; Harris and Barraclough, 1997; Juurlink et al., 2004). The most prudent approach is to assume a high suicide risk in both bipolar and unipolar patients.

Bipolar-I versus Bipolar-II Disorder

Identifying diagnostic subgroups with an increased incidence of suicide or suicide attempts is one of the first steps toward identifying individual bipolar patients who are at particularly high risk. Several investigations over the last three decades have found that patients with bipolar-II disorder have a higher risk of suicide attempts than those with bipolar-I. These studies were reviewed by Rihmer and Kiss (2002) (see Table 8–1).

In addition, Bulik and colleagues (1990) studied 67 patients with a history of recurrent depression and suicide attempts. In comparison with 163 patients with recurrent major depression and no suicide attempts, they found that attempters were distinguished by a history of bipolar-II depression. The findings of these studies suggest that bipolar-II depression confers a particularly high risk of suicide in patients presenting with major depression. A recent retrospective study of 90 bipolar-I and 10 bipolar-II patients, however, did not find a significant difference in rates of suicide attempts between the two groups (Valtonen et al., 2006).

TABLE 8–1. **History of Prior Suicide Attempts in Patients with Unipolar Major Depression and Bipolar-I and Bipolar-II Disorder**

Study	Patients with Unipolar Depression Rate (%)	Patients with Bipolar-I Disorder Rate (%)	Patients with Bipolar-II Disorder Rate (%)
Dunner et al., 1976	2/23 (9)	11/29 (38)	9/16 (56)
Endicott et al., 1985	26/204 (13)	30/122 (25)	15/56 (27)
Coryell et al., 1987	31/303 (10)	7/29 (24)	7/40 (18)
Cassano et al., 1992	60/558 (11)	9/35 (26)	17/94 (18)
Vieta et al., 1997	—	12/38 (32)	6/22 (27)
Tondo et al., 1999	24/126 (19)	34/353 (10)	7/25 (28)
TOTAL	143/1234 (12)	103/606 (17)	68/253 (24)

Note: Bipolar-I + bipolar-II versus unipolar: $X^2 = 21.32$, degrees of freedom $(df) = 1$, $p < .001$; bipolar-I versus unipolar: $X^2 = 9.41$, $df = 1$, $p < .01$; bipolar-II versus unipolar: $X^2 = 26.59$, $df = 1$, $p < 0.001$; bipolar-II versus bipolar-I: $X^2 = 5.85$, $df = 1$, $p < .02$.

Source: Rihmer and Kiss, 2002. Reprinted with permission from Blackwell Publishing.

In their review, MacQueen and Young (2001) noted a particularly high liability for comorbidity with personality disorders, substance abuse disorders, and anxiety disorders in bipolar-II patients with an elevated risk of suicide (see Chapter 7). Bipolar-II patients, who have higher rates of comorbid substance abuse and personality disorders than bipolar-I patients, may be at increased risk in large part because of the comorbidity. Rihmer and Kiss (2002) found that when lifetime prevalence in the general population is the comparator, bipolar-II patients have the highest prevalence of attempted and completed suicides. The evidence strongly suggests that bipolar-II patients have—relative to the general population and to those with bipolar-I or unipolar depression—the highest rate of suicide.

Differences by Gender

In the general population of the United States, approximately three times as many women as men attempt suicide; however, four times as many men actually kill themselves (NCIPC, 2005). The patterns of suicidal behavior among women and men with manic-depressive illness show both similarities to and differences from this pattern.

Like the general female population, bipolar women attempt suicide more often than bipolar men. In contrast to the general population, however, there is no clear predominance of males among bipolar patients who actually commit suicide; the completed suicide rate for males is generally equivalent to or lower than that for females.

Reviewing 28 studies conducted from 1945 to 2001, Tondo and colleagues (2003) found that among bipolar patients, the average SMR for suicide was 14.9 for males and 21.1 for females. And a recent Swedish study of mortality outcomes in 15,386 bipolar patients found very similar SMRs for suicide—15.0 for men and 22.4 for women (Osby et al., 2005). It may be that the risk of suicide associated with manic-depressive illness is so powerful that it overrides the male–female differences in the general population. With regard to suicide attempts, Tondo and colleagues (2003) found that the rate among females within the bipolar subgroup (15 to 48 percent) was about double that for men (4 to 27 percent). Evidence of differences by gender among suicide attempters may be distorted by reporting biases, however. When patients are asked about past suicidal behavior, women may be more likely than men to admit to or remember attempts; men, on the other hand, may be more prone to suicidal equivalents, such as extreme risk taking, involvement in car accidents, and substance abuse. These behaviors are less often explored in surveys.

In summary, women with manic-depressive illness attempt suicide more often than men. In contrast to the general population, the suicide rate in women with manic-depressive illness is higher than or equivalent to that in men.

Seasonality

Seasonality affects the timing of manic and depressive affective episodes (see Chapter 16). It also has a profound effect on suicide. There is a robust literature on suicide and seasonality, in part because it is easier to date a suicide than the onset of an affective episode accurately and precisely. Most of the literature reviewed here does not specify diagnosis, but at the end of the section we discuss studies that deal expressly with bipolar disorder and seasonal suicide patterns related to mood states.

We reviewed dozens of seasonality studies for the first edition of this text. Since that time, many more such studies have been published. Taken as a whole, this literature affirms a striking peak incidence of suicide in late spring–early summer. Many studies have also found a smaller peak in October, generally for women rather than men. Both peaks, however, have lessened in amplitude over time (Fig. 8–2). Findings of more recent studies add considerably more nuance to the overall pattern of a spring-to-summer peak in suicides.

Seasonality and Suicide Rates

Granberg and Westerberg (1999) analyzed suicide data from Sweden (1911–1993) and New Zealand (1975–1995) and found that suicides peaked in the spring months— May in Sweden and November in New Zealand. In other studies, carried out in the southern hemisphere (Takahashi, 1964; Parker and Walter, 1982), the seasonality of suicide was consistent with the pattern seen in the northern hemisphere (i.e., peaks in the spring), although for New South Wales, Parker and Walter (1982) found two peak suicide periods (in May and November) among women rather than one. Chew and McCleary (1995), using time-series and cross-sectional data for 28 countries and employing bivariate plots and simple correlation techniques, found a sizable spring peak in suicide only in the temperate zones. More recently, Lee and colleagues (2006), utilizing the nationwide mortality database in Taiwan 1997–2003, found that suicides peaked in spring, regardless of gender or age. Ambient temperature was positively associated with suicide after adjustment for seasonality.

Fisher and colleagues (1997), studying 16,389 nationally registered suicide deaths between 1980 and 1989, found a peak in the spring in South Africa. Retamal and Humphreys (1998), reviewing 5,386 suicides in Chile for the period 1979–1994, found the highest rates in the "warm months" (i.e., the southern hemisphere's spring and summer), particularly December, and the lowest rates in the colder months, particularly June. Morken and colleagues (2002) studied all admissions in Norway for mania and depression during 1992–1996 ($N = 4,341$) and all 14,503 suicides in the years 1969–1996. They observed a significant peak in depression for women in November, with a secondary peak in April, and a peak for men in admissions for both depression and mania in April. Both genders showed a trough in admissions in July. Among men, the monthly occurrence of suicides correlated with the rate of admissions

Figure 8–2. Seasonal patterns of suicide. (*Source:* Jamison, 1999, *Night Falls Fast.* Reprinted with permission.)

for depression and mania (a spring peak); no such correlation was found in women. It may be that women were admitted earlier in the course of their depressive episode and that the peak severity occurred later; men may have been more severely depressed at the time of their admission. This issue has not been studied systematically.

Maes and colleagues (1993a) found significant spring seasonality for violent suicides but not for nonviolent suicides in Belgium. They also noted seasonality in the severity of depressive symptomatology as measured by the Zung self-rating scale, with greater severity reported in the spring months. Preti and colleagues (1998, 2000), examining violent suicide attempts in Italy, found a peak in the spring months, but only for violent suicide attempts in males. No seasonal trend was observed in nonviolent suicides among males or females during 1984–1995.

Findings reported by Maes and colleagues (1994) and Linkowski and colleagues (1992) suggest that violent suicides and perhaps violent attempts may be more common in sunny weather or higher temperatures. It is known that violent suicides and attempts are much more common in males than in females, a fact that is consistent with the greater occurrence of seasonality patterns in males.

Rasanen and colleagues (2002) investigated the seasonal distribution of the specific suicide method for both genders ($N = 20,234$) in Finland for the years 1980–1995. In summer, significant peaks occurred in suicides by drowning, jumping, and gassing among males. In autumn, there were peaks in female suicides by poisoning and drowning. Traffic suicides showed substantial winter troughs for both genders. The results demonstrated that specific violent and nonviolent methods for suicide formed their traditional clusters on the basis of seasonality, except for suicides by gassing and shooting.

Gender differences in seasonal patterns of suicide in Italy were examined by Micciolo and colleagues (1989). They found cyclic fluctuations in the number of suicides in both sexes, but only one significant peak per year for men and two for women. The most significant peak for both men and women was in May; women had a second peak in October and November. Hakko and colleagues (1998) studied seasonal patterns of suicide in Finland using a database of 21,279 suicides and found a peak for males from April to July; the distribution for females was bimodal, with peaks in May and October. In the elderly, they found a significant excess of suicides in autumn. Violent suicides showed a single spring peak, whereas nonviolent suicides displayed a bimodal distribution. Marion and colleagues (1999) found that in British Columbia, suicides among the young were associated with a spring–summer peak, whereas those among the elderly appeared to be related to deviations from expected temperatures for the

time of year. Salib (1997), studying suicide in an elderly population of 40,000 in Cheshire, England, over a 5-year period, found a positive relationship of suicide with hours of sunshine and humidity, rather than with extreme weather conditions. The findings of more recent studies have raised the question of whether the elderly may be affected more by rapid shifts in weather conditions than by seasonal effects. These findings raise the possibility that studies of seasonality should take into account age as well as violent versus nonviolent suicide methods, rather than simply merging groups of suicide cases.

There have also been suggestions that seasonal variation is greatest in rural as opposed to urban areas (e.g., Micciolo et al., 1991); one possible explanation for this difference is that urban living conditions, such as less direct exposure to natural light and more exposure to artificial light, may somehow reduce the seasonal effect. In their analysis of seasonal patterns of suicide in farmers and nonfarmers, Simkin and colleagues (2003) observed no significant seasonal patterns in violent suicides among nonfarmers.

The often-raised possibility of the effect of lunar cycles on suicide was addressed in a review of 20 studies by Martin and colleagues (1992), who found no evidence to support such a relationship. Likewise, Maldonado and Kraus (1991) found no effect of lunar phase in 4,190 suicides occurring between 1925 and 1983 among residents of Sacramento County, California. They did find that suicide occurred most frequently on Monday for both genders across age groups, and least frequently between the hours of 4:00 and 8:00 AM.

In short, it appears that seasonal variation in suicide applies most consistently to males, to the use of violent methods, and to those living in temperate zones. Seasonality may not be as much of a factor for females and males using nonviolent methods.

As noted earlier, a significant weakening of the association between seasonality and suicide over time has been observed in a number of studies. Rihmer and colleagues (1998), for example, found a link with seasonality in a (relatively small) sample of suicides from 1981–1986, but no such link in a sample from 1990–1996. Likewise, Hakko and colleagues (1998) found a decreasing frequency of seasonality in suicides in Finland after 1990. A reevaluation of seasonal variation in suicide in Australia and New Zealand led Yip and colleagues (1998) to conclude that seasonality was less of a determining factor than it had been. Tietjen and Kripke (1994) found no seasonal peaks in suicide in California's Los Angeles and Sacramento counties. Rock and colleagues (2003), on the other hand, found that seasonal amplitude had increased over time in Australia, contrasting this finding with those of contemporary European reports showing a decrease in seasonal amplitude over time. A recent study of suicides and seasonality in the Austrian prison system ($N = 412$), conducted over a 53-year period by Fruehwald and colleagues (2001), found no seasonal fluctuation in suicide rates. Parker and colleagues (2001) found no seasonal variation in 2,013 male and 1,382 female suicides in the equatorial region of Singapore.

Given the strength and breadth of the early findings of a strong seasonal component to suicide, an obvious question is why the seasonal effect has abated. In a review of the international literature on the seasonal incidence of suicide, Aschoff (1981) proposed that environmental factors play a role in the seasonal patterns observed. He found that during the nineteenth century, seasonal variation in suicide rates was greatest in the least industrialized nations and declined with greater industrialization. It is likely that certain aspects of industrialization (e.g., artificial light, central heating) may partially insulate patients from environmental risk factors for affective episodes. Seasonal variation in suicide rates, as we have seen, is greatest in the temperate latitudes as opposed to the north, with its extremes of light and temperature. Seasonal variation also is most correlated with hours of clear sunshine (not day length per se). Petridou and colleagues (2002), evaluating the traditional peak occurrence of suicide in June in the northern hemisphere and in December in the southern hemisphere, found an association between the seasonal amplitude of suicide and total sunshine. They suggested that suicide may be triggered by sunlight, perhaps through seasonally determined hormones such as melatonin (see later discussion). Papadopoulos and colleagues (2005) studied Greek suicide patterns and solar radiance data for a 10-year period and found that the solar radiance on the day preceding suicide was positively correlated with suicide risk, as was average solar radiance during the 4 days preceding that. They hypothesized that "sunshine acts as a natural antidepressant, which first improves motivation, then only later improves mood, thereby creating a potential short-term increased risk of suicide initially upon its application" (pp. 287–288).

Another likely explanation for the trend toward diminishing amplitude of the spring-to-summer peak in suicide rates is the greater use of mood-stabilizing medications. Rihmer and colleagues (1998) hypothesized that the link between seasonality and suicide has been weakened by the widespread use of lithium and antidepressants. Likewise, Oraveez and colleagues (2006) attributed the decrease in the seasonality of suicides in Slovenia to improvements in access to and effectiveness of psychiatric treatment following the 1991 war. Because major depression has such a strong seasonal component, the investigators argued that the decrease in the seasonality of suicide occurred as a result of improved treatment.

Neurobiological Factors in Seasonality

Clearly, profound biological changes occur in response to seasonal variations in light and temperature. Many neurobiological systems of relevance to mood disorders and suicide—including neurotransmitters, sleep and temperature regulators, melatonin, cholesterol, testosterone, estrogen, and thyroid hormone (summarized in Jamison, 1999; Institute of Medicine [IOM], 2002)—show pronounced seasonal fluctuation in their levels.[3]

A number of measures of serotonin function (see the later discussion of serotonin and suicide) have been reported to be correlated with the seasons.[4] This correlation may reflect a biological variable related to violent suicides, the effect of which may be diminished by older age, as well as urban living and perhaps even antidepressant treatment (see earlier discussion). Relating seasonal patterns in suicide to seasonal changes in various biological systems could thus yield greater insight into biological factors in susceptibility to suicide.

Timonen and colleagues (2004), studying 1,296 males and 289 females during the years 1988–2000, found the proportion of suicides in atopic (allergic) patients to be significantly higher than that in nonatopic patients. They further found that 72 percent of suicides in atopic patients occurred during the first 6 months of the year, and 28 percent during the second 6 months. By contrast, the distribution across the two periods was even in nonatopic patients. De Vriese and colleagues (2004) found a correlation between monthly variations in levels of the n-3 polyunsaturated fatty acids arachidonic acid and eicopentanoic acid and the mean weekly number of violent (but not nonviolent) suicides. A seasonal effect on factors likely to change levels of omega-3 essential fatty acids—such as fluctuating availability of foods and increased intake of fat-rich foods during the winter months—has been suggested by Hibbeln (1998, personal correspondence, 1999).

Seasonality in Bipolar Disorder

The seasonal pattern of suicide appears to run counter to that of bipolar depression, which is more likely to occur in the winter months in the temperate zones. (See Chapter 16 for extensive discussion of the seasonal patterns of mania and depression.) It may be that the increased activation associated with longer periods of light in the late spring months brings to a suicidal climax depressive episodes that begin in the winter months, particularly among those bipolar patients who are prone to developing dysphoric manic states. Cassidy and Carroll (2002a) analyzed the seasonal occurrence of 304 hospital admissions for mixed or manic bipolar states. They found that the frequency of all admissions for mania peaked in early spring, with a nadir in late fall. Admissions for mixed mania had a significantly different pattern, with a peak in late summer and a nadir in late November. Whitney and colleagues (1999) likewise found that mixed-state admissions in Canada peaked in the summer, but they did not find a seasonal pattern for mania and depression. D'Mello and colleagues (1995), studying the admissions of 377 bipolar patients in Michigan over a 6-year period, observed that women had a bimodal seasonal distribution, with peak admission rates in the spring and fall. They found that aggressive behavior peaked in the spring for both men and women. Several other investigators (Parker and Walter, 1982, in New South Wales; Mulder et al., 1990, in New Zealand; and Takei et al., 1992, in London) found a peak in admissions for mania in spring and summer.

These findings suggest a seasonal pattern in activation levels in bipolar disorder. Wehr (1992) observed that the risk for depression peaked at two opposite times of the year—spring/early summer and fall/early winter. These two periods are associated with opposite vegetative symptoms: sleep and appetite increases in winter depressions and decreases in spring/summer depressions. Maes and colleagues (1993b) observed that the severity of depression as measured by the Zung Self-Rating Depression (ZD) and Anxiety (ZA) scales showed a significant increase in the spring (April–May), with lows occurring in August–September; up to 31 percent of the variance in the weekly average of ZA scores could be explained by a circannual rhythm. In a subsequent study, Maes and colleagues (1995) noted a correlation between seasonal variations in serum L-tryptophan and suicide. Taken together, the studies reviewed here suggest an activation of manic-depressive illness (including mixed states, as well as unipolar recurrent depression) in the spring/summer months that roughly parallels the seasonal increase in suicides reported in the temperate zones, especially in males.

The second suicide peak in October may reflect an increase not only in unipolar depressive episodes, but also in suicidal depressions following the pronounced increase in manic episodes among bipolar patients during the summer months. That is, this second peak may represent suicidal postmanic depressions. It also may reflect the impact of mixed, transitional mood states. As patients recover from summer or autumn hypomania or mania, or as they switch from hypomania or mania into depression, mixed states are not uncommon. A recent study of depressed patients with mixed states found that the depressive episodes peaked in autumn (Sato et al., 2006). In vulnerable individuals, this may lead to periods of an acute, agitated suicidal state.

CAUSES OF SUICIDE

In this section, we review what is known about the biological, psychological, and social factors associated with suicide

in bipolar illness. This growing body of research is focused on determining what role these factors play—as underlying causes, risk factors, or protective factors—and on ascertaining whether they can be modified through treatment. To date, while it is clear that suicide is caused by a potent combination of biological and psychosocial risk factors, research has not yet reached the point where any particular combination of factors can be identified as predictive of suicide.[5]

Genetic and Family Transmission

The tendency for suicides to run in families has been noted in writings dating back many hundreds, if not thousands, of years. Using modern methods, researchers have shown that suicidal behavior does indeed have heritable contributions. This has been demonstrated through three lines of inquiry: family studies, studies of suicide in monozygotic (MZ) versus dizygotic (DZ) twins, and studies of adoptees (for reviews see Roy et al., 1999; Baldessarini and Hennen, 2004). These types of studies allow us to draw inferences about heritability and genetic contributions to suicide. Yet while they help narrow the search for genes that may be implicated, they cannot, by design, be used to identify particular genes (candidate gene identification is discussed in the next section).

Family studies compare the risk of suicidal behavior (i.e., suicides or suicide attempts) in close relatives of index cases versus the risk in close relatives of nonsuicidal cases or normal controls. Tsuang (1977, 1983) was among the first of modern scientists to report clustering of suicide in families. Since the 1970s, dozens of such investigations have been undertaken. In a recent meta-analysis of 22 studies, Baldessarini and Hennen (2004) found a nearly three-fold higher risk of suicidal acts among relatives of index cases compared with controls (Fig. 8–3). The investigators used random-effects regression modeling with weighting for study size and interstudy variances.

In the original studies on which the meta-analysis was based, the index suicide cases were not limited to a particular psychiatric diagnosis; a few studies were limited to major depression, but only one to bipolar illness (with comorbid alcoholism) (Potash, 2000). This latter study found bipolar disorder, alcoholism, and attempted suicide to be clustered in some families. Among subjects with bipolar disorder, 38 percent of those with comorbid alcoholism had made a suicide attempt; 22 percent of those without alcoholism had attempted suicide ($p < .005$).

Family transmission of suicidal behavior is not necessarily tantamount to genetic transmission, for any linkage between suicide and families also could be through learned behaviors or shared environment (e.g., parenting, physical or sexual abuse). Identifying genetic transmission requires piecing together of additional evidence, such as studies of

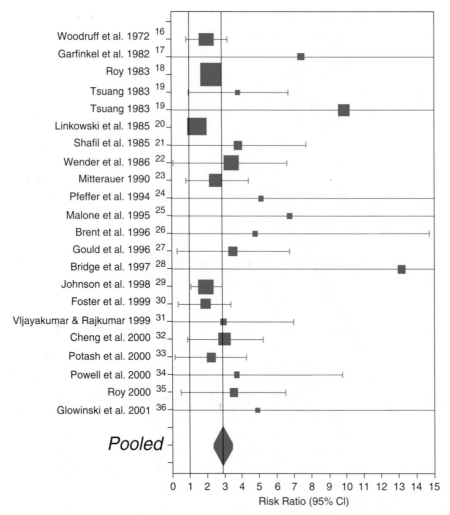

Figure 8–3. Meta-analysis of 22 studies of familial risk of suicide behavior based on random effects of modeling of relative risk (size of shaded squares reflects approximate weighting by sample size and variance measures) among families of suicidal probands versus controls and their 95% confidence intervals (CI; horizontal bars), with a pooled risk ratio and its CI (diamond). All 22 studies found increased familial risk associated with suicidal probands. The pooled risk ratio (vertical line with diamond) is 2.86 (CI, 2.32–3.53), which is highly significantly ($p < .0001$) greater than the null of 1.0 (vertical line). (*Source*: Baldessarini and Hennen, 2004.)

concordance rates in twins and adoptees, biological markers, and genetic polymorphisms, as well as linkage analysis.

Twin studies are designed to separate genetic from environmental contributions by comparing risks in MZ and DZ twins. Roy and colleagues (1999) compared concordance rates in 176 twin pairs with a suicide and found a greatly elevated rate among MZ (13.2 percent) versus DZ (0.7 percent) twins. His review examined only completed suicides, not attempts. In an analysis pooling seven twin studies, the rate of suicide or suicide attempts in MZ twin pairs (23 percent) was found to be much higher than that in DZ (0.1 percent) twin pairs (Table 8–2) (Baldessarini and Hennen, 2004). These rates yielded a relative risk of 175, but the investigators considered this figure to be unreliably high because the 0.1 percent rate in DZ pairs was calculated from only 2 suicides among more than 1,000 pairs. The investigators concluded that case ascertainment was likely to have been incomplete because the rate among DZ twins should have been comparable to that found among siblings, which typically runs about 9 percent in most family studies. Substituting this expected rate of 9 percent for the actual rate of 0.1 percent among DZ twins, they found a more modest relative risk of 2.6 in MZ compared with DZ twins. The increased risk is similar in magnitude to that found in a large study of 3,416 female adolescent twins (relative risk [RR] =1.9) (Glowinski et al., 2001).

Adoption studies compare the risk of suicidal behavior in biological versus adoptive relatives of index cases of suicide. This design gives adoption studies the advantage of controlling for shared environmental factors. Three adoption

TABLE 8–2. **Summary of Twin Studies of Suicidal Risk**

Study	REPORTED CO-TWIN SUICIDAL RATES		
	Identical (MZ)	Fraternal (DZ)	Risk Ratio
Kallman and Anastasio, 1947[a]	0/11	0/8	Not estimable
Haberlandt, 1967[b]	14/51	0/98	>27
Juel-Nielson and Videbach, 1970[a]	4/15	0/58	>15
Zair, 1981[a]	1/1	Not reported	Not estimable
Roy et al., 1991[a]	7/62	2/114	6.41 (95% CI, 1.38–30.0)
Statham et al., 1998[c]	365/1,538	0/1,199	>285
Roy et al., 1999[c]	10/26	0/9	>133
Total (7 studies)	401/1,704	2/1,486	174.8 (95% CI, 43.6–700.5)
Twin rates	23.5%	0.135%	175[d]
Family risk	Not applicable	8.98%[e]	2.62

Notes: The estimated risk (concordance) among DZ co-twins (0.135%) is 67 times lower than the average rate (8.98%) among the combined pool of first- and second-degree relatives in family studies summarized in Table 1 of Baldessarini and Hennen (2004), suggesting a more-plausible estimate of the MZ/DZ risk ratio of 2.62 (23.5%/8.98%; X^8 [1 df] = 276; p <.0001). Even with DZ and family rates pooled, the MZ/DZ risk ratio would be 23.5%/7.40%, or 3.18. For most studies, CIs are not provided because zero values appear in several numerators.

[a]Based on rate of suicides.
[b]Based on rate of suicides plus attempts.
[c]Based on rate of attempts only.
[d]Overall, Fisher's exact p <.0001 for the 7 studies.
[e]Based on raw data pooled from Table 1, column 3 (612/6811, or 8.98%), in Baldessarini and Hennen (2004).
CI = confidence interval; DZ = dizygotic; MZ = monozygotic.
Source: Baldessarini and Hennen, 2004. Reprinted from *Genetics of Suicide: An Overview* by Baldessarini and Hennen. Copyright 2004. Reproduced by permission of Taylor & Francis Group, LLC, http://www.taylorandfrancis.com.

studies have been undertaken, all of which used the same register of 5,483 adoptions in greater Copenhagen from 1924 to 1947 (Kety et al., 1968; Schulsinger et al., 1979; Wender et al., 1986). Pooling the data from these studies, Baldessarini and Hennen (2004) found that biological relatives of suicide cases are nearly five times more likely than adoptive relatives to commit suicide (risk ratio of 4.8) (Table 8–3).

What is being transmitted in the subjects of family, twin, and adoption studies? Is it the genes for a particular psychiatric disorder or some other factor (e.g., impulsivity, aggression) that may act independently of, or in an overlapping, additive, or catalytic manner with, a psychiatric disorder? For there to be overlap, some traits (and the genes underlying those traits) might be hypothesized to confer vulnerability to affective disorder as well as to suicidal behavior. Most of the research addressing the latter questions has not focused specifically on manic-depressive illness, however.

Several family studies have found that a higher risk of suicidal behavior holds true even after controlling for the effects of psychiatric disorders.[6] One of the largest and most recent studies was reported by Qin and colleagues (2002), who conducted a nested case-control study of 4,262 people who committed suicide between the ages of 9 and 45 during 1981–1997 and 80,238 population-based controls (matched for age, sex, and date of suicide). They found that a family history of suicide and psychiatric illness significantly and independently increased the suicide risk ratio by 2.58 and 1.31, respectively. This and the preceding studies are widely interpreted to suggest that there is an independent contributor to suicide risk beyond psychiatric illness.

In comprehensive reviews, Roy and colleagues (1999) and Mann (1998, 1999) and their colleagues proposed a stress–diathesis model of suicide in which an independent genetic/biologic factor predisposes to suicide risk only in

TABLE 8–3. **Summary of Adoption Studies of Suicide Risk**

Groups	REPORTED SUICIDE RATES IN RELATIVES		
	Biological	Adoptive	Risk Ratio (95% CI)
A. Kety et al., 1968[a]			
Suicides	5/156 (3.20%)	1/83 (1.20%)	2.67 (0.32–22.4)[b]
B. Schulsinger et al., 1979[c]			
Suicides	12/269 (4.46%)	0/148 (0.00%)	4.46[d]
C. Wender et al., 1986[e]			
Suicides+attempts	28/387 (7.24%)	8/180 (4.44%)	1.63 (0.76–3.50)
Suicides	15/387 (3.88%)	1/180 (0.56%)	6.93 (0.93–52.4)
Attempts	13/387 (3.36%)	7/180 (3.89%)	0.86 (0.32–2.13)
D. Pooled data from studies A and C	20/543 (3.68%)	2/263 (0.76%)	4.84 (1.14–20.6)

Notes: All three studies are based on a single Danish database. Study A data are for rates of suicides or attempts in biological or adoptive first-degree relatives of early-adopted probands who were diagnosed with schizophrenia-like disorders ($n=33$), committed suicide ($n=57$), or were diagnosed with an affective disorder (definite or probable DSM-III major depression or bipolar disorder; $n=71$), compared with early-adopted controls matched for number, gender, socioeconomic class of adoptive parents, age at adoption, current age compared with proband age at suicide, and time living with biological mother. Study B data (involving suicidal adopted probands), although complementary to other analyses, are probably not independent and are therefore not included in D (pooled data from studies A and C).
[a]Schizophrenia-like probands.
[b]Fisher's exact $p=0.0056$.
[c]Suicidal probands.
[d]CI is indeterminate because of zero numerator.
[e]Mood-disordered probands.
CI=Confidence interval.
Source: Baldessarini and Hennen, 2004. Reprinted from *Genetics of Suicide: An Overview* by Baldessarini and Hennen. Copyright 2004. Reproduced by permission of Taylor & Francis Group, LLC, http://www.taylorandfrancis.com.

association with psychiatric disorders or major life stressors. Psychiatric disorders and major life stressors, in other words, may trigger the genetic susceptibility to suicidal behavior.

Kety (1987) was among the first to hypothesize that a genetically influenced inability to control impulsive behavior might be a specific and independent susceptibility factor. Several family studies have lent support to the hypothesis that impulsive aggression, independently of psychiatric illness, increases suicide risk.[7] Impulsive aggression has been linked to low serotonin function (see reviews by Linnoila and Virkkunen, 1992; Oquendo and Mann, 2000), which is a biological marker of suicidal behavior (see later discussion).

Aggressiveness/impulsivity was one of a number of potential suicide risk factors studied by Oquendo and colleagues (2004). They tested the stress–diathesis model for suicidal behavior in a prospective investigation of 308 patients with major depressive or bipolar disorder. They found that the three strongest predictors of future suicidal acts were a history of suicide attempt(s), severe depression (according to subjective self-reports), and, for unknown reasons, cigarette smoking (although the National Comorbidity Survey—Replication [2001–2003] found no causal effect of smoking on suicidal behavior). Each of these factors posed an additive risk. The authors also determined that the tendency toward pessimism, as well as the presence of aggressive/impulsive traits, heightened future suicide risk in an additive manner. Swann and colleagues (2005) found that a history of severe suicidal behavior in 48 patients with bipolar disorder was associated with impulsivity, manifested as a tendency toward rapid, unplanned responses (as measured by impulsive errors on an immediate memory task and shorter response latencies).

Diathesis–stress models of suicide often assume that a predisposition to impulsive behavior provides the "diathesis" and the acute depressive or manic symptoms the "stress" that result in suicide.[8] However, there are virtually no longitudinal data on measures of impulsivity or aggression in bipolar disorder, and at the clinical level, rather than being invariant, impulsivity would be expected to be accentuated during manic and mixed states. Further, characterization of the essential deficit as being in the domain of impulsivity or aggressivity may be too narrow. An especially comprehensive neuropsychological study recently contrasted the profiles of medication-free depressed patients who had a history of a high-lethality suicide attempt, a low-lethality suicide attempt, or no suicide attempt with the profiles of healthy controls (Oquendo et al., 2003). The cognitive domains sampled included general intellectual functioning, motor functioning, attention, memory, and executive functioning. A discriminant analysis indicated that separate dimensions distinguished the total depressed sample from the healthy controls and the high-lethality attempters from the other patient groups. Impairment in attention and memory segregated the patients from controls, highlighting that a basic attentional disturbance may be a key factor in determining the cognitive sequelae of mood disorders, both unipolar and bipolar (see Chapter 9). Impaired executive function distinguished high-lethality attempters, with the executive function measures not restricted to indices of impulsivity. This work raised the possibility that a more broad-based deficit in executive function, perhaps related to self-monitoring functions, was disturbed in individuals with a history of a high-lethality suicide attempt.

In summary, there are strong genetic influences on suicidal behavior according to the findings of family, twin, and adoption studies. The findings of these studies also suggest that a family history of suicide and impulsivity/aggressiveness may increase the risk of suicide independently of transmission of psychiatric disorders. The possibility of independent risk factors should motivate clinicians, during their assessment of suicidal patients, to ask about family history of suicide, impulsivity, and aggression (see Chapter 25).

Neurobiological Factors

Serotonin Hypofunction

Many studies conducted over several decades have found an association between suicide and serotonin hypofunction. The first investigators to observe the association were Asberg and colleagues (1972), who found, in particularly violent suicide cases, low levels of 5-hydroxyindolacetic acid (5-HIAA)—the principal serotonin metabolite—in cerebrospinal fluid (CSF). A meta-analysis of 20 studies involving 1,002 psychiatric patients found that those with a history of attempted suicide, particularly violent attempts, had lower levels of 5-HIAA in CSF than did psychiatric controls (Lester, 1995). Lower serotonergic activity has

been localized to the prefrontal cortex in imaging studies of high-lethality suicide attempters (Oquendo et al., 2003). A recent prospective study of 27 bipolar depressed patients found that six subjects made suicide attempts during the 2-year follow-up period. These patients had higher aggression and hostility scores than the patients who did not make an attempt; CSF 5-HIAA, homovanillic acid (HVA), and MHPG levels were negatively correlated with the maximum lethality of the suicide attempts (Sher et al., 2006).

The robust finding of serotonin hypofunction, combined with the research discussed earlier pointing to genetic contributions to suicide, led to a search for candidate genes whose products control serotonin biosynthesis, degradation, or reuptake. Studies have sought to link higher prevalence of polymorphisms in serotonin-related genes to suicidal behavior.

Although serotonin hypofunction remains an important finding, studies of candidate genes have produced conflicting results and are beset by methodological problems (for reviews see Mann, 1998, 2002; Baldessarini and Hennen, 2004); moreover, few studies have focused specifically on bipolar patients. Consequently, a complete review of this subject is beyond the scope of this chapter. The recent studies highlighted here are illustrative of the complex range of findings regarding the enzyme tryptophan hydrolyase (TPH; the rate-limiting enzyme in serotonin synthesis), serotonin receptor subtypes, and the promoter region of the serotonin transporter. The serotonin transporter gene is responsible for reuptake of serotonin into the presynaptic neuron.

One explanation for finding low serotonin metabolites in individuals who have committed suicide is that less serotonin is being produced as a result of genetic defects affecting serotonin synthesis. Studying TPH, Turecki and colleagues (2001) found that one haplotype for the gene was significantly more prevalent among suicides involving violent methods than among living controls. Pooley and colleagues (2003) also found that a variation in the TPH gene was associated with deliberate self-harm. Other investigators, however, found no association between several TPH polymorphisms and suicidal behavior (Kunugi et al., 1999; Ono et al., 2000).

One of the earliest findings in autopsy studies was the higher number of serotonin 5-HT$_{1A}$ receptors, particularly in the prefrontal cortex, in suicide cases (Arango et al., 1995). Pandey and colleagues (2002) found an increase in another receptor subtype, the 5-HT$_{2A}$ receptor, in the prefrontal cortex and hippocampus of teenage suicide victims. In another study, one of the few with a distinct subgroup of bipolar patients, a polymorphism in the 5–HT$_{2A}$ receptor was found in this subgroup to be associated with a *lower* risk of suicidal behavior (Bonnier et al., 2002). On the other hand, Turecki and colleagues (2003), studying genes for seven serotonin receptor subtypes, found no differences in allelic or genotypic distributions. Schmauss (2003) found evidence of altered transcripts of the 5-HT2$_C$ gene in the brains of depressed suicide victims and hypothesized that the alteration reflects defects in regulation of ribonucleic acid (RNA) editing by synaptic serotonin.

The promoter region of the serotonin transporter gene has been found to be altered in several studies of suicidal behavior or violent suicides. Bondy and colleagues (2000) found increased frequency among suicide victims (with unknown diagnoses) of one or two short alleles of the serotonin transporter gene promoter (5-HTTLPR). The short allele, as compared with the long allele, has been linked to lower transcriptional efficacy (Lesch et al., 1996). In prior studies, the alleles were found to be associated with anxiety-related personality traits, affective disorders, or severe alcohol dependence. In a meta-analysis, Lin and Tsai (2004) also found a significant relationship between the short allele of 5-HTTLPR and suicidal behavior, especially violent suicide. But many studies have not found a relationship between the serotonin transporter polymorphism and completed suicide (Mann et al., 2000; Fitch et al., 2001) or suicide attempts (Geijer et al., 2000; Baca-Garcia et al., 2004) or in suicidal inpatients (Russ et al., 2000).

Two key studies sought to determine the predictive value of possessing the homozygous short (S/S) allele. Courtet and colleagues (2004) followed 133 patients hospitalized for a suicide attempt after first genotyping them for both A218C TPH and the functional S/L 5-HTTLPR polymorphism. Of the 76 patients they followed for 1 year, 20 reattempted suicide. The frequencies of the S or S/S allele were higher in those who had reattempted suicide, with elevated odds ratios (in comparison with the homozygous long [L/L] allele group) of 2.8 and 6.5, respectively. Impulsivity scores on the Baratt Impulsivity Scale (BIS) were significantly higher in patients carrying the S/S genotype than in those carrying the S/L genotype ($p = .026$). No differences were found in the TPH gene. The authors concluded that the SS genotype is a risk factor for future suicide attempts among those who have made a previous attempt.

A related study by Caspi and colleagues (2003) prospectively followed a cohort to test whether genetic vulnerability, as manifested by the short allele of 5-HTTLPR, would lead to depression or suicidality in individuals exposed to serious life stressors. Their hypothesis was supported by the finding that individuals with one or two copies of the short allele displayed, after exposure to stressful life events, more depressive symptoms, diagnosable depression, and

suicidal ideation or attempts compared with individuals homozygous for the long allele. This study provides evidence of a gene–environment interaction, insofar as an individual's response to stressful life events is moderated by a particular aspect of his or her genetic makeup (in this case, the short allele of the promoter region of the serotonin transporter gene). It is noteworthy that the study found a relationship of genotype not only with depressive symptoms, but also with suicidal ideation or attempts.

While few studies of candidate genes have looked at possible gender differences, Baca-Garcia and colleagues (2003) published pilot data suggesting that females with the L/L allele are less likely to make suicide attempts than those with the S/S or S/L alleles. This protection may be lost, however, during life phases characterized by lower estradiol, such as menses or menopause.

The brain's serotonin system is highly complex. Although the findings of studies reviewed here point to genetic alterations in the serotonin system as having a relationship to suicidal behavior, the findings with respect to manic-depressive illness and suicide remain inconclusive.

Low Cholesterol

A number of studies have suggested a possible relationship between low cholesterol and impulsive aggression, including higher death rates from suicide. The link is hypothesized to occur through cholesterol's effect on serotonin activity (Mann, 1998). The findings of these studies, however, which include both large epidemiologic surveys and studies of suicidal individuals, have been mixed.[9] In some cases, an association was found only in violent suicide attempters (Alvarez et al., 2000). (See reviews by Boston et al., 1996; Hillbrand and Spitz, 1997.)

In those studies looking specifically at bipolar patients, the findings have again been mixed. Bocchetta and colleagues (2001) studied 783 consecutive patients admitted to a lithium clinic. They found that the proportion of men with a lifetime history of suicide attempts or a history of a suicide by a first-degree relative was significantly higher in the group with low cholesterol levels (in the lowest 25th percentile) than in those with higher levels. Cassidy and Carroll (2002a) found low fasting cholesterol in manic patients, particularly during mixed manic episodes, and hypothesized that this condition is secondary to immune activation. On the other hand, Tsai and colleagues (2002), studying 43 bipolar patients who died by suicide in Taiwan between 1985 and 1996, found no difference in cholesterol levels compared with controls, who were bipolar patients still living.

In summary, if there is a relationship between low cholesterol and suicide, it is likely to apply to violent suicide attempts and completed suicides. However, lowering cholesterol with statin medications does not appear to have increased suicide risk in the large samples studied (Manfredini et al., 2000; Muldoon et al., 2001), and it is unclear whether the association between low cholesterol and suicide risk will hold true in bipolar patients.

Hypothalamic–Pituitary–Adrenal Axis Hyperactivity

Hyperactivity of the hypothalamic–pituitary–adrenal (HPA) axis has long been hypothesized as a biochemical marker of suicide. The HPA axis is the preeminent modulator of the relationship between acute stress exposure and physiological activation. In studies dating back to the 1960s, researchers observed that, within days before suicide, patients with major affective disorders had elevated levels of urinary 17-hydroxycorticosteroid and serum cortisol.[10] Not all studies of suicide found these elevations, however (Levy and Hansen, 1969).

In a related finding, individuals who died from suicide had enlarged adrenal glands compared with controls who died from accidents (Dorovini-Zis and Zis, 1987; Szigethy et al., 1994). Findings of increased levels of corticotropin-releasing factor (CRF) in the CSF of suicide victims (Arato et al., 1989; Brunner and Bronisch, 1999), as well as evidence of downregulation of CRF receptors in the frontal cortex (Nemeroff et al., 1988), suggested increased CRF release prior to suicide. Hucks and colleagues (1997) found no decrease in CRF receptors, even when they compared those taking and not taking antidepressants before suicide. More recently, Hiroi and colleagues (2001) found a shift in the ratio of corticotropin-releasing hormone receptor 1 (CRH-R1) to corticotropin-releasing hormone receptor 2 (CRH-R2) in the pituitary gland of suicide victims.

Another measure of HPA hyperactivity studied in relation to suicide is the dexamethasone suppression test (DST), which shows a failure of exogenous dexamethasone to suppress levels of cortisol secreted by the adrenal glands. Most studies have found a relationship between DST nonsuppression and suicide completion, but the relationship to suicide attempts is not as strong.

Studying 65 patients with major depression, Brown and colleagues (1986) found no relationship between DST nonsuppression and suicide attempts. In contrast, Coryell (1990) observed that 76 depressed inpatients who were nonsuppressors at inpatient admission were more likely over a 5-year follow-up period to develop mania or hypomania and to make serious suicide attempts. Studying depressed inpatients, Norman and colleagues (1990) matched 13 patients who had committed suicide with depressed inpatients who had made suicide attempts before admission ($n = 25$) and those who had not made attempts ($n = 28$). More than half of the patients committing suicide were nonsuppressors, compared with lower proportions of

suicide attempters and nonattempters. Likewise, a meta-analysis found that DST nonsuppression was predictive of completed suicide (Lester, 1992).

Findings of a more recent study strengthened the relationship between nonsuppression and completed suicide. Coryell and Schlesser (2001) found that nearly half of 78 inpatients with affective disorders were DST nonsuppressors at admission. After being followed for 15 years, 26.8 percent of nonsuppressors eventually died by suicide, compared with only 2.9 percent of DST suppressors. Within this sample, a comparatively small number of bipolar patients had received a DST because most had been admitted in a manic state, which made cooperation in taking the DST more difficult. Data from studies of abused children and patients with post-traumatic stress disorder also suggest that these overwhelming stressors can persistently alter the responses of the HPA axis (Heim and Nemeroff, 1999, 2002).

Norepinephrine Function

Several studies have identified alterations in norepinephrine transmission in relation to suicide. Ordway (1997) and others (Arango et al., 1997; Gonzalez-Maeso et al., 2002) found reductions in norepinephrine levels in the locus caeruleus (LC) of suicide victims, as well as increased levels of tyrosine hydroxylase and supersensitivity of alpha-2 adrenoceptors. Ordway characterized the changes he found in suicide victims as being similar to those found in rats after LC activation. He hypothesized that suicide victims experience chronic activation of the LC, leading to depletion of norepinephrine and other compensatory changes. Recently, Ono and colleagues (2004) found evidence suggesting that a Val/Val polymorphism for the catecholamine-metabolizing enzyme, catechol-O-methyltransferase, may be protective against suicide.

Psychological Traits and Temperament

A passive sense of hopelessness is a chronic risk factor for suicide. This conclusion is supported by the findings of a 20-year prospective study (Beck et al., 1999; Brown et al., 2000); another large-scale prospective investigation, the National Institute of Mental Health's (NIMH) Collaborative Program on the Psychobiology of Depression-Clinical Studies, which studied 954 patients with affective disorders, including more than 300 with bipolar illness (Fawcett et al., 1990); and a meta-analysis of case-control, cohort, and cross-sectional investigations of attempted suicides (23 studies) or completed suicides (13 studies) in bipolar patients (Hawton et al., 2005). While hopelessness has generally been conceptualized as a symptom specific to depression, the NIMH study found baseline hopelessness to be trait-like (Young et al., 1996). The study also found that baseline hopelessness predicted a suicide attempt. In the 20-year prospective study, researchers found that severity of suicidal ideation at its worst point is predictive of suicide. The patients who scored in the high-severity category on this measure were far more likely to ultimately kill themselves than those in the lower-severity group (odds ratio [OR] = 13.8) (Beck et al., 1999). We are unaware of any studies concerning familial transmission of hopelessness. Hostility, which in an acute way is often associated with mixed states, is also associated with increased rates of attempted and completed suicide (so, too, relatedly, are impulsivity and aggression) (Michaelis et al., 2004; Rutter and Behrendt, 2004; Galfalvy et al., 2006).

Certain temperaments, such as novelty seeking and harm avoidance, have been hypothesized to show familial or genetic transmission. Such temperaments may also be related to suicide risk. According to Cloninger and colleagues (1993, 2000), novelty seeking is related to impulsiveness, while harm avoidance tends to be related to anxiety and anhedonia. Studying 758 sibling pairs from 177 nuclear families of alcoholics, Cloninger and colleagues (1998) demonstrated significant heritability for proneness to anxiety and harm avoidance. Likewise, the capacity for pleasure in an individual may be trait-like and connected to temperament (Clark, 1991). A strong harm avoidance trait could be related to both vulnerability to anhedonia and comorbid anxiety disorders. Engstrom and colleagues (2003) measured personality characteristics of bipolar patients with the Temperament and Character Inventory (TCI) and found that patients with early-onset bipolar illness scored significantly higher on harm avoidance than those with late onset. Suicide attempts also were significantly more common among patients with early onset. Bondy and colleagues (2000), as noted earlier, observed that the presence of one or two short alleles of the serotonin transporter gene was associated with anxiety-related personality traits as well as affective disorder. Caspi and colleagues (2003) found that individuals with one or two copies of the short allele exhibited more diagnosable depression and suicidality in response to stressful life events. Their study yielded evidence of a gene–environment interaction, in which the individual's response to major life stresses is mediated by his or her genetic makeup. As more evidence becomes available, vulnerability to suicide may be manifest in detectable familial–genetic traits associated with other biological markers that are triggered by psychiatric illness and major life stresses.

Social Factors

The impact of social factors, such as losing an important relationship or a job or facing legal or criminal proceed-

ings, can be devastating to anyone; this is particularly true, however, for those with a major psychiatric illness such as bipolar disorder. Although rarely sufficient by themselves to cause suicide, social stressors can precipitate or determine the timing of the act. In this way, they act as risk factors that increase the likelihood of suicide. They may trigger suicide in individuals with certain biological vulnerabilities and psychological traits (e.g., Caspi et al., 2003, discussed earlier), but most studies have not teased apart their precise role in manic-depressive illness. Social stressors may also precipitate sleeplessness; this, in turn, has been shown in bipolar patients to increase the risk of an affective relapse.

Social factors not only can increase risk, but also may buffer individuals from suicide. For example, supportive families and friends and religious beliefs may, to a point, deter suicide by acting as protective factors (IOM, 2002). Religious beliefs and devotion—as opposed to practice and affiliation—have been shown to be protective for African-American women (Neeleman et al., 1998; Greening and Stoppelbein, 2002; Kaslow et al., 2004), the ethnic group with the lowest suicide rate in the United States (Kaslow, 2000). The potentially protective role of religious belief and practice has not been studied in relation to individuals with bipolar illness, however.

Social and cultural factors also shape an individual's willingness to seek help, styles of coping with adversity, and social support structures. On a societal level, social and cultural factors influence laws, regulations, and health policies that dictate the availability of resources for treatment and prevention (U.S. Department of Health and Human Services, 2000; IOM, 2002). Indeed, awareness of the potency of cultural and social factors prompted the U.S. Surgeon General, Dr. David Satcher, to mobilize clinicians, public health professionals, communities, families, and the media as part of a comprehensive strategy for suicide prevention (U.S. Public Health Service, 1999).

CLINICAL CORRELATES OF SUICIDE

In this section, we review research findings on correlations between suicide and various features of bipolar disorder: mixed states, depression, rapid cycling, and severe anxiety or agitation. We then examine suicide in bipolar disorder in relation to comorbid personality disorders, substance abuse, psychosis, and course of illness.

History of Suicide Attempts

There is an extensive literature documenting the strong correlation between a history of suicide attempts and subsequent completed suicide (see, for example, Nordstrom et al., 1995a,b; Tsai et al., 2002; Joiner et al., 2005). Harris and

Barraclough, in their extensive meta-analysis, found that a suicide attempt created a 37-fold risk for completed suicide; several large prospective studies also demonstrated a substantial increased risk for suicide in those who had previously attempted it (Jawcett et all., 1990; Marangell et al., 2006). In their meta-analysis of 13 studies of completed suicide and 23 studies of attempted suicide, Hawton and colleagues (2005) found that past suicide attempts were the factor most predictive of future suicidal behavior. In the Finnish Jorvi Bipolar Study, 191 bipolar patients were followed for 18 months, during which time 20 percent attempted suicide (Valtonen et al., 2006). Baseline previous suicide attempts were the most significant predictor (odds ratio [OR] = 3.8; 95 percent confidence interval [CI] = 1.7–8.8; p = 0.001) of a subsequent attempt.

During a 2-year follow-up period, 12 of 64 bipolar patients studied at Columbia University made at least one suicide attempt. All attempters had a history of past suicide attempts; none of the previously nonattempters made an attempt (Galfalvy et al., 2006).

Mixed States

Mixed states are a significant risk factor for suicide. Among the first to study the relationship between agitated, dysphoric states and suicide was Jameison (1936), who concluded that mixed states were the most dangerous clinical phase of illness for suicide risk.[11] In his investigation of 100 suicides (half with manic-depressive psychosis), he noted that the combination of depressive symptoms, mental alertness, and tense, apprehensive, and restless behavior was particularly lethal. Mixed states represent a potentially deadly combination of depressive affect and cognition, linked to dysphoric state, heightened energy level, and increased impulsiveness. Jameison's clinical account of mixed states and their association with suicide remains apt, as does his observation that those patients who were both tense and restless were at the greatest risk for suicide:

> Finally there are the patients with mixed manic-depressive states. The majority of these show the usual depression, numerous self-accusations, ideas of guilt and punishment and a varying degree of hypochondriasis. At the same time there is a mental alertness, associated with tense, apprehensive and restless behavior. The retardation of thought and action that paralyzes the acting out of the wish for death in the average depressed patient is entirely absent in these persons. They are, therefore, the most dangerous types of patients with mental disease, so far as suicide is concerned. The records of the fifteen patients in the group emphasize this strikingly. Three of these patients committed suicide twenty-four hours after leaving the hospital, two within forty-eight hours, another

within a week and still another within two weeks. The patient who was longest outside the hospital lived two months, and the average period for this group was fifteen days! (Jameison, 1936, p. 4)

Winokur and colleagues (1969) found that suicidal thoughts or attempts occurred in 13 percent of depressive episodes following mania and in a strikingly high proportion of mixed states (43 percent), although the latter finding applied only to women. Kotin and Goodwin (1972) also described the coexistence of suicidal behavior and mixed states, as did Kraepelin (1921) in his original clinical monograph.

In a series of studies, Dilsaver and colleagues (1994, 1997; Dilsaver and Chen, 2003) found that, compared with patients with pure mania, patients with depressive mania had significantly higher rates of suicidality. Suicidality was defined as a severity level of 3 to 7 on the suicide subscale of the SADS, which ranges from mild suicidality (frequent ideation, but without a specific method or plan) to suicide attempts. More recently, Dilsaver and colleagues (2005) studied suicidality in adolescents and determined that mixed states increased the probability of attempting suicide for girls only, in whom the increased risk was four-fold. In a study of 100 bipolar-I manic patients, Goldberg and colleagues (1998, 1999) found a significant relationship between dysphoric mania and suicidal ideation. They also noted that multiple suicide attempts were associated with nonremission of mixed mania. Sato and colleagues (2004), using the criteria for dysphoric mania developed by McElroy and colleagues (1992, 1995) and Strakowski and colleagues (1996), studied 576 patients hospitalized with acute mania. They found that mixed mania was strongly associated with suicidality.

Depression

It has long been known that depression is strongly correlated with suicide and suicide attempts (Jameison and Wall, 1933; Barraclough et al., 1974; Weeke, 1979). More recent findings strengthen the early clinical observations. Isometsa and colleagues (1994) studied a sample of 31 bipolar patients who committed suicide in Finland within a 12-month period, 74 percent of whom had been receiving psychiatric care at the time of their suicide. Among these patients, 79 percent were depressed at the time of death, 11 percent were in a mixed state, and 11 percent died during or immediately after remission of psychotic mania. Dilsaver and colleagues (1997) found bipolar depression to have been associated with suicidality somewhat more frequently than were mixed states, although both conditions were associated with greater suicidality than was pure mania. Grunebaum and colleagues (2004) compared suicide attempts among 347 patients with melancholic versus nonmelancholic major depression. They found that melancholic features during depression were correlated with more serious past attempts and the probability of suicide at follow-up.

The severity of depression is a factor as well (Arato et al., 1988; Henriksson et al., 1993; Isometsä et al., 1994). Swedish researchers psychiatrically assessed an entire rural population and then kept track of its mental health for the next 15 to 25 years (Hagnell et al., 1981). Virtually all of the men who committed suicide during the follow-up period had been diagnosed during their initial evaluations as having depressive illness. The suicide rate for men with no psychiatric diagnosis at all was 8.3 per 100,000, but for those with depression it escalated to 650. No one with mild depression committed suicide, but the rate rose to 220 per 100,000 for those who had been diagnosed with moderate depression and to 3,900 per 100,000 for those with severe depressive illnesses.

Weeke (1979) found that at the time of death, 58 percent of manic-depressive patients who committed suicide had been in a constant or worsening depressive state. Fully 30 percent of the patients, however, had been classified as "depressive state, recovering." Keith-Spiegel and Spiegel (1967) compared the clinician-rated mood states of 61 psychiatric patients immediately preceding their suicides with those of 51 matched control patients of comparable age and diagnoses who had not committed suicide or had no history of a suicide attempt. Those who killed themselves had histories of more frequent and more severe depressions, as well as more suicide attempts, threats, and suicidal ideation. Of particular significance, however, was that just before death, those who committed suicide had been assessed by their clinician as being calmer and in better spirits than members of the control group. An apparently unwarranted mood shift had been observed in those who killed themselves.

These findings add weight to the clinical observation, dating back hundreds of years, that improvement in depression is associated with an increased risk for suicide.[12] Several factors may account for this counterintuitive observation. The improvement may reflect a sense of calm once the decision has been made to die, a genuine calm before the storm brought about by biological changes, or a transition from one phase of the illness to another (e.g., from depression to hypomania, mania, or a mixed state). It also may reflect true clinical improvement, with a concomitant level of frustration when symptoms recur. In some instances, an improved clinical state enables a previously indecisive and lethargic patient to become more able to make an unambivalently lethal decision and to act on that decision. Finally, "improvement" may in fact be a patient's deliberate deception of physicians, hospital staff, and family so a suicide plan can be carried out. Problems

in assessing clinical improvement were described decades ago by Jameison (1936, p. 4):

> It is only when the depression is lifting, often some weeks before the morbid and self-accusatory ideas have disappeared, that the possibility of suicide is less remote. Unfortunately, at this time a tendency to project the inner distress on the environment leads to complaints and pleadings, so that relatives, noting the improvement, agree with the patient that the hospital restrictions are prolonging the illness. The patient is then removed at a time when he is potentially more suicidal than at any time before.

Rapid Cycling

Rapid cycling increases the risk of suicide and suicidal behavior. One of the first large studies to examine the relationship between suicide and rapid cycling was NIMH's Collaborative Study on the Psychobiology of Depression-Clinical Studies (Fawcett et al., 1987). Of the study's 954 patients, 569 had unipolar depression,[13] 185 had bipolar-I, 114 had bipolar-II, and the remaining 80 had schizoaffective disorder. The incidence of suicide over the 4-year study period was 3 percent. The rate did not differ by diagnosis. What did distinguish patients who died by suicide from those who did not was mood cycling during the index episode ($p < .002$). Mood cycling in this study meant that the patient had been admitted in one mood state, such as mania, and cycled into the other before recovery. While this is not synonymous with the classic definition of rapid cycling (i.e., four or more affective episodes in 1 year), there is overlap between the two groups. The authors of the study concluded that mood cycling, which is a feature of bipolar or schizoaffective disorder, is associated with suicide, particularly in men.

In a 5-year prospective study of 345 patients with bipolar-I or -II disorder, 89 patients were identified, using DSM-IV criteria, as having a pattern of rapid cycling for 1 year or more (Table 8–4; Coryell et al., 2003). The rapid-cycling patients were significantly more likely than the rest of the patients to have had onset of illness before age 17 and were twice as likely to attempt, but not to complete, suicide.[14] The differences between the groups were most pronounced for attempts rated as being of high lethality.

Brodersen and colleagues (2000) conducted a 16-year follow-up study of 133 patients with major affective disorders (defined as having two to three affective episodes in a 5-year period) treated with lithium. Most of the 11 suicides occurred among the "atypical" patients (those with schizoaffective disorder, bipolar-II disorder, mixed episodes, and/or rapid cycling). MacKinnon and colleagues (2005), in a study of 1,574 family members with bipolar disorder, also found that a history of rapid mood switching was

TABLE 8–4. **Relationship between Rapid Cycling, Suicide, and Suicide Attempts before Intake and during Follow-Up**

	Any Rapid Cycling (n=89)	No Rapid Cycling (n=256)
Before Intake, No. (%)		
Any attempt	51 (57.3)[a]	85 (33.2)
Any attempt of high intent	31 (34.8)[a]	38 (14.8)
Any attempt of high lethality	36 (40.4)[a]	35 (13.7)
After Intake, No. (%)		
Completed suicide	3 (3.4)	11 (4.3)
Any attempt	46 (51.7)[a]	70 (27.3)
Any attempt of high intent	27 (30.3)[a]	33 (12.9)
Any attempt of high lethality	30 (33.7)[a]	36 (14.1)

[a]Significant differences by chi square, $p < .001$.
Source: Adapted from Coryell et al., 2003. Copyright American Medical Association. All rights reserved.

associated with increased suicidality. Two other studies found trends for suicidal behavior and rapid cycling (Bauer et al., 1994; Maj et al., 1994). On the other hand, using retrospective chart reviews of 100 rapid-cycling and 120 non-rapid-cycling outpatients, Wu and Dunner (1993) found no association between suicide attempts and rapid cycling. Still, most studies have found that rapid cycling increases the risk of suicide and suicidal behaviors.

Anxiety and Agitation

Studies have shown high rates of comorbid anxiety disorder in bipolar patients, often reaching at least 40 percent (McElroy et al., 2001; Simon et al., 2004). The high incidence of comorbid anxiety disorders in both bipolar-I and bipolar-II patients calls for special attention to severe symptoms of anxiety in the assessment and management of suicide risk in bipolar patients (see Chapter 25).

Anxiety figured prominently in a major study of time-related risk factors for suicide. In their prospective study of 955 bipolar and unipolar patients, Fawcett and colleagues (1990) delineated a cluster of risk factors that were better predictors of suicide over the short term (acute risk factors) and others that were better over the long term (chronic risk factors). They found that anxiety symptoms were predictive both acutely (within 1 year of study entry) and chronically (after the first year of study entry). Among the 14 patients who committed suicide within 1 year of assess-

ment, suicide was related to symptoms of severe psychic anxiety, panic attacks, anhedonia, and moderate alcohol abuse; the abuse of alcohol with another drug was a significant risk factor, especially in males (see later discussion). No difference was found between bipolar and unipolar depressed patients with regard to severe psychic anxiety, panic attacks, and suicide. Over the next 4 years, another 13 patients killed themselves. These later suicides were most commonly associated with severe hopelessness, somatic anxiety, suicidal ideation, and a history of one or more suicide attempts. These findings underscore the importance of assessing patients in terms of acute versus long-term suicide risk (see Chapter 25).

The identification of time-related factors helps address the difficult problem of predicting a relatively infrequent behavior in the midst of subtle and fluctuating mood states. This point is illustrated by the predictive role of past suicide attempts. While attempts carry a high chronic risk for suicide—with an SMR of 37, according to Harris and Barraclough (1997)—they do not confer a significant acute risk.

Numerous other studies underscore the role of comorbid anxiety/agitation in relation to suicide. Among a sample of 209 outpatients who had attempted suicide or been identified as being at high risk for continued suicidal behavior or eventual suicide, Rudd and colleagues (1993) noted a statistically significant incidence of comorbid panic disorder and post-traumatic stress disorder among suicidal bipolar patients. Likewise, MacKinnon and colleagues (2005) found that comorbid panic disorder increased the risk of suicidality in individuals with bipolar disorder. Among patients with major depression, Reich (1998) found that suicide attempts were correlated with higher levels of comorbid anxiety. Hall and colleagues (1999) found that severe anxiety was present in 90 percent and panic attacks in 80 percent of suicide attempters. Schnyder and colleagues (1999) reported similar findings showing the presence of severe anxiety in a study of 30 consecutive emergency room suicide attempters who were later admitted to a psychiatric inpatient unit (diagnoses not specified in the study). Likewise, Angst and colleagues (1998) found the presence of anxiety to be a suicide risk factor in a 5-year follow-up sample of 186 patients with unipolar and 220 patients with bipolar depression. And in an analysis of 76 inpatient suicides, Busch and colleagues (2003) found that 79 percent of patients had chart notes indicating severe anxiety/agitation within 1 week of their suicide.

One study attempted to ascertain what features of bipolar illness, including panic disorder, are related to suicidality. Dilsaver and colleagues (1997) divided their sample of 125 bipolar patients into three groups—those with bipolar depression, those with depressive mania, and those with pure mania. They examined the incidence of suicidality (rated using the SADS), psychosis, and intra-episode panic disorder (IEPD). IEPD was highly prevalent in the bipolar depression (79 percent) and depressive mania groups (56 percent) but rare (2.3 percent) in the pure mania group. Overall, the findings suggest a high degree of overlap among suicidality, IEPD, and bipolar depression or depressive mania, as opposed to pure mania.

Taken together, these studies argue for the assessment of severe anxiety or agitation and for aggressive anxiolytic treatment in the management of suicide risk in affective disorders (see Chapter 25).

Insomnia and excessive concern about sleep disturbances have been noted as correlates of increased potential for suicide,[15] as has pervasive hopelessness (see earlier discussion). The body of evidence has led to widespread acceptance that insomnia and hopelessness are risk factors for suicide. Global insomnia is considered an acute risk factor because it was found, in a prospective study, to be associated with suicide within the first year of study entry (Fawcett et al., 1990).

Comorbidity and Axis II Disorders

Suicide among individuals with comorbid psychiatric conditions is so prevalent that it is the norm rather than the exception. This point is best illustrated by a population-based study from Finland, which found that a small fraction—only 12 percent—of all 229 suicide victims had only one Axis I diagnosis with no comorbidity (Henriksson et al., 1993). Comorbid conditions and certain behavioral states dramatically increase the risk of suicide. Most of the studies reviewed here, however, did not study bipolar disorder separately. This may be an important limitation on the conclusions that can be drawn about the role of comorbid conditions in suicide among bipolar patients.

In a psychological autopsy study of 117 suicides, Foster and colleagues (1999) found that, in comparison with deceased community controls without a mental disorder, the risks were extraordinarily high for two groups of patients: those with comorbidity (an Axis I and Axis II disorder; OR=346.0) and those with a single Axis I disorder (OR=52.4). Kim and colleagues (2003), studying the records of 115 male suicides, found that the most common comorbidities in suicide completers were depressive disorders plus cluster B disorders[16] and substance dependence plus cluster B disorders (27.8 percent). In this study, those who committed suicide, compared with controls, were 22 times more likely to have three or more diagnoses (OR=22.38, $p < .0000001$). Heikkinen and colleagues (1997) compared 56 suicides who had both Axis I disorders (most commonly major depression) and comorbid personality disorders with an equal number who had no comorbidity. The patients with personality disorders, cluster B type, had experienced multiple life events preceding their suicide compared with the noncomorbid patients who had died by suicide. It appears clear from these studies that comorbidity of Axis I and Axis II disorders strikingly increases the risk of suicide.

Substance Abuse

Comorbid substance abuse is another risk factor for suicide in both bipolar and unipolar patients, particularly in the young (Fawcett et al., 1987; Murphy, 1988). In their large, prospective study, Fawcett and colleagues (1987) found a significant increase in long-term risk with so-called "double abuse" (alcohol plus any other abused substance). They also found recent, moderate alcohol abuse to be a short-term (acute) risk factor (see Chapter 25).

Like Fawcett and colleagues, others have noted an association between alcohol abuse and suicide. Barraclough and colleagues (1974) found that as the number of suicide attempts increased, so did the chances that the attempter was alcohol dependent. In a study of 204 suicides, Rich and colleagues (1988) noted substance abuse and affective disorders to be the most frequent diagnoses for men and women. Morrison (1975) found that bipolar patients who were also alcohol dependent had a higher rate of suicide in their family histories than did nondependent bipolar patients. In a study of suicide among adolescents and young adults, Runeson (1989) observed a 47 percent rate of co-morbid substance abuse with any Axis I or II diagnoses. Depressive disorders were diagnosed in 64 percent of those who committed suicide (major depressive disorder = 41 percent).

Tondo and colleagues (1999) found an association between substance abuse disorders and suicide attempts in hospitalized patients, with substance abuse raising the suicide risk more than two-fold regardless of the disorder. In a study of 307 male veterans, Waller and colleagues (1999) noted that comorbidity of alcohol abuse and bipolar-I or unipolar depressive disorder was always associated with an increased risk of suicidality.

Pini and colleagues (1999) found that among 125 bipolar patients with psychotic features, the subgroup having substance abuse associated with other Axis I comorbidities had an earlier age at onset of their bipolar disorder, more frequent onset with a mixed state, and a higher risk of suicide. Oquendo and Mann (2001) observed that bipolar patients who attempted suicide had higher levels of aggression and comorbid substance abuse than nonattempters. Vieta and colleagues (2000) noted that among 40 patients with bipolar-II disorder, 21 percent had substance abuse comorbidity, and this group had significantly higher rates of suicidal ideation and attempts. Vieta and colleagues (2001) studied 129 bipolar outpatients in remission, finding comorbidity in 31 percent; these patients also had higher rates of mixed states, depressive episodes, and suicide attempts. Cornelius and colleagues (1995) found that suicidality was disproportionately higher among patients with comorbid depression and substance abuse than among those with either disorder alone.

The connection between suicide and substance abuse may be attributable to increased impulsivity or aggressiveness, impaired sleep, or destabilization of illness. As we have seen, low levels of the serotonin metabolite 5-HIAA are correlated with aggression and impulsivity, and it has been shown that patients making the most violent and impulsive suicide attempts have low 5-HIAA levels (see also Chapter 14). It is of interest that Rosenthal and colleagues (1980) found significantly lower levels of 5-HIAA among depressed patients with a family history of alcoholism than among those without such a family history. Low 5-HIAA levels also have been found in alcoholics after recovery (Ballenger et al., 1979; Linnoila and Virkkunen, 1992; Virkkunen and Linnoila, 1993). Therefore, not only do substance abusers have impaired judgment and decreased inhibition from the drugs themselves, but they may also bear a biological risk for suicide. Bipolar patients who are impulsive or more temperamentally prone to agitated states may be more inclined to use alcohol and other drugs than those who are not. Swann and colleagues (2004)

compared scores on a measure of impulsiveness (the BIS) in interepisode bipolar patients with and without substance abuse. Trait impulsivity was increased in interepisode bipolar disorder only in the case of current substance abuse.

Psychosis

The relationship between psychosis and suicide in mood disorders is unclear. An early, often-cited retrospective analysis of patients with unipolar depression hospitalized at the New York State Psychiatric Institute between 1955 and 1980 found an unusually high rate of delusions among those who committed suicide (Roose et al., 1983). Bipolar patients were not considered separately in this study, but the findings were suggestive of symptom patterns associated with a high risk of suicide. The authors noted that depressed inpatients who were delusional were five times more likely than those who were nondelusional to commit suicide, and that delusional males were particularly vulnerable. Two recent studies found that bipolar children and adolescents with a history of psychotic features were more likely to be suicidal than those who did not have such a history (Papolos et al., 2005; Caetano et al., 2006). The recent study from the Juvenile Bipolar Research Foundation (Papolos et al., 2005) also found that bipolar children and adolescents who threatened to commit suicide were far more likely to report having hallucinations than those who did not threaten suicide.

On the other hand, several studies suggest no such relationship. A study of 1,593 affectively ill patients revealed no increased risk of suicide among the 27.8 percent who had been psychotic at the time of their index hospitalization (Black et al., 1988). Likewise, Fawcett and colleagues (1987) found that psychotic patients diagnosed with affective illness did not have higher prospective rates of suicide over a 10-year follow-up. Dilsaver and colleagues (1997) found no association between the presence of psychosis and mild suicidality; a subsequent study found no association between psychotic features and suicidality in adolescents (Dilsaver et al., 2005). Similarly, Coryell and Tsuang (1982) and Frangos and colleagues (1983) found no increased risk of suicide in patients with delusional depression.

Course of Illness

There is consistent evidence of an increased risk of suicide and suicide attempts early in or just after the first episode of affective illness,[17] as well as in bipolar disorder more specifically. Among the first to study the time course of suicide attempts in bipolar patients were Johnson and Hunt (1979). They found in their very small sample that 30 percent of suicide attempts (90 percent of which warranted hospitalization) occurred at the onset of the illness or

TABLE 8–5. **Suicide in Bipolar Patients with a Hospital Diagnosis of Bipolar Disorder (N=15,386) in Sweden, 1973–1995**

Age	STANDARDIZED MORTALITY RATIO	
	Males	Females
All ages	15.0	22.4
<30 yr[a]	81.6	71.7

[a]Age at first admission and in the first year of follow-up.
Source: Reprinted with permission from Osby et al., 2001. Copyright, American Medical Association. All rights reserved.

during the first episode of depression. Half of the serious suicide attempts occurred within 5 years of the onset of illness. In a related finding, Balazs and colleagues (2003), studying 100 suicide attempters in Hungary, observed that 60 percent were experiencing their first depressive episode. (Of this group, 35 percent had had mania or hypomania symptoms in the past.) In the largest study, Osby and colleagues (2001) documented suicide rates among all hospitalized patients in Sweden from 1973 to 1995, including more than 15,000 with bipolar disorder. The SMR was found to be especially high in patients whose age at first admission was less than 30 (81.6 for males and 71.7 for females) (Table 8–5).

Recent discharge from a hospital also carries a higher risk (Geddes and Juszczak, 1995, 1997; Appleby et al., 1999). A study was conducted of all suicides (N=481) among discharged patients who had been receiving care in 128 Veterans Affairs hospitals in the United States from 1994 to 1998 (Desai et al., 2005). The patients had been diagnosed as having depression, bipolar disorder, schizophrenia, or post-traumatic stress disorder. The study found suicide deaths to be concentrated in the first 6 months after discharge, with almost 50 percent occurring within 3 months after discharge. Bipolar and unipolar rates were similarly high. A comprehensive investigation of all suicides committed in Denmark from January 1, 1981, to December 31, 1997 (N=21,169) found that there were two sharp peaks of risk for suicide in relation to psychiatric hospitalization (Qin and Nordentoft, 2005). The highest peak, which was strikingly elevated in those patients with affective illness, was in the week immediately following discharge from the hospital. The second peak was in the week following admission to the hospital. Suicide was substantially more likely in patients who had shorter hospitalizations.

Several studies have examined suicide risk in relation to age at onset. Perlis and colleagues (2004) studied 983 subjects diagnosed with bipolar disorder on entry into the multicenter Systematic Treatment Enhancement Program for Bipolar Disorder (STEP-BD). For patients whose age at onset could be determined, the authors found that earlier onset of illness was associated with a greater likelihood of suicide attempts (Table 8–6). Based on multiple regression, the risk of making at least one suicide attempt was 2.85 times greater for those diagnosed with very early onset (before age 13) relative to those diagnosed after age 18. Early onset (ages 13 to 18) was also associated with higher rates of comorbid anxiety disorders and substance abuse, themselves risk factors for suicide (see earlier discussion). Grunebaum and colleagues (2006) found that suicide attempts in 96 patients with bipolar illness correlated with an earlier age at onset.

Engstrom and colleagues (2003) studied patients with bipolar-I and -II disorders and reported that in early-onset patients, treatment response was significantly lower ($p=.005$), and suicide attempts were more common

TABLE 8–6. **Comorbid Conditions and Suicide Attempts in Bipolar Disorder by Age at Onset (percent)**

	Onset Age <13 yr (n=272)	Onset Age 13–18 yr (n=370)	Onset Age >18 yr (n=341)	Wald X^2 (2 df)	p Value
Suicide attempts[a]	49.8	37.0	24.6	32.58	<.0001[b,c,d]
Any anxiety disorder	69.2	53.9	38.3	48.87	<.0001[b,c,d]
Alcohol abuse/dependence	47.3	46.6	31.9	15.89	.0004[b,c]
Drug abuse and dependence	34.2	33.4	15.1	40.86	<.0001[b,c]

[a]These were past suicide attempts reported at study entry.
[b]p <.05 for pairwise comparison of prepubertal and adult-onset groups.
[c]p <.05 for pairwise comparison of adolescent and adult-onset groups.
[d]p <.05 for pairwise comparison of prepubertal and adolescent-onset groups.
Source: Adapted from Perlis et al., 2004, with permission from the Society of Biological Psychiatry.

($p = .001$). Leverich and colleagues (2002, 2003) showed that a history of childhood sexual or physical abuse was associated with earlier age at onset; increased Axis I, II, and III comorbid disorders; more rapid cycling; and a higher rate and greater severity of suicide attempts (see Chapter 6). Similarly, Goldberg and Ernst (2004) found that a history of poor adjustment in childhood and adolescence was associated with both substance abuse and dependence and increased suicide attempts in adult patients with bipolar disorder.

The course of affective illness may have different effects on men and women. Johnson and Hunt (1979), in a very small but intriguing study, found that more men than women attempted suicide at the onset of manic-depressive illness (42 versus 17 percent), but that this gender difference later disappeared. Attempts by women were distributed more evenly across time. Although all attempts by women occurred within approximately 15 years after the onset of illness, those by men were distributed more extremely and bimodally: 60 percent of men who attempted suicide did so within 2 years after the onset of illness, and the other 40 percent 23 years or more after onset.

These findings underscore the importance of early recognition of bipolar disorder, accurate diagnosis, and aggressive treatment. They also highlight the need for ongoing reappraisal of suicidal risk (see Chapter 25).

CONCLUSIONS

Suicide is still far too common in manic-depressive illness. Patients diagnosed today face a lifetime suicide risk of at least 5 percent. While this figure is lower than in previous eras—a result in part of better treatments and in part of the inclusion of less severely ill patients in outcome studies—several groups of patients continue to bear a disproportionately high risk burden, including those who are hospitalized or recently discharged and those who are untreated, inadequately treated, or treatment resistant. Further, the suicide rate remains strikingly high early in the course of illness.

The precise causes of suicide remain elusive, although they most certainly entail an interaction between the underlying affective illness and additional biological and psychosocial risk factors. But research has not yet found any particular combination of risk factors to be sensitive or sufficient enough to predict a suicide. Salient risk factors include rapid cycling, mixed states, and severe depressive episodes. A significant advance has come with the identification of which of many risk factors operate in the short term (e.g., agitation, severe hopelessness, global insomnia) versus the long term (e.g., past suicide attempt, various comorbidities). Risk factors and their identification, moreover, while far from perfect predictors of suicide, can serve as guideposts for clinicians confronting a complex clinical picture of an illness that encompasses the extremes of human emotions.

NOTES

1. National statistics tend to underestimate suicide deaths because of the difficulty of establishing suicidal intent in single-car accidents and other "accidental" deaths and because of cultural, financial, and religious disincentives to label a death as a suicide.
2. For example, Fawcett et al., 1987, 1990; Black et al., 1988; Angst et al., 1999.
3. Wetterberg et al., 1978; Carlsson et al., 1979; Oddie et al., 1979; Perez et al., 1980; Aschoff, 1981; Behall et al., 1984; Losonczy et al., 1984; Gordon et al., 1987; Lacoste and Wirz-Justice, 1989; Sarrias et al., 1989; Souêtre et al., 1989; Modai et al., 1992; Maes et al., 1995; Pine et al., 1995; Verkes et al., 1996; Zajicek et al., 2000.
4. Mann et al., 1992; D'Hondt et al., 1994; Maes et al., 1995; Pine et al., 1995.
5. Pokorny, 1983, 1991; Goldstein et al., 1991; IOM, 2002.
6. For example, Egeland and Sussex, 1985; Brent et al., 1996; Johnson et al., 1998; Statham et al., 1998; Johnson and Cameron, 2001; Fu et al., 2002.
7. Pfeffer et al., 1994; Brent et al., 1996, 2003; Johnson et al., 1998.
8. Mann et al., 1999; Keilp et al., 2001; Oquendo and Mann, 2001; Oquendo et al., 2004.
9. Fawcett et al., 1997; Partonen et al., 1999; Tanskanen et al., 2000; Ellison and Morrison, 2001; Golomb et al., 2002; Lester, 2002; Lalovic et al., 2004.
10. Bunney and Fawcett, 1965; Fawcett and Bunney, 1967; Bunney et al., 1969; Krieger, 1970.
11. Koukopoulos and Koukopoulos (1999) traced the history of the conceptualization of mixed states back to Kraepelin, who conceived them as a form of manic-depressive insanity; before that to the state of melancholia agitata described by Richarz (1858); and still further back to Hippocrates, who described the anxiety seen in agitated melancholia in *Diseases II*. This state, characterized by anxiety and agitation as primary symptoms, has gradually been separated from manic-depressive illness, appearing today as a subtype of major depression-agitated type.
12. Rush, 1812; Kraepelin, 1921; Clouston, 1915; Henderson and Gillespie, 1927; Jameison and Wall, 1933; Stengel, 1955; Copes et al., 1971; Copas and Fryer, 1980; Barner-Rasmussen, 1986; Schweizer et al., 1988.
13. Of the 569 with unipolar major depression, 210 were in first episodes, and 359 were in recurrent episodes.
14. There were too few completed suicides to permit meaningful comparisons.
15. Jameison and Wall, 1933; Slater and Roth, 1969; Barraclough et al., 1974; Motto, 1975; Fawcett et al., 1987, 1990.
16. Cluster B disorders are antisocial personality disorder, borderline personality disorder, histrionic personality disorder, and narcissistic personality disorder.
17. Guze and Robins, 1970; Tsuang and Woolson, 1977, Weeke, 1979; Inskip et al., 1998.

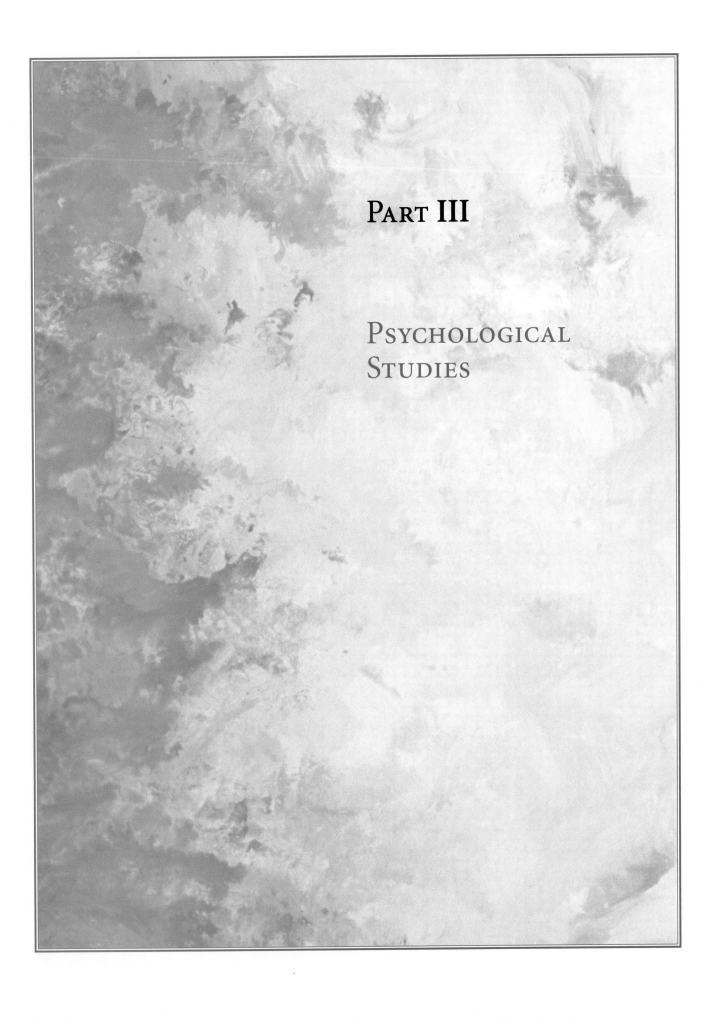

PART III

PSYCHOLOGICAL STUDIES

Neuropsychology

I seem to be in perpetual fog and darkness. I cannot get my mind to work; instead of associations "clicking into place" everything is an inextricable jumble; instead of seeming to grasp a whole, it seems to remain tied to the actual consciousness of the moment. . . . I could not feel more ignorant, undecided or inefficient. It is appallingly difficult to concentrate.

—*John Custance (1952, p. 62)*

In this chapter, we examine what can be learned from studies of the neuropsychology of manic-depressive illness. Two streams of neuropsychological investigation can be distinguished. One uses a battery of objective measures, focusing largely on the sensorimotor and cognitive functions, to characterize profiles of strength and weakness in the various phases of bipolar or recurrent unipolar illness. The other generates hypotheses about how affective states, normal and abnormal, are represented in the brain and what factors mediate their expression. We consider the contributions of this second stream of investigation after reviewing what has been learned from the first, the evaluation of sensorimotor and cognitive function in manic-depressive illness, with an emphasis on the bipolar form. In the final section, we assess the overall contribution of neuropsychology to the conceptualization of mood disorders.

CONTRIBUTIONS OF NEUROPSYCHOLOGICAL EVALUATION

The contributions of traditional neuropsychological testing to our understanding of manic-depressive illness pertain to four issues. Such investigation can (1) provide an empirical basis for and clarification of clinical phenomenological concepts; (2) determine which abnormalities are state dependent and which are state independent; (3) characterize the neuropsychological functions that appear to be most persistently impaired, providing a clue to pathophysiology; and (4) determine the burden of the illness and its treatments with respect to cognitive functioning in terms of both cross-sectional and longitudinal outcomes.

Objectifying Clinical Constructs

First, neuropsychological investigation can identify the constituent processes impaired in some of the classic symptoms of the disorder. For example, psychomotor disturbance is common in major depression and bipolar disorder, and depressed bipolar patients may be especially likely to manifest psychomotor retardation (Sobin and Sackeim, 1997). In turn, this motor disturbance is viewed by some as having special prognostic significance with respect to treatment outcome (Hickie et al., 1990a, 1996; Parker and Hadzi-Pavlovic, 1993). However, the term "psychomotor retardation" is itself an amalgam, and the slowness of movement seen in depressed patients may reflect slowing in any of a variety of cognitive or motor processes. Indeed, some success has been achieved in using objective measures to dissect the constituent processes of such retardation and to identify those disturbed in affective disorders (Sobin and Sackeim, 1997). Thus in principle, neuropsychological evaluation can determine just what is slowed in psychomotor retardation and quantify the extent of abnormality.

Similarly, disturbances in attention are rife in mood disorders, yet they can pertain to distinct cognitive processes such as vigilance or sustained attention, freedom from distraction, divided attention, and capacity to shift set.[1] Neuropsychological investigation can clarify the nature of what is typically referred to as impaired concentration.

Identifying State-Related and State-Independent Abnormalities

The above contribution involves clarifying and quantifying deficits described more generally by clinical characterization of key features of the disorder. However, neuropsychological evaluation also yields information on strengths and weaknesses that go beyond clinical phenomenology. For the past 40 years, there has been an unresolved debate about whether the bipolar subgroup of manic-depressive illness is overrepresented in individuals with higher levels of intelligence and/or creativity (Richards et al., 1983; Andreasen, 1987; Jamison, 1993) (see Chapter 12). This issue can be addressed by determining whether premorbid intelligence in individuals with bipolar disorder exceeds population norms, and whether such individuals exceed normative values on indicators of creativity, such as those assessed by measures of cognitive flexibility and idiosyncratic thought. In turn, findings in this area may be helpful in considering sociobiological questions, such as why the genes for bipolar disorder have been preserved.

More generally, through comparison of individuals in remission and in the depressed or manic state of bipolar disorder, neuropsychological investigation can provide new information on the sensorimotor and cognitive abnormalities that fluctuate with affective state or are invariant across the disorder. As noted above, the state of depression or mania can introduce serious confounds in neuropsychological evaluation. Therefore, a number of recent investigations have placed special emphasis on detailing the deficits characteristic of bipolar patients in remission,[2] of children at risk for the disorder (Decina et al., 1983; Dickstein et al., 2004; Meyer et al., 2004), and of other first-degree relatives (Sobczak et al., 2002; Ferrier et al., 2004; Zalla et al., 2004), including discordant monozygotic twins (Gourovitch et al., 1999). Indeed, the identification of abnormalities that persist across the phases of the illness or that precede its first expression as a mood disorder may provide markers of disease vulnerability and suggest neurobiological abnormalities responsible for disease expression.

Establishing Differential Deficits of Relevance to Pathoetiology

Perhaps the most common goal of neuropsychological evaluation is to identify the sensorimotor or cognitive processes that are most disturbed in patients with bipolar disorder, in contrast to either normative values or individuals with other neuropsychiatric disorders. The peaks and especially the nadirs of neuropsychological profiles are taken as evidence that certain neuropsychological processes are particularly disturbed, and therefore of particular relevance when considering pathoetiology.

The methods needed to establish such "differential deficits" were reviewed by Chapman and Chapman (1973) in the context of determining what aspect of information processing is most relevant in accounting for thought disorder in schizophrenia. Although there is intuitive appeal to a focus on abnormalities of greatest magnitude, what appears

to be most broken is not necessarily that which is in greatest need of repair. For example, intermittent dysfunction of the electrical system in a car may short out the radio, but the broken radio is not the fundamental problem. Other conceptual reservations concern the fact that cognitive processes are interdependent. Attention has a widespread impact on neuropsychological function. When one cannot attend adequately to information, encoding, learning, and memory are all impaired and, depending on other factors, perhaps more so than the attentional measures themselves. At a methodological level, the validity of comparisons across tests depends on the equivalence of the tests with regard to psychometric properties, particularly internal reliability (the extent to which one dimension is assessed) and difficulty level (overall performance level in the sample). These properties are partly intrinsic to a test and partly a function of the sample being assessed. Thus while it is common to view findings of differential deficit as indicating that one process is more impaired than another, such findings are commonly a psychometric artifact due to the fact that tests with greater power to discriminate among individuals detect larger differences. Thus, it can be argued that the prevalence of particular neuropsychological deficits, their persistence, and/or the extent to which particular deficits account for symptom severity may be as or more important than a gauge of the absolute level of deficit.

Documenting Neuropsychological Burden

Finally, neuropsychological evaluations have practical value in documenting the burden of the illness. Here as well, multiple approaches can be taken. Current theorizing suggests that states of depression and mania, especially when untreated, result in a destructive, atrophic process in the hippocampus due to excessive release of glucocorticoids (Brown et al., 1999; Lupien et al., 1999; MacQueen et al., 2003) (see Chapter 14). In turn, this progressive structural abnormality should be expressed in progressive deficits in declarative, episodic memory, the neuropsychological functions that are especially tied to hippocampal integrity. Indeed, it has been reported that, independently of age, hippocampal volume in euthymic unipolar women covaries with duration of lifetime exposure to the depressed state, as well as with verbal memory performance (Sheline et al., 1996, 1999).

Episode frequency is higher in bipolar than in most unipolar samples, and bipolar patients tend to express the most virulent forms of affective disturbance (e.g., psychotic depression). Thus it is possible that the neuropsychological consequences of manic-depressive illness are especially severe in bipolar relative to recurrent unipolar patients. In a recent study, performance on five tests of learning and memory was compared in young and elderly depressed unipolar and bipolar inpatients (Burt et al., 2000). Unipolar and bipolar patients within each age group had equivalent scores on the verbal and performance intelligence indices of the Wechsler Adult Intelligence Scale-Revised (WAIS-R) (Wechsler, 1981) and on the modified Mini-Mental State (mMMS) exam (Stern et al., 1987). All patients were tested during a major depressive episode, and symptom severity was found to be similar across the groups. The elderly bipolar patients were distinguished by a higher number of prior affective episodes and psychiatric hospitalizations compared with the other three groups. There was a tendency for the young bipolar group to outperform the young unipolar group on several memory measures. As illustrated by the findings obtained with the Complex Figure Test (Fig. 9–1), elderly bipolar patients decidedly showed the most marked deficits on four of the five tests.

While limited by a cross-sectional design, these findings suggest that deterioration in memory function may be a more prominent characteristic of bipolar than unipolar illness, broadly defined. It would be interesting to know whether there would be unipolar–bipolar differences in memory measures if the two groups were matched on total number of episodes. Given the neuroprotective effects posited for lithium (Manji et al., 2000a,b; Moore et al., 2000) and possibly other mood stabilizers (see Chapter 18), it becomes especially important to determine the impact of treatment on these putative longitudinal effects.

Neuropsychological burden not only results from disease expression and progression, but may also be an inadvertent outcome of treatment (as may neuroprotection). An especially frequent complaint of patients treated with lithium is that, in concert with a dampening of the peaks and valleys of mood fluctuation, creative processes are inhibited. Some individuals report that they are not as original or forward thinking when treated with lithium, or are less quick to see connections and less spontaneous (see Chapter 12). These claims have been tested in neuropsychological investigations, whose results have revealed adverse cognitive effects of lithium that are dose dependent and appear to reverse shortly after discontinuation of the drug (Shaw et al., 1986, 1987).

META-ANALYSIS OF FINDINGS ON NEUROPSYCHOLOGICAL DEFICITS IN MOOD DISORDERS

In the following sections, we present a critical evaluation of what has been learned from neuropsychological evaluations of samples of manic-depressive patients. Much of the literature on neuropsychological function in mood disorders, especially in the depressed phase, has failed to distinguish between bipolar and unipolar subgroups. Necessarily, some of the discussion of neuropsychological deficits in depression

Figure 9–1. Findings obtained with Complex Figure Test. Unmedicated unipolar (UP) and bipolar (BP) patients in an episode of major depression were divided into young and elderly groups. Across multiple measures of memory, the elderly BP patients were greatly impaired, while the young BP patients tended to have the best performance. Shown are scores for copying a complex figure and also for later reproduction of the figure from memory. The delayed reproduction scores show the special deficit in the bipolar elderly. (*Source*: Burt et al., 2000. Reprinted with permission from Lippincott Williams & Wilkins.)

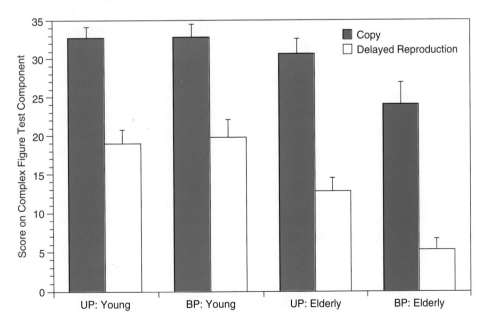

may not be specific to bipolar disorder, but to the extent that recurrent unipolar patients are included, these studies address the broader concept of manic-depressive illness. However, the major focus here is on those neuropsychological abnormalities that are consistent across manic, depressed, and euthymic phases of the bipolar form of the illness.

For the purposes of this chapter, we conducted a new meta-analysis of studies comparing neuropsychological functions in bipolar and healthy comparison samples. We identified 74 studies published since 1975 that entailed neuropsychological evaluations in a bipolar sample as compared with a healthy control or a psychiatric comparison sample (e.g., schizophrenia), and that met high methodological standards. For a study to be included, patients in the bipolar sample had to be described as predominantly in a depressed or manic state or in remission, and sufficient quantitative values had to be reported so that effect size could be computed. In addition, studies were labeled "mixed" if the bipolar sample included patients with a mix of manic, depressed, or euthymic states; did not specify the affective state; or provided no clear classification of state. Nonetheless, few of the studies classified as "mixed" actually focused on patients in a mixed state, and it is fair to assume that the bulk of patients in these studies were in a depressed state. The 74 studies thus identified yielded 1,216 statistical comparisons of a bipolar sample with another group on neuropsychological outcome measures. These comparisons pertained to multiple neuropsychological domains, sometimes with multiple tests sampling the same domain, and often with multiple outcome measures within a test.

The comparisons reported here concern only the performance of bipolar patients relative to normal control participants, and statistical comparisons were used in the meta-analysis only if they pertained to a major cognitive domain, such as attention. This filter reduced the number of studies examined to 52, and the number of neuropsychological comparisons to 614.[3] For each test, all outcome measures were examined so that the effect size assigned a test was the average of these measures. In our meta-analysis, effect sizes for different tests representing the same domain within any study (e.g., attention) were also averaged.[4]

Global Intellectual Functioning

Several key questions have been posed about general intellectual functioning in manic-depressive illness, a literature that focuses primarily on the bipolar subgroup. Most of the research in this area has centered on whether intelligence or global neuropsychological status is invariant across symptomatic states and remission, or the state of depression or mania is associated with deficits or enhancements. There has also been considerable interest in whether premorbid

levels of intelligence, or surrogate measures such as occupational achievement, differ from population norms.

Figure 9–2 presents a meta-analysis of recent studies contrasting the full-scale intelligence quotient (IQ) scores of bipolar patients and healthy volunteers obtained with the WAIS-R. Despite the relatively small number of studies, significant deficits were observed in the remitted, manic, and mixed samples relative to controls. (Only one study [Deptula et al., 1991] was classified as exclusively examining bipolar depressed patients.) Thus, preliminary evidence indicates that intelligence, as assessed by a well-validated measure, is reduced in bipolar illness in both the remitted and manic states. This conclusion is supported by a variety of early studies that found evidence for general intellectual impairment in symptomatic bipolar patients.

The above findings do not imply that variations in state have no impact on intelligence scores. Cross-sectional comparison with control samples can establish whether each state manifests abnormality, but can give only a rough indication of the magnitude of changes that may occur within the same individuals in different states. Indeed, there is evidence that some patients have higher intellectual functioning when hypomanic than when depressed (Donnelly et al., 1982). Furthermore, a variety of longitudinal studies have found the remitted state to be associated with higher IQ than the depressed state.[5] While such findings have been interpreted as indicating a state-dependent deterioration in IQ (Miller, 1975), much of this work was subject to the same confound: repeat IQ testing generally results in a modest increase in scores attributable to practice effects (Matarazzo et al., 1980). Most studies tested patients in a depressed or manic state, with later retesting during euthymia. Such an invariant order would bias results toward higher scores in the euthymic or remitted state relative to depression or mania.

The firmest conclusion that can be drawn from this literature is that samples of bipolar patients, whether remitted or not, show modest global cognitive impairment as reflected by diminished IQ scores. This conclusion is strengthened by findings obtained using broad-based clinical neuropsychological batteries, such as the Halstead-Reitan or Luria-Nebraska. Summary impairment scores on these batteries correlate highly with IQ scores. Several studies have found gross impairment, on a level comparable to that in schizophrenia, in manic samples, and moderate-to-severe impairment in unipolar and/or bipolar depressed samples.[6]

Interpretation of a global intellectual deficit in bipolar disorder is highly contingent on beliefs about the level of premorbid functioning. For example, an IQ deficit in the remitted state may reflect an impairment that preceded the expression of bipolar disorder, or may represent a form of deterioration resulting from the disorder or its treatments. On the other hand, it has been suggested that bipolar patients

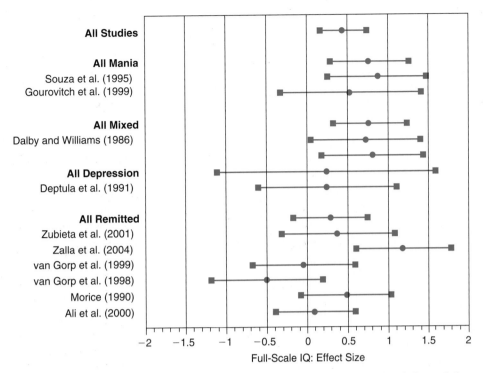

Figure 9–2. Meta-analysis of full-scale intelligence quotient (IQ) scores obtained with the Wechsler Adult Intelligence Scale-Revised (WAIS-R). Effect sizes (Hedges' G) are presented for individual study comparisons of a bipolar sample with healthy controls, as well as for samples of bipolar patients in remission, depression, mixed state, or mania and across all studies. Squares = confidence interval; circles = mean.

may be premorbidly advantaged; that is, their level of intelligence prior to disease expression tends to be above average. Were this the case, it would indicate that the deficits observed in comparisons with healthy volunteers underestimate the deterioration from premorbid values.

Unfortunately, while often discussed, this issue has received limited research attention. Mason (1956) contrasted the prerecruitment IQs of Army veterans hospitalized for schizophrenia and what was termed manic-depressive illness, which no doubt included some patients with recurrent unipolar depression. The schizophrenia sample had premorbid IQs below control values, whereas the IQs of mood disorder patients were significantly better than those of healthy subjects. Woodruff and colleagues (1968, 1971) found that bipolar patients and their brothers had higher levels of occupational and educational achievement than unipolar patients and their brothers, with the latter group not differing from healthy volunteers. Other work has similarly indicated that the families of individuals with bipolar disorder have an advantage relative to population norms for educational and occupational achievement (Petterson, 1977; Waters et al., 1981), as well as creativity (see Chapter 12). Indeed, limited research with children of bipolar probands before the first manifestation of frank mood disorder supports the possibility of an IQ elevation in the premorbid state (Decina et al., 1983).

This possibility of an elevation in premorbid intellectual abilities relative to population norms is reinforced by the literature on the relationship between social class and bipolar disorder. A number of studies, starting at the beginning of the twentieth century, have generally found that bipolar disorder is overrepresented in individuals with middle and high income levels and among business and other professionals. It is possible that these associations reflect an ascertainment bias. Individuals of a higher socioeconomic level may be especially likely to be diagnosed with a mood disorder instead of schizophrenia or schizoaffective disorder, with the reverse pertaining to those of lower socioeconomic levels. However, the fact that these associations are also observed among the family members of bipolar probands undercuts this hypothesis (Woodruff et al., 1971; Monelly et al., 1974; Eisemann, 1986; Coryell et al., 1989).

Thus there is reason to suspect that as a group, individuals with bipolar disorder are endowed with general intellectual abilities superior to the distribution in the general population and may be more likely to have backgrounds of middle and upper socioeconomic levels. Yet it also appears that bipolar disorder is characterized by poorer general intelligence across all phases of illness. If both of these views are correct, it would suggest that the disorder is associated with significant deterioration in general intellectual abilities or that there are compensatory cognitive advantages in a subgroup of individuals with bipolar illness (see Chapter 12). Studies contrasting patient samples with healthy volunteers likely underestimate the extent of deterioration because they do not account for the premorbid baseline.

Contexts in which a group differs in premorbid intellectual abilities present significant problems in interpreting comparisons with patients with other disorders or healthy volunteers. Neuropsychological tests differ in their sensitivity to the generalized effects of brain insult. For example, vocabulary and comprehension subtests of the WAIS-R are traditionally viewed as "hold" scales because of their relative immutability in providing an indication of premorbid ability in the face of brain damage. However, samples of patients with bipolar disorder have usually been matched to comparison groups on the basis of current demographic and neuropsychological features (e.g., age, sex, current IQ). This design may entail, therefore, that the two groups are mismatched with respect to premorbid levels. Thus patterns of apparently specific deficits seen in remitted or symptomatic states may be reflecting only the varying sensitivity of tests to a generalized destructive process.

Verbal and Performance IQ

The full-scale IQ score of the WAIS-R encompasses two composite scores: one for verbal IQ (VIQ) and one for performance (nonverbal) IQ (PIQ). It is well established that patients with mood disorders have a pattern of higher VIQ than PIQ. For example, a review by Kluger and Goldberg (1990) compared the VIQ–PIQ discrepancy in patients with bipolar disorder, right-hemisphere damage, left-hemisphere damage, and bilateral damage and healthy volunteers. Lower PIQ than VIQ was found in 19 of 22 studies of mood disorder patients (14 studies of bipolar and unipolar depressed patients, 4 of manic patients, and 4 of mixed groups), in 20 of 20 studies of patients with right-hemisphere lesions, and in 28 of 30 studies of patients with bilateral injuries. In contrast, PIQ exceeded VIQ in 15 of 20 studies of patients with left-hemisphere lesions. (See also our review of 25 studies in the first edition of this text.)

These effects were examined in the studies of bipolar samples included in our meta-analysis. Figure 9–3a presents the findings for VIQ and Figure 9–3b those for PIQ. Across studies and within studies grouped by state examined (mania, depression, mixed, remission), bipolar patients and normal controls evidenced no difference in VIQ. In contrast, across all studies ($z = 3.36$, $p < .001$) and within studies grouped by state, bipolar samples showed a marked deficit in PIQ; the effect size (Hedges' G) across studies for PIQ was 0.71 (standard error [SE] = 0.21), near the threshold for a strong effect. Specifically, the three studies of

bipolar patients in remission produced an effect size of 0.56 (SE = 0.25).

The nature of the VIQ–PIQ discrepancy was closely examined in a study by Sackeim and colleagues (1992). They administered the full WAIS-R to 100 inpatients who were experiencing an episode of major depressive disorder and had been referred for electroconvulsive therapy (ECT), along with 50 matched healthy volunteers. In addition to age, gender, and race, the groups in this study were matched on indicators of premorbid function, specifically education and highest lifetime occupational level (sustained for 2 years). Based on an algorithm developed by Barona and colleagues (1984), estimates of premorbid full-scale IQ, VIQ, and PIQ were computed for all participants. A subset of patients was readministered the WAIS-R within 1 week ($n = 26$) or 8 weeks after termination of ECT ($n = 33$). Of the 100 patients, 25 were diagnosed with bipolar disorder, and 75 were unipolar. According to the Research Diagnostic Criteria (RDC) (Spitzer et al., 1978), 36 percent of the patient sample were psychotically depressed, 46 percent were of the retarded subtype, and all were of the endogenous subtype. Using a cap of 10, the bipolar patients averaged 5.3 (standard deviation [SD] = 3.2) prior affective episodes and 3.1 (SD = 2.7) prior hospitalizations. In contrast, the unipolar patients averaged 3.3 (SD = 3.4) prior affective episodes and 1.8 (SD = 2.6) prior psychiatric hospitalizations. Of the unipolar patients, 79 percent had recurrent illness.

Figure 9–4 presents the estimated premorbid IQ scores and IQ scores obtained with the WAIS-R for the total patient and healthy volunteer samples. The two groups did not differ in any of the three premorbid estimates. There was no consistent difference between estimated premorbid VIQ and PIQ in either group. In contrast, analyses of obtained IQ scores indicated that the patient group had significantly lower full-scale IQ. This result was attributable to low PIQ scores: the two groups did not differ in VIQ, but showed a marked difference in PIQ.[7] While the VIQ scores of the healthy comparison group averaged 4.7 points higher than their PIQ scores, the comparable figure in the patient sample was 12.7 points. The obtained VIQ among patients was less than 4 points lower than the premorbid estimate, while the obtained PIQ was more than 15 points lower than the premorbid estimate.

These effects pertained to patients with both unipolar and bipolar depression. Figure 9–5 plots the cumulative distribution of VIQ–PIQ discrepancy scores for the healthy control and bipolar and unipolar subgroups. Throughout the range of discrepancy scores, the two patient groups were generally shifted to the right of healthy controls by approximately 10 points. The only indication of a difference between unipolar and bipolar patients was a higher

Figure 9–3. Meta-analysis of (a) verbal and (b) performance intelligence quotients (IQ). Effect sizes (Hedges' G) are presented for individual study comparisons of a bipolar sample with healthy controls, as well as for samples of bipolar patients in remission, depression, mixed state, or mania and across all studies. Squares = confidence interval; circles = mean.

frequency of marked discrepancies favoring VIQ in the bipolar group. However, the mean discrepancy in bipolar patients (14.52 ±14.22) was not different from that in unipolar patients (12.04 ±10.78).

Starting with Wechsler (1944), a common explanation for this discrepancy in mood disorder patients has concerned the effects of psychomotor retardation on task performance. Four of the PIQ subtests (picture arrangement, picture completion, object assembly, and block design) are timed tests, while this is true of only one VIQ subtest (arithmetic). Therefore, slowed processing or motor execution could conceivably lead to diminished performance. This issue was addressed in four ways. One approach involved testing the first 34 patients in the sample under conditions in which both timed and untimed performances were scored. In other words, the subtests were administered and scored in the usual manner, except that patients were allowed to complete each subtest after the standard time limit had expired. Scoring without time constraints had little impact on discrepancy scores, either before or after the course of ECT. The baseline discrepancy in the untimed condition averaged 11.35 (SD=11.06). Patients who met the RDC for retarded subtype ($n=46$) did not differ from the other patients ($n=54$) on this discrepancy score (retarded, 12.78±12.03; nonretarded, 12.56±11.54).

Another approach taken to this issue was to examine more broadly the relationships of symptom severity and other clinical features to the VIQ–PIQ discrepancy. A regression analysis was conducted on baseline discrepancy scores, with age, Hamilton Rating Scale for Depression (HAM-D) score (depression severity), duration of current depressive episode (chronicity), duration since onset of first affective episode, and number of previous affective episodes (recurrence) as predictors. Only baseline HAM-D scores showed a relationship. Greater symptom severity at baseline was associated with a smaller VIQ–PIQ discrepancy and lower VIQ scores. There were no other effects. Thus factors that varied with depression severity did

not appear to be responsible for the VIQ–PIQ difference, and marked severity tended to diminish the discrepancy. There was no evidence of an association with chronicity or frequency of recurrence.

Compatible with these findings were those of analyses conducted after readministration of the WAIS-R 1 and 8 weeks after completion of ECT. The 1-week group ($n = 26$) showed a slight decrease in the discrepancy at retesting, with average scores decreasing from 12.12 ± 11.16 to 9.64 ± 13.22. Virtually no change was seen at the 8-week follow-up ($n=33$), with the average discrepancy decreasing from 13.48 ± 13.01 to 12.24 ± 12.86. Restricting the follow-up sample to patients in remission had no impact.

These findings suggest that the VIQ–PIQ discrepancy was manifested independently of affective state and characterized patients in remission. Indeed, it is possible that the discrepancy is expressed before the first episode of mood disturbance. This possibility is supported by the results of studies of children of bipolar probands aged 7 to 14 (Decina et al., 1983; Sackeim and Decina, 1983). None of the children had yet expressed bipolar disorder, and relatively few had other diagnosable mood disorders, although behavioral disturbance was common. Nonetheless, a marked VIQ–PIQ discrepancy was observed on the Wechsler Intelligence Scale for Children-Revised (WISC-R) in the high-risk sample relative to healthy comparison volunteers. Similar

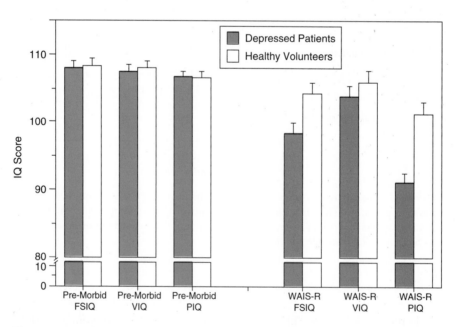

Figure 9–4. Premorbid intelligence quotient (IQ) estimates and IQ scores obtained with the Wechsler Adult Intelligence Scale-Revised (WAIS-R) in unmedicated patients with major depression and healthy controls. Premorbid estimates were identical in the patient ($n=100$) and control ($n=50$) groups. The patient group showed a marked discrepancy between verbal and performance IQ (VIQ > PIQ). FSIQ=full-scale IQ; PIQ=performance IQ; VIQ=verbal IQ. (*Source*: Sackeim et al., 1992. Reproduced with permission of Psychology Press.)

Figure 9–5. Cumulative distribution of verbal and performance IQ discrepancy scores for healthy controls and bipolar and unipolar depressed patients. Both patient groups are shifted to the right of healthy controls and have an average discrepancy favoring a verbal IQ approximately 10 points higher across the distribution in controls. (*Source*: Sackeim et al., 1992. Reproduced with permission of Psychology Press.)

results had been reported in an earlier, uncontrolled study of children at high risk (Kestenbaum, 1979).

Thus the notion that bipolar disorder is associated with a global intellectual impairment that is state independent should be revised. The reductions in full-scale IQ seen in mood disorders appear to be largely attributable to a decrement in PIQ, with preservation of VIQ. This differential deficit is relatively constant across states of euthymia, depression, and mania and may precede syndromal expression.

In interpreting this effect, it is important to consider whether the discrepancy arises from one or two subtests on the WAIS-R or WISC-R or reflects a more uniform difference in verbal and nonverbal task performance. In the study by Sackeim and colleagues (1992), a descriptive (canonical) discriminant analysis was conducted with diagnostic group (patient versus healthy volunteer) as the classification variable and scaled scores on the 11 subtests as the dependent measure. This analysis produced a single significant discriminant function, providing a description of the profile of subtests that distinguishes maximally

between the groups. Structure coefficients were determined for this linear function. These coefficients are more stable than the original weighting of subtests in the discriminant function (Huberty, 1984), and reflect the association between scores on a subtest and total scores on the composite discriminant function. The median structure coefficient for the five PIQ subtests was 0.53, with a range of 0.43 to 0.70. In contrast, the median structure coefficient for the six VIQ subtests was 0.13, with a range of 0.03 to 0.38. All five PIQ subtests made strong contributions to the differentiation between patients and controls. The comprehension (0.29) and digit span (0.38) VIQ subtests also contributed, but more weakly. Therefore, the results of this analysis suggest that the PIQ deficit in mood disorders is not specific to a particular PIQ subtest, but is expressed uniformly across all five PIQ subtests.

Thus the relative deficit in PIQ is uniform across the various subtests assessing this form of intelligence. The magnitude of this discrepancy appears to be independent of the phase of affective disorder, and may be a marker of a bipolar diathesis. Early work on children at risk indicated that children with behavioral disturbances suggestive of early signs of bipolar disorder, such as grandiosity, conduct disorder, or separation anxiety, are especially likely to manifest the discrepancy (Decina et al., 1983; Sackeim et al., 1983a). While many researchers attributed this phenomenon to a differential impact of psychomotor slowing on PIQ, this hypothesis can now be rejected given the discrepancy's persistence in remission, manifestation in at-risk samples, and persistence even when performance is not constrained by timing.

In this light, two hypotheses have been advanced. One posits that the PIQ deficit reflects a fundamental disturbance in visuospatial processing and implies a differential right hemisphere deficit (Flor-Henry, 1979). The second hypothesis is that the discrepancy has little localizing value and reflects the greater sensitivity of PIQ and other forms of "fluid" intelligence to generalized impairment, in contrast to the "crystallized" intelligence reflected in VIQ subscales (Kluger and Goldberg, 1990; Bearden et al., 2001).

Were the discrepancy to reflect a fundamental deficit in visuospatial processing, it could be compatible with a right-hemisphere insult, especially in parietal cortex. This classic formulation is compatible with evidence that manifestation of mania without a history of major depression (i.e., unipolar mania) is seen principally in the context of brain insult and most commonly with right-hemisphere damage, generally involving parietal tissue. Thus, bipolar illness would be viewed as especially likely to manifest a form of right-hemisphere dysfunction. However, the evidence in mood disorders clearly reveals that the discrepancy is also manifested in unipolar depression, at least in samples with severe and/or recurrent disorder. Thus if this discrepancy indeed reflects a lateralized insult, it must be viewed as characteristic of recurrent mood disorders—that is, manic-depressive illness in Kraepelin's terminology.

The second hypothesis is that the discrepancy per se has limited lateralizing value. It is seen with both bilateral and right-hemisphere brain damage. The effect size seen in mood disorder samples is comparable to that seen in patients with bilateral brain damage, itself a notable fact, and below that seen in patients with right-hemisphere lesions (Kluger and Goldberg, 1990). There is no reason to suspect, for example, that the pathophysiological process resulting in right-hemisphere dysfunction in mood disorders would produce the same level of differential deficit as that seen in patients with gross brain lesions.

A broader perspective on the neuropsychological profiles of mood disorder patients may help resolve this issue. The laterality hypothesis would stipulate that mood disorder samples show especially marked deficits in tests that rely heavily on visuospatial processing. The view that the discrepancy arises from generalized brain impairment would

suggest that the deficit in PIQ is of the same magnitude as deficits across a host of cognitive functions, including attention and memory.

Indeed, our examination of the profile of cognitive deficits in bipolar disorder raises a third, novel hypothesis. There is indeed evidence of widespread and generally uniform cognitive deficit across the phases of bipolar disorder, with little indication that visuospatial abilities are especially impaired. Rather, verbal skills appear to be consistently preserved. The implication is that the cognitive systems subserving language are spared with respect to an otherwise generalized disease process, are constitutionally endowed at higher capacity, or are complemented by compensatory cognitive advantages of an as-yet undetermined nature.

Psychomotor Functioning

The domain of psychomotor functioning reflects the integrity of processes determining the speed of information processing and the speed and organization of motor behavior. Individuals may appear to be "slowed" because of dysfunction in motor output and/or in the speed of thought. Alternatively, individuals may appear to be "dull" or "slow" because of poverty of mental content, in essence a lack of thought. This domain pertains to functions as diverse as manual dexterity, reaction time, and levels of spontaneous activity. As reviewed by Sobin and Sackeim (1997), a variety of experimental techniques have been developed to assess the component processes that may underlie psychomotor disturbance in mood disorders.

Disturbances of motility and speed of processing have long been considered central to the phenomenology of mood disorders. Psychomotor disturbance has generally been regarded as a cardinal feature of endogenous or melancholic depression, and some have contended that careful assessment of psychomotor disturbances has predictive value with respect to treatment outcome. The racing thoughts of the manic state suggest dysregulation in speed of processing that is opposite to that often seen in the depressed state. Thus psychomotor function, like mood and sleep, may be one of the few domains to show opposite symptom manifestations depending on phase of illness.

Some theorists have taken this overlap between the mood and motor output systems to suggest that mood disorders are essentially disorders of motility (Flor-Henry, 1983). While this is clearly an overstatement, it is noteworthy that mood disturbance occurs at especially high rates in patients with movement disorder. This observation is especially well documented for Parkinson's and Huntington's diseases. As indicated earlier, Huntington's disease is of special note as perhaps the only neurological illness to produce both depression and mania at some frequency. In contrast, imaging research has yet to relate psychomotor disturbance in mood disorders to basal ganglia dysfunction. Instead, the Hammersmith group found that psychomotor symptoms covary with the magnitude of regional cerebral blood flow deficits in prefrontal regions (Dolan et al., 1993). Indeed, they suggested that the prefrontal deficits commonly seen in both major depression and schizophrenia reflect a common psychomotor disturbance. Presumably, this disturbance pertains to executive functions that regulate the flow and speed of information processing.

Cognitive and Motor Speed

In a substantial literature over the last five decades, slowed reaction time has been documented in mood disorder patients during episodes of major depression relative to healthy participants (Marvel and Paradiso, 2004). The subgroups most likely to manifest this slowing were variously described in this work as manic-depressive, bipolar, psychotic, or presenting with endogenous depression compared with subgroups classified as neurotic, nonpsychotic, or reactive. Thus, there was a general impression that severity of illness was associated with psychomotor slowing. Frequently in this work, depressed samples had slower performance relative to healthy participants, nondepressed neurotic patients, and patients with acute schizophrenia. Nonetheless, the depressed samples were often less slowed than patients with chronic schizophrenia or brain damage. The investigators also found that clinical improvement was usually linked to improved speed of responding, suggesting that psychomotor slowing is largely a state-dependent phenomenon. In much of this work, time to complete tasks, such as the digit symbol subtest of the WAIS-R, was used to assess psychomotor slowing. Consequently, disturbances in cognitive processes and motor execution were confounded, and the source of the slowing was not identified.

While this issue is the subject of increasing attention (Sobin and Sackeim, 1997), it remains unresolved and may not have a simple answer. Cornell and colleagues (1984) varied cognitive load in a series of reaction-time measures when comparing patients who met diagnostic criteria for melancholia with nonmelancholic, nonendogenous depressed patients. They found that both groups manifested slow motor performance, and that this was a key abnormality independent of melancholia. In contrast, the melancholic subgroup was especially sensitive to the effects of cognitive load in further slowing motor response. This result was interpreted as reflecting an impairment in cognitive processing—a cognitive slowing—in melancholic patients.

Other dimensions to consider in studies of psychomotor speed concern the effects of distraction and the distinction between preferred rates of response and response speed when one is working at one's best. In a comprehensive study, Blackburn (1975) contrasted six groups of patients:

acutely symptomatic bipolar manic, bipolar depressed, and unipolar depressed and the same three groups at rest. Blackburn used separate tasks thought to measure principally mental and motor speed, although the motor task had more than nontrivial cognitive components. The mental task was administered with patients working both at their own speed (preferred speed) and as quickly as possible. The motor task was administered under conditions of no distraction, internal distraction (the patient counting), and external distraction (a news program played loudly during task performance). Acutely ill bipolar depressed patients were slower than all other groups on the motor task with no distraction. Surprisingly, both internal and external distraction resulted in improved performance among the bipolar depressed group but in deterioration among the unipolar patients, while results with the manic patients were equivocal. In contrast, on the mental speed test at the preferred rate of responding, the acutely ill manic patients were faster than the other two groups, but did not differ from the manic patients in remission. With instructions to respond as quickly as possible, the six groups had comparable scores.

The results of this study illustrate two points. First, most neuropsychological evaluations call for patients to perform at their best, which may obscure deficits in routine information processing. Second, this study provided evidence that bipolar depressed patients are especially likely to manifest marked psychomotor slowing. It has long been contended that psychomotor retardation is characteristic more of bipolar than of unipolar depression (Kotin and Goodwin, 1972; Dunner et al., 1976). We revisit this issue in reviewing the literature on spontaneous activity (see the later discussion).

Recent studies using reaction time measures have demonstrated that psychomotor disturbance is characteristic of elderly patients with bipolar disorder. Pier and colleagues (2004) manipulated task difficulty and contrasted speed of figure copying in 12 elderly depressed patients and matched healthy controls in an attempt to isolate cognitive from motor slowing. Pronounced psychomotor retardation was seen in the patient group, which reflected a cognitive and more pronounced motor slowing. However, patients were studied while medicated, and medication effects on psychomotor speed are commonly observed (Caligiuri et al., 2003).

Surprisingly, three recent studies of psychomotor speed in bipolar adolescents failed to find differences from controls or other clinical groups (DelBello et al., 2004; Dickstein et al., 2004; McCarthy et al., 2004). Furthermore, there is only equivocal evidence for psychomotor disturbance in the first-degree relatives of bipolar probands. Zalla and colleagues (2004) compared euthymic bipolar patients, patients with schizophrenia, the unaffected first-degree relatives of both patient groups, and healthy controls in performance on tests of verbal fluency—the Stroop Word Color Interference Test, the Wisconsin Card Sorting Test, and the Trail Making Test. Compared with healthy controls, patients with schizophrenia performed poorly on all measures. The only abnormality seen in the euthymic bipolar group and the two groups of unaffected relatives reflected increased slowness on the Stroop test. This deficit could have been attributable to an increased susceptibility to interference and/or psychomotor slowing in the context of increased cognitive demand. In contrast, Ferrier and colleagues (2004) found no evidence of psychomotor disturbance when contrasting the neuropsychological performance of 17 unaffected first-degree relatives of bipolar patients with that of matched controls. Instead, the relatives were significantly impaired in backward digit span, spatial span, and tasks of visuospatial declarative memory, while verbal declarative memory was intact.

It is premature to conclude that psychomotor disturbance is infrequent in children and adolescents manifesting bipolar disorder or in first-degree family members. These issues have been studied infrequently, and the extant research used relatively small samples, a key limitation in studies of familial transmission given heterogeneity in genetic diathesis. Furthermore, while there is substantial evidence that reaction time improves with clinical remission in mood disorders, as reviewed in the next section, there is also substantial evidence for persistent psychomotor disturbance in remitted bipolar patients on tasks that make significant motor demands in terms of both dexterity and speed (e.g., Purdue Pegboard). Little information exists on potential impairments in pediatric bipolar patients or first-degree relatives in the aspects of psychomotor dysfunction most persistent in adult patients with bipolar disorder.

There has been limited investigation of the neurobiological correlates of impairments in cognitive and motor speed in bipolar disorder. Caligiuri and colleagues (2003) conducted functional magnetic resonance imaging (fMRI) while patients in the manic or depressed phase of bipolar illness and healthy controls performed a manual reaction-time task. The study results implicated both basal ganglia disturbance and a dimension of laterality. Manic patients had higher blood oxygen level–dependent (BOLD) responses in the left globus pallidus and significantly lower activity in the right globus pallidus, while depressed patients showed the reverse pattern of asymmetry. Level of activity within the globus pallidus and caudate was associated with the severity of manic symptoms. Notably, patients not receiving antipsychotic or mood-stabilizing medications had higher BOLD responses throughout the motor cortex, basal ganglia, and thalamus. These findings suggest that the depressed and manic states are related to excessive and lateralized activity within the basal ganglia, and that antipsychotics and mood stabilizers suppress cortical and subcortical hyperreactivity.

The results of subsequent research focused on the supplementary (SMA) and primary (M1) motor areas underscore the possibility of a disturbance in lateralized control over motor processes. Using fMRI and several reaction time tasks, Caligiuri and colleagues (2004) showed that healthy controls differentially activated the left and right SMA on right- and left-hand trials, respectively. In contrast, in the small samples of bipolar manic and depressed patients, the latter failed to suppress the ipsilateral right SMA in right-hand trials, while the former had bilateral SMA activation for both left- and right-hand trials. Both depressed and manic patients had greater activity in the left M1, and antipsychotic or mood-stabilizing medications were associated with increased reaction time, lower BOLD response in M1 and SMA, and a loss of normal hemispheric asymmetry. In addition to again raising the issue of a lateralized disturbance, the results of this work suggest that the psychomotor disturbance in bipolar disorder may be an outcome of excessive excitability in mediating brain regions. This formulation contrasts with the hypothesis, derived from resting positron emission tomography (PET) studies (Bench et al., 1992; Dolan et al., 1994), that psychomotor retardation reflects reduced activity in specific prefrontal cortical structures.

Recent work has also clarified the extent to which psychomotor disturbance in bipolar disorder reflects cognitive dysfunction that may interfere with the planning or initiation of movement and/or disturbance in the execution of movement. Caligiuri and Ellwanger (2000) administered a traditional psychomotor battery, as well as a measure of the integrity of motor programming, to 36 patients who met *Diagnostic and Statistical Manual* (DSM)-IV criteria for psychomotor retardation. The programming task assessed capacity to adjust velocity scaling of movement relative to movement distance. Compared with healthy controls, the patient group evidenced longer reaction time and impairment in velocity scaling. A significant subgroup had deficits that were akin to those observed with the bradykinesia associated with parkinsonian conditions. Thus the retardation was viewed as encompassing both the planning and the execution of movement. An earlier detailed review of this literature likewise suggested that psychomotor disturbance usually involves a mix of cognitive and motor deficits (Sobin and Sackeim, 1997).

Finally, limited attention has been given to the neurochemical imbalances that may result in disturbances in cognitive and motor speed. Swann and colleagues (1999) compared unipolar and bipolar depressed patients and manic and mixed-state patients with healthy controls in tests of psychomotor speed and accuracy of tracking. The depressed groups were impaired on all behavioral measures, whereas the manic and mixed patients did not differ from the controls. Cerebral spinal fluid (CSF) and urinary measures of catecholamines and their metabolites were obtained. For virtually all behavioral measures, increased catecholamine function was associated with poorer performance in bipolar but not unipolar patients. Further, psychomotor function was related to depression severity in bipolar but not unipolar depression. The results of this preliminary study raise the possibility that psychomotor retardation in bipolar disorder is accompanied by, if not an outcome of, catecholamine overdrive. This view may be congruent with imaging findings that suggest excessive excitability or failure of inhibition in the motor control systems of bipolar patients. Indeed, at a speculative level, it has long been thought that catatonia, which may be viewed as an extreme form of psychomotor retardation, reflects an internal state of excessive arousal, rapidly reversed by interventions with sedative or barbiturate properties (amobarbital, lorazepam, ECT).

Motor Skills

Traditional neuropsychological evaluations have placed little emphasis on assessment of reaction time per se. This situation is changing rapidly with the increasing use of computerized neuropsychological batteries, which allow more readily for trial-by-trial computation of reaction time. Instead, psychomotor function has typically been assessed with a range of performance measures that are sensitive to the dexterity or accuracy of motor execution, as well as speed. In the studies contributing to our meta-analysis, the psychomotor tasks employed included the Purdue Pegboard, Pursuit Rotor, mirror writing, and motor sequencing tasks, among others. Given this diversity of tasks, a deficit in psychomotor function may reflect some fundamental or general impairment in motor execution or output.

Figure 9–6 presents the findings on psychomotor function from our meta-analysis. It is evident that despite the diversity of tasks, there was a consistent effect across all studies, with bipolar samples showing impaired performance relative to healthy participants (overall effect size = 0.55, SE = 0.18, z = 3.12, p = .002). This effect is significant when the analysis is restricted to studies of patients in remission; the magnitude of the deficit in psychomotor function is near that for PIQ.

The source of the motor abnormalities seen in mood disorders is still unknown. In fact, relatively little work has been done to better characterize the phenomenology of this motor disturbance. Exquisite methodologies have been

Figure 9–6. Meta-analysis of psychomotor measures. Effect sizes (Hedges' G) are presented for individual study comparisons of a bipolar sample with healthy controls, as well as for samples of bipolar patients in remission, depression, mixed state, or mania and across all studies. Squares = confidence interval; circles = mean.

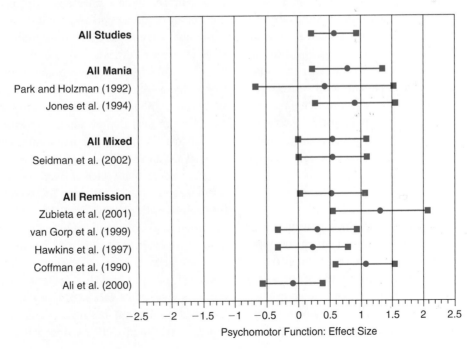

developed to assay components of motor control, but they have rarely been applied to mood disorder samples.

There are suggestions of a lateralized component to the motor disturbances seen in mood disorders. Indeed, there have been isolated reports of individuals whose handedness covaried with the phase of bipolar illness (depression, euthymia, mania). However, the relationship between handedness and bipolar illness is far from clear. Various researchers have reported that the frequency of left-handedness in mood disorders is increased (Fleminger et al., 1977), decreased (Merrin, 1984; Yan et al., 1985), or unchanged (Merrin, 1984; Yan et al., 1985). Sackeim and Decina (1983) took a different approach to this issue. They examined the possibility that handedness moderates genetic factors in the transmission of bipolar disorder. They found that the handedness of bipolar patients was associated with family history of affective disorder and not with family history of sinistrality. Among the bipolar-I subgroup, for example, 49 percent of strongly right-handed patients had a positive family history of affective disorder, compared with 89 percent of weakly right-handed and left-handed patients.

The possibility of a lateralized dimension to the motor disturbance of bipolar disorder is supported by the results of studies examining grip strength. Flor-Henry and Yeudall (1979) found that patients in either the manic or depressive phase of mood disturbance showed greater right-hand than left-hand grip strength, implicating right hemisphere dysfunction. They also found that speed of finger tapping was reduced primarily in the left hand. Merrin (1984) obtained similar results with respect to grip strength, and the asymmetry distinguished mood disorder patients from both patients with schizophrenia and normal controls. Merrin observed that patients with bipolar disorder and psychotic features were most likely to show the asymmetry. More recently, it was found that instability in maintaining stable force with the index finger placed on a strain gauge was greater for the left than the right hand in patients with bipolar disorder, whereas the opposite was true in patients with schizophrenia (Lohr and Caligiuri, 1995, 1997). These scattered results, along with the imaging findings in bipolar patients showing lateralized disturbances in activation patterns during motor tasks (Caligiuri et al., 2003, 2004), point to the need for systematic study of motor asymmetry.

Spontaneous Activity

Routine clinical evaluations of psychomotor disturbance and those conducted using formal rating instruments typically address a different level of behavior from that assessed with neuropsychological or information processing measures. For example, the CORE is a well-studied instrument that quantifies the extent of psychomotor disturbance. Box 9–1 lists the 18 behavioral manifestations assessed by

---

BOX 9–1.   Items in the CORE Measure of Psychomotor Disturbance

- Facial immobility (average across the interview)
- Postural slumping (average across the interview)
- Noninteractiveness (ability to respond to the social cues in the interview)
- Nonreactivity (rate any episode, not duration through the interview)
- Facial apprehension (rate any episode or fixed expression)
- Delay in responding verbally (average across the interview)
- Length of verbal responses
- Inattentiveness
- Facial agitation (movement; rate any episode—intensity rather than duration)
- Body immobility (amount, not speed; average across the interview)
- Motor agitation (rate any episode; intensity rather than persistence)
- Poverty of associations (ability to elaborate)
- Slowed movement (speed, not amount; average across the interview)
- Verbal stereotypy (rate any episode)
- Delay in motor activity (average across the interview)
- Impaired spontaneity of talk (ability to initiate conversation)
- Slowing of speech rate (average across the interview)
- Stereotyped movements (rate any episode)

---

the CORE. These aspects of psychomotor function are considerably more diverse than those assessed with the more atomistic approach of neuropsychological measurement. Further, these abnormalities are assessed in the normal course of interaction and not in relation to specific test demands. Of course, this sign- or symptom-based approach to assessment assumes a conceptualization of the boundaries and constituents of psychomotor disturbance. There would likely be strong consensus that some of the signs or symptoms in Box 9–1, such as facial immobility, delay in responding verbally, and slowed movement, reflect aspects of the construct. On the other hand, there could be considerable debate about the inclusion of other signs or symptoms, such as nonreactivity (lack of interest or pleasure), inattentiveness, and verbal stereotypy, in assessing the severity of psychomotor disturbance.

Parker and colleagues (1993, 1995a, 2000) contended that the assessment of signs and symptoms of psychomotor disturbance is of special importance in mood disorders. Specifically, they argued that such disturbance accounts for the lion's share of the variance in the diagnosis of melancholia. Melancholic and nonmelancholic depressed patients differ markedly in CORE scores, with the endogenity of symptoms accounting for a smaller portion of the variance.[8] Parker and colleagues claimed that the fundamental symptomalogical characteristic of the melancholic patient is psychomotor disturbance. They also found that the severity of psychomotor disturbance has predictive value with regard to treatment outcome with ECT and medications (Hickie et al., 1990b, 1996; Parker and Hadzi-Pavlovic, 1993), and that the psychomotor disturbance in melancholic unipolar patients shares features with the bradykinesia of Parkinson's disease in demonstrating difficulties with the initiation of movement in the absence of external cues (Austin et al., 2000; Rogers et al., 2000). The theoretical importance of some of these findings is challenged by the notion that the broad definition of psychomotor disturbance incorporates assessment of cardinal features of melancholia (such as lack of mood reactivity) that may not reflect psychomotor abnormalities. Thus the associations between the CORE and melancholic diagnosis may be partly tautological, and the linkage to treatment outcome could conceivably be associated with items influenced by melancholic manifestations that do not reflect psychomotor disturbance (e.g., inattentiveness).

A recent study contrasted the CORE ratings of bipolar and unipolar depressed patients. Parker and colleagues (2000) compared 904 unipolar and 83 bipolar patients using three methods for subtyping melancholia (DSM, clinical classification, and CORE). With all three methods, bipolar patients were considerably more likely to be diagnosed with melancholia and psychotic depression. Prevalence of psychomotor disturbance and pathological guilt were the signs or symptoms that distinguished the groups.

While it can be argued that studies of reaction time and other aspects of information processing may provide too narrow a view of psychomotor disturbance, it is also true that the use of rating scales such as the CORE is limited in that ratings may be contaminated by patient behavior reflective of domains other than psychomotor disturbance. Patient reports of lack of interest, loss of pleasure, or marked psychic anxiety may affect ratings of psychomotor disturbance. An alternative approach is to examine objective measures that reflect broader aspects of psychomotor function. Two such measures examine spontaneous activity and speech rate.

Various devices are available for continuous recording of the amount of motor activity. For example, activity monitors, worn like a wrist watch, can provide 24-hour data on fluctuation in movements of the wrist or arm. The potential utility of this approach is illustrated by findings in movement disorders. Although Huntington's disease is characterized by chorea, patients with this disorder have shown less daytime spontaneous movement than healthy controls. Further, this hypokinesia correlates cross-sectionally with impairment in voluntary movement, with disturbed posture and gait, and most robustly with reduced functional capacity (van Vugt et al., 2001). Over a 2-year follow-up period, van Vugt and colleagues (2001) also found that spontaneous activity remained unchanged in clinically stable patients, but worsened in those who deteriorated in functional capacity. Thus in this context, hypokinesia, as assessed by activity monitoring, showed a strong relationship with functional impairment.

A set of small-group comparisons reported by Kupfer and colleagues led to a number of explicit hypotheses about the patterns of gross motor activity in depression and mania.[9] These investigators suggested that (1) manic patients have higher activity levels than severely agitated depressed patients; (2) unipolar depressed patients have higher activity levels than bipolar depressed patients; (3) clinical remission in depression is accompanied by an increase in activity levels; and (4) manic patients manifest their highest activity levels in the late evening and early nighttime, whereas hypomanic patients peak during the daytime (see Chapter 2 for a discussion of the overlap between agitated depressive and mixed hypomanic states). These observations were based on small subgroups; lacked comparison with a normal control group; and were derived from work on a specialized inpatient unit at the National Institutes of Health (NIH), where hospital routine and regimentation may have affected activity levels. While there has been surprisingly limited further research in this area since the mid-1970s, the additional studies that have been done have substantially clarified the nature of the deficit in spontaneous activity during episodes of major depression.

In a study by Wolff and colleagues (1985), a group of 18 normal controls was housed on the same ward and shared in the same activities as a group of 30 euthymic patients (25 bipolar, 5 unipolar). In addition, 27 patients were studied through at least two phases of illness (depression, euthymia, or mania); the depressed state was consistently associated with lower 24-hour levels of activity than euthymia. This difference was significant for the within-subject comparison during daytime but not nighttime periods. Mania was associated with higher activity levels than depression, with the difference seen mainly in the late evening and nighttime hours (7:00 PM to 4:00 AM). Although mania tended to be associated with higher levels than euthymia, none of these comparisons were significant; however, the sample size for comparisons with euthymia was substantially smaller for mania ($n=11$) than for depression ($n=23$). Of special note is that, in comparison with controls, euthymic patients still manifested lower 24-hour activity levels, attributable mainly to the daytime period (2:00 PM to 12:00 AM).

Royant-Parola and colleagues (1986) followed a group of 12 patients with major depression, monitoring their activity throughout a hospital stay. In addition to the amount of activity, they assessed duration of immobility. Activity troughs and immobility peaks were bunched before noon and around 3:00 PM. With remission, activity levels increased, and immobility decreased. The authors suggested that immobility is a particularly sensitive measure, especially for patients with agitated depression, and that daytime manifestation may reflect release of an ultradian sleep–wake rhythm in major depression (see Chapter 16).

A reduction in daytime spontaneous activity does not appear to be an artifact of concomitant medications. Volkers and colleagues (2003) compared 67 unmedicated unipolar depressed patients with 64 matched healthy controls. Relative to the control sample, the patient group showed lower activity levels in daytime and higher activity levels and reduced immobility during sleep. It is not known whether this shift toward increased activity levels at night in depressed and manic samples contributes to or is an outcome of disrupted sleep, or both phenomena reflect the same underlying disturbance in rhythmicity.

As noted, these studies of spontaneous activity in mood disorders were conducted in inpatient samples, often with highly treatment-resistant patients. The generalizability of their findings to broader clinical populations was recently tested. Iverson (2004) conducted activity monitoring among 48 depressed patients being seen in primary care and 25 controls with general medical conditions. The depressed group was divided by a median split in scores on the Beck Depression Inventory (BDI) II (Beck et al., 1996). Patients with higher BDI scores had lower activity levels than the other depressed patients and the control group; this effect was most marked during 12:00 PM to 6:00 PM, in line with previous findings in the depressed state. However, the possibility of distinct subgroups was raised in a pilot study of geriatric patients with unipolar major depression. Teicher and colleagues (1988) compared eight geriatric depressed inpatients with eight elderly controls studied in similar settings and found that the depressed group had 29 percent higher mean total 24-hour activity levels, with no difference in circadian amplitude or frequency. Daily peak activity averaged slightly more than 2 hours later in the depressed sample, and the degree of this delay correlated with serum cortisol levels at 4:00 PM after earlier administration of dexamethasone. The heightened activity levels in this small geriatric sample contrast with the findings in unipolar and bipolar adult samples.

Overall, the findings in this area are consistent in indicating that episodes of major depression, whether bipolar or unipolar, are associated with reduced 24-hour activity, especially during daytime hours, and perhaps most markedly during the period 12:00 PM to 6:00 PM. There are suggestions in the study findings that bipolar depressed patients

manifest greater reductions in spontaneous activity than do unipolar patients, but work in this area with bipolar disorder has been limited in recent years. The evidence is robust and consistent that spontaneous activity levels improve with remission from the depressed state, although it is possible that this improvement fails to reach the levels of healthy controls. It is unknown whether the putative residual deficit is associated with the severity of residual depressive symptoms or is independent. The limited evidence indicates that mania is associated with increased activity levels relative to those of depressed patients, especially during the nighttime. However, it is not clear that the increase associated with mania exceeds the values obtained in healthy controls.

Clinical observation of psychomotor disturbance led to the original hypothesis that psychomotor retardation is more common and/or more severe in bipolar than unipolar patients (Kotin and Goodwin, 1972; Dunner et al., 1976). However, the need to ground such observations in objective measures is reflected in conflicting results obtained with the CORE. Mitchell and colleagues (1992) compared 27 age- and sex-matched pairs of unipolar and bipolar patients who met criteria for melancholia based on several diagnostic schemes. Bipolar patients were less likely to have slowed movement. In general, items reflecting psychomotor retardation were less common and agitation was more common in the bipolar cohort. In contrast, almost a decade later, Mitchell and colleagues (2001) compared the clinical features of 39 pairs of bipolar and unipolar patients using a similar methodology. The bipolar patients were more likely than the unipolar patients to manifest psychomotor-related melancholic features and symptoms of atypical depression. The authors suggested that psychomotor retardation, atypical features, and, less commonly, psychosis constitute the clinical signature of bipolar depression.

Speech Rate

Speech is a motor act. Clinically, it is common to observe severely depressed patients speaking in a halting, slow manner with frequent pauses, and often with a weak or raspy voice. It is also clear that manic patients often have racing speech along with racing ideas. Thus it is an empirical matter whether objective analysis of speech and voice characteristics will reveal abnormalities associated with mood disorders and/or provide information of prognostic significance.

The small literature in this area has presented consistent findings. The most common paradigm has been to examine automatic speech, as in counting from 1 to 10, where cognitive load is minimal,[10] although there have also been studies that involved taking samples of natural speech, as might occur during a diagnostic interview (Bouhuys and Mulder-Hajonides van der Meulen, 1984; Alpert et al.,

2001; Cannizzaro et al., 2004). The most common dependent measure has been speech pause time (SPT), the duration of the silent interval between phonations. Szabadi and colleagues (1976) and later Greden and colleagues (Greden and Carroll, 1980; Greden et al., 1981; Greden, 1982) first claimed that SPT was elongated in major depression without a change in phonation time, and that SPT shortened with clinical remission. These claims have received substantial support and have been extended to bipolar depressed patients. SPT has shown significant associations with depression severity, the Widlocher scale (Widlocher, 1983) for assessing psychomotor retardation, and reaction time.[11] Other aspects of speech, including total speaking time, various quantitative features of fundamental frequency and pitch, and speed of voice change, have shown less consistent associations with mood disorders. There is surprisingly little information on the impact of manic states on these measures, and comparisons of unipolar and bipolar depressed patients have shown limited power.

Attention

Impaired attention and insufficient motivation are the two most common reasons given for the pattern of widespread neuropsychological deficit in mood disorders (Miller, 1975; Bearden et al., 2001). To the extent that motivational impairments resolve with remission of depression or mania, persistent neuropsychological impairments are unlikely to be due to motivational factors. Attentional processes are in many respects the gateway to learning, memory, and other higher cognitive processes. While some forms of learning (e.g., procedural learning) undoubtedly occur outside of awareness and do not depend on the integrity of attentional processes, such is not the case for much of our knowledge of ourselves and the world.

Attention is a complex concept that encompasses multiple distinct processes. The concept of working memory denotes the capacity to hold in awareness for a limited time a limited number of visual or auditory representations. This type of attentional process, as in "keeping in mind" a telephone number, can be assessed with various "span" tasks, in which patients recall or recognize a serial list of digits, letters, or shapes just presented. In contrast, the capacity to detect a rarely occurring target is the form of attention commonly referred to as vigilance. The classic example here is the air traffic controller who monitors a screen for representations of two aircraft on a collision course. Although this event is infrequent, detecting its occurrence is of obvious importance. In psychiatric research, vigilance is commonly assessed with the Continuous Performance Test (CPT), originally developed by Beck and colleagues (1956) to detect lapses in attention among epilepsy patients. Another form of attention concerns freedom from distraction

or interference. The capacity to carry out more than one task simultaneously requires that one split attention between tasks (e.g., speaking on the phone while driving) or rapidly shift attention from one task to another. One method of assessing distractibility involves using dichotic listening; individuals must monitor for the occurrence of a target embedded in information delivered to one ear (as in vigilance tasks) but with other, sometimes conflicting, information presented to the other ear. In this context, freedom from distractibility involves the capacity to disattend to irrelevant but competing information channels. A similar phenomenon is tapped by the Stroop test. In one condition of this test, individuals identify the color of nonmeaningful stimuli, such as a series of X's. In another condition, they report the color of visual stimuli that are color names. These names may be in conflict with the appearance of the stimuli. For example, the word "green" may be presented for a stimulus in the color blue. The interference produced by such color–color word conflict is assessed by comparing reaction time in this condition with that for simple color naming. Disattending to the meaning of the word and focusing only on the color would optimize performance on the Stroop test.

It has long been thought that attentional processes are impaired in episodes of major depression in a state-dependent fashion (Cronholm and Ottosson, 1961; Sternberg and Jarvik, 1976) and that attentional deficits limit the extent to which learning may occur. Meta-analyses have consistently shown that attention and learning are among the most markedly impaired functions in episodes of major depression (Zakzanis et al., 1998).

Figure 9–7 presents the results of our meta-analysis of attentional measures in studies of bipolar disorder. The effect size (Hedges' G)[J] across all studies was 0.64 (SE = 0.063, $p < .001$) and was significant for studies of depression (effect size = 0.61, SE = 0.28, $p < .03$), mania (effect size = 0.75, SE = 0.15, $p < .001$), mixed states (effect size = 0.74, SE = 0.12, $p < .001$), and remission (effect size = 0.54, SE = 0.10, $p < .001$). While the effect size was smallest for studies of remitted patients and highest for studies of the manic state, formal testing failed to reveal a significant difference among the groups. Indeed, contrary to the notion that attentional disturbance is purely state dependent, deficits in this domain relative to healthy controls were seen in virtually all studies of patients in remission. This has been demonstrated in more recent studies of attentional deficits in euthymic patients as well.[12] A similar pattern of attentional deficits has been found in bipolar children and adolescents (see the review by Kyte et al., 2006; Kolur et al., 2006).

Our analysis of effects on attention involved 212 comparisons from 39 studies. Given that attentional processes are heterogeneous and are sampled by tasks differing radically

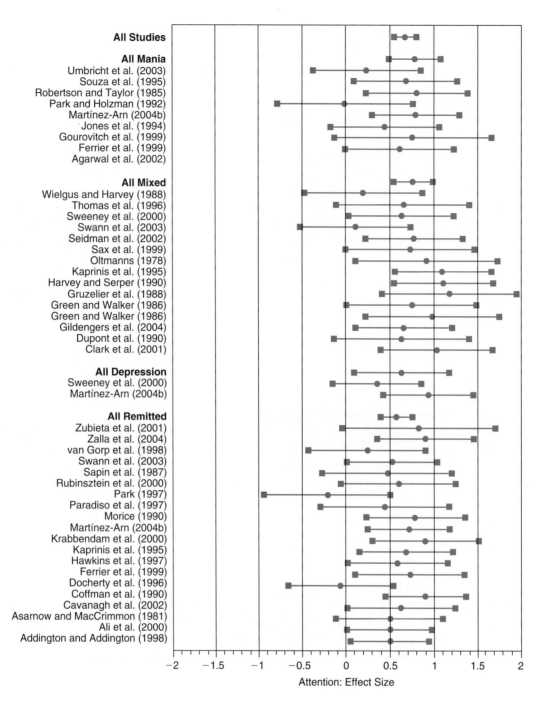

Figure 9–7. Meta-analysis of attention measures. Effect sizes (Hedges' G) are presented for individual study comparisons of a bipolar sample with healthy controls, as well as for samples of bipolar patients in remission, depression, mixed state, or mania and across all studies. Squares = confidence interval; circles = mean.

in their cognitive demands, averaging across distinct attentional measures could obscure more discrete patterns of deficit. Therefore, the analyses were predated for studies of patients in remission and for all studies as a function of the specific neuropsychological procedure used to evaluate attention. As seen in Figure 9–8, although the number of studies contributing to results for individual tests is often small, a consistent pattern is evident. Except for working-memory

tasks, all other tests showed a consistent deficit in both the remitted state and across remission and the phases of bipolar illness. Indeed, except for cancellation tasks, the effect sizes are uniform for the remaining tasks and essentially equivalent both for studies restricted to remission and for all studies. The failure to find a deficit in working memory may be related to the small number of studies that addressed this area and to the use of simple tasks, such as matching to sample (which may produce floor effects), to assess working memory. On the other hand, Harmer and colleagues (2002) noted that disturbance in sustained attention is a consistent finding in remitted bipolar patients, but that many vigilance tasks contain working components. By using tests of sustained attention that did and did not draw on working memory, they were able to demonstrate that the impairment in sustained attention did not derive from or depend on impairment in working memory.

Cancellation procedures require that targets embedded in an array of targets and foils be crossed out, with the rates of target identification (hits) relative to false identification (commission errors or false alarms) as the measure of performance accuracy. In brain-damaged individuals, right parietal injury is especially likely to disrupt cancellation performance, often producing a pattern of hemispatial neglect whereby failure to identify targets (false-negative errors) is overrepresented on the left side of arrays (Mesulam, 2000). While there was a robust effect size for deficits on cancellation tasks in patients in remission (effect size = 0.87, SE = 0.20, $p < .001$), the effect was even more robust when studies of patients in symptomatic

states were included (effect size = 0.1.34, SE = 0.37, $p < .001$). This difference is due to the three studies of mania, which produced an especially high effect size (1.96, SE = 0.84). Again, the small number of studies providing cancellation test data calls for caution in placing emphasis on this specification. Rather, the conclusion most justified from the findings summarized in Figures 9–7 and 9–8 is that attentional disturbance is broadly manifested in bipolar disorder across multiple instantiations of this cognitive domain. Not only is the magnitude of deficit relatively uniform across tasks, but it is surprisingly uniform across the phases of bipolar illness, including remission. Furthermore, given the centrality of attentional processes to the integrity of many higher-order cognitive processes, the findings of attentional deficits in remission imply that broad or diffuse cognitive impairment should characterize many individuals with bipolar disorder in remission.

Learning and Memory

Disturbances in learning and memory may be divided into at least six categories of disturbance, each with its own pathoanatomical correlates (Kopelman, 2002; Stern and

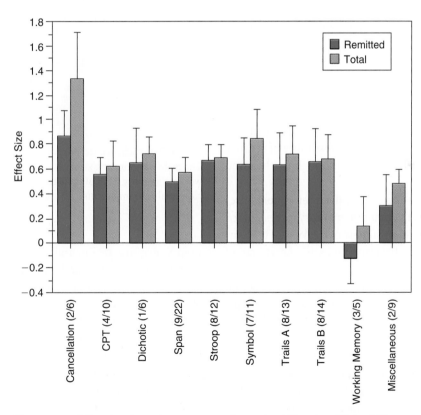

Figure 9–8. Effect sizes for various measures of attention. Effect sizes (Hedges' G) are shown for comparisons of bipolar patients in remission with healthy controls and for the total set of comparisons of bipolar patients across phases of illness with healthy controls. The numbers in parentheses indicate for each attentional measure the number of comparisons of remitted bipolar patients, followed by the total number of comparisons. CPT = Continuous Performance Test.

Sackeim, 2002; Squire et al., 2004): (1) Sensory memory deficits, involving modality-specific failures of preattentive information registration, at times associated with impairment of the reticular activating system or temporal or occipital neocortex; (2) Short-term or primary memory deficits, involving failures of acquisition and brief retention in a limited-capacity store, also associated with disturbance in prefrontal and temporal neocortex; (3) Abnormalities in acquisition and retention of long-term episodic memory, associated with prefrontal, medial temporal, and diencephalic impairment; (4) Disturbances of access to semantic memories, involving failures of storage or retrieval of language or knowledge that is not linked to temporal, sequential, or other contextual (episodic) information, and associated with disruption of posterior association cortex; (5) Deficits in the acquisition and retention of nondeclarative information, as reflected in procedural learning, priming, and classical conditioning (impairments in distinct neural systems are linked to the type of deficit, with striatal impairment tied to deficits in procedural learning and memory); and (6) Disturbances in the use of strategies mediating the acquisition and retention of information, with frontal cortex dysfunction linked to abnormalities in planning, encoding, and retrieval strategies.

When cast in this way, it is apparent that much of the landscape in learning and memory remains unexplored with respect to modulation by mood disorders. Although there has been some work suggesting subtle impairments of sensory and perceptual processes in major depression, including bipolar disorder, especially with respect to auditory processing (Yovell et al., 1995), investigation in this area has been extremely limited. The possibility of sensory memory deficits is largely untested, although not believed to be likely.

There is no evidence that mood disorder patients present with impairments of semantic memory, as tested, for example, by the information subtest of the WAIS-R. Memory for facts appears to be impervious to the effects of mood disorders.

In recent years, nondeclarative aspects of learning and memory, especially procedural learning, have been increasingly represented in neuropsychological batteries (Fig. 9–9). The preliminary evidence in bipolar disorder does not suggest impairment in procedural learning or memory, especially when remitted samples are examined (van Gorp et al., 1999; Altshuler et al., 2004). Preservation in this area may suggest that conscious awareness of mental contents is a property of the cognitive systems disrupted in mood disorders.

Of the six categories of memory disturbance, the focus of research in mood disorders has been on short-term memory, long-term episodic memory, and the strategies

Figure 9–9. Schematic representation of the structure of memory. The main component systems are declarative, nondeclarative, and working memory. Each of these components comprises more elemental subcomponents. (Adapted from Stern and Sackeim, 2002).

used to acquire, retain, and recall declarative information. This focus has concerned almost exclusively the learning and retention of new information. Recall of information about the past, whether pertaining to autobiographical or public events, has rarely been assessed outside of studies of retrograde amnesia after brain insult. To establish a baseline for assessing the extent of amnesia following ECT, the Columbia University group compared unmedicated patients in episodes of major depression (bipolar and unipolar) with healthy controls on the "productivity" of memory for the past. Whether assessed in terms of autobiographical or public events and in terms of remembrance of the event itself versus details about the event, the depressed samples showed small but statistically significant deficits at baseline (McElhiney et al., 1995). The fact that these patients reported slightly fewer memories about themselves or the world could reflect little more than an impairment of the acquisition of information during the affective episode, since what was not learned cannot be remembered. Alternatively, it is also true that what has not taken place cannot be remembered. Relative to the experience of healthy controls, reduced activities during episodes of illness may lead to a relative paucity of events about which to have recent memories. In any case, these data suggest that mood disorder patients are unlikely to have a fundamental or clinically significant deficit in the recall of past events or the details of past events. Furthermore, McElhiney and colleagues (1995) found no indication of a bias in depressed samples toward differential recall of negatively charged events.

Short-Term Memory

The distinction between short-term and long-term memory is arbitrary, and is usually taken as representing the methodological distinction between memory for new information tested after a very short delay (usually less than 10 seconds) and after longer delays (tens of seconds to years) (Wickelgren, 1973). This distinction is consequential because holding information in short-term memory is thought to be mediated by prefrontal working-memory processes, while the consolidation and retention of this information are determined by the integrity of the medial temporal lobe and other structures. The distinction is reflected in the common experience of not being able to reproduce a phone number when attention is directed away. In the absence of continual rehearsal, some information is lost, and in the case of bilateral hippocampal damage, retention of new declarative information may be limited to the period of rehearsal. Retention of new information over delays greater than tens of seconds depends on the integrity of consolidation and retrieval processes that are thought to involve initially the hippocampus and other structures.

By far the most common method for assessing short-term memory has involved forward and backward auditory digit span procedures, although word, letter, block, and shape span tasks are also available (Lezak, 1995; Spreen and Strauss, 1998). The early literature is not consistent in addressing the elemental question of whether auditory digit span performance is abnormal in mood disorders.[13] However, as seen in Figure 9–8, more recent studies comparing patients with bipolar disorder and healthy controls have revealed a consistent deficit in the performance of span tasks, auditory or visual, and pertaining to digits, words, or shapes. Across 22 studies and all phases of bipolar disorder, the pooled effect size for this comparison was moderate: 0.58 (SE = 0.12, $p < .001$). In the 9 studies contrasting patients in remission, the effect size was 0.50 (SE = 0.11, $p < .001$).

It is conceivable that the impairment of span performance is specific to procedures not involving auditory presentation of digits. Baddeley (1986) proposed that the phonological loop challenged by digit span tasks is distinct from a visuospatial scratch pad, with both being key aspects of working or short-term memory (see Fig. 9–9). However, no differences are seen in a comparison of effect sizes in studies using digit span and those using other span procedures. Thus the conclusion is justified that bipolar patients, whether in remission or not, have a deficit in short-term memory, as reflected in span performance. This deficit is interpreted as reflecting impaired attention.

Verbal learning tasks present another context for assessing the integrity of short-term memory. However, recall or recognition after a single presentation of a list relies on both short- and long-term processes. This point is supported by the serial position effect, in which recall is best for the early (primacy effect) and late (recency effect) items in a list and poorest for the middle ones (Bayley et al., 2000). The recency effect reflects the integrity of short-term memory given the minimal interval between presentation of the last items on the list and recall. The primacy effect reflects the contribution of transfer to long-term memory and the consolidation process. Since many of the reports on learning in bipolar illness concern cumulative performance in recalling a list during repeated testing over several trials, such procedures, while involving minimal retention intervals since the last presentation of a list, nonetheless rely heavily on long-term memory.

Figure 9–10 illustrates the effect sizes obtained in comparisons of patients with bipolar disorder and healthy controls on learning tasks, both verbal and nonverbal. Across all studies, the effect size is 0.91 (SE = 0.11, $p < .001$). In comparisons restricted to remitted patients, the effect size is 0.81 (SE = 0.15, $p < .001$).

Without question, bipolar disorder is associated with a marked deficit in the acquisition of new information. This deficit is seen in all phases of the illness, and its magnitude does not appear to be lessened among patients in remission. However, cross-sectional comparison should be used only to establish the existence of deficits in specific phases of the disorder. Whether the deficits are truly comparable in mania, depression, or remission requires within-subject longitudinal investigation. For example, the reduced noise of measurement involved in neuropsychological assessment of remitted as opposed to acutely ill patients can inflate effect sizes indicating deficits in remission. Furthermore, it is common to evaluate clinical samples in a medication-free state when acutely ill at baseline, but to evaluate patients in remission who are medicated. Such a confound could also intensify the deficits observed in remitted patients.

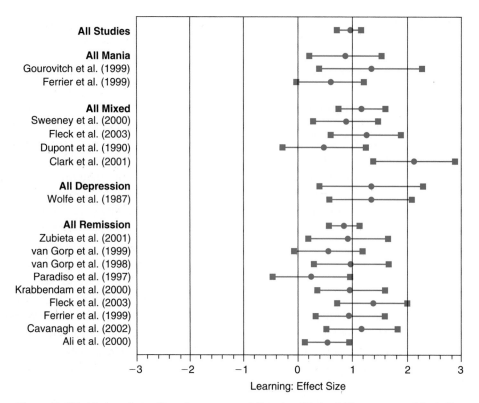

Figure 9–10. Meta-analysis of learning measures. Effect sizes (Hedges' G) are presented for individual study comparisons of a bipolar sample with healthy controls, as well as for samples of bipolar patients in remission, depression, mixed state, or mania and across all studies. Squares = confidence interval; circles = mean.

There has been very little investigation into bipolar-I vs. bipolar-II differences in attention, verbal learning and memory, and executive functioning. Recently, Torrent and colleagues (2006) compared 71 euthymic bipolar patients (38 bipolar-I, 33 bipolar-II) with 35 healthy controls on a battery of cognitive tasks. Both bipolar groups showed significant deficits in working memory, attention, and executive functions, with bipolar-II patients performing at a level between the bipolar-I patients and the healthy controls. Possibly confounding the results, bipolar-I patients were more likely to be taking lithium, carbamazepine, and/or antipsychotics; bipolar-II patients were more likely to be taking antidepressants. It is unclear which patients were taking more than one medication or what effects the medications may have had on performance.

Long-Term Memory

In recent years, it has been claimed that memory is the domain demonstrating the greatest impairment in mood disorders. Literature reviews and meta-analyses have indicated that relative to healthy controls, patients in an episode of major depression (bipolar or unipolar) manifest markedly inferior performance on tests involving the recall or recognition of information over a substantial delay or after

substantial training (Burt et al., 1995; Zakzanis et al., 1998). Further, it has been suggested that in recurrent unipolar disorder, lifetime duration of the depressive state is associated with both hippocampal atrophy and verbal memory deficits (Sheline et al., 1996, 1999). In line with this view, there is preliminary evidence that elderly bipolar patients show greater deterioration in memory processes than do elderly unipolar patients (Burt et al., 2000). Thus it would appear safe to conclude that long-term memory is especially impaired, that the impairment intensifies with disease progression, and that the impairment likely reflects dysfunction in medial temporal lobe structures.

The classic formulation of deficits in learning and memory in mood disorders presents a quite different view. Cronholm and Ottosson (1963) asserted that the depressed state is associated with a reduced capacity to acquire new information, but with no impact on the capacity to retain the information once it has been acquired. Thus in their work, patients were found to be notably deficient in learning verbal and nonverbal paired associates, but did not show proportionately greater loss of what was originally learned over a delay. In another influential study, Sternberg and Jarvik (1976) used similar tasks and also found that patients in an episode of major depression performed more poorly than controls on learning but not on retention, as measured by a "forgetting score," the mathematical difference in the number of items recalled before and after a delay. Following a pharmacological trial, the extent of clinical improvement covaried with improved learning (immediate memory).

One difficulty with this early work is that the integrity of long-term memory was assessed using a forgetting score that did not account for differences in the amount of material learned. Clearly the more one learns, the more material is available for forgetting. Steif and colleagues (1986a) raised conceptual and empirical issues in the assessment of these constructs. Despite more stringent controls, they also found that the primary deficit distinguishing unmedicated, depressed patients from controls was the learning or acquisition of new information, as opposed to the retention of what had been learned. Indeed, with retesting after a course of ECT, the authors were able to demonstrate a double dissociation. Whereas the state of depression involved impairment in learning and not retention, after ECT patients had a deficit in the retention of newly learned information, with no impact on learning. This type of effect is illustrated in Figure 9–11.

Figure 9–11. Dissociation in the effects of electroconvulsive therapy (ECT) on learning and retention of new information. Patients were randomly assigned to low- or high-dosage bilateral (BL) or right unilateral (RUL) ECT. Before and immediately after the course, they were administered a test of verbal list learning and retention using the selective reminding procedure (Buschke, 1973). Little change in immediate learning was seen when post-ECT values were compared with baseline values, with the exception of possible improvement in the low-dose RUL ECT group. In contrast, both low- and high-dose BL ECT resulted in clear-cut deficits in free recall of the list after a delay. The results illustrate the selective effect of ECT on the retention of newly learned information, which is thought to be due to a deficit in consolidation. (*Source*: Sackeim et al., 1993.)

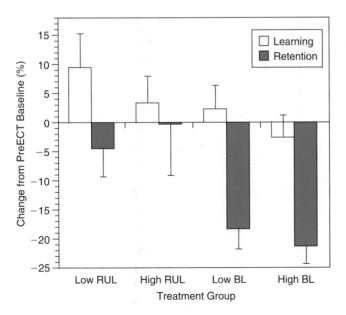

Why, then, are there conflicting views, with some recent work emphasizing long-term memory as a source of impairment and earlier work emphasizing impaired learning? It is quite likely that this apparent conflict stems from the fact that attentional deficits compromise the intake of information and disrupt learning. In turn, if little is learned, little can be remembered. For the most part, the work on impaired memory in depression has not taken into account the earlier stages of processing and their contributions. Thus in a concrete sense, being able to report only 3 of 15 items on a list after a 2-hour delay could reflect anterograde amnesia if 12 items were recalled during learning. On the other hand, if only 4 or 5 items were learned, impaired acquisition of the information would be the central deficit.

Figure 9–12 presents the effect sizes for comparisons of bipolar patients with healthy controls on a variety of memory measures. While the effect sizes for the subgroups and across all studies are substantial, they are virtually identical to the values obtained when assessing learning only (see Fig. 9–9). Again, it is hazardous to draw conclusions about within-subject effects using cross-sectional data. Nonetheless, the most parsimonious account of this literature is that impaired attention, which persists in remitted patients, is the major factor determining the adequacy of learning and memory.

Mediational Processes

Many processes determine whether a particular memory will be retrieved. Some of these processes relate to the infrastructure of memory, so that there is a contrast, for example, between deficits in the storage of information as assessed by recognition tasks and in the active retrieval of information as assessed by recall performance. Other processes, such as the organization imposed on newly presented information and the resultant depth of encoding, may determine whether information is learned and/or stored. Still other factors affect not so much whether new information will be retained, but how the choice is made whether to recall events from the past. For example, the issue is hotly debated as to whether being in the depressed or manic state biases retrieval toward memories that share the same affective valence. This form of mood-congruence effect addresses the question of whether depressed patients have preferential access to or are biased to retrieve negatively evaluated information.

Storage Versus Retrieval. Assuming that information is acquired, failure to recall can be due to a breakdown either in consolidation or storage or in retrieval. Because recognition of information is far less demanding of retrieval processes but is dependent on the adequacy of storage, an

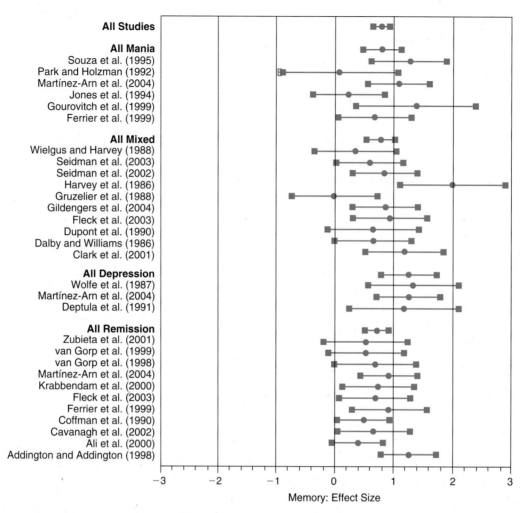

Figure 9–12. Meta-analysis of memory measures. Effect sizes (Hedges' G) are presented for individual study comparisons of a bipolar sample with healthy controls, as well as for samples of bipolar patients in remission, depression, mixed state, or mania and across all studies. Squares=confidence interval; circles=mean.

asymmetry whereby retrieval is impaired but recognition is intact could suggest a specific impairment in retrieval strategies—either the way information is organized for later retrieval or the way the search strategy is organized. However, recognition is intrinsically easier than retrieval, at least when the same information is tested, and claims of differential deficit are easily confounded with task differences in discriminating power and other psychometric properties.

A few authors have claimed that patients in an episode of major depression have a greater deficit in recall relative to recognition (Weingartner et al., 1977; Frith et al., 1983; Deptula et al., 1991). This work is problematic, however, because of the failure to compare recognition and recall paradigms directly or the lack of psychometric matching. These limitations were overcome by Calev and Erwin (1985), who used a matched-task paradigm. They found that depressed patients performed better on verbal recognition than on recall tasks, whereas healthy controls performed

similarly on both (demonstrating the adequacy of the matching). The recall disturbance was attributable to a reduced ability to organize the retrieval system. Thus, very limited data suggest the possibility of a particular deficit in retrieval processes in mood disorders. This deficit may be an example of a failure to engage in active, effortful processing.

Attention, Effort, and Levels of Processing. The deficits manifested by patients with mood disorders in tasks of learning and memory appear to be attributable largely to attentional dysfunction. Relevant here are well-established models from cognitive psychology that distinguish between automatic and effortful processing[14] and models of depth or levels of processing.[15] In the former models, attention is conceptualized as a limited-capacity resource. Automatic operations make minimal use of this resource and take place without intention or awareness. They do not interfere with ongoing cognitive operations and do not benefit from rehearsal. For example, remembering where one put one's keys is typically an instance of automatic or incidental learning. Typically, one does not consciously attempt to remember this information, and one is usually unaware of learning it. Skill or procedural learning and other nondeclarative forms of memory do not involve explicit, consciously mediated cognitive rehearsal. In contrast, effortful processes require the use of limited attentional capacities and interfere with other cognitive activities. The cognitive operations are initiated voluntarily and benefit from practice.

Similarly, a levels-of-processing approach emphasizes that the amount of attentional capacity allocated to the initial steps of information processing (e.g., encoding) influences the later retrievability of the information. The deeper the level of processing, the greater is the attentional allocation and the better the retrieval. For example, if one's task in listening to a set of words is to determine which words rhyme with a target (acoustic or shallow processing), later memory of the list will be poorer than if the task is to determine whether each word has the same meaning as a target (semantic or deep processing). The two models are convergent in that engaging in greater depth of processing is often an effortful, attention-demanding process.

The notion that individuals in episodes of major depression have a deficit in engaging spontaneously in effortful or deeper levels of processing has received substantial, although not unequivocal (Christensen et al., 1997), support. In a now-classic study, Weingartner and colleagues (1981) found that depressed patients did not differ from healthy controls in recalling words that had been acoustically (shallowly) processed, but were inferior in remembering semantically (deeply) processed words. The control group showed the typical advantage of better recall of the deeply processed words. In contrast, the patient group had equivalent scores on the two tasks, suggesting that despite the difference in task requirements, the patients' encoding on both tasks was shallow.

A second study reported by Weingartner and colleagues (1981) demonstrated that when deep encoding was provided externally on a verbal memory task, depressed patients performed similarly to healthy controls. Essentially, when given a list of random words, a depressed sample was shown to have markedly impaired recall. When presented a word list drawn from discrete semantic categories in which the word order was clustered, however, patients were not distinguishable in recall from healthy controls. Both the extent of categorization of words and the overt clustering within categories determined the magnitude of the difference in recall between patients and controls.

The implication of this work is that depressed patients, when exposed to new material, are less likely than healthy

controls to apply preexisting knowledge and impose the organization that facilitates learning and memory. In this respect, the locus of abnormality is at the encoding stage and results in diminished learning. Fundamentally, the depth of encoding and the automatic versus effortful distinctions converge. Imposing organization is an effortful process, and in most circumstances, the automatic versus effortful distinction maps to shallow versus deep processing. This deficit pertains to the set of mediational processes termed by Moscovitch (1994) "working with memory." These processes involve the selection and execution of strategies used to enhance information processing and are thought to be heavily represented in prefrontal cortex. Further, effortful or deeper processing requires the allocation of attentional resources. Thus it is conceivable that the fundamental abnormality resides in an inflexibility or limited capacity of attentional mechanisms rather than difficulties with selecting or applying appropriate strategies for encoding or retrieval. Put another way, it would appear that the depressed state is characterized by a cognitive impairment likely to be most manifest on tasks that require complex processing, effortful processing, and/or independent structuring of information relative to preexisting knowledge.

This remains an active area of investigation, with repeated demonstrations that depressed patients are more likely than healthy controls to engage in shallow and/or noneffortful processing.[16] However, almost all of this work has focused on demonstrating the phenomenon and establishing its boundaries. There is little clarity regarding the neurobiological basis of this abnormality or its implications for therapeutics. Roy-Byrne and colleagues (1986) suggested that the deficit in effortful processing is dopaminergically mediated, but this hypothesis has yet to receive substantial investigation.

One thread in this literature ties the lack of effortful processing to an entirely different domain of behavioral limitation. Cohen and colleagues (1982) found that severity of depressive symptomatology correlated negatively with grip strength, as assessed with a hand dynamometer. Both symptom scores and grip strength correlated with performance on a verbal memory test, with less effort on the motor task being associated with poorer memory scores. The results of this work suggest that in major depression, there is a parallel between the diminished effort in physical activity and the diminished mental effort that results in inattention and lack of structuring of incoming information. Certainly, it would be noteworthy were this the case. While the effort expended in voluntary activity has a voluntary quality, as in how strongly one grips a dynamometer, this is not the conception regarding the mental effort leading to more extensive encoding. The failure to impose organization and process at deeper levels should be viewed as unconscious or automatic. Furthermore, the lack-of-effort analogy does not accord with what may be the most common reason for shallow processing in mood disorders. Under conditions of marked agitation or psychic pain, patients will often indicate that it is a struggle to get through the next 5 minutes, let alone attend to a task. With internal ruminations and marked distress, even reading a newspaper headline can be difficult. Thus it is probable that in some circumstances, the lack of effortful processing is due to the fact that the effort is being expended elsewhere.

It might be thought that this type of deficit in mediational processes should be fully state dependent. Otherwise, we would have to posit that patients with mood disorders engage in "shallow" processing even when in remission. Further, were this defect purely state dependent, it would have a rather limited role in accounting for the learning and memory deficits in patients with mood disorders. As described earlier, there is substantial evidence that attentional, learning, and memory deficits continue largely unabated during remission. Longitudinal investigation in this area has been limited, however. Hammar and colleagues (2003b) found that unipolar patients in a state of major depression were impaired in an effortful but not automatic visual search task. The deficit persisted for at least 6 months despite substantial clinical improvement. Further work of this type is needed.

Mood Congruence.   *Mood congruence* refers to the notion that the efficiency of mnemonic processing is biased by the congruence between the current affective state and the affective tone of the material being remembered. In general, it is believed that dysphoric or negative life events are recalled more easily when individuals are in a depressed state than when they are in a euthymic or manic state (Blaney, 1986).

This phenomenon has been examined mainly in studies using laboratory manipulations, such as rigged experiences of success and failure in completing laboratory tasks. These studies have yielded some evidence that depressed patients can be biased in recalling negative events or can exercise a mnemonic selectivity that emphasizes neutrality over positivity.[17] This type of mediational process, if of general consequence, would affect the content of remembrances, with the implication that this bias toward greater negativity in content may contribute to the monolithic experience of depression, and perhaps also to its maintenance. However, subtle demonstrations of bias in laboratory or real-world settings do not mean that this phenomenon is of general consequence. In intensive interviews regarding autobiographical events, severely depressed patients differ little from healthy controls in the richness of their reports of positive or negative events in their recent and remote past (McElhiney et al., 1995).

Summary

Deficits in learning and memory characterize unipolar depression and bipolar disorder through all its phases. The effect sizes for these deficits are the largest among neuropsychological domains. While it has been common in recent years to assert that episodes of major depression are associated with a memory deficit, there is little evidence that the deficits seen in learning and/or memory processes extend beyond attentional disturbance. This attentional disturbance may be structural in the sense of dysfunction in a limited-capacity store, or perhaps more likely, a disturbance in the allocation of attentional resources. The substantial literature on bipolar patients in remission indicates that the deficits in learning and memory persist during euthymia. There are compelling findings that mood disorder patients in episodes of major depression are more likely to engage in shallow processing and to fail to impose the organization on incoming information that assists in acquisition and retention. This "cognitive laziness" results from a failure of executive function—in this case, the utilization of strategies that facilitate learning and memory. Thus it becomes especially germane to inquire whether there is a more general impairment of executive functions.

Executive Functions

The concept of executive functions became a driving force in much thought about the core deficits in psychopathology, especially schizophrenia and bipolar disorder, starting in the 1980s. Fundamentally, disruption of these functions is deemed responsible for the lack of self-regulation on a variety of dimensions in patients with these disorders. Executive functions perform the brain's housekeeping, strategizing, and oversight roles, and come closest in principle to the neuropsychological concept of a neural homunculus in charge of neural resource allocation and other administrative functions or, perhaps, the concept of will.

The vagueness of definitions and descriptions of executive functions is to be expected given the vast and complex aspects of psychic functioning likely devoted to strategic, integrative, planning, inductive, and deductive activities. Indeed, at one level the type of executive functions involved in optimizing learning strategies by imposing conceptual organization (chunking) on incoming information automatically and without awareness must be quite distinct from the processes involved in making career choices, anticipating danger while driving, or inhibiting a prepotent response. Thus executive functions address our capacity to reason, to anticipate, to shift conceptual or perceptual sets, to solve problems, and so on.

Despite this richness of possibilities, a very limited range of executive functions has been studied in bipolar disorder. Figure 9–13 presents the results of our meta-analysis of comparisons involving executive functions other than reasoning. Tests of reasoning or concept formation were examined separately, partly because they are so strongly dependent on language and verbal abilities; these findings are presented in Figure 9–14. The instruments used most commonly to test the integrity of executive functions are the Wisconsin Card Sort Test (WCST) and the Category Test of the Halstead-Reitan battery. Both involve complex procedures in which individuals derive rules or abstractions from experience. The WCST also assesses the capacity to shift sets upon recognizing that the rules have changed. It is considered a test of executive functions in part because it requires strategic planning,

organized searching, use of feedback to shift conceptual set, goal-oriented behavior, and the capacity to inhibit impulsive responding (Spreen and Strauss, 1998). Other instruments used to test executive functions include the Tower of London, which places heavy emphasis on planning (Shallice, 1982) and involves the rearrangement of balls in a vertical column to match a prespecified order using a minimum of moves, attentional set-shifting tasks, and decision-making tasks.

As seen in Figure 9–13, substantial deficits in executive functions were observed in all phases of bipolar disorder. Across the 25 studies contributing data, the overall effect size was 0.79 (SE = 0.13, $p < .001$). In the 14 studies that examined remitted bipolar patients, the effect size was 0.75 (SE = 0.18, $p < .001$), hardly suggestive of a state-dependent effect. Two recent studies also have found pervasive deficits in executive

Figure 9–13. Meta-analysis of executive function measures. Effect sizes (Hedges' G) are presented for individual study comparisons of a bipolar sample with healthy controls, as well as for samples of bipolar patients in remission, depression, mixed state, or mania and across all studies. Squares = confidence interval; circles = mean.

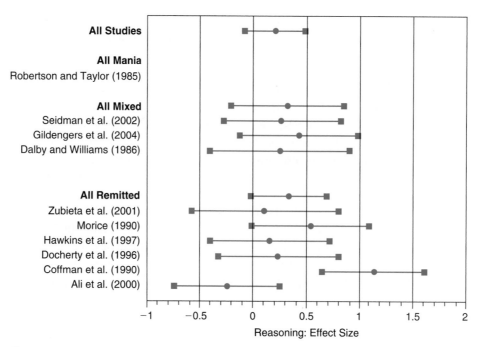

Figure 9–14. Meta-analysis of reasoning measures. Effect sizes (Hedges' G) are presented for individual study comparisons of a bipolar sample with healthy controls, as well as for samples of bipolar patients in remission, depression, mixed state, or mania and across all studies. Squares = confidence interval; circles = mean.

functioning in bipolar patients (Nehra et al., 2006; Robinson et al., 2006).

As in unipolar disorder, then, there is substantial evidence that periods of acute illness in bipolar disorder are associated with diminished executive functions, especially with respect to concept formation and set shifting. Recent studies have demonstrated this as well (Frangore et al., 2005; Goswami et al., 2006), including one that looked at executive functioning in patients with pediatric bipolar disorder (Pavuluri et al., 2006). Imaging studies have shown that, in healthy samples, the procedures examined in this domain result in activation of the dorsolateral prefrontal cortex (DLPFC). Abnormalities in DLPFC function in mood disorders have been reported from the earliest brain imaging studies of cerebral blood flow (CBF) or cerebral metabolic rate (CMR$_{glu}$), and more than 20 imaging studies have reported inverse relationships between depression severity and DLPFC, CBF, or CMR$_{glu}$.[18] It is noteworthy that these studies did not include significant sampling of ventral or orbital prefrontal cortex functions, notably inhibition of prepotent responses, as in "go–no go" tasks. In terms of what was studied, there is strong evidence for persistent impairment of executive functions despite remission. Indeed, it is noteworthy that the effect size for remitted patients is equivalent to that for patients in acute affective episodes.

However, inspection of Figure 9–14 suggests that the deficit in executive functions may not be uniform across various component processes. Values for one study (Robertson and Taylor, 1985) were omitted from the figure because they reflected an extreme outlier, in this case manic patients having clearly superior performance on a reasoning task compared with healthy participants. Inclusion of these values would further reduce the evidence for a deficit in reasoning. As it stands, the overall effect size is small, 0.21 (SE = 0.14, p = .15), and for studies of remitted patients is 0.33 (SE = 0.18, p = .07). A deficit in reasoning relative to controls was not significant within any of the four subgroups.

The tests that contributed to our meta-analysis on reasoning included the similarities and arithmetic subtests of the WAIS-R and tests of abstraction and concept attainment. Commonly, results of tests of reasoning correlate substantially with verbal abilities. The relative preservation of reasoning skills against a backdrop of marked deficits in other executive functions may reflect a pattern in which cognitive operations that are heavily dependent on language are among the least affected of the higher cognitive functions.

Verbal and Visuospatial Skills

The final cognitive domains subjected to this meta-analysis were verbal and visuospatial skills. Work in the verbal domain has been dominated by tasks assessing controlled oral word association (COWA). Such tests assess the spontaneous production of words beginning with a given letter, usually F, A, or S (FAS test), within a stipulated period of time. Alternatively, the tests may assess production of words as instances of a concept, such as animal naming. Verbal fluency, especially letter fluency, has often been taken as another type of executive function. Indeed, there is evidence that COWA is one of the last measures of prefrontal function to mature, with developmental improvement extending beyond age 12, whereas adult levels are achieved considerably earlier for many other measures (Lewis, 1983). There is some evidence from both imaging and lesion studies that temporal lobe regions may make more of a contribution to category than to letter fluency. However, this distinction and the stronger claim that letter fluency is subserved largely by prefrontal regions are supported only partially by lesion analysis and imaging

activation effects, with exceptional findings suggesting more widely distributed representations.[19]

The copy portion of the Complex Figure Test (Rey, 1941) is the task used most commonly to represent visuospatial functions. This task involves copying a detailed and complex figure, with accuracy of reproduction being scored for 18 portions of the figure. The copying portion of the procedure is followed by delayed reproduction purely from memory. To focus on visuospatial constructional ability, as opposed to visual memory, we included only copy procedures in this domain. Other tests commonly used to sample visuospatial functions are the WAIS-R block design subtest and tests of perceptual organization, such as line orientation, gestalt completion, and embedded figures.

Figures 9–15 and 9–16 present results of our meta-analysis for the verbal and visuospatial domains, respectively. The deficits seen in verbal skills are moderate at best

Figure 9–15. Meta-analysis of verbal skill measures. Effect sizes (Hedges' G) are presented for individual study comparisons of a bipolar sample with healthy controls, as well as for samples of bipolar patients in remission, depression, mixed state, or mania and across all studies. Squares = confidence interval; circles = mean.

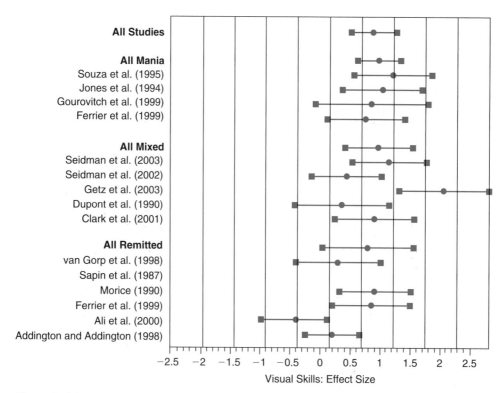

Figure 9–16. Meta-analysis of visual skill measures. Effect sizes (Hedges' G) are presented for individual study comparisons of a bipolar sample with healthy controls, as well as for samples of bipolar patients in remission, depression, mixed state, or mania and across all studies. Squares = confidence interval; circles = mean.

(see Fig. 9–15). The effect size (Hedges' G) for the comparison of bipolar and healthy control groups across all studies ($n = 26$) is 0.35 (SE = 0.09, $p < .001$). However, the effect is not significant across 12 studies of remitted bipolar samples (effect size = 0.22, SE = 0.12, $p = .064$) or 5 studies in mania (effect size = 0.495, SE = 0.31, $p = .11$). Relative to the pattern of widespread impairment across symptomatic and remitted states, verbal skills appear to have been preserved. In the few cases in which bipolar samples had inferior verbal fluency performance relative to healthy controls, the patient groups tended to make more incorrect responses (e.g., repeating the same word) and did not differ in number of responses (Wolfe et al., 1987; Coffman et al., 1990).

A different level of deficit is manifest in Figure 9–16, which summarizes our meta-analysis of visuospatial performance measures. One study (Sapin et al., 1987) was excluded because of an outlying value that only accentuated the deficit in remitted patients. Across all studies, the effect size is 0.65 (SE = 0.18, $p < .001$), and in remitted bipolar patients it is 0.57 (0.28, $p < .01$).

Comparisons across Domains: The Topography of Cognitive Deficit in Bipolar Disorder

Figure 9–17 combines the values on effect size reported for the various cognitive domains and presents the cognitive

deficit profiles for the comparisons of depressed, mixed-state manic, and remitted samples with healthy controls, as well as the comparisons across all phases of illness. The profile is relatively invariant across the phases of illness. Three central points can be made.

First, the same pattern of strengths and weaknesses is seen in remission and during episodes of affective disturbance. This invariance suggests that the core disturbance is state independent. Second, it is often claimed that the magnitude of deficit is generally greatest during mania, still marked during major depression, and least evident in remission. The deficit noted by investigators as residual during remission varied considerably among the studies included in our meta-analysis. Indeed, limited power, differences in the reliability of measurement, and other factors make it likely that different tasks would achieve statistical significance in separating remitted patients from controls. By combining these findings in a meta-analysis, it became evident that the remitted samples generally had the same level of deficit as the acutely ill groups in the areas most disturbed, and perhaps somewhat less marked deficits in the areas most disturbed in the acutely ill groups (e.g., learning and memory). The larger point is that the cognitive deficits observed in remitted patients were not a pale shadow of the deficits seen during affective disturbance, but were substantial, reliable, and of the same distribution as those seen during acutely ill states.

The third point is that against a background of generalized deficit, verbal processes as reflected in VIQ, verbal skills (i.e., verbal fluency), and reasoning are relatively preserved. This novel observation recasts the initial question about the meaning of the VIQ–PIQ discrepancy in bipolar disorder. The deficit in PIQ may not be of special note, and it may not signal, per se, a right-hemisphere abnormality. Rather, the effect sizes for PIQ and visuospatial skills are in the range of those for motor disturbance, attentional deficits, and other domains. What may be consequential is that verbal processes are preserved and, across the phases of illness, show less deterioration than virtually all other higher cognitive processes.

Why might this be, or better yet, what can this tell us about the neurobiology of bipolar illness? First, the fact that deficits in attention and concentration are reliably observed across the phases of bipolar illness means that cognitive impairment must be generalized. This point is underscored by the findings suggesting consistent impairment of executive functions. Attention and concentration may be seen as the fuel of higher cognitive processes, determining the capacity and efficiency limitations on processing. Executive functions determine resource allocation and thus also broadly shape the integrity of cognitive processing. Indeed, with respect to learning, memory, and visuospatial skills, there is little evidence that deficits reflect more than an attentional disturbance. Therefore, rather than positing multiple specific deficits in bipolar disorder, one could hypothesize that a persistent noradrenergic or dopaminergic disturbance gives rise to attentional impairment that in turn produces the widespread, more generalized pattern (Swanson et al., 1998; Cools and Robbins, 2004).

But why do we see the preservation of verbal processes? Surely attentional mechanisms also drive performance in this area. There are several possibilities. First, some of the areas of preservation concern aspects of cognition that are relatively protected against the effects of brain injury. The WAIS-R vocabulary and information subtests are often considered "hold" scores, indices more likely to reflect premorbid abilities than are tests more sensitive to the effects

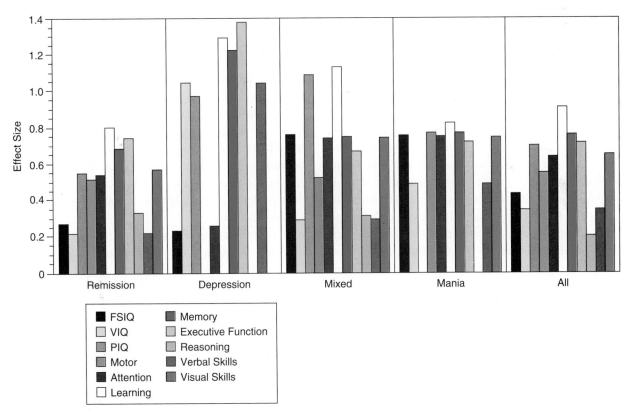

Figure 9–17. Profile of neuropsychological impairment in bipolar disorder. Effect sizes are shown for comparisons of a bipolar group (in remission or in a phase of depression, mixed state, or mania) with healthy controls for 11 cognitive domains. All bipolar subgroups, including remission, show deficits relative to controls. These impairments are most accentuated for the learning, memory, and executive function domains and are pronounced for all domains except those heavily involving verbal skills (verbal IQ, reasoning, and verbal skills). The preservation of verbal skills against a background of generalized impairment may be the salient dissociation. FSIQ = full-scale IQ; PIQ = performance IQ; VIQ = verbal IQ.

of brain damage (Lezak, 1995). These subtests assess semantic memory, or knowledge of facts, which has not been found to be impaired in bipolar disorder. Specifically, these subtests, by posing specific questions, may place few demands on attention or any form of new learning. This view posits, therefore, that the relative preservation of verbal skills is due to their escaping the deleterious and otherwise generalized impact of the core cognitive disturbance, presumably in the area of attention. However, the findings regarding verbal fluency and reasoning may belie this view since it is difficult to argue that attentional processes do not contribute to their performance.

A second alternative is to view this preservation of verbal processes as indicating a disassociation in the cognitive neural systems dysregulated in bipolar disorder. At the grossest level, this view would suggest preservation of left-hemisphere subsystems involved in verbal processing. How this could come about and the neurochemical and/or neurodevelopmental processes responsible for such a dissociation are a matter of speculation.

Finally, this asymmetry may be an endophenotype of bipolar disorder. We should not assume that the topography of cognitive function is a flat playing field in this patient population. As discussed at the outset, there is good reason to suspect that intellectual endowment is distributed differently in the families of bipolar probands than in the general population. Indeed, one of the earliest studies of children at risk found that the VIQ–PIQ discrepancy was robust before the onset of the first affective episode and was most common in children with prodromal symptoms (Decina et al., 1983; Sackeim and Decina, 1983). Thus the genetic transmission of bipolar disorder may confer a relative advantage for verbal processes. The insult that results in manifestation of the disorder may have a rather generalized effect, leading to impairments in multiple domains. This decrease in function is shared relatively equally, and verbal functions appear to be preserved only because their baseline was elevated. Research on the neuropsychological profiles of first-degree relatives of bipolar probands (Keri et al., 2001a) and of monozygotic twins discordant for bipolar disorder (Gourovitch et al., 1999) is in its infancy, but has indicated that impairments are evident in tests of learning and memory but not in verbal skills.

Other Neuropsychological Domains

A number of other cognitive functions have been studied in bipolar disorder, but with insufficient frequency to be included in our meta-analysis. These functions include auditory perception, somatosensory function, pain perception, impulsivity, processing of facial affective displays, and the extent of thought disorder. The paucity of research in these domains indicates a parochialism in the mapping of cognitive functions in this disorder, with a strong focus on measures of attention, executive functions, and learning and memory. For example, rates of suicide are elevated in bipolar disorder, and diathesis–stress models of suicide often assume that a predisposition for impulsive behavior provides the "diathesis" and acute depressive or manic symptoms the "stress" that results in the act[20] (see Chapter 8). However, there are virtually no longitudinal data on measures of impulsivity or aggression in bipolar disorder, and at the clinical level, impulsivity would not be expected to be invariant, but to be accentuated during manic or mixed states. Further, characterization of the essential deficit as being in the domain of impulsivity or aggressivity may be too narrow.

An especially comprehensive neuropsychological study recently compared the profiles of medication-free depressed patients with a history of a high-lethality suicide attempt, a low-lethality suicide attempt, and no history of suicide attempt, and healthy controls. The cognitive domains sampled included general intellectual functioning, motor functioning, attention, memory, and executive functioning. A discriminant analysis indicated that different dimensions distinguished the total depressed sample from the healthy controls and distinguished the high-lethality attempters from the other patient groups. Impairment in attention and memory distinguished the patients from the controls, again highlighting that a basic attentional disturbance may be a key factor in determining the cognitive sequelae of mood disorders, both unipolar and bipolar. Impaired executive function distinguished high-lethality attempters, with the executive function measures not being restricted to indices of impulsivity. The results of this work raise the possibility that a more broad-based deficit in executive function, perhaps related to self-monitoring functions, is disturbed in individuals with a history of high-lethality suicide attempts.

Recent years have seen a movement away from the study of "cold" cognition to the study of "hot" cognition in bipolar disorder.[21] This distinction is thought to make neuropsychological investigation more ecologically valid and more likely to address core deficits in bipolar disorder. The movement to assess hot cognition is instantiated in studies in which the information being processed, such as facial emotional expression or the meaning of affectively laden words, has affective significance. Thus in both bipolar disorder and schizophrenia, there has been a significant increase in reports on facial emotion discrimination and other aspects of the processing of emotionally laden information. A particular emphasis in this work has been the extent to which such processing is biased by the affective state of patients (depressed versus manic) (Murphy et al., 1999).

Work in this area is insufficiently developed to yield conclusions. A cautionary note is in order, however, especially in light of the enthusiastic recommendations being made to incorporate affective processing tasks in studies of mood disorders. The processes involved in the regulation of mood appear to be wholly independent of the processes that subserve the "reception" of emotion (i.e., the processing of emotionally laden information). As noted earlier, brain injury can result in highly specific deficits in aspects of emotional processing and have no impact on the regulation of mood or emotional expression. Alternatively, there can be marked disturbance in mood without apparent impact on emotional processing. It is unclear to what extent determining that the intonation of a voice is sad differs fundamentally from determining that the speaker is male, that the voice is raspy, and so on. It is clear that the presentation of such stimuli rarely has an impact on affective state. Determining that a voice is sad does not require that one feel sad, and thus these procedures cannot be said to be indirect mood manipulations.

Often the outcome of such investigation is an indication of biased processing on the part of patient subgroups. Using an affective go–no go task, Murphy and colleagues (1999) alternated happy and sad words in blocks as either targets requiring response or distracters requiring inhibition of response. Compared with healthy controls, manic patients were slower to respond to sad but not to happy targets, whereas depressed patients were slower when responding to happy but not to sad targets. Manic patients also had an excess of response inhibition errors (responding to a distracter). Thus, the results of this study suggest a difference between depressed and manic patients in attentional bias as a function of affective valence. This effect was not seen in remitted patients in a subsequent study (Rubinsztein et al., 2000). Note that this effect can be distinguished from mood congruence effects. In the study by Murphy and colleagues (1999), patients were impeded in processing targets that did not correspond to their affective state. Mood congruence phenomena reflect privileged access to evaluations, memories, and so on that are congruent in emotional content with the current mood state.

Nonetheless, there is evidence that current affective state impacts the processing of ongoing affectively charged information. More broadly, mood congruence effects also pertain to the differential retrieval of memories, the attributions made for ongoing positive and negative events, and other aspects of complex cognitive function. For example, the depressed state is frequently characterized by a marked cognitive bias, referred to as depressive realism. When healthy controls, or for that matter patients with schizophrenia, are confronted with success, the tendency is to assume that they caused this outcome, they should be praised, and the outcome was very good. In contrast, when confronted with failure, healthy controls will often state that the outcome was uncontrollable, they should not be blamed, and it was not so bad anyway. While patients with major depression might be expected to show a reverse bias, to overaccentuate the negative, their attributions tend to be much more even-handed than those of controls, and thus by most accounts, more realistic (Sackeim and Wegner, 1986). Therefore, it is fair to say that the states of depression and euphoria are characterized by a gross alteration in cognitive schema, reflecting diminished or absent self-serving biases in the depressed state (Taylor and Brown, 1988, 1994; Colvin and Block, 1994). If the objective of recent work on hot cognition in mood disorders is to address state-related biases in information processing, it is far from clear that studies of facial emotional identification provide the optimal models.

FACTORS AFFECTING COGNITIVE FUNCTION

Treatment

In many of the studies included in our meta-analysis, bipolar patients were tested in an unmedicated state when depressed or manic, but were medicated when studied in the remitted state. This convention arises from the fact that a period of medication withdrawal in acutely ill patients is considered acceptable before starting a new treatment. Indeed, in some cases such withdrawal is of clinical value. On the other hand, the risks of relapse are so high that withdrawal of treatment in recently remitted patients is unacceptable. Consequently, this pattern introduces a potentially serious confound in much of the neuropsychological and neurobiological investigation of state-independent phenomena in bipolar disorder. Specifically, could the widespread neuropsychological impairment seen in remitted patients be a result of an adverse and generalized cognitive effect of continuation and maintenance treatment? Could lithium, the anticonvulsant medications, or the antidepressants be responsible for this cognitive profile? To the extent that patients in some studies are abruptly withdrawn from psychotropics, what impact does drug withdrawal have on cognitive function?

For example, Martinez-Arán and colleagues (2004a) conducted a comprehensive study of cognitive impairment in euthymic bipolar patients, contrasting 40 such patients with 30 healthy controls and accounting for the effects of subsyndromal symptomatology. After controlling for age, premorbid IQ, and subsyndromal symptomatology, the patient sample still manifested deficits on several measures of memory and executive functions. The extent of verbal memory impairment was related to a longer duration of illness, a higher number of manic episodes, and prior psychotic symptoms. However, 38 of the 40 patients were receiving psychotropic medications at the time of testing: 33 of the 40 were being treated with lithium carbonate, 12 with carbamazepine, and 7 with valproate; 11 patients were receiving more than one mood stabilizer; 23 were also being treated with antipsychotic medications (15 of which were on atypical antipsychotics), 17 were being given benzodiazepines, and 8 were receiving antidepressants. The complexity of these medication regimens is characteristic of the long-term treatment of bipolar disorder and illustrates the difficulty of ruling out adverse medication effects or interactions in naturalistic studies.

The most rigorous way of addressing this question is to conduct a randomized, placebo-controlled trial. Given the possibilities of state-related changes in cognition, fluctuating clinical symptomatology, effects of ancillary medications (e.g., benzodiazepines), practice and order effects, and other factors, adverse cognitive effects of primary mood-stabilizing or adjunctive sedative medications could easily be falsely accentuated or underestimated. Especially in clinical populations, however, the feasibility and ethics of such a study are questionable.

The best alternative in such a circumstance is longitudinal investigation using an ABA design, with patients being tested while on (A) and off (B) medication. Perhaps the most critical study in this area used such a design. Shaw and colleagues (1987) studied 28 outpatients with mood disorders maintained on lithium prophylaxis. Of these 28, 22 completed the protocol, 6 being dropped because of clinical deterioration; a criterion for participation was maintaining euthymia throughout. On average, patients had been maintained on lithium for 9.4 years (SD = 5.8 years), with an average level of 0.80 mEq/L (SD = 0.23 MEq/L). Patients were tested at the same time each week at each of five weekly sessions. The first session took place while patients continued to receive lithium, the second and third while they received substituted placebo, and the fourth and fifth after they had returned to lithium. Motor speed was assessed using the finger-tapping procedure, and the Buschke Selective Reminding Test was used to evaluate effects on learning and memory.

Over the 5 weeks of this study, depression and mania symptom scores were flat and in the euthymic range. Lithium levels went from a mean of 0.83 mEq/L at the first session to 0.05, 0.04, 0.71, and 0.74 at sessions 2 through 5, respectively. Figure 9–18 presents the results for the finger-tapping task and Figure 9–19 those for the memory test. Motor speed was quantified as the mean number of taps per five 10 s trials with both the dominant and nondominant hand. There was a significant difference in tapping performance across the 5 weeks, with motor speed improving after

Figure 9–18. Tapping rate with lithium discontinuation and reinstatement. Twenty-two patients were retested for tapping speed weekly for 5 weeks. Lithium was discontinued after the first week and reinstated by the fourth week. Tapping speed improved in weeks 2 and 3 off lithium and slowed with lithium reinstatement. (*Source*: Shaw et al., 1987.)

discontinuation of lithium and deteriorating with its reintroduction. The magnitude of this effect, while consistent, was small. For example, the deterioration between weeks 3 and 5 (*p* < .02) averaged a 4.2 percent reduction in tapping rate.

The study by Shaw and colleagues (1987) constituted the first report of reversible lithium-induced motor speed impairment. Several previous studies of patients and healthy participants had suggested that lithium had a negative effect on performance of the WAIS-R digit symbol test and possibly on perceptual-motor tasks (Demers and Heninger, 1971; Judd, 1979; Squire et al., 1980). The digit symbol subtest is usually regarded as an attentional measure. Given its timed nature, however, motoric slowing would have a negative impact. Thus the findings of the Shaw et al. (1987) study raise the possibility that lithium resulted in a subtle slowing of basic motor movement, which could affect any timed procedure.

The findings obtained with the Buschke Selective Reminding Test are illustrated in Figure 9–19. This test produces a variety of indices of the adequacy of short- and long-term memory, and a representative index of each is plotted in the figure. Short-term recall is heavily influenced by attention and reflects the recall of items just recently presented, as in the reminding procedure. Long-term recall concerns the number of words recalled at some interval since original presentation or reminding. No impact of

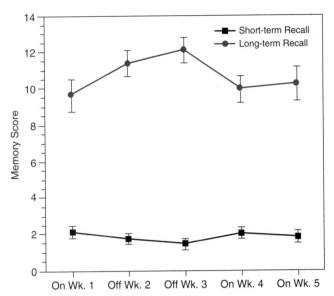

Figure 9–19. Short- and long-term recall on a verbal learning and memory test with lithium discontinuation and reinstatement. Lithium was discontinued after the first week and reinstated by the fourth week. Short-term or immediate memory was unaffected by lithium status. Long-term recall was reduced when patients were given lithium. (*Source*: Shaw et al., 1987. Reprinted with permission.)

lithium withdrawal or reintroduction on the short-term memory measures was observed. Instead, substantial improvement in long-term memory measures occurred when lithium was removed, and deterioration when it was reintroduced. At face value, these data suggest that lithium had little impact on the attentive processes involved in the immediate recall of new information, but produced a significant compromise (about 20 percent) in the amount of information that could be recalled with a delay since presentation. In other words, these data suggest that lithium produced a mild anterograde amnesia.

In fact, although negative findings have been reported regarding lithium's effects on memory (Squire et al., 1980), a substantial literature is consistent with these effects. Reus and colleagues (1979) compared 17 bipolar manic patients receiving lithium with 7 other patients who had discontinued lithium for at least 3 weeks (5 because of pregnancy). Using procedures similar to those of Shaw and colleagues (1987), they found that the lithium group had a deficit in long-term recall. Specifically, this deficit pertained to the capacity to recall consistently material for which earlier learning had been established. This finding supports the possibility that lithium has negligible effects on attention and the intake or encoding of new information, but interferes with the retrieval of what has been learned. Were this the case, it would represent a neurocognitive profile distinct from that which appears to characterize bipolar patients in

remission, in whom learning and memory appear to be equally disrupted (see Fig. 9–17). Other research has yielded findings that support this framework. Two studies of healthy participants found that retrieval of information after a long delay (7 to 14 days) was impaired by lithium (Karniol et al., 1978; Kropf and Muller-Oerlinghausen, 1979). And in a study of 18 bipolar patients, Christodoulou and colleagues (1981) found no effect of a 16-day placebo period on short-term memory measures.

In this light, the findings of naturalistic studies of cognitive impairment in bipolar disorder may take on different meaning. Lund and colleagues (1982) found that chronic bipolar patients stabilized on lithium performed in the low-average range on tests of attention and memory, below expectations given their educational achievement. This pattern in remitted patients could reflect both a trait-level deficit in attentional and executive functions and a specific deleterious effect of lithium on long-term retrieval. Kessing (1998) found that both the number of affective episodes and treatment with lithium were associated with inferior performance on two of five tests of diffuse cognitive function. In this case, exposure to lithium and the effects of chronicity could not be separated. Finally, Engelsmann and colleagues (1988) conducted a longitudinal cognitive investigation of bipolar patients treated with lithium. They found little evidence of a cumulative deleterious effect, as there was significant decline over a 6-year follow-up period in only 1 of 10 memory subtests. However, evidence from discontinuation and reinstatement studies indicates that adverse effects of lithium on cognition are expressed immediately, and reverse at least partially with discontinuation. The findings of Engelsmann and colleagues (1988) are critical in suggesting that any short-term negative impact is not cumulative.[22]

Cognitive impairment is a common complaint of patients treated for bipolar disorder, and undoubtedly contributes considerably to nonadherence to treatment regimens (see Chapter 21). It has been common for clinicians to dismiss such complaints of clouded thinking, slowed processing, or memory impairment as reflecting the ravages of the illness, somatization and negativism on the part of the patient, and the like. Teasing out which if any cognitive effects reflect disease processes and which indicate adverse pharmacological effects is next to impossible for any individual patient. Given the neurotoxicity of lithium at high doses, it should not be unexpected if some individuals show cognitive sensitivity and experience a range of cognitive impairments while receiving the drug. In some cases, these effects can be addressed through dosage reduction. However, especially for patients in whom lithium is clearly more effective than alternative maintenance agents, there may be no choice but to accept these side effects as part of the price of maintaining remission. In this respect, the absence of evidence that lithium per se has a cumulative deleterious influence and the clear evidence of reversal of deficits once the drug is discontinued should be reassuring. So, too, should the accumulating body of evidence indicating that lithium exerts a neuroprotective effect (see Chapter 14).

As noted earlier, an especially common complaint of patients receiving long-term treatment with lithium is blunting of creativity. Similar to the notion that lithium can blunt the peaks of extreme dysphoric and euphoric states, some patients report that lithium interferes with the highest levels of creativity. Given the apparent overrepresentation of bipolar illness among individuals in the creative arts, the frequency of this complaint is not surprising (see Chapter 12).

Evaluating the validity of this claim is difficult, however. Enhanced creativity is frequently reported in hypomanic states, with a concomitant increase in productivity. Rather than a reduction in creativity being attributable to lithium, effective treatment of bipolar disorder and the maintenance of sustained remission may have this untoward consequence. Were this the case, however, complaints about reduced creative abilities should be reported for any agents that produce or sustain remission. Yet experience indicates that such complaints are especially common among those being treated with lithium as opposed to other mood stabilizers. Indeed, a preliminary and, as far as we know, as yet unreplicated case study, has been reported in which complaints of diminished creativity were reduced by switching from lithium to sodium divalproex (Stoll et al., 1996).

The obvious difficulty here involves operationalizing the construct of creativity. No single neuropsychological test fully captures this construct. Shaw and colleagues (1986) conducted a critical study in this area, which is one of the only controlled studies to date of lithium's effects on the creative process. When given a word association task, such as providing associations for the word "camera," individuals will differ in the number and in the novelty or idiosyncrasy of the associations they report. Norms in fact exist for the frequency of particular associations. "Photograph" would be a highly common association for the stimulus "camera," whereas "chamber," "private," "stealth," or "sub-rosa" would be understandable but idiosyncratic responses. Using the same methodology over a 5-week testing period involving discontinuation and reinstatement of lithium, Shaw and colleagues (1986) found that upon discontinuation, remitted patients were more generative and also showed an increase in idiosyncrasy of association. Both effects reversed when lithium was reinstituted (see Chapter 12 for further discussion of this and related studies). In a subsequent study, this effect of discontinuation was reaffirmed (Kocsis et al., 1993). Therefore, the extremely limited data available suggest that lithium may result in a diminution of unusual associations, making the case for an impact on creativity more plausible. The effect may be complicated in those patients in whom discontinuation of lithium precipitates a rapid relapse to hypomania and thus an increase in associational fluency secondary to mood state.

This focus on the cognitive sequelae of lithium should not be taken as implying that the major alternatives to lithium, anticonvulsant mood stabilizers, do not present similar issues. Rather, it is only in the case of lithium that there is a substantial empirical literature on potential adverse cognitive effects. Indeed, examination of the neuropsychological effects of the anticonvulsants is standard in evaluating their use in seizure disorders.

Clinical Features

A good deal of medical research involves searching for clinical–pathological correlations in an effort to identify individuals at heightened risk or to further our understanding of disease processes. Once it has been accepted that manic-depressive illness, especially its bipolar form, is associated with a profile of cognitive deficits, a host of questions arise regarding the factors that influence the expression of such neuropsychological disturbances. For example, do all individuals manifest the cognitive deficits characteristic of bipolar illness, or do subgroups manifest these effects more intensely? Alternatively, does the manifestation of cognitive deficits change with development? In particular, does chronicity of illness affect the expression of such deficits? Is the adult pattern of cognitive deficit seen in pediatric bipolar disorder or in children at risk for the disorder? If so, does this obviate the potential confound of medication effects? And to what extent does the severity of cognitive deficits covary with structural abnormalities of the brain, especially the burden of hyperintensities as revealed by fMRI?

Psychotic Features

A number of studies have found a link between the presence of psychotic features and a more chronic and severe course of bipolar illness with respect to both symptomatic and functional outcomes.[23] Especially since cognitive impairment is linked to poorer functional outcomes in bipolar disorder (Zarate et al., 2000), one might surmise that psychotic features are predictive of poorer neuropsychological outcome. This conjecture has received some empirical support. Albus and colleagues (1996) failed to find differences in cognitive performance between first-episode nonpsychotic patients with mood disorders and healthy controls. In contrast, mood disorder patients with psychotic features performed as poorly as patients with first-episode schizophrenia. Thus in this study, the presence of psychosis was found to be a greater determinant of neuropsychological profile than the diagnosis of mood disorder or schizophrenia. In light of the neuropsychological deterioration often seen early after the onset of psychosis in first-episode schizophrenia and the hypothesis that psychotic states are intrinsically toxic (Wyatt, 1991, 1995), it is especially important to examine the validity of this association and to determine whether early intervention can improve cognitive and other long-term outcomes in patients with bipolar disorder with psychotic features. The duration of untreated psychosis in patients with first-episode schizophrenia is associated with both the quality of symptomatic outcomes and the extent of cognitive deterioration (Norman and Malla, 2001; Amminger et al., 2002).

Chronicity and Other Developmental Effects

An active effect of psychiatric illness on brain structure and function need not be restricted to psychotic subtypes. Altshuler (1993) and others have contended that episodes of depression and mania may have similar consequences. Indeed, a particularly popular view is that the release of excessive glucocorticoids during such episodes leads to hippocampal atrophy and consequent disruption of declarative memory processes (Brown et al., 1999) (see Chapter 15). This possibility accords with data indicating that the lifetime duration of depression is associated with hippocampal volume and verbal memory performance in euthymic women with recurrent major depression (Sheline et al., 1996, 1999). A role for interventions is supported by recent evidence that the linkage between lifetime duration of days depressed and structural and functional outcomes holds only for periods without active antidepressant treatment (Sheline, E., personal communication, May 2004).

Bipolar patients can vary in the chronicity of their disorder, differing in the number of episodes, type of episodes, number of hospitalizations, duration of episodes, and severity of symptoms. The directions of these effects are not necessarily uniform. An unremitting, continuous episode of illness may indicate greater chronicity than a history of recurrent but responsive episodes. Adequate metrics by which to evaluate the course of bipolar illness are unavailable. Nonetheless, patients with more severe symptomatic presentations and with courses of illness lacking long periods of remission (e.g., chronic and/or recurrent) tend to have poorer neuropsychological outcomes.[24] Cognitive outcomes in bipolar patients have been linked to a rapid-cycling course (McKay et al., 1995), number of prior hospitalizations (Tham et al., 1997), and lifetime duration in episodes of mania or depression (van Gorp et al., 1998). Denicoff and colleagues (1999) found that number of episodes, longer duration of illness, and more frequent hospitalizations were each associated with performance on tests of attention, abstraction, and memory. Kessing (1998), using regression techniques, found a linkage to cognitive dysfunction for number of episodes and not for duration of illness (see Chapter 4).

While the consensus on this issue is impressive, each of the supportive studies used a cross-sectional design. Two observations illustrate the problem: (1) a more virulent course is associated with neuropsychological deterioration, and (2) patients in remission manifest a profile of cognitive dysfunction, noteworthy mainly for the relative sparing of verbal functions, but otherwise widespread. It is conceivable that the abnormalities seen in remitted patients reflect the deterioration associated with chronicity and are not present from the onset of illness. If so, longitudinal evaluation should detect this change over time. Unfortunately, longitudinal investigation of cognitive function in bipolar disorder has rarely been conducted. An exception in this regard is a study conducted by Dhingra and Rabins (1991). They followed for 5 to 7 years 25 bipolar patients who initially presented in a manic state with no signs of cognitive impairment. At long-term follow-up, approximately one third of the sample had clinically significant cognitive impairment.

Another approach can be taken to determine whether the cognitive deficits seen in euthymia precede the classic expression of illness, accompany the onset of the first affective episode, or are a result of the expression of the disorder. Evaluating family members of bipolar probands, children at risk for bipolar disorder, or pediatric manifestations of bipolar disorder can provide clues to the unfolding of cognitive deficits in this illness. For example, Dickstein and colleagues (2004) compared 21 bipolar children with 21 age- and gender-matched controls on the Cambridge Neuropsychological Test Automated Battery. The bipolar children had a profile of deficits similar to that seen in adults, with deficits in attention, set shifting, and visuospatial memory. Post hoc analyses indicated that these deficits could not be attributed to manic symptoms or the presence of attention-deficit disorder. The average age of the bipolar sample was 12.7 years (range 6 to 17 years), and it is conceivable that the medications used to treat the condition or other ancillary factors distorted cognitive performance. Clarification of the neuropsychological profiles of children at risk (as well as family members) could help clarify these issues while minimizing the confounding effects of illness expression and treatment.

Results of a study by Burt and colleagues (2000) suggest that neuropsychological course may be quite different in bipolar and unipolar patients. The authors compared young and elderly unipolar and bipolar patients in an episode of major depression on the performance of a variety of memory measures. No differences in performance were found between the young bipolar and unipolar groups, while the elderly bipolar patients had markedly inferior performance compared with all other groups. The authors speculated that the history of more frequent affective episodes and the earlier age at onset in the bipolar group resulted in a more pronounced deteriorative process.

The evidence, reviewed earlier, that lithium has negative but quickly reversible cognitive effects does not contradict the possibility that the drug also exerts neuroprotective effects (Manji et al., 2000a,b) (see Chapter 14). To date, there is no evidence that long-term exposure to lithium, as opposed to any other agent, has a specific or general impact on the cognitive deficits characteristic of bipolar disorder. Research to address these issues is essential.

Structural Brain Abnormalities

The fact that some neurocognitive effects reverse with the discontinuation or reinitiation of lithium demonstrates a causal pathway. However, medication effects are unlikely to account for the bulk of the deficits seen during symptomatic or remitted states. There appears to be a core pattern of cognitive deficit that is manifested across the phases of illness. Some evidence indicates that duration of lifetime exposure to major depression covaries with hippocampal volume and a measure of verbal memory. More generally, the evidence for persistent cognitive deficit raises the issue of neuroanatomical correlates (see Chapter 15). There are particular reasons for investigating the relations of MRI hyperintensities (HI) to cognitive manifestations in bipolar disorder.

In comparison with healthy controls and other neuropsychiatric groups, elderly patients with major depressive disorder have consistently shown high rates of abnormality in MRI evaluations. These abnormalities appear as areas of increased signal intensity in both balanced, T_2-weighted and fluid-attenuated inversion recovery (FLAIR) images. T_1-weighted sequences maximize the contrast between gray and white matter and provide fine anatomic detail. In contrast, T_2-weighted and FLAIR sequences are particularly sensitive in identifying fluid-filled areas, which appear as areas of high signal intensity.

The abnormalities can be classified into three types. Periventricular hyperintensities (PVH) are a halo or rim adjacent to ventricles that in severe forms invades surrounding deep white matter. Alternatively, single, patchy, or confluent foci may be observed in deep white matter hyperintensities (DWMH), with or without PVH. HI may also be found in deep gray structures, particularly the basal ganglia, thalamus, and pons. These abnormalities have been referred to as leukoencephalopathy, leukoariosis, subcortical arteriosclerotic encephalopathy, encephalomalacia, and unidentified bright objects (UBOs). Because the HI in major depression are not restricted to white matter and their etiology has not been established, we use the term encephalomalacia.

Figure 9–20 illustrates a moderate-to-severe case of encephalomalacia. FLAIR images are presented for a patient with late-onset, first-episode major depression. The image on the left illustrates PVH, with thick bands of high signal intensity (white) adjacent to the lateral ventricles. Note that on the left side of this image, the HI are extending into the deep white matter. The image on the right is of a higher MRI slice from the same patient and shows multiple confluent HI through the DWMH. In patients presenting with these MRI findings, clinicians typically receive radiological reports that emphasize ischemic small-vessel disease.

In one of the largest prospective MRI series in major depression, all 51 elderly patients (aged >60) referred for ECT presented with HI, more than half rated moderate to severe, and 51 percent had lesions of subcortical gray nuclei (Coffey et al., 1990). These rates of abnormality greatly exceeded those found in a healthy control sample, with basal ganglia abnormalities being most discriminative (Fig. 9–21). The depressed samples studied to date have often included patients with comorbid medical illnesses, without adequate controls for risk factors for cerebrovascular disease (CVD), medications being taken, or drug abuse. Nonetheless, in the work of Coffey and colleagues (1990), when depressed patients with preexisting neurological conditions were excluded, the rate of encephalomalacia greatly exceeded that found in normal controls. In a replication study, patients with major depression showed marked increases in the frequency of PVH, DWMH, and basal ganglia and thalamic HI relative to controls matched for CVD risk factors (Coffey et al., 1993). The age-adjusted odds ratio for PVH was 5.32. In other, often large population studies of elderly healthy controls, when the halos or caps commonly seen at the top and bottom of the lateral ventricles were excluded, approximately 10 to 30 percent presented with MRI white matter abnormalities, with typically mild severity and low rates of subcortical gray matter abnormalities (Breteler et al., 1994).

The rate or severity of encephalomalacia in geriatric depression may equal or exceed that in Alzheimer's disease (Erkinjuntti et al., 1994) and may be comparable to that in multi-infarct dementia (Zubenko et al., 1990; see Sackeim et al., 2000a, for a review). Meta-analyses have supported the excess of HI in geriatric unipolar depression (Videbech, 1997). These abnormalities tend to be overrepresented in frontal lobe white matter and in the basal ganglia, perhaps with a left-sided predominance (Greenwald et al., 1998). For instance, Greenwald and colleagues (1998) found that left frontal DWHI and left putamen HI discriminated between an elderly unipolar sample and a matched healthy comparison group.

Figure 9–20. Fluid-attenuated inversion recovery (FLAIR) images of a patient with late-onset major depression. White or bright areas show magnetic resonance imaging (MRI) hyperintensities. The image on the left demonstrates periventricular hyperintensities, with a broad band of increased signal adjacent to the lateral ventricles and invading the deep white matter. The image on the right, from the same patient at a higher level, shows multiple, confluent foci of hyperintensities in the deep white matter (centrum semiovale).

Several correlates of HI burden have been suggested in studies of elderly unipolar patients. The excess of HI appears to be most marked in patients with late- as opposed to early-onset mood disorder.[25] In turn, this association may be due to a greater rate of cerebrovascular risk factors in the late-onset population. Indeed, as in normal and neurological samples, the strongest predictors of encephalomalacia in unipolar depression are age and cerebrovascular risk factors. There are also suggestions that, in addition to late onset, absence of a family history of mood disorder is predictive of HI burden (Krishnan et al., 2004). This finding regarding transmission of mood disorder would suggest determination of whether family history of CVD is overrepresented in unipolar or bipolar patients with significant encephalomalacia, an issue yet to be resolved.

In unipolar patients, the presence of encephalomalacia has predictive power with respect to treatment outcome and subsequent course. In naturalistic studies, greater HI burden has been associated with poorer acute response to antidepressant medications and ECT.[26] The limited information on longitudinal follow-up suggests that encephalomalacia in unipolar disorder may be a marker for cognitive decline and the development of dementia (Hickie et al., 1997; Baldwin et al., 2000).

In normal, nonsymptomatic subjects, some degree of encephalomalacia may be observed, and its prevalence and extent are linked to aging. It is unclear whether the limited encephalomalacia in normal samples is associated with cognitive impairment, and there may be threshold effects for HI volume (Boone et al., 1992). Nonetheless, in normal and neurological samples, there is a body of replicated findings associating encephalomalacia specifically with deficits in attention, motor speed, and executive function (e.g., Breteler et al., 1994; see Sackeim et al., 2000a, for a review). As noted earlier, these are hallmark deficits in unipolar and bipolar depression. In nonpsychiatric patient samples, the most common neurological abnormalities associated with encephalomalacia are gait disturbances, tendency to fall, extensor plantar reflex, and primitive reflexes.[27]

There has been limited investigation of the neuropsychological correlates of encephalomalacia in unipolar major depression. Ebmeier and colleagues (1997) found that the severity of DWMH was inversely related to global cognitive function (Mini-Mental State scores) in elderly depressed patients. In an especially comprehensive study, Lesser and colleagues (1996) compared 60 late-onset (>50 years of age) unipolar depressed patients, 35 early-onset (<35 years of age) depressed patients, and 165 normal controls. All subjects were at least 50 years of age. The late-onset group had greater DWMH than either of the other groups. Cognitive deficits were most marked in the late-onset group and pertained to nonverbal intelligence, nonverbal memory, constructional ability, executive function,

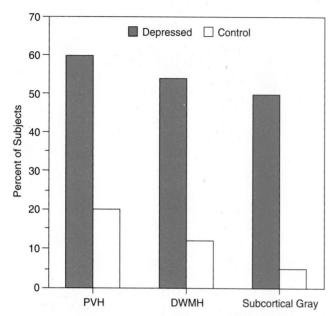

Figure 9–21. Representation of the findings of Coffey and colleagues (1990). The percentages of patients with major depression and control subjects are contrasted in rates of periventricular hyperintensities (PVH), deep white matter hyperintensities (DWMH), and hyperintensities in subcortical gray matter structures.

and speed of processing. Patients with greater severity of DWMH had significantly poorer executive function.

Jenkins and colleagues (1998) found that elderly depressed patients with HI showed poorer performance on a number of learning and memory indices, with the pattern of deficits resembling that observed in subcortical degenerative disorders (i.e., Huntington's and Parkinson's diseases). Simpson and colleagues (1997b) conducted neuropsychological assessment after treatment of an elderly unipolar depressed sample. Signal abnormalities in the pons were associated with reduced psychomotor speed, basal ganglia HI were linked to impaired category productivity (executive function), and PVH were associated with recall deficits. It should be noted that since the severity of encephalomalacia in this study was also associated with clinical outcome, the findings regarding neuropsychological correlates may have been confounded with clinical state. Yet the findings of these and other studies indicate that in general, encephalomalacia in elderly unipolar patients is associated with impairments of psychomotor function, attention, executive function, and learning and memory. There is also evidence that specific cognitive domains may be affected by the anatomic location of HI (deep white matter, periventricular, or subcortical gray matter structures).

The characterization of encephalomalacia in bipolar disorder is less certain, in part because it has received less research attention. Nonetheless, encephalomalacia clearly has different meanings in bipolar and unipolar disorder.

In considerably younger samples than those studied in unipolar disorder, several groups have reported that MRI HI are more common among young bipolar patients than controls.[28] Aylward and colleagues (1994) found that older (> age 38) and not younger bipolar patients had an excess of HI. Brown and colleagues (1992) failed to detect an excess in young bipolar patients, although they did observe that severe HI were overrepresented in elderly patients with major depression. In a sample of 600 psychiatric patients who underwent MRI, Breeze and colleagues (2003) failed to observe a difference in rates of DWMH in bipolar patients compared with other psychiatric groups. However, in the same sample, this group reported that bipolar patients had a clear excess of *severe* DWMH compared with other groups (Lyoo et al., 2002). In relatively small samples, Silverstone and colleagues (2003) compared bipolar depressed, unipolar depressed, and healthy participants and found that the bipolar patients had twice the rate of severe DWMH relative to unipolar patients or healthy controls. Ahn and colleagues (2004) recently confirmed an excess of DWMH in bipolar adults relative to healthy controls, with the discrimination being strongest for more severe structural abnormality.

The findings of two recent studies are particularly revealing. Pillai and colleagues (2002) compared rates of white matter HI in adolescents with bipolar disorder and schizophrenia and matched healthy controls. These HI were more common in the bipolar group (67 percent) relative to the schizophrenic (37 percent) and comparison (32 percent) groups. HI occur in individuals with early-onset bipolar disorder and have been reported at first psychiatric contact. Ahearn and colleagues (1998) conducted MRI examinations of the affected and unaffected first-degree relatives of bipolar probands. Of the 21 family members examined, 15 had HI, including 6 of 10 family members with no history of mood disorder and all of those with bipolar disorder. Lesions of both white matter and subcortical gray nuclei were seen. The authors raised the possibility that these HI serve as a biomarker of bipolar disorder.

The literature on encephalomalacia in bipolar disorder is somewhat less consistent than that in unipolar disorder in demonstrating this structural abnormality. On the other hand, some authors claim that encephalomalacia is especially marked in bipolar disorder. The reasons for this discrepancy are not well understood. Nonetheless, reports demonstrating differences from healthy participants and other psychiatric groups are sufficient for us to conclude that bipolar disorder is characterized by an excess of these structural abnormalities. In their meta-analysis, Bearden and colleagues (2001) found a pooled odds ratio of 7.2 for the likelihood of HI in bipolar patients relative to healthy participants.

The striking thing is that the correlates of these abnormalities appear to differ in bipolar and unipolar disorder. There is a dramatic difference in age at manifestation. In all populations studied to date, HI burden increases with advancing age. This may also be true in bipolar disorder. What is exceptional, however, that adolescents with bipolar disorder show the abnormality (Botteron et al., 1995; Lyoo et al., 2002; Pillai et al., 2002). In unipolar patients and neurological samples, the presence and severity of HI are linked to CVD. Indeed, the predominant view is that encephalomalacia is an outcome of ischemic changes in white matter watershed areas that are fed by tiny arterioles and have limited collateral vascular supply. Rigidification of these small vessels or blockage through arteriosclerosis will result in ischemic damage. Not surprisingly, then, age and cerebrovascular risk factors would be key determinants. Further, given this hypothesized vascular etiology, it is not surprising that encephalomalacia is especially prevalent in late-onset depression in patients without a family history of mood disorder. It is CVD that is the primary agent, and not a genetic liability to depression. Indeed, the invasion of fibers in the white matter by HI must be a random process. If the right fibers are damaged, major depression may result as disconnection syndrome (Geschwind, 1965). Further, it makes sense that encephalomalacia, by reflecting ischemic brain changes, is associated with specific forms of cognitive impairment and predicts future course.

The young age at which many bipolar patients show this abnormality makes it unlikely that these HI are the outcome of an ischemic disease process. Indeed, the notion that the severity of the MRI abnormalities covaries with cerebrovascular risk factors has not been established in bipolar samples. Excluding patients or controlling for CVD risk factors still results in an excess of HI in bipolar samples relative to controls (Altshuler et al., 1995; Hickie et al., 1995). Thus while a vascular, age-related etiology for encephalomalacia is most likely in unipolar disorder, a different etiology may be at play in bipolar disorder. In turn, it cannot be assumed that HI burden is associated with neuropsychological impairment in bipolar disorder.

Limited investigation has been done in this area. In a small sample, Dupont and colleagues (1990) found that bipolar patients with HI were more impaired than bipolar patients without HI or healthy controls on tests of attention, letter fluency, visuospatial skills, and memory. In contrast, Krabbendam and colleagues (2000) compared matched groups of remitted patients with bipolar disorder, patients with schizophrenia, and healthy controls. The groups did not differ in the presence or severity of HI. More surprisingly, no differences in cognitive performance were found between patients with and without white matter lesions. Clearly, this area needs further attention, and the pathoetiology of encephalomalacia in bipolar disorder remains a mystery.

NEUROPSYCHOLOGY AND THE CONCEPTUALIZATION OF MOOD DISORDERS

However revealing about the disorder, a detailing of the areas of cognitive strength and weakness in manic-depressive illness is a highly incomplete account of the neuropsychological contribution to theories of the nature of the illness. The application of psychometrics to affective processes lags considerably behind advances in cognitive assessment. However, the study of brain–behavior relationships with respect to the regulation of emotion draws on a vast clinical and experimental literature involving psychiatric, neurological, and healthy samples to derive conclusions about how emotional states are represented in the brain and what may go wrong such that some individuals are subject to recurrent bouts of depression or mania. The remainder of this chapter is devoted to a brief review of some of the key questions addressed in this literature.

Are Mood Disorders Deficit States or Release Phenomena?

Theorists such as Donald Klein have viewed major depression as a deficit state, the affective equivalent of an aphasia (Klein et al., 1980). The depressed patient is characterized by an inability to feel pleasure, lack of interest, sleep and appetite disturbance, lack of energy, immobility, and so on. By this view, then, basic appetitive, motoric, and hedonic functions are disturbed, much as sensation, movement, or speech is lost in neurological disorders resulting from destructive brain lesions.

An alternative view is that these affective states are manifested as highly integrated behaviors with mood, motor, cognitive, and conative components. Normal states of sadness and euphoria or, by extension, depression and mania are "positive symptoms" in the sense of Hughlings Jackson (1985), reflecting "hyperfunction" more than "hypofunction," and are expressed through excitatory or disinhibitory mechanisms (Head, 1921). By this view, depression and mania are more akin to automatic speech than to speech arrest (Sackeim, 1986).

What type of evidence might support such a view? First, complex affective states can reliably be provoked by stimulating specific regions of the brain. Indeed, they can be turned on and off by changing the electrical stimulation. During the course of deep-brain stimulation for movement disorders, it has become clear that stimulation at a particular contact on an electrode in the subthalamic nucleus (or elsewhere) can provoke an overwhelming feeling of depression, accompanied by crying, beliefs of worthlessness or hopelessness, and other classic phenomena associated with the depressed state.[29] Turning the stimulation off turns off the emotional display. The importance of such demonstrations lies not so much in the hints about localization, but more in the fact that the immediacy of the depressive mood and of the changes in emotional expression and worldview indicate the triggering of an integrated "depressive system" that alters the content of both mood and thought. Thus the brain, at least in this context, behaves in a way envisaged neither by James (1890) nor by Schachter (Schachter and Singer, 1962). We do not come to have a feeling because we are expressing the emotion (e.g., we know we are afraid because we are running), as suggested by James. Nor do we come to have a feeling because of an appraisal we have made about our surroundings that explains why we are aroused, as suggested by Schachter. In the case of deep-brain stimulation, mood, expression, and thought present simultaneously as integrated psychic phenomena triggered by a manipulation of brain tissue. None has primacy, as would be demanded by these earlier theories.

Depressive-catastrophic reactions during the Wada procedure are another example of provoked and transient mood disorder. This procedure involves injecting a barbiturate into the internal carotid artery to temporarily "barbiturate" the ipsilateral hemisphere (Snyder and Harris, 1997; Wada, 1997). Contralateral flaccid hemiplegia or hemiparesis and homonymous hemianopsia soon result. The procedure is used to establish laterality of language and verbal memory in individuals scheduled for neurosurgery (Branch et al., 1964; Cohen-Gadol et al., 2004; Takayama et al., 2004). At a point when sensorimotor function and cognition return toward baseline, some patients report depressed mood and catastrophic beliefs (e.g., their lives are ruined, the world is coming to an end). Since the 1950s, some investigators have claimed that left-side injections are more likely to produce this outcome, whereas right-side injections are more likely to result in a euphoric reaction.[30] While this idea is subject to controversy (Kolb and Milner, 1981; Kurthen et al., 1991), results of a recent study using masked ratings of facial expression during the Wada procedure support the notion that depressive reactions are more common with left-side injection.

Normal functioning is characterized by its own mood swings. Profound sadness, as during mourning or other losses, is a normal variant and shares virtually all the symptoms of the clinical disorder. What distinguishes major depressive episodes from the normal experience of intense dysphoric states is not so much the phenomenology of these presentations as the fact that major depression does not resolve as quickly. Viewing these phenomena in normal individuals as a deficit state strains credibility. Furthermore,

states of euphoria and mania also involve integrated manifestations in mood, motor function, cognition, and conation, with many of these functions appearing to be in overdrive.

Another argument regarding the status of depression and mania as release phenomena concerns the fact that the disorders most clearly reflecting deficits in emotional processes are distinct from depression and mania. Individuals may have agnosias for emotional communications. In other words, they may be incapable of identifying affective intonation or emotional facial expressions. For example, prosopoaffective agnosia refers to the inability to discern facial emotional expression without an accompanying deficit in processing of facial identity (Vuilleumier et al., 1998). Other neurological disorders can result in an incapacity to display emotions, either voluntarily or spontaneously (Borod et al., 1988; Ghacibeh and Heilman, 2003). And alexithymia is a disorder involving the capacity to feel or process affectively laden information (Becerra et al., 2002; Kano et al., 2003; Larsen et al., 2003); some refer to this condition as emotional blunting or emotion blindness. If affective disorders have a form of negative symptoms reflecting a fundamental defect or incapacity, these conditions would be exemplars.

Are We Wired to Be Depressed, and What Are the Therapeutic Implications?

The difference in conceptualization discussed above is not academic. The release model essentially claims that we are wired to be depressed and euphoric. Depressive or manic states do not arise because of a disruption of various discrete functions, such as sleep and appetite, but represent the expression of excitatory or disinhibitory release of distributed networks that subserve the integrated features of mood disorder (Tanaka and Sumitsuji, 1991). Concretely, this conception posits that there are depression and euphoria circuits in the brain, just as there are circuits for fear.

By positing that excessive excitation or disinhibition leads to release of the affective states, this perspective also has implications for our understanding of therapeutics. ECT is the most effective short-term treatment for both the depressed and manic phases of bipolar disorder. As reviewed in Chapter 19, bipolar depressed patients remit at the same rate as unipolar patients but require fewer treatments (Daly et al., 2001). Regardless of the form of ECT that was used in a series of randomized, controlled trials at Columbia University, bipolar patients on average required about 1.5 fewer treatments than unipolar depressed patients, with optimal forms of ECT resulting in immediate remission rates of 60 to 80 percent (Fig. 9–22). The immediate remission rate in mania is also on the order of 80 percent, and improvement is often

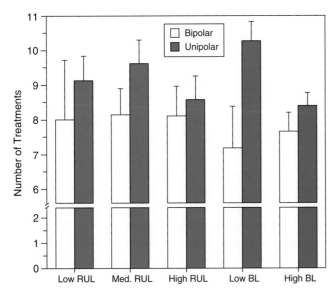

Figure 9–22. Number of electroconvulsive therapy (ECT) treatments for bipolar and unipolar depressed patients. Based on data pooled across four studies at the New York State Psychiatric Institute/Columbia University, 78 bipolar patients required on average about 1.5 fewer treatments than 185 unipolar depressed patients. Patients were randomly assigned to forms of ECT that differed in electrical dosage (low, medium, and high) and electrode placement (right unilateral [RUL] versus bilateral [BL]). An analysis of variation (ANOVA) was conducted on the number of treatments administered, with diagnosis (bipolar versus unipolar), treatment condition (five levels), and the interaction of those two factors as between-subject terms, and age and pre-ECT Hamilton Rating Scale for Depression (HAM-D) score as covariates. The main effects of diagnosis ($p = .0008$) and pre-ECT HAM-D score ($p = .0002$) were significant. (*Source*: Adapted from Sackeim et al., 1987, 1993, 2000b, and Sackeim, 2004.)

brisker than in major depression (Mukherjee et al., 1994). Why is ECT unique among therapeutics in both the breadth of its therapeutic action and its success rate? Why is a treatment that results in a hyperexcited state of the brain effective in treatment conditions that we posit reflect the release of function?

ECT is a profound anticonvulsant.[31] The induction of the seizure initiates a set of endogenous inhibitory processes that terminate the seizure (Madsen et al., 2000); the leading theories on what mediates this anticonvulsant effect involve increased transmission of gamma-aminobutyric acid (GABA), endogenous opioids (Sanacora et al., 2003), or other peptides (Tortella and Long, 1985). ECT raises the seizure threshold for itself and all agents that trigger seizures through GABAergic antagonism (Green et al., 1982). It also results in progressive shortening of seizure duration and weakening of seizure expression (Sackeim, 1999). Increasing the threshold for seizures and blocking or weakening seizure expression are the two conditions to be satisfied in determining whether a drug has anticonvulsant

properties. In a variety of animal models, including kindling, electroconvulsive shock (ECS) exerts more powerful anticonvulsant properties than drugs such as carbamazepine or valproate. In this light, it is not surprising that ECT has been of value in the treatment of resistant seizure disorders, including status epilepticus (Sackeim et al., 1983b; Lisanby et al., 2001).

The therapeutic properties of ECT have been linked to its anticonvulsant effects. Forms of ECT that result in the most marked increases in seizure threshold tend to be the most effective (Sackeim, 1999). The strength of the inhibitory process immediately after the seizure can be indexed by the presence or absence of postictal suppression of the electroencephalogram (EEG). Postictal suppression (bioelectric silence) is predictive of a favorable outcome (Nobler et al., 1993; Suppes et al., 1996; Perera et al., 2004). Most critically, since Kety's work initiated the field of brain imaging (Kety et al., 1948), it has been clear that ECT results in marked reductions in CBF (and CMR_{glu}).[32] Recent work has revealed powerful relationships between the extent of this suppression in prefrontal regions and clinical outcome in both major depression and mania (Nobler et al., 1994, 2000b, 2001). Consonant with this perspective, ECT results in a marked increase in slow-wave (delta) activity. The efficacy of the procedure has been linked to a topography dominated by increased slow-wave activity in prefrontal regions (Sackeim et al., 1996a). Thus depressed and manic patients may have "bad brakes," resulting in a failure to diminish activation in the released mood circuitry. ECT, at least temporarily, enhances inhibitory tone, reducing expression of the released mood circuitry.

The large imaging literature on antidepressant effects is mainly in keeping with this view (Mayberg et al., 1999; Drevets et al., 2002; Seminowicz et al., 2004). Although there are disagreements about the sites of inhibition that are most critical, the antidepressant effects of ECT, sleep deprivation, and antidepressant medications have commonly been tied to reductions of regional cerebral blood flow (rCBF) or CMR_{glu} in specific brain regions. Frontal pole, medial orbital prefrontal cortex, anterior cingulate, and amygdala have been identified as primary in reflecting the covariation between reduced CBF or CMR_{glu} and clinical outcome.[33]

Of course, this view readily accommodates the fact that several anticonvulsant agents have mood-stabilizing properties. Thus to the extent that depressed or manic patients can be said to have "bad brakes," treatments with prophylactic properties may exert tonic inhibition.

Does the Brain Regulate Depression and Mania Differently?

Bipolar disorder is one of the few illnesses in which polar-opposite symptoms (euphoria and depression) are experienced as part of the same illness. It is tempting to view these abnormal states as the ends of a seesaw, such that when one side is up, the other is down. This analogy presumes that some force is tilting a balance toward or away from depression or mania, thus regulating both. However, the nature of regulatory control probably differs for euphoric and dysphoric states. Take the example of uncontrollable laughing and crying. In the context of destructive, silent (nonepileptic) lesions, pathological crying is more frequent than pathological laughing (Mills, 1912; Davison and Kelman, 1939; Tateno et al., 2004). Uncontrollable outbursts of laughter as a prodrome or during seizures are referred to as gelastic epilepsy (Daly and Mulder, 1957; Gascon and Lombroso, 1971). As peri-ictal manifestations, these highly organized behavioral displays occur in the context of excessive cerebral excitability, during states of hypersynchronous neuronal firing (Arroyo et al., 1993). Dacrystic epilepsy refers to the occurrence of crying as a prodromal or ictal event. When we collected the world literature on gelastic and dacrystic epilepsy, we found a pattern with pathological laughing and crying: there were 91 cases of laughing as a peri-ictal event, but only 6 cases of crying outbursts and 6 cases that presented laughing and crying outbursts to an equal extent (Sackeim et al., 1982b).

It is unlikely that the paucity of dacrystic epilepsy and excess of gelastic epilepsy case studies reflects only a reporting bias. As noted, in the context of silent, nonirritative lesions, reports of pathological crying are common. Taken at face value, this difference in rates of occurrence suggests that uncontrollable crying is released more readily through disinhibitory mechanisms as opposed to an excitatory process, while laughter is readily released through "irritative" or excitatory as well as disinhibitory mechanisms.

Even granting such a possibility, it is not evident that the pattern of neural control over these emotional displays is of consequence for the regulation of mood. At issue is whether these examples of dysregulation of spontaneous emotional expression should serve as a model for the pathophysiology of abnormal mood states. Three key arguments support the validity of this model.

First, as noted earlier, in a substantial minority of patients with pathological laughing and/or crying, mood is altered during the outbursts in a manner that is consonant with the expressive outburst. Thus these individuals report marked sadness during pathological crying and euphoria during pathological laughter. This same pattern holds for gelastic and dacrystic epilepsy. This would suggest that in some cases, the physiological state that results in release of the expressive outbursts also releases these organized mood states (Black, 1982). Precise data are lacking on the prevalence of mood alterations during ictal events. It is noteworthy that fear and euphoria are commonly reported.

For example, Dostoyevsky stated that he would give up 10 years of his life for the brief period of ecstasy he experienced as a peri-ictal event.

Second, the therapeutics of pathological laughing and crying supports the concept that mood and emotional expression are part of an integrated emotion circuit. In controlled trials, antidepressant medications, including tricyclic antidepressants and selective serotonin reuptake inhibitors (SSRIs), have been found to be effective.[34]

Third, the lateralization of brain damage (or seizure foci) in these cases of uncontrollable emotional display matches that seen for depressive and euphoric mood changes that occur after destructive, silent lesions. As with the Wada procedure, and also not without controversy, a significant body of research has linked acute depressive reactions following brain insult to damage in left-sided regions, especially in frontal cortex, and euphoric mood changes to right-sided damage.[35] Figure 9–23 presents ratings of the predominant side of lesion in cases of pathological laughing and crying; the raters were blinded to the nature of the affective display (Sackeim et al., 1982a). As in the literature on mood change, crying outbursts are associated with an excess of left-sided lesions, and laughing outbursts with an excess of right-sided lesions.

Sackeim and colleagues (1982b) hypothesized that the opposite pattern would obtain when these outbursts occurred in the context of epilepsy as prodromal or ictal events. Focal seizure activity has unique localizing value. For example, lateralized somatosensory alterations have 100 percent correspondence to contralateral seizure activity in somatosensory cortex. Hughlings Jackson (1985) described the "homunculus," the ordered representation of the body in motor and somatosensory cortex based on the march of motor symptoms during Jacksonian seizures, a description later validated by Penfield with direct electrical stimulation of motor cortex (Penfield and Jasper, 1954). Sackeim and colleagues had further hypothesized that depressive and euphoric mood states following lateralized silent (nonepileptic) lesions reflect disinhibition in contralateral brain regions that subserve depressed or euphoric states—that is, breaking a brake over contralateral regions. Thus, for example, they posited that euphoria results from right-sided brain damage due to release of the left-sided regions that subserve this affective state. This hypothesis derived partly from data indicating that right hemispherectomy (removal of the anterior two thirds of the cerebral hemisphere) often results in a syndrome of increased jocularity, poor judgment, lack of responsibility, and so on (Sackeim et al., 1982b). These affective changes cannot be mediated by the broad expanse of cortex that has been removed, but only by remaining subcortical regions in the ipsilateral hemisphere or by release of the

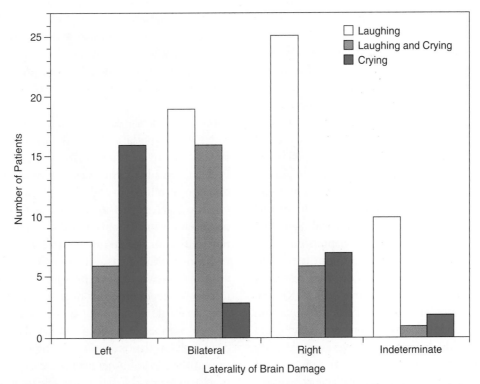

Figure 9–23. Distribution of primarily left-sided, right-sided, bilateral, and indeterminate nonirritative lesions in patients with pathological laughing only, laughing and crying, and crying only. Left-sided and right-sided lesions are associated with pathological crying and laughing, respectively, whereas bilateral lesions are associated with presentation of both uncontrollable laughing and crying. (*Source*: Sackeim et al., 1982b.)

regions in the contralateral hemisphere. Likewise, the affective changes seen after barbituration of the left or right hemisphere suggest that contralateral disinhibition may be at play.

Figure 9–24 presents findings regarding the lateralization of epileptic foci in cases of gelastic epilepsy. There was an overwhelming excess of left-sided foci, as predicted—the opposite of what was seen with pathological laughing in the context of silent lesions. Thus, the model offered by Sackeim and colleagues (1982b) stipulated that depressed and euphoric states are under reciprocal inhibitory control. Depressive phenomena are released mainly by disinhibitory mechanisms, while euphoric mood changes and laughter are released by disinhibition or direct excitation. The model did not require that the inhibitory control mechanisms be reciprocal. Including this element implied a partial seesaw effect. Reciprocal regulation would mean that depression and euphoria cannot be experienced simultaneously, an issue that is key to the conceptualization of mixed states.

Our conceptions of how emotional processes are represented in the brain are rudimentary. Undoubtedly the model of Sackeim and colleagues is overly broad and, at best, an echo of the true state of affairs. Nonetheless, the evidence that led to this model was consistent and illustrated the power of using experimental invasive techniques (e.g., deep brain stimulation, Wada test, hemispherectomy), along with experiments in nature (lateralization of epileptic foci and silent lesions), to constrain theorizing

Figure 9–24. Distribution of left-sided, right-sided, and indeterminate epileptic foci in patients with gelastic (laughing) epilepsy. Foci were more than twice as likely to be left-sided than right-sided. (*Source*: Sackeim et al., 1982b.)

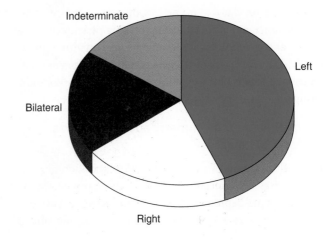

about fundamental mechanisms in the regulation of emotion.

There are other speculative grounds for postulating a fundamental difference in the neural control of euphoric and dysphoric states or, as some have suggested, emotional states involved in approach or avoidance (Davidson, 1995). A long list of pharmacological agents, including laughing gas, stimulants, opioids, cocaine, and others, can reliably induce euphoric mood in the majority of people. Many of these effects are immediate, occurring within seconds or minutes after exposure. In contrast, despite intensive research efforts and standard surveillance techniques during drug screening, not a single pharmacological agent has been identified that can reliably induce depression in the majority of naïve individuals. In only a minority of individuals with a family history of mood disorder, reserpine will elicit a depressive reaction (Kraemer and McKinney, 1979). Similarly, tryptophan depletion has no impact on mood in healthy individuals, except for a small change in a minority of individuals with a positive family history (Ellenbogen et al., 1996; Shansis et al., 2000). This discrepancy in the likelihood that pharmaceutical agents can provoke depression or mania is curious, and its significance is reinforced by the psychometrics of psychological mood manipulation.

Symbolic representations can drive mood change. Being told that one is deficient, unloved, corrupt, or ineffective affects mood. Clearly, we are built such that our ideas about the world and ourselves can alter our mood. Indeed, a small industry has developed that uses psychological manipulations to produce mood changes in specific directions (e.g., from sadness to euphoria) (Velten, 1968; Bouhuys et al., 1995; Richell and Anderson, 2004). This literature suggests that the range or intensity of affect produced by psychological manipulations is often greater for inductions of sadness than those of happiness. In other words, it appears to be much easier to induce clear-cut sadness as opposed to euphoria through words or music (symbolic representations).

If these observations are valid—and much work needs to be done on the psychometrics of mood change—they may advance our understanding of how pharmacological agents and psychological manipulations constitute intrinsically different types of triggers or pathways for mood alteration, perhaps because of intrinsic differences in modulating disinhibitory versus excitatory processes.

Functional Brain Asymmetry and the Localization of Mood Systems

In the first edition of this text, laterality and kindling were identified as key concepts in theories about the neural origins of manic-depressive illness. At the time, it was common to hypothesize that schizophrenia was an outcome of left-hemisphere dysfunction, while manic-depressive illness derived from right-hemisphere deficits (Flor-Henry, 1976). Another view was that a cumulative history of stress, affective episodes themselves, and biological predisposition fueled a kindling process that resulted in manifestation of mood disturbance and progressively more frequent and intense episodes of illness (Post, 1990, 2002).

Neither hypothesis has remained the focus of mainstream research. In both cases, this shift in attention reflects in part advances in basic neuroscience that have produced research tools and concepts with the potential to provide great explanatory power with respect to fundamental abnormalities in clinical populations, as well as opportunities for designing new interventions. Understanding of intracellular cascades and the factors that promote cellular resilience or the expression of neurogenesis has led to new conceptualizations of pathoetiology and potential avenues for treatment (see Chapter 14).

In a number of respects, the lateralization view was a dead end. On the one hand, linking disorders to dysfunction at the level of a hemisphere, even if true, was hardly precise in terms of localization. The total right hemisphere could not be abnormal in mood disorders. Furthermore, this hypothesis was imprecise as to whether this right-hemisphere dysfunction is the core problem resulting in periodic manifestations of depression and mania or in an expression of these affective states.

Perhaps the greatest limitation of the laterality hypothesis was its lack of practical application for diagnosis or treatment or for the development of a direct method for testing validity. Until recently, psychiatry had no means other than ECT of targeting biological treatment to specific brain areas. Systemic administration of medications allows no control over the neural systems being modulated. In contrast, left and right unilateral ECT produce profound asymmetries in the physiology and function of the brain. Unilateral ECT produces marked decreases in CBF and CMR_{glu} and marked increases in EEG slow-wave activity in the hemisphere ipsilateral to the side of stimulation (Kriss et al., 1978; Nobler et al., 1994; Sackeim et al., 1996b). It also produces marked disjunctions in neuropsychological measures. For example, assessment of orientation and language functions in the postictal period immediately following left and right unilateral ECT is as reliable as the Wada test in identifying laterality of language (Pratt et al., 1971; Pratt and Warrington, 1972). Thus the view that euphoric and depressed states reflect release of function in the left and right hemispheres, respectively, would imply that left unilateral ECT is more effective than right unilateral ECT in the treatment of mania, with the reverse holding true for depression. Although some findings in the ECT literature support both predictions (Small et al.,

1993), the larger point is that left and right unilateral ECT both show considerable efficacy in the treatment of mania and depression, and that any difference in therapeutic effects is relatively minor compared with the shared variance. Given the asymmetrical physiological and cognitive effects of unilateral ECT, the efficacy data largely contradict a prominent role for functional brain asymmetry in treatment mechanisms and, by extension, in the pathophysiology of depression and mania.

A key observation that promoted interest in lateralization effects was the association between localization of stroke and other forms of brain damage and manifestation of mood disturbance. Clinically, as mentioned earlier, it has long been noted that "unipolar mania" (i.e., manifestation of mania without prior or subsequent episodes of major depression) occurs almost exclusively in the context of coarse brain injury (Jorge et al., 1993; Fujikawa et al., 1995; Robinson, 1997). Further, it is generally agreed that such lesions are predominantly right-sided (Cummings and Mendez, 1984; Starkstein et al., 1988a).

In contrast, the relationships between location of brain lesion and manifestation of depression have become less certain with additional research. Interest in the laterality of emotion was sparked by findings relating side of brain injury to affective state (Gainotti, 1972) and to uncontrollable emotional expressions (Sackeim et al., 1982a), by the demonstration of asymmetry in the emotional expressions of the human face (Sackeim et al., 1978), and by the linkage of disturbances in the processing of affectively laden information to right-sided brain damage (Heilman et al., 1975). However, the relevance of a laterality dimension to mood disorders was contingent on reliable associations between side of brain damage and manifestations of mood disturbance.

Gainotti (1969, 1972) was the first to examine systematically the distinct differences in emotional reactions of patients with left- and right-hemisphere stroke. Right-sided damage was associated with anosognosia (denial of illness) or anosodiaphorie (lack of concern about illness, i.e., a carefree attitude) and a "euphoric-indifference reaction." Robinson's research, however, catalyzed interest in this area. In a seminal paper, Robinson and colleagues (1984) linked the severity of depressive symptoms shortly after stroke to damage to left-sided prefrontal regions. The closer the lesions were to the left frontal pole, the more severe was the depressive syndrome. Right parietal lesions were also linked to depression, but at lower incidence and with lesser intensity of depressive manifestations. This work had important methodological limitations, such as the exclusion of patients with significant aphasia, which possibly distorted the sample of patients with left-sided injury, and problems in the blinding of assessment given the motor,

sensory, and cognitive deficits that reveal the side of lateralized brain damage. Most of the subsequent studies failed to replicate Robinson's core findings, and some meta-analyses of this literature contested the existence of an association between lesion location and depressive manifestations (Carson et al., 2000; Narushima et al., 2003; Yu et al., 2004).

Missing from this perspective were the results of long-term follow-up of individuals with penetrating head wounds after World War II. Mood disturbance was common in such patients. In particularly careful work, Lishman (1968) noted that right posterior head wounds were far more likely to be associated with depressive and manic manifestations than were injuries to any of the remaining three quadrants. It hardly appeared likely that different forms of nonirritative brain insult—stroke versus head wound—could fundamentally alter the linkage between side of brain insult and depressive symptoms.

One possibility accounting for the discrepancies in this literature concerns the issue of time since stroke. Robinson's early work involved patients who were examined very soon after stroke, recruited at emergency room presentation. Later studies often examined patients months to years after their cerebrovascular accident. There has been little longitudinal work addressing whether localization of damage is related to the persistence (chronicity) and/or late emergence of depressive symptoms. Nelson and colleagues (1994) evaluated affective symptoms in patients with lateralized stroke at 2-week, 2-month, and 6-month time points. Initially, the group with left-hemisphere stroke experienced a slower rate of recovery from depressive symptoms. At the 6-month time point, however, the emotional functioning of the right-hemisphere group worsened. The evidence regarding temporal interval as a moderator of the relationship between lesion location and affective disturbance is not consistent, and considerably more work is necessary (Carson et al., 2000). Nonetheless, the positive findings in this area introduce a dynamic element to the relationships between brain injury and altered affective states.

One interpretation of this literature would be to argue that in the acute poststroke period, depressive symptoms are most severe when the lesion is closest to the left frontal pole. The most recent meta-analysis (Narushima et al., 2003) supports this association. However, manifestation of this syndrome is time-limited, and depressive symptoms spontaneously remit within a few months. In contrast, right parietal lesions result in milder depressive symptoms in the acute period. Yet this disturbance is more likely to be chronic, and these lesions may also result in late-emerging affective disturbance. Following the disinhibition model for nonirritative lesions, both left anterior and right posterior stroke may disinhibit right prefrontal areas critical to the manifestation of depressed mood. Prefrontal-parietal connectivity is well established, and reciprocal inhibitory pathways have been demonstrated (Goldman-Rakic, 1987; Woods et al., 1993). Thus this view, albeit post hoc in accounting for discrepancies, leads to the assertion that the functional consequences of brain lesions are time dependent, and this temporal effect may differ based on laterality. That such temporal effects can occur is amply demonstrated in the neurosurgical literature on the treatment of highly resistant mood disorders. Therapeutic benefit from psychosurgery usually is manifest only months after the intervention.

Dissociating Therapeutics and Pathophysiology

Although the linkage of right-sided damage to mania remains uncontested, there is uncertainty about the role of lateralized brain damage in the manifestation of depressed states. Indeed, one possibility yet to be raised is that the strength of association for lateralized effects is stronger for euphoric or manic than for dysphoric or depressed states. As seen in Figure 9–22, the association between pathological laughing and right-sided silent lesions is stronger than that between pathological crying and left-sided lesions. As seen in Figure 9–24, there is also a robust association between laterality of epileptic focus and uncontrollable laughter as a peri-ictal phenomenon.

Until recently, data-driven formulations of this type had little possibility of being tested experimentally. The common denominator in this sort of theorizing is that disinhibition of right prefrontal structures is the common final pathway for depressive manifestation. If that were the case, selective suppression of such activity would be expected to have antidepressant properties, and left prefrontal suppression to have antimanic effects.

The development of noninvasive methods for focal neuromodulation resulted in new life for this area of research. For example, repetitive transcranial magnetic stimulation (rTMS) offers a means of suppressing or enhancing activity in regions under the coil or at a distance through patterns of connectivity. Because the scalp and skull are transparent to the magnetic field, it is possible through use of appropriate coil geometry to restrict stimulation to target brain areas. There is considerable evidence that slow-frequency rTMS (one or fewer pulses per second) produces an inhibitory effect, whereas fast-frequency rTMS (five or more pulses per second) has a poststimulation excitatory effect (Wassermann et al., 1993; Terao and Ugawa, 2002; Wu et al., 2002).

There is now a substantial literature on sham-controlled studies testing the efficacy of rTMS in major depression, and the meta-analyses of this literature have all reached the same conclusions (Holtzheimer et al., 2001; McNamara et al.,

2001; Burt et al., 2002). The active rTMS conditions compared with sham have been fast-frequency left DLPFC stimulation and slow-frequency right DLPFC stimulation. Both interventions yield moderate to large effect sizes for antidepressant properties; in other words, both are consistently superior to sham. However, these findings are of greater theoretical than practical importance. In absolute magnitude, the therapeutic effects in the active conditions, although superior to those in sham, have commonly been modest, and the durability of the benefit derived has rarely been tested. For rTMS to have a role in routine practice, these issues must be addressed (Sackeim, 2000b).

From a theoretical perspective, however, it is extraordinary that a highly lateralized intervention can display these antidepressant properties, and moreover, that antidepressant effects can be achieved with opposite physiological alterations (inhibition versus excitation) that are dependent on the laterality of the brain region stimulated. Taken at face value, for example, these effects could indicate that the key to exerting antidepressant properties is the state of the "seesaw": any intervention that tips the seesaw toward greater left prefrontal or reduced right prefrontal expression in the DLPFC will have antidepressant properties. This formulation could mean that mood states are not attributable to the physiological status of a specific brain region, but are an emergent property reflecting the balance of activity among regions in a distributed network. Another possibility is that different individuals benefit from slow right or fast left rTMS, and that left-sided hypofunction and right-sided hyperfunction are alternative routes to major depression (Kimbrell et al., 1999; Speer et al., 2000).

Focal brain stimulation offers an experimental means of testing key concepts about the neuroanatomy and neurophysiology of mood disorders and their treatment. Two caveats are in order about the state of knowledge in this area. First, while it is established that slow right and fast left rTMS have antidepressant properties, however modest, it is assumed that fast right and slow left rTMS are ineffective, something that has never been adequately tested. For example, were slow left DLPFC to exert equal antidepressant properties, a fundamental role for laterality in generating therapeutic effects would be seriously questioned. The key experiment, in which depressed patients are randomly assigned in a 2×2 design to slow- or fast-frequency stimulation and left or right DLPFC, has not been conducted, and is essential to further understanding of the effects of this intervention on mood.

The second caveat is more general. It is often assumed that knowledge of the mode of action of a therapeutic agent (e.g., serotonin reuptake blockade) dictates conceptualization about the underlying pathophysiology (or vice versa). However, there are many examples in medicine in which the optimal treatment for a condition acts through a mechanism distinct from the pathoetiology of the illness. It is doubtful that anyone ever became depressed because of lack of a seizure, and yet ECT is the most effective antidepressant. Put more forcefully, many of our pharmacological interventions produce chronic alterations in brain neurochemistry and other aspects of physiology that are simply not seen otherwise in nature and do not restore the brain to a normative state. Thus the circuitry involved in achieving an antidepressant effect may be distinct from that responsible for manifestation of the mood disorder. The therapeutic properties of interventions such as rTMS may reveal a great deal about the pathways that modulate or ameliorate the experience of major depression. However, these pathways may be distinct from those that generate the abnormal mood state.

Ultimately, progress in genetics and molecular biology is likely to produce breakthroughs in our understanding of the pathoetiology of bipolar disorder and recurrent unipolar depression and in our ability to provide more effective therapeutic interventions. Nonetheless, these disorders need to be understood at a system level. Discrete aspects of emotional life have neural representation. System theories draw on evidence from neurological, psychiatric, and normal populations to constrain hypotheses about the neuroanatomy and physiology that subserve abnormal mood states and that mediate therapeutic outcomes. We are just entering an era in which these hypotheses can be tested through the controlled use of anatomically targeted alterations of physiology and neurochemistry. It can be anticipated that the formulations presented here will be refined or undone, and that the next edition of this text will offer superior descriptions of the neural networks dysregulated in manic-depressive illness.

CONCLUSIONS

Normal Findings in Bipolar Patients

Bipolar patients have normal VIQ, a finding that challenges the idea that bipolar disorder is associated with pervasive intellectual impairment. One possible explanation is that the cognitive systems underlying language are spared from the otherwise generalized bipolar disease process; or they may be constitutionally endowed at higher capacity. Likewise, preliminary evidence indicates that procedural learning and memory are not significantly affected by bipolar illness, while limited data suggest that the ability to recall past events, or details of past events, is not significantly impaired in bipolar patients.

Alone among the executive functions, reasoning remains relatively preserved in bipolar illness. Because the results of tests of reasoning correlate substantially with the results of tests of verbal ability, this finding may reflect a pattern in which cognitive operations heavily dependent on language are among the higher cognitive functions least affected by bipolar disorder.

Neuropsychological Deficits in Bipolar Patients

Intelligence is somewhat reduced in bipolar illness in both the remitted and manic states as reflected in diminished IQ scores. Reasoning remains intact. The marked deficit in PIQ among bipolar patients is commonly ascribed to the effects of mood-dependent psychomotor retardation on task performance, but the presence of the deficit during remission and in individuals at risk for bipolar disorder, as well as its persistence when performance is untimed, argues otherwise. It now appears that the discrepancy is independent of the affective state and may even be present before the first episode of mood disturbance. The above proposed explanation for normal VIQ scores in bipolar patients can also help account for the deficit in PIQ: although the cognitive systems underlying language are spared by the disease or are constitutionally endowed at higher capacity, those underlying other components of intelligence, including performance, are not.

Attention comprises several distinct processes, and its overall integrity is central to the normal functioning of higher cognitive processes such as learning and memory. Disturbances of attention ("impaired concentration") are typical of bipolar disorder, and attention is among the most dramatically impaired functions in patients during episodes of major depression, and indeed across all phases of the illness, including remission. With respect to learning, memory, and visuospatial skills, there is little evidence that deficits reflect more than an attentional disturbance. Short-term memory deficits are typical of bipolar patients, even in remission. It is possible that these deficits result from impaired attention. Bipolar patients also have decided and uniform difficulty in acquiring new information during all phases of the illness, including remission.

Executive functions come closest to the idea of a neural homunculus in charge of administering neural resources. Only a very limited range of executive functions in bipolar disorder has been studied, however. The studies that have been conducted have found substantial deficits in all phases of bipolar disorder. Severe illness has been associated in particular with difficulty in concept formation and set shifting.

NOTES

1. Corwin et al., 1990; Rubinsztein et al., 2000; Sweeney et al., 2000; Murphy and Sahakian, 2001; Quraishi and Frangou, 2002; Martinez-Arán et al., 2004b; Marvel and Paradiso, 2004.

2. Martinez-Arán et al., 2000, 2002a,b, 2004a,b; Rubinsztein et al., 2000; Zubieta et al., 2001; El-Badri et al., 2001; Yen et al., 2002; Altshuler et al., 2004; Dixon et al., 2004.

3. The 52 studies that contributed to the meta-analysis were Oltmanns, 1978; Savard et al., 1980; Asarnow and MacCrimmon, 1981; Robertson and Taylor, 1985; Dalby and Williams, 1986; Green and Walker, 1986; Harvey and Brault, 1986; Sapin et al., 1987; Wolfe et al., 1987; Gruzelier et al., 1988; Wielgus and Harvey, 1988; Coffman et al., 1990; David and Cutting, 1990; Dupont et al., 1990; Harvey and Serper, 1990; Morice, 1990; Deptula et al., 1991; Park and Holzman, 1992; Jones et al., 1994; Kaprinis et al., 1995; Souza et al., 1995; Docherty et al., 1996; Thomas et al., 1996; Hawkins et al., 1997; Lohr and Caligiuri, 1997; Paradiso et al., 1997; Park, 1997; Addington and Addington, 1998; van Gorp et al., 1998, 1999; Ferrier et al., 1999; Gourovitch et al., 1999; Sax et al., 1999; Ali et al., 2000; Krabbendam et al., 2000; Rossi et al., 2000; Rubinsztein et al., 2000; Sweeney et al., 2000; Clark et al., 2001; Zubieta et al., 2001; Agarwal et al., 2002; Cavanagh et al., 2002; Seidman et al., 2002, 2003; Fleck et al., 2003; Getz et al., 2003; Kremen et al., 2003; Swann et al., 2003; Umbricht et al., 2003; Gildengers et al., 2004; Martínez-Arán et al., 2004b; Zalla et al., 2004.

4. The effect size measure used throughout was Hedges' G, and the z-value associated with the point estimate (effect size across studies) and the variance of this estimate were computed to determine significance. All computations were conducted with a beta version of Comprehensive Meta-Analysis II. Dr. Michael Borenstein made upgrades to the program that enabled this meta-analysis.

5. Davidson, 1939; Fisher, 1949; Callagan, 1952; Miller et al., 1981; Donnelly et al., 1982.

6. Flor-Henry and Gruzelier, 1983; Rush et al., 1983; Silverstein and Meltzer, 1983; Taylor and Abrams, 1983.

7. This specification was supported by a significant interaction between group (patient vs. normal control) and IQ component (VIQ vs. PIQ) in a repeated measure analysis of covariance (ANCOVA).

8. Ashton et al., 1995; Parker et al., 1995a,b; 2000; Mitchell et al., 1996.

9. Kupfer and Foster, 1973; Kupfer et al., 1974, 1975; Weiss et al., 1974a,b; Foster and Kupfer, 1975; McPartland et al., 1975; Goode et al., 1979.

10. Szabadi et al., 1976; Greden and Carroll, 1980; Greden et al., 1981; Godfrey and Knight, 1984; Hardy et al., 1984; Hoffmann et al., 1985; Nilsonne, 1987, 1988; Alpert et al., 2001.

11. Bouhuys and Mulder-Hajonides van der Meulen, 1984; Hardy et al., 1984; Hoffmann et al., 1985; Alpert et al., 2001; Cannizzaro et al., 2004.

12. Clark et al., 2002, 2005; Liu et al., 2002; Strakowski et al., 2005.

13. Whitehead, 1973a,b; Strömgren, 1977; Breslow et al., 1980; Gass and Russell, 1986.

14. Hasher and Zacks, 1979; Roy-Byrne et al., 1986; Thomas et al., 1999; Hammar, 2003.

15. Craik and Tulving, 1975; Craik and Jennings, 1992; Mandzia et al., 2004; Newell and Andrews, 2004.

16. Roy-Byrne et al., 1986; el Massioui and Lesevre, 1988; Hartlage et al., 1993; Christensen et al., 1997; Thomas et al., 1999; Den Hartog et al., 2003; Hammar, 2003; Hammar et al., 2003a,b; Politis et al., 2004.

17. Nelson and Craighead, 1977; Breslow et al., 1981; Gotlib, 1981; Clark and Teasdale, 1982; Coyne and Gotlib, 1983; Gotlib and Olson, 1983; Yang and Rehm, 1993; Murray et al., 1999; Winter et al., 2000.

18. Sackeim and Prohovnik, 1993; Soares and Mann, 1997; Haldane and Frangou, 2004; Rogers et al., 2004.

19. Joanette and Goulet, 1986; Bayles et al., 1993; Schlosser et al., 1998; Spreen and Strauss, 1998; Spence et al., 2000.

20. Mann et al., 1999; Keilp et al., 2001; Oquendo and Mann, 2001; Oquendo et al., 2004.

21. Phillips et al., 2003a,b; Schaefer et al., 2003; Tavares et al., 2003; Chamberlain and Sahakian, 2004.

22. One study (Joffe et al., 1988) found no difference among bipolar patients treated with lithium, carbamazepine, or no medication on tests of attention, visuomotor function, and memory. However, this study also failed to find differences between the bipolar groups and healthy controls on the cognitive measures, raising doubt about the sensitivity or reliability of the neuropsychological assessment. Other studies yielding negative findings on the cognitive effects of lithium include Telford and Worrall, 1978; Kjellman et al., 1980; and Ghadirian et al., 1983.

23. Tohen et al., 1990a,b, 2000; Albus et al., 1996; Atre-Vaidya et al., 1998.

24. McKay et al., 1995; Tham et al., 1997; Kessing, 1998; van Gorp et al., 1998; Denicoff et al., 1999.

25. Lesser et al., 1993; Salloway et al., 1996; Dahabra et al., 1998; Kumar et al., 1998.

26. Hickie et al., 1995, 1997; Simpson et al., 1997a, 1998; Baldwin et al., 2000.

27. Steingart et al., 1987; Junqué et al., 1990; Cadelo et al., 1991; Baloh et al., 1995.

28. Dupont et al., 1987, 1990, 1995; Swayze et al., 1990.

29. Bejjani et al., 1999; Berney et al., 2002; Stefurak et al., 2003; Okun et al., 2004.

30. Terzian and Cecotto, 1959; Alema and Donini, 1960; Terzian, 1964; Rosadini and Rossi, 1967; Rossi and Rosadini, 1967.

31. Sackeim et al., 1983a, 1987b; Sackeim, 1999, 2004.

32. Engel et al., 1982; Rosenberg et al., 1988; Volkow et al., 1988; Silfverskiöld and Risberg, 1989; Nobler et al., 1994, 2001; Henry et al., 2001.

33. Wu et al., 1992, 1999; Mayberg et al., 1999; Teneback et al., 1999; Nobler et al., 2000a; Drevets et al., 2002.

34. Andersen et al., 1993; Benedek and Peterson, 1995; Jeret, 1997; McCullagh and Feinstein, 2000; Kaschka et al., 2001; Smith et al., 2003; House et al., 2004.

35. Hommes, 1965; Gainotti, 1970, 1972; Robinson and Szetela, 1981; Robinson et al., 1984; Narushima et al., 2003.

10 Personality, Personality Disorders, and Interpersonal Functioning

Those only, who lived for some time with [Lord Byron], could believe that a man's temper, Proteus like, was capable of assuming so many shapes. It may literally be said, that at different hours of the day he metamorphosed himself into four or more individuals, each possessed of the most opposite qualities; for, in every change, his natural impetuosity made him fly into the furthermost extremes. In the course of the day he might become the most morose, and the most gay; the most melancholy, and the most frolicsome . . . the most gentle being in existence, and the most irascible.

—Julius Millingen (Byron's physician), 1831

The intense emotions and troubling thoughts and behaviors of manic and depressive states often confound the person who has bipolar disorder and family members alike: What is due to the illness? What is due to personality? Where does one end and the other begin? Will treatment alter not only the disorder, but also personality? Do pathological mood states reflect the real self, or is there a coherent self despite the mood swings that characterize the disorder? Scientists and clinicians ask related questions: Are there unique and characteristic personality styles associated with bipolar disorder, and are they present when the person is not affectively ill? Are there predisposing or precursor "traits"? Do personality characteristics affect the course of the disorder? (Related questions concerning the mild forms of bipolar disorder that may be continuous with personality patterns are discussed separately in Chapter 2.)

Questions about "personality" are both personally meaningful and clinically and theoretically important because they may help shed light on the enormous variability among individuals with bipolar disorder and aid in achieving a fuller understanding of the disorder's development. Issues of personality have been addressed in various ways by psychologists and psychiatrists, and in the first section of this chapter we review both the complexities of the questions examined and the research results.

We next address the issue of personality disorders, the enduring and dysfunctional patterns of behaviors and traits defined by Axis II of the *Diagnostic and Statistical Manual* (DSM), that may accompany Axis I diagnoses of any kind. Personality disorders may profoundly color the experience of the coexisting psychological disorder, as well as affect both the clinical and social adjustment of the individual and the success of treatment. They have been the focus of many recent studies in the field of bipolar research, and the results of these studies may help inform patients and clinicians about how individuals with a diagnosis of bipolar illness can be so different from one another in presentation and prognosis.

Finally, we discuss the interpersonal functioning of individuals with bipolar disorder in major role areas, such as intimate relationships, social behavior, and family relations. There is increasing interest not only in the clinical manifestations of bipolar disorder, but also in the ways in which individuals with the disorder live their lives and cope with their condition. What are the unique interpersonal patterns and challenges for the bipolar patient, and what does the social milieu itself contribute to the understanding of the course of the disorder? Of particular importance is growing awareness of the discrepancies that sometimes exist between social functioning and clinical status.

Prior to DSM-III the term "manic-depressive illness" could either mean what we now call bipolar disorder or include all recurrent affective disorders. When the context of the older literature makes clear that it is referring to bipolar disorder, we use that term. Because the literature relevant to this chapter rarely distinguishes recurrent from nonrecurrent forms of unipolar depression, we focus on the bipolar subgroup of manic-depressive illness.

PERSONALITY AND BIPOLAR DISORDER

In this section, we begin by reviewing a number of conceptual and methodological issues associated with studies of the relationship between personality and bipolar disorder. We then examine, in turn, the findings of studies addressing personality during mania and depression, comparisons of two major dimensions of personality—neuroticism and extraversion–introversion—among remitted bipolar patients and normal groups, comparisons of the personality traits of bipolar and unipolar patients, effects of medication on personality, and predictive associations between personality characteristics and the development and outcome of bipolar disorder.

Conceptual Issues and Key Definitions

The terms *personality, character,* and *temperament* are sometimes used interchangeably. They differ in important ways, however.

Personality generally refers to the unique aspects of an individual, especially those most distinctive or likely to be noticed by others in social interactions. Personality theorist Gordon Allport (1961, p. 35) suggested that personality is simply "what a person 'really is' "—his or her most typical and deeply characteristic features. Yet there are as many psychological definitions of personality as theorists writing about the subject. Two prominent theorists summarized these many definitions succinctly as focusing on one or more of the following facets: "the individual's social stimulus value; the integrative or organizational function of personality; an individual's general adjustment; the unique or individual aspects of behavior; and the essence of man" (Hall and Lindzey, 1970, p. 8). In the absence of any universally accepted definition, most personality theorists define the construct by the assessment instruments they use to measure it. Clearly, some theories of personality lend themselves more readily to empirical research than others.[1]

Personality has traditionally been viewed as having several qualities: it is stable across time and situations; it encompasses an organized set of traits forming a coherent personality style; and it is the underlying psychological "cause" of a person's specific behaviors and beliefs. These assumptions have been challenged because we have learned that behaviors and beliefs are overtly and subtly determined by experiences, by current environmental demands, by cognitive capacities and styles, by genetic and constitutional factors, and certainly by affect and emotion. Nevertheless, researchers are increasingly attempting to account for the complexities involved by defining a few traits that can be used to describe most people and by taking into account the biological, temperamental features of personality and the environmental determinants that greatly shape its expression.

Character has been defined as "personality evaluated"—that aspect of an individual which bears a moral stamp and reflects the person's integrative and organizing functions. The concept of character is employed less frequently in the United States than in Europe, although it is often used interchangeably with that of personality. In part, the concept of personality disorder addresses the issue of a person's character traits.

Temperament has always been viewed as having a more constitutional, genetic, and biological basis than either personality or character. Hippocrates and Galen, for example, based their theories of temperament on the four humors of the body. According to Allport (1961, pp. 33–34), "Temperament refers to the characteristic phenomena of an individual's emotional nature, including his susceptibility to emotional stimulation, his customary strength and speed of response, the quality of his prevailing mood, and all peculiarities of fluctuation and intensity in mood, these phenomena being regarded as dependent upon constitutional make-up, and therefore largely hereditary in nature."

The affective temperaments that reflect the milder manifestations of the bipolar spectrum are discussed extensively in Chapter 2. Although there is overlap between the topics of personality and the bipolar spectrum, we attempt in this chapter to limit the discussion to several specific issues detailed in the following sections.

Relationship of Personality to Affective Disorders

Several researchers (Akiskal et al., 1983; Clark et al., 1994) have noted the complex relationship and interactions between personality and affective illness, especially depression. From their work and that of many others, four major models have been formulated:

- Personality is a *predisposition* to affective illness. This model assumes that personality patterns precede and therefore predispose an individual to develop affective illness. This view, fundamental to psychoanalytical thought and writing, also is reflected to varying degrees in the writings of cognitive and behavioral psychologists who have formulated various theories about predisposing characteristics for depression, such as negative views of the self and depressive attributional style. There is a relatively small literature on personality antecedents of bipolar disorder.
- Personality is an *expression* of affective illness. Personality patterns are viewed as manifestations of mild to moderate forms of the underlying affective illness. The individual's temperament is assumed to be intricately bound up with the genetic predisposition to mania and depression. This view, integral to the work of Kraepelin and Kretschmer, is shared in part by most of the modern researchers who posit a continuum of affective states (see Chapters 1 and 2).
- Personality is a *modifier* of affective illness. Many investigators (Chodoff, 1972; Klerman, 1973; von Zerssen, 1977) have emphasized the role of personality in determining the clinical presentation of affective symptom patterns (especially in obsessive, dependent, or hysterical person-

ality types), the response to psychotherapy and medication, the tendency to become dependent on alcohol or other drugs, and adherence to prescribed treatment regimens. They have also identified personality as an important determinant of the nature and extent of interpersonal relationships. These relationships, in turn, can affect both precipitating events and the likelihood of emotional support during and after affective episodes. The ability to handle the enormous stress and complications of affective illness is assumed to be strongly influenced by premorbid personality and character structure.

• Personality is *altered* by affective illness. In this model, personality is assumed to be altered by the experience of affective illness. Various consequences of the illness—including changes in self-esteem and social interaction patterns; difficulties in sustaining meaningful relationships and employment; and frequent fluctuations in mood, energy, perception, and thinking—are all thought to both cause and reflect short- or long-term personality changes that may be reversible or irreversible. The obvious importance and impact on personality of such illness variables as frequency, duration, severity, and nature of episodes have not been well studied.

These models of the association between affective illness and personality are not mutually exclusive, and they may be difficult to disentangle in practice. Moreover, research has not tested all of the models with respect to bipolar disorder, leaving many questions unanswered. Recent research has generally addressed several largely descriptive issues. One such issue concerns the stability of personality traits and whether they vary by manic or depressed state. A related issue is whether there are unique personality characteristics of bipolar patients that differ from those of unipolar depressed or well individuals. Still another set of issues has to do with the predictive association between personality features and clinical course. Before turning to a review of studies that address these matters, however, a further caution concerning methodological issues is in order.

Methodological Issues

In addition to the conceptual issues raised above, many specific methodological problems are intrinsic to the study of personality and bipolar disorder. The most central of these is the problem of *trait and state*, or disentangling manifestations of illness from the more stable and lasting structures of personality. Specific problems include the substantial difficulties of separating the current clinical state from measured personality traits, of assessing the effects of medications on personality (independently of their effects on the underlying affective illness), of sorting through the personality effects of previous manic and depressive episodes, and of delineating the effects of subclinical episodes on personality. Fundamental issues of measurement and philosophy emerge when two pivotal questions are posed. First, what aspects of personality are being studied when one is assessing the successfully treated person with bipolar illness—true premorbid ones or affectively changed and attenuated ones? Second, to what extent is personality a function of medication level or of the cumulative effects of disease?

Another set of problems concerns issues of *diagnostic and illness heterogeneity*. Heterogeneity is well recognized in the unipolar depressive disorders (in symptom patterns, etiology, severity, episodic patterning, and frequency). Although bipolar illness is more homogeneous, it, too, can be confusingly varied. Few investigations of personality distinguish between bipolar-I and bipolar-II, and fewer still consider other issues related to the full spectrum of bipolarity, such as the stage or severity of manic and depressive illness at the time of testing, the ratio of manic to depressive episodes, the age at illness onset, the frequency and nature of mixed states, the duration and patterning of episodes, and the characteristic nature of the manic episodes (euphoric and expansive, for example, rather than paranoid and dysphoric). All of these variables are likely to have both long- and short-term effects on the expression of personality. Other variables generally not controlled for in personality studies of affective illness include seasonal factors of importance to studies done during both remission and illness (see Chapter 4); the competence and sophistication of clinical care, including such common problems as prescribing incorrect medications or dosages; and selection factors intrinsic to the nature of remission studies—that is, a selection bias favoring healthier, more normal bipolar patients.

Measurement and design also are problematic. Until recently, comparison groups were inadequate. Early studies compared manic-depressive (predominantly bipolar) with schizophrenic patients; more recent studies have used unipolar depressed patients as controls. Studies using subjects from the general population as controls, although a clear improvement, too often have not controlled for family history of affective illness or for important demographic variables, such as age, IQ, socioeconomic status, and gender. Standard problems of measurement, such as the reliability and validity of the psychometric tests used, are well reviewed elsewhere. We note here, however, that much of the earlier research employed assessment methods based on questionable assumptions and validity (e.g., Rorschach), or on instruments that may no longer be widely used now that newer and more empirically and conceptually based approaches are available. In the sections to follow, older work is noted briefly, with greater emphasis on more contemporary methods.

Several study designs have been used to investigate personality and bipolar illness, including studies of patients across different mood states. In addition, comparisons have been made between affectively ill bipolar and unipolar patients, remitted bipolar and unipolar patients, and remitted bipolar patients and members of the general population. These design strategies are generally appropriate to address simple, descriptive questions, but more complex designs, including longitudinal studies, are greatly needed to pursue questions relating personality characteristics to the clinical and course features of bipolar disorder and social adjustment. Heterogeneity of comparison groups (for example, the tendency not to distinguish melancholic from nonmelancholic unipolar depression) is a significant problem (Parker et al., 2004).

Psychoanalytic Perspectives

Prior to the psychoanalytic era, most early clinical investigators assumed that personality structure in bipolar disorder reflected the underlying disease process.[2] Psychoanalytic theorists considered two major issues in their writings on manic-depressive illness: the etiology of mania and depression and the underlying personality structure of patients with bipolar illness. Most psychoanalysts focused primarily on the origins and nature of depression rather than mania. Their findings on this subject are well known and are not presented here. Instead, we briefly outline psychoanalytic concepts of mania and the manic-depressive personality. Although neither time nor research has supported the psychoanalytic perspective on bipolar illness, it is historically important, especially in the United States, because it deeply influenced generations of psychiatrists, psychologists, and social workers.

From a psychoanalytic perspective, mania can best be understood as a defense against underlying depressive affect. This fundamental concept has been stated in different ways by many authors.[3] Although interesting, the psychoanalytic perspective suffers from the usual difficulties involved in analyzing open-ended, clinical observations: such observations are retrospective, interpretative, and highly speculative. Comparison groups are lacking, and there are few, if any, ways of subjecting the theory to test. Finally, as (Kotin and Goodwin, 1972, p. 684) concluded from their data-based studies of mania:

> Our data suggest that if mania is a defense against depression, it is often an inadequate defense, since depressive symptoms remain prominent during the manic phase.

The manic-depressive personality has been viewed by psychoanalysts as narcissistic (Freud, 1917; Fenichel, 1945), masochistic (Gerö, 1936; Jacobson, 1953; Garma 1968), extraverted,[4] and highly conventional.[5] Rado (1928) discussed at length the belief that manic-depressive individuals have an "obsessive need for the approval of others."[6] Alexander (1948) described the manic-depressive individual as warm, outgoing, and practical—a person who prefers the concrete to the abstract. Not surprisingly, he noted a tendency for the emotions to rule reason. English (1949) characterized the manic-depressive patient as perfectionist, egocentric, logical, wise, talented, afraid to hate (except when manic), and rigid. Other writers (Dooley, 1921; Wilson, 1951; Cohen et al., 1954) highlighted somewhat different constellations of traits and the problems they pose for the therapist and others.[7] Obviously inadequate as an etiological model, what psychoanalysts have historically viewed as "personality" often appears from our modern perspective to be the expression of symptoms of bipolar illness.

Personality during Mania and Depression

Studies contrasting personality functioning during manic or hypomanic and depressive states often—not surprisingly—reveal dramatic differences. Rather than a core, stable personality as assumed by psychoanalytically oriented theorists, observations made during episodes reflect the powerful influence of fluctuating mood and energy levels, as well as behavioral changes, brought about by the illness.

Comparisons between Manic/Depressive Episodes and Periods of Remission

Bipolar patients tested during remission show clear changes relative to personality profiles obtained during depressive episodes. Early studies focused in particular on neuroticism as measured by Eysenck's (1959) Maudsley Personality Inventory (MPI) (e.g., Perris, 1971; Liebowitz et al., 1979; Hirschfeld et al., 1983). The majority of studies showed significant decreases in neuroticism during remission, as well as increases in extraversion. A review of the stability of neuroticism scores during clinical states of depression and remission (mainly among unipolar depressed patients) suggested that neuroticism captures two elements: (1) a depressive-state influence and (2) an underlying vulnerability dimension that predicts the development and severity of depression (Clark et al., 1994). Neuroticism has also been conceptualized as a general factor termed *negative affectivity*, defined as a temperamental sensitivity to stimuli associated with a range of negative emotional states, negative perceptions and expectations, and low self-esteem (Clark et al., 1994).

In a combined sample of bipolar and unipolar patients, Hirschfeld and colleagues (1983) found that impulsivity scores were unchanged from depression to remission, and that no state-dependent changes occurred in measures of rigidity, obsessionality, restraint, reflectiveness, demandingness, and dominance. They also found, however, that patients who had recovered from a depression scored lower than when depressed on measures of emotional lability, neuroticism, passivity, hypersensitivity, and interpersonal dependency and higher on measures of emotional strength, resiliency, and extraversion. For a subgroup of patients who had not recovered from depression at the time of follow-up, scores on the personality tests did not change, lending credence to the authors' interpretation that "the changes recorded for the recovered patients reflect the influence of the depressed state" (Hirschfeld et al., 1983, p. 698).

A few studies have examined personality profiles across all three major affective states: mania, depression, and euthymia. Researchers (Lumry et al., 1982) administered the Minnesota Multiphasic Personality Inventory (MMPI) to a small sample of bipolar-I patients. The MMPI profiles obtained from 12 patients when manic or hypomanic and from 10 of these patients when depressed were classic manic and depressive profiles. The mean profile for the 12 euthymic patients was entirely within normal limits. The mean MMPI profiles obtained during hypomania or mania and depression are shown graphically in Figure 10–1. The authors concluded that the normal profile pattern obtained during euthymia in most of their lithium-stabilized patients indicated "complete restitution of normality."

Perceptions of Self across Affective States

Widely discrepant views of the self emerge during mania, depression, and normal functioning. Indeed, these differences in self-perception have been incorporated into the DSM-IV diagnostic criteria for mania and depression ("inflated self-esteem or grandiosity" and "feelings of

worthlessness or excessive or inappropriate guilt," respectively). In an attempt to study alternating views of the self in depression and mania, Platman and colleagues (1969) administered the Emotions Profile Index weekly to 11 bipolar patients. This psychological measure was designed to assess eight primary emotions: fear, anger, acceptance, rejection, surprise, exploration, joy, and deprivation. Twelve staff members were asked to provide their conceptions of mania and depression. This collective profile was then compared with the profiles produced by patients while manic or depressed.

The staff's and patients' conceptions of depression were strikingly similar on all eight dimensions. For both groups, depression was characterized by decreases in sociability, in interest in new experiences, and in feelings of acceptance, as well as by increases in feelings of deprivation, in aggression, and in rejection of others. Mania, on the other hand, was perceived in very different ways by staff and patients, with seven of eight mean scores showing highly significant differences (at the $p < .01$ level). Patients while manic saw themselves as sociable, trusting, moderately impulsive, and cautious and not at all stubborn or aggressive. Staff members, however, saw them as only moderately sociable, somewhat distrustful, extremely impulsive and aggressive, quite rejecting of others, and completely incautious and unafraid. Response patterns from patients were far more variable than those from staff members, suggesting a more stereotypical (or accurate) view from the latter group.

Patients were asked, when normal, to recall their previous manic and depressive episodes. Their recalled depressive profiles were similar to those produced while actually depressed, and both resembled the staff-generated depressive profile. By contrast, profiles of recalled manic episodes did not resemble those actually obtained during mania. The patients' recall of mania was far more highly correlated with staff perceptions of mania ($r = .95$) than with their own ratings produced while manic ($r = .35$). The authors concluded:

> These facts imply that the self-critical judgmental process is severely impaired in the manic state but not in the depressed state. This is consistent with the well-known fact that manic patients do not usually admit to any illness, or that they deny the maladaptive nature of their behavior. This is also why it is difficult to detect the presence of manic states by means of self-description type inventories; these usually show that the manic patient is normal.

One interesting theoretical question posed by these findings is whether the manic patient is deliberately misrepresenting his feelings and behavior, or whether he is simply unable to discriminate the specific feelings and behaviors which are judged by an outside observer as pathognomonic of mania (Platman et al., 1969, p. 213).

Figure 10–1. Mean Minnesota Multiphasic Personality Inventory (MMPI) profiles of bipolar probands during a hypomanic/manic phase (blue circles; $n = 12$) and during a depressive phase (black circles; $n = 10$); 5 cases overlap. (*Source:* Adapted from Lumry et al., 1982.)

Jamison and colleagues (unpublished data) examined self-perceptions across affective states in 69 euthymic bipolar patients using the Semantic Differential, a combination of associational and scaling procedures. Patients were tested with 22 pairs of opposite adjectives (e.g., good–bad, strong–weak, complex–simple), shown as the polar ends of a seven-point continuum. Patients indicated their perceptions of themselves when manic, hypomanic, depressed, and normal by marking the most descriptive point between each polar pair. Analyses of variance by gender, with repeated measures of mood phase, were performed on the adjective pairs. The phase of illness affected virtually all pairs, indicating that changes in self-perception across the affective states of bipolar illness were consistent and widespread (Fig. 10–2). Statistical comparisons, conducted to identify significant differences between each pair of different mood phases, revealed a number of consistent patterns, particularly for the adjective pairs reflecting a positive–negative, or valuative, dimension.

For all these pairs, self-perceptions in the depressed phase were significantly more negative than those in the other phases. More interesting, for all except two pairs (serious–humorous and cautious–rash), the ratings for the hypomanic phase did not differ significantly from those for the euthymic phase. Compared with men, women rated themselves overall as less active and as more "cold" and "boring" during the depressed phase, and more "exciting" and "warm" during the manic phase. Women also perceived themselves as more changeable overall relative to men.

Of interest, men's and women's perceptions of their masculinity–femininity in various phases of illness also changed (not shown). Women felt less feminine and men less masculine in the depressed than in the euthymic phase; the opposite was true for the hypomanic and manic phases. In other words, depression had a neuterizing effect and hypomania or mania a polarizing or enhancing effect on sexual identity.

Figure 10–2. Perceptions of self in 69 bipolar patients as a function of affective state. Squares = normal state; diamonds = depressed state; circles = hypomanic state. (*Source:* Jamison et al., unpublished data.)

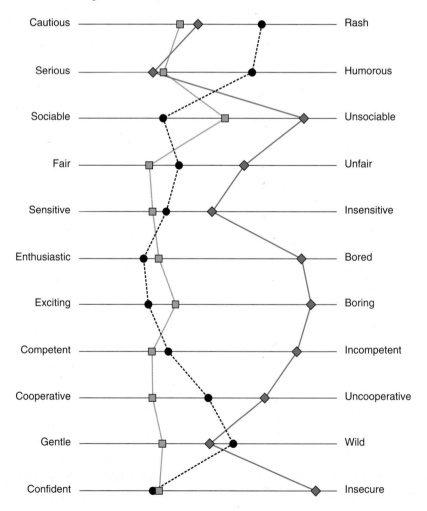

Throughout their bipolar cycles, patients underwent not only mood swings, but also substantial changes in their perception of self, self-esteem, energy expenditure, and interpersonal conduct. The study revealed that, as expected, bipolar patients had high self-esteem in the hypomanic or manic phase and low self-esteem in the depressive phase. Of more interest, self-esteem in the euthymic state did not differ substantially from that in the hypomanic phase. That is, bipolar patients generally held themselves in high regard; their apparently low self-esteem during the depressive phase was encapsulated, without perceived long-term adverse effects. Interpersonal conduct was perceived by patients to be less socially desirable in the hypomanic phase than during euthymia. Such findings are especially revealing in light of the common conception that bipolar patients are outgoing and socially engaging during their highs; this suggests that patients may have some insight into the one-sidedness of their social engagement in the manic and hypomanic phases.

Comparisons of Remitted Bipolar Patients and Normal Groups

Two major dimensions of personality—neuroticism and extraversion—have been compared between remitted bipolar patients and normal groups.

Neuroticism

Measures of neuroticism, typically using the MPI (or its later version, the Eysenck Personality Inventory [EPI]), identify significant differences between each pair of different mood phases (e.g., Clark et al., 1994). The neuroticism scale of the MPI/EPI is more likely to reflect changes in clinical state than is the extraversion scale. Several investigators have shown that neuroticism scores decrease following recovery in patients with endogenous depression (Crookes and Hutt, 1963; Coppen and Metcalfe, 1965; Ingham, 1966). In normal populations, neuroticism and extraversion are independent factors, but in psychiatric patients, the correlation between the two is usually quite high.

Eysenck and colleagues (Eysenck and Eysenck, 1963a,b) have defined neuroticism as "a largely inherited lability of the autonomic nervous system" and as a general measure of emotionality. Its principal components include mood swings, a sense of inferiority, poor emotional adjustment, lack of social responsibility, suspiciousness, lack of persistence, social shyness and hypochondriasis, and lack of relaxed composure. Moodiness, which has the single highest loading on the neuroticism factor in the EPI, is illustrated by positive answers to the following sample items: "Do you sometimes feel happy, sometimes depressed, without any apparent reason?" "Are you inclined to be moody?" and "Do you have frequent ups and downs

in mood, either with or without apparent cause?" Because of this measure of affective lability, the construct has frequently been investigated as a potential indicator of bipolar disorder.

Only one of several early studies[8] comparing neuroticism scores on the MPI/EPI found significant differences between remitted bipolar patients and normal populations (Hirschfeld and colleagues [1986] found lower neuroticism among never-ill relatives of bipolar patients than among the patient group). This apparently anomalous finding was replicated in a more recent study conducted within the same program (the Collaborative Program on the Psychobiology of Depression). Solomon and colleagues (1996) compared 30 individuals diagnosed with bipolar-I disorder who were first-degree relatives or spouses of the patients in the Hirschfeld study and 974 never-ill relatives. They found that the bipolar patients, who were currently in remission, scored significantly higher on neuroticism than did the controls. Thus although most of the early studies indicated no stable traits of elevated neuroticism for remitted bipolar patients, results of more recent investigations suggest that some samples of such patients may in fact show elevated levels of the trait.

Extraversion–Introversion

As with neuroticism, the primary psychological measure of the extraversion–introversion dimension used in research on affective illness is the MPI/EPI. Extraversion was originally characterized in the MPI/EPI by impulsivity (typical item: "Are you inclined to be quick and sure in your actions?") and sociability (typical item: "Would you be very unhappy if you were prevented from making numerous social contacts?"). In normal populations, impulsivity and sociability correlate at 0.5, producing a second-order factor of extraversion. More recently, impulsivity has been recognized as a separate factor, and it is not included in contemporary assessments of extraversion. Thus there may be some discrepancy between results of older and newer studies (Watson et al., 1994). Introversion can be further subdivided into social introversion (characteristic of those who prefer not to have much social contact with others) and neurotic introversion (characteristic of those who are afraid to have contact with others and are basically unsure of themselves and their interpersonal competence) (Eysenck, 1956). Just as neuroticism has been conceptualized as negative affectivity (as discussed earlier), extraversion has been conceptualized as positive affectivity—a stable, heritable, temperamental trait (Clark et al., 1994).

Based on the typical conceptualization of extraversion, many researchers have expected to find greater levels of this trait among bipolar patients. The authors of the MPI/

EPI (Eysenck, 1959; Eysenck and Eysenck, 1963a,b) described a typical extravert as one who:

> [is] sociable, likes parties, has many friends, needs to have people to talk to . . . craves excitement, takes chances . . . is generally an impulsive individual . . . [is] easy going, optimistic . . . prefers to keep moving and doing things . . . and [loses] his temper quickly.

A typical introvert, on the other hand:

> [is a] quiet, retiring sort of person, introspective, fond of books rather than people . . . reserved and distant except to intimate friends . . . tends to plan ahead . . . distrusts the impulse of the moment . . . does not like excitement . . . likes a well-ordered mode of life . . . keeps his feelings under close control . . . does not lose his temper easily . . . [and is] reliable, somewhat pessimistic.

As noted earlier, the extraversion–introversion scale of the MPI/EPI, unlike the neuroticism scale, is relatively impervious to the effects of mood or clinical state. Most studies comparing extraversion in remitted bipolar patients and normal individuals have found no significant differences between the two groups. One study of 45 bipolar patients, using the Cattell 16 Personality Factor Inventory, reported that remitted bipolar patients were more extraverted than the general population (Popescu et al., 1985). Two studies, however, found remitted female bipolar patients to be less extraverted (more introverted) than published norms or never-ill relatives (Hirschfeld, 1985; Hirschfeld et al., 1986). There was no significant difference for men (Hirschfeld et al., 1986).

Cyclothymia and Hyperthymia

Several investigators have found that an underlying cyclothymic temperament is particularly associated with bipolar-II disorder (Hartouche et al., 1998; Benazzi and Akiskal, 2005), as well as being elevated in healthy relatives of bipolar probands (Mendlowicz et al., 2005). Other investigators have confirmed Kraepelin's observation of a high rate of hyperthymic temperament in both bipolar-I and bipolar-II patients (Cassano et al., 1992; Perugi et al., 1998), although the interpretation of this observation is confounded by the fact that elevated rates of hyperthymic temperament have been demonstrated in control subjects as well (Evans et al., 2005; Matsumoto et al., 2005; Mendlowicz et al., 2005). Other researchers have found that individuals with bipolar disorder score significantly higher than controls on measures of novelty seeking (a tendency to seek out new situations, to be curious and impulsive, a trait discussed further in the next section) (Cronin and Zuckerman, 1992; Young et al., 1995; Nowakowska et al., 2005). A similar elevation in novelty-seeking behavior has been shown to occur in pediatric bipolar patients and in the offspring of bipolar patients (Chang et al., 2003).

In summary, there are few significant differences between remitted bipolar patients and normal individuals on the two most frequently assessed personality dimensions, neuroticism and extraversion–introversion. Other studies that have included different measures of personality traits have also failed to find significant differences (e.g., Lepkifker et al., 1988). However, Solomon and colleagues (1996) found that the bipolar-I group scored significantly lower than never-ill controls on measures of emotional stability, ego resiliency, and ego control. They cautioned that their comparison group had been screened for absence of psychopathology, whereas prior disorders may not have been ruled out for control groups in other studies. They also noted that nearly 50 percent of their bipolar group had a history of substance abuse. The results of early studies require caution as well because their samples were small, and probably differed as to the extent of their predominance of mania and depression, as well as their social role functioning. Thus some samples of bipolar patients may indeed differ from normal controls during remission, perhaps depending on the composition and clinical features of the sample. In particular, it is likely that elevated neuroticism and introversion characterize those with prominent depressive episodes. (See Savitz and Ramesar, 2006, for an excellent review of personality research in bipolar disorder.)

Significant differences are found between bipolar patients and controls on measures of temperament. Several studies have found that cyclothymia and novelty seeking are more elevated in bipolar samples.

Comparisons of Bipolar and Unipolar Patients

Of historical interest in the pursuit and eventual recognition of the unipolar–bipolar distinction was a series of studies conducted in the 1970s comparing depressed unipolar and bipolar patients. Donnelly and colleagues (e.g., Donnelly and Murphy, 1973, 1974; Donnelly et al., 1976) found several differences between the groups: when acutely depressed, bipolar patients exhibited a greater social desirability response set with more "normal" profiles and less neuroticism, less impulse control, and less anxiety relative to unipolar patients. Many other studies found that unipolar patients scored higher in the direction of neuroticism and low self-esteem, or emotional instability.[9] Two studies using alternative measures of neuroticism concluded that bipolar patients were more neurotic than unipolar patients (Abou-Saleh and Coppen, 1984; Popescu et al., 1985). However, many studies that specifically pursued comparisons of unipolar and bipolar patients in remission on neuroticism using the MPI/EPI failed to show differences between the groups.[10]

In several studies of extraversion using the MPI/EPI[11] and two using the extraversion factor from the Cattell 16 Personality Factor Questionnaire (Murray and Blackburn, 1974; Popescu et al., 1985), remitted bipolar patients scored higher on extraversion than did remitted unipolar patients. More recent and more tightly designed studies also found that remitted bipolar patients scored significantly higher on extraversion than remitted unipolar patients (e.g., Sauer et al., 1997; Janowsky et al., 1999). Preliminary findings suggest that not only bipolar–unipolar differences but also differences between bipolar subtypes may be associated with specific temperamental and personality profiles. Akiskal and colleagues (2006) administered a large battery of self-report personality scales to 78 bipolar-I, 64 bipolar-II, and 251 unipolar patients, all remitted. Most of the bipolar-I patients described themselves as essentially normal in emotional stability and extraversion, and they scored low on measures of neuroticism. In contrast, both the bipolar-II and unipolar patients scored high on neuroticism, although in the bipolar-II subgroup, the neuroticism scores were elevated as a result of mood lability, while in the unipolar group, the elevation was due to subdepressive traits. Two studies (Bech et al., 1980; Hirschfeld et al., 1986) found no significant differences in extraversion between the two groups. Hirschfeld and colleagues (1986) found no significant bipolar-unipolar differences in women, but they did find that bipolar men scored higher on extraversion measures than did unipolar men. Three studies of dominance, a closely related personality factor, found that bipolar patients were more dominant than unipolar patients (Strandman, 1978; Abou-Saleh and Coppen, 1984; Popescu et al., 1985).

A more recent comparison of depressed unipolar and bipolar patients failed to find greater "normality" in the bipolar group (Wetzler et al., 1995). In general, across testing with the MMPI and the Millon Clinical Multiaxial Inventory-II (MCMI) (Millon, 1987), few consistent differences were observed. Bipolar patients scored higher on indicators of narcissism, antisocial behaviors, and compulsive personality style, but Wetzler and colleagues (1995) noted that such elevated scores could be due to residual aspects of mania, such as grandiosity.

Cloninger (1987) developed a personality assessment system (the Tridimensional Personality Questionnaire [TPQ]) purporting to link heritable temperaments with underlying brain monoaminergic pathways. Three dimensions—harm avoidance (HA; pessimistic and shy versus carefree and outgoing), reward dependence (RD; sentimental and tender-hearted versus insensitive and practical), and novelty seeking (NS; curious and impulsive versus stoical and orderly) are presumed to relate to, and perhaps predict, forms of psychopathology.

A consistent finding in the literature, for example, is an association between elevated HA and unipolar depression (Strakowski et al., 1992), even during remission. Strakowski and colleagues (1993) found that bipolar patients, by contrast, scored significantly lower on HA than did unipolar depressed patients, and did not differ from controls. Young and colleagues (1995) suggested, however, that the patients in the Strakowski sample were not recovered from mania at the time of testing, and they therefore undertook a study of carefully defined "remitted" bipolar patients compared with recovered unipolar patients and controls. They found no significant differences between unipolar and bipolar patients on HA, and both patient groups had significantly higher HA than did the controls. Bipolar patients scored significantly higher on the NS scale than did unipolar and control subjects. The results suggest that HA may be a nonspecific indicator of mood disorders (perhaps like neuroticism), whereas NS may be more specific to bipolar disorder. The cross-sectional design of the Young et al. study makes it impossible to determine whether the traits result from manic episodes, are subsyndromal symptoms, or represent premorbid personality characteristics. There is suggestive evidence that bipolar patients with an earlier age at onset are more harm avoidant (Engström et al., 2003). A recent study of type A behavior in 23 bipolar-II and 42 unipolar patients found that the bipolar patients had significantly higher scores, largely attributable to greater impatience, time urgency, and irritability (Oedegaard et al., 2006).

Another study employing the TPQ compared 50 bipolar patients considered to be euthymic with U.S. norms. Like Young and colleagues (1995), Osher and colleagues (1996) found that the patients had significantly elevated scores on HA, as well as on RD, including the "persistence" subscale of RD. Unlike Young's group, however, Osher and colleagues found no differences on NS.

Overall, few general conclusions can be drawn. Although bipolar patients in remission may differ from unipolar patients on extraversion, there is little indication that they are "healthier" than unipolar patients, and there is mixed evidence on normalcy during remission compared with well controls. Inconsistencies in study findings derive in part from heterogeneity among populations (due to use of differing diagnostic or inclusion criteria), variations in type and degree of illness (including manic/depressive states and response to treatment, as well as degree of recurrence within unipolar patients), inconsistent criteria for "remission," and inclusion or exclusion of patients with "double depressions" (concurrent major depressive episode and dysthymia). The search for descriptive differences therefore appears unproductive, at least at this point in time, and more interesting questions of prediction and the implications of various traits are increasingly the focus of research, as discussed in the next section.

Predictive Associations between Personality Features and Clinical Outcome

Premorbid Traits and Vulnerability

Although the topic of premorbid traits and vulnerability is a well-developed area of research in unipolar depression, it is rarely addressed in bipolar samples, perhaps because of the general assumption of a genetically based biological predisposition to bipolar disorder. Nevertheless, as suggested in Chapter 2, there may be early traits that portend the development of bipolar illness, or characteristics that might be viewed as risk factors given the appropriate biological vulnerability. An obvious research strategy would be assessment of premorbid characteristics, ideally in longitudinal studies involving subjects who are at high risk by virtue of having one or both parents with bipolar disorder. As indicated in Chapter 6, however, such work is in its infancy.

Although several studies have attempted to evaluate personality characteristics or subsyndromal symptoms of mood disorders,[12] there is little consensus on the best methods and instruments to use for the purpose. Several early studies identified personality traits associated with high-risk children: aggressiveness (e.g., Worland et al., 1979; Kron et al., 1982); extraversion, introversion, and impulsiveness (Kron et al., 1982); and sensation seeking (e.g., Nurnberger et al., 1988). Long-term follow-up studies are needed to determine whether such traits predict eventual bipolar disorder in high-risk populations. One such study of premorbid functioning was conducted by Clayton and colleagues (1994), who reviewed military records of performance on the Freiburg Personality Inventory of men who were later diagnosed with bipolar disorder. No differences in premorbid personality were observed as compared with controls who did not develop bipolar disorder.

Temperament and Vulnerability

As noted earlier, neuroticism may be conceptualized as a broad temperamental construct of negative affectivity, which has been linked empirically to general emotional distress (anxiety and depression) reflecting both current mood state and vulnerability to developing depression (Clark et al., 1994). Extraversion, conceptualized as positive affectivity, may be predictive of depression (with low positive affectivity being associated with depression and introversion). Persons with high positive affectivity/extraversion "feel joyful, enthusiastic, energetic, friendly, bold, assertive, proud, and confident," whereas those with low positive affectivity/introversion "tend to feel dull, flat, disinterested, and unenthusiastic" (Clark et al., 1994, p. 107). While low positive affectivity/

introversion has been linked to depression, other theorists have recently proposed that high positive affectivity/extraversion may be linked to a biologically based approach system that activates behavior in response to signals for reward—also called the behavioral activation system (Gray, 1982). According to Depue and Iacono (1988), the behavioral activation system is similar to what they term the behavior facilitation system, which they believe underlies bipolar disorder. The latter system is believed to include locomotor behavior, incentive motivation, interest and alertness, and level of pleasure or excitement seeking. Poor regulation and the tonic level of the system have been speculated to predict mood disorders and their specific manifestations. Depue and colleagues (1994) also proposed a link between temperament and neurotransmitter functioning, and found preliminary evidence of an association between dopaminergic functioning and positive emotionality. The association among positive affectivity, bipolar temperament, and emotional resilience was addressed at length by Jamison (2004).

Johnson and colleagues developed a polarity-specific model of mood states and hypothesized that behaviors and traits consistent with the behavioral activation system may differentially predict manic symptoms (see, e.g., Johnson et al., in press). They specifically tested the hypothesis that extraversion and achievement striving would predict manic symptoms over time in bipolar-I patients, whereas neuroticism would predict increases in depressive symptoms (Lozano and Johnson, 2001). Using a version of the NEO Five-Factor Inventory (Costa and McCrae, 1992) that includes all of these constructs, Lozano and Johnson (2001) followed 39 bipolar patients over a 6-month period. Controlling for initial manic symptoms, they found that achievement striving predicted increased manic symptoms (although extraversion did not); likewise, controlling for initial depressive symptoms, they found that level of neuroticism predicted increases in depression. Thus their findings provided some support for their polarity-specific model.

Partially consistent data were obtained by Strakowski and colleagues (1993) in investigating their hypothesis regarding recovery from first-episode mania among 27 bipolar patients. They found that, although personality measures in the form of TPQ scores did not predict time to clinical recovery, *functional* recovery (which was uncorrelated with symptom status) was predicted by level of novelty seeking on the TPQ. Novelty seeking was significantly higher among those who failed to attain premorbid levels of adjustment, a finding consistent with the view that this dimension reflects impulsiveness and pleasure seeking. The authors noted, however, that they could not rule out the possibility that high scores on novelty seeking reflected subsyndromal symptoms. (Although bipolar patients score higher than unipolar patients on novelty seeking, Parker and colleagues

[2004] made the critical point that the heterogeneity among unipolar depressed patients is a confusing and confounding source of inconsistency in studies.)

An additional predictive study, by Carpenter and colleagues (1999), examined the association between neuroticism and affective symptoms, self-confidence, and marital satisfaction among a sample of married bipolar patients. Using the NEO Five-Factor Inventory of personality (Costa and McCrae, 1985), administered when the patients were not in an episode, they found that greater neuroticism predicted more severe illness during the 2 years before entry into the study and during the first year of treatment, worse Global Assessment Scale (GAS) scores during treatment, and lower self-confidence. Neuroticism also predicted Axis II (personality disorder) dimensional scores. Of interest, extraversion—but not neuroticism—predicted marital distress. The authors noted that in general, the personality scores were not especially deviant as a group, although there was considerable variability; they also observed that extremely high neuroticism scores could be indistinguishable from personality disorder.

Effects of Medication on Personality

Evidence for a strong effect of medication on personality functioning relates almost entirely to lithium and comes from several sources: studies of lithium's effects on normal subjects; prima facie evidence derived from both clinical and systematic observation of the drug's profound effects on behavior, mood, and personality in affectively ill patients; and comparisons of personality studies completed in the prelithium era with those completed after lithium treatment became widespread. Results of the latter studies indicate that personality differences between bipolar patients and other groups pale considerably, and often entirely, when lithium is used effectively.

We raise here several important philosophical and treatment issues. Does lithium make the personality of a bipolar individual revert to pre-illness levels, or does it decrease variability in mood and personality functioning beyond those levels? Does lithium create an abnormally stable personality and mood system? To what extent is personality in lithium-treated patients a function of blood level? Does a patient who is inadequately treated with or only partially responsive to lithium show premorbid personality or subsyndromal disease? How does lithium's influence on personality affect medication adherence?

Several authors have examined the effects of lithium on personality function in normal subjects. Schou (1968) was the first to describe systematically the cognitive, behavioral, and personality effects of the drug in normal people. At relatively low blood levels, lithium had minimal effects on personality functioning in medical student volunteers.

In three researchers taking lithium at higher levels, however, effects were more pronounced. They noted occasional hypersensitivity but also decreased responsivity to their environment, increased indifference and malaise, greater passivity, and cognitive changes (discussed further in Chapters 12 and 21). Judd and colleagues (1977a), studying lithium's effects on normal male volunteers, found that in addition to reporting a mood-lowering effect, their subjects cited less inclination and desire to "deal with the demands of the environment." Normal men studied by Kropf and Müller-Oerlinghausen (1979) showed, while on lithium, decreased social involvement, activity, and concentration, as well as increased boredom and lethargy. When White and colleagues (1979) administered the Profile of Mood States (POMS) to 10 normal volunteers treated with lithium, the subjects reported a reduced sense of well-being and fewer social interactions; they also complained of fatigue, anxiety, lack of initiative, and decreased efficiency. In an indirect measure of lithium's ability to attenuate emotional responsiveness, Belmaker and colleagues (1979) found that, while taking lithium, neither normal subjects nor patients experienced the predicted increased heart rate generally caused by participation in cognitive tasks. Both of these studies, although intriguing, were relatively short-term trials (1–3 weeks and 2 weeks, respectively), and there is some indication that longer periods of time on lithium result in at least partial accommodation to some of these effects.

The most clear-cut influences of lithium on bipolar personality were evident in personality studies done on euthymic, lithium-stabilized patients. Additionally, a few studies have examined personality and mood stabilization over time in lithium-treated, affectively ill patients. Bonetti and colleagues (1977) administered the EPI and the Marke-Nyman Temperament Scale to 33 recurrent (minimally three episodes) unipolar and 28 bipolar patients at the end of the index episode and at least 3 months later. They found that personality changes were more pronounced in the bipolar patients, especially on measures of sociability, initiative, and impulsiveness. Neuroticism scores decreased most dramatically within the unipolar group (test–retest differences, $p < .001$). The authors speculated that lithium both reduced symptoms and altered habitual patterns of personality, such as high activity levels and impulsiveness in bipolar patients and anxious–neurotic traits in unipolar patients.

In an interesting and important study of the relationship between lithium blood level and personality change, Kropf and Müller-Oerlinghausen (1985) conducted a double-blind study of lithium dose reduction (20 percent) in 14 long-term lithium-treated patients (5 unipolar, 9 bipolar), all of whom were euthymic when tested. Eleven patients (3 unipolar, 8 bipolar) maintained at their regular lithium levels served as controls. The patients receiving higher levels of lithium tended to be less active, less obsessive, and less elated. Specifically, those taking lower levels of lithium scored higher on Von Zerssen's measures of initiative and assertiveness ($p < .05$) and of social resonance (social acceptance and assertiveness), transparency (social openness and sensitivity), and social potency (sociability and "ability for devotion"). However, a significant proportion (29 percent) of the patients in the experimental group became affectively ill at a reduced lithium level.

Mood stability in lithium-treated patients, although not a direct measure of personality, clearly is related to personality functioning. Folstein and colleagues (1982) administered the Visual Analogue Mood Scale (VAMS) for 30 days to 65 euthymic bipolar patients on chronic lithium therapy and to 36 nonpatient control subjects. The mean mood ratings for the two groups were similar; the patients, however, reported significantly less mood variability. The authors attributed this unusual degree of mood stability to the effects of lithium treatment and suggested that euthymic patients might view this change as an undesirable aspect of lithium therapy. DePaulo and colleagues (1983) administered the VAMS to 17 euthymic bipolar patients and 21 nonpatient controls. Like Folstein and colleagues (1982), they found that the mean mood ratings were similar in the two groups and that the patients' moods were less variable than those of the controls. Three bipolar patients were studied separately, during and after lithium treatment. Two became manic, and the third, who remained euthymic while off lithium, showed markedly increased variability in daily mood ratings. The authors were uncertain whether these results reflected baseline differences in reporting between affectively ill patients and normal controls, lithium's therapeutic effects, or a medication effect.

PERSONALITY DISORDERS

Axis II (personality) disorders occur relatively frequently in clinical populations (with a range of about 5 to 40 percent, varying by personality disorder type) (Widiger and Rogers, 1989). Although epidemiologic studies of personality pathology in community samples have been infrequent and limited in scope, Weissman's (1993) review of such studies suggests that the population prevalence is 10 to 23 percent. Researchers have raised the question of the rates of personality disorders in bipolar samples and explored the correlates of Axis II pathology.

Early studies of the comorbidity of personality disorder with bipolar illness were hampered by methodological shortcomings, such as shifting diagnostic criteria for assessing Axis II disorders, assessment methods of uncertain validity, unclear or mixed samples of bipolar patients (e.g.,

comingling bipolar-I and -II), and small patient samples. A particularly serious problem was the failure to evaluate bipolar patients during euthymic states, so that reported "personality disorders" may have reflected largely mood state–related symptoms rather than stable underlying personality pathology.

Table 10–1 presents recent studies that attempted to verify bipolar-I diagnoses in patients while making an effort to control for mood state at the time of the assessment of Axis II disorders. For the most part, these studies used validated structured interview methods for assessing personality disorders. The samples included outpatients as well as inpatients, and those of varying ages and social/cultural circumstances. However, these studies employed relatively small samples, and some failed to control for other comorbid conditions, such as substance abuse. It is important to note that age at onset of bipolar disorder has not been explored (see Chapter 6), and early age at onset may be a significant predictor of Axis II symptomatology. Moreover, many of the studies were based on samples in tertiary care treatment, and may therefore reflect relatively more severe or complex cases of bipolar disorder.

Despite the significant variability in sample characteristics among these studies, however, they yield evidence of rates of comorbid personality disorders that, although relatively consistent with those of other diagnostic groups in clinical populations, exceed the rates in the general population. Several studies involved a unique sample not generalizable to the overall population of persons with bipolar-I disorder; for example Kutcher and colleagues (1990) included only adolescents, Carpenter and Hittner (1995) only married patients, and Kay and colleagues (1999) only male veterans. Overall, the rates of personality disorders across all the samples ranged from 22 to 62 percent, as listed in Table 10–1.

According to the studies reported in Table 10–1, somewhat higher rates of personality disorders were found among bipolar patients who had experienced more previous episodes and those who had a history of alcohol abuse, and when self-report questionnaires or informant reports (rather than clinician interviews) were used as the basis for symptom assessment. At least two studies found an association between greater levels of depressive symptoms and personality disorders (Brieger et al., 2003; George et al., 2003). One additional study—not included in the table because it appears to have combined bipolar-I, bipolar-II, and cyclothymic patients in unknown proportions—found that participants with dysthymia or bipolar disorder were more likely to have personality disorders (70 percent) than patients in treatment for other disorders, such as anxiety disorder (Flick et al., 1993). A recent study of young adults with affective illness found significantly higher median levels of

Table 10—1. Personality Disorders in Bipolar-I Patients

Study	Sample	Method	Clinical State	Comparison Group	Overall Rate[a] (%)	Most Common Diagnoses
Kutcher et al., 1990	20 adolescents/outpatients[b]	Personality Disorders Examination (PDE) (interview)	Euthymic		35	Borderline, narcissistic
Pica et al., 1990	26 inpatients (16 bipolar-I, 10 bipolar schizoaffective)	Structured Interview for DSM-III Personality Disorders (SIDP-III)	Current symptoms not controlled	33 patients with schizophrenia	62	Histrionic, antisocial, borderline
O'Connell et al., 1991	50 outpatients	Personality Diagnosis Questionnaire-Revised (PDQ-R)	Current symptoms not controlled but "stable"		58	Borderline, histrionic
Carpenter et al., 1995	23 outpatients (married or cohabiting)	PDE	Few or no current symptoms		22	Dependent, borderline, obsessive-compulsive
Peselow et al., 1995	66 patients	Structured Interview for DSM-III-R Personality Disorders (SIDP-III-R)	Interviewed when manic or hypomanic, then again when euthymic		53 manic or hypomanic, 45 euthymic	Borderline, schizoid, histrionic
Dunayevich et al., 1996	33 first-episode, 26 multiple-episode inpatients	Structured Clinical Interview for DSM (SCID-II)			48	Avoidant, Cluster B (mixed)[c]
Barbato and Hafner, 1998	42 outpatients	International Personality Disorders Examination (IPDE) (interview)	"In remission"		45	Histrionic, borderline, avoidant, compulsive
Ucok et al., 1998	90 outpatients	SCID-II	Euthymic	58 normal controls	48 bipolar patients, 16 controls	Histrionic, compulsive, paranoid
Kay et al., 1999	61 Veterans Affairs (VA) outpatients	SCID-II PDQ-R	Euthymic	Compared patients with and without history of alcohol abuse disorder	38[d]	Cluster A, Cluster C[c]
Brieger et al., 2003	60 inpatients	SCID-II NEO Five Factor Personality Inventory	"Mostly in remission"	117 unipolar depressed inpatients	38 bipolar, 51 unipolar	Compulsive, narcissistic, borderline
George et al., 2003	52 outpatients	PDE	"In remission"		29	Histrionic, compulsive

[a]Estimates of personality disorders in general clinical populations range from 5 to 40 percent (Widiger and Rogers, 1989), and in community samples from 10 to 23 percent (Weissman, 1993).

[b]There were no differences in rates of Axis II disorders between bipolar-I and schizoaffective patients, so the authors combined the groups in their analysis.

[c]Cluster A: paranoid, schizoid, schizotypal; Cluster B: antisocial, borderline, histrionic, narcissistic; Cluster C: avoidant, dependent, obsessive-compulsive.

[d]Highest in patients with history of alcohol abuse.

borderline characteristics in the bipolar patients than in those with major depression (Smith et al., 2005). Three of the borderline characteristics differentiated bipolar from unipolar depression: "I've never threatened suicide or injured myself on purpose"; "I have tantrums or angry outbursts"; and "Giving in to some of my urges gets me into trouble." A study of 40 bipolar-II patients (Vieta et al., 1999) found that 33 percent met diagnostic criteria for a personality disorder. Overall, therefore, the typical bipolar patient sample appears to have relatively high rates of Axis II comorbidity.

Table 10–1 also indicates the most frequent individual personality disorder diagnoses. A number of studies found multiple disorders in bipolar patients, as is generally typical of diagnoses on Axis II. Viewed individually, however, the Cluster B disorders—especially borderline and histrionic—were most common among the bipolar samples. Rossi and colleagues (2001) also reported high rates of borderline as well as compulsive personality disorders; however, their bipolar sample included only those with recent depressive episodes, excluding those with recent mania.

Despite the general consistency in frequency and types of personality disorders observed across studies, the meaning of the results remains elusive. Conceptually, it is widely recognized that rates of comorbidity may be inflated because of the overlap of symptoms across disorders. Despite various efforts to assess for personality pathology during euthymic states, it is nonetheless possible that the personality disorders reported may reflect the symptoms of hypomania or depression. For instance, histrionic or borderline pathology may be difficult to distinguish from attention seeking, intense or exaggerated emotional expression, intense irritability, impulsive or provocative behaviors, and affective instability and rapidly changing mood. (See MacKinnon et al., 2006, for an excellent review of the centrality of affective instability to both bipolar illness and borderline personality disorder.) Peselow and colleagues (1995), comparing personality pathology assessed in the same patients during hypomania and euthymia, found a reduction in such pathology when the patients had recovered from the hypomanic state. Thus personality pathology may be inflated as a result of overlapping symptoms in Axis I and II categories containing manic, mixed, and depressive symptoms and behaviors.

A related conceptual question, noted previously, is the issue of whether personality pathology may be a consequence of bipolar disorder. Thus, for example, the unstable self-image or identity disturbance or the recurrent suicidal or parasuicidal behaviors of the borderline personality may be a reaction to the cumulative unpredictable and massively destructive mood swings of bipolar illness. It is possible that the onset of bipolar disorder in childhood or early adolescence may exacerbate identity difficulties

and impair the ability to form solid and sustaining relationships, thereby contributing to diffuse Axis II symptomatology. Thus the maladaptive behaviors reflected in personality disorders may in some cases be dysfunctional coping methods or adaptations to the illness.

A third conceptual consideration concerns sampling: patients included in the studies reported in Table 10–1 may reflect those who are most disturbed, and who are seen in research-oriented settings that may draw more difficult patients not readily managed in community or private care. As noted, clinical samples in general (compared with epidemiologic samples), and especially those in tertiary care settings, may not be representative in terms of comorbidity because they are likely to be sicker.

Finally, as discussed in Chapter 3, some would argue against conceptualizing Axis II disorders as conditions comorbid with bipolar disorder. Instead, it is argued, they may represent forms of disorder in the bipolar spectrum (e.g., Akiskal et al., 1985, 2000; Deltito et al., 2001). Gunderson and colleagues (2006) recently reported the results of a 4-year prospective investigation of 196 patients with bipolar disorder and 433 patients with personality disorders. They found that bipolar-I and bipolar-II disorders were significantly more common in patients with borderline personality disorder (19.4 percent) than in patients with other types of personality disorder (7.9 percent). The presence of co-occurring bipolar disorder had no significant effect on the course of the borderline personality disorder, as measured by remission rates, functional adjustment, or treatment utilization rates (hospitalization and medication usage). The investigators concluded that there was only a modest association between bipolar disorder and borderline personality disorder, "thereby making a strong spectrum relationship with bipolar disorder extremely unlikely" (p. 1177). We do not know enough at the present time to draw firm conclusions on this question.

Despite uncertainty about the conceptualization of personality disorder comorbidity, one meaning of comorbid Axis II pathology is not ambiguous: bipolar (or any psychiatric) patients who have personality pathology typically have worse outcomes. Kay and colleagues (2002) found significantly lower rates of employment, more complex medication regimens, and greater likelihood of substance and alcohol abuse among bipolar-I male veterans who had diagnosed personality disorders (but no differences between the groups in age at onset or duration of disorder). Over time, Carpenter and colleagues (1995) found that patients with personality disorder had significantly more symptoms and worse social adjustment scores than those without such disorder. Others have also found this to be the case (Bieling et al., 2003). Kutcher and colleagues (1990) found that adolescent bipolar patients without personality disorder had a better response to lithium treatment.

Although Ucok and colleagues (1998) did not find differences in lithium responsiveness among their bipolar patients with and without personality disorder, they did find that patients with Axis II comorbidity had made more severe suicide attempts. Barbato and Hafner (1998) found that bipolar-I patients with personality disorder had significantly more lifetime days hospitalized and more severe symptomatology than those without personality disorder, and were more likely to report that their medications were "unhelpful." Others (Dunayevich et al., 1996) have reported that patients with multiple episodes were more likely than first-episode patients to have personality disorder. Moreover, in a 12-month follow-up of these patients, those diagnosed with personality disorder were less likely to show syndrome or symptom recovery and had achieved significantly less functional recovery (Dunayevich et al., 2000). The authors speculated that poor medication adherence may mediate the link between personality disorder and poor outcome (see Chapter 21). Poor adherence, in turn, may reflect poorer response to treatment. Finally, Vieta and colleagues (1999) reported that those in their bipolar-II sample with personality disorder had earlier age at onset of bipolar disorder and more severe suicidal ideation. In general, these findings are consistent with those of research on other psychiatric populations, indicating that, whether true "comorbidity" is involved or mainly more severe general symptomatology, patients with Axis II disorders typically have worse illness course and are more difficult to treat effectively.

INTERPERSONAL FUNCTIONING

No one has the slightest idea of what I've been through with Cal [Robert Lowell]. In 4½ years, counting this present breakup, he has had four collapses! Three manic, and one depression. These things take time to come and long after he is out of the hospital there is a period which can only be called "nursing." The long, difficult pull back—which does not show always to others. I knew the possibility of this when I married him, and I have always felt that the joy of his "normal" periods, the lovely time we had, all I've learned from him, the immeasurable things I've derived from our marriage made up for the bad periods. I consider it all a gain of the most precious kind. But he has torn down this time everything we've built up . . . how difficult these break-ups are for both of us. (Elizabeth Hardwick[13])

Moods are by nature compelling, contagious, and profoundly interpersonal. Mania and depression alter the perceptions and behaviors not only of those who have them, but also of those who are related or closely associated. Bipolar illness—marked as it is by extraordinary and confusing fluctuations in mood, personality, thinking, and behavior—inevitably has powerful and often painful effects on relationships. Violence, poor judgment, and indiscreet financial and sexual behavior are almost always destructive and embarrassing to spouses, children, family members, and friends. Trust is not easily restored in the wake of mania, nor are goodwill and love always regenerated after months of severe, depleting, and unremitting depression.

Mood-related changes in interpersonal functioning are not the whole story, however; increasing evidence points to persisting social, marital, and family difficulties even when individuals are not in the throes of an episode. Such impairments in interpersonal relationships may affect subsequent clinical functioning in a complex, reciprocal pattern. In this section, we review issues and studies concerned with bipolar patients and their relationships with other people. It should be emphasized that the studies reviewed focused exclusively on the impaired functioning associated with symptoms and episodes. As is typical of most psychopathology studies, little research has been conducted on aspects of marital and family functioning that may be associated with positive moods and behaviors, such as optimism, energy, and infectious enthusiasm (Jamison, 2004).

Social Functioning

Impairment during Mania and Depression

The complex, subtle, and potentially infuriating aspects of manic interpersonal behavior were observed by most early clinical investigators (see Chapter 1). Hypomanic behavior, especially, was noted for its powerful and confusing influence on others. The positive, engaging, and occasionally charismatic qualities of many individuals with bipolar illness are discussed at length in Chapters 2 and 12. Here we describe some of the more detrimental interpersonal features of bipolar illness.

Kraepelin (1921, p. 61) wrote of the skill of hypomanic patients in manipulating fellow patients:

It is just the peculiar mixture of sense and maniacal activity, frequently also an extensive experience of institutions, which makes them extremely ingenious in finding out means to satisfy their numerous desires, to deceive their surroundings, to procure for themselves all kinds of advantages, to secure the property of others for themselves. They usually soon domineer completely over their fellow-patients, use them for profit, report about them to the physician in technical terms, act as guardian to them, and hold them in check.

Psychoanalytic writers, with rare exceptions, regarded the interpersonal lives of bipolar patients as unstable and chaotic, narcissistically based, bereft of empathic regard for the rights of others, too dependent or independent, singularly rigid, and full of rage. These conclusions are not surprising given that they were based substantially on experiences with patients in the prepharmacotherapy era. Understandably, such perceptions led most psychoanalysts to be wary of and reluctant to treat these patients. Since the psychoanalytic relationship with bipolar patients was seen as superficial and distant, countertransference was the subject of considerable discussion and writing about such patients (see Chapter 22). Most psychoanalytic writers were interested primarily in the origins of the illness and the personality structure of bipolar patients, but we present here a brief review of their observations and interpretations of interpersonal behavior.

Abraham (1911, 1924), one of the earliest writers to formulate psychodynamic principles in bipolar illness, described what he perceived to be the patients' abnormal character development and inability to maintain good relationships. These features, he speculated, were coupled with an ongoing sense of impending loss of objects, which produced a "rageful" stance toward these objects and their inability to "gratify narcissistic demands." Freud (1917), for the most part, concurred: "Manic-depressives show simultaneously the tendency to too-strong fixations to their love-object and to a quick withdrawal of object cathexis. Object choice is on a narcissistic basis."

The attitude of bipolar individuals toward others was described by Blalock (1936, p. 342) as "a selfish one serving in its several aspects the narcissistic needs of the patient." Equally critical in his views, Fenichel (1945) regarded bipolar patients as "love addicts," narcissistic, and incapable of love. To English (1949, p. 131), the bipolar patient was egocentric, incapable of relating warmly to others, rigid, afraid to hate except when manic, and powerfully influenced by the intensity of feelings:

> The manic-depressive is afraid of extremes of emotion, of great love, or of hostility, and yet these are the very things he may show in his illness. One patient . . . said, "To live is like opening all my pores on a cold day and subjecting myself to a catastrophe." The manic-depressive therefore has a defect in catching the feelings of others. He ignores what others feel and want as long as he can. Thus in trying to avoid being hurt he avoids the strengthening influence of friendship.

Fromm-Reichmann (1949), in a similar vein, described a "lack of subtlety," a "lack of any close interpersonal relatedness," and a tendency to exaggerate the intensity of interactions with other people. While describing manic-depressive

patients as manifesting a "particular kind of narcissistic dependency on their love objects," Jacobson (1953, p. 66) provided a perspective at variance with that of the earlier psychoanalytic writers:

> We are also surprised to see that as long as they are not sick, they may be delightful companions or marital partners, a feature that Bleuler mentioned especially. In their sexual life they may show a full . . . response, and emotionally, in contradistinction to schizoid persons, a touching warmth and unusual, affectionate clinging to people they like . . . [they] are potentially able to function extraordinarily well.

Cohen and colleagues (1954, p. 119), however, commented on what they viewed as the illusion of normal relationships in manic-depressive patients:

> The appearance of closeness is provided by the hypomanic's liveliness, talkativeness, wittiness, and social aggressiveness. Actually, there is little or no communicative exchange between the hypomanic and any one of his so-called friends. . . . The concept of reciprocity is missing; the needs of the other for similar experiences are not recognized.

Finally, Gibson and colleagues (1959, p. 1,102) stressed the dependent nature of the manic-depressive patient—the difficulties in dealing with feelings of envy and competition and the "common use of denial as a defense, there being a notable lack of subtlety, and of awareness of their own or the feelings of others in their interpersonal relations."

Janowsky and colleagues (1970, 1974), in an attempt to measure more objectively the interpersonal behavior of patients during the manic phase of their illness, assessed the interactional style of acutely manic patients with tape recordings of psychotherapy sessions (both group and individual), physician and social worker notes, observations of milieu therapy, and nurses' behavioral descriptions and ratings of patients. The manic person's interpersonal maneuvers are, according to these authors, "simultaneously cementing and distancing." Although their study presumes too much conscious control and manipulation on the part of the patient, it is one of the few clinical reports to describe in detail the interpersonal behavior of hospitalized manic patients. We quote, as an example, from their work on the manic patient's perceptiveness with regard to vulnerability and conflict (Janowsky et al., 1970, p. 254):

> Intimately related to the manic's ability to appeal to the self-esteem systems of others is his extraordinary perceptiveness. In interpersonal encounters, the manic possesses a highly refined talent for sensing an individual's vulnerability or a group's area of conflict, and exploiting this in

a manipulative fashion. This sensitivity may be utilized in dealing directly with a given individual or in focusing on areas of conflict between others. In either case, the manic patient is able to make covert conflicts overt, causing the person or group with whom he is dealing to feel discomfort. . . . What he says cannot be dismissed as untrue or unreal, for the areas attacked truly do exist and, indeed, are areas of vulnerability.

The playful, high-energy, and extraverted behaviors associated with mania are often irritating. So, too, are the interpersonal qualities usually present during depression. Interviews with roommates of college students identified by clinical assessments as falling in the bipolar spectrum (cyclothymia as well as bipolar-I or -II) found that bipolar students were perceived as excessively excitable, showed poor judgment, were argumentative when hypomanic, and were irritable and socially withdrawn when depressed (Depue et al., 1981). It is not surprising, given the number of negative social behaviors exhibited by the bipolar students, that 58 percent of the roommates reported that they avoided the subject, finding him or her "noxious."

Fluctuations in levels of sociability almost define bipolar illness. Energetic seeking out of other people and uninhibited social behavior are common features of mania. Winokur and colleagues (1969, p. 63) described this in their monograph:

A most characteristic sight when the patient is brought to the hospital is a frightened and exhausted family, which has frequently been awake for 1 or more nights being lectured to by a bright-eyed and excited patient.

In their study of 30 bipolar patients, Murphy and colleagues (1974) found two distinctive behavioral characteristics of mania: noticeably increased psychomotor activity and, of relevance here, a need for increased interpersonal contact ("people seeking"). Akiskal and colleagues (1977) reported that half of their cyclothymic patients alternated periods of uninhibited people seeking with periods of introverted self-absorption.

During depressive episodes, maladaptive patterns of relating to others are common, including social withdrawal, loss of enjoyment and pleasure, irritability, increased criticism of and negativism toward others, and sensitivity to criticism or rejection by others (see Chapter 2; Benazzi, 2000). Depressed people are often highly dependent on others for reassurance and support, yet appear paradoxically to reject the support or view it as untrustworthy and insufficient. Friends and family may be frustrated by the exaggerated dependence of the depressed patient, especially when they seem unable to relieve his or her despondency. Moreover, the depressed person may be particularly sensitive to perceived rejection or criticism, and minor or even nonexistent slights are exaggerated or interpreted inaccurately. All of these common symptoms of depression can thwart the best intentions and efforts of friends and family members.

Interpersonal tension may be further intensified by the depressed individual's marked guilt and feelings of worthlessness and self-blame for real or perceived negative social encounters. Indeed, when depressed, individuals may correctly perceive that they are a burden to others, a reality that may serve to heighten their depression (e.g., Coyne et al., 1987). Moreover, depression tends to elicit negative reactions even from strangers or acquaintances; many studies (reviewed in Gurtman, 1986) have demonstrated that others tend to reject depressed persons and express preferences for avoiding interactions with them.

Impairment despite Remission and Treatment

Compared with the clinical states and symptomatology of individuals with bipolar disorder, relatively little attention has been devoted to understanding social and interpersonal aspects of the disorder. Increasingly, however, research supports prior clinical observations of the extent to which social impairment persists even during stable, euthymic periods. For instance, Cooke and colleagues (1996) identified a sample of bipolar patients who were euthymic as well as free of recent substance abuse, personality disorder, or medical illness. The patients were administered the self-report functioning scales of the Medical Outcomes Study, and their results were compared with those previously obtained for a large number of individuals in treatment for a variety of chronic medical illnesses. Cooke and colleagues found that the bipolar patients scored lower on social functioning than did the medically ill patients. Similarly, Romans and McPherson (1992) interviewed remitted bipolar-I patients about their social functioning, and found that they scored significantly lower on availability and perceived adequacy of close relationships and had significantly fewer general social contacts and interactions than did a random community sample. A recent multicenter European study of 144 remitted bipolar patients found that, compared with normal subjects, patients were less well adjusted in general and, more specifically, in their leisure activities, relationships with extended family, marital relationships, and work activities (Blairy et al., 2004).

A study comparing outpatients in treatment for schizophrenia or bipolar disorder found that the two patient groups showed relatively similar levels of cognitive and social impairment on a battery of measures (Dickerson et al., 2001). Although the schizophrenic patients generally performed worse on most measures, the bipolar group was nearly as impaired. However, the clinical state of the bipolar patients at the time of testing was not specifically noted. Coryell and colleagues (1993) reported on 5-year follow-ups of patients from the National Institute of Mental Health (NIMH) Psychobiology of Depression sample, including 148 bipolar patients. Both unipolar and bipolar probands showed deficits in their relationships with friends, children, and relatives, and they also displayed less involvement in and enjoyment of social and recreational activities compared with non-ill controls. Although Coryell and colleagues did not report on the clinical status of the bipolar probands during the follow-up period, they noted that the majority were being treated for their disorder. Thus despite treatment and variations in the course of the disorder, the bipolar patients fared relatively poorly compared with matched controls. It may be noted that several studies comparing unipolar and bipolar probands on social functioning have yielded inconsistent results, probably because of variability in clinical histories, mood states during assessment, premorbid functioning and temperament, age and demographic factors, and methods of measuring interpersonal functioning.[14]

Overall, therefore, it appears that bipolar disorder is associated with a variety of general indicators of social impairment. Even when the individual is not in an affective episode, these interpersonal difficulties appear to persist. The direction of causality remains unclear, however. Are the maladjustments in social functioning due to bipolar disorder, or might they be related to clinical variables such as comorbid substance abuse or early age at onset? In the following sections, we review research addressing the predictors of social functioning and the predictive relationship between social functioning and subsequent clinical status.

Clinical Predictors of Social Functioning

The relatively sparse literature aimed at understanding the conditions under which bipolar disorder is associated with good or poor interpersonal functioning is also limited by relatively small samples, varying definitions and methods of assessing functioning, and a narrow range of potentially key variables. Nevertheless, these studies provide intriguing glimpses of issues warranting further study.

O'Connell and colleagues (1991) evaluated predictors of general functioning in 248 bipolar patients using the GAS. Several variables correlated with outcome and were evaluated in a multiple-regression equation. Number of prior admissions was the strongest predictor, followed by family attitudes and social class. Family attitudes of hostility and criticism imply poor interpersonal relationships in the family, suggesting in turn poor general functioning associated with interpersonal difficulties. Bauwens and colleagues (1991) explored correlates of social adjustment in 27 remitted bipolar patients. They found that a composite overall measure of social adjustment was significantly related to

episode frequency, and poorer social/leisure activity was associated with more episodes and hospitalizations. Scores on depression symptomatology were also associated with lower levels of social/leisure activity.

Several studies have found that depression is more linked to difficulties in functioning than is mania. In a study aimed at exploring the mutual influence of social and clinical functioning, Gitlin and colleagues (1995) evaluated the impact of both past episode history and subclinical symptoms on indicators of social functioning in a sample of 82 bipolar patients followed for at least 2 years. Social (close relationships) and family functioning were significantly related to number of past and recent depressive episodes but not to manic or hypomanic episodes. In all the analyses, subclinical symptoms were more strongly predictive of poorer social functioning than was number of clinical episodes. The researchers also determined that depressive episodes were significantly more (negatively) predictive of the quality of relationships with family members than were manic episodes, with a similar trend toward a greater association of depression with social (close) relationships. In contrast, occupational functioning was negatively associated with both depressive and manic episodes.

A recent review and investigation of functional outcomes in bipolar patients revealed depression to be one of the few fairly consistent predictors of social, family, and marital (as well as occupational) functioning (Bauer et al., 2001). This study is noteworthy for its careful assessment of symptoms and functioning over 48 weeks in a sample of 43 male Veterans Affairs outpatients. The amount of time depressed and average depression symptom scores—but not mania scores—were significantly correlated with social and work functioning. Other researchers (Cooke et al., 1996) also found that bipolar patients' low scores on social functioning were associated with subclinical depressive symptoms (subclinical mania/hypomania was not assessed), and social functioning was lower in bipolar-II than in bipolar-I patients. Different investigators (Romans and McPherson, 1992), in contrast, found that a subgroup of patients with a predominantly manic course reported less adequate close relationships and less available social contacts than did those with depressive episodes, although the effect was not statistically significant. Perhaps consistent with the previously cited studies, Romans and McPherson found that patients with a longer history of illness reported fewer close and general social contacts.

A study of 40 bipolar-I patients' social functioning (Lam and Wong, 1997) included ratings of relationships with intimate partners and friends and "social presentation." The investigators evaluated recognition of prodromes of mania and depression and scored the patients' reports of how they coped with prodromal symptoms of depression and mania. Generally, those with good awareness of pro-dromal symptoms and good coping methods had better overall social functioning. A multiple-regression analysis to predict overall social functioning indicated that lower current subclinical depression scores and good reported coping with prodromes of mania and depression signifi-cantly predicted good functioning, whereas number of past hospitalizations and current subsyndromal manic symptoms did not.

Social Predictors of Clinical Outcomes

The question of the origins of and contributors to social ad-justment in those with bipolar disorder takes on particular urgency in view of studies now beginning to demonstrate a functional link between social and clinical outcomes. As ev-idence accumulates of enormous variability in the clinical course of bipolar disorder, even in those who are adequately or aggressively treated pharmacologically,[15] studies have in-creasingly been exploring predictors of diverse clinical out-comes by including social variables.

Among recent longitudinal outcome studies, several in-dicate the importance of interpersonal functioning. Table 10–2 summarizes several studies of social predictors of clin-ical outcomes in patients with bipolar disorder. In all of these studies, patients were in treatment, and many of the studies controlled for medication adherence. The studies differ considerably in the social functioning variables as-sessed, but they are consistent in finding that indicators of interpersonal adjustment play an important role in clinical outcomes, independently of clinical history factors. Note that several of the studies found social impairment to be es-pecially predictive of depressive symptoms. Coryell and col-leagues (1998) hypothesized that a "prevailingly depressive subtype" of bipolar patients may mark a particularly poor prognosis group with considerable social dysfunction.

Several of the studies listed in Table 10–2 identified family discord or negative family attitudes toward the patient with bipolar disorder as a predictor of worse clinical outcomes (Miklowitz et al., 1988; see also O'Connell et al., 1991). Re-search on the effect of family attitudes (particularly those of the caretaker or spouse) on the course of bipolar disorder, including "expressed emotion" and related constructs, is re-viewed below in the section on marital functioning.

A particular focus of several of the studies in Table 10–2 is the role of the quality and availability of social support in predicting clinical outcomes among individuals with bipolar disorder. Generally, social support refers to individuals' per-ceptions of the extent to which others are available to pro-vide emotional and material assistance and to their satisfac-tion with the perceived supportiveness offered by others. O'Connell and colleagues (1985) found that a global mea-sure of social support was the strongest correlate of clinical outcome, social adjustment, and overall GAS score. Other researchers (Stefos et al., 1996) found that social support and social functioning variables predicted outcome, but clinical factors did not. They observed that 69 percent of patients with good social support, compared with 25 percent of those with low support, remained episode-free during a 4-year period of assessment. Similar results have been reported more recently.[16] Of interest, several investigators[17] have found the effects of social support to be polarity-specific, with lower social support at baseline predicting more in-crease in depressive symptoms over time, but no significant association with changes in manic symptoms was found. The relationship between social support and clinical out-come is complicated by the likelihood that support is more likely to be given to those who are less overtly or chronically ill. It may well be that patients who experience primarily eu-phoric manias or hypomanias garner more support than those who have predominantly mixed states. This issue has not been adequately addressed in the research conducted to date. Clearly, premorbid functioning and temperament are relevant, albeit poorly studied, factors in predicting how in-dividuals will cope with their illnesses and maintain or de-velop personal relationships.

Conceptualization and Methodology

Although the studies discussed above generally indicate a link between clinical and interpersonal functioning, there is clearly a need for more exploration of the origins of poor or good social functioning. One promising pattern concerns the role of depression, with most studies indicat-ing an association between depressive symptoms and so-cial functioning. While several studies suggest that depres-sive symptoms may be especially impairing, however, the specific contributors and features of social functioning are not known. For instance, do symptoms prevent individu-als from engaging in social relationships and activities, or do symptoms affect the quality (and eventually the avail-ability) of such pursuits? Do symptoms emerge subclini-cally during developmentally important periods of life to an extent sufficient to impair normal acquisition of social skills and attributes, or are the social impairments conse-quences of repeated episodes that devastate the individ-ual's coping capacities?

There is a need to explore the origins of social impair-ments, as the question of whether they predate or follow bipolar episodes is unresolved. The topic of "premorbid social adjustment," although well established in schizophre-nia research and a potent predictor of disorder and func-tioning, is relatively less well studied in bipolar samples. An exception is the work of Cannon and colleagues (1997), who clearly demonstrated that the social functioning of bipolar patients when they were children and adolescents

TABLE 10–2. **Social Predictors of Clinical Outcomes**

Study	Sample	Significant Predictors of Poorer Outcome
O'Connell et al., 1985	60 bipolar-I outpatients	Episode intensity–duration score over a 1-yr period was correlated with less social support and worse social adjustment scores. Social factors were correlated more strongly with outcome than were demographic or clinical variables.
Miklowitz et al., 1988	23 bipolar inpatients	Relapse during a 9-mo follow-up was associated with family negative expressed emotion and negative interactions (affective style). Social variables predicted outcome independently of demographic and clinical factors.
Gitlin et al., 1995	52 bipolar-I outpatients	Relapse over a mean follow-up period of 4 yr was associated with both clinical features (prior episodes) and worse social adjustment. Strongest associations were between depressive symptoms and prior depressive episodes and poor family and social functioning.
Stefos et al., 1996	14 bipolar-I and 7 bipolar-II patients	A higher rate of major recurrences over a 4-yr follow-up period was associated with less social support, impaired social and leisure activities, and poor quality of relationships with the extended family, but clinical predictors were not significant.
Coryell et al., 1998	113 bipolar (with mania) inpatients and outpatients	Depression at 15-year follow-up was predicted by poor social (functional) adjustment before the study and persisting depression in the first 2 yr of follow-up. Earlier manic symptoms were generally unrelated to functional or clinical outcomes at 15-yr follow-up.
Kulhara et al., 1999	118 bipolar-I outpatients	A higher rate of recurrence over the follow-up period was associated with more depressive episodes before lithium treatment, more life events, and less social support.
Johnson et al., 2000	59 bipolar-I patients	Longer time to recovery over a 2-yr follow-up period was associated with lower social support. Depressive symptoms over time were predicted by life events and lower social support, but manic symptoms were not predicted by lower social support or stressors.
Johnson et al., 2003	94 bipolar patients	Those who relapsed over a 12-mo follow-up period had significantly lower perceived social support. Those with lower perceived support were also more likely to have partial rather than complete remission before relapse.
Cohen et al., 2004	52 bipolar-I outpatients	Episode recurrence over a 1-yr follow-up period, after controlling for clinical variables, was predicted by low social support and life events. Depressive episodes were more strongly predictive than manic episodes.

(continued)

TABLE 10–2. **Social Predictors of Clinical Outcomes** (*continued*)

Study	Sample	Significant Predictors of Poorer Outcome
Kim and Miklowitz, 2004	125 bipolar outpatients (116 bipolar-I, 9 bipolar-II)	Patients from families with high expressed emotion (EE) relatives did not experience higher rates of relapse over 2-yr follow-up, but they did experience higher levels of depression.
Yan et al., 2004	47 bipolar-I outpatients	High EE in collaterals (romantic partners, parents, friends) predicted depressive but not manic recurrence. After controlling for prior symptom severity, patients with high EE were five times more likely to have a depressive recurrence than those with low EE.

(as reported retrospectively by their mothers) was significantly worse than that of normal comparison subjects of similar age. Appropriate social behavior, quality of peer relations, and pursuit of interests appeared to be impaired in the prebipolar lives of patients. It is unclear, however, whether these individuals were actually symptomatic at young ages. Moreover, variability in reported adjustment suggests differing subgroups, including some with exceptionally good functioning. Such patterns warrant further study—as does clarification of the role of childhood disorders (see Chapter 7) in later social adjustment.

In view of the apparent impact of depressive symptoms on social adjustment, it may be noted that research on unipolar depression is focused increasingly on interpersonal functioning. Social variables are seen as playing a role in vulnerability to onset of the disorder and in the prediction of relapse, recurrence, and chronicity, and also as resulting from the impact of depression on the relationships of the depressed person with others. A large body of research has begun to document the role of social factors in depression, presumably operating both as cause and consequence of the disorder (e.g., reviews in Hammen and Brennan, 2002; see also Joiner and Coyne, 1999). This research may provide guidelines for further studies of bipolar samples.

There is a related need for further study of the specific effects of depression and mania on interpersonal relationships. Are there conditions under which manic and hypomanic symptoms portend decrements in social connections, as appears to be the case with depression? Or can they under some circumstances facilitate social contacts and friendships? Can the optimism and positive affectivity often associated with bipolar patients who have an underlying hyperthymic temperament lead to more opportunity for relationships that may prove to be sustaining and meaningful?

Marriage

I am tired of papering over the cracks and pretending to friends and relatives that life is wonderful. It is the nearest and dearest who come in for the bulk of the barrage.... It is the Jekyll and Hyde syndrome. I never know which is going to walk in through the door, and the unpredictability is most unnerving. It is like living on a knife-edge. You can never relax or take anything for granted and any thought of lapsing into "placid serenity" is completely out of the question. (Anonymous[18])

To understand some of the important clinical as well as research issues that arise in addressing the topic of bipolar disorder and marital relationships, a brief discussion of research on unipolar depression and marital functioning is useful. This is followed by a review of descriptive studies of bipolar disorder and marital functioning and a consideration of the complex and reciprocal relationship between marital and clinical functioning. The section ends with a review of the literature on sexual behavior in bipolar illness, assortative mating among bipolar patients, and effects on marriage of treatment of bipolar spouses.

Unipolar Depression and Marital Functioning

There has been considerable research on depression and marital functioning in recent years, corresponding to a growing focus on the interpersonal causes and consequences of depression, as well as the development of effective psychotherapies aimed at treating interpersonal and marital dysfunction in depressed individuals. Two themes and sets of findings in particular are potentially relevant to bipolar disorder.

First, the phenomenology of depression may contribute to problematic marriages. Weissman and Paykel (1974) were among the first to characterize the marriages of depressed women as fraught with friction, inadequate communication, dependency, overt hostility, resentment and guilt, poor sexual relationships, and a lack of affection. For both men and women, depressive symptoms such as irritability, loss of energy and enjoyment, heightened sensitivity to criticism, and defeatist and pessimistic attitudes all may erode the initial concern and patience of the spouse. The depressed person's exaggerated negative interpretations of self, the world, and the future may seem irrational and inexplicable, while an unwillingness to engage in typical or enjoyable pursuits and unresponsiveness to encouragement may be frustrating to the spouse and may even appear to reflect willfulness or resistance. Spouses and partners often are especially troubled by the restrictions on social and leisure activities and by the depressed person's withdrawal, worry, and suicidal thoughts (e.g., Coyne et al., 1987; Fadden et al., 1987).

As Coyne (1976) noted, there may be a deteriorating marital process in which initial concern and caring by the spouse is eventually replaced by resentment and impatience—reactions likely perceived by the depressed person as rejection and lack of sympathy, provoking further depression. As might be expected, observed communications between depressed individuals and their partners are characterized by relatively more negativity and fewer positive interactions than those of nondepressed couples (Johnson and Jacob, 1997). Such patterns have been found to be particularly pronounced among depressed women compared with depressed men (Gotlib and Whiffen, 1989; Johnson and Jacob, 1997). Over time, depression in a spouse may be perceived as a significant burden, and may even cause distress and symptoms in the nondepressed spouse (Coyne et al., 1987). Not surprisingly, depressed individuals are less likely than nondepressed controls to be married, and if they are married, they are more likely to divorce or to report the marriage as being of poor quality (Fadden et al., 1987; Coryell et al., 1993; Whisman, 2001).

A second set of findings in the unipolar field that is salient for bipolar disorder indicates that depressive episodes often result from environmental precipitants, among which marital conflict and difficulties may be especially common and potent. For example, Weissman (1987) noted a 25-fold increase in the relative risk for major depressive episodes among those in unhappy marriages, based on Epidemiological Catchment Area data for 3,000 respondents (see also Brown and Harris, 1986; Coryell et al., 1992; Anderson et al., 1999). Thus the consequences of depression for relationships may include the creation of a context that is stressful and unfulfilling, contributing to increased risk for further symptomatology.

The self-perpetuating cycle of depression and marital distress may be further complicated by some individuals' vulnerabilities in the form of maladaptive dependency or the need for frequent reassurance, dysfunctional skills in resolving interpersonal problems and conflicts, and maladaptive mate selection (Hammen, 1997, 1999). Moreover, there is evidence that the impaired interpersonal relationships of depressed persons may not be confined to periods of depression. For instance, several studies have shown that even in remission, formerly depressed patients and community members continue to show social impairment, including marital dissatisfaction and conflict (Weissman and Paykel, 1974; Billings and Moos, 1985; Hammen and Brennan, 2002).

The link between depression and marital distress may be reciprocal: some individuals may be particularly vulnerable to developing depressive reactions because of dysfunctional needs and skills with regard to intimate relationships. As suggested earlier, increased recognition of the link between depression and marital distress has led to the development of several therapeutic approaches based on addressing marital difficulties as a way to treat depressive disorders. Interpersonal psychotherapy (Klerman et al., 1984; Weissman et al., 2000) and behavioral marital therapy (Beach and Jones, 2002), for example, have proven successful both in reducing depression and in improving marital functioning.

Bipolar Disorder and Marital Functioning

The marriages of untreated, inadequately treated, or treatment-nonresponsive bipolar patients tend to be turbulent, fluctuating, and uncertain. An overall clinical description was given by Janowsky and colleagues (1970, p. 259):

> Diametrically opposed styles of marital relating, occurring during depressed or manic phases respectively, seem intolerable to the spouse. The depressive phase is usually viewed by the spouse as an illness over which the patient has little control. Here, spouses offer significant physical care and emotional support. The patient, during the depressive phase, often expresses much guilt and self-blame and sometimes speaks of the spouse in laudatory and absolving terms. . . .
>
> In contrast, the attitude of the spouse undergoes a marked change when the patient is manic. The manic phase is perceived as a willful, spiteful act. Lip service only is given to seeing the mania as an illness. There is always an underlying feeling that the manic can control his actions, and does not do so out of maliciousness, selfishness, and lack of consideration. This impression is fostered by the fact that the manic often has periods of seeming reasonableness. . . .
>
> Related to the issue of the spouse feeling betrayed and experiencing diminished self-esteem is the problem of marital infidelity. Often, manic patients speak of divorce, make sexual advances to other people, become engaged in affairs. . . .

> In all these situations, the spouses felt trapped in what they perceived as an impossible situation. They felt caught in a whirlwind of activity, personally threatened, powerless to enforce limits. . . . Their moods and feelings were intimately related to the disease state of the sick partner.

Not all would agree with this characterization of spousal perceptions. Nevertheless, the turmoil associated with marriage to someone who undergoes unpredictable severe mood shifts clearly is highly stressful and challenges the coping capabilities of the partner. As we shall see, the attitudes expressed within the intimate relationship may also create conditions that may influence the course of bipolar illness.

At present, research on and conceptualization of marital functioning is less well developed for patients with bipolar disorder than for those with unipolar depression. Some of the earliest bipolar studies simply compared the marital functioning of unipolar and bipolar patients, yielding mixed findings as to which group had the "worse" outcomes (Janowsky et al., 1970; Brodie and Leff, 1971; Ruestow et al., 1978). The more crucial questions, however, concern marital functioning in treated patients, the impact of clinical features of bipolar disorder on intimate relationships, and effects of the quality of relationships on outcomes among bipolar patients.

Studies of treated patients provide ample but perhaps unsurprising evidence that marital functioning is often impaired among those with bipolar disorder. For instance, in one of the largest follow-up studies (5 years) of bipolar patients, Coryell and colleagues (1993) found that 148 such patients were only half as likely to be married by the end of the follow-up period as matched well controls (32 percent never married, compared with 15 percent of controls). Those who had married were twice as likely to be divorced as controls (45 percent divorced, compared with 18 percent of controls). Similarly, the Stanley Foundation Bipolar Network reported rates of divorced/separated or single status exceeding U.S. national norms (Suppes et al., 2001). It should be noted, however, that there is no evidence of higher divorce rates among those with bipolar disorder than among those with unipolar depression.

Corresponding to the high rates of divorce and reduced frequency of marriage among bipolar patients, couples in which one spouse is bipolar commonly report dissatisfaction. Several studies have obtained such information from the patient. For instance, Radke-Yarrow (1998) interviewed bipolar women in a study of offspring and family interactions. She found that women with bipolar disorder (a mix of bipolar-I and -II) reported higher rates of marital disorder at all follow-up assessments (62 to 76 percent) compared with non-ill women (7 to 13 percent) or women with

unipolar depression (53 to 59 percent). She speculated that psychiatric illness in many of the fathers of bipolar women may have contributed in part to the high rates of marital discord. Bauwens and colleagues (1991) collected Social Adjustment Scale information on 27 remitted bipolar, 24 remitted unipolar, and 25 control individuals. They found that bipolar patients scored midway between the unipolar (worst) and control (best) subjects in overall marital adjustment. Frequency of hospitalizations per year tended to be correlated with poorer marital adjustment, but there was no indication of the specific features of the course of illness that might have a particular association with marital difficulties.

A limited number of studies have examined the perceptions of spouses of bipolar patients. Hoover and Fitzgerald (1981) compared reported marital interactions of 42 bipolar and depressive inpatients and their spouses with those of 30 normal couples from the community. Using the 67-item Conflict in Marriage Scale (designed to measure resolution of conflicts, ways of dealing with anger, and content of disputes), they found that couples with an affectively ill spouse scored significantly higher on expressed conflict than did the community controls. Within the affectively ill group, couples with a bipolar-I member expressed more conflict than those with a unipolar or bipolar-II member, but the effects were not statistically significant. Of interest, there was low agreement between spouses in couples that included a member with mood disorder, with the ill member typically reporting much higher levels of conflict. Hoover and Fitzgerald (1981, p. 67) proposed several possible explanations for this discrepancy:

> It may be that conflict with an ill partner is more difficult to acknowledge and express. . . . Another possibility is that the spouses of manic-depressive patients derive some personality reinforcement, a tested sense of ability or moral fulfillment, from caring for a recurrently sick partner. Or perhaps some spouses need to be a trifle oblivious and not too sensitive to remain with a manic-depressive patient through the years. . . . Finally, there remains the possibility that, in a complementary sense, mercurial persons seek out cheerful, denying persons to marry whereas stolid maintainers of the peace search for more spontaneous, mood-varying types.

Levkovitz and colleagues (2000) collected reports from 34 spouses of bipolar and unipolar patients during remission and from 34 non-ill control spouses. Unfortunately, results were not reported separately for the two diagnoses. Overall, however, patients' spouses perceived significantly more negative characteristics in their marriage, lower marital satisfaction, and more negative and fewer positive traits in their partner. There was some suggestion that these more negative views were associated with unemployment status and prior history of suicide attempts on the part of the ill spouse, but generally there were no associations with clinical features of the disorder.

Few studies have attempted to shed light on the particular concerns of the spouse married to a bipolar patient. In a small-scale study, researchers administered the Family Attitudes Questionnaire to 19 bipolar patients and their well spouses to determine their attitudes and beliefs about the etiology, familial risk, and long-term burden of bipolar illness, as well as their attitudes toward marriage and childbearing (Targum et al., 1981). The reported long-term burdens of the illness included financial difficulties, home and child neglect, marital problems, loss of status and prestige, tension, and fears of recurrence of acute illness. The researchers concluded that the bipolar patients compared with their spouses tended to minimize problems associated with their illness and were more likely to deny the role of genetic factors in the disorder.

When the investigators asked the couples whether they would have married their spouses if they had known more about bipolar illness, 5 percent of the bipolar patients but fully 53 percent of their spouses said they would not have, a statistically significant difference. Similarly, when asked whether they would have had children, 5 percent of the bipolar patients and 47 percent of their spouses said they would not have. Both patients and spouses perceived violent behavior as the most troubling characteristic of mania. Patients also were especially worried by their poor judgment during mania. Spouses were particularly concerned about impulsive spending, overtalkativeness, and decreased need for sleep. Both groups saw suicide threats and attempts as the most troubling aspect of depression, and patients were also bothered by the hopelessness and poor concentration accompanying that state; spouses, on the other hand, were most disturbed by the patient's lowered self-esteem and withdrawal from others. Overall, the most troublesome long-term social problems resulting from bipolar illness were financial difficulties, unemployment, marital problems, recurrences of illness leading to rehospitalization, and social withdrawal due to depression. The researchers concluded:

> Well spouses who have coped with affective illness for many years perceived bipolar illness as a profound burden that had seriously disrupted their lives. . . . The regrets of the well spouse are a most striking feature of this study. . . . Whereas affective episodes may not be directly associated with major persistent psychological deficits, the damaging effects of these episodes may still yield psychological and economic consequences, particularly for the spouse. The spouse is the person who bears the brunt of manic episodes. . . . In depression, the spouse is the most frequent target of demands and hostility, and often feels inordinate responsibility for the mood state of the patient. (Targum et al., 1981, p. 568)

Targum and colleagues (1981) were the first to examine and compare systematically the attitudes of bipolar patients and their spouses and to highlight spousal distress. Yet other studies (e.g., Frank et al., 1981, in a study of 16 couples) have not found such negative effects. It should be noted that the study by Targum and colleagues did not employ a comparison group; moreover, most of the couples had been married for many years, increasing the chances that the bipolar spouse had not been treated with lithium or another mood stabilizer. In a study conducted in India, Chakrabarti and Gill (2002) found that caregivers (mainly spouses) of bipolar patients reported experiencing less of a burden than that reported by caregivers of people with schizophrenia; the burden they did experience involved mainly physical and mental health problems.

Perlick and colleagues (1999) studied perceived burden in a large sample of caregivers of 266 bipolar-I and -II and schizoaffective (manic) patients. Patients' depression was perceived as being associated with a greater burden relative to mania; caregiver distress was especially pronounced when the patient displayed symptoms of "misery, irritability, and withdrawal." The authors also found that the association between severity-of-illness factors and perceived burden was mediated by caregivers' beliefs and attitudes. Specifically, perceived burden was higher among those who believed the patient with bipolar disorder could control his or her symptoms whereas the caregiver could not, and among those with an accurate awareness of the nature and prognosis of the disorder.

Others have likewise speculated that a critical factor in attitudes toward partners with bipolar disorder is the extent to which the patient is perceived as willfully causing or controlling the symptoms. A study conducted by Hooley and colleagues (1987), which included both schizophrenic and bipolar patients and their spouses or family members, revealed that spouses or family of patients with florid, positive symptoms (auditory or visual hallucinations; grandiosity; agitation; speech disorganization; delusions; elated mood; silliness; or inappropriate affect, appearance, or behavior) reported significantly higher levels of marital satisfaction than spouses of patients with negative symptoms (social isolation, depression, lack of emotion, or routine or leisure-time impairment). The authors attributed this difference to the fact that the more bizarre and flagrant positive symptoms, unlike the negative ones, were perceived by the spouse as being caused by an illness and thus beyond the patient's volition. It is likely that milder symptoms of hypomania and depressive symptoms are especially likely to be attributed erroneously to the patient's personality and behaviors. As discussed later, the attitudes of spouses and family members may play a significant role in clinical outcomes and therefore may be an important factor in treatment effectiveness.

A study of caregiver burden among spouses of bipolar patients was conducted in New Zealand (Dore and Romans, 2001). The caregivers were, for the most part, partners or parents of 41 bipolar patients. Virtually all reported that the patient was difficult and irritable or more distant during an affective episode, and that this caused the caregiver considerable distress. Nearly half reported experience with or concern about violence when the patient was in the midst of an episode. Marital difficulties were common and sometimes persistent. Fully 62 percent of the partners said they would probably not have entered into the relationship had they had more knowledge and understanding of the illness beforehand. Nevertheless, most caregivers felt that the relationship was good when the patient was in remission, and few were experiencing significant distress symptoms themselves at the time of the assessment.

Marital Functioning, Family Attitudes, and Predictors of Outcome

Clinical experience suggests that mood stabilizers have a positive effect on marriages involving bipolar individuals because the drugs partially or totally eliminate both highly volatile and disruptive manic episodes and frightening and depleting depressive episodes. These benefits appear to be corroborated by the few existing studies of marital interaction among adequately treated bipolar patients (McKnight et al., 1989). As the results of one early study suggest, however, improvements may be perceived differently by the spouse and the patient. Demers and Davis (1971) found that most of the well spouses participating in their study perceived improvements associated with lithium treatment, including enhanced marital satisfaction, as well as observed decreases in nervousness, violent or threatening behavior, withdrawn or demanding behavior, and sadness. Yet only a minority of the patients themselves perceived such positive changes—perhaps because they were still experiencing subsyndromal episodes or, in some instances, because of their perceived loss of the positive experiences associated with hypomania.

Although the improved clinical status of a bipolar spouse may greatly relieve the patient's partner and family, there is, as noted earlier, a reciprocal impact: increasing evidence indicates that the quality of marital and family functioning may contribute to the patient's clinical outcome during treatment. Results of several studies suggest that good marital functioning or just being married may contribute to the effectiveness of treatment in reducing episodes. For instance, Yazici and colleagues (1999) found that being married was associated with good response to lithium; 27 percent of good-response patients and 48 percent of poor-response patients were unmarried. Similar results have been reported by others (O'Connell et al., 1991). It is important to note, however, that these findings cannot clarify the direction of causality of effects, inasmuch as good response to lithium may be more likely among more well-functioning individuals, as well as those whose manic episodes are relatively more euphoric in nature (see Chapter 18). Likewise, medication adherence and stable sleep may be more likely in the context of a good marriage.

Several studies have found that the "expressed emotion" or "affective style" of partners (the overall negativity or positivity of attitudes toward the patient) may predict relapse and outcome in treated patients over time (Mundt et al., 2000). Miklowitz and colleagues (1988), for example, first demonstrated that bipolar patients whose spouses or parents expressed negative attitudes about them during hospitalization for mania were significantly more likely to have a relapse in the ensuing 9 months than were those patients whose spouses or parents expressed more benign or positive attitudes. O'Connell and colleagues (1991) also found that attitudes of family members, including those of spouses, were significantly related to outcome in a lithium treatment outpatient clinic. More negative attitudes were expressed by partners of patients with poor outcomes (40 percent) than by partners of patients with good outcomes (12 percent). Perlick and colleagues (2001) found that greater perceived caretaker burden, which, as noted, reflects in part attitudes toward the patient and the illness, predicted depressive relapse at follow-up, even after controlling for baseline symptoms. Furthermore, over a 15-month period of mood stabilization, those patients who had fewer symptoms but whose caretakers reported a high perceived burden were more likely to experience a recurrence of their illness. The investigators suggested that stressful family environments contribute to caretaker burden and possibly to depression, as well as to patient relapse.

A family-focused psychoeducational treatment program was devised by Miklowitz and Goldstein (1997) to improve the attitudes of spouses and family members toward the bipolar patient by increasing their knowledge and understanding of the disorder and improving their skills in communicating and solving family-related problems. An evaluation of the treatment suggested that it was effective in improving positive nonverbal communication, and that such improvements accounted in part for the progress seen in patients' symptoms over a 1-year period (Simoneau et al., 1999; Miklowitz et al., 2003) (see Chapter 22). The effectiveness of psychosocial treatments that include spouses is increasingly being demonstrated (e.g., Clarkin et al., 1998), including their potential role in helping to extend the duration and quality of the beneficial effects of medication on the outcome of bipolar disorder (see Chapter 22).

Sexual Behavior

> Again judging from my own experience, the sexual symptoms of the manic state seem to be the most powerful and important of all. . . . The normal inhibitions disappear, and sexual activity, instead of being placed, as in our Western Christian civilization, in opposition to religion, becomes associated with it. This release of the underlying sexual tension . . . seems to me to be the primary and governing factor of all the ecstasies and many other experiences of the manic state. (John Custance, 1952)

Changes in sexual desire, thought, and behavior during depression and mania were observed centuries ago. Aretaeus of Cappadocia (150 AD), for example, observed that "a period of lewdness and shamelessness exists with the highest type of [manic] delirium" (Jelliffe, 1931, p. 20). In the nineteenth and twentieth centuries, Tuke (1892), Kraepelin (1921), Bleuler (1924), Campbell (1953), and Mayer-Gross and colleagues (1955) also described heightened sexuality during mania and decreased sexuality during depression (see Chapter 2).

Fluctuations in sexual drive are sufficiently important in bipolar illness to warrant inclusion as diagnostic criteria in DSM-III and/or DSM-IV ("sexual indiscretions" for manic episodes and "decrease in sexual interest or drive" for depressive episodes). Items pertaining to sexual behavior are on most self- and observer-rating instruments for both mania and depression (see Chapter 12). Beigel and colleagues (1971), for example, required nurses to judge 26 items most characteristic of manic behavior, thought, and affect. Of those items, the 2 pertaining to sex ("talks about sex" and "is sexually preoccupied") had high concordance with independent ratings on both a psychiatrists' global mania scale and a nurses' manic-symptom checklist.

The actual data on changes in sexual behavior and thinking during different phases of bipolar illness are relatively limited. Quantified observational data are presented in Chapter 2 and can be summarized here. Hypersexuality was observed or reported in 57 percent of manic patients (averaged across seven studies, with a range of values from 25 to 80 percent), and actual nudity or sexual exposure was reported in 29 percent (averaged across three studies, with a range of values from 23 to 33 percent). Akiskal and colleagues (1977) reported that 40 percent of their cyclothymic patients had "episodic or unexplained promiscuity or extramarital affairs." Allison and Wilson (1960) studied the sexual behavior of 24 manic patients using data based on physician observations and on historical information from patients and their relatives. They found no relationship between

sexual display during mania and age, religion, duration of illness, previous episodes, or social class. Women were far more sexually provocative and seductive than men (58 and 0 percent, respectively) on a 5-point rating scale. However, women and men were equally likely to have both increased "libidinal drives" and increased frequency of sexual relations. In 78 percent of the patients, the frequency of sexual intercourse increased substantially during manic episodes.

A recent study of sexual satisfaction in 37 partners of bipolar patients found that partners were less satisfied when the patient was affectively ill (Lam et al., 2005). The investigators attributed this finding to illness-related changes in sexual interest, affection, and responsiveness.

Winokur and colleagues (1969) found that 65 percent of manic episodes were characterized by increased sexuality. In 32 percent of cases, the sexuality was of a socially approved type, that is, within marriage or a long-lasting relationship. In 10 percent of patients, the increased sexuality was in thought or discussion only, and in 11 percent it was manifested in socially disapproved behavior. In this latter group, patients were homosexually or heterosexually promiscuous or both; in all cases, the hypersexuality was clearly associated with being ill. Like those patients studied by Allison and Wilson (1960), the women (18 percent) in the study of Winokur and colleagues were more likely to have increased sexual contacts (noncoital) than the men (3 percent), but women and men were equally likely to have an increased frequency of intercourse (30 and 35 percent, respectively).

Spalt (1975) studied lifetime sexual behavior in 42 patients with unipolar depression, 19 with bipolar illness, 56 with secondary affective illness, and 38 with nonaffective illness. Extramarital sexual experiences were more frequent among bipolar patients (29 percent had more than 10 experiences) than among unipolar patients (12 percent). Bipolar patients (21 percent) also were more likely than unipolar patients (10 percent) to have had more than 10 sexual partners during their lifetime. These figures almost certainly reflect many other behavioral differences between the two groups, including hypersexuality and differences in sexual drive during normal periods, as well as differences in levels of gregariousness, sociability, and interpersonal turmoil.

Jamison and colleagues (1980) studied changes attributed to affective illness in 35 bipolar and 26 unipolar patients. Twice as many women (41 percent) as men (20 percent) reported that sexual intensity was "very much increased" during hypomania; 40 percent of the men and 18 percent of the women stated that sexual intensity during hypomania was "somewhat increased." Women rated increased sexual intensity as the most important or enjoyable change they experienced during hypomania.[19] Bipolar patients were significantly more likely than unipolar patients ($p < .01$) to feel that increased sexual intensity was a lasting characteristic attributable to their mood disorder.

As noted, bipolar illness also can be associated with decreased sexual drive. For example, Winokur and colleagues (1969) reported that 63 percent of patients with bipolar mixed states reported decreased sexual interest. Indeed, approximately three-fourths of bipolar depressed patients have been found to experience a loss of sexual interest: 73 percent reported by Winokur and colleagues (1969) and 77 percent by Casper and colleagues (1985).

Sexual responsiveness can also be dampened in patients taking lithium.[20] Sheard (1971, 1975) and Lion (1975) attributed this phenomenon to a common effect on aggressive and sexual behaviors, both often occurring together in bipolar patients. Lorimy and colleagues (1977) reported that half of their patients taking prophylactic lithium experienced troublesome side effects affecting their sexual activities, including decreases in sexual intensity, frequency of sexual drive, and frequency of sexual intercourse. However, patients reported that once intercourse began, there was no decrement in enjoyment or orgasmic ability.

What accounts for these lithium-induced changes is unclear. Among the possible explanations are lithium-induced hypothyroidism, decreased frequency or intensity of hypomanic episodes, or the direct effect of lithium on the central mechanisms underlying sexual drive and behavior. Yet another possible reason for these changes is vacillation in interpersonal relationships brought about by lithium, with secondary manifestation in the sexual domain.

Assortative Mating among Bipolar Patients

An additional challenge to marital adjustment among individuals with bipolar disorder is the increased likelihood of nonrandom mate selection. Specifically, research, although limited, suggests that bipolar individuals have an increased likelihood of marrying a partner with affective illness (see Chapter 13). For instance, in a sample of 56 married inpatients with mood disorders, Merikangas and Spiker (1982) found a higher degree of assortative mating among bipolar than unipolar patients. They noted high diagnostic concordance between patients and spouses for both affective disorders and alcoholism. The effects could not be attributed to spouses' symptomatic reactions to marriage to an ill spouse because the spouses appeared to have a predisposition to the disorders based on elevated rates of psychiatric and mood disorders in their own relatives. Colombo and colleagues (1990) studied assortative mating in a large sample of more than 1,000 patients with mood or anxiety disorders. They observed that while patients with bipolar illness were less likely to marry overall than were those with unipolar disorder, there was a specific assortative mating pattern such that bipolar men were more likely than controls to have wives with mood disorders.

Most of the few studies examining assortative mating have had methodological limitations, such as small sample sizes, lack of direct comparison groups, and differing diagnostic criteria. A meta-analysis approach is especially helpful for evaluating pooled effects across several small studies. One such analysis (Mathews and Reus, 2001), based on the six best-designed studies, confirmed the commonly reported finding of assortative mating for bipolar individuals, with higher rates than for those with unipolar depression. Specific analyses based on husbands and wives were inconclusive because of limited data, but suggested that data supporting the marriage of bipolar men to women with mood disorders are much more robust than is the case for the marriage of bipolar women to men with mood disorders. The authors also noted the paucity of evidence of mood disorders in mates before the marriage; thus depressive reactions to stress in marriage to a bipolar partner cannot be ruled out.

Although these studies raise a number of questions to be pursued in further research, they support the often-observed pattern of the marriage of bipolar individuals to those who also have mood disorders. Such dual-disorder pairings may promote shared understanding, but may also give rise to marital discord and instability by contributing to stressful home environments and potentially to limited skills for resolving interpersonal disputes. While not confined to bipolar disorder, such pairings may present a treatment challenge requiring family or couple interventions. Obviously if confirmed, assortative mating also has considerable genetic significance.

Effects on Marriage of Treatment of Bipolar Spouses

Clinical experience suggests that lithium, the only mood stabilizer that has been studied systematically for its effect on marital stability, has a highly stabilizing effect on the marriages of patients with bipolar illness because it partially or totally eliminates both highly volatile and disruptive manic episodes and frightening and depleting depressive ones. These benefits appear to be corroborated by the few marital studies of adequately treated bipolar patients,[21] although they were not observed in the study by Targum and colleagues (1981).

Demers and Davis (1971) administered the Marital Partner Attribute Test to 14 married bipolar patients and their spouses. Lithium produced a highly significant decrease in spouses' negative ratings of the patients but no significant changes in patients' ratings of their spouses. In fact, 13 (93 percent) of 14 bipolar patients were rated by their spouses as improved and as having significantly fewer undesirable attributes ($p < .01$) after lithium treatment. Spouses particularly noted decreases in nervousness; bizarre, threatening, and violent behavior; withdrawn or demanding behavior; guilt; sadness; and undue exaggeration of abilities. But they also reported missing the enthusiasm and heightened sexuality associated with hypomanic phases:

> Hypomanic joviality, enthusiasm, and spontaneity are often regarded as social pluses; and manic-depressives and their spouses complain about the loss of these valued attributes. When pressed to discuss the sexual compatibility of the marriage, frequently they will say it is worse since lithium treatment started, as the lithium-treated spouse has less libidinal strivings. (Demers and Davis, 1971, p. 352)

Although 77 percent of the spouses rated the marriage as considerably improved, only 43 percent of the bipolar patients expressed this opinion. Patients may be more sensitive to the loss of positive experiences associated with bipolar illness, whereas their spouses may be more aware of lithium's beneficial effects. Such a possibility would be consistent with the discrepancies in perceptions reported by Targum and colleagues (1981). These results again underscore the importance of sophisticated clinical management and subtle titration of lithium to the lowest possible level consistent with efficacy.

O'Connell and Mayo (1981) studied the effects of lithium treatment on 12 bipolar patients and their families. They found that lithium increased the direct care of children by both patients and spouses, significantly alleviated marital friction, and resulted in increased cooperative planning, communication, and trust.

Holinger and Wolpert (1979) found that the majority (59 percent) of their 56 manic-depressive patients showed improvement in their relationships with spouses, families, or friends as a result of taking lithium; slightly more than one-third (39 percent) showed no change. The primary changes observed by the authors were decreases in impulsivity, fragility, and erratic behavior; confidence in relationships increased. The bipolar patients were far more likely than the lithium-treated unipolar patients to demonstrate a change in interpersonal behavior (59 and 11 percent, respectively). In a study by Lepkifker and colleagues (1988), psychiatrists' ratings of marital and other interpersonal relationships were significantly higher for the 50 bipolar and 50 unipolar patients (all of whom were euthymic and lithium-treated) than for 50 psychiatric controls with personality disorders. There were no significant bipolar–unipolar differences.

Finally, Ruestow and colleagues (1978), in a study cited earlier, suggested that bipolar manic-depressive patients, especially men, could have good marriages if stabilized by lithium. While emphasizing the importance of adjunctive use of marital therapy, they also suggested "that patients be treated with medication . . . prior to the initiation of marital therapy and that the need for intensive marital therapy be reassessed after the patient's illness has been stabilized."

Bipolar Disorder and Family Functioning

In addition to the genetic risk imparted by bipolar parents to their children, there is a potential risk due to the children's exposure to parents' moods and maladaptive child rearing. This is an understudied research topic in bipolar samples; however, there is an important and well-developed literature linking the effects of parental depression and the commonly associated environmental conditions with diagnosable disorders in children and disturbances in their functioning.[22] The vast majority of these studies involved mothers with diagnosed unipolar depression or nondiagnosed women who displayed elevated symptoms of depressed mood; the samples included children of all ages, from infancy to young adulthood. Across the wide array of samples with varying demographic characteristics in these studies, the results have been quite consistent. Infants display a variety of indicators of distress and discomfort while interacting with depressed mothers. School-age children with clinically depressed mothers show high rates of major depression, as well as anxiety and disruptive behavior disorders, with studies indicating that 50 percent or more of such children may have diagnosable disorders during childhood and adolescence (Hammen, 1991; Beardslee et al., 1998). The offspring of depressed parents have also been found to be impaired in academic and social functioning, and indicators of maladjustment and psychopathology appear to suggest further dysfunction over follow-up periods of several years (Anderson and Hammen, 1993; Weissman et al., 1997; NICHD Early Child Care Research Network, 1999).

While children's maladjustment may in part reflect genetically transmitted disorder, it has been widely speculated that depressed parents, particularly depressed mothers, are impaired in their parental roles in ways that have substantial negative impacts on their children, ways likely to be linked to the chronicity and severity of and perhaps the timing of the child's exposure to the parent's depression. Depressed women may be apathetic and withdrawn, display less physical affection, or be irritable and critical with their children. Not only do the symptoms of depression interfere with the kinds of warm, consistent, responsive, and available nurturing believed to be optimal for children's development, but the depressed parent may also be unable to assist the child in coping with stressful life events that befall the child or family and may fail to model effective strategies for coping with interpersonal and stressful challenges. In addition, the lives of depressed women are commonly characterized by a variety of factors that may have a negative impact on the developing child, including marital conflict or divorce, as well as work and financial difficulties that create stressful conditions in the family.

As noted, far less research has been conducted on the parenting characteristics of women with bipolar disorder than on those of women with depression. Moreover, parenting behaviors are likely to differ as a function of mood state. While depressive symptoms may be associated with maladaptive parenting, it is less clear that bipolar parents who are euthymic or even hypomanic display dysfunctional behaviors. Additionally, significant changes in parenting style, perhaps resulting from mood shifts, may themselves have important effects on children. It is also important to distinguish the potentially detrimental effect on children of such cofactors of bipolar disorder as exposure to violence, psychosis, and substance abuse from outcomes associated with typical functioning while not in the midst of episodes. Thus parenting characteristics should be explored as a function of current, typical, and potentially changing clinical status, with attention to the considerable differences in outcomes that may be associated with each.

As noted in Chapter 7, relatively few studies addressing high risk for bipolar disorder have examined psychosocial mechanisms of children's risk in bipolar families. Radke-Yarrow (1998), reporting the results of an approximately 10-year follow-up of children of unipolar and bipolar mothers, summarized the results of several observational sessions involving mothers and their children. She and her colleagues attempted to characterize two mechanisms by which a mother's disorder affected her children—maternal symptomatology, and socialization and caregiving functions. Both unipolar and bipolar women were frequently observed to be irritable and angry with their youngsters (42 percent), and some of the bipolar women displayed an overall uninvolved or unavailable style (19 percent). Bipolar women also evidenced boundary issues, "unstable enthusiasms," and impulsive behavior in their interactions (61 to 69 percent). Overall, the maternal styles observed were fairly stable over the years of the study and were predictive of maladaptive outcomes in the children. It should be noted that because most of the bipolar women in the study had bipolar-II disorder, their symptoms were chiefly depressive, and the specific role of mania was not examined.

A study of the family environments of bipolar parents of 56 children aged 6 to 18 was conducted by Chang and colleagues (2001). They collected parents' reports on the Family Environment Scale, and found significantly lower scores on the cohesion and organization subscales and higher scores on the conflict subscale compared with normative data. The scores were unrelated to whether the children had diagnoses of Axis I disorders, however, so child psychopathology was not directly associated with family functioning.

One of the rare studies of mother–infant behavior involving women with bipolar disorder compared ratings of mother–child interactions during hospitalization among unipolar, bipolar, and schizophrenic women (Hipwell and Kumar, 1996). All groups displayed erratic or dysfunctional interactions at first, but improved over time. While the scores of the bipolar women were initially similar to those of the schizophrenic women, they showed greater improvement over the course of hospitalization: by the time of discharge, 77 percent of bipolar and 86 percent of unipolar mothers fell within the normal range, compared with only 33 percent of schizophrenic women. It appeared that the impairments associated with bipolar disorder were symptom related and became normalized with clinical improvement.

The University of California-Los Angeles (UCLA) High Risk Study observed mother–child interactions among bipolar, unipolar, and medically ill and well women during discussions involving typical family disagreements. The researchers found that the bipolar women largely resembled the normal comparison women in their interaction styles, whereas the unipolar depressed women were significantly more negative, critical, and withdrawn from the discussion task with their children (Gordon et al., 1989). Analysis of the findings of this study revealed that overall, depressive mood was a strong predictor of maternal behavior, as well as of children's symptoms (Hammen, 1991). Regardless of diagnosis, women with more severe depressive symptoms had more disturbances in their interactions with their children, and their children were less well adjusted in various roles. Bipolar women had significantly fewer depressive episodes over the course of the study (3 years) than did unipolar women, and thus the phenomenology of the family experiences was quite different for the two groups. Anderson and Hammen (1993) reported that the offspring of bipolar mothers had better social adjustment and academic achievement relative to those of unipolar depressed mothers; indeed, their adjustment resembled that of children of normal community women. Similar results were reported by Klein and colleagues (1986), who found normal social adjustment in the adolescent offspring of parents with bipolar disorder. However, if the offspring themselves had cyclothymic behavior and mood disturbances, they tended to have impaired social adjustment. Thus the sparse evidence available suggests relatively good adjustment in children of bipolar parents (unless the children themselves are symptomatic) and provides little indication of significant parenting impairment, except among those with chronic depression.

One hypothesis that should be pursued in future research is that the reactions of children and other family members to depression, mania, and mixed states are almost certainly quite different. As discussed earlier, a manic episode may be viewed as being more clearly beyond the individual's control than a depressive episode and therefore may be more likely to elicit alternative caretaking for children. The predominant mood state of the parent's mania—euphoric versus angry and highly volatile—is certainly relevant but has not been studied in this context. Also, of course, the parent's psychological and social functioning between episodes is likely to be a strong predictor of children's adjustment, inasmuch as stable and euthymic periods may help repair disruptions caused by periods of symptomatology. Not only the specific effects of depression and mania, but also the level of chronicity or recovery between major episodes, are of considerable predictive significance in understanding the overall effects of parenting behavior.

Clearly, further studies are needed to evaluate the parental functioning of adults with bipolar disorder. Of particular importance is the quality of parenting when the patient is not in the midst of a major episode. As in research on the effects of unipolar depression on children's risk, it is also important to measure and evaluate the environment in which families live, including parents' marital status, economic conditions, and the spouse's mental health and adjustment, as well as general resources for coping with the illness.

CONCLUSIONS

Personality

Contemporary research generally dispels the idea that the personalities of bipolar patients are fundamentally different from those of people without mood disorders. Descriptive studies comparing bipolar patients with other groups have yielded few consistent results and clearly suggest enormous variability, depending in part on the instruments used and individuals' current mood status. The major drawback of such studies is their limited utility. Nevertheless, the close and likely bidirectional association between personality and mood disorders suggests that many behaviors and attitudes we regard as personality may in fact be somewhat unstable and highly colored by affective experiences. The field now appears ready to proceed to more conceptually and practically challenging questions and prospective methods concerning the predictive utility of personality constructs: Do they tell us something important about the course of disorder, treatment responsiveness, and functional outcome

beyond that attributable to symptoms or psychosocial context? Are there premorbid signs of eventual bipolar disorder that might help in both understanding the risk for illness and altering its course? What are the underlying neurobiological processes of normal mood and temperament that may help us understand mood disorders?

Personality Disorders

Research on personality disorders—the enduring, pervasive, and dysfunctional styles measured on Axis II of the DSM—has increased in sophistication in the bipolar field. As with most Axis I disorders, studies of bipolar patients evaluated during remission indicate relatively high rates of personality disorders, and such disorders generally predict a relatively worse course of illness and functional adjustment. However, the overlap among bipolar symptoms, mood states, and personality pathology may obscure the question of whether a bipolar patient truly has an Axis II disorder.

Interpersonal Functioning

Interpersonal functioning is commonly a casualty of bipolar disorder, although there is tremendous variability in individuals' abilities to sustain close friendships and family relationships. It is unclear whether the effects of bipolar disorder on interpersonal functioning are the result of episodes or of underlying impairment of social skills. There is, however, ample evidence that poor social functioning may negatively affect clinical outcomes. Thus interventions targeting social and family relationships may potentiate the effects of psychopharmacology and, of course, benefit the loved ones greatly affected by their relative's disorder.

NOTES

1. These differences were well summarized by Hall and Lindzey (1970): the relative importance of the uniqueness of the individual (the idiographic-nomothetic controversy), whether man should be viewed as possessing purposive or teleological qualities, the importance of group membership, the relative importance of conscious and unconscious determinants of behavior, the number of motivational concepts, the importance of the principles of reward and association, the relative emphasis on stable structures or the process of change in personality, the functional independence of personality structure at any particular point in time, the relative importance of genetic factors in determining behavior, and the relative importance of early developmental experiences.

2. Thus Kraepelin (1921) delineated four fundamental types of temperament: *depressive, manic, irritable,* and *cyclothymic.* Kretschmer (1936) stressed the overlap among these personality types in the prepsychotic, *cycloid personality* of manic-depressive patients: "they form layers or patterns in individual cases, arranged in the most varied combinations." Campbell

(1953), too, described a cycloid personality, which could occur in one of three forms—*hypomanic, depressive,* and *cyclothymic*—"with innumerable gradations and mixtures between the three." He, like Kraepelin, regarded all of these personality types as "part of the same disease process, and that any one of these may change into any other." Leonhard (1957), who separated major affective illness into unipolar and bipolar types, also regarded many personality patterns in manic-depressive patients as subclinical, or "diluted," forms of the primary illness itself. Mayer-Gross and colleagues (1955) derived personality topologies similar to those of Kraepelin (1921), Kretschmer (1936), and Campbell (1953): *cyclothymic* (social, good-hearted, kind, and easy-going), *hyperthymic* (elated, humorous, lively, and hot-tempered), and *hypothymic* (quiet, calm, serious, and gentle). Rowe and Daggett (1954) and Von Zerssen (1977) summarized premorbid personality traits of manic and depressed patients, which are quite consistent with the earlier clinical topologies.

3. Dooley (1921, p. 167) wrote:

> The behavior found in the manic attack, in which the patient throws himself with almost equal vim into every possible avenue of expression, is in itself a defense reaction. By thus taking the offensive he keeps himself safe from the approach of the painful thought or feeling which is usually a realization of some failure or degradation, or fundamental inferiority of his own. When he is depressed his defense is no longer possible and he is weighed down by the pain of the acknowledged defect.

More specifically, Schwartz (1961, p. 244) described the dynamic purpose for hyperactive behavior and grandiose thought:

> The hypermotility in mania may have a twofold purpose. First, it may serve as a method for distracting attention from the perception of deprivation; second, it is a diffuse and multidirectional effort to obtain pleasure, in which some realistic basis for the denial of deprivation may be grasped.... Grandiosity as a defense by denial against emptiness, however ... may even represent, additionally, an intellectual attempt at a further regression, in the service of the ego, to the stage of omnipotence.

Grotstein (1986) described the manic mechanism of denial in terms of power and self-regulation:

> The psychical state which is set up to regulate this primal state of powerlessness is that of a fraudulent state of power, including that of a severe superego and/or compulsive and/or hypomanic defenses which seek to create an artificial "floor" over a "floorless" psyche.

4. Dooley, 1921; Wilson, 1951; Arieti, 1959; Stone, 1978.
5. Cohen et al., 1954; Arieti, 1959; Gibson et al., 1959; Smith, 1960.
6. This concept was explained in a different way by Arieti (1959, p. 431):

> The receptiveness to others and willingness to introject the others determines, at this early age, some aspects of the personality of the patient. He tends to become

an "extrovert"; at the same time he tends to become a conformist, willing to accept what he is given by his surroundings (not only in material things but also in terms of habits and values).

7. According to Dooley (1921, p. 39, 166):

> The personality of the manic depressive individual also presents an obstacle. Those who manifest frequent manic attacks are likely to be headstrong, self-sufficient, know-it all types of persons who will not take suggestions or yield to direction. They are "doers" and managers, and will get the upper hand of the analyst and everyone else around them if given the opportunity .... The manic-depressive character is extroverted, he tries always to relate himself to his environment, he minimizes the subjective element and makes use of every object in the range of his senses.

Wilson (1951, p. 362) further discussed the therapist's problems in treating the manic-depressive patient:

> From the psychiatrist's point of view he is uninteresting because he is hard to get at. He is friendly and superficially cooperative, but soon personality investigation ceases because the patient refuses to be self analytical. When the patient is depressed or manic, his illness seems to explain his unapproachableness, and when he is well he will have nothing to do with you except in a very superficial way. This impenetrable shell is characteristic of persons with this illness and sets them apart from those having other forms of depression.

Cohen and colleagues (1954, p. 120) described the manic-depressive personality as dependent, even during states of normal functioning:

> We see, then, in the adult cyclothymic, a person who is apparently well adjusted between attacks, although he may show minor mood swings or be chronically overactive or chronically mildly depressed. He is conventionally well-behaved and frequently successful, and he is hardworking and conscientious; indeed, at times his overconscientiousness and scrupulousness lead to his being called obsessional. He is typically involved in one or more relationships of extreme dependence, in which, however, he does not show the obsessional's typical need to control the other person for the sake of power, but instead seeks to control the other person in the sense of swallowing him up. His inner feeling, when he allows himself to notice it, is one of emptiness and need. He is extremely stereotyped in his attitudes and opinions, tending to take over the opinions of the person in his environment whom he regards as an important authority. Again this contrasts with the outward conformity but subtle rebellion of the obsessional. It should be emphasized that the dependency feelings are largely out of awareness in states of well-being and also in the manic phase; in fact, these people frequently take pride in being independent.

8. Frey, 1977; Hirschfeld and Klerman, 1979; Liebowitz et al., 1979; Bech et al., 1980; Hirschfeld, 1985, 1986.

9. Perris, 1966; Murray and Blackburn, 1974; Hirschfeld and Klerman, 1979; Liebowitz et al., 1979; Winters and Neale, 1985.

10. Perris, 1971; Frey, 1977; Bech et al., 1980; Matussek and Feil, 1983; Hirschfeld, 1985; Hirschfeld et al., 1986.

11. Frey, 1977; Hirschfeld and Klerman, 1979; Liebowitz et al., 1979; Abou-Saleh and Coppen, 1984.

12. Kron et al., 1982; Gershon et al. 1985; Klein and Depue, 1985; Nurnberger et al., 1988; Grigoroiu-Serbanescu et al., 1989, 1991.

13. Cited in Hamilton, 1982, p. 214.

14. See, e.g., Bauwens et al., 1991; Coryell et al., 1993; Mundt et al., 2000; Dorz et al., 2002.

15. Harrow et al., 1990; Tohen et al., 1990; Keller et al., 1993; Gitlin et al., 1995.

16. Kulhara et al., 1999; Johnson et al., 2000, 2003; Cohen et al., 2004.

17. Johnson et al., 2000; Cohen et al., 2004; Kim and Miklowitz, 2004; Yan et al., 2004.

18. Published in *The Times* (London), January 24, 1986.

19. Stoddard and colleagues (1977) studied eight affective episodes in a 39-year-old rapid-cycling woman. They collected systematic behavioral data twice a day and observed that she became sexually provocative during mania. Conversely, a significant predictor of her switch into depression was a decrease in sexual preoccupation ($p < .05$).

20. In addition to the references in this paragraph, see Demers and Davis (1971).

21. Demers and Davis, 1971; Ruestow et al., 1978; Frank et al., 1981; O'Connell and Mayo, 1981.

22. Downey and Coyne, 1990; Gelfand and Teti, 1990; Hammen, 1991; Goodman and Gotlib, 1999; NICHD Early Child Care Research Network, 1999.

11   Assessment

Our customary grouping into manic and melancholic attacks does not fit the facts, but requires substantial enlargement, if it is to reproduce nature.

—Emil Kraepelin (1921, p. 191)

Standardized measures of mania and depression provide the common language by which clinicians and researchers can communicate. By minimizing differences in the way clinicians record their observations, such instruments contribute to the widespread sharing of information and provide yardsticks for a variety of observers in very different settings. The measures discussed in this chapter vary in their goals and uses. Some help in determining the severity of episodes or symptom states, providing information about treatment response, and ascertaining the incidence of different types of affective states. Quantitative rating scales for mania and depression can be especially important in longitudinal studies (e.g., to describe the natural course of the illness and individual manic and depressive episodes) for identifying the progression and resolution of symptom patterns; studying euthymic states in bipolar patients; and correlating manic and depressive states with other aspects of behavior, cognition, personality, and neurobiology. The assessment literature focuses on bipolar disorder or major depression; there are no measures of depression that focus on the highly recurrent forms that, along with bipolar disorder, make up what we mean by manic-depressive illness. Accordingly the focus of this chapter is on the bipolar subgroup.

There are several additional uses of assessment instruments in the field of bipolar disorder. With the abundance of longitudinal studies of bipolar course, as well as treatment outcome studies, procedures for systematic mapping of the course of the disorder have been developed. Less focused on symptoms as such than measures of severity of mood states, such procedures have the primary aim of capturing changes in and patterns of mood episodes over time. Another relatively new development is the search for measures of risk for bipolar disorder. The potential utility of procedures that could be used to assess subsyndromal or preclinical states lies in their ability to predict who will develop bipolar disorder over time. Because those with the disorder may be untreated and underdiagnosed, it would be useful to have screening measures to identify such individuals in general psychological, psychiatric, or medical settings. Also discussed in this chapter are measures of functional outcomes in work and social relationships; we note the paucity of such approaches relative to those with a clinical focus. Gaining a fuller understanding of bipolar disorder—as well as helping patients improve in key areas that affect the quality of their lives—requires attention to the development and application of such measures.

Several general types of measures have been developed to classify and quantify changes in affective states. The major categories, delineated by von Zerssen and Cording (1978), are (1) self-ratings, made by patients; (2) observer ratings, usually made by clinicians; (3) analyses of behavior (including linguistic analyses of speech or written productions); and (4) objective measurements, either of spontaneous activities (physical activity) or of reactions within a standardized situation (objective psychometric tests). This chapter necessarily is limited to an overview of self-rating and observer rating scales constructed to measure manic, depressive, mixed, and cyclothymic states. Measurement issues specific to particular topics are covered in the relevant chapters of this volume. For example, diagnostic evaluation is covered in Chapter 3, assessment of course and outcome in Chapter 4, assessment of neuropsychological functioning in Chapter 9, and measures of personality in Chapter 10. This chapter includes those generic rating scales that have been used or replicated most widely, as well as several instruments with potential utility for specific goals, such as screening for bipolar disorder.

We begin by describing conceptual and methodological issues involved in the assessment of manic and depressive states. We then review in turn instruments used for assessment of the two states, and analyze and compare the scales used for both purposes. The following sections describe instruments used for combined assessment of manic and depressive states, assessment of bipolar risk and screening for bipolar disorder, charting of the course of bipolar disorder, assessment of psychosocial adjustment, and assessment of bipolar symptoms in children and adolescents.

CONCEPTUAL AND METHODOLOGICAL ISSUES

Conceptual Challenges

There are a number of difficulties associated with the measurement of manic and depressive conditions. Moods may be highly unstable, fluctuating rapidly over days or even hours. Bipolar conditions by definition include patterns over time, requiring longitudinal data gathering, which is fraught with its own pitfalls. Moods may be mixed, including both manic and depressive elements, and may include or reflect other emotional states and comorbid conditions, such as anxiety, substance abuse, and Axis II disorders (see Chapters 7 and 10). Bipolar conditions themselves are highly heterogeneous, including a wide range of syndromal and subsyndromal states, which vary in course and episode features. Continuing changes and refinements in diagnostic criteria and elucidation of potential subtypes suggest that no "gold standard" criteria currently exist against which to validate new instruments. Generally, there is reliance on convergent validation—agreement between the results of two instruments or of newer and older instruments. Additionally, most measures attempt to include a multitude of clinical symptoms of the syndromes of mania or depression. However, refinements of models of etiology and targeted treatment-related functional outcomes will likely require greater attention to specific clusters of symptoms—such as anhedonia, excessive activity, or distractibility—that are poorly conceptualized and lack adequate measures. Most of the instruments described in this chapter are used largely for clinical assessment and may not be sufficient for other research purposes. Finally, a further challenge, even for well-established measures, is the need for empirically derived endpoints that would be widely accepted and consistently employed as markers of meaningful clinical change in treatment outcome studies (Baldessarini, 2003).

Methodological Issues

Added to these conceptually challenging issues are numerous psychometric hurdles that must be overcome by any good measure, including establishment of various forms of reliability and validity. As discussed later, clinical activity and research in the field of bipolar disorder have brought to light a number of gaps in existing tools for measuring manic and depressive states, indicating that much progress has yet to be made.

One methodological challenge is clarification of the goals of assessment. What do we mean, for example, by the measurement of "depression," a term that variously denotes a mood state, a constellation of symptoms, and a diagnostic entity? Instruments designed to assess a constellation of symptoms of depression, such as the Beck Depression Inventory (BDI), are sometimes used erroneously as diagnostic tools, identifying "depression" if respondents score beyond a certain cutoff point. Yet a diagnostic instrument, such as the Structured Clinical Interview for DSM (SCID), used to identify major depressive episodes, may do a limited job of measuring the mood state "depression." Numerous instruments, as we shall see, purport to assess syndromic features of depression or mania. Nonetheless, they may differ considerably in their item content, with varying emphases on cognitive, behavioral, mood, and somatic features (e.g., Snaith, 1993). The goals and limitations of each instrument must be clearly conceptualized so its uses will be appropriate to the purposes at hand, and conclusions based on a particular assessment strategy must be specific to that instrument.

Selection of appropriate instruments for specific purposes also requires determination of the validity of an assessment approach for a particular goal. Instruments appropriate for selecting patients for a treatment study or investigating an etiological mechanism may not be valid for measuring changes in mood state or evaluating outcomes over time. Thus different assessment procedures may be required to diagnose, measure severity, observe course features, and assess elements of a particular symptom.

In addition to such issues regarding the goals and meaning of various instruments, methodological challenges are inherent in the very assessment of manic and depressive mood states. Mood states color subjective reports of experiences and behavior, as well as memory of the past and expectations of the future; when depressed, for example, an individual may report having "always" been depressed and may exaggerate symptoms of past depressive episodes. Transient mood states may not only vary with clinical conditions, but also be affected by seasonal, diurnal, menstrual, and other cyclic variations. As noted, moreover, mixed states are more common than previously believed, and they confound the utility of bipolar scales—those constructed on the assumption that mania and depression are, in all respects, opposite states. Mood states also are often highly nonspecific across diverse clinical populations. It has been demonstrated that depressed patients, although distinguishable from normal populations on most scales, may not be readily distinguished by mood symptoms from other clinical populations, such as general medical patients, schizophrenic patients, or other psychiatric patients (Mendels et al., 1972; Murphy et al., 1982). Similarly, certain manic symptoms, such as impulsivity, irritability, and distractibility, may occur in various diagnostic groups.

In the discussion that follows, these and related methodological problems are examined in greater detail. As a first step, we outline the advantages and disadvantages of the two major methods for measuring manic and depressive states: self-rating and observer rating.

Self-Rating of Affective States

There are obvious advantages to using self-ratings by affectively ill patients. Foremost, as Murphy and colleagues (1982) pointed out, patients are in a unique position to provide information about their feelings and moods—key symptoms in any assessment of mood disorders. The value of self-ratings was confirmed by Raskin and colleagues (1970), who found that a mood scale completed by patients was one of the best measures of significant treatment effects. The patient is also, for the most part, free of the theoretical biases that affect the development and use of observer ratings, and "has access to the totality of his experience, rather than only a subset of behavior that the observer views" (Murphy et al., 1982). For example, in an early study, Zealley and Aitken (1969) analyzed independent mood recordings made by patients and nursing staff; an example of the results of their analysis is shown in Figure 11–1, which illustrates the lag between a patient's self-ratings and a nurse's ratings of the patient. The results of this study indicate that patients' mood symptoms changed from depressed to normal to hypomanic more rapidly than the staff detected, and suggest that the staff may have been unaware of patients' mood states day to day. In addition to improved accuracy, there are several practical advantages to using patient self-report measures: they require relatively little professional time and expense, can be completed rapidly, and can be used for repeated measurement (Hamilton, 1976; Murphy et al., 1982).

Self-ratings have obvious disadvantages, however. Patients must be literate, cooperative, not too depressed or too manic, and able to concentrate (Hamilton, 1976; Snaith, 1981; Murphy et al., 1982). Other difficulties derive from patients' idiosyncratic interpretations of the language of rating scales, their highly variable degrees of insight, and the scales' inability to differentiate clearly between symptoms (e.g., mood and energy changes) when they occur simultaneously (Pinard and Tetreault, 1974; Snaith, 1981). Finally, there is some evidence that severely depressed patients tend to underestimate the severity of their psychopathology (see, e.g., Paykel et al., 1973). For instance, Prusoff and colleagues (1972b) assessed 200 depressed patients using semistructured clinical interviews and self-reports. They found that self-report ratings, although useful in measuring the presence or

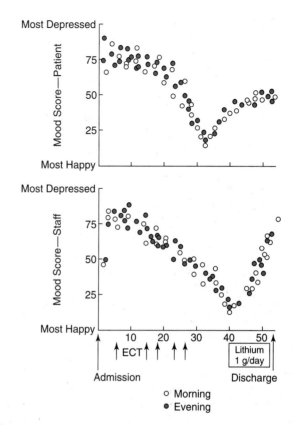

Figure 11–1. Visual analogue scale scores obtained from nursing staff and from a patient with manic-depressive illness. ECT = electroconvulsive therapy; open circles = morning observations; filled circles = evening observations. (*Source*: Adapted from Zealley and Aitken, 1969.)

absence of symptoms, were not a reliable index of symptom severity. Self-reports and clinically obtained measures were far more highly correlated at follow-up than during an acute episode. In a related study, Prusoff and colleagues (1972a) examined the nature of the discrepancy in scores derived from self- and clinician ratings. They found that patients whose ratings of symptoms were higher than those of clinicians tended to be younger, less severely depressed, and more histrionic. Conversely, those who minimized their symptoms tended to be older, more severely depressed, and obsessive. These results may reflect in part variations among patients with differing clinical and demographic characteristics, ranging from acute emotional turmoil with exaggerated subjective suffering to withdrawn, perhaps passive detachment and more physical manifestations.

Observer Rating of Affective States

In summarizing the advantages of observer ratings, Hamilton (1976, p. 158) cited the observer's ability to:

> evaluate the intensity of any one symptom by comparing it against the background of experience which he has . . .

penetrate the mask which the patient holds up, whether deliberately or unintentionally . . . [and] rate and assess certain manifestations of illness which the patient would find impossible or extremely difficult to do. [These include] loss of insight . . . mild retardation . . . [and] hypochondriasis and delusions. An observer can rate all grades of severity of an illness . . . whereas a patient can be too ill to complete a questionnaire.

At the same time, however, observer ratings have significant potential drawbacks, as discussed at length by both Lorr (1974) and Bech (1981). Lorr noted that variability in the degree of the patient's disturbance from one interview to another affects both self- and observer ratings. Furthermore, observers may differ in efficiency and their manner in relating to the patient, and rating scales may be worded ambiguously or require too much inference. Bech (1981) stressed sources of variance in observer ratings, including differences that occur because information is not gathered from the same sources, differences in multiple observers' perceptions of the same phenomena, and variations in the terminology used to report results of observations of the same phenomena. Variations in the mood of the observer also affect ratings for some items (Bunney and Hamburg, 1963); this is the case especially for anger and anxiety ratings, which may be distorted if the observer confuses his own feelings with those of the patient.

ASSESSMENT OF MANIC STATES

Self-Rating Scales

Self-rating scales have rarely been used to measure manic states. Poor judgment, uncooperativeness, cognitive impairment, distractibility, and denial combine to make meaningful measurement problematic. Platman and colleagues (1969), for instance, found a very low correlation (0.35) between self-ratings of patients during manic episodes and ratings by staff. After recovery, however, the patients' recall of mania was highly correlated (0.95) with staff perceptions. An early instrument designed to assess the less severe, hypomanic range of symptoms was the M-D Scale, developed by Plutchik and colleagues (1970). It had 16 items scored in a yes/no format (e.g., "Lately I feel like breaking things"; "I've been telephoning a lot of friends recently"). This instrument demonstrated discrimination of hypomania from normality, but little reliability or validity information is available.

Recently, renewed attempts have been made to develop and employ self-rating scales for mania because of their obvious advantages. Shugar and colleagues (1992; see also Braunig et al., 1996) reported on the development and

initial validation of a Self-Report Mania Inventory (SRMI). This instrument currently consists of 47 items rated true or false. Its developers based the scale on behavioral items indicative of severity and DSM-III-R criteria, on the assumption that these would be reported more accurately than would inferences about symptoms. Examples include the following: "I started things I didn't finish"; "I partied more"; "I was getting into arguments"; and "I thought I could change the world."

Braunig and colleagues (1996) found that manic patients were able to report reliably on such behaviors over various intervals on the SRMI. Self-report scores correlated highly with results of the Young Mania Rating Scale (YMRS) assessed by observers, and also reflected clinical improvement in hospitalized manic patients. In one study of 20 rapid-cycling bipolar patients, the SRMI results correlated with YMRS ratings, but the SRMI was found to be more sensitive than the latter scale to milder mood fluctuations in the euthymia to hypomania range (Cooke et al., 1996). A study of manic inpatients by Altman and colleagues (2001) found that the SRMI showed good sensitivity in detecting severe cases (86 percent) and was also sensitive to post-test treatment effects; however, its results did not correlate significantly with interviewer-based ratings at initial evaluation. The authors suggested as one possible explanation for this discrepancy that at least eight of the items on the SRMI refer to behaviors that would be prohibited in an inpatient setting (e.g., drinking alcoholic beverages), and thus the instrument might underestimate the severity of manic symptoms in such settings.

Altman and colleagues (1997) reported on the development and preliminary psychometric characteristics of the Altman Self-Rating Mania Scale (ASRM). Five content items based on DSM-IV criteria (cheerful, self-confident, sleep less, talk more, and activity) remained after specificity analyses, and each is presented with five response options. In a later study, Altman and colleagues (2001) compared the ASRM with the SRMI and a visual analogue scale (VAS) (the Internal State Scale [ISS], discussed later, used to record patients' subjective impressions of their mood states) in a sample of manic patients. The ASRM was found to have the highest sensitivity (93 percent) for detecting acute manic symptoms, showed good agreement with an interviewer-rated severity scale, and was also sensitive to treatment-related changes. The authors noted that further studies of patients with mixed states are needed.

Visual analogue scales are discussed later in the section on combined assessment of depression and mania. We note here, however, an application of the VAS methodology to self-reported manic symptoms in a French study using the Ahearn and Carroll (1996) Multiple Visual Analog

Scales of Bipolarity (MVAS-BP) (Akiskal et al., 2001). This instrument, based on a model of mania proposed by Carroll and Klein (Carroll, 1991), comprises 26 VAS items on global mood state; anger; and subscales of "consummatory reward," "incentive reward," "psychomotor pressure," and "central pain." A study of 104 hospitalized manic patients found that patient self-reports were especially likely to correlate with clinician reports on emotional factors of depression and elation. In a related analysis of the same sample, Hantouche and colleagues (2001) found that the MVAS-BP was particularly useful in detecting dysphoric mania, with such patients scoring significantly lower than euphoric manic patients on the psychometrically derived subtypes of symptoms.

The examples cited here provide evidence of the utility of self-reported manic symptoms. Further work is needed, however, to develop the psychometric features of the scales, as well as to identify their limitations.

Observer Rating Scales

Considerably more effort in assessment of manic states has focused on observer ratings, including methods based on patient interviews and behavioral observations. The following sections describe several of the more commonly used instruments and their historical predecessors. Readers are referred to a review by Livianos-Aldana and Rojo-Moreno (2001) for psychometric details and reproduction of various instruments. We begin by discussing observation-based scales (typically used by medical and nursing staff in inpatient settings) and then turn to clinician-administered interview-based scales (which may also include observations of the individual during the interview).

Early Efforts to Develop Rating Scales for Observations of Mania

One of the first systematic observer rating scales for the measurement of mania—the Manic State Rating Scale (MSRS)—was developed at the National Institute of Mental Health (NIMH) (Beigel et al., 1971; Murphy et al., 1974). The scale is made up of 26 items, rated from 0 to 5 on both frequency and intensity dimensions. It was designed to be used by trained research nursing staff in inpatient settings (Table 11–1). The nine superscripted items in Table 11–1 were found to be core features of mania—elements present in all patients and most characteristic of manic severity. The reliability and validity of the MSRS are generally good (Livianos-Aldana and Rojo-Moreno, 2001), and the evidence suggests that the scale can easily be taught to new nursing staff. On the other hand, the MSRS has been criticized as being too extensive to be practical. It is also thought to contain inadequately defined items and scale steps; to require too much time to complete; and to exclude certain core features of mania, such as sleep changes (Petterson et al., 1973; Tyrer and Shopsin, 1982).

The Modified Manic Rating Scale (MMRS) (Blackburn et al., 1977; Loudon et al., 1977) was based largely on the MSRS. It comprises 28 items and uses a six-point rating scale for information derived from interviews and from nursing staff and case notes. The authors found good validity when using a global rating scale as an independent measure, and the scale was highly reliable when employed in a structured interview by several independent raters.

Attempting to develop a shorter but still reliable observation-based rating scale for mania, Petterson and colleagues (1973) devised a seven-item scale that uses a five-point severity system. The behaviors assessed are motor activity, pressured speech, flight of ideas, noisiness, aggressiveness, orientation, and elevated mood. As with the other scales that measure only mania, the Petterson Scale is flawed both theoretically and empirically in not assessing mixed (simultaneous manic and depressed) states. Although the scale rates fewer symptoms of mania than does the MSRS, its measures of severity are far more precisely defined, and because of its relative brevity, it can be readministered easily to obtain serial ratings. Interrater reliability is good, and validity measures generally indicate good correspondence with other measures of mania and treatment outcome. However, several salient aspects of mania, such as sleep and work disturbances, are not assessed.

Young Mania Rating Scale

Presently, the YMRS is the most commonly used interviewer-based measure of severity of manic symptoms. Young and colleagues (1978) sought to develop a mania rating scale broader than the Petterson Scale but shorter and with more explicit ratings of severity than the MSRS. To this end, they devised an 11-item checklist, modeled on the Hamilton Rating Scale for Depression (HAM-D) (discussed later in the section on observer rating scales for depressive symptoms). They based their choice of items on published descriptions of the core symptoms of mania—those cutting across the entire spectrum of illness severity, although dysphoria is not included. Items assessed during the 15- to 30-minute interview are elevated mood, increased motor activity (energy), sexual interest, sleep changes, irritability, speech (rate and amount), language–thought disorder, language content, disruptive–aggressive behavior, appearance, and insight. Ratings are based on subjective reports by patients and on behavioral observations made by the clinician during the interview. Seven of the items are rated on an explicitly defined severity scale of 0 to 4. Four items (irritability, speech rate and amount, language content, and disruptive–aggressive behavior) are scored on a broader scale of 0 to 8. The authors reported that, based on their published results for relatively

Table 11–1. **Manic State Rating Scale**

Part A—Frequency (How much of time?)	The Patient	Part B—Intensity (How intense is it?)
0 to 5		0 to 5
—	1. Looks depressed	—
—	2. Is talking[a]	—
—	3. Moves from one place to another[a]	—
—	4. Makes threats	—
—	5. Has poor judgment[a]	—
—	6. Dresses inappropriately	—
—	7. Looks happy and cheerful	—
—	8. Seeks out others	—
—	9. Is distractible[a]	—
—	10. Has grandiose ideas	—
—	11. Is irritable[a]	—
—	12. Is combative or destructive	—
—	13. Is delusional	—
—	14. Verbalizes depressive feelings	—
—	15. Is active[a]	—
—	16. Is argumentative	—
—	17. Talks about sex	—
—	18. Is angry[a]	—
—	19. Is careless about dress and grooming	—
—	20. Has diminished impulse control[a]	—
—	21. Verbalizes feelings of well-being	—
—	22. Is suspicious	—
—	23. Makes unrealistic plans	—
—	24. Demands contact with others[a]	—
—	25. Is sexually preoccupied	—
—	26. Jumps from one subject to another	—

[a]Core feature of mania.

Source: Adapted from Beigel et al., 1971. Reprinted with permission from the *American Journal of Psychiatry*. Copyright 1971, American Psychiatric Association.

small samples, the scale is a reliable, valid, and sensitive measure of mania. More recent data showed that interrater reliability averaged .68 across items (Altman et al., 1994). The YMRS is increasingly being employed in bipolar clinical trials and treatment outcome studies because of its ease of use (e.g., Tohen et al., 2000; Leverich et al., 2001). The following is a sample from the YMRS developed to assess elevated mood:

Elevated Mood

0 = absent

1 = mildly or possibly increased on questioning

2 = definite subjective elevation; optimistic, self confident; cheerful; appropriate to content

3 = elevated, inappropriate to content; humorous

4 = euphoric; inappropriate laughter; singing

Bech-Rafaelsen Mania Scale

The main purpose of the Bech-Rafaelsen Mania Scale (MAS) (Bech et al., 1979; Bech, 2002) is to assess the severity of current manic symptoms. There are 11 items rated on a five-point scale, with highly specific ratings of severity; for example, a score of 1 on the sleep item represents a reduction of sleep by 25 percent, and a score of 2 represents a reduction by 50 percent. To control for diurnal variation in mood and behavior, the investigators specified that the 15- to 30-minute interview should always take place at a fixed hour. The scale items are motor activity, verbal activity, flight of thoughts, voice/noise level, hostility/destructiveness, mood (feelings of well-being), self-esteem, contact with others, sleep changes, sexual interest, and work activities. Data demonstrating the scale's adequate interrater reliability and a high degree of item homogeneity were presented in an article by Bech and colleagues (1986). An example of the motor activity item follows:

0: Normal motor activity, adequate facial expression.
1: Slightly increased motor activity, lively facial expression.
2: Somewhat excessive motor activity, lively gestures.
3: Outright excessive motor activity, on the move most of the time. Rises one or several times during interview.
4: Constantly active, restless, energetic. Even if urged, patient cannot sit still.

The MAS is commonly used in treatment outcome trials. For instance, it is being used in ongoing trials of adjunctive interpersonal and social rhythm therapy for bipolar patients (Frank et al., 1999). Results of recent research also indicate the scale's validity and internal consistency (e.g., as reviewed by Bech [2002]), as well as its sensitivity to changes in bipolar patients participating in a drug trial (e.g., Licht and Jensen, 1997). It might be noted that Bech (2002; see also Rossi et al., 2001) has recommended using the MAS in conjunction with the Bech-Rafaelsen Melancholia Rating Scale (reviewed later) to capture the frequent co-occurrence of depressive and manic symptoms.

Clinician-Administered Rating Scale for Mania

The Clinician-Administered Rating Scale for Mania (CARS-M) (Altman et al., 1994) was derived from the Schedule for Affective Disorders and Schizophrenia (SADS) and DSM-III-R to characterize the severity of manic symptoms. The 15 items are each rated on a six-point severity scale ("insight" is rated on a five-point scale). Preliminary validity data were based on comparisons with the YMRS; the correlation with the latter was .94. Test–retest and internal consistency reliabilities were found to be adequate. Factor analyses revealed two subscales, mania and psychoticism, which are scored separately.

Additional Interviewer-Based Scales for Mania

Several additional scales for rating mania have been developed, but appear to be used relatively infrequently and may be limited in their testing of psychometric properties. The Manic Diagnostic and Severity Scale (MADS) was developed by Secunda and colleagues (1985) as part of the NIMH Collaborative Program on the Psychobiology of Depression-Clinical Studies. The authors aggregated previously developed items from physician- and nurse-rated instruments to create the MADS. Two subscales taken from physician-rated scales—the Schedule for Affective Disorders and Schizophrenia–Change (SADS-C) Scale 17 and the Global Severity Scale (Katz and Itil, 1974)—correspond, respectively, to the elated–grandiose

and paranoid–destructive indices proposed by Beigel and Murphy (1971). Two factors derived from the nurse-rated Affective Disorder Rating Scale (ADRS) (Murphy et al., 1982) also address items designed to measure these two major subtypes of manic symptoms. The MADS subscales measure elevated mood, sleep and energy changes, grandiosity, guardedness, anger, disturbances in insight and judgment, negativism, restlessness, impulsivity, and distractibility. Detailed reliability and validity data have not yet been published (see Livianos-Aldana and Rojo-Moreno [2001] for further discussion).

Several general rating scales measure features of mania even though they were not developed specifically for that purpose. These scales include the Inpatient Multidimensional Psychiatric Scale, the Brief Psychiatric Rating Scale, and the Clinical Global Inventory. The Differential Diagnostic Scale, Bellevue Differential Inventory, and SADS, devised for differentiating mania from schizophrenia and not directly relevant to the measurement of mania per se, are not reviewed here.

ASSESSMENT OF DEPRESSIVE STATES

Self-Rating Scales for Depressive Symptoms

Several self-report instruments are available for assessment of depressive symptoms, syndromes, and mood states. A few of those most widely used in clinical and research applications are discussed here. Further information on these and numerous other measures was provided by Ronan and colleagues (2000). Many additional instruments have been developed for use with specific populations, such as children and adolescents and the elderly, and for assessment of specialized content areas related to depression, such as hopelessness, suicidality, and self-esteem. These instruments are beyond the scope of the current discussion.

Beck Depression Inventory

The Beck Depression Inventory (BDI) is the most widely used self-rating scale for depression for both research and clinical purposes. Developed by Beck and colleagues (1961) and revised as the BDI-II for consistency with DSM-IV (1996), the scale consists of 21 items, each containing four response options with content ranging in severity from not depressed to severely depressed. Individuals select the one response per item that best corresponds to their current clinical state "over the past 2 weeks," and the options are scored on a scale of 0 to 3, yielding a total across all items. For the BDI-II, a score below 13 suggests minimal depression, a score of 14 to 19 mild depression, and so on. Like all self-report scales in which a cutoff is used to indicate significant symptoms, the scale is not a diagnostic instrument, and scores may be elevated temporarily as a result of environmental, medical, or other difficulties. The items assessed include mood, guilt, irritability, social withdrawal, indecisiveness, fatigability, sleep and appetite changes, and loss of libido. The original BDI tended to emphasize the mood and cognitive features of depression, with less assessment of the more somatic symptoms, whereas the BDI-II includes modifications that permit individuals to indicate whether they have experienced an increase or decrease in sleep and appetite. The following sample item illustrates the range of severity assessed:

14. Worthlessness
   0 I do not feel that I am worthless.
   1 I don't consider myself as worthwhile and useful as I used to.
   2 I feel more worthless as compared to other people.
   3 I feel utterly worthless.

The original BDI had excellent psychometric properties, including internal consistency and test-retest reliability. It was shown to be a valid indicator of severity of depressed mood, having good correspondence with other measures and diagnostic criteria for depression (e.g., Beck et al., 1988). The BDI-II likewise has been well tested. It shows good correspondence with the HAM-D (Hamilton, 1960) and with other measures of depression-related constructs (Beck et al., 1996).

Zung Self-Rating Depression Scale

The Zung Self-Rating Depression Scale (Zung SDS), a 20-item scale with a four-point severity range, measures somatic, psychological, and mood aspects of depression. It is a modified version of the earlier Zung Depression Scale (Zung et al., 1965; Zung, 1974). For an item such as "I have trouble sleeping through the night," the patient is expected to indicate which of the following responses is most appropriate: "none or a little of the time," "some of the time," "good part of the time," or "most or all of the time." Note that the graded response to this question applies only to frequency, not to the extent of sleep loss. Further, the scale does not rate hypersomnia, a frequent symptom among patients with bipolar depression.

The Zung SDS does not show consistently high correlation with the HAM-D (Murphy et al., 1982). It has been criticized on the grounds that depressed patients have difficulty judging the degree and frequency of their symptoms, and endogenous symptoms are underrepresented (Rush et al., 1986). Hamilton (1988) also reported as a major shortcoming of the Zung SDS its relative insensitivity to clinical improvement after treatment (Rickels et al., 1968; Feighner et al., 1984). However, its brevity may enhance its value as a quick screen for severity of depressive symptoms.

Carroll Depression Rating Scale-Revised

The original Carroll Rating Scale was developed to parallel closely in item content the observer-scored HAM-D (Carroll et al., 1981; Feinberg et al., 1981; Smouse et al., 1981). The Carroll Depression Rating Scale-Revised (CDS-R) (Carroll, 1998) is a 61-item self-report questionnaire with items concerning 17 areas of depressive symptoms over the past few days, each rated yes or no. The revised version attempts to make the scale more compatible with DSM-IV. Examples include the following:

2. I have dropped many of my interests and activities.
7. I feel worthless and ashamed of myself.

Both the original and revised scales were based on Carroll's observation that neither existing self-report nor clinician-based scales were adequate for diagnosis of depressive symptoms (Carroll et al., 1981).

Most empirical evaluation of the Carroll scales has been based on the original version, but the author has indicated that the evaluation results are also applicable to the CDS-R. The scales appear to have excellent convergent validity with both self-report and clinician-based measures (e.g., correlation with the BDI, $r = .86$; correlation with the observer-rated HAM-D, $r = .71$ [Carroll, 1998]). Because it is similar in structure and content to the HAM-D and is less time-consuming and less expensive to administer, it may be a good alternative (see Smouse et al., 1981; Tandon et al., 1986). Correlations with other depression scales suggest that it is as sensitive to bipolar as to unipolar depression. Carroll and colleagues (1981) suggested that a cutoff of 10 can serve as a screen for the presence of significant depression.

Hamilton Depression Inventory

A different self-report instrument based on the observer-rated HAM-D was developed by Reynolds and Kobak (1995). The Hamilton Depression Inventory consists of 38 questions covering the original items of the HAM-D; there is also a melancholia subscale for evaluating the severity of DSM-IV melancholia symptoms. The instrument attempts to measure both the frequency and severity of symptomatology over the preceding 2 weeks. Its psychometric properties are promising, including a correlation of .94 with scores on the clinician-administered HAM-D in a sample of 403 adults (Reynolds and Kobak, 1995). It has not been extensively used in research or clinical settings, however, and its value therefore awaits confirmation.

A briefer version (19 items) of the same scale, the Reynolds Depression Screening Inventory (RDSI) (Reynolds and Kobak, 1998), is intended to take only 5 to 10 minutes to complete. Using a clinical cutoff score of 16, it has the potential to identify major depression among nonreferred community adults with a high degree of sensitivity and specificity. Therefore, it may serve as a useful screening instrument. Its research uses have been limited to date, however.

Inventory of Depressive Symptomatology

Another recent addition to self-report measures of depression is the self-report version of the Inventory of Depressive Symptomatology (IDS-SR), devised by Rush and colleagues (1986, 1996b). It was based on the authors' clinician-rated scale (IDS-C, discussed later), which was developed to improve on the HAM-D and was recently revised to include symptoms compatible with DSM-IV. The IDS-SR includes 30 items assessed over the preceding week, rated 0 to 3, measuring three factors: a cognitive/mood factor; an anxiety/arousal factor; and a sleep, appetite, and leaden paralysis factor (confirmed by Corruble et al., 1999). Both the self-report and clinician-administered versions take approximately 30 to 45 minutes to complete. Excellent psychometric properties have been reported, including good convergent validation with other measures of self- and clinician-reported symptoms (Rush et al., 1996b; see also Trivedi et al., 2004). Research has demonstrated that the measures are sensitive to treatment-related changes. Recently, Rush and colleagues (2003) developed a shortened form of the two versions of the IDS, called the Quick IDS (QIDS, with self-report and clinician versions), consisting of 16 items from the original 30-item scale—those needed to assess DSM-IV criteria for major depression. Trivedi and colleagues (2004) reported on the use of these shorter versions with a large sample of outpatients with major depression or bipolar disorder. They concluded that the brief instruments corresponded closely to the longer IDS measures, had solid psychometric properties, and were sensitive to treatment-related change.

Additional Self-Report Scales

Several additional self-report scales for depressive symptoms merit mention. The Center for Epidemiologic Studies-Depression (CES-D) scale (Radloff, 1977) is used extensively in community surveys and as a screening measure for depression. It was designed to be administered quickly and easily in research and epidemiologic settings, but has limited clinical utility. Normative information on its use in various samples was reported by Weissman and colleagues (1977). Furukawa and colleagues (1997) reviewed studies of the CES-D and the limitations of its psychometric properties, and presented data on potential cutoff scores to be used in various settings to predict the probability of depressive disorder given a specific individual score.

The Inventory to Diagnose Depression (Zimmerman et al., 1986) was developed to serve as a self-report diagnostic

instrument for assessing the attainment of syndromic features of major depressive disorder based on DSM-III features; the authors presented initial evidence of its validity. Recently, noting changes in the DSM-IV criteria, Zimmerman and colleagues (2004a) developed a new 38-item self-report measure called the Diagnostic Inventory for Depression (DID), which includes symptoms, severity, duration, and impairment due to depressive symptoms. The authors reported on initial psychometric evaluation of the measure based on 626 psychiatric outpatients. The DID showed significant agreement with the SCID on diagnoses of depression, as well as convergent and discriminant validity. The instrument also showed sensitivity to change in symptom severity in follow-up assessments.

Bech and colleagues (2001) similarly developed a self-report scale for diagnosing major depressive episodes. A preliminary study based on 43 psychiatric patients and controls indicated a sensitivity of 1.0 and a specificity of .82 in comparison with DSM-IV/*International Classification of Diseases 10* (ICD-10) diagnoses. Further work is warranted to determine the validity of the procedure for screening and other clinical purposes.

Depressed Mood Self-Rating Scales

There are a number of scales for measuring depressed mood state, not including associated symptoms and syndromic features of depression. Such scales have been widely used in research on moods and emotions, may capture short-term changes in mood, and in some cases may be useful for limited clinical purposes.

- Visual analogue scales, mentioned earlier, are used to measure both manic and depressive states, and therefore are discussed in the section on combined measurement instruments (Hayes and Patterson, 1921; Zealley and Aitken, 1969).
- The Depression Adjective Check Lists (DACL) have both state and trait versions and have been studied extensively, including among clinical populations (Lubin, 1994).
- The Medical Care Outcomes Study (MOS) Screener (Burnam et al., 1988) was developed as an eight-item scale to screen for symptoms of depression in the MOS, in order to identify those with likely depressive disorders. It is not suitable as a measure of severity, and its use for diagnosis requires application of a complex formula for weighting items. Nevertheless, it appears to have acceptable validity and has been used extensively in epidemiologic and health policy research.

Observer Rating Scales for Depressive Symptoms

It is often argued that, while self-report instruments are uniquely suited to capturing the subjective experiences of depression, certain aspects of the depressive syndrome may be characterized more accurately by observers. As suggested earlier, self-reports may be biased not only by the cognitive capabilities or awareness, as well as mood-related perceptions, of depressed individuals, but also by their motives to present themselves in certain lights. Thus, for instance, evaluation of treatment outcomes may require objective ratings by trained clinicians. The drawback of such methods—and the reason for the relative paucity of such instruments compared with self-report questionnaires—is the requirement for training and the establishment of adequate expertise and reliability.

Hamilton Rating Scale for Depression

The HAM-D remains the most widely used observer-rated scale for depression. It was developed by Hamilton (1960) to measure severity and changes over time in the clinical state of depressed patients, and has been amended several times over the years. Although not developed as a diagnostic tool, it has been used with success in making retrospective diagnoses from chart reviews (Thase et al., 1983). It has been widely used as well to evaluate treatment response, correlate depression severity with biological parameters, and evaluate depression subtypes.

The HAM-D is focused much more on somatic and behavioral symptoms than on mood and cognitive symptoms. In its most commonly administered form, it consists of 17 items (9 on a five-point scale [0 to 4] and 8 on a three-point scale [0 to 2]) that measure mood, guilt, suicidal ideation, sleep disorders, changes in work and interests, psychomotor agitation and retardation, anxiety, somatic symptoms, hypochondriasis, loss of insight, and loss of weight. In later versions, additional items were added, so that it is essential to indicate which version is being reported. Note that, in contrast with most depression assessment instruments, the content includes several items pertaining to anxiety states. These features may be somewhat less relevant to bipolar than to unipolar depression.

Interobserver reliability is good, although various factor analyses have extracted inconsistent numbers and types of factors (see Hedlund and Vieweg, 1979). The HAM-D's high reliability, ease of administration (taking approximately 30 minutes), and emphasis on somatic symptoms have been cited as reasons for its enormous popularity (Murphy et al., 1982). On the other hand, critics believe that somatic symptoms are disproportionately represented in the HAM-D, that the differential weighting of symptoms is arbitrary, and that anchor points are ambiguous. Furthermore, certain symptoms, such as hypersomnia, increases in weight and appetite, and changes in quality of mood, are not assessed (Bech, 1981; Rush et al.,

1986). This last point may be an especially important limitation in the assessment of bipolar depression. As noted earlier, Rush and colleagues (1996a) developed a clinician-administered version of what they believe is an improved HAM-D addressing several of the shortcomings noted. The IDS-C is currently being used in the multisite NIMH–Stanley Foundation Bipolar Network study (Leverich et al., 2001), and its scores correlate highly with those on the HAM-D. A study of depressed inpatients reported by Corruble and colleagues (1999) confirmed the IDS-C's strong psychometric properties and suggested that it is more sensitive to treatment-related changes than the Montgomery-Asberg Depression Rating Scale (MADRS) (discussed later). The brief, 16-item clinician version of the QIDS was also found to have excellent psychometric properties in a large-scale study of unipolar depressed and bipolar outpatients (Trivedi et al., 2004). Finally, there is a Revised HAM-D (Warren, 1994). It remains to be seen whether alternatives to the HAM-D will flourish in clinical research over time.

Bech-Rafaelsen Melancholia Rating Scale

The Bech-Rafaelsen Melancholia Rating Scale, developed to combine the HAM-D and the Cronholm-Ottosson Depression Scale, comprises 11 items rated at five degrees of severity (Bech et al., 1979; Bech and Rafaelsen, 1980; Rafaelsen et al., 1980). Items are decreased motor activity, decreased verbal activity, intellectual and emotional retardation, psychic anxiety, suicidal impulses, lowered mood, self-depreciation, sleep disturbances, tiredness and pains, decreased motivation, and decreased productivity in work and interests. The interview is designed to be completed within 15 to 30 minutes, and to control for possible diurnal variation, is to be administered at approximately the same time of day each time. Guidelines for ratings are highly specific; for example, the guidelines for intellectual retardation are as follows:

0   Normal intellectual activity.
1   The patient has to make an effort to concentrate on his work.
2   Even with a major effort it is difficult for the patient to concentrate or make decisions. Less initiative than usual. The patient easily experiences "brain fatigue."
3   Marked difficulties with concentration, initiative and decision-making. For example, can hardly read a newspaper or watch television. Score 3 as long as the retardation has not clearly influenced the interview.
4   When the patient during the interview has shown marked difficulties in following normal conversation.

The interobserver reliability of the Bech-Rafaelsen Melancholia Rating Scale has been found to be as high as that of the HAM-D (Rafaelsen et al., 1980), and the item–total score correlations are adequate (Bech and Rafaelsen, 1980).

Montgomery-Asberg Depression Rating Scale

Yet another observer rating scale for depression is the MADRS of Montgomery and Asberg (1979), developed to measure changes in depression after antidepressant treatment. Easily administered by clinicians, the scale's 10 items measure the major components of clinical depression: apparent sadness, reported sadness, inner tension, reduced sleep, reduced appetite, concentration difficulties, lassitude, inability to feel, pessimistic thoughts, and suicidal thoughts. Items are rated on a seven-point scale (0 to 6), with illustrative anchor points given for ratings of 0, 2, 4, and 6. For example, ratings for the item measuring pessimistic thoughts are as follows:

Representing thoughts of guilt, inferiority, self-reproach, sinfulness, remorse and ruin

0 No pessimistic thoughts.

1

2 Fluctuating ideas of a failure, self-reproach or self-depreciation.

3

4 Persistent self-accusations, or definite but still rational ideas of guilt or sin. Increasingly pessimistic about the future.

5

6 Delusions of ruin, remorse or unredeemable sin. Self-accusations which are absurd and unshakable.

The MADRS exhibits construct validity and concurrent validity relative to the HAM-D (Davidson et al., 1986; Khan et al., 2004). Further, it is easily and relatively quickly administered, has well-defined items, and provides for equal weighting of symptoms (Rush et al., 1986). The MADRS has been shown to demonstrate considerable clinical relevance as well (Williamson et al., 2006). On the other hand, its unidirectional rating of sleep change (i.e., decreased sleep) may be a disadvantage in rating bipolar patients. It may be noted that a self-report version of the MADRS (the MADRS-S) has been developed and shown to correlate highly with the BDI (Svanborg and Asberg, 2001).

Additional major observer rating scales for depression include the Cronholm-Ottosson Depression Scale (Cronholm and Ottosson, 1960); the Inpatient Multidimensional Psychiatric Scale (Lorr, 1974); the Physicians' Global Assessment Scale (GAS) (Carney et al., 1965; Endicott et al., 1976); and the Newcastle Rating Scales (Roth et al., 1983), which have been of special interest in biological studies because of their sensitivity to endogenous or melancholic items. As one might expect from the symptomatic differences

reviewed in Chapters 1 and 2, bipolar and unipolar depressed patients show different patterns of response to some of the same standard rating instruments (Paykel and Prusoff, 1973). In this light, it is unfortunate that there have been no systematic studies of the differential sensitivity of rating scales to bipolar depression. To our knowledge, the only scale designed specifically with bipolar patients in mind is the ADRS (Murphy et al., 1982), described later.

Instruments for assessment of depression are being refined and developed with increasing frequency and psychometric sophistication. The tension between having well-developed and empirically sound measures on the one hand and the capacity for widespread use and communicability on the other will doubtless grow. Most of today's instruments continue to be validated by comparison with older instruments (e.g., the HAM-D) without sufficient consideration of sources of invalidity of the latter. A further significant problem is the heterogeneity of the scales' contents, with some being far more focused on somatic or cognitive symptoms than others (see the later discussion). This variation leads to discrepancies in the results of treatment and clinical studies. Moreover, given the heterogeneity among clinical presentations of depressive syndromes, there have been calls for the development of more "narrow-band" instruments that can be used to assess individual or clusters of symptoms, such as energy and fatigability, sleep difficulties, and hopelessness. Such more narrowly focused assessments could potentially facilitate advances in treatment or in understanding of depressive subtypes.

Perhaps the greatest limitation of most well-established self-report and observer rating scales for depression is their failure to capture potentially unique aspects of bipolar depression. This shortcoming, discussed at length in Chapter 2, is of obvious concern to most researchers in the field (see Berk et al., 2004, for a review of the subject). Further research on the clinical features of bipolar depression is needed to help identify factors that should be developed or refined in assessment instruments.

ANALYSIS AND COMPARISON OF SCALES FOR MANIA AND DEPRESSION

There are many ways of comparing rating scales; here we focus primarily on differences in item content. Content profiles of the items included in observer rating scales for mania and in self-report and observer rating scales for depression are presented in Figures 11–2 through 11–5. The classification of items is, of necessity, occasionally arbitrary. For example, symptoms of mood and cognition (hopelessness and pessimism) often overlap, as do symptoms of behavior and activity level. Working within these and

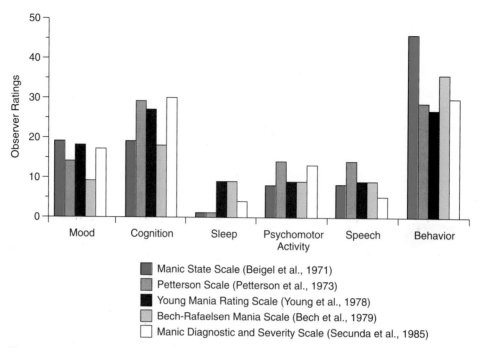

Figure 11–2. Relative weighting of item content: Observer rating measures of mania.

other constraints, it is possible to develop item-content profiles—that is, the items in each scale that are designed to assess a particular feature of mania or depression.

Content of Mania Scales

Figure 11–2 illustrates relative weightings for mood, cognition, sleep, psychomotor activity, speech, and behavior in observer rating scales for mania. The CARS-M (Altman et al., 1994) is not included; its 10 mania items are based on DSM-III-R and SADS criteria, with a separate psychoticism–insight subscale. Figure 11–3 portrays content profiles for more specific types of manic behavior—aggression and hostility, hypersexuality, impaired judgment, seeking out others, impulsivity, and appearance. Mood items represent approximately 15 percent of the total number of observer-rated mania items. The greatest emphasis is placed on euphoric and expansive mood, although all but two scales (the Petterson Scale and the Bech-Rafaelsen MAS) also include items measuring dysphoric, angry, irritable, or negativistic mood.

Despite the frequency of depression during mania (see Chapter 2), this mixed mood state is assessed in only one scale—the MSRS. The proportion of cognitive items is high on all scales, especially the MADS and the Petterson Scale. Sleep disorder symptoms, although integral to the diagnosis and pathophysiology of mania, are the least represented of all symptoms on the various scales; indeed, two scales do not inquire about sleep changes at all. Psychomotor activity and speech symptoms are measured by all of the mania scales. Behavior changes, like cognitive symptoms, are widely represented, especially on the MSRS. The breakdown of behavior symptoms shown in Figure 11–3 reveals that the symptoms represented most widely and consistently are aggression and hostility, followed by hypersexuality and seeking out others. Impaired judgment, impulsivity, and appearance are assessed less consistently.

The decision to use a particular rating scale for mania is based not only on the item content, but also on the nature of the patient population and the training of the raters administering the scale. The YMRS and the MAS, for example, are more appropriate for less severely ill patients and require a less experienced rating staff, whereas the MSRS is more comprehensive, but also requires sophisticated nurse raters. If patients are only hypomanic rather than manic, additional useful subjective information may be obtained by using self-rating forms.

Content of Depression Scales

Relative weightings for item content in self-rating scales for depression are shown in Figure 11–4 and for item content in observer rating scales in Figure 11–5. Mood and cognitive symptoms are the best represented of symptom groups in both types of scales. The BDI is particularly weighted toward cognitive items, and the MADRS toward both mood and cognition. Somatic and sleep symptoms are represented most strongly on the HAM-D and on its self-rating parallel, the CDS-R. There are no other major differences in relative weightings of item content. Behavior items are not substantially represented on either self-rating

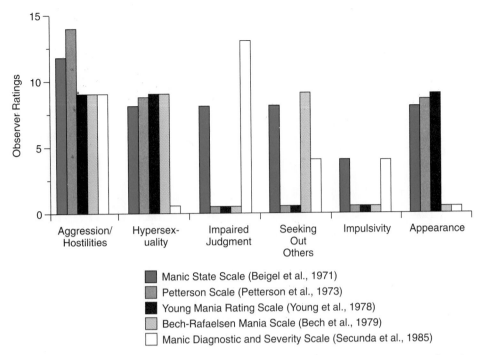

Manic State Scale (Beigel et al., 1971)
Petterson Scale (Petterson et al., 1973)
Young Mania Rating Scale (Young et al., 1978)
Bech-Rafaelsen Mania Scale (Bech et al., 1979)
Manic Diagnostic and Severity Scale (Secunda et al., 1985)

Figure 11–3. Relative weighting of item content for behavior items: Observer rating measures of mania.

Figure 11–4. Relative weighting of item content: Self-rating measures of depression.

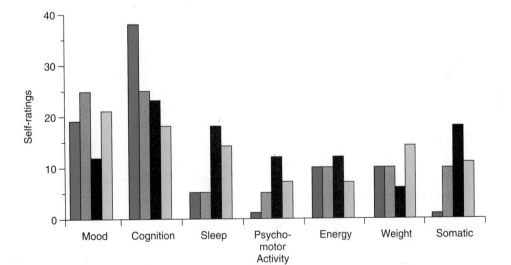

Beck Depression Inventory (Beck et al., 1961)
Zung Self-Rating Depression Scale (Zung, 1974)
Carroll Depression Rating Scale-Revised (Carroll, 1998)
Inventory for Depressive Symptomatology (Rush et al., 1986, 1996b)

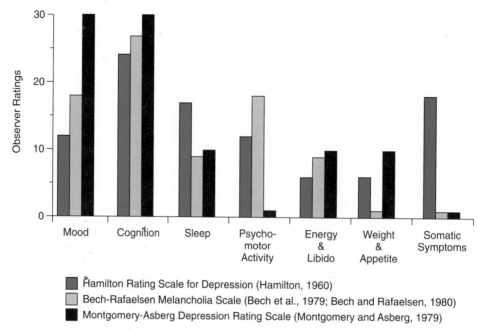

Figure 11–5. Relative weighting of item content: Observer-rating measures of depression.

or observer rating scales with the exception of work activities and interests, which together make up 7 percent of the total self-rating and 6 percent of the total observer rating items (all of the latter are on the HAM-D). As in the assessment of mania, the choice of instruments for assessment of depression depends on the patient population being evaluated, the level of interviewer training required, and the nature of the clinical or research issue being addressed. It is often useful to combine a self-rating with an observer rating measure.

COMBINED ASSESSMENT OF MANIC AND DEPRESSIVE STATES

A single rating scale that measures depression and mania along one continuum creates both theoretical and practical difficulties because it implies that depression and mania are opposite states—an assumption clearly contrary to what is known about the nature and expression of bipolar disorder (see Chapter 2). Monopolar scales (e.g., Bech, 1981) also generally preclude the measurement of mixed and transition states, rapid-cycling states, and diurnal or other cyclic variations in mood, behavior, and activity. A combination of individual measures of depression and mania or other combined measures, such as those discussed later, can be used to mitigate these problems.

Visual Analogue Scales

In their most commonly administered form, visual analogue scales (Hayes and Patterson, 1921; Zealley and Aitken, 1969) are composed of a 100-mm line anchored at either end with opposite descriptors (e.g., "Worst I have ever felt" and "Best I have ever felt"). The patient is asked to place a mark or line across the point on the scale that best characterizes his or her mental state. Ratings are made frequently, typically once or twice a day, a characteristic that makes visual analogue scales especially appropriate for longitudinal studies of mood and treatment effects. Further advantages include the rapidity of assessment, economic feasibility, involvement of patients in their research and treatment protocols, a relative lack of cultural and educational bias, and good reliability and validity (Zealley and Aitken, 1969; Folstein and Luria, 1973; Luria, 1975). The simplicity of the test makes it ideal for depressed patients who are very ill or indecisive.

Moderately high correlations exist between visual analogue scales and the Zung SDS, the HAM-D, and global ratings by psychiatrists (Folstein and Luria, 1973; Luria, 1975), although correlations with clinical judgment tend to decrease after acute treatment (Zealley and Aitken, 1969). Moreover, such scales are not sensitive at lower levels of depression and other types of psychopathology. The most important limitation of the simple versions of these scales is that they are global measures not designed to assess specific psychopathological states or symptoms. As noted previously, however, Ahearn and Carroll's bipolar scales use the VAS format for self-report across a variety of symptoms (e.g., Akiskal et al., 2001).

A more recent application of the VAS format, involving development and rescaling of the Internal State Scale (ISS), was reported by Bauer and colleagues (2000). The 15-item self-report covers items from subscales called "activation," "well-being," a "depression index," and "perceived conflict," measuring patients' subjective impressions of mood states. In a Veterans Affairs medical center study of bipolar patients, scores on the subscales were able to identify and distinguish among groups that were euthymic, manic/hypomanic, mixed, and depressed. Glick and colleagues (2003) recently developed a Likert-based scoring system that they believe is easier to use than the VAS method and results in characteristics similar to those of the original ISS. With respect to its use for self-rating of mania, however, Altman and colleagues (2001) found that the ISS well-being scale was not sensitive to treatment effects in manic inpatients, although the activation scale did show significant changes from pre- to post-treatment. Most important, the ISS had relatively poor sensitivity, detecting only 45 percent of patients with moderate or severe symptomatology at baseline.

Affective Disorder Rating Scale

The ADRS (Murphy et al., 1982) comprises 34 specific items assessing mania and depression, using a 6-point scale for the frequency and intensity of the behavior and global ratings (on a 15-point scale) of mania, depression, psychosis, anxiety, and anger. For the global ratings, specific guidelines for assigning scores are provided. For example, in the mild range (within normal limits), scores of 2 or 3 on the mania scale reflect "especially talkative, active, enthusiastic, gregarious or boisterous behavior," while at the extreme end of the scale, scores of 13 to 15 reflect "nearly continuous manic activity and other symptoms, with uncontrolled, impulsive behavior requiring close supervision and often seclusion for the majority of the day." Although preliminary psychometric data suggest good convergent validation with other scales of depressive and manic symptoms, little information exists about the properties and use of this instrument.

Comprehensive Psychopathological Rating Scale

The Comprehensive Psychopathological Rating Scale (CPRS) was developed in 1971 by the Swedish Medical Research Council to measure treatment effects (Asberg et al., 1978). Four scale steps, each described in detail, are allocated for each item. The scale, designed for use by all trained mental health workers, can be used to assess both reported and observed behaviors. Items include elevated and sad mood states, indecision, lassitude, fatigability, concentration difficulties, reduced or increased sexual interest, ideas of grandeur, and ecstatic experiences. Reliability studies among depressed patients in the United Kingdom (Montgomery et al., 1978a) and among cross-cultural populations

of Swedish and British depressed patients (Montgomery et al., 1978b) indicated that the CPRS is "highly reliable and highly sensitive [and] easily communicable" (Perris, 1979).

ASSESSMENT OF BIPOLAR RISK AND SCREENING INSTRUMENTS

Risk for Bipolar Disorder

There is considerable interest in detecting risk for bipolar disorder. The aim is to enable early intervention to alter the course of the illness and prevent the severe psychosocial consequences of the disruption of normal social development typically associated with the disorder. Several such instruments have been developed for use in research studies.

General Behavior Inventory

The General Behavior Inventory (GBI), a self-report inventory for nonpatients, was developed to identify individuals at high risk for developing bipolar disorder, particularly adolescents and young adults (Depue et al., 1981). Five dimensions of bipolarity are defined as characterizing the disorder: its core behaviors and symptoms; their intensity, frequency, and duration; and rapid shifts in mood and behavior. Sample questions (taken from a longitudinal mood-rating study), with their extreme polar descriptors, are presented in Table 11–2. Each item is rated on a four-point frequency scale.

The GBI, uniquely designed to measure subsyndromal variants of bipolar disorder (see Chapter 1), was validated in an initial series of studies through interview-derived diagnoses, interviews with college roommates, family histories of affective illness, clinical characteristics, and longitudinal mood-rating investigations (Depue et al., 1981). The GBI was originally viewed as a measure of subsyndromal cyclothymia or prodromal signs of bipolarity. Klein and colleagues (1986) predicted that it would identify youths at risk for bipolar disorder in a sample of offspring of bipolar-I parents; they found that half of the offspring had significant cyclothymic features identified by the GBI. The authors noted that offspring with cyclothymic features had significantly poorer social adjustment relative to noncyclothymic offspring and children of control parents. A follow-up study of 45 college students identified by the GBI as being at risk for bipolar disorder was conducted 19 months later (Klein and Depue, 1984); the investigators found that high scorers continued to exhibit significant impairment of functioning. Two patients had been hospitalized for major depressive episodes, and overall, the group reported higher suicidal ideation and treatment seeking.

Table 11–2. **Sample Items from the General Behavior Inventory**

Question Content	Extreme Polar Descriptions
Stimulus-seeking/excitement (receptivity toward and stimulation by the world)	• Passionately absorbed in the world's excitement; my sensations and feelings incredibly intensified; I seek out novel stimulations. • Life is too much trouble; sick of everything.
Flight of ideas/thought retardation (thought processes)	• Brilliant penetrating ideas emerging spontaneously and with great rapidity. • My mind is cold, dead; nothing moves.
Decisiveness/doubt	• Supremely confident in my judgment and strength of mind; I can instantly see problems which confuse others and solve them. • Utterly immobile, frozen by doubts; nothing is certain or solid for me.

Source: Depue et al., 1981. Reprinted with permission from the *American Journal of Psychiatry*. Copyright 1981, American Psychiatric Association.

Noting that the GBI appeared to identify those at risk for unipolar as well as bipolar depressive conditions, Depue and colleagues (1989) subsequently revised the GBI specifically to identify subgroups of unipolar (46 items) and bipolar (hypomanic/biphasic, 26 items) affective conditions. They reported that in a university sample, high scorers for the two conditions were identified and diagnosed by blind interviewers. The GBI's unipolar and bipolar scales showed adequate sensitivity (.78 and .76, respectively) and high specificity (.99 for both) for research use in nonclinical samples.

Hypomanic Personality Scale

Eckblad and Chapman (1986) developed the Hypomanic Personality Scale (HPS), a self-report scale for use in identifying those with gregarious and overactive behavior styles characteristic of episodes of hypomanic euphoria and hypothesized to indicate potential risk for developing bipolar disorder. The scale consists of 48 true–false items, such as "Sometimes ideas and insights come to me so fast that I cannot express them all" and "I would rather be an ordinary success in life than a spectacular failure" (scored in hypomania direction if false-rated). Internal consistency and test–retest reliabilities were shown to be high among a student population. The scale was validated among a university population against standardized diagnostic assessments; high scorers were significantly more likely to have experienced hypomanic episodes and depressive symptoms, drug and alcohol use, and psychotic-like symptoms. A longitudinal study of 36 high scorers on the HPS and 31 controls followed the groups for 13 years (Kwapil et al.,

2000). As predicted, significantly more high scorers than controls developed bipolar disorder (25 percent versus none) and experienced major depressive episodes (28 versus 19 percent); this was the case in particular for those who also scored high on the impulsive–nonconformity scale (Chapman et al., 1984). High scorers also had more severe psychotic-like symptoms, borderline personality disorder symptoms, and substance abuse disorders relative to the controls. A more recent study of 224 German university students found that the HPS was more effective in ascertaining individuals with a history of hypomanic or manic episodes than those with a history of depressive episodes (Meyer and Hautzinger, 2003).

An abbreviated version of the HPS was included in the Oregon Adolescent Depression Project (Klein et al., 1996), where it was found to be predictive of a wide range of psychosocial impairments; mood, disruptive, and substance abuse disorders; and suicide attempts. Among youths with a history of depressive disorders, the HPS appeared to predict for high scorers significantly more severe symptoms of depression and worse functional outcomes. Hofmann and Meyer (2006) studied three groups of young adults with high (n=17), medium (n=19), and low (n=18) scores on the Hypomanic Personality Scale. Those at elevated risk for bipolar disorder reported greater mood instability, as well as higher levels of both positive and negative affect. Although the sample has not yet been followed long enough to validate use of the HPS as a predictor of bipolar disorder, the scale appears to be valid for predicting mood and behavioral dysfunction that is potentially indicative of the disorder.

More recently, researchers have developed measures to assess bipolar spectrum disorder on the assumption that categorical measures are intrinsically limiting. These assessment systems—the Bipolar Affective Disorder Dimension Scale (Craddock et al., 2004) and the Bipolar Spectrum Diagnostic Scale (Ghaemi et al., 2005)—are promising but need further validation and replication. Also promising but preliminary are measures developed to assess dysfunctional beliefs that may predispose to bipolar disorder (Mansell and Jones, 2006) and positive self-dispositional appraisals linked to both hypomanic personality and bipolar disorder (Jones et al., 2006). Measures of temperament, beyond the scope of this chapter, have been studied by many groups[1] (see Chapter 10).

Screening for Bipolar Disorder

Noting that many cases of bipolar spectrum disorder may go undetected and undiagnosed, Hirschfeld and colleagues (2000, 2002) developed the Mood Disorder Questionnaire (MDQ), a brief self-report screening instrument for use in primary care, community agency, and psychiatric settings (Table 11–3). Based on DSM-IV criteria, it contains 13 yes–no items, as well as 2 additional questions designed to verify whether symptoms occurred during the same time period and caused significant problems. The questionnaire originated with a sample of 198 patients from five outpatient mood disorders clinics, who were then interviewed by telephone using the SCID for bipolar-I, bipolar-II, and bipolar–not otherwise specified (NOS) disorders. Using a threshold of seven or more yes responses, along with an indication that the symptoms occurred during the same time period and caused moderate or severe problems, the sensitivity was .73 and the specificity .90. This suggests a basis for the instrument's use in psychiatric settings, but how useful it will prove to be in general medical or community settings (where screening instruments should have the most utility) remains to be seen. When the same investigators conducted a population-based replication study, for example, the sensitivity of the MDQ (identification of true positive cases) was found to be .28, much lower than that found in the original study (Hirschfeld et al., 2003b). A recent study of 1,157 patients at a general medicine clinic found that although the specificity of the MDQ was lower than found in mood disorders clinics, the measure was helpful in identifying bipolar patients who would not otherwise have been recognized (Das et al., 2005). On the other hand, in a review of studies of screening instruments, Phelps and Ghaemi (2006) concluded that where there is likely to be a low prevalence of bipolar disorder, such as in community or primary care settings, screening measures such as the MDQ can rule out bipolarity but do not effectively rule it in.

As discussed, Hirschfeld's group reported on a population-based replication study in which the sensitivity of the MDQ was found to be much lower than that found in the original study (Hirschfeld et al., 2003b). Replication and further validation studies are well-warranted in view of the overlap of bipolar symptoms with those of other mood, substance, and behavioral disorders.

Despite ongoing concerns about its utility outside of mood disorders clinics, the MDQ has been widely disseminated, appearing in psychiatric publications and on Web sites, in the hope that it can facilitate the identification and treatment of bipolar disorder. It was tested in a French population of bipolar patients, with the investigators finding much greater sensitivity in bipolar-I than in bipolar-II patients (90 and 52 percent, respectively) (Rouget et al., 2005). It also served as the basis for an epidemiologic survey of bipolar spectrum disorder (see Chapter 5) (Hirschfeld et al., 2003a). But given the evidence to date that the MDQ appears to be insufficiently accurate to be used as a case-finding measure in community studies or as a screening scale in clinical practice, further research and refinement of the instrument are needed (Zimmerman et al., 2004b). Given that many bipolar patients lack insight into the hypomanic and manic phases of their illness, one helpful refinement might be a version of the instrument that could be filled out by family members. We recommend that the MDQ, while promising, be viewed with some skepticism until further validation and replication studies have been completed.

A somewhat similar scale, the Manic Depressiveness Scale, was documented by Thalbourne and colleagues (1994). The 19-item questionnaire, assessing manic and depressive experiences, was administered to normal college students and to a sample of bipolar patients. Despite significant mean differences between the groups and relatively good internal consistency and reliability, however, the scale showed overlapping distributions between the two populations, apparently precluding its use to identify bipolar disorder among nonpatient samples. A later revision (9 manic experience items and 9 depressive experience items) was found to correlate with severity of illness and number of hospitalizations for bipolar patients, but not for unipolar depressed patients (Thalbourne and Bassett, 1998).

Recently, Solomon and colleagues (2006) reported the development of a brief instrument to screen for bipolar disorder in patients acutely ill with major depression. The Screening Assessment of Depression-Polarity (SAD-P) consists of 3 items demonstrating the greatest disparity between bipolar-I and unipolar depression: presence of delusions during the current episode of major depression, number of prior episodes of major depression, and family

TABLE 11–3. **Sample Items from the Mood Disorder Questionnaire**

Question	Response	
1. Has there ever been a period of time when you were not your usual self and . . .		
• you felt so good or so hyper that other people thought you were not your normal self or you were so hyper that you got into trouble?	○ yes	O no
• you were so irritable that you shouted at people or started fights or arguments?	○ yes	○ no
• you felt much more self-confident than usual?	○ yes	○ no
• you got much less sleep than usual and found you didn't really miss it?	○ yes	○ no
• you were much more talkative or spoke much faster than usual?	○ yes	○ no
• thoughts raced through your mind or you couldn't slow your mind down?	○ yes	○ no
• you were so easily distracted by things around you that you had trouble concentrating or staying on track?	○ yes	○ no
• you had much more energy than usual?	○ yes	○ no
• you were much more active or did many more things than usual?	○ yes	○ no
• you were much more social or outgoing than usual; for example, you telephoned friends in the middle of the night?	○ yes	○ no
• you were much more interested in sex than usual?	○ yes	○ no
• you did things that were unusual for you or that other people might have thought were excessive, foolish, or risky?	○ yes	○ no
• spending money got you or your family into trouble?	○ yes	○ no
2. If you checked YES to more than one of the above, have several of these ever happened during the same period of time?	○ yes	○ no
3. How much of a problem did any of these cause you—like being unable to work; having family, money, or legal troubles; getting into arguments or fights?		
• No problem		
• Minor problem		
• Moderate problem		
• Serious problem		

Source: Adapted from Hirschfeld et al., 2000. Reprinted with permission from the *American Journal of Psychiatry*, Copyright 2005, American Psychiatric Association.

history of major depression or mania. The investigators found that the screening instrument was easy to use and, in a cross-validation sample, correctly identified a substantial proportion of subjects with bipolar or unipolar illness (bipolar major depression was identified in the bipolar-I index sample with a sensitivity of 0.82 and in the cross-validation sample with a sensitivity of 0.72).

Screening for Bipolar Spectrum Disorders in Youths

As noted previously, the GBI (Depue et al., 1981) was initially developed for use with college-age young adults. Recently, it has been used in younger samples. A study of clinically diagnosed children and adolescents, for instance, found that both youth- and parent-reported symptoms on the bipolar scale of the GBI were sensitive to the detection of actual bipolar disorder (Youngstrom et al., 2001; Findling et al., 2002). Results of various studies suggest that a cutoff score of 13 and higher for adults, and of 17 and higher for children and adolescents may be useful in screening for bipolar spectrum disorder or risk. Reichart and colleagues (2005) in the Netherlands used the GBI to assess psychopathology among 129 adolescent and young adult children of a bipolar parent over a 5-year follow-up period. They found that the depression scale of the GBI discriminated well between the development of new bipolar disorder and no disorder or unipolar disorder.

Also as noted previously, a version of the HPS (Eckblad and Chapman, 1986) was used in the Oregon Adolescent Depression Project (Klein et al., 1996), where it identified youths with clinical features and functional impairment who may have been in the bipolar spectrum. Further research is needed, however, to validate diagnostic status over time.

CHARTING THE COURSE OF BIPOLAR DISORDER

Because bipolar disorder is recurrent by definition, it is essential to have methods for capturing the phenomenology of the course of the illness to supplement methods used to characterize individual episodes. Indeed, Kraepelin (1921) used life charts with many of his patients and, from the study of these charts, made critical observations about the course of manic-depressive illness. Figure 11–6 is a case history used by Kraepelin to illustrate periodic mania with isolated episodes of depression. Such procedures yield charts of the past or recent history of changes in the illness, permitting examination of both clinical and research issues based on details of

those patterns. There are several methods for systematically assessing—either retrospectively or prospectively—the details of the topology and course of bipolar disorder.

Longitudinal Interval Follow-Up Evaluation

The contribution of the Longitudinal Interval Follow-up Evaluation (LIFE) to characterization of the course of bipolar disorder is noted only briefly here because this method is a procedure widely used for all DSM-related disorders. Developed by Keller and colleagues (1987), it is a semistructured interview procedure whose purpose is to provide a continual (e.g., weekly) charting of symptomatology, psychosocial functioning, and treatment based on regular follow-up evaluations. Severity of psychopathology is rated on a six-point Psychiatric Status Rating (PSR) scale tied to Research Diagnostic Criteria symptoms; several areas of psychosocial functioning (e.g., employment, relationships with family members) are also rated on five- or seven-point scales. The PSR scale and psychosocial ratings have been shown to have high interrater reliability (e.g., Keller et al., 1987). The LIFE charts provide an excellent basis for characterizing landmark clinical events, such as time to recovery or duration of episodes. The LIFE methods are widely used, especially in research on unipolar depression, as in the NIMH Collaborative Program on the Psychobiology of Depression-Clinical Studies (e.g., Judd et al., 2000; Solomon et al., 2000); they are also used to study anxiety disorders (e.g., Warshaw et al., 1994).

Life Chart Method

The Life Chart Method (LCM) was designed as a brief, easily administered, and flexible approach for mapping the course

Figure 11–6. Relapsing mania with isolated periods of depression. Light blue = depression; dark blue = manic excitement. (*Source*: Kraepelin, 1921, p. 143) Reprinted with permission.

of bipolar disorder. In the original development of the approach, Post and colleagues (e.g., Squillace et al., 1984; Roy-Byrne et al., 1985) identified several goals for such a methodology: to systematize retrospective clinical history data; to capture meaningful episodes that might be missed because of incomplete memory; and, of course, to provide detailed phenomenological and descriptive information about the clinical course of mood disorders. The methodology bases the definition of an episode on functional impairment rather than symptomatic criteria, on the assumption that the former information is recalled more readily than whether a particular symptom occurred during a given time frame. Moreover, definitions based on functional impairment may capture a more detailed picture of variations in mood than can definitions based on strict adherence to DSM criteria. Accordingly, manic and depressive episodes are each measured on a three-point scale: mild, with only subjective distress and no or minimal functional impairment; moderate, with clear impairment in functioning in usual roles; and severe, involving incapacitation or resulting in hospitalization. Manic episodes are defined by any level of severity, and depressive episodes by moderate or severe ratings. The investigators noted that subjective reports were supplemented by the observations of others, especially for mild mania, a state often overlooked or denied by patients themselves.

The LCM has the advantage that it can be applied flexibly, so that different studies or contexts may involve different duration criteria (e.g., Kramlinger and Post, 1996; Denicoff et al., 1997), may be prospective or retrospective (or both), and may include staff ratings as well as patient reports. Denicoff and colleagues (1997) presented reliability and validity data on a prospective version of the LCM, developed during 2 years of a clinical trial on bipolar-I and -II outpatients. Daily ratings of mood severity based on functional impairment were provided by patients, supplemented by information from other sources (including spouses). Interrater reliabilities were very high. Validity was supported by significant associations with both self- and clinician-rated mood measures that included the BDI, YMRS, HAM-D, and GAS.

It may be noted that daily administration of the LCM using a palmtop handheld device is under investigation. Initial feasibility data indicate that this approach is useful and might greatly facilitate frequent monitoring of mood states and psychosocial functioning (Scharer et al., 2002). In a related development, Whybrow and colleagues (2003) devised the ChronoRecord, software patients can use on their home computers to record mood, sleep, life events, and medication intake. They found that 83 percent of the 96 patients they studied expressed high acceptance of the computer format.

Average Mood Symptom Score

The Average Mood Symptom Score (AMSS) is a somewhat similar method of prospective charting of mood patterns, adapted from the LCM (Gitlin et al., 1995). Hammen and colleagues (1989) first reported use of the procedure as a method for characterizing the timing and features of changes in symptoms of unipolar depression and bipolar disorder in relation to stressful life events. The goal is to systematize the severity and duration of mood states over time during ongoing follow-up. To this end, clinicians' chart notes of clinical status and dates of changes are translated into a time line, with dates on the horizontal axis and a vertical axis indicating nine levels of severity of mania or depression (where the zero midpoint is euthymia). Based on DSM criteria, manic states are rated as M1 (only one or two symptoms) through M4 (severe, hospitalized mania) above the zero point, or D1 (only one or two symptoms) through D4 (severe major depressive episode involving hospitalization or suicide attempt) below the zero point; mixed states can also be indicated. Figure 11–7 presents an example.

In addition to time lines that can be used to identify dates of onset or significant changes in severity or polarity of symptoms, the method yields a quantitative score of symptomatology per unit of time. A total mood score for a defined period may be calculated as level of symptoms multiplied by duration in days; the AMSS is the total mood score divided by days in the period of interest. A series of studies has employed such methods in samples of both unipolar and bipolar patients to characterize course of illness in relation to psychosocial factors, such as role functioning and episodic stressful life events (Ellicott et al., 1990; Hammen et al., 1992, 2000).

ASSESSMENT OF PSYCHOSOCIAL ADJUSTMENT

There has been increasing emphasis on the need for characterization of psychiatric patients' functional outcomes as a critical supplement to the relatively exclusive focus on clinical status. As Weissman (1997) noted, since the 1960s there has been a growing appreciation that for all disorders, it is necessary to understand individuals in their social contexts because family, social, and occupational adjustment all have an impact on clinical course. Moreover, social role functioning is a crucial marker by which individuals, their families, and the community at large judge the success of treatment in general and the effectiveness of specific interventions. Further impetus for studying functional outcomes in bipolar populations comes from the commonly noted discrepancy between clinical state and role functioning among people with mood disorders. For instance, many individuals who have recovered from

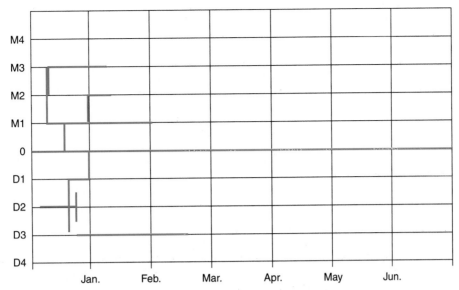

Figure 11–7. Example of time line for characterizing the timing and features of changes in symptoms of unipolar depression and bipolar disorder (see text for explanation).

episodes or have not experienced recurrences nonetheless display functional impairment,[2] especially in family and work adjustment. Maladjustment in important roles, moreover, may contribute—presumably as a stressor—to further clinical episodes and debility. Consequently, interest in the measurement of functioning in major roles and the use of such data to evaluate treatment outcomes has grown. In this section, we briefly review some of the methods used for these purposes and the resultant findings, noting that such issues are by no means specific to bipolar illness.

Unfortunately, actual progress in mapping social adjustment among those with mood disorders has been relatively limited, owing to the complexity of the constructs involved and the resulting problems in collecting reliable and valid information in relevant areas. The widely used GAS or its variant, the Global Assessment of Functioning (GAF) scale, employed as Axis V of DSM-IV, has been criticized for confounding clinical symptoms and psychosocial functioning (Williams, 2000). The single-item GAS and GAF scales provide no specificity in ratings for different areas of functioning. Similarly, the Clinical Global Impressions Scale for Bipolar Illness (CGI-BP) (Spearing et al., 1997), while providing clinician judgments specifically of illness severity and changes in mania, depression, and overall bipolar illness, does not yield information about functioning and changes in particular roles. Similar concerns may arise with regard to many "quality-of-life" scales, which provide general information about the adverse effects of clinical and medical states but less information about particular areas of discomfort (e.g., Vojta et al., 2001).

Weissman and colleagues (1981) reviewed a number of scales that specifically address social functioning and found

their quality and utility to be relatively poor. Thus although many such scales exist, few have provided the utility and psychometric qualities necessary for their survival (see Williams, 2000).

Currently, three patient-report scales are used relatively widely in research on quality-of-life issues for those with mood disorders. The Social Adjustment Scale-Self Report (SAS-SR) (Weissman and Bothwell, 1976; Weissman et al., 1978) assesses instrumental and emotional role functioning in six areas: work, social and leisure, marital–sexual, relationships with extended family, parenting, and family unit. It includes a total of 54 items and yields both subscale and overall adjustment scores. An example is the following:

> How have you been getting along with the children during the last 2 weeks?
> 1. I had no arguments and got along very well.
> 2. I usually got along well but had minor arguments.
> 3. I had more than one argument.
> 4. I had many arguments.
> 5. I was constantly in arguments.

The SAS-SR has been shown to have excellent reliability and validity (reviewed by Williams, 2000). The initially developed clinician-rated version of the SAS employs a semi-structured interview format and is especially suitable for use when there is concern that patients' mood status may distort their responses and perceptions.

The Social Adaptation Self-Evaluation Scale (SASS) (Bosc et al., 1997) was developed for use in clinical trials. It contains 21 self-report items covering current functioning in various psychosocial domains. As noted by Weissman (1997), its content emphasizes subjective aspects of functioning, including motivation and self-perception, drive, and mastery, but focuses less on role performance. Instrumental functioning, such as work behavior and family and parental role functioning, is not specifically included. However, to the extent that the scale taps interest and enjoyment in functional roles, it adds an important dimension beyond clinical status.

The Short-Form Health Survey (SF-36) (Ware and Sherbourne, 1992) of the MOS includes several items specific to role functioning, such as loss of work functioning due to medical or depressive conditions. Data from the MOS have provided an important comparison between people with depressive conditions and those experiencing a variety of major medical syndromes (e.g., Wells et al., 1989; Hays, 1995). However, what is measured is largely global functioning, and the self-report format makes it difficult to disentangle actual psychosocial behavior and adjustment from depressive mood state.

Clinician-rated social adjustment scales include the Weissman Social Adjustment Scale (the precursor to the SAS-SR) and the social functioning scales of the LIFE method discussed previously (e.g., Keller et al., 1987). Both scales have solid psychometric properties but generally lack sufficient behavioral detail to fully characterize functioning in specific domains, such as work, parenting, and marital life.

ASSESSMENT OF BIPOLAR SYMPTOMS IN CHILDREN AND ADOLESCENTS

Measurement of Mania

As noted in Chapter 6, there is considerable controversy regarding the diagnosis of mania and manic symptoms in children (see also Chapter 3). The NIMH Bipolar Child Roundtable (2001) recommended the use of well-established interview diagnostic procedures for this purpose. One such instrument is the Kiddie Schedule for Affective Disorders and Schizophrenia (KSADS), specifically the Washington University version (WASH-U-KSADS), which contains items developed to assess childhood mania and other syndromes, including onset and offset of individual items and syndromes for current and lifetime disorders. Geller and colleagues (2001) reported excellent interrater reliability, including high kappa values between expert observers and offsite blind evaluators on ratings of mania and rapid cycling. At this time, the majority of NIMH-funded studies of bipolar disorder in children use the WASH-U-KSADS sections on mania and rapid cycling.

There is obviously a long way to go in developing an array of measures of mania symptoms in children that will parallel those available for adults. Considerable work is still needed to assess individual manic symptoms in children validly and reliably; to establish developmentally appropriate indicators; and to distinguish them from those of other disorders, such as attention-deficit hyperactivity disorder (ADHD). For instance, it is necessary to address symptoms that occur in bipolar children but not in those with ADHD, including hypersexuality and grandiosity, while also distinguishing overlapping symptoms, such as distractibility and hyperactivity. Parents of 268 subjects (93 with a prepubertal or early-adolescent form of bipolar disorder, 81 with ADHD, and 94 healthy controls) completed the 10-item Conners' Abbreviated Parent Questionnaire before the WASH-U-KSADS was administered (Tillman and Geller, 2005). The results are shown in Table 11–4. Items 7, 8, 9, and 10 significantly distinguished between those children and adolescents with bipolar illness and those with ADHD. The authors concluded that the Conners' Abbreviated Parent Questionnaire (sensitivity = 0.73, specificity = 0.86) is a promising tool as a screen for early- and adolescent-onset bipolar disorder. The NIMH Research Roundtable on Prepubertal Bipolar Disorder (2001) recommended that researchers develop operational criteria for frequency and severity of various behaviors and symptoms potentially relevant to juvenile mania and the co-occurring disruptive behavior disorders and impairing symptoms.

To date, little information exists on the use of adult rating scales for manic symptoms with children. Gracious and colleagues (2002) reported on a parent-completed version of the YMRS, noting that it discriminated well among diagnostic groups aged 5 to 17, including those with ADHD. They found good psychometric properties for an eight-item version (eliminating three items, such as sexual interest, that did not contribute to the total scores) (see also Youngstrom et al., 2002, 2003). The agreement between the reports of children and adolescents and those of parents is problematic, however. Children, for example, are more likely than parents to report racing thoughts and decreased need for sleep (Tillman et al., 2004), and adolescents with bipolar disorder tend to underreport manic symptoms (Youngstrom et al., 2004).

Measurement of Depression

The assessment of depressive symptoms and syndromes in children and adolescents has been well described elsewhere (e.g., Nezu et al., 2000). In general, self-report questionnaires about symptoms and diagnostic interviews can be administered reliably and yield valid conclusions about symptom severity and the presence of depressive disorders. For example, a Children's Depression Inventory (CDI) was developed by Kovacs (1981); it has a three-response options format with content appropriate for those aged 7 to 17. The BDI, discussed earlier, is suitable for most patients aged 13 and older.

TABLE 11–4. Scores on Items of the Conners' Abbreviated Parent Questionnaire for Subjects with a Prepubertal and Early Adolescent Bipolar Disorder (BP) Phenotype, Subjects with Attention-Deficit Hyperactivity Disorder (ADHD), and Healthy Comparison Subjects

Questionnaire Item	SUBJECTS WITH A BP PHENOTYPE ($n=92$)		SUBJECTS WITH ADHD ($n=80$)		HEALTHY COMPARISON SUBJECTS ($n=92$)	
	Mean	Std. Dev.	Mean	Std. Dev.	Mean	Std. Dev.
1. Restless or overactive	2.9[a]	0.9	3.0[a]	0.8	1.2	0.5
2. Excitable, impulsive	3.2[a]	0.8	3.1[a]	0.8	1.3	0.5
3. Disturbs other children	2.7[a]	1.0	2.5[a]	0.8	1.1	0.3
4. Fails to finish things he or she starts—short attention span	2.9[a]	1.0	2.9[a]	0.9	1.2	0.4
5. Constantly fidgeting	2.7[a]	1.0	3.1[a]	0.8	1.2	0.4
6. Inattentive, easily distracted	3.2[a]	0.9	3.3[a]	0.7	1.2	0.4
7. Demands must be met immediately—easily frustrated	3.3[a,b]	0.9	2.9[a]	1.0	1.2	0.4
8. Cries often and easily	2.5[a,c]	1.0	1.9[a]	0.9	1.2	0.5
9. Mood changes quickly and drastically	3.2[a,c]	0.9	2.3[a]	1.0	1.2	0.4
10. Temper outbursts, explosive and unpredictable behavior	3.1[a,c]	1.0	2.3[a]	1.0	1.2	0.4

Note: See Tillman and Geller (2005) for a scoring algorithm and age-specific cutoffs for use of the Conners' Abbreviated Parent Questionnaire as a screening tool. Std. Dev. = standard deviation.
[a]Significant difference compared with the healthy comparison group ($p<.0001$).
[b]Significant difference compared with the ADHD group ($p<.003$).
[c]Significant difference compared with the ADHD group ($p<.0001$).
Source: Tillman and Geller, 2005. Reprinted with permission from the *American Journal of Psychiatry*, Copyright 2005, American Psychiatric Association.

Two major issues are associated with assessment of depression in children. First, most diagnostic interview procedures assume that children's reports of their symptoms should be supplemented by information collected from caretakers. Most diagnostic methods for assessing depression, such as the clinician-administered KSADS (Ambrosini, 2000) or the Diagnostic Interview Schedule for Children (DISC), which is administered by trained laypersons (Shaffer et al., 2000), prescribe separate interviews for children and parents. KSADS commonly uses a "best clinical estimate" method, combining information from the child and the parent weighted by the type of information given, according to the clinician's judgment. For example, internal symptoms, such as depressed feelings and negative thoughts, cannot readily be detected by parents, and there-

fore the child's report on these symptoms might be given greater weight in a diagnosis of depression. The DISC is a highly structured interview, with a computer-based scoring algorithm often being used to combine information about diagnostic criteria.

A second, related issue concerns the relatively low agreement among informants (the child or adolescent, parents, and teachers). This problem occurs for all childhood disorders, not just depressive illnesses. It has been speculated, however, that reports of depression may be associated with systematic biases in the reports of certain informants. Specifically, some research has indicated that relatively depressed women may distort or exaggerate their children's behavior as more negative than it actually is. However, a review of 22 studies by Richters (1992) revealed that such claims were based largely on inadequate designs, including simple associations between mothers' and children's symptoms that could be accurate given the common finding of disorders in offspring of depressed women. Subsequent studies using sophisticated methods, such as covariance structure analysis with latent variables formed from different informants, have supported the hypothesis that depressed mothers may report more negative behaviors. As these studies have shown, the fact that maternal depression truly is associated with more child disorder makes the conclusion of "bias" unclear (Fergusson et al., 1993; Boyle and Pickles, 1997). Other researchers who have evaluated parent–child concordance over time (Renouf and Kovacs, 1994; Boyle and Pickles, 1997) have suggested that maternal bias, if any, may be more pronounced for younger than for older children.

CONCLUSIONS

The status of assessment methods in bipolar disorder varies by topic:

- Diagnostic procedures, not specifically discussed in this chapter, are administered relatively reliably but are only as valid as our evolving conceptualization of bipolar disorder.
- Evaluation of states of depression has been a significant achievement in recent years, making use of a number of well-supported self-report and clinician-rated procedures that measure the presence and severity of various depressive symptoms. Instruments vary, however, in their coverage of particular symptoms.
- Measurement of states of mania is less well developed. The experience of manic symptoms interferes with obtaining valid self-reports by questionnaire, but even clinician-based measures are relatively sparse. Several self-report and clinician-rated instruments for measuring mania are currently available, but psychometric studies of their merits lag behind those used for depressive symptoms.
- There is a significant potential gap in measurement of particular symptoms or clusters. This gap is particularly pronounced in the assessment of mixed states. It might be anticipated that further developments in both conceptualization and instrumentation for specific symptoms would improve evaluation of the treatment of bipolar conditions (e.g., sleep disturbances, mixed states, cognitive–intellectual functioning).
- Several methods are for characterizing the course of bipolar disorder, based on symptom levels, episode status, and functional impairment. These methods of longitudinal or retrospective charting have proved valuable for understanding features of the course of the disorder, and potentially they can play an important role in treatment decision making.
- Preliminary steps have been taken to evaluate hypomanic personality, or risk for future bipolar disorder. Similarly, there have been some positive steps toward the development of screening instruments to help identify in nonclinical populations those who are at risk or have already experienced bipolar states.
- Initial steps have also been taken to describe functioning in important roles—areas of living that may be relatively independent of symptom levels. Further work is needed to provide scales that capture both objective features of how individuals live their lives and the contexts in which they struggle with their illness, as well as methods for capturing the motivations and perceptions of people with bipolar disorder.
- Research on the assessment of mania and manic symptoms in children is at a relatively preliminary stage. Diagnostic assessments require careful attention to clinical and course features, such as rapid cycling and mixed states, that differ between children and adults with bipolar disorder. There is a great need for developmentally appropriate indicators of symptoms, as well as for indicators that can distinguish among groups with overlapping disorders, such as ADHD.

NOTES

1. Many of these studies were reported in a special issue of the *Journal of Affective Disorders* in 2005: Akiskal et al., 2005a,b,c; Akiyama et al., 2005; Erfurth et al., 2005a,b; Matsumoto et al., 2005; Mendlowicz et al., 2005.
2. Paykel and Weissman, 1973; Harrow et al., 1990; Mintz et al., 1992; Gitlin et al., 1995.

[Edgar Allan Poe's alcoholism] was one of the methods by which he fought the intolerable morbidity of his manic-depressive state of mind . . . Had this been his only weapon to relieve the depressions that overtook him, he would, like thousands of others similarly affected, have lived his life unknown and gone unsung by posterity. But he had a second weapon—his pen.

—*W. R. Bett (1952, pp. 74–75)*

HISTORICAL BACKGROUND

The notion of a relationship between creativity and extremes in mood states is an ancient one, described in pre-Grecian myths and later by Plato and Socrates. Divine madness and inspiration were thought to be obtainable only during particular states of mind, such as loss of consciousness, affliction with illness, or fits of "possession." In his speech on divine madness in *Phaedrus*, Socrates said:

> Madness, provided it comes as the gift of heaven, is the channel by which we receive the greatest blessings . . . [T]he men of old who gave things their names saw no disgrace or reproach in madness; otherwise they would not have connected it with the name of the noblest of all arts, the art of discerning the future, and called it the manic art. (Plato, 1974, pp. 46–47)

He went on to discuss artistic "madness" in particular (p. 48): "If a man comes to the door of poetry untouched by the madness of the Muses, believing that technique alone will make him a good poet," he proclaimed, "he and his sane compositions never reach perfection, but are utterly eclipsed by the performances of the inspired madman."

Madness, as understood by Plato and Socrates, encompassed a wide range of states of thought and emotion, not just psychosis, but the emphasis was on a profoundly altered state of thinking, awareness, and feeling. Aristotle, writing in the 4th century BC, focused more specifically on the relationship among melancholia, madness, and inspiration. "Why is it," he asked, "that all men who are outstanding in philosophy, poetry or the arts are melancholic?" This was true of Ajax and Bellerophontes, he said: "The former went completely insane. . . . And many other heroes suffered in the same way as these. In later times also there have been

Empedocles, Plato, Socrates and many other well-known men. The same is true for most of those who have handled poetry" (1936, pp. 155–157).

The Renaissance saw a resurgence of interest in the relationship among genius, melancholy, and madness, but an important distinction was made between sane melancholics of high achievement and individuals whose insanity prevented them from using their gifts. The eighteenth century witnessed a sharp change in attitude, with rational thought seen as essential to genius, a view then sharply reversed by the nineteenth-century Romantics, who once again emphasized extremes in mood and experience as critical to artistic inspiration and expression. In 1812—the same year that Byron, the personification of Romantic, melancholic intensity, published *Childe Harold's Pilgrimage*—physician Benjamin Rush, author of the first major psychiatric treatise in the United States, recorded his clinical observations about the relationship between acute manic and creative states (Rush, 1812, pp. 153–154):

> From a part of the brain preternaturally elevated, but not diseased, the mind sometimes discovers not only unusual strength and acuteness, but certain talents it never exhibited before. . . . Talents for eloquence, poetry, music and painting, and uncommon ingenuity in several of the mechanical arts, are often involved in this state of madness. . . . The disease which thus evolves these new and wonderful talents and operations of the mind may be compared to an earthquake, which, by convulsing the upper strata of our globe, throws upon its surface precious and splendid fossils, the existence of which was unknown to the proprietors of the soil in which they were buried.

An ironic exception to the nineteenth-century writers who emphasized deep, mysterious, and irrational forces giving rise to genius was the essayist Charles Lamb, himself institutionalized for what would now be called bipolar illness, and companion to a sister intermittently insane with the same illness. In *The Sanity of True Genius*, Lamb argued for a balance of faculties, much as the eighteenth-century writers had done (Lamb, 1987, pp. 212–213):

> Far from the position holding true, that great wit (or genius, in our modern way of speaking), has a necessary alliance with insanity, the greatest wits, on the contrary, will ever be found in the sanest writers. It is impossible for the mind to conceive a mad Shakespeare. The greatness of wit, by which the poetic talent is here chiefly to be understood, manifests itself in the admirable balance of all faculties. Madness is the disproportionate straining or excess of any one of them. . . . The ground of the mistake is, that men, finding in the raptures of the higher poetry a condition of exaltation, to which they have no parallel in their own experience, besides the spurious resemblance of it in dreams and fevers, impute a state of dreaminess and fever to the poet. But the true poet dreams being awake. He is not possessed by his subject, but has dominion over it.

The late nineteenth and early twentieth centuries saw a moderation of earlier Romantic views, due in part to the inevitable swing from any extreme and in part to the more circumspect reasoning of academic psychologists and psychiatrists. William James and Emil Kraepelin, for example, emphasized positive features associated with certain kinds of madness, or "psychopathy," and speculated on how these features might combine with other talents in some instances to produce an extraordinarily creative or accomplished person. They also stressed, however, the debilitating extremes of mental illness—psychosis or morbid depressions, for example—in addition to the milder, potentially productive hypomanias and more reflective, philosophical melancholias. These scholars underscored the need for sustained attention, discipline, and balance in the truly accomplished individual. This more moderate view has characterized most modern thinking about the relationship between psychopathology and genius.

Kraepelin, a contemporary of William James, was acutely aware of the dire consequences of untreated manic-depressive illness. But like many who had observed and studied it, he wrote of its occasional positive aspects as well (Kraepelin, [1921] 1976, p. 17):

> The volitional excitement which accompanies the disease may under certain circumstances set free powers which otherwise are constrained by all kinds of inhibition. Artistic activity namely may, by the untroubled surrender to momentary fancies or moods, and especially poetical

activity by the facilitation of linguistic expression, experience a certain furtherance.

Swiss psychiatrist Eugen Bleuler concurred, and further drew the parallel between manic and artistic thought (Bleuler, 1924, pp. 466, 468):

> The *thinking* of the manic is flighty. He jumps by by-paths from one subject to another, and cannot adhere to anything. With this the ideas run along very easily and involuntarily, even so freely that it may be felt as unpleasant by the patient. . . .
>
> Because of the more rapid flow of ideas, and especially because of the falling off of inhibitions, artistic activities are facilitated even though something worthwhile is produced only in very mild cases and when the patient is otherwise talented in this direction. The heightened sensibilities naturally have the effect of furthering this.

William James, like his brother Henry and other members of their family, was subject to profound, debilitating depressions. Nonetheless, he wrote about the potentially valuable combination of an ardent, excitable temperament with talent (James, 1902):

> The psychopathic temperament [by which James meant "border-line insanity, insane temperament, loss of mental balance"], whatever be the intellect with which it finds itself paired, often brings with it ardor and excitability of character. . . . His conceptions tend to pass immediately into belief and action . . . [W]hen a superior intellect and a psychopathic temperament coalesce—as in the endless permutations and combinations of human faculty, they are bound to coalesce often enough—in the same individual, we have the best possible condition for the kind of effective genius that gets into the biographical dictionaries. Such men do not remain mere critics and understanders with their intellect. Their ideas possess them, they inflict them, for better or worse, upon their companions or their age.

Myerson and Boyle, writing from Boston's McLean Hospital in the 1940s, reiterated the basic position of William James; as Kraepelin and Rush had done, they focused on manic-depressive illness. In discussing affective psychosis in socially prominent families, they concluded (Myerson and Boyle, 1941):

> It does not necessarily follow that the individuals who appear in these records were great because they had mental disease, although that proposition might be maintained with considerable cogency and relevance. It may be that the situation is more aptly expressed as follows. The manic drive in its controlled form and phase is of value *only* if joined to ability. A feebleminded person of hypomanic temperament would simply be one who carried on

more activity at a feebleminded level, and this is true also of mediocrity, so the bulk of manic-depressive temperaments are of no special value to the world, and certainly not of distinguished value. If however, the hypomanic temperament is joined to high ability, an independent characteristic, then the combination may well be more effective than the union of high ability with normal temperament and drive might be. The indefatigability, the pitch of enthusiasm, the geniality and warmth which one so often sees in the hypomanic state may well be a fortunate combination and socially and historically valuable.

EVIDENCE FOR A LINK BETWEEN MANIC-DEPRESSIVE ILLNESS AND CREATIVITY

Any relationship between manic-depressive illness and creativity would appear to be unlikely, especially in light of recent and overwhelming evidence that pervasive cognitive deficits mark many if not most individuals afflicted by the bipolar form of the disorder (see Chapter 9), although it should be noted that standard measures of intellectual functioning, such as IQ tests, show only a modest association with creativity (see, e.g., Ochse, 1990; Piirto, 1994; Simonton, 1994). (Anecdotally, it is of interest that scientists Richard Feynman and James Watson scored 120 on their respective IQ tests.) It is counterintuitive that such a destructive illness could be associated with imagination or great works of art. Yet the perceived association is a persistent cultural belief and one that is backed by data from many studies. All of these studies are limited by their methods, but as we shall see, their findings—converging as they do from across varied methodologies and different populations—are certainly suggestive. It may be, of course, that there is no relationship. Or there may be a link, but not a causal one. If there is a link, it may be that creativity or the creative lifestyle leads to instability (for example, through highly irregular sleep patterns, financial and other stresses, alcohol and drug abuse, or a social milieu with an excessive tolerance for erratic behavior), rather than the instability's facilitating creativity. Indeed, there may be a selection factor for those who choose a life within the arts.

We argue here that there is a causal link whereby the cognitive styles, temperaments, and intense, cyclic moods associated with bipolar spectrum disorders cause some who are already creative and productive to be even more so. The argument is not that manic-depressive illness and its related temperaments are essential to creative work; clearly they are not. Nor do we argue that most people who have bipolar or recurrent depressive illness are creative; they are not. The argument is, rather, that a *disproportionate* number of eminent writers and artists have suffered from bipolar spectrum disorders and that, under some circumstances, creativity can be facilitated by such disorders. Indeed, great creative accomplishment is by definition a rare merging of temperament, intellect, imagination, happenstance, energy, and discipline.

While we focus here on mood, cognitive, and temperamental aspects of great achievement, the role of hard work and discipline cannot be overemphasized. Lord Byron is a good example of this point. There can be little question that his poetry was strongly affected by his extreme moods and indisputable mental anguish, but his personal discipline was extraordinary. Byron's extensive reworking of a single stanza from *Don Juan*, for example, is illustrated in Figure 12–1 and Box 12–1. "His reason was punctuated, even disturbed, by passion," wrote another poet, "but whatever he was in person he was not, as an artist, passion's slave. In the poetry Byron masks his passion and makes it into endurable art" (Bold, 1983, p. 13). Byron himself wrote: "Yet, see, he mastereth himself, and makes / His torture tributary to his will."[1]

Methodological Issues

There are several ways to examine the relationship between manic-depressive illness and creativity, but until recently, apocryphal speculation far outweighed systematic study. Criticism of work purporting to find a link has been justified. Biographical studies—while intrinsically fascinating, irreplaceable, and deeply instructive sources of information about moods, their extremes, and their roles in the lives of artists—are fraught with difficulties (Jamison, 1993).[2] This criticism has been discussed at length elsewhere (see, e.g., Jamison, 1993; Post, 1994; Ludwig, 1995).

Writers and artists, for example, however brutally honest they may be in some of their self-assessments, are of necessity subjective and biased as well. The reliability of letters, journals, and memoirs can be limited because they are written from a single perspective or because the writer was fully mindful of future biographers and posterity. Biographers, too, write with biases and under the influence of prevailing or idiosyncratic viewpoints. Historical context and existing social customs also determine which behaviors are culled or emphasized for comment. Certain lifestyles provide cover for deviant and bizarre behavior, and the arts, especially, have long given latitude to extremes in behavior and mood. The assumption is prevalent that within artistic circles, madness, melancholy, and suicide are somehow normal, making it difficult at times to distinguish truth from expectation.

Biographical or posthumous research poses other problems as well. Any historical perspective dictates that a listing of highly accomplished, affectively ill individuals will be illustrative, but by no means definitive. Always in the analysis of individual lives, problems arise. It is fairly easy

Figure 12–1. Autograph page from stanza 9, canto III, of Byron's *Don Juan* (reduced by one-third). (*Source*: Reproduced by permission of the Pierpont Morgan Library, New York. MA56-57.)

to identify any number of major nineteenth-century British or American poets who were manic-depressive, for example, but it is more difficult to determine what proportion of the total pool of "great poets" they represent. (In many instances, of course, the individuals under study are sufficiently important to be interesting in their own right, independently of any general grouping.) Also, more detailed information exists for some individuals than for others (for example, those more in the public eye, those living in relatively recent times, those institutionalized, or those writing more extensively about themselves).

The tendency for highly accomplished individuals to be, almost by definition, inordinately productive and energetic creates a problem of another sort—a bias toward underdiagnosis of the manic side of bipolar illness. Biographical studies indicate that writers, artists, and composers often describe their periods of melancholy or depression in great detail, but that other aspects of mood swings, such as hypomania and even at times overt psychosis, are subsumed under "eccentricity," "creative inspiration," or "artistic temperament." Thus many individuals with clear histories of profound or debilitating depressions are

BOX 12–1. Reworking by Byron of Stanza 9, Canto III, from *Don Juan*

1. ~~Life is a play and men~~
   All tragedies are finished by a death,

2. All Comedies are ended by a marriage,

3. ~~For Life can go no further~~
   ~~These two form the last gasp of Passion's breath~~

4. ~~All further is a blank—I won't disparage~~

5. ~~That holy state—but certainly beneath~~

6. ~~The Sun—of human beings~~

3. ~~These two are lovellers, and human breath~~
   ~~So~~   ~~These point the epigram of human breath,~~
   ~~Or any~~ The future states of both are left to faith,

4. ~~Though Life and love I like not to disparage~~
   ~~The~~ For authors ~~think~~ description might disparage
              fear

5. ~~'Tis strange that poets never try to wreathe~~ [sic?]
   ~~With eith~~   ~~'Tis strange that poets of the Catholic faith~~

6. ~~Neer go beyond~~   ~~and~~   ~~but seem to dread miscarriage~~

7. ~~So dramas close with death or settlement for life~~
   ~~Veiling~~   ~~Leaving the future states of Love and Life~~
   ~~The paradise beyond like that of life~~

8. ~~And neer describing either~~
   ~~To mere conjecture of a devil—and—or wife~~

5. The worlds to come of both ~~—&~~ or fall beneath,

6. And ~~all—both the worlds would blame them for miscarriage~~
   And then both worlds would punish their miscarriage—

7. ~~So leaving both with priest & prayerbook ready~~
   So leaving ~~Clerg both a~~ each their Priest and prayerbook
        ready,

8. They say no more of death or of the Lady.

Source: Steffan, 1971, p. 345. Reprinted from Byron's *Don Juan: Volume 1, The Making of a Masterpiece*, 2nd Edition, edited by Truman Guy Steffan, Copyright 1957, 1971, renewed 1985. Courtesy of the University of Texas Press.

labeled "melancholic" rather than manic-depressive, despite their episodic (and often seasonal) histories of extremely high energy, irritability, enthusiasm, and increased productivity (periods often accompanied by costly lapses in financial, social, and sexual judgment). Paradoxically, the more chronically hypomanic the individual, the more noticeable and relatively pathological the depression will be. Diagnostic biases in the opposite direction also occur. Some researchers tend to overdiagnose bipolar illness because they observe patterns of behavior common to both hypomania and normal accomplishment (for example, enthusiasm, high energy, and the ability to function with little sleep) and then label as manic-depressive anyone displaying these "symptoms."

Despite the difficulty of conducting diagnostic studies based on biographical material, valid and useful research can be carried out by using in a systematic way what is known about bipolar illness: its symptomatic presentation (for example, pronounced changes in mood, energy, sleep, thinking, and behavior); associated behavior patterns (such as alcohol and drug abuse, pathological gambling, violence, pronounced and repeated financial reversals, and chaotic interpersonal relationships); its association with suicide[3]; its natural course[4]; and a family history, especially in first-degree relatives (parents, siblings, or children), of depression, mania, psychosis, or suicide. Psychiatric and medical conditions that can have similar symptoms (for example, thyroid and other metabolic disturbances, drug-induced states, or complex partial seizures and related epileptic conditions) need to be considered, and ruled out, as well. Making a retrospective diagnosis is, in many ways, like putting together the pieces of a three-dimensional puzzle or solving a mystery by a complicated but careful marshaling of evidence. Biographical diagnoses must ultimately, of course, be more tentative than diagnoses made on living individuals, being circumstantial by nature, but they can be made, reliably and responsibly and with an appreciation for the complexities of anyone's life, especially that of an artist.

Studies of living artists, writers, and composers have had serious methodological flaws as well, including small sample sizes, inconsistent definitions of creativity and psychiatric illness, and nonrandom or nonspecified selection of subjects. These issues are discussed in greater detail later in the chapter.

Biographical Studies

Many case-history studies of psychopathology in eminent writers and artists were conducted during the late nineteenth and early twentieth centuries. Lombroso (1891) found an overrepresentation of manic-depressive illness in his study of geniuses and attributed it to his belief that those who suffered from the illness "feel and notice more things and with greater vivacity and tenacity than other men, their recollections are richer, and their mental combinations more fruitful" (p. 27). Babcock (1895), writing a few years later, observed that the geniuses he had studied were more likely to be emotionally unstable and given to extremes in moods. Jacobson (1912), White (1930), and Lange-Eichbaum (1932) found high general rates of insanity in their biographical studies of genius. The latter concluded that within the group defined as geniuses, artists and poets tended more to insanity than scientists and statesmen. Reid (1912) and Onuf (1918) found that manic-depressive illness was strongly overrepresented in their eminent subjects.

In a more quantitative analysis, Juda (1949) studied 113 German artists, writers, architects, and composers; she was one of the first to undertake an extensive, in-depth investigation of not only artists and writers but also their relatives.

TABLE 12–1. **Biographical Studies of Depression, Mania, and Suicide in Eminent Writers, Composers, and Artists**

Study	Subjects	Findings
Juda, 1949	113 German artists and writers	Two-thirds were "psychically normal"; more suicides and "insane and neurotic" individuals in artistic group than general population. Highest rates of psychiatric abnormalities in poets (50%), musicians (38%), painters (18%), and architects (17%). First-degree relatives of artists and writers were more likely to be cyclothymic, commit suicide, or have manic-depressive illness. Psychosis was much more common in grandchildren of artists and writers.
Martindale, 1972	21 eminent English poets (born 1670–1809); 21 eminent French poets (born 1770–1909)	55% of English poets and 40% of French poets had significant psychopathology ("nervous breakdown," suicide, and/or alcoholism). One in 7 had been placed in asylum or had suffered from severe "recurring and unmistakable symptoms," such as hallucinations or delusions.
Trethowan, 1977	60 eminent composers	Mood disorders "easily the commonest and most important of psychiatric illnesses" in composers; approximately 50% had a "melancholic temperament."
Jamison, 1993	36 eminent/most anthologized British and Irish poets (born 1705–1805)	17% had been committed to insane asylum; 22% had a history of psychosis; 39% had a strong family history of psychosis, suicide, and/or melancholia; 6% committed suicide.
Schildkraut et al., 1994	15 abstract expressionist artists (New York School)	More than 50% had a depressive illness; 40% received treatment; 20% hospitalized; 13% committed suicide; 2 paternal suicides.
Post, 1994	100 eminent American and British writers	5% had history of bipolar psychosis; 2% unipolar psychosis; 16% severely disabled by depression; 8% committed suicide. Total of 82% with "affective abnormalities."

(continued)

TABLE 12–1. **Biographical Studies of Depression, Mania, and Suicide in Eminent Writers, Composers, and Artists** (continued)

Study	Subjects	Findings
Ludwig, 1995	1,004 eminent individuals across all fields of accomplishment	Compared with other professions (business, science, public life), artistic group had 2–3 times the rate of psychosis, suicide attempts, mood disorders, and substance abuse. Those in the artistic group were 6–7 times more likely to have been involuntarily hospitalized.
Post, 1996	45 scientists, 52 composers, 48 artists, 50 writers	Severe depressive illness: scientists (18%); composers (15%); artists (8%); writers (36%).
Czeizel, 2001	21 eminent Hungarian poets (born 1554–1925)	Bipolar-I (14%); bipolar-II (53%); major depression (9%); committed suicide (9%).
Wills, 2003	40 eminent American modern jazz musicians	Psychotic illness (7.5%); major affective illness (28.5%); inpatient treatment for depression (10%); committed suicide (2.5%).

She found a high rate of what she called manic-depressive psychosis (4.3 percent) in her comparison sample of scientists (a broadly defined group), but no manic-depressive illness in the artists. (Not uncommon for the times, there was diagnostic confusion between schizophrenia and manic-depressive illness.) The artists, instead, showed a disproportionate rate of "undetermined psychoses" (2.7 percent) and schizophrenia (2.7 percent). First-degree relatives of the artists and writers, however, were disproportionately likely to be cyclothymic, to commit suicide, or to have manic-depressive illness. Juda's findings, together with those from more recent systematic biographical studies, are presented in Table 12-1. The methods and populations used across these studies varied enormously, as did the selection criteria and means used for diagnostic ascertainment.

The inconsistencies and methodological flaws in these studies were substantial, but the individuals studied were of indisputable artistic ability, and most had made lasting contributions to their fields. What is of interest is the consistency of the findings—the strikingly increased rates of psychosis, institutionalization, and suicide in eminent artists and writers. The markedly elevated rates for depressive illnesses are particularly noteworthy given that the overwhelming majority of the subjects were men, who have a considerably lower rate of depression than women.

To study the occurrence of mood disorders and suicide in a consecutive sample of all of the most eminent British and Irish poets born within a 100-year period (the most frequently represented poets in 15 anthologies of eighteenth- and nineteenth-century verse), Jamison (1993) examined autobiographical sources, contemporary accounts, and medical records (where available) for poets born between 1705 and 1805. She examined the available letters, journals, and medical records for symptoms of depression, mania, and mixed states; seasonal or other patterns in moods, behavior, and productivity; the nature of the course of the illness (for example, age at onset, duration, and patterns of recurrence); and evidence of other psychiatric or medical illnesses (for example, substance abuse or syphilis) that might confound the diagnostic picture. She placed a strong emphasis on both the severity and the recurrence of symptoms. In all cases it was the *patterning* of mood, cognitive, energy, sleep, and behavior symptoms that formed the focus of the study. The results are summarized in Table 12–2. Jamison's findings—a disproportionately high rate of psychosis, manic-depressive illness, institutionalization, and suicide—are consistent with those of other biographical studies, such as Martindale's (1972) of eminent English and French poets; Trethowan's (1977) of composers; Schildkraut and colleagues' (1994) of visual artists; Ludwig's (1992) of artists, writers, composers, and eminent nonartists (see Table 12–3); Post's (1994, 1996) of American and British writers and of scientists, composers, artists, and writers, respectively;

TABLE 12–2. **Mood Disorders and Suicide in Eminent British and Irish Poets Born 1705–1805**

Poets	Comments
Samuel Johnson 1709–1784	Severe recurrent melancholia. Perceived himself as intermittently mad and had a terror of insanity. First serious breakdown at 20, lasting more than 2 years. Experienced tics, obsessions, and phobias as well. Felt he had inherited his "vile melancholy" from his father.
Thomas Gray 1716–1771	"Habitual melancholy" and attacks of depression that grew more frequent over time. Father "subject to intermittent fits of insanity"; extravagant, alcoholic, and violent.
Williams Collins 1721–1759	Psychotic melancholia and possible mania. First complete breakdown at 29. Confined to lunatic asylum; "accustomed to rave much and make great moanings." Dissipation, intemperance, and excess while undergraduate at Cambridge. Little known about family history.
Christopher Smart 1722–1771	Ecstatic, grandiose, and religious mania. First confined to asylum in his early thirties, but financial extravagance, instability, and dissipation apparent while an undergraduate at Cambridge. Spent several years in "madhouse" on "incurable ward."
Joseph Warton 1722–1800	No indication of a significant mood disorder.
Oliver Goldsmith 1730–1774	Violent temper, fitfully melancholic, financially extravagant, compulsive gambler. Increasingly irritable, melancholic, and subject to "violent alternations of mood" as he grew older. Little known about family history except that Goldsmiths were perceived as "strange" and "eccentric."
William Cowper 1731–1800	Recurrent psychotic melancholia and repeated suicide attempts. Delusions and hallucinations. First signs of mental instability while in his twenties; confined to asylum in his early thirties. Family history of melancholia.
James Macpherson 1736–1796	No indication of a significant mood disorder.
Robert Fergusson 1750–1774	Cyclothymic temperament progressed to psychotic melancholia and then maniacal excitement (possibly exacerbated by head trauma). Died "furiously insane," at age 24, in the Edinburgh Bedlam.
Thomas Chatterton 1752–1770	Committed suicide at age 17. Extremely moody even as a child. Subject to severe melancholia as well as periods of frenzied energies, occasionally incoherent enthusiasms, and extreme grandiosity. "Wild" fluctuations in mood. Sister confined to asylum, and niece suffered from unspecified psychiatric condition.
John Bampfylde 1754–1796	Confinement in private "madhouse" for 20 years. "Fell into dissipation" after Cambridge studies. Little known about nature of his psychiatric problems. "A disposition to insanity in the family," including a sister who became insane.

(continued)

Poets	Comments
George Crabbe 1754–1832	By age 24 described an "annual woe and dread"; suffered throughout his life from fits of depression. Daily opium use (initially prescribed for tic douloureux) for more than 40 years. Father, described as "a man of imperious temper and violent passions," became increasingly and more irrationally violent as he became older.
William Blake 1757–1827	Hallucinations and delusions from an early age. Periods of exaltation and grandiosity, as well as periods he described as "a deep pit of melancholy—melancholy without any real reason." Excessive irritability and attacks of rage, suspiciousness, and paranoia. Little information about family history although one brother, who spoke of visions of Moses and Abraham, was described as a "bit mad."
Robert Burns 1759–1796	Severe, recurrent, often seasonal melancholia (described by Burns as "the miseries of a diseased nervous system" and a "deep incurable taint which poisons my existence"). Mercurial, agitated, and volatile temperament. Both parents described as "subject to strong passions," fiery, and irascible.
Joanna Baillie 1762–1851	No indication of a significant mood disorder.
William Lisle Bowles 1762–1850	No indication of a significant mood disorder.
Samuel Rogers 1763–1855	No indication of a significant mood disorder.
William Wordsworth 1770–1850	Self-described as "of a moody and violent temper." Subject to hypochondriacal aches and pains. Described by some biographers as suffering from severe depressions "to the verge of a mental breakdown," but their nature and severity are unclear. Sister's "insanity" likely to have been due to dementia rather than to a psychiatric illness.
Sir Walter Scott 1771–1832	At various times described himself as suffering from a "disposition to causeless alarm—much lassitude—and decay of vigor and intellect," a *morbus eruditorum*, and a "black dog" of melancholy.
Samuel Taylor Coleridge 1772–1834	Extended and recurrent melancholia. Mercurial, restless, extravagant, grandiose, and agitated. Fitful enthusiasms and despairs. Opiate addiction. Visionary states. Family history of affective illness and suicide.
Robert Southey 1774–1843	Described as unduly excitable, with a history of "nervous fever" and an unbalanced state of "nerves"; however, unclear indication of recurrent mood disorder of any significant severity.
Walter Savage Landor 1775–1864	Violent, restless, and unstable temperament. Litigious and impulsive. "Very much disposed" to melancholy. Expelled from both Rugby and Oxford. Thought by others to have had "at least a touch of insanity." "Ungovernable temper" and financially extravagant.

(continued)

Poets	Comments
Thomas Campbell 1777–1844	Recurrent and severe melancholia, "aggravated fits of despondency." First attack when 18. Violently irritable, financially extravagant, and "alternately excited and depressed within short-periods of time." Insanity in his and his wife's families. Son placed in asylum, suffering from melancholia, "capricious fits of temper," paranoia, and "leap-frog play of thoughts."
Leigh Hunt 1784–1859	Autobiography describes a "nervous condition," a "melancholy state," which lasted, the first time, for several months. "I experienced it twice afterwards, each time more painfully than before, and for a much longer period . . . for upwards of four years, without intermission, and above six years in all."
Thomas Love Peacock 1785–1866	No indication of a significant mood disorder.
George Gordon, Lord Byron 1788–1824	Recurrent, often agitated, melancholia. Volatile temperament with occasional "paroxysms of rage." Mercurial and extravagant; worsening depressions over time. Strong family history of mental instability and suicide.
Percy Bysshe Shelley 1792–1822	Recurrent, agitated, and occasionally suicidal melancholia. "Hysterical attacks" followed by periods of listlessness; often seasonal. Ecstatic episodes and "violent paroxysms of rage." Self-described as "tormented by visions," the psychiatric nature of which remains unclear. Probable transient delusions. Intermittent laudanum use for "nerves."
John Clare 1793–1864	Spent 25 years in insane asylum. Long periods of inertia and melancholia interspersed with episodes of frenzied, violent, and extravagant activity. Hallucinations, as well as delusions of persecution and grandeur. Cause of madness listed as "hereditary" by asylum physician.
John Keats 1795–1821	"Violent and ungovernable as a child"; described by brother as nervous, "morbid," and suffering from "many a bitter fit of hypochondriasm" [melancholy]; periods of depression often followed by periods of intense activity and "exhilaration." Described himself as having a "horrid Morbidity of Temperament." Rapidly shifting moods predated symptoms and diagnosis of tuberculosis.
George Darley 1795–1846	Recurrent, occasionally suicidal melancholia. Increasing periods of depression and social withdrawal. Described extreme mood swings, ranging from "causeless and unreasonable" periods of "frolic, extravagance, and insane" actions to "crazed" periods of despair.
Hartley Coleridge 1796–1849	Recurrent melancholia; severe mood swings alternating between "depression and extravagant hilarity." Lifelong struggles with alcoholism, "heavings of agony," and "paroxysms of rage." Expelled from Oxford for dissipation. Eccentric and visionary. Under conservatorship toward end of life. Insanity on both sides of his family.

(*continued*)

TABLE 12–2. **Mood Disorders and Suicide in Eminent British and Irish Poets Born 1705–1805** (continued)

Poets	Comments
Thomas Hood 1799–1845	Periods of morbidity, melancholia, and lethargy, but diagnosis complicated by severe, recurrent physical illness.
Thomas Lovell Beddoes 1803–1849	Committed suicide at 45 after at least one earlier attempt. Volatile, extravagant, eccentric, and subject to severe recurrent melancholia. Father, also a physician, was highly eccentric and of an "extremely ardent" temperament.
Robert Stephen Hawker 1803–1875	"Fits" of depression throughout his life. Deep depression and "brain fever" after wife's death; possible psychosis. Volatile, extravagant, and eccentric. Intermittent opium habit. Physician had "never encountered in all his practice so excitable a tissue as that which held [his] Brain." "My Grandfather and Father," Hawker wrote, "were both of the same excitable temperament."
James Clarence Mangan 1803–1849	Recurrent and prolonged psychotic depressions. Hallucinations, agitation, "great overcurtaining gloom." Extreme eccentricity: "with one voice they all proclaimed me mad." Probable opiate abuse. Father described as extravagant, financially dissolute, and of "quick and irascible temper."

Note: Poets selected for inclusion were the most frequently represented in 15 anthologies of eighteenth- and nineteenth-century British and Irish verse.
Source: Adapted from Jamison, 1993.

Czeizel's (2001) of Hungarian poets;[5] and Wills' (2003) of the lives of American jazz musicians. These studies are necessarily subjective in many respects—although suicide, psychosis, and institutionalization are relatively objective phenomena—but they are notable for the eminence of the subjects involved and for the consistency of their findings. Suicide rates were markedly elevated in all of the studies (see Fig. 12–2).

Studies of Living Writers and Artists

There have been fewer studies of psychopathology in living writers and artists. Andreasen and colleagues undertook the first such inquiries into the relationship between creativity and mental disorders (Andreasen and Canter, 1974; Andreasen and Powers, 1975; Andreasen, 1987). These studies, using structured interviews, the Research Diagnostic Criteria (RDC), and matched control groups,

TABLE 12–3. **Rates of Suicide, Depression, Mania, and Psychosis in a Sample of Writers, Artists, and Composers**

		LIFETIME RATES (%)			
	Sample Size	Depression	Mania	Psychosis	Suicide
Poets	53	77	13	17	20
Fiction writers	180	59	9	7	4
Nonfiction writers	64	47	11	8	1
Artists	70	50	9	4	6
Composers	48	46	6	10	0

Source: Adapted from Ludwig, 1992.

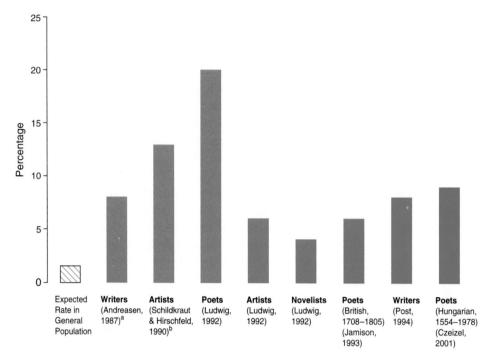

Figure 12–2. Suicide rates in writers and artists. [a]Suicide rate at the time of study completion. [b]Two other artists died in single car accidents.

represented significant methodological advances over prior, anecdotally based research. The size of the sample of writers was relatively small (N = 30), however, and the subjects were of varying levels of creative accomplishment (all were participants in the University of Iowa Writers' workshop, but some were nationally acclaimed writers, while others were graduate students or teaching fellows not nationally or internationally recognized). Andreasen noted that because she studied only writers, her results could not be generalized to other groups of creative individuals, such as philosophers, scientists, or musicians. Although this is true, and writers may be disproportionately likely to have affective disorders, the homogeneity of the sample is valuable in its own right.

The results of the Iowa research are summarized in Table 12–4. Clearly, the writers had an exceptionally high rate of affective illness and alcoholism. Fully 80 percent of the study sample met standardized (RDC) diagnostic criteria for a major affective disorder. In contrast, 30 percent of the control sample (individuals outside the arts who were matched for age, education, and gender) met the same criteria ($p < .001$). Although this is a much lower figure relative to the study sample, it still represents a rate greater than that expected for the general population. It is unclear whether this discrepancy reflects an overrepresentation of affective illness in the control sample, or the diagnostic criteria were overly inclusive for both the

creative and control groups. Almost one-half (43 percent) of the creative sample met the diagnostic criteria for bipolar-I or bipolar-II disorder.

In a study of eminent British writers and artists, Jamison (1989) examined rates of treatment for affective illness within these groups and looked at seasonal patterns of moods and productivity, the nature of intense creative episodes and the similarities between such episodes and hypomania, and the perceived role of very intense moods in the writers' or artists' work. Subjects were chosen for the study on the basis of having won at least one of several specified top prizes or awards in their fields. Thus, all painters and sculptors were either Royal Academicians or Associates of the Royal Academy, and the work of 9 of the 18 poets in the study sample had already been anthologized in *The Oxford Book of Twentieth Century English Verse*. Six of the eight playwrights had won the New York Drama Critics Award and/or the Evening Standard Drama Award (the London Critics' award); several had won both or had won one of these awards more than once.

The artists and writers were asked whether they had ever received treatment for a mood disorder and, if so, what that treatment had consisted of. The results, shown in Figure 12–3, indicate that a large proportion of the total sample (38 percent) had been treated for an affective illness. Three-fourths of those treated had been given antidepressants or lithium or

TABLE 12–4. **Lifetime Prevalence of Mental Illness in Writers and Control Subjects**

Diagnosis (Research Diagnostic Criteria)	Writers (n = 30) (%)	Controls (n = 30) (%)	p
Any affective disorder	80	30	.001
Any bipolar disorder	43	10	.01
Bipolar-I	13	0	NS
Bipolar-II	30	10	NS
Major depression	37	17	NS
Schizophrenia	0	0	NS
Alcoholism	30	7	.05
Drug abuse	7	7	NS
Suicide	7	0	NS

NS = not significant.
Source: Adapted from Andreasen, 1987. Reprinted with permission from the *American Journal of Psychiatry*, American Psychiatric Association.

had been hospitalized. Poets were most likely to have received medication for depression (33 percent) and were the only ones to have received medical intervention (hospitalization, electroconvulsive therapy, and/or lithium) for mania (17 percent). Thus, one-half of the poets had been treated with drugs or hospitalized for mood disorders. This rate is strikingly high when compared with rates in the general population (see Chapter 5). It is even higher when one considers the fact that the proportion of those in the general population so seriously ill as to actually seek and receive treatment is much lower, perhaps one-third to one-half the rates reported in prevalence studies using diagnostic criteria alone (Andreasen and Canter, 1974; Robins et al., 1984). A further probable underestimate of the total rate of affective illness in the study sample derives from the sample's being comprised largely of men, who, as noted, are less likely than women to suffer from depression, as well as less likely to seek treatment. The playwrights had the highest total rate of treatment for mood disorders (63 percent), but a very high percentage (38 percent) had been treated with psychotherapy alone; it is unclear whether this was due to a difference in illness severity or in treatment preference. Visual artists and biographers had relatively lower rates of treatment (13 and 20 percent, respectively); all treatment was with antidepressants.

Although, with the exception of the poets, the subjects reported being treated for depression, not mania or hypomania, the design of the study did not allow systematic inquiry into hypomanic or manic episodes. About one-third of the writers and artists reported histories of severe mood swings, however, and one-fourth reported histories of extended elated mood states. The novelists and poets most frequently reported elated mood states, whereas the playwrights and artists were the most likely to report severe mood swings. Biographers reported no history of severe mood swings or elated states, an interesting finding since of the five groups, they were the least likely to be associated with creativity and thus provide a natural comparison group (i.e., one highly proficient in writing but perhaps less outstandingly creative by the nature of their work).

One of the major purposes of the British study was to look at the similarities and dissimilarities between periods of intense creative activity and hypomania. Hypothesized similarities were based on the episodic nature of both; the overlapping nature of the behavioral, mood, and cognitive changes associated with both; and a possible link between the duration and frequencies of the two types of experiences. The vast majority of the subjects (89 percent) reported having had experienced intense creative episodes (100 percent of the poets, novelists, and artists; 88 percent

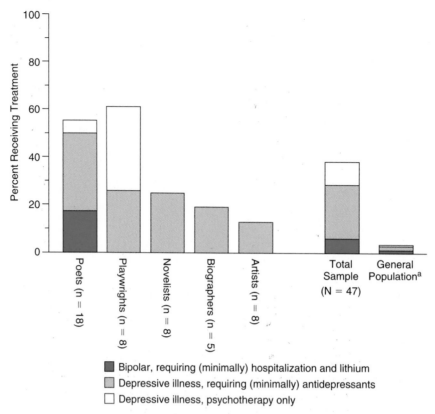

Figure 12–3. Rates of treatment for affective illness in a sample of British writers and artists. The percentages for the general population are based on Epidemiological Catchment Area data. They indicate that less than one-third of those individuals with bipolar or unipolar disorder receive treatment in any 6-month period. (*Source*: Jamison, 1989.)

of the playwrights; and, consistent with results reported earlier, only 20 percent of the biographers). The modal duration of these episodes was 2 weeks (35 percent); 55 percent of the episodes lasted 1 to 4 weeks, 20 percent 1 to 24 hours, and 25 percent longer than 1 month. The episodes were characterized by increases in enthusiasm, energy, self-confidence, speed of mental associations, fluency of thoughts, elevated mood, and a sense of well-being. Mood and cognitive changes showed the greatest degree of overlap with the episodes characterized as "intense creativity." Approximately half of the subjects described a decreased need for sleep and increased sensory awareness, but several of the more behavioral changes typically associated with hypomania (hypersexuality, increased talkativeness, and spending of money) were reported by only a minority of subjects.

When asked open-ended questions about changes before these intense creative episodes, 89 percent reported less need for sleep. (Coincident with the timing of the switch process in bipolar illness, 28 percent spontaneously reported waking abruptly at 3:00 or 4:00 AM and being unable to return to sleep.) Fifty percent of the subjects reported a sharp increase in mood just

before the beginning of an intensely creative period; for example, "I have a fever to write, and throw myself energetically into new projects"; "excited, anticipatory, energetic"; "more optimistic"; "elated"; "uplifted"; "euphoric"; and "ecstatic." Dysphoria preceded creativity in 28 percent of the subjects; that is, subjects reported feeling "more anxious"; "near suicide"; "increased irritability and tension"; "fearfulness, general mood of distress and slight paranoia"; and "irritable, antisocial." Finally, 22 percent reported mixed mood changes and psychomotor restlessness; for example, "mixture of elation together with some gloominess, feeling of isolation, sexual pressure, fast emotional responses"; "restlessness"; "low ebb bordering on despair often precedes good phase when work will flow almost as though one is a medium, rather than an originator"; "restless, dissatisfied." When asked specifically about the importance of very intense feelings and moods in their work, almost 90 percent stated that such feelings and moods were either integral and necessary (60 percent) or very important (30 percent). More poets than any other group regarded these intense moods as integral and necessary to what they did and how they did it.

Yet another link between creativity and affective illness may be the seasonal patterns underlying both moods and artistic productivity (as discussed more extensively by Jamison, 1993). Subjects rated their moods and productivity over a period of 36 months. Figures 12–4 and 12–5 show mood and productivity curves for the study sample (broken down by those writers and artists with a history of treatment for an affective illness and those with no such history). Very different seasonal patterns emerged. Those with a history of treatment demonstrated inversely related curves for summer productivity and moods, whereas those in the group with no history of treatment showed mood and productivity curves more directly covarying. In the treatment group, the peaks for productivity preceded and followed the mood peak by 3 to 4 months.

There are several possible explanations for these differences. First, increased productivity associated with elevated mood is almost certainly less likely to lead to treatment-seeking behavior than low productivity associated with elevated or any other mood. Second, the elevated mood of the treatment group may reflect more true hypomania (i.e., greater distractibility, increased stimulus and people seeking), which may well lead to less productivity in the acute phase. Indeed, Andreasen (1980, p. 381) found this in several of the writers in her study: "Some of their periods of hypomania were clearly counterproductive. The increased energy that they experienced could not be focused and controlled so that it could be expressed creatively, and so that energy was dissipated in social or personal outlets."

The British study of writers and artists revealed many overlapping mood, cognitive, and behavioral (especially sleep) changes between hypomania and intense creative

Figure 12–5. Mean mood and productivity ratings (36 months) in British writers and artists with no history of treatment for affective illness (N=32). (*Source*: Jamison, 1989.)

states. Cognitive and mood changes showed far more overlap than behavioral ones, indicating that the milder forms of hypomania may represent the more productive phase. The affective continuum that ranges from normal states through hypomania and then mania is very important, but poorly understood (Jamison, 2004). It remains unclear whether the overlap in cognitive and mood changes represents etiologically related syndromes or phenomenologically similar but causally unrelated patterns of expression. It also remains unclear to what extent writers and artists are simply more sensitive than the general population to their own mood states and are therefore more able, and perhaps also more willing, to articulate and report them.

In the no-treatment group, the periods of intensified mood and increased productivity may represent a milder form of hypomania, with cognitive and mood changes only. These milder forms of hypomania or intensified normal functioning may result in simultaneous peaks for mood and productivity. In the treatment group, the execution of work may have preceded and lagged behind the mood component.

In another study of psychiatric disorders in living writers, Ludwig (1994), using the *Diagnostic and Statistical Manual* (DSM)-III-R and the Lifetime Creativity Scales developed by Richards and colleagues (1988, discussed below), compared 59 female writers with 59 female nonwriters matched for age, educational level, and father's occupational status. The writers were far more likely to meet the diagnostic criteria for depression and mania, and five times more likely to have made a suicide attempt (see Fig. 12–6). They were also more likely to have had a history of panic attacks, drug abuse, or an eating disorder.

Figure 12–4. Mean mood and productivity ratings (36 months) in British writers and artists with a history of treatment for affective illness (N=15). (*Source*: Jamison, 1989.)

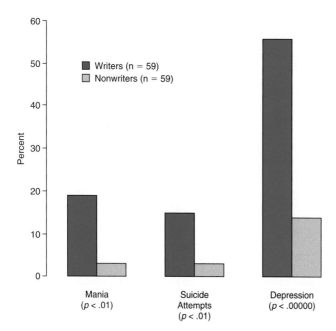

Figure 12–6. Lifetime rates of mood disorders in female writers and nonwriters. (*Source*: Adapted from Ludwig, 1994. Reprinted with permission from the *American Journal of Psychiatry*, American Psychiatric Association.)

Family Studies

A familial association between psychopathology and creativity has been found in several studies. Early biographical work by Lombrosa (1891), Galton (1892), and Lange-Eichbaum (1932) suggested that both psychopathology and creative accomplishment ran in the families of eminent writers, artists, and composers. Juda (1949), as we have noted, found that first-degree relatives of artists and writers were more likely to have had manic-depressive illness, committed suicide, been cyclothymic, or been psychotic. This finding is supported by the results of Jamison's (1993) study of first-degree relatives of eminent British and Irish poets, as well as by the extensive family history (often multigenerational) of suicide, manic-depressive illness, and psychosis in the pedigrees of, among others, George Gordon, Lord Byron; Alfred Lord Tennyson; Robert Schumann; William and Henry James; Herman Melville; Samuel Taylor Coleridge; Virginia Woolf; Ernest Hemingway; Mary Shelley and Mary Wollstonecraft; James Boswell; Samuel Johnson; Vincent van Gogh; Théodore Géricault; Gustav Mahler; Robert Lowell; John Berryman; Anne Sexton; August Strindberg; Tennessee Williams; and Eugene O'Neill.

More systematic investigations have provided a valuable supplement to these case studies. Karlsson (1970), at the Institute of Genetics in Iceland, showed that first-degree relatives of psychotic patients, as well as the patients themselves, were far more likely than the general popula-

tion to be eminent across many fields of artistic and intellectual endeavor. He also showed that there was a significantly increased risk of mental illness in distinguished Icelandic scholars and their relatives. Although Karlsson posited a familial relationship between schizophrenia and creativity, later investigators have concluded that his data actually show a very strong relationship between mood disorders, especially bipolar illness, and creativity (Richards, 1981; Andreasen and Glick, 1988; George et al., 1988).

Other researchers have looked at familial patterns of creativity and mood disorders in living artists and writers. Andreasen (1987) investigated the family histories of the University of Iowa Writers' Workshop writers and controls discussed earlier (see Table 12–5). Consistent with the elevated rate of affective illness in the writers, there was a significantly higher rate of affective illness in the primary relatives of the writers than in the primary relatives of the controls ($p < .001$). The overall prevalence for any type of psychiatric disorder was also much higher in the relatives of the writers (42 percent) than in the relatives of the controls (8 percent). Additionally, more first-degree relatives of writers than of controls showed histories of creative accomplishment (20 versus 8 percent).

Using a very different research design to study the relationship between creativity and psychopathology, Richards and colleagues (1988) at Harvard investigated creativity broadly defined in a sample of patients and their relatives. They hypothesized that a genetic vulnerability to manic-depressive illness may be accompanied by a predisposition to creativity, which may be more prominent among close relatives of patients with bipolar spectrum disorders than among the patients themselves. Such a compensatory advantage, they speculated, would be roughly analogous to the resistance to malaria found among unaffected carriers of the gene for sickle-cell anemia. To test their hypothesis, the researchers selected 17 bipolar and 16 cyclothymic patients, along with 11 of their normal first-degree relatives, using criteria that would ensure inclusion of a spectrum of disorders. These patients and their relatives were compared with 15 normal control subjects and with 18 controls who had a psychiatric diagnosis but no personal or family history of major affective disorder, schizophrenia, or suicide. Unlike other studies in the field, which limited the definition of creativity to significant, socially recognized accomplishment in the arts or sciences, these investigators attempted to measure the disposition toward originality manifested in a wide range of everyday endeavors. They administered the Lifetime Creativity Scales, a previously validated instrument that assesses the quality and quantity of "everyday" creative involvement in both work and leisure activities.

TABLE 12–5. **Mental Illness in First-Degree Relatives of 30 Writers and 30 Control Subjects**

Family History Diagnosis (Research Diagnostic Criteria)	ALL RELATIVES			PARENTS			SIBLINGS		
	Of Writers (n=116) (%)	Of Controls (n=121) (%)	p	Of Writers (n=60) (%)	Of Controls (n=60) (%)	P	Of Writers (n=56) (%)	Of Controls (n=121) (%)	p
Any affective disorder	18	2	.001	7	2	.001	20	3	.001
Bipolar disorder	3	0	.056	2	0	NS	5	0	NS
Major depression	15	2	.01	5	2	.05	14	3	.05
Alcoholism	7	6	NS	8	7	NS	5	5	NS
Suicide	3	0	NS	3	0	NS	2	0	NS
Any illness	42	8	.0001	42	8	.00003	43	8	.001

NS = not significant.
Source: Adapted from Andreasen, 1987. Reprinted with permission from the *American Journal of Psychiatry*, American Psychiatric Association.

Richards and colleagues found significantly higher combined creativity scores among the bipolar and cyclothymic patients and their normal first-degree relatives than among the control subjects (see Fig. 12–7). The normal index relatives showed suggestively higher creativity relative to the bipolar patients, and the cyclothymic patients were close to the normal relatives. Modifying their original hypothesis, the authors concluded (p. 287):

Overall peak creativity may be enhanced, on the average, in subjects showing milder and, perhaps, subclinical expressions of potential bipolar liability (i.e., the cyclothymes and normal first-degree relatives) compared either with individuals who carry no bipolar liability (control subjects) or individuals with more severe manifestations of bipolar liability (manic-depressives). . . . There may be a positive compensatory advantage . . . to genes associated with greater liability for bipolar disorder. The possibility that normal relatives of manic-depressives and cyclothymes have heightened creativity may have been overlooked because of a medical-model orientation that focused on dysfunction rather than positive characteristics of individuals. Such a compensatory advantage among the relatives of a disorder affecting at least 1% of the population could affect a relatively large group of people.

Figure 12–7. Mean creativity in selected diagnostic groups. Mean overall peak creativity scores for controls with a diagnosis (DX), normal controls (N), normal first-degree biological relatives of cyclothymes and manic-depressives (NC Rel), cyclothymes (CYC), and manic-depressives (MDI). (*Source*: Richards et al., 1988.)

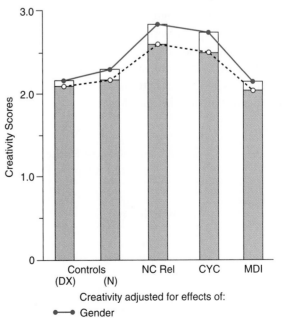

More recently, Simeonova and colleagues (2005) examined the potential familial connection between bipolar illness and creativity in a different way. They compared creativity in bipolar parents (n=40), their offspring with bipolar disorder (n=20), and bipolar offspring with attention-deficit hyperactivity disorder (ADHD) (n=20) with healthy control adults (n=18) and their healthy control children (n=18). The investigators found that parents with bipolar disorder and their bipolar offspring scored higher than healthy controls on measures of creativity. They suggested several interpretations for their findings, which are consistent with those of studies discussed earlier: bipolar disorder could "cause" creativity; bipolar disorder and creativity could be transmitted independently from parents to children; family environment may affect the putative familial cotransmission of creativity and bipolar disorder; or the genes for bipolar disorder and creativity may be "linked and co-segregate through generations, accounting for their co-occurrence in people with BD [bipolar disorder]" (p. 624). The study was unable to ascertain which of these hypotheses was the most viable, and its measure of creativity (the Barron-Welsh Art Scale) is not commonly used for that purpose, but the findings suggest that children with familial bipolar illness are more creative than healthy control children. The researchers also found that creativity in bipolar children was negatively correlated with duration of illness, which they attributed to the deleterious effects of prolonged illness and/or protracted exposure to medications.

In earlier, related research, Coryell and colleagues (1989) found that, although affectively ill groups (major depression, n=442; bipolar-I, n=64; bipolar-II, n=88) did not differ from one another in occupational or educational achievement, the first-degree relatives of the probands with bipolar disorder had significantly higher mean levels of achievement compared with the first-degree relatives of the probands with major depression. Earlier, Woodruff and colleagues (1971) had shown that bipolar probands and their brothers had higher status ratings than probands with major depression and their brothers.

The results of these studies suggest that creativity and mental illness, especially bipolar disorder, may tend to aggregate in certain families and not in others, but they do not show decisively that genetic factors are operating; that is, they demonstrate that there is a familial association, but not necessarily that the characteristics under discussion are heritable. It could be, for example, that the family and its environment, rather than the genetic inheritance itself, are exerting the primary influence. McNeil (1971), using an adopted-offspring research design, attempted to clarify this nature-versus-nurture problem. All of his subjects were adults who had been adopted shortly after birth and were part of a larger Danish psychiatric genetics study. They were classified as being "high creative" (most of the individuals in this group had achieved national prominence in the arts), "above average," or "low creative." Their rates of mental illness were then compared with those found in their biological and adoptive parents. The results are summarized in Table 12–6. The rates of mental illness were highest in the "high creative" group and their biological parents. The rates of psychopathology in the adoptive parents did not vary significantly from one level of adoptee creativity to another. Although the size of the sample was necessarily small, and the type of psychopathology was not rigorously ascertained, the study is both an interesting and an important one; its significance lies in the reasons given by McNeil in his summary remarks (p. 405):

> Mental illness rates in the adoptees were positively and significantly related to their creative ability level, substantiating the hypothesized relationship between creative ability and mental illness. The mental illness rates of the biological parents were positively and significantly related to the creative ability of the adoptees. Mental illness rates among the adoptive parents and the adoptive and biological siblings were independent of the adoptees' creative ability level. The data were interpreted as evidence for the influence of prebirth factors on the relationship between creative ability and mental illness. No evidence of family-related postbirth influence was found.

TABLE 12–6. **Rates of Mental Illness in Adoptees and their Biological and Adoptive Parents**

Adoptee Group	Adoptees (%)	Biological Parents (%)	Adoptee Parents (%)
High creative	30	27.7	5.3
Above average	10	8.3	5.0
Low creative	0	12.1	5.1

Source: Adapted from McNeil, 1971. Reproduced with permission from Blackwell Publishing Ltd.

Hypothesized Relationships between Manic-Depressive Illness and Creativity

In hypothesizing possible relationships between manic-depressive illness and creative accomplishment, several general areas need to be explored: characteristics of the illness, such as acute and long-term cognitive, temperamental, and mood changes; experiences due to having the illness; and the relative importance of different aspects of the illness to various types of accomplishment.

Characteristics of the Illness

Profound changes in mood, cognition, personality, sleep, energy, and behavior can occur during all phases of manic-depressive illness. Even during normal states, many individuals experience subtle and not-so-subtle fluctuations in the intensity of their perceptions and feelings. All of these changes have potentially important effects on creativity and productivity, but perhaps most relevant to our discussion here are those changes that occur during the milder manic states. The DSM-IV-R criteria for hypomania are given in Chapter 3; even the most casual review suggests prima facie reasons for a possible connection between hypomania and accomplishment. There is some truth in the easy, glib question that often arises in clinical teaching situations: Who would not want an illness that numbers among its symptoms elevated and expansive mood, inflated self-esteem, more energy than usual, decreased need for sleep, and enhanced sexuality? (Notably, DSM-III criteria for hypomania also included "sharpened and unusually creative thinking" and "increased productivity" as diagnostic criteria.)

Many creative individuals describe their mood states during moments of greatest inspiration and productivity as elated, expansive, and, on occasion, ecstatic. Although it is unclear whether these mood changes precede or follow creative thought, there is some evidence that expansiveness of thought and grandiosity of both mood and thought—common features of mild mania—can result in an increased fluency and frequency of ideas that is highly conducive to creative achievement. The similarities between intense creative episodes and hypomania were discussed earlier; these are periods when many successful artists and writers report powerful mood and sleep changes, often just preceding times of intense creative activity. This period of elated and expansive mood is described by many individuals as a time of faster and more fluid thinking, new ideas, and novel connections between thoughts. The fluency of thought common to hypomania and creative activity was reported by Kraepelin (1921, p. 15) in his citation of the experimental work of Isserlin:

> Isserlin has specially investigated the duration of ideas in manic patients. He found that their associations show

heightened distractibility in the tendency to "diffusiveness," to spinning out the circle of ideas stimulated and jumping off to others, a phenomenon which in high degree is peculiar to mania.

The increase in speed of thoughts—ranging from a very mild quickening, to flight of ideas, to psychotic incoherence—may exert its influence on creative production in several ways. Speed per se, or the quantity of thoughts and associations, may be enhanced. Also significant, however, may be the effect of this increased quantity on the qualitative aspects of thought; that is, the sheer volume of thought may produce unique ideas and associations.

Guilford's (1957) systematic psychological studies of the nature of creativity led to the conclusion that creative thinking encompasses several components (many of which relate directly to cognitive changes that take place during mild manias as well). *Fluency of thinking* is defined operationally by Guilford through several related concepts, each with tests to measure it: (1) word fluency, or the ability to produce words each containing a specified letter or combination of letters; (2) associational fluency, or the production of as many synonyms as possible for a given word in a limited amount of time; (3) expressional fluency, or the production and rapid juxtaposition of phrases or sentences; and (4) ideational fluency, or the ability to produce ideas to fulfill certain requirements in a limited amount of time. In addition to fluency of thinking, Guilford developed two other concepts important to creativity: *spontaneous flexibility*, or the ability and disposition to produce a great variety of ideas, with freedom to switch from category to category, and *adaptive flexibility*, or the ability to devise unusual types of solutions (relative to the frequency of response occurrences in the general population). Guilford (1959) also concluded, as did Hudson (1966) in his later work, that creative individuals are far more characterized by "divergent" thinking ("a type of thinking in which considerable searching about is done and a number of answers will do") than by "convergent" thinking ("thinking toward one right answer").

More recently, several researchers have shown that manic patients, unlike normal individuals or patients with schizophrenia, tend to exhibit pronounced *combinatory thinking*. Characterized by the merging of "percepts, ideas, or images in an incongruous fashion," the ideas formed in this way become "loosely strung together and extravagantly combined and elaborated" (Shenton et al., 1987; Solovay et al., 1987). Manic subjects show highly combinatory thought patterns—often characterized by humor, flippancy, and playfulness—in sharp contrast to the response patterns exhibited by normal subjects and by patients with schizophrenia (see Chapter 2, particularly Table 2–4).

Andreasen and Powers (1975) compared manic patients, schizophrenic patients, and writers from the University of Iowa Writers' Workshop on measures of conceptual overinclusiveness (the tendency to combine test objects into categories in a way that tends to "blur, broaden, or shift conceptual boundaries"). They hypothesized that creative writers might show thinking styles similar to those seen in schizophrenic individuals, but this notion was found to be groundless; instead, they observed that the writers showed conceptual styles quite like those of the manic patients: "Both writers and manics tend to sort in large groups, change dimensions while in the process of sorting, arbitrarily change starting points, or use vague distantly related concepts as categorizing principles" (p. 72). The subjects differed primarily in the degree of control they were able to exert over their patterns of thought, with the writers able to carry out "controlled flights of fancy during the process of sorting, while the manics tend to sort many objects for bizarre or personalized reasons" (p. 72).

Schuldberg (1990) found that several hypomanic traits contributed to performance on tests measuring creativity; of particular relevance here, he found that creative cognition was far more similar to hypomanic flight of ideas than to the loose associations that are characteristic of schizophrenia. Relatedly, people having strong emotional responses in general, who also tend to score higher on measures of being at risk for developing bipolar illness, often have more elaborate and generalizing cognitive operations (Larsen et al., 1987). Early studies had found that rhymes, punning, and sound associations increase during mania, and that many patients spontaneously start writing poetry while manic (Kraepelin, 1921; Murphy, 1923). Welch and colleagues (1946), in an early study of associational fluency in 101 inpatients at the Payne Whitney Psychiatric Clinic, found that patient groups that would today be called bipolar scored higher when elated than other clinical groups; all patient groups scored higher when elated than when less elated (see Table 12–7).

Nearly 150 years ago, Richarz noted that "in mania thoughts tend to form strings of ideas...that link together by their content, alliteration, or assonance. In racing thoughts, the ideas come and go rapidly as if they were hunting each other or continuously overlapping without any link between them" (1858; quoted in Koukopoulos and Koukopoulos, 1999, pp. 557–558). The predominant difference between the two states described is mood; that is, the elated mood of mania probably is more likely to result in a linking of ideas than is the dysphoria associated with racing thoughts.

Likewise, in studies of word-associational patterns, researchers have found that the number of original responses

TABLE 12–7.   **Average Score on the Association Test for Elated and Nonelated Patients When Classified According to Clinical Groups**

Clinical Group	Mean Score When Elated	Mean Score When Not Elated
Anxiety neurosis	—	3.5
Depression	—	2.3
Manic excitement	8.8	—
Manic-depressive	9.9	4.2
Manic-depressive, psychopathic	7.6	3.1
Paranoid reaction	—	5.4
Psychopathic personality	4.3	2.8
Schizophrenia	6.9	3.8
All groups	7.9	3.2

Source: Adapted from Welch et al., 1946.

to a word-association task (in which an individual is asked to give as many associations as possible for a particular word) increases three-fold during mania; the number of statistically common, or predictable, responses falls by approximately one-third (Henry et al., 1971; Pons et al., 1985). Henry and colleagues (1971) found that the change in word-association patterns was directly proportional to the severity of manic symptoms. Other researchers have found that acutely manic patients score much higher on a word-association task than patients acutely ill with schizophrenia or control subjects (Levine et al., 1996) (see Fig. 12–8). Hypomania also has been found to increase intellectual functioning on the Wechsler Adult Intelligence Scale (Donnelly et al., 1982). Many mood-induction studies have shown that a strongly positive, or "up," mood facilitates creative problem solving[6]; relatedly, the majority of the British writers and artists in Jamison's (1989) study reported pronounced elevations in mood just prior to their periods of intensive creative activity. Richards and Kinney (1990) at Harvard found that the overwhelming majority of bipolar patients they studied reported being in a mildly or very elevated mood when experiencing their greatest periods of creativity. Several features closely linked to elevated mood states in their subjects clearly overlapped with those found in the British writers and artists; these included

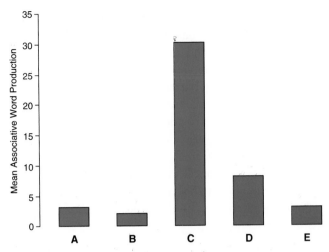

Figure 12–8. Mean associative word production—differential findings in acute manic versus acute schizophrenic patients. Given for each group are mean (± standard error [SE]) of associative words produced to 12 stimulus words. Mean associative word production by bipolar patients with acute mania (C) was higher in a statistically significant manner than in patients with acute schizophrenia (D) ($t = 2.43$, $p < .05$). Both patients with mania and patients with acute schizophrenia showed significantly higher associative word production than control subjects (A) ($t = 4.5$, $p < .001$; $t = 4.5$, $p < 0.001$, respectively). Patients with unipolar depression (B) or residual schizophrenia (E) showed mean associative word production similar to the control values. (*Source*: Levine et al., 1996. Reproduced with permission from Karger Publishing.)

increased speed of association, ease of thinking, new ideas, and expansiveness. Although the tendency has been to assume that creative periods lead to "high" or elevated moods and noncreative periods to depressed ones, the results of these studies suggest that the reverse may be true. It may be that elevations in mood such as those caused by hypomania result in more creative thought; likewise, depressed mood and thinking usually lead to periods relatively bereft of creative work.

In all these facets of creative thought, the elements of fluency and flexibility of cognitive processing are emphasized. Clearly, the mere quickening and opening up of thought in an otherwise unimaginative person will not result in creative achievement. If the cognitive processes of an otherwise creative individual are hastened and loosened by hypomania, however, a qualitatively different result may well emerge. Hyperacusis, so often experienced during manic states, may contribute to creativity as well. Characteristics of a noncognitive nature—such as boldness, grandiosity of spirit and vision, disinhibition, impatience, abandonment of normal judgment and restraint, and recklessness—also link bipolar illness and creative accomplishment. The temperamental characteristics observed to be common in highly creative individuals—persistence, wit, self-confidence, a

pleasure in taking risk, high energy, independence, exuberance, rebelliousness, and playfulness[7] are also characteristic of many who have hypomanic and cyclothymic temperaments. Stanford researchers, for example, found that bipolar patients and highly creative individuals have more personality traits in common than do healthy normal controls and creative individuals (Nowakowska et al., 2005; see also Jamison, 2004).

It may be that the combination of experience, potentiating personality characteristics (see Chapter 10), and cognitive changes that occur during hypomania and may facilitate original thought gives rise to a subgroup of individuals with bipolar illness that is unusually creative. Two critical components of creativity—an independent, risk-taking, restless, and enthusiastic personality, and a fluent, disinhibited cognitive style—are found at an increased frequency in the bipolar population, thus producing some of the conditions that may lead to a disproportionate rate of creativity in a group otherwise characterized by damaging moods and behavior. Recent research lends credence to the importance of disinhibition, or an openness to incoming stimuli from the surrounding environment, to creativity. Carson and colleagues (2003), for example, found that highly creative Harvard students were seven times more likely to have low inhibition scores than less creative Harvard students. The investigators hypothesized that low inhibition, when coupled with extreme flexibility of thought, may lead to mental illness in some individuals and to creative accomplishment in others. Presumably it could also lead to the coexistence of creativity and mental illness in yet others. Likewise, the ability to function well on a few hours of sleep and to work at a high energy level are integral to most hypomanic states; they are also integral to putting ideas into action. In her studies of outstanding artists and scientists, for example, Anne Roe (1946, 1951, 1952) found one trait that stood out: the willingness and ability to work hard and to work long hours.

Throughout this book, we stress the recurrent, cyclic nature of manic-depressive illness—its natural course, pathophysiology, subjective experience, and seasonal and diurnal patterns. Integrally linked to this conception and of particular consequence here is the significance of contrasting, recurrent mood states. Cyclic patterns are common to both mood disorders and the nature of creative work. The ebbing and flowing character of inspiration, described so often, bears a striking resemblance to changes from the vitality to nonvitality of different seasons, death and rebirth, and the antithetical qualities of the bipolar mood states.

Clinical characteristics such as changes in mood, thinking, energy, and behavior are usually opposite in mania and depression. This is true for linguistic and artistic patterns as well. Manic patients, for example, tend not only to speak more and more rapidly, but also to use more colorful and powerful speech, including more action verbs and adjectives (see Chapter 2). Artistic expression also changes across mood states (see Table 12–8 and Plates 15–18). Manic patients tend to use vivid and highly contrasting colors; depressed patients, on the other hand, use primarily black and cold, darker colors (when the depression begins to clear, the palette tends to lighten accordingly). The content of paintings produced during mania tends to be more sexual, filled with motion and bright portrayals of natural phenomena such as fires, waterfalls, and landscapes; in contrast, paintings done during the depressed phase tend to show a paucity of ideas, a lack of motion, and themes of death and decay. Paintings produced by manic patients are usually done rapidly and impulsively and often have an agitated or swirling quality; paintings produced by depressed patients are relatively barren, are painted slowly, and exhibit less imagination. The contrasting nature of the elated and depressive states provides, for those with artistic or literary ability, a rich variety of experiences and sensations from which to create.

The ability to reconcile opposite states, whether they are of mood, thought, or vitality, is critical to any creative act.[8] Thomas Moore (1832), himself a poet, described this ability in his friend Byron:

TABLE 12–8. **Artistic Expression during Mania and Depression**

Feature	Mania	Depression
Color	Vivid, hot, sharply contrasting (Zimmerman and Garfinckle, 1942); wild (Reitman, 1950); highly colored, without the time to use a variety of colors (Dax, 1953); vivid (Plokker, 1965); bright, warm, optimistic (Enâchescu, 1971); color did not differentiate manic patients as a diagnostic group (Wadeson and Carpenter, 1976).	Somber (Reitman, 1950); somber, usually black with upper portion darkest (Dax, 1953); dark colors, upper portion of picture generally darker than lower, lightening of palette as depression begins to clear (Plokker, 1965); dark, dirty, cold, somber (Enâchescu, 1971); bipolar more colorful than unipolar (Wadeson and Carpenter, 1976).
Content	Sexual, setting sun, orifices (Zimmerman and Garfinckle, 1942); often obscene (Dax, 1953); flowers, landscapes, sunrises, fires, waterfalls, animals, people, dance scenes (Enâchescu, 1971).	Poverty of ideas (Reitman, 1950); immobile figures with sunken heads, signs of death, starless nights rather than days, trees broken off, no flowers (Dax, 1953); representations of delusions (sin, poverty, hypochondriasis), torture, suicide (Plokker, 1965); mourning scenes, physical or moral disaster, abandonment, physical decompensation (Enâchescu, 1971).
Affect	Positive, assured (Zimmerman and Garfinckle, 1942); excitement (Reitman, 1950); careless (Dax, 1953); euphoric (Enâchescu, 1971).	Useless, depressive, cold, gloomy (Enâchescu, 1971).
Form and activity	Extreme agitation, productive, fluid composition, swirl-like forms (Zimmerman and Garfinckle, 1942); restless, disordered, incoherent lines (Reitman, 1950); rapidly produced, lacking in restraint (Dax, 1953); deterioration in composition (Plokker, 1965); rapid and expansive, far more productive than in depressed phase; lines are rash, thick, and crossed (Enâchescu, 1971).	Bareness and lack of detail (Dax, 1953); rarely engaged in artistic activity (Plokker, 1965); less creative activity (Enâchescu, 1971).

It must be perceived by all endowed with quick powers of association how constantly, when any particular thought or sentiment presents itself to their minds, its very opposite, at the same moment, springs up there also; if anything sublime occurs, its neighbour, the ridiculous, is by its side; across a bright view of the present or the future, a dark one throws its shadow; and, even in questions respecting morals and conduct, all the reasonings and consequences that may suggest themselves on the side of one of two opposite courses will, in such minds, be instantly confronted by an array just as cogent on the other. A mind of this structure—and such more or less, are all those in which the reasoning is made subservient to the imaginative faculty—though enabled, by such rapid powers of association, to multiply its resources without end, has need of the constant exercise of a controlling judgment to keep its perceptions pure and undisturbed between the contrasts it thus simultaneously calls up.

The manic-depressive, or cyclothymic, temperament carries with it the capacity to react strongly and quickly; it is, in a biological sense, an alert and excitable system. It responds to the world with a wide range of emotional, perceptual, intellectual, behavioral, and energy changes, and it creates around itself both the possibilities and chaos afforded by altered experiences and fluctuating tempos. The constant transitions can be painful and confusing. Such chaos in those able ultimately to transcend it or shape it to their will can, however, result in an artistically useful comfort with transitions, an ease with ambiguities and with life on the edge, and an intuitive awareness of the coexisting and oppositional forces at work in the world.

Of interest, two recent studies found increased cyclothymia in creative individuals (Akiskal et al., 2005; Nowakowska et al., 2005). The relationship between the cyclic and contrasting nature of manic-depressive illness and creative work is discussed in much further detail by Jamison (1993).

Experiences Derived from Having the Illness

I do strongly feel that among the greatest pieces of luck for high achievement is ordeal. Certain great artists can make out without it, Titian and others, but mostly you need ordeal. My idea is this: The artist is extremely lucky who is presented with the worst possible ordeal which will not actually kill him. At that point, he's in business. Beethoven's deafness, Goya's deafness, Milton's blindness, that kind of thing. And I think that what happens in my poetic work in the future work will probably largely depend not on my sitting calmly on my ass as I think, "Hmm, hmm, a long poem again? Hmm," but on being

knocked in the face, and thrown flat, and given cancer, and all kinds of other things short of senile dementia. At that point, I'm out, but short of that, I don't know. I hope to be nearly crucified.—John Berryman (1976, p. 322)

Berryman, a contemporary of Robert Lowell and Theodore Roethke, was, like them, a winner of the Pulitzer Prize for poetry and someone who suffered from bipolar illness. At the end of a full but highly painful and tumultuous life, he committed suicide (as had his father and aunt before him). He was far from alone in believing that suffering could be conducive to creative work. Learning through intense and deep emotional experiences and using that learning to add meaning and depth to creative work is probably the aspect of the relationship between mood disorders and accomplishment most widely accepted and written about. The influence of pain's dominion fills novels, biographies and autobiographies, sermons, and canvases; there is no shortage of portrayals.

Profound depression or the suffering of psychosis can, and often does, fundamentally change expectations and beliefs about the nature and length of life, God, and other people. Many writers have described the impact of their long periods of depression, how they have dealt with them, and how they have used them in their work. Anne Sexton, a contemporary of Lowell, Roethke, and Berryman, was also a Pulitzer Prize winner in poetry and someone who almost certainly had bipolar illness. After many hospitalizations for both mania and depression, she, like Berryman, committed suicide. She described the importance of using pain in her work:

I, myself, alternate between hiding behind my own hands, protecting myself any way possible, and this other, this seeing ouching other. I guess I mean that creative people must not avoid the pain that they get dealt. . . . Hurt must be examined like a plague. (Sexton and Ames, 1977, p. 105)

Robert Lowell, who wrote of depression, "I don't think it a visitation of the angels but a weakening in the blood," also wrote:

Depression's no gift from the Muse. At worst, I do nothing. But often I've written, and wrote one whole book—*For the Union Dead*—about witheredness. . . . Most of the best poems, the most personal, are gathered crumbs from the lost cake. I had better moods, but the book is lemony, soured and dry, the drought I had touched with my own hands. That, too, may be poetry—on sufferance. (quoted in Giroux, 1987, p. 287)

Both Lowell and Sexton wrote of their heightened psychological sensitivity and vulnerability in graphic and quite similar physical metaphors: "seeing too much and feeling it/with one skin-layer missing" (Lowell) and "even illusion breaks its filament wings/on the raw skin of all I wouldn't know" (Sexton).

Hypomania and mania often generate ideas and associations, propel contact with life and other people, induce frenzied energies and enthusiasms, and cast an ecstatic, rather cosmic hue over life. Melancholy, on the other hand, tends to force a slower pace; cools the ardor; and puts into perspective the thoughts, observations, and feelings generated during more enthusiastic moments. Mild depression can act as ballast; it can also serve a critical editorial role for work produced in more fevered states. Depression prunes and sculpts; it also ruminates and ponders and, ultimately, subdues and focuses thought. It allows structuring, at a detailed level, of the more expansive patterns generated during hypomania.

Relative Importance of Different Aspects of the Illness to Various Types of Accomplishment

Changes brought about by bipolar illness—during hypomania, mania, depression, and normal states—produce different advantages and disadvantages in various fields of creative work and other types of accomplishment. Although there are no systematic data, a review of available studies strongly suggests that the actual prevalence of bipolar illness is distributed unequally across professions; for example, poets appear to have an unusually high rate, scientists a lower one. To a poet, the cognitive, energy, mood, and experiential advantages of the elated and depressive states may outweigh the disruptions, chaos, turmoil, and inconsistent productivity that would be insurmountable to most scientists. Pragmatic issues of education and job requirements also probably affect the rates of bipolar illness in various occupations. Composers and poets, while increasingly likely to obtain graduate levels of education or professional training, do not absolutely require it. On the other hand, medical and graduate schools—particularly those with highly structured programs, such as those for medicine and law—tend to select students who, by and large, have demonstrated an ability to conform to strict requirements for consistently high levels of performance over long periods of time. This may well exclude many individuals at risk or those with an actual history of bipolar illness, since they are more likely to show greater variability in their performance across seasons and years.

The risk period for a first manic or depressive episode overlaps considerably with the period of advanced education, eliminating some bipolar individuals from being selected. Further selection bias exists in the decisions made about those individuals who have actually had an affective episode, especially a manic one, while in training. The professional consequences of a psychotic break are generally different for those in medicine, clinical psychology, nursing, or law school than they are for those writing poetry or composing music.

Even within the field of literary accomplishment, differences in the characteristics of bipolar illness are likely to produce relative gains and losses for various types of writers. Poets may benefit much more than novelists from mood and cognitive changes, for example, because the language and rhythms of poetry are more akin to primitive thought processes and psychosis and because the nature of sustained work is probably different in poetry and fiction.

Certain aspects of bipolar illness probably are important and helpful in other fields of accomplishment as well. It is likely that mood changes (elevated and expansive mood, inflated self-esteem, increased enthusiasm, increased emotional intensity, and infectious mood) are equally, if differently, important to those who create and to those in business or positions of leadership. This is probably true as well for increased energy levels and a decreased need for sleep. On a very general level, however, cognitive changes (sharpened and unusually creative thinking, flight of ideas, and hyperacusis) are likely more useful to those in the arts and sciences than to those in positions of political and military leadership. Conversely, interpersonal changes brought about by hypomania (enhanced liveliness, uninhibited people seeking, interpersonal charm, the ability to find vulnerable spots in others and to make use of them, increased perceptiveness at the subconscious or unconscious level, and increased social ease) are probably more likely to benefit those in leadership positions than those in the arts and sciences.

IMPORTANCE OF STUDYING POSITIVE ASPECTS OF MANIC-DEPRESSIVE ILLNESS

Although it certainly is possible to exaggerate or romanticize the positive aspects of mood disorders, it is important not to minimize their beneficial features or deal with them in only a perfunctory way. Understanding the assets that may accompany manic-depressive illness—the characteristics linking it to the arts, leadership, and society at large—is important to a thorough understanding of the illness. Three principal areas of consideration are relevant to the study of the positive features of manic-depressive: theoretical, clinical, and social–ethical.

Theoretical Considerations

Positive aspects of manic-depressive illness, including associations with accomplishment, are, of course, interesting in their own right. At first glance, the notion of advantage gained from an otherwise catastrophic illness may appear counterintuitive, yet both history and clinical experience affirm the reality of this paradox. The association may be an infrequent one, but it is important. Most clinical research understandably has focused on the depressive spectrum and given relatively little emphasis to the manic continuum. There has been next to no study of the spectrum of elated states most relevant to the discussion here. Of the many still unexamined aspects of bipolar illness that could profitably be studied, its positive features are particularly germane. There has been little research into subtle oscillations in perception, mood, behavior, and cognition across the elated states. Quantitative and qualitative differences between the milder hypomanias and manias also require more study. Likewise, we need to learn to differentiate characteristics of high-functioning normal individuals—those with decreased need for sleep coupled with high energy, productivity, and mood—from the characteristics of individuals with hyperthymia, cyclothymia, or bipolar illness.

The existence of elated states also provides an opportunity for cognitive psychologists to study a long-standing theoretical question: Does cognition precede or follow mood change? The considerable body of literature on this question is based on studies of depression and, because of psychological assumptions about etiology, tends to assume that cognitive changes precede—indeed cause or facilitate—depressive affect. Similarly, many creative individuals and students of creativity assume that inspiration, creative ideas, and fluency of thinking precede euphoric affect. That is, many believe that the creative act generates euphoria, not that heightened mood facilitates the increased flow of thoughts and ideas. Notwithstanding these assumptions, evidence indicates that in a sizable proportion of highly creative writers and artists, elevated mood changes precede cognitive and behavioral changes, and that intense creative episodes are, in many instances, indistinguishable from hypomania (Richards and Kinney, 1990; Schuldberg, 1990; Jamison, 1993, 2004).

Yet another important theoretical issue, one with enormous practical ramifications, centers on the highly seductive, if not actually addictive, qualities of the elated or euphoric states. Such altered states of consciousness and mood can be highly potent reinforcers during euthymic or depressed periods, creating in some patients a strong desire to induce or recreate such conditions. This phenomenon is roughly analogous to drug self-administration, in which a highly pleasurable and often immediate state can be obtained. Thus for some patients, the positive aspects of the illness may be similar to stimulant addiction.

Clinical experience suggests that patients may attempt to induce mania by discontinuing lithium not just at times when they are depressed but also when they face problematic decisions and life events. Because the negative consequences are delayed, it is not always clear to the patient that the costs outweigh the benefits. The clinical implications of this phenomenon are discussed in the next section and in Chapters 21 and 22. Here it is important to mention that the addictive or addictive-like qualities of the elated states raise fascinating issues about the means used to self-induce these states (sleep deprivation, medication nonadherence, or psychological means), the relevance of this phenomenon to kindling models, and, of course, the use of cocaine and other stimulants to self-medicate or to induce euphoric and high-energy states. The high rate of affective illness in cocaine abuse (see Chapter 7) may reflect not only self-medication per se, but also an attempt to recapture a known, previously experienced and highly pleasurable mood state, a reality that makes bipolar individuals perhaps uniquely vulnerable to cocaine addiction on both psychological and biological grounds.

Clinical Considerations

The existence of potentiating positive features in bipolar illness, perceived to be or actually associated with increased creativity and productivity, affects the willingness of some afflicted with the illness to seek and comply with treatment. Many highly accomplished individuals in the arts, the sciences, and business are reluctant to seek treatment for their mood disorders because they are reluctant to give up the edge they feel they obtain from it. Others view their serious mood problems as part of the human condition, the price one pays for being "too sensitive," having an artistic temperament, or leading an artistic lifestyle. Indeed, many such individuals see emotional turmoil as essential to their identity as performing or creative artists. Additionally, many writers and artists are concerned that psychiatric treatment will erode or compromise their ability to create. An appreciation of the potentially productive or "up" side of mood disorders may lead to greater credibility on the part of the treating clinician, as well as a stronger therapeutic bond. Strict adherence to an often arbitrary distinction between psychopathology on the one hand and a chaotic, tumultuous, and artistic lifestyle on the other can lead to unnecessary suffering and treatment resistance.

Writers and artists frequently express concern about the effects of psychiatric treatment on their ability to create and produce; these concerns are especially pronounced when it comes to taking medication. Some of this mistrust no doubt reflects unfounded preconceptions, fears of altering long-established work patterns and rituals, or simple resistance to treatment. In some instances, however, these concerns are grounded in reality. A review of the literature on mood-stabilizing medications reveals disturbingly little research on the effects of the drugs on productivity and creativity.

Even the early lithium researchers were well aware of problems created by lithium's effects on certain useful or enjoyable qualities of the illness (e.g., decreasing or eliminating the highs of hypomania, decreasing sexuality and energy levels), as well as by the drug's untoward side effects (possible cognitive slowing and memory impairment) (see Chapters 9 and 21). Schou (1968, p. 78) described the subjective effects of lithium in three "normal" subjects (medical researchers). This description has relevance to highly creative individuals who are dependent on the mind and the senses for their work:

> The subjective experience was primarily one of indifference and slight general malaise. This led to a certain passivity. . . . The subjective feeling of having been altered by the treatment was disproportionately strong in relation to objective behavioral changes. The subjects could engage in discussions and social activities but found it difficult to comprehend and integrate more than a few elements of a situation. Intellectual initiative was diminished and there was a feeling of lowered ability to concentrate and memorize; but thought processes were unaffected, and the subjects could think logically and produce ideas.

It should be noted that Schou's study involved a relatively short-term trial of lithium, and there is some indication that patients partially accommodate to lithium's cognitive effects. Many patients, of course, experience no significant cognitive side effects, and for those who do, the risks of no treatment must always be weighed against those side effects.

What is actually known about the specific effects of lithium and other medications on productivity and creativity? Polatin and Fieve (1971, p. 864) described their clinical experience of using lithium in creative individuals:

> In the creative individual who does his best work in the course of a hypomanic period, the complaint regarding the continued use of lithium carbonate is that it acts as a "brake." These patients report that lithium carbonate inhibits creativity so that the individual is unable to express himself, drive is diminished, and there is no incentive. These patients also indicate that when they are depressed, the symptoms are so demoralizing and so uncomfortable that they welcome the "mild high" when the depression disappears and prefer to settle for a cyclothymic life of highs and lows rather than an apathetic middle-of-road mood state achieved through the use of lithium carbonate.

> Their argument is that if lithium carbonate prevents the high and may possibly prevent the "low," they prefer not to take lithium carbonate, since never to have a high as a result of the drug seems equivalent to being deprived

of an "addictive-like" pleasurable and productive state. Some of these patients are terrified of having a low again, but insist on taking their chances without lithium carbonate therapy, knowing that sooner or later they will be compensated by the high, even if they do go into a low state.

No controlled studies of lithium's effects on productivity have been conducted, but Marshall and colleagues (1970) and Schou (1979) studied a total of 30 artists, writers, and businessmen taking lithium. Their findings are summarized in Table 12–9. More than three-quarters (77 percent) of the patients reported no change or an increase in their productivity while on lithium. Approximately one-quarter reported a decrease. In 17 percent, lithium was seen as leading to problems sufficient to warrant refusal to take it. It is not known how accurately these figures reflect artists and writers at the upper end of creative accomplishment. Most of these subjects, although earning their living by their creative work, were not at that level. Schou (1979) pointed out that lithium may affect inspiration, the ability to execute, or both, and saw the following as contributing factors in a creative individual's response to lithium: the severity of illness, the type of illness, the artist's habits of using manic periods of inspiration, and individual sensitivity to the pharmacological action of the drug.

Three other studies of particular relevance for artistic creativity yielded conflicting results. Judd and colleagues (1977) found no effects of short-term lithium treatment on creativity in normal subjects. A study using bipolar patients as their own controls, however, found substantial detrimental effects of the drug on associational productivity and originality of responses (Shaw et al., 1986; see Fig. 12–9). These differing results may be due in part to the fact that lithium's effect on cognition is probably quite different in bipolar patients and normal controls (Pons et al., 1985). Lithium exerts effects not only on cognition, but also on drive and personality (see Chapter 10); although cognitive side effects are undeniably important to creative work, so, too, are these noncognitive effects. Kocsis and colleagues (1993) found that lithium discontinuation resulted in improvement on memory and creativity measures (although not idiosyncratic word associations), as well as motor performance. In an open, nonrandom case series of seven bipolar patients who reported cognitive dulling during lithium therapy, Stoll and colleagues (1996) concluded that the partial or full substitution of divalproex sodium for lithium as the primary mood stabilizer "reduced the cognitive, motivational, or creative deficits attributed to lithium" (p. 359). To our knowledge,

TABLE 12–9. **Productivity While Taking Lithium**

	Marshall et al. (1970)	Schou (1979)	Combined Number	%
Subjects	6 artists and businessmen	24 artists and writers	30	
Productivity on lithium				
Increased	5	12	17	57
No change	0	6	6	20
Decreased	1	6	7	23
Refused to continue lithium treatment	1	4	5	17

however, there has been no replication of this preliminary finding. Individual differences in clinical state, serum lithium levels, sensitivity to cognitive side effects, and the severity, frequency, and type of affective illness clearly affect the degree to which an individual will experience impairment in intellectual functioning, creativity, and productivity. Artists, writers, and many others who rely on their initiative, intellect, emotional intensity, and energy for their life's work underscore the need for a reexamination of this problem.

Artists and writers represent a group at high risk for affective illness and should be assessed and counseled accordingly. Ideal treatment requires a sensitive understanding

Figure 12–9. Associational patterns and lithium level. (*Source:* Adapted from Shaw et al., 1986. Reprinted with permission from the *American Journal of Psychiatry*, American Psychiatric Association.)

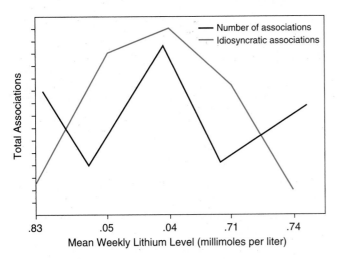

of the possible benefits of mood disorders to creativity and also the severe liabilities of untreated depression and mania, including the risk of suicide, hospitalization, and substance abuse. Moreover, the clinician must be aware of available medications and side effects that could potentially be damaging to the creative process. Physicians should minimize medication levels whenever possible.

Social and Ethical Considerations

As noted in Chapter 13, genetic research has progressed to the point that ethical issues are now arising about prenatal screening and selective abortion, as well as the identification and treatment of individuals at high risk for developing bipolar illness. It becomes particularly important under these circumstances to have at least some broad notion of the possible benefits, as well as catastrophic outcomes, of bipolar illness not only for potential parents and the unborn child, but also for society at large. The implications of losing societal variance in such basic characteristics as drive, cognitive style, energy, risk taking, and temperament have not yet been examined in any systematic way, although evolutionary perspectives on depression and bipolar illness have been discussed at some length.[9] Ironically, these issues were considered, to some extent, in the 1930s; in one study, carried out in Germany, the advisability of sterilizing manic-depressive individuals was examined. Luxenburger (1933) found manic-depressive illness to be greatly overrepresented in the higher occupational classes and recommended against sterilizing these patients, "especially if the patient does not have siblings who could transmit the positive aspects of the genetic heritage." Myerson and Boyle (1941, p. 20), in their study of manic-depressive psychosis in socially prominent American families, concurred:

> Perhaps the words of Bumke need to be taken into account before we embark too whole-heartedly on any sterilization program: "If we could extinguish the sufferers from manic-depressive psychosis from the world, we would at the same time deprive ourselves of an immeasurable amount of the accomplished and good, of color and warmth, of spirit and freshness. Finally only dried up bureaucrats and schizophrenics would be left. Here I must say that I would rather accept into the bargain the diseased manic-depressive than to give up the healthy individuals of the same heredity cycle."

Treatable common illnesses such as bipolar illness—ones that may confer societal and individual advantage and that vary greatly in the nature of their expression and their severity—are particularly problematic. Francis Collins (1990), director of the U.S. National Human Genome Research Institute and a scientist who was instrumental in identifying the genes for cystic fibrosis and neurofibromatosis, was asked in an interview about prenatal testing for diseases that vary in severity or that first occur only later in life:

> This is where it gets muddy, and everyone is going to draw the line differently. Consider the situation with manic-depressive illness, a reasonably common disorder. It is clearly genetically influenced, though not in a simple way. Now, manic-depressive illness can be a terrible cross to bear. The swings into depression are awful, and the highs can be very destructive. Yet a substantial number of highly creative people have suffered from this disease. Suppose we find the gene responsible for manic depression. If every couple has a prenatal test to determine if a fetus is at risk for manic depression, and if every time the answer is yes that fetus is done away with, then we will have done something troubling, something with large consequences. Is this what we want to do?

CONCLUSIONS

There is strong scientific and biographical evidence linking mood disorders to artistic creativity. Biographies of eminent poets, composers, and artists attest to the prevalence of extremes of mood in creative individuals. Systematic studies are increasingly documenting the link as well. It should be emphasized, however, that most creative writers, artists, and musicians have no significant psychopathology. Conversely, most individuals with manic-depressive illness are not unusually creative.

We have considered the issue of the reliability—indeed, the advisability—of making a posthumous diagnosis of manic-depressive illness. This concern is important and valid. Labeling as manic-depressive anyone who is unusually creative, accomplished, energetic, intense, moody, or eccentric both diminishes the notion of individuality within the arts and trivializes a very serious, often lethal illness. We have been careful to base our conclusions and suggestions on what is known clinically and scientifically about depression and bipolar disorder.

That the illness and its related temperaments are associated with creativity appears clear; the clinical, ethical, and social implications of this association are less so. We have tried to convey that bipolar disorder and depression are destructive, painful, sometimes fatal, and yet intriguing and important illnesses. In the great majority of instances, the effective treatments now available will not hinder creative ability. Indeed, treatment almost always results in longer periods of sustained productivity. One of our concerns, however, remains the study, public discussion, and development of treatments that will minimize the side effects of currently available medications.

The neurochemical and anatomical processes responsible for the cognitive changes occurring during manic and highly creative states are poorly understood. It remains for molecular biology, neuropsychology, and quickly evolving neuroimaging techniques to provide us with a more sophisticated understanding of the underlying changes in thought and behavior that are enhanced, left unaffected, or impaired by shifting patterns of mood (see, e.g., Hoffman et al., 2001; Folley et al., 2003; Ghacibeh et al., 2006).

Perhaps some suffering must always accompany great artistic achievement. Certainly, depth and intensity of human feeling must be a part of creation in the arts. But modern medicine now allows relief of the extremes of despair, turmoil, and psychosis. It allows choices not previously available. Most of the writers, artists, and composers discussed in this chapter had no such choices.

NOTES

1. George Gordon, Lord Byron. "Manfred," act II, scene 4, lines 160–161. *Lord Byron: The Complete Poetical Works*, vol. 4, p. 86. Edited by Jerome J. McGann. Oxford: Clarendon Press, 1986.
2. Much of the discussion of manic-depressive illness and creativity in this chapter is based on Jamison's elaboration, in *Touched with Fire*, of the arguments originally presented in the first edition of *Manic-Depressive Illness*.
3. Fully 70 to 90 percent of all suicides are associated with bipolar or depressive illness; therefore, if an individual has died by suicide, it is usually the case that a mood disorder was at least contributory.
4. An episodic, cyclic course of symptoms with normal functioning in between; usual onset of symptoms in the late

teens or early twenties, with temperamental signs often exhibited much earlier; seasonal aspects to the mood and energy changes; and if untreated, a worsening of the illness over time. (See Chapter 4.)

5. This study was brought to the attention of the authors by Dr. Zoltán Rihmer.

6. Isen and Daubman, 1984; Isen et al., 1985, 1987; Greene and Noice, 1988; Fodor, 1999; Isen, 1999; Fodor and Laird, 2004.

7. Roe, 1946, 1951, 1952; MacKinnon, 1962; Getzels and Jackson, 1963; Hudson, 1966; Barron, 1968; Welsh, 1977, Gardner, 1993; Winner, 1996; Jamison, 2004.

8. Among the many writers who have emphasized the importance of the reconciliation of opposite states in the creative process are Aristotle, "On the Art of Poetry," *Classical Literary Criticism*, translated by T. S. Dorsch, London: Penguin, 1965; Percy Bysshe Shelley, "A Defence of Poetry," *Shelley's Critical Prose*, edited by B.R. McElderry (1821; reprint, Lincoln: University of Nebraska Press, 1967); Maurice Bowra, *The Romantic Imagination*, Cambridge: Harvard University Press, 1950; J.P. Guilford, Traits of creativity, in H.H. Anderson (Ed.), *Creativity and its Cultivation*, New York: Harper, 1959; F. Barron, *Creative Person and Creative Process*, New York: Holt, Rinehart & Winston, 1969; A. Koestler, *The Act of Creation*, New York: Dell, 1971; A. Storr, *The Dynamics of Creation*, London: Penguin, 1972; A. Rothenberg, *The Emerging Goddess*, Chicago: University of Chicago Press, 1979; J. Carey, *John Donne: Life, Mind and Art*, London: Faber and Faber, 1981; K. Miller, *Doubles: Studies in Literary History*, Oxford: Oxford University Press, 1985.

9. Price, 1967, 1972; Gardner, 1982; Jamison, 1993; Wilson, 1993; Price et al., 1994; Brody, 2001; Watson and Andrews, 2002; Gilbert, 2004, 2006; Keller and Nesse, 2005; Keller and Miller, 2006.

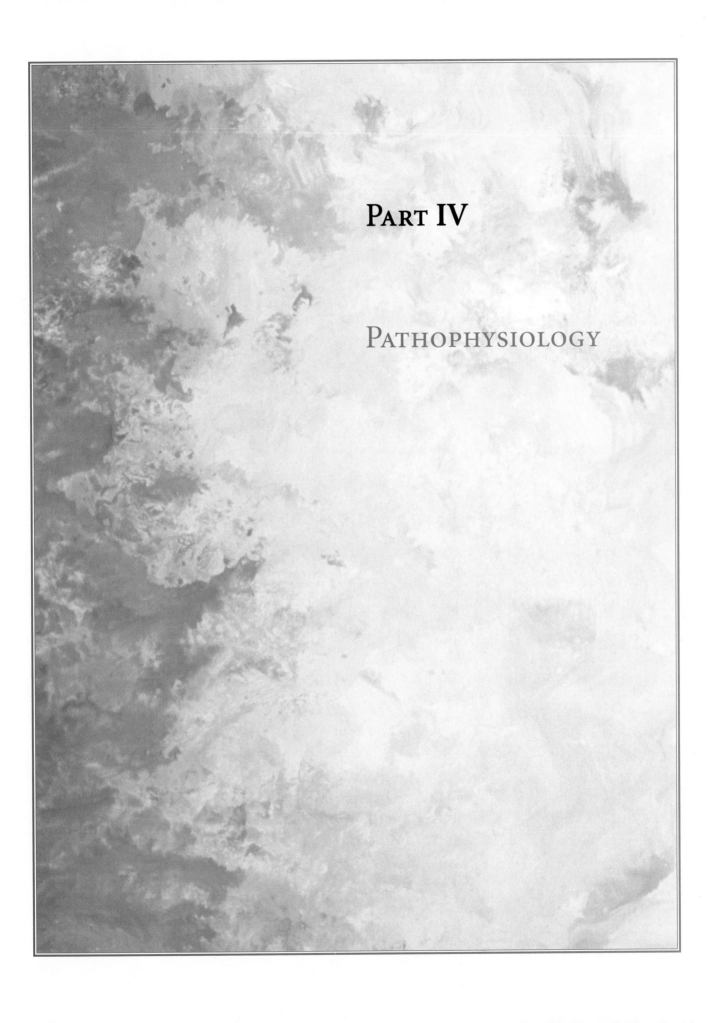

PART IV

PATHOPHYSIOLOGY

13 Genetics

That other inward, inbred cause of melancholy is our temperature, in whole or part, which we receive from our parents . . . such as the temperature of the father is, such is the son's, and look what disease the father had when he begot him, his son will have after him, "and is as well inherited of his infirmities as of his lands."

—Robert Burton (1621, p. 211)

A generation ago, few mental health professionals believed that inherited vulnerabilities could be central to the development of psychiatric illness. Fearing that discovery of a genetic diathesis might cast a stigma on patients and lead to therapeutic nihilism, many clinical observers found social and developmental reasons to explain the inescapable fact that mental illness runs in families. Gradually, the genetic evidence became too compelling to ignore. Recent advances in the molecular genetics of several neuropsychiatric diseases, particularly the discovery of linkage and association of deoxyribonucleic acid (DNA) markers with the bipolar subtype of manic-depressive illness, appear to reaffirm the older evidence. If, as expected, particular gene variants are definitively implicated in manic-depressive susceptibility, better understanding of pathophysiological mechanisms should follow.

Along with its theoretical importance, knowledge of genetics has practical relevance, and the new discoveries could result in new diagnostic tests and improved treatment methods. Clinicians now use family histories to help diagnose an illness correctly and to manage psychotropic medications properly. They also need a familiarity with the most up-to-date evidence to answer the questions of an increasingly sophisticated population of patients, relatives, spouses, and prospective spouses requesting genetic counseling.

At present, the most clinically useful evidence for genetic transmission continues to be the traditional genetic–epidemiological findings from twin, family, and adoption studies. In addition to demonstrating genetic transmission, the genetic–epidemiological data suggest the degree to which illness in the population is familial, and they help specify diagnoses that aggregate together. The role of age, gender, and other demographic and sociocultural vari-

ables can also be clarified from this evidence. Genetic–epidemiological studies of diagnosis do not, however, allow one to identify the mode of genetic transmission in recurrent affective disorder. And neither they nor pedigree studies illuminate other important genetic issues: Is there biological heterogeneity? What is the pathophysiological inherited process in an illness? Where on the gene map is the disease locus (or loci)? What are the gene defects? To answer these questions, pathophysiological and genetic linkage studies are needed.

The focus here is on bipolar forms of manic-depressive illness, but we consider the central question of the genetic relationship between bipolar and recurrent unipolar subgroups, particularly the more highly recurrent forms. A common genetic diathesis for both bipolar and recurrent unipolar disorders would suggest that the correct conceptual model for these illnesses is the spectrum or continuum model in which recurrence (cyclicity) is fundamental to what is being transmitted. Different risk genes, however, would argue for a categorical model of discrete and independent affective disorders defined by clinical diagnosis (see Chapters 1 and 3). More careful quantification of the degree of recurrence in bipolar and (especially) unipolar samples might allow one to address new questions such as whether the genetic diathesis for bipolar disorder has more to do with recurrence (cyclicity) or polarity (as is often simply assumed) (see Chapter 1).

This chapter begins with a brief review of major developments in the history of the study of genetics. We then turn to a summary of the findings of family, twin, and adoption studies that make up the literature on the genetic epidemiology of manic-depressive illness, studies that attempt to determine whether the illness is heritable, as well as the mode of its inheritance. Next we summarize recent advances made in understanding the human genome and the nature of genes to set the stage for an examination of the various molecular methods used in attempting to locate the genes for manic-depressive illness and the results stemming from their use. Four such methods are then reviewed: (1) the linkage method, used to identify a chromosomal region that harbors a susceptibility gene; (2) alternative phenotypic definition, which attempts to identify homogeneous clinical subtypes of manic-depressive illness; (3) the association method, an alternative to the linkage method for identification of disease genes; and (4) consideration of alternative genetic mechanisms, an approach that uses clues, both biological and clinical, to home in on genes with unique features potentially relevant to manic-depressive illness. We follow this review with a discussion of gene expression and pathogenesis—a topic that takes the argument for the involvement of a gene in manic-depressive illness beyond statistical association to the field of neurobiology. Next we address pharmacogenetics, or the clinical observation of inherited differences in drug effects, and genetic counseling, which is aimed at helping concerned parents address vulnerabilities they may pass on to their children. Finally, we look to the future, examining research directions and prospects for patients as the study of the role of genetics in manic-depressive illness builds on the work reviewed in this chapter.

HISTORY OF THE STUDY OF GENETICS

Early Observations

Though the twisted, or helical, structure of DNA was not discovered until 1953, the observation that traits run "in the blood," or in families, was first made in antiquity. Lucretius, a Roman who lived from 94 BC to 55 BC, wrote, for example, that "children are born like the mother, thanks to the mother's seed, just as the father's seed makes them like the father. But those whom you see with the form of both, mingled side by side the features of both parents, spring alike from the father's body and the mother's blood" (quoted in Mellon, 1996, p. 13).

The recognition of a hereditary component to mental illness dates back at least as far as the Renaissance. In 1520 the Swiss physician Paracelsus wrote *Diseases Which Lead to a Loss of Reason*, in which he described a subgroup of the "truly insane," which he called the *insani*: "*Insani* are those who have been suffering from it since birth and have brought it from the womb as a family heritage . . . [T]he circumstance is such that if there is insanity in the brain, the child's mother also has some deficiency in her brain, for the brain of the parents is continued in the brain of the son." Paracelsus went on to make note of the apparent complexities of the hereditary influence on insanity: "This [hereditary transmission] does not always happen because the sperma become mixed, and either the man or the woman may or may not be insane, and the child may follow the insanity or take after the one who has the greater influence. It may even happen that if both [parents] are insane they still would give birth to a healthy child" (quoted in Mellon, 1996, p. 21).

In his book *The Anatomy of Melancholy*, published in 1621, Robert Burton wrote of the familial nature of depression in particular: "Their voice, pace, gesture, looks, is likewise derived with all the rest of their conditions and infirmities; such a mother, such a daughter . . . I need not therefore make any doubt of Melancholy, but that it is a hereditary disease" (quoted in Mellon, 1996, p. 25). The familial nature of mania was evident to some early observers as well. Philippe Pinel, a French psychiatrist who is considered one of the founders of modern psychiatry, wrote in his 1809 textbook on mental illness: "It would be difficult not to concede a hereditary transmission of mania, when one recalls that everywhere some members of certain families are struck in several successive generations" (quoted in Shorter, 1996, p. 29).

The Birth of Genetics

The birth of modern genetics dates to 1865. In that year the Austrian monk Gregor Mendel presented the results of his studies of traits in pea plants under the title *Experiments in Plant Hybridization*. His experiments led to the following conclusions: (1) distinct traits, such as length of the stem and color of the seed, assort themselves independently; (2) each trait exists in alternative forms, and each individual has two forms (or factors), such as that for tall and for short, or for purple and for white, and these factors separate (or segregate) independently rather than blending together; and (3) one factor is dominant over the other (which is recessive), so that if the dominant factor is present, it will be expressed. Though ignored for many years, this work was rediscovered and confirmed in 1900.

The first demonstration of a Mendelian trait in man was the report in 1902 by Archibald Garrod at St. Bartholomew's Hospital in London that alkaptonuria, a disease characterized by dark urine, followed a recessive pattern of inheritance. Garrod later described this as an "inborn error of metabolism." The field of medical genetics—founded in England by, for example, Ronald Fisher, J.B.S. Haldane, Lionel Penrose, and John Roberts and developed in the United States by others, such as James Neel (University of Michigan) and Victor McKusick (Johns Hopkins)—was built on Garrod's conception of genetic disease.

From the 1860s through the turn of the century, DNA and chromosomes were discovered, and it was proposed that chromosomes could bear the Mendelian factors. What Mendel called factors would come to be known as *genes*, and the alternative forms of each factor were dubbed *alleles*. (An allele is defined as an alternative form of a genetic locus; a single allele for each locus is inherited from each parent.) In the same period, the Englishman Francis Galton pioneered the application of statistical methods to the study of biological and mental phenomena, creating a new field called *biometrics*. He first suggested that studies of twins could be employed to disentangle the genetic and environmental contributions to physical and mental traits such as height and intelligence; this work would give rise to the field of statistical genetics.

The German School of Psychiatric Genetics

Emil Kraepelin was a German psychiatrist who gave definition to the current conception of manic-depressive illness in the 1899 edition of his classic textbook on mental disorder, which he wrote during his years as professor at the University of Heidelberg (see Chapter 1). In his chapter on the causes of manic-depressive illness (which included bipolar and recurrent unipolar depression), he stated: "The causes of the malady we must seek, as it appears, essentially in morbid predisposition.... Hereditary taint, I could demonstrate in about 80 per cent of the cases [I] observed in Heidelberg" (Kraepelin, 1899, p. 165). He went on to declare that "compared to innate predisposition external influences only play a very subordinate part in the causation of manic-depressive insanity" (p. 127).

Kraepelin founded what has been called the German school of psychiatric genetics (Kallman, 1953, p. 34). Ernst Rudin, a student of Kraepelin's who later became his deputy, developed this school. Rudin, who conducted and directed family and twin studies of mental illness from about 1913 until the late 1930s, presided over family studies of manic-depressive illness (Banse, 1929; Slater, 1936a,b, 1938), as well as the first twin study to shed light on the illness (Luxenburger, 1928).

Eugenics

Eugenics had its origins in the work of Francis Galton, who believed that genetic selection could be employed to improve the genetic fitness of "the race." The eugenics movement took hold in many countries around the world, including the United States, where the Cold Spring Harbor Eugenics Records Office was set up in 1905 to gather data on family histories of the "feebleminded" (among other subjects). The aim of this effort was to reduce the societal load of these illnesses by preventing procreation of the "eugenically undesirable" and limiting their immigration into the country (Kevles, 1995, pp. 56, 92). In Germany, the Society for Race Hygiene was established in 1905, and Ernst Rudin

served the society in numerous roles, including president. Rudin also was an editor of *Archives of Racial and Social Biology* (Weber, 1996). In 1934, after the Nazis' rise to power, Rudin played a role in shaping the "Law for the Prevention of Progeny with Hereditary Defects," which allowed for the forced sterilization of people with a number of hereditary diseases, including manic-depressive illness. Over the next 5 years, hundreds of thousands of sterilizations were performed in Germany, and by 1940 mass executions of mental patients had begun, based on selections made by physicians, including psychiatrists (Mellon, 1996, p. 111).

Post–World War II Era

Because the atrocities committed by the Nazis had in part grown out of eugenics principles, there was a massive recoiling away from eugenics and, by extension, from genetics, among the psychiatric community in the post–World War II era. This development coincided with the rise of psychoanalysis, which was perceived as offering the possibility of treatment and even cure. By contrast, genetics, and biological psychiatry more broadly, were perceived by some as treating patients like guinea pigs—research subjects from whom something could be learned but for whom little could be done.

Despite this general turning away from psychiatric genetics, a few investigators persisted in their efforts at defining the genetic contribution to manic-depressive illness. Among them were Elliot Slater in England and Franz Kallman, who had left Germany for the United States in 1936, both of whom published family and twin studies of manic-depressive illness in the 1950s. In the late 1960s, interest began to revive in the genetics of manic-depressive illness, as it did in biological psychiatry and in medical genetics generally. This interest has grown enormously in the past decade as the computer-based and molecular tools available to study heredity and the genome have multiplied exponentially.

GENETIC EPIDEMIOLOGY OF MANIC-DEPRESSIVE ILLNESS

The first stage in the study of the genetics of an illness involves defining who is and is not to be considered ill (see Fig. 13–1). In the language of genetics, the question is: "What is the phenotype, or trait, under study?" Clear criteria must be applied in defining the phenotype to maximize the homogeneity of the sample. While the field has in recent years focused mainly on the bipolar-I (BP-I) phenotype, much work has also focused on the broader concept of manic-depressive illness, which encompasses the BP-I, bipolar-II (BP-II), and recurrent major depression phenotypes, along with some studies including schizoaffective

Figure 13–1. The sequence of genetics research on manic-depressive illness (MDI). This figure demonstrates both the historical sequence through which research on the genetics of manic-depressive illness has progressed and the logical sequence of reasoning about gene discovery in the illness. See text for details. (*Source:* Haines and Pericak-Vance, 1998. Reprinted with permission of John Wiley & Sons, Inc.)

disorder, manic or bipolar type. Systematic case definitions were lacking until the 1970s, when the Research Diagnostic Criteria (RDC) first came into widespread use (Spitzer and Endicott, 1975). Since the 1980s, the *Diagnostic and Statistical Manual* (DSM) has provided the standard diagnostic criteria for genetic studies. We note that while researchers in genetic epidemiology (the term applied to these kinds of studies) have emphasized recurrent unipolar depression when they have studied the relationship of unipolar to bipolar illness, the DSM-III and -IV definitions of major depressive disorder do not require recurrence. Indeed, by separating bipolar disorder out as a separate illness "from the top," with recurrent unipolar depression (defined perhaps too broadly as simply more than one episode) becoming a tertiary category under depressive disorders, DSM-III and -IV have made it more difficult to conceptualize the relationship between bipolar

disorder and the more recurrent forms of unipolar depression.

The second stage of inquiry involves determining whether the illness is heritable. Only when heritability has been firmly established does it make sense to begin looking for the particular genes responsible for this inheritance. Determination of heritability starts with studies of familial aggregation and proceeds with twin and adoption studies (see Fig. 13–1). Study of the genetic epidemiology of manic-depressive illness also includes research on the mode of inheritance of the illness, through which investigators try to determine how many genes are involved and how they are transmitted within families.

Family Studies

If a disease has a genetic basis, it is expected to run in families. Studies of familial aggregation typically begin with individuals who have manic-depressive illness—the first such person identified in a family is referred to as a *proband*—and assess whether family members of this proband have unexpectedly high rates of illness. Ideally, to ensure good sensitivity, the needed information is obtained through direct interviews of relatives rather than through family history and/or medical records alone (Andreasen et al., 1986). Clear diagnostic criteria enhance reliability and allow for comparability in replication. Use of a set of families ascertained through a control proband helps reduce diagnostic bias and provides rates against which the ill families can be appropriately compared.

Early studies assessed the morbid risk for manic-depressive illness. Prior to the 1960s, about 14 studies demonstrated the substantial risk of manic-depressive illness in first-degree relatives of probands with the disorder (see Table 13–1). Only since the late 1960s have studies assessed the independent morbid risk for bipolar disorder and for major depression (see Table 13–2).[1] There have been many studies using bipolar probands; the 12 in which the majority of subjects were directly interviewed are summarized in Table 13–2.[2] These studies have found rates of 10.7 percent for bipolar illness in relatives of ill probands and 1.0 percent for the illness in relatives of control probands. It is interesting that in the families of bipolar individuals, rates not only of bipolar illness but also of major depression are elevated. Relatives of bipolar probands have a 15.9 percent risk of major depression, while the risk in relatives of controls is 7.3 percent.

The first study to report systematically on manic-depressive illness subtypes essentially as they are currently delineated was that of Gershon and colleagues in 1982. They documented the lifetime prevalence of illness in 1,254 adult first-degree relatives of probands with schizoaffective (11 families), BP-I (96 families), BP-II (34 families), and major depressive (30 families) disorders and in relatives of normal control probands (43 families). This study, performed

TABLE 13–1. **Family Studies of Manic-Depressive Illness before 1960**

Study	First-Degree Relatives (Sample Size)	Risk of MDI in First-Degree Relatives (%)
Hoffman, 1921	139	13.8
Banse, 1929	452	15.5
Humm, 1932	92	4.4
Roll and Entres, 1936	298	12.0
Weinberg and Lobstein, 1936	505	7.4
Slater, 1936	704	15.5
Strömgren, 1938	489	9.7
Pollock et al., 1939	—	—
Luxenburger, 1942	1398	15.8
Hoffman and Wagner, 1946	—	—
Sjogren, 1948	253	4.8
Schulz and Rudin, 1951	—	—
Kallman, 1952	306	23.2
Stenstedt, 1952	979	13.9

Note: Many of the original papers are in German; —— = not available; MDI = manic depressive illness.
Source: Based on tables in Tsuang and Faraone (1990, p. 38) and Rosenthal (1970, p. 207).

TABLE 13–2. Family Studies of Bipolar Illness and Major Depression Since 1960

Proband/Study	Sample Size (Relatives)	Age-Adjusted Lifetime Prevalence in First-Degree Relatives (%)				
		BP	BP-I	BP-II	SA	MDD
Bipolar Disorder						
Winokur and Clayton, 1967	167	10.2	—	—	—	20.4
Mendlewicz and Rainer, 1974	781	17.7	—	—	—	22.4
James and Chapman, 1975	260	6.4	—	—	—	13.2
Johnson and Leeman, 1977	213	15.5	—	—	—	19.8
Abrams and Taylor, 1980	47	8.5	—	—	—	6.4
Baron et al., 1982	135	14.5	—	—	1.5	16.3
Tsuang et al., 1980	223	3.6	—	—	—	11.9
Jakimow-Venulet, 1981	804	11.8	—	—	—	6.1
Maier et al., 1993	389	7.0	—	—	0.5	21.9
Weighted mean	*3,019*	*11.9*	—	—	*0.8*	*15.6*
Bipolar-I Disorder						
Gershon et al., 1982	548	—	4.5	4.1	1.1	14.0
Andreasen et al., 1987	569	—	3.9	4.2	0.5	22.8
Pauls et al., 1992	408	—	8.7	3.7	0.4	11.6
Heun et al., 1993	166	—	3.6	1.8	0	16.3
Weighted mean	*1,691*		*5.2*	*3.8*	*0.6*	*16.6*
Bipolar-II Disorder						
Gershon et al., 1982	191	—	2.6	4.5	0.6	17.3
Andreasen et al., 1985	267	—	1.1	8.2	0.4	26.2
Heun and Maier, 1993	115	—	3.5	6.1	0.9	18.3
Weighted mean	*573*		*2.1*	*6.5*	*0.6*	*21.6*
Major Depression						
Smeraldi et al., 1977	185	0.6	—	—	—	8.0
Tsuang et al., 1980	483	2.0	—	—	—	13.6
Abrams and Taylor, 1980	106	4.7	—	—	—	7.5

(continued)

TABLE 13–2. Family Studies of Bipolar Illness and Major Depression Since 1960 *(continued)*

Proband/Study	Sample Size (Relatives)	Age-Adjusted Lifetime Prevalence in First-Degree Relatives (%)				
		BP	BP-I	BP-II	SA	MDD
Jakimow-Venulet, 1981	306	0.5	—	—	—	9.5
Gershon et al., 1982	166	—	1.5	1.5	0.7	16.6
Baron et al., 1982	143	2.2	—	—	3.0	17.7
Weissman et al., 1984	810	—	0.9	1.9	0.3	17.6
Andreasen et al., 1985	1,171	—	0.6	2.9	0.2	28.4
McGuffin et al., 1987	315	—	—	—	—	24.7
Maier et al., 1993	697	1.8	—	—	0.5	21.6
Weissman et al., 1993	651	—	—	—	—	24.4
Weighted mean	*5,033*	*1.7*	*0.8*	*2.4*	*0.5*	*20.5*
Schizoaffective Disorder						
Scharfetter, 1981	263	4.4	—	—	2.5	4.4
Gershon et al., 1982	84	—	10.7	6.1	6.1	14.5
Baron et al., 1982	64	1.6	—	—	3.2	26.5
Kendler et al., 1986	84	3.9	—	—	—	7.1
Andreasen et al., 1987	138	—	3.6	5.8	0.7	25.4
Goldstein et al., 1993	149	3.1	—	—	2.3	7.7
Maier et al., 1993	204	8.0	—	—	3.9	20.6
Kendler et al., 1993a	152	4.8	—	—	1.8	44.9
Weighted mean	*1,138*	*4.8*	*6.3*	*5.9*	*2.7*	*17.8*
Controls						
Tsuang et al., 1980	541	0.3	—	—	—	7.5
Gershon et al., 1982	265	—	0	0.5	0.5	5.8
Weissman et al., 1984	521	—	0.2	1.1	0.2	5.9

(continued)

Table 13–2. Family Studies of Bipolar Illness and Major Depression Since 1960 (continued)

Proband/Study	Sample Size (Relatives)	Age-Adjusted Lifetime Prevalence in First-Degree Relatives (%)				
		BP	BP-I	BP-II	SA	MDD
Maier et al., 1993	419	1.8	—	—	0.4	10.6
Weissman et al., 1993	255	—	—	—	—	5.5
Weighted mean	*2,001*	*1.0*	*0.1*	*0.9*	*0.3*	*7.3*

Note: The mix of highly recurrent and minimally recurrent patients in the MDD group can obscure the relationship between bipolar disorder and some forms of unipolar depression.

BP = bipolar disorder; MDD = major depressive disorder; SA = schizoaffective disorder; — = not studied or reported.

at the National Institute of Mental Health (NIMH), involved direct interviews of most first-degree relatives using the Schedule for Affective Disorders and Schizophrenia—Lifetime Version, a semistructured interview (Endicott and Spitzer, 1978). Two independent clinicians used a modified version of the RDC to make diagnoses based on these interviews, along with family informant data and medical records. A consensus diagnosis was then established. In calculating the lifetime risk of mood disorders in relatives, the raw data were modified to account for the variable age at onset of the disorders. This was done using the Stromgren method, which weighs the number of people at risk by the proportion of the risk period through which they have passed.

The findings of Gershon and colleagues (1982, 1985, 1986, 1988, 1989) and Gershon and Goldin (1989) provide among the best accounts available of the familial aggregation of affective disorders. The lifetime risk of BP-I among relatives in the BP-I proband families was elevated at 4.5 percent (versus 0 percent in controls). The risk for BP-II among relatives was also elevated in BP-I proband families at 4.1 percent (versus 0.5 percent in controls). Similarly, the risk for major depressive disorder in these families was increased at 14.0 percent (versus 5.8 percent in controls). There was an overall lifetime risk of 23.7 percent for an affective disorder in the first-degree relatives of the BP-I probands compared with a risk of 6.8 percent in the control families. Of interest, the risk for BP-I was also increased in relatives of the schizoaffective probands (10.7 percent); the risk for BP-II was elevated as well in relatives of the BP-II probands (4.5 percent) and schizoaffective disorder probands (6.1 percent); and the risk for major depression was substantial—two to three times that of controls—in relatives of all affected probands. When all families were taken together, children of one affectively ill parent had a 27 percent lifetime risk of affective disorder, compared with a risk of 74 percent among children of two ill parents (Gershon et al., 1982).

A useful way of estimating the strength of the genetic contribution to illness is to apply the concept of *relative risk* to siblings, which entails comparing the rate of illness in siblings of ill probands with that in the general population. The family studies shown in Table 13–2 demonstrate a relative risk of 10.7 for bipolar disorder in first-degree relatives of bipolar probands.[3] This risk is roughly the same as that for schizophrenia, but far below that for single-gene diseases such as phenylketonuria, for which the relative risk to siblings is 2,500.0. The magnitude of the relative risk to siblings suggests that while there is an important genetic contribution to bipolar disorder, other, presumably environmental, factors play a role as well. The comparable relative risk for major depression is 2.8, suggesting a more modest genetic component, though the risk for early-onset recurrent depression (part of Kraepelin's manic-depressive illness) is probably at least 4.0–5.0 (Levinson, 2006).

Family studies can do more than simply reveal the presence or absence of aggregation; they can also be useful in segregation analysis for assessing whether the pattern of transmission of an illness favors one mode of inheritance (e.g., single major locus or gene) over another (e.g., polygenic or multifactorial). Several segregation analyses of bipolar disorder have provided support for a major locus effect (Rice et al., 1987; Pauls et al., 1995; Spence et al., 1995), but other analyses have not found such evidence (Bucher et al., 1981; Goldin et al., 1983).

Models of the mode of inheritance have also been constructed using the relative risk metric. The increased risk for illness in relatives may be conferred by either one or multiple genes. If multiple genes are responsible, each has its own locus-specific relative risk, which contributes some fraction of the total increased risk. Risch (1990) defined both a heterogeneity model, in which a variety of single genes act independently in different families to cause disease, and a multiplicative multilocus model, in which multiple genes interact to cause disease. Using this metric, Craddock and colleagues (1995b) showed that the heterogeneity model is not consistent with the relative risk data available for bipolar disorder. Instead, the multiplicative model with at least three, and more likely four or more, risk genes provides the best fit with the data. Craddock and colleagues concluded that, although there may be occasional families with a single-gene form of bipolar illness, such families must be rare and cannot explain the majority of familial occurrence of the disorder. These results are consistent with the idea of manic-depressive illness, even in its more homogeneous bipolar form, as a genetically complex disorder (see the discussion below of the linkage method).

Twin Studies

Familial aggregation of disease suggests, but does not prove, a genetic contribution to disease. Environmental factors, such as exposure to toxins or emotionally traumatic family experiences, could in theory also lead to familial aggregation. Twin studies have been the approach used most widely to attempt to disentangle these contributions. The logic of twin studies is this. Identical or *monozygotic* (MZ) twins are 100 percent genetically the same, whereas fraternal or *dizygotic* (DZ) twins share just 50 percent of their genes; yet the two twin types are assumed to be no different in the degree to which they share environments.[4] Therefore, any increased similarity in manifestation of manic-depressive illness detected in MZ twins compared with that in DZ twins should be due to the greater genetic similarity of the former. The main measure in these studies is the *concordance rate* for illness; that is, starting with an ill twin as the proband, what is the rate of illness in the co-twin?

Early studies tested for manic-depressive illness (see Table 13–3). Six such studies found concordance rates of 77 percent for MZ twins and 23 percent for DZ twins, with a heritability of .71 (where 1.00 would be complete heritability and 0 would be none). More recent studies have used the bipolar and major depressive disorder phenotypes.[5] Three studies assessed bipolar disorder; they found a 63 percent concordance rate for MZ twins and a 13 percent rate for DZ twins, with a heritability of .78. Seven studies assessed major depressive disorder; they found concordance rates of 34 percent in MZ twins and 26 percent in DZ twins, with a heritability of .34, although this estimate would be higher if the studies had focused on those patients with more highly recurrent forms of the disorder (see below).

Among the most meticulously conducted twin studies of manic-depressive illness is that of Bertelsen and colleagues (1977), which drew on the Danish Central Psychiatric Register and the Danish Twin Register to identify 126 probands with the disorder from among 110 twin pairs. The work was done in the 1960s and 1970s using a database of Danes born during 1870–1920. A single psychiatrist conducted an unstructured interview of 133 of the 138 living twins and made diagnoses in conjunction with a second psychiatrist using the interview results and information available through the registers. Zygosity was determined in about half of the twins using serological examination of 16 to 25 different red blood cell types, tissue types, serum protein variants, and enzymes. In the other half of the twins, zygosity was assessed anthropometrically from information gathered through questions about pronounced similarity of general appearance and mistaken identity by others. For three twin pairs, zygosity could not be determined, and these pairs were dropped from the analysis.

Bertelsen and colleagues presented their findings in two ways. In the first, all identified ill twins are counted as probands. This method, called the *proband-wise concordance*, is considered the most epidemiologically correct, though it has the intuitive flaw of counting some pairs twice, as both affected members of a twin pair may occasionally be assessed independently as probands. The other method, called the *pair-wise concordance*, counts all twin pairs only once and is more conservative as it yields lower estimates of heritability. The following results are the proband-wise concordance rates. They are presented by proband diagnosis, with *concordance* defined as the likelihood of the co-twin having either major depression or bipolar disorder. Results are expressed as percentages; perfect concordance would be 100 percent, while no concordance would be 0 percent. The rates of concordance for BP-I are MZ=80, DZ=13; for BP-II, MZ=78, DZ=31; and for major depression, MZ=54, DZ=24. Heritability is calculated most simply as (concordance rate in MZ twins—concordance rate in DZ twins) divided by (100—concordance rate in DZ twins). Using this metric, the heritability for each disorder is as follows: BP-I=.77, BP-II=.68, and major depression=.39. Notably, of 32 concordant MZ pairs, 7 included one subject with bipolar disorder and one with major depression (Bertelsen et al., 1977).

Many observers have cited the lack of complete concordance between MZ twins as evidence that environmental factors must play a role in the etiology of bipolar disorder. More recently, others have suggested that this lack of complete concordance could be due to epigenetic factors—that is, factors that affect the control of gene expression—and that these factors may or may not be influenced by the environment (Petronis, 2001). In support of this hypothesis, there is evidence that MZ twins, despite having identical DNA sequence for all their genes, may differ in the way their genes are expressed (Weksberg et al., 2002).

TABLE 13–3. **Twin Studies of Manic-Depressive Illness and Bipolar Disorder**

Proband/Study	Sample Size (Pairs)	Concordance (%) MZ	Concordance (%) DZ	Heritability[a]
Manic-Depressive Illness				
Luxenburger, 1928, 1930	17	80	0	.80
Rosanoff et al., 1935	90	70	16	.64
Slater and Shields, 1953	39	73	32	.60
Kallman, 1953, 1954	82	100	26	1.00
Da Fonseca, 1959	60	71	38	.53
Kringlen, 1967	26	50	0	.50
Weighted mean	*314*	*77*	*23*	*.71*
Bipolar Disorder				
Bertelsen et al., 1977	71	79	19	.74
Torgersen, 1986	10	75	0	.75
Weighted mean	*81*	*79*	*17*	*.74*
Bipolar-I Disorder				
Bertelsen et al., 1977	49	80	13	.77
Cardno et al., 1999	49	36	7	.84
Weighted mean	*98*	*59*	*10*	*.80*
Bipolar-II Disorder				
Bertelsen et al., 1977	22	78	31	.68
Major Depression				
Bertelsen et al., 1977	44	54	24	.39
Torgersen, 1986	92	27	12	.54
Andrews et al., 1990	82	7	9	0
McGuffin et al., 1996	177	46	20	.48
Lyons et al., 1998	3,372	23	14	.36
Bierut et al., 1999	2,662	33	26	.30

(continued)

TABLE 13–3. **Twin Studies of Manic-Depressive Illness and Bipolar Disorder** *(continued)*

Proband/Study	Sample Size (Pairs)	Findings Concordance (%) MZ	DZ	Heritability[a]
Kendler et al., 2000	3,790	44	39	.34
Weighted mean	*10,219*	*34*	*26*	*.34*

Note: DZ = dizygotic; MZ = monozygotic. For studies since 1960, only those in which a majority of subjects were directly interviewed are included. DZ, dizygotic; MZ, monozygotic.

[a]Where authors calculate heritability, these figures are provided. If heritability is not provided in a report, Holzinger's heritability (MZ concordance – DZ concordance/100 – DZ concordance) has been calculated.

Patterns of concordance can be converted to a heritability value—often thought of as the percentage of the liability to illness that is genetic—in several ways. Current twin studies employ a liability threshold model (Falconer, 1965), which simultaneously tests the heritability of and environmental contribution to illness. When individuals cross the liability threshold, they develop illness. The model requires the specification of a population prevalence of illness to indicate how many people in the population lie on the ill side of the threshold. Moreover, heritability estimates will vary with the prevalence figures used, an issue of particular importance for major depression, for which population estimates have varied dramatically. For example, one depression study reported that heritability was 48 percent when one estimate was used and 75 percent when another was used (McGuffin et al., 1996).[6]

Adoption Studies

A second paradigm for separating genetic from environmental effects is the adoption study. The conceptual basis for this approach is that in adoptees, the genetic inheritance occurs through one set of parents, while the cultural and environmental experience occurs through a different set. The two sets of factors and their potential association with illness can therefore be disentangled.

There are several possible ways to conduct an adoption study. One that has been used for manic-depressive illness is the adoptees' relatives method. In this method, ill and control adoptees are identified as probands, and rates of illness are then compared in the biological and adoptive relatives of each group. If genetics plays a role, the biological relatives of ill adoptees will have elevated rates of illness compared with those in the other three relative groups.

Only four adoption studies have addressed manic-depressive illness (see Table 13–4). The most methodologi-

cally rigorous such study is that of Mendlewicz and Rainer (1977), who reported on a cohort of patients identified in Belgium. This study employed four proband groups with a total of 102 probands: bipolar adoptees, bipolar non-adoptees, control adoptees, and individuals who had contracted polio in their youth. The latter group was included to control for the effect on parents of bringing up a disabled child. Clinicians who were blind to the status of the proband interviewed biological and adoptive parents of adoptees and parents of nonadoptees. A total of 299 parents were included in the study. Parents were instructed at the beginning of the interview not to speak about their children unless specifically asked. A semistructured interview was used, as well as standardized diagnostic criteria. The principal finding was that the biological parents of bipolar adoptees had a 31 percent rate of affective disorder—significantly higher than the 12 percent rate in the adoptive parents of these adoptees, the 2 percent rate in the biological parents of the control adoptees, and the 10 percent rate in the parents of the polio probands. Conversely, the 31 percent rate of affective disorder in the parents of the bipolar adoptees was quite similar to the 26 percent rate in parents of bipolar nonadoptees.

Inclusion of the control groups in the Mendlewicz and Rainer study was important, as it helped address some of the criticisms of this method. Adoptive parents are often screened for stability and therefore might be expected to have a lower-than-average rate of affective disorder. The rates in these adoptive parents were not lower than those in the polio proband parents. Conversely, biological parents of adoptees may be more likely to be unstable, but the biological rates of affective disorder in parents of normal adoptees were not higher than those in the polio proband parents. The results strongly support a genetic basis for the bipolar form of manic-depressive illness.

TABLE 13–4. **Adoption Studies**

Proband/Study	Sample	Rate of Manic-Depressive Illness		
		Biological III Proband Group	Biological Control Group	Adoptive Relatives
Manic-Depressive Illness				
Cadoret et al., 1985	443 adoptees	22.2	10.1	—
Wender et al., 1986	1,080 relatives	5.2	2.3	2.8
Bipolar-I				
Mendlewicz and Rainer, 1977	299 parents	31.6	2.3	12.2
Unipolar Depression				
von Knorring et al., 1983	—parents	5.1	5.4	2.7

Note: —=not studied or reported.

Adoption studies are not easy to conduct because they require access to large databases, and there are barriers of confidentiality involved whose breach can be a highly sensitive matter. Two such studies that have been done have used national registries, those of Sweden and Denmark. In these studies, direct interviews were not performed. In these two studies, moreover, probands had diagnoses including "affect reaction" and "neurotic depressive reaction," which are not readily reconcilable with current diagnostic nomenclature. The results of one of these studies supported genetic transmission of depression (Wender et al., 1986), while those of the other did not (von Knorring et al., 1983). Another adoption study used relatives as probands and measured rates of depression in the adoptees of those relatives who were affectively ill compared with those who were not. The results supported genetic transmission (Cadoret et al., 1985). Thus, of the four adoption studies of manic-depressive illness, three provide support for a genetic vulnerability, and one does not.

ADVANCES IN UNDERSTANDING THE HUMAN GENOME

In the next section, on the linkage method, the discussion shifts from the question of whether there is a genetic component to susceptibility to manic-depressive illness to the question of where the disease genes are located in the human genome. Before examining the progress made in answering that question, however, we must review the remarkable advances that have occurred in our understanding of the nature of those transmissible "factors," first identified by Mendel, that we now call "genes." We begin by tackling some basic genetic and biological concepts. Two analogies may be helpful.

First, think of the human genome as being like the *Oxford English Dictionary*. The *genome* refers to the full complement of human DNA. Just as the *Oxford English Dictionary* is a compendium of all the words that can create meaning in the English language, the genome is a collection of all the genes that can create things in the human body. The *Oxford English Dictionary* has 23 volumes, and the human genome has 23 chromosomes. Each volume contains many word entries, and each *chromosome*—a long stretch of DNA—contains many genes. Each of the 405,000 words is spelled using the 26-letter English alphabet, and each of the 20,000 genes is spelled using the four-nucleotide genetic alphabet. The four nucleotides (or *bases*) are *A* for adenine, *T* for thymine, *G* for guanine, and *C* for cytosine; each is a molecule that conveys information much as a letter does. The human genome contains 3 billion of these nucleotide letters. Just as there can be normal variant spellings of a word—e.g., "organization" versus "organisation" (the British spelling)—there can be variant nucleotide sequences for a gene that make no difference for the gene. And just as there can be typographical errors that change word meanings—"well" versus "hell" or "hype" versus "hope"—there can be mistakes in the gene sequence that change gene function. Functionally significant variations are the ones that concern us when we consider vulnerability to manic-depressive illness.

What does gene function have to do with such vulnerability? Consider a second analogy. Genes are like blueprints that direct the workings of cells, including brain cells. Genes made of DNA code for messengers made of a molecule called *ribonucleic acid* (RNA). The messenger RNA directs the production of specific proteins. Proteins are the molecules that do the work in brain cells. They act as building blocks, signal receptors, and chemical switches. So if the blueprint for a gene is misdrawn, aberrant proteins will result, and brain cells may misfire or malfunction. Francis Crick, codiscoverer of the structure of DNA, called this conception—DNA makes RNA, and RNA makes proteins—the central dogma of molecular biology.

The investigation of differences in *DNA sequence* among individuals became possible in the late 1970s to early 1980s with the discovery of *restriction fragment length polymorphisms* (RFLPs). These are single nucleotide variations among individuals, or polymorphisms, in the DNA sequence that occur at greater than 1 percent frequency and result in differential susceptibility to being cleaved by bacterial enzymes called *restriction enzymes*. These enzymes can thus be used as tools for establishing the sequence at points in the DNA where variability exists.

In the late 1980s to early 1990s, *microsatellite DNA markers* were discovered and exploited to assess DNA variation among individuals. These markers generally are not located within the coding regions of genes, called *exons*. These regions code for the production of messenger RNA, with every three nucleotides forming a *codon*, which ultimately directs production of a particular *amino acid*, a building block for a specified protein. Exons are like islands in a vast sea; only about 3 percent of DNA takes this form. The noncoding regions of DNA can lie within genes; between the exons, in which case they are called *introns* (an intron thus interrupts the protein-coding sequence of a gene, being transcribed into RNA but cut out of the message before being translated into protein); or between genes, in which case they are called *intergenic* regions. The microsatellite markers are generally located in these noncoding regions. They comprise stretches of DNA with two-, three-, or four-nucleotide repeat sequences, such as CACACACA or GATAGATAGATA, where the repeat occurs a variable number of times. For example, the CA repeat at a given location in the DNA might occur 7 consecutive times, 18 consecutive times, or somewhere in between. This variability allows two copies of a chromosome to be distinguished from each other. This DNA variability in microsatellite markers is extremely useful in linkage studies.

Beginning in the late 1990s, extensive sequencing of the human genome began to reveal very large numbers of single nucleotide differences, or polymorphisms—called *single nucleotide polymorphisms* (SNPs)—across the genome (see Fig. 13–2). These polymorphisms have been found to exist at about 1 of every 200 nucleotides. This finding suggests that people are about 99.5 percent the same in terms of DNA sequence, and that it is in the 0.5 percent difference that the factors influencing vulnerability to bipolar disorder lie. About 10 million SNPs have been identified in the public SNP database (dbSNP); it is expected that 15 million SNPs should exist, of which about 6 million should be common. Studies of bipolar disorder that take advantage of this understanding of SNPs began to appear in 2002 (Sklar et al., 2002).

The explosion of sequence information has largely been a product of the Human Genome Project, a U.S. government–funded initiative begun in 1987. The project's mandate was initially to provide a dense map of the human genome, and eventually to provide the full sequence. As of this writing, the sequence is considered more than 99 percent complete. To return to the *Oxford English Dictionary* analogy, the word entries have been largely spelled out. Much work remains to be done, however, particularly in clarifying the functions of genes, a task analogous to defining the meanings for each word entry in the dictionary.

Advances in computer science have been of great help in this enterprise, generating the new field of bioinformatics. These advances have enabled the creation of large and complex Web-based databases cataloguing the genes on each chromosome, the sequence of the genes, their variations, their functions, and more.[7] On each of these sites, information can be obtained in a matter of minutes or hours that would have taken scientists months or years to obtain just a decade ago.

THE LINKAGE METHOD

The Method

The goal of a linkage study is to identify a chromosomal region that harbors a susceptibility gene (see Fig. 13–1). There are three stages to this type of study: (1) clinical assessment of subjects to determine whether they have manic-depressive illness (either the bipolar or recurrent unipolar subtype) (phenotype); (2) testing of DNA from the subjects (from their white blood cells) to determine their genetic profile at a series of markers; and (3) use of statistical techniques to test whether bipolar or recurrent unipolar disorder and DNA markers travel independently or together (*cosegregation*). If they cosegregate, we say that the DNA marker is located close to the disease gene on the same chromosome. Because the locations of the DNA markers on chromosomes are established, the observation of cosegregation or linkage tells us roughly where a disease gene should lie. The usefulness of linkage hinges on the recombination

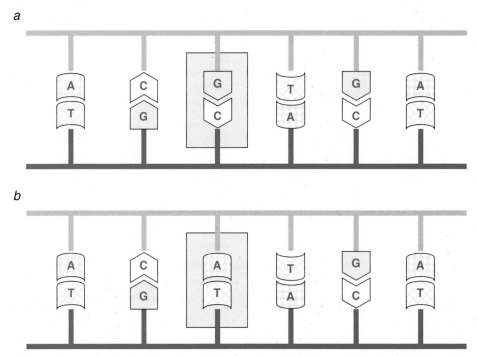

Figure 13–2. Single nucleotide polymorphisms (SNPs): the most common form of genetic variation. SNPs occur about once every 200 nucleotides. They typically have two allelic variants consisting of one of two nucleotides. *a* and *b* here represent an individual's two copies of a segment of chromosome 11 that is part of the coding sequence for the BDNF gene. Note that each chromosome has two strands, called either *forward* and *reverse* or *sense* and *antisense*. The sequence of one strand determines the sequence of the other because A and T are always paired, as are G and C. Sequence *a* contains a G allele on the forward strand, shown as the top strand, which is the one that codes for the gene. Sequence *b* contains an A allele on the top strand in the same position, so that this individual is a heterozygote for this SNP. The third, fourth, and fifth bases in the sequence form a codon, which codes for an amino acid. GTG codes for valine, while ATG codes for methionine. Some evidence suggests the G allele confers risk for bipolar disorder, while the A allele is protective.

between pairs of similar, or *homologous*, chromosomes during meiosis, which increases as a function of the distance between marker and gene (see Fig. 13–3). The rate of recombination is measured in centimorgans (cM), with each cM corresponding to a 1 percent likelihood of recombination and to roughly 1 million base pairs of DNA (1 Mb).

Thomas Hunt Morgan first employed the linkage method in the development of gene maps of the fruit fly in the early twentieth century. The method was used to link presumed genes for one fly trait to presumed genes for another. The first linkage study of manic-depressive illness was reported in 1968, before DNA markers were available. ABO blood types were used as markers, so that the presumed genes for the blood types were tested for linkage to the illness (Tanna and Winokur, 1968).

The linkage method has since been widely applied in mapping of human disease genes, especially since the 1980s, after Botstein and colleagues (1980) suggested that RFLPs (the DNA markers discussed in the preceding section) distributed across the genome could be used to detect linkage to disease genes. The first published genetic studies of the bipolar form of manic-depressive illness to use DNA markers, all in the same issue of *Nature* in 1987, were conducted by three groups that focused on chromosome 11 (Detera-Wadleigh et al., 1987; Egeland et al., 1987; Hodgkinson et al., 1987b). The first study of bipolar illness to employ microsatellite markers was conducted by the Gershon group at NIMH in 1990 (Berrettini et al., 1990). These researchers used markers on the X-chromosome in an attempt to verify prior reports of linkage in the region.[8]

The more variable or *polymorphic* a marker is—the larger the number of alleles—the more genetically informative it becomes for linkage studies. The variations among individuals can easily be detected using laboratory methods that reveal which of two variants, or *alleles*, an individual has at a given point, or *locus*, along the chromosome. The characterization of the two alleles is referred to as the *genotype* for that DNA marker. A standard genomewide scan today would use 400 microsatellite DNA markers at an average spacing of 10 cM to genotype individuals at locations across all 23 chromosomes. Newer genomewide scans employing 5,800 SNP DNA markers at an average spacing of .64 cM are just becoming available.

A positive result in a linkage study implicates a chromosomal region that is typically quite broad—as much as 30 cM from a linkage peak—which means as much as 60 cM in total (Roberts et al., 1999). A linkage region is indicated by the identity of the chromosomal arm (short [p] or long [q]) and the segment of that arm (numerical designation) on which the linkage peak falls (see Fig. 13–4).

LOD Score Approach

One statistical method used to test for linkage of markers to illness phenotype is the logarithm of the odds of linkage (LOD) score approach, which is mode of inheritance–based; that is, it requires specifying whether transmission is dominant, recessive, or X-linked. This approach has been highly successful in isolating genes for Mendelian diseases. The *odds* here refer to the ratio between the likelihood that the inheritance pattern observed in a pedigree or set of pedigrees would result from a particular amount of linkage between the genetic marker and the phenotype being investigated and the likelihood that the observed data would

result if there were no linkage. When a single locus and a single illness phenotype are tested, an LOD score of 3.0 is sufficient to claim linkage because this score indicates a 5 percent likelihood that a linkage finding is due to chance. However, genome scans employ tests of multiple markers and test further for linkage using multiple definitions of the disease phenotype. To guard against the possibility of *type I error*, or false positive linkage claims, Lander and Kruglyak (1995) calculated new statistical thresholds. These often-cited criteria raised the bar for declaring an initial linkage finding significant, requiring an LOD threshold of 3.3 (the threshold for "suggestive" linkage is 1.9). A more recent approach uses simulation to determine the statistical significance of a finding. Computer programs can employ the set of families and DNA markers used in a given study to calculate the likelihood of a given LOD score's arising by chance in thousands of simulated genome scans. An empirical *p* value for a linkage finding is derived by comparing actual results with these simulated results.

The virtue of such a mode of inheritance–based method is that with a correct model, the test is very powerful and gives both an LOD score and an estimate of the genetic distance between the marker and the disease gene or locus.

Figure 13–3. Recombination: the basis for linkage studies. Genetic linkage between a disease and markers is determined for each chromosome by identifying how frequently a DNA marker and a presumed bipolar gene are passed together from parent to child. Circles are females, and squares are males. The solid shapes represent those affected with bipolar illness, and the open shapes are unaffected individuals. In *a*, there is a DNA marker, M, that is on the same chromosome as the disease gene, D, but is physically far from it. For the top-left individual, the father, the thick line represents copy 1 of chromosome 13, and the thin line represents copy 2 of chromosome 13. During meiosis, as sperm cells are being formed, these two copies of chromosome 13 pair, and parts of each are exchanged with the other. This process, which occurs for every chromosome in egg as well as in sperm, is called *recombination*. Because of recombination, the disease gene and the marker are not necessarily inherited together; the two are thus not linked. In *b*, the marker under consideration is physically close to the disease-causing gene, so that recombination does not separate them. All three children who inherit the bipolar gene also inherit the nearby marker. If the pattern in *b* were seen in many families, it would suggest linkage. Note that in linkage, D is not actually observed; D is presumed to be present when the subject is affected with bipolar illness.

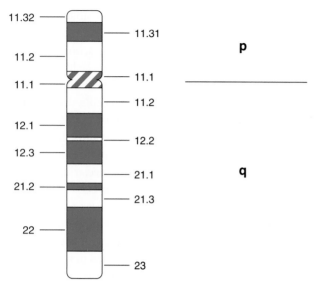

Figure 13–4. Schematic of a human chromosome (chromosome 18) depicting nomenclature based on cytogenetic banding patterns. Each human chromosome has a short arm (*p* for *petit*) and long arm (*q* for *queue*), separated by a *centromere*. The ends of the chromosome are called *telomeres*. Each chromosome arm is divided into regions, or *cytogenetic bands*, that can be seen using a microscope and special stains. The cytogenetic bands are labeled p1, p2, p3, q1, q2, q3, etc., counting from the centromere out toward the telomeres. At higher resolutions, sub-bands can be seen within the bands. The sub-bands are also numbered from the centromere out toward the telomere. (*Source:* National Center for Biotechnology Information Web site: http://www.ncbi.nlm.nih.gov/Class/MLACourse/Original8Hour/Genetics/chrombanding.html)

However, the LOD score approach requires a number of assumptions about the mode of transmission, as well as other factors.[9]

Affected Sibling Pair Method

So-called model-free or *nonparametric* approaches, such as the affected sibling pair method, require few assumptions and are thus more robust than a mode of inheritance–based method. The affected sibling pair method measures sharing of alleles at various DNA markers. Siblings are expected to share 50 percent of their alleles at any locus; significantly increased allele sharing among siblings with illness at a given marker constitutes evidence for linkage. Those without illness (unaffected) are not included in the analysis to avoid the uncertainty created by the possibility that they will become ill later. Such model-free methods can also be applied to affected relatives. The Lander and Kruglyak (1995) threshold for significance using model-free methods is a *p* value of 2.2×10^{-5}, corresponding to a nonparametric LOD score of 3.6 (the threshold for "suggestive" linkage is 7.4×10^{-4} or a nonparametric LOD score of 2.2). The first bipolar study published using

the affected sibling pair method was reported in 1994 (de Bruyn et al., 1994).

A drawback of the affected sibling pair method is that it is not as powerful for localizing disease genes as mode of inheritance–based methods. To minimize the likelihood of failing to detect linkage in a region where a susceptibility gene of modest effect (relative risk of 2.0) exists, a large sample of sibling pairs is required. In fact, if a nonparametric LOD score of greater than 3.0 is the criterion for detection, a sample size of about 400 affected sibling pairs is required to achieve adequate power (Hauser et al., 1996). The first study to achieve a sample size of this magnitude was published in 2003; the NIMH Bipolar Disorder Collaborative completed its Wave 3 study with 446 affected sibling pairs (see the discussion below).

Findings

There have been 21 genomewide linkage scans for bipolar illness published to date, and these studies have identified a number of regions potentially harboring genes for susceptibility to the disorder (see Fig. 13–5). Note that these findings were sometimes obtained using the bipolar subtype of manic-depressive illness, but in other instances the broad definition incorporating recurrent major depression was used. At least five bipolar linkage findings (and perhaps more, depending on the interpretation of statistical thresholds) have reached genomewide statistical significance in multifamily samples: 6q22 (Middleton et al., 2004), 8q24 (Cichon et al., 2001), 15q14 (Turecki et al., 2001), 21q22 (Liu et al., 2001b), and 22q12 (Kelsoe et al., 2001). Promising though they are, these findings have not been replicated consistently across studies. Other regions that have been repeatedly implicated in bipolar disorder include 1q41, 4p16, 4q32–35, 12q23–24, 13q31–33, 16p12–13, 18p11, 18q12–23, and Xq24–28.

Meta-analyses

Three meta-analyses of linkage studies have been performed, with results differing because of differences in the studies included and the techniques employed. A 2002 meta-analysis of 11 genome scans for bipolar illness used the multiscan probability technique, which combines *p* values across scans in regions with clusters of positive scores. This analysis revealed that two regions reached genomewide significance across the studies: 13q32 ($p < 6 \times 10^{-6}$) and 22q12–13 ($p < 1 \times 10^{-5}$) (Badner and Gershon, 2002). Despite this suggestion of a convergence of findings in these two regions, however, a second meta-analysis was less encouraging. This latter analysis used data from 18 genome scans, supplemented by unpublished data when the published data were incomplete (see Table 13–5). The authors used a rank-based method to ensure that the meta-analysis would not be biased by statistical methodology. They found

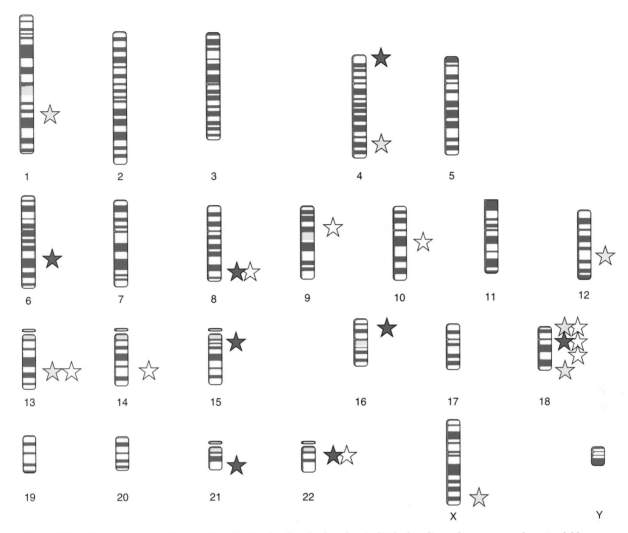

Figure 13–5. Chromosomal regions implicated in bipolar disorder, based on individual studies and two meta-analyses. Dark blue stars represent regions where a genomewide significant linkage has been found. Light blue stars are regions with more than one suggestive linkage finding. White stars are regions with the strongest evidence for linkage in either of two meta-analyses of genomewide bipolar disorder linkage scans.

that no region reached genomewide significance across the combined studies. The strongest regions were 9p21–22, 10q11–22, 14q24–32, 18p–18q21, and to a lesser extent 8q24 (Segurado et al., 2003). The most recent meta-analysis differed from the two earlier ones in using original genotype data rather than published results. The authors combined data on 1,067 families from 11 studies and found genomewide significant results for chromosomal regions 6q and 8q (Mc-Queen et al., 2005).

These data add to the evidence from mode of transmission studies that no single gene accounts for the susceptibility to bipolar disorder in a majority of affected families. Thus, multiple susceptibility genes may contribute to the risk. Indeed, it is likely that multiple genes contribute cumulatively to susceptibility in each family, a notion referred to as *epistasis* (see the discussion below).

Promising Linkage Regions

Chromosome 4

Two regions of chromosome 4 have been implicated in bipolar illness. On 4p16, Blackwood and colleagues (1996) initially reported significant linkage in a single large Scottish family, with an LOD score of 4.8. Supporting data have come from several other studies (see Evans et al., 2001, for references). Of interest, one study in four large Amish families reported evidence for a protective locus in this same chromosomal region. Using "never mentally ill" family members as the "affected" phenotype, an LOD score of 4.05 was obtained (Ginns et al., 1998).

On the opposite end of the chromosome, 4q35, there is also some evidence for a susceptibility gene for bipolar disorder. Suggestive evidence of linkage—an LOD score of

TABLE 13–5. **Genome Scans for Bipolar Disorder with More Than 20 Affected Subjects**

Study	Center	Sample Size (Affected)	Strongest Findings
Coon et al., 1993	Utah	51	5q
McInnes et al., 1996	Costa Rica	24	11p13–14, 18p11.3, 18q22–23
NIMH1: Detera-Wadleigh et al., 1997; Edenberg et al., 1997; Stine et al., 1997; Willour et al., 2003	National Institute of Mental Health (NIMH) Collaborative	424	10p12, 16p12–13
Detera-Wadleigh et al., 1999	NIMH–Intramural Research Program	160	13q32, 18p11
Morissette et al., 1999a	Quebec	56	12q24
Friddle et al., 2000; McInnis et al., 2003	Johns Hopkins Psychiatry/Stanford	301	8q24, 18q21–22
Cichon et al., 2001	Bonn	128	8q24
Kelsoe et al., 2001	University of California, San Diego	76	22q11–12
Turecki et al., 2001	Toronto	106	15q14
Badenhop et al., 2002	Sydney	69	3q25–26
Bennett et al., 2002	UK/Irish	367	2q37.3, 18p11
NIMH2: Dick et al., 2002; Willour et al., 2003; Zandi et al., 2003	NIMH Collaborative	228	4q35, 11p15.5, 16p12–13, Xp11.3
Liu et al., 2003	Columbia	297	2p13–16
NIMH3: Dick et al., 2003; Schulze et al., 2004	NIMH Collaborative	741	6q16–22, 17q25
Curtis et al., 2003	University College–London	39	12q23–24
Ekholm et al., 2003	Finland	132	4q32, 16p12
Maziade et al., 2005	Montreal	72	15q11.1, 16p12.3, 18q12–21
Macgregor et al., 2004	Edinburgh	41	1q42
Middleton et al., 2004	State University of New York, Syracuse	75	6q22
Fallin et al., 2004	Johns Hopkins Epidemiology	97	1q23.3, 3p23, 11q12, 18q22.2
Venken et al., 2005	Antwerp	46	6q23–24, 9q31–33

3.19—was first obtained for this region in a single very large Australian pedigree (Adams et al., 1998). Subsequently, McInnis and colleagues (2003) found suggestive evidence of linkage in this region in 65 Johns Hopkins pedigrees, and Willour and colleagues (2003) found a nonparametric LOD score of 2.49 in the same region in 56 NIMH Wave 2 families.

Chromosome 6q16–22

This region was first implicated in bipolar disorder in 2003, when the results of the largest bipolar genome scan to date were analyzed (Dick et al., 2003). The sample, the third to come out of the NIMH Bipolar Disorder Collaborative (Wave 3), contained 245 families and 741 affected subjects. This region was the strongest in the genome for this scan, with a peak LOD score of 3.05 (Schulze et al., 2004). Similarly, a study of 25 Portuguese bipolar families found the strongest signal in the genome at 6q22, with a maximum nonparametric linkage (NPL) score of 4.2 (Middleton et al., 2004). As noted, this region reached genomewide significance in the McQueen and colleagues (2005) meta-analysis.

Chromosome 8q24

Cichon and colleagues (2001) implicated this region at the significant level in a study of 75 German, Israeli, and Italian families (the Bonn sample). They found a parametric

LOD score of 3.62 using a dominant model of inheritance and a narrow phenotype definition that included only BP-I as affected. The region had been implicated earlier by Friddle and colleagues (2000), who used the first 50 families of the Johns Hopkins sample. In an expanded Hopkins sample of 65 families, McInnis and colleagues (2003) found an NPL score of 3.13. When further markers were genotyped in this region in the 65 families, a parametric LOD score of 3.32, which is genomewide significant, was obtained (Avramopoulos et al., 2004). As noted, this region reached genomewide significance in the McQueen and colleagues (2005) meta-analysis.

Chromosome 12q24

This region became interesting after investigators reported the cosegregation of bipolar illness with Darier disease, a rare dominantly inherited skin disorder located on chromosome 12q24 in one family (Craddock et al., 1994). In a genome scan of a Quebec region genetic isolate, Morissette and colleagues (1999b) reported suggestive linkage in the region, while Ewald and colleagues (1998) found an LOD of 3.37 in two Danish families using a DNA marker located nearby. Of interest, the d-amino acid oxidase (*DAO*) gene, recently implicated in schizophrenia (Chumakov et al., 2002), is in this region, about 1.4 Mb from the Darier disease gene.

Chromosome 13q31–33

The 22-family genome scan of Detera-Wadleigh and colleagues (1999) identified 13q32 with a nonparametric LOD of 3.5, just short of genomewide significance. Subsequent genotyping narrowed the interval, but did not improve the LOD score (Liu et al., 2001a). The 13q31–33 region has also been implicated at the suggestive level by Kelsoe and colleagues (2001), and by Potash and colleagues (2003b) in a subset of Johns Hopkins bipolar families characterized by multiple members with psychotic features (see the discussion below of alternative phenotypic definition). Several groups have detected association with a pair of overlapping genes in this region, *G72* and *G30* (see the later section on the association method). As noted, this region reached genomewide significance in the Badner and Gershon (2002) meta-analysis.

Chromosome 16p12–13

Six independent studies have implicated this region. Ewald and colleagues (1995a) reported an LOD of 2.5 on 16p13, and McInnes and colleagues (1996) reported an LOD of 1.46 on 16p13. The NIMH Collaborative found modest evidence of linkage to 16p12–13 in its Wave 1 sample (Edenberg et al., 1997) and stronger evidence for the same region in its Wave 2 sample (Dick et al., 2002).

Maziade and colleagues (2004) and Ekholm and colleagues (2003) each found evidence of linkage to 16p12 in their genome scans. The findings from these six studies are spread over 50 cM.

Chromosome 18

Chromosome 18 may harbor several regions of interest. Evidence of possible linkage was first reported in the pericentromeric region, an area straddling the short and long arms of the chromosome (Berrettini et al., 1994). This linkage was later narrowed to 18p11.2, with an LOD score of 2.32 being obtained (Detera-Wadleigh et al., 1999). Evidence for pericentromeric linkage was also reported in the Johns Hopkins sample, in which suggestive linkage was detected in the 18q21 region as well (Stine et al., 1995). These results are notable for a parent-of-origin effect, the evidence for linkage being derived primarily from families with paternal inheritance of bipolar illness and from paternally transmitted DNA marker alleles. The Johns Hopkins group followed up on its original report with evidence from an entirely new set of 30 families that again supported linkage on 18q (McMahon et al., 1997). A combined analysis of the 58 Johns Hopkins families showed the strongest evidence for linkage on 18q21–22, as did an analysis of a slightly expanded sample of 65 families (McInnis et al., 2003).

Other groups have also found evidence for linkage on chromosome 18, though in varying regions, including 18p11.3 (McInnes et al., 1996), 18q12 (Ewald et al., 1997; Maziade et al., 2001), 18q22 (de Bruyn et al., 1996), and 18q23 (Coon et al., 1996; Freimer et al., 1996; Nothen et al., 1999). The meta-analysis by Segurado and colleagues (2003) divided chromosome 18 into four parts for purposes of the study. Three of the four parts were significantly linked to bipolar disorder, at least nominally, when the results from 18 genome scans were pooled.

Chromosome 21q22

Investigators initially reported linkage on chromosome 21q22 based on a single large multigenerational pedigree with an LOD score of 3.41 (Straub et al., 1994). The same group subsequently documented an analysis of this chromosomal region involving 56 families, which yielded an LOD score of 3.48 (Liu et al., 2001b). In two different datasets, Detera-Wadleigh and colleagues (1996, 1997) found evidence for linkage on 21q. Smith and colleagues (1997) obtained an LOD score of 1.29 in this region. However, when they used a model that simultaneously incorporated the effects of two loci—the 21q locus and the tyrosine hydroxylase locus on 11p15—the LOD score increased to 3.87, suggesting that genes in these two regions may interact to cause disease.

Chromosome 22q11–13

In a genome scan of 20 families, Kelsoe and colleagues (2001) found a parametric LOD score of 3.84 at 22q12, which was genomewide significant. In this same study, the authors reported results from the NIMH Wave 2 sample, which yielded LOD scores of 1.58 at 22q12 and 2.72 at a marker on the border between 22q11 and 22q12. Other suggestive findings in this region include that of Detera-Wadleigh and colleagues (1999), who reported a nonparametric LOD score of 2.1, and that of Potash and colleagues (2003b), who studied a subset of Johns Hopkins bipolar families characterized by multiple members with psychotic features and found an NPL score of 3.06 in the 22q12 region (see the discussion below of alternative phenotypic definition). As noted, this region reached genomewide significance in the Badner and Gershon (2002) meta-analysis.

X-Chromosome

Rosanoff and colleagues (1935) first proposed the idea that a gene on the X-chromosome might be implicated in manic-depressive illness. A number of subsequent studies of the bipolar subgroup found evidence for linkage in the Xq28 region using markers for color blindness and G6PD deficiency, but this evidence has not proven replicable, even within the same families.[10] However, there have also been reports of linkage in the q24–27 region, starting with the Factor IX locus (Mendlewicz et al., 1987). Another study found an LOD score of 3.9 at the same locus in one pedigree (Lucotte et al., 1992). And a Finnish group reported an LOD score of 3.54 at a DNA marker in the Xq24–27 region, also based on one pedigree (Pekkarinen et al., 1995). Thus, the existence of a bipolar susceptibility gene on Xq24–27 remains a possibility.

Complex Disorders

The linkage method has yielded spectacular successes in medicine, with detection of linkage being followed by the discovery of a disease gene for Huntington's disease, cystic fibrosis, and Duchenne muscular dystrophy, among others. These illnesses, which are all uncommon, are called *simple mendelian disorders* because they follow the relatively simple rules laid out by Mendel. Like many illnesses currently under study, however, including asthma, hypertension, and diabetes mellitus, manic-depressive illness is common and does not follow these mendelian rules. For these illnesses, referred to as *complex genetic disorders*, there is not a one-to-one correspondence between gene and disease; rather, these disorders may result from the actions of any one of several genes. A variant of one gene may cause the illness in one family, while a variant of a different gene may cause it in another family (*genetic heterogeneity*). Many people may carry the susceptibility gene, but not manifest the illness (*incomplete penetrance,* penetrance being defined as the proportion of individuals of a particular genotype that express its phenotypic effect in a given environment). Many others may have the illness, but not carry the susceptibility gene (*phenocopy*).[11] Additionally, as mentioned earlier, two or more genes may interact to cause disease (*epistasis*).[12] These types of inheritance complexities have contributed to the difficulty of establishing linkage for bipolar disorder.

For common diseases such as bipolar illness, geneticists have hypothesized that common gene variants likely play a role, rather than rare variants (Reich and Lander, 2001). The common disease–common variant hypothesis has implications for how gene hunting will proceed in the future, including the kinds of samples collected and the kinds of DNA markers studied.

ALTERNATIVE PHENOTYPIC DEFINITION[13]

Given that manic-depressive illness is likely to be *oligogenic*—a term denoting a phenotypic trait produced by two or more genes working together, each with modest but detectable effect—the question arises of whether it is possible to identify clinical and biological features of the illness that might define more genetically homogeneous subtypes. Clinical subtyping has borne fruit in the study of other illnesses. In breast cancer research, for example, restricting the gene search to families with early onset of the disease led researchers to a gene—*BRCA1*—that turned out to be common in families with comorbid ovarian cancer (Miki et al., 1994), as well as a second gene—*BRCA2*—that is less likely than *BRCA1* to be associated with ovarian cancer and more likely than *BRCA1* to cause male carriers to develop disease (Wooster et al., 1994). In Alzheimer's disease research as well, identification of families with early onset of the illness led to detection of the genes presenilin-1, presenilin-2, and amyloid precursor protein, all of which can cause the illness when abnormal (mutated) (St. George-Hyslop, 2000). This section first reviews clinical subtypes of major depressive disorder and then of bipolar disorder for which there is evidence of familial aggregation and in some cases, for which there is molecular evidence. A discussion of potential biologically defined phenotypes, or *endophenotypes*, follows.

Clinical Subtypes of Major Depressive Disorder

Genetic studies have tended not to focus exclusively on major depressive disorder because of its lower heritability relative to bipolar disorder. Instead, as noted earlier, many linkage studies have employed a broad phenotype model that includes recurrent major depressive disorder along with bipolar disorder. Findings derived from such a broad model should implicate genes predisposing to both bipolar disorder and recurrent unipolar depression, which might properly be considered manic-depressive illness genes. The first three genomewide linkage scans of major depressive disorder were published in 2003–2004. To address the lower-heritability problem, these studies all employed clinical subtyping strategies, with the idea that a restricted phenotype might have greater heritability than major depressive disorder generally.

Recurrent, Early Onset

Two features of many patients with major depression—recurrent episodes and early age at onset—have a robust association with increased familial risk, with the former association perhaps having been found more consistently (Sullivan et al., 2000). In a study of 763 first-degree relatives of 75 probands with major depression, for example, Bland and colleagues (1986) found that relatives of probands with recurrent depression and early age at onset had a 17.4 percent risk of depression, while relatives of probands with single-episode depression and late age at onset had a 3.4 percent risk.

Two groups have ascertained families through a strategy of selecting for recurrent early-onset cases of major depression. The Zubenko group performed linkage analysis in 81 families ascertained through probands with recurrent, early-onset major depression. They detected linkage in several regions, the strongest being 11p15 (Zubenko et al., 2003). The Genetics of Recurrent Early-onset Depression (GenRED) project, a multicenter collaborative project on the genetics of depressive illness, has recruited 680 families that include 971 affected sibling pairs—a sample large enough to have the power to detect linkage even for a susceptibility gene of modest effect. The families were recruited through probands with recurrent major depressive disorder who experienced their first episode prior to age 31. Linkage analysis of about half of the sample revealed a significant signal on chromosome 15q25–26 (Holmans et al., 2004).

Investigators in the primarily European Depression Network (DeNT) study are recruiting probands whose major depressive disorder is recurrent, though they are not screening for early onset. In the initial phase of the study, they recruited 414 families with 470 affected sibling pairs (Farmer et al., 2004); the aim is to recruit a total of 1,200 families.

Gender-Specific

Because rates of major depressive disorder in women are about twice those in men, investigators have wondered whether susceptibility genes may differ to some extent by gender. One study estimated that the genetic effects for males and females were just over half correlated (Kendler and Prescott, 1999), while another estimated they were entirely correlated (Kendler and Walsh, 1995). Data from three family studies are consistent with partial overlap (Merikangas et al., 1985; Faraone et al., 1987; Reich et al., 1987). Sullivan and colleagues (2000) concluded that "although the data are limited, the most parsimonious explanation appears to be that men and women share most but not all genetic influences for major depression."

One study found significant parametric evidence of linkage to markers in 2q33–34 in 170 affected female sibling pairs, but not in male pairs (Zubenko et al., 2002). The region between the markers that yielded the peak LOD score includes the *CREB1* gene, which encodes a cyclic adenosine monophosphate (cAMP)-responsive element-binding protein (CREB), an attractive candidate gene because CREB has been implicated in depression and antidepressant response. This protein appears to be important for many aspects of neuronal functioning. Levels of CREB have been found to be abnormally low in persons with major depression and in the brain tissue of suicide victims, and have been observed to be altered by exposure of rat neurons to antidepressants and lithium (see Chapter 14).

A second study found evidence of linkage uniquely in families with at least four affected males (Abkevich et al., 2003). This linkage, in chromosomal region 12q22–23.2, was detected in a sample of Mormon families in Utah in which ascertainment was restricted to families with a minimum of four affected relatives. In addition to subjects with recurrent major depressive disorder, individuals with only a single episode of major depression were considered affected, as were those with bipolar disorder (who made up about 15 percent of the individuals with mood disorder in these families).

Clinical Subtypes of Bipolar Disorder

Psychotic Features

The term *psychosis* has been used in a variety of ways. Here we use it to refer to the presence of hallucinations and/or delusions, as does the specifier for psychotic features in the mood disorders section of DSM-IV. By this definition, psychosis occurs in about two-thirds of manic episodes (see Chapter 18) (Coryell et al., 2001). In two samples of families with bipolar illness, Potash and colleagues (2001, 2003a) found evidence for familial aggregation of psychotic symptoms in manic-depressive illness generally and BP-I specifically. Taken together, results of these studies showed that the odds of having psychotic features were about three times greater for a BP-I relative of a psychotic BP-I proband than for a BP-I relative of a nonpsychotic BP-I proband. Another study found a significant correlation ($p < .001$) between bipolar sibling pairs for scores on a psychosis rating scale (Omahony et al., 2002), while still another showed that delusional thinking aggregated in families of psychotic bipolar subjects (Schurhoff et al., 2003). Potash and colleagues (2001) hypothesized that psychotic symptoms in bipolar disorder may be a clinical manifestation of a shared genetic vulnerability to bipolarity and schizophrenia.

In the chapter on genetics in the first edition of this book, we hypothesized the existence of some shared genetic liability between bipolar disorder and schizophrenia, based on results of family studies of the two disorders (Gershon et al., 1982, 1988). Those studies showed an excess of major depression and schizoaffective disorder in the relatives of both bipolar and schizophrenic probands. The excess of major depression in both groups has been a consistent finding (Maier et al., 1993), although the excess of schizoaffective disorder has been less so. Most studies have not found an excess of schizophrenic relatives in bipolar proband families or an excess of relatives with bipolar disorder in schizophrenic proband families. Studies using three large datasets have addressed the issue of overlap between psychotic mood disorder (both bipolar and unipolar) and schizophrenia (see Table 13–6). Two of the datasets showed higher-than-expected rates of psychotic mood disorder in relatives of schizophrenic probands and vice versa[14]; the third dataset also suggested shared liability

TABLE 13–6. Family Studies Comparing Schizophrenia and Psychotic Affective Disorder

Study	Sample Size (First-Degree Relatives)	Risk in First-Degree Relatives (%)		
		Psychotic Affective Disorder	Schizoaffective Disorder	Schizophrenia
Probands with Psychotic Affective Disorder				
Kendler, 1986 (Iowa)	50	—	0	4.3
Kendler et al., 1993a,b,c (Roscommon)	214[a]	6.5	5.7	3.3
Ehrlenmeyer-Kimling, 1997[b]	67	7.5	6.0[c]	0
Weighted mean	*331*	*6.7*	*4.9[d]*	*2.8[e]*
Probands with Schizophrenia				
Kendler, 1985 (Iowa)	723	2.5	1.4	3.7
Kendler et al., 1993a,b,c (Roscommon)	350	4.9	3.0	8.0
Erlenmeyer-Kimling et al., 1997	84	3.6	2.4[f]	13.1
Weighted mean	*1,157*	*3.3[g]*	*2.0[h]*	*5.7*
Control Probands[i]				
Kendler, 1985 (Iowa)	1,056	1.0	0.1	0.2
Kendler et al., 1993a,b,c (Roscommon)	710[a]	1.0	1.1	1.1
Erlenmeyer-Kimling et al., 1997	136	0	0.7	0
Weighted mean	*1,902*	*0.9*	*0.5*	*0.5*

Note: — = not studied or reported.
[a]These numbers are approximations as exact figures are not available.
[b]This study examined only children of probands, whereas the other two studies examined all first-degree relatives.
[c]Schizoaffective, mainly schizophrenic type.
[d]This is significantly higher than the controls (odds ratio [OR] = 9.6, chi-square = 41.8, $p < .001$).
[e]This is significantly higher than the controls (OR = 7.7, chi-square = 22.8, $p < .001$).
[f]Schizoaffective, mainly affective.
[g]This is significantly higher than the controls (OR = 3.3, chi-square = 16.1, $p < .001$).
[h]This is significantly higher than the controls (OR = 3.8, chi-square = 13.1, $p = .001$).
[i]The Roscommon study used unscreened controls, while the other two studies used screened controls.

between the two disorders (Erlenmeyer-Kimling et al., 1997). In addition, some twin studies have found evidence of shared heritability between psychotic mood disorder and schizophrenia (Farmer et al., 1987; Cardno et al., 2002).

Linkage studies of bipolar disorder and schizophrenia have implicated overlapping chromosomal regions that could harbor susceptibility genes shared by the two disorders (Berrettini, 2000). On chromosome 10p12–14, three studies found evidence of linkage for schizophrenia (Faraone et al., 1998; Straub et al., 1998; Schwab et al., 2000). In the NIMH Bipolar Disorder Collaborative study (Wave 1), the strongest signal in the genome was found at 10p12 (Foroud et al., 2000). On chromosome 18p11.2, three studies found evidence of linkage for bipolar disorder (Berrettini et al., 1994; Stine et al., 1995; Nothen et al., 1999), and one study uncovered suggestive evidence of linkage and evidence of linkage disequilibrium for schizophrenia (Schwab et al., 1998). The latter study found a stronger signal when the phenotype was broadened to include mood disorder. On chromosome 13q32, two significant findings (Blouin et al., 1998; Brzustowicz et al., 1999) and a more modest one (Lin et al., 1997) were reported for schizophrenia. Two suggestive findings were reported for bipolar disorder (Detera-Wadleigh et al., 1999; Kelsoe et al., 2001). On chromosome 22q11–13, modest evidence of linkage for schizophrenia was found (Gill et al., 1996; Schizophrenia Collaborative Linkage Group for Chromosome 22, 1998). One group reported significant linkage for bipolar disorder in the same region (Kelsoe et al., 2001). Of interest, the meta-analysis of 11 genome scans for bipolar disorder that identified 13q31–33 and 22q11–13 as the two strongest linkage regions in the genome for the disorder also identified these two regions as the strongest across 18 genome scans for schizophrenia (Badner and Gershon, 2002).

Potash and colleagues (2003b) tested the hypothesis that those bipolar pedigrees most enriched for psychotic symptoms would show increased evidence of linkage to the regions of prior overlap in linkage between bipolar disorder and schizophrenia. Linkage in the four regions was assessed for the full family set and for subsets of families defined by the presence of psychotic symptoms in affectively ill family members. The 10 (of 65) families in which three or more members had psychotic mood disorder showed suggestive evidence of linkage to 13q31 (NPL score = 3.56) and 22q12 (NPL score = 3.32). These results differed significantly from those for the full 65 families, which showed little or no evidence of linkage in the two regions. The 10 families did not show evidence of linkage to 10p12–14 or 18p11.2. These findings suggest that bipolar illness with psychotic features may be a genetically meaningful subtype and that this subtype may share some susceptibility genes with schizophrenia.

Data from a genome scan for bipolar disorder were reanalyzed by Park and colleagues (2004) according to the presence or absence of psychotic features. Some evidence of linkage to psychotic bipolar disorder was obtained on chromosome 13q32, though the strongest results were on chromosomes 9q31 and 8p21. No signal emerged for chromosome 22q11–13.

The hypothesis of etiologic overlap suggests the existence of either psychosis genes (within an oligogenic model) or joint mood and psychosis genes. This latter possibility implies that examination of mood-related subtypes of schizophrenia would further illuminate the issue of etiologic overlap. Indeed, results of four studies suggest that elevated familial rates of mood disorder may occur in a subset of schizophrenic subjects.[15] Pulver and colleagues (2000) tested the hypothesis that some families with schizophrenia may carry genes predisposing to both psychotic and mood symptoms. In an effort to reduce genetic heterogeneity in schizophrenia, they analyzed a subset of 6 families (from a set of 54) in which at least one relative had a psychotic mood disorder. The strongest linkage signal in the genome for this family subset was on chromosome 22q12, where results were suggestive; linkage evidence was also suggestive for 13q33.

Bipolar-II

Results of several studies conducted in the 1980s indicated that the diagnosis of BP-II in genetic studies was unreliable (Andreasen et al., 1981). A more recent study, however, found that the reliability of the Research Diagnostic Criteria BP-II diagnosis was extremely good in the genetic study done at Johns Hopkins, with a kappa value of .72 for hypomania (Simpson et al., 2002). One possible explanation for this difference is that at Johns Hopkins, academic psychiatrists specializing in affective disorders conducted the interviews. The three studies that examined the familial aggregation of BP-II and used a methodology that included direct examination of the majority of subjects are summarized in Table 13–2. These studies showed that this form of the disorder appears to breed true, as rates of BP-II are elevated in relatives of BP-II probands. In the one twin study that specifically analyzed probands with BP-II, a high heritability was observed (Bertelsen et al., 1977).

Interest in BP-II at Johns Hopkins derived from the observation that it was the most common phenotype in the first set of 28 BP-I proband families ascertained (Simpson et al., 1993). Subsequent analyses of the Johns Hopkins linkage data on chromosome 18q21–22 in these families showed that linkage depended mainly on BP-II–BP-II sibling pairs. Sharing of DNA markers was demonstrated among 18 of 22 pairs in which both siblings had BP-II in the original dataset. When a second dataset of 30 more families was prospectively examined, 9 of 11 BP-II pairs showed significant DNA marker sharing at 18q21–22. When the 15 of 58 families that contained BP-II–BP-II pairs were analyzed for linkage, they generated an LOD score of 4.67[16] (McMahon et al., 2001), which was significantly higher than that for the overall sample. Subsequent genotyping of more markers increased the LOD score to 5.42 (Schulze et al., 2003).

Bipolar Disorder with Comorbid Panic and Anxiety Disorders

Using two independent datasets, MacKinnon and colleagues (1997, 2002) found that affectively ill relatives of BP-I probands with comorbid panic disorder are more likely to have comorbid panic disorder themselves than are similar relatives of BP-I probands without this comorbidity. This finding suggests that comorbid panic disorder may define a genetically meaningful subtype of bipolar disorder. This hypothesis was tested using linkage data from chromosome 18, a region where the Johns Hopkins group had previously found bipolar linkage. MacKinnon and colleagues found that bipolar families having at least one member with panic disorder showed stronger linkage in this region than did other bipolar families. Another study stratified bipolar families by the presence of comorbid anxiety disorders generally and found that among relatives of children with bipolar and anxiety disorders, the two disorders appeared to cosegregate. However, this result was based on a small dataset, as there were only seven relatives with bipolar disorder (Wozniak et al., 2002).

Early Onset

As with depression, several studies have found a higher rate of bipolar disorder among relatives of early-onset bipolar probands than among relatives of later-onset probands (Strober et al., 1988; Coryell et al., 2001; Grigoroiu-Serbanescu et al., 2001). Other studies have revealed significant correlation between bipolar sibling pairs for age at onset (Baron et al., 1981; Leboyer et al., 1998; Omahony et al., 2002). Faraone and colleagues (2004) studied the correlation between relatives with bipolar illness for age at onset of mania. They found a significant correlation, with an estimated heritability for age at onset of .41. They went on to use age at onset of mania as a quantitative trait for linkage analysis—a powerful approach because it provides a finer-grained assessment of the phenotype than is derived from a simple dichotomous depiction of the data. The results showed suggestive evidence for linkage in three regions that had not emerged in the conventional phenotype linkage analysis of their dataset: 12p, 14q, and 15q. A similar approach was taken by the Johns Hopkins group, which showed that age at onset was familial (Lin et al., 2005, 2006) and that early onset was correlated with linkage

on 21q22.13 in two distinct datasets. This region of chromosome 21 is one previously implicated in bipolar disorder (see above).

Bipolar Disorder with Comorbid Attention-Deficit Hyperactivity Disorder (ADHD)

Results of three studies from Massachusetts General Hospital suggest that comorbid ADHD in childhood-onset bipolar disorder may mark a genetically meaningful subtype of the illness (Wozniak et al., 1995; Faraone et al., 1997, 2001a). In these studies, 143 first-degree relatives of probands with bipolar disorder and comorbid ADHD were examined. Among the 33 relatives with ADHD, 14 had bipolar disorder (42 percent), whereas among the 110 relatives without ADHD, only 6 had bipolar disorder (5 percent). These results suggest that the two disorders occur together, or *co-segregate*, within families. Further support for the familial connection between the two disorders comes from a meta-analysis, performed by the same group, of five studies comparing rates of ADHD in children of bipolar parents (15 percent) with rates in children of controls (5 percent) (Faraone et al., 1997). A subsequent study found that 28 percent of children of bipolar probands had ADHD (Chang et al., 2000). In the converse meta-analysis, examining rates of bipolar disorder in the relatives of children with ADHD and of controls, rates were 2.6 percent in the former group and 1.3 percent in the latter. Although the difference was not as dramatic as that found in the meta-analyses examining rates of ADHD, it did reach statistical significance (Faraone et al., 1997). A major methodological issue in this work concerns the overlapping diagnostic criteria for childhood onset bipolar disorder and ADHD (see also Chapter 7). Symptoms such as distractibility, increased activity, and increased talkativeness are shared by the two criteria sets, which makes conclusions about the true biological relationship between the disorders more difficult to draw (Kent and Craddock, 2003).

Cognitive Features

Cognitive decline was one of the defining features of Kraepelinian dementia praecox (schizophrenia); by definition, Kraepelinian manic-depressive illness was a disorder in which such decline was not seen. Although the issue has not been resolved, some evidence from studies of euthymic bipolar patients supports the hypothesis that residual neuropsychological impairments persist in a subgroup of patients (Ferrier and Thompson, 2002). Studies of this kind are potentially confounded, however, by the possibility of residual symptoms in patients and by the potential cognitive effects of medications (see Chapter 9). The presence of cognitive abnormalities in unaffected family members can provide a more definitive answer to the question of whether cognitive deficits are a heritable bipolar trait in some cases.

The potential genetic overlap between bipolar disorder and schizophrenia was discussed earlier; we noted that psychotic symptoms (hallucinations and/or delusions) have been proposed as a possible clinical manifestation of this overlap. Cognitive impairment may plausibly represent another phenotypic aspect of the same overlap. Such deficits may define a subgroup of patients. In one study (Decina et al., 1983), children of bipolar probands had significantly higher verbal than performance IQ. In another study, children of psychotic manic-depressive parents were significantly impaired on a digit span test compared with controls (Erlenmeyer-Kimling and Cornblatt, 1992). In the only neuropsychological study of identical twins discordant for bipolar illness, seven unaffected twins demonstrated mild impairments in several tests of learning and memory, as did their affected twins (Gourovitch et al., 1999). More research is needed to clarify these results.

Rapid Cycling

Three studies of familial aggregation of rapid-cycling bipolar disorder yielded negative results (Nurnberger et al., 1988; Coryell et al., 1992; Lish et al., 1993). One recent study assessed a related clinical variable—the rapid switching of mood—and found modest evidence for the familial clustering of this trait in a large sample (MacKinnon et al., 2003a). In a related study, rapid switching was found to be more common in bipolar families in which multiple members also had panic attacks (MacKinnon et al., 2003b). More research is needed to determine whether this variable will prove valuable in resolving the genetic heterogeneity of bipolar disorder.

Endophenotypes

Lithium Responsiveness

Three types of studies have investigated lithium responsiveness as a potentially genetically informative trait: studies of family history of manic-depressive illness, studies of the familial aggregation of lithium response, and molecular studies. The family history studies have yielded mixed results: some found a positive family history of bipolar disorder or more broadly defined manic-depressive illness to be associated with a good response to lithium, while others did not (see Coryell et al., 2000, for references). Studies of the familial aggregation of lithium response have been few and small. These studies, discussed below in the section on pharmacogenetics, generally support the hypothesis that lithium response in one family member is predictive of lithium response in others. Given the biological plausibility of lithium response as an endophenotype in bipolar disorder, Turecki and colleagues (2001) ascertained 31 Canadian bipolar families through excellent lithium responders.

A complete genome scan of these families revealed parametric linkage support for chromosome 15q14 at a genomewide significant level. Further testing with positive lithium response as the phenotype implicated a locus on chromosome 7q11.2.

White Matter Hyperintensities

A number of brain imaging abnormalities have been reported to be associated with bipolar disorder and major depression (see Chapter 15). An increase in white matter hyperintensities may be the most consistent of the abnormalities seen in bipolar patients. While the heritability of these changes in bipolar subjects has not been assessed, a study of elderly male twins in the cardiovascular literature found a heritability of 73 percent for white matter hyperintensities in 514 twin pairs (Carmelli et al., 1998). One large extended family has been documented in which all 9 members with bipolar illness and 6 of 10 members without affective disorder had white matter hyperintensities (Ahearn et al., 2002). The investigators performed a linkage study employing white matter hyperintensities as an endophenotype and using DNA markers near the *NOTCH3* candidate gene. No evidence for linkage was found. There have also been suggestions of abnormalities in volume or metabolism in the prefrontal cortex, hippocampus, and amygdala in patients with manic-depressive illness. The extent to which these abnormalities represent inherited traits is currently unclear, however. Only one small study has assessed brain region volumes in twins discordant for the bipolar subgroup (Noga et al., 2001).

Evoked Potentials

The auditory P300 event-related potential is a "brain wave" that appears on an electroencephalogram (EEG) when subjects monitor series of stimuli for rarely presented targets. The P300 is thought to reflect the operations of short-term working memory. Results of one study suggest that aspects of P300 abnormality have a genetic basis. There is a large Scottish family in which 7 members have schizophrenia, 1 has bipolar disorder, and 10 have major depression. All 18 of these family members, as well as 11 others, carry a balanced chromosomal translocation resulting in chromosomal breakpoints on 1q and 11q. (See the later section on testing gene- and allele-specific function for a discussion of cytogenetics and these breakpoints.) When 12 family members carrying the translocation were tested on the P300 along with noncarriers and normal controls, the carriers were abnormal by two measures—prolonged latency and elevated amplitude—in comparison with the other two groups (Blackwood et al., 2001). Further studies are needed to determine whether other families show cosegregation of P300 abnormalities.

FROM THE BOOK OF NUMBERS TO THE BOOK OF GENESIS: THE ASSOCIATION METHOD

The Method

Association is an approach to disease gene identification that provides an alternative to the linkage method. While linkage is a property of genes or loci and occurs within families, association is a property of alleles and occurs across a population. An association study can be used for two different purposes. The first is to test directly whether a gene variant may be implicated in manic-depressive illness (most, though not all, such studies focus on the bipolar subgroup). An association between a phenotype and an allele at a locus may mean that the allele in question leads to susceptibility to the phenotype. The second use of association studies is for the narrowing of linkage regions through linkage disequilibrium mapping. This indirect approach can provide information about the location of a disease gene with resolution that is roughly 1,000-fold greater than that of a linkage study. An association between a phenotype and an allele at a locus may mean that the allele is in linkage disequilibrium (discussed below) with a susceptibility allele either within the same gene or at a nearby gene.

One can test candidate genes for their association with bipolar disorder by determining whether a particular allele occurs more commonly in those with bipolar illness (cases) than in controls. The choice of controls in a case–control association study can be problematic, however, as differences in allele frequency between the disease and control groups due to differing genomic backgrounds and unrelated to the phenotype (population stratification) may confound the study results. This problem is often addressed by selecting controls thought to be ethnically identical to the cases. A more rigorous approach to handling this problem is now available, in which genotypes at random DNA markers are used as a way of testing the similarity in genomic background between cases and controls. Failure to find significant differences in genomic background suggests that the controls are adequate. Relatively few studies to date have used this method, however.

The preferred method for avoiding the stratification problem is to use family-based association. The most widely used test of this kind—the transmission disequilibrium test—counts the number of times an allele is transmitted by parents to affected probands and compares this result with the number of times that allele is not transmitted by parents to affected probands (Spielman et al., 1993) (see Fig. 13–6). This family constellation—a proband and his or her parents—is referred to as a *trio*, and these data are being collected by many groups for association studies. It is important to note that family-based association may be less prone to false-positive findings than the approach of selecting ethnically identical controls, but because of potentially reduced power, it may be more prone to false negative results (Risch, 2000).

There are two types of candidate genes—functional candidates and positional candidates. In the 1990s, tests of association were typically applied to *functional candidate genes*—those coding for a protein thought to have some biological role in manic-depressive illness. Because of neurobiological data implicating the neurotransmitters, particularly serotonin, norepinephrine, and dopamine, in bipolar disorder and depression, most studies focused on functional candidate genes from these systems. Results have been mixed, with a number of genes yielding both negative and weakly positive results (see Table 13–7). A subset of functional candidate genes that has been studied in relation to

Figure 13–6. Family-based association: the transmission disequilibrium test. The test is performed using trios composed of an affected individual and his or her parents. It does not matter for this test whether the parents are affected. The test determines whether a particular allele is transmitted to affected individuals more often than it is not transmitted. In this example, there are four heterozygous parents—the father in *a*, the mother in *b*, and both parents in *c* (squares are males, circles are females, and filled-in symbols are affected). Each of these four parents could have transmitted either the G or T allele to his or her affected child. In all four cases, the G was transmitted. Note that the mother in *a* and the father in *b* could transmit only a T because they are homozygous for this allele. Thus, they are not informative for this test. A consistent pattern of overtransmitting the G allele across a large number of trios would implicate this allele in association with disease.

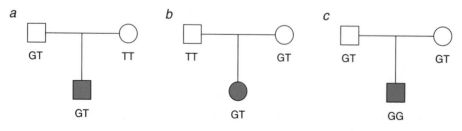

TABLE 13–7. Genes That Have Been Tested for Association in Bipolar Disorder

Serotonin System

Gene	Function	Chromosome Location	Positive[a]	Negative[a]	Studies
5-HTT	Transporter	17q11.2	Promoter length polymorphism +++++ Intron 2 repeat polymorphism ++++++	– – – – – – – –	Battersby et al., 1996; Collier et al., 1996a,b; Kunugi et al., 1997a; Oruc et al., 1997b; Rees et al., 1997; Bellivier et al., 1998a; Esterling et al., 1998; Furlong et al., 1998c; Gutierrez et al., 1998; Hoehe et al., 1998; Mendes de Oliveira et al., 1998; Bocchetta et al., 1999; Kirov et al., 1999c; Liu et al., 1999; Vincent et al., 1999; Mundo et al., 2000; Mynett-Johnson et al., 2000; Ospina-Duque et al., 2000; Saleem et al., 2000a; Dimitrova et al., 2002; Rotondo et al., 2002; Serretti et al., 2002b; Yen et al., 2003; Mendlewicz et al., 2004
5-HT1A	Receptor	5q12.3		– –	Erdmann et al., 1995; Vincent et al., 1999
5-HT1B	Receptor	6q14.1		– – –	Vincent et al., 1999; Mundo et al., 2001b; Huang et al., 2003
5-HT1D	Receptor	1p36.12		–	Vincent et al., 1999
5-HT2A	Receptor	13q14.2	++	– – – – – – –	Gutierrez et al., 1995; Arranz et al., 1997; Mahieu et al., 1997; Zhang et al., 1997; Tsai et al., 1999; Vincent et al., 1999; Massat et al., 2000; Tut et al., 2000; Chee et al., 2001; Ni et al., 2002a; Ranade et al., 2003; Etain et al., 2004
5-HT2C	Receptor	Xq23	+	– – – –	Gutierrez et al., 1996; Oruc et al., 1997b; Vincent et al., 1999b; Gutierrez et al., 2001; Lerer et al., 2001
5-HT4	Receptor	5q32	+		Ohtsuki et al., 2002
5-HT6	Receptor	1p36.13	+	–	Hong et al., 1999; Vogt et al., 2000

(continued)

TABLE 13–7. **Genes That Have Been Tested for Association in Bipolar Disorder** (*continued*)

Gene	Function	Chromosome Location	Positive[a]	Negative[a]	Studies
5-HT7	Receptor	10q23.31			Erdmann et al., 1996; Vincent et al., 1999
TPH	Synthesis enzyme	11p15.1	+	– –	Bellivier et al., 1998b; Furlong et al., 1998b; Vincent et al., 1999; Rietschel et al., 2000; Souery et al., 2001; Rotondo et al., 2002
MAOA	Degradation enzyme	Xp11.3	+ + + +	– – – –	Craddock et al., 1995a; Kawada et al., 1995a; Lim et al., 1995; Nothen et al., 1995; Rubinsztein et al., 1996; Muramatsu et al., 1997; Parsian and Todd, 1997; Furlong et al., 1999a; Kirov et al., 1999b; Kunugi et al., 1999; Turecki et al., 1999; Preisig et al., 2000; Syagailo et al., 2001
Dopamine System					
DAT1	Transporter	5p15.33	+	– –	Gomez-Casero et al., 1996; Manki et al., 1996; Souery et al., 1996b; Waldman et al., 1997; Georgieva et al., 2002
DRD1	Receptor	5q35.2	+	– –	Nothen et al., 1992; Cichon et al., 1994, 1996; Savoye et al., 1998; Ni et al., 2002b
DRD2	Receptor	11q23.2	+ + + +	– – – –	Nothen et al., 1992; Craddock et al., 1995c; Perez de Castro et al., 1995; Arinami et al., 1996; Manki et al., 1996; Oruc et al., 1996; Souery et al., 1996b; Furlong et al., 1998a; Savoye et al., 1998; Stober et al., 1998; Bocchetta et al., 1999; Kirov et al., 1999a; Li et al., 1999b; Heiden et al., 2000; Massat et al., 2002b
DRD3	Receptor	3q13.31	+	– –	Rietschel et al., 1993; Shaikh et al., 1993; Parsian et al., 1995; Gomez-Casero et al., 1996; Manki et al., 1996; Souery et al., 1996b; Piccardi et al., 1997; Savoye et al., 1998; Massat et al., 2002b

Gene	Function	Location			References
DRD4	Receptor	11p15.5	+++	– – – – – –	Lim et al, 1994; Perez de Castro et al., 1994; Di Bella et al., 1996; Manki et al., 1996; Weiss et al., 1996; Oruc et al., 1997a; Bocchetta et al., 1999; Serretti et al., 1999a, 2002b; Muglia et al., 2002D
RD5	Receptor	4p16.1		– – –	Asherson et al., 1998; Kirov et al., 1999a; Muir et al., 2001
Norepinephrine System					
NET	Transporter	16q12.2		– –	Stober et al., 1996; Leszczynska-Rodziewicz et al., 2002
Monoamine Metabolism					
COMT	Monoamine degradation	22q11.21	+++++	– – – – – –	Biomed European Biopolar Collaborative Group, 1997; Gutierrez et al., 1997; Kunugi et al., 1997b; Lachman et al., 1997; Li et al, 1997; Kirov et al., 1998; 1999a; Mynett-Johnson et al., 1998; Ohara et al., 1998b; Papolos et al., 1998; Geller and Cook, 2000; Rotondo et al., 2002; Serretti et al., 2003
DBH	Converts dopamine to norepinephrine	9q34.2		–	Kirov et al., 1999a
DDC	Monoamine synthesis	7p12.2	+	– –	Borglum et al., 1999; Speight et al., 2000; Jahnes et al., 2002
TH	Norepinephrine and dopamine synthesis	11p15.5	+++++	– – – – – – – –	Todd and O'Malley, 1989; Korner et al., 1990; Leboyer et al., 1990; Nothen et al., 1990; Gill et al., 1991; Inayama et al., 1990; Korner et al., 1994; Kawada et al., 1995b; Meloni et al., 1995; Perez de Castro et al., 1995; Souery et al., 1996b; Todd et al., 1996; Malafosse et al., 1997; Oruc et al., 1997a; Serretti et al., 1998; Burgert et al., 1998; Furlong et al., 1999b; McQuillin et al., 1999; Souery et al., 1999; Muglia et al., 2002; Serretti et al., 2003

(continued)

TABLE 13–7. Genes That Have Been Tested for Association in Bipolar Disorder (*continued*)

Gene	Function	Chromosome Location	Positive[a]	Negative[a]	Studies
MAOB	Degradation enzyme	Xp11.3		–	Parsian and Todd, 1997
GABA					
GABRA1	Receptor	5q34	+		Horiuchi et al., 2004
GABRA3	Receptor	Xq26	+	– –	Puertollano et al., 1995; Duffy et al., 2000; Massat et al., 2002a
GABRA5	Receptor	15q12	+	–	Papadimitriou et al., 1998; Duffy et al., 2000
GABRB1	Receptor	4p12		–	Puertollano et al., 1997
GABRB3	Receptor	15q12		– –	Duffy et al., 2000; Papadimitriou et al., 2001
Other					
ACE	Angiotensin-converting enzyme	17q23.3	+	– –	Meira-Lima et al., 2000; Pauls et al., 2000; Segman et al., 2002
A1AR	Adenosine receptor	1q32.1		–	Deckert et al., 1998
BDNF	Brain-derived neurotrophic factor	11p14	+ + +	– – – –	Neves-Pereira et al., 2002; Sklar et al., 2002; Hong et al., 2003; Nakata et al., 2003; Geller et al., 2004; Kunugi et al., 2004; Oswald et al., 2004
BZRP	Benzodiazepine receptor	22q13.2		–	Kurumaji et al., 2001
CART	Neuropeptide	5q13.2		–	Jung et al., 2004
CCK	Cholecystokinin	3p22–21.3		–	Hattori et al., 2002
CNR1	Cannabinoid receptor	6q15		–	Tsai et al., 2001
CRH	Corticotropin-releasing hormone	8q13.1		–	Alda et al., 2000
CTLA4	Immunoglobulin	2q33.2		–	Jun et al, 2004
DRP2	Regulator of axonal growth	8p21.2		–	Nakata et al., 2003
ESR1	Estrogen receptor	6q25.1		–	Jones et al., 2000

Gene	Function	Location			Reference
ESR2	Estrogen receptor	14q23.2	–		Kealey et al., 2001
FZD3	Wnt receptor	8p21.1	–		Hashimoto et al., 2005
GNB3	G-protein	12p13.31	– –		Lin et al., 2001; Kunugi et al., 2002
IMPA1	Myo-inositol monophosphatase	8q21.13	–		Sjoholt et al., 2004
INPP1	Inositol phosphate 1-phosphatase	2q32.2	–		Piccardi et al., 2002
NCAM1	Neural cell adhesion	11q23.1		+	Arai et al., 2004
NTF3	Neurotrophic factor	12p13.31	–		Tadokoro et al., 2004
PENK	Proenkephalin	8q12.1	–		Alda et al., 2000
PLA2G4A	Phospholipase	1q31.3	–		Meira-Lima and Vallada, 2003
PLCG1	Phospholipase	20q12		+	Turecki et al., 1998
TNFA	Cytokine	6p21.33		+	Meira-Lima et al., 2003; Pae et al., 2004
Trinucleotide Repeat Containing					
KCNN3	Potassium channel	1q22	– – – – – – –		Chandy et al., 1998; Guy et al., 1999; Hawi et al., 1999; McInnis et al., 1999; Rohrmeier et al., 1999; Bowen et al., 2000; Saleem et al., 2000b; Jin et al., 2001; Meira-Lima et al., 2001; Ujike et al., 2001
SCA2	Spinocebellar ataxia 2	12q24.12	–		Franks et al., 1999
ASH1	Transcription factor	12q23.2	–		Franks et al., 1999
TCF4	Transcription factor	18q21.1	– – –		McInnis et al., 2000; Meira-Lima et al., 2001; Del Favero et al., 2002
MAB21L	Protein regulator	13q13.3	–		Meira-Lima et al., 2001
NOTCH4	Developmental signaling factor	6p21.3	– –		Swift-Scanlan et al., 2002; Prathikanti et al., 2004
Positional					
DISC1	Cytoskeletal protein	1q42.2		+	Hodgkinson et al., 2004

(continued)

TABLE 13–7. Genes That Have Been Tested for Association in Bipolar Disorder *(continued)*

Gene	Function	Chromosome Location	Positive[a]	Negative[a]	Studies
WFS1	Wolframin	4p16.1	+	– – –	Middle et al., 2000; Kato et al., 2003; Serretti et al., 2003; Koido et al., 2005
DAO	D-amino acid oxidase	12q24.11		–	Schumacher et al., 2004
DUSP6	MAP kinase phosphatase	12q21.33		–	Toyota et al., 2000
PLA2A	Phospholipase	12q24.23	+	–	Dawson et al., 1995; Jacobsen et al., 1996
PLA2G1B	Phospholipase	12q24.23		–	Meira-Lima et al., 2003a
G72/G30	Possible NMDA receptor regulation	13q33	+ + + +		Hattori et al., 2003; Chen et al., 2004; Schumacher et al., 2004; Schulze et al., 2005
ADCY9	Adenylate cyclase	16p13.3		–	Toyota et al., 2002
SSTR5	Somatostatin receptor	16p13.3	+	–	Nyegaard et al., 2002
GRIN2A	NMDA receptor subunit	16p13.3	+		Itokawa et al., 2003
GOLF	G-protein	18p11.21		–	Turecki et al., 1996
IMPA2	Myo-inositol monophosphatase	18p11.21	+		Sjoholt et al., 2004
NDUFV2	Mitochondrial protein	18p11.22	+		Washizuka et al., 2003
PACAP	Pituitary adenyl cyclase activating peptide	18p11.32		–	Ishiguro et al., 2001
ABCG1	Transporter	21q22.3		–	Kirov et al., 2001
XBP1	Transcription factor	22q12.1	+	– –	Kakiuchi et al., 2003; Cichon et al., 2004; Hou et al., 2004
PLA2G6	Phospholipase	22q13.1		–	Meira-Lima et al., 2003b

Notes: The phenotype here is defined narrowly as bipolar only for some studies, while it is defined as bipolar plus major depression for others. The relatively few studies examining only major depression are not included.

[a]A positive result indicates a finding that was statistically significant; a negative result represents a finding that was not statistically significant. This determination is based on overall results, and does not take account of secondary analyses.

bipolar disorder is the group of genes that contain trinucleotide repeat sequences. This structural feature has been implicated in numerous neuropsychiatric diseases and has been hypothesized to play a role in bipolar disorder (see the later section on consideration of alternative genetic mechanisms).

The *positional candidate genes* are those that reside in linkage regions and are thus in a chromosomal position of interest. Studies of positional candidate genes conducted in the 1990s were confined primarily to work on genes that were both positional and biological candidates. Work is currently under way on larger-scale association testing of many positional candidate genes in linkage regions. Genes with at least three positive association findings are discussed below.

Promising Candidate Genes

Serotonin Transporter

The serotonin transporter gene, *5-HTT*, is the most heavily studied gene in research on manic-depressive illness because of the importance of serotonin in depression, the central role of 5-HTT in serotonergic function at the synapse, and the demonstration of a functionally meaningful DNA variation in the promoter region of the gene. The promoter region plays a crucial role in the expression of the gene, and *5-HTT* has a stretch of promoter DNA that exists in a short and a long form. The short form has been found to result in decreased levels of gene expression compared with the long form. Four studies of bipolar disorder have found a positive association between the short variant and illness,[17] while 13 studies have found no significant difference (see Table 13–7). Of these studies, 5 were family based, and only 1 of these 5 showed positive association.[18] A meta-analysis of 15 case–control samples found evidence for a significant, though quite small, effect of this polymorphism in bipolar disorder, reporting an odds ratio of 1.13 for having the short versus the long allele among the cases as compared with the controls (Lasky-Su et al., 2005).

A second polymorphism in the gene, a repeat in intron 2, has also been heavily studied, and there is evidence as well from a transgenic mouse model that this polymorphism may influence gene expression (MacKenzie and Quinn, 1999) (see the later section on testing gene- and allele-specific function). There have been 6 positive and 10 negative studies of this polymorphism. Five of these were family-based studies, and of these five, one was positive and three were negative.[19]

Several studies have used the alternative phenotypic definition approach (discussed previously) in testing association with these markers. Two studies found modest evidence of association between the short promoter variant and violent suicide attempters with manic-depressive illness

(Bellivier et al., 2000; Courtet et al., 2001), and a third found an association between the short variant and completed suicide (Bondy et al., 2000). One negative study for the phenotype of violent suicidal behavior in a primarily manic-depressive sample has been reported (Rujescu et al., 2001) (see Chapter 8).

MAOA

This gene encodes monoamine oxidase A (MAOA), an enzyme that degrades monoamine neurotransmitters, such as dopamine, norepinephrine, and serotonin. There are several reasons why MAOA may have a role in manic-depressive illness. First, monoamine oxidase inhibitor (MAOI) medications, such as tranylcypromine, treat depression. Second, in a large Dutch kindred with a form of X-linked mild mental retardation, all affected males showed aggressive, impulsive, and sometimes violent behavior, including arson, attempted rape, exhibitionism, and attempted suicide (Brunner et al., 1993). Each of the affected males in the family was shown to carry a mutation in the *MAOA* gene. The behavioral phenotype in this family was believed to bear some resemblance to a manic syndrome.

Thirteen studies have examined the possible association of four *MAOA* polymorphisms with either bipolar disorder or bipolar disorder combined with major depression. Four of these studies yielded statistically significant positive findings, while nine failed to show an association (see Table 13–7). However, two meta-analyses that examined pooled data from seven and five studies, respectively, found significant associations for the two polymorphisms they examined (Furlong et al., 1999a; Preisig et al., 2000). One of these polymorphisms, a microsatellite marker in intron 2, had an allele that was 1.55 times more likely to be found in Caucasian bipolar subjects than in controls and an allele that was 2.65 times more likely to be found in Japanese bipolar subjects than in controls. For a single base variant in the coding sequence, one allele was 1.30 times more likely in Caucasian cases than in controls (Furlong et al., 1999a). An important caveat is that these meta-analyses, like all of the positive studies, used the case–control method. The only two studies to use family-based methods both failed to show evidence for an association (Nothen et al., 1995; Parsian and Todd, 1997), so the possibility that the positive findings for this gene are due to undetected population stratification cannot be ruled out.

TH

This gene encodes tyrosine hydroxylase, the rate-limiting enzyme in the synthesis of dopamine and norepinephrine. A total of 21 studies have sought an association between bipolar disorder and *TH* polymorphisms, including four RFLPs and one microsatellite repeat within intron 1; of these, 5 yielded positive results and 16 negative (see Table 13–7). A meta-analysis of 11 studies using the microsatellite marker showed no evidence for association with bipolar disorder in the pooled data (Furlong et al., 1999b). Current evidence does not support involvement of the *TH* gene in bipolar disorder.

COMT

This gene codes for an enzyme involved in the degradation of dopamine and norepinephrine. It has been much studied in relation to schizophrenia in part because it lies in a chromosomal region within 22q11 that has been implicated in psychotic illness through velocardiofacial syndrome (VCFS). This syndrome, which is often accompanied by psychotic symptoms, results from microdeletion or loss of a segment from the 22q11.2 region. Another interesting feature of *COMT* is the existence of an SNP shown to be functionally significant, with the variant coding for methionine having a three- to four-fold lower level of enzymatic activity than the one coding for valine. There have been five positive and seven negative studies of this variant (see Table 13–7). A meta-analysis of seven case–control reports, representing 910 bipolar cases and 1,069 controls, found a statistically significant, though very modest, effect whereby the low-activity methionine variant was 1.18 times more likely in subjects with bipolar disorder than in controls (Craddock et al., 2001). None of the three family-based studies showed significant evidence for an association (Mynett-Johnson et al., 1998; Kirov et al., 1999a; Geller and Cook, 2000).

DRD2

The dopamine D2 receptor (DRD2) has been the subject of intense interest because of its critical role in the mechanism of action of antipsychotic medications. There have been 4 positive and 11 negative association studies of this gene in relation to bipolar disorder (see Table 13–7). Notably, the most recent study had three to four times more patients than any of the prior studies. This study found that one allele of a microsatellite marker within intron 2 was 1.7 times more common in bipolar cases than in controls ($p = .00035$) (Massat et al., 2002b). While this finding might be construed as indicating that when the sample is sufficiently large, a real though modest association can be found with *DRD2*, again one would like to see confirmatory evidence from family-based association studies. Two such studies have been done to date; both were negative. Thus, firm conclusions about an etiologic role for *DRD2* in bipolar disorder cannot be drawn at present.

DRD4

The dopamine D4 receptor (DRD4) has been of interest in psychiatric genetics since its discovery as a dopamine receptor with a high affinity for clozapine and the discovery

shortly thereafter of multiple variants in the population (Van Tol et al., 1991, 1992). The most studied variant is a repeat polymorphism in exon 3, encoding the third intracellular loop of the gene. One of the variants, the 7-repeat variant, was shown to be less potent at inhibiting dopamine-stimulated cAMP formation in cells as compared with the other two common variants (Asghari et al., 1995). This variant has been shown to be significantly associated with ADHD in separate meta-analyses of 8 case–control studies and 14 family-based studies (Faraone et al., 2001b). There have been 3 positive and 7 negative studies of association of bipolar disorder with *DRD4* (see Table 13–7). Three of these studies were family based; 2 were negative (Bocchetta et al., 1999; Serretti et al., 2002a), and 1 was positive (Muglia et al., 2002). Of interest, the latter positive study was associated with a parent-of-origin effect (see the section below on alternative genetic mechanisms).

BDNF

At the start of the new century, armed with greater awareness of the neurobiology of manic-depressive illness, a wider array of identified SNPs, and a greater technical capacity to perform SNP genotyping, Sklar and colleagues (2002) undertook a family-based association study of 76 functional candidate genes located in diverse regions of the genome. The study yielded two nominally positive associations with the bipolar subgroup, and only one of these—brain-derived neurotrophic factor (*BDNF*)—was supported, albeit weakly at a nonstatistically significant level, in two replication samples. The authors found that two samples shared an undertransmitted haplotype (an ancestral chromosomal fragment) marked by two SNPs. A second study (Neves-Pereira et al., 2002) also found an association between *BDNF* and bipolar disorder using the same SNP identified in the Sklar et al. screen, which in its G form leads to synthesis of the amino acid valine, but in its A form results in methionine. As in the study by Sklar and colleagues, the A allele was found to be undertransmitted in this family-based study. Replication attempts in one European (Oswald et al., 2004) and three Asian (Nakata et al., 2003) case–control datasets were negative, however (Nakata et al., 2003). Further support for the Sklar group's finding comes from a report that the G allele of *BDNF* was shown to be preferentially transmitted to people with prepubertal and early-adolescent bipolar disorder (Geller et al., 2004). Similarly, the G allele was associated with neuroticism, a personality trait correlated with depression (Sen et al., 2003), although a Chinese case–control study of major depression was negative (Tsai et al., 2003). The potential genetic role of *BDNF* in mood disorder is intriguing because of the part it plays in the brain's response to stress, in the treatment of animal models of depression, and in the putative mechanism of action of antidepressant medications (Licinio and Wong, 2002; see also Chapter 9).

G72/G30

The genes discussed above were all studied because they were thought to have a biological role in bipolar disorder. Yet our lack of fundamental understanding of bipolar pathophysiology may mean that positional candidate genes with no known biological relationship to bipolar disorder, or perhaps no currently known function at all, may be real susceptibility genes for the disorder. One intriguing new finding concerns two genes of unknown function—G72 and G30—that overlap each other on the same stretch of DNA. A group studying schizophrenia genetics discovered these genes as positional candidates in the 13q32 linkage region. They reported an association of SNPs in and around these genes with schizophrenia (Chumakov et al., 2002). In the same study, the protein product of G72 was found to interact with DAO; DAO is expressed in the human brain, where it oxidizes d-serine, a potent activator of the N-methyl-D-aspartate–type glutamate receptor.

The Gershon group, which first reported linkage to this same region in bipolar disorder, tested for association of SNPs in G72/G30 in the NIMH Clinical Neurogenetics 22-family bipolar sample and in the NIMH Wave 1 and 2 bipolar samples. Using the transmission disequilibrium test to assess family-based association, they obtained positive results for both samples (Hattori et al., 2003). A second study of G72/G30, by Chen and colleagues (2004), employed the Johns Hopkins bipolar sample. Using a case–control approach, they found that two G72/G30 SNPs were associated with illness. A third study also found evidence for an association of SNPs in G72/G30 with both schizophrenia and bipolar disorder (Schumacher et al., 2004). Yet another study examined the G72 gene in two bipolar samples and, in the context of looking at psychosis in general and individual psychotic symptoms, found an association specifically with persecutory delusions (Schulze et al., 2005). While promising, the results of these studies cannot be regarded as conclusive because the associated variations within the genes differ from one study to the next, and no functional variation has yet been implicated. Nonetheless, G72/G30 does constitute the first positional candidate gene(s) for bipolar disorder to be associated with illness in independent reports.

Linkage Disequilibrium

In addition to testing for whether a candidate gene is associated with disease, it is possible to test for such an association with random marker alleles in noncoding regions of DNA. When an association is found, the marker allele is in linkage disequilibrium with the disease locus, reflecting the common inheritance of an ancestral chromosomal fragment, or *haplotype*, among affected individuals. (A haplotype denotes the collective genotype of a number of closely linked DNA markers or loci on a chromosome.) This approach can be viewed as a linkage test in one enormous family. Because the family is so big, with numerous generations and thus numerous recombinations of chromosomal fragments, the chromosomal region implicated by a positive finding—the region left unrecombined, or intact—is much smaller than the region implicated by linkage.

The chromosomal distance across which linkage disequilibrium can be detected in a European population ranges from a few thousand to 100,000 bases, with an average of about 22,000 bases (Gabriel et al., 2002). The distance is smaller for African populations. These regions, called *haplotype blocks*, are roughly 1,000-fold smaller than the typical size of a linkage region (Roberts et al., 1999). These short distances have been an obstacle to the use of linkage disequilibrium mapping because they necessitate large numbers of very tightly spaced DNA markers to detect association with a disease gene. Only since the turn of the century have large numbers of SNPs become available, allowing for the conduct of very dense marker studies. A number of projects are currently using SNPs to narrow the localization of a linkage region, although no study employing this method in a general bipolar population, as opposed to a population isolate, has yet been published. It is thought that 300,000 or more SNPs would be required to conduct a genomewide association study in a genetically mixed population (Gabriel et al., 2002). Studies that would test 500,000 SNPs in a large bipolar sample are currently being planned.

Population Isolates

Linkage disequilibrium studies have been published for a population isolate. Such populations are thought to be more genetically homogeneous than ethnically mixed populations; moreover, linkage disequilibrium may exist over a larger chromosomal region in these isolates than in a mixed population, potentially facilitating detection. Population isolates that have been studied in relation to bipolar disorder include the Amish, Ashkenazi Jews, the population of the Central Valley of Costa Rica, inhabitants of eastern Finland, and families from the Saguenay–Lac-St-Jean region in Quebec. A genome scan on the Costa Rican sample yielded several strong linkage findings, including one on 18p11.3. SNP genotyping across the region yielded a strong association with markers in a 19,000-base region that contains just two genes, with the most strongly implicated gene being CLUL1, clusterin-like 1 (retinal), for which the function is not known (McInnes et al., 2001). Another study from the same group included a genomewide linkage disequilibrium scan using 1,186 microsatellite markers on 109 unrelated Costa Rican BP-I subjects. This study found evidence for increased sharing of an ancestral chromosomal fragment among ill subjects on 8p23.1, suggesting the possibility of a susceptibility gene in this region (Ophoff et al., 2002).

There are caveats to the population isolate strategy. The necessary homogeneity may exist only if the isolate has a particular history, that is, a small number of unrelated founders (10–100) and slow population growth during the early generations following the initial bottleneck. Some populations currently regarded as isolates may not meet these criteria (Wright et al., 1999). Further, the age and frequency of the sought-after disease mutation affect the ability to detect linkage disequilibrium with neighboring markers. In particular, if the disease mutation is significantly older than the marker mutation, little or no association may be detected even when the physical distance between the two is small (Chakravarti, 1999). If gene variants leading to susceptibility to bipolar disorder are common variants, they probably developed a very long time ago. Because of their age, they are likely to have been scrambled by the many recombinations that have occurred during the numerous meioses between then and now. In this setting, linkage disequilibrium between the marker and the disease allele may not exist over any greater distance in an isolate than in the general population.

CONSIDERATION OF ALTERNATIVE GENETIC MECHANISMS

Earlier we discussed alternative phenotypic definition as a potential means of achieving greater genetic homogeneity in a bipolar sample. Another promising route to gene discovery involves considering alternative genetic mechanisms that underlie disease. Whereas previously we focused on "rethinking the phenotype," we now turn to "rethinking the genotype." Clinical observations of the patterns of illness and inheritance in families can provide important clues to the underlying genetic mechanism.

Anticipation and Trinucleotide Repeats

The phenomenon of *anticipation*, in which successive generations of afflicted individuals suffer from an earlier and more severe form of the disease, implicates a unique pathogenetic mechanism. Anticipation has been observed in a number of neurologic and neuropsychiatric diseases, including myotonic dystrophy, fragile X syndrome, and Huntington's disease—all caused by genes with trinucleotide repeat sequences that expand in successive generations. In 34 Johns Hopkins families, evidence for anticipation in bipolar disorder was observed (McInnis et al., 1993). Anticipation in bipolar illness was also seen in Swedish families, Japanese families,

and a Romanian sample, in which it was restricted to subjects inheriting the disorder from the paternal side (Nylander et al., 1994; Grigoroiu-Serbanescu et al., 1997; Ohara et al., 1998a). In a Canadian bipolar sample, evidence for anticipation was also found, although the authors suggested that a censoring bias may have been partially responsible for this result (Merette et al., 2000). This bias is due to having apparently normal subjects in the younger generation who might eventually develop the disorder, though their potentially later age at onset is not evident at the time of the study. Other potential biases can also influence analyses of anticipation (Goossens et al., 2001). Anticipation studies of bipolar disorder have attempted to control for these biases, but the possibility of false positive findings cannot be ruled out.

In support of the clinical findings, a few reports have suggested that expanded trinucleotide repeat sequences may exist in bipolar disorder; however, the majority of studies have been negative in this regard (see Table 13–7 for trinucleotide repeat–containing genes that have been tested for association with bipolar disorder; see Goossens et al., 2001, for further references). Although the anticipation and trinucleotide repeat hypothesis has not yet yielded strong candidate bipolar genes, the possibility remains that types of repeats not yet carefully examined may play a role in the etiology of bipolar disorder.

Parent-of-Origin Effect

Among 34 Johns Hopkins pedigrees, an excess of maternal transmission of bipolar disorder was observed, a finding consistent with those of a number of prior studies (summarized by McMahon et al., 1995). Some subsequent findings (Lin and Bale, 1997), though not all (Kato et al., 1996b), have been consistent with this observation. One study found that the rate of the disorder among the offspring of affected fathers was significantly higher than that among those with affected mothers (Kornberg et al., 2000).

If there is a clinical parent-of-origin effect, there are a number of possible explanations. In some cases, bipolar disorder could be inherited through mitochondrial genes. In other cases, the illness could be accounted for by an imprinted gene, for which alleles are expressed differentially based on the gender of the transmitting parent. Other possibilities include X-linkage; the psychosocial consequences of being reared by an affected mother; and intrauterine maternal factors, such as differential susceptibility to infectious agents. It is also possible that ascertainment bias accounts for the clinical parent-of-origin findings. The first two possibilities are discussed below.

Mitochondrial Inheritance

The *mitochondria* are organelles within cells; they have their own unique genome, composed of 16,569 nucleotides coding for 37 genes. The inheritance of this genome is strictly maternal. Thus mitochondrial inheritance would be a good explanation for maternal inheritance of disease. McMahon and colleagues (2000) examined the mitochondrial genome in a Johns Hopkins bipolar sample and found no evidence of an association between any SNPs examined and the illness. One group has, however, reported modest evidence of an association between two mitochondrial SNPs and bipolar disorder (Kato et al., 2000, 2001), while another group found evidence for a nonspecific weak effect of mitochondrial gene variants on the disorder (Kirk et al., 1999).

Genomic Imprinting

When heritable differences in gene expression between individuals exist and are not accounted for by variation in the DNA sequence, epigenetic factors are said to be involved. One important epigenetic mechanism is *genomic imprinting*—the parent-of-origin–specific silencing of one allele of a given gene with a corresponding parent-of-origin–specific expression of the other allele. Imprinting has been demonstrated for about 25 genes to date (Morison and Reeve, 1998), and imprinted genes have been implicated in such diseases as Angelman syndrome, Prader-Willi syndrome, and Beckwith-Weidemann syndrome. Although imprinted genes are thought to play an important role in growth, they can also be involved in maternal behavior (Li et al., 1999a) and in social behavior (Skuse et al., 1997). Mouse studies of the developing brain employing genetically engineered mice with predominantly maternal or predominantly paternal genomes have indicated that maternal genes play a disproportionate role in the development of the cortex, while paternal genes play a disproportionate role in hypothalamic development (Keverne et al., 1996).

Two bipolar genome scans have examined parent-of-origin–specific linkage. Reporting on the Bonn sample, Cichon and colleagues (2001) identified two regions—2p21–24 and 2q31–32—that showed suggestive evidence for linkage when only maternal transmission was examined, and two regions—14q32 and 16q21–23—that showed suggestive linkage when only paternal regions were examined (Cichon et al., 2001). Of interest, the 14q32 linkage region is immediately adjacent to a known imprinted gene, *DLK1*. Because imprinting is thought to occur in clusters, there may be other imprinted genes in the region. McInnis and colleagues (2003), examining the Johns Hopkins sample, found two regions—1q42 and 13q12—that showed linkage with maternally transmitted alleles and one region—18q21–22—that showed linkage with paternally transmitted alleles (McInnis et al., 2003). The 13q12 region contains $5\text{-}HT_{2A}$, reported to be imprinted in fibroblasts (Kato et al., 1996a) and in brain tissue from some subjects but not others (Bunzel

et al., 1998). One association study of $5\text{-}HT_{2A}$ examined whether parent-of-origin–specific association could be detected in bipolar subjects; results were negative (Murphy et al., 2001).

Earlier studies of chromosome 18 in the Johns Hopkins sample found that linkage to chromosome 18q21–22 came predominantly from paternally inherited alleles. A subsequent study, focusing on a phenotypically defined subgroup of families (see the earlier section on alternative phenotypic definition), obtained a nonparametric LOD score of 4.67 for paternally transmitted alleles (which rose to 5.42 in a more recent analysis [Schulze et al., 2003]) and near zero for maternally transmitted alleles. This result suggested the possibility that an imprinted gene in the region could account for the linkage in the 18q22 region. Of note, one imprinted gene, *TCEL2*, has been reported on 18q12, although that is the only identified imprinted human gene to date on chromosome 18.

Two association studies have found parent-of-origin–specific evidence for association with bipolar disorder: one study of *DDC*, which codes for dopa-decarboxylase (Borglum et al., 2003), and one study of *DRD4* (Muglia et al., 2002). Both genes are biologically plausible candidates, and both lie adjacent to known imprinted genes. A study assessing imprinting of *DRD4*, however, found evidence for normal, nonimprinted expression of the gene.

A more complex scenario of brain region–specific, developmental stage–specific, or alternative transcript–specific imprinting cannot be ruled out at present. An example of brain region–specific imprinting is the *UBE3A* gene, which is thought to cause Angelman syndrome. In a mouse model, this gene was expressed in an imprinted fashion in Purkinje cells, hippocampal neurons, and mitral cells of the olfactory bulb, but not clearly imprinted in other brain regions (Albrecht et al., 1997). *Transcripts* are expressed genes, encoded as messenger RNA. A single gene may give rise to several different, or alternative, transcripts, as a result of cutting and pasting (*splicing*) of the exons that form the gene. One striking example of alternative transcript–specific imprinting is the *GNAS* gene. It is expressed normally with one transcript, only from the maternal copy with another transcript, and only from the paternal copy with still another transcript (Hayward et al., 1998).

TOWARD THE PROMISED LAND: GENE EXPRESSION AND PATHOGENESIS

In this section we review work that moves the argument for the involvement of a gene in manic-depressive illness beyond the realm of statistical association and into the realm of neurobiology. Establishing causal relationships between gene variants and disease depends first on being able to show that the susceptibility variant alters the structure or function of the messenger RNA and/or protein product. Establishing causality also depends on demonstrating a relationship between a susceptibility variant and other intermediate features of disease pathology or disease phenotype, such as neuronal structure and function, brain structure and function, and intermediate neuropsychological variables. Figure 13–7 illustrates the many intervening levels that come between genotype and phenotype. The discussion that follows focuses on studies of gene expression in the bipolar subgroup of manic-depressive illness and on the few studies that have examined candidate gene variants in relation to intermediate phenotypes. These studies have been carried out in brain samples and in white blood cell samples from bipolar patients, as well as in experimental cell lines and in mouse models.

Expression in the Brain

Gene expression studies ideally employ brain tissue from patients. For obvious reasons, these must be postmortem tissues. Several collections of such brains exist, including the collections of the Stanley Medical Research Institute and the Harvard Brain Tissue Resource Center. The Stanley collection has been widely distributed, and many investigators have studied changes in gene expression levels in the 50 bipolar brains available. A challenge in these studies lies in the selection of the brain area to study. Investigators would like to choose the area with known pathology in bipolar disorder, though this cannot yet be done with certainty (see Chapter 15). Studies have focused on the prefrontal and frontal cortex, the amygdala, and the hippocampus as the most likely candidate brain regions (see Table 13–8).

In studies focusing on the role of one or a few specific genes in bipolar disorder, decreased levels of the following messenger RNAs were found: prodynorphin in the amygdaloid complex, GAD65 and complexin I and II in the hippocampus, and Ca^{2+}/calmodulin-dependent protein kinase II and neuropeptide Y in the prefrontal cortex (see Table 13–8).

Four published studies employed broad approaches that can be used to measure changes in many gene transcripts

Figure 13–7. Genetic to pathogenic pathway to manic-depressive illness. Many levels of pathogenesis intervene between genetic etiology and the syndrome of manic-depressive illness. Study of the relationship between a potential susceptibility gene variant and manic-depressive illness requires examination of the impact of the variant on a number of these disease components. An interaction of environmental factors with gene expression or function, or protein expression or function, is also possible. (*Source:* Adapted from McHugh and Slavney, 1998.)

TABLE 13–8. Gene Expression Studies of Bipolar Brain Samples

Study	Sample Size[a]	Gene	Change	Brain Region
Findings in Bipolar Samples Only				
Young et al., 1996	20	G protein α (s)	No change	Frontal, temporal, occipital
Caberlotto et al., 1999	30 (Stanley)	Neuropeptide Y	Decreased	Prefrontal
Eastwood et al., 2000	30 (Stanley)	Complexin I and II	Decreased	Hippocampus
Sun et al., 2001	34 (Stanley)	Serotonin transporter and NF-κB	Increased	Frontal
Bezchlibnyk et al., 2001	30 (Stanley)	TGF-β1	Decreased	Frontal
		CASP8	Increased	
		TOB	Increased	
Heckers et al., 2002	30 (Harvard)	GAD65	Decreased	Hippocampus
		GAD67	No change	
Xing et al., 2002	30 (Stanley)	CaMKII	Decreased	Prefrontal
Hurd, 2002	29 (Stanley)	Prodynorphin	Decreased[b]	Amygdaloid complex
Woo et al., 2004	34 (Harvard)	GRIN2A	No change	Anterior cingulate
Konradi et al., 2004	19 (Harvard)	43 genes, including 18 mitochondrial, GAD67, and somatostatin	Decreased	Hippocampus
Iwamoto et al., 2004	26 (Stanley)	53 genes, including LIM1 and HSPF1	Increased and decreased	Prefrontal
Iwamoto et al., 2005	70 (Stanley2[c])	27 genes	Increased for 23 of 27	Prefrontal
Findings in Bipolar Samples Also Found in Schizophrenia Samples in Same Study				
Guidotti et al., 2000	30 (Stanley)	RELN and GAD67	Decreased[d]	Prefrontal and cerebellum
Vawter et al., 2002	19	Synapsin Ia, IIa, IIIa	Decreased	Hippocampus
Mimmack et al., 2002	30 (Stanley)	APOL2	Increased	Prefrontal
Koh et al., 2003	30 (Stanley)	Neuronal calcium sensor-1	Increased	Dorsolateral prefrontal
Tkachev et al., 2003	30 (Stanley)	8 oligodendrocyte- and myelin-related genes	Decreased	Prefrontal
Iwamoto et al., 2004	26 (Stanley)	9 genes, including serotonin receptor 2C	Decreased	Prefrontal

[a]Bipolar plus control samples.
[b]Decrease also found in major depression brain sample in the same study.
[c]This sample, though from the Stanley Medical Research Institute, differs from those in the other studies.
[d]Decrease found in psychotic bipolar samples.

simultaneously without regard to prior hypotheses about the gene's biological role. One used a technique called *serial analysis of gene expression* (SAGE), while the other used a microarray approach. SAGE generates short sequence tags for many of the transcripts present in a tissue sample and identifies them by comparison with the public gene sequence database. Three studies employed *microarrays*, which use large numbers of short sequences from genes as bait to detect matching transcripts from tissue samples. The totality of the expressed genes, or *transcripts*, is sometimes referred to as the *transcriptome* (by analogy with the word *genome*). The SAGE and microarray methods have the potential to be transcriptome-wide, to assess all transcripts at once, though at present their coverage is more limited.

The SAGE study, conducted by Sun and colleagues (2001), covered 1,856 sequence tags, although some of these may have come from the same transcript, so that this figure represents some smaller number of transcripts. This study yielded evidence that two transcripts—for the serotonin transporter gene and for the NF-κB transcription factor—were significantly overexpressed in the frontal cortex of 19 bipolar subjects as compared with 15 controls. Essentially the same sample was used in a second study, conducted by Bezchlibnyk and colleagues (2001), which employed the microarray approach and examined the same brain region, the frontal cortex. However, the results of the two studies do not coincide. Instead, the microarray study, which assessed 1,200 genes simultaneously, found decreased levels of transforming growth factor beta 1 (TGF-β1) and increased levels of caspase-8 precursor (CASP8) and transducer of erbB2 (TOB).

Another microarray study assessed 12,558 genes, using hippocampal tissue from the Harvard Brain Tissue Resource (Konradi et al., 2004). In this study, the expression of 43 genes was found to be decreased in bipolar disorder; 18 of these genes coded for mitochondrial proteins. Expression of GAD67 and somatostatin were decreased as well. A third microarray study assessed about 12,000 genes using prefrontal cortex (Iwamoto et al., 2004). The investigators found altered expression of 53 genes in bipolar disorder, 7 of which overlapped with schizophrenia and 8 with major depressive disorder. The study focused on two genes, *HSPF1* and *LIM*, whose expression was also altered in lymphoblastoid cells from bipolar subjects. This same group conducted an expression study of 676 mitochondria-related genes (Iwamoto et al., 2005). They found a global decrease in expression of these genes in the prefrontal cortex of bipolar subjects, but they also found evidence that the decrease was correlated with both sample pH and medication use. When these factors were accounted for, there were 27 genes with altered expression, 23 of which showed up-regulation.

Other studies, like that of Iwamoto and colleagues (2005) noted above, have found changes in expression levels of genes in both bipolar and schizophrenic samples. One of these studies found a reduction in eight oligodendrocyte- and myelin-related genes in both bipolar and schizophrenic subjects (Tkachev et al., 2003). Two of these genes—*OLIG2* on 21q22.11 and *SOX10* on 22q13.1—are in bipolar disorder linkage regions; another, *ERBB3*, is particularly interesting functionally as it codes for the receptor of neuregulin 1, a gene strongly implicated in schizophrenia.

In subjects with both disorders, the expression levels of the genes coding for neuronal calcium sensor-1 (Koh et al., 2003) and apolipoprotein L2 (Mimmack et al., 2002) were found to be increased in the prefrontal cortex, and the expression levels for synapsin IIa and IIIa were decreased (the expression levels for synapsin Ia were decreased only in the bipolar brains) (Vawter et al., 2002). Expression levels of RELN, coding for the reelin protein, and GAD67, coding for a form of glutamate decarboxylase, were decreased in the brains of subjects with psychotic bipolar disorder and with schizophrenia when prefrontal cortex and cerebellum were assayed (Guidotti et al., 2000). The decrease in RELN expression appears to be mediated through an epigenetic change known as *hypermethylation* in the promoter region of the gene. The addition of a methyl group to the C nucleotide residing in this region may result in reduced binding of transcription factors (which facilitate gene expression), leading in turn to decreased expression of the gene. In a mouse model of reelin expression, investigators found that when mice were injected with methionine, an amino acid that provides methyl groups, the mice showed a decrease in reelin expression; further, they displayed poorer performance on a test of prepulse inhibition, which is thought to be a neurophysiological endophentype for schizophrenia (Tremolizzo et al., 2002).

Studies of gene expression in the bipolar brain face a number of important difficulties. One is simply the limited access to tissues. Although samples are available, the number of samples remains small, limiting the power to detect modest changes. Second, the quality of the available tissue varies, as samples undergo varying postmortem delay prior to autopsy and varying pH due to differences in the agonal period prior to death—both of which affect RNA quality (Johnston et al., 1997). Third, samples studied typically come from patients who have been treated with psychiatric medications, which may themselves alter gene expression. Fourth, there may be microbrain region-specific expression alterations that are not readily detected or replicated in gross samples. Finally, although transcriptome-wide approaches hold great promise, the technology is still evolving, so that aspects of data analysis, reliability, and validity remain to be fully resolved.

Expression in White Blood Cells

Studies using lymphoblast cells or granulocytes from patients have the great advantage that these samples are much more readily obtainable than brain tissue. A recent study demonstrates the value of using lymphoblastoid cell lines to examine variation in gene expression levels. Cheung and colleagues (2003) examined expression levels in lymphoblastoid cells from normal individuals, including some sibling pairs and some MZ twin pairs. They found that for some genes, expression levels varied significantly among the subjects. For five genes that were intensively studied, the variance among individuals was 3–11 times greater in unrelated individuals than among MZ twins, and the variance among sibling pairs was 2–5 times greater than among these twins. These results suggest that heritable factors that vary among individuals contribute to differences in levels of gene expression.

Although studies have indicated that functional abnormalities exist in the lymphocytes of bipolar patients, there have been few efforts to examine gene expression. The major weakness of this approach to studying bipolar disorder is that it is not clear that expression in these white blood cells mirrors expression in neurons, as control of expression may be tissue- and cell type–specific.

On the other hand, some abnormalities that have been detected in lymphocytes appear to mirror changes detected in postmortem brain tissue from bipolar subjects. For example, low inositol levels have been found in the frontal cortex of patients, as well as in lymphocytes (Shimon et al., 1997; Belmaker et al., 2002). A crucial component of the inositol pathway is inositol monophosphatase (IMPase). A report examining IMPase activity in drug-free bipolar patients using quantitative reverse transcription–polymerase chain reaction (RT-PCR) on lymphocytes found an approximately two-thirds reduction in IMPase-relative messenger RNA levels compared with control subjects (Nemanov et al., 1999). Yoon and colleagues (2001) found decreased IMPA2 messenger RNA levels in lymphoblasotid cell lines from BP-I patients, though only in males with decreased basal levels of intracellular calcium. Inositol system genes have been considered leading candidates for involvement in bipolar etiology because of this system's central involvement in response to mood-stabilizing medications (Williams et al., 2002). One study examined messenger RNA levels of three G protein alpha subunits and of phosphatidylinositol-3 kinase (PI-3K) regulatory subunit p85 in the granulocytes of bipolar patients compared with controls. One of the G protein alpha subunits, alpha(s), was markedly increased in bipolar patients; this increase was observed in both lithium-treated and unmedicated patients.

Testing Gene- and Allele-Specific Function

Functional studies of the impact of an allele associated with bipolar disorder can be performed using cell culture. A copy of the gene containing the candidate allele can be inserted (transfected) into cells in culture. These cells can then be compared with control cells. Gene expression in these cells can be measured, as can relevant consequences of gene function, such as binding capacity for a receptor. For example, the serotonin transporter promoter polymorphism was studied in this way. Lymphoblast cell lines were transfected with genes encoding the long variant and genes encoding the short variant. The transcriptional activity of the long variant was found to be twice that of the short variant (Lesch et al., 1996). The observation that this variant is functionally significant has helped make the serotonin transporter promoter polymorphism the object of intense study.

Another example of the use of cell culture to study candidate gene function comes from a report on the gene *DISC-1*. To understand why *DISC-1* is a candidate gene for manic-depressive illness requires a brief digression to discuss a method called *cytogenetics*. Cytogenetics is the third method—linkage and linkage disequilibrium being the other two—that can provide evidence for particular genes as positional candidates. This approach involves detecting chromosomal aberrations in families with manic-depressive illness and determining whether the aberration travels with the illness across generations. A chromosomal aberration, referred to as a *balanced translocation*, between chromosomes 1 and 11 has been reported, in which a portion of each chromosome has broken off and joined onto the broken end of the other. This phenomenon can be tolerated, except to the extent that the breakpoints result in the disruption of genes. In a large family containing 87 members, 37 were found to carry the translocation, including 7 individuals with schizophrenia, 1 with bipolar disorder, and 10 with recurrent major depression. The breakpoint on chromosome 1 has been found to disrupt two genes—*DISC-1* and *DISC-2*. Researchers have shown that the DISC-1 protein normally associates with another protein, NUDEL, which is associated with cortical development and is linked to *LIS-1*, the disease gene for a form of lissencephaly, a disorder of cortical development. The abnormal form of DISC-1, the form predicted to occur in individuals with the translocation, failed to bind NUDEL. Neuronal cells were transfected with either normal or abnormal *DISC-1* genes. While neuronal outgrowth was normal in the normal DISC-1 cells, it was reduced in the abnormal DISC-1 cells (Ozeki et al., 2003). These results support the potential involvement of *DISC-1* in the etiology of recurrent affective illness, and schizophrenia.

An even more powerful approach to the study of gene function is to create mouse models for the gene under study. A variety of approaches exist for genetically altering the mouse. The *knockout* approach allows for the creation of a mouse lacking one or both copies of the gene. Tissue-specific knockout methods allow even more narrowly defined gene effects to be examined. In the conditional knockout, the mouse carries the gene, but investigators can turn it off at will. Transgenic approaches allow for the introduction of extra copies of normal genes or copies of altered genes. The *knockin* approach allows for the simultaneous knockout of the normal gene and transgenic insertion of an altered version of the gene. With these mouse models, gene effects in the brain and on behavior can be studied. For example, a mouse model of Huntington's disease was created using a transgenic *huntingtin* gene, which was altered to carry the disease mutation (abnormal variant) and was under conditional control using a tetracycline-responsive system. The mouse exhibited Huntington's disease–like motor symptoms because of the action of the mutant gene. When the investigators administered tetracycline to the mice and thus turned off the mutant gene, the symptoms abated (Yamamoto et al., 2000). These methods have not yet been applied to the study of bipolar disorder, though they have been applied to depression.

The glucocorticoid receptor (GR) has been much studied in mouse models of depression and anxiety. The following lines of mice have been generated: those with disrupted *GR* alleles; those with nervous system–specific knockout of *GR*; transgenic mice with increased GR expression; transgenic mice that express an antisense RNA, which results in decreased GR expression by binding to and neutralizing the normal GR RNA; and knockin mice, in which the normal gene is knocked out while abnormal *GR* genes are introduced and then expressed (Gass et al., 2001). Behaviors thought to model depression—such as performance on the Porsolt forced swim test, the tail suspension test, or the learned helplessness paradigm—can be measured in these genetically altered mice as a way of gauging the impact of the gene, and these behaviors may have relevance for manic-depressive illness. Attempts at creating animal models of depression with these mice have yielded mixed results, however. Behaviorally, none of these mouse lines has consistently exhibited depression-like impairment. The transgenic line with decreased GR expression did, however, show an enhanced stress-associated adrenocorticotropic hormone (ACTH) response, which was normalized by antidepressant medication treatment. This finding suggests that the endocrinological component of depression might be partially modeled in this mouse line (Montkowski et al., 1995).

Other genes studied in this way include *BDNF* and the serotonin transporter gene. A line of mice carrying a knockout of one of two *BDNF* alleles was developed and studied for depressive-like behaviors. The knockout mice generally did not show significant differences from wild mice in their propensity to these behaviors; thus they may not constitute a model for depression (MacQueen et al., 2001). A serotonin transporter gene knockout mouse line has also been developed. When investigators studied this knockout using two genetically disparate mouse lines, they found that in one line, the knockout mice showed decreased immobility on the tail suspension test, whereas in the other, the knockout mice did not differ on this test. The former group showed a reaction consistent with an antidepressant-like effect, which would be expected because these mice had an increased extracellular level of serotonin, but the other group did not. It is possible that the behavioral difference was mediated by an interaction of the serotonin transporter gene with other, as yet unknown, genes that vary between the two mouse lines (Holmes et al., 2002).

Although no genetically engineered mouse models for mania exist, one team of investigators suggested using rats administered amphetamine for such a model (Niculescu et al., 2000). They argued that the euphoric and stimulated state that results in humans who ingest this drug is reminiscent of mania, and the hyperactive state that results in rats may be a reasonable proxy. The researchers gave rats amphetamines and then a day later sacrificed them and extracted RNA from their amygdala and prefrontal cortex. The expression levels of 8,000 genes were assessed simultaneously in these samples by means of a microarray. The investigators were particularly interested in the altered expression of genes having human homologues that mapped to regions of prior linkage interest in bipolar disorder and schizophrenia. They found altered expression of eight genes that met this criterion, one of which—*GRK3* (G-protein receptor kinase 3)—was expressed 14-fold more in the prefrontal cortex of the amphetamine-treated rats than in that of the control samples. The human homologue maps to chromosome 22q11, where the same investigators had suggestive evidence for linkage with bipolar disorder.

Reports are beginning to emerge from studies examining aspects of allele-specific functions of genes in the human brain. For example, the serotonin transporter promoter region polymorphism was assessed in relation to amygdala activation in a functional magnetic resonance imaging paradigm. Subjects carrying a short variant of the polymorphism had greater amygdala activation in response to fearful stimuli compared with those having only the long variant. This result was consistent with a prior observation of greater anxiety associated with carrying the short allele (Hariri et al., 2002).

FROM GENE TO BEDSIDE: PHARMACOGENETICS AND GENETIC COUNSELING

Pharmacogenetics

Pharmacogenetics is a field that first developed in the 1950s with clinical observations of inherited differences in drug effects. In the early 1960s, a few studies of familial correlation in response to antidepressants were published. One such study found that of 41 pairs of relatives treated with the antidepressant imipramine, 38 had a concordant response: both responded in 34 pairs, neither responded in 4 pairs, and one responded in 3 pairs (Angst, 1961, 1964, cited in Pare and Mack, 1971). A second study, by Pare and colleagues (1962), found that in 8 relative pairs, there was concordance for 6 of 6 pairs of tricyclic antidepressant trials and for 6 of 6 pairs of MAOI antidepressant trials. Pare and Mack (1971) later reported concordance in 10 of 12 new pairs of related patients treated with antidepressants from the same class, making the total 22 of 24 (92 percent) for the Pare et al. and Pare and Mack studies. By contrast, analysis of relatives' responses to antidepressants of different classes from the two studies revealed concordance in just 7 of 18 pairs (39 percent) (Pare and Mack, 1971).

The first study to report on familial correlation in lithium response involved just six children of lithium-responsive relatives. The two children in the study who had bipolar disorder both had clear responses to lithium (McKnew et al., 1981). In the only sizable study of familiality of lithium response, 24 bipolar relatives of lithium responders were assessed, along with 40 lithium-treated patients from an outpatient clinic. The prevalence of unequivocal response among the relatives was 67 percent, compared with a response rate of 35 percent in the comparison clinic group (Grof et al., 2002).

More recent studies have analyzed the relationship of allelic variation in biological candidate genes to drug response. At least nine studies have examined lithium response in bipolar disorder in this way. Negative findings have been reported for the dopamine type 2, 3, and 4 receptors; for the serotonin type 1A, 2A, and 2C receptors; and for the GABAA-α1, INPP1, and PLC-γ1 genes (Serretti et al., 2002c). A study of the tryptophan hydroxylase gene found a worse lithium response for those with the A/A variant of the gene, though this difference was only marginally significant (Serretti et al., 1999b). One published study of the serotonin transporter gene found a significantly worse response in subjects carrying two copies of the short allele in the promoter region polymorphism (Serretti et al., 2001). Another study found that people carrying a particular version of a variant within their mitochondrial DNA had a better response to lithium than those without this version (Washizuka et al., 2003).

At least 14 studies have examined antidepressant response in relation to gene variants. The serotonin transporter gene promoter region variant has been studied most extensively because the selective serotonin reuptake inhibitor (SSRI) antidepressants are known to work through the protein product of this gene (and because the variant is functionally significant). Eight of eleven published studies have suggested a better response to SSRIs in patients with long alleles and a slower or worse response in subjects with short alleles. Of interest, one study included a group treated with nortriptyline as well as one treated with paroxetine. Those with the long allele in that study did not respond as quickly to nortriptyline as they did to paroxetine (Pollock et al., 2000), a result suggesting the possibility of an SSRI-specific effect. The findings of three studies, however, were not consistent with those of the other eight, showing a better response to SSRIs for carriers of the short allele or no association (see Table 13–9). It may be significant that two of the three negative studies involved Asian populations, while seven of the eight positive studies involved populations of European ancestry. The short and long alleles have been shown to be composed of subtypes, and these subtypes have been found to vary between Japanese and Caucasian populations (Nakamura et al., 2000). Given that one study in a Chinese sample was positive for the long variant, however, this explanation may be incomplete. Further uncertainty stems from the observation by Mundo and colleagues (2001a) that bipolar patients who had experienced antidepressant-induced mania were more likely to carry the short allele than those who did not have this response to antidepressants. The authors hypothesized that the short allele may be associated with an exaggerated response to antidepressants, which is difficult to reconcile with the findings noted above.

A number of other gene variants have been studied in relation to antidepressant response. Variants of the tryptophan hydroxylase gene were found to be associated with slower or poorer response to SSRIs in two studies (Serretti et al., 2001; Peters et al., 2004), while variants of the serotonin 2A receptor and of the G-protein beta-3 gene were associated with response to mixed antidepressants in one study each. A variant of the norepinephrine transporter gene was associated with response to milnacipran, a serotonin and norepinephrine reuptake inhibitor, in a small sample (Yoshida et al., 2004). No association with antidepressant response was found in studies of the dopamine 2 and 4 receptors or of the *MAOA* gene.

Genetic Counseling

Studies of the familial aggregation of manic-depressive illness (especially the bipolar form) have provided valuable data that can be used by clinicians to help educate concerned

Table 13–9. Studies of the Association of the Serotonin Transporter Gene Promoter Region Variant with Response to Selective Serotonin Reuptake Inhibitor (SSRI) Antidepressants

Study	Sample Size	Medication	Result
Positive			
Smeraldi et al., 1998	99	Fluvoxamine	L allele associated with better response, $p = 017$
Zanardi et al., 2000	64	Paroxetine	L allele associated with more favorable and faster response, $p < .0001$
Pollock et al., 2000	95	Paroxetine	L/L genotype associated with more rapid response, $p = .028$
Zanardi, 2001	155	Fluvoxamine	L allele associated with better response, $p = .002$
Yu et al., 2002	121	Fluoxetine	L/L allele carriers had better response, $p = .013$
Rausch et al., 2002	51	Fluoxetine	L allele associated with better response, $p < .03$
Serretti et al., 2004	220	Fluvoxamine or paroxetine	L allele associated with better response, $p = .034$
Murphy et al., 2004	255	Paroxetine	L/L genotype associated with better response, $p = .04$
Negative			
Kim et al., 2000	120	Fluoxetine/paroxetine	S/S genotype associated with better response, $p = .007$
Yoshida et al., 2002	66	Fluvoxamine	S allele associated with better response, $p = .01$
Peters et al., 2004	96	Fluoxetine	No association reported

Source: Based on Serretti et al., 2002a.

patients who wonder what vulnerabilities they may be passing on to their children. Particularly when they are considering conceiving a child, patients often ask clinicians for information and sometimes advice concerning their plans. On the one hand, some patients may be unaware of the increased likelihood that their children will develop manic-depressive illness (see the above section on family studies). On the other hand, some people have exaggerated fears about the risk of illness. One of the authors of this text counseled a healthy woman who was considering having her first child. She was concerned because her brother-in-law had bipolar disorder, and she feared that her child might develop it as well. When she was informed that the risk for developing bipolar disorder in a second-degree relative was just 2–3 percent, she felt more at ease.

Although risk data from genetic epidemiology are of some value in providing a sense of the magnitude of risk for developing bipolar or recurrent unipolar disorder, it is also important to bear in mind that enormous variation in the rates of illness among family members will be evident in any collection of pedigrees. This observation illustrates an important weakness of counseling based on averages. Genetic counseling for such illnesses as cystic fibrosis, Huntington's disease, and Tay-Sachs disease is based on a genetic assay that can yield a fairly precise prediction of risk. In contrast, because the genes for bipolar disorder remain largely unidentified and unstudied in terms of risk, counselors and clinicians do not yet have available the kind of data that would allow for more exact predictions.

Additional complexities affect the potential benefits of genetic counseling: manic-depressive illness is for the most part not a fatal condition; there are several available treatments, and there is good reason to believe that many patients can lead full and meaningful lives with treatment; and the risk data that exist do not distinguish between those in whom the illness would be severe and those who would respond well to standard treatments. What is quite predictable in a family at high risk seeking counseling is that the delay in recognition and diagnosis of manic-depressive illness in all affected children will likely be brief compared with the usual decade-long delay encountered by those with the bipolar form of the illness. There are many reasons to believe that much morbidity can be prevented by such early diagnosis.

Our practice has been to ask common clinical psychiatric questions as well as standard family-history questions of couples seeking counseling. For example: "Why do you want a child now as opposed to at some other time? What are your plans for child care?" And for a mother with bipolar disorder: "What are the risks and plans if a postpartum (puerpual) depression or mania ensues?" These standard clinical questions usually lead to the most fruitful discussions of the prospective parents' expectations. A sensible determination of the wisdom of proceeding with childbearing can often be made in the current era in which precise DNA tests are lacking.

Couples who come for counseling reveal scenarios both common and worrisome. Some have difficult marriages and want a child to bring them closer together. Other couples present a situation in which the prospective mother had bipolar disorder. In one instance she was also the prime breadwinner in the family, and had a brittle illness in which pregnancy and changes of medication had led to severe relapses. The couple had not formulated a plan for what they would do if the mother became ill before, during, or after childbirth. On the other hand, very (financially and emotionally) secure couples express worries about modest risks of illness. In some cases, the parent's illness is under excellent control with simple monotherapies. These couples often have not fully considered the pragmatic aspects of their prospective child's potential functional level. When asking such couples about their concerns, one might ask: "Well, what if he or she turns out exactly like you (the ill parent)?" When the answer is "OK, I think that would be wonderful," the question of risk levels can become moot again.

Three studies have attempted to assess how genetic counseling might proceed in the future. These studies examined the attitudes of patients and their families toward genetic testing for bipolar genes, should such tests become available. One study found that the overwhelming majority of patients and spouses said they would take advantage of genetic tests for bipolar disorder if such tests were to become available, primarily to ensure that they would obtain treatment to prevent episodes of illness. A majority of respondents said they would "definitely not" abort a fetus that carried a bipolar gene, and a majority agreed that the knowledge that one of them carried such a gene would not have deterred them from marriage or childbearing (Trippitelli et al., 1998). The results of another study were similar: the vast majority of respondents supported genetic testing for adults and children, but 70 percent did not support prenatal testing as a means of deciding whether abortion would be indicated (Jones et al., 2002).

Smith and colleagues (1996), however, painted a more complex picture. In their study of members of a bipolar support group, medical students, and psychiatry residents, a clear majority of respondents said they would have their children tested for a bipolar gene if prophylactic treatment were available, though interest was more mixed in the absence of such treatment. The proportion of subjects who said they would choose termination of pregnancy depended on both the likelihood and the severity of illness indicated by a positive test. With a 25 percent likelihood of illness or a mild course of illness, fewer than 10 percent preferred termination, whereas with a 100 percent chance of illness or a severe course, the proportion who said they would terminate was much higher—40–55 percent and 70–85 percent, respectively.

LOOKING TO THE FUTURE

Research Directions

From Linkage to Association

Linkage studies, the workhorse of research in bipolar genetics since the late 1980s, will move from center stage as association studies assume a greater role. The chromosomal regions implicated by bipolar linkage studies will be studied using large case–control and trio (case–parents) samples. This shift is occurring because linkage studies can identify the general chromosomal localization of a gene, but only association can truly pinpoint the location of the disease gene and, even more specifically, the location of the particular variant within the gene that is responsible for disease susceptibility. By analogy, think of searching for a needle in 23 enormous haystacks. Linkage is analogous to figuring out which haystack and which general area of that haystack holds the needle. Once that has been accomplished, a more fine-grained approach is needed to sort through the pieces of straw. Association is that fine-grained method.

Association Methods and Strategies

The feasibility of performing association studies is advancing rapidly as SNP genotyping methodologies become faster, more accurate, and less expensive. Several good methodologies exist, though no single one has yet emerged as the definitive best option. The number of SNPs available on Web-based databases is in the millions already and still growing. Further, biotechnology companies have genotyping assays prepared for SNPs within tens of thousands of genes, making these studies even more readily available to researchers.

The recent discovery that haplotype blocks exist in the genome across broad populations has led to the proposal that association could be performed more cost-effectively using these blocks than was previously thought possible. Most individuals might share one of just four or five variants of a given block. Thus characterizing the variation across most individuals for the block to determine which haplotype they have might require genotyping 15–20 SNPs rather than all 200 or so that would be predicted to exist in the block. This proposal rests on the assumption of the common disease–common variant hypothesis, under which the common haplotype blocks would likely harbor the common alleles that predispose some people to manic-depressive illness. An alternative position holds that testing gene-related SNPs is much more efficient. This approach would require genotyping only one-tenth as many SNPs, and those tested would stand a far greater chance of being the functionally relevant variants. This approach would also allow for the possibility of detecting lower-frequency disease alleles (Botstein and Risch, 2003).

Power

Very large samples are now being gathered for bipolar studies. The NIMH Bipolar Disorder Collaborative study has already ascertained and assessed a linkage sample of 644 families with 921 affected sibling pairs. The collaborative is currently in the process of acquiring a sample of 5,000 cases for association studies, including, potentially, studies that would assay 500,000 SNPs simultaneously across the genome (whole-genome association). Very large samples have the power to detect the modest gene effects likely to play a role in susceptibility to bipolar disorder. Large samples also provide sufficient power to employ new analytical techniques that can test for interactions between genes.

Genetic Homogeneity

Use of phenotypic subtypes and endophenotypes may allow linkage and association to be performed on more genetically homogeneous subgroups within bipolar disorder. This capability would prevent the dilution of individual gene effects that occurs when all bipolar subjects are considered jointly if multiple genes are contributing to the broad phenotype. Potential examples of relevant subgroups are BP-II, BP-I with psychotic features, bipolar disorder with comorbid panic disorder, BP-I with an early age at onset, and lithium-responsive bipolar disorder. More work is needed to define genetically meaningful clinical subtypes and to determine familial endophenotypic measures. Conversely, genetic findings may help clarify the validity of potential subtypes. For example, we may come to better understand how early-onset recurrent major depression differs from less recurrent severe forms of depression; such understanding could allow us to differentiate the genetics of recurrence or cyclicity from that of polarity. Population isolates may also be of use in limiting genetic heterogeneity.

Gene Expression and Pathogenesis

Findings of statistical association between a gene variant and manic-depressive illness will need to be complemented by functional studies of the relevant gene and its potentially pathogenic alleles. Given its greater homogeneity relative to the very broad category of recurrent unipolar as defined by DSM-IV, the bipolar subgroup provides the most fruitful phenotype for such studies. For example, postmortem brain samples from bipolar subjects will be a valuable resource for testing gene expression levels. Brain tissue is, of course, not available on subjects who are studied for linkage and association, but lymphoblastoid cell lines are. Although these cells express only about one-half of all genes, and potential tissue-specific regulation of gene expression may limit their usefulness, the existence of such cell lines in the very bipolar subjects who show association could provide investigators with a useful means of studying the expression of some candidate genes.

In the best-case scenario, a smoking-gun genetic lesion will be found that is clearly and obviously an etiologic factor in bipolar disorder. Such a lesion might be a nonsense mutation leading to a truncated and entirely dysfunctional protein product. This hypothesis would be most persuasive if the mutation occurred in a large percentage of cases and in no subjects who were not cases. If, in addition, the gene coded for a protein that had a known role in neurotransmission or neuronal migration, the case for an etiologic role would be exceedingly strong. An example of this situation is the Duchenne's muscular dystrophy gene, where the majority of mutations result in truncation of the dystrophin protein. Similarly, researchers studying Crohn's disease found a gene, *NOD2*, with a truncating mutation in some cases (Ogura et al., 2001). This gene codes for a protein involved in the immune response to bacterial lipopolysaccharides, a process previously implicated in the disease.

Perhaps more likely is that assembly of the smoking gun will be required. We are likely to find variations in genes that have subtle effects, such as the substitution of one amino acid for another, or the increased or decreased level of expression of the gene and, hence, the protein product. These variations may occur more often than expected in patients, though they may also occur in nonpatients. We will need to see multiple replications, and these may have to occur in large samples for the small effects to be detectable. A potential complication here is that a given genetic variation may be clearly associated with disease in one population, but may be rare and thus only minimally associated with disease in another population. The finding of an association between calpain-10 and non-insulin–dependent diabetes in Mexican Americans illustrates the difficulties involved in demonstrating a cause–effect relationship between a gene of small effect and disease (Horikawa et al., 2000). Studies of association in other ethnic populations have not been obviously supportive, with a negative association being reported in Japanese subjects (Horikawa et al., 2003) and four nonsignificant results in Europeans (see Rasmussen et al., 2002). When the four European samples were pooled, however, a significant result with an odds ratio for the risk haplotype of 1.62 was obtained.

Ultimately, determination of the relationship between a gene and bipolar illness will require studies that go beyond

DNA to look at gene expression (RNA), the protein product, and pathogenesis as well. It may be possible to study genotype–endophenotype correlations. If a gene is involved in bipolar illness, it should be possible to demonstrate the effect the disease allele has on, for example, P300 deficits and white-matter hyperintensities. Given the likelihood of relatively modest effects for bipolar susceptibility alleles, a conclusive case for the involvement of an implicated gene may require demonstration of a pathogenic pathway.

Gene–Environment Interactions

Once bipolar genes have been discovered, researchers will want to know whether the illness occurs more often when people carrying the susceptibility allele are exposed to particular factors or experiences. A number of environmental exposures that have been suggested as causative factors in manic-depressive illness, whether bipolar or recurrent depressive, such as loss of a parent at an early age or obstetrical complications, could be assessed to determine whether they increase the risk of illness in conjunction with the risk genotype. For example, the interaction between the short variant of the serotonin transporter promoter polymorphism and stressful life events may play a role in the predisposition to major depressive episodes (Caspi et al., 2003).

Future Prospects for Patients

Pharmacogenetics

Pharmacogenetic studies could provide the first exciting clinical benefits to come from genetic investigations of manic-depressive illness. If the illness is genetically heterogenous, some of its genetic forms could predict response to one treatment, such as lithium, while other forms could predict response to another treament, such as carbamazepine, valproate, or lamotragine. For treating nonrecurrent depression, there may be some genetic vulnerabilities associated with good SSRI response, and other genetic vulnerabilities associated with a better response to noradrenergic medications such as bupropion or desipramine. These findings could allow clinicians to optimize the use of already-effective medications by choosing the drug most likely to work for a given patient with a particular genetic profile.

Rational Drug Development

Fundamental benefit will come from an improved understanding of the pathophysiology of manic-depressive illness in both its bipolar and recurrent unipolar forms. Finding a gene will lead to an examination of the functions of its protein product in the neuron. This examination could lead in turn to the elucidation of a cascade of neuronal events at work in the disorder. Understanding of these basic processes would guide the search for treatments of bipolar and/or recurrent unipolar disorder, and could illuminate the mechanisms and functions of mood regulation generally. The gene product or another protein with which the gene product interacts could be a target for conventional pharmacology, such as receptor blockade or inactivation of an enzyme. Alternatively, the gene product could be cloned and introduced, as has been done with blood clotting factor VIII (for hemophilia A) and growth hormone (for growth hormone deficiency).

Gene Therapy

Even variations on gene therapy, where the aim is to modify gene function directly, could be conceived. The gene itself could be directly targeted by gene augmentation therapy if loss of function of a gene were the problem, with extra copies of the normal gene being introduced. Alternatively, targeted inhibition of gene expression could be employed if there were a novel gene product or inappropriate expression of a gene; this could be accomplished using antisense therapeutics, whereby gene-specific antisense sequences block the effects of a given susceptibility gene. The desirability of such an intervention is less than clear when a "susceptibility" gene rather than a "causative" gene is at issue, however, because a susceptibility gene may have important positive as well as negative effects (see the section below on pitfalls).

Diagnosis

There are currently no laboratory methods for diagnosing bipolar or recurrent unipolar disorder; rather, these diagnoses rest solely on clinical data. Identification of a causative gene could clarify the diagnostic process by providing physical evidence of the disorder (though see the discussion of pitfalls for a cautionary note). Presymptomatic diagnosis may also become possible and could lead to preventive treatments. Greater precision in prognosis may come from genotype–phenotype correlations, whereby particular symptom clusters and natural course are found to be associated with specific gene variants. This could be especially helpful in sharpening the definitions within the broad category of "recurrent unipolar," which in DSM-IV can range from two episodes in a lifetime to highly cyclic cases with as many lifetime episodes as are typically seen in untreated bipolar disorder.

Prevention

The role of life events and other environmental factors in the causation of bipolar or early-onset recurrent unipolar disorder may be defined more clearly by epidemiologic studies when groups homogeneous for the presence of a bipolar or recurrent unipolar susceptibility gene can be ascertained.

Preventive efforts targeted at reducing these factors in vulnerable individuals would logically follow. This has been done most effectively for phenylketonuria, a rare genetic disease in which failure to metabolize dietary phenylalanine leads to severe mental retardation. This devastating outcome is now largely prevented through identification of newborns with the mutation and the implementation of a phenylalanine-restricted (and tyrosine-supplemented) diet.

Stigma

Finding a gene for manic-depressive illness would accelerate efforts at destigmatizing the condition by establishing it even more firmly as a disease rather than a frightening mystery or a weakness of character. It may also be possible to define a relationship between disease-promoting gene variants and adaptive psychological functions, such as creativity (Jamison, 1993), which would further destigmatize the disorder by illuminating positive aspects of the genetic endowment.

Pitfalls

Though the promise of genetics is great, expectations have far outpaced actual progress in the minds of some. Study participants sometimes ask when they will get back their results because of the mistaken belief that genetic testing for manic-depressive illness (especially bipolar disorder) is already available. Not only is such testing currently unavailable, but it is also not clear that a useful genetic test will emerge even when a bipolar gene is found. Because risk alleles for the disorder may elevate risk only to a relatively small degree, they may prove to be of questionable predictive value. The *APOE4* allele of the *APOE* gene, which confers increased risk for Alzheimer's disease, provides an illustrative example. The risk of Alzheimer's across the population is 9 percent. Having a copy of the *APOE4* allele increases the lifetime risk to 17 percent. It is difficult to know whether this information would be useful to people. Indeed, experts have generally recommended against performing diagnostic genetic tests for this gene (Liddell et al., 2001). On the other hand, a study of three susceptibility genes for deep venous thrombosis showed that, while having a single disease gene variant increased the disease risk to only a minor degree, having disease variants in all three genes led to an eight-fold increase in risk (Yang et al., 2003). Similarly with bipolar disorder, diagnostic and predictive testing may become valuable after several disease genes have been identified.

Another area of concern is the possibility of unintended consequences of obtaining genetic information about manic-depressive illness. At the beginning of this chapter, the misuse of genetics in the form of the eugenics movement, and eventually in the form of the mass murder of mental patients, was described. This history suggests the need to think carefully about what people will do with the knowledge generated by genetic studies. One major concern is whether parents would choose to abort fetuses known to carry, for example, bipolar susceptibility genes. Might there be a price to pay for this kind of intervention? What if Abraham Lincoln or Winston Churchill, both of whom had mood disorders, had never been born?

The temptation may also arise to modify germ cells to purge the germ line of susceptibility alleles. The technical danger here stems from uncertainty about the biological results of such manipulations. For example, while the celebrated cloning of Dolly the sheep and other mammals appeared initially to be a great success, these efforts were subsequently plagued by the development of an overgrowth syndrome in many of the cloned animals (Young et al., 1998). Similarly, there is some evidence that in vitro fertilization procedures used by infertile couples may increase the risk of altered gene programming that can lead to disease (DeBaun et al., 2003).

Beyond biological concerns regarding germ-line manipulation, there are ethical concerns. As Billings and colleagues (1999, p. 1874) noted:

> Choices about . . . programmes for enhancement would . . . reflect prejudices, socioeconomic and political inequalities, and even current fashion. . . . [G]ermline intervention would intentionally subject later generations to modifications undertaken on the basis of existing values and conditions. The chance that 'desirable' manipulations might later be viewed as disastrous makes germline enhancement 'therapies' unacceptable.

While we can envision a time when we may have a comprehensive understanding of manic-depressive illness genes, their interactions, their role in the brain, and their role in behavior, as well as a full understanding of the technical requirements for adroitly manipulating the germ line, that time is a very long way off.

CONCLUSIONS

Genetic Epidemiology of Manic-Depressive Illness

For the bipolar subgroup, the risk of illness in a first-degree relative of an ill person is roughly 10 times the risk in a random person. The risk of having the illness if an identical twin has it is about 63 percent. The calculated heritability for bipolar disorder from twin studies is about .78. For major depression, the risk to first-degree relatives of depressed probands is about three times higher than the overall population risk. The risk in identical twins of depressed probands is about 34 percent, and the calculated heritability is also about 34 percent. These numbers are higher when probands with the highly recurrent forms of depression are examined. There have been fewer adoption studies of manic-depressive illness; the studies that have been done modestly support a genetic contribution to the illness. Taken together, the data indicate a strong genetic component to susceptibility to bipolar disorder and a less strong, though still significant, genetic component to susceptibility to major depression, especially the more recurrent forms. Modeling of disease transmission through family studies has suggested that bipolar disorder is most likely caused by at least three interacting susceptibility genes, and maybe more. Furthermore, family and twin studies clearly demonstrate a genetic relationship between bipolar disorder and major depression.

Advances in Understanding the Human Genome

About 20,000 genes exist in the human genome. The information they contain is spelled out in a nucleotide alphabet made up of four letters—the nucleotides G, C, A, and T. There are about 3 billion of these nucleotides spread over 23 chromosomes, and most of the sequence does not vary among people throughout the world. There is some variability, however, and it is in this occasional variability that potential differences in susceptibility to manic-depressive illness may be found. The capacity to investigate genes has benefited enormously from advances in genetic technology and information. Microsatellite markers have made possible highly informative linkage studies aimed at identifying chromosomal regions where disease genes might lie. The Human Genome Project has provided a wonderfully detailed roadmap of the genome, allowing those investigating manic-depressive illness to select genes to study from chromosomal regions of interest, and to choose SNPs to study from candidate genes or candidate regions.

The Linkage Method

The linkage method has been the major focus of genetic investigation of bipolar disorder since the mid-1980s. As of this writing, however, attempts to localize bipolar genes through linkage have had only limited success, as the findings obtained have not converged as consistently as might be hoped on one or a small number of chromosomal regions. The most likely reasons for this are that bipolar illness is a genetically complex disorder, meaning a number of different genes confer susceptibility to the disorder; that these genes may each individually confer only a modest increase in the risk of illness; and that differing combinations of susceptibility genes may cause disease in differing groups of people. Though the pace of progress has been slower than expected, the 20 or so genome scans of bipolar illness conducted to date have yielded some strong linkage

signals, some of which have been identified in a number of studies. The more promising linkage regions—including 4p16, 4q35, 6q22, 8q24, 12q24, 13q31–33, 16p12, 18p11–q12, 18q22–23, 21q22, and 22q11–13—are worthy of further study to clarify whether they do, in fact, harbor bipolar genes. The lack of definitive success in discovering bipolar genes has prompted some investigators to consider other approaches to the problem, including redefining the phenotype (such as focusing first on highly recurrent mood disorders and only secondarily on polarity) and rethinking potential genetic mechanisms that may underlie the disease.

Alternative Phenotypic Definition

Use of alternative methods of phenotypic definition may help define more genetically homogeneous groups of manic-depressive and bipolar subjects. Familial aggregation and linkage data exist for bipolar disorder to support the utility of subtyping by the presence of psychotic symptoms, of comorbid panic disorder, and of BP-II in families. Similar support exists for using age at onset as a phenotypic variable and for selecting families on the basis of lithium-responsive probands. Familial aggregation has been demonstrated for bipolar disorder with comorbid anxiety disorders and comorbid ADHD, but no correlation with linkage evidence has been reported. Little evidence exists at present for familial aggregation of cognitive impairments or temperamental vulnerabilities in bipolar disorder. Finally, the biological variables, or endophenotypes, of white-matter hyperintensities and abnormal P300 evoked potential have been found to be familial in individual pedigrees.

The Association Method

Association studies can be used for two different purposes. The first is to test directly whether a gene variant may be implicated in illness. Studies of this kind have until recently focused on monoamine system genes. Studies of genes encoding the serotonin transporter, the monoamine oxidase type A enzyme, the catechol-O-methyltransferase enzyme, and the type 2 and type 4 dopamine receptors have yielded some weakly positive, along with some negative findings. Small effects for variants of these genes in bipolar disorder are a possibility. More recently, an association has been found for three other genes—one coding for BDNF and two overlapping genes of unknown function, called *G72* and *G30*. The BDNF finding is promising, particularly because of biological evidence for the role of BDNF in depression and in antidepressant response, but cannot be viewed as conclusive because the effect is small, and replication has not been consistent. The *G72/G30* finding is notable for reproducing an association first seen with schizophrenia, for showing positive findings across six bipolar samples, and for being the only replicated positional candidate finding in bipolar studies. The second use of association studies is for the narrowing of linkage regions through linkage disequilibrium mapping. This approach was taken using a population isolate with linkage to 18p11.3, and the result was to narrow the region of interest to 19,000 bases, a stretch containing just two genes.

Alternative Genetic Mechanisms

Exploration of alternative genetic mechanisms of disease may aid in the process of gene discovery. Clinical observations have suggested some of these mechanisms. Anticipation, or worsening severity of illness in successive generations, has been observed, suggesting the trinucleotide repeat hypothesis, though subsequent clinical studies have not consistently confirmed the initial clinical observation. An excess of clinically defined maternal transmission of bipolar disorder has also been observed, indicating mitochondrial inheritance or genomic imprinting, though again, subsequent clinical studies have not consistently replicated the initial observation.

Of the genetic avenues pursued to date in the study of bipolar disorder, the trinucleotide repeat hypothesis and the mitochondrial inheritance hypothesis have been studied extensively but have not yielded bipolar genes to date, although work continues in these areas. The genomic imprinting hypothesis has generated some interesting leads that are currently being pursued. These include modest evidence of parent-of-origin–specific linkage on chromosomes 1q, 2p, 2q, 13q, 14q, 16q, and 18q, as well as modest evidence for parent-of-origin–specific association with bipolar disorder for the dopamine receptor type 4 gene and the dopamine decarboxylase gene, both of which lie near known imprinted genes.

Gene Expression and Pathogenesis

Proving that a gene—or more specifically a particular gene variant, an allele—is causally related to manic-depressive illness will require more than simply demonstrating a statistical association between the allele and the disease; an important piece of evidence would be the demonstration that the allele causes meaningful alteration in the structure or expression level of messenger RNA. A number of genes have been shown to have abnormal expression levels in the prefrontal cortex, hippocampus, or amygdala of bipolar subjects, though none of these findings have yet been replicated. Allelic variation, however, has not yet been shown to correlate with any of these changes. Studies in lymphoblastoid cell lines from the general population show inherited variation in the expression of a number of genes, but few studies of gene expression in white blood cells derived from bipolar subjects have been done.

Candidate genes and candidate allelic variants can be studied in cell culture and in genetically engineered mice. Cell culture has been employed to demonstrate that the serotonin transporter gene promoter polymorphism differentially affects transcriptional activity. No genetically engineered mice provide a clear animal model for depression or bipolar disorder at present. BDNF heterozyogous knockout mice did not show depressive-like behavior. Serotonin transporter knockout mice did show depressive-like behavior when the mice derived from one genetic background, but not when they derived from a second background. Transgenic mice with decreased glucocorticoid receptor expression showed endocrine abnormalities of the kind seen in depression, and these abnormalities were reversible with antidepressant administration, but the mice did not show depressive-like behavior.

Ultimate proof of a causal relationship between a gene variant and manic-depressive illness will depend on investigations that go beyond the study of nucleic acids. Changes in structure and/or function will need to be shown in the protein product of the putative disease gene. Further, the proposed disease allele should result in observable changes in aspects of biochemical pathway processes, in neuronal and/or glial function, in brain region structure or function, and in intermediate phenotype measures. Again, study of the promoter region polymorphism of the serotonin transporter gene provides an example of this kind of study. The short variant was shown to be associated with greater amygdala activation in response to fearful stimuli in a functional magnetic resonance imaging study.

Pharmacogenetics and Genetic Counseling

There is modest evidence suggesting that response to antidepressants and to lithium may be inherited traits. This finding implies that when a choice of medications must be made for patients with new-onset mood disorders, selecting one that has worked for a family member may be a sensible practice. While the familiality of lithium response suggests that genetic variation is responsible for differences in the drug's effectiveness, no particular gene has yet been clearly associated with these differences. A number of studies have suggested that the long promoter variant of the serotonin transporter gene may confer a greater likelihood or speed of response to SSRIs than the short promoter variant, though this result cannot yet be considered definitive.

Genetic counseling is a feature of current clinical practice. It should be informed by results of family studies, which suggest that on average, the risk to children of those with manic-depressive illness is elevated to a modest degree. There are no genetic tests available at present to provide precise estimates of the risk to children in specific cases. Should such tests become available, they are likely to be used in particular to aid in early diagnosis. Even without these tests, the attention paid by ill parents to the possibility of illness in their children can help ensure prompt diagnosis and treatment, which may stave off more substantial morbidity.

Looking to the Future

While linkage studies of major depression are just getting under way, work in bipolar genetics is moving toward association studies designed to narrow the localization of disease genes and to test gene variants for a role in bipolar disorder. These studies rely on a rapidly developing set of technologies for the detection, screening, and analysis of SNPs. The ongoing recruitment of large numbers of patients and families is creating study samples with the power to enable detection of relatively small gene effects and examination of the interactions between genes. The discovery of susceptibility genes will also be enhanced by approaches that decrease genetic heterogeneity, such as the study of phenotypic subtypes and endophenotypes. It is possible that the first genes for bipolar disorder have already been discovered, though ultimately proving that a particular gene plays an etiologic role in the illness will require studies that extend beyond DNA to demonstration of the gene's role in a pathogenic pathway.

The discovery of bipolar genes (and ultimately those associated with recurrent unipolar depression) will open the door to a number of potential benefits to patients. An intangible benefit may be the reduced stigma that would result from demonstrating that manic-depressive illness has a physical basis. Moreover, pharmacogenetics could allow clinicians to optimize their choice of medications based on a patient's genetic profile. The discovery of biochemical pathways of disease could lead to the development of novel medications. Gene therapy, in which unhelpful alleles are turned off or helpful ones turned on, might even become possible. Genetic testing could become a possibility as well for purposes of diagnosis, prognosis, prevention, or early intervention.

Despite these reasons for optimism about the future of genetic medicine in manic-depressive illness, there are also grounds for caution and pitfalls of which to be aware. Because of the possibility that alleles for the illness or any of its subgroups will have only small effects, the use of each individually in genetic testing may be limited. Even if the tests were useful, it is not clear that employing them in prenatal testing would ultimately be desirable. Though some people might be tempted to eliminate susceptibility alleles for manic-depressive illness from germ-line cells, this kind of manipulation is fraught with technical hazards and ethical dangers.

NOTES

1. Only studies that employed direct interviews of the majority of relatives are included here.

2. The 12 studies are those in the bipolar and BP-I sections of Table 13–2, with the exception of Heun and Maier because that study used the same sample as Maier et al.

3. This calculation incorporates data from both the bipolar proband studies and the BP-I proband studies. Heun and Maier is not counted since the subjects in this study are accounted for by the Maier et al. study.

4. One criticism of twin studies is that the equal-environment assumption is not necessarily true; rather, MZ twins are more likely to seek out similar environments or be treated more similarly by people in the environment than are DZ twins. The validity of the assumption has been tested in several ways. For example, some studies have refuted this criticism (Kendler et al., 1993c; Hettema et al., 1995; Xian et al., 2000) by failing to find differences in phenotypic similarity for psychiatric disorders based on perceived versus actual zygosity. A more direct approach to the question is that taken by Lytton and colleagues (1977), who observed young twins and their parents. They found that parents did respond more similarly to MZ than to DZ twins, but that this difference was in reaction to the behavior exhibited by the twins.

5. Only studies that employed direct interviews of the majority of relatives are included here.

6. Another important aspect of heritability is that it is not expected to be a constant figure, but to be population and environment dependent. Kendler (2001) summarized 10 studies of behavioral traits that demonstrate changing heritability over time. For example, Heath and colleagues (1985) showed that in Norway, heritability of educational attainment was about 40 percent for men born before World War II and about 70 percent for men born after. This result is thought to be due to increased equality of educational opportunity after the war, leading to a more merit-based system in which the innate potential of individuals could be expressed more fully (Heath et al., 1985).

7. As of this writing, the best-known of these websites are those of the National Center for Biotechnoloy Information (NCBI) (http://www.ncbi.nlm.nih.gov/), the University of California at Santa Cruz (UCSC) (http://www.genome.uscs.edu/), and Celera (proprietary).

8. An earlier study, from an Icelandic and English group, was the first to use repeat-length polymorphisms to test linkage in manic-depressive illness, employing markers derived from larger repeats, called *minisatellites* (Hodgkinson et al., 1987a).

9. A well-known example of the problems inherent in the approach is the case of the chromosome 11p linkage finding by Egeland and colleagues (1987), who originally reported an impressive LOD score of 4.08 at a DNA marker in a single large Amish family from southeastern Pennsylvania. However, restudy of the same family provided evidence against the linkage, with the LOD score dropping to −9.31. In the later reanalysis, additional subjects were included, and the diagnosis of some of the original subjects changed from unaffected to affected (Kelsoe et al., 1989). This reevaluation led to recognition of several pitfalls in the traditional linkage methods, including the precariousness of using unaffected

family members in an analysis, and contributed to a shift toward a different analytic approach.

10. Reich et al., 1969; Mendlewicz et al., 1972, 1979, 1980; Baron et al., 1987, 1993.

11. The complex phenotype of nonsyndromic hearing loss—deafness without nonauditory symptoms—provides a dramatic example of genetic heterogeneity: 12 different genes have been identified that each can cause the disorder independently, with more likely to follow (Griffith and Friedman, 1999).

12. This appears to be the case, for example, with Hirschsprung's disease; in this case, the gene EDNRB, encoding a G protein–coupled receptor, and the gene RET, encoding a receptor tyrosine kinase, may interact to contribute to disease susceptibility (Carrasquillo et al., 2002).

13. Suicide in people with manic-depressive illness has been studied as an alternative phenotype, and a genetic component to suicidal behavior has been established. This work is described in Chapter 9.

14. Kendler et al., 1985, 1986, 1993a,b.

15. DeLisi et al., 1987; Sham et al., 1994, 1996; Kendler et al., 1997.

16. Both the LOD score noted here and the subsequent score described by Schulze and colleagues (2003) are nonparametric and paternal allele–specific. The latter refers to an LOD score calculated only on the basis of alleles inherited from fathers, omitting the alleles that come from mothers. (See the discussion below of genomic imprinting.)

17. In one additional positive study, the variant was not specified (Vincent et al., 1999).

18. Esterling et al., 1998; Kirov et al., 1999c; Mundo et al., 2000; Mynett-Johnson et al., 2000; Serretti et al., 2002a.

19. Bocchetta et al., 1999; Kirov et al., 1999c; Mynett-Johnson et al., 2000; Dimitrova et al., 2002.

Neurobiology

The madness results from an aberrant biochemical process. . . . With all of this upheaval in the brain tissues, the alternating drenching and deprivation, it is no wonder that the mind begins to feel aggrieved, stricken, and the muddied thought processes register the distress of an organ in convulsion.

—*William Styron (1990, p. 47)*

Attempts to comprehend the brain's role in mania and depression—a quest the ancients could undertake only in rhetorical flight—began in earnest as clinically effective mood-altering drugs began to appear in the late 1950s and early 1960s. The psychopharmacological revolution fortuitously coincided with the arrival of new techniques that made it possible to characterize neurotransmitter function in the central nervous system. Over the next three decades, clinical studies attempted to uncover the biological factors mediating the pathophysiology of manic-depressive illness through a variety of biochemical strategies. Studies were, by and large, designed to detect relative excess or deficiency associated with pathological states; not surprisingly, progress in unraveling the unique neurobiology of recurrent mood disorders was slow using such strategies in isolation.

The last decade of the twentieth century marked the start of a truly remarkable period for biomedical research. The "molecular medicine revolution" has brought to bear the power of sophisticated cellular and molecular biologic methodologies to tackle many of society's most devastating illnesses. The rate of progress has been exciting indeed, and hundreds of G protein–coupled receptors and more than a dozen G proteins and effectors have been identified and characterized at the molecular and cellular levels. As a result, it has become possible to study a variety of human diseases caused by abnormalities in cell-to-cell communication; these studies are offering unique insights into the physiologic and pathophysiologic functioning of many cellular transmembrane signaling pathways.

Psychiatry, like much of the rest of medicine, has entered a new and exciting age resulting from the rapid advances in and the promise of molecular and cellular biology as well as

neuroimaging (discussed in Chapter 15; Cowan et al., 2002). Although we have yet to identify the specific abnormal genes or proteins associated with manic-depressive illness, there have been major advances in our understanding of the illness, particularly in the bipolar subgroup and in the mechanisms of action of the most effective treatments. These advances have generated considerable excitement among the clinical neuroscience community and are reshaping views about the neurobiological underpinnings of the disorder. It is our firm belief that the impact of molecular and cellular biology—which has been felt throughout clinical medicine—will have major repercussions for understanding the fundamental pathophysiology of bipolar and recurrent unipolar disorders and that we will see the development of markedly improved treatments for these devastating illnesses.

In this chapter, we begin by discussing some fundamental, unique facets of manic-depressive illness that have made a true understanding of its core pathophysiology so challenging. We then trace the evolution of the models that have guided biochemical and pharmacological studies, with emphasis on bipolar disorder. Next we review findings of the literature on the potential involvement of several major neurotransmitter and neuropeptide systems. We then turn to an area that has witnessed the greatest advances in biomedical science in recent years—the molecular and cellular mechanisms underlying long-term neuroplasticity and gene expression. Finally, we attempt to synthesize the findings from molecular, cellular, biochemical, systems, circuitry, neuroimaging, postmortem, and behavioral studies to propose an integrated model.

As is the case throughout this volume, we focus primarily on the bipolar subgroup of manic-depressive illness. Where recurrent unipolar disorder (especially the highly recurrent forms) is salient, however, it is included in the discussion. We also note when data for unipolar depression (unfortunately all too often broadly defined without respect to recurrence) may shed light on the underlying pathophysiology of manic-depressive illness or highly recurrent unipolar depression.

The approach taken in this chapter reflects the explosion of information since we published the first edition of this volume:

- Our emphasis in the chapter is on findings of the literature on bipolar disorder. To supplement this discussion, we provide additional information on the Web site for this volume: (1) a summary of older but important biological findings in manic-depressive illness that have not been extensively pursued in recent years for reasons that are not always clear (these investigations include electrolytes, sodium, magnesium, and calcium; membrane transport studies including red blood cells/plasma lithium ratio, Na/K ATPase studies, and red blood cell cation transport); (2) investigations of neurotransmitter-related enzymes, including monoamine oxidase (MAO), catechol-O-methyltransferase (COMT), and dopamine-β-hydroxylase (DBH); and (3) additional discussion of biological correlates of the switch process, focusing on the hypothalamic–pituitary–adrenal and hypothalamic–pituitary–thyroid axes, the serotonergic, dopaminergic, and noradrenergic systems, and related neuropeptides. Additional details on various other topics in this chapter are provided on the accompanying Web site as well.
- We present a considerable amount of material in table form; in general, when we extensively covered a topic in the first edition of this volume (e.g., biogenic amines), we present a summary table of the major findings that have stood the test of time, as well as a table of findings from more recent studies.
- When discussing the effects of medication on various biochemical pathways, we focus in general (with notable exceptions) on the well-established mood stabilizers—lithium, carbamazepine, and valproate.

THE UNIQUE NEUROBIOLOGY OF RECURRENT MOOD DISORDERS (ESPECIALLY BIPOLAR): CONSTRAINTS FOR CLINICAL STUDIES

It is likely that in individuals with manic-depressive illness, perhaps especially in its bipolar form, altered expression of critical proteins ensuing from a series of interacting susceptibility genes predisposes to a dysregulation of signaling in regions of the brain, resulting in a periodic loss of homeostasis and clinical manifestation of affective symptomatology—that is, mania and/or depression (Goodwin

and Ghaemi, 1998; Manji and Lenox, 1999; Payne et al., 2002). Thus the biological processes underlying the risk for mood cycling may even be quite distinct from the biology driving the clinical symptoms of mania or depression per se (Goodwin and Ghaemi, 1998). In this regard, it should be noted that there is increasing evidence for a shared genetic risk for both bipolar and recurrent unipolar disorders (see Chapter 13), suggesting that the underlying pathophysiological processes predisposing to recurrent mood disturbance may share common features. Furthermore, the clinical picture and system response are the result of a complex, dynamic interaction between the dysregulated signaling systems and activation of existing physiological feedback mechanisms designed to compensate for extreme changes. In this manner, the constellation of symptoms—including not only mood but also autonomic, endocrine, sleep/wake, and circadian activity determinants—reflects both the stage and progression of illness and unique individual characteristics conferring heterogeneity in clinical presentation and diagnosis.

In light of this complexity and the dynamic properties of the system, we would expect research strategies examining biochemical and endocrine variables to be subject to a high degree of inherent variability, using not just cross-sectional analyses among patients but even longitudinal designs over time within individual patients. Furthermore, the use of peripheral sources and postmortem brain to address biochemical and neuroendocrine activity within the brains of patients introduces another set of variables inherent in the experimental design, most often placing significant constraints on the interpretation of data. Additionally, when patient groups cannot be matched for comparison on a particular variable, the appropriate statistic may be an analysis of covariance, used to control for the influence of confounding variables. These characteristics may be associated (confounding) or not (independent) with the phenomenon under study (e.g., the observed outcome of an illness after a specific intervention), thereby making a simple analysis of variance problematic. Even age matching can introduce distortions. For example, in age-matched unipolar and bipolar depressed patients, the latter group's earlier age of onset means their average duration of illness will have been longer, and this parameter should be evaluated independently despite the general homogeneity of the population (Goodwin et al., 1978).

We should also keep in mind that a true understanding of the pathophysiology of manic-depressive illness in either its bipolar or highly recurrent unipolar form, must address its neurobiology at different physiological levels—molecular, cellular, systems, and behavioral (see Fig. 14–1); unfortunately, most studies to date have examined these levels in isolation.

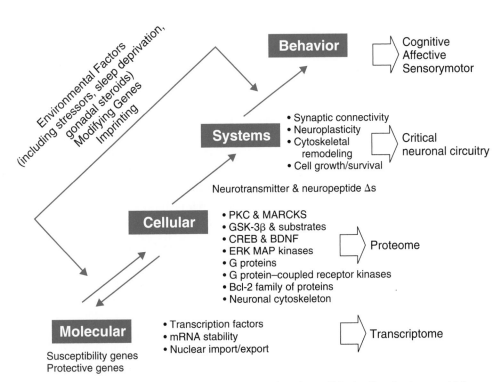

Figure 14–1. For a complete understanding of the pathophysiology of bipolar disorder, its neurobiology must be addressed at different physiologic levels (i.e., molecular, cellular, systems, and behavioral levels). Bcl-2 = B-cell leukemia/lymphoma; BDNF = brain-derived neurotrophic factor; CREB = cAMP response element binding protein; ERK = extracellular receptor-coupled kinase; GSK-3 = glycogen synthase kinase-3; MAP kinase = mitogen-activated protein kinase; MARCKS = myristoylated alanine-rich C kinase substrate; PKC = protein kinase C; proteome = the population of cellular protein species and their expression level; transcriptome = the population of cellular messenger RNA species and their expression level. (*Source*: Manji and Lenox, 2000a. Reprinted with permission from Elsevier.)

As discussed in Chapter 13, it is clear that manic-depressive illness arises from the interaction of multiple susceptibility (and likely risk) genes. These genes (and the proteins for which they code) are undoubtedly related much more closely to specific biochemical processes and thus specific symptoms than to "bipolar disorder or recurrent depression" as defined by the *Diagnostic and Statistical Manual*, 4th edition (DSM-IV) (Manji et al., 2003a).

One strategy that may have considerable utility in elucidating the complex neurobiology of the bipolar form of the illness is an endophenotype-based approach (Lenox et al., 2002; Gottesman and Gould, 2003; Manji et al., 2003a; Hasler et al., 2006). Such an approach may allow for the enrichment of study populations based on pathophysiological considerations, and may ultimately lead to a greater understanding of the illness. It is our strong belief that conceptualizing the disorder through an endophenotypic approach will also enable a more biologically relevant classification of patients along dimensional properties of the disorder, rather than the traditional categorical classifications imposed by our diagnostic manuals and reimbursement systems.

Additional major problems in the interpretation of biological data are associated with the diagnostic specificity of patient populations and the lack of comparability of patient states across studies even in those who truly have the same diagnosis. Are they studied at the same point in their recurrent illness? Are the effects "primary" to the illness, or do they represent the individual's compensatory adaptations to the illness? How long have patients been drug-free? It is now clear, for instance, that withdrawal from the high therapeutic doses of antidepressants currently employed produces biochemical changes that persist for at least 3 and up to 8 weeks following discontinuation. For more than a decade, the bulk of psychiatric patients available for biochemical studies have been those recently or currently on medication at the beginning of an investigation. None of the studies reported here, for example, specify a minimum withdrawal over 3 weeks, and most involve only a 1- to 2-week drug-free period. Indeed, as we discuss later, it is quite likely that medication has major effects on brain structure as well, calling into question many of the volumetric brain imaging studies conducted without regard to medication status. Indeed, there are only a few studies in which a parameter is followed longitudinally over different states in one or two untreated subjects. From a research point of view, such studies are particularly valuable,

BOX 14–1.   **The Pathophysiology of Manic-Depressive Illness: Constraints for Experimental Design**

* Complex disease with diagnostic heterogeneity
* Episodic nature of symptoms and distinct symptom clusters
* The biology underlying recurrence and cyclicity may be distinct from that responsible for specific symptom clusters
* Disease progression dictates changes over the course of the illness
* Dynamic interaction between compensatory and adaptive changes in brain and primary neurobiology of the disorder
* Effect of treatment and treatment withdrawal on measures
* Potential circadian rhythm abnormalities suggest that single time-point studies may be inadequate
* Relative inaccessibility of target organ and dependence on peripheral models
* Lack of suitable animal models
* Characterization of "mood" as a quantitative trait (QTL analysis) has not yet been accomplished

Source: Bachmann et al., 2005.

although they clearly must be generalized with caution since investigated patients are those able and willing to tolerate prolonged periods without drugs, and therefore may be atypical.

Our task becomes even more daunting when one considers the possibility that a major component of the pathophysiology of bipolar disorder (and perhaps also the more highly recurrent forms of unipolar depression) may stem from discordant biological rhythms, ranging from ultradian to infradian, that ultimately drive the periodic recurrent nature of the disorder. Not only do data collected at different times of the day (or seasons) lack comparability, but a free-running rhythm can produce epiphenomena that may be misinterpreted as correlates of the mood cycle. These problems are of more than passing interest, since rhythm disturbances have been hypothesized to be central to the pathophysiology of the illness (see Chapter 16).

In summary, constraints on experimental design in the study of recurrent mood disorders include the diagnostic heterogeneity of a complex disease; the biology underlying recurrence and cyclicity (which may be distinct from that responsible for specific symptom clusters); and potential circadian rhythm abnormalities. Thus simple time-point studies may be inadequate. Another constraint for research on bipolar disorder is posed by the lack of suitable animal models for use in biochemical and pharmacological studies. The evolution of such models is the subject of the next section. For additional constraints on experimental design, see Box 14–1.

ANIMAL MODELS OF MOOD DISORDERS

The need to use caution in applying animal models to complex neuropsychiatric disorders has been well described (McKinney, 2001; Weiss and Post, 1994). It is unlikely we will ever develop rodent models that display the full range of validity criteria. Modeling in animals is a valuable tool for exploring the underlying pathologies of human diseases and developing better therapies. Yet, modeling psychopathology is more difficult than modeling other somatic diseases, primarily because of three major considerations (Einat et al., 2002a; Nestler et al., 2002a):

* The diagnosis of psychiatric disorders is based on evaluation of diverse symptoms rather than on specific, objective measures.
* There are no fully validated biological markers for psychiatric disorders.
* Many features of major psychiatric illnesses can be totally observed only in humans, in whom the cortical mantle has evolved to a much greater extent than in other species.

Despite these limitations, however, animal models have been used for many years as the basis for experimental efforts to reproduce in nonhuman species the essential features of human disorders (Suomi, 1982; McKinney, 1988). Animal models of psychiatric disorders can also be defined operationally as unusual behavioral states in animals that are specifically reversed by the same pharmacological treatments that reverse symptoms of the human disorder (Petty and Sherman, 1981). An homologous animal model for a human mental disorder ideally should be simple, reproducible, and similarly quantifiable, compared to the human disorder in these paradigms: symptoms, postulated etiology, mediating mechanisms, and treatment responses.

In considering an animal model of depression or of any other illness seen in humans, it is critical to be clear on the validity criteria of that model (McKinney, 2001). The best animal model of a disease is theory driven (McKinney, 2001; Einat et al., 2002b, 2003a; Nestler et al., 2002a). An animal model of depression, for example, is expected to replicate the etiological factors and many of the symptoms associated with depression in humans. A related approach is to model a disease mechanism in a laboratory animal and recreate particular features of the disorder. Both approaches have been used recently with considerable success in creating animal models for several neurological conditions (e.g., Huntington's disease, familial Alzheimer's and Parkinson's diseases) in which the underlying genetic abnormalities are known.

An alternative approach is to reproduce in animals particular symptoms of mood disorders. Integrated in the concepts of face and construct and predictive validity, these models can then be used to study the biological mechanisms underlying those symptoms and to develop new treatments that alleviate the symptoms. The main limitation of these models is that they may poorly reflect mechanisms involved in the human situation. Thus the biological basis of the animal symptoms may be different from that of human symptoms, and drugs that treat the former may not treat the latter. Another approach is to simply develop models that can be used to screen for new treatments. Such models may not have face validity for the human disease, but this does not matter as long as the models have predictive value for identifying new treatment agents. Several such screening tests are available, as outlined below, but the value of these tests in identifying treatments with novel mechanisms of action will remain unknown until such treatments are identified (Einat et al., 2002b; Nestler et al., 2002b).

Models of Depression

It should be noted at the outset that, while many of the depression models do show construct, face, or predictive validity for depression, none model recurrence. The only paradigms that models recurrence, at least to some extent, are the kindling models discussed later and circadian/ultradian rhythm models discussed in Chapter 16.

The Primate Separation Paradigm

In its earliest version, the primate separation paradigm consisted of rearing monkeys from birth either in total isolation, completely deprived of social contact with other animals, or in wire cages with only visual and auditory contact permitted. Animals reared in either environment for the first 6 to 12 months of life, then tested socially with other animals, spend most of their time manifesting a despair syndrome: huddled alone in a corner, rocking, clasping themselves, and refraining from play or social encounters with peers (McKinney, 1988). Subchronic treatment with tricyclic antidepressants, such as imipramine, can significantly reduce elements of this despair syndrome, such as huddling (Suomi et al., 1978). Certain elements of the syndrome have been reversed by other categories of drugs, including a neuroleptic (chlorpromazine) and an anxiolytic (diazepam) (McKinney et al., 1973; Noble et al., 1976). In a few studies, even electroconvulsive therapy (ECT) has been shown to reverse this depressive-like behavior (McKinney, 1986). Endogenous neurochemical changes noted during the separation period include reduced cerebrospinal fluid levels of norepinephrine, which were shown to be reversed by antidepressant treatment (Kraemer et al., 1984).

Although some of the observed behaviors are roughly analogous to major depression in humans, the fact remains that the onset of depressive illness typically occurs in adulthood. These infant monkeys are probably displaying a response more analogous to the "anaclitic depression" observed by Spitz (1946) among newborn human infants suffering from maternal deprivation. Aware of these limitations, some investigators of primates have attempted to model depression using juvenile monkeys separated from their peer groups (Kraemer et al., 1984). Of course, one of the fundamental realities of depressive illness is that it clusters in genetically predisposed individuals. Thus, the observation of considerable individual variability in the development of despair behavior among rhesus monkeys is of special importance and has prompted cross-fostering studies, which are beginning to tease apart environmental and genetic factors in individual vulnerability to separation (Mineka and Suomi, 1978; McKinney, 1988).

Several rodent models involving manipulation of early life environment have also been used, including prenatal stress, early postnatal handling, and maternal separation (Meaney et al., 1994; Caldji et al., 2000; Ladd et al., 2000). Environmental enrichment has been used as a reciprocal stimulus. In some of these models, early life stress produces neuroendocrine and behavioral changes in rats and mice that persist into adulthood. For example, animals subjected to early stress show a hyperactive hypothalamic–pituitary–adrenal (HPA) axis, as indicated by elevated corticotropin-releasing factor (CRF) and glucocorticoid levels in response to stress. They also exhibit increased locomotor responses to novelty and, in some studies, greater vulnerability to learned helplessness (see below) and drug self-administration.

Overall, separation models of depression are generally good in terms of their replicability, and have been used successfully with a variety of species, from rodent to non-human primate. In addition, many of the resulting abnormalities can be reversed by antidepressant treatment, although negative reports have also appeared.

The Learned Helplessness Model of Depression

The learned helplessness model is based on exposing animals to uncontrollable, aversive stressors (Seligman and Maier, 1967). Variations of the original paradigm include inescapable tailshock or footshock, which is varied and random, and behavioral despair, as evidenced in a test involving swimming to exhaustion. The former produces a more naturalistic situation, whereas the latter is essentially a version of learned helplessness.

Rats subjected to various forms of stress, such as shock or forced swimming, are subsequently unable to acquire and perform a simple escape task. The effect lasts up to 1 week after the inescapable stress (Weiss et al., 1984). The interpretation is that any behavioral or other difference found between groups can be attributable to the psychological variable of control over shock termination. Animals that have acquired learned helplessness show several neurovegetative changes that are reminiscent of depression, such as rapid eye movement (REM) sleep alterations, reduced body weight, diminished sexual behavior, and elevated CRF and corticosterone levels. Repeated dosing with antidepressants, as well as repeated electroconvulsive seizures (the animal model of ECT), reduces the latency to escape and decreases the number of animals that show learned helplessness (Willner, 1984; Hitzemann, 2000).

The attractiveness of the learned helplessness model is that it is based on a plausible theory linking cognitive function to visceral sequelae. On the other hand, these models suffer from some of the same limitations as the separation models:

- Compared with the relatively low frequency of clinical depression in the populations studied, the behavior is produced in a substantially larger proportion of the individual animals tested.
- The animals require a considerable amount of stress, and severe stress does not uniformly play a critical role in the onset of major depressive episodes in humans. In recurrent mood disorders, stress may be more important to the onset of the initial episode than to subsequent episodes. Thus, the extent to which learned helplessness is a superior model for post-traumatic stress disorder and other conditions in which stress is a clear etiological factor remains unknown.
- These syndromes generally can be reversed rather quickly by restoring the animal to a normal environment. This is certainly not the case in major depressive illness.
- Controversy has centered on whether the effects of learned helplessness are truly cognitive or simply products of stress-induced inactivity.
- As noted above, while these models have utility in reproducing some facets of the depressive syndrome, they do very little to address the recurrent nature of manic-depressive illness.

Forced Swim Test

The forced swim test, also known as the Porsolt test, is the most widely used animal model in depression research, more specifically as a screen for antidepressant treatments (Borsini and Meli, 1988; Lucki, 1997; Porsolt, 2000). The test involves placing a rat or mouse in a tank filled with water and measuring the amount of time the animal is immobile. Acute or short-term treatment with most antidepressants increases the latency to immobility and decreases the period of immobility, and in most cases this occurs at drug doses that are not activating on their own. Although this test is used mainly as an empirical test, one interpretation is that antidepressants may increase active coping responses to swim stress. A variant of the forced swim test, used in mice, is the tail suspension test. Here, mice are suspended by their tails, and the time it takes each animal to become immobile (to hang passively upside down) is measured. Acute administration of most antidepressants decreases immobility.

The major advantage of the forced swim test (or tail suspension test) is its relatively high throughput and ease of use. However, there are also disadvantages. Antidepressants decrease immobility in the test animals even after single doses, despite the fact that the clinical effects of these agents require administration for several weeks at least. Thus, the test is sensitive to the immediate effects of these agents and may not be capturing per se the true mood-elevating changes produced by these medications in the brain.

Chronic Mild Stress

Several tests related to learned helplessness and based on exposure of animals to uncontrollable stress have been used in rats. In general, it has been much more difficult to establish equivalent tests in mice.

In the chronic mild stress paradigm, rodents are exposed to a variety of relatively mild stresses (isolation housing, disruption of light–dark cycles, brief food or water deprivation, tilting of home cages) intermittently for relatively prolonged periods of time (e.g., several weeks). Another stress-based model is social defeat. Here, an animal is exposed repeatedly to an aggressive and dominant animal. In some laboratories, no physical contact is involved, while in others the defeated animals experience mild physical duress.

The advantage of these tests is that they have greater face validity than many other tests because they involve more naturalistic stresses. Stressed animals are reported to exhibit "anhedonia" as inferred from a reduction in sucrose drinking, as well as a variety of cardiovascular or neuroendocrine sequelae, which are reported to be reversed by longer-term antidepressant treatment in some studies. The major disadvantage of the chronic stress models is their poor reproducibility. Both the behavioral abnormalities produced by chronic stress and the palliative effects of antidepressants in these paradigms have been difficult to replicate across laboratories, which has reduced their general application.

Models of Bipolar Disorder

An ideal model for bipolar disorder should include spontaneous and progressive behavior that oscillates between increased and decreased manifestations of the model behavior and that may be similar to a human behavior phenotypic to mania or depression (face validity). The model behavior should also be normalized by chronic, but not acute, treatment with mood stabilizers such as lithium and several anticonvulsant drugs, but react in the manic-like direction to treatment with antidepressants (predictive validity).

Additionally, a well-validated model should be based on one of the mechanistic theories of the disease.

The progressive and cycling nature of the disease presents a unique difficulty in any attempts to model it. Indeed, most models tend to focus on one pole of the disorder, either mania or depression, whereas a number of models employ other examples of oscillatory physiology or behavior even if they do not overtly resemble any symptoms of bipolar disorder.

Hyperactivity Models

Because models for major depression are relatively available, there have been more attempts to develop valid animal models for the manic state that is a unique feature of bipolar disorder. Since hyperactivity is one of the simpler behaviors to detect, monitor, and quantify, a number of models for mania have focused on this aspect of the disorder. Some of these models are reviewed by Einat and colleagues (2000, 2002b) and are briefly described here.

Baseline Locomotor Activity

Locomotor activity in a novel environment is affected by many factors, such as the time of day, environmental stimuli, and the history of the animal. The effects of mood stabilizers on spontaneous activity are equivocal, but more effects have been reported for chronic lithium use (Lerer et al., 1984; Berggren, 1985) than for acute treatment with this drug (Ushijama et al., 1986). Interestingly, a clearer reduction in basal activity following lithium treatment has been observed during the dark phase (when rodents are more active), which suggests that the drug may suppress only high levels of activity (similar to the manic state) without affecting low baseline activity levels (Lerer et al., 1984; Kofman and Belmaker, 1990).

Psychostimulant-Induced Hyperactivity

Acute treatment with appropriate doses of psychostimulants can produce a range of mania-like behaviors, including hyperactivity, heightened sensory awareness, alertness, insomnia, and changes in sleep patterns (Gessa et al., 1995; Einat et al., 2000). The hyperactivity induced by psychostimulants can be easily detected (Antoniou et al., 1998) and is sensitive to lithium treatment[1] and possibly to anticonvulsant mood stabilizers (Kuruvilla and Uretsky, 1981; Maitre et al., 1984; Maj et al., 1985). Yet the sensitivity of this model to mood stabilizers is not universal; rather, it is dependent on the mode of administration or the specific type of activity measured (see Einat et al., 2000, 2002a).

Sleep Deprivation

Sleep deprivation has a rapid therapeutic effect in both unipolar and bipolar depression (see Post et al., 1987; Szuba et al., 1994; Barbini et al., 1998; see also Chapters 16 and 19), which can be maintained by treatment with lithium or antidepressant drugs (Szuba et al., 1994). At the same time, sleep deprivation can induce manic episodes in euthymic bipolar patients and has been suggested as a final common pathway in the genesis of mania (Wehr et al., 1987).

With the clinical phenomenon in mind, Gessa and colleagues attempted to examine the effects of sleep deprivation in animals. In their studies, they demonstrated that rats exposed to 72 hours of sleep deprivation exhibit a variety of behaviors that have face validity for modeling a manic episode. These behaviors include insomnia (for about 30 minutes, after rats are permitted to sleep), hyperactivity, irritability (Albert et al., 1970; Fratta et al., 1987; Gessa et al., 1995), aggressive behavior (Hicks et al., 1979), and hypersexuality (Morden et al., 1968). Furthermore, Gessa and colleagues (1995) demonstrated that lithium treatment alleviates the insomnia and hyperactivity elements of the behavior, thereby adding predictive validity to the face validity of the proposed model.

Gessa and colleagues (1995) suggest that sleep deprivation in the rat may be a valid model for mania and that this model can offer new directions for the study of the pathological mechanism of the disorder. They attempted to study the brain mechanisms underlying these manic-like behaviors. Their findings indicate that treatment with the dopaminergic D2 antagonist haloperidol or with the dopamine D1 receptor antagonist SCH 23390 significantly reduces the sleep latency (time to the onset of sleep after sleep deprivation) in the model (Fratta et al., 1987), whereas treatment with the dopamine D1 agonist SKF 38393 prolongs the period of insomnia (Gessa et al., 1995). Interestingly, the dopamine D2/D3 agonist quinpirole produces a biphasic effect in small doses, possibly acting presynaptically (Eilam and Szechtman, 1990) to reduce sleep latency, whereas at higher doses, acting postsynaptically, it was shown to prolong sleep latency (Gessa et al., 1995). Furthermore, naloxone (an opioid antagonist) reduces sleep latency, whereas morphine, beta-endorphin, and [D-Ala2, D-Leu5] enkephalin prolong the period of insomnia (Fratta et al., 1987). Neurochemical studies of this model demonstrated that sleep deprivation induces only small effects related to adrenergic or serotonergic receptors (Siegel and Rogawski, 1988) but has stronger effects on the dopaminergic (DeMontis et al., 1990) and opioid (Fadda et al., 1991, 1992) systems in the brain (Gessa et al., 1995).

Recent molecular and cellular biology studies have renewed interest in sleep deprivation as a possible model. Thus there is now incontrovertible evidence that the expression of selected critical genes varies dramatically during sleep and waking events, a variation that likely plays a major role in regulating various long-term neuroplastic events. Messenger ribonucleic acid (mRNA) differential display, microarray, and biochemical studies have shown that short-term sleep deprivation (short-term sleep deprivation has no clear definition regarding number of hours) is associated with a rapid increase in various plasticity-related genes. Notably, these are precisely the plasticity-related molecules whose expression is increased by chronic antidepressant treatment.

In an extension of the gene expression studies, Cirelli and colleagues (Cirelli and Tononi, 2000; Cirelli et al., 2002) hypothesize that a key factor responsible for the induction of the plasticity genes may be the level of activity of the neuromodulatory noradrenergic and serotonergic systems. Both of these systems project diffusely to most of the brain, where they regulate gene expression, and are quiescent only during REM sleep (Cirelli et al., 2002). Thus sleep deprivation may be capable of rapidly activating "antidepressant/mania-inducing" genes (Payne et al., 2002), and despite the technical difficulties inherent in establishing this model, it is clearly worthy of further study.

Sensitization and Kindling

Most longitudinal studies of the course of manic-depressive illness indicate that recurrences are not simply random. Rather they show, on average, that its course presents a pattern of increasing frequency over time, a phenomenon most extensively studied in the bipolar subgroup (see Chapter 4). Post and colleagues (Post and Kopanda, 1976; Post et al., 1984d,e; Post and Weiss, 1989) have focused on two intriguing animal models that attempt to account for this tendency of episodes to accelerate: behavioral sensitization and electrophysiological kindling. These models are of considerable interest, even though they do not provide full homologies for other aspects of the illness.

Behavioral Sensitization to Psychostimulants.   Repeated, intermittent administration of many psychostimulants results in a gradual increase in behavioral response termed *reverse tolerance* or *sensitization* (e.g., Robinson and Becker, 1986; Stewart and Badiani, 1993; Einat et al., 1996). This clearly progressive phenomenon, used in the past to model psychosis (see Robinson and Becker, 1986), has frequently been proposed and used as a model for the development of bipolar illness, since the development of sensitized behavior is similar to the progression of manic episodes, with a gradual increase in severity and progressively more rapid onset (Post et al., 1981, 1982). This model offers not only face validity but also some construct validity, considering the involvement of the dopaminergic system in manic psychosis (e.g., Jimerson et al., 1982; Carli et al., 1997). Moreover, cocaine mimics several of the pharmacological effects of stress, and one of the proposed models for bipolar

disorder suggests that the clinical course of the disorder is exacerbated by psychosocial stressors that interact with effector genes and immediate early genes (Post and Weiss, 1996).

Intriguingly, recent studies have shown that cocaine sensitization and reward are under the influence of circadian genes and rhythm (see Chapter 16). Abarca and colleagues (2002) found that mPer1 and mPer2 mutant mice, as well as wild-type mice, exhibited an approximately five-fold increase in activity after an acute cocaine injection compared with controls, showing that there is no initial difference in sensitivity to acute cocaine administration in Per mutants. After repeated cocaine injections, however, wild-type mice exhibited a sensitized behavioral response that was absent in mPer1 knockout mice. By contrast, mPer2 mutant mice exhibited a hypersensitized response to cocaine (Abarca et al., 2002). Conditioned place preference experiments revealed similar behavioral reactions: mPer1 knockout mice showed a complete lack of cocaine reward, whereas mPer2 mutants showed a strong cocaine-induced place preference. Finally, in another set of experiments, these investigators tested C57/BL6J mice at different zeitgeber times and found that cocaine-induced behavioral sensitization and place preference are under the control of the circadian clock. These studies are highly complementary to those of Nikaido and colleagues (2001), who found that methamphetamine augmented the expression of mPer1 in the caudate-putamen. Together, these studies suggest that processes involved in some of the actions of psychostimulants that may be of particular relevance to bipolar disorder (sensitization and reward) are under the influence of circadian rhythms and modulated in a complex manner by clock genes.

Despite the many strengths of this model, it should be noted that its predictive (pharmacological) validity is equivocal. Some studies have found inhibition of the phenomenon by lithium (Post et al., 1984c), but others have not (Poncelet et al., 1987; Cappeliez and Moore, 1990). Moreover, in contrast with the kindling model (see below), carbamazepine treatment has not been found to have any clear-cut effects (Post et al., 1984c; Weiss et al., 1990). An additional problem with the model is the gradual transition in behaviors across injections of most psychostimulants, from hyperactivity that is easily monitored and quantified to locally oriented stereotypic movements that may be difficult to interpret (see Ellinwood et al., 1972; Kilbey and Ellinwood, 1977; Eilam and Szechtman, 1990).

Amygdala Kindling.   The amygdala kindling model was the first major attempt to develop a model on the basis of its progressive nature rather than on a clear behavioral similarity with bipolar disorder. As a nonhomologous model it should be emphasized that the model is not based on the notion that bipolar disorder is a seizure disorder, but reflects the progressive nature of the illness and has considerable heuristic value (see also Chapter 4). In kindling of the amygdala, for example, repeated once-daily stimulation for 1 second initially produces no observable behavioral or electrophysiological effects. Upon repetition, however, afterdischarges increase in frequency, duration, and complexity of waveform, and eventually the animal develops a full-blown major motor seizure in response to a stimulus that was previously below the threshold. If the stimulation is repeated frequently enough, the animal will eventually develop a spontaneous seizure disorder, in which seizures occur without any exogenous stimulation (e.g., Racine, 1978; for a review see Post and Weiss, 1997).

Because of the gradual intensification of the response and the ongoing transition from stressor vulnerability to autonomous episodes, Post and colleagues suggest that although the behavioral response is different from that observed during manic episodes (Weiss et al., 1995), kindling may be an appropriate model for bipolar disorder (Post and Ballenger, 1981; Post et al., 1984b; Post and Weiss, 1997). Support for the model comes from studies demonstrating reduced seizure response after pretreatment with lithium, anticonvulsant mood stabilizers,[2] or electroconvulsive shock (the animal model of ECT) (see Post et al., 1984b; Minabe et al., 1987, 1988). Moreover, in the course of treatment of amygdala-kindled animals with anticonvulsant drugs, the drugs show tolerance episodically with breakthroughs of seizures; this appearance of seizures during treatment may be similar to the periodic outbursts of bipolar episodes (Post and Weiss, 1996).

Interestingly, the kindling model was a key factor for the study of the anticonvulsant drug carbamazepine as an effective mood stabilizer (Post et al., 1984b; Post and Weiss, 1997). The model is also supported by some mechanistic findings (construct validity) as it induces changes in immediate early genes, gene expression, and synaptic structure that may be similar to changes in bipolar disorder (see Post and Weiss, 1997).

The kindling model therefore offers strong predictive validity, some face validity, and partial construct validity. Unfortunately, the model is quite complicated to induce and demands special equipment and conditions. These technical problems, combined with the theoretical difficulty of a clear dissimilarity between the observed behavior (seizures) and the behavioral manifestation of manic-depressive illness in patients, have led to less than enthusiastic acceptance of the model in recent years.

Nevertheless, it is important to point out that both the sensitization and kindling models, while not directly analogous to the behavioral or affective disturbances of manic-depressive patients, have helped clarify the mechanisms underlying the accelerating longitudinal course of the illness, especially in its bipolar form. Thus when one reviews the parallels between the two models and bipolar disorder, the following features are notable:

- For each model, evidence exists for the predisposing effects of both genetic factors and early environmental stress.
- These models show threshold effects (mild alterations eventuating in full-blown episodes).
- Each model can show similarity of episodes through repeated occurrences.
- With each model, a maximum disturbance occurs earlier in the episode as the number of recurrences increases.
- In both models, early episodes may require precipitants, whereas later ones can occur spontaneously.
- With each model, repeated episodes of one phase may lead to emergence of the opposite phase.
- Younger animals appear to be more vulnerable to sensitization and kindling, a finding suggesting a parallel with the young age of onset of bipolar disorder.
- As we discuss later, a growing body of data has shown that both psychostimulant sensitization and kindling are associated with activation of the protein kinase C (PKC) signaling cascade, a pathway whose activity is inhibited by mood stabilizers.

Thus, these models serve to broaden the conceptual framework for linking clinical phenomenology to neurobiological mechanisms. The average pattern of cycle acceleration over time could reflect a mix of patients with a variety of patterns. Some might accelerate dramatically over time, whereas others might do so moderately or not at all. In patients having a dramatically shorter cycle with each episode, the form of the illness may be analogous to the pattern of increasingly rapid onset of hyperactivity and stereotypy following repeated administration of a psychomotor stimulant. The role of environmental stress in enhancing behavioral sensitization may resemble its postulated role in the onset of affective episodes. These findings may help integrate psychosocial and neurobiological perspectives. Specifically, if one postulates that a psychosocial stress can precipitate manic or depressive episodes, the sensitization and kindling models would suggest that, after a certain amount of repetition, the episodes will develop spontaneously (see Chapter 4). This chain of events fits the clinical histories of many patients with bipolar disorder, in which clear-cut psychosocial or physical stresses are associated with the onset of early episodes, but in time the episodes become more autonomous. By the time patients are seen in treatment settings, they may indeed have an autonomous illness.

As Post and Weiss (1989) point out, however, sensitization and kindling phenomena in animals do not yet represent precise models of human cyclic mood disorders. In addition to the respective time frames being quite different, the models imply a close similarity between stress-precipitated and pharmacological-induced events, a similarity that needs to be demonstrated experimentally.

Extreme Sensitization.   An extension of the psychostimulant sensitization model was recently suggested by Antelman and colleagues (Antelman et al., 1995; Antelman and Caggiula, 1996; Caggiula et al., 1998), who demonstrated that when animals reach a level of extreme sensitization to cocaine, some of their behavioral and biochemical responses begin to oscillate. The oscillations can be detected in some measures—such as the efflux of striatal and nucleus accumbens dopamine, hippocampal serotonin, and plasma levels of corticosterone and glucose—and in one behavioral measure—shock-induced hypoalgesia. Moreover, both biochemical and behavioral oscillations are completely prevented by chronic lithium pretreatment, adding predictive validity to the model (Antelman et al., 1998).

The extreme sensitization model appears to have more similarities with bipolar disorder than is the case for other models because it incorporates features of progressive and oscillating responses. Moreover, a recent study demonstrates that the behavioral response can be conditioned (Kucinski et al., 1999); that is, the behavior can be influenced by the environment, just as a manic or depressive episode can be triggered or precipitated by the environment. However, the measures used in the model are far removed from changes observed in bipolar patients, whereas other measurable changes induced by extreme sensitization, such as hyperactivity and reward-related behaviors, that are more homologous with human behavior and appear to model mania do not show cyclicity. These latter behaviors are not easily normalized by mood stabilizers. Moreover, the cycling measures were normalized by lithium, but further validation will require additional studies testing the effects of other mood stabilizers as well as other psychiatric drugs. Still, the notion of a cycling phenomenon is important, and additional study of this model might be useful.

A different derivative of the psychostimulant-induced models focusing on the response to the direct D2/D3 agonist quinpirole has been studied. Unlike other dopamine agonists, quinpirole (in appropriate doses) induces a biphasic response over time, starting with hypolocomotion and developing into a hyperlocomotion state (Eilam and Szechtman, 1989). This biphasic response can have face validity as a model for the two states of bipolar disorder—depression and mania. To assess this possibility, researchers examined the effects of mood stabilizers on the biphasic response.

They found that treatment with lithium or valproate affected the hyperactivity but not the hypoactivity phase (Shaldubina et al., 2002). Accordingly, this model has no advantage over the other psychostimulant-induced models.

Conclusions

If animal models are to realize their promise, they must incorporate certain cardinal features of recurrent mood disorders, especially the bipolar subgroup. The first is spontaneous, progressive behavior that oscillates between increased and decreased manifestations of the model behavior that is similar to the human phenotypic expression of mania or depression (face validity). The model behavior should also be normalized by chronic, but not acute, treatment with mood stabilizers such as lithium and several anticonvulsant drugs, but react in the manic-like direction to treatment with antidepressants, psychostimulants, and sleep deprivation (predictive validity). Finally, the models should involve both genetic vulnerability and cyclicity.

Ideal animal models for bipolar disorder are not available, but a variety of behaviors in animals may represent certain facets of the disease. Beyond the long-standing debate over the value of models that are not a comprehensive reflection of a disorder, or its underlying pathophysiology (Kilts, 2001; Machado-Vieira et al., 2004), it is accepted that partial models are helpful (McKinney 2001). Furthermore, there is a growing appreciation that bipolar disorder may represent a heterogeneous group of disorders that may be more amenable to study with an endophenotypic approach (Lenox et al. 2002; Hasler et al., 2006; discussed in greater detail later in this chapter). Accordingly, changes in behavior that are related to any facet of the depression–mania *continuum* may be relevant as models of these components of bipolar disorder. Behavioral tests for many such components are available and used in different contexts. Animals are tested for activity, response to drugs, hedonistic properties, resilience and despair, anxiety and risk-taking behaviors, judgment, sexual behavior, distractibility, sleep patterns, and more, all behaviors that may be relevant to bipolar disorder. Not all these models may be valid for components of bipolar disorder, and the process of validating models requires significant work (Willner, 1991; Einat et al., 2003a). However, experimentation done in different contexts may still help gain insight into possible mechanisms involved in bipolar disorder.

An increasing number of methodologies are now available that allow for the targeted manipulation of a specific gene (and protein) in a precise temporal and spatial (brain region–specific) manner. These evolving methodologies represent a new horizon for modeling the disorder, as it is now possible to attempt and create models that are hypothesis driven and have a sound theoretical base, rather than being based on behavioral similarity. Moreover, the availability of new molecular techniques makes it possible to explore connections between specific molecules and behavior, as well as gene–environment interactions. These advances will undoubtedly allow for the creation of improved animal models of arguably one of the most complex human neuropsychiatric disorders.

MAJOR NEUROTRANSMITTER AND NEUROPEPTIDE SYSTEMS IN MANIC-DEPRESSIVE ILLNESS

The impetus for the study of the biogenic amines in patients with manic-depressive illness was provided largely by the discovery of effective pharmacologic treatments for depression and mania. These treatments led to the formulation of the so-called pharmacological bridge between depressive illness and neurotransmitter systems in the brain. Unfortunately, as a rule, the studies of neurotransmitters and neuropeptides in depressed patients have not separately analyzed those patients with the more recurrent forms, that is, those who are a part of the manic-depressive spectrum. An initial foundation for this pharmacological bridge was formed by the following observations:

- Reserpine—an antihypertensive later shown to deplete amine transmitters in rodents—is associated with an unexpectedly high incidence of depression.
- Effective antidepressant drugs increase intrasynaptic concentrations of serotonin and norepinephrine.
- Antihypertensives that deplete these monoamines sometimes precipitate depressive episodes in susceptible individuals.
- Psychostimulants and dopamine agonists are capable of triggering manic episodes in susceptible individuals.
- Cholinomimetics (e.g., intravenous physostigmine, a central cholinesterase inhibitor) briefly but dramatically reduce symptoms in manic patients and precipitate depression in euthymic bipolar patients maintained on lithium.

Even more striking pharmacological findings go beyond effects on a single episode of depression or mania to indicate the effects of drugs on the long-term course of manic-depressive illness, particularly the bipolar subgroup. As discussed in Chapter 19, antidepressants in general and tricyclics in particular may increase the frequency of cycles and worsen long-term outcome. Finally, the monoaminergic systems are extensively distributed throughout the network of limbic, striatal, and prefrontal cortical neuronal circuits thought to support the behavioral and visceral manifestations of mood disorders.

Given these compelling pharmacological data, it is not surprising that investigators have postulated that

dysregulation of the major monoaminergic systems may play a major role in the pathophysiology of manic-depressive illness. We now review biological studies related directly or indirectly to the hypotheses generated by various pharmacological bridges, addressing in turn the noradrenergic, dopaminergic, serotonergic, cholinergic, GABAergic, and glutamatergic systems, and finally neuroendocrine systems and neuropeptides.

The Noradrenergic System

The noradrenergic system was one of the first neurotransmitter systems examined in studying the pathophysiology of affective disorders. Early theories of depression postulated that an imbalance in the metabolism of norepinephrine (NE) was responsible for mood disorders (Bunney and Davis, 1965; Schildkraut, 1965). This postulate has been extensively investigated but has proven difficult to study experimentally, in part because of the formidable methodological difficulties involved in assessing central nervous system (CNS) noradrenergic function in humans. Here we briefly review, critically appraise, and integrate the research findings to date on NE in manic-depressive illness, with a focus on the bipolar subgroup. (See Figure 14–2 for a depiction of the regulatory processes involved in NE neurotransmission.)

Studies of Norepinephrine and MHPG in Plasma

The principal metabolite of NE, 3-methoxy-4-hydroxyphenylglycol (MHPG), has been extensively measured in cerebrospinal fluid (CSF), plasma, and urine. In earlier studies, MHPG was found to be elevated in CSF in patients with depression, mania, and schizoaffective disorder (Schildkraut, 1965). The 1980s saw a series of investigations of plasma NE, the majority of which revealed some degree of elevation, interpreted as evidence of increased peripheral sympathetic nervous system activity in patients with major depression.[3] Several studies using radioenzymatic and radiotracer assay techniques also demonstrated elevated plasma NE concentrations under presumed resting conditions in patients with major depression, in particular unipolar patients fulfilling criteria for melancholia (Roy et al., 1985, 1987; Veith et al., 1985). In well-controlled studies, Rudorfer and colleagues (1985) found that supine plasma NE levels were significantly lower in bipolar patients than in either unipolar depressive patients or normal volunteers.

Going beyond the study of plasma NE levels under resting conditions, studies of the responsiveness of plasma NE to various provocative challenge tests provide evidence for dysregulation of the noradrenergic system in depression. Thus, using an orthostatic challenge paradigm, it was demonstrated that the increase in plasma NE is consistently greater in depressed unipolar or bipolar patients than in age- and

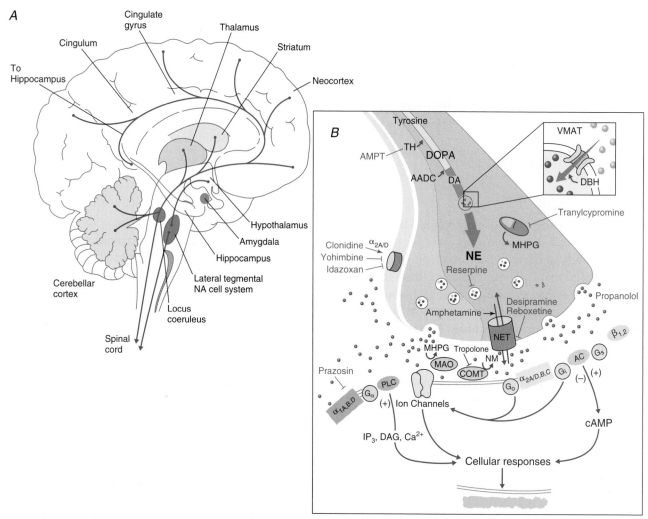

Figure 14–2. *A*: Gross anatomical relationships. *B*: The various regulatory processes involved in norepinephrine neurotransmission. The amino acid L-tyrosine is actively transported into presynaptic norepinephrine (NE) nerve terminals, where it is ultimately converted into NE. The rate-limiting step is conversion of L-tyrosine to L-dihydroxyphenyalanine (L-DOPA) by the enzyme tyrosine hydroxylase (TH). AMPT (α-methyl-para-tyrosine) is a competitive inhibitor of TH and has been used to assess the impact of reduced catecholaminergic function in clinical studies. Aromatic amino acid decarboxylase (AADC) converts DOPA to DA. DOPA then becomes decarboxylated by decarboxylase to form dopamine (DA). DA is then taken up from the cytoplasm into vesicles, by vesicular monoamine transporters (VMATs) and hydroxylated by DAβ-hydroxylase (DBH) in the presence of O^2 and ascorbate to form NE. Normetanephrine (NM) is formed by the action of catechol-O-methyltransferase (COMT) on NE. NE can be further metabolized by monoamine oxidase (MAO) and aldehyde reductase to 3-methoxy-4-hydroxyphenylglycol (MHPG). Reserpine causes a depletion of NE in vesicles by interfering with uptake and storage mechanisms (depressive-like symptoms have been reported with this agent). Once released from the presynaptic terminal, NE can interact with a variety of presynaptic and postsynaptic receptors. Presynaptic regulation of NE neuron firing activity and release occurs through somatodendritic (not shown) and nerve terminal α_2-adrenoceptors, respectively. Yohimbine potentiates NE neuronal firing and NE release by blocking these α_2-adrenoceptors, thereby disinhibiting these neurons from a negative feedback influence. Conversely, clonidine attenuates NE neuron firing and release by activating these receptors. Idazoxan is a relatively selective α_2-adrenoceptor antagonist primarily used for pharmacologic purposes. The binding of NE to G protein–coupled receptors, which are coupled to adenylyl cyclase (AC) and phospholipase C beta (PLC-β produces a cascade of second messenger and cellular effects (see diagram). NE's action is terminated in the synapse by rapidly being taken back into the presynaptic neuron through NE transporters (NET). Once inside the neuron it can either be repackaged into vesicles for reuse or it undergoes enzymatic degradation. The selective NE reuptake inhibitor and antidepressant reboxetine and older-generation tricyclic antidepressant desipramine are able to interfere with or block the reuptake of NE. Amphetamine is able to facilitate NE release by altering NET function. Note: Grey spheres = DA neurotransmitters; blue spheres = NE neurotransmitters. DAG = diacylglycerol; IP_3 = inositol (1,4,5) trisphosphate. (*Source*: Schatzberg and Nemeroff, 2004. Reprinted with permission from *The American Journal of Psychiatry*. Copyright 2004 by the American Psychiatric Association.)

gender-matched controls (Rudorfer et al., 1985). Depressed patients have been shown to produce an exaggerated release of NE in response to a variety of stressors, including orthostatic, cold pressor, and mental arithmetic stressors (Roy et al., 1985; Rubin et al., 1985; Veith et al., 1988).

Taken together, the studies of plasma NE provide strong evidence for dysregulation of peripheral release of NE in affective illness, with a difference in the pattern of dysregulation between unipolar and bipolar patients. Stated another way, bipolar patients appear to have reduced to average resting output of NE with a highly exaggerated NE response to standing, while unipolar patients (especially a subgroup of anxious, melancholic patients with dexamethasone nonsuppression) have an average to elevated resting NE, with moderately exaggerated response to standing (and perhaps "stressors" in general) (Rudorfer et al., 1985; Potter and Manji, 1994). Whether these differences can be attributed to the difference in polarity or cyclicity cannot be known since the unipolar and bipolar groups were not matched for the frequency of recurrence.

As we reviewed in the first edition of this text, studies of plasma MHPG have yielded variable results and do not generally support the concept of a unipolar–bipolar distinction (Potter and Linnoila, 1989). Plasma MHPG in unipolar depressive patients tends to be similar to that of controls, albeit with greater variance (Siever and Uhde, 1984). Similar to the association with plasma NE, depressed dexamethasone-nonsuppressors have higher levels of plasma MHPG (Jimerson et al., 1983; Roy et al., 1986). Plasma MHPG levels tend to be lower in bipolar than in unipolar depressed patients (Siever, 1987; Goodwin and Jamison, 1990) and are higher in bipolar patients when manic than when depressed (Halaris, 1978; Jimerson et al., 1981; Maj et al., 1984) or euthymic (Maj et al., 1984).

Studies of Norepinephrine and MHPG in Cerebral Spinal Fluid

For some years, measures of NE and its metabolites in CSF were thought to directly reflect brain NE "activity." This assumption is, however, problematic, since high correlations have been found between plasma and CSF NE and MHPG (Kopin, 1985; Goldstein et al., 1987). Pharmacological studies in dogs have revealed parallel changes in plasma and CSF NE following ganglion blockade, suggesting that sympathetic outflow may determine (at least in part) NE concentrations in both compartments (Goldstein et al., 1987). Plasma MHPG is the major source of CSF MHPG, which readily crosses the blood–brain barrier (Kopin, 1985). Given the high correlation between plasma and CSF MHPG observed in comparisons of high and low catecholamine output states, an equation has been derived to "correct" for the contribution of plasma MHPG to that of CSF (Kopin, 1985;

Goldstein et al., 1987). In the relatively narrow range of values observed in depressed patients and controls, however, such an equation is of questionable utility for identifying "brain MHPG" (Linnoila et al., 1986), and to date has not provided new insights in studies of depression.

Certain other methodological problems are unique to CSF measures. First, standards for obtaining spinal fluid, such as elapsed time between needle insertion and sample collection, have not been established. Therefore, subjects may not have the same degree of accommodation to the stress of the needle stick. Moreover, sampling at a single point in time may not reflect the biochemical process of depression or mania, but a state-dependent fluctuation from a recent external or internal stress.

CSF concentrations of NE have been reported to be elevated in depressed patients with an atypical presentation, higher scores for nurse-rated anxiety, and a longer duration of hospitalization (Post et al., 1984b). Earlier investigations showed that CSF NE is higher in mania than in depression (Post et al., 1978; Gerner et al., 1984). Moreover, in dysphoric mania, defined by the coexistence of high depression ratings, NE in CSF correlates modestly but significantly ($r \approx .5$) with ratings for dysphoria and anxiety but not with ratings for mania (Post et al., 1989). Post and colleagues suggest that CSF NE may be positively correlated with the degree of anxiety across a variety of psychopathologic syndromes, including depression, mania, and perhaps anxiety.

Reports suggest that CSF MHPG is lower in bipolar-I depressed patients than in unipolar patients, but as is the case for CSF NE, variables other than overall diagnosis may influence values (Potter et al., 1987). Thus, for instance, within a group of depressed patients, those with increased anxiety, agitation, somatization, and sleep disturbance were found to have significantly elevated levels of CSF MHPG (Redmond et al., 1986). CSF MHPG has been reported to be elevated in manic patients compared with controls (Post et al., 1984b; Redmond et al., 1986; Swann et al., 1986). In one study of mania, CSF MHPG concentration correlated with certain dysphoric elements of the manic syndrome—namely total manic severity and hostility (Swann et al., 1987). Moreover, this study found a significant reduction in CSF MHPG with lithium treatment, even when the treatment was unsuccessful.

Swann and colleagues have conducted the most comprehensive studies of catecholamine function in mania since publication of the first edition of this text. When they compared biogenic amines in mixed manic (n = 8) and in pure and nonagitated bipolar depressed (n = 27) inpatients, they found that MHPG was higher in CSF from mixed manic than that from agitated depressed patients (Swann et al., 1994). Moreover, patients in a mixed state had higher urinary excretion of NE and elevated output of NE relative to its metabolites, suggesting that mixed manic patients combine certain biological abnormalities considered to be characteristic of both mania and depression.

More recently, the same group investigated relationships between performance on psychomotor tests of motor speed (reaction time and tapping speed) and visual tracking (trail making and dot placement) and catecholamine system function, including CSF or urinary concentrations of catecholamines or their metabolites (Swann et al., 1999). They found that both unipolar and bipolar depressed patients were impaired in motor speed, dexterity, and visual tracking, whereas manic and mixed patients did not differ from controls in these areas. Furthermore, increased catecholamine function correlated with slowing on all other measures for patients with bipolar disorder; relationships between catecholamines and psychomotor function were weaker in unipolar depressed subjects, and psychomotor function was related to severity of depression only in bipolar patients. These latter findings add to the data suggesting that catecholamine systems are associated with increased arousal and psychomotor impairment in patients with bipolar disorder (Goodwin and Ghaemi, 1998).

Taken together, findings from CSF studies of NE and its metabolite MHPG suggest that NE output is higher in mania than in depression and that there may be relatively higher values in unipolar than in bipolar depression. Relative elevation within patient groups may, in turn, be related to anxiety or the overall severity of the condition. As noted previously, it is possible that the CSF findings reflect events occurring in the sympathetic nervous system as much as those occurring in the brain. It is therefore not surprising that the pattern of findings is similar in CSF and plasma. Nevertheless, in some studies, CSF NE or MHPG was found to be correlated with dysphoric elements of the manic syndrome, while urinary measures tended to be associated with euphoric components (Swann et al., 1986; Post et al., 1989), suggesting that studies examining multiple measures and components of the noradrenergic system allow for the most meaningful interpretations.

Studies of Postmortem Brain

Numerous postmortem studies have investigated the role of monoaminergic functioning in major depressive disorder and suicide. Yet there has been a dearth of studies examining the status of monoamine transmitters in autopsy specimens from subjects specifically with bipolar disorder. A study by Young and colleagues (1994c) found that NE turnover (MHPG/NE ratio) was markedly elevated in autopsied frontal, temporal, and occipital cortex of individuals with an antemortem diagnosis of bipolar disorder. In comparison, serotonin (also known as 5-hydroxytryptamine [5-HT]) and dopamine (DA) turnover (5-hydroxy-indoleacetic acid

[5-HIAA]/5-HT and homovanillic acid [HVA]/DA, respectively) were found to be significantly reduced in temporal and occipital cortex, respectively. In an intriguing preliminary study, Baumann and colleagues (1999a) investigated a possible unipolar–bipolar dichotomy by performing a morphological comparison of the locus coeruleus (LC) obtained postmortem. They found that bipolar patients (n=6) had significantly more neurons on both sides of the LC as a whole than did patients with unipolar depression (n=6). Furthermore, topographical analysis revealed that this difference was restricted to the rostral two-thirds and the dorsal portion of the LC, in which bipolar patients showed at least a trend to higher neuron numbers than those of unipolar patients or controls. However, as is characteristic of most unipolar–bipolar comparisons, the two groups were not matched for frequency of recurrence, so that one cannot know whether the differences reflect a difference in polarity or cyclicity.

Studies of Norepinephrine and Its Metabolites in Urine

Since the catecholamine hypothesis of affective disorders was proposed, attempts to characterize the output of the noradrenergic system in depressed patients have focused on measurements of MHPG in urine more than any other single parameter (Potter et al., 1987; Filser et al., 1988). These studies were fueled (at least to some extent) by early data interpretations suggesting that about 50 percent of MHPG in urine was derived from the CNS. However, subsequent work indicated that MHPG readily crosses the blood–brain barrier to the CSF; earlier estimates of the CNS contribution to urinary MHPG have thus been revised to approximately one-third their original values (see Kopin, 1985).

The conclusions in the literature vary, but some authors emphasize that there is (albeit modestly) decreased 24-hour urinary excretion of MHPG in depressed patients compared with that of controls. Also with regard to urinary excretion of MHPG, unipolar depressed patients are more heterogeneous than bipolar-I patients (Maas, 1972). When one examines the studies more closely, it appears that the reduced excretion of MHPG is accounted for exclusively by bipolar patients—although a more recent study, in which subsequent patients in the same center were examined, does not replicate this finding, perhaps suggesting a change in the patient population over time (Grossman and Potter, 1999). Moreover, reduced urinary MHPG may be present only in bipolar-I and not in bipolar-II patients (Muscettola et al., 1984; Schatzberg et al., 1989), with MHPG levels in the former group being similar to those of patients with unipolar depression (Schatzberg et al., 1989). Patients with unipolar depression generally have greater urinary MHPG concentrations than those of bipolar-I patients. Average urinary MHPG is not reduced in unipolar populations taken as a whole; rather, there may be a subgroup of such patients who have elevated MHPG compared with that of controls and bipolar subjects (Schatzberg et al., 1982). Furthermore, pretreatment levels of urinary MHPG have correlated with improvement in manic syndrome scores (Swann et al., 1999). Consistent with an overall activation of the noradrenergic system during mania, manic patients also exhibit significantly increased urinary concentrations of NE compared with those of depressed patients or control subjects (Swann et al., 1987).

Low levels of urinary MHPG in depressed patients have been reported to approach normal values with clinical improvement, thus this measure may be state-dependent (Pickar et al., 1978). Similarly, longitudinal studies of bipolar patients suggest increased MHPG excretion in manic compared with depressed states (Post et al., 1984b; Potter et al., 1987). It has also been noted that manic patients responding to lithium have decreased MHPG and increased NE excretion relative to the total excretion of NE and its metabolites, a finding suggesting that lithium response is associated with an alteration of catecholamine metabolism pathways (Swann et al., 1987). Overall, however, urinary MHPG by itself has not proven to be a sufficiently robust and consistent measure to warrant general acceptance as a useful tool in diagnosis or in prediction of treatment response (Davis and Bresnahan, 1987).

Subsequent investigators have attempted to go beyond the "too little or too much" hypotheses of affective disorders. One approach has been to measure the 24-hour concentrations of urinary catecholamines and their metabolites in an effort to identify possible abnormalities in the relative activity of NE metabolic pathways in depression and mania. Since all major metabolites are measured, 24-hour urinary measures of NE and its metabolites can account for differences among individuals in the relative metabolism of NE, as well as its turnover (amount formed and excreted per 24 hours at steady state) (Manji and Lenox, 1994, 1998).

Consistent with the findings of elevated basal and/or stress-induced plasma NE, several investigators have observed elevated urinary excretion of NE and its major extraneuronal metabolite, normetanephrine (NMN), in depressed patients (Roy et al., 1985, 1986, 1988; Maas et al., 1987; Davis et al., 1988). Moreover, this finding appears more impressive when the excretion of NE and NMN in depressed patients is examined relative to total NE excretion. Thus in the study by Maas and colleagues (1987), a modest increase in total urinary catecholamine excretion (16 percent) was accompanied by marked increases in urinary NE (57 percent) and NMN (42 percent) in depressed patients. These results suggest a shift toward extreneuronal metabolic pathways and are consistent with findings suggesting increased NE release and "spillover" in depression.

More recently, Grossman and Potter (1999) compared the urinary excretion of NE, NMN, MHPG, and vanillylmandelic acid (VMA) in age- and gender-matched unipolar and bipolar depressed patients with that of healthy volunteers hospitalized in an inpatient unit at the National Institute of Mental Health (NIMH). Only depressed subjects with a minimum 4-week drug-free period were included. Total turnover (NE + NMN + MHPG + VMA) was reduced in these patients. In contrast with previous reports, MHPG concentration did not distinguish unipolar from bipolar depressed patients and was not significantly different from that in healthy volunteers. A construct of the average fractional extraneuronal concentration of NE (NE + NMN/NE + NMN + MHPG + VMA) was significantly higher in unipolar and bipolar depressed patients than in healthy volunteers. These findings, which suggest that both unmedicated unipolar and bipolar depressed patients have a "hyperresponsive" noradrenergic system, provide a framework linking plasma and urinary findings. Interestingly, total turnover of NE (NE + NMN + MHPG + VMA) was significantly lower in both unipolar and bipolar depressed patients than in healthy volunteers, suggesting a reduction of tyrosine hydroxylase (TH) activity in sympathetic neurons; these findings are noteworthy in view of lithium's effects on TH (see below).

The relationship between sympathoadrenal and HPA axis activity has also been investigated in patients with unipolar depression. Some investigators (Schatzberg et al., 1989) but not all (Maes et al., 1987) have reported significant positive correlations between urinary cortisol and urinary MHPG concentrations in depressed patients. A similar positive correlation has been reported for plasma cortisol and epinephrine concentrations (Stokes et al., 1981). Previous studies examining the levels of CSF NE and CSF corticotropin-releasing hormone (CRH) receptor found normal, reduced, and increased levels (Nemeroff et al., 1984b; Roy et al., 1988; Potter and Manji, 1994; Geracioti et al., 1997). Subsequently, Wong and colleagues (2000) found that around the clock, patients with melancholic depression had elevated levels of CSF NE and plasma cortisol, but not CSF CRH or plasma adrenocorticotropic hormone (ACTH).

In summary, although the data suggest that measures of catecholamines in CSF, plasma, and urine have provided important information, these types of studies have fallen into disuse over recent years. Rather, there has been a steady shift toward the use of less invasive, in vivo, high-resolution methods (functional magnetic resonance imaging [MRI], positron emission tomography [PET], and single photon emission computed tomography [SPECT]). Yet while some progress has been made in visualizing specific molecules, such as receptors and transporter sites, these brain imaging modalities do not yet permit detailed examination of brain biochemistry.

Clinical Studies of Adrenergic Receptors

The future development of selective receptor ligands for PET studies may eventually permit the direct assessment of CNS adrenergic receptors in humans. To date, studies of NE receptors in affective disorders have been limited to indirect research strategies. Two strategies are most commonly used: (1) characterization of receptor number and function in readily accessible blood elements, and (2) pharmacological challenge strategies whereby alterations in biochemical, neuroendocrine, cardiovascular, or behavioral parameters in response to various receptor agonists and/or antagonists are measured.

Receptors on Blood Cells.   Because of the accessibility of platelets and lymphocytes, both α_2 and β_2 adrenergic receptors have been studied extensively in affective disorders, and elaborate hypotheses about CNS adrenergic receptor dysfunction have been generated solely on the basis of such studies. There are several problems with the assumption that changes in adrenergic receptors on peripheral cells reflect similar alterations in the CNS.[4] This caveat notwithstanding, we now turn to a discussion of adrenergic receptors in manic-depressive illness.

α_2-Adrenergic Receptors.   Numerous studies have measured the binding of α_2-agonist or -antagonist ligands to platelets obtained from patients with affective illness and normal individuals. Yet while human platelets and cerebral cortex contain homogeneous populations of the same α_{2A} receptors (Bylund et al., 1988), radioligand studies across groups are confounded by numerous methodological problems, such as patient populations that vary in gender, age, frequency of recurrence, and current clinical state, as well as differing drug washout periods and assay techniques (see Piletz et al., 1986).

A review of 13 studies using yohimbine-alkaloid radioligands revealed no significant differences in the B_{MAX} of platelet α_2-adrenergic receptors between depressed patients and controls (see Kafka and Paul, 1986; Piletz et al., 1986; Katona et al., 1987). Most studies using partial or full agonists, however, have observed increased B_{MAX} in the platelets of depressed patients compared with controls (Garcia-Sevilla and Fuster, 1986; Pandey et al., 1989; Garcia-Sevilla et al., 1990; Piletz et al., 1990). These results have frequently been interpreted as evidence for the α_2 hypersensitivity theory of depression (Garcia-Sevilla et al., 1986b, 1990; Piletz et al., 1990). Yet these studies have used the imidazoline compounds clonidine, para-aminoclonidine (PAC), and UK-14,304 as radioligands, and it is now known that these ligands also bind to imidazoline sites (Bousquet

and Feldman, 1987; Michel et al., 1990). In one of the few studies of bipolar disorder, bipolar depressed patients were found to show a trend toward a higher density of α_2-adrenergic receptors (Karege et al., 1992). In this study, platelet α_2 receptor measures were related to plasma MHPG. Moreover, stress-induced desensitization of α_2-adrenergic receptors in human platelets (Freedman et al., 1990), accompanied by significant increases in plasma catecholamines and subjective anxiety, suggests that the circulating environment may be the prime determinant of platelet α_2 numbers.

In general, direct study of CNS adrenergic receptors has been limited to comparison of receptor density and affinity in suicide victims (generally unipolar depressive patients) and "appropriate controls." Notwithstanding the numerous methodological pitfalls associated with the study of postmortem tissues (e.g., postmortem delay, cause of death, morbid and premorbid drug history), preliminary data indicate alterations in the density and/or affinity of β- and possibly α_2-adrenergic receptors in depressed suicide victims. Similar to the findings observed in platelets, there are elevations in the binding of the imidazolinic "α_2 ligands," such as clonidine and UK-14,304 (Meana and Garcia-Sevilla, 1987). Whether these sites represent α_2 receptors or imidazoline sites remains to be established, however, although more recent data indicate that both classes of receptors and sites are elevated (Garcia-Sevilla et al., 1996).

β-Adrenergic Receptors.   It is now well documented that different classes of antidepressants, when administered chronically, desensitize β-adrenergic receptors (Banerjee et al., 1977; Sulser 1978; Bergstrom and Kellar, 1979). Thus peripheral β receptors, if they indeed mirror changes in central β-adrenergic receptors, would clearly represent useful tools for defining the role of β-adrenergic receptors in depressive illness and in the effects of treatment. However, alterations in β-adrenergic receptor density in rat brain induced by antidepressants appear to be restricted to the β_1 subtype (Minneman et al., 1979), while human mononuclear leukocytes (MNLs) contain only the β_2 subtypes (Meurs et al., 1982).

Despite these caveats, several groups have investigated the density of β-adrenergic receptors in untransformed lymphocytes or leukocytes of untreated or treated mood disorder patients, with fairly inconsistent results. Some report a decrease in numbers of β-adrenergic receptors in depressed patients,[5] whereas others describe an increase or no change in comparison with healthy volunteers.[6]

In contrast to the inconsistent results of binding studies described above, most studies measuring MNL β-adrenergic receptor–stimulated adenylyl cyclase (AC) activity have found decreased responsiveness in depressed patients compared with that in healthy volunteers.[7] The consistently observed decrease in leukocyte β-adrenergic receptor function in depression could reflect an inherited abnormality of the β-adrenergic receptor/(Gs)/AC complex, as suggested by the findings of a study by Wright and colleagues (1984) using Epstein-Barr virus (EBV)-transformed lymphocytes from manic-depressive patients and controls. However, these findings need to be replicated and a number of additional confounding factors considered (Werstiuk et al., 1990; Manji et al., 1997a).

In another study, Kay and colleagues (1993, 1994) examined β-adrenergic receptor binding and AC activity in lymphoblast cell lines established from 12 patients with bipolar disorder and 10 unrelated healthy controls. The use of immortalized lymphoblasts offers the theoretical advantage of being able to grow the cells for several months away from the potentially confounding effects of circulating factors (catecholamines, hormones, drugs); thus the cells are presumed to reflect closely the individual's genetic contribution to the receptor system in question. It should be noted, however, that the immortalized cells are not "normal," and display a markedly altered β-receptor density relative to fresh, circulating lymphocytes. Nevertheless, unless the immortalization process affects the patients' lymphocytes differently from those of the controls, the model can be used to provide useful information. In Kay and colleagues' study, no significant differences were found in [^{125}I] iodocyanopindolol binding affinity or capacity or in β-adrenergic receptor agonist–stimulated cyclic adenosine monophosphate (cAMP) response. As expected, incubation of lymphoblasts with a β-adrenergic receptor for 24 hours prior to assay reduced both the number of receptors and adenylyl cyclase activity. There was significantly less receptor downregulation in cells of bipolar patients, suggesting that agonist downregulation of receptor number may be less efficient than in control cells. Although these results are clearly quite preliminary, they are intriguing because the inability to downregulate receptors in the face of excessive stimulation has been postulated as representing a fundamental defect in bipolar disorder.

Initial measurements of these β-adrenergic receptors in postmortem brain tissue from mood disorder patients (±individuals who committed suicide) have yielded mixed results. Biegon and Israeli (1988) reported a significant, 50 percent increase in β-adrenergic receptor density in prefrontal cortical homogenates in postmortem brain tissue of suicide victims. They noted that the increased binding was selective, appearing in some cortical regions but not in basal ganglia or white matter areas. Mann and colleagues also found increased β-adrenergic receptor density in the postmortem brain tissue of suicide victims (Arango et al., 1990; Mann et al., 1986). However, Crow and colleagues

(1984) demonstrated decreased density of hippocampal β-adrenergic receptor in the postmortem brain tissue of depressed patients who had been hospitalized. In this latter group, previous antidepressant treatment may have induced β-adrenergic receptor downregulation.

Pharmacological Challenge Strategies

Pharmacological challenge paradigms, which employ agents known to stimulate receptor sites directly or indirectly, have been used extensively to test pathophysiological hypotheses about noradrenergic dysfunction in affective illness (Siever, 1987). The α$_2$-adrenergic agonist clonidine (which may also exert effects at imidazoline sites; see above) has been administered to depressed patients, and the responses of plasma MHPG, blood pressure, heart rate, sedation, growth hormone (GH), and cortisol have been measured. Clonidine-induced decreases in plasma MHPG have been found to be somewhat more marked (Siever et al., 1984) or unchanged (Charney et al., 1983) when using oral or intravenous (IV) clonidine, respectively. Similarly, the plasma MHPG response to yohimbine (an α$_2$-adrenergic antagonist) is unchanged in depressed patients (Heninger et al., 1988). Price and colleagues (1986) reported that the cortisol response to yohimbine was significantly greater in depressed patients than in controls despite similar MHPG responses between groups. Clonidine-induced decreases in blood pressure and increases in sedation have been found to be not significantly different in depressed patients compared with normal controls (Checkley et al., 1981; Charney et al., 1982). Similarly, responses of cortisol and ACTH to acute clonidine administration in depressed patients vary, with levels increased, decreased, or unchanged (Siever, 1987).

In contrast, a series of studies has consistently shown a significantly reduced GH response to clonidine (presumably mediated by postsynaptic hypothalamic α$_2$-adrenergic receptors) in depressed patients.[8] These findings generally have been interpreted as evidence for subsensitive central postsynaptic α$_2$-adrenergic receptors in depression, perhaps secondary to elevations in NE.

A much smaller number of studies have investigated the GH response to adrenergic challenge in bipolar disorder. Ansseau and colleagues (1987) investigated the GH response to clonidine in seven manic patients who had been medication-free for 3 months, age- and gender-matched to seven inpatients with major depression and seven with minor depression inpatients who had been drug-free for at least 2 weeks. Both the manic patients and those with major depression showed a blunting of the GH response relative to patients with minor depression. Additionally, Dinan and colleagues (1991) reported a significant blunting of the desipramine-induced GH release in medication-free manic patients (n=7) compared with controls. Finally, in a longitudinal study of a single 64-year-old rapidly cycling patient, Gann and colleagues (1993) reported that GH secretion after clonidine stimulation was blunted on depressed and hypomanic days. It is now clear, however, that this response is not specific to depression and mania, since a blunted GH response to clonidine has been reported in patients with panic disorder (Charney and Heninger, 1986; Uhde et al., 1986; Nutt, 1989), generalized anxiety symptoms, and obsessive-compulsive disorder (Siever et al., 1983). Thus, a blunted α_2-adrenergic response may be observed in any condition characterized by tonic or episodic abnormally elevated central NE.

Catecholamine Depletion Challenges

Additional evidence for noradrenergic dysfunction in the pathophysiology of depression comes from studies that use α-methylparatyrosine (AMPT) to deplete central NE stores (Miller et al., 1996). In these studies, administration of AMPT to depressed patients who had been successfully treated with desipramine or mazindol (both of which are NE uptake inhibitors) resulted in a rapid return of depressive symptoms. Interestingly, administration of AMPT to depressed patients did not worsen the core symptoms of depression but did cause worsening of some neurovegetative symptoms, in particular anergia and tiredness. Even more interesting is a study that investigated the effects of AMPT on lithium-treated, euthymic bipolar patients (Anand et al., 1999). Intriguingly, the authors did not observe any mood-lowering effects of AMPT, but did observe a "rebound hypomania" in a significant percentage of the patients. Although preliminary, these results are compatible with the notion of a dysregulated signaling system in which the compensatory adaptation to catecholamine depletion results in an "overshoot" due to impaired homeostatic mechanisms. We come back to this study in our discussion of dopamine below.

Lithium and the Noradrenergic System

In view of the long-standing interest in the role(s) of the noradrenergic system in manic-depressive illness, it is not surprising that extensive research has been conducted on lithium's effects on that system. Overall, lithium's effects on NE appear to be temporally and brain region–specific.[9]

Use of both acute and chronic lithium has been reported to increase (Schildkraut et al., 1966, 1969) or not to change (Ho et al., 1970; Ahluwalia and Singhal, 1980) the turnover of NE in some but not all regions of the brain. As is the case with the other neurotransmitters (see below), effects of lithium on NE receptor binding in studies in rodent brain have generally been inconclusive (Treiser and Kellar, 1979;

Maggi and Enna, 1980; Schultz et al., 1981). However, significant effects have been consistently observed on βAR-mediated cAMP accumulation, with lithium inhibiting the response both in vivo and in vitro (discussed in detail below). Lithium is unable to block antidepressant-induced β-adrenergic receptor downregulation (Rosenblatt et al., 1979) and in fact produces a greater subsensitivity (cAMP response) (Mork et al., 1990), but it does prevent reserpine or (6-OHDA)–induced βAR supersensitivity (Pert et al., 1978; Treiser and Kellar, 1979; Hermoni et al., 1980).

Additional data from preclinical and clinical studies suggest that lithium treatment results in subsensitive α_2 receptors.[10] In preclinical studies, long-term lithium was found to attenuate α_2-adrenergic–mediated behavioral effects (G. Goodwin et al., 1986a; Smith, 1988) and presynaptic α_2 inhibition of NE release (Moises et al., 1986), while enhancing (K^+)-evoked NE release (Ebstein et al., 1983). While lithium has been reported to reduce high-affinity platelet [^{3}H] clonidine binding (Wood and Coppen, 1983; Garcia-Sevilla et al., 1986b; Pandey et al., 1989), compatible with a functional "uncoupling" of the receptor from the G protein (Kim and Neubig, 1987; Neubig et al., 1988), interpretation of these data is confounded by the coexistence of the imidazoline binding site discovered later.

In clinical investigations, both increases and decreases in plasma and urinary NE metabolite levels have been reported after lithium treatment.[11] Lithium has been reported to reduce excretion of NE and metabolites in manic patients while increasing excretion in depressed patients, associated with higher plasma NE concentrations in some cases.[12] As discussed earlier, however, there is evidence that urinary excretion of MHPG is low during bipolar depression and elevated during mania/hypomania.[13] In part, these inconsistencies may be related to the inability to control adequately for state-dependent changes in affective states, with associated changes in activity level, arousal, and sympathetic outflow. Subsequent studies have demonstrated that 2 weeks of lithium administration in normal subjects results in increases in urinary NE and NMN, fractional NE release, and a trend toward significantly increased plasma NE, suggesting an enhanced neuronal release of NE (Manji et al., 1991a). These data are compatible with similar observation of increased levels of plasma dihydroxyphenylglycol (DHPG), a major extraneuronal NE metabolite (Poirier-Littre et al., 1993), raising the possibility that lithium may regulate (TH) (discussed later).

Thus current evidence supports lithium's action in facilitating the release of NE, possibly through effects on the presynaptic α_2 "autoreceptor" and through upregulation of TH, while concurrently reducing the β-adrenergic–stimulated AC response. This action may contribute to lithium's attenuation of the euphorigenic effects of amphetamine.

Carbamazepine and the Noradrenergic System

Carbamazepine's effects on noradrenergic metabolism are complex, including decreases in NE turnover (Maitre et al., 1984), weak reuptake blockade (Purdy et al., 1977), and, contrary to the action of most other putative antidepressant substances, upregulation rather than downregulation of β_2 adrenergic receptors following chronic administration (G. Chen et al., unpublished results). Similar to antidepressants and lithium, however, carbamazepine decreases β_2 adrenergic receptor–stimulated AC activity, an effect due largely to direct inhibition of the catalytic subunit of AC (Chen et al., 1996b). Parenthetically, this effect could account for carbamazepine's atypical antidepressant properties in some patients, including those who are unresponsive to more traditional tricyclic and related compounds.

Carbamazepine's effects on noradrenergic metabolism are nonetheless intriguing from several perspectives. For one thing, determining which actions of carbamazepine are important to its antimanic effects, including its ability to decrease stimulated-induced release of NE as well as inhibit NE turnover, remains an open issue (Waldmeier et al., 1984; Post et al., 1985). It is of considerable interest that while noradrenergic tone is necessary to carbamazepine's anticonvulsant effects in some models (Quattrone and Samanin, 1977; Quattrone et al., 1978; Crunelli et al., 1979), it is unnecessary in others (Quattrone et al., 1981). The α_2-adrenergic agonist clonidine blocks the anticonvulsant effects of carbamazepine on electroconvulsive shock (the animal model of ECT) (Crunelli et al., 1979; Fischer and Muller, 1988), while the α_2-adrenergic agonist yohimbine blocks carbamazepine's effects on amygdala-kindled seizures (Weiss et al., 1993). Thus it is clear that even when a putative biochemical effect of the drug is linked to its mechanism of action in one type of seizure or psychiatric syndrome, this may not be the case for all the subcategories and subtypes of that syndrome. However, Post and colleagues (1985) found no changes in plasma or CSF NE or MHPG with carbamazepine treatment in affectively ill patients.

Valproate and the Noradrenergic System

Few studies have directly investigated the effects of valproate on the NE system. Khaitan and colleagues (1994) found that chronic (21 days of treatment in rats with valproate) did not significantly alter the density of β_2 adrenergic receptors in rat cortex. By contrast, Chen and colleagues (1996a) found that chronic (6-day) incubation of C6 glioma cells with valproate (.5 mM) resulted in a 33 percent reduction in B_{MAX} and a marked and selective 41 percent reduction in β_1 without having any significant effects on β_2. Chronic (6-day) incubation of C6 cells with valproate (.5 mM) also was found to markedly attenuate isoproterenol-stimulated cAMP production in intact cells at a rate of approximately 50 percent.

In a more recent study, Sands and colleagues (2000) examined changes in mRNA expression for TH, the NE transporter (NET), and the α_{2A} autoreceptor in rat LC after treatment with valproate. TH mRNA increased slightly (16 percent) following acute treatment, and more so after chronic valproate treatment (26 percent), while neither NET nor α_{2A} mRNA expression changed. Further, chronic valproate treatment attenuated the elevation in TH mRNA expression induced in the LC in response to acute restraint. This result is quite consistent with those of Manji and colleagues (unpublished observations). They investigated the effects of chronic valproate on TH protein levels and found that chronic administration of valproate increased TH protein levels in human neuroblastoma cells in vitro and in rat frontal cortex and hippocampus ex vivo.

The Noradrenergic System in Manic-Depressive Illness: Summary

Considerable evidence suggests that depressed patients excrete disproportionately greater amounts of NE and its major extraneuronal metabolite, NMN, relative to total catecholamine synthesis compared with controls. This is particularly true of melancholic unipolar depressed subjects, but more recent data suggest that under adequately controlled (>4 weeks) study, drug-free bipolar depressed subjects may exhibit a similar dysregulation of the noradrenergic system. At least with regard to mania, the original catecholamine hypothesis has withstood the test of time, with increased noradrenergic function consistently observed in mania, although this finding may ultimately reflect a secondary effect. The intriguing recent findings that CSF and urinary NE measures may be associated with the dysphoric and euphoric components of the manic syndrome, respectively, deserve further investigation and suggest that something other than mania per se may be producing the changes. Findings of increased fractional urinary output of NE and NMN and of an exaggerated rise in plasma NE upon orthostatic challenge in depressed unipolar and bipolar patients are compatible with findings of increased "leakiness" of presynaptic NE terminals (Esler 1982; Veith et al., 1985). Boxes 14–2 and 14–3 summarize overall major findings and findings of newer studies supporting the involvement of the noradrenergic system in the pathophysiology and treatment of bipolar disorder and recurrent unipolar depression.

The Dopaminergic System

It is perhaps surprising that the role of the dopaminergic system in the pathophysiology of manic-depressive illness

BOX 14–2.   A Summary of Major Findings Supporting Involvement of the Noradrenergic System in the Pathophysiology and Treatment of Bipolar Disorder and Recurrent Unipolar Disorder

- CSF, urinary NE, and MHPG: Mania > depression in BP; UPd > BPd
- Plasma NE: Basal levels: BPd < N < UPd (for UPd, especially melancholic, DST+ve)
- Plasma NE: Upon challenge: BPd > UPd > N
- CSF NE: Correlated with dysphoric symptoms and severity in bipolar patients
- Effects of AMPT: Reversal of antidepressant effects in unipolar patients, but "rebound hypomania" in lithium-treated bipolar patients
- Blunted growth hormone response to α_2 agonists and increases in platelet α_2 binding density (most studies in recurrent UP, but likely to occur in both BP and UP)
- Antidepressant efficacy of agents whose biochemical effects include increasing NE
- Agents that increase NE release or block reuptake are capable of triggering mania
- Effective antidepressant treatments generally reduce NE turnover (even those whose primary biochemical target is not the NE system)
- Antidepressant and lithium reduce β adrenergic receptor density and/or function (cAMP formation) in limbic and limbic-related areas of rat brain

α-methyl paratyrosine; BPd = bipolar depressed; CSF = cerebrospinal fluid; DST+ve = dexamethasone nonsuppressors; MHPG = 3-methoxy-4-hydroxyphenylglycol; N = normal; NE = norepinephrine; UP = unipolar patients; UPd = unipolar depressed.

has not received greater study, since it represents a prime candidate on a number of theoretical grounds. For example, the opposite motoric changes seen in the bipolar subgroup are perhaps the most defining characteristics of the illness, ranging from near catatonic immobility to the profound hyperactivity of manic states. Similarly, loss of motivation is one of the central features of depression, while anhedonia and "hyperhedonic states" are among the most defining characteristics of bipolar depression and mania, respectively. In this context, it is noteworthy that the midbrain dopaminergic system is known to play critical roles in regulating not only motoric activity but also motivational and reward circuits. It is clear that motivation and motor function are closely linked, and that motivational variables can influence motor output both qualitatively and quantitatively. Furthermore, there is considerable evidence that the mesolimbic dopaminergic pathway plays a crucial role in the selection and orchestration of goal-directed behaviors, particularly those elicited by incentive stimuli.

CSF Homovanillic Acid Levels

It should be noted that of the three monoamine neurotransmitters evaluated most extensively in preclinical studies, two—serotonin and DA—have been studied in depressed patients almost exclusively in terms of concentrations of their respective metabolites, 5-HIAA and HVA (the major DA metabolite), in CSF. Under carefully controlled conditions, the neurotransmitter metabolites will, in part, reflect relative differences in the output and metabolism of DA and serotonin in those brain regions that contribute the most to CSF concentrations. In humans, however, the relative contributions of different brain areas are not well understood. Moreover, it is really not possible to study the responsiveness of 5-HT and DA neuronal systems with a single-point measure of transmitter metabolite in CSF; at most, longer-term changes can be reflected in CSF studies. Thus, CSF studies of 5-HIAA and HVA in untreated depressed patients can identify some relative differences but cannot directly address the source of any alteration, even to the extent of distinguishing changes of output from those of metabolism and/or elimination.

When considering actual studies, it is also important to recognize that limitations of assay methodology make it difficult to be confident about many earlier studies. The technique of performing two lumbar punctures within a few days of each other, before and after the administration of probenecid to block the active acid transport of 5-HIAA and HVA out of CSF, was an ingenious approach to obtaining an estimate of 5-HT and DA function and release (that is, the amount of accumulation of 5-HIAA and HVA between the period of probenecid administration and the lumbar tap). Such probenecid-induced accumulations sometimes revealed group differences not seen when so-called baseline measures were used (Goodwin et al., 1973). Findings of lower levels of DA metabolite, HVA in CSF, and increased peripheral prolactin levels under both basal and challenge conditions in depressed patients indicated hypofunction of DA in the brain (Willner, 1995; Nicholas et al., 1998).

The strongest finding from clinical studies implicating DA in depression is reduced HVA in CSF; indeed, this is one of the most consistent biochemical findings in depression (Goodwin and Sack, 1974; Asberg et al., 1984; Manji et al., 1995b). There is also evidence for a decreased rate of CSF HVA accumulation in subgroups of depressed patients, including those with marked psychomotor retardation compared with patients with agitation. (Willner, 1983). Furthermore, low levels of HVA may be associated with cognitive impairment in both depressed patients and patients suffering from Parkinson's disease (Wolfe et al., 1990).

Genetic Studies

- COMT low-activity allele (MET 158; COMTL) reported to be a risk factor to BPD (Li et al., 1997; Rotondo et al., 2002)
- COMT low-activity allele showed a tendency to be transmitted among female BPD probands (Mynett-Johnson et al., 1998)
- Increased presence of COMT LL (low-activity allele) in BPD ultrarapid cycling (Kirov et al., 1998; Papolos et al., 1998)
- Apparent association between COMT 158val (low-activity allele) in velocardiofacial syndrome and ultrarapid cycling (Lachman et al., 1996)
- Tyrosine hydroxylase gene variant subjects (TH*2/2) have lower depressive scores in mood disorder patients (Serretti et al., 1998)
- Decrease in depressive symptoms in mood disorder patients when tyrosine hydroxylase (TH) *2/2 gene is present (Serretti et al., 1998)
- Weak association between TH gene with BPD (Perez de Castro et al., 1995)
- Dopa decarboxilase gene reported to be a minor susceptibility gene for BPD (odds ratio 1.48 patients vs. control) (Borglum et al., 1999)

Norepinephrine and its Metabolites

Postmortem brain	• Increase in NE turnover (cortex and thalamus) in BPD (postmortem) (Vawter et al., 2000)
	• Increase in NE turnover in frontal-temporal-occipital and temporal areas in BPD (Young et al., 1994b)
CSF	• Changes in NE CSF primarily associated with psychomotor component of depressed state in affective patients (Katz et al., 1994)
	• Increase in MHPG CSF in mixed manic vs. agitated depressed (Swann et al., 1994)
	• Increased NE CSF in manic patients (Post et al., 1989)
Plasma	• Increased NE excretion in "environment-sensitive" manic patients (Swann et al., 1990)
	• Increased NE (standing and supine) in bipolar depressed patients (Rudorfer et al., 1991)
Urinary	• Increased urinary NE in mania (single rapid-cycling case) (Juckel et al., 2000)
	• Pretreatment urinary MHPG related to improvement of mania (Swann et al., 1999)
	• Decreased total NE turnover (NE + NMN + MHPG + VMA) and an increase in average fractional extraneuronal concentration of NE in bipolar depressed patients (Grossman and Potter, 1999). Previously reported only in unipolar patients
	• Urinary NE correlated with severity of current mood in one rapid-cycling patient (Joyce et al., 1995)
	• Increased urinary NE in mixed bipolar patients (Swann et al., 1994)
	• 24 hour urinary excretion of NE correlated with agitation; 24 hour excretion of epinephrine relative to its metabolite levels correlated with severity of manic symptoms and agitation with NE (Swann et al., 1991)
	• Increased catecholamine function correlates with slowing in performance on psychomotor tests of motor speed in BPD; psychomotor function was related to severity of depression in bipolar, but not in unipolar patients (Swann et al., 1999)

Other Findings

Different distribution of neurons in LC in bipolar patients vs. unipolar patients vs. controls (Baumann et al., 1999a)

Treatment Related

Preclinical	• Valproate treatment increases tyrosine hydroxylase mRNA in LC (Sands et al., 2000)
	• Chronic lithium or valproate increases tyrosine hydroxylase protein levels in limbic and limbic-related areas of rat brain and human neuroblastoma cells (Chen et al., 2000)
	• Lithium (1.0 mM) increases the number of TH-positive neurons derived from a human teratocarcinoma (hNT) approximately six-fold. Moreover, even after withdrawal of lithium chloride (LiCl) on day 5, the number of TH-positive neurons in cultures remained significantly increased (Zigova et al., 1999)
	• Transplantation studies with TH-positive neurons derived from a human hNT showed that all animals with LiCl-pretreated hNT-DA neuronal grafts had TH immunoreactive cells (100%) compared to only 43% of animals with the non-lithium-treated hNT-DA neuronal grafts (Baker et al., 2000)
	• Excessive α_1 stimulation (phenylephrine) in rats produces impairment of cognitive function reminiscent of that seen in mania (Arnsten et al., 1999)

(continued)

BOX **14–3.** Newer Studies Supporting Involvement of the Noradrenergic System in the Pathophysiology and Treatment of Manic-Depressive Illness (Primarily Bipolar) *(continued)*

* Valproate reduces β-adrenergic receptor density and/or function (cAMP formation) in C6 glioma cells; in vivo data not available (Chen et al., 1996a)

Clinical

α_2-AR

* Idaxozan, an α_2 antagonist, shown to have efficacy in treatment of BPD in small studies (Grossman and Potter, 1999)
* Clonidine, an α_2 agonist, shown to have efficacy in treatment of acute mania in small studies (Bakchine et al., 1989; Kontaxakis et al., 1989; Diacicov and Tudorache, 1990; Tudorache and Diacicov 1991)

* Increased α_2-adrenoreceptor sensitivity with CBZ in BPD (Dilsaver et al., 1993)
* Increased (trend) density of α_2-adrenoreceptor in platelet in bipolar depressed patients (Karege et al., 1992)
* Increased cortisol and GH in bipolar depression in single rapid-cycling case, normalized with valproate treatment (Juckel et al., 2000)

β-AR

* Decreased melatonin levels during light night in BP-I patients (β-adrenoreceptor mediated?) (Nurnberger et al., 2000)

AR = adrenoreceptor; BPD = bipolar disorder; BP-I = bipolar-I; CBZ = carbamazepine; COMT = catechol-O-methyltransferase; CSF = cerebrospinal fluid; DA = dopamine; GH = growth hormone; LC = locus coeruleus; MHPG = s-methoxy-4-hydroxyphenylglycol; NE = norepinephrine; NMN = normetanephrine; VMA = vanillylmandelic acid.

By contrast, levels of HVA in the CSF of manic patients have been found to be increased compared with controls in four studies and not significantly different in three studies. When manic patients are compared with depressed patients, the results are more consistent: five studies of bipolar depressed patients found higher HVA in mania, and one other yielded insufficient data to make this comparison. These studies confirm the evidence from older studies with mixed depressed groups.

The Dopaminergic System and the Switch Process

There is arguably the strongest pharmacological support for the dopaminergic system among all the neurotransmitter systems with regard to potential involvement in the switch process to hypomania/mania:

* The DA precursor L-dopa almost uniformly produces hypomania in bipolar patients (Goodwin et al., 1970; Murphy et al., 1971; Van Praag and Korf, 1975).
* Amphetamine, which promotes DA release and inhibits its uptake, can precipitate hypomania in bipolar patients and induce a hypomania-like state in normal people (Jacobs and Silverstone, 1986), but is generally not considered an antidepressant in unipolar patients (Goodwin and Sack, 1973).
* The direct DA agonists bromocriptine and piribedil appear to be effective antidepressants in some bipolar patients and capable of precipitating mania (Gerner et al., 1976; Silverstone, 1978, 1984). Interestingly, antidepressant response to piribedil has been associated with low pretreatment levels of HVA in CSF (Post et al., 1978).
* Neuroleptics that selectively block DA receptors (such as pimozide) are effective against severe mania.

Catecholamine Depletion Strategies

Earlier we described the work of Anand and colleagues (1999) who examined the effects of catecholamine depletion with AMPT in lithium-treated euthymic bipolar subjects. The rebound hypomania noted earlier was not associated with changes in iodobenzamide (IBZM) binding, suggesting that the "overshoot" was not mediated by enhanced "recovery-associated DA release." Rather, the overshoot was most likely mediated by sensitized postsynaptic dopaminergic mechanisms (due to DA depletion) or noradrenergic mechanisms.

Most recently, McTavish and colleagues (2001) administered a tyrosine-free mixture that lowered both subjective and objective measures of the psychostimulant effects of methamphetamine, as well as manic scores. These preliminary findings suggest that tyrosine availability to the brain attenuates pathological increases in DA neurotransmission following methamphetamine administration and putatively in mania.

Neuroreceptor Imaging Studies of the Dopaminergic System

PET Studies. Compared with the number of studies in schizophrenia and depression, very few neurochemical studies of the dopaminergic system have been conducted in manic-depressive illness. One PET study with [^{11}C]-SCH23390 investigated D1 binding in medication-free bipolar subjects. The authors found reduced binding potential in the frontal cortex in patients compared with normal controls, and no significant difference in striatum (Suhara et al., 1992). This study included a small sample (n = 10) of euthymic, depressed, and manic patients. This work needs to be extended to unipolar patients and replicated independently in bipolar individuals.

A PET study with N-[^{11}C]methylspiperone found increased binding potential (B_{max}) for striatal D2 receptors in psychotic bipolar patients compared with nonpsychotic bipolar patients and healthy individuals (Pearlson et al., 1995). Patients were neuroleptic-naïve or neuroleptic-free for at least 6 months. These findings are similar to those previously reported by this group for schizophrenia, and thus may be related to psychotic status.

In a subsequent study, the concentration of the vesicular monoamine transporter protein (VMAT2) was quantified with (+)[^{11}C]dihydrotetrabenazine (DTBZ) and PET (Zubieta et al., 2000). This study included 16 asymptomatic patients with bipolar-I disorder and a prior history of mania with psychosis (9 men and 7 women) and individually matched healthy subjects. VMAT2 binding in the thalamus and ventral brain stem of the bipolar patients was found to be higher than that in the comparison subjects.

In a follow-up study, the same research group attempted to assess the diagnostic specificity of these findings by comparing VMAT2 concentrations in euthymic bipolar-I patients (15), schizophrenic patients (12), and age-matched healthy volunteers (15) (Zubieta et al., 2001). It was found that VMAT2 binding in the thalamus was higher in the bipolar-I patients than in the schizophrenic and control groups. The authors interpret the intriguing findings of increased VMAT2 expression in euthymic bipolar-I patients as representing trait-related abnormalities in the concentration of monoaminergic synaptic terminals. However, chronic lithium treatment has recently been demonstrated to increase VMAT protein in rat FCx (the only region examined) (Zucker et al., 2001), raising the possibility that the PET human studies may have been confounded by treatment effects.

Most recently, Yatham and colleagues (2002) assessed presynaptic DA function in 13 neuroleptic- and mood stabilizer–naive nonpsychotic first-episode manic patients by measuring [^{18}F]6-fluoro-L-dopa ([^{18}F]DOPA) uptake in the striatum by means of PET. No significant differences were found between [^{18}F]DOPA uptake rate constants in the striatum in the manic patients and comparison subjects; however, treatment with valproate significantly reduced the [^{18}F]DOPA uptake rate.

SPECT Studies. In major depression, SPECT studies performed using [^{123}I]-IBZM, a DA D2 receptor ligand that is sensitive to endogenous DA concentrations, have found increased striatal DA D2/D3 receptor availability during the depressed phase, which could potentially be accounted for by a reduction of endogenous DA release (Drevets et al.,

2002). Two studies (D'Haenen and Bossuyt, 1994; Shah et al., 1997) found that patients with unipolar depression have increased striatal uptake of [^{123}I]-IBZM compared with controls. Ebert and Ebmeier (1996) found a nonsignificant trend toward increased [^{123}I]-IBZM binding in depressed patients versus controls, which became significant in a subgroup that displayed overt psychomotor retardation. Consistent with this latter observation, Shah and colleagues (1997) found that striatal [^{123}I]-IBZM binding correlated inversely with movement speed and verbal fluency measures, implying that the elevation of DA D2/D3 receptor availability correlated with psychomotor slowing in depression; however, interpretation of these data was confounded by the presence of drug effects (Drevets et al., 2002).

Anand and colleagues (1999, 2000b) have used SPECT to study dynamic changes in the DA synapse in response to pharmacological challenges with drugs such as amphetamine and AMPT that alter synaptic DA levels. The initial study included 13 patients with bipolar disorder (7 medication-free, 6 on mood stabilizer therapy) who at the time had been in a euthymic state for more than 4 weeks and 13 age- and gender-matched healthy controls. SPECT scans of the striatal D2/D3 receptor radiotracer [^{123}I]-IBZM were performed before and after an amphetamine challenge (.3 mg/kg IV). Reduction in striatal [^{123}I]-IBZM binding potential from the first scan to the second was used as an indirect measure of the amount of DA released. Bipolar patients and healthy subjects did not differ on baseline mood state and baseline striatal D2 receptor binding. Amphetamine challenge led to a significantly greater behavioral response in bipolar patients than in healthy subjects. However, there was no significant difference between the two groups in striatal [^{123}I]-IBZM binding following amphetamine challenge. Thus, this study did not find evidence for increased striatal DA release in euthymic bipolar patients. Instead, these data are consistent with enhanced postsynaptic DA responsivity in bipolar patients (discussed later).

Enhancing Dopamine Function in the Treatment of Depression

Interestingly, monoamine oxidase inhibitors (MAOIs) represent the only pharmacological monotherapy that is reported to be effective in 50 percent or more of patients who fail to respond to the full range of tricyclic antidepressants. Nolen and colleagues (1988) reported on a controlled trial, indicating the superior efficacy of tranylcypromine (average dose of approximately 80 mg/day) in such patients. As reviewed in Chapter 19, tranylcypromine is superior to imipramine in chronic, mild unipolar depression (McGrath et al., 1987) and in "anergic" bipolar depression (Himmel-hoch et al., 1991; Thase et al., 1992), and phenelzine is superior in unipolar patients refractory to imipramine (McGrath et al, 1993). An open-label study of high-dose tranylcypromine (average 120 mg/day) in 14 unipolar patients with a clear history of nonresponse to at least two prior medication treatments yielded an impressive 50 percent "complete" response rate on the Hamilton Depression Rating Scale (HAM-D) (Amsterdam, 1991). The authors speculate that higher plasma concentrations of tranylcypromine enhance the drug's sympathomimetic (amphetamine-like) activity. In other words, at higher doses, one may actually recruit a pharmacodynamic effect of the drug beyond MAO inhibition.

Identifying multiple specific effects in humans, however, is not simple. Studies with DA reuptake inhibitors such as nomifensine have shown clear antidepressant effects in major depression. Similarly, bromocriptine, a postsynaptic DA receptor agonist, has been reported to have efficacy comparable with that of standard tricyclic antidepressants (Silverstone, 1984) and to be useful in antidepressant-resistant depression (Inoue et al., 1996) and in relapses that occur with selective serotonin reuptake inhibitor (SSRI) treatment (McGrath et al., 1995).

In a small pilot study of depressed patients, Schaefer and colleagues (1996) found that 69 percent (9/13) of patients taking pramipexole (a D2/ D3 agonist) had a greater than 30 percent reduction in (HAM-D) total scores relative to baseline scores. DeBattista and colleagues (2000) reported the successful augmentation of an SSRI when pramipexole was added in treatment-resistant major depression. In a retrospective chart review, Sporn and colleagues (2000) found that pramipexole (mean dose .70 mg/day) was effective in 50 percent (6/12) of subjects with bipolar depression and 40 percent (8/20) of subjects with unipolar depression. Lattanzi and colleagues (2002) reported that pramipexole in the dose range of .375–1.0 mg/day was effective in treatment-resistant depression (14 unipolar, 17 bipolar patients) when used adjunctively with other antidepressants. Pramipexole was also tested in a double-blind 8-week, placebo-controlled study involving 174 subjects with unipolar depression without psychotic features (Corrigan et al., 2000). In patients with bipolar depression, two double-blind, placebo-controlled trials found pramipexole to be superior to placebo in the treatment of depressive symptoms (Goldberg et al. 2004; Zarate et al. 2004b,c). In the bipolar II depression study (Zarate et al. 2004b,c), 21 patients treated with lithium or valproate were randomized to receive add-on pramipexole $1.7 \pm .9$ mg/day (n=10) or placebo (n=11) for 6 weeks. All subjects except for one in each group completed the study. At the endpoint, changes in both Montgomery-Asberg Depression Rating Scale (MADRS) and 24-item HAM-D scores in the pramipexole group were significantly larger compared with those in the placebo group. Response rates were significantly higher among patients taking pramipexole than those taking placebo, 60 percent versus 9 percent.

In another study, the efficacy of pramipexole augmentation was assessed in patients who had treatment-resistant bipolar depression. Twenty-two patients (bipolar-I n=15, bipolar-II n=7) treated with lithium, divalproex, carbamazepine, lamotrigine, and/or topiramate at stable doses for a month, with HAM-D scores of ≥18, were randomized to receive pramipexole (1.7 ± 1.3 mg/day) or placebo for 6 weeks. The mean change from baseline in HAM-D scores was significantly greater in patients taking pramipexole than in those taking placebo. The proportion of responders was significantly higher in patients taking pramipexole, 67 percent versus 20 percent.

Lithium and the Dopaminergic System

The effect of lithium on DA synthesis and transmission has been investigated extensively in preclinical studies by directly determining changes in DA or HVA and indirectly examining lithium-induced changes in DA-linked behaviors (Bunney and Garland-Bunney, 1987). Lithium administration has also been found to cause a dose-dependent decrease in DA formation,[14] which occurs at 25 percent lower doses in the striatum than in the limbic forebrain (Poitou and Bohuon, 1975; Segal et al., 1975; Laakso and Oja, 1979).

Based on the heuristic hypothesis that supersensitive DA receptors underlie the development of manic episodes, it has been postulated that lithium would prevent DA receptor supersensitivity (Bunney and Garland, 1983; Bunney and Garland-Bunney, 1987). In a series of studies, it was found that lithium prevented haloperidol-induced DA receptor upregulation (Rosenblatt et al., 1980; Verimer et al., 1980; Bunney and Garland, 1982) and supersensitivity to iontophoretically applied DA or IV apomorphine (Gallager et al., 1978). Indeed, lithium appears to be effective in blocking both the behavioral and biochemical manifestations of supersensitive DA receptors induced by receptor blockade.

A proposed site of action for lithium's ability to block behavioral supersensitivity is the postsynaptic receptor and the prevention of haloperidol-induced increases in DA receptors. Despite significant functional evidence, however, DA receptor binding studies have remained inconclusive, suggesting a possible postreceptor site of lithium action, potentially related to receptor–effector coupling. Interestingly, a number of studies have reported a lack of effect if lithium is administered after the induction of DA supersensitivity (Klawans et al., 1977; Staunton et al., 1982a,b; Bloom et al., 1983), suggesting that in this model, lithium exerts its greatest effects prophylactically.

Among the numerous behavioral effects of lithium in animals, perhaps the best studied are those on stimulant-induced activity. Lithium's ability to antagonize increases in amphetamine-induced locomotor activity without having major effects on basal activity has gained much attention, in part because it tends to mimic the clinical situation in which lithium does not have major effects on "baseline" activity levels, but has a profound effect on the hyperactivity observed in manic states. It is also of interest that lithium has been reported to attenuate the euphoriant and motor-activating effects of oral amphetamine in depressed patients, although equivocal results have been observed upon methylphenidate challenge (Huey et al., 1981; Van Kammen et al., 1985).

Studies of DA and its metabolites in patients' CSF before and after lithium treatment have yielded conflicting results.[15] A longitudinal study of one unipolar and seven bipolar women found that lithium reduced the levels of DA, DOPAC, and HVA in all the patients (Linnoila et al., 1983b), but the possible role of alterations in mood state and motor activity remained a confounding variable, as it does for all clinical investigations using this research strategy.

Overall, although the data from human investigations are sparse, lithium's postulated ability to reduce both pre- and postsynaptic aspects of DA transmission represents an attractive mechanism for its antimanic therapeutic action. Subsequent studies have investigated the effects of lithium on putative postreceptor components of dopaminergic signaling. Thus, lithium has been shown to potentiate the hyperactivity induced by intra-accumbens cholera toxin administration (which activates the stimulatory G proteins, G_s and G_{olf}) (Kofman et al., 1998). Another study found that the G protein coupled to D1 stimulation was upregulated after chronic lithium, presumably as a compensatory mechanism due to reduced DA throughput. Interestingly, chronic antidepressants have also been associated with enhanced D1 signaling, suggesting that these compensatory effects of lithium may play a role in the "rebound" increase in manic episodes observed after abrupt lithium discontinuation (see Chapter 18).

Studies in the last few years have demonstrated that lithium at therapeutically relevant concentrations increases gene expression through the activator protein-1 (AP-1) transcription factor pathway in vitro (Yuan et al., 1998). Follow-up studies investigated the ability of lithium to increase the expression of endogenous genes known to be regulated by AP-1, in particular TH (Chen et al., 1998). Chronic lithium treatment resulted in significant increases in TH levels in rat frontal cortex, hippocampus, and striatum. Lithium

(1.0 mM) also increased TH levels in human SH-SY5Y neuroblastoma cells in vitro, indicating that the drug increases TH levels in both rodent and human tissues, likely through a direct cellular effect.

In subsequent studies, lithium's potential utility in a Parkinson's disease transplantation model was investigated. In this context, neurons derived from a human teratocarcinoma (hNT) were shown to survive and integrate within the host brain following transplantation and to provide functional recovery in animal models of stroke and Huntington's disease. To maximize the likelihood of success following transplantation (i.e., DA synthesis), researchers have recently investigated lithium's effects on TH expression in these derived neurons (Zigova et al., 1999). Therapeutically relevant doses of lithium chloride (1.0 mM) were found to increase the number of TH-positive neurons approximately six-fold (Zigova et al., 1999). In addition, the TH-positive hNT neuron mean soma profile area and neurite length were significantly larger than in controls by 60 and 70 percent, respectively. Moreover, even after withdrawal of lithium chloride on day 5, the number of TH-positive neurons in cultures remained significantly increased. These data suggest that hNT cells are indeed responsive to lithium exposure and may serve as a continual source of TH-expressing neurons in new therapeutic approaches to degenerative brain disease.

In additional follow-up work, researchers investigated the potential use of hNT neurons for transplantation into the substantia nigra (SN) and striatum of the rat model for Parkinson's disease (Baker et al., 2000). Twenty-seven rats were grafted with one of three hNT neuronal products— hNT neurons, hNT-DA neurons, or lithium chloride (LiCl)–pretreated hNT-DA neurons. Immunostaining for TH expression revealed no TH-immunoreactive (THir) neurons in any animals with hNT neuronal grafts. Interestingly, THir cells were observed in 43 percent of animals with hNT-DA neuronal grafts but in all the animals with LiCl-pretreated hNT-DA neuronal grafts.

Valproate and the Dopaminergic System

Few preclinical studies have examined the effects of valproate on the dopaminergic system after chronic administration, that is, in paradigms likely to reflect the biochemical effects of the drug most relevant for the treatment of bipolar disorder. Acute valproate administration has been demonstrated to increase or decrease HVA levels in caudate (Biggs et al., 1992; Vriend and Alexiuk, 1996), to increase HVA levels in brain stem and frontal cortex (Loscher and Honack, 1996), and to increase HVA levels in CSF of freely moving rats (MacMillan et al., 1987). Interestingly, Ichikawa and colleagues (2001) found that both carbamazepine and valproate increased extracellular DA levels in rat medial prefrontal cortex, effects also seen with clozapine. Moreover, increased prefrontal DA was completely abolished by the selective 5-HT$_{1A}$ receptor antagonist N-[2-[4-(2-methoxyphenyl)-1-piperazinyl]ethyl]-N-2-pyridinylcyclo-hexanecarboxamide (WAY100635, .05 mg/kg).

To elucidate possible mechanisms underlying the effects of carbamazepine and valproate on neurotransmitter exocytosis, the effects of these neuroleptic drugs and botulinum toxins (BoNTs) on basal, Ca^{2+}- and K^+-evoked release of DA and serotonin were determined by microdialysis in the hippocampus of freely moving rats (Murakami et al., 2001). Perfusion with low and high concentrations of carbamazepine and valproate increased and decreased basal DA release, respectively. On the basis of additional studies, these investigators postulated that carbamazepine and valproate affect both the enhancement of syntaxin-mediated monoamine release during the resting stage and the inhibition of synaptobrevin-mediated release during the depolarizing stage.

In animal behavioral studies, valproate was found to attenuate the acute locomotor effects of methylphenidate and, at higher doses, to block the development of sensitization to subsequent administration (Eckermann et al., 2001). Chronic valproate pretreatment also produced a borderline significant reduction in quinpirole-induced hyperactivity without effects on the hypoactive phase (Shaldubina et al., 2002).

Carbamazepine and the Dopaminergic System

In Maitre and colleagues' (1984) review of the literature, they conclude that carbamazepine decreases DA turnover through unknown mechanisms. Later, Baptista and colleagues (1993) found that carbamazepine blocks cocaine-induced increases in DA overflow in the n. accumbens as measured by in vivo dialysis. This effect could account for the observation of Aigner and colleagues (1990) that carbamazepine inhibits cocaine intake in self-administration in the rhesus monkey, a process thought to be mediated by accumbens dopaminergic mechanisms.

The Dopaminergic System in Manic-Depressive Illness: Summary

Overall, indirect evidence for the involvement of recurrent mood disorder is provided by the involvement of that system in circuits known to regulate motivation, reward, and motoric activity, as well as pharmacological data demonstrating that dopaminergic agonists trigger hypomanic/manic episodes and that drugs that reduce dopaminergic throughput (including mood stabilizers and antipsychotics) are antimanic. However, there are fewer data suggesting *primary* dopaminergic abnormalities in manic-depressive illness. It is our contention that the

---

BOX 14–4.   A Summary of Major Findings Supporting Involvement of the Dopaminergic System in the Pathophysiology and Treatment of Bipolar Disorder and Recurrent Unipolar Depression

- Reduced CSF HVA in depressed patients
- Blunted neuroendocrine and temperature responses to DA agonists
- Reduced internal jugular venoarterial HVA concentration gradients
- Antidepressant efficacy of agents whose biochemical effects include increasing intrasynaptic dopamine
- ECT consistently enhances DA function
- Depressogenic effects of AMPT and reserpine in susceptible individuals
- Medications that block D2 receptors have antimanic efficacy
- Lithium-treated euthymic bipolar patients show a rebound hypomania following AMPT
- Depression very common in Parkinson's disease
- Prominent anhedonia, amotivation, and psychomotor retardation in bipolar depression
- Critical role of DA in reward, motivation, and motoric circuits

CSF = cerebrospinal fluid; DA = dopamine; ECT = electroconvulsive therapy; HVA = homovanillic acid.

---

primary abnormality in manic-depressive illness, and perhaps especially in its bipolar form, is a compromised ability to regulate multiple signals (including those generated by the dopaminergic system). Indeed, supporting this contention are recent data suggesting that bipolar disorder may be associated with polymorphisms affecting the functioning of the G protein–coupled receptor kinase 3 (GRK-3).

The GRKs are a family of proteins whose cellular function is to turn off or dampen the signal when receptors are exposed to high levels of neurotransmitters. These proteins are involved in rapidly phosphorylating receptors that are overstimulated, thereby uncoupling the receptors from their second messenger systems. Thus, a faulty desensitization system due to a mutation in GRK is of considerable interest with respect to the pathophysiology of bipolar disorder, as it would result in overshooting in response to multiple neurotransmitter systems, thereby producing excessive excursions from the norm. These observations, if replicated, would suggest that bipolar disorder is associated with an abnormality of DA function, but is not due to defects in the dopaminergic system itself, rather in the machinery involved in dampening and fine-tuning dopaminergic signals. Boxes 14–4 and 14–5 summarize overall major findings and findings of newer studies supporting the involvement of the dopaminergic system in the pathophysiology and treatment of bipolar disorder and recurrent unipolar depression.

Genetic Studies

Receptors
- DA receptor D2 S311C variant associated with disorganization and delusion features in psychosis (Serretti et al., 2000)
- Reduced novelty seeking in carriers of *DRD3* allele 1 in BPD (Staner et al., 1998)
- D3 receptor (homocygous for the (2-2)Bal I polymorphism) reported to exhibit manic symptomatology in monopolar form (Chiaroni et al., 2000)
- Increase in DA D3 receptor gene allele 1 reported in BPD families (Parsian et al., 1995)
- Association between DA D4 receptor gene and mood disorders (Manki et al., 1996)

Transporter
- *DAT* (DA transporter) gene (single nucleotide polymorphism), linkage desequilibrium with BPD (Greenwood et al., 2001)
- *DAT1* with a missense substitution inherited between a BPD father and his BPD son (Grunhage et al., 2000)
- Linkage desequilibrium reported between *DAT1* gene and BPD (Waldman et al., 1997)

Enzymes
- Dopa decarboxylase gene reported to represent a minor susceptibility gene for BPD (odds ratio 1.48 patients. vs. control) (Borglum et al., 1999)
- COMT low-activity allele showed a trend toward being transmitted among female BPD probands (Mynett-Johnson et al., 1998)
- COMT low activity (MET 158; COMTL) reported to be a risk factor for BPD (Li et al., 1997; Rotondo et al., 2002)
- Increased presence of COMT LL (low activity allele) in BPD ultrarapid cycling (Kirov et al., 1998; Papolos et al., 1998)
- Apparent association between COMT 158val (low activity allele) in velocardiofacial syndrome and ultrarapid cycling (Lachman et al., 1996)
- Decrease in depressive symptoms reported in mood disorder patients when tyrosine hydroxylase (TH) *2/2 gene is present (Serretti et al., 1998)
- Weak association reported between *TH* gene and *DRD2* gene with BPD (Perez de Castro et al., 1995)
- Mutation of *NURR1* in BPD, single case (*NURR1*-deficient animals fail to develop mesencephalic DA neurons) (Buervenich et al., 2000)

Other Observations

- Reduced frontal cortex D1 receptor binding (PET) reported in medication-free BPD (Suhara et al., 1992)
- Increased D2 receptor B_{max} reported in psychotic BPD (Pearlson et al., 1995)
- Increased levels of immunoglobulin G with affinity for DA reported in CSF of psychotic patients (12 of 20 were BPD) (Bergquist et al., 1993)
- Increased urinary DA reported to predict manic mood in one rapid-cycling patient (Joyce et al., 1995)
- Increase of episodic parkinsonism, before onset of depression, that disappeared during mania, in 3 cases of rapid-cycling patients (Scappa et al., 1993). Consistent with hypo- and hyperdopaminergic DA functioning in bipolar depression and mania, respectively
- Higher vesicular monoamine transporter (VMAT2) binding in the thalamus and ventral brain stem of bipolar patients than in controls. Unclear whether due to primary disease, lithium treatment, or a combination of these

Treatment Related

Mood stabilizers
- Reduction of platelet MAO activity and increase in dopamine β-hydroxylase activity with Li treatment in BPD (Sofuoglu et al., 1995)
- Reduction in prolactin with long-term Li treatment in euthymic BPD (Basturk et al., 2001)
- Increase in DA metabolism (increase in HVA) when Li is added to a neuroleptic in acute psychosis (Bowers et al., 1992)
- Decrease in presynaptic DA after valproate in BP-I patients (Yatham et al., 2002)
- Decrease by carbamazepine (and not by Li) of chronic imipramine-induced supersensitivity to locomotor response to quinpirole (D'Aquila et al., 2000, 2001) and decrease in quinpirole-induced biphasic locomotion (D2 D3 agonist) by anticonvulsants (Shaldubina et al., 2002)
- Valproate treatment increases tyrosine hydroxylase mRNA in locus coeruleus (Sands et al., 2000)
- Chronic lithium or valproate increases tyrosine hydroxylase protein levels in limbic and limbic-related areas of rat brain and human neuroblastoma cells (Chen et al., 2000)

(continued)

BOX **14–5.** **Newer Studies Supporting Involvement of the Dopaminergic System in the Pathophysiology and Treatment of Manic-Depressive Illness (Primarily Bipolar)** *(continued)*

- Lithium increases the number of TH-positive neurons derived from a human teratocarcinoma approximately six-fold. Moreover, even after withdrawal of LiCl on day 5, the number of TH-positive neurons in cultures remained significantly increased (Zigova et al., 1999)
- Transplantation studies with TH-positive neurons derived from a human teratocarcinoma (hNT) showed that all the animals with LiCl-pretreated hNT-DA neuronal grafts had TH immunoreactive cells (100%) compared to only 43% of animals with the non–lithium-treated hNT-DA neuronal grafts (Baker et al., 2000)

Antidepressants
- Resistant bipolar depression responds to addition of drugs increasing intrasynaptic DA (Erfurth et al., 2002)
- Pramipexole, roniprole are effective add-on treatment for resistant BP-II depression (Perugi et al., 2001)
- Pramipexole augmentation effective in bipolar or unipolar depression (Sporn et al., 2000)

Psychostimulants
- Attenuation of behavioral effects of methamphetamine in dietary tyrosine-depleted manic patients (McTavish et al., 2001)
- Increased behavioral response to amphetamine challenge without changes in D2/D3 binding in striatum in euthymic BP patients (Anand et al., 2000b)

BP = bipolar; BPD = bipolar disorder; BP-I = bipolar-I; COMT = catechol-O-methyltransferase; CSF = cerebrospinal fluid; DA = dopamine; HVA = homovanillic acid; Li-lithium; LiCl = lithium chloride; MAO = monoamine oxidase; TH = tyrosine hydroxylase.

The Serotonergic System

Interest in the role of the serotonergic system in mood disorders derived from a long-standing tradition of research into the role of this indoleamine in the therapeutic mechanisms of action of antidepressants and lithium. There is considerable evidence of abnormalities in the serotonergic neurotransmitter system in patients suffering from depression; however, the data for bipolar disorder are much less extensive, and for recurrent unipolar, data are virtually nonexistent (Meltzer and Lowy, 1987; Shiah and Yatham, 2000; Mahmood and Silverstone, 2001). The serotonergic dysfunction in the pathophysiology of depression has been reported to occur at many different levels, including precursor availability, neurotransmitter synthesis, storage, release, presynaptic autoreceptor function, neurotransmitter reuptake, metabolism, and postsynaptic neurotransmitter receptors.

Studies of Serotonin Metabolites in CSF

As we reviewed in the first edition of this text, earlier findings on 5-HIAA in CSF were in the direction of reductions in depressed patients, but with much less consistency than more recent findings, perhaps because of reliance on fluorometric assay. There was also a trend in those data toward lower 5-HIAA in bipolar than in unipolar patients. Investigators have been unable to demonstrate convincing evidence for group differences in the CSF levels of 5-HIAA (with or without probenecid) between unipolar and bipolar patients; there appears, however, to be a subgroup of patients with low levels of 5-HIAA, which may be associated with certain illness characteristics (impulsivity, aggression, and suicide attempts [Van Pragg, 1982; Meltzer and Lowy, 1987; Virkkunen et al., 1989]). Findings of studies of baseline 5-HIAA in CSF of unmedicated depressed patients are inconsistent: the NIMH Collaborative Study reports increased 5-HIAA in depressed women (Koslow et al., 1983). In 83 patients with melancholia diagnosed and treated at the Karolinska Institute in Sweden, by contrast, 5-HIAA was found to be modestly but significantly reduced (Asberg et al., 1984). In the former study, there was a trend toward lower 5-HIAA in female bipolar than female unipolar patients; in the latter study, there were no unipolar–bipolar differences in this measure.

Studies of CSF 5-HIAA in manic patients have generally produced variable and inconsistent results (Goodwin and Ghaemi, 1998; Shiah and Yatham, 2000). Baseline CSF 5-HIAA levels in manic patients compared with nondepressed controls have been reported to be decreased in four studies, unchanged in nine studies, and increased in three studies; by contrast, most studies found no difference in the levels of CSF 5-HIAA between manic and depressed patients. Of four studies that examined CSF 5-HIAA accumulation following administration of probenecid in manic and depressive patients as well as controls, two found that both manic and depressed patients had diminished CSF 5-HIAA formation compared with that in controls, and one that manic patients had significantly lower CSF 5-HIAA accumulation than that in depressive patients and controls.

Mixed-State, Well-State, and Longitudinal Studies   As discussed in Chapter 1, mixed states are now recognized as common, and it is likely that the biochemical studies already reviewed included such patients among subjects diagnosed as manic. To our knowledge, there has still been only one CSF study focused on mixed states—that of Tandon and colleagues (1988), who compared mixed bipolar patients with pure manic and unipolar depressive patients. Whereas both HVA and 5-HIAA were higher in the patients with pure mania than in those with depression, the mixed group could be biochemically divided into two subgroups whose metabolite levels resembled those of the pure manic and pure depressive groups, respectively. In addition, these authors compared their metabolite data with published normal control values obtained by the same method. They noted that all three groups had 5-HIAA levels significantly below normal, a finding they interpreted as consistent with the permissive hypothesis (discussed below).

In a few CSF amine metabolite studies, measurements were repeated after recovery in an attempt to assess the well state. In most studies of the well state, however, it is virtually impossible to tease drug effects apart from the recovered state itself. The study of spontaneous or ECT-induced recovery is one approach to this problem, but only preliminary data are available. Coppen and colleagues (1972), Ashcroft and colleagues (1973), and Van Praag and De Haan (1979) reported that their depressed patients with low levels of CSF 5-HIAA failed to normalize with recovery. Berrettini and colleagues (1985b), by contrast, found no difference in CSF 5-HIAA (and HVA) in recovered bipolar patients compared with healthy controls, although this study did not compare the well state with the illness phase in the same patients. The persistence of low 5-HIAA levels reported by Coppen and colleagues and by Van Praag and De Haan is of interest in light of the suggestion that CSF 5-HIAA is similar in both manic and depressive phases of the illness. Relevant to these questions are two small longitudinal studies of 5-HIAA (Asberg et al., 1973; Post et al., 1980a), which demonstrated reasonable stability of 5-HIAA levels over time. The issue of postrecovery metabolite data reemerges when we review drug effects.

To our knowledge, no group of bipolar patients has been studied with serial measurement of CSF metabolites through the depressive and manic phases. A few scattered cases of rapid-cycling patients have been presented, although it is not clear just how representative such patients are. Post and colleagues (1977) and Cutler and Post (1982) followed CSF amine metabolites through seven depressive phases and eight manic phases in three patients. Baseline and probenecid-induced accumulation of 5-HIAA were not significantly different during mania and depression, but NE levels were significantly higher in mania. Additional longitudinal studies are discussed in the next two sections.

In postmortem studies, low concentrations of 5-HT and its metabolite 5-HIAA have been reported in the brain stem of depressed patients who completed suicide (Traskman et al., 1981). In brains from nine subjects with a DSM-III-R diagnosis of bipolar disorder who died while depressed, a significant reduction in levels of 5-HIAA was found in frontal (−54 percent) and parietal cortex (−64 percent) (Young et al., 1994c).

Overall, however, findings on CSF and brain 5-HIAA tend to support the permissive hypothesis of Prange, which suggests that, in bipolar disorder, a background state independent deficit in central 5-HT function is associated with impaired buffering so that bidirectional changes in other systems (perhaps involving norepinephrine and/or dopamine) are "permitted" to occur and produce abnormal excursions in mood and behavior.

Platelet 5-HT Uptake

Rausch and colleagues (1986) measured 5-HT uptake in depressed patients, manic bipolar patients, and patients with other affective disorders and nonaffective psychiatric disorders using a randomized block factorial analysis of variance. They found that the depressed patients had significantly lower maximal velocity (V_{max}) of serotonin uptake in comparison with matched controls, without a statistically significant difference in affinity (i.e., the tightness of binding of the transmitter to the reuptake site). No statistically significant difference was found for any of the other diagnostic groups in comparison with controls for V_{max} or Km.

By contrast, Meltzer and colleagues (1981) noted a tendency for a decrease in 5-HT uptake in four manic patients and an increase in seven manic patients, although manic patients as a group did not differ significantly from healthy controls. Similarly, Scott and colleagues (1979) reported no difference in 5-HT uptake in 8 manic patients compared with 26 healthy controls. Meagher and colleagues (1990) found increased 5-HT uptake in 15 manic patients compared with 19 healthy controls. In this study, however, manic patients as a group had a large variation in their 5-HT uptake compared with the control group that could very well have been due to the effects of medication. Indeed, when five drug-free manic patients in this study were compared with controls, there was no difference in 5-HT uptake between the two groups. Marazziti and colleagues (1991), by contrast, reported decreased 5-HT uptake in 7 manic patients compared with 12 healthy controls. Of these seven patients, only three were drug-free, which confounds the interpretation of results.

Challenge Studies

Tryptophan Depletion Challenge Studies. Serotonin is synthesized from tryptophan, an essential amino acid derived from the diet. The rating-limiting step in serotonin synthesis is the hydroxylation of tryptophan by the enzyme tryptophan hydroxylase to form 5-hydroxytryptophan. Under normal circumstances, this rating-limiting enzyme is not saturated by substrate; thus, tryptophan concentration can impact the rate of synthesis. Tryptophan is then taken up into the brain via a saturable carrier mechanism. Tryptophan actively competes with other large neutral amino acids for transport, and brain uptake of tryptophan is thus determined by both the amount of circulating tryptophan and the ratio of tryptophan to the other large neutral amino acids. (See Figure 14–3 for a diagram of the effects of tryptophan depletion.)

Pretreatment plasma tryptophan has been reported to be lower in depressed patients than in healthy controls and to be able to differentiate certain subgroups of depression (Meltzer and Lowy, 1987; Maes et al., 1990). Depressed patients exhibit reduced plasma concentrations of 5-hydroxytryptophan after ingestion of test doses of oral L-tryptophan (Deakin et al., 1990). Lower pretreatment plasma tryptophan has been reported to be predictive of response to antidepressant treatment (Moller et al., 1986;

Lucca et al., 1992). The depletion of dietary L-tryptophan has also been reported to induce relapse in recently remitted depressed patients (Delgado et al., 1990; Neumeister et al., 1997).

In contrast to these findings, several studies have recently found that the effect may be less consistent than previously reported. Moore and colleagues (1998) observed no effect on mood in fully remitted patients medicated with SSRIs. Leyton and colleagues (1997) also reported that acute tryptophan depletion did not induce relapse or change in mood in fully remitted, medication-free former patients with major depression. Neumeister (2003) summarized the behavioral data for healthy controls with and without genetic risk for depression and for patient populations during the symptomatic phase of depression and in remission. Overall, these data indicate a trait abnormality of serotonin function in depression and suggest that antidepressants may compensate for the underlying deficit.

Of the 15 tryptophan depletion studies that have been conducted in depression, only 3 included some patients with bipolar depression (Delgado et al., 1990, 1999; Leyton et al., 1997). Only three such studies have been conducted specifically in bipolar disorder (Benkelfat et al., 1995; Capiello et al., 1997; Johnson et al., 2001). In one study, tryptophan depletion was found to be associated with increased manic symptoms for 3 days (Cappiello et al., 1997). Two patients met criteria for a relapse. In two other studies, euthymic patients who were being treated with lithium were unaffected by tryptophan depletion (Cassidy et al., 1998b; Johnson et al., 2001). Patients in these studies had been in a long remission. In the study by Johnson and colleagues, tryptophan depletion was induced in 30 patients with manic-depressive illness (20 bipolar and 10 unipolar), all stabilized on lithium treatment for at least 1 year. The study was performed using a randomized, double-blind, controlled design. Plasma tryptophan was reduced by 80 percent in the experimental group and 16 percent in the control group. However, no clinically relevant mood changes were observed. Transient reduction in serotonergic function does not appear to affect mood in patients with affective disorders stabilized on lithium treatment.

Many of these studies are limited in that they included mixed samples of patients with major depression (recurrence not specified) or bipolar disorder (depressed phase, treated with antidepressants). Furthermore, most of these studies do not present results for bipolar and unipolar patients separately. Bipolar depressed patients treated with antidepressants do not appear to be more or less vulnerable to tryptophan depletion than unipolar patients; however, currently available studies suggest that tryptophan depletion does not produce a lowering of mood in lithium-treated euthymic patients.

Figure 14–3. The mechanisms by which tryptophan depletion reduces central nervous system serotonin. CSF = cerebrospinal fluid; LNAA = large, neutral amino acid; Try = tryptophan; 5-H$_{1AA}$ = 5-hydroxy-indoleacetic acid. (*Source*: Fernstrom and Wurtman, 1997.)

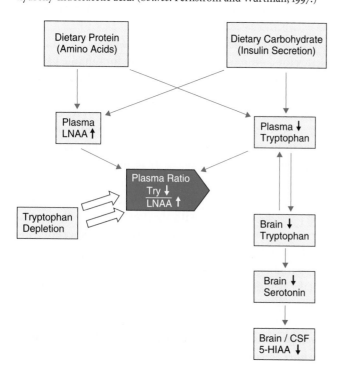

Most recently, investigators have studied unaffected relatives of bipolar patients to examine the possibility that sensitivity to the deleterious mood and cognitive effects of lowered serotonin may represent an endophenotype for bipolar disorder. In a double-blind, crossover design, 20 unaffected relatives (URs) from multiplex bipolar families and 19 control subjects underwent acute tryptophan depletion (ATD) (Quintin et al., 2001). Unlike the control subjects, URs experienced a lowering of mood during ATD but not during the placebo. Furthermore, URs tended to show increased impulsivity in the ATD condition. Measurements obtained before ingestion of the amino acid (AA) drink indicated that, relative to control subjects, URs exhibited lower serotonin platelet concentrations, lower affinity, and fewer binding sites of the serotonin transporter for imipramine; these differences were unaffected by tryptophan depletion.

In a more recent study, Sobczak and colleagues (2002) investigated the effects of ATD on cognitive performance in healthy first-degree relatives of bipolar patients (FHs) (n=30) and matched controls (n=15) in a placebo-controlled, double-blind, crossover design. Performance on planning, memory, and attention tasks was assessed at baseline and 5 hours after ATD. The authors found that speed of information processing on the planning task following ATD was impaired in the FH group but not in the control group. Furthermore, FH subjects with a bipolar-I relative (FH-I) showed impairments in planning and memory independent of ATD. In all subjects, ATD impaired long-term memory performance and speed of information processing; it did not affect short-term memory or focused and divided attention. These results suggest serotonergic vulnerability affecting frontal lobe areas in FH subjects, indicated by impaired planning.

Taken together, the above results suggest that vulnerability to reduced tryptophan availability may represent an endophenotype for bipolar disorder, a notion that warrants further investigation; also future studies should include a group with highly recurrent unipolar depression.

Neuroendocrine Challenge Studies.   A series of neuroendocrine challenge paradigms has been investigated to examine more closely the presynaptic serotonergic neurons in patients with mood disorders (Shiah and Yatham, 2000; Mahmood and Silverstone, 2001). In healthy subjects, the IV infusion of tryptophan increases prolactin plasma levels (Price et al., 1991). In depressed patients, however, this release of prolactin to IV tryptophan is blunted compared with that in healthy controls (Price et al., 1991; Cappiello et al., 1996). As with most of the other serotonergic measures, only a few studies have been undertaken in bipolar patients, perhaps reflecting the difficulty of maintaining

bipolar patients medication-free for a sufficiently long period of time so as to be confident of the lack of confounding residual medication-related effects. The serotonin precursor tryptophan has been used to test neuroendocrine responses in patients and controls. In a placebo-controlled study, the cortisol and ACTH responses to tryptophan was blunted in remitted bipolar patients compared with those in controls (Nurnberger et al., 1990).

Neuroendocrine challenge with the appetite suppressant fenfluramine produces similar results to the IV infusion of tryptophan. The administration of fenfluramine causes a rapid increase in the plasma levels of prolactin in normal subjects. When fenfluramine is administered to depressed patients, however, the prolactin release is blunted (Mitchell and Smythe, 1990; Shapira et al., 1993). This blunted prolactin response has been reported to normalize with successful treatment and has been proposed as a test for predicting response to antidepressant treatment (Malone et al., 1993; Shapira et al., 1993).

Only two studies have employed the fenfluramine challenge test in homogeneous samples of manic patients (Newman et al., 1998). One found that the prolactin and cortisol responses of manic patients to either fenfluramine (n=10) or sumatriptan (n=9) did not differ from those of normal controls (discussed in Shiah and Yatham, 2000; Mahmood and Silverstone, 2001). Thakore and colleagues (1996), by contrast, found increased basal cortisol levels and reduced prolactin response to fenfluramine in nine manic patients compared with nine healthy controls matched for age and gender. They suggest that mania is associated with a state of decreased 5-HT responsiveness, similar to that found in the depressed state and reminiscent of the permissive hypothesis of bipolar disorder discussed earlier.

The growth hormone (GH) response was found to be blunted in depressed patients in a study using sumatriptan, a 5-HT$_{1D}$ agonist, as the challenge agent (Yatham et al., 1997). Mahmood and colleagues (2002) found a blunted GH response to sumatriptan in bipolar patients with migraine compared with bipolar patients without migraine, "pure" migraine patients, and healthy controls.

Investigation of Serotonin Receptors

Several different serotonin receptor subtypes have been identified in recent years. Subtyping is based in part on the characteristics of binding to serotonin, other agonists, or antagonists. Three main classes—5-HT$_1$, 5-HT$_2$, and 5-HT$_3$ receptors—are further subdivided into subtypes 5-HT$_{1A}$, 5-HT$_{1B}$, 5-HT$_{1D}$, 5-HT$_{1E}$, and 5-HT$_{1F}$. The 5-HT$_2$ receptors may be divided into 5-HT$_{2A}$, 5-HT$_{2B}$, and 5-HT$_{2C}$ subtypes.

The 5-HT$_{1A}$ Receptor.   The 5-HT$_{1A}$ receptor has been implicated in the pathophysiology and treatment of mood disorders on the basis of evidence that patients with major depression have blunted physiological responses to 5-HT_{1A} receptor agonists in vivo and abnormal 5-HT_{1A} receptor binding postmortem (Bowden et al., 1989; Lopez et al., 1998; Stockmeier et al., 1998). During 5-HT_{1A} receptor agonist challenge, physiological increases in plasma concentrations of ACTH and cortisol are attenuated in unmedicated subjects with unipolar depression (recurrence not specified) (Cowen, 2000). Postmortem studies of cerebral 5-HT_{1A} receptor binding and mRNA expression in unipolar depression and bipolar disorder suggest 5-HT_{1A} receptor dysfunction in mood disorders, but these data are limited to two studies with small sample sizes (Bowden et al., 1989; Lopez et al., 1998). Lopez and colleagues (1998) found that 5-HT_{1A} receptor mRNA levels were abnormally reduced in the hippocampus in six subjects with major depressive disorder who died by suicide, and Bowden and colleagues (1989) found reduced 5-HT_{1A} receptor binding to [^{3}H] 8-hydroxy-2-(di-n-propyl)aminotetralin (8-OH-DPAT) in the temporal polar and posterior ventrolateral prefrontal cortex in seven patients with unipolar depression or bipolar disorder dying of natural causes.

Supporting the above postmortem findings, recent PET studies have yielded in vivo evidence of reduced pre- and postsynaptic 5-HT_{1A} receptor binding in both unipolar and bipolar depressed patients. Drevets and colleagues (2000) reported that the regional 5-HT_{1A} receptor binding of depressed subjects with primary, recurrent, familial mood disorders (i.e., part of the manic-depressive spectrum) as determined with PET was significantly reduced relative to healthy controls. The investigators found that the mean 5-HT_{1A} receptor binding potential was reduced by 42 percent in the midbrain raphe and 25–33 percent in the limbic and neocortical areas in the mesiotemporal, occipital, and parietal cortex. These findings are consistent with those of Sargent and colleagues (2000), who found decreased 5-HT_{1A} receptor binding, measured with PET and [carbonyl-^{11}C]WAY 100635, in 15 unmedicated depressed patients relative to 18 healthy controls in the raphe, medial temporal cortex, insula, anterior cingulate, temporal polar cortex, ventrolateral prefrontal cortex, and orbital cortex. Seven of the unmedicated subjects were naive to antidepressant drugs, and the other eight had been untreated for a mean of 63 weeks. No differences were found between depressed patients and controls in the inferior occipital cortex or angular gyrus. Ten of the subjects were scanned both before and after paroxetine treatment; it was found that 5-HT_{1A} receptor binding had not significantly changed in any area.

Cortisol Hypersecretion and 5-HT_{1A} Receptor Abnormalities.

One factor that may contribute to the reduction in 5-HT_{1A} receptor binding in depression is increased cortisol secretion (known to occur in many depressed patients, as discussed below), since postsynaptic 5-HT_{1A} receptor mRNA expression is under tonic inhibition by corticosteroid receptor stimulation in some brain regions. The magnitude of the reduction in 5-HT_{1A} receptor density and mRNA levels due to stress-induced glucocorticoid secretion in rodents is similar to the magnitude of the differences seen between depressed and healthy humans. In rats, for example, chronic unpredictable stress was found to reduce 5-HT_{1A} receptor density an average of 22 percent across hippocampal subfields, similar to the 25 percent reduction in hippocampal 5-HT_{1A} receptor binding found in depression. Similarly in tree shrews, chronic social subordination stress (for 28 days) was found to decrease the density of 5-HT_{1A} receptors in posterior cingulate, parietal cortex, prefrontal cortex, and hippocampus by 11–34 percent, similar to the magnitude of reduced 5-HT_{1A} receptor binding found in other studies in these regions (Drevets et al., 2000; Sargent et al., 2000).

These findings are particularly noteworthy since chronic lithium has recently been demonstrated to attenuate the cytosol-to-nucleus translocation of the glucocorticoid receptor (Zhou et al., 2005). Movement (translocation) of the glucocorticoid receptor from the cytosol to the nucleus is required for its ability to regulate gene expression. By inhibiting this movement, lithium would be expected to attenuate the ability of glucocorticoids to regulate gene expression. This is precisely what has been observed in preclinical studies (Zhou et al., 2005). Furthermore, Drevets and colleagues (personal communication, 2003) have found that chronic lithium normalizes 5-HT_{1A} receptor binding potential in bipolar patients, an effect entirely consistent with an attenuation of glucocorticoid effects.

5-HT_2 Receptors.

Mann and colleagues (1986) have reported an increased number of postsynaptic 5-HT_2 receptors in the brains of depressed patients, which is consistent with the work of Matsubara and colleagues (1991) who found an increase in the number of 5-HT_1 and 5-HT_2 receptors in the prefrontal cortex of suicide victims; however, another group did not replicate this finding (Stockmeier et al., 1997). Investigators have also used platelets from patients with mood disorders to study 5-HT_2 receptor binding to platelet membranes and serotonin-induced changes in platelet shape and aggregation to study 5-HT_2 receptors in patients with mood disorders.

There have been at least 12 independent studies in which the B_{max} for the 5-HT_{2A} receptor on platelets from depressed patients has been measured.[16] One of these studies found no difference in this measure between patients suffering from depression and controls. All of the others found a significant increase in the B_{max} value for platelet 5-HT_{2A} receptors for depressed and suicidal patients compared with controls. Most of these studies either did not study bipolar patients or did not clearly separate unipolar and bipolar depressed patients. In one of the only studies of manic subjects, Velayudhan and colleagues (1999) used 125I-ketanserin as the radioligand for platelet 5-HT_2 receptors. They found no difference in the density or affinity of platelet 5-HT_2 receptors obtained from 29 manic patients and 29 healthy controls; moreover, 2 weeks of lithium treatment had no significant effect on these parameters.

Using SPECT, D'Haenen and colleagues (1992) found increased uptake of a 5HT_2 receptor antagonist, 2-ketaserin labeled with iodine 123 [^{123}I], in parietal cortex bilaterally and right greater than left asymmetry in the inferofrontal region of depressed patients compared with controls. A PET study (Biver et al., 1997) revealed a decrease in uptake of another 5HT_2 antagonist, altanserin labeled with fluorine [^{18}F], in the right anterior portion of insular cortex and right posterolateral orbitofrontal cortex of depressed patients compared with controls. PET studies have yielded mixed results: two studies (Attar-Levy et al., 1999; Yatham et al., 2000) found a decrease in [^{18}F] setoperone (5HT_2 antagonist) binding in the frontal cortex of depressed patients compared with controls, whereas one (Meyer et al., 1999) found no difference between the two groups. As with most studies of unipolar depression, the category itself is so heterogenous (including nonrecurrent, minimally recurrent, and highly recurrent), that nonreplications are to be expected.

An exciting recent pharmacogenetic study searched for genetic predictors of treatment outcome in 1,953 patients with recurrent major depressive disorder (a mean of six previous episodes) who were treated with the antidepressant citalopram in the Sequenced Treatment Alternatives for Depression (STAR*D) study and prospectively assessed (McMahon et al., 2006). In a split-sample design, a selection of 68 candidate genes was genotyped with 768 single nucleotide polymorphism markers chosen to detect common genetic variation. A significant and reproducible association was found between treatment outcome and a marker in HTR2A ($p = 1 \times 10^{-6}$ to 3.7×10^{-5} in the total sample). Other markers in HTR2A also showed evidence of association with treatment outcome in the total sample. HTR2A encodes the serotonin 2A receptor, which is down-regulated by citalopram. Participants who were homozygous for the A allele had an 18 percent reduction in absolute risk of failing to respond to treatment, compared to those homozygous for the other allele. The A allele was six times more frequent in white than in black participants, for whom treatment was also less effective in this sample (McMahon et al., 2006). The A allele may thus contribute to racial differences in outcomes of antidepressant treatment. Taken together with prior neurobiological findings, these new genetic data make a compelling case for a key role of HTR2A in the mechanism of antidepressant action.

Serotonin Transporter Binding.   As discussed in Chapter 13, polymorphisms and variable tandem repeats in the serotonin transporter (*SERT*) gene have been the focus of extensive research in a variety of psychiatric disorders. Furlong and colleagues (1998) undertook a meta-analysis of over 1,400 individuals of European Caucasian origin. They used 772 controls and 375 bipolar and 299 unipolar patients to investigate the 5-HT transporter variable number tandem repeat (VNTR) polymorphism, and 739 controls and 392 bipolar and 275 unipolar patients to study the promoter polymorphism. They found a significant association with promoter allele 2 in the bipolar groups (estimated odds ratio 1.21; 95 percent confidence interval 1.00–1.45), unipolar groups (odds ratio 1.23; 95 percent confidence interval 1.01–1.42), and combined bipolar and unipolar groups (odds ratio 1.22; 95 percent confidence interval 1.04–1.42). These results raise the possibility that the promoter allele 2, previously shown to result in lower levels of SERT transcription, may be associated with risk for affective disorder. Preliminary reports have also linked *SERT* gene variants with antidepressant-induced mania (Mundo et al., 2001) and antidepressant response to sleep deprivation in bipolar patients (Benedetti et al., 1999).

Another method for evaluating presynaptic serotonergic function is measurement of SERT binding. A number of studies of postmortem brain tissue have been conducted to investigate SERT in projection regions of serotonergic cell bodies in suicide victims with depressive disorder. The results of these studies have been mixed. Early studies focused primarily on suicide victims and used [^{3}H] imipramine, a less-than-optimum radioligand for measuring SERT. Those studies found increases, decreases, or no change in [^{3}H] imipramine binding to frontal cortex in suicide victims (Stanley et al., 1982; Crow et al., 1984; Arora and Meltzer, 1989a). More recently, other radioligands, including [^{3}H] paroxetine, [^{3}H] citalopram, and [^{125}I]cyanoimipramine, have been identified as superior ligands for measuring SERT (Gurevich and Joyce, 1996). Unfortunately, the results obtained with these newer ligands in subjects with depression have also been mixed. Studies have found either significant decreases (Joyce et al., 1993; Arango et al., 1995) or no changes (Mann et al., 1996a; Bligh-Glover et al., 2000).

Since SERT is transcribed from a single copy gene, the platelet and CNS SERT are identical. Thus, abnormalities in platelet SERT may reflect abnormalities in CNS SERT (Owens and Nemeroff, 1998). A number of studies of platelet SERT density have been undertaken using [^{3}H]-imipramine binding or [^{3}H]-paroxetine binding. Although the results of these studies are not entirely consistent, they suggest overall that the B$_{max}$ value for platelet is significantly lower in depressed subjects than in healthy subjects (Ellis and Salmond, 1994; Owens and Nemeroff, 1998).

Ichimiya and colleagues (2002) studied 13 antidepressant-naive or antidepressant-free patients with mood disorders and 21 age-matched healthy control subjects. The patients consisted of seven with unipolar depression and six with bipolar disorder. PET scans were performed using a selective ligand for SERT, [^{11}C](+)McN5652. Binding potential in the thalamus was found to be significantly increased in patients with mood disorders compared with controls, whereas binding potential in the midbrain did not differ between the groups. Subgroup comparison showed that unipolar depressed patients had significantly higher binding potential in the thalamus than that in controls.

In another endophenotype study, Leboyer and colleagues (1999) measured plasma 5-HIAA, platelet 5-HT, and [^{3}H] imipramine in 20 unaffected relatives (URs) from families having at least two members with bipolar disorder and in 19 controls. They found that the URs manifested lower platelet SERT function than that in controls as revealed both by reduced number and diminished affinity of imipramine binding sites and diminished platelet 5-HT content. These preliminary results once again raise the possibility that reduced SERT function may represent an endophenotype in bipolar disorder and perhaps also in highly recurrent unipolar depression.

Lithium and the Serotonergic System

Preclinical studies show that lithium's effects on 5-HT function may occur at a variety of levels, including precursor uptake, synthesis, storage, catabolism, release, receptors, and receptor–effector interaction (Bunney and Garland-Bunney, 1987; Price et al., 1990). Overall, there is reasonable evidence from these studies that lithium enhances serotonergic neurotransmission, although its effects on 5-HT appear to vary depending on brain region, length of treatment, and 5-HT receptor subtype.[17]

In contrast to short-term studies, most long-term studies tend to show that 5-HT and 5-HIAA levels decrease with lithium administration.[18] Treiser and colleagues (1981) found that long-term lithium increased basal and K$^+$-stimulated 5-HT release in hippocampus but not cortex, while Friedman and Wang (1988) found that lithium increased 5-HT release in parietal cortex, hypothalamus, and hippocampus after 2–3 weeks, but not after a single injection or 1 week of treatment.

Taken together, these studies suggest that, rather than simply increasing or decreasing 5-HT release, lithium may be serving to prevent excursions from the mean, thereby stabilizing 5-HT function (Knapp and Mandell, 1973).

Receptor binding studies have shown complex, regionally specific effects of acute or chronic lithium on the density of 5-HT$_1$ and 5-HT$_2$ receptors, although most findings suggest decreases in both sites, at least in hippocampus.[19] Similarly, findings on the effects of both short- and long-term lithium treatment on 5-HT$_2$-mediated head-twitch behavior, as well as hyperactivity responses to the serotonin precursor 5-hydroxytryptophan, have been inconsistent.[20]

The prolactin (PRL) response to 5-HT is, however, more consistently reported to be increased after short-term lithium use (Meltzer et al., 1981; Koenig et al., 1984; Meltzer and Lowy, 1987). Investigators using a variety of methodologies have provided evidence that lithium produces a subsensitivity of presynaptic inhibitory 5-HT$_{1a}$ receptors,[21] which may result in a net increase in the amount of 5-HT released per impulse.

In a series of important preclinical investigations, de Montigny and colleagues used electrophysiological recordings to measure the effects of lithium on the 5-HT system. They found that short-term lithium did not affect the responsiveness of the postsynaptic neurons to 5-HT or the electrical activity of the 5-HT neurons, but enhanced the efficacy of the ascending (presynaptic) 5-HT system (Blier and de Montigny, 1985; Blier et al., 1987). These observations led de Montigny and colleagues to propose that lithium may increase the efficacy of other antidepressant treatments (Blier and de Montigny, 1985; Blier et al., 1987). As reviewed in Chapter 19, several open and double-blind clinical investigations have now demonstrated that approximately 50 percent of nonresponders are converted to responders upon lithium administration within 2 weeks (de Montigny et al., 1981, 1983; Heninger et al., 1983). A number of the early human CSF studies are difficult to interpret, however, because of their methodology and study design, and their findings are most often confounded by concomitant alterations in mood state and neurovegetative symptomatology. Small increases in CSF 5-HIAA levels have been reported after subchronic lithium treatment in bipolar patients.[22] Several studies have indicated that long-term lithium treatment "normalizes" previously low platelet 5-HT uptake in bipolar patients, an effect that may persist for several weeks after discontinuation (Born et al., 1980; Coppen et al., 1980; Meltzer et al., 1983; Poirier et al., 1988). Findings on the effects of lithium treatment on [^{3}H] imipramine binding in platelets remain inconclusive.[23] Findings of neuroendocrine studies in patients have been more consistent, showing that acute or subacute lithium treatment results in augmented prolactin and/or cortisol responses to various challenges (fenfluramine, tryptophan, 5-hydroxytryptophan) in affectively ill patients. These findings suggest that lithium does indeed facilitate serotonergic throughput in discrete brain areas.[24] However, recent studies in normal volunteers after 2 weeks of "therapeutic" lithium did not indicate increased neuroendocrine responses, suggesting that lithium's effect on the serotonergic system may depend on its underlying activity (Manji et al., 1991a).

Overall, current evidence from both preclinical and clinical studies supports a role for lithium in enhancing presynaptic activity in the serotonergic system in the brain. Direct studies of lithium's effects on serotonergic neurotransmission in humans have been limited in the past by the complexity of the widespread distribution of different types of serotonergic fibers throughout the brain, the only recently recognized multiple receptor subtypes, the relative lack of serotonin-specific pharmacological agents and outcome variables reflecting selective serotonergic responses, and inadequate attention to effects dependent on duration of treatment and affective and physiological state of the patient. Given the current understanding of the molecular neurobiology of both receptor subtypes and the transporter in the serotonergic system, we anticipate new, more specific pharmacological probes for future preclinical and clinical investigations.

Valproate and the Serotonergic System

Khaitan and colleagues (1994) found that chronic treatment (21 days in rats) with valproate did not significantly alter the hypothermia induced by 8-OH-DPAT, an agonist at 5-HT_{1A} receptors. Treatment with valproate also had no effect on radioligand binding to 5-HT_{1A} or 5-HT_2.

Maes and colleagues (1997) measured plasma cortisol response to l-5-hydroxytryptophan in 10 drug-free manic patients before and after treatment with valproate for 3 weeks. They found that administration of l-5-hydroxytryptophan produced an increase in cortisol responses both before and after valproate treatment; however, the l-5-hydroxytryptophan–induced cortisol response was significantly higher after treatment with valproate than before it. Their findings suggest that chronic treatment with valproate may enhance central 5-HT function in manic patients and appear to be consistent with the hypothesis that increasing 5-HT function plays a role in the antimanic effects of the drug.

Two other studies also have shown that valproate treatment leads to an increase in central 5-HT activity in humans. Fahn (1978) reported that treatment with valproate increased CSF levels of 5-HIAA in a patient with postanoxic intentional myoclonus. And Shiah and colleagues (1997) reported that 1 week of treatment with valproate significantly attenuated the hypothermic response to ipsapirone, a 5-HT_{1A} receptor agonist, in 10 healthy human males. This finding suggests that valproate enhances 5-HT neurotransmission

by causing a subsensitivity of presynaptic 5-HT_{1A} autoreceptors, because the hypothermic response to 5-HT_{1A} receptor agonists has been suggested to be mediated by those autoreceptors (although mixed pre- and postsynaptic activation has also been suggested for mediation of hypothermia in rats).

In contrast to the positive results of the above studies, Kusumi and colleagues (1994a) found no in vitro effect of valproate (100 M) on basal calcium or 5-HT–induced intracellular calcium mobilization in the platelets of 7 healthy subjects. Although the body of data investigating valproate's effects on the serotonergic system is much smaller than that for lithium, it does tend to suggest nonidentical effects of the two drugs. Whether these differences account for observed clinical differences between the two drugs requires further study.

Carbamazepine and the Serotonergic System

Carbamazepine enhances serotonin levels in hippocampus in epilepsy-prone rats (Yan et al., 1992; Dailey et al., 1995) with a magnitude and time course suggesting a significance to its anticonvulsant effects. Moreover, depletion of serotonin inhibits carbamazepine's actions in these animals (Dailey et al., 1995), although the mechanism of this effect is unknown. To our knowledge, no study to date has examined the effects of carbamazepine on 5-HT activity in manic patients. However, some human studies have shown evidence for an increase in 5-HT function during carbamazepine treatment.

For example, Elphick and colleagues (1990) studied plasma prolactin response to IV administration of tryptophan in seven healthy human males before and after a 10-day course of carbamazepine. They found that after the carbamazepine treatment, the prolactin response to tryptophan was significantly enhanced. Moreover, carbamazepine treatment has been reported to increase plasma total and free tryptophan in epileptic patients (Fernstrom, 1983), which could lead to an increase in brain 5-HT function.

In contrast, Post and colleagues (1984a) found no significant effect of carbamazepine on CSF levels of 5-HIAA in affectively ill patients. Likewise, Kusumi and colleagues (1994a) reported no in vitro effect of carbamazepine (10 M) for 1 or 4 hours on basal calcium or 5-HT–induced intracellular calcium mobilization in the platelets of seven healthy subjects.

Subsequently, Mannel and colleagues (1997) administered d, l-fenfluramine challenge tests to 30 mixed affective disorder patients after a mean period of 9.2 months of prophylactic treatment with either lithium or carbamazepine. Of the 30 patients, 15 were treated with lithium and the other 15 with carbamazepine. The authors found that the cortisol response to d, l-fenfluramine was significantly increased in the lithium-treated patients compared with those receiving carbamazepine, whereas there was no significant difference in the prolactin response to d, l-fenfluramine between the two groups. These findings are in keeping with the enhancing effect of lithium, but not carbamazepine, on 5-HT function. However, interpretation of the study data was limited by a lack of placebo control, heterogeneity of diagnostic groups, and some patients taking neuroleptics within 72 hours before d, l-fenfluramine challenge testing.

The Serotonergic System in Manic-Depressive Illness: Summary

In summary, data from a variety of studies—including CSF 5-HIAA, neuroendocrine challenge, platelet and brain SERT, 5-HT receptor binding, and PET studies—suggest that abnormalities of the serotonergic system are present in depression. There have been far fewer studies of bipolar disorder in this regard, but the available data suggest the possibility of similar abnormalities. Most interesting are the PET studies demonstrating reduced 5-HT$_{1A}$ binding in bipolar depressed patients and in unipolar depressed patients with bipolar relatives. Equally intriguing are recent reports that vulnerability to the deleterious effects of reduced tryptophan may represent an endophenotype for bipolar disorder. Boxes 14–6 and 14–7 summarize overall major findings and findings of newer studies supporting the involvement of the serotonergic system in the pathophysiology and treatment of bipolar disorder and recurrent unipolar depression.

The Cholinergic System

There has been a long-standing interest in the potential involvement of the cholinergic system in manic-depressive illness, based primarily on studies indicating the prominent mood and behavioral effects of cholinergic agonists and antagonists. Identification of this association initially stemmed from observations that industrial poisoning with cholinesterase inhibitors (which enhance acetylcholine [ACh] function by inhibiting its degradation) produced a depression-like clinical picture (Rowntree et al., 1950). In 1973, Janowsky and colleagues noted that physostigmine, a central cholinesterase inhibitor, caused brief but dramatic decreases in manic symptoms, a finding replicated by Modestin and colleagues (1973a,b) and Davis and colleagues (1978). These observations led Janowsky and colleagues to propose the cholinergic–aminergic balance hypothesis: that an increased ratio of cholinergic to adrenergic activity underlies the pathophysiology of depression, whereas the reverse occurs in mania. Because physostigmine made the patients in the study sick, questions were raised about the specificity of this finding. Yet proponents of the

---

BOX **14–6.**   **A Summary of Major Findings Supporting Involvement of the Serotonergic System in the Pathophysiology and Treatment of Bipolar Disorder and Recurrent Unipolar Depression**

- Reduced CSF 5-HIAA appears to be characteristic of both suicidal and impulsive/aggressive patients, whether unipolar or bipolar
- Reduced CSF 5-HIAA may be found in both depressive and manic states (consistent with a permissive hypothesis)
- Blunted neuroendocrine and temperature responses to various 5-HT agonists
- Reduced [³H]IMI binding in platelets and postmortem brain
- Reduced 5-HT$_{1A}$ receptor binding in living brain and postmortem brain tissue
- Antidepressant efficacy of agents that increase intrasynaptic 5-HT
- Agents that increase intrasynaptic 5-HT are capable of triggering manic episodes, albeit less so than catecholamine-enhancing agents
- Tryptophan depletion induces a rapid depressive relapse in SSRI-treated patients (but not lithium-treated patients)
- Chronic antidepressants generally reduce 5-HT turnover in patients, even agents whose primary biochemical target is not the 5-HT system
- Chronic SSRIs reduce cell body 5-HT$_{1A}$ density, thereby increasing 5-HT neuron firing
- Antidepressants generally decrease 5-HT$_2$ density in rat frontal cortex, but ECS increases it

CSF = cerebrospinal fluid; ECS = electroconvulsive stimulation; SSRI = selective serotonin reuptake inhibitor.

ACh hypothesis point out that the effect—inhibition of behavior and reduction of mania—generally precedes the associated nonspecific nausea and vomiting.

Physostigmine administration can also precipitate depression in euthymic bipolar patients maintained on lithium (Oppenheim et al., 1979) and in normal volunteers (Janowsky and Risch, 1984). Likewise, the direct muscarinic agonist arecoline produces depressive symptoms in euthymic bipolar patients off lithium and in normal volunteers (Nurnberger et al., 1983, 1989). And depressive symptoms, including psychomotor retardation and depressed mood, are often a complication of acetylcholinesterase inhibitor treatment of Alzheimer's disease. Such sensitivity to the mood-lowering effects of cholinergic drugs appears dependent on the presence of an underlying psychiatric disorder.

As described in Chapters 18 and 19, the cholinesterase inhibitor donepezil was added to various existing therapies in treatment-resistant bipolar patients in an open study, with benefits reported in over half the patients (Burt et al., 1999). However, manic episodes have also been associated with the

Genetic Studies

Enzymes
- TPH (tryptophan hydroxylase) gene intron 7 A218C polymorphism associated with BPD (Bellivier et al., 1998b)
- TPH*A-containing variant may be a protective factor for depressive symptoms in male mood disorder patients (Serretti et al., 2001)
- Differences in distribution of alleles for the MAO-A–CA repeat in female BPD (meta-analysis) (Preisig et al., 2000)
- Increased frequency of COMT met158 and the short 5-HTTLPR (linked functional polymorphic region) alleles and genotypes in BPD without panic disorder (Rotondo et al., 2002)

Transporter
- Increased frequency of allele 12 of VNTR (variable number tandem repeat) polymorphism intron 2 of 5-HTT gene in BPD (Collier et al., 1996a)
- 5-HTTLPR homozygous low-activity genotype reported to be associated with affective disorder (Collier et al., 1996b)
- VNTR in the second intron of 5-HTT gene reported to be associated with BPD (Kunugi et al., 1997; Rees et al., 1997)
- Polymorphism in $5-HT_{2C}$ receptor gene and 5-HTT gene reported to be found in BP-I females may represent a minor increase in susceptibility (Oruc et al., 1997)
- Homozygocity for the short variant of the 5-HTTLPR reported to be more frequent in BPD (Bellivier et al., 1998a)
- Promoter allele 2 of 5-HTT gene (that results in lower level of 5-HT transporter transcription) may be associated with risk for affective disorder (meta-analysis) (Furlong et al., 1998)
- The 12 repeat of the VNTR in intron 2 of the 5-HTT gene reported to be a susceptibility (although small) factor in BPD (Kirov et al., 1999)
- Individuals homozygous for the long variant 5-HTTLPR had better mood symptom amelioration after total sleep deprivation (Benedetti et al., 1999)
- Increased 5-HTTLPR 3′UTR G/T polymorphism associated with BPD (Mynett-Johnson et al., 2000)
- 5-HTT gene variations associated with susceptibility to puerperal psychosis in BPD (Coyle et al., 2000)
- Increased 5-HTTLPR long allele reported in rapid cycling (Cusin et al., 2001)

- 5-HTTLPR short variant associated with poor response to fluoxamine in MDD and BPD (Zanardi et al., 2001)
- Increased 5-HTTLPR short-allele gene and higher rate of homozygosity for the short variant in patients with history of induced mania by serotonergic antidepressants (Mundo et al., 2001)

Receptors
- $5-HT_{2C}$ receptor gene, Ser23 allele, may increase susceptibility to BPD in females (Gutierrez et al., 1996)
- 5-HT5A gene allelic association was found with the −19 G/C polymorphism and BPD, MDD, and schizophrenia (Birkett et al., 2000)
- Variation in the $5-HT_6$ gene may be associated with BPD (Vogt et al., 2000)
- $5-HT_{2A}$ receptor gene promoter polymorphism 1438 A/G may be causally related to BPD (Chee et al., 2001)
- Increase of $5-HT_{2C}$ receptor gene (Cys 23 Ser) allele in MDD-BPD (Lerer et al., 2001)
- $5-HT_{3A}$ receptor C178T missense mutation may represent susceptibility to BPD (Niesler et al., 2001)
- Increased frequency of A allele of $5-HT_{2A}$ receptor gene in subgroup of BP-I patients with low suicidal risk (Bonnier et al., 2002)

Serotonin and metabolite levels
- Increased plasma free 5-HT and 5-HIAA in BPD patients treated chronically with Li (Artigas et al., 1989)
- Reduced 5-HIAA in frontal-parietal and 5-HIAA/5-HT ratio in temporal cortex in bipolar postmortem studies (Young et al., 1994b)
- Increased 5-HT platelet levels in bipolar depressed patients (Shiah et al., 1999)

Challenge Studies

- Blunted response of prolactin to fenfluramine in manic patients inconsistently reported (Thakore et al., 1996) (Yatham 1996)
- Blunted GH response to sumatriptan ($5-HT_{1D}$ agonist) reported in BPD patients who also suffered migraine (Mahmood et al., 2002)
- Sumatriptan-induced GH response reported to be blunted in depressed but not manic patients (Yatham et al., 1997)
- Decreased planning and memory function reported in first-degree relatives of BP-I patients after acute tryptophan depletion. Double-blind crossover trial (Sobczak et al., 2002)

(continued)

BOX 14–7. Newer Studies Supporting Involvement of the Serotonergic System in the Pathophysiology and Treatment of Manic-Depressive Illness (Primarily Bipolar) *(continued)*

Intracellular Signaling Related to 5-HT

- Increased basal membrane/cytosol PKC portioning, and increased 5-HT-elicited platelet PKC translocation and membrane/cytosol portioning in mania. Li (2 weeks) normalized the changes (Friedman et al., 1993; J. Wang et al., 1999)
- Decrease of 5-HT-induced Ca mobilization by pretreatment with PKC activator (PMA) (Suzuki, 2001)
- Enhanced 5-HT-receptor-mediated G protein coupling in frontal cortical membranes from postmortem BPD patients (Friedman and Wang, 1996)
- Increase in 5-HT-induced Ca mobilization of untreated manic patients (Yamawaki et al., 1996; Suzuki et al., 2001). Restored to control levels in treated euthymic BPD patients (Okamoto et al., 1995)
- Increased Ca response to 5-HT in platelets from BPD patients; 5-HT-induced intraplatelet Ca response reported to represent a good predictor of mood stabilizer response in a 5-year follow-up (Kusumi et al., 2000)

Treatment Related

Challenge studies
- Increased prolactin response to tryptophan infusion after short-term Li treatment (Price et al., 1989)
- Increase in plasma cortisol response to L-5-HTP (5-hydroxytryptophan) after treatment with valproate in manic patients (Maes et al., 1997)
- Acute tryptophan depletion did not reverse beneficial effects of Li on mood and suicidality in BPD patients (Hughes et al., 2000)
- TCA and MAOIs had higher rate of switch to mania than fluoxetine in BPD patients (Boerlin et al., 1998)

- IMI and PXT had better antidepressant response than placebo only in patients with low plasma Li levels in bipolar depression. Possibly supportive of serotonergic effects of Li (Nemeroff et al., 2001)
- Potentiation of antidepressant effect of total sleep deprivation and prevention of short-term relapse reported to be produced by pindolol (5-HT$_{1A}$ antagonist) in bipolar depression (Smeraldi et al., 1999). Overall, the pindolol augmentation strategy remains controversial

Receptor and transporter studies
- Increased potency of 5-HT in a platelet shape change velocity paradigm (May represent a contributory factor in the cardiovascular risk associated with mood disorders); reduced after antidepressant treatment in unipolar and bipolar depression (Brusov et al., 1989)
- Increased 5-HT platelet uptake in mania patients; normalized at discharge (Meagher et al., 1990)
- Reduced V$_{max}$ of 5-HT uptake in platelets in BPD patients (Marazziti et al., 1991)
- Reduced (trend) 5-HT uptake sites in frontal cortex in BPD depressed patients (Leake et al., 1991)
- Reduced platelet 5-HTT function in unaffected relatives of BPD patients (Leboyer et al., 1999)
- Reduced 5-HT$_{1A}$ receptor binding potential in raphe and hippocampus-amygdala (PET), more marked in bipolar and unipolar depressive patients with bipolar relatives (Drevets et al., 1999)
- Increased binding potential of 5-HTT in thalamus in mood disorder patients (Ichimiya et al., 2002)

BPD = bipolar disorder; BP-I = bipolar-I; Ca = calcium; COMT = catechol-O-methyltransferase; GH = growth hormone; IMI = imipramine; Li = lithium; MAOI = monoamine oxidase inhibitor; MDD = major depressive disorder; PKC = protein kinase C; PXT = paroxetine; TCA = tricyclic antidepressant.

---

use of donepezil in case reports (Benazzi, 1998, 1999). A recent small, 6-week double-blind, placebo-controlled trial involving 11 patients with treatment-resistant mania found no difference in the efficacy of add-on donepezil compared to placebo in the treatment of manic symptoms in patients with treatment-resistant mania (Evins et al., 2006).

In a small open study, Stoll and colleagues (1996) gave choline bitartrate to six lithium-treated outpatients with rapid-cycling bipolar disorder. Five of the six patients were reported to have a reduction in manic symptoms and four to have a marked reduction in all mood symptoms during the choline therapy. Although these findings are intriguing, the small sample size and open nature of this study suggest that caution is required in the interpretation of the results.

Finally, the muscarinic agonist xanomeline has been reported to decrease mood swings and psychotic-like behaviors in Alzheimer's patients (Bodick et al., 1997). In preclinical studies, muscarinic agonists have been found to increase and antagonists to decrease immobility or "despair" in the forced swim test model of depression. Thus, the cholinesterase inhibitor physostigmine, but not the peripherally acting neostigmine, increases immobility in the forced swim test, suggesting depressogenic activity. Interestingly, the enhanced immobility produced by physostigmine was reversed by the α_1-adrenergic agonist metoprolol, supporting the contention that a balance between the cholinergic and adrenergic systems may play an important role in modulating mood. The hypercholinergic Flinders

Resistant Line of rats has exaggerated immobility in the forced swim test, as do rats after chronic treatment with muscarinic antagonists to produce cholinergic supersensitivity (Janowsky et al., 1994).

The cholinergic hypothesis is also supported by a number of indirect observations documenting differences in the responses of patients and controls after specific interventions, such as cholinergic-induced REM sleep (Sitaram et al., 1982; Janowsky et al., 1994). REM occurs during discreet periods of sleep, but its onset can be induced earlier in normal volunteers by cholinergic agents.[25] Sitaram and colleagues (1980) found faster induction of REM sleep with arecoline (a cholinergic agonist) in two groups of drug-free euthymic patients with affective disorders (primarily bipolar disorder). The same research team followed up with a second report on 14 euthymic bipolar patients, again finding that the second REM period occurred significantly earlier (Sitaram et al., 1982). Two groups replicated these results nearly a decade later (Berger et al., 1989; Nurnberger et al., 1989).

A few studies have addressed the heritability of this trait. Nurnberger and colleagues (1983) investigated the cholinergic induction of REM during sleep in seven sets of identical twins. Overall, they found an intraclass correlation of .69 for REM latency time after cholinergic stimulation, suggesting a genetic component to REM latency findings.

Sitaram and colleagues (1987) studied REM latency after cholinergic exposure in 35 ill and 34 healthy first-degree relatives of 34 unipolar depressed probands, selected on the basis of their supersensitivity to cholinergics. Supersensitivity was observed in 66 percent of the ill relatives and 22 percent of the well relatives, again suggesting that REM latency tracks with affective illness. Unfortunately for our current goal of identifying subclinical endophenotypes in nonaffected relatives, these studies did not compare their findings with a control population.

In sum, findings on cholinergic-induced REM sleep in bipolar subjects have been consistent among studies. However, there is incongruence regarding the state versus trait status of this phenotype: some studies have identified state independence (Sitaram et al., 1980; Nurnberger et al., 1989), while others have not (Berger et al., 1989).

Although less extensively than for the serotonergic or noradrenergic systems, investigators have also used neuroendocrine challenge tests to examine the acetylcholine system in depression. An exaggerated GH response to pyridostigmine in major depression has been reported, an observation (with 63 percent sensitivity) that distinguished these patients with unipolar depression from those with schizophrenia and alcohol dependence syndrome (Cooney et al., 1997). Dinan and colleagues (1994) used the same test to investigate the cholinergic system in seven male manic patients and seven male healthy controls. They found that the GH response to pyridostigmine (120 mg) was significantly enhanced in the manic patients. They conclude that the enhanced pyridostigmine/GH responsiveness in mania may be due to enhanced somatostatin tone or increased cholinergic receptor responsivity.

Sokolski and DeMet (1999, 2000) have used pupillary constrictions following application of the cholinergic agonist pilocarpine as a means to investigate the cholinergic system. Cholinergic sensitivity was assessed prior to and following treatments by means of graded concentrations of pilocarpine eyedrops (.03–2.0 percent). Pupil size changes were quantified with an infrared pupillometer. The same group also found that lithium and valproate both potentiated the cholinergic responses, and that improvements in mania were closely correlated with decreases in ED50 (i.e., amount of pilocarpine necessary to bring about half-maximal responses). These results are consistent with the suggestion that the antimanic effects of lithium and valproate may involve (at least in part) increasing cholinergic activity in relation to monoaminergic neurotransmission.

Investigators have also used magnetic resonance spectroscopy (MRS) to investigate "choline resonance." The first reported in vivo proton MRS study of choline compounds in affective disorders found that elderly depressed patients had increased choline/chromium (Cho/Cr) ratios in basal ganglia compared with controls (Charles et al., 1994). Subsequently, a similar difference was found between muscular dystrophy and controls (Renshaw and Cohen, 1993; Charles et al., 1994). Early studies in bipolar patients (Sharma et al., 1992; Lafer et al., 1994) also indicated that Cho/Cr resonance was elevated in basal ganglia compared with that in controls. Two studies of cortical regions found that there were no choline-level differences in either the parietal or occipital regions in affective disorder patients compared with controls (Sharma, 1992; Stoll et al., 1992), suggesting that the finding of increased Cho/Cr may be limited to the subcortical region.

A number of studies have attempted to investigate the effects of medication on choline levels in affective disorder patients. Again examining the basal ganglia, studies by two groups have found elevated Cho/Cr levels in depressed subjects which normalized with therapy (Renshaw, 1993; Charles et al., 1994). A larger controlled study by the Renshaw group (Sonawalla et al., 1999) found that basal ganglia Cho/Cr levels increased compared with baseline in outpatients with unipolar depression treated for 8 weeks with fluoxetine. In bipolar patients, an early cross-sectional investigation by Lafer and colleagues (1994) found no difference in basal ganglia Cho/Cr levels between a group of lithium-treated and lithium-free bipolar subjects; however, other medications may have been an important confound.

A more recent longitudinal study of lithium's effects on medication-free bipolar patients, measured with quantitative MRS methods (G. Moore et al., 1999), found a significant decrease compared with baseline in frontal lobe choline concentration after 7 days of lithium treatment, an effect that persisted with chronic lithium treatment (4 weeks).

This study is interesting in several respects. Recent in vitro studies suggest that lithium, potentially through its effects on PKC, stimulates phospholipase D, resulting in the breakdown of phosphatidylcholine (PTC) to diacylglycerol (DAG) (discussed below). A mobile head group on the PTC molecule may make this compound partially visible by MRS, contributing in part to the total brain Cho signal observed through proton MRS.

Lithium and the Cholinergic System

Neurochemical, behavioral, and physiological studies have all indicated that the cholinergic system is involved in affective illness (Dilsaver and Coffman, 1989) and that lithium alters the synaptic processing of ACh in rat brain. The addition of up to 1 mM of lithium in vitro has no effect on ACh synthesis or release, but chronic in vivo lithium treatment appears to increase ACh synthesis, choline transport, and ACh release in rat brain (Simon and Kuhar, 1976; Jope, 1979). While some investigators have reported reductions in ACh levels in rat brain following subchronic administration (Krell and Goldberg, 1973; Ho and Tsai, 1975; Ronai and Vizi, 1975), Jope (1979) reported increased synthesis of ACh in cortex, hippocampus, and striatum following 10 days of lithium administration.

With respect to the density of muscarinic receptors, chronic lithium has been reported to increase (Kafka et al., 1982; Levy et al., 1982; Lerer and Stanley, 1985), decrease (Tollefson et al., 1982), or not change (Maggi and Enna, 1980) the binding of the cholinergic ligand [^{3}H]quinuclidinyl benzilate (QNB) in various areas of rat brain. In human caudate nucleus, lithium is reported to reduce the affinity of [^{3}H]QNB binding. The effects of lithium on both up- and downregulation of muscarinic receptors in brain have also been investigated. There have been reports that lithium is able to abolish the increase in [^{3}H]QNB binding produced by atropine, but is without effect on the downregulation induced by the cholinesterase inhibitor diisopropylfluorophosphate (DFP); these data are variable and inconclusive, however (Levy et al., 1982; Lerer and Stanley, 1985). Ellis and Lenox (1990) examined both receptor binding and muscarinic receptor–coupled phosphoinositide (PI) response in rat hippocampus during atropine-induced upregulation. They found that chronic treatment with atropine results in an upregulation of muscarinic receptors and a supersensitivity of the PI response

in the hippocampus. Coadministration of chronic lithium prevented the development of supersensitivity of the muscarinic receptor PI response without significantly affecting the extent of upregulation of receptor binding sites. These findings suggest that lithium's actions are exerted at a point beyond the receptor binding site, possibly affecting the coupling of the newly upregulated receptors at the level of the signal-transducing G proteins. Thus, similar to the case for dopaminergic and fl-adrenergic receptors, it appears that lithium can block the development of cholinergic receptor supersensitivity. Chronic lithium has also been reported to increase intraerythrocyte concentrations of choline more than 10-fold.[26] This appears to be the result of not only inhibition of choline transport but also enhanced phospholipase D–mediated degradation of phospholipids, which may as well be mediated via PKC activation.

In behavioral studies, chronic lithium in clinically relevant doses is reported to enhance a number of cholinergically mediated responses, including catalepsy and hypothermia. The effect of lithium on pilocarpine-induced catalepsy and hypothermia was found to be of the same order of magnitude as the enhancement induced by chronic scopolamine pretreatment. Combined administration of both pretreatments resulted in additive effects, suggesting that different mechanisms may be involved (Russell et al., 1981; Lerer and Stanley, 1985; Dilsaver and Hariharan, 1988). Of interest in this regard is a study by Dilsaver and Hariharan (1989), who reported that chronic lithium treatment results in a supersensitivity of nicotine-induced hypothermia in rats.

Perhaps the most striking example of lithium's ability to potentiate muscarinic responses comes from the lithium–pilocarpine seizure model.[27] In large doses, pilocarpine and other muscarinic agonists cause prolonged, usually lethal seizures in rats. Although lithium alone is not a convulsant, pretreatment with lithium increases the sensitivity of pilocarpine almost 20-fold.[28] Interestingly, this behavioral effect of lithium is markedly attenuated by intracerebroventricular administration of myoinositol in both rats and mice (Kofman et al., 1991; Tricklebank et al., 1991), representing perhaps the best correlation between a biochemical and behavioral effect of lithium (see later discussion of phosphoinositide turnover). A synergism with the cholinergic system also occurs in electrophysiological studies in hippocampal slices, in which pilocarpine and lithium together, but not alone, produce spontaneous epileptiform bursting (Jope et al., 1986; Ormandy and Jope, 1991). Elegant studies in rat hippocampus have demonstrated that lithium can reverse muscarinic agonist–induced desensitization, an effect that is mediated through PI hydrolysis and can be reversed by inositol (Pontzer and Crews, 1990). Studies by Evans and colleagues (1990) have indicated that lithium's role in lithium–pilocarpine seizures is to increase excitatory transmission through a presynaptic facilitatory effect. Lithium alone was also found to augment synaptic responses; this effect of the drug could be blocked by a PKC inhibitor. These results suggest that lithium's effects in this model may occur through a PKC-mediated presynaptic facilitation of neurotransmitter release (discussed later). Biochemical, electrophysiological, and behavioral data suggest that chronic lithium administration stimulates ACh synthesis and release in rat brain and potentiates some cholinergic-mediated physiological events. Interestingly, similar to the situation observed with the catecholaminergic system, pharmacological studies indicate that chronic lithium prevents muscarinic receptor supersensitivity, most likely through postreceptor mechanisms. Overall, the preponderance of the data suggests that chronic lithium enhances cholinergic throughput.

By contrast, very few studies have examined the effects of valproate or carbamazepine on the cholinergic system. However, existing data suggest that carbamazepine, like lithium, may enhance cholinergic function. Zhu and colleagues (2002) showed through in vivo microdialysis that therapeutically relevant concentrations of carbamazepine increased basal ACh release in frontal cortex of freely moving rats, effects regulated by N-type voltage-sensitive Ca^{2+} channels. Acute administration of modest doses of carbamazepine (25 mg/kg) has been shown to increase both striatal and hippocampal extracellular levels of ACh, whereas both acute and chronic administration of carbamazepine (25 and 50 mg/kg, respectively, per day) were found to increase intracellular ACh levels in striatum and hippocampus (Mizuno et al., 2000).

The Cholinergic System in Manic-Depressive Illness: Summary

Overall, although not extensively, the data are consistent with Janowsky's original proposal that cholinergic–adrenergic balance may play a role in modulating affective behavior.

Although lithium clearly potentiates cholinergic responses, the therapeutic activity of other antidepressant and antimanic drugs does not consistently parallel effects on the cholinergic system, and a number of these agents, including MAOIs and various "second-generation" antidepressants, lack any interaction with cholinergic receptors (Rudorfer et al., 1984). Together these findings suggest that, although manipulation of the cholinergic system is capable of modulating affective state, it does not clearly represent a relevant therapeutic action of currently available agents. The possibility that additional means of augmenting the functioning of the cholinergic system may have utility is an interesting avenue that has not been extensively studied. Unfortunately, there have been few follow-up

---

BOX 14–8. Newer Studies of the Cholinergic System in the Pathophysiology and Treatment of Manic-Depressive Illness (Primarily Bipolar)

Clinical Studies

- Increased pilocarpine required to elicit 50 percent reduction in pupil size; correlated with severity of mania (Sokolski and DeMet, 2000)
- Increased pupillary responsiveness to pilocarpine (cholinergic agonist) after valproate and lithium treatment in mania (DeMet and Sokolski, 1999; Sokolski and DeMet, 1999)
- Increased pyridostigmine (acetylcholine esterase inhibitor)-induced release of GH in manic patients (Dinan et al., 1994)
- Increased erythroyte choline concentration in patients with mania (Stoll et al., 1991)
- RS 86 (cholinergic agonist) exhibited antimanic and REM sleep–inducing properties (Berger et al., 1991)

In Vitro Studies

- Chronic valproate, but not lithium or carbamazepine, reduced carbachol-stimulated early growth response-1 (Egr-1) DNA binding activity by 60 percent in SH-SY5Y cells (Grimes and Jope, 1999)
- Lithium inhibited carbachol stimulation AP-1 gene expression in SH-SY5Y cells (Jope and Song, 1997)
- Selective effect of lithium on M1-mediated muscarinic neurotransmission in hippocampal slices in CA3 pyramidal neurons of guinea pigs (Muller et al., 1989)

GH = growth hormone; REM = rapid eye movement.

---

studies to investigate more fully the role of specific muscarinic receptor subtypes in mediating the antimanic effects of nonselective cholinomimetics. The poor selectivity and tolerability of muscarinic agonists and other cholinomimetics and the low efficacy of agonists for putative target receptors have precluded extensive study and development of these agents for affective disorders. Box 14–8 summarizes findings of newer studies supporting the involvement of the cholinergic system in the pathophysiology and treatment of manic-depressive illness, principally the bipolar subgroup.

The GABAergic System

Gamma aminobutyric acid (GABA), widespread in the CNS, is the major inhibitory neurotransmitter, diminishing the activity of its many target neurons. (See Figure 14–4 for a depiction of the various regulatory processes involved in GABAergic neurotransmission.) GABAergic neurons are much more diffusely located than catecholaminergic neurons, with similar GABA concentrations being found in diverse brain regions. Since GABA exerts a general inhibitory

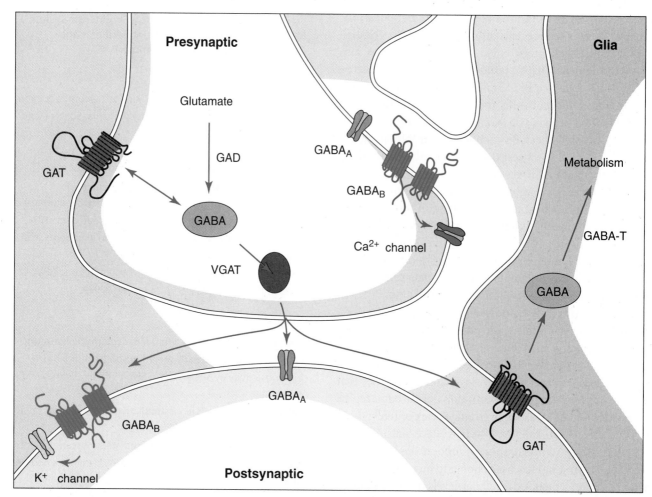

Figure 14–4. The various regulatory processes involved in GABAergic neurotransmission. The amino acid (and neurotransmitter) glutamate serves as the precursor for the biosynthesis of gamma-aminobutyric acid (GABA). The rate-limiting enzyme for the process is glutamic acid decarboxylase (GAD), which utilizes pyridoxal phosphate as an important cofactor. Furthermore, agents such as L-glutamine-γ hydrazide and allylglycine inhibit this enzyme and thus the production of GABA. Once released from the presynaptic terminal, GABA can interact with a variety of presynaptic and postsynaptic receptors. Presynaptic regulation of GABA neuron firing activity and release occurs through somatodendritic (not shown) and nerve terminal GABA$_B$ receptors, respectively. Baclofen is a GABA$_B$ receptor agonist. The binding of GABA to ionotropic GABA$_A$ receptors and metabotropic GABA$_B$ receptors mediates the effects of this receptor. The GABA$_B$ receptors are thought to mediate their actions by being coupled to Ca^{2+} or K$^+$ channels via second messenger systems. Many agents are able to modulate GABA$_A$ receptor function. Benzodiazepines, such as diazepam, increase chloride (Cl) permeability and there are numerous antagonists available directed against this benzodiazepine-binding site. There is also a distinctive barbiturate-binding site on GABA$_A$ receptors, and many psychotropic agents are capable of influencing the function of this receptor (see diagram). GABA is taken back into the presynaptic nerve ending by a high-affinity GABA uptake transporter (GAT) similar to that of the monoamines. Once inside the neuron, GABA breakdown can occur by GABA-transaminase (GABA-T), which is localized in the mitochondria; GABA that is not degraded is sequestered and stored into secretory vesicles by vesicular GABA transporters (VGAT), which differ from vesicular monoamine transporters in their bioenergetic dependence. (*Source*: Owens and Kriegstein, 2002. Reprinted with permission from Macmillan Publishers, Ltd.)

role on brain excitability, it is not altogether surprising that it has been postulated to be involved in a variety of disorders presumed to be associated with phasic regional neuronal hyperexcitability. Furthermore, the increased use of valproate as a treatment for mania in recent years has led to a resurgence of interest in the potential role of GABA in bipolar disorder.

Several investigators have reported significantly lower CSF and plasma GABA levels in patients with major depression (predominantly unipolar) than in controls (Petty and Schlesser, 1981; Petty et al., 1990). In three other studies, however (Post et al., 1980b; Gerner and Hare, 1981; Joffe et al., 1986), investigators sampled a later aliquot higher up in the rostrocaudal gradient for GABA and found no significant difference between depressed patients and controls. Berrettini and colleagues (1986) sampled euthymic bipolar depressed patients and found them to be not significantly different from controls. Even in studies finding low levels of GABA, the findings were not specific to cases of depression or mania but were also seen in alcoholism (Petty et al., 1993).

In a longitudinal study of one patient with rapid cycles, Joffe and colleagues (1986) found CSF GABA to be significantly higher during the patient's five manic episodes than in the four depressed episodes. Two well-state studies of CSF GABA (Berrettini et al., 1986; Joffe et al., 1986) produced conflicting results; the former noted lower levels compared with controls whereas the latter did not.

The relationship between GABA in plasma and in CSF is not clear. In one small study, no correlation was found (Berrettini and Post, 1984). In contrast, Petty and Sherman (1984) reported that plasma GABA levels were significantly lower than normal in a group of 62 medicated depressed patients. Only four of these patients were bipolar, however, and their mean levels were very close to those of the controls. Combining data from their four previous studies, Coffman and Petty (1986) found that manic and remitted bipolar patients had significantly higher levels of plasma GABA than those of control subjects, but when the patients were depressed, the plasma GABA levels did not differ from the controls. Of three studies of GABA in recovered bipolar patients, one, using lithium-treated patients, showed GABA levels significantly higher than normal levels (Petty and Sherman, 1984; Coffman and Petty, 1986), whereas the other two, using patients off all medication for 2 weeks, showed significantly lower than normal levels (Berrettini et al., 1983, 1985b). This apparent discrepancy might be explained by the longitudinal finding of the Berrettini group that plasma GABA levels fall significantly after lithium is discontinued. Interestingly, a small study of identical twins revealed that plasma GABA levels show a close intrapair correspondence (Berrettini and Post, 1984). However, it is too early to assess whether this measure will be useful as a trait marker for bipolar disorder. Low plasma GABA differentiates well from ill subjects in about one-third of bipolar patients (Petty et al., 1993) and is also seen in euthymic unmedicated bipolar patients (Berrettini et al., 1982). Plasma GABA levels do not correlate with severity of symptoms for either depression or mania (i.e., are state-independent); however, the key research for identifying whether the marker is familial and segregates with illness in families with affective disorders has not yet been done.

In a large multicenter trial of valproate in the treatment of mania (Bowden et al., 1994; see Chapter 18), plasma concentrations of GABA were measured before and after treatment in a subset of 63 patients. Interestingly, although treatment with both lithium and valproate resulted in reductions in plasma GABA levels, pretreatment levels of plasma GABA predicted response to valproate but not to lithium. However, it was the patients with higher levels of plasma GABA who were more likely to show an antimanic response to valproate. Since valproate is believed to enhance GABA function (discussed below), these observations suggest a more complex relationship between the manic state and "too little GABA."

Krystal, Sanacora, and colleagues undertook a series of in vivo MRS studies to measure GABA in patients with mood disorders (Sanacora et al., 1999; Krystal et al., 2002). Measurement of GABA levels in occipital cortex (the only brain region demonstrated thus far to allow for reliable GABA quantitation using MRS) appeared to discriminate between unipolar and bipolar depressed patients. Thus, these investigators found significant reductions in occipital cortex GABA levels in unipolar but not bipolar depressed patients. Interestingly, among unipolar depressed patients, reductions were most prominent in patients with melancholic or psychotic depression compared with those meeting criteria for atypical depression, a form of depression with features that overlap considerably with bipolar depression.

Recently, Dean and colleagues (2005) measured the density of GABA ([^{3}H] muscimol) and benzodiazepine ([^{3}H] flumazenil) binding sites on the GABA(A) receptor in hippocampi, obtained postmortem, from schizophrenic, bipolar-I disorder and control subjects. In addition, they measured the amount of [^{3}H] flumazenil binding that could be displaced with zolpidem and clonazepam. There were complex, regionally specific changes in [^{3}H] muscimol binding in the hippocampus from subjects with bipolar disorder. Notably, there were also significant decreases in zolpidem-sensitive and increases in zolpidem-insensitive [^{3}H] flumazenil binding in most regions of the sections of the hippocampal formation studied in bipolar disorder. Unlike [^{3}H] flumazenil, zolpidem does not bind to the $\alpha 5$ subunit of the GABA(A) receptor; these findings therefore raise the possibility that there is an increase in GABA(A) receptors containing $\alpha 5$ subunit in the hippocampus from subjects with bipolar-I disorder.

Postmortem Brain Studies of GABA Synthetic Enzymes

In postmortem brain studies, Guidotti and colleagues (2000) identified unexpected abnormalities in the levels of reelin and the GABA synthetic enzymes glutamic acid decarboxylase (GAD_{65} and GAD_{67}) in schizophrenia and bipolar disorder. Reelin is a glycoprotein secreted preferentially by cortical GABAergic interneurons (layers I and II) that binds to integrin receptors located on dendritic spines of pyramidal neurons or on GABAergic interneurons of layers III through V expressing the disabled-1 gene product (Dab-1), a cytosolic adaptor protein that mediates reelin action (Guidotti et al., 2000). The authors found that prefrontal cortex and cerebellar expression of reelin mRNA, GAD_{67} protein and mRNA, and prefrontal cortex reelin-positive cells was significantly decreased by 30–50 percent in patients with schizophrenia or bipolar disorder with psychosis, but not in those with unipolar depression without psychosis, when compared with nonpsychiatric subjects.

Benes and colleagues (2000) developed techniques for immunolocalizing GAD_{65} and applied these techniques to anterior cingulate and prefrontal cortices of 12 normal controls, 12 schizophrenic subjects, and 5 bipolar subjects. They found that in the bipolar subjects, the density of GAD65-IR terminals was significantly reduced in all four layers of anterior cingulated cortex (layers II–VI), but these differences were most significant in layers II (27.8 percent) and III (37.2 percent), regardless of whether the subjects had been treated with neuroleptics. In prefrontal cortex, the bipolar subjects showed similar differences in terminal density for pyramidal neurons and nonpyramidal neurons but not neuropil in the four laminae examined. The bipolar group showed no differences in either the size of cell bodies or GAD_{65} immunoreactive terminals; given the small sample size, however, the possibility of a Type II error cannot be excluded.

The same group (Heckers et al., 2002) investigated hippocampal sections from 15 bipolar subjects, 15 schizophrenic subjects, and 15 controls through an in situ hybridization for GAD_{65} and GAD_{67} mRNA. These investigators found that the density of GAD_{65} and GAD_{67} mRNA-positive neurons was decreased by 45 and 43 percent, respectively, in subjects with bipolar disorder, but only 14 and 4 percent, respectively, in subjects with schizophrenia. The decreased density of GAD_{65} mRNA-positive neurons in subjects with bipolar disorder was significant in sectors CA2/3 and dentate gyrus, and that of GAD_{67} mRNA-positive neurons was significant in CA4 but not other hippocampal sectors. Cellular GAD_{65} mRNA expression was significantly decreased in subjects with bipolar disorder, particularly in CA4, but not in schizophrenic subjects. Cellular GAD_{67} mRNA expression was normal in both groups.

Studies of Reelin

As discussed above, postmortem studies have revealed that an unexpected molecule may be involved in the pathophysiology of severe neuropsychiatric disorders, including bipolar disorder and schizophrenia (Impagnatiello et al., 1998; Fatemi et al., 2000a, 2001a,b; Guidotti et al., 2000). Reelin is a member of a growing group of diverse proteins whose absence is associated with an almost identical phenotype—inversion of cerebral cortical layers and reduction or absence of cerebellar foliation.

Costa and colleagues first showed that reelin protein and mRNA were reduced in several brain areas in both schizophrenic and psychotic bipolar patients, leading to their suggestion that reelin deficiency may be a vulnerability factor for psychosis independent of diagnosis (Guidotti et al., 2000; Costa et al., 2001, 2002). Subsequently, Fatemi and colleagues confirmed Costa's findings, but found similar reductions in reelin protein in hippocampi of nonpsychotic bipolar and depressed patients, suggesting that reelin deficiency alone is not a marker of psychosis (Fatemi et al., 2000b, 2001a,b, 2002).[29]

Recent results from Fatemi's group (unpublished observations) revealed that reelin 410 and 180 kilodalton species were significantly reduced in cerebellum of subjects with bipolar disorder (with and without psychosis) compared with normal controls. Bipolar subjects also demonstrated significant deficits in GAD proteins of 65 and 67 kilodalton (GAD_{65} and GAD_{67}) compared with controls. In contrast, reelin deficiency was limited to the 180 kilodalton species in cerebella of schizophrenic subjects. All schizophrenic and depressed subjects also showed significant reductions in GAD_{65} and GAD_{67} proteins compared with levels in controls. These results confirm the findings of a recent study by Benes and colleagues (Heckers et al., 2002) showing a global deficit in levels of GAD_{65} and GAD_{67} in hippocampus of subjects with bipolar disorder. Interestingly, some brain GABAergic interneurons share the synthetic machinery for production of reelin and GAD_{65} and GAD_{67} proteins (Pesold et al., 1998a,b) and appear to be dysfunctional in bipolar subjects. Finally, deficits in hippocampal and cerebellar reelin levels in bipolar subjects (Fatemi et al., 2000b; unpublished observations; Guidotti et al., 2000) correlate well with decreases in levels of blood reelin in patients with bipolar disorder (Fatemi et al., 2001a). Future larger studies should aim to correlate the extent of reelin deficiency observed in hippocampus and cerebellum of subjects with bipolar disorder with blood and CSF levels of the same protein to better define the role of reelin in the etiology of bipolar disorder, recurrent depression, and other neurodevelopmental disorders, such as schizophrenia and autism.

Lithium and the GABAergic System

In contrast to the abundant literature on lithium's effects on monoamine neurotransmitters, much less work has been conducted on the amino acid neurotransmitters and neuropeptides (Bernasconi, 1982; Lloyd et al., 1987; Nemeroff, 1991). Studies have indicated that previously low levels of plasma and CSF GABA are normalized in bipolar patients being treated with lithium (Berrettini et al., 1983, 1986), paralleling reported GABA changes observed in several regions of rat brain (Gottesfeld et al., 1971; Maggi and

Enna, 1980; Ahluwalia et al., 1981). Interestingly, following withdrawal of chronic lithium, GABA levels return to normal in striatum and midbrain, but remain elevated in pons-medulla (Ahluwalia et al., 1981), possibly as a result of elevated levels of the GABA-synthesizing enzyme GAD.

Lithium has also been postulated to prevent GABA uptake, and chronic lithium has been shown to significantly decrease low-affinity [³H]GABA sites in corpus striatum and hypothalamus. Since lithium has no effect on in vitro [³H]GABA binding, these receptor changes have been interpreted as downregulation secondary to activation of the GABAergic system (Maggi and Enna, 1980). Although the clinical relevance of these findings remains unclear, it is noteworthy that decreases in CSF GABA have been reported in unipolar depressed patients (Post et al., 1980b; Berrettini et al., 1982).

In the GABAergic system, the chronic administration of lithium, valproate, or carbamazepine exerts important effects, decreasing GABA turnover in frontal cortex (Bernasconi, 1982). In addition, all three mood stabilizers are reported to increase GABA(B) receptors in hippocampus following chronic, but not acute, administration (Motohashi et al., 1989). These findings are interesting given that the GABA(B) agonist baclofen appeared to exacerbate depression in a small group of patients, and its discontinuation was associated with improvement in mood and behavior (Post et al., 1991). The data suggest the possibility that GABA(B) antagonists rather than agonists could have a useful antidepressant effect, and that the effect of mood stabilizers on GABAergic tone could be related to some of the drugs' psychotropic properties.

Valproate and the GABAergic System

A leading hypothesis of how valproate exerts its anticonvulsant effect is that it increases the availability of GABA in GABAergic synapses (Johannessen, 2000). GABA, an inhibitory amino acid neurotransmitter, would be expected to inhibit excessive firing of synapses, thus inhibiting epileptogenic activity. A number of studies show that valproate, at therapeutic concentrations, is an inhibitor of succinate semialdehyde dehydrogenase (SSADH).[30] This enzyme is critical for the GABA shunt, an enzymatic series of reactions that produces both glutamate and GABA by circumventing a portion of the tricarboxylic acid (TCA) cycle. GABA transaminase (GABA-T) converts GABA to succinate semialdehyde (SSA), which is then converted to succinate by SSADH. Valproate's effect on SSADH would be expected to increase levels of SSA, which has a strong inhibitory effect on GABA-T activity. Thus, GABA concentration should

increase as GABA-T is inhibited by an increasing SSA concentration.

Indeed, numerous studies have documented an increase in GABA concentration in rodent brain after valproate administration (Johannessen, 2000). It is possible that valproate exerts its antimanic effects through inhibition of SSADH. However, since the long-term effects of the drug are seen only following long-term treatment, the effect of SSADH on other cellular processes (perhaps not related to GABA concentration) may be related to the long-term changes in gene expression, protein concentration, and protein phosphorylation that are postulated to be the ultimate reason for valproate's mood-stabilizing effects (G. Gould et al., 2003, 2004c).

Farther downstream of SSADH, the GABA shunt reenters the TCA cycle; thus, inhibition of the GABA shunt could lead to lower overall activity of the TCA cycle. Indeed, lower TCA activity—or perhaps increased GABA—may explain the decreased glucose metabolism observed during valproate treatment (Leiderman et al., 1991; Gaillard et al., 1996; Johannessen, 2000). Valproate also inhibits SSA reductase, the enzyme that converts SSA to γ-hydroxybutyrate (GHB) with a Ki (the concentration of the drug required to inhibit enzymatic activity by 50 percent) of 85 micromolar (μM) (Whittle and Turner, 1978; Johannessen, 2000). Valproate increases plasma (Loscher and Schmidt, 1980), CSF (Loscher and Siemes, 1984), and brain GABA (Patsalos and Lascelles, 1981) GABA, theoretically by inducing GAD (Nau and Loscher, 1982) as well as inhibiting GABA aminotransferase (Loscher, 1993). In addition, valproate increases GABA release (Gram et al., 1988) and interacts with GABA transporters (Nilsson et al., 1990).

The GABAergic System in Manic-Depressive Illness: Summary

Since GABA is the major inhibitory neurotransmitter and exerts a major effect on neuronal excitability, it is not surprising that abnormalities in the GABAergic system have been reported in mood disorders. However, the body of biochemical data is not very strong, and recent MRS studies suggest a GABAergic deficit (albeit only in occipital cortex) in unipolar but not bipolar patients. More intriguing are the several postmortem studies that have demonstrated a decrease in GAD$_{65}$ mRNA-positive neurons in CA2 and CA3 dentate gyrus and of GAD-67 mRNA-positive neurons in CA4 dentate gyrus in bipolar disorder (Heckers et al., 2002); decreased GAD-67 protein and mRNA and reelin (secreted by GABAergic interneurons) mRNA in prefrontal cortex and cerebellum of psychotic bipolar patients (Guidotti et al., 2000); and decreased immunoreactive density of GAD$_{65}$ in layers II and III of anterior cingulate cortex in bipolar disorder (Benes et al., 2000). These findings raise the possibility of a GABAergic deficit in limbic and limbic-related areas (potentially due to loss of GABAergic neurons) in bipolar disorder, and warrant further study. Box 14–9 summarizes the findings of newer studies supporting the involvement of the GABAergic system in bipolar disorder.

The Glutamatergic System

It is surprising that the glutamatergic system has only recently undergone extensive investigation for its possible involvement in the pathophysiology of mood disorders, since it is the major excitatory neurotransmitter in the CNS, known to play a role in regulating the threshold for excitation of most other neurotransmitter systems. (For the regulatory processes involved in glutamatergic neurotransmission, see Figure 14–5.) Although much of the evidence for the potential involvement of the glutamatergic system in manic-depressive illness—derived from plasma, CSF, and postmortem studies—must be considered indirect, a growing body of data suggests that direct and indirect glutamate modulators may exert antidepressant effects, perhaps particularly so in bipolar depression (Krystal et al., 2002; Zarate et al., 2002).

Plasma and CSF Glutamate Levels

Altamura and colleagues (1993) reported that glutamate plasma levels were significantly higher in patients with mood disorders (n = 15) than in neurological patients with tension headache (n = 10). Glutamate plasma levels were also found to be higher for patients with mood disorders than for healthy volunteers and patients with schizophrenia,

---

BOX 14–9.   Newer Studies Suggesting a Role for the GABAergic System in the Pathophysiology and Treatment of Manic-Depressive Illness (Primarily Bipolar)

Genetic Studies

- Increased genotype 1-1 GABRA3 gene (α_3 subunit GABA receptor) in Xq28 in females with bipolar disorder (Massat et al., 2002)
- GABA(A) receptor α_5 subunit gene polymorphism in cr 15 (GABRA5) associated with bipolar disorder (Papadimitriou et al., 1998)

Plasma Level Studies

- Higher pretreated GABA plasma levels in bipolar disorder are correlated with response to valproate (but not lithium); decrease after treatment (Petty et al., 1996)
- Decreased GABA plasma levels in manic and depressive phases of bipolar disorder (Petty et al., 1993)

Postmortem Studies

- Decreased glutamic acid decarboxidase (GAD_{65}) mRNA-positive neurons in CA2 CA3 dentate gyrus and GAD_{67} in CA4 in bipolar disorder (Heckers et al., 2002)
- Decreased GAD67 protein and mRNA, and reelin (secreted by GABAergic interneurons) mRNA in prefrontal cortex and cerebellum of psychotic bipolar patients (Guidotti et al., 2000)
- Decreased immunoreactive density of GAD65 in layers II and III of anterior cingulate cortex in bipolar patients (Benes et al., 2000)
- Increased density of flumazenil binding to GABA(A) in area 9 in bipolar disorder (Dean et al., 2001)
- Decreased density of calbindin-D28K-labeled neuron in layer 2, and increased clustering among parvalbumin-labeled neurons (markers of GABA populations) in cingulate cortex in bipolar patients (Cotter et al., 2002a)

Figure 14–5. The various regulatory processes involved in glutamatergic neurotransmission. The biosynthetic pathway for glutamate involves synthesis from glucose and the transamination of α-ketoglutarate; however, a small proportion of glutamate is formed more directly from glutamine by glutamine synthetase. The latter is actually synthesized in glia, and via an active process (requiring ATP) is transported to neurons where glutaminase is able to convert this precursor to glutamate (see upper part of diagram). (In astrocytes glutamine can undergo oxidation to yield α-ketoglutarate, which can also be transported to neurons and participate in glutamate synthesis.) Glutamate is either metabolized or sequestered and stored into secretory vesicles by vesicular glutamate transporters (VGluTs) (see inset in upper left corner of diagram). Glutamate can then be released by a calcium-dependent excitotoxic process. Once released from the presynaptic terminal, glutamate is able to bind to numerous excitatory amino acid (EAA) receptors, including both ionotropic (e.g., NMDA) and metabotropic receptors. Presynaptic regulation of glutamate release occurs through metabotropic glutamate receptors ($mGluR_{2/3}$) that subserve the function of autoreceptors. The middle part of the diagram shows glutamate receptors; in the upper left are ionotropic receptors. Activation of the AMPA receptor (AMPA R) by glutamate permits the depolarization of the membrane (1). When glutamate and glycine are present, this depolarization results in the release of magnesium from the NMDA receptor (NMDAR) channel (2). Calcium also enters through the NMDAR pore (3). Interchange of cations additionally occurs via NMDAR and the kainate glutamate receptor (KAR). In the upper right of the diagram metabotropic receptors are shown. Activation of Group I metabotropic glutamate receptors (mGlu 1), which are coupled with a G protein ($G_{q/11}$), produces activation of phospholipase C-β (PLC-β). Activation of Group II metabotropic glutamate receptors (mGlu 2), which are coupled with G_i or G_o, produces either inhibition of adenylyl cyclase (AC) or opening of potassium channels (not shown) respectively. At the bottom of the figure the subunit composition of known receptor subtypes are shown. It is now known that there are a number of important intracellular proteins able to alter the function of glutamate receptors (see middle section of diagram). Also, growth factors like GDNF and S100β secreted from glial cells have been demonstrated to exert a tremendous influence on glutamatergic neurons and synapse formation. Of note, 5-HT_{1A} receptors have been documented to be regulated by antidepressant agents and to modulate the release of S100β. (*Source*: Schatzberg and Nemeroff, 2004. Reprinted with permission from *The American Journal of Psychiatry*. Copyright 2004 by the American Psychiatric Association.)

anxiety disorders, and organic mental disorders. In addition, Mauri and colleagues (1998) found elevated plasma and platelet levels of glutamate in depressed patients compared with controls. Conversely, Maes and colleagues (1998) found no difference in the plasma glutamate levels of treatment-resistant depressed patients and age- and gender-matched controls. Berk and colleagues (2001) suggest that the platelet glutamate receptors may be supersensitive in schizophrenia and depression with psychotic features but not in mania with psychotic features, com-

pared with controls. At this point, however, the relationship between plasma and platelet indices of glutamatergic function and central neurotransmission is unclear.

Brain Imaging Studies

Magnetic Resonance Spectroscopy.   The past decade has seen rapid advances in MRS and its application to the study of recurrent mood disorders (reviewed in Glitz et al., 2002; Moore and Galloway, 2002). It should be emphasized that although some investigations refer to measuring "glutamate,"

Receptor Subunit Types

Ionotropic			Metabotropic		
NMDA	AMPA R	Kainate	Group I	Group II	Group III
NR1	GluR 1	GluR 5	mGlu 1 a-b-c-d	mGlu 2	mGlu 4 a-b
NR2 A-B-C-D	GluR 2	GluR 6	mGlu 5 a-b	mGlu 3	mGlu 6
NR3 A-B	GluR 3	GluR 7			mGlu 7 a-b
	GluR 4	KA 1			mGlu 8 a-b
		KA 2			

the spectral resolution at the field strength used suggests that "Glx" (a peak containing glutamate and additional compounds, including glutamine) may be more appropriate. Using in vivo proton MRS and tissue segmen-tation in 19 patients with major depression and 18 age-matched controls, Auer and colleagues (2000) found a significant decrease in absolute concentrations of anterior cingulate cortex glutamate (10–40 percent) in severely depressed patients compared with the controls, whereas in occipital cortex Sanacora and colleagues (2004) found MRS glutamate increased. In an MRS study of 10 children with bipolar disorder aged 6 to 12 elevated levels of glutamate/glutamine were found in both frontal lobes and basal ganglia compared with controls (Castillo et al., 2000).

Positron Emission Tomography.   As discussed in Chapter 15, the glucose metabolic signal (which correlates closely with cerebral blood flow [CBF] during physiological activation) is thought to reflect primarily glutamatergic transmission (Magistretti and Pellerin, 1996). Thus, the findings of PET imaging studies of major depressive disorder and bipolar depression indicating abnormalities in regional CBF and glucose metabolism are compatible with those indicating abnormalities in glutamatergic transmission. Other types of experimental evidence suggest a consistent pattern of abnormalities in the neural circuitry implicated in emotional processing. Specifically, major depressive episodes are associated with elevated glucose metabolism in thalamus, amygdala, insula, pregenual anterior cingulate cortex, posterior orbital cortices, and ventral lateral prefrontal cortex (Drevets, 2000). Since the projections from the orbital frontal cortex to the limbic structures are glutamatergic, depression- and mania-related hypo- and hyperactivity may be suggestive of either decreased (depression) or increased (mania) activation of glutamatergic corticolimbic pathways. Thus, the hypothesis that a mood-stabilizing drug (for example, lamotrigine) might modulate glutamate release or the consequences of glutamate release could be consistent with these data from functional neuroimaging studies.

Postmortem Studies.   Holemans and colleagues (1993) found no difference in the number of *N*-methyl-D-aspartate (NMDA) receptors in various brain regions of 22 suicide victims compared with age- and gender-matched controls; each of the suicide victims had a retrospective psychiatric diagnosis of depression and had not recently been treated with medication. Similarly, Palmer and colleagues (1994) examined the [^{3}H] MK-801

binding characteristics of glycine and zinc and found no significant differences between suicide victims and controls; this assay theoretically measures allosteric modulatory sites on the NMDA receptor. Since the NMDA receptor is a target for drugs of abuse, such as PCP, it is noteworthy that toxicology screens were negative.

By contrast, Nowak and colleagues (1995a) found downregulation of the high-affinity glycine binding to the NMDA receptor in frontal cortex of suicide victims, of whom almost a third had a positive toxicology screen. It remains unclear, however, whether the subjects included in the study had received psychotropic medications. Finally, the diagnoses of the victims were also unclear; thus the relationship of these findings to patients with clinical depression remains unknown. The authors suggest that their finding supports the hypothesis that glutamatergic dysfunction is involved in the psychopathology underlying suicide and potentially in human depression.

Perhaps the greatest impetus for the recent interest in studying the glutamatergic system in severe, recurrent mood disorders has been a growing appreciation that these disorders, while neurochemical, are also characterized by impairments of neuroplasticity and cellular resilience. Although the precise mechanisms underlying the cell atrophy and death that occur in recurrent mood disorders are unknown, considerable data have shown that impairments of the glutamatergic system play a major role in the morphometric changes observed with severe stresses. Thus, microdialysis studies have shown that stress increases extracellular levels of glutamate in hippocampus, and NMDA glutamate receptor antagonists attenuate stress-induced atrophy of CA3 pyramidal neurons (McEwen, 1999; Sapolsky, 2000b).

Although a variety of methodological issues remain to be fully resolved, the preponderance of the evidence to date suggests that the atrophy, and possibly death, of CA3 pyramidal neurons arises at least in part from increased glutamate neurotransmission (McEwen, 1999a; Sapolsky, 2000a). (For a graphic of the cellular mechanisms by which stress and mood disorders may impair structural plasticity, see Figure 14–6.) It should be noted, however, that although NMDA antagonists block stress-induced hippocampal atrophy, no studies have demonstrated that they are able to block the cell death induced by severe stress. This suggests that the mechanisms underlying atrophy and death may lie on a continuum, with severe (or prolonged) stresses "recruiting" additional pathogenic pathways in addition to enhanced NMDA-mediated neurotransmission. As discussed earlier, stress increases extracellular levels of glutamate, and sustained activation of NMDA as well as of non-NMDA ionotropic receptors

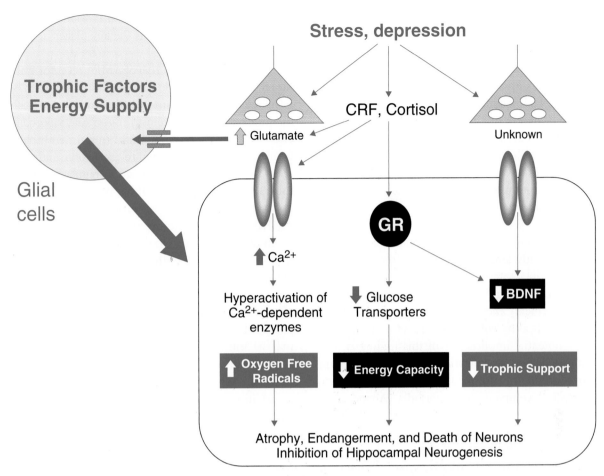

Figure 14–6. The multiple mechanisms by which stress and potentially affective episodes may attenuate cellular resiliency, resulting in atrophy, death, and endangerment of hippocampal neurons. The primary mechanisms appear to be (1) excessive NMDA and non-NMDA glutamatergic throughput; (2) downregulation of cell surface glucose transporters, which are involved in bringing glucose into the cell—reduced levels of glucose transporters thus reduce the neuron's energetic reservoir, making it susceptible to energy failure when faced with excessive demands; and (3) reduction in the levels of brain-derived neurotrophic factor (BDNF), which is essential for the neuron's normal trophic support and synaptic plasticity. The well-documented reduction in glial cells may contribute to impairments of neuronal structural plasticity by reducing the neuron's energy supply and reduced glial-mediated clearing of excessive synaptic glutamate. CRF = corticotrophin releasing factor; GR = glucocorticoid receptor. (*Source*: Manji et al., 2003b.)

could result in high intracellular levels of calcium. Overactivation of the glutamate ionotropic receptors is known to contribute to the neurotoxic effects of a variety of insults, including repeated seizures and ischemia. Neurotoxicity follows as a response to overactivation of calcium-dependent enzymes and the generation of oxygen free-radicals. Stress or glucocorticoid exposure also compromises the metabolic capacity of neurons, thereby increasing the vulnerability to other types of neuronal insults. Activation of the HPA axis appears to play a critical role in mediating these effects, since stress-induced neuronal atrophy is prevented by adrenalectomy and duplicated by exposure to high concentrations of glucocorticoids (Sapolsky, 1996, 2000b; McEwen, 1999b). The role

of the corticotropin-releasing hormone (CRH) and glucocorticoid signaling system is discussed in greater detail later.

Somatic Treatments and the Glutamatergic System

Findings of early studies suggested that D-cycloserine and amantadine, both of which have NMDA antagonistic effects, exert antidepressant effects (Krystal et al., 2002; Zarate et al., 2002). Berman and colleagues (2000) conducted a small placebo-controlled, double-blind trial assessing the treatment effects of a single dose of the NMDA receptor antagonist ketamine in seven patients with depression. The authors report that subjects with depression experienced significant improvement in depressive symptoms shortly (within 72 hours) after taking ketamine but not placebo.

Perhaps the greatest evidence that glutamate modulation may be important in the pathophysiology and treatment of bipolar disorder comes from the clinical use of the anticonvulsant lamotrigine. It is particularly noteworthy that lamotrigine may be one of the few agents shown to have preferential efficacy in the treatment and prevention of bipolar depression (see Chapters 19 and 20).

Although the exact mechanism of action of lamotrigine is unknown, inhibition of an excessive release of glutamate is postulated as a likely candidate (Leach et al., 1986; Calabrese et al., 1996; J. Wang et al., 1996). Lamotrigine also exerts a cerebroprotective effect after focal ischemia (Smith et al., 1996). Recently, lamotrigine has been reported to reduce the hyperglutamatergic consequences of NMDA receptor dysfunction (cognitive dysfunction [learning and memory impairment] and psychomimetic effects) caused by ketamine in healthy volunteers (Anand et al., 2000a). One of the potential implications of this finding is that, in addition to having thymoleptic properties, lamotrigine may prove useful in treating the psychotic symptoms that frequently accompany mood episodes (Anand et al., 2000a).

Lithium and the Glutamatergic System

In view of the evidence that excessive synaptic glutamate may contribute to neuronal atrophy and loss, it is noteworthy that chronic treatment with lithium (plasma levels ~.7 mM) has been shown to upregulate synaptosomal uptake of glutamate in mice (Dixon and Hokin, 1998). Furthermore, chronic treatment with therapeutically relevant concentrations of LiCl in cultured rat cerebellar, cortical, and hippocampal neurons protected against glutamate-induced excitotoxicity involving apoptosis mediated by NMDA receptors (Nonaka et al., 1998). The investigators reported that the protection could be attributed at least in part to inhibition of NMDA receptor–mediated Ca^{2+} influx (Nonaka et al., 1998; Hashimoto et al., 2002).

A growing body of data suggests that AMPA (alpha-amino-3-hydroxy-5-methyl-4-isoxazolepropionic acid) glutamate receptor trafficking, including receptor insertion and internalization and delivery to synaptic sites, provides an elegant mechanism for activity-dependent regulation of synaptic strength. AMPA receptor subunits undergo constitutive endocytosis and exocytosis; however, the process is highly regulated, with a variety of signal transduction cascades being capable of producing short- or long-term changes in synaptic surface expression of AMPA receptor subunits. Indeed, although the mechanisms of long-term potentiation (LTP) and long-term depression (LTD) have not been completely elucidated, it is widely accepted that AMPA receptor trafficking is the key player in these phenomena.

In view of the critical role of AMPA receptor trafficking in regulating various forms of plasticity, recent studies have sought to determine whether two structurally very dissimilar antimanic agents, lithium and valproate, exert effects on AMPA receptor trafficking. Interestingly, these two agents have been shown to exert robust effects on the same signaling pathways known to regulate AMPA receptor trafficking (see below). It has been shown that lithium and valproate have a common effect on downregulating AMPA GluR1 synaptic expression in hippocampus after prolonged treatment with therapeutically relevant concentrations, as assessed both in vitro and in vivo (Du et al., 2003). In cultured hippocampal neurons, lithium and valproate were found to attenuate surface GluR1 expression after long-term treatment. Further supporting the therapeutic relevance of this finding, an agent that provokes mania, the antidepressant imipramine, has an opposite effect as it upregulates AMPA synaptic strength in hippocampus (Du et al., 2003).

Additional support for the therapeutic relevance of these data is provided by studies indicating that AMPA receptor antagonists attenuate several "manic-like" behaviors produced by amphetamine administration. Thus, AMPA antagonists have been demonstrated to attenuate psychostimulant-induced development or expression of sensitization and hedonic behavior without affecting spontaneous locomotion. Additionally, some studies have demonstrated that AMPA receptor antagonists reduce amphetamine- and cocaine-induced hyperactivity.[31]

As discussed earlier, one current model of mania that has been used extensively and has reasonable heuristic value in the study of mood disorders involves the use of psychostimulants in appropriate paradigms. Psychostimulants such as amphetamine and cocaine are known to induce manic-like symptoms in healthy volunteers and to trigger frank manic episodes in individuals with bipolar disorder. The best-established animal models of mania therefore use the administration of amphetamine or cocaine to produce hyperactivity, risk-taking behavior, and increased hedonic drive—all important facets of the human clinical condition of mania. Moreover, these psychostimulant-induced behavioral changes are attenuated by the administration of chronic lithium in a therapeutically relevant time frame. Thus, the fact that AMPA receptor antagonists are capable of attenuating psychostimulant-induced sensitization, hyperactivity, and hedonic behavior provides compelling behavioral support for our contention that AMPA receptors play important roles in regulating affective behavior.

Taken together, findings of biochemical and behavioral studies investigating the effects of antimanic (lithium and valproate) and promanic (antidepressants, cocaine, amphetamine) agents on GluR1 suggest that AMPA receptor trafficking is an important target in the pathogenesis and treatment of certain facets of bipolar disorder. The mechanisms by which glutamate receptors are actively recruited to synapses have long intrigued the neuroscience community; the findings reviewed here suggest that they may also play important roles in the pathophysiology and treatment of complex neuropsychiatric disorders.

Valproate and the Glutamatergic System

In addition to the effects on AMPA receptor trafficking described above, valproate appears to affect glutamatergic neurotransmission through other mechanisms. Acute administration of valproate in vitro has been shown to augment the release of glutamate (Dixon and Hokin, 1997). Ueda and Willmore (2000) reported on the effect of valproate on glutamate transporter expression in hippocampus. With a dose of 100 mg/kg/day of valproate given for 14 days, they found an increase in EAAT1 levels and a decrease in EAAT2 levels. Hassel and colleagues (2001) reported that chronic treatment of rats with valproate (200 or 400 mg/kg/day for 90 days) led to a dose-dependent increase in hippocampal glutamate uptake capacity as measured by uptake of [^{3}H]glutamate into proteoliposomes by increasing the levels of the glutamate transporters EAAT1 and EAAT2 in hippocampus. It is of note that the doses of 200 or 400 mg/kg/day used in this study are much higher than those used in humans, approximately 20–50 mg/kg/day. Thus overall, chronic valproate likely decreases instrasynaptic glutamate levels through a variety of mechanisms.

In rodent models, valproate has been shown to reduce seizure activity induced by AMPA glutamate receptor agonists (Turski, 1990; Steppuhn and Turski, 1993). In postmortem human brain tissue, Künig and colleagues (1998) found that therapeutic levels of valproate decreased binding of AMPA to the AMPA glutamate receptors, thus effectively blocking them. Findings from a series of studies from different laboratories that used various preparations suggest that valproate blocks synaptic responses mediated by NMDA glutamate receptors as well (Loscher, 1999). As disussed above, lithium and valproate, at therapeutically relevant concentrations, also appear to share a common target in regulating AMPA receptor trafficking.

Carbamazepine and the Glutamatergic System

Carbamazepine has been shown to reduce NMDA-evoked depolarizations in preclinical studies (Davies, 1995) and has been found to have antagonistic properties on the NMDA receptor subtype of glutamate receptors (Hough et al., 1996). In this latter study, therapeutically relevant concentrations of carbamazepine inhibited the rise in intracellular free Ca^{2+} concentration induced by NMDA and glycine in a rapid, reversible, and concentration-dependent manner. This inhibition produced by carbamazepine was noncompetitive with respect to NMDA and glycine.

The Glutamatergic System as an Indirect and Direct Target for Antidepressants

NMDA receptor antagonists, such as MK-801 and AP-7, and an AMPA receptor potentiator, the biarylpropylsulfonamide LY392098, have demonstrated "antidepressant" effects in animal models of depression. These studies have included the application of inescapable stressor, forced swim, and tail suspension–induced immobility tests; learned helplessness models of depression; and exposure of animals to a chronic mild stress procedure (Li et al., 2001). Furthermore, antidepressant administration has been shown to affect NMDA receptor function (Nowak et al., 1993, 1995b) and receptor binding profiles (Paul et al., 1992). Also consistent with the putative role of the glutamatergic system in the mechanism of action of antidepressants is the fact that repeated antidepressant administration regionally alters expression of mRNA that encodes multiple NMDA receptor subunits and radioligand binding to these receptors (see Fig. 14–7) within circumscribed areas of the CNS (Skolnick, 1999). According to two recent open-label studies, riluzole (U.S. Food and Drug Administration [FDA] approved for amyotrophic lateral sclerosis [ALS]), which is an inhibitor of glutamate release, was found to have antidepressant effects in patients with treatment-resistant unipolar and bipolar depression (Zarate et al. 2004a, 2005). See Figure 14–8 for an overview of the target receptors of new antidepressant drugs that act on the glutamatergic system. As noted above, NMDA receptor antagonists such as MK-801 and AP-7 have been shown to have antidepressant properties in animal models of depression, leading to two studies of IV ketamine in depression (Berman et al., 2000; Zarate et al., 2006b). Ketamine, a high-affinity noncompetitive NMDA antagonist, has been used as a standard anesthetic agent for many years in both pediatric patients and adults, with doses as high as 2 mg/kg IV. There is abundant preliminary evidence that ketamine has anxiolytic and antidepressant effects in animal models and may have rapid antidepressant properties (Zarate et al., 2006b). These studies in treatment-resistant unipolar major depressive disorder showed robust and rapid antidepressant effects resulting from a single IV dose of an NMDA antagonist. Interestingly, onset of antidepressant

Figure 14–7. Schematic illustrating pathway convergence among conventional (biogenic amine-based) antidepressants, NMDA antagonists, and AMPA receptor potentiators (ARPs). BDNF = brain-derived neurotrophic factor; MAP = mitogen-activated protein; pCREB = phosphorylated cAMP response element-binding protein; PDE = phosphodiesterase; PKA = protein kinase A. (*Source*: Skolnick et al., 2001. Reprinted with permission from Elsevier.)

effects was seen very rapidly (occurring within 2 hours post-infusion) and remained significant for 1 week; studies in bipolar patients are ongoing (Zarate et al., 2006b). In contrast to the dramatic effects observed in this study, a previous controlled study did not show antidepressants effects of the low- to moderate-affinity noncompetitive NMDA antagonist memantine when administered orally (Zarate et al., 2006a). While it is likely that higher-affinity NMDA antagonists are necessary for antidepressant effects to occur, it must be acknowledged that IV administration may also be an important factor. Overall, the intriguing results observed with ketamine support the hypothesis that directly targeting the NMDA receptor complex may bring about rapid and relatively sustained antidepressant effects. This line of research holds considerable promise for developing new treatments for depression (see Fig. 14–8), with the potential to alleviate much of the morbidity and mortality associated with the delayed onset of action of traditional antidepressants.

Based largely on the observation that AMPA receptor activation increases expression of brain-derived neu-

rotrophic factor (BDNF, discussed in detail later), Skolnick and colleagues have undertaken a series of studies investigating the putative antidepressant efficacy of AMPA receptor potentiators in models of depression (Legutko et al., 2001; Li et al., 2001; Skolnick et al., 2001). AMPA receptors are a subfamily of ionotropic glutamate receptors mediating fast excitatory transmission in the CNS. As with most other ligand-gated ion channels, AMPA receptors possess multiple, allosteric modulatory sites that represent targets for fine-tuning the activity of the receptor by pharmacological means. In addition to their ionotropic properties, AMPA receptors have been functionally linked to a variety of signal transduction events involving G proteins and the mitogen-activated protein kinase (MAPK) (Bahr et al., 2002). This raises the possibility that more subtle modulation of AMPA receptors may be a useful strategy to activate MAPK neurotrophic cascades. One class of compounds, AMPA receptor potentiators (ARPs), dramatically reduces the rate of receptor desensitization and/or deactivation (Skolnick et al., 2001).[32]

Figure 14–8. Receptors that may represent a target for novel agents for the treatment of depression. Glutamate (glu) is synthesized in neuron from α-ketoglutarate through the tricarboxylic acid (TCA) cycle. After release, glutamate is reuptaken by glutamate transporters (EAAT1/2/3), shown in glia and a presynaptic neuron (EAAT3). In the glia, glutamate is catabolized to glutamine (through the enzyme glutamine synthetase), diffuses to the neurons, and is then metabolized back to glutamate (through the enzyme glutaminase). The different glutamate receptors and the presumed antiglutamatergic drug sites of action are presented. Memantine is a noncompetitive antagonist at the NMDA receptor (NMDA R). Felbamate is a noncompetitive NMDA receptor antagonist (glycine NR1 and glutamate NR2B), an AMPA receptor (AMPA R) antagonist, an mGlu group I receptor antagonist, and a glutamate release inhibitor (acting through blockade of Ca^{2+} and Na^+ voltage-dependent channels). Riluzole is a glutamate release inhibitor (acting through blockade of Ca^{2+} and Na^+ voltage-dependent channels), a GABA(A) agonist and probably an AMPA and kainate antagonist. The sites for second-generation mGlu group II and III receptor agonists are also depicted. KA R = kainate glutamate receptor. (*Source*: Manji et al., 2003b.)

The Glutamatergic System in Manic-Depressive Illness: Summary

At present, the evidence for abnormalities in the glutamatergic system in manic-depressive illness is quite indirect. As we discuss in detail later, a growing body of data suggests that recurrent mood disorders, especially the bipolar subgroup, are associated with impairments of neuroplasticity and cellular resilience, but the direct evidence for glutamatergic excitotoxicity is lacking. The strongest support comes from pharmacological data, with lithium, valproate, carbamazepine, and lamotrigine all regulating facets of glutamatergic functioning. Perhaps the most

exciting recent preclinical finding is that lithium and valproate downregulate the synaptic expression of the AMPA receptor subunit GluR1, whereas the opposite effect is seen with promanic agents (psychostimulants and imipramine). These studies suggest that regulation of glutamatergically-mediated synaptic plasticity may play a role in the treatment of mood disorders. Indeed, one recent and very attractive hypothesis is that alterations in neural plasticity in critical limbic and reward circuits, mediated by increasing the postsynaptic AMPA to NMDA throughput, may represent a convergent mechanism for antidepressant action (Zarate et al., 2006b). Box 14–10 summarizes direct and indirect evidence supporting the involvement of the

BOX **14–10.**   Direct and Indirect Evidence Supporting a Role for the Glutamatergic System in the Pathophysiology and Treatment of Manic-Depressive Illness (Primarily Bipolar)

CSF, Plasma, and Platelet Studies

- CSF glutamine levels elevated in medication-free depressed patients vs. controls (2 BPD, 16 MDD) and correlated with CSF magnesium levels (Levine et al., 2000)
- Glutamine plasma levels higher in 59 depressive patients (MDD, BPD) vs. controls (Mathis et al., 1988)
- Increased plasma glutamate and decreased platelet levels in medication-free depressed patients (4 MDD, 11 BPD) vs. controls (Altamura et al., 1993)

MRS Studies

- Increased Glu/gln ratio in frontal lobe and basal ganglia in bipolar children (Castillo et al., 2000)
- Decreased Glu levels in anterior cingulate cortex of depressed patients vs. controls (7 patients were medication-free and 12 were under antidepressant treatment; 1 BPD and 18 MDD) (Auer et al., 2000)

Postmortem Brain Studies

- Decreased neuronal EAAT3 and 4 mRNA expression in striatum in BPD (McCullumsmith and Meador-Woodruff, 2002)
- NR2D (a subunit of NMDA receptor) mRNA higher in striatum in BPD (n = 15) than in MDD (15) (Meador-Woodruff et al., 2001)
- gluR1 (a subunit of AMPA receptor) mRNA lower in BPD (n = 15) than in controls (15) (Meador-Woodruff et al., 2001)
- (^{3}H)AMPA binding higher in BPD than in MDD (Meador-Woodruff et al., 2001)
- Reduced glutamate decarboxilase immunoreactive marked terminals in anterior cingulate cortex (most in layer II–III) (Benes et al., 2000)

Treatment Related

Preclinical studies
- Reduced tricarboxylic acid cycle and reduced ATP with valproate in mice (Johannessen et al., 2001)
- Chronic lithium upregulates and stabilizes glutamate uptake by presynaptic nerve endings in mouse cerebral cortex (Dixon and Hokin, 2002)
- Chronic antidepressants regulate NMDA receptor mRNA and binding (Boyer et al., 1998)
- Imipramine and phenelzine decreased potassium-stimulated glutamate outflow in rat prefrontal cortex and not in striatum (Michael-Titus et al., 2000)
- AMPA receptor potentiator LY392098 (a biaryl-propylsulfonamide) produces antidepressant-like effect in rats and mice (Li et al., 2001)

Clinical studies
- Lamotrigine is effective in treatment-resistant BPD (Sporn and Sachs, 1997)
- Lamotrigine has significant antidepressant efficacy in 195 depressed BP-I patients (double-blind, placebo-controlled study) (Calabrese et al., 1999)
- Lamotrigine showed 52–63 percent response in depressed, manic, mixed, and rapid-cycling bipolar patients (Hurley, 2002)
- Increased density of flumazenil binding site GABA(A)R (γ_2 receptor subunit) in BA 9 (Dean et al., 2001)
- Ketamine improves depressive symptoms in depressed patients (8 MDD, 1 BPD), lasting longer (3 days) than euphoric effects (hours), in double-blind, placebo-controlled study (Berman et al., 2000)

Source: Manji et al., 2003.

AMPA = α-amino-3-hydroxy-5-methyl-4-isoxazolepronionic acid; BPD = bipolar disorder; BP-I = bipolar-I; CSF = cerebrospinal fluid; MDD = major depressive disorder; NMDA = N-methyl-D-aspartate.

glutamatergic system in the pathophysiology and treatment of bipolar disorder.

Neuroendocrine Systems and Neuropeptides

Neuroendocrine Systems

The contribution of altered endocrine function to pathological mood states was among the earliest themes in biological psychiatry. The modern era of clinical neuroendocrinology began in the early 1960s, spurred by the development of simple, reliable assay methods for hormones in blood and urine; in due course this field became one of the most prolific research areas in biological psychiatry. Affective disorders became the major focus as it became increasingly apparent that hypothalmic function was intimately involved in many of depression's core symptoms, such as poor regulation of appetite and sleep and decreased sex drive (Gold et al., 1988; Holsboer et al., 2001; Gold and Chrousos, 2002). However, with the revolution in molecular medicine and a much greater focus on intracellular events, there has been much less emphasis on neuroendocrine systems in research on recurrent mood disorders. Furthermore, there is a growing appreciation that simply measuring plasma levels of various hormones—regardless of how precisely the new technologies allow—does not provide a true window into the brain as was once hoped because of the large number of variables (e.g., hypothalamic/pituitary blood flow, degree of stress, sleep, diet, activity levels) that are likely to be altered with these disorders and are difficult to control for. Nevertheless, the study of peptide hormones of the hypothalamic–pituitary axis measured in body fluids under both baseline and challenge conditions has provided some important clues, and these findings are reviewed here.

The emerging animal data on the effects of neurohormones on brain function (i.e., the brain as a gland) have added impetus for the trend toward evaluating neuroendocrine findings in their own right, not simply as a reflection of amine neurotransmitter changes. The actions of a single neurohormone peptide on a wide range of brain receptors characteristically span a much longer time period than the actions of monoamines. The influence of neurohormones on neurons may have been elaborated for teleological reasons. Also, the possibility that one substance effectively commands and organizes multiple coordinated physiological and behavioral responses is consistent with the importance of certain peptides in the long-term phasic changes typical of manic-depressive illness.

One new and intriguing approach to interpreting neuroendocrine data is to assess their variability, either within individual patients or across patient groups. The study of neuroendocrine variability may bring us closer to the pathophysiology of bipolar illness and recurrent depression.

With the isolation of the specific peptide factors responsible for release of individual hormones from the pituitary, clinical endocrinology has developed increasingly sophisticated challenge tests for assessing the dynamics of hypothalamic–pituitary function, and these new techniques have spurred renewed interest in neuroendocrine research in affective disorders. Knowledge has developed rapidly on the hypothalamic neurotransmitter systems that regulate the release of trophic factors to the pituitary. This growing knowledge has increased the potential of neuroendocrine strategies as a window into midbrain neurotransmitter function, particularly of the biogenic amines. It is fair to say that the amine hypotheses is still the major conceptual prism through which neuroendocrine data in affective illness are viewed.

To reiterate, the neuroendocrine literature can be divided into two distinct but overlapping categories. The first includes studies that have used baseline neuroendocrine measures and provocative challenge tests to unravel subclinical endocrine abnormalities in depressed patients. The second encompasses studies in which neuroendocrine measures have been used as a window into central neurotransmitter function (e.g., as a measure of receptor activity or neurotransmitter turnover).

The Hypothalamic–Pituitary–Thyroid Axis. Of all the endocrine systems hypothesized to be linked to recurrent mood disorders, the hypothalamic–pituitary–thyroid (HPT) axis is a prime candidate. In 1864, Graves noted that patients with endemic goiter often showed a markedly "morbid and melancholic turn of mind." Since that time, it has repeatedly been noted that disorders of thyroid function frequently are accompanied by changes in mood (Prange et al., 1974; Joyce, 1991; Styra et al., 1991), and patients with recurrent mood disorders (particularly those with rapid bipolar cycles) frequently have HPT axis abnormalities (Wehr et al., 1988; Zach and Ackerman, 1988; Hendrick et al., 1998). Thyroid hormones reportedly alter the clinical course of some forms of cyclic depressive illness, potentiate the actions of various antidepressants (Goodwin et al., 1982), and can precipitate mania in bipolar patients (Josephson and Mackenzie, 1979, 1980; Wehr and Goodwin, 1987a). The more recent and carefully controlled reports of HPT axis function in depressed patients have, in fact, revealed subtle but significant abnormalities in many manic-depressive patients. Finally, both lithium and carbamazepine have been shown to alter HPT axis function, and some investigators have suggested that the therapeutic effects of these drugs may correlate with their effects on this axis.

The regulation of thyroid hormone secretion—triiodothyronine (T_3) and thyroxine (T_4)—is initiated by the release of a hypothalamic tripeptide, thyrotropin-releasing hormone (TRH). TRH is released into the portal circulation from axons that originate in the median eminence of the hypothalamus. It is then transported to the pituitary, where it binds to specific thyrotropic cells, which release thyroid-stimulating hormone (TSH). This hormone, in turn, is released into the general circulation and stimulates the thyroid gland to synthesize and release T_3 and T_4. Thyroid hormones have widespread metabolic effects and can directly alter many aspects of the peripheral nervous system, as well as CNS function.[33]

Clinically, it was observed that hypothyroidism was often associated with depression. Less frequently, hyperthyroidism (or the administration of thyroid hormone) was associated with euphoric states, including full manic reactions. In pioneering studies during the 1930s, Gjessing substantially ameliorated periodic catatonia in some patients through sustained use of hypermetabolic doses of thyroid hormone, one of the earliest prophylactic treatments in psychiatry. In his classic monograph, Gjessing (1938) speculated that reduced or poorly regulated thyroid function is important to the pathophysiology of various cyclic mental disturbances, including manic-depressive illness. Although Gjessing's studies did not have widespread influence at the time, recent developments have rekindled interest in his work.

As noted above, most neuroendocrine researchers view the phenomena they study as secondary to disturbances in brain neurotransmitters—occurring downstream in a cascade of neuronal events. A major exception to this view is the relationship between decreased thyroid function and rapid cycling in bipolar patients. Here, the endocrine dysfunction itself may cause the increased cycling. This hypothesis led to evaluation of high-dose thyroid as a treatment for rapid cycling, and some positive results have been reported; unfortunately, cardiovascular side effects, along with a lack of industry support, for research on compounds that are generic, have precluded more extensive study (see Chapter 18).

Despite the existence of numerous studies, the status of peripheral thyroid indices in affective illness remains unclear. Bauer and Whybrow (1988) concluded that the most frequent thyroid abnormality associated with major depression (although not specific to this diagnosis) is a relative increase in plasma T_4 without accompanying changes in its active (T_3) or inactive (rT_3) metabolites. In contrast, Gold and colleagues (1981a) found mild hypothyroidism in 9 percent of their large unipolar sample (usually reflected by slight increases in TSH), and antithyroid antibodies have been reported in up to 20 percent of patients with depression.[34] If T_4 actually is increased in depression, disagreement exists as to whether this is part of the pathophysiology of the depressive symptoms (Joffe et al., 1984) or is a compensatory peripheral increase to "allow delivery of more thyroxine to a brain whose homeostatic mechanisms have gone awry—an effect achieved without subjecting the organism to increased metabolic demands due to increased circulating levels of T_3" (Bauer and Whybrow, 1988, p. 82).

Styra and colleagues (1991) found a 12 percent prevalence of elevated T_4 levels in 99 bipolar and unipolar patients. No statistically significant difference in response to antidepressant treatment was observed between the hyperthyroxinemia group and the normal serum T_4 group. In another study, free T_4 index (FT_4I) and T_4 levels were measured in 31 manic patients shortly after admission to a psychiatric hospital (Joyce, 1991). Over one-third had elevated thyroid hormone levels (due to increases in FT_4I). Low FT_4I levels prospectively predicted more hospital admissions in the 12 months from index admission. Joffe and colleagues (1994) reported that the overall frequency of Grade II subclinical hypothyroidism was 20 percent in 66 bipolar patients, with no difference in frequency of subclinical hypothyroidism or in mean thyroid hormone levels between the mixed-state and non–mixed-state groups. Interestingly, somewhat akin to the results seen with the HPA axis discussed later, Zarate and colleagues (1997) found in a study of first-episode patients that TSH was higher in mixed than in manic bipolar patients.

This latter finding may be most applicable to bipolar illness, where there is some evidence of a subtle decrease in thyroid function, especially among those with rapid cycles,[35] although not all studies agree on this.[36] Evidence of thyroid dysfunction in bipolar illness may have emerged because of the antithyroid effects of lithium, in effect unmasking subtle preexisting thyroid pathology.

The association between lithium-induced hypothyroidism and rapid cycling is observed predominantly in women. As noted in Chapter 18, women may also be more sensitive to the cycle-inducing effects of tricyclic antidepressants. If hypothyroidism (either in the presence or absence of lithium treatment) is related to the development of rapid-cycling bipolar depression, it is not yet clear how. Several individual case reports have described cyclical mood disturbances developing in patients following subtotal thyroidectomy (Hertz, 1964). However, thyroidectomy per se is not sufficient for the development of rapid cycling; clearly, other predisposing factors must be present. In Chapter 16, we suggest that the effects of thyroid hormones on the periodicity of biological clocks in animals, coupled with altered circadian pacemaker function in bipolar patients, may explain the apparent inductive effect of hypothyroidism in rapid-cycling patients. Almost all rapid-cycling bipolar patients are female (Wehr et al., 1988). Likewise, thyroid dysfunction, including the antithyroid effects of lithium, is much more common among women (Joffe et al., 1988). These observations link female sex, hyperthyroidism, and rapid cycling.

Hatterer and colleagues (1988) propose that relatively reduced thyroid function among bipolar patients on lithium may be associated with poor outcome. They report that plasma T_3 levels were significantly lower among patients who relapsed on lithium, although all values remained in the normal range (see Frye et al., 1999a). As discussed earlier, Gjessing (1938) described a group of patients with periodic catatonia who, when given large doses of thyroid hormone, responded with rapid (less than 1 week) and long-lasting improvement. In a somewhat larger group of patients with periodic psychoses, Wakoh and Hatotani (1973) found similar beneficial effects of treatment with large doses of thyroid hormone. As noted in Chapter 3, these patients share many clinical features with rapid-cycling bipolar patients, and their conditions probably represent the same illness.

In a later study, Stancer and Persad (1982) gave hypermetabolic doses of T_4 (300 to 500 µg/day) to 10 rapid-cycling bipolar patients. Of the seven women, five responded dramatically, whereas two men and an adolescent did not. Consistent with this finding are reports that thyroid hormone in combination with standard mood-stabilizing drugs can attenuate cycles in bipolar patients (Goodwin, 1982; Bauer and Whybrow, 1988). High-dose T_4 ($482\pm72\,\mu g$/day) proved to have excellent antidepressant effects in approximately 50 percent of severely therapy-resistant depressed patients (5 unipolar and 12 bipolar) in an 8-week open label and 27.2 ± 22.0-month follow-up of responders (Bauer et al., 1998a).

In another study, six resistant bipolar patients (non-rapid-cycling) were treated with supraphysiological doses of T_4 (250 to 500 μg/day) adjunctively and followed up for 27.8 ± 12.8 months. The mean number of relapses declined from 5.3 ± 3.1 to $.8\pm.8$, compared with the number of relapses during the same length of time for each patient before the start of treatment with high-dose T_4 (Bauer et al., 1998a,b).[37]

Another approach to the HPT axis involves the study of circadian patterns of TSH release. Normally, TSH secretion peaks during the night (Weeke, 1973), but this peak is absent in some patients with affective disorders (Weeke and Weeke, 1978; Goldstein et al., 1980), including those with rapid-cycling bipolar disorder (Kasper et al., 1988; Sack et al., 1988). Sleep deprivation represents another challenge test in that it is associated with an increase in nocturnal TSH. Both bipolar (Sack et al., 1988) and unipolar depressed patients (Kasper et al., 1988) have been shown to have blunted TSH response to total sleep deprivation.[38]

Potential Involvement of Thyrotropin-Releasing Hormone. Preclinical studies have shown that TRH has an extensive extrahypothalamic distribution including the limbic system, amygdala, and frontal cortex, and in addition to its neurohormonal role, appears to act as a neurotransmitter (Griffiths, 1985). Thus in preclinical animal studies, administration of TRH appears to have a mild stimulant effect including increased arousal and motor activity (Nemeroff et al., 1984a).

In humans, at least two clinical studies have reported elevated levels of CSF TRH in patients with acute depression (Kirkegaard et al., 1979; Banki et al., 1988), while a third found no difference from control subjects (Roy et al., 1994). A more recent and larger study included both bipolar and unipolar medication-free depressed patients ($n=56$) compared with normal controls ($n=34$) and again found no differences in CSF TRH. However, there was a gender difference, with females having, on average, lower TRH levels than men—a finding most significant in the bipolar group (Frye et al., 1999b).

The TRH stimulation test uses a challenge dose and measures the plasma TSH concentration at baseline and at 30-minute intervals. Multiple studies have used this test in depressed patients, and all have found that approximately 25–30 percent have a blunted TSH response despite being euthyroid at the time.[39] Using a modified TRH stimulation test in which TRH is administered at 8 AM and then again at 11 PM, Duval and colleagues (1990) were able to achieve a 95 percent specificity and 89 percent sensitivity for the diagnosis of major depression in patients who had a markedly blunted nocturnal TSH response. An attempt to correlate low CSF TRH with a blunted TSH response to TRH stimulation was negative (Frye et al., 1999b).

TRH analogues have been shown to have antidepressant properties, effects that have been postulated to occur independently of thyroid hormone secretion (Redei et al., 1999; Lloyd et al., 2001). Furthermore, in rodents, electroconvulsive shock (the animal model of ECT) was shown to induce the synthesis of TRH in multiple subcortical limbic and frontal cortical regions (Sattin, 1999). Early studies that tested TRH as an antidepressant were quite promising. Prange and colleagues (1972) found that IV TRH given in a double-blind, crossover design produced a striking improvement in mood that lasted for a few hours and then faded; however, subsequent studies found no such improvement (Amsterdam et al., 1981).

To determine whether these variable results were due at least in part to the presumed poor blood–brain barrier permeability, a study of intrathecal TRH administration was conducted (Marangell et al., 1997). The investigators administered TRH (500 μg) to eight medication-free inpatients with refractory depression by means of a lumbar intrathecal injection and an identical sham lumbar puncture procedure, separated by 1 week, in a double-blind, crossover design. They found that five of the eight patients responded to intrathecal TRH. The responses were rapid and clinically robust, but they were short-lived.

The same laboratory also compared the antidepressant effect of intrathecal and IV TRH administered in a double-blind design to two treatment-refractory patients with bipolar-II disorder (Callahan et al., 1997). Each patient experienced a robust antidepressant response by both routes; subsequent open trials also showed IV TRH to be effective until apparent tolerance developed. Intrathecal TRH was readministered, and both subjects again experienced robust antidepressant responses. These preliminary data suggest that there is a differential mechanism of tolerance to the two routes of administration and that IV TRH may exert antidepressant effects by indirect, secondary mechanisms. In a recent study, 20 patients with bipolar type I or type II major depressive episode (MDE) were given nocturnal IV TRH 500 μg ($n=10$) or saline ($n=10$) at midnight in a randomized, double-blind fashion. Sixty percent of the TRH group and 10 percent of the saline group showed a greater than or equal to 50 percent reduction in baseline total HAM-D score within 24 hours ($p=.03$).

BOX **14–11.**   **Recent Studies Investigating Abnormalities of the Hypothalamic–Pituitary–Thyroid Axis in Manic-Depressive Illness**

- Unipolar and bipolar patients were studied for 1 year, either continuing usual lithium dosage or reduced dosage by up to 50 percent. There was an association between lower dosage/level of lithium and lower side effects, including lower TSH levels (with no association between affective morbidity and lithium dosage/level) (Abou-Saleh and Coppen, 1989)

- Depressive and manic symptoms decreased significantly compared with baseline in 11 refractory rapid-cycling bipolar disorder patients treated with high-dose levothyroxine as add-on therapy. (Supranormal circulating levels of free thyroxine were necessary to induce clinical response) (Bauer and Whybrow, 1990)

- The diagnostic value of the TRH test was not conclusive for any subgroups of depressed patients including bipolar patients (Vanelle et al., 1990)

- A 12 percent prevalence of elevated thyroxine levels was found in 99 bipolar or unipolar patients. No statistically significant difference in response to antidepressant treatment was observed between the hyperthyroxinemia group and the normal serum thyroxine group (Styra et al., 1991).

- Euthymic bipolar patients were studied after lithium discontinuation. Significant increases ($p < .001$) in plasma thyroxine (T_4) levels and a decrease ($p < .01$) in TSH levels were observed 1 month after lithium withdrawal. No relationship could be demonstrated between the magnitude of the change in hormone levels and the probability of relapse of manic symptoms (Souza et al., 1991).

- Free thyroxine index (FTI) and thyroxine (T_4) levels were measured in 31 manic patients shortly after admission to a psychiatric hospital. Over one-third had elevated thyroid hormone levels (due to increases in FT4I). Low FT4I levels prospectively predicted more hospital admissions in the 12 months from index admission (Joyce, 1991).

- The overall frequency of Grade II subclinical hypothyroidism was 20 percent in 66 bipolar patients. There was no difference in frequency of subclinical hypothyroidism or in mean thyroid hormone levels between the mixed state and non-mixed-state group (Joffe et al., 1994)

- In 20 female patients (major depression, schizophrenia, mania), TRH tests were administered before, during, and after a course of ECT. No significant changes in the mean TSH response were found over the course of ECT and the initial TSH response did not predict the treatment outcome (Hofmann et al., 1994).

- Six resistant bipolar patients (non-rapid-cycling) were treated with supraphysiological doses of thyroxine (250–500 micrograms/day) as add-on and followed up for 27.8 ± 12.8 months. The mean number of relapses declined from 5.3 ± 3.1 to $.8 \pm .8$ compared to the same length of time for each patient before the start of treatment with high-dose T_4 (Baumgartner et al., 1994).

- TSH was higher in a first-episode study in mixed vs. manic bipolar patients (Zarate et al., 1997)

- High-dose T_4 (482 ± 72 micrograms/day) proved to have excellent antidepressant effects in approximately 50% of severely therapy-resistant depressed patients (5 unipolar and 12 bipolar) in an 8-week open-label study and at 27.2 ± 22.0 months follow-up of responders (Bauer et al., 1998)

- In 30 bipolar patients in a 3-year study (CBZ and/or Li), a low level of fT_4 during lithium treatment was associated with more affective episodes and greater severity of depression (Frye et al., 1999)

- There was no correlation between CSF TRH and TSH and the severity of depression (Frye et al., 1999)

- The switchover rate to mania in bipolar depressed patients (16 of 158 inpatients) was significantly higher in patients with lower basal TSH (15.4%) than in the group of patients with higher basal TSH (5.1 %) (Bottlender et al., 2000).

CBZ = carbamazepine; CSF = cerebrospinal fluid; ECT = electroconvulsive therapy; Li = lithium; TRH = thyrotropin-releasing hormone; TSH = thyroid-stimulating hormone.

HAM-D ratings fell by an average of 52 percent after TRH administration versus 12 percent after saline administration ($p = .038$). Antidepressant effects of TRH lasted up to 48 hours. There was no correlation between ΔTSH, ΔT_4, or ΔT_3 measures after TRH (or saline) administration and the change in HAM-D scores (Szuba et al., 2005).

In summary, while there are many suggestions that the HPT axis is altered in mood disorders, many of the clinical studies of TRH have yielded mixed results. The extent to which there is a subgroup of patients having alterations in the HPT axis that may have clinical and ultimately treatment significance remains unclear. There are important gaps in the literature on TRH, including comparisons of unipolar and bipolar patients, studies of bipolar patients while in a manic state, and postmortem and receptor studies of TRH—subjects that should be further explored. Box 14–11 summarizes findings of recent studies implicating abnormalities of the HPT axis in bipolar disorder.

Corticotropin-Releasing Factor and the Hypothalamic-Pituitary-Adrenal Axis.   Evidence of HPA axis activation in bipolar disorder is suggested by multiple lines of evidence. Cushing's syndrome secondary to chronic high levels of endogenous glucocorticoids is associated with a number of psychiatric and psychological disturbances, regardless of its etiology. Major depression, mania, anxiety disorders, cognitive dysfunction and delirium, and hippocampal atrophy have commonly been reported (Krystal et al., 1990; Sonino and Fava, 2001). In a prospective study, for example, 81 percent of subjects diagnosed with Cushing's syndrome developed a psychiatric disorder, most frequently a mood disorder (Kelly et al., 1996). Interestingly, treatment with antiglucocorticoid therapeutics has been reported to result in an improvement in mood and cognitive dysfunction (Kelly et al., 1996), as well as an increase in hippocampal volume in proportion to the treatment-associated decrement in urinary-free cortisol after corrective surgery (Starkman et al., 1999; Simmons et al., 2001).

In subjects without Cushing's, multiple case reports, as well as pharmaco-epidemiological studies, have noted the effects of exogenous steroids on mood (Brown et al., 1999). In a recent review, Sirois (2003) found that 75 percent of patients treated with exogenous corticosteroids exhibited affective symptoms, including mania and depression. At least one study found that mania or hypomania occurred on the day of treatment with corticosteroids, and depression was seen on nontreatment days (Sharfstein et al., 1982).

Measurements of HPA activity in patients are also overwhelmingly supportive. Indeed, overactivity of the HPA axis in depression (either unipolar or bipolar) is among the most consistently replicated biological findings in psychiatry. The anatomical sites and neurohumoral mediators involved in the regulation of this complex neuroendocrine cascade, defined largely in the past decade, are among the best characterized of all neuroendocrine systems (Owens and Nemeroff, 1998; Holsboer, 2000; Gold and Chrousos, 2002).

Discovery of the physiological regulation of human cortisol secretion was soon challenged by further evidence clarifying interactions among adrenal steroids, neuropeptides, and catecholamines. These interactions, which determine the absolute level and periodicity of cortisol secretion from both the hypothalamus and the pituitary, are considerably more complex than had previously been suspected (Axelrod and Reisine, 1984). Such complexity must be kept in mind when relating clinically observed abnormalities in the function of the HPA axis to a specific neuroendocrine defect.

Despite these complexities, the HPA abnormalities reviewed can probably be traced to central (i.e., hypothalamic) rather than peripheral dysregulation of cortisol secretion (Gold et al., 1984b). In brief, the secretion of cortisol from the adrenal cortex is initiated in the CNS through a neurotransmitter-mediated release of hypothalamic CRF, which in turn stimulates pituitary corticotropin (ACTH)

secretion. Various neurotransmitters and neuromodulators, including acetylcholine, NE, serotonin, and GABA, have been implicated in stimulating CRF release (Pepper and Krieger, 1984); different ones predominate at different times, depending on environmental stress, circadian periodicity, and other physiological conditions. Human cortisol secretion can be inhibited by corticosteroids, such as dexamethasone, and this feedback inhibition can readily be demonstrated at both central and pituitary locations. Preliminary data indicate that the central components of the axis are ordinarily more sensitive to glucocorticoid negative feedback than are those in the pituitary gland (P. Gold, unpublished observations). Such distinctions become important in interpreting clinical data on cortisol secretion (with and without dexamethasone).

The earliest studies showed that depressed patients had elevated plasma cortisol levels, which decreased after recovery in most but not all patients (Board et al., 1957; Gibbons, 1964). By and large, these studies included a mixed population of depressive patients and used rather primitive techniques for assaying cortisol. More recent studies, using highly specific radioimmunoassays, more frequent sampling of cortisol (to take into account the well-known diurnal rhythm in cortisol secretion), and more homogeneous groups of patients, including children (Weller and Weller, 1988), have consistently shown significant cortisol hypersecretion in many but not all depressed patients.

Although cortisol hypersecretion has been reported in both bipolar and unipolar patients (Sachar et al., 1973), whether it occurs with the same frequency in both groups remains an open question. Several investigators have examined bipolar patients longitudinally and observed significant hypercortisolemia (and/or elevations of urinary cortisol metabolites) during the depressed but not manic phase (Rizzo et al., 1954; Bunney et al., 1965; Kennedy et al., 1989). These results were confirmed and extended by Rubinow and colleagues (1984), who found that both unipolar and bipolar depressed patients have higher urinary free cortisol levels than patients in the manic phase or healthy controls. The urinary free cortisol levels in Rubinow's manic patients were significantly lower than those of normal controls.

Dexamethasone Suppression Test. In addition to cortisol hypersecretion, other state-dependent abnormalities in HPA function have been reported in affective illness. The most common finding is an early escape, or rebound, of cortisol from the suppression induced by dexamethasone (Carroll et al., 1968; Stokes et al., 1975). This phenomenon, the basis for the dexamethasone suppression test (DST), has been used extensively in psychiatric patients (Goodwin and Jamison, 1990; Rush et al., 1996).

As we reviewed in the first edition of this text, the DST is an indicator of the sensitivity of the HPA axis to feedback suppression by exogenously administered steroid (dexamethasone). Approximately 40–50 percent of endogenously depressed patients respond abnormally to the test (Brown et al., 1979; Carroll, 1980). The specificity of the test in depression is questionable, however, since several confounding variables, such as weight loss and various medications, can produce false-positive (abnormal) results. Also arguing against specificity is evidence that other psychiatric disorders (particularly in their acute phases) may be associated with abnormal dexamethasone suppression. Nevertheless, even a conservative analysis of the many studies of dexamethasone suppression must conclude that positive tests occur far more frequently among severely depressed patients than among those with other major psychiatric diagnoses, even when the known confounding factors are taken into account. Among depressed patients, correlations have been found among dexamethasone suppression, levels of anxiety, somatization (Greden et al., 1984), guilt, anorexia, and weight loss (Feinberg and Carroll, 1984).

At first glance, abnormal dexamethasone suppression would appear to be consistent with the hypercortisolemia seen in depression, which might downregulate functional receptors for glucocorticoids at either the hypothalamic or pituitary level. However, hypercortisolemia and dexamethasone nonsuppression are apparently independent—one can be present without the other (Asnis et al., 1981). This finding suggests that the two may not be causally related or may be separate phenomena stemming from the same process but separated in time. For example, dexamethasone suppression may persist for a short time after a brief episode of hypercortisolemia has passed.

Dexamethasone suppression has been relatively well studied in bipolar illness. During depression, between 25 and 60 percent of bipolar patients have abnormal DST results. According to some investigators (Carroll, 1976; Greden, 1982), but not all (Graham et al., 1982; Godwin et al., 1984; Deshauer et al., 1999), these results revert to normal during the hypomanic and manic phases. The large variability in the rates of abnormal DST results among bipolar patients is also seen in unipolar patients (Stokes et al., 1984). Most investigators have found no significant difference in the rates of abnormal DST results among bipolar and unipolar depressed patients, but some do report that unipolar depressed patients have significantly higher postdexamethasone cortisol values than those of bipolar patients (see Rothschild et al., 1982), primarily because of the very high values in psychotic unipolar patients.

In the initial DST findings for manic patients, the rates of nonsuppression were not significantly greater than those reported in controls (Carroll, 1976; Greden, 1982). Subsequent studies, however, found that variable proportions of manic patients failed to suppress.[40] In fact in some studies, nonsuppression in mania is as frequent as it is in bipolar depression (Graham et al., 1982; Arana et al., 1983; Godwin et al., 1984).

How can we account for these discrepancies? Patients with dysphoric manias—that is, mixed manic-depressive states—frequently have abnormal DST results (Evans and Nemeroff, 1983; Krishnan et al., 1983). If the proportion of such manias differed substantially from one study to another, variable nonsuppression in the manic groups might be expected. However, some reports of dexamethasone nonsuppression in mania specify that the patients were not simultaneously depressed (Graham et al., 1982; Arana et al., 1983). Of special interest is a small group of longitudinal studies in which the DST was used during both phases of the illness in the same patient. In one of these studies (Godwin et al., 1984), most of the bipolar patients showed similar DST results (either abnormal or normal) in both the manic and depressive phases. This finding suggests that there may be a subgroup of bipolar patients in whom HPA axis dysregulation underlies both phases of illness.

When the entire literature on the DST in bipolar disorder is examined critically, it becomes clear that nonsuppression occurs more frequently in the depressive and mixed phases of the illness, but is also not at all uncommon in mania. Clearly, if one considers all studies measuring some aspect of cortisol secretion in manic-depressive patients, the evidence indicates that hypercortisolemia occurs more frequently in the depressed phase than in the hypomanic, manic, or euthymic phases. When cortisol hypersecretion clearly differentiates depression from mania, why does dexamethasone suppression not do the same?

Studies by Meltzer and colleagues (1982), Klein and colleagues (1984), and Atkinson and colleagues (1986) may shed some light on this question. These investigators showed that dexamethasone administration also decreases pituitary prolactin secretion and that, in psychiatric patients with affective symptoms, there is a significant association between nonsuppression of both cortisol and prolactin. Thus, abnormal dexamethasone suppression could indicate a nonspecific abnormality in the feedback sensitivity of the pituitary gland rather than a specific limbic system disturbance, as was previously postulated. This interpretation is not, however, consistent with findings of subsequent studies employing CRF infusions (Gold et al., 1984b, 1986; Gold and Chrousos, 1985), which found normal feedback at the pituitary level.

Virtually all studies agree that both hypercortisolemia and DST results become more normal after recovery from manic or depressive episodes (Carroll, 1982; Joyce and Paykel, 1989). Such evidence indicates that the abnormalities are state-dependent and do not provide a marker for the underlying vulnerability to bipolar disorder or recurrent depression. Also, the fact that these HPA axis abnormalities are not specific to manic-depressive illness or even to major affective illness means they probably reflect downstream physiological concomitants of depression and arousal. It is possible that recurrent affective disorders involve some episodic vulnerability in these systems, perhaps initially requiring activation by stress.

Detailed studies of glucocorticoid receptor (GR) and mineralocorticoid receptor (MR) in subjects with mood disorders are still ongoing. In this context, one postmortem brain study suggested that decreased GR mRNA may be present in the hippocampus of individuals with bipolar and unipolar disorder (Webster et al., 1999). Additionally, another postmortem brain study found significantly lower GR and MR protein and mRNA levels in prefrontal cortex of patients with major depressive disorder compared with those in controls (Lopez et al., 2004). GR mRNA levels were reported to be decreased in layers III and VI in the entorhinal cortex in patients with mood disorders (Webster et al., 2002). As discussed below, Nemeroff and colleagues (1988) have additionally shown a marked decrease in CRF binding sites in the frontal cortex of suicide victims. In an in vivo study using spirinolactone to assess MR function in subjects with depression (an MR antagonist), Young and colleagues (2003) found that subjects with depression had higher functional activity of the MR system, with an increased secretion of cortisol in response to spirinolactone in comparison with matched controls. Furthermore, transgenic mice with reduced GR have HPA axis and cognitive disturbance that may parallel depression in humans and that normalizes with antidepressant exposure. Antisense oligonucleotides targeted to GR (a genetic strategy to reduce the levels of GR mRNA and protein) were found to reduce immobility on the forced swim test, as did the antiglucocorticoid drug mifepristone (RU-486) (Korte et al., 1996). As discussed below, these observations have led to clinical trials of novel therapeutics targeting the glucocorticoid system. Xing and colleagues (2004) determined MR mRNA expression in the postmortem prefrontal cortex of patients with major depression (recurrence not specified) bipolar, and schizophrenic disorders and nonpsychiatric controls (n = 15 for each patient group, and n = 14 for controls) by in situ hybridization. In the dorsolateral prefrontal cortex Brodmann's area 9 (BA 9), MR mRNA was significantly lower ($p < .05$) in all laminae (I–VI) in bipolar disorder patients, and in laminae I, III, IV and VI in patients with schizophrenia than in the controls. MR mRNA in BA 9 was negatively correlated with the duration of psychiatric illnesses. Whether these findings may be linked to the abnormal prefrontal function, HPA axis activation, or the deficits in slow-wave sleep (SWS) found in these major psychiatric illnesses remains to be further explored. In another study, GR mRNA expression was reduced in the basolateral/lateral nuclei in schizophrenia and bipolar disorder patients (n = 15/per group) compared to that in controls (Perlman et al., 2004). To determine if the GR modulates these features of emotional responsiveness, Wei and colleagues (2004) generated transgenic mice overexpressing GR specifically in forebrain. These mice displayed a significant increase in anxiety-like and depressant-like behaviors relative to wild-type (control) mice. Intriguingly, the mice were also supersensitive to antidepressants and showed enhanced sensitization to cocaine. These intriguing findings parallel the human observation that glucocorticoids are capable of inducing both manic and depressive symptomatology. Furthermore, as we describe in greater detail below, very recent microarray studies have shown that both lithium and valproate robustly upregulate the expression of a chaperone protein BAG-1, (Bcl-2 associated atahanogene) that inhibits GR function. Together, these results suggest the forebrain overexpressing GR in mouse may represent a very useful model to delineate some of the circuitry and molecular mechanisms underlying the range of behavioral phenotypes observed in manic-depressive disorder and is worthy of further study.

Role of Corticotropin-Releasing Factor. CRF has become one of the most extensively studied of all the neuropeptides in relation to its potential role in affective disorders. CRF is a 41–amino acid peptide and is a direct regulator of secretion of ACTH from the anterior pituitary. In addition, it acts as a neurotransmitter in extrahypothalamic brain areas. CRF is thought to mediate the neuroendocrine, autonomic, and behavioral response to stress and to underlie some of the observed abnormalities, such as hypercortisolemia, dexamethasone nonsuppression, and stress intolerance, found in depressed patients.

There have been numerous studies of the CSF concentration of CRF in untreated depressed patients, most of which have replicated elevated levels (Nemeroff et al., 1984b; Banki et al., 1987; France et al., 1988; Arato et al., 1989). Elevated levels have also been observed in the CSF of suicide victims (Arato et al., 1989). In contrast to somatostatin, elevated CRF in the CSF appears to be secondary to increased production of the peptide, as elevated levels of mRNA have also been found in the hypothalamus of depressed suicide victims (Plotsky et al., 1995). In addition, the mean number of CRF immunoreactive neurons in the hypothalamus were increased in a postmortem study of depressed patients (Raadsheer et al., 1994). The elevated CSF levels appear to normalize after treatment with ECT or antidepressants (Nemeroff et al., 1991), and failure of normalization may be predictive of relapse (Banki et al., 1992). CSF levels of CRF in patients with mania are not significantly different from those in control subjects (Banki et al., 1992).

Nemeroff and colleagues (1988) found a 23 percent reduction in the number of CRF binding sites in the frontal cortex of suicide victims compared with that in controls; these reductions in CRF binding sites have been postulated to represent a compensatory downregulation in the face of sustained CRF elevations. In contrast, Leake and colleagues (1991) found no differences in CRF immunoreactivity or receptor binding in a small group of depressed patients who died from natural causes. In addition, Hucks and colleagues (1997) found no difference between both medicated and medication-free suicide victims and matched controls. Whether these differences are secondary to differences in postmortem time or in clinical sample characteristics remains unclear.

The CRF stimulation test uses a standard dose of CRF and measures the ACTH response. A subset of depressed patients (both unipolar and bipolar) displayed a suppressed ACTH response to CRF (Holsboer et al., 1987; Young et al., 1990). These results have been interpreted as downregulation of CRF receptors as a result of CRF hypersecretion.

In a study by Gold and colleagues (1984b), the CRF-induced release of ACTH was found to be normal in a group of manic and euthymic bipolar patients, further supporting the findings above of normal or low HPA axis function in manic patients as reflected by urinary free cortisol. Apparently, the central mechanisms responsible for the hypersecretion of CRF in depression revert to normal following the switch to mania or euthymia. As noted previously, several major neurotransmitter systems (noradrenergic, adrenergic, serotonergic, cholinergic, and GABAergic) have been implicated in the regulation of CRF release from the paraventricular nucleus of the hypothalamus. In studies of CRF release by hypothalamic organ culture, Gold's group showed that GABA is inhibitory, whereas NE, acetylcholine, and serotonin are excitatory (Calogero et al., 1988, 1989). Drugs that mimic the actions of acetylcholine have been reported to increase ACTH and cortisol secretion in animals and humans, and there is evidence that cholinergic agonists work on the HPA axis through a receptor-mediated release of hypothalamic CRF. In animals, atropine (a muscarinic–cholinergic antagonist) has been shown to block both stress-induced elevations of ACTH and cortisol (Hedge and Smelik, 1968; Hedge and de Wied, 1971) and the normal circadian rhythm of cortisol secretion (Krieger et al., 1968; Ferrari et al., 1977). The previously discussed depressive-like behavioral effects of physostigmine (a reversible cholinesterase inhibitor) are highly correlated with increased blood levels of ACTH, beta-endorphin, cortisol, and prolactin (Risch et al., 1980, 1981). These same investigators also report that depressed bipolar and unipolar patients secrete significantly more ACTH and

beta-endorphin after physostigmine administration than do controls (Risch et al., 1983).

To test the hypothesis of increased cholinergic sensitivity in major depression, Rubin and colleagues (1999) administered physostigmine (PHYSO) to patients and control subjects at a dose that elevated plasma ACTH, cortisol, and arginine vasopressin (AVP) concentrations but produced few or no side effects. These hormone increases following PHYSO occurred primarily in female depressive patients and male controls and were not significantly related to the presence or absence of side effects. These preliminary results support the hypothesis of heightened cholinergic sensitivity in premenopausal female but not in male patients with major depression.

Preclinical studies using animal behavior models have indicated that CRF receptor antagonists, specifically of the CRF receptor-1 subtype, have anxiolytic and antidepressant activity (Mansbach et al., 1997). These results led to the testing of a CRF receptor-1 antagonist, R121919, in an open trial in 24 patients with depression (Zobel et al., 2000). Initial results were encouraging, and further clinical studies are anticipated. Given the number of abnormalities in the HPA axis, as well as the strong evidence for CRF hypersecretion in both unipolar and bipolar depression, an associated abnormality in the CRF gene might be hypothesized. However, at least two genetic linkage and association studies have failed to support the linkage of CRF polymorphisms to bipolar illness (Stratakis et al., 1997; Alda et al., 2000).

Combined Dexamethasone/Corticotropin-Releasing Hormone Test. The combined dexamethasone (DEX)/CRH challenge test has increasingly been used to assess the dysregulation of the HPA axis because of its purported greater sensitivity than that of either the DST or CRH test used alone. The sensitivity of the DEX/CRH test for major depressive episodes is about 80 percent, exceeding the 44 percent sensitivity of the standard DST reported in a meta-analysis of the literature (Heuser et al., 1994). Furthermore, the DEX/CRH test has been reported to be more closely associated with the diurnal activity of the HPA axis than the standard DST in healthy and depressed subjects (Deuschle et al., 1998).[41]

Recent studies have shown that the ACTH response to the DEX/CRH test is significantly higher in patients with unipolar depression than in controls (Holsboer et al., 1995; Rybakowski and Twardowska, 1999; Oshime et al., 2000). As a prognostic tool, this test showed that remitted patients previously suffering from unipolar depression with a high cortisol response at admission and discharge or with a substantially increased cortisol response at discharge were at much greater risk for relapse within the next 6 months (four- to six-fold higher than individuals with a normal cortisol response) (Zobel et al., 1999, 2000).

This test has also been investigated as a vulnerability marker in a population of first-degree relatives of affectively ill patients. It was found that these relatives released more cortisol after stimulation with the DEX/CRH test than a control group, but less than a group of patients with an acute major depressive episode (Holsboer et al., 1995). Furthermore, 4 years later, the same test results were obtained in this vulnerable group of subjects (Modell et al., 1998).

After the DEX/CRH test, significantly higher cortisol release has been described in patients with depression in the course of bipolar illness than in those with unipolar depression, with both groups having higher release than control subjects (Rybakowski and Twardowska, 1999). Both manic and depressed patients have been reported to have an increased release in response to the DEX/CRH test. Remitted patients have had a significant decrease in cortisol release, but still higher than normal controls (Schmider et al., 1995). A potential confounding variable here is medication. Thus recent studies have shown that chronic lithium and valproate increase the levels of a protein that inhibits GR function; such effects would be entirely consistent with the recent observations of enhanced DEX/CRH responses after chronic lithium treatment (Bschor et al., 2002, 2003).

Role of Stress and Glucocorticoids in Modulating Neural Plasticity.

As noted earlier, there has been a growing appreciation that stress and glucocorticoids are capable of causing atrophy and death of neurons in a variety of brain areas (McEwen, 1999, 2001; Sapolsky, 2000). Indeed, one of the most consistent effects of stress on cellular morphology is atrophy of hippocampal neurons (McEwen, 1999b; Sapolsky, 2000).[42] As discussed in Chapters 9 and 15, some data suggest that the magnitude of hippocampal atrophy observed in individuals with unipolar depression may be related to the duration of illness. This finding suggests that ongoing illness-related neurochemical changes may contribute to impairments of cellular plasticity and resilience. Study of the effects of stressors that bring about some of the behavioral and biochemical abnormalities seen in depression is therefore highly pertinent.

To date, most studies of atrophy and survival of neurons in response to stress, as well as hormones of the HPA axis, have focused on the hippocampus, in part because of the well-defined and easily studied neuronal populations of this limbic brain region, including the dentate gyrus granule cell layer and the CA1 and CA3 pyramidal cell layers. (See Figure 14–9 for the effects of stress on this area.) These cell layers and their connections (mossy fiber pathway and Schaffer collateral) have also been used as cellular

models of learning and memory (i.e., long-term potentiation). Another major reason the hippocampus has been the focus of stress research is that the highest levels of glucocorticoid receptors are expressed in this brain region (Lopez et al., 1998). However, it is clear that stress and glucocorticoids also influence the survival and atrophy of neurons in other brain regions (e.g., prefrontal cortex; see below) that have not yet been studied in the same detail as the hippocampus.

Caution in the interpretation of clinical findings is suggested by the results of recent longitudinal studies undertaken to investigate the effects of early life stress and inherited variation in monkey hippocampal volumes (Lyons et al., 2001). In these studies, paternal half-siblings raised apart from one another by different mothers in the absence of fathers were randomized to one of three postnatal conditions that disrupted diverse aspects of early maternal care. The researchers found that paternal half-siblings with small adult hippocampal volumes responded to the removal of all mothers after weaning with initially larger relative increases in cortisol levels (Lyons et al., 2001). Plasma cortisol levels 3 and 7 days later and measures of cortisol-negative feedback in adulthood were not, however, correlated with hippocampal size. Thus, these studies suggest that small hippocampi also reflect an inherited characteristic of the brain, and their findings highlight the need for caution in attributing causality in cross-sectional human morphometric studies of the hippocampus.

Although not as extensively studied as the hippocampus, recent research has demonstrated histopathological changes in rat prefrontal cortex after corticosterone administration (Wellman, 2001).[43] An intriguing finding of this study, similar to the hippocampal findings summarized above, was a strong heritability of the right ventral medial prefrontal volume. Thus in this study, certain fathers produced offspring with large right ventral medial prefrontal volumes, whereas others produced offspring with small right ventral medial prefrontal volumes (Lyons, 2002). Since the paternal half-siblings were raised apart by different mothers in the absence of fathers, the phenotypic similarities in right ventral medial prefrontal volumes likely represent a major genetic contribution, effects not seen for other prefrontal regions.

Mechanisms Underlying Stress-Induced Morphometric Changes.

As discussed earlier, considerable data suggest that abnormal activation of the glutamatergic system plays a major role in mediating stress-induced morphological changes. Furthermore, it is clear that activation of the HPA axis plays a critical role in mediating these effects, since stress-induced neuronal atrophy is prevented by adrenalectomy and duplicated by exposure to high concentrations

Figure 14–9. Molecular and cellular determinants underlying the opposing actions of stress and antidepressant treatment on hippocampal structure. Stress can have multiple effects depending on the subregion of the hippocampus examined. In the dentate gyrus, acute or chronic stress results in decreased neurogenesis of new neurons. In the CA3 pyramidal cell layer, repeated stress results in atrophy or remodeling of pyramidal neurons, decreasing the number and length of apical dendrites. Glucocorticoid administration causes a similar effect, and decreased expression of brain-derived neurotrophic factor could contribute to pyramidal cell atrophy. Chronic antidepressant administration can reverse the atrophy of CA3 neurons. The effects of antidepressant treatment occur via acute regulation of 5-HT and norepinephrine and the regulation of intracellular signaling and gene expression. GABA-BZ = gamma amino butyric acid-benzodiazepine; GR = glucocorticoid receptors; MR = mineralocorticoid receptors. (*Source*: Adapted from Warner-Schmidt and Duman, 2006. Reprinted with permission.)

of glucocorticoids (Sapolsky, 1996, 2000b; McEwen, 1999a). More recent data also suggest a critical role for CRF in the long-term effects of early-life stress on hippocampal integrity and function. Thus, the administration of CRF to the brains of immature rats has been demonstrated to reduce memory function throughout life; these deficits are associated with progressive loss of hippocampal CA3 neurons and chronic upregulation of hippocampal CRF expression, effects that do not require the presence of stress levels of glucocorticoids (Brunson et al., 2001).[44]

In addition to directly causing neuronal atrophy, stress and glucocorticoids appear to reduce cellular resilience, thereby making certain neurons more vulnerable to other insults, such as ischemia, hypoglycemia, and excitatory amino acid toxicity (Sapolsky, 2000a). Thus recurrent stress (and presumably recurrent mood disorder episodes, which are often associated with hypercortisolemia) may lower the threshold for cellular death and atrophy in response to a variety of physiological (e.g., aging) and pathological (e.g., ischemia) events. The potential functional significance of these

effects is supported by the finding that overexpression of the glucose transporter blocks the neurotoxic effects of neuronal insults (Sapolsky, 2000a; Manji and Duman, 2001). Such processes may conceivably play a role as well in the relationship between mood disorders and cerebrovascular events, considering that individuals who develop their first depressive episode in later life have an increased likelihood of showing MRI evidence of cerebrovascular disease (see Chapter 15).

The precise mechanisms by which glucocorticoids exert these deleterious effects remain to be fully elucidated, but likely involve the inhibition of glucose transport (thereby diminishing the capability for energy production and augmenting susceptibility to hypoglycemic conditions) and the aberrant, excessive facilitation of glutamatergic signaling (Sapolsky, 2000a). The reduction in the resilience of discrete brain regions, including hippocampus and potentially prefrontal cortex, may also reflect the propensity for various stressors to decrease the expression of BDNF in this region (Smith et al., 1995; Nibuya et al., 1999). The mechanisms underlying the downregulation of BDNF by stress have not been fully elucidated, however. Adrenal-glucocorticoids do not appear to account for these actions of stress, since administration of a high dose of glucocorticoid is not sufficient to decrease BDNF, and adrenalectomy does not block the effect of stress.

Role of Stress and Glucocorticoids in Impairing Hippocampal Neurogenesis. The finding that neurogenesis occurs in the adult human brain has reinvigorated research into the cellular mechanisms by which the birth of new neurons is regulated in the mammalian brain (Eriksson et al., 1998). The localization of pluripotent progenitor cells and neurogenesis occurs in restricted brain regions. The greatest density of new cell birth is observed in the subventricular zone and the subgranular layer of the hippocampus. Cells born in the subventricular zone migrate largely to the olfactory bulb and those born in the subgranular zone to the granule cell layer. The newly generated neurons send out axons and appear to make connections with surrounding neurons, indicating that they are capable of integrating into the appropriate neuronal circuitry in hippocampus and cerebral cortex.

Neurogenesis in the hippocampus is increased by enriched environment, exercise, and hippocampal-dependent learning (Kempermann et al., 1997; Van Praag et al., 1999; Gould et al., 2000). Upregulation of neurogenesis in response to these behavioral stimuli and the localization of this process to hippocampus have led to the proposal that the birth of new cells is involved in learning and memory (Gould et al., 2000). Subsequent studies have shown that decreased neurogenesis occurs in response to both acute and chronic stress (Gould et al., 2000). Removal of adrenal steroids (i.e., adrenalectomy) increases neurogenesis, and treatment with high levels of glucocorticoids reproduces the downregulation of neurogenesis that occurs in response to stress. Aging also influences the rate of neurogenesis; although neurogenesis continues into late life, the rate is significantly reduced (Cameron and McKay, 1999). The decreased rate of cell birth may result from upregulation of the HPA axis and higher levels of adrenal-steroids that occur in later life. Lowering glucocorticoid levels in aged animals restores neurogenesis to levels observed in younger animals, a finding indicating that the population of progenitor cells remains stable but is inhibited by glucocorticoids (Cameron and McKay, 1999).

Studies have examined the effects of knocking out the glucocorticoid receptor or mineralocorticoid receptors on neurogenesis in mice (Gass et al., 2000). A reduction of granule cell neurogenesis (to 65 percent of control levels) was found in mineralocorticoid receptor mice (MR−/− mice), whereas glucocorticoid receptor mice (GR−/− mice) did not show neurogenic disruption, a finding that eventually related the mineralocorticoid receptor to the pathogenesis of hippocampal changes observed in chronic stress and affective disorders (Gass et al., 2000). These observations raise the interesting possibility that CRF and GR antagonists, currently being developed for the treatment of mood and anxiety disorders, may have particular utility in the treatment of elderly depressed patients.

Also of potential relevance for our understanding of the neurobiology and treatment of mood disorders is the finding that ovariectomy decreases the proliferation of new cells in the hippocampus, effects that are reversed by estrogen replacement. The rate of neurogenesis fluctuates over the course of the estrus cycle in rodents, and the total rate of cell birth is higher in female rodents than in males. In addition to potentially playing a role in the beneficial cognitive effects of estrogen, the regulation of neurogenesis by this gonadal steroid may provide important clues about certain sexually dimorphic characteristics of mood disorders.

Targeting of the HPA Axis as a Strategy for the Treatment of Severe Mood Disorders. Given the evidence reviewed above, there is a growing appreciation of the potential role of abnormalities of the HPA axis in mediating the phenotypic expression of certain affective states (Gold and Chrousos, 2002). Not surprisingly, then, there is increasing interest in targeting this system for the development of novel therapeutics (see also Chapter 19). Published double-blind, placebo-controlled clinical studies aimed at modulating the HPA axis have employed inhibitors of glucocorticoid synthesis (Malison et al., 1999; Wolkowitz et al., 1999a), antagonists of the glucocorticoid receptor (Belanoff et al., 2001; Young, 2006), hydrocortisone to downregulate the HPA axis (in a proof-of-concept study reported by DeBattista et al., 2000), and dehydroepiandrosterone (Bloch et al., 1999; Wolkowitz et al., 1999b). Some of these drugs have been investigated for proof of concept rather than for use as a standard of care, and it is expected that modified and improved medications would lack some of the limiting side effects observed with these compounds. We describe below some of the drugs currently under investigation in clinical and/or preclinical trials.

CRF1 Receptor Antagonist. A number of small-molecule CRF 1R antagonists have been evaluated using in vivo paradigms in animal models to attenuate CRF-induced ACTH release (Saunders and Williams, 2003). Several classes of CRF 1R inhibitors have been identified, including peptides (astressin, α-helCRF) and small-molecule nonpeptides (CP-154526, antalarmin, DMP-695, DMP-696, CRA-1000, R-121919, SSR-125543, NBI 35965, NBI 27914) (Holmes et al., 2003; Saunders and Williams, 2003). Preclinical studies have shown that CRF 1R antagonists reduce CRF-induced ACTH release and CRF-induced cAMP production (Saunders and Williams, 2003).

Antalarmin, a novel pyrrolopyrimidine compound (Webster et al., 1996), administered to primates in oral doses of 20 mg/kg, significantly diminished CRF-stimulated ACTH release and the pituitary–adrenal, sympathetic, and adrenal medullary responses to stress, and also reversed stress-induced inhibition of exploratory and sexual behaviors (Habib et al., 2000). In the chronic stress model in mice, both antalarmin (10 mg/kg) and fluoxetine (10 mg/kg) were found to improve measures of physical state, weight gain, and emotional response in the light–dark test compared with those of stressed, untreated animals (Ducottet et al., 2003).

CP-154,526, developed by Pfizer, has been evaluated in animal paradigms for treatment of anxiety. It has high penetrability like antalarmin and decreases synthesis of CRF in the paraventricular nucleus (Seymour et al., 2003). Mansbach and colleagues (1997) showed its efficacy in the learned helplessness model of depression in rats. SSR125543A, a 2-aminothiazole derivative that displays a high affinity for human CRF 1 receptors, showed efficacy in the forced swim test and chronic mild stress models in rats in a study comparing it with antalarmin and fluoxetine (Griebel et al., 2002). In other studies, CRA 1000, a nonpeptide pyrimidine CRF 1R antagonist being developed by Taisho Pharmaceuticals (Okuyama et al., 1999), reduced immobility in the learned helplessness paradigm in male wistar rats when given by intraperitoneal injection (Harro et al., 2001). DMP696, developed by Dupont, is a selective, potent, and highly bioavailable nonpeptide CRF 1R antagonist that has been tested in behavioral models of anxiety and is being tested in behavioral paradigms for depression (Li et al., 2003).

Interestingly, R-121919 reduced anxiety and depressive symptoms in patients with unipolar depression in an open-label clinical trial (Zobel et al., 2000). Its clinical development was discontinued, however, probably in response to two cases of healthy volunteers with elevated liver enzymes receiving a high dose of the compound (Kunzel et al., 2003). Yet in an extended data report of the clinical study in major depression patients, no serious side effects were noted in the hypothalamic–pituitary–gonadal system, the HPT axis, the renin–angiotensin system, and prolactin or vasopressin secretion. In addition, no effects on clinical laboratory parameters (including liver enzymes) were observed, encouraging the development of CRF 1R antagonists as antidepressant medications (Kunzel et al., 2003).

Dehydroepiandrosterone.   Dehydroepiandrosterone (DHEA) serves as a precursor for both androgenic and estrogenic steroids and, together with its sulphated form (DHEA-S), is secreted by the adrenal gland and produced in the CNS. Thus, DHEA and DHEA-S are neuroactive steroids having a number of effects that can be described as "functional antagonism" of the actions of glucocorticoids (although DHEA does not directly interact with the glucocorticoid receptor, and there is no known receptor for DHEA in any tissue) (McEwen, 2003). Among its effects, DHEA counteracts the actions of glucocorticoids to inhibit memory and primed-burst potentiation (a form of long-term potentiation) and antagonizes oxidative damage in brain (and in other organs) produced by acute hyperglycemia. Although mediated by an unknown cellular and molecular mechanism, DHEA also interacts with neurotransmitters (serotonin, GABA, excitatory amino acids, and DA), in addition to its glucocorticoid antagonism (reviewed by McEwen, 2003).

DHEA's antidepressant efficacy has been suggested by clinical trials in dysthymic and depressed patients. Wolkowitz and colleagues (1997) reported on a case series comprising six middle-aged and elderly patients with unipolar depression and low basal plasma DHEA and/or DHEA-S levels who received DHEA 30–90 mg/day for 4 weeks. A decrease in depression ratings and an improvement in memory performance, correlated with increases in plasma levels of DHEA and DHEA-S, were observed. The effects of DHEA were also investigated in a double-blind, placebo-controlled, randomized crossover treatment study using 90 and 450 mg of DHEA in patients with midlife-onset dysthymia (a total of 6 weeks on medication and 6 weeks on placebo). The study was completed by 15 of 17 patients; 60 percent of those patients responded to DHEA, compared with 20 percent on placebo (Bloch et al., 1999). Finally, a double-blind, placebo-controlled study was conducted in 22 patients with unipolar depression (medication-free or on stabilized antidepressant regimens) using DHEA at a maximum dose of 90 mg/day or placebo for 6 weeks. A decrease of 50 percent or greater in depressive symptoms was seen in 45 percent of the patients and none in the placebo group (Wolkowitz et al., 1999b). In a recent double-blind, randomized, placebo-controlled crossover study involving 23 men and 23 women with midlife-onset major or minor depression, 6 weeks of DHEA (90–450 mg/day) was found to be superior to placebo in reducing depressive symptoms (Schmidt et al., 2005).

Glucocorticoid Receptor Antagonists.   Mifepristone (RU-486) is a nonselective antagonist of the GR receptor that has shown efficacy in treating psychotic depression (Murphy et al., 1993; Belanoff et al., 2001, 2002) and is being used in ongoing trials in bipolar disorder (Manji et al., 2003b). Young and colleagues (2004) have reported preliminary data on mifepristone (600 mg) compared with placebo in 19 subjects with bipolar depression. They found a beneficial effect on mood and neurocognitive functioning. In a separate study not yet published, 208 patients were randomized to receive 7 days of mifepristone or placebo in addition to their ongoing treatment for psychotic unipolar depression. Although both groups improved significantly, there was no statistical difference between them. A post hoc analysis indicated that the mifepristone patients improved more rapidly than the placebo group (DeBattista et al., 2003). In a recent study, 20 bipolar patients were treated with 600 mg/day of the corticosteroid receptor antagonist mifepristone (RU-486) or placebo for 1 week in a double-blind crossover design (Young et al., 2004). Following treatment with mifepristone, selective improvement in neurocognitive functioning was observed. Spatial working memory performance was significantly improved compared to that of placebo. Hamilton Depression Rating Scale scores and Montgomery-Asberg Depression Rating Scale scores were also improved. These data provide preliminary evidence that glucocorticoid receptor antagonists may have useful cognitive-enhancing and possibly antidepressant properties in bipolar disorder and perhaps also in recurrent depression.

Other GR antagonists being developed are ORG 34517 (Organon), AL082D06 (Abbott), and cyproterone acetate (Schering). Bachmann and colleagues (2003) synthesized three derivatives of mifepristone with higher selectivity for binding to the glucocorticoid receptor, secondary to decreased binding to progesterone receptors (ORG 34517, ORG 34850, and ORG 34116). Among these agents, ORG 34517 is highly potent at the glucocorticoid receptor. Preliminary data for its antidepressant efficacy were presented at the 2002 Collegium Internationale Neuro-psychopharma-cologicum (CINP) meeting by Hoyberg and colleagues (2002). This compound is now in Phase III trials.

Miner and colleagues (2003) have reported on a new compound, AL082D06 (D06), discovered by screening compound libraries, that binds specifically to the glucocorticoid receptor with no measurable binding affinity to the progesterone receptor. This compound was found to antagonize glucocorticoid-mediated transcriptional regulation in in vitro cell-based models of transcriptional activation.

Cyproterone acetate is available outside the United States as an antiandrogen approved for paraphilias. It is used as a contraceptive agent added to an estradiol combination that is also widely used for hair growth. Honer and colleagues (2003) report on its GR antagonism properties, and while it could be tested in depression, it is unlikely to be clinically useful because of its antiandrogenic properties and risk of severe liver damage.

Inhibition of glucocorticoid synthesis has also been investigated as an antidepressant strategy in unipolar and bipolar patients. This research has included the compounds ketoconazole (which poses a risk for hepatotoxicity and drug interaction), metyrapone, and aminogluthethimide.

Recently, in a double-blind, randomized, placebo-controlled study, 63 inpatients with major depression were randomized to receive either placebo or metyrapone (1 g/day) for the first 3 weeks of a 5-week trial with nefazodone or fluvoxamine. A higher proportion of patients receiving metyrapone showed a positive treatment response at day 21 and at day 35 compared with placebo patients. The clinical course of patients treated with metyrapone showed an earlier onset of action beginning in the first week. The plasma concentrations of corticotropin and deoxycortisol were significantly higher during metyrapone treatment, whereas cortisol remained largely unchanged (Jahn et al., 2004).

Corticotropin-Releasing Factor and the Hypothalamic–Pituitary–Adrenal Axis in Manic-Depressive Illness: Summary.

In summary, there is a great deal of support for alterations in the HPA axis, as well as in CRF, in affective disorders. HPA axis hyperactivity in mood disorder patients is generally manifested by increased cortisol levels in plasma (especially at the circadian nadir), urine, and CSF; increased cortisol response to ACTH; blunted ACTH response to CRH challenge; enlarged pituitary and adrenal glands; and postmortem downregulation of frontal cortical CRH. Reduced corticosteroid receptor feedback has been implicated in this process by challenge studies using the DST and the DEX/CRH test.

With respect to bipolar disorder, increased HPA axis activity has been associated more consistently with mixed manic states and depression and less with classic manic episodes (Garlow et al., 1999). As we discuss in greater detail later, a growing body of data suggests that recurrent mood disorders are associated with impairments of neuroplasticity and cellular resilience. The potential contribution of abnormalities of glucocorticoid secretion to these effects and the therapeutic utility of CRF and GR antagonists is an area of extensive current research. Box 14–12 summarizes evidence supporting the involvement of the HPA axis in bipolar disorder and unipolar depression.

Gonadal Steroids

Gonadal steroids as a group have wide-ranging neuromodulatory actions. In fact, gonadal steroids play a role in all stages of neurodevelopment, including neurogenesis, synaptogenesis, neural migration, growth, differentiation, cell survival, and death (Pilgrim and Hutchison, 1994). These various actions, in general, stem from the fact that gonadal steroids are able to modulate genomic transcription and therefore direct and modulate the synthesis of various enzymes and receptor proteins. These actions are tissue-specific and are directed by the presence or absence of tissue-specific coactivators or corepressors (Katzenellenbogen et al., 1996). Further, gonadal steroid actions on

BOX **14–12.**   Evidence Supporting the Involvement of the Hypothalamic–Pituitary–Adrenal Axis in Severe, Recurrent Mood Disorders

- Increased CRF in the CSF
- Blunted ACTH hormone, beta-endorphin, to CRF stimulation
- Reduced CRF receptors in frontal cortex in suicide (may represent compensatory downregulation in the face of overstimulation)
- Pituitary gland enlargement in depressed patients
- Adrenal gland enlargement in depressed patients and suicide victims
- Increased cortisol production during depression
- DST nonsuppression in UP depression
- DST nonsuppression in BP depression and mixed states
- Increased urinary free cortisol concentrations in depression
- Depressogenic and anxiogenic behavioral effects of CRF agonists in rodents
- Preliminary data suggest efficacy of CRF antagonists and GR-blocking drugs in depression

ACTH = adrenocorticotropic hormone; BP = bipolar; CRF = corticotropin-releasing factor; CSF = cerebrospinal fluid; DST = dexamethasone suppression test; GR = glucocorticoid receptor; UP = unipolar.

the brain may be dependent on context and developmental stage. In addition, classic neurotransmitters and other chemicals can directly activate gonadal steroid receptors in the absence of the steroid ligand, and conversely, gonadal steroids have been shown to have modulatory effects on classic neurotransmitter receptors. Thus there appears to be an avenue of "cross talk" between the two systems. Unbound steroid receptors have also been shown to have transcriptional activator and repressor actions. In summary, gonadal steroids appear to have widespread effects that are contextually dependent.

Testosterone.   To date there have been relatively few studies examining potential links between testosterone and affective disorders. Early studies focused on group differences between those with affective illness, including depression and mania, and those with schizophrenia. For example, Mason and colleagues (1988) found higher testosterone levels in patients with paranoid schizophrenia than in those with affective disorders, including mania. Subsequent reports have confirmed that testosterone levels are not elevated in patients with mania compared with controls, although luteinizing hormone concentrations do appear to be elevated (Whalley et al., 1985, 1987; Hunter et al., 1989). An early small study by Sanchez and colleagues (1976) indicated that lithium may lower levels of testosterone, but findings of a more recent and larger study indicate that most patients treated with lithium for 5 years

have normal testosterone levels (Kusalic and Engelsmann, 1996).

Most recent work has focused on the exogenous use of anabolic–androgenic steroids both in medical treatment and illicitly in the bodybuilding and sports industries. Several studies have indicated that the exogenous use of testosterone can increase manic ratings and aggression in some normal men (Pope et al., 2000), as well as affectively vulnerable individuals (Weiss et al., 1999). Pope and Katz (1988) interviewed 41 bodybuilders and football players who had used steroids and were able to retrospectively diagnose manic episodes in 12.2 percent and a major depressive episode in another 12.2 percent, specifically while withdrawing from steroids. Thus, although the preponderance of the evidence supports the induction of affective symptoms by the exogenous use of testosterone, there is little evidence to date to support any role of testosterone in "naturally" occurring affective syndromes.

Estradiol.   The rates of unipolar depression in male and female children are roughly equal until puberty. At that time, the rate for females becomes double that for males. The Epidemiologic Catchment Area (ECA) Study and the National Comorbidity Study (NCS) both report the highest 12-month prevalence ratio for major depression in women during their reproductive years, compared with premenarchal girls, postmenopausal women, and men of all ages (Weissman et al., 1988; Kessler et al., 1993). The difference in prevalence does not appear to be secondary to differences in course, recurrence rates, or number of episodes, as evidenced by a study (Simpson et al., 1997) that followed 96 men and 101 women for 8.4 years. Thus it appears that women are at greater risk for a first episode of major depression during their reproductive years (Joffe and Cohen, 1998). This observation has led some to propose that the monthly hormonal fluctuations experienced by women beginning at puberty somehow play a role in the pathophysiology of depression in vulnerable individuals (Nolen-Hoeksema, 1987; Joffe and Cohen, 1998).

By contrast, the rate of bipolar disorder is very close to equal in men and women—.9 percent 1-year prevalence rates of .9 and 1.1 percent, respectively, according to the ECA (see Chapter 5). The question of whether hormonal fluctuations play a role in the pathophysiology of bipolar disorder does not appear at first glance to be as pertinent as in major depression. However, the risk of postpartum (puerperal), premenstrual, and even menopausal affective symptoms seem to be increased in bipolar disorder. For example, in the NIMH Genetics Initiative study (Blehar et al., 1998), almost half of women with bipolar-I disorder reported severe emotional disturbances in relation to childbearing, with one-third reporting episode onset during pregnancy. In addition, two-thirds of women with bipolar-I disorder reported frequent premenstrual mood disturbances, and 20 percent reported emotional disturbances during the menopause transition. Reich and Winokur (1970) found that 20 percent of women with bipolar disorder suffered from postpartum mania. Dean and colleagues (1989) found a 50 percent relapse rate (both depression and mania) in the 6 weeks following childbirth in women with bipolar disorder. Thus, although hormonal fluctuations may not play a role in the risk of onset of bipolar disorder, they may in fact influence the course and exacerbation of the illness.

Rapid-cycling bipolar disorder is generally defined as four or more affective episodes (depression, mania, or hypomania) in 1 year. As discussed in Chapter 4, the majority of patients with rapid-cycling bipolar disorder are female. In reviewing the available studies on rapid cycling, Leibenluft (1996) calculated that approximately 71–74 percent of patients in these studies were female. Further, when the definition is made more stringent to require 12 or more cycles per year, the proportion of women in a sample increases dramatically (Bauer and Whybrow, 1990).

It does not appear that fluctuations in mood symptoms are correlated with menstrual cycle phase in rapid-cycling patients. For example, although a retrospective study found that 60 percent of 25 rapid-cycling patients experienced severe premenstrual symptoms (Price and DeMarzio, 1986), a prospective study of 47 women found no relationship between mood fluctuations and menstrual cycle phase (Wehr et al., 1988). This latter finding is supported by a subsequent prospective study involving 25 women with rapid-cycling bipolar disorder (Leibenluft et al., 1999). The fact remains, however, that women with bipolar disorder appear to be more vulnerable to rapid cycling. There is some evidence to suggest that rapid cycling can be induced by antidepressant treatments. It is unclear, however, whether the vulnerability in women is secondary to an interaction between antidepressants and the female hormonal system or women being more likely to receive antidepressants (Leibenluft et al., 1999).

What potential role, then, do estrogen and progesterone play in the underlying pathophysiology of bipolar and recurrent depressive disorders? Both have been shown to modulate serotonin function, and estrogen, as well as other gonadal steroids, may influence the effects of antidepressant treatment.[45]

Estrogen has also been shown to increase the expression of nerve growth factors as well as their receptors (Sohrabji et al., 1994). Preclinical studies in rats indicate that ovariectomy reduces the expression of BDNF in parts of the hippocampus as well as the frontal and temporal cortex, and that estrogen replacement increases BDNF expression in some but not all of these areas (Singh et al., 1995; Simpkins et al., 1997). As we discuss later, BDNF has recently been hypothesized to be involved in the mechanism of action of antidepressants, thus estrogen's effect on BDNF parallels BDNF's antidepressant action.

There are several case reports of estrogen-induced mania or rapid cycling in bipolar patients and at least one case of late-life mania associated with estrogen administration in a patient with no previous history of bipolar illness (Young et al., 1997). Further, Chouinard and colleagues (1987) reported on two cases of bipolar disorder that were stabilized by the addition of an estrogen–progesterone combination in addition to mood stabilizers.

Several preclinical studies have found that estrogen increases the expression of PKC, an important intracellular messenger (Maizels et al., 1992; Rebas et al., 1995). As noted below, both lithium and valproate have been shown to be inhibitors of PKC. Further, a pilot study using tamoxifen (a potent PKC inhibitor) in the treatment of mania was significantly positive.

Taken together, the findings of these studies suggest that in general, estrogen may have a more positive effect on mood and progesterone a more negative effect. Both of these gonadal steroids exert significant intracellular effects as well as more global effects on neurotransmitter levels that may ultimately affect mood and mood regulation. Thus women with an inherent vulnerability to a mood disorder, whether depression or bipolar disorder, may be affected by the monthly fluctuations of estrogen and progesterone or by the more rapid changes induced by delivery. Obviously, the situation is a complex one that deserves further exploration.

Neuropeptides

The Endogenous Opioid System. The discovery of the opiate receptor and its endogenous ligand provided the tools for characterizing endogenous opiate systems involving the endorphins and enkephalins. The fact that these systems modulate behavior related to mood, such as pleasure, pain, and self-stimulation, suggests that they may be involved in affective illness. One straightforward hypothesized formulation involves decreased endogenous opiate function in depression and increased opiate function in mania. Such alterations could occur either in the endogenous opiate neuromodulator or in the density or sensitivity of opiate receptors.

Evaluation of these hypotheses has been approached through several experimental paradigms, such as administrating opiate agonists or antagonists to patients, assessing endorphins and related opiate-binding activity in spinal fluid and plasma, conducting neuroendocrine tests following a challenge with exogenous opiates, and examining the effects of mood-altering drugs on opiate systems (see Stengaard-Pedersen and Schou, 1982).

Trials of Opiate Antagonists in Mania.   Endorphins have been studied more extensively than any other group of peptides, not only because they were among the first peptides localized in brain after the discovery of their receptors (Pert and Snyder, 1973), but also because the availability of the relatively pure opiate antagonist naloxone facilitated clinical dissection of the opiate system's function in manic-depressive illness. Despite this scientific activity, however, only tenuous links have been drawn between opiate systems and recurrent affective disorder.

In light of morphine's obvious effects on mood and motor activity in animals and humans, the strategy of blocking endogenous opiate receptors with naloxone in manic patients was viewed with considerable anticipation. The initial study (Janowsky et al., 1978) showed small but significant decreases in manic symptoms following a daily 20 mg IV infusion of naloxone, but subsequent studies have not been as positive.[46]

These negative results were later replicated by the World Health Organization Collaborative Study (Pickar et al., 1982b), a double-blind, placebo-controlled, crossover study of 26 manic patients, although this group did observe significant naloxone-associated reduction in psychotic symptoms in schizophrenic patients concurrently treated with neuroleptics. Emrich and colleagues (1979) actually found exacerbation of manic symptoms in one of two bipolar patients. Thus, the initial observations of antimanic effects with high-dose naloxone have not held up to more extensive efforts at replication. Naloxone-sensitive mania, if it exists, appears to be relatively rare and may require very large doses. It should be noted that several opiate-receptor subsystems in the brain are relatively resistant to blockade by naloxone, so that even with high doses, the naloxone strategy does not provide an unequivocal test of the theory that mania is associated with excess function of some endogenous opiate system in a localized region of the brain.

Trials of Opiates and Opiate Analogs in Depression.   The complementary strategy, administering opiates to depressed patients, has also been pursued. Synthetic opiates were among the earliest drugs used in the treatment of depression (see Chapter 19), and work in this area has begun anew with trials of the endogenous opiate-like peptides, p-endorphin, and enkephalin analogs. The bipolar–unipolar distinction was, understandably, not used in the classic opiate literature. Surprisingly, some recent peptide studies also failed to distinguish these groups, and none of these studies focused on recurrent depression, per se.[47]

Three case reports from different patient populations have noted euphoric or confusional states with opiate administration (Foley et al., 1979; Oyama et al., 1982; Pickar et al., 1984). The fact that large amounts of an endogenous opiate substance administered directly into the CNS can produce a manic-like state does not, however, really bear on the question of whether disturbances in the endogenous opiate systems are involved in the pathophysiology of bipolar disorder. More recently, there have been sporadic reports of mania associated with tramadol (Watts and Grady, 1997), with a tramadol–fluoxetine combination (Gonzalez-Pinto et al., 2001), and with codeine and paracetamol (Orr et al., 1998). However, acute or chronic naloxone has little positive effect or even a negative effect in depressed patients (Terenius et al., 1977; Davis et al., 1979; Janowsky et al., 1979).

Measurement of Opiates in Body Fluids and Postmortem Brain Tissue.   The role of opioid substances in mood disorders has been assessed by measuring their concentrations in CSF. These studies have not revealed any consistent abnormalities.[48]

Peckys and Hurd (2001) examined the prodynorphin and kappa opioid receptor mRNA expression levels in the anterior cingulate and dorsolateral prefrontal cortices of subjects diagnosed with schizophrenia, bipolar disorder, or major depression compared with controls without a psychiatric diagnosis. Multivariate analyses failed to reveal any differences in mRNA expression levels among the four diagnostic groups, though a group trend (nonsignificant) was evident for expression of the kappa opioid receptor and prodynorphin mRNAs in the prefrontal cortex.

More recently, Hurd (2002) used in situ hybridization histochemistry to characterize the anatomical distribution and expression levels of prodynorphin mRNA within amygdaloid complexin postmortem brain obtained from patients with depression, bipolar disorder, schizophrenia, and controls. Individuals with major depression had significantly reduced (41–68 percent) expression of prodynorphin mRNA in the accessory basal (both parvicellular and magnocellular divisions) and amygdalohippocampal areas compared with that in controls. The bipolar group also showed a significant reduction in mRNA expression levels in the amygdalohippocampal area and in the parvicellular division of the accessory basal area.

Lithium administration has been reported to produce time- and dose-dependent increases in met-enkephalin and leu-enkephalin levels in the basal ganglia and nucleus accumbens. It has also been found to increase dynorphin levels (as determined by immunoreactive dynorphin A [1-8] peptide) in the striatum (Sivam et al., 1986, 1988).[49]

In one of the few applicable clinical studies, CSF levels of various pro-opiomelanocortin (POMC) peptides were examined in euthymic bipolar patients before and during lithium treatment. No significant effects of lithium on the CSF levels of any of the peptides were observed (Berrettini et al., 1985b, 1987).

In summary, trials of opiate agonists and antagonists in depression and mania have thus far failed to produce any convincing evidence that these systems are significantly involved in the pathophysiology of affective illness. The same can be said about the study of these peptides in body fluids, and postmortem studies are too preliminary. By contrast, preclinical studies suggest that lithium does regulate the opioidergic systems.

Somatostatin. Somatostatin is a hypothalamic tetradecapeptide originally identified as an inhibitor of GH release. Since then it has been found in the gastrointestinal tract and the pancreatic islet cells; it is also widely distributed throughout the CNS. Somatostatin has been implicated in sleep, eating behaviors, activity state, memory, and concentration, as well as nociception.[50]

Five of six studies of CSF somatostatin of depressed patients (N = 167) compared with normal controls or other patient populations showed significantly lower levels among the depressed patients. In a study by Rubinow and colleagues (1983), lowered somatostatin levels were observed in both unipolar and bipolar depressed patients. Low somatostatin levels in depression appear to be state-dependent, increasing to normal levels with improvement to a euthymic state or a switch to mania. These findings are consistent with those of Berrettini and colleagues (1987), who reported that in 30 euthymic bipolar patients (10 free of medication and 20 receiving lithium), somatostatin levels in CSF did not differ from those of 20 normal volunteers.

Initial studies (Doran et al., 1986), confirmed by Rubinow (1986), suggest that somatostatin is lower in patients who have abnormal DST results regardless of diagnosis, a finding consistent with a role for this peptide in the regulation of ACTH secretion (Reisine, 1984). Also, somatostatin in CSF is lower in patients with Cushing's disease (Kling et al., 1993), suggesting that elevated cortisol levels may suppress somatostatin release.

Carbamazepine is associated with significantly decreased levels of somatostatin in CSF compared with medication-free values (Rubinow, 1986). Whether this lowered level of somatostatin is in any way related to the clinical effects of carbamazepine is not clear. Lithium and antidepressants do not appear to have this effect.

Vasopressin. Extensive animal data indicate that central vasopressin is involved in regulating memory, pair sensitivity, sleep, the synchronization of circadian rhythms, and fluid and electrolyte balance. Noting the parallel between these functional roles of vasopressin and the syndrome of affective illness, Gold and colleagues (1978) hypothesize that a deficiency in central vasopressin function is involved in the pathophysiology of depression, especially alterations in cognitive functioning, circadian rhythms, and fluid and electrolyte balance.[51]

Subsequently, abnormalities in vasopressin expression or receptor activity have been found in both major depression and rodent genetic models of depression (Zhou et al., 2001; Keck et al., 2003). The nonpeptide V 1b receptor antagonist SSR149415 has been reported to exert marked anxiolytic-like and antidepressant-like effects in rodents (Griebel et al., 2002). In contrast to the marked effects of pharmacological V 1b receptor antagonism, mice with a targeted mutation in the V 1b receptor show reduced aggression but normal anxiety-like behavior and neuroendocrine stress responses, postulated to arise from a compensatory change at the level of the V 1a receptor or CRF system (Wersinger et al., 2002). Taken together, the findings of current research suggest that blockade of central V 1b receptors may represent a novel therapeutic strategy for the treatment of stress-related psychiatric disorders (Holmes et al., 2003). A recent study found that orally active vasopressin V1a receptor antagonist, SRX251, selectively blocks aggressive behavior (Ferris et al., 2006).

Two important drugs for recurrent affective disorders, lithium and carbamazepine, affect vasopressin function in apparently opposite directions. Lithium is associated with the induction of diabetes insipidus, presumably by inhibiting renal vasopressin-induced adenylate cyclase activity, and carbamazepine has been used in treating hypothalamic diabetes insipidus (even though it will not reverse the condition when induced by lithium) (Post et al., 1984a). A study of the effects of ECT on vasopressin levels in depressed patients showed a sharp rise in plasma vasopressin levels after treatment, which continued in most patients 4–8 days thereafter (Devanand et al., 1987).

Substance P. Substance P is an undecapeptide neurotransmitter that appears to play an important role in pain sensation and analgesia. It acts as an excitatory neurotransmitter in primary afferent (dorsal root) nerve terminals in the mammalian spinal cord and regulates sympathetic noradrenergic function. Substance P is also found in discrete areas in the CNS, including the substantia nigra, caudate-putamen, amygdala, hypothalamus, and cerebral cortex, where it is thought to act as an excitatory neurotransmitter. It is usually colocated with one of the more classic neurotransmitters, frequently serotonin. Early reports indicated elevated CSF substance P immunoreactivity in depressed and schizophrenic patients (Rimon et al., 1984). However, these results were not confirmed by Berrettini and colleagues (1985c), who found no differences in immunoreactivity between unmedicated acutely manic, euthymic, or depressed unipolar and bipolar subjects and normal volunteers.

Substance P receptors, also known as neurokinin-1 (NK-1) receptors, are highly expressed in brain regions that regulate affective behavior and response to stress, such as the limbic system. An examination of NK-1 receptors in postmortem brain of subjects with bipolar disorder (n=13), unipolar depression (n=13), and schizophrenia (n=14) and normal controls (n=14) (Burnet and Harrison, 2000) found no differences in autoradiographic binding in the anterior cingulated gyrus among the four groups, although the possibility of a Type II error cannot be excluded. However, the ratio of superficial to deep laminar binding was lower in the group with unipolar depression, which the authors theorize could reflect alterations in specific neural circuits expressing the NK-1 receptor. Given the important role of the amygdaloid complex in the regulation of emotional behavior, Carletti and colleagues (2005) compared the mRNA levels of preprotachykinin A (PPT-A, a precursor of both substance P and neurokinin A [NKA]) and 3H-SP binding sites in the amygdala of patients affected by bipolar disorder, major depression, or schizophrenia with those of matched controls. A significant reduction in PPT-A mRNA expression levels was detected in all three diagnostic groups, mainly in the basal, lateral, and accessory basal amygdaloid nuclei, but not in the temporal cortical area proximal to the amygdala. While these results support the involvement of the tachykinins in bipolar disorder, they suggest that there is a generalized impairment of the substance P system in the amygdala in mood disorders and schizophrenia rather than this being a disease-related phenomenon.

Lithium has been shown to increase the substance P content of striatum when administered chronically to rats, an effect antagonized by the concurrent administration of haloperidol (Hong et al., 1983). More recent studies have demonstrated a lithium-induced increase in tachykinin levels that appears to be associated with an increase in transcription of the rat preprotachykinin gene (Sivam et al., 1989). Studies of the effects of subchronic lithium on regional brain concentrations of substance P, neurokinin A, and neuropeptide Y have demonstrated a regionally specific increase in the immunoreactivity of all the peptides (Mathe et al., 1990; Husum et al., 2001).

Preclinical studies have suggested that NK-1 antagonists may have anxiolytic effects (File, 1997) and that substance P agonists have anxiolgenic properties (Aguiar and Brandao, 1996). These findings have led to the development of potential antidepressants, such as MK-869, an NK-1 antagonist. MK-869 was shown to be as effective as paroxetine in treating depressive symptoms in a double-blind, placebo-controlled study (Kramer et al., 1998). Unfortunately, the further development of MK-869 as an antidepressant has been suspended because of side effects. At any rate, subsequent large clinical studies, which included an active SSRI comparator, showed no efficacy of an NK-1 antagonist in the treatment of depression.

Neuropeptide Y.   Neuropeptide Y (NPY) is a 36 amino-acid peptide synthesized in the arcuate nucleus of the hypothalamus and found in the raphe nucleus. It is stimulated by stress and corticosteroids. Preclinical studies have indicated that antidepressants, lithium, and ECT all increase the concentration of NPY (by immunoreactivity) (Stenfors et al., 1989; Wahlestedt et al., 1990) and mRNA expression (Weiner et al., 1992; Zachrisson et al., 1995) in many brain regions in rats. Further, reduced concentrations of NPY have been observed in the CSF (Widerlöv et al., 1988b) and plasma (Hashimoto et al., 1996; Nilsson et al., 1996) of patients with major depression. There have been some results conflicting with the hypothesis that NPY is downregulated in depression; for example, Berrettini and colleagues (1987) found no difference in CSF NPY immunoreactivity among diagnostic groups, and Irwin and colleagues (1991) actually found an increase in plasma NPY immunoreactivity in depressed patients. Widdowson and colleagues (1992) found reduced immunoreactivity of NPY in the prefrontal cortex and caudate nucleus of suicide victims, particularly in those with a diagnosis of major depression. Caberlotto and Hurd (1999) studied NPY mRNA levels in the prefrontal cortex of patients diagnosed with schizophrenia, bipolar disorder, and unipolar depression, as well as in normal controls. NPY mRNA levels were found to be reduced in bipolar patients only, with no correlation with suicide.

NPY acts through at least five distinct receptor subtypes, with the Y1 and Y2 subtypes being most abundant in the CNS. Preclinical studies in animal models of depression have indicated that the Y1 receptor mRNA is decreased in specific limbic and cortical regions, while the Y2 receptor mRNA appears to be unaltered. Caberlotto and Hurd (2001), however, found no alterations of the expression of either Y1 or Y2 mRNA levels in the prefrontal cortex in subjects with bipolar disorder, unipolar depression, or schizophrenia compared with matched controls. Thus, despite the conflicting findings on NPY levels in CSF, further exploration of NPY mRNA levels, receptor levels, and clinical effects is warranted.

Studies from the Mathe laboratory (Zachrisson et al., 1995; Husum et al., 2001) have demonstrated that lithium, electroconvulsive treatments (ECT in humans and electroconvulsive shock in rodents), and antidepressants affect NPY in a specific temporal manner and in specific brain regions. More recently, the same laboratory investigated brain NPY-like immunoreactivity (NPY-LI) under basal conditions and following a series of electroconvulsive shocks in both male and female Flinders Sensitive Line (FSL) rats, an animal model of depression, and their controls, Flinders Resistant Line (FRL) rats (Jimenez-Vasquez et al., 2000). Hippocampal NPY-LI in both sexes was significantly lower in the "depressed" FSL rats than in the control FRL rats. Electroconvulsive shock increased NPY-LI in both male and female rats of both strains in hippocampus, frontal cortex, and occipital cortex. In the hypothalamus, the increase was found only in the FSL rats. In both FSL and control rats, basal NPY-LI was lower in the hippocampus of female rats than in male rats. Overall, although the data are limited, NPY remains a neuropeptide with potential involvement in the pathophysiology and treatment of manic-depressive illness, and warrants additional study.

Cholecystokinin. The peptide cholecystokinin (CCK) is of interest in affective illness primarily as a potential mediator of appetite disturbance, since it can produce anorexia in various animals. Moreover, in light of the previously reviewed evidence that DA may be involved in bipolar disorder (and perhaps also in recurrent depression), it is of interest that CCK has been found to coexist with DA in individual neurons.

Some but not all clinical trials of CCK or its analogs in psychotic patients suggest that these peptides can alter psychotic symptomatology. Gemer and Yamada (1982) and Gjerris and colleagues (1984) found no significant differences among normal volunteers and depressed or manic patients in CSF levels of CCK. In contrast, Verbanck and colleagues (1984) reported a significant decrease in CCK in the CSF of patients with bipolar depressive illness compared with controls. In examining the range of values in their control group, however, it appears that the bipolar patients were well within the normal range, although they lacked the relatively greater high tail of values observed in the normal volunteers. Zachrisson and colleagues (1996) showed that both chronic lithium and electroconvulsive shock inhibit CCK synthesis in the caudate-putamen.

Neurotensin. Neurotensin has complex interactions with mesolimbic dopaminergic systems and displays neuroleptic-like properties in some animals, making it an interesting peptide for study in affective illness. Indeed, clinical studies in schizophrenia have shown low levels of CSF neurotensin concentration, effects that were normalized by effective antipsychotic drug treatment. Furthermore, the behavioral and biochemical effects of centrally administered neurotensin resemble remarkably those of systemically administered antipsychotic drugs, and antipsychotic drugs increase neurotensin neurotransmission (Binder et al., 2001). In cultured cells (with a catecholamines phenotype), lithium has been demonstrated to dramatically potentiate increases in intracellular levels of neurotensin and

the mRNA encoding it, caused by combinations of nerve growth factor, dexamethasone, and the adenylate cyclase activator forskolin (Dobner et al., 1988). To date, the few clinical studies of neurotensin in CSF in bipolar disorder have indicated no abnormalities (Berrettini et al., 1983). Furthermore, Austin and colleagues (2000) found no association between three sequence variants of the proneurotensin gene and bipolar disorder.

Vasoactive Intestinal Polypeptide. Vasoactive intestinal polypeptide (VIP), a peptide with very high concentrations in the cerebral cortex, is thought to have important interactions with muscarinic–cholinergic receptors (Hedlund et al., 1983). VIP is also of interest because it is an agonist in the release of ACTH cortisol secretion. In two separate studies, Gjerris and colleagues (1981, 1984) found that VIP levels in the CSF of patients with endogenous depression or mania did not differ from those of controls. However, they found decreased levels in patients with nonendogenous atypical depression characterized by dysphoric hysterical features, reversed diurnal variation, and lack of clearly circumscribed past depressive episodes. Berrettini and Post (1984) reported no difference in VIP levels between euthymic bipolar patients and controls.

Oxytocin. Oxytocin is similar to vasopressin in its structure, anatomical distribution, and wide-ranging effects in the CNS. Secretion of these peptides into CSF has been demonstrated to be independent of their secretion into plasma (Perlow et al., 1982; Kalin et al., 1985). Thus, CSF measures may provide a window into the brain that cannot be obtained by peripheral sampling.

Demitrack and Gold (1988) measured oxytocin in the CSF of patients with affective illness and normal volunteers, with findings roughly comparable to those for vasopressin: manic patients had lower levels of oxytocin than depressed patients. If this interesting finding is replicated, it may be relevant to the opposite effects of oxytocin and vasopressin on learning and memory in animals; that is, oxytocin produces effects resembling amesia (Bohus et al., 1978). More recently, Purba and colleagues (1996) found elevated numbers of oxytocin immunoreactive neurons in the paraventricular nucleus of the hypothalamus in eight patients with either unipolar or bipolar depression compared with controls.

Calcitonin. Animal studies indicate that calcitonin is involved in regulating a variety of functions, including motor activity, appetite, and pain. It is for this reason, as well as its effects on calcium metabolism, that calcitonin is an interesting candidate for study in affective disorders.

Carman and colleagues (1984) observed significantly lower levels of immunoreactive calcitonin in the CSF of

Figure 14–10. Signal transduction pathways provide good explanatory power for understanding the complex neurobiology of manic-depressive illness. CRF = corticotropin-releasing factor; FDG = fluorodeoxyglucose; GH = growth hormone; rCBF = regional cerebral blood flow; SST = serum sialyl transferase; TRH = thyrotropin-releasing hormone.

manic versus bipolar depressed or euthymic patients or normal controls. Carmen's group followed up its preliminary CSF investigations with a double-blind clinical trial of calcitonin in mania and observed a significant and substantial reduction in hyperactivity in 85 percent of the manic patients. A later study found that calcitonin gene-related peptide immunoreactivity (CGRP-LI) concentrations in CSF were increased in depressed patients compared with schizophrenic and control subjects (Mathe et al., 1994).

Most recently, Buervenich and colleagues (2001) investigated the frequency of four novel polymorphisms in the calcitonin/CGRPα (CALCA) gene in a number of neuropsychiatric disorders. They found that a 16–base pair microdeletion polymorphism was present in a family with multiple cases of unipolar or bipolar depressive disorder. Furthermore, using this polymorphism as a marker, cosegregation with the phenotype was observed in the majority of individuals. These intriguing findings await independent replication.

Neurotransmitter and Neuropeptide Systems in Manic-Depressive Illness: Summary

Overall, there is a growing appreciation that while abnormalities in these multiple neurotransmitter and neuropeptide systems are involved in mood disorders,[52] they likely represent the downstream effects of other, more primary

abnormalities.[53] Signal transduction pathways are in a pivotal position in the CNS, able to affect the functional balance among multiple neurotransmitter systems, and have therefore been postulated to play a role in mediating the more-downstream abnormalities in multiple neurotransmitter systems and physiological processes (Manji et al., 2000a; Warsh et al., 2000; Bezchlibnyk and Young, 2002). (Figure 14–10 illustrates the pivotal position of signal transduction pathways.) Moreover, as we discuss in greater detail below, signaling pathways are clearly targets for our most effective pharmacological treatments for recurrent mood disorders.

SIGNALING NETWORKS: THE CELLULAR MACHINERY

Multicomponent, cellular signaling pathways interact at various levels, thereby forming complex signaling networks that allow cells to receive, process, and respond to information (Bourne and Nicoll, 1993; Bhalla and Iyengar, 1999) (see Fig. 14–11). These networks facilitate the integration of signals across multiple time scales and the generation of distinct outputs, depending on input strength and duration, and regulate intricate feedforward and feedback loops (Weng et al., 1999). These properties of signaling networks suggest that they play critical roles in cellular memory; thus, cells with different histories, and therefore expressing a different repertoire of signaling molecules and interacting at different levels, may respond quite differently to the same signal over time. Given their widespread and crucial role in the integration, regulation, amplification, and fine-tuning of physiological processes, it is not surprising that abnormalities in signaling pathways have now been identified in a variety of human diseases (Milligan and Wakelam, 1992; Weintraub, 1995; Spiegel, 1998). Pertinent for the present discussion is the observation that a variety of diseases manifest relatively circumscribed symptomatology despite the widespread, often ubiquitous expression of the affected signaling proteins.

Complex signaling networks are likely present in all eukaryotic cells and control various metabolic, humoral,

Figure 14–11. Four major signaling pathways in the postsynaptic region of a neuron that combine to form a local signaling network. The major linear routes of signal flow are depicted by the thick arrows of four different colors: light grey (phospholipase C [PLC]) pathway), light blue (Ras pathway), dark grey (adenylyl cyclase pathway), and dark blue (Ca²⁺/calmodulin [CaM] pathway). The interactions between different pathways are represented by black lines with arrows (representing activation) or dots (representing inhibition). Although most major interactions in the network are shown, these connections are not meant to be all-inclusive; additional connections could exist. The three different shades of background represent three different cell compartments: the plasma membrane (top level), cytosol (middle level), and nucleus (bottom level). Some of the signaling proteins that translocate between different compartments are shown in both compartments. Examples include mitogen-activated protein kinase (MAPK), which when activated translocates from the cytoplasm to the nucleus to phosphorylate and activates transcription factors; and the transcription factor CREB, which upon phosphorylation by protein kinase A (PKA) translocates to the nucleus. AA = anachiclonic acid; AC = adenylate cyclase; AMPAR = AMPA-type glutamate receptor; βAR = beta-adrenergic receptor; BDNF = brain-derived neurotrophic factor; Ca = Calcium; CaM = calmodulin; CaMK = CaM kinase; cAMP = cyclic AMP; CaN = calcinerinn; CREB = cAMP-responsive element-binding protein; DAG = diacylglycerol; GEF/SOS = guanine nucleotide exchange factor/SOS; GLU = glutamate; IP₃ = inositol triphosphate; MEK = MAP kinase kinase; mGluR = metabotropic glutamase receptor; NE = norepinephrine; NMDA = NMDA-type glutamate receptor; PDE = phosphodiesterase; PKA = protein kinase A; PKC = protein kinase C; PLA₂ = phospholipase A₂; PLC-β = phospholipase C-beta; PPI = protein phosphatase-1; RTK = receptor tyrosine kinase. (Source: Weng et al., 1999. Reprinted with permission from AAAS.)

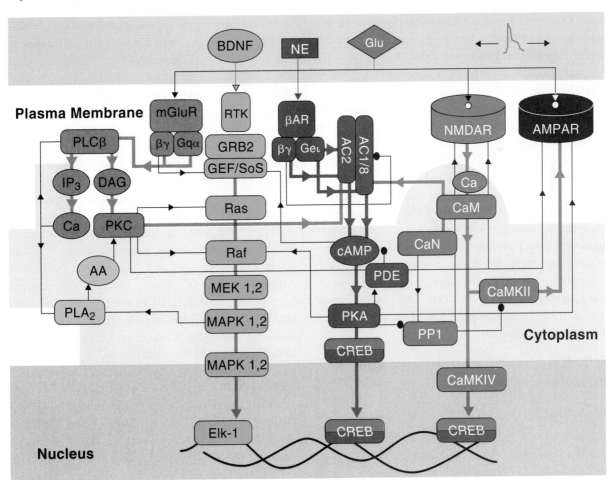

BOX 14–13.   Putative Roles for Signaling Pathways in Mood Disorders

- Amplify, attenuate, and integrate multiple signals, the basis of intracellular circuits and cellular modules
- Regulate multiple neurotransmitter and peptide systems, the basis of neuronal circuits and systems modules
- Critical role in cellular memory and long-term neuroplasticity
- Dynamic regulation of complex signaling networks form the basis for higher-order brain function, mood, and cognition
- Major targets for many hormones implicated in mood disorders, including gonadal steroids, thyroid hormones, and glucocorticoids
- Abnormalities are indeed compatible with life—many human diseases arise from defects in signaling pathways
- Brain regional dysregulation and circumscribed symptoms are possible despite the relatively ubiquitous expression of signaling proteins
- Signaling proteins have been identified as targets for medications that are most effective in treatment of mood disorders

and developmental functions. Yet they may be especially important in the CNS, where they serve the critical roles of first amplifying and "weighting" numerous extracellularly generated neuronal signals and then transmitting these integrated signals to effectors, thereby forming the basis for a complex information processing network (Manji, 1992; Bourne and Nicoll, 1993). The high degree of complexity generated by these signaling networks may be one mechanism by which neurons acquire the flexibility required for generating the wide range of responses observed in the nervous system. These pathways are thus undoubtedly involved in regulating such diverse vegetative functions as mood, appetite, and wakefulness, and are therefore likely to be involved in the pathophysiology of manic-depressive illness. We now turn to a discussion of the direct and indirect evidence supporting a role for abnormalities in signaling pathways in the pathophysiology and treatment of this illness with an emphasis on the bipolar subgroup. Box 14–13 summarizes findings to date on the putative roles of signaling pathways in mood disorders. Table 14–1 presents findings of studies examining the role of signaling abnormalities in bipolar disorder.

Evidence for the Involvement of the G_s/cAMP-Generating Signaling Pathway

G Proteins Regulating AC Activity

Several independent laboratories have examined G proteins in patients with mood disorders.[54] (Figure 14–12 shows the effects of G proteins on the AC system.) Young

and colleagues were the first to report increased levels of $G\alpha_s$ in bipolar patients in two separate studies (Young et al., 1993; Wang et al., 1997). Compared with controls matched for age, postmortem interval, and brain pH, increased levels of $G\alpha_s$ were found in frontal, temporal, and occipital cortex, but not in hippocampus, thalamus, or cerebellum, in postmortem brain tissue from patients with bipolar disorder. This group also found increases in forskolin (FSK)-stimulated AC activity in postmortem brain, compatible with a postreceptor abnormality in bipolar disorder. The findings of elevated $G\alpha_s$ levels and/or function are also supported by recent work of Wang and Friedman (1996), who noted increased agonist-activated [^{35}S]GTPγS binding to G protein α subunits in frontal cortical membrane preparations from postmortem brain of bipolar patients. Garcia-Sevilla and colleagues (1999) reported increased levels of $G\alpha_{i1/2}$ in prefrontal cortical samples obtained postmortem from depressed patients who committed suicide, effects that were apparently attenuated by antemortem antidepressant treatment. Overall, the findings in postmortem brain tissue in unipolar depression have been less consistent perhaps related to the heterogenity of unipolar patient samples with respect to recurrence (Warsh et al., 2000; Bezchlibnyk and Young, 2002).

In keeping with the G protein abnormalities in brain tissue obtained postmortem from bipolar patients, Schreiber and colleagues (1991) reported "hyperfunctional" G protein function in leukocytes of untreated manic patients, demonstrating that agonist-stimulated binding of [^{3}H]Gpp(NH)p (a stable, nonhydrolysable analog of guanosine triphosphate [GTP]) was enhanced in leukocyte membranes of untreated manic patients compared with controls. These findings suggest the presence of increased levels of G proteins and/or enhanced receptor-mediated activation of G proteins in leukocytes from untreated manic subjects.

Subsequent studies have found significantly higher levels of $G\alpha_s$ in mononuclear leukocytes from depressed bipolar but not unipolar patients (Young et al., 1994a). Manji and colleagues (1995b) quantitated the levels of the major G protein α subunits in leukocytes and platelets from both untreated (predominantly manic) and lithium-treated, euthymic bipolar patients. In both platelet and leukocyte membranes, there were higher levels of the 45 kilodalton form of $G\alpha_s$ in the overall group of bipolar patients (treated or untreated) than in the controls. A recent study found elevated levels of $G\alpha_s$ mRNA in granulocytes obtained from bipolar but not unipolar patients (Spleiss et al., 1998). This study also found nonsignificant elevations in the levels of $G\alpha_{is}$ in unmedicated bipolar patients, which intriguingly were modulated by lithium in bipolar (but not unipolar) patients (Spleiss et al.,

TABLE 14–1. Clinical Studies of Second Messenger System Abnormalities in Patients with Manic-Depressive Illness (Primarily Bipolar)

Intracellular Messengers	Tissue	Physiological Change	Study
G protein–coupled cyclic AMP system	Postmortem cerebral cortex	↑ $G\alpha_s$ and forskolin-stimulated cAMP production	Young et al. 1993
		No change in $G\alpha_s$ mRNA levels	Young and Woods, 1996
		↑Coupling of 5-HT receptors to membrane G proteins	Wang and Friedman, 1996
		↓[^{3}H]-cAMP binding	Rahman et al., 1997
		↑ cAMP-dependent PKA activity	Fields et al., 1999
		↓ $G\alpha_s$ levels in Li-treated subjects	Dowlatshahi et al., 1998
		↓ forskolin-stimulated AC activity	
		↓ CREB levels in anticonvulsant-treated subjects	
	Mononuclear leukocytes (MNLs)	↓ Isoproterenol-stimulated cAMP production in depressed subjects	Mann et al, 1985
		Mania: ↑ agonist-induced Gpp(NH)p binding, $G\alpha_s$ and $G\alpha_i$ levels	Halper et al., 1988
		Depression: ↓ agonist-induced Gpp(NH)p binding, $G\alpha_s$ and G_i levels	Schreiber et al., 1991
		↑ $G\alpha_s$ and $G\alpha_i$ levels in depressed subjects	Avissar et al., 1996
		↑ $G\alpha_s$ levels	Young et al., 1994b
		↓ $G\alpha_s$ levels in Li-treated patients; no change in haloperidol-treated subjects	Manji et al., 1995b
			Karege et al., 1999
			Mitchell et al., 1997
	Platelets and MNLs	↑ $G\alpha_s$ levels in platelets of euthymic BP-I and -II patients on medication; no change in MNLs	
	Platelets	↑ cAMP-dependent protein phosphorylation in euthymic BPD patients	Perez et al, 1995, 2000
		↑ Basal and cAMP-stimulated protein phosphorylation in Li-treated subjects	Zanardi et al., 1997
		↑ PKA catalytic subunit levels in manic and depressed vs. euthymic BPD patients and controls	Perez et al., 2000
		↑ Rap1 levels	
Phosphoinositide-generated second messenger system	Postmortem occipital cortex	↑ $G\alpha_{q/11}$ and phospholipase C-β immunoreactivity	Mathews et al., 1997
		↓ GTPγS and NaF-stimulated [^{3}H]PI hydrolysis	Jope et al., 1996
	Postmortem frontal cortex	↑ PKC activation	Wang and Friedman, 1996
	Platelets	↑ PMA and phorbol-ester-induced PKC translocation	Shimon et al., 1997
		↓ Inositol levels	Friedman et al., 1993
		↑ Basal, and membrane-bound vs. cytosolic PKC activity in manic vs. depressed and control	H. Wang et al., 1999
		↑ 5-HT-elicited PKC translocation	
		↓ PKC responsiveness to PMA/thrombin in depressed BPD patients	Brown et al., 1993
		↑ PIP_2 levels in manic subjects	Soares and Mallinger, 1997
		↑ PIP_2 levels in mania vs. untreated euthymia	Soares et al., 1997, 1999
		↓ PIP_2 after Li treatment vs. manic BPD patients	

AC=adenyl cyclase; BPD=bipolar disorder; BP-I=bipolar-I; Li=lithium; PI=phospoinositide; PIP$_2$=phosphatidylinositol biphosphate; PKA=protein kinase A; PKC=protein kinase C; PMA=phorbol 12-myristate 13-acetate.

Figure 14–12. The cAMP signaling pathway. Receptors can be both positively (e.g., β-adrenergic, D_1) or negatively (e.g., 5-HT_{1A}, D_2) coupled to adenylyl cyclase (AC) to regulate cAMP levels. The effects of cAMP are mediated largely by activation of protein kinase A (PKA). One major downstream target of PKA is CREB (cAMP-responsive element-binding protein). After activation, the phosphorylated CREB binds to the cAMP-responsive element (CRE), a gene sequence found in the promoter of certain genes. Recent data suggest that antidepressants may activate CREB, bringing about increased expression of a major target gene, BDNF. Phosphodiesterase is an enzyme that breaks down cAMP to AMP. Some antidepressant treatments have been found to upregulate phosphodiesterase. Drugs such as rolipram, which inhibit phosphodiesterase, may be useful as adjunct treatments for depression. Forskolin is an agent used in preclinical research to stimulate AC. (*Source*: Schatzberg and Nemeroff, 2004. Reprinted with permission from *The American Journal of Psychiatry.* Copyright 2004 by the American Psychiatric Association.)

1998). (See Table 14–2 for a list of findings from studies involving G protein signaling in bipolar disorder.) Similar to what has been observed in the CNS, one recent study evaluated the role of platelet G proteins as "signal coincidence detectors," and found this function to be impaired in depressed patients (Mooney et al., 1998).[55]

Another G protein subunit ($G\alpha_{olf}$) is located at a "linkage hotspot" on chromosome 18, identified by several groups (see Chapter 13). $G\alpha_{olf}$ is highly homologous to $G\alpha_s$ and is now known to be expressed in DA-rich areas of the brain, including caudate-putamen, nucleus accumbens, and olfactory tubercle (Herve et al., 1993). Using double in situ hybridization, Corvol and colleagues (2001) showed that virtually all striatal efferent neurons, identified by the expression of preproenkephalin A, substance P, or D1

receptor mRNA, contained high amounts of $G\alpha_{olf}$ mRNA and undetectable levels of $G\alpha_s$ mRNA. Interestingly, heterozygous $G\alpha_{olf}$ knockout mice, which have half the normal $G\alpha_{olf}$ levels, showed a markedly reduced locomotor response to psychostimulants (Corvol et al., 2001). As discussed earlier, there is unquestionable evidence for the involvement of the dopaminergic system in bipolar disorder, thus the possibility of an abnormality in a G protein coupled to D1 receptors and regulating behavioral responses to psychostimulants has generated considerable interest. To date, however, no mutations have been identified in the $G\alpha_{olf}$ gene, although studies are ongoing.

Overall, the most consistent finding to emerge is that in both peripheral cells and postmortem brain tissue from bipolar patients, elevations are observed in the predominant

Table 14–2. G Protein Signaling in Manic-Depressive Illness (Primarily Bipolar)

Tissue	Physiological Change	Study
Postmortem cerebral cortex	$\uparrow G\alpha_s$; $\leftrightarrow G\alpha_i$, $G\alpha_o$, and $G\alpha$ levels	Young et al., 1993
	$\leftrightarrow G\alpha_s$ mRNA levels	Young and Woods, 1996
	$\uparrow$ Coupling of 5-HT receptors to membrane G proteins	Friedman and Wang, 1996
	$\uparrow G\alpha_s$ levels	
	$\uparrow$ ADP-ribosylation of $G\alpha_i$ and $G\alpha_o$	
	$\uparrow G\alpha$ coprecipitation with $G\alpha$	
	$\downarrow G\alpha_s$ levels in Li-treated subjects	Dowlatshahi et al., 1998
Leukocytes and platelets	$\uparrow G\alpha_s$ and $G\alpha_i$ levels in depressed patients	Young et al., 1994b
	$\uparrow G\alpha_s$ levels in leukocytes of BPD patients	Manji et al., 1995b
	$\downarrow G\alpha_{q/11}$ and $\uparrow$ ADP ribosylation in platelets from Li-treated patients	
	$\downarrow$ Agonist-induced Gpp(NH)p binding in depression	Avissar et al., 1996
	$\downarrow G\alpha_s$ levels	Avissar et al., 1997
	$\downarrow$ Agonist-induced Gpp(NH)p binding, and $G\alpha_s$ and $G\alpha_i$ levels $\uparrow$ in mania and $\downarrow$ in depression	
	$\uparrow G\alpha_s$ levels in platelets of BP-I and -II patients, irrespective of treatment; $\leftrightarrow$ in MNLs	Mitchell et al., 1997
	$\uparrow G\alpha_s$ levels in depressed and Li-treated patients	Spleiss et al., 1998
	$\downarrow G\alpha_s$ levels in Li-treated patients	Karege et al., 1999
	$\leftrightarrow G\alpha_s$ levels in Li-treated BP-I patients	Alda et al., 2001

BPD = bipolar disorder; BP-I = bipolar-I; Li = lithium; MNLs = mononuclear leukocytes.
Source: Bezchlibnyk and Young, 2002.

subspecies of $G\alpha_s$ present in the tissues examined. Since $G\alpha_s$ is a ubiquitously expressed protein, it may appear counterintuitive that an abnormality in this protein may play a role in the pathophysiology of bipolar disorder. However, there is already a precedent for clinical disorders arising from abnormalities in the levels of $G\alpha_s$, which present with limited clinical manifestations despite the ubiquitous expression of the protein (Spiegel, 1998). These heterogeneous clinical effects and tissue-specific manifestations have been postulated to arise from differences in receptor, G protein, and effector stoichiometries in different tissues, as well as from tissue-specific differences in the ability of various cells to compensate for the abnormality.

It should be emphasized, however, that there is at present no evidence to suggest that the alterations in the levels of $G\alpha_s$ are due to a mutation in the $G\alpha_s$ gene itself (Ram et al., 1997). Indeed, there are numerous transcriptional and posttranscriptional mechanisms that regulate the levels of G protein α subunits, and the elevated levels of $G\alpha_s$ could potentially represent the sequelae of alterations in any one of these other biochemical pathways. Thus, at this point, considerable caution is required in interpreting the data, since they derive primarily from peripheral cell models and may not adequately reflect CNS pathology. The possibility of the presence of aberrant biochemical pathways that regulate $G\alpha_s$ levels in bipolar

disorder is currently undergoing further study (Warsh et al., 2000).

cAMP/Protein Kinase A Signaling

The most commonly used strategy has been to characterize receptor function in readily accessible blood elements, and much clinical research has focused on the activity of the cAMP-generating system in mood disorders. Overall, the preponderance of the evidence suggests altered receptor and/or postreceptor sensitivity of the cAMP-generating system in the absence of consistent alterations in the number of receptors themselves (Wang et al., 1997; Warsh et al., 2000).

Higher levels of cAMP-stimulated phosphorylation of a protein with a molecular weight of ~22 kilodaltons have been found in platelets obtained from 10 treated euthymic bipolar patients compared with controls; by contrast, no significant difference was found in basal phosphorylation between the groups (Perez et al., 2000). Follow-up studies identified the approximately 22 kilodalton protein as Rap1, and once again found higher cAMP-stimulated phosphorylation in the bipolar patients (Perez et al., 2000).

Warsh and colleagues have undertaken the most thorough series of studies investigating the cAMP/protein kinase A (PKA) system in postmortem human brain in bipolar disorder. They found that the levels of PKA regulatory subunits (as assessed by [3H]cAMP binding) were significantly lower in cytosolic fractions of frontal, temporal, occipital and parietal cortex, cerebellum, and thalamus of bipolar patients than in matched controls (Rahman et al., 1997). Furthermore, preliminary findings indicate that the reduction of regulatory subunits of PKA in the cytosolic fractions of temporal cortex of bipolar patients is accompanied by higher basal kinase activity in the cytosolic fractions of those patients' temporal cortex (Fields et al., 1999). These observed changes in PKA provide additional important evidence for dysregulation in the $G\alpha_s$-mediated cAMP cascade in bipolar disorder. (See Table 14–3 for findings related to cAMP signaling in bipolar disorder.)

Finally, as discussed in more detail in Chapter 13, genetic abnormalities in cAMP response element binding protein (CREB) and BDNF may also occur in depression. Sequence variations in the CREB1 gene have been reported to cosegregate with major depression in women. To our knowledge, similar studies have not yet been undertaken in bipolar disorder.

TABLE 14–3. **Cyclic AMP Signaling in Manic-Depressive Illness (Primarily Bipolar)**

Tissue	Physiological Change	Study
Postmortem cerebral cortex	↑ Forskolin-stimulated cAMP production	Young et al., 1993
	↓ [³H]-cAMP binding	Rahman et al., 1997
	↔ AC levels	Reiach et al., 1999
	↑ Maximal and basal cAMP-dependent PKA activity	Fields et al., 1999
	↓ PKA EC50 for cAMP	
	↓ Forskolin-stimulated AC	Dowlatshahi et al., 1998
	↓ CREB levels in anticonvulsant-treated subjects	
Leukocytes and platelets	↓ PGE1-stimulated cAMP in depressed MDD and BPD patients; ↓ NE	Siever et al., 1984
	Inhibition of PGE1-stimulated cAMP production ↓ Isoproterenol-stimulated cAMP production in depressed MDD and BPD patients	Mann et al., 1985
		Halper et al., 1988
	↓ Forskolin-stimulated AC activity subsequent to Li treatment	Ebstein et al., 1987
	↓ Basal and stimulated AC activity in Li-treated patients	Ebstein et al., 1988
	↑ Agonist-induced Gpp(NH)p binding in manic patients	Schreiber et al., 1991
	↑ cAMP-dependent protein phosphorylation in euthymic patients	Perez et al., 1995, 2000
	↑ Basal and cAMP-stimulated protein phosphorylation after Li treatment	Zanardi et al., 1997
	↑ Basal and NaF stimulated	Emamghoreishi et al., 2000
	↓ Isoproterenol-induced cAMP formation in subjects with high Ca^{2+} levels	
	↑ PKA catalytic subunit levels vs. untreated euthymic BPD patients and controls	Perez et al., 2000
	↔ PKA regulatory subunit levels	
	↑ Rap1 levels	

AC = adenyl cyclase; BPD = bipolar disorder; Li = lithium; MDD = major depressive disorder; PKA = protein kinase A.

Effects of Mood Stabilizers and Antidepressants on the G$_s$/cAMP-Generating Signaling Pathway

Lithium and G Proteins

Although it appears that lithium (at therapeutic concentrations) does not affect G proteins directly, considerable evidence indicates that chronic lithium administration affects G protein function indirectly.[56] Interestingly, for both G$_s$ (the G protein stimulating cAMP production) and G$_i$ (the G protein inhibiting cAMP production), lithium's major effects in both humans and rodents are most compatible with a stabilization of the heterotrimeric, undissociated, inactive alpha beta gamma ($\alpha\beta\gamma$) conformation of the G protein.[57] Lithium also exerts complex effects on the activity of AC, with the preponderance of the data demonstrating an elevation of basal AC activity but an attenuation of receptor-stimulated responses in both preclinical and clinical studies.[58] It has been postulated that these elevations of basal cAMP and dampening of receptor-mediated stimulated responses may play an important role in lithium's ability to prevent "excessive excursions from the norm" (Manji et al., 1995a; Jope, 1999). These complex effects likely represent the net effects of direct inhibition of AC, upregulation of certain AC subtypes, and effects on the stimulatory and inhibitory G proteins (Chen et al., 1996a; Li and El-Mallahk 2000; Manji and Lenox, 2000a).[59]

Consistent with this hypothesis, lithium has been shown to potentiate the hyperactivity induced by intra-accumbens cholera toxin administration (which activates the stimulatory G proteins, G$_s$ and G$_{olf}$) (Kofman et al., 1998). An investigation of the effects of lithium on the striatum revealed that 2 weeks (but not 1 week) of lithium increased the protein levels by about 50 percent (Miki et al., 2001). Furthermore, it was found that G$_{olf}$ returned to baseline levels 1 week after withdrawal of lithium. These investigators postulated that the increased G$_{olf}$ expression after chronic lithium represents a compensatory adaptation to the suppression of the AC system by lithium (see below) and may be responsible (at least in part) for the "rebound" increase in manic episodes observed after abrupt lithium discontinuation (see Chapter 19). These results suggest that direct inhibitors of AC (such as carbamazepine) may have utility in the prevention of lithium-discontinuation emergence of mania.

Overall, many of the long-term effects of chronic lithium on G proteins are likely attributable to an indirect post-translational modification of the G protein(s) and a relative change in the dynamic equilibrium of the active and inactive states of protein conformation. In this context, it is noteworthy that investigators have demonstrated that lithium alters the levels of endogenous ADP-ribosylation in C6 glioma cells (Young and Woods, 1996) and in rat brain (Nestler et al., 1995), suggesting another mechanism by which chronic lithium may indirectly regulate the activity of these critical signaling proteins.

Lithium and the AC System

As stated above, lithium has been demonstrated to exert complex effects on AC activity, with the preponderance of data demonstrating an elevation of basal AC activity along with attenuation of a variety of receptor-mediated responses (Manji et al., 1995b; Wang et al., 1997). Lithium in vitro inhibits the stimulation of AC by guanyl imidodiphosphate, or Gpp(NH)p (a poorly hydrolyzable analogue of GTP), and calcium-calmodulin, both of which can be overcome by Mg^{2+} (Andersen and Geisler, 1984; Newman and Belmaker, 1987; Mork and Geisler, 1989). Lithium also competes with both Mg^{2+} and Ca^{2+} for membrane-binding sites, and lithium's inhibition of solubilized catalytic units of AC can be overcome by Mg^{2+}. These findings suggest that lithium's inhibition of AC in vitro may be due to competition with Mg^{2+} on a site on the catalytic unit of AC (Andersen and Geisler, 1984; Newman and Belmaker, 1987). However, the inhibitory effects of chronic lithium treatment on rat brain AC are not reversed by Mg^{2+}, and these effects still persist after washing of the membranes but are reversed by increasing concentrations of GTP (Mork and Geisler, 1989). These results suggest that the physiologically relevant effects of lithium (i.e., those seen on chronic drug administration and not reversed immediately with drug discontinuation) may be exerted at the level of signal-transducing G proteins at a GTP-responsive step (discussed below).[60]

More recently, lithium's effects on the phosphorylation and activity of CREB have been examined in rodent brain and in cultured human neuroblastoma cells, with somewhat conflicting results (Ozaki and Chuang, 1997; Wang et al., 1999b). As we discuss later, however, CREB is now known to be phosphorylated and regulated by the MAPK signaling cascade, which is also a target for lithium's actions (see below). Thus lithium's effects on CREB levels and phosphorylation may be temporally and spatially specific, and reflect the relative contributions of these two major signaling pathways in different tissues.

A series of studies have also examined lithium's effects on AC in humans. In a longitudinal study of healthy volunteers, 2 weeks of lithium administration was found to significantly increase platelet basal and postreceptor-stimulated AC activity (Risby et al., 1991), effects strikingly similar to those observed in rodent brain. Consistent with a lithium-induced increase in basal cAMP and AC levels, a subsequent study found that platelets obtained from lithium-treated euthymic bipolar patients showed an enhanced basal and cAMP-stimulated phosphorylation into Rap1 (a PKA substrate) as well as into a 38 kilodalton phosphoprotein (Perez et al., 2000). Interestingly, these investigators did not find similar effects of lithium in healthy subjects, raising the possibility of a perturbed phosphorylation/dephosphorylation homeostatic mechanism in bipolar disorder.

Carbamazepine and the AC System

In contrast to the effects observed with lithium, carbamazepine has very modest effects on G proteins (H. Manji, unpublished observations). It has, however, been demonstrated to have many effects on the cAMP signaling pathway, which plays a major role in the regulation of neuronal excitability and has been postulated to play a role in the pathophysiology of both seizure disorders (Kuriyama and Kakita, 1980; Ludvig and Moshe, 1989) and bipolar disorder. It is thus noteworthy that carbamazepine decreases the basal concentrations of cAMP in mouse cerebral cortex and cerebellum, and reduces cAMP production induced by NE (Palmer, 1979), adenosine (Palmer, 1979; Van Calker et al., 1991), and the epileptogenic compounds ouabain and veratridine in brain slices (Lewin and Bleck, 1977; Ferrendelli and Kinscherf, 1979). In manic patients, carbamazepine was found to decrease elevated CSF levels of cAMP (Post et al., 1982). Recent studies have also demonstrated that carbamazepine inhibits FSK-induced c-fos gene expression in cultured pheochromocytoma (PC-12) cells (Divish et al., 1991). Thus overall, considerable evidence indicates that carbamazepine inhibits cAMP formation.

More recent studies have investigated the possible mechanisms by which carbamazepine inhibits the cAMP-generating system. It was found that carbamazepine, at therapeutically relevant concentrations, inhibited both basal AC and FSK-stimulated cAMP accumulation in C6 glioma cells (Chen et al., 1996b). Within the clinical therapeutic range (~50 μM), carbamazepine inhibited basal cAMP levels by 10–20 percent and FSK-stimulated cAMP production by 40–60 percent. Taken together, these data indicate that carbamazepine is more effective in inhibiting the activated AC system, although the possibility of "floor effects" (that is, an inability to lower basal cAMP levels beyond certain levels in this system) cannot be ruled out. To further characterize the site at which carbamazepine exerts its inhibitory effects, ACs were purified from rat cerebral cortex with an FSK affinity purification column. It was found that, similar to the situation observed in intact C6 cells and in C6 cell membranes, carbamazepine inhibited both basal and FSK-stimulated activity of purified AC (Chen et al., 1996b).

Taken together, the data suggest that carbamazepine inhibits cAMP production by acting directly on AC and/or through factor(s) that are closely associated with and copurify with AC. Consistent with these results, it has been demonstrated that carbamazepine attenuates FSK-induced expression of c-fos (an immediate early gene) in PC-12 cells and inhibits FSK-induced phosphorylation of CREB in C6 glioma cells. Since c-fos and CREB are known to be involved in mediating a number of long-term neuronal responses, these effects might be postulated to play a role in the delayed therapeutic effect of carbamazepine.

Valproate and the G$_s$/AC System

Recent studies have examined the effects of valproate on components of the β-adrenergic receptor–coupled cAMP-generating system (Chen et al., 1996b). Chronic valproate has been shown to produce a significant alteration of the β-adrenergic receptor–coupled cAMP-generating system in cultured cells in vitro; these effects were observed at concentrations of valproate similar to those attained in plasma in the clinical treatment of neuropsychiatric disorders. In contrast to what has been observed with chronic lithium treatment (discussed above), it was found that chronic valproate produced a significant reduction in the density of β-adrenergic receptors. Interestingly, the decrease in number of β-adrenergic receptors (approximately 30 percent) was accompanied by an even greater decrease in receptor- and postreceptor-mediated cAMP accumulation, suggesting that chronic valproate also exerts effects at the β-adrenergic receptor/G$_s$ interaction, or at postreceptor sites (e.g., G$_s$, AC). Consistent with this contention, it was indeed found that chronic but not acute valproate incubation induced a marked decrease in the levels of Gα_s 45 but not any other G protein α subunits examined (Gα_s 52, Gα_{i1-2}, Gα_o, or G$\alpha_{q/11}$). In view of the suggested involvement of G$_s$ in the pathophysiology of bipolar disorder (discussed above), as well as the effects of lithium on the β-adrenergic receptor/G$_s$/AC system, these effects may play a role in valproate's therapeutic effects and are worthy of further study.

Antidepressants and the G$_s$/AC System

The cAMP signaling cascade appears to be a major target for the action of chronic antidepressant treatments. Recent studies have demonstrated an enhanced coupling between Gα_s and the catalytic unit of AC (Rasenick et al., 2000) and activation of cAMP-dependent protein kinase enzyme activity (Nestler et al., 1989; Popoli et al., 2000). Antidepressants have also been demonstrated to activate cAMP-dependent and calcium/calmodulin-dependent protein kinases, effects that are accompanied by increases in the endogenous phosphorylation of selected substrates (microtubule-associated protein 2 and synaptotagmin) (Popoli et al., 2000).

Duman and colleagues (1997, 2000) have undertaken an elegant series of studies demonstrating that the chronic treatment of rats with a variety of antidepressants increases the levels of CREB mRNA, CREB protein, and CRE (cyclic AMP response element) DNA binding activity in hippocampus. Furthermore, the same group has demonstrated that chronic antidepressant treatment increases the expression of two important genes known to be regulated by CREB—BDNF and its receptor TrkB (Duman et al., 1997, 2000). Preliminary postmortem human brain studies have also indicated increased levels of CREB and hippocampal BDNF (B. Chen et al., 2001) in patients treated with antidepressants, providing indirect support for the rodent and cell culture studies (Dowlatshahi et al., 1998).

Interestingly, recent studies have shown that short-term sleep deprivation brings about changes in pCREB and BDNF similar to those seen with chronic antidepressants. This finding raises the intriguing possibility that antidepressant- or sleep deprivation–induced activation of these plasticity cascades may play a role not only in the antidepressant effect but also in the mania-inducing effect of these modalities. This possibility is discussed in greater detail later.

The Phosphoinositide Signaling Cascade

The impetus for the study of this major second messenger system in bipolar disorder was the seminal observation by Allison and Stewart (1971) that lithium reduces brain levels of inositol. Subsequently, Hallcher and Sherman (1980) showed that this reduction was due to inhibition of the enzyme inositol monophosphatase, an effect that occurred at therapeutically relevant concentrations (the enzyme was inhibited by 50 percent at a lithium concentration of ~.8 mM). Because the mode of lithium's inhibition is uncompetitive (that is, the more active the system, the greater the inhibition), Berridge and colleagues (1982, 1989) suggested that lithium selectively inhibits PI-derived second messengers of systems that are "overly activated" in mania without interfering with basal function. Furthermore, since inositol depletion is presumed to occur more readily in the CNS than in the periphery, Berridge's inositol depletion hypothesis of lithium action has gained considerable attention.

Although inositol phospholipids are relatively minor components of cell membranes, they play a major role in receptor-mediated signal transduction pathways and are involved in a diverse range of responses in the CNS (Berridge and Irvine, 1989; Chuang, 1989; Fisher et al., 1992). Furthermore, several subtypes of adrenergic, cholinergic, and serotonergic receptors are coupled to phosphatidylinositol-4,5-bisphosphate (PIP_2) hydrolysis in the brain, resulting in the production of two very important second messengers— IP3 (which mobilizes calcium) and diacylglycerol (which activates PKC). Thus, the inositol depletion hypothesis offers a very attractive explanation for lithium's therapeutic efficacy in treating multiple aspects of bipolar disorder and highly recurrent depressive disorders.

As we discuss in greater detail below, it is indeed quite likely that some of lithium's effects do indeed stem from inhibition of inositol monophosphatase, and this initiates a cascade of signaling and gene expression changes that ultimately produce many of the drug's therapeutic effects. Does lithium, in fact, correct an underlying abnormality in the PI signaling pathway in recurrent mood disorders? The data relevant to this question must be considered preliminary; nevertheless, converging data from peripheral cell studies and postmortem brain studies suggest that the PI/PKC signaling system may play a role in the pathophysiology of cyclic mood disorders, perhaps especially bipolar disorder. (See Table 14–4 for study findings related to PI signaling.)

One study measured membrane phospholipids in platelets of seven medication-free patients in the manic phase of bipolar disorder and seven healthy controls. It was found that the relative percentage of platelet membrane PIP_2 was significantly higher in the manic patients than in the controls (Brown, 1993). In a more recent study of nine medication-free bipolar depressed patients, the same group showed that these patients had significantly increased levels of platelet membrane PIP_2 compared with levels in controls (Soares et al., 2001). Studies have also investigated inositol monophosphatase (IMPase) mRNA levels in lymphocytes. It was found that a small group of medication-free bipolar patients exhibited a reduction in IMPase mRNA levels, whereas mood stabilizer–treated patients had normalized values (Nemanov et al., 1999).

Investigators have also attempted to determine whether there are any abnormalities in the PI signaling system in postmortem brain in bipolar disorder. In a postmortem study by Shimon and colleagues (1997), free inositol levels were found to be lower in prefrontal cortex from bipolar patients than in controls. Another postmortem study found increased $G\alpha_{q/11}$ immunoreactivity in postmortem occipital cortex from patients with bipolar disorder (Mathews et al., 1997). However, these elevated levels of $G\alpha_{q/11}$ were accompanied by reduced agonist-induced PI turnover (Jope et al., 1996), although the potential effects of long-term lithium treatment remained to be fully delineated. A number of studies have also investigated the mediators of PI signaling—Ca^{2+} and PKC.

Protein Kinase C in the Pathophysiology of Recurrent Mood Disorders

Protein Kinase C Signaling in Animal Models of Mood Disorders

As discussed earlier, two current models of mania that have been used and have reasonable heuristic value in the study of mood disorders are kindling and behavioral sensitization

TABLE 14–4. Phosphoinositide Signaling in Manic-Depressive Illness (Primarily Bipolar)

Tissue	Physiological Change	Study
Postmortem cerebral cortex	↑ $G\alpha_{q/11}$ and PLC-β immunoreactivity; ↔ Gβ	Matthews et al., 1997
	↓ GTPγS and NaF-stimulated [^{3}H]PI hydrolysis in BPD vs. Li-treated and controls	Jope et al., 1996
	↔ Ca^{2+}-stimulated PLC activity	
	↑ PKC activation	
	↑ PMA and phorbol ester–induced PKC translocation	Wang and Friedman, 1996
	↑ Cytosolic α and membrane–associated γ- and ε-PKC isozyme levels	
	↓ Cytosolic ε-PKC levels	
	↔ IMPase activity in depressed patient samples	Atack, 1996
	↓ Inositol levels in frontal cortex; ↔ IMPase activity	Shimon et al., 1997
Platelets	↓ PLC activity in Li-treated euthymic patients	Ebstein et al., 1988
	↑ Membrane-bound vs. cytosolic PKC activity	Friedman et al., 1993
	↑ 5-HT elicited PKC translocation	
	↓ Basal and 5-HT-elicited PKC activity following 2 weeks of Li treatment	
	↑ PIP_2 levels in manic patients	Brown et al., 1993
	↑ PIP_2 levels manic vs. untreated euthymic patients	Soares and Mallinger, 1997
	↓ Li-treated vs. manic; ↔ between Li-treated vs. untreated euthymic patients	Soares et al., 1997
	↓ PIP_2 in Li-treated euthymic patients; ↔ in other phospholipids	Soares et al., 1999
	↑ Basal PKC activity in mania	H. Wang et al., 1999
	↓ PKC responsiveness to PMA/thrombin in depression	
	↑ PKC responsiveness to 5-HT	
	↔ PMA-induced translocation	
	↔ PKC-α levels	Young et al., 1999
	↓ PIP_2 following Li treatment; ↔ in other phospholipids	Soares et al., 2000a
	↓ PIP_2 in Li-treated patients	Soares et al., 2000b
	↓ Cytosolic PKC-α levels	
	No correlation between PLC and PIP_2 measures	
	↑ Membrane PIP_2 levels in depressed patients; ↔ in other phospholipids	Soares et al., 2001
Erythrocytes	↓ Inositol 1-phosphatase activity in Li-treated patients	Moscovich et al., 1990

BPD = bipolar disorder; Li = lithium; PIP_2 = phosphatidylinositol biphosphate; PKC = protein kinase C; PLC = phospholipase C.

Source: Bezchlibnyk and Young, 2002.

BOX **14–14.** Protein Kinase C and the Pathophysiology of Manic-Depressive Illness (Primarily Bipolar)

- Amphetamine produces increases in protein kinase C (PKC) activity, and GAP-43 phosphorylation (implicated in neurotransmitter release)
- PKC inhibitors block biochemical and behavioral responses to amphetamine and cocaine and also block cocaine-induced sensitization
- Increased membrane/cytosol PKC partitioning in platelets from manic subjects; normalized with lithium treatment
- Increased PKC activity and translocation in bipolar disorder patients' brains compared to controls
- Increased levels of RACK-1 (receptor for activated C kinase) in bipolar patients' brains compared to controls
- Lithium and valproate regulate PKC activity, PKC α, PKC ε, and myristoylated alanine-rich C kinase substrate (MARCKS)
- Preliminary data suggest that PKC inhibitors may have efficacy in treatment of acute mania

Source: Manji and Lenox, 1999.

(Lyon, 1991; Post and Weiss, 1992). Considerable evidence implicates long-term alterations in midbrain dopaminergic transmission in the development of behavioral sensitization, but the cellular mechanism(s) underlying the long-term changes in excitability observed in kindled or stimulant-sensitized animals have not been fully elucidated. A growing body of evidence implicates alterations in both PKC and certain G proteins (especially G_i and G_o).[61] In particular, dramatic increases in membrane-associated PKC have been observed in the bilateral hippocampus at up to 4 weeks and in the amygdala/pyriform cortex at 4 weeks after the last kindled seizure (Daigen et al., 1991).

Studies have also implicated alterations in PKC activity as mediators of long-term alterations in neuronal excitability in the brain following chronic stimulant use. Several independent laboratories have now demonstrated that both acute and chronic amphetamine exposure produces an alteration in PKC activity and its relative cytosol-to-membrane distribution, as well as the phosphorylation of a major PKC substrate, GAP-43, which has been implicated in long-term alterations of neurotransmitter release (Giambalvo, 1992a,b; Gnegy et al., 1993; Iwata et al., 1997a,b). (See Box 14–14 for a summary of research findings related to PKC activity.) In a few studies, pharmacological inhibition of PKC results in behavioral changes similar to mood stabilizers. Direct injection of the specific PKC inhibitor RO31-8220 into the nucleus accumbens inhibited amphetamine hyperactivity (Browman et al., 1998). Inhibition of PKC in the ventral tegmental area (VTA) with the PKC inhibitor H7 reduced cocaine hyperactivity (Steketee, 1994)

and a similar injection to A10 area (where the VTA is located) disrupted cocaine sensitization (Steketee, 1994).

Increased hedonistic drive and increased tendency to abuse drugs are well known facets of manic behavior. Two models of such behaviors are consumption of reward and conditioned place preference (CPP) (Papp et al., 1991). PKC inhibition with H7 in the A10 area blocked the development of cocaine CPP (Steketee, 1994), ICV injections of the PKC inhibitor calphostine blocked morphine CPP (Narita et al., 2001), and intra-accumbens injections of the PKC inhibitor NPC-15437 blocked amphetamine CPP (Aujla and Beninger, 2003). Furthermore, PKC inhibition in the accumbens inhibited the development of morphine dependence, a measure that may be related to increased drug craving (Valverde et al., 1996).

PKC-related targeted mutations also support the involvement of PKC in affective-like behaviors. PKC γ knockout (KO) mice show reduced morphine-induced CPP (Narita et al., 2001) and PKC ε KO mice demonstrate reduced ethanol self-administration (Olive et al., 2000).

Indeed, abundant evidence has now accumulated to show that activation of PKC enhances both depolarization-mediated and basal release of DA (Robinson, 1991; Cowell and Garrod 1999), a neurotransmitter implicated in the manic syndrome (as discussed above). Release of DA by PKC activation has been demonstrated in a variety of tissues, including striatal synaptosomes, effects that have been demonstrated to be independent of extracellular calcium. The ability of amphetamine to produce heightened locomotor activity is thought to be due to its ability to enhance DA release from mesolimbic DA neurons. Furthermore, PKC inhibitors have been demonstrated to markedly reduce amphetamine-induced DA release (Giambalvo, 1992a,b). It is now believed that in addition to blocking the reuptake of NE and DA, psychostimulants facilitate the release of these neurotransmitters in large part by activation of PKC (Giambalvo, 1992a,b; Gnegy et al., 1993; Iwata et al., 1997a,b). Finally, recent nonhuman primate studies investigating cognitive deficits similar to those observed in mania have also demonstrated the efficacy of a selective PKC inhibitor. Birnbaum and associates (2004) have demonstrated that excessive activation of PKC dramatically impaired the cognitive functions of the prefrontal cortex, exposure to stress activated PKC and resulted in prefrontal dysfunction, and inhibition of PKC (including indirectly with mood stabilizers) protected cognitive function. These data suggest that PKC may play an important role in some of the cognitive features of mania.

As noted earlier, abnormalities of circulating glucocorticoids are well known to be associated with affective symptomatology (Banki et al., 1987), and interestingly, elevated glucocorticoids have been associated with both depressive and manic symptomatology (Haskett, 1985; Banki et al., 1987; Ur et al., 1992). It is noteworthy that a recent study found the repeated administration of dexamethasone for 10 days caused a significant increase in B_{max} of phorbol dibutyrate ([^{3}H]PDBu) binding to PKC, increased PKC activity, and increased levels of PKC α and ϵ in rat and hippocampus (Dwivedi and Pandey, 1999).

It is indeed striking that behavioral sensitization and kindling (which have been postulated as models for bipolar disorder and mania), as well as dexamethasone administration, produce robust alterations in the PKC signaling pathway in critical limbic structures, given that lithium and valproate aim for these same biochemical targets. Although considerable caution obviously must be employed when extrapolating results from rodent brain, the fact that these two models and glucocorticoid administration are associated with effects on PKC signaling opposite to those observed with chronic lithium or valproate is compelling indeed. Interestingly, there is also evidence suggesting that chronic antidepressants may modulate PKC activity in limbic and limbic-associated areas of rat brain (Nalepa, 1993, 1994). Moreover, PKC was recently demonstrated to regulate the activity of NE, DA, and serotonin transporters (Apparsundaram et al., 1998; Blakely et al., 1998; Zhang et al., 1998). Whether these complex effects of antidepressants on PKC activity underlie their apparent ability to trigger manic episodes and perhaps promote rapid cycling in susceptible individuals (Goodwin and Jamison, 1990) remains to be determined.

Human Studies Implicating Protein Kinase C in the Pathophysiology of Recurrent Mood Disorders

To date, only a limited number of studies have directly examined PKC in bipolar disorder (Hahn and Friedman, 1999). Although undoubtedly an oversimplification, particulate (membrane) PKC is sometimes viewed as the more active form of PKC; thus an examination of the subcellular partitioning of this enzyme can be used as an index of the degree of activation. Friedman and colleagues (1993) investigated PKC activity and translocation in response to serotonin in platelets obtained from bipolar subjects before and during lithium treatment. They found that ratios of platelet membrane-bound to cytosolic PKC activities were elevated in the manic subjects compared with the euthymic, lithium-treated bipolar patients. In addition, serotonin-elicited platelet PKC translocation was enhanced in those subjects.

In postmortem brain tissue from bipolar patients, Wang and Friedman (1996) measured PKC isozyme levels, activity, and translocation. They found increased PKC activity and translocation in the brains of the bipolar patients compared with controls, effects accompanied by elevated levels of selected PKC isozymes in the cortex of the bipolar subjects.

More recently, the same group found that postmortem brains of bipolar subjects showed increased association with receptor for activated C kinase 1 (RACK1) (Wang and Friedman, 2001). Since PKC is anchored to the membrane by RACK1, these results suggest that increased association of RACK1 with PKC isozymes may be responsible for the increases in membrane PKC and its activation previously observed in frontal cortex of brains of bipolar patients.

In comparison with the studies in bipolar disorder discussed above, two recent studies used [^{3}H]PDBu, a radioligand that binds to PKC, to investigate particulate and cytosolic PKC in postmortem brain samples obtained from depressed patients and/or individuals who had committed suicide. Pandey and colleagues (1997) found that the B_{max} of [^{3}H]PDBu binding sites was significantly decreased in both membrane and cytosolic fractions from Brodmann's areas 8 and 9 in teenage suicide subjects compared with matched controls; no unipolar–bipolar distinctions were made and there was no quantification of recurrence among the unipolar patients. Coull and colleagues (2000) found increased [^{3}H]PDBu binding in the soluble fraction (suggesting less in the active membrane fraction) in antidepressant-free suicides compared with controls in frontal cortex. The results of these two studies could potentially be interpreted as reflecting reduced PKC function, due either to a reduction in the absolute levels or a reduction in the particulate/soluble fractions. Considerable additional research is required, however, to adequately justify such a conclusion.

Abnormalities of Calcium Signaling in Bipolar Disorder

Acting through intracellular proteins such as myristoylated alanine-rich C kinase substrate (MARCKS) and calmodulin and enzymes such as PKC, AC, and CaM kinase, calcium ions have been shown to regulate the synthesis and release of neurotransmitters, neuronal excitability, cytoskeletal remodeling, and long-term neuroplastic events. Thus it is not surprising that a large number of studies have investigated intracellular Ca^{2+} in peripheral cells in bipolar disorder (Dubovsky et al., 1992b; Emamghoreishi et al., 1997; Wang et al., 1997; see Tables 14–5, 14–6, and 14–7). In view of the caveats associated with studies of peripheral circulating cells, the remarkable consistency of the findings of this research is surprising indeed. Studies have consistently shown elevations in both resting and stimulated levels of intracellular Ca^{2+} in platelets, lymphocytes, and neutrophils of patients with bipolar disorder. These calcium abnormalities have been postulated to represent state-dependent findings (Dubovsky et al., 1992b), but recent studies using transformed lymphoblasts from bipolar patients have revealed similar abnormalities, suggesting that they may be trait-dependent (Emamghoreishi et al., 1997).

TABLE 14–5. **Intracellular Calcium in Blood Elements of Manic-Depressive Illness (Primarily Bipolar): Platelets**

Study	Stimulation	Intracellular Ca level	Treatment Status
Bowden et al., 1988	Basal	BPd (14) > UPd (29)	Untreated[a]
		Note that BPd = C (10) and UP = BPm (11)	
Dubovsky et al., 1989	Basal	BPm (15) > C (15)	Untreated and recovered
	PAF/thrombin	BPm, BPd (15) > BPe (13), UP (13), C	
Tan et al., 1990	Basal	BPe (6) > C (7)	Li-treated
	Thrombin	BPe > C (with or without in vitro Li incubation)	
Dubovsky et al., 1991	Basal	BPd (15) > UPd (9), C (13) = BPe (9)	Untreated and treated
	Thrombin	BPd > UP, C	
Dubovsky et al., 1992b	Basal	BPm (4), BPd (5) > C (7)	Untreated
Kusumi et al., 1994a	Basal	BPd (16) = UPm (26) = UPn (18) = C (30)	Untreated
	5-HT	BPd, UPm > UPn, C	Untreated and remitted[b]
Berk et al., 1994	Basal	BPm (21), BPd (19), BPe Li-treated (20) > C (20)	
		(DSS only in BPe > C)	
	Dopamine	Elevated in all groups	
		(DSS), no differences among groups	
Dubovsky et al., 1994	Basal	Plasma of patients does not alter Ca in platelets	
		of C BP or SA BPM	
Bothwell et al., 1994	Basal	BP (17) = UPd (27) = C (44)	
	5-HT/PAF	Li-treated > TCA-treated and C (in any group)	
		BP (17) = UPd (27) = C (44)	
Tan et al., 1995	Basal	BPm (7) > C (26)[b]	Haloperidol-treated
	Thrombin	BPm (7) > C (26)[b]	
Okamoto et al., 1995	Basal	Untreated BPm (10) > BPe Li-CBZ–treated (10), C (14)	[b]
	5-HT	Untreated BPm > BPe Li-CBZ–treated, C	
Yamawaki et al., 1996	Basal	BP (13) > UPd (12) > C (15)	Untreated[b]
	5-HT	BP, UPd > C	
Hough et al., 1999	Basal	BP > C (14)	Treated and untreated[b]
	Thrombin/	BP > C	
	5-HT/TGN		
Kusumi et al., 2000[c]	5-HT	BP (24), UPm (51), UPn (23)	
		BPd lower basal Ca and higher Ca response = better	
		response to MS	
Suzuki et al., 2001	Basal	BP (20) = UPm (26) = UPn (16) = C (30)	Untreated
	5-HT	BP > C	

BP = bipolar patients; BPd = BP depressed; BPe = BP euthymic; BPm = BP manic; C = controls (healthy volunteers); CBZ = carbamazepine; DSS = difference statistically significant; Li = lithium; MS = mood stabilizer; PAF = platelet activator factor; SA = schizoaffective patients; TCA = tricyclic antidepressant; UP = unipolar patients; UPd = unipolar depressed patient; UPm = UP melancholic; UPn = UP not melancholic.

[a]Statistical significance not calculated.
[b]Difference not statistically significant.
[c]Follow-up of 5 years.

The regulation of free intracellular Ca^{2+} is a complex process involving extracellular entry, release from intracellular stores following receptor-stimulated PI hydrolysis, uptake into specific organelles, and binding to specific proteins (see Fig. 14–13). Thus, the abnormalities observed in bipolar disorder could arise at a variety of levels, and recent studies suggest that they lie beyond the receptor (Hough et al., 1999). In this context, since PKC is known to regulate calcium signaling at multiple levels (Shibata et al., 1996; Si-Tahar et al., 1996; Ozaki and Chuang, 1997), more recent studies have investigated its putative role in mediating the calcium abnormalities in bipolar disorder. Preliminary analysis suggests that alterations in tonic PKC activity may play an important role in mediating the abnormal intracellular calcium responses observed in bipolar patients (H. Manji and R. Post, unpublished observations).

Table 14–6. Intracellular Calcium in Blood Elements of Manic-Depressive Patients (Primarily Bipolar): Lymphocytes

Study	Stimulation	Intracellular Ca level	Treatment Status
Dubovsky et al., 1992b	Basal	BPm (4), BPd (5) > C (7)	Untreated
van Calker et al., 1993	Basal not shown	BPe (9) Li-treated, BP (14) untreated, C (10)	
	fMPL	BPe > C > BP	
Dubovsky et al., 1994	Basal	BP (26) > C (7)	[a]
	PHG, concavalin A	BP > C	[a]
		CBZ lowered Ca basal and Ca-stimulated in BP, not in C	
Forstner et al., 1994	Basal in neutrophils	C (14) = Li-treated (14) BP or UP	
	fMLP	Li treatment lowered Ca response	
Emamghoreishi et al., 1997	Basal in BLCL	BP-I (28) > C (20) but not BP-II (11), UP (14)	[b]
	PHG in T ly		
Hough et al., 1999	Basal	BP > C (14)	Treated and untreated[b]
	Thrombin, 5-HT, TGN	BPm > C only with TGN	

BLCL = immortalized B lymphoblasts cell line; BP = bipolar patients; BPd = BP depressed; BPe = BP euthymic; BPm = bipolar patient manic; C = controls (healthy volunteers); CBZ = carbamazepine; fMLP = formylmethionylleucylphenalanin; Li = lithium; PHG = phytohemaglutinin; UP = unipolar patients; TGN = thapsigargin; T ly = T lymphocytes.
[a]Statistical significance not calculated.
[b]Difference not statistically significant.

In an effort to understand the relationship between possible abnormalities of the PI cascade and intracellular calcium, Warsh and colleagues (2000) have investigated IMPA1 and IMPA2 gene expression and calcium homeostasis in B lymphoblast cell lines (BLCLs) from bipolar-I patients (Yoon et al., 2001). They found that IMPA2 mRNA levels were significantly lower in BLCLs from male bipolar-I patients with high [Ca^{2+}] (n = 6) than in healthy male subjects (n = 5), male bipolar-I patients with normal BLCL [Ca^{2+}], and female bipolar-I patients with high [Ca^{2+}]. Furthermore, they found a negative correlation between IMPA2 mRNA levels and [Ca^{2+}] in the male patients.

In view of the extensive cross talk between calcium (Ca^{2+})- and cAMP-mediated signaling systems, Emamghoreishi and colleagues (1997) have postulated that abnormalities in Ca^{2+} homeostasis in bipolar disorder may be linked to disturbances in the function of G proteins that mediate cAMP signaling. To investigate this hypothesis, they phenotyped bipolar-I patients on the basis of basal intracellular Ca^{2+} and then investigated the cAMP system. They found that isoproterenol-stimulated cAMP formation was lower in intact B lymphoblasts from bipolar-I patients with high Ca^{2+} (greater than or equal to 2 standard deviations above the mean concentration of healthy subjects) compared with patients having normal B lymphoblast Ca^{2+} and healthy subjects. Furthermore, although basal and NaF-stimulated cAMP production was found to be greater in B lymphoblast membranes from male bipolar-I patients with high versus normal Ca^{2+}, there were no differences in the percent stimulation. These findings raise the intriguing possibility that trait-dependent disturbances in G protein–mediated cAMP signaling occur in conjunction with altered Ca^{2+} homeostasis in those bipolar-I patients with high B lymphoblast Ca^{2+} and are worthy of further study. The possible basis for a gender difference in the responses also warrants more extensive investigation.

The Phosphoinositide/Protein Kinase C Signaling Pathway as a Target

Lithium and the Phosphoinositide Cycle: The Inositol Depletion Hypothesis

As discussed earlier, lithium at therapeutically relevant concentrations is an uncompetitive inhibitor of the intracellular enzyme inositol monophosphatase (concentration of lithium required to inhibit enzymatic activity by 50 percent (Ki) ~.8 mM). This inhibition results in an accumulation of inositol monophosphate (IP) and a reduction in the generation of free inositol (Allison and Stewart, 1971; Hallcher and Sherman, 1980; Sherman et al., 1986)[62] (see Fig. 14–14).

A number of studies have been conducted to examine the effects of lithium on receptor-mediated PI response in brain in a variety of neurotransmitter systems (e.g., cholinergic, serotonergic, noradrenergic, and histaminergic). Although some investigators have found a reduction in agonist-stimulated PIP_2 hydrolysis in brain slices from rats exposed acutely and chronically to lithium, these findings have often been small, inconsistent, and subject to methodological differences.[63,64]

TABLE 14–7. **Calcium Signaling in Manic-Depressive Illness (Primarily Bipolar)**

Cells	Activity	Study
Erythrocytes	↓ Na$^+$/K$^+$-ATPase activity in depressed patients	Hokin-Neaverson et al., 1974; Johnson, 1980; Naylor et al., 1980
	↑ Ca^{2+}-ATPase activity in mania and depression ↔ Ca^{2+} response; ↑ Ca^{2+}-ATPase levels in mania and depression	Linnoila et al., 1983a Bowden et al., 1988
Neutrophils	↑ fLMP-stimulated Ca^{2+} responses in untreated mania and depression; ↓ stimulated Ca^{2+} responses in Li-treated patients	van Calker et al., 1993
	↓ fLMP-stimulated Ca^{2+} responses in Li-treated patients	Forstner et al., 1994
Leukocytes and platelets	↑ Basal and stimulated Ca^{2+} levels in mania and depression	Dubovsky et al., 1989, 1991, 1992a,b
	↑ 5-HT-stimulated Ca^{2+} response in mania and depression	Yamawaki et al. 1996
	↑ Basal Ca^{2+} levels in Li-treated patients; ↑ thrombin-stimulated Ca^{2+} response; ↑ stimulated Ca^{2+} response in vitro with Li	Tan et al., 1990
	↑ 5-HT-stimulated Ca^{2+} response in depressed patients	Kusumi et al., 1991, 1994a; Eckert et al., 1994
	↔ Basal or stimulated Ca^{2+} in Li-treated patients; ↑ serum and 5-HT-stimulated intracellular Ca^{2+} levels	Bothwell et al., 1994
	↔ Basal or stimulated Ca^{2+} with chronic Li treatment or in vitro	Kusumi et al., 1994b
	↓ Basal Ca^{2+} in euthymic patients	Berk et al., 1994
	↑ 5-HT-stimulated Ca^{2+} responses in manic patients	Okamoto et al., 1995
	↔ Ca^{2+} uptake in mania or depression; ↑ Ca^{2+} uptake following in vitro Li treatment	Berk et al., 1996
	↑ Basal Ca^{2+} concentration; ↓ percent change in phytohemagglutinin-stimulated vs. basal Ca^{2+} levels in BP-I patients	Emamghoreishi et al., 1997
	↑ Basal and stimulated Ca^{2+} concentration; ↔ between types, medication state, or severity	Hough et al., 1999
	↑ Basal and NaF-stimulated and ↓ isoproterenol-stimulated cAMP formation in BPD subjects with high basal Ca^{2+} levels	Emamghoreishi et al., 2000
	↑ 5-HT-induced Ca^{2+} response correlated with response to mood stabilizer treatment in a longitudinal study	Kusumi et al., 2000
	↔ Basal or 5-HT-induced Ca^{2+}	Suzuki et al., 2001

BPD = bipolar disorder; BP-I = bipolar-I; fMPL = formylmethionylleucylphenalanin; Li = lithium.
Source: Bezchlibnyk and Young, 2002.

A number of recent studies have investigated the possibility that lithium and other putative mood stabilizers may regulate the PI system independently of inhibiting IMPase. In this context, investigators have examined lithium's effects on the PI system distal to the receptor since, as noted above, experimental evidence has shown that lithium may alter receptor coupling to PI turnover.[65]

A most interesting potential new target for the actions of structurally dissimilar mood stabilizers is a high-affinity myoinositol transport system (called "SMIT"—Sodium sensitive high-affinity *Myo-Inositol Transporter*) that has been characterized in various cell types, including those of neural origin (van Calker and Belmaker, 2000). Thus it was recently demonstrated that the activity of the SMIT and the expression of its mRNA in astrocytes are downregulated after chronic treatment with therapeutic concentrations of lithium (van Calker and Belmaker, 2000). Interestingly, downregulation of the SMIT was also observed after administration of valproate and carbamazepine. If replicated in vivo, these findings suggest that the SMIT may represent a novel target for the development of new drugs. Most recent finding implicating PI signaling in the actions of mood stabilizers comes from Benes and colleagues (2000), who used a novel tissue-culture assay that measures sensory neuron growth-cone stability to infer that mood stabilizers have a common mechanism of action—depletion of neuronal inositol (1,4,5) trisphosphate (IP$_3$).[66]

In human studies, researchers have used MRS to investigate lithium's effects on brain myoinositol levels in bipolar patients undergoing chronic lithium treatment. In a longitudinal study, Moore and colleagues (1999c) quantitated myoinositol in medication-free bipolar depressed

Figure 14–13. In neurons, Ca^{2+}-dependent processes represent an intrinsic, nonsynaptic feedback system that provides the competence for adaptation to different functional tasks. Ca^{2+} is generally mobilized in one of two ways in the cells: either by mobilization from intracellular stores or from the outside of the cell via plasma membrane ion channels and certain receptors (e.g., NMDA). The external level of Ca^{2+} is approximately 2mM, yet resting intracellular Ca^{2+} levels are in the range of 100nM (2×10^4 lower). Local high levels of calcium result in activation of enzymes, signaling cascades, and at extremes, cell death. Release of intracellular stores of calcium is primarily regulated by IP_3 receptors, which are activated upon generation of IP_3 by phospholipase C activity, and the ryanodine receptor that is activated by the drug ryanodine. Ca^{2+} is sequestered in the endoplasmic reticulum (the vast web and framework for Ca^{2+}-binding proteins to capture and sequester Ca^{2+}). Ca^{2+}-buffering and triggering proteins are nonuniformly distributed—thus the considerable subcellular variation of Ca^{2+} concentrations (e.g., near a Ca^{2+} channel). The primary mechanism for Ca^{2+} calcium exit from the cell is via sodium calcium exchange or by means of a calcium pump. (*Source*: Schatzberg and Nemeroff, 2004. Reprinted with permission from *The American Journal of Psychiatry*. Copyright 2004 by the American Psychiatric Association.)

patients at baseline and after acute (5-day) and chronic (4-week) blinded lithium adminstration. They found that therapeutic administration of lithium produces significant reductions in myoinositol levels in bipolar patients in brain regions previously implicated in the pathophysiology of bipolar disorder. However, the major lithium-induced myoinositol reductions are observed after only 5 days of lithium administration, at a time when the bipolar patient's clinical state is completely unchanged. Similar results have been obtained in independent studies of both child and adult bipolar patients (Davanzo et al., 2001; Yildiz et al., 2001).

The evidence reviewed here suggests that the PI signaling cascade is a target for the action of mood stabilizers and that IMPase inhibition likely represents an important primary biochemical target for the actions of lithium. However, the therapeutic actions of lithium occur only after chronic treatment and usually remain in evidence for some time after discontinuation—actions that cannot be attributed only to inositol reductions evident in the presence of lithium. Thus, although the preponderance of the data suggests that the initial actions of lithium may occur with a relative depletion of inositol and thereby alterations in receptor-coupled PI response, the effects of chronic lithium

(and likely the therapeutically relevant ones) are more likely to be mediated by resultant changes at different levels of the signal transduction processes, including the level of PKC (Jope and Williams, 1994; Manji et al., 1995a,b; Manji and Lenox, 1998). We now turn to the growing body of evidence implicating PKC as a target for the actions of mood stabilizers.

Protein Kinase C in the Treatment of Bipolar Disorder

In view of the pivotal role of the PKC signaling pathway in the regulation of neuronal excitability, neurotransmitter release, and long-term synaptic events (Conn and Sweatt, 1994; Chen et al., 1997; Hahn and Friedman, 1999), it has been postulated that the attenuation of PKC activity

Figure 14–14. Effects of lithium on the phosphoinositide (PI) cycle. A number of receptors in the central nervous system (including M_1, M_1, M_1, $5\text{-}HT_2$) are coupled, via $G_{q/11}$, to activation of PI hydrolysis. Activation of these receptors induces phospholipase C hydrolysis of phosphoinositide 4,5-bisphosphate (PIP_2) to diacylglycerol (DAG) and inositol-1,4,5-triphosphate (Ins 1,4,5P_3). DAG activates protein kinase C (PKC), an enzyme that has many effects including the activation of phospholipase A-2 (PLA_2; an activator of arachidonic acid signaling pathways). IP_3 binds to the IP_3 receptor, resulting in the release of intracellular calcium from intracellular stores, most notably the endoplasmic reticulum (ER). Calcium, an important signaling molecule, initiates a number of downstream effects such as activation of calmodulins and calmodulin-dependent protein kinases. IP_3 is recycled back to PIP_2 by the enzymes inositol monophosphate phosphatase (IMPase) and inositol polyphosphatate phosphatase (IPPase), both of which are targets of lithium. Thus, lithium may initiate many of its therapeutic effects by inhibiting these enzymes, bringing about a cascade of downstream effects involving PKC and gene expression changes. A = agonist; BBB = blood–brain barrier; G = protein; R = receptor. (*Source*: Schatzberg and Nemeroff, 2004. Reprinted with permission from *The American Journal of Psychiatry*. Copyright 2004 by the American Psychiatric Association.)

may play a role in the antimanic effects of lithium and valproate. Recently, a pilot study found that tamoxifen (a nonsteroidal antiestrogen known to be a PKC inhibitor at higher concentrations [Baltuch et al., 1993]) may indeed possess antimanic efficacy (Bebchuk et al., 2000). Clearly these results must be considered preliminary because of the small sample sizes thus far. In view of preliminary data suggesting the involvement of the PKC signaling system in the pathophysiology of bipolar disorder, however, these results suggest that PKC inhibitors may be very useful agents in the treatment of mania. Larger double-blind, placebo-controlled studies of tamoxifen are currently under way, and if positive, may soon lead to the development of completely novel, potentially very rapidly acting antimanic agents.

Evidence from various laboratories has clearly demonstrated that lithium at therapeutically relevant concentrations exerts major effects on the PKC signaling cascade (see Fig. 14–15). Currently available data suggest that acute lithium exposure facilitates a number of PKC-mediated responses, whereas longer-term exposure results in an attenuation of phorbol-ester-mediated responses, which is accompanied by downregulation of specific PKC isozymes (Manji and Lenox, 1999; J. Wang et al., 1999). Studies in rodents have demonstrated that chronic (but not acute) lithium produces an isozyme-selective reduction in PKC α

and ε in frontal cortex and hippocampus in the absence of significant alterations in the β, γ δ, or ζ isozymes (Manji et al., 1993; Manji and Lenox, 1999; Chen et al., 2000). Concomitant studies carried out in immortalized hippocampal cells in culture exposed to chronic lithium show a similar reduction in the expression of both the PKC α and ε isozymes in the cell, as determined by immunoblotting (Manji and Lenox, 1999). Furthermore, chronic lithium has been demonstrated to dramatically reduce the hippocampal levels of a major PKC substrate, MARCKS, a protein implicated in regulating long-term neuroplastic events (Lenox et al., 1992; see Table 14–8).

Although the effects of lithium on PKC isozymes and MARCKS are striking, a major problem inherent in neuropharmacological research is the difficulty of attributing therapeutic relevance to any observed biochemical finding. It is thus noteworthy that the structurally dissimilar antimanic agent valproate produces effects very similar to those of lithium on PKC α and ε isozymes and MARCKS protein.[67] Interestingly, lithium and valproate appear to have their effects on the PKC signaling pathway through distinct mechanisms (Manji and Lenox, 1999; Lenox and Hahn, 2000). These biochemical observations are consistent with the clinical observations that some patients show preferential response to one or the other of the agents, and that

Figure 14–15. The potential mechanisms by which chronic lithium (Li$^+$) or valproate (VPA), or direct-acting protein kinase C (PKC) inhibitors, may be useful in the treatment of acute mania. Activation of PKC, which is known to occur through psychostimulants or stress, results in the phosphorylation of key substrates, notably GAP-43 (growth-cone-associated protein) and MARCKS (myristoylated alanine-rich C kinase substrate), facilitating the release of neurotransmitters. Chronic lithium or valproate attenuates PKC signaling, an effect that may be responsible for the treatment of various facets of the manic syndrome. (*Source*: Bachman et al., 2005. Reprinted with permission.)

TABLE 14–8. Effects of Lithium and Valproate on Protein Kinase C (PKC) Signaling

	Lithium	Valproate
PKC activity	▼	▼
PKC α	▼	▼
pPKC α	▼	▼
PKC ε	▼	▼
MARCKS levels	▼	▼
Inositol-responsive	+	−

additive, or even synergistic therapeutic effects are often seen in patients when the two agents are coadministered.

As discussed in Chapters 18, 19, and 20, a growing body of data suggests that omega-3 fatty acids (ϖ-3 FA) may have some benefit in the treatment of bipolar disorder (see below). It is thus noteworthy that the ϖ-3 FA eicosapentaenoic acid (EPA) and docosahexaenoic acid (DHA), as well as the combination of DHA and EPA, were found to inhibit PKC activity at concentrations as low as 10 μM (Kim et al., 2001). By contrast, arachidonic acid had no effect on PKC activity. Thus, in toto, the biochemical data indicate that structurally dissimilar antimanic agents—lithium, valproate, and ϖ-3 FA—attenuate PKC function in a therapeutically relevant time frame, whereas promanic psychostimulants activate PKC. These findings suggest that PKC modulation may indeed play a critical role in the treatment of mania. However, one of the major difficulties inherent in neuropharmacological research is the attribution of therapeutic relevance to any observed molecular or cellular findings. This difficulty is exacerbated in the case of mood stabilizers, since the prototypical drugs for bipolar disorder were developed serendipitously and exert multiple biochemical and cellular effects, but also some, such as lithium, have therapeutic effects in the prevention and treatment of recurrent depression as well.

With respect to the treatment of mania, attempts to develop improved, potentially more rapidly acting medications are dependent on identifying therapeutically relevant targets, and one of the most important routes to linking cellular and therapeutic effects is by studying final outcomes—behavior (Holmes et al., 2003; Williams et al., 2003). A series of studies was therefore undertaken to assess more directly the possible involvement of PKC inhibition in manic-like behavior in established animal models for the manic syndrome (Einat et al., 2000, 2003b). To explore a wide range of manic-like behaviors, three different behavioral models were used, all induced by amphetamine: (1) hyperactivity, (2) increased risk-taking, and (3) increased hedonic behavior. As we noted in the first edition of this text, these behaviors were chosen because they reflect some of the most important and consistently observed facets of mania in patients. Amphetamine-based models were used because of their ability to trigger manic episodes in susceptible humans.

Given the desire to extrapolate the findings—if positive—directly to large-scale clinical research, the studies were undertaken using the only compound with appreciable CNS PKC inhibitory activity that has been approved for human use—tamoxifen (O'Brian et al., 1988; Baltuch et al., 1993). Tamoxifen has been widely used in the treatment of breast cancer (Catherino et al., 1993; Jordan, 1994). A number of its effects are due to estrogen receptor antagonism (Jordan, 1994), but recent research has shown that it is also a potent and selective PKC inhibitor at therapeutically relevant concentrations (Horgan et al., 1986; O'Brian et al., 1988; Couldwell et al., 1993). Tamoxifen clearly crosses the blood–brain barrier and has already been used safely in women, men, and children (Pollack et al., 1997; Jordan, 2003), including for the treatment of a CNS disorder, malignant glioma (Couldwell et al., 1996; Mastronardi et al., 1998). It was found that acute tamoxifen significantly reduced acute or chronic amphetamine-induced hyperactivity in a large open field without affecting spontaneous activity levels. Furthermore, the same treatment normalized amphetamine-induced increase in visits to the center of an open field (representing risk-taking behavior) and reduced hedonic-like amphetamine-induced conditioned place preference. Biochemical results were consistent with the behavioral changes, and tamoxifen attenuated amphetamine-induced phosphorylation of GAP-43, consistent with PKC inhibition.

The Role of Fatty Acids

As noted above, the possible involvement of fatty acids (in particular the ϖ-3 FA) in the treatment of mood disorders has recently received considerable attention. The predominant naturally occurring ϖ-3 FA are DHA, EPA, and linolenic acid. The ϖ-3 FA appear to cross the blood–brain barrier easily and are incorporated into neuronal membranes. Because of their highly folded chemical structure, ϖ-3 FA increase the fluidity of the membrane lipid bilayer, thereby changing transmembrane protein function. This has been proposed to represent the mechanism by which membrane phospholipids become more resistant to hydrolysis by phospholipases.[68]

In a series of studies, investigators have used in vivo brain-imaging methodologies to investigate the potential effects of mood-stabilizing agents on CNS fatty acids. It was found that lithium and valproate produce selective reductions in the turnover rate of the phospholipid arachidic acid (AA) in rat brain (Chang et al., 1996, 2001). Lithium produced a reduction of 80 percent accompanied by a reduction in the expression of the gene and protein of an AA-specific phospholipase A2 (cPLA2). Valproate decreased the turnover of AA by 33 percent with no effect on cPLA2 protein levels, and was postulated to act directly in the incorporation of AA into brain phospholipids. Ongoing studies should serve to delineate the facets of recurrent mood disorders (perhaps especially bipolar disorder) that these membrane changes may modulate.

The Role of Synaptic Vesicle Proteins

Because synaptic proteins are downstream targets of many signaling pathways implicated in the pathophysiology and/ or treatment of mood disorders, and because alterations in presynaptic function could modulate synaptic plasticity and therefore CNS information flow, the role of these proteins in mood disorders merits attention. The presynaptic machinery controls the processes of exocytosis and endocytosis at the synapse, and is composed of a large number of proteins interacting in complex ways. These proteins are phosphoregulated by many major serine/threonine kinases and phosphatases, including PKC, PKA, calcium/ calmodulin-dependent kinases (CaMK) I and II, MAPK, casein kinase II (caskII), cyclin-dependent kinase (cdk), and the protein phosphatases 2a and 2b (PP2A and calcineurin, respectively). Some of these phosphorylations appear to reflect presynaptic mechanisms of synaptic plasticity (Turner et al., 1999). Expression-level regulation is also effected by many processes and pathways, including spatial learning (Gomez-Pinilla et al., 2001), stress (Thome et al., 2001), estrogen (Brake et al., 2001), BDNF (Tartaglia et al., 2001), CREB (Hoesche et al., 1995; Ryabinin et al., 1995), and POU-family transcription factors (Morris et al., 1996; Deans et al., 1997).

Evidence of Pathological Alterations in the Presynaptic Release Machinery

Postmortem studies have shed much light on the potential dysfunction of the synapse in psychiatric disorders. Most studies have focused on schizophrenia, although similar results have often been found in bipolar disorder when included. Eastwood and Harrison (2001) recently reviewed findings on synaptic markers in schizophrenia and mood disorders and assayed several proteins in anterior cingulate cortex. They found that GAP-43, synaptophysin, and complexin II were reduced in bipolar disorder, correlated with length of illness. In general, however, the results were more suggestive of an overall atrophy of excitatory synaptic connections rather than a specific pathology related to the machinery of neurotransmitter release.[69]

Overall, many suggestive findings implicate presynaptic proteins in the pathophysiology of schizophrenia and severe mood disorders. It remains to be seen, however, whether these changes are directly related to the psychopathology of the disease, or are epiphenomena of altered neurotrans-

mission, impaired cellular growth and survival, substance abuse, and/or some other causative factor. Suggestive of the former hypothesis, three genes encoding synaptic proteins have been identified with possible risk-conferring alleles. Several variant alleles of synaptojanin (at the 21q22 locus) appeared to be more frequent in bipolar patients (Saito et al., 2001a). Synaptojanin is a polyphosphoinositide 5-phosphatase and is believed to have a role in clathrin uncoating in the final stages of slow synaptic vesicle endocytosis. Homozygous synaptojanin-null mutant mice display abormal phosphoinositide metabolism and a large increase in clathrin-coated vesicles, which may be related to the observation of enhanced long-term depression (Cremona et al., 1999). A mutant splice acceptor in the gene encoding synaptobrevin (at the Xq28 locus) may occur with greater frequency in male bipolar patients (Saito et al., 2000). Synaptobrevin (also called VAMP) is part of the SNARE (N-ethylmaleimide-sensitive fusion factor attachment protein receptor) complex, which is essential for docking of vesicles prior to release. Knockout mice display large deficits in spontaneous and particularly calcium-evoked release of synaptobrevin (Schoch et al., 2001). Finally, a mutation in the promoter of SNAP-29, a SNAP-25 homologue mapping to the velocardiofacial syndrome (VCFS) critical region at 22q11, was demonstrated to be more common in schizophrenic patients (Saito et al., 2001b).

Presynaptic Proteins as Targets of Psychiatric Drugs

CaMKII is highly enriched in both presynaptic and postsynaptic terminals. Chronic, but not acute, treatment with paroxetine or fluvoxamine (both SSRIs) or with venlafaxine (a dual 5-HT/NE reuptake inhibitor) was found to increase CaMKII activity in vesicle-enriched fractions of rat hippocampus (Popoli et al., 1995). This effect may be attributable at least in part to an increase in tyrosine autophosphorylation. Treatment with desmethylimipramine, imipramine, electroconvulsive shock (the animal model of ECT), and s-adenosylmethionine (a methyl doner with putative antidepressant properties with an unknown mechanism) was found to produce similar effects on CaMKII activity in hippocampus and/or frontal cortex (Pilc et al., 1999; Consogno et al., 2001a,b).[70]

The involvement of presynaptic proteins in mood-stabilizer treatment is much less well studied. An increase in synapsin in cultured cerebellar granule cells has been reported (Lucas and Salinas, 1997), and it has been shown that lithium stimulation of synapsin expression probably occurs through the inhibition of glycogen synthase kinase 3β (GSK-3β), a fairly well-documented effect of lithium. Further work by this group revealed that lithium and valproate induced the clustering of synapsin into bright punctae in a variety of primary neurons (Hall et al., 2002).

Changes in the mRNA of several synaptic proteins following lithium treatment were found in a microarray study of nerve growth factor (NGF)-differentiated PC12 cells (Cordeiro et al., 2000). Likewise, preliminary data from this group demonstrated an increase in the expression of several synaptic proteins following treatment with valproate in rat hippocampal slices. Published findings suggest, however, that synapsin is unchanged or downregulated following in vivo chronic treatment with lithium (Vawter et al., 2002) or valproate (Hassel et al., 2001), respectively. Additional data from the Manji group suggest no effect of lithium or valproate on synapsin levels (N.A. Gray et al., unpublished observations). The observation that effects are distinct in cell culture and in vivo suggests that the increase seen in culture may be a function of increased synaptogenesis (an effect that would presumably be more apparent in a growth-intensive environment such as cell culture).[71]

Current work by the Manji group indicates that phosphorylation of synapsin at site 1 is increased following chronic treatment with lithium or valproate in rat hippocampus. Site 1 of synapsin is phosphorylated by PKA and/or CaMKI, and dephosphorylated by PP2A. While we could find no study exploring effects of mood stabilizers on CaMKI, many studies have investigated PKA activity following lithium treatment. In general, the effects appear to be quite complex and dependent on brain region, subcellular fraction, stimulation, and length of treatment. There is some indication that the catalytic PKA and adenylate cyclase type 1 may be somewhat increased in soluble fractions of rat hippocampus following chronic lithium treatment (Mori et al., 1998; Jensen et al., 2000), although stimulated phosphorylation may be reduced (Jensen and Mork, 1997). This observation parallels that of earlier work suggesting elevated basal but reduced stimulated cAMP levels in cortex of treated rats (Manji et al., 1991b). The effects of lithium and valproate on serine/threonine phosphatases have not been demonstrated. The authors of a recent study hypothesize that lithium's rescue of (PKB/Akt) dephosphorylation under low-K^+ conditions may be due to inhibition of a protein phosphatase (Mora et al., 2001); however, they do not rule out an upstream increase in phosphorylation.

Glycogen Synthase Kinase-3 as a Target

Recently, considerable excitement has been generated by the identification of a completely unexpected and novel target for lithium—a crucial kinase that functions as an intermediary in numerous intracellular signaling pathways called glycogen synthase kinase-3 (GSK-3).[72] GSK-3 plays a critical role in the survival of neurons, and this role has been postulated to be the target of lithium and valproate (Gould and Manji, 2002a; Li et al., 2002). As discussed later, a growing body of data has demonstrated neuroprotective effects

of lithium in many preclinical models. It is possible that the effect of lithium on GSK-3 plays a role in these phenomena.[73] (See Figure 14–16 for more details on the effects of lithium and valproate on the GSK-3 cascade.)

At this point, it is critical to note that evidence suggests an association between mood disorders and impairments of neuroplasticity and cellular resilience, with both in vivo and postmortem studies suggesting neuron and/or glial cell loss or atrophy in circumscribed brain areas. Importantly, lithium has effects suggestive of neuroprotection clinically, as well as in rodent and cell-based models. Lithium may exert these neuroprotective effects, at least in part, by inhibition of GSK-3. (See Box 14–15 for findings related to the neuroprotective effects of GSK-3 inhibition.)

A second putative target pathway resulting from GSK-3 inhibition is suggested by research exploring the underlying circadian cycle of drosophila. The *Drosophila* orthologue of GSK-3 (SHAGGY or ZW3/Sgg) regulates circadian rhythms in this species. A decrease in SHAGGY activity results in a longer circadian period (Martinek et al., 2001)—precisely the effect noted in numerous species, including *Drosophila*, after treatment with lithium (Klemfuss, 1992). While there are many differences between the molecular components of circadian cycles in mammals and *Drosophila*, there are also many similarities (Wager-Smith and Kay, 2000; Reppert and Weaver, 2001; Williams and Sehgal, 2001). Thus it is interesting to speculate that GSK-3 has a similar general action in the function of the mammalian circadian clock (Gould and Manji, 2002a; Lenox et al., 2002). This putative function of GSK-3 in mammals therefore represents another possible therapeutic target for the actions of lithium on GSK-3. In fact, longer circadian periods after lithium exposure have been observed in unicellular organisms, plants, invertebrates, and vertebrates, including such mammals as mice, rats, squirrel monkeys, and humans.[74] (See Figures 14–17 for the circadian cycles in *Drosophila* and mammals, Figure 14–18 for the effects of lithium on the circadian cycle, and see Chapter 16.)

Very recent data from a variety of leading laboratories have greatly strengthened the case for an important role for GSK-3 in the pathophysiology and treatment of recurrent mood disorders, especially bipolar disorder (see Gould and Manji, 2005, and references therein):

- GSK-3 is markedly regulated by serotonin, dopamine, psychostimulants, and antidepressants, and is at the nexus of multiple neurotransmitter and signaling cascades putatively involved in these disorders.
- GSK-3 is a major regulator of apoptosis and cellular plasticity and resilience. Generally, increased activity of GSK-3 is pro-apoptotic, while inhibiting GSK-3 attenuates or prevents apoptosis (see Gould and Manji, 2005,

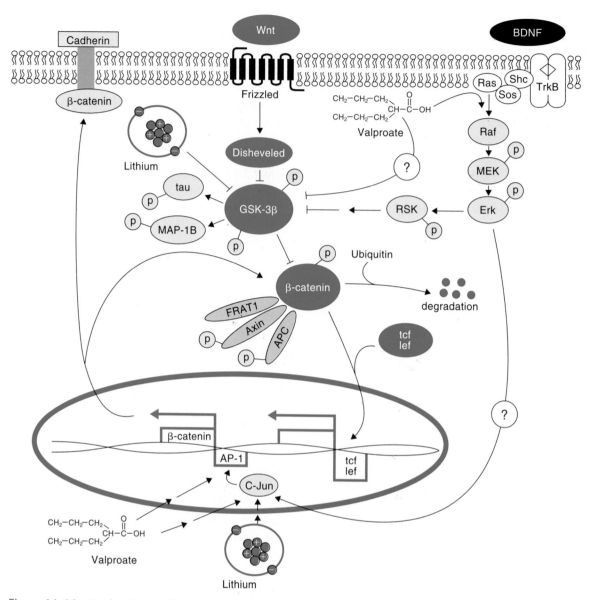

Figure 14–16. Signaling through Wnt glycoproteins and frizzled receptors activates disheveled, resulting in inhibition of glycogen synthase kinase-3β (GSK-3β). Phosphorylation of β-catenin by GSK-3β results in its degradation by ubiquitin. Non-degraded (nonphosphorylated) β-catenin binds to lef/tcf transcription factors, targeting transcription of specific genes. Lithium competes with Mg^{2+} to inhibit GSK-3β (Ryves and Harwood, 2001). Valproate may be an inhibitor of GSK-3β. Alternately, it may exert its action on Wnt signaling through inhibition of histone deacetylase, by its known actions on C-Jun, through upregulation of β-catenin mRNA, or by its action on the Ras/RSK pathway (Chen et al., 1997, 1999; Phiel and Klein, 2001; Yuan et al., 2001). BDNF = brain-derived neurotrophic factor; MAP = mitogen-activated protein kinase; MEK = MAP kinase kinase. (*Source*: Gould and Manji, 2002b. Reprinted by permission of SAGE Publications, Inc.)

for review). (See Figure 14–19 for details on the GSK-3 signaling convergence.)

- As noted above, GSK-3 has a major effect on regulating the circadian period in diverse species, an effect it shares with lithium (Gould et al., 2004a,b). Notably, treatment strategies are being developed that derive from a chronobiological model of recurrent mood disorders.

- Recent animal behavioral data (from pharmacologic and genetic models) have shown that manipulation of the GSK-3 signaling cascade produces both antidepressant and antimanic effects in models of depression or mania. To the best of our knowledge, other than lithium, this is the only manipulation that has been demonstrated to exert both antidepressant and antimanic effects.

BOX 14–15.   GSK-3β Inhibition is Neuroprotective

- GSK-3β activity required for β-amyloid-induced neurotoxicity in primary hippocampal cultures (Takashima et al., 1995)
- GSK-3β overexpression induces apoptosis in Rat-1 and PC-12 cells (Pap and Cooper, 1998)
- Dominant negative GSK-3β prevents apoptosis following inhibition of PI3K (Pap and Cooper, 1998)
- FRAT-1 (a protein that interacts with the β-catenin/axin/GSK-3β complex) rescues primary sympathetic neurons from PI3K inhibition–induced cell death (Crowder and Freeman, 2000)
- Dominant negative form of GSK-3β or an inhibitory GSK-3β binding protein attenuates serum deprivation of PI3K-induced apoptosis (Hetman et al., 2000)
- Synthetic GSK-3β inhibitors protect primary sensory and granule neurons from potassium deprivation of PI3K-induced cell death (Cross et al., 2001)
- Rat-1 cells stably overexpressing Wnt-1 are resistant to vincristine and vinblastine apoptosis (B. Chen et al., 2001)

In view of their therapeutic effects not only in bipolar disorder but also in Alzheimer's disease and other neurodegenerative disorders, it is not surprising that specific, brain-penetrant GSK-3 inhibitors are actively under development by numerous pharmaceutical companies. Unless side effects prove to be prohibitive, GSK-3 inhibitors may represent a completely novel class of treatments for bipolar disorder (Gould and Manji, 2005).

We now turn to discussion of an emerging field of research in manic-depressive illness that has generated considerable excitement in the clinical neuroscience community and is reshaping our views about the pathophysiology of severe mood disorders: the critical role of impairments of cellular plasticity and resilience.

The Role of Cellular Plasticity Cascades

Although traditionally viewed exclusively as a neurochemical disorder, recent evidence suggests the possibility that the underlying primary pathophysiology of bipolar disorder may involve intracellular signaling cascades that produce not only functional but also morphological impairments, rather than specific alterations in a particular neurochemicals per se. In this regard, it is noteworthy that increasingly neuroimaging, neuropathologic, and biochemical studies suggest impairments in cellular plasticity and resilience in patients who suffer from severe, recurrent mood disorders.

Atrophic Changes in Manic-Depressive Illness: Primary Illness Pathology or the Ravages of Illness Progression?

As discussed in Chapters 9 and 15, recent morphometric MRI and postmortem investigations have demonstrated abnormalities of brain structure that persist independently of mood state and may contribute to corresponding abnormalities in metabolic activity (Manji and Duman, 2001; Manji et al., 2001a). Structural imaging studies have demonstrated reduced gray matter volumes in areas of the orbital and medial prefontal cortex, ventral striatum, and hippocampus and enlargement of the third ventricle in patients with mood disorders relative to controls (Drevets, 2001; Beyer and Krishnan, 2002; Strakowski et al., 2002). Also consistent is the presence of white matter hyperintensities in the brains of elderly depressed patients and patients with bipolar disorder; these lesions may be associated with poor treatment response.[75]

Postmortem Morphometric Findings.   In addition to the accumulating neuroimaging evidence (see Chapter 15), several postmortem brain studies now provide direct evidence for reductions in regional CNS volume, cell number, and cell body size (see Box 14–16).

Baumann and colleagues (1999a, 1999b) reported reduced volumes of the left nucleus accumbens, the right putamen, and bilateral pallidum externum in postmortem brain samples obtained from patients with unipolar major depressive disorder or bipolar disorder. Several recent postmortem stereological studies of the prefrontal cortex have also demonstrated reduced regional volume, cell numbers, and/or cell sizes. Morphometric analysis of the density and size of cortical neurons in the dorsolateral prefrontal cortex (DLPFC) and orbitofrontal cortices has revealed significant reductions in mood disorder patients compared to control subjects (Rajkowska et al., 1999; Rajkowska, 2000; see Table 14–9). The neuronal reductions have generally been more subtle than the corresponding glial alterations (see below) and detected only when specific morphological size-types of neurons were analyzed in individual cortical layers. For example, marked reductions in the density of large neurons (corresponding to pyramidal glutamatergic excitatory neurons) were found in layers III and V of the DLPFC in bipolar disorder and major depressive disorder. In other prefrontal regions such as rostral orbitofrontal cortex, the most prominent neuronal reductions in major depressive disorder are confined to layer II cells (mostly corresponding to nonpyramidal inhibitory local circuit neurons). Reductions in the density of specific populations of layer II nonpyramidal neurons containing the calcium binding protein calretinin have also been reported in the anterior cingulate cortex in subjects with a history of mood disorders.

Decreases in laminar neuronal densities have also been reported in the dorsolateral prefrontal cortex (Rajkowska et al. 2001) and anterior cingulate cortex (Benes et al., 2001; Bouras et al., 2001; Cotter et al., 2002a) in bipolar disorder, although not all studies have observed these findings

Figure 14–17. Schematic of genes involved in the circadian cycles of *Drosophila* (*a*) and mammals (*b*). The molecular mechanism regulating circadian rhythms relies on a daily cycle of interactions between positive and negative regulators. In *Drosophila* (*a*), CYCLE (*Drosophila* BMAL1) and CLOCK help mediate transcription of TIMELESS and PERIOD genes. PERIOD binds to TIMELESS in the cytoplasm. These proteins then enter the nucleus and act as negative regulators of CLOCK and CYCLE (Allada et al., 2001). SHAGGY (the *Drosophila* orthologue of GSK-3β) appears to phosphorylate TIMELESS, advancing the entry of this protein into the nucleus (Martinek et al., 2001). Lithium is a direct inhibitor of SHAGGY (Klein and Melton, 1996; Stambolic et al., 1996), suggesting a method by which lithium lengthens the circadian period in diverse species, including *Drosophila* (Klemfuss, 1992). The mammalian circadian cycle (*b*) has many similarities (Allada et al., 2001) as well as notable differences, for example, lack of a true TIMELESS orthologue (Reppert and Weaver, 2001). The role of GSK-3β in mammalian circadian cycles is unknown (see also Chapter 16). (*Source*: Gould and Manji, 2002b. Reprinted by permission of SAGE Publications, Inc.)

(Ongur et al., 1998; Cotter et al., 2001; see Table 14–9). Moreover, reduced density of pyramidal neurons in cortical layers III and V (Rajkowska et al., 2001) and nonpyramidal neurons in layer II (Benes et al., 2001) have been observed in the same regions. This last observation coincides with reports on reductions in the density of layer II nonpyramidal neurons that are identified with specific antibodies against the calcium binding protein calbindin in the anterior cingulate cortex (Cotter et al., 2002a) and dorsolateral prefrontal cortex (Reynolds et al., 2002) in bipolar disorder. (Calbindin-immunoreactive neurons are known to colocalize with GABA). Elegant detailed studies from the Rajkowska laboratory have undertaken measurements of the density and size of calbindin-immunoreactive neurons in layers II and upper part of layer III of the dorsolateral prefrontal cortex, revealing a 43 percent reduction

b   # The circadian cycle in mammals

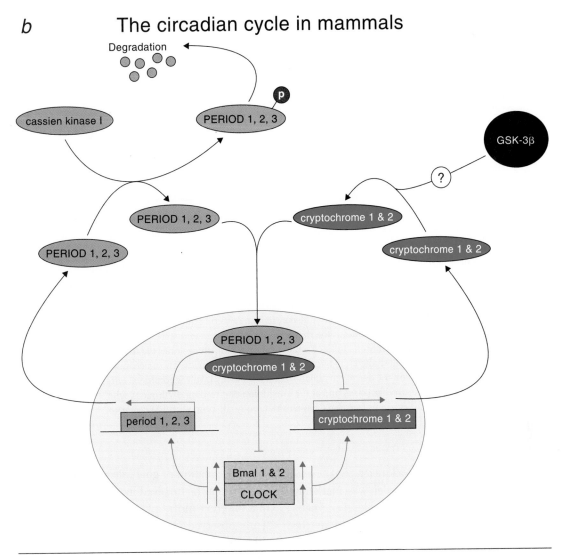

Figure 14–17. *(continued)*

in the density of these neurons in major depressive disorder compared with controls (Rajkowska, 2002a,b). Notably, in the rostral orbitofrontal cortex there was a trend for a negative correlation between the duration of depression and sizes of neuronal cell bodies (Rajkowska et al., 1999). The longer the duration of illness, the smaller the neurons were, suggesting changes associated with disease progression. More subtle than in major depressive disorder, reductions in neuronal soma size have been observed in bipolar disorder by some investigators (Rajkowska et al., 2001; Chana et al., 2003) but not by all (Ongur et al., 1998; Bouras et al., 2001; Cotter et al., 2001). In one other study a minor increase in the size of small nonpyramidal neurons was noted in the anterior cingulate cortex in bipolar subjects (Benes et al., 2001). However, given the major trophic effects of lithium and valproate, it is quite possible that the more modest findings in bipolar disorder actually represent a long-term protective effect of these medications.

Additional morphometric studies have also reported layer-specific reductions in interneurons in the anterior cingulate cortex) and reductions in nonpyramidal neurons (~ 40 percent lower) in CA2 of the hippocampal formation in bipolar subjects compared with controls (Benes et al., 1998). Overall, the layer-specific cellular changes observed in several distinct brain regions, including the prefrontal cortex, anterior cingulate cortex, and hippocampus, support the contention that multiple neuronal circuits underlie the neuropathology of mood disorders. (Manji and Lenox, 2000b; Rajkowska et al., 2004). Notably, some disorganization in neuronal clusters in layers II and III of the entorhinal cortex was also observed (Beckmann and Jakob, 1991; Bernstein et al., 1998). In a large study in which neuronal and glial cell packing density and soma size were estimated in the hippocampal subfields in 19, patients with major depression and 21 age-matched controls, prominent abnormalities in the CA regions and dentate gyrus were

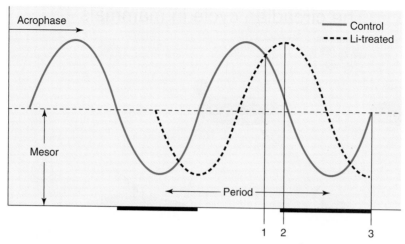

Figure 14–18. Chronic lithium treatment and circadian rhythms. The most prominent rhythmic component under normal conditions has a period of 24 hours. This rhythm usually reflects a complex interaction between endogenous rhythmic and other mechanisms (homeostatic, adaptive, pathological, etc.). The 24-hour rhythms with a proven endogenous component are called *circadian*, reflecting the observation that under constant external conditions the rhythms free run with an endogenous period that is close to 24 hours. Chronic (but not acute) lithium treatment prolongs the free-running period in almost all studied biological systems, including humans. The mechanism of lithium's action on the diverse circadian rhythms probably involves combined effects at the level of the circadian clock and at the integration of circadian rhythmicity with other regulatory systems (see also Chapter 16). (*Source*: Ikonomov and Manji, 1999.)

found in major depressive subjects (Stockmeier, 2003). Neuronal density in major depressive disorder was markedly increased by 30–40 percent above the control level and neuronal cell body size was significantly decreased in the CA1–3 subfields and dentate gyrus. An increase in packing density paralleled by smaller cell sizes in major depressive disorder suggests a decrease in neuropil consisting of neuronal and glial processes and their synapses (Stockmeier, 2003).

Glial Cell Pathology.   In addition to neuronal pathology, unexpected reductions in glial cell number and density have recently been found in postmortem brains of both patients with major depression and bipolar disorder. Marked decreases in overall and laminar (layers III–IV) glial cell packing densities were found in subjects with major depressive disorder compared with nonpsychiatric control subjects (Rajkowska et al., 1999). Comparable reductions in glial densities were also detected in DLPFC from subjects with bipolar disorder across all cortical layers except layer IV (Rajkowska 1997, 2000). Further immunohistochemical examination of PFC glial cells in major depressive disorder indicated that the reductions in the population of astroglial cells account at least in part for the global glial deficit that has also been found in this disorder (Miguel-Hidalgo et al., 2000). In bipolar disorder, however, it is possible that a different population of glial cells (oligodendroglia and/or microglia) may be involved in this pathology, since reductions in a different morphological type of glial cell were consistently observed in all cortical layers of DLPFC in bipolar subjects (Rajkowska, 2000). An independent histological study of area sg24 located in the subgenual prefrontal cortex also found striking reductions in glial cell numbers in patients with familial major depressive disorder (24 percent reduction) and bipolar disorder (41 percent reduction) compared to controls (Ongur et al., 1998). However, when familial and nonfamilial subgroups of depressed patients were combined, the reductions were not found; these intriguing findings raise the possibility that the subgenual prefrontal coretx glial cell findings may be most apparent in a particularly strongly genetic form of the illness. This observation is consistent with this group's neuroimaging report on reductions in cortical gray matter volume found in the same brain region in a similar diagnostic group. While these results are intriguing, further immunohostochemical and molecular studies are needed to definitively determine if the same types of glial cells underlie the glial deficit that has been observed in both major depressive disorder and bipolar disorder, and if this glial loss occurs via similar mechanisms. While the most prominent findings thus far have been from the frontal cortex, a growing body of data suggests that glial pathology extends beyond the frontal

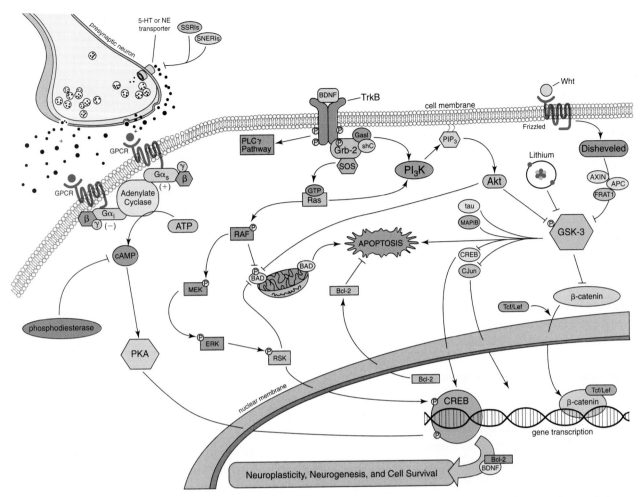

Figure 14–19. Glycogen synthase kinase-3 (GSK-3) is a component of diverse signaling pathways. These include G protein–coupled receptor signaling (left), neurotrophic factor signaling (center), and the Wnt signaling pathway (right). Neurotrophins such as brain-derived neurotrophic factor (BDNF) act through Trk receptors A, B, and C to activate phosphoinositide-3 kinase (PI₃K) and Akt and inhibit GSK-3. Many effectors have been implicated in GSK-3's neurotrophic effects, including transcription factors (e.g., C-Jun, p53, CREB) and recently the proapoptotic Bcl-2 family member BAX. In the Wnt signaling pathway, secreted Wnt glycoproteins interact with the frizzled family of receptors and through disheveled-mediated signaling inhibit GSK-3. Stability of this process requires the scaffolding proteins axin and adenomatous polyposis coli (APC). Normally, active GSK-3 phosphorylates β-catenin, leading to its ubiquitin-dependent degradation. However, when GSK-3 is inhibited in the Wnt pathway, β-catenin is not degraded, allowing for its interaction with T-cell-specific transcription factor (Tcf) to act as a transcription factor. (*Source*: Gould and Manji, 2005. Reprinted with permission from Macmillan Publishers, Ltd.)

cortex to the hippocampus. A recent study of the hippocampus in 40 patients with major depression and aged-matched control subjects reported marked increases in glial cell density and unchanged sizes of glial nuclei in all hippocampal CA subfields and the granule cell layer of the dentate gyrus (Stockmeier et al., 2004). Increases in glial cell packing density detected postmortem in patients with major depression are suggestive of reduction in surrounding neuropil (see above) and may be related to decreases in hippocampal volume noted by neuroimaging studies in major depression disorder (see Chapter 15).

Glial Cell Type Affected in Mood Disorders. Glial cells do not represent a single subtype, and in addition to their traditional roles in neuronal migration (radial glia), myelin formation (oligodendrocytes), and inflammatory processes (astrocytes and microglia), glia (predominantly astrocytes) are now accepted to have roles in providing trophic support to neurons, neuronal metabolism, and the formation of synapses and neurotransmission. To date, the exact identity of the glial cell subtypes most affected in mood disorders remains to be fully established, but considerable data suggest the involvement of several subtypes. Alterations in glial fibrillary acidic protein (GFAP) (generally considered to represent a marker for astrocytes in areas of the brain such as frontal cortex) in both bipolar disorder and major depressive disorder are suggested by a proteomic study in which different forms of GFAP displayed

BOX 14–16. Postmortem Morphometric Brain Studies in Mood Disorders Demonstrating Cellular Atrophy and/or Loss

Reduced Volume or Cortical Thickness

- Cortical thickness rostral oribitofrontal cortex, major depressive disorder (MDD)
- Laminar cortical thickness in layers III, V, and VI in subgenual anterior cingulate cortex (area 24) in bipolar disorder (BPD)
- Volume of subgenual prefrontal cortex in familial MDD and BPD
- Volumes of nucleus accumbens (left), basal ganglia (bilateral) in MDD and BPD
- Parahippocampal cortex size (right) in suicide

Reduced Neuronal Size and/or Density

- Pyramidal neuronal density, layers III and V in dorsolateral prefrontal cortex in BPD and MDD
- Neuronal size in layer V (−14%) and VI (−18%) in prefrontal cortex (area 9) in BPD
- Neuronal size in layer VI (−20%) in prefrontal cortex (area 9) in MDD
- Neuronal density and size in layer II–IV in rostral oribitofrontal cortex, in layer V/VI in caudal oribitofrontal cortex, and in supra- and infragranular layers in dorsolateral prefrontal cortex in MDD
- Neuronal size in layer VI (−23%) in anterior cingulate cortex in MDD
- Neuronal density in layers III, V, and VI in subgenual anterior cingulated cortex (area 24) in BPD
- Layer-specific interneurons in anterior cingulate cortex in BPD and MDD
- Nonpyramidal neuronal density in layer II (−27%) in anterior cingulate cortex in BPD
- Nonpyramidal neurons density in the CA2 region in BPD

Reduced Glia

- Density/size of glia in dorsolateral prefrontal cortex and caudal oribitofrontal cortex in MDD and BPD—layer-specific
- Glial cell density in sublayer IIIc (−19%) (and a trend to decrease in layer Va) in dorsolateral prefrontal cortex (area 9) in BPD
- Glial number in subgenal prefrontal cortex in familial MDD (−24%) and BPD (−41%)
- Glial cell density in layer V (−30%) in prefrontal cortex (area 9) in MDD
- Glial cell density in layer VI (−22%) in anterior cingulate cortex in MDD
- Glial cell counts, glial density, and glia-to-neuron ratios in amygdala in MDD

disease-specific abnormalities (Johnston-Wilson et al., 2000). Another type of glial cell, oligodendroglia, may also be involved in the general glial pathology, as reduced density, immunoreactivity, and ultrastructural changes in oligodendrocytes were found in the dorsolateral prefrontal and anterior frontal cortex in patients with bipolar and major depressive disorder (Orlovskaya et al., 2000; Uranova et al., 2001). Moreover, a reduction of key oligodendrocyte-related and myelin-related gene expression was reported in the dorsolateral prefrontal cortex in bipolar disorder (Tkachev et al., 2003). Recently, Aston and associates (2005) undertook a microarray study examining approximately 12,000 genes in temporal cortex in 12 patients with major depression (recurrence not qualified) and 14 controls (bipolar subjects were not included in this study). They found that 17 genes related to myelination were significantly reduced. Eight of these genes encode for structural components of myelin, whereas five other genes encode enzymes that are involved in the synthesis of myelin or are essential in the regulation of myelin formation and metabolism. These intriguing findings support the neuroimaging data for abnormalities of white matter in critical circuits in manic-depressive illness (see Chapter 15).

It is clear that considerably more work is needed to fully elucidate the precise pathophysiological significance of the glial cell findings in major depressive disorder and bipolar disorder. There has nonetheless been tremendous progress in our understanding of the critical roles of glial cells in the regulation of neuronal function and in their involvement in a variety of neuropsychiatric diseases. Compelling evidence now exists that radial glial cells have the potential to not only guide newly born neurons but also self-renew and generate *both neurons and astrocytes*. Furthermore, recent data have shown that astrocytes increase the number of mature, functional synapses on CNS neurons seven-fold, demonstrating that CNS synapse number can be profoundly regulated by glia. Glial cells are also known to play critical roles in the regulation of synaptic glutamate levels, CNS energy homeostasis, and the liberation of trophic factors, and they indeed form dynamic, complex synaptic networks with neurons.[76] All of these findings suggest that the prominent glial loss observed in major depressive and bipolar disorders may be integral to the pathophysiology of the disorders and worthy of further study.

While total reproducibility does not exist among either the neuroimaging or postmortem studies, the differences likely represent variations in experimental design (including medication effects—see below), and in patient populations (as would be expected in heterogenous conditions such as mood disorders). Overall, the data suggest that although clearly not classic degenerative disorders, severe mood disorders are illnesses associated with atrophic brain

TABLE 14–9. Morphological Abnormalities in the Cerebral Cortex in Mood Disorders

Disease (No. of Subjects)	Area; Hemisphere	Methods	Neurons	Glia	Study
Prefrontal Cortex					
MDD (12)/C (12)	DLPFC (BA 9); left	Nissl	↓ Density of large neurons (20–60% LII, III, VI); ↑ Density of small neurons; ↓ Size (5% LIII, 7% LVI)	↓ Density (20–30% in LIII, V); ↑ Size (6% LIIIa)	Rajkowska et al., 1999
BPD (10)/C (11)	DLPFC (BA 9); left	Nissl	↓ Density of all (19% LIII) and pyramidal neurons (17–30% LIII, V)	↓ Density (19% LIIIc; 12%LVb); ↑ Size (9% LI, 7% LIIIc)	Rajkowska et al., 2001
MDD (15)/BPD (15)/C (15)	DLPFC (BA 9) left + right	Nissl	↓ Size (20% LVI in MDD); ↓ Size (14% LV, 18% LVI in BPD)	↓ Density (30% LV, MDD); = Size (MDD, BPD)	Cotter et al., 2002a
MDD (14)/C (15)	DLPFC (BA 9); left	GFAP-IHC	Not examined	↓ Area fraction and ↓ density (LIII–V; in subgroup of young MDD subjects); = Area and density (young and old subjects combined)	Miguel-Hidalgo et al., 2000
MDD (12)/C (12)	ORB (BA 10–47); left	Nissl	↓ Density of large neurons (20–60% LII–IV); ↑ density of small neurons (LIII); ↓ size (9% LII, III)	= Density	Rajkowska et al., 1999
	ORB (BA 47); left		↓ Density (LIIIa, Va); ↓ size (6% LII)	↓Density (15–18%, LIIIc–VI)	
Anterior Cingulate Cortex					
MDD (4f)/BPD (4f)/C (5f)	Subgenual (BA 24) left+right	Nissl	= Density (MDD, BPD); = Number (MDD, BPD); = Size (MDD, BPD)	↓ Number (24% overall, MDD); ↓ Number (41% overall, BPD); = Size (MDD, BPD)	Ongur et al., 1998
MDD (15)/BPD (15)/C (15)	Supragenual (BA 24) left+right	Nissl	↓ Size (18% LVI in MDD); = Density (MDD, BPD)	↓ Density (22% LVI, MDD); = Density (BPD)	Cotter et al., 2001
MDD (20)/BPD (21)/C (55)	Supra- and subgenual (BA 24) left	Nissl	↓ Density (LIII, V, VI in BPD but not in MDD); = Size (MDD, BPD)	Not examined	Bouras et al., 2001
BPD (10)/C (12)	Pregenual (BA 24) (no hemisphere specified)	Nissl	↓ Density (27% LII) and ↑ size (LII, III) of nonpyramidal neurons	= Density	Benes et al., 2001

(continued)

Table 14–9. **Morphological Abnormalities in the Cerebral Cortex in Mood Disorders** (*continued*)

Disease (No. of Subjects)	Area; Hemisphere	Methods	Neurons	Glia	Study
MDD (15)/ BPD (15)/C (15)	Supragenual (BA 24) left + right	Nissl	↓ Size (9% LV in MDD and 16% in BPD) ↓ Neuronal clustering in BPD ↑ Density (LV in MDD; LVI in BPD)	↑ Size (13% LI, 10% LII in MDD) = Density (MDD, BPD)	Cotter et al., 2002b
MDD (15)/ BPD (15)/C (15)	Supragenual (BA 24) left + right	CB, PV, CR IHC	↓ Density of CB neurons (LII, BPD) ↑ Clustering of PV neurons in BPD = Density of CB, PV, CR in MDD	Not examined	Cotter et al., 2002a

BA = Brodmann's area; BPD = bipolar disorder; C = control; CB = calbindin; CR = calretinin; DLPFC = dorsolateral prefrontal cortex; f = familial; GFAP = glial fibrillary acidic protein; IHC = immunohistochemistry; L = layer; MDD = major depressive disorder; ORB = orbitofrontal cortex; PV = paravalbumin; ↓, ↑ indicate significantly different from control; = indicates not significantly different from control.

Source: Reproduced with permission from Rajkowska et al., 2004.

changes. Thus research is required to understand whether more rigorously defined subtypes of depression or mood disorders are associated with any particular abnormality (Lenox et al., 2002; Hasler et al., 2006). Nevertheless, the marked reduction in glial cells in these regions has been particularly intriguing. Abnormalities of glial function could thus prove integral to the impairments of structural plasticity and overall pathophysiology of mood disorders.

It must be acknowledged that it is not currently known if these impairments of structural plasticity (cell loss, cell atrophy, white matter changes) constitute developmental abnormalities conferring vulnerability to severe mood episodes, compensatory changes to other pathogenic processes, or the sequelae of recurrent affective episodes (Carlson et al., 2006). Indeed, data suggest that multiple factors may be operative. In support of the potential primary etiologic role of cellular plasticity cascades, some studies have observed reduced gray matter volumes and enlarged ventricles in mood disorder patients at first onset and in children (see Chapter 9). Moreover, in contrast to the situation seen in unipolar patients, studies suggest that some young bipolar patients exhibit white matter hyperintensities on T2-weighted MRI scans. White matter hyperintensities are associated with a number of events, most notably aging and cerebrovascular disorders, thus their presence in some young bipolar patients is noteworthy (since they would not be expected to have overt cerebrovascular disease).

While these studies do not demonstrate that the changes precede illness onset, they certainly suggest that these changes do not simply represent the toxic sequellae of decades of illness. Resolving these issues will depend partly on experiments that delineate the onset of such abnormalities within the illness course and determine whether they precede depressive episodes in individuals at high familial risk for mood disorders. In this context, a recent report showed that individuals at high risk of developing mood disorders exhibited reduced subgenual prefrontal cortical volumes, raising the possibility that this endophenotype may constitute a heritable vulnerability factor in these patients (discussed in Carlson et al., 2006). Additional studies of high-risk individuals are currently under way.

There are, however, data to suggest that some of the brain changes may be associated with duration of illness and the consequences of affective episodes per se. Sheline and colleagues (1996) measured hippocampal volumes of subjects with a history of major depressive episodes but currently in remission and with no known medical comorbidity and compared them to matched normal controls. Subjects with a history of major depression had significantly smaller left and right hippocampal volumes; moreover, the degree of hippocampal volume reduction correlated with total duration of major depression. In a follow-up study, the same research group found that longer durations during which depressive episodes went untreated with antidepressant medication were associated with reductions in hippocampal volume (Sheline et al., 2003). MacQueen and associates (2003) compared 20 never-treated depressed subjects in a first episode of depression with matched healthy control subjects. They also compared 17 depressed subjects with multiple past episodes of depression with matched healthy controls and with the first-episode patients. Notably, although both first- and multiple-episode depressed groups (who were therefore part of the manic-depressive spectrum) had hippocampal dysfunction apparent on several tests of recollection memory, only depressed subjects with multiple depressive episodes had hippocampal volume reductions (MacQueen et al., 2003). Finally, curve-fitting analysis revealed a significant logarithmic association between illness duration and hippocampal volume. These data suggest that in unipolar depression, hippocampal volumetric changes may be related to the number and duration of depressive episodes. It is noteworthy that similar changes have not been reported in bipolar patients. While this may represent distinct pathophysiologies, it is our contention that this more likely reflects the fact that, compared to recurrent unipolar patients, most bipolar patients are on neuroprotective mood stabilizers (see below). In studies of other brain regions (subgenual prefrontal cortex or amygdala), bipolar patients do not show atrophic changes when treated chronically with mood stabilizers.

It is perhaps most useful to conceptualize the cell death and atrophy that occur in mood disorders as arising from an impairment of "cellular resiliency." McEwen (2000) has elegantly elaborated on the concept of allostatic load and its potential involvement in mood disorders. Many factors that are essential for survival can, over long time intervals, exact a cost (allostatic load) that can accelerate disease processes (McEwen, 2000). At this point, it is unclear whether the regional cellular atrophy in mood disorders occurs because of the magnitude and duration of biochemical perturbations, an enhanced vulnerability to the deleterious effects of these perturbations (due to genetic factors and/or early life events), or a combination thereof. In this context, a growing body of data demonstrates that early stress can have a major impact on brain development (Graham et al., 1999). Furthermore, while there are undoubtedly genetic contributions (conferring both susceptibility and protection) to the impact of neonatal stresses on brain development, it is noteworthy that it has also been demonstrated that nongenomic transmission can occur across generations not only of maternal behavior but also stress responses (Francis et al., 1999). The possibility that these neurochemical alterations produce a state of neuroendangerment (see above) that contributes to the subsequent development of morphological brain changes in adulthood requires further investigation. A growing body of data is also demonstrating a relationship (potentially bidirectional) between mood disorders and cardiovascular and cerebrovascular disease (see Chapter 7), suggesting that at least in a subset of patients (perhaps those who have been "primed" for impairments of cellular resiliency by genetic factors), CNS vascular insufficiency may be a contributory factor.[77]

Overall, it seems likely that the impairments of cellular plasticity represent both etiologic factors and the consequence of disease progression. Furthermore, there is almost no doubt that these atrophic brain changes contribute to illness pathophysiology by disrupting the circuits that mediate normal affective, cognitive, motoric and neurovegetative functioning. We now turn to one of the most exciting recent advances in manic-depressive illness research—the observations that neurotrophic signaling cascades represent the targets for mood-stabilizing agents.

Neurotrophic Signaling Cascades: Critical Targets in Treatment

Neurotrophins are a family of regulatory factors that mediate the differentiation and survival of neurons, as well as the modulation of synaptic transmission and synaptic plasticity. They can be secreted constitutively or transiently, and often in an activity-dependent manner. Recent observations support a model in which neurotrophins are secreted from the dendrite and act retrogradely at presynaptic terminals to induce long-lasting modifications. Within the neurotrophin family, BDNF is a potent physiological survival factor that has also been implicated in a variety of pathophysiological conditions. The cellular actions of BDNF are mediated through two types of receptors: a high-affinity tyrosine receptor kinase (TrkB) and a low-affinity pan-neurotrophin receptor (p75). TrkB is preferentially activated by BDNF and NT4/5, and it appears to mediate most of the cellular responses to these neurotrophins.

BDNF and other neurotrophic factors are necessary for the survival and function of neurons, which implies that a sustained reduction of these factors could affect neuronal viability. What is sometimes less appreciated, however, is the fact that BDNF also has a number of much more acute effects on synaptic plasticity and neurotransmitter release and facilitates the release of glutamate, GABA, DA, and serotonin.[78]

As discussed earlier, BDNF is best known for its long-term neurotrophic and neuroprotective effects, which may be very important for its putative role in the pathophysiology and treatment of mood disorders. In this context, it is noteworthy that although endogenous neurotrophic factors have traditionally been viewed as increasing cell survival by providing necessary trophic support, it is now clear that their survival-promoting effects are mediated largely by inhibition of cell death cascades. Increasing evidence suggests that neurotrophic factors inhibit cell death cascades by activating the extracellular receptor-coupled kinase (ERK) MAPK signaling pathway (Chen and Manji, 2006). The best characterized molecular mechanisms of this pathway include upregulation of expression of anti-apoptotic proteins such as B-cell CLL/lymphoma/leukemia-2 (Bcl-2) through a transcriptional mechanism, direct phosphorylation-inactivation of pro-apoptotic proteins such as BAD, and direct phosphorylation-inactivation of key enzymes in the apoptosis process such as caspase-9. Many of these pathways converge at the level of mitochondrial function. We now turn to a discussion of the possibility of neurotrophic signaling-mediated mitochondrial dysfunction in bipolar disorder.

Neurotrophic-Signaling-Mediated Mitochondrial Function

Kato and colleagues anticipated recent developments in the field when they first proposed that mitochondrial dysfunction may play an important role in the pathophysiology of bipolar disorder (Kato and Kato, 2000; Murashita et al., 2000; Kato, 2001). Since then, findings of a host of human neuroimaging and postmortem brain studies, as well as preclinical molecular and cellular biology studies, have strongly supported the contention that mitochondria play a central role in the impairments of plasticity and cellular resilience manifest in bipolar disorder.

It is not our contention that bipolar disorder is a classic mitochondrial disorder. Individuals with mitochondrial dysfunction often manifest psychiatric symptoms, but the vast majority of bipolar patients do not show the symptoms of classic mitochondrial disorders, such as optic and retinal atrophy, seizures, dementia, ataxia, myopathy, exercise intolerance, cardiac conduction defects, diabetes, and lactic acidosis (Fadic and Johns, 1996).

Studies of fibroblasts from patients with mitochondrial encephalomyopathy, lactic acidosis, and stroke-like episodes (MELAS, frequently caused by a mutation in the mitochondrial transfer RNA) have shown an elevated basal level of ionized Ca^{2+}, with impairments in normal sequestration of Ca^{2+} influxes induced by depolarization and alterations in maintaining normal mitochondrial membrane potentials (Moudy et al., 1995; Rothman, 1999). This inability to buffer intracellular Ca^{2+} may cause toxic cell injury and compromise the long-term viability of neurons in patients with mitochondrial encephalomyopathies. It is thus clear that dysregulation of Ca^{2+} homeostasis is an essential component of the pathophysiology of classic mitochondriopathies. As discussed above, calcium is a very common signaling element and plays a critical role in the CNS by regulating the activity of diverse enzymes and facilitating neurotransmitter release (Szabo et al., 2003). Excessively high levels of calcium are also a critical mediator of cell death cascades within neurons, necessitating diverse homeostatic mechanisms to regulate intracellular calcium levels very precisely.

Interestingly, impaired regulation of Ca^{2+} cascades has been found to be the most reproducible biological measure of abnormalities described in research on bipolar disorder. For this reason, mechanisms involved in Ca^{2+} regulation have been postulated to underlie aspects of the pathophysiology of bipolar disorder. To date, 15 studies have consistently revealed elevations in basal intracellular Ca^{2+} levels in platelets, lymphocytes, or neutrophils of patients with bipolar disorder. By contrast, there have been only four negative studies. Although this may partly represent publication bias, elevation in basal Ca^{2+} represents one of the most replicated findings in research on bipolar disorder. More exaggerated platelet intracellular Ca^{2+} elevations have also been found in bipolar patients in response to stimulation with thrombin, platelet-activator factor (PAF), serotonin, DA, and thapsigargin (see Tables 14–5 and 14–6).

Most recently, Kato and colleagues (2003) investigated cytosolic and mitochondrial Ca^{2+} responses to PAF, carbonyl cyanide m-chlorophenylhydrazone (CCCP) (a mitochondrial uncoupler that abolishes mitochondrial Ca^{2+} uptake), and thapsigargin in lymphoblastoid cells from bipolar subjects. They found that the thapsigargin-induced cytosolic Ca^{2+} response was significantly higher in patients with bipolar disorder, a result not seen when the effects of Ca^{2+} influx from outside the plasma membrane were eliminated with a Ca^{2+}-free measurement buffer. By contrast, response to thapsigargin tended to be higher in patients with bipolar disorder when in the Ca^{2+}-free condition. Furthermore, CCCP-induced Ca^{2+} responses differed significantly between mitochondrial DNA 5178/10398 haplotypes that had previously been reported to be associated with bipolar disorder (Kato et al., 2003).

Taken together, these results clearly suggest that the mitochondrial–endoplasmic reticulum (ER) calcium regulation system contributes to the Ca^{2+} abnormalities seen in bipolar disorder. In an elegant series of recent studies, Kakiuchi and colleagues (2003) identified XBP1, a pivotal gene in the ER stress response, as contributing to the genetic risk for bipolar disorder. Using DNA microarray analysis of lymphoblastoid cells derived from two pairs of twins discordant with respect to the illness, they found downregulated expression of genes related to ER stress response in both affected twins. Furthermore, polymorphism (−116C→G) in the promoter region of XBP1, affecting the putative binding site of XBP1, was not only significantly more common in Japanese patients but also overtransmitted to affected offspring in trio samples of the NIMH Bipolar Disorder Genetics Initiative. This research group further showed that XBP1-dependent transcription activity of the −116G allele was lower than that of the −116C allele, and furthermore, in cells with the G allele, induction of XBP1 expression after ER stress was markedly reduced (Kakiuchi et al., 2003). Finally, it was found that valproate at therapeutically relevant concentrations rescued the impaired response by inducing ATF6, the gene upstream of XBP1.

Overall, these findings are of great importance in view of the growing body of evidence demonstrating the potential toxic effects of elevated intracellular Ca^{2+} in neuronal and glial cerebral cells. In fact, it has been demonstrated that both the subcellular compartmentalization of Ca^{2+} and the source of the Ca^{2+} may be greater determinants of neurotoxicity than the absolute intracellular Ca^{2+} levels per se (Sapolsky, 2000b), and that there are major relationships between Ca^{2+} released from IP_3-sensitive ER stores and mitochondrial Ca^{2+} uptake (Mattson et al., 2000). As discussed in Chapter 15, there is also a growing body of data from neuroimaging and postmortem studies demonstrating impairments of cellular plasticity and resilience in recurrent mood disorders.

Konradi and colleagues (2004) undertook an elegant series of postmortem brain microarray studies, providing additional evidence for mitochondrial dysregulation processes in bipolar disorder. They found that nuclear mRNA coding for mitochondrial proteins was decreased in bipolar disorder compared with schizophrenia. These findings involved expression of genes regulating oxidative phosphorylation in the mitochondrial inner membrane and the ATP-dependent process of proteasome degradation. Most recently, Benes and associates (2006) performed a post hoc analysis of an extant gene expression profiling database obtained from the hippocampus using a novel methodology with improved sensitivity. Postmortem brain tissue from bipolar disorder patients showed a marked upregulation of 19 out of 44 apoptosis genes; by contrast, the schizophrenia patients showed a downregulation of genes associated with apoptotic injury and death. Additionally, antioxidant genes showed a marked downregulation in bipolar disorder patients, suggesting that accumulation of free radicals might occur in the setting of a previously reported decrease of the electron transport chain in this disorder. Notably, the changes seen in bipolar disorder and schizophrenia patients did not appear to be related to exposure to either neuroleptics or mood stabilizers.

Since a growing body of indirect clinical, genetic and neuroimaging studies implicate mitochondrial dysfunction in the pathophysiology of bipolar disorder and schizophrenia, Kakiuchi and colleagues (2005) assessed mtDNA deletion(s) by comparing the copy number of two regions in mtDNA—nd1 and nd4—by means of real-time quantitative

PCR in the frontal cortex of 84 subjects (30 control, 27 with bipolar disorder, and 27 with schizophrenia). Although they observed no association between mtDNA deletions and the two major mental disorders in the frontal cortex, they found that the relative amount of mtDNA decreased with age in bipolar disorder ($p = .016$); these results suggest inherited or acquired abnormalities in the system maintaining replication of mtDNA may play a role in the pathophysiology of bipolar disorder.

We have outlined here evidence to support the contention that neurotrophic signaling (and its downstream effects on mitochondrial function) is integral to many facets of bipolar disorder. It needs to be reiterated that although some studies suggest a parent-of-origin effect, we are not suggesting that bipolar disorder is a classic mitochondrial disorder, rather, that many of the upstream abnormalities (likely nuclear genome codes) converge to regulate mitochondrial function implicated in both abnormalities of neurotransmitter synaptic plasticity and long-term cellular resilience. Indeed, Stork and Renshaw (2005) have also posited that the many facets of the complex neurobiology of bipolar disorder can be fit into a more cohesive bioenergetic and neurochemical model. Specifically—similar to what we are proposing here—they propose that the existence of mitochondrial dysfunction in bipolar disorder involves impaired oxidative phosphorylation, a resultant shift toward glycolytic energy production, a decrease in total energy production and/or substrate availability, and altered phospholipid metabolism.

How then is one to conceptualize neurotrophic signaling and mitochondrial-associated impairments of cellular plasticity and resilience in the pathophysiology and treatment of severe mood disorders (bipolar disorder and major depression)? There is growing appreciation of the diverse functions that mitochondria play in regulating integrated CNS function. Mitochondria are intracellular organelles best known for their critical roles in regulating energy production via oxidative phosphorylation, regulation of intracellular Ca^{2+}, and mediation of apoptosis. However, increasing evidence suggests that mitochondria may be integrally involved in the general processes of synaptic plasticity. Indeed, increased synaptic activity has been shown to induce the expression of mitochondrial-encoded genes, indicating that the regulation of metabolism is an important component in the long-term regulation of synaptic strength. All in all, these findings suggest that mitochondrial Ca^{2+} sequestration has a key role in modulating the tone of synaptic plasticity in a variety of neuroanatomical regions, including those implicated in the pathophysiology of anxiety disorders. Regulation of mitochondrial function is likely to play important roles in regulating synaptic strength and in neuronal circuitry–mediating complex behaviors. In support of this contention, Hovatta and associates (2005) have

used a combination of behavioral analysis of six inbred mouse strains with quantitative gene expression profiling of several brain regions. Intriguingly, they found that genes involved in oxidative stress metabolism were related to complex affective behaviors. Together, these results suggest that the mitochondrially mediated impairments of plasticity observed in bipolar disorder may have ramifications for not only long-term disease progression, course of illness, and functional impairments but also "here-and-now" symptomatology. Indeed, it has recently been demonstrated that short-term lithium-induced increases in subgenual prefrontal cortex gray matter were related to treatment response (see below). These observations raise the interesting possibility that enhancing mitochondrial vigor may represent an important adjunctive strategy for the optimal long-term treatment of bipolar disorder and perhaps of highly recurrent depression as well. Novel molecular targets to improve mitochondrial function include pharmacological attempts to bypass defects in the respiratory chain, scavenging excessive oxygen radicals and enhancers of mitochondrial membrane stabilization, including, theoretically, inhibitors of the permeability transition pore (PTP). In addition, strategies already being investigated or under consideration include MAPK phosphatase inhibitors that increase expression of the anti-apoptotic protein Bcl-2, presynaptic glutamate receptor subtypes that attenuate glutamate release, AMPA potentiators that increase BDNF expression, and NMDA antagonists that enhance cellular plasticity.

Next we discuss the consistent body of data demonstrating that mood stabilizers (most notably lithium and valproate) robustly regulate the expression and function of genes and proteins associated with major roles in neuronal plasticity and resilience.

Activation of the Extracellular Receptor-Coupled Kinase Signaling Cascade by Lithium and Valproate

In view of the important role of the ERK signaling cascade in mediating long-term neuroplastic events (see Fig. 14–20), a series of studies has been undertaken to investigate the effects of lithium and valproate on this signaling cascade.[79] These studies have shown that lithium and valproate, at therapeutically relevant concentrations, robustly activate the ERK MAPK cascade in human neuroblastoma SH-SY5Y cells (Yuan et al., 2001; Chen et al., 2002). Follow-up studies have recently shown that, similar to the effects observed in neuroblastoma cells in vitro, chronic lithium and valproate also robustly increase the levels of activated ERK in areas of brain that have been implicated in the pathophysiology and treatment of bipolar disorder—the anterior cingulate cortex and hippocampus (Chen et al., 2002; Einat et al., 2003b; Hao et al., 2004). In animal behavioral studies it was found that chemical inhibition of the brain

Neurotrophins and the ERK MAP Kinase Signaling Cascade

Figure 14–20. The influence of neurotrophic factors on cell survival, as mediated by activation of the mitogen-activated protein (MAP) kinase cascade. Activation of neurotrophic factor receptors, also referred to as Trks, results in activation of the MAP kinase cascade via several intermediate steps, including phosphorylation of the adaptor protein SHC and recruitment of the guanine nucleotide exchange factor SOS. This results in activation of the small guanosine triphosphate–binding protein Ras, which leads to activation of a cascade of serine/threonine kinases. This includes Raf, MAP kinase kinase (MEK), and MAP kinase (also referred to as extracellular response kinase, or ERK). Ras also activates the PI$_3$ kinase pathway, a primary target of which is the enzyme glycogen synthase kinase (GSK-3). Activation of the PI$_3$ kinase pathway deactivates GSK-3. GSK-3 has multiple targets in cells including transcription factors (β-catenin and C-Jun) and cytoskeletal elements such as tau. Many of the targets of GSK-3 are pro-apoptotic when activated. Thus, deactivation of GSK-3 via activation of the PI$_3$ kinase pathway results in neurotrophic effects. Lithium inhibits GSK-3 and this may be partially responsible for lithium's psychotrophic effects. One target of the MAP kinase cascade is RSK, which influences cell survival in at least two ways. Rsk phosphorylates and inactivates the pro-apoptotic factor BAD. RSK also phosphorylates CREB and thereby increases the expression of the anti-apoptotic factor Bcl-2 and brain-derived neurotrophic factor (BDNF). (*Source*: Manji et al., 2003a.)

ERK pathway in rats reduces immobility in the forced swim test and increased locomotive and explorative activity in the large open field test. These studies also showed that ERK1 (one of two ERK subtypes) knockout mice have brain region-specific functional deficits of the ERK pathway and exhibit reduced immobility in the forced swim test, increased activity in the open field test, persistently increased home-cage wheel running activity for at least 30

days, and enhanced response to psychostimulants (reviewed in Chen and Manji, 2006). Very recent studies have therefore examined the role of the ERK pathway as a behavioral modulator in left anterior cingulate cortex, one of the brain regions being implicated in the pathophysiology of mood disorders by human brain imaging and postmortem studies (Chen and Manji, 2006). Rats chronically infused with an ERK pathway inhibitor directly to left anterior cingulate cortex showed significant reduction of immobility in the forced swim test, increase in locomotive activities in the open field test, and enhancement of locomotive response to amphetamine. To further verify these findings, a method was developed to regionally express dominant negative ERK1 (to inhibit function of endogenous ERK) in left anterior cingulate cortex by injection of lentiviral vectors. Compared to the controls, rats injected with a dominant negative ERK1 expression vector showed reduced immobility in the forced swim test, significant increases in activity in the open field test, significant increases in numbers of arm entries (without changing overall time spent in either open or closed arms) in the elevated plus maze test, and a significantly higher response to amphetamine. These rats also consumed more sweetened water in the sucrose and saccharin preference tests than did control rats. Taken together, this body of data supports the role of the anterior cingulate in modulation of behaviors relevant to mood disorders; furthermore, the ERK pathway in the left anterior cingulate cortex is one of the intracellular loops of neuronal circuitry that mediates hedonic and locomotive and explorative activities.

As dicussed above, one of the major downstream targets of the ERK MAP kinase cascades is arguably one of the most important neuroprotective proteins, Bcl-2. Bcl-2 is the acronym for the B-cell lymphoma/leukemia-2 gene. This gene was first discovered because of its involvement in B-cell malignancies, where chromosomal translocations activate the gene in the majority of follicular non-Hodgkin's B-cell lymphomas (discussed in Manji et al., 1999b, and references therein). Although the precise mechanisms of action of Bcl-2 are unknown, it is now clear that Bcl-2 is a protein that inhibits both apoptotic and necrotic cell death induced by diverse stimuli. Indeed, it is likely that Bcl-2 is very effective against diverse insults because many different several cellular mechanisms are involved in its protective effects; these likely include sequestering of the proforms of caspases, inhibition of the effects of caspase activation, antioxidant effects, enhancemenet of mitochondrial calcium uptake, and attenuation of the release of calcium and cytochrome c from mitochondria (reviewed in Adams and Cory, 1998).

A role for Bcl-2 in protecting neurons from cell death is now supported by abundant evidence; Bcl-2 has been shown to protect neurons from a variety of insults in vitro including growth factor deprivation, glucocorticoids, ionizing radiation, and oxidant stressors such as hydrogen peroxide, tert-butylhydroperoxide, reactive oxygen species, and buthionine sulfoxamine (Adams and Cory, 1998; Bruckheimer et al., 1998). In addition to these potent in vitro effects, Bcl-2 has also been shown to prevent cell death in numerous studies in vivo. In the absence of pharmacological

means of increasing CNS Bcl-2 expression until recently (see below), all the studies up to this time have used transgenic mouse models or viral vector–mediated delivery of the Bcl-2 gene into the CNS. In these models, Bcl-2 overexpression has been shown to prevent motor neuron death induced by facial nerve axotomy and sciatic nerve axotomy, save retinal ganglion cells from axotomy-induced death, protect against the deleterious effects of MPTP or focal ischemia, and protect photoreceptor cells from two forms of inherited retinal degeneration. Interestingly, neurons that survive ischemic lesions or traumatic brain injury in vivo show upregulation of Bcl-2.[80] Overexpression of Bcl-2 has also been shown to prolong survival and attenuate motor neuron degeneration in a transgenic animal model of amyotrophic lateral sclerosis (Kostic et al., 1997).

Most recently, it has been clearly demonstrated that not only does Bcl-2 overexpression protect against apoptotic and necrotic cell death, it can also promote *regeneration* of axons in the mammalian CNS, leading to the intriguing postulate that Bcl-2 acts as a major regulatory switch for a genetic program that controls the *growth* of CNS axons (Chen et al., 1997). Since Bcl-2 has also recently been shown to promote neurite sprouting, it has been convincingly argued that increasing CNS Bcl-2 levels may represent a very effective therapeutic strategy for the treatment of many neurodegenerative diseases (Chen et al., 1997). As articulated already, the only means of therapeutically increasing CNS Bcl-2 levels in the adult brain has been by the use of complex gene transfer methodologies. Thus pharmacological means of robustly increasing CNS Bcl-2 levels represents a major potential advance for the long-term treatment of certain neurodegenerative disorders. In the next section we discuss the exciting findings demonstrating that Bcl-2 is robustly increased by lithium and valproate.

Robustly Increased Expression of Bcl-2 with Lithium and Valproate

Chronic treatment of rats with therapeutic doses of lithium and valproate produced a doubling of Bcl-2 levels in the frontal cortex, effects due primarily to a marked increase in the number of Bcl-2-immunoreactive cells in layers II and III of the anterior cingulated cortex (Chen et al., 1999; Manji et al., 1999a, 2000a; see Fig. 14–21). Interestingly, the importance of neurons in the anterior cingulate has recently been emphasized, since these areas are important for providing connections with other cortical regions and are targets for subcortical input (Chapter 9). Chronic lithium was also found to markedly increase the number of Bcl-2 immunoreactive cells in the dentate gyrus and striatum (Manji et al., 1999b), and detailed immunohistochemical studies following chronic valproate treatment are currently under way.

Saline Control

Valproate

Lithium

Bcl-2 Peptide Blocking

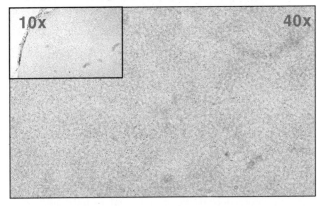

Figure 14–21. Effects of chronic lithium and valproate treatment on Bcl-2 immunolabeling in frontal cortex. Rats were chronically treated with saline, lithium, or valproate, and immunohistochemistry of Bcl-2 was performed in parallel for each of the groups. Chronic lithium and valproate treatment resulted in a doubling of Bcl-2 levels in FCx. (*Source*: Manji et al., 1999b. Reprinted with permission.)

Subsequent to these findings, lithium was demonstrated to increase Bcl-2 levels in C57BL/6 mice (Chen et al., 1999), human neuroblastoma SH-SY5Y cells in vitro (Manji and Chen, 2000), and rat cerebellar granule cells in vitro (Chen and Chuang, 1999). This latter work was undertaken as part of research investigating the molecular and cellular mechanisms underlying the neuroprotective actions of lithium against glutamate excitotoxicity (see below). The investigators found that lithium produced a remarkable increase in Bcl-2 protein and mRNA levels. Moreover, lithium was found to reduce levels of the pro-apoptotic protein p53 in both cerebellar granule cells (Chen and Chuang, 1999) and SH-SY5Y cells (Lu et al., 1999).

Overall, then, the data clearly show that chronic lithium exposure robustly increases levels of the neuroprotective protein Bcl-2 in areas of rodent frontal cortex, hippocampus, and striatum in vivo, and in cultured cells of both rodent and human neuronal origin in vitro. Furthermore, at least in cultured cell systems, lithium has been demonstrated to reduce levels of the pro-apoptotic protein p53. Most recently, it has been demonstrated that repeated ECT significantly increases precursor cell proliferation in the dentate gyrus of the adult monkey, effects that appear to be due to increased expression of Bcl-2 (Perera et al., submitted). These results suggest that stimulation of neurogenesis and enhanced expression of Bcl-2 may contribute to the therapeutic actions of ECT. Behavioral studies have also been undertaken to determine if Bcl-2 plays a role in the pathogenesis and treatment of depression (Yuan et al., 2005). Bcl-2 +/− mice and wild-type littermates were studied in the learned helplessness paradigm. Bcl-2 +/− mice and wild-type littermates were also treated with antidepressant citalopram (10 mg/kg/day) acutely and chronically, and responses in the tail suspension and learned helplessness tests were examined. In the learned helplessness test, there was a significantly higher rate of escape failures in the Bcl-2+/− mice. Furthermore, while chronic citalopram increased escape failures in the wild-type mice, it was without effect in the Bcl-2 +/− mice. Similarly, citalopram was effective in the tail suspension test but was without effect in the Bcl-2 +/– mice. These data demonstrate that Bcl-2 +/– mice are insensitive to the SSRI antidepressant citalopram in two animal models of depression, indicating that some of the therapeutic effects of antidepressants may be mediated through actions of Bcl-2. In total, these observations suggest that regulation of Bcl-2-mediated plasticity is likely to play important roles in regulating synaptic strength and neuronal circuitry–mediating complex behaviors (Yuan and Manji, unpublished observations).

Neuroprotective Effects of Lithium: Compelling Preclinical Evidence

Lithium's robust effects on Bcl-2 and GSK-3β in the mature CNS indicate that it may possess significant neuroprotective properties. Indeed, several studies conducted before the identification of Bcl-2 or GSK-3β as targets for lithium's actions had already demonstrated the drug's neuroprotective properties.[81] The protective effects of lithium have been investigated in a number of in vitro studies, particularly those using rat cerebellar granule cells, PC12 cells, and human neuroblastoma SH-SY5Y cells. In these studies, lithium was shown to protect against the deleterious effects of glutamate, NMDA receptor activation, low potassium, and toxic concentrations of anticonvulsants (see Box 14–17). Lithium also protected PC12 cells from serum and nerve growth factor deprivation (Volonte and Rubenstein, 1993), protected both PC12 cells and human neuroblastoma SH-SY5Y cells from ouabain toxicity (Li et al., 1994), and protected SH-SY5Y cells from cell death induced by both thapsigargin (which mobilizes intracellular Ca^{2+}) and MPP^+. Most recently, lithium has been shown to protect cultured neurons from beta-amyloid-induced cell death (Alvarez et al., 1999) and to protect against the deleterious effects of GSK-3fl overexpression coupled with staurosporine addition (Bijur et al., 2000).

In addition to studies demonstrating lithium's protective effects in vitro, there have been a number of investigations of its neuroprotective effects in vivo. In this context, the effects of lithium on the biochemical and behavioral manifestations of excitotoxic lesions of the cholinergic system have been investigated (Pascual and Gonzalez, 1995; Arendt et al., 1999). These studies have demonstrated that lithium pretreatment attenuates both the behavioral deficits (passive avoidance and ambulatory behavior) and the reduction in choline acetyl transferase activity associated with forebrain cholinergic system lesions (Pascual and Gonzalez, 1995).[82]

In another study investigating lithium's effects against excitotoxic insults, it was demonstrated that lithium attenuated the kainic acid–induced reduction in glutamate decarboxylase levels and [³H]D-aspartate uptake (Sparapani et al., 1997). Chronic lithium has also been shown to exert dramatic

---

BOX 14–17.   Neurotrophic and Neuroprotective Effects of Lithium

Protects cultured cells of rodent and human neuronal origin in vitro from

- Glutamate, NMDA
- High concentrations of calcium
- MPP^+
- β-amyloid
- Aging-induced cell death
- HIV regulatory protein, Tat
- Glucose deprivation
- Growth factor or serum deprivation
- Toxic concentrations of anticonvulsants
- Platelet activating factor (PAF)
- Aluminum toxicity
- Low K^+
- C2-ceramide
- Ouabain
- GSK-3β + staurosporine/heat shock

Enhances hippocampal neurogenesis in adult mice

Protects rodent brain in vivo from

- Cholinergic lesions
- Radiation injury
- Middle cerebral artery occlusion (stroke model)
- Quinolinic acid (Huntington's model)

Human Effects

- No subgenual prefrontal cortex gray matter volume reductions in cross-sectional MRI studies
- No reductions in amygdala glial density in postmortem cell counting studies
- Increased total gray matter volumes on MRI compared to untreated bipolar disorder patients in cross-sectional studies
- Increased NAA (marker of neuronal viability) levels in bipolar disorder patients in longitudinal studies
- Increased gray matter volumes in bipolar disorder patients in longitudinal studies

Source: Gould and Manji, 2002b.

---

protective effects against middle cerebral artery occlusion, reducing not only the infarct size (by 56 percent) but also the neurological deficits (abnormal posture and hemiplegia) (Nonaka and Chuang, 1998). Most recently, the same group found that chronic in vivo lithium treatment robustly protected neurons in the striatum from quinolinic acid–induced toxicity in a putative model of Huntington's disease (Senatorov et al., 2004; see Fig. 14–22).

In addition to its effects on ERK MAPK, Bcl-2, and GSK-3fl, lithium's effects on other signaling pathways and

Middle Cerebral Artery Occlusion

Quinolinic Acid Infusions

Control

Lithium

Figure 14–22. Chronic lithium protects against quinolic acid (QA)–induced toxicity and against middle cerebral artery occlusion. *Left panel*: Sixteen days of lithium pretreatment decreases the size of QA-induced striatal lesion determined by GAD_{67} mRNA in situ hybridization. Rats (n = 10) were subcutaneously pre-injected with lithium chloride (LiCl) for 16 days and then intrastriatally infused with QA (30 nmol). Control rats (n = 8) received subcutaneous injections of normal saline instead of LiCl. Animals were killed 7 days after QA infusion and brains were sectioned for in situ hybridization using a ^{33}P-labeled antisense oligonucleotide probe complementary to 67 kDa GAD mRNA. Shown here are autoradiograms of GAD_{67} mRNA in situ hybridization from a typical saline control and lithium-pretreated experiment. *Right panel*: Chronic lithium treatment protects against ischemic brain damage in a focal cerebral ischemia model in rats. Representative photomicrographs show ischemic brain damage in a saline-treated control (top) and LiCl-treated rat (bottom) 24 hours after left middle cerebral artery (MCA) occlusion. Note that ischemic damage was observed in the cerebral cortex of the frontal, sensorimotor, and auditory areas and in the lateral segment of the caudate nucleus. Chronic lithium reduced the area of ischemic brain damage. (*Source*: Nonaka and Chuang, 1998; Wei et al., 2001. Reprinted with permission from Lippincott Williams & Wilkins.)

transcription factors (Manji et al., 1995a; Jope, 1999) may contribute to its neuroprotective effects. In this context, it is noteworthy that recent studies have shown that modulation of Akt-1 activity is involved in glutamate excitotoxicity and may play a role in lithium's neuroprotective effects in rat cerebellar granule cells (Chalecka-Franaszek and Chuang, 1999).

Neurotrophic and Neuroprotective Effects of Valproate

Valproate's effects on Bcl-2 and GSK-3fl suggest that this mood stabilizer may also possess neuroprotective/ neurotrophic properties. Additionally, it has been

demonstrated that valproate increases the expression of the molecular chaperone GRP78, a protein that binds Ca^{2+} in the endoplasmic reticulum and protects cells from the deleterious effects of damaged proteins (J. Wang et al., 1999). Although valproate has not been as extensively studied as lithium, a growing body of data suggests that it does indeed exert neuroprotective effects (Bruno et al., 1995; Mark et al., 1995; Mora et al., 1999).

More recent studies have used the SH-SY5Y model system to investigate the protective effects of valproate and lithium. SH-SY5Y cells were incubated with lithium (1.0 mM) or valproate (.6 m) for 3 days. Cells were then exposed to two different toxins—thapsigargin (which mobilizes intracellular calcium; .5 mM for 16 hours) or MPP$^+$ (25 mM for 16 hours). The mitochondrial dehydrogenase activity that cleaves 3-(4,5-dimethylthiazol-2-yl)-2,5-diphenyl tetrazolium bromide (MTT) was used to determine cell survival in a quantitative colorimetric assay. It was found that treatment with lithium and valproate exerted significant protective effects against both toxins.

In an extension of their studies, Ren and colleagues recently sought to determine whether valproate, like lithium, exerts protective effects in a middle cerebral artery occlusion (MCAO) stroke model. They found that post-insult treatment with valproate reduced brain infarct size when measured at 24 or 48 hours after the onset of MCAO-induced ischemia (Ren et al., 2004). Valproate also facilitated functional recovery from neurological deficits under these experimental conditions; these effects occurred at a dose (300 mg/kg) similar to that used in animal studies to control seizures. Valproate-induced neuroprotection was further demonstrated by a reduction in MCAO-induced caspase-3 activation in the ischemic area, as shown by immunohistochemistry and western blotting analysis (Ren et al., 2004). These results suggest that valproate neuroprotection in the MCAO model involves anti-apoptotic actions in the ischemic penumbra. It is noteworthy that lithium-induced neuroprotection in the rat MCAO/reperfusion model is also associated with suppression of ischemia-induced caspase-3 activation (Ren et al., 2003; Xu et al., 2003).

Facilitation of Retinal Ganglion Cell Survival and Axon Regeneration with Lithium

Based on the remarkable neurotrophic and neuroprotective effects of lithium, studies were undertaken to determine whether lithium supports the survival and axon regeneration of retinal ganglion cells (RGCs), a model that has been used to study glaucoma, optic nerve neuritis, and the degeneration of RGCs (Chen et al., 1995, 1997; Quigley et al., 1995). In general, following injury, the postnatal mammalian optic nerve, like many other axonal pathways in the CNS, regenerates poorly; most often, injured RGCs undergo apoptotic cell death (Chen et al., 1995, 1997; Quigley et al., 1995). While this regenerative failure has long been attributed to extrinsic inhibitors in the environment of the mature brain, seminal research by the Chen and Tonegawa group (Chen et al., 1995, 1997) demonstrated that mature RGCs lack an intrinsic component to initiate axonal growth following injury, and that this intrinsic component is the neurotrophic protein Bcl-2. Investigators have therefore postulated that a prerequisite for successful regeneration of severed optic nerves in adult mammals is the activation of an intrinsic regenerative mechanism of RGC axons—namely, the induction of Bcl-2 expression in neurons.

Lithium was the first medication demonstrated to robustly upregulate Bcl-2 in rodent brain in vivo and in cells with a human neuronal phenotype (see above). Furthermore, these effects of lithium occur well within its therapeutic range (indeed, robust effects occur at levels less than those required to treat acute mania). Studies were therefore undertaken to determine whether lithium would not only prevent injury-induced degeneration of RGCs and other CNS neurons but also promote the regeneration of their axons (Huang et al., 2002) (see Fig. 14–23). These studies showed that lithium, acting directly on RGCs, supports both neuronal survival and axon regeneration at its established therapeutic concentrations (.5–1.2 mM) (Huang et al., 2002). These intriguing results not only offer new clues to a better understanding of the regulation of retinal and CNS regeneration but also suggest that lithium may have considerable utility in treating retinal and optic nerve neurodegeneration (e.g., glaucoma and optic nerve neuritis) and conditions involving optic nerve damage and/or RGC loss. In view of lithium's well-established safety profile in humans and the fact that robust effects are observed at well-tolerated levels, clinical trails should be undertaken for treatment of these devastating illnesses.

Increases in Hippocampal Neurogenesis with Lithium

As discussed already, through use of a method for labeling cell division directly in the adult human brain, it has been shown that the dentate gyrus (an area where robust lithium-induced increases in Bcl-2 levels are observed) can produce new neurons during adulthood in humans. A large number of the newborn daughter cells are known to die rapidly, likely through apoptosis (Kempermann and Gage, 1999). Thus increasing Bcl-2 levels could enhance the survival of the newborn cells, allowing them to differentiate into neurons. Additionally, Bcl-2 has been shown to have robust effects on the regeneration of CNS axons (Chen et al., 1997).

Programmed cell death is present in neurogenic regions of the adult brain, and a significant portion of the adult-born cells is eliminated during the first months of maturation. Kuhn and colleagues (2005) therefore investigated if overexpression of the anti-apoptotic protein Bcl-2 would improve the survival of neural progenitor cells and, as a consequence, increase neurogenesis in the adult hippocampus. They found that transgenic animals, which express human Bcl-2 under the neuron-specific enolase promoter (NSE-huBcl-2), show a significant reduction of apoptotic cells in the hippocampal granule cell layer to about half of the wild-type level. Furthermore, they found that the rate of adult neurogenesis is doubled in the dentate gyrus of Bcl-2-overexpressing mice, as demonstrated by quantification of progenitor cells with DCX and of new neurons through bromodeoxyuridine (BrdU)/neuronal nuclei antigen (NeuN) double-labeling.

Figure 14–23. Li$^+$ promotes retinal ganglion cell (RGC) axon regeneration in a dose-dependent manner in culture. *A:* Epifluorescence photomicrographs of representative retina-brain slice cocultures in the absence and presence of lithium chloride (LiCl). Regenerating axons were labeled by placing DiI (a lipophilic fluorescent label) into retinal explants and were visualized by fluorescence microscope. Arrows indicate labeled axons growing into the brain slices. *B, C:* Dose–response curve of Li$^+$ on axon regeneration. *B:* The number of labeled axons extending into the brain slices. *C:* Quantification of the longest distances of axon regeneration into the brain slices, measured from the interfaces of the retinal explants and brain slices. *$p < .05$ compared with control. (*Source:* Huang et al., 2003. Reproduced with permission of *Investigative Ophthalmology and Visual Science.*)

In view of Bcl-2's major neuroprotective and neurotrophic role, a study was undertaken to determine whether lithium, administered at therapeutically relevant concentrations, affects neurogenesis in adult rodent brain. To investigate the effects of chronic lithium on neurogenesis, mice were treated with therapeutic lithium (plasma levels .97±.20 mM) for approximately 4 weeks. After treatment with lithium for 14 days, the mice were administered single doses of BrdU, a thymidine analog that is incorporated into the DNA of dividing cells, for 12 consecutive days. Lithium treatment continued throughout the duration of the BrdU administration. Following BrdU immunohistochemistry (Chen et al., 2000), three-dimensional cell counting was performed with a computer-assisted image analysis system (see Rajkowska, 2000). This system is based on the optical disector method and estimates the number of cells independent of section thickness and cell shape. It was found that chronic lithium administration does in fact result in an increase in the number of BrdU-positive cells in the dentate gyrus (Chen et al., 2000) (see Fig. 14–24). Moreover, approximately two-thirds of the BrdU-positive

cells also double-stained with the neuronal marker NeuN, confirming their neuronal identity. Double-staining of BrdU and Bcl-2 was also observed; studies with Bcl-2 transgenic animals are currently under way to delineate the role of Bcl-2 overexpression in the enhanced hippocampal neurogenesis. These results have also been replicated by Kim and associates (2004), who have demonstrated that lithium selectively increases neuronal differentiation of hippocampal neural progenitor cells both in vitro and in vivo. Most recently, Perera and colleagues (2006, submitted) examined the effects of repeated electroconvulsive shock (the animal model of ECT) on dentate neurogenesis in nonhuman primates. Similar to the effects observed with chronic lithium (see above), they found that ECS-induced neurogenesis was accompanied by increases in Bcl-2 levels.

The ability of valproate to promote neurogenesis from embryonic rat cortical or striatal primordial stem cells was recently examined; 6 days of valproate increased by up to five-fold the number and percentage of tubulin β III–immunopositive neurons, increased neurite outgrowth, and decreased by five-fold the number of astrocytes

Figure 14–24. Effects of chronic lithium neurogenesis in the dentate gyrus of adult mice. C57BL/6 mice were treated with lithium for 14 days and then received once-daily bromodeoxyuridine (BrdU) injections for 12 consecutive days while lithium treatment continued. Twenty-four hours after the last injection, the brains were processed for BrdU immunohistochemistry. Cell counts were performed in the hippocampal dentate gyrus at three levels along the dorsoventral axis in all the animals. BrdU-positive cells were counted using unbiased stereological methods. Chronic lithium produced a significant 25% increase in BrdU immunolabeling in both right and left dentate gyrus (*p* < .05). Many BrdU-labeled neurons also stained with NeuN, a neuron-specific marker. (*Source*: Chen et al., 2000; Gray et al., 2003. Reprinted with permission from Blackwell Publishing Ltd.)

Figure 14–25. Valproate promotes neurite growth in a time- and concentration-dependent manner. The photographs from a representative experiment were taken after 1-, 4-, 8-day treatments with valproate (VPA). Data shown in bar graph are mean ± standard error of 30–100 cells measured in the photographs. Similar results were obtained from two additional independent experiments. Arrow in right panel indicates growth cone. (*Source*: Adapted from Yuan et al., 2001. Reproduced with permission of American Society for Biochemistry and Molecular Biology.)

without changing the number of cells (Laeng et al., 2004). Valproate also promoted neuronal differentiation in human fetal forebrain stem cell cultures. Intriguingly, the neurogenic effects of valproate on rat stem cells exceeded those obtained with BDNF or NT-3. Similar effects were observed with lithium, but not carbamazepine. Most of the newly formed neurons were GABAergic, as shown by 10-fold increases in neurons that immunostained for GABA and the GABA-synthesizing enzyme GAD65/67. The enhancement of GABAergic neuron numbers, neurite outgrowth, and phenotypic expression via increases in the neuronal differentiation of neural stem cells may contribute to the therapeutic effects of valproate in the treatment of bipolar disorder. (Figure 14–25 shows valproate's promotion of neurite outgrowth.)

Increased N-acetylaspartate and Gray Matter with Lithium

To investigate the potential neurotrophic effects of lithium in humans more definitively, a longitudinal clinical study was undertaken with proton MRS to quantitate N-acetylaspartate (NAA) levels. NAA is a putative neuronal marker, localized to mature neurons and not found in mature glial cells, CSF, or blood. A number of studies have now shown that initial abnormally low brain NAA measures may increase and even normalize with remission

of CNS symptoms in disorders such as demyelinating disease, amyotrophic lateral sclerosis, mitochondrial encephalopathies, and HIV dementia. NAA is synthesized within mitochondria, and inhibitors of the mitochondrial respiratory chain decrease NAA concentrations, effects that correlate with reductions in ATP and oxygen consumption (Manji et al., 2000a). Thus, NAA is now generally regarded as a measure of neuronal viability and function, rather than strictly as a marker for neuronal loss per se (for an excellent review of NAA, see Tsai and Coyle, 1995).

It has been found that chronic lithium administration at therapeutic doses increases NAA concentration in the human brain in vivo (Moore et al., 2000). This finding provides intriguing indirect support for the contention that, similar to observations in rodent brain and in human neuronal cells in culture, chronic lithium increases neuronal viability and function in the human brain. Furthermore, a striking correlation of approximately .97 between lithium-induced NAA increases and regional voxel gray matter content was observed (Moore et al., 2000), thereby providing evidence for colocalization with the region-specific Bcl-2 increases observed (e.g., gray versus white matter) in rodent brain cortices. These results suggest that chronic lithium may exert not only robust neuroprotective effects (as has been demonstrated in a variety of preclinical paradigms) but also neurotrophic effects in humans (see Fig. 14–26).

In follow-up studies to the above work on NAA, it was hypothesized that, in addition to increasing functional neurochemical markers of neuronal viability, lithium-induced increases in Bcl-2 would lead to neuropil increases and thus to increased brain gray matter volume in bipolar patients. In this clinical investigation, brain tissue volumes were examined with high-resolution three-dimensional MRI and validated quantitative brain tissue segmentation methodology to identify and quantify the various components by volume, including total brain white and gray matter content. Measurements were made at baseline (medication-free, after a minimum 14-day washout) and then repeated after 4 weeks of lithium at therapeutic doses. This study showed that chronic lithium significantly increases total gray matter content in the human brain of patients with bipolar disorder (see Fig. 14–27). No significant changes were observed in brain white matter volume or in quantitative measures of regional cerebral water content, thereby providing strong evidence that the observed increases in gray matter content are due to neurotrophic effects and not to any possible cell swelling and/or osmotic effects associated with lithium treatment. Most recently, to investigate the clinical significance of these findings, a longitudinal study was performed exploring neurotrophic effects of the mood stabilizer lithium via high-resolution volumetric MRI in well-characterized bipolar depressed subjects (n = 28) at baseline (medication-free) and following chronic lithium administration (4 weeks) (Moore et al., 2006). Total brain gray matter, prefrontal gray matter, and left subgenual prefrontal gray matter were determined by means of validated semiautomated segmentation and region-of-interest methodology. Significant increases in total brain gray matter in bipolar subjects were observed following chronic lithium administration, confirming the previous preliminary study. Regional analyses in the bipolar subjects revealed significant differences between responders (greater than 50 percent decrease in HAM-D) and nonresponders; only responders showed increases in gray matter in the prefrontal cortex and left subgenual prefrontal cortex (Moore et al., 2006). The increase in gray matter in these areas that are specifically implicated in the neuropathophysiology of bipolar disorder in various neuroimaging and postmortem neuropathology investigations suggests that the observed effects may be linked to clinical response. The findings also support the notion that future development of treatments more directly targeting molecules in critical CNS pathways regulating cellular plasticity hold promise as novel, improved long-term treatments for mood disorders (see Fig. 14–28).

It is striking that lithium has such robust effects on the cytoprotective protein Bcl-2, exerts neuroprotective effects in

Figure 14–26. Mechanism by which lithium may increase *N*-acetyl-aspartate (NAA) levels. Lithium, via its effects on Bcl-2 and glycogen synthase kinase 3β (GSK-3β), may exert major neurotrophic effects, resulting in neuropil increases, accompanied by increases in NAA levels. ERK = extracellular receptor-coupled kinase. (*Source*: Manji et al., 2000b. Reprinted with permission from Elsevier.)

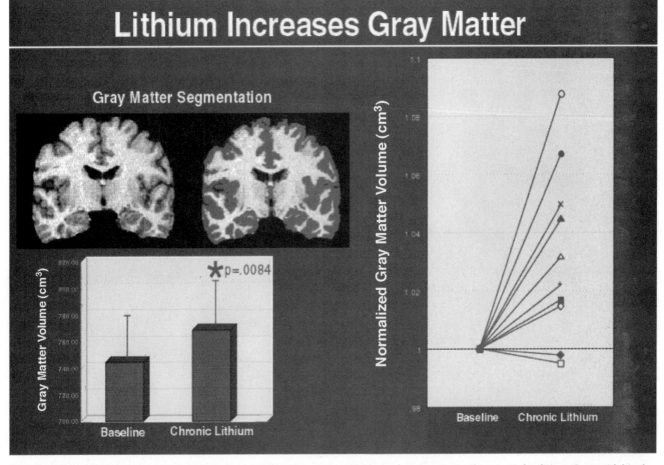

Figure 14–27. Brain gray matter volume is increased following 4 weeks of lithium administration at therapeutic levels in patients with bipolar disorder. Brain tissue volumes were examined by means of high-resolution three-dimensional MRI and validated quantitative brain tissue segmentation methodology to identify and quantify the various components by volume, including total brain white and gray matter content. Measurements were made at baseline (medication-free, after a minimum 14-day washout) and then repeated after 4 weeks of lithium at therapeutic doses. Chronic lithium significantly increases total gray matter content in the human brain of patients with bipolar disorder. No significant changes were observed in brain white matter volume or in quantitative measures of regional cerebral water. (*Source*: Gould and Manji, 2002b. Reprinted by permission of SAGE Publications, Inc.)

a variety of paradigms, and actually increases gray matter volume in humans. These exciting results suggest that lithium may have utility in the treatment of a variety of neuropsychiatric disorders associated with cell atrophy and loss and impairment of cellular resilience. One obvious concern, however, is lithium's tolerability, especially in patients with neurodegenerative disorders. A series of studies was therefore undertaken to determine whether the chronic administration of lithium at low doses also regulates Bcl-2 expression. These studies found that chronic lithium administration (4 weeks) at doses that produce plasma levels of approximately .35 mM (below the threshold for CNS-mediated side effects) robustly increased Bcl-2 levels in rat frontal cortex and hippoxampus (see Fig. 14–29) and hippocampus. Furthermore, there is accumulating evidence suggesting that lithium exerts neuroprotective effects at low doses. Thus, 0.5 mM lithium has been shown to protect cultured cerebellar gran-

ule cells from glutamate excitotoxicity and to decrease levels of the pro-apoptotic protein p53. In middle cerebral artery occlusion, an in vivo model of stroke, lithium has also been shown to offer significant protection at .5 milliequivalents (mEq)/kg. Of particular interest, a recent study demonstrated that cortical neurons are even more potently protected from excitotoxicity, with significant increases in viability occurring as low as .1 mM. Overall, the data clearly suggest that lower than traditional antimanic doses of lithium have neurotrophic and neuroprotective effects, and may thus have utility as adjunctive treatment for neuropsychiatric disorders associated with cell loss and atrophy.

Regulation of Cell Survival Pathways with Antidepressants

Seminal studies from the Duman group have investigated the possibility that the factors involved in neuronal atrophy

Figure 14–28. Neurotrophic mechanisms in depression. Severe stress causes several changes in hippocampal pyramidal neurons, including a reduction in their dendritic arborizations, and a reduction in brain-derived neurotrophic factor (BDNF) expression (which could be one of the factors mediating the dendritic effects). Antidepressants increase dendritic arborizations and BDNF expression of these hippocampal neurons via growth factor cascades. By these actions, antidepressants may reverse and prevent the actions of stress on the hippocampus and ameliorate certain symptoms of depression. VPA = valproate. (*Source*: Adapted from Nestler et al., 2002a. Reprinted with permission from Elsevier.)

and survival could be the target of antidepressant treatment (Duman et al., 1999; D'Sa and Duman, 2002) (see Fig. 14–30). These studies demonstrated that one pathway involved in cell survival and plasticity, the cAMP–CREB cascade, is upregulated by antidepressant treatment (Duman et al., 1999).

Preclinical studies have also demonstrated that antidepressant treatment in vivo increases CREB phosphorylation and cAMP response element–mediated gene expression in mouse limbic brain regions (Thome et al., 2000). Upregulation of CREB and BDNF occurs in response to several different classes of antidepressant treatments, including norepinephrine- and serotonin-selective reuptake inhibitors and electroconvulsive shock, indicating that the cAMP–CREB cascade and BDNF are common postreceptor targets of these therapeutic agents (Nibuya et al., 1995, 1996) (see Fig. 14–31). In addition, upregulation of CREB and BDNF is dependent on chronic treatment, consistent with the therapeutic action of antidepressants (reviewed in

Nestler et al., 2002b; Duman, 2004; Berton and Nestler, 2006). A role for the cAMP–CREB cascade and BDNF in the actions of antidepressant treatment is also supported by studies demonstrating that upregulation of these pathways increases performance in behavioral models of depression (Duman et al., 1999). It has been observed as well that induced CREB overexpression in the dentate gyrus results in an antidepressant-like effect in the learned helplessness paradigm and the forced swim test in rats (A. Chen et al., 2001). Indirect human evidence comes from studies showing increased hippocampal BDNF expression in postmortem brain of subjects treated with antidepressants at the time of death compared with untreated subjects (B. Chen et al., 2001).

In elegant studies from the Nestler laboratory, mice were administered chronic social defeat stress followed by chronic imipramine (a tricyclic antidepressant) (Tsankova et al., 2006). Adaptations at the levels of gene expression and chromatin remodeling of five BDNF splice variant mRNAs

(I–V) and their unique promoters in the hippocampus were then studied. Defeat stress induced lasting downregulation of BDNF transcripts III and IV and robustly increased repressive histone methylation at their corresponding promoters. Chronic imipramine reversed this downregulation and increased histone acetylation at these promoters (Tsankova et al., 2006). As we discuss in greater detail later, these experiments underscore an important role for epigenetic factors in the pathophysiology of mood disorders, and they highlight the therapeutic potential for histone methylation and deacetylation inhibitors.

The data reviewed here clearly show that molecules in neurotrophic signaling cascades are regulated by both antidepressants and mood stabilizers. Where, then, is the specificity? Are these agents simply nonspecific plasticity enhancers?

At the outset, it should be emphasized that BDNF and the ERK pathway are not synonymous. BDNF uses at least three major signaling cascades to bring about its biological effects through TrkB: ERK MAPK, PI-3-kinase/Akt, and phospholipase C; BDNF, at higher concentrations, also stimulates p75NTR. The ERK MAPK pathway is regulated by several mechanisms. Thus, in addition to the neurotrophins, a variety of neurotransmitters and other neuroactive molecules also regulate the ERK pathway in stage- and other region-specific manners in the brain. It is also

Figure 14–29. Effects of low-dose lithium treatment on Bcl-2 levels in rat frontal cortex and hippocampus. Chronic lithium was shown to robustly increase the levels of the major neuroprotective protein Bcl-2 at therapeutic levels (.6–1.0mM). A series of studies was undertaken to determine if low-dose lithium also produced Bcl-2 upregulation. Inbred male Wistar Kyoto rats were treated with Li_2CO_3 at "full dose" (resulting in plasma levels of ~.8mM) or "half dose" (resulting in plasma levels of ~.35mM) for 3 to 4 weeks. *Left panel*: Quantification of immunoblotting of Bcl-2 in frontal cortex, which was conducted by established methods with monoclonal antibodies directed against Bcl-2. *Right panel*: Immunohistochemistry in rat hippocampus. Treatment of rats with either full-dose or half-dose lithium for 3 to 4 weeks resulted in significant increases in the levels of Bcl-2. * $p < .05$ compared with control. These results suggest that low-dose lithium may also confer neuroprotective effects, even in those patients who are intolerant of full-dose lithium because of side effects.

Figure 14–30. Influence of antidepressant treatment on the cAMP–CREB cascade. Antidepressant treatment increases synaptic levels of norepinephrine (NE) and 5-HT by blocking the reuptake or breakdown of these monoamines. This results in activation of intracellular signal transduction cascades, one of which is the cAMP–CREB cascade. Chronic antidepressant treatment increases Gs coupling to adenylyl cyclase (AC), particulate levels of cAMP-dependent protein kinase (PKA), and CREB. CREB can also be phosphorylated by Ca^{2+}-dependent protein kinases, which can be activated by the phosphatidylinositol pathway (not shown) or by glutamate ionotropic receptors (e.g., NMDA). Glutamate receptors and Ca^{2+}-dependent protein kinases are also involved in neural plasticity. One gene target of antidepressant treatment and the cAMP–CREB cascade is brain-derived neurotrophic factor (BDNF), which contributes to the cellular processes underlying neuronal plasticity and cell survival. (*Source*: Manji and Duman, 2001.)

likely that the stoichiometries, coupling efficiencies, and subcellular compartmentalization vary in different brain regions. Not altogether surprisingly, different behavioral effects have been reported when different brain regions were involved. It is likely that the differential effects are modulated not only by the region-specific expression of specific signaling but also by the network properties of vulnerable structures. The dynamics of the impairments of cellular plasticity and resilience are thus also likely to be determined by intrinsic properties of the affected areas.

Cellular and Neurotrophic Actions of Antidepressants

Findings of several studies support the hypothesis that antidepressant treatment produces neurotrophic-like effects (see Box 14–18). One early study found that antidepressant treatment induced regeneration of catecholamine axon

terminals in the cerebral cortex (Nakamura, 1990). Another study examined the influence of antidepressant treatment on the atrophy of hippocampal neurons in response to stress (Watanabe et al., 1992). Chronic administration of an atypical antidepressant, tianeptine, was found to block the stress-induced atrophy of CA3 pyramidal neurons, measured as a blockade of the decrease in the number and length of apical dendrite branch points. Additional studies are needed to further characterize the influence of these and other classes of typical and atypical antidepressants on the atrophy of CA3 neurons. The neurotrophic and neuroprotective effects of antidepressants in other models of cell damage or atrophy also need to be examined.

Czeh and colleagues (2001) conducted some interesting preclinical studies in which stress-induced changes in brain structure and neurochemistry were found to be counteracted

**Antidepressant Treatment Increases
CREB Expression in Hippocampus**

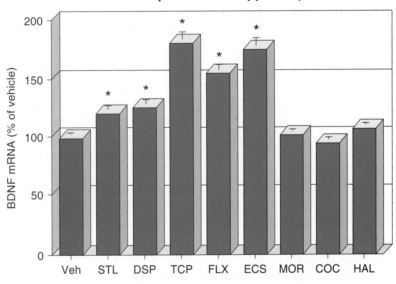

**Chronic Antidepressant Treatment Increases
BDNF Expression in Hippocampus**

Figure 14–31. Chronic antidepressant treatment increases CREB and BDNF expression in rat hippocampus. Upregulation of CREB mRNA (*a*) occurs in response to several different classes of antidepressant treatments, including norepinephrine- and serotonin-reuptake inhibitors, and electroconvulsive seizure, indicating that the cAMP–CREB cascade is a common postreceptor target of these therapeutic agents (Nibuya et al., 1995, 1996). Notably, CREB mRNA increases were not observed with several nonantidepressant psychoactive agents (including morphine, cocaine, or haloperidol), indicating specificity of effects. Upregulation of BDNF mRNA (*b*) also occurs in response to several different classes of antidepressant treatments, including a norepinephrine/NE reuptake inhibitor, SSRIs, and electroconvulsive seizure. Notably, BDNF mRNA increases were not observed with several nonantidepressant psychoactive agents (including morphine, cocaine, or haloperidol), indicating specificity of effects. In addition, upregulation of both CREB and BDNF is dependent of chronic treatment, consistent with the therapeutic action of antidepressants. As discussed in the text (not shown here), lithium and valproate have also been shown to upregulate CREB and BDNF mRNA and protein levels. Indirect human evidence comes from studies showing increased hippocampal BDNF and CREB expression in postmortem brain of subjects treated with antidepressants at the time of death compared with that of antidepressant-untreated subjects. COC = cocaine (a psychostimulant); DSP = desipramine (a noradrenergic antidepressant); ECS = electroconvulsive shock (an animal model of ECT); FLX = fluoxetine (an SSRI); HAL = haloperidol (a typical antipsychotic); MOR = morphine (an opioid); STL = sertraline (an SSRI); TCP = tranylcypromine (an MAOI); Veh = vehicle control. (*Source*: Unpublished data from Ronald S. Duman, Ph.D. Professor of Psychiatry and Pharmacology, Director, Abraham Ribicoff Research Facilities Yale University School of Medicine.)

BOX **14–18.** **Summary of the Differences in Neurotrophic Properties of Antidepressants and Lithium: Evidence from Contemporary Studies**

- Antidepressants exert major effects on cAMP-responsive element binding protein (CREB) and brain-derived neurotrophic factor (BDNF) expression in rat hippocampus.
- Antidepressants *may* exert modest effects on extracellular response kinase (ERK) activation in rat brain.
- Lithium exerts major effects on ERK activation in rat frontal cortex and hippocampus.
- Lithium exerts major effects on Bcl-2 in rat frontal cortex.
- Cross-sectional neuroimaging studies suggest that patients treated with chronic lithium or valproate do not show subgenual prefrontal cortex atrophy; patients treated with selective serotonin reuptake inhibitors (SSRIs) show atrophy similar to that in untreated patients.
- Longitudinal studies show that chronic lithium increases the levels of N-acetylaspartate (NAA) in areas of brain in bipolar patients; there are no similar published studies with valproate or antidepressants.
- Longitudinal studies show that chronic lithium increases gray matter volumes in bipolar patients; there are currently no similar published studies with antidepressants.

by treatment with tianeptine. In their study, male tree shrews subjected to a chronic psychosocial stress paradigm were found to have decreased NAA, a putative marker of neuronal viability (Tsai and Coyle, 1995; Moore and Galloway, 2002), measured in vivo by proton magnetic resonance spectroscopy (^{1}H-MRS); decreased granule cell proliferation in the dentate gyrus of the hippocampus; and a reduction in hippocampal volume compared with non-stressed animals. These stress-induced effects were prevented and reversed in shrews treated concomitantly with tianeptine (Czeh et al., 2001). Once again, however, the generalizability of these effects to other classes of antidepressants is unclear. (See Figure 14–32 on the neurotrophic effects of antidepressants.)

Relevance of Antidepressant Regulation of Hippocampal Neurogenesis

Recent studies have shown that chronic, but not acute, antidepressant treatment also increases the neurogenesis of dentate gyrus granule cells (Jacobs et al., 2000; Manev et al., 2001; D'Sa and Duman, 2002). These studies found that chronic administration of different classes of antidepressant treatment, including norepinephrine- and serotonin-selective reuptake inhibitors and electroconvulsive shock (the animal model of ECT), increases the prolif-

eration and survival of new neurons. In contrast to what has been observed with mood stabilizers, increased neurogenesis is not observed in response to chronic administration of nonantidepressant psychotropic drugs. Studies demonstrating that neurogenesis is increased by conditions that stimulate neuronal activity (e.g., enriched environment, learning, exercise) suggest that this process is also positively regulated by and may even be dependent on neuronal plasticity (Kempermann, 2002).

The enhancement of hippocampal neurogenesis by antidepressants serves to highlight the degree to which these effective treatments are capable of regulating long-term neuroplastic events in the brain. In view of the opposite effects of stress and antidepressants on hippocampal neurogenesis, it is quite plausible that alterations in hippocampal neurogenesis are fundamental to the clinical syndrome of depression. To further investigate this hypothesis, Santarelli and colleagues (2003) conducted an important series of experiments. Mice were administered a variety of antidepressants or vehicle for 28 days, and their responses on a novelty-suppressed feeding were investigated. A 35 percent improvement in the speed of retrieving food or water was observed in mice taking antidepressants. In a second experiment, a 60 percent increase in BrdU-positive cells in the dentate gyrus was found after 11–28 days of treatment with fluoxetine. To test whether hippocampal neurogenesis was necessary for the antidepressants' behavioral effects, mice were exposed to x-rays directed at the hippocampus, leading to an 85 percent reduction in BrdU-positive cells in the subgranular zone. These mice were then treated with fluoxetine, imipramine, or vehicle for 28 days. The previously noted effect of antidepressants on the novelty-suppressed feeding test was not seen in irradiated mice, suggesting that these behavioral effects of chronic antidepressants may be mediated by new neuronal growth in the hippocampus (see Fig. 14–33). However, novelty-suppressed feeding behavior is generally regarded as a test of anxiety behavior and also responds to benzodiazepines (generally not regarded as having antidepressant efficacy). Thus it may be premature to infer that inhibition of the antidepressant effect of these drugs also occurs as a result of the suppression of neurogenesis; studies with genetic strategies to regulate hippocampal neurogenesis are under way and should delineate the role of hippocampal neurogenesis in the pathophysiology and treatment of mood disorders.

A problem to be addressed with the neurotrophic hypothesis of antidepressant drug action is the "tryptophan depletion conundrum." It is now well established that patients successfully treated with SSRIs show a rapid depressive relapse following experimental procedures that deplete tryptophan and serotonin (Delgado et al., 1991, 1999; Aberg-Wistedt et al., 1998). How are such rapid effects to

Figure 14–32. Neurotrophic effects of antidepressants. *Left*: Antidepressant treatment increases synaptic levels of norepinephrine (NE) and serotonin (5-HT) by blocking the reuptake or breakdown of these monoamines. This results in activation of intracellular signal transduction cascades, one of which is the cyclic adenosine monophosphate–cAMP-responsive element-binding protein (cAMP–CREB) cascade. Chronic antidepressant treatment increases Gs coupling to adenylyl cyclase (AC), particulate levels of cAMP-dependent protein kinase (PKA), and CREB. CREB can also be phosphorylated by Ca^{2+}-dependent protein kinases, which can be activated by the phosphatidylinositol pathway or by glutamate ionotropic receptors (e.g., NMDA, not shown). One gene target of antidepressant treatment and the cAMP–CREB cascade is brain-derived neurotrophic factor (BDNF), which contributes to the cellular processes underlying neuronal plasticity, and restoration/enhancement of neural connectivity mechanisms, which are essential for healthy affective functioning. *Right*: At the dendritic level, antidepressants increase synapse formation and neural outgrowth, restoring critical circuitry function. AR = adrenoreceptors; DAG = diacylglycerol; IP, inositolmonophosphate; NMDA = N-methyl-D-aspartate; P = phosphorylated; PIP_2 = phosphoinositide 4,5-biphosphate; PLC, phospholipase C; TrkB, specific tyrosine kinases receptor. (*Source*: Manji et al., 2003b.)

be reconciled with the postulated neurotrophic actions of antidepressants? It is our contention that treatment of depression is attained by providing both trophic and neurochemical support; the trophic support restores normal synaptic connectivity, thereby allowing the chemical signal to reinstate the optimal functioning of critical circuits necessary for normal affective functioning. Thus, tryptophan depletion diets are capable of inducing a depressive relapse in SSRI-treated patients through reduced neurotransmitter synthesis and release, although they are not likely to have acute major effects on brain structure per se (see Fig. 14–34).

Long-term Clinical Implications of the Neurotrophic Effects of Mood Stabilizers and Antidepressants

As discussed earlier, there is now a considerable body of work both conceptually and experimentally suggesting that impairments in cellular plasticity and resilience may play an important role in the pathophysiology of recurrent mood disorders. Does the long-term administration of agents such as lithium and valproate actually retard disease- or affective episode–induced cell loss or atrophy? The distinction between disease progression and affective episodes per se is an important one, since it is quite possible that the neurotrophic effects of lithium or valproate may even be independent of their ability to treat or prevent affective episodes. We are aware of no longitudinal studies that fully address this question, but it clearly represents a very important and fundamental issue worthy of investigation.

Findings that lithium administration increases brain NAA levels and gray matter volumes, as well as cross-sectional results demonstrating "normalized" subgenual prefrontal cortex volumes in patients treated with lithium and valproate, do provide indirect support for such a contention. The evidence also suggests that, somewhat akin to the treatment of conditions such as hypertension and diabetes, early and potentially sustained treatment may be necessary to adequately prevent many of the deleterious long-term sequelae associated with mood disorders.

For many refractory depressed patients, there may be a limited benefit to new drugs that simply mimic many traditional drugs that directly or indirectly alter neurotransmitter levels or bind to cell surface receptors. Such strategies implicitly assume that the target circuits are functionally intact and that altered synaptic activity will thus be transduced to modify the postsynaptic throughput of the system. However, the evidence presented here suggests that, in addition to neurochemical changes, many patients also have pronounced structural alterations (e.g., reduced spine density, neurite retraction, overall neuropil reductions) in critical neuronal circuits. Thus, optimal treatment may be attained only by providing more direct trophic support. The trophic support would be envisioned as enhancing and maintaining normal synaptic connectivity, thereby allowing the chemical signal to reinstate the optimal functioning of critical circuits necessary for normal affective functioning.

While lithium and valproate clearly exert neurotrophic effects, they do so through indirect mechanisms—that is, many of their direct biochemical targets are considerably upstream of neuroprotective proteins such as GSK-3, ERK, and Bcl-2. Thus many patients with endogenous or acquired defects in the machinery involved in mediating the effects of mood stabilizers on neurotrophic proteins would

Figure 14–33. Antidepressant treatment increases neurogenesis in adult hippocampus. *Left panel*: A typical section of dentate gyrus that has undergone immunohistochemical analysis for bromodeoxyuridine (BrdU), the thymidine analog used to label newborn cells. The darker cells in the subgranular zone (SGZ) represent BrdU-positive cells. Chronic antidepressant treatment increases the number of BrdU-positive cells, determined 24 hours after BrdU administration. *Right panel*: Quantification of immunocytochemical data, showing antidepressant treatments increase the number of BrdU-labeled cells in dentate gyrus. Con = control; ECS = electroconvulsive shock; Fluox = fluoxetine, a 5-HT selective inhibitor; Reb = a norepinephrine selective reuptake inhibitor reboxetine; TCP = a monoamine oxidase inhibitor tranylcypromine. (*Source*: Gray et al., 2003; unpublished data from Ronald S. Duman, Ph.D. Professor of Psychiatry and Pharmacology, Director, Abraham Ribicoff Research Facilities, Yale University School of Medicine.)

Figure 14–34. Resolution of the tryptophan depletion conundrum of the neurotrophic hypothesis of antidepressant drug action. Treatment of depression is attained by providing both trophic and neurochemical support; the trophic support restores normal synaptic connectivity, thereby allowing the chemical signal to reinstate the optimal functioning of critical circuits necessary for normal affective functioning. Brain-derived neurotrophic factor (BDNF) also facilitates the release of neurotransmitters that act on this restored, intact circuit. Acute reduction in synaptic serotonin levels via its effects on reducing BDNF levels is capable of rapidly reducing the release of a number of neurotransmitters. Thus, tryptophan depletion diets are capable of inducing a depressive relapse in selective serotonin reuptake inhibitor–treated patients via the effects on neurotransmitter release, although likely not having major effects on structural brain changes. AC = adenylyl cyclase; cAMP = cyclic adenosine monophosphate; CREB = cAMP-responsive element-binding protein; DAG = diacylglycerol; GABA = gamma-aminobutyric acid; Glu = glutamate; IP, inositolmonophosphate; NE = norepinephrine; NMDA = N-methyl-D-aspartate; P = phosphorylated; PIP_2 = phosphoinositide 4,5-biphosphate; PKA = protein kinase A; PLC, phospholipase C; TrkB, specific tyrosine kinases receptor. (*Source:* Manji et al., 2003b.)

be expected not to display marked neurotrophic effects from the drugs. Optimal long-term treatment for refractory patients may require the early use of agents that enhance neuroplasticity and cellular resilience.

In this context, it is noteworthy that there are a number of pharmacological "plasticity-enhancing" strategies that may be of considerable utility in the treatment of mood disorders (Quiroz et al., 2004; Gould et al., 2004). Among the most immediate of these are NMDA antagonists, glutamate-release-reducing agents such as lamotrigine, AMPA potentiators, and cAMP phosphodiesterase inhibitors. An increasing number of strategies are being investigated for developing small-molecule agents to regulate the activity of growth factors, MAPK cascades, and the Bcl-2 family of proteins. This work holds much promise for the development of novel therapies for the long-term treatment of severe, refractory mood disorders. Table 14–10 summa-

rizes findings to date on potential targets for the development of new agents for the treatment of mood disorders (see Fig. 14–35).

CONCLUSIONS

The first edition of *Manic-Depressive Illness* was published in 1990; since then, there have been tremendous advances in our understanding of both the normal and abnormal functioning of the brain. Indeed, it is our firm belief that the impact of molecular and cellular biology–which has been felt in every corner of clinical medicine–will ultimately also have major repercussions for our understanding about the fundamental core pathophysiology of manic-depressive illness, and will lead to the development of improved treatments. Recent years have witnessed a more wide-ranging understanding of the neural circuits and the

TABLE 14–10. Potential Targets for the Development of New Antidepressants and Antibipolar Agents

Molecule	Hypothesized Involvement in Mood Disorders or Treatment	Function Plausibly Relevant to Mood Disorders	Findings from Animal Models	Direct or Surrogate Human Evidence	Observations from Clinical Treatment Studies
5-HT$_{1A}$/5-HT$_{1B}$ antagonists	5-HT$_{1A}$/5-HT$_{1B}$ antagonists may augment AD response.	Somatodendritic 5-HT$_{1A}$ receptors regulate 5-HT neuron firing; nerve terminal 5-HT1B receptors facilitate 5-HT release. Blockade increases 5-HT throughput via two mechanisms.	Coadministration of 5-HT$_{1A}$/5-HT$_{1B}$ antagonists facilitates AD-induced 5-HT throughput.	Both PET and neuroendocrine studies suggest reduced 5-HT$_{1A}$ levels/function in depression. However, these studies have not investigated somatodendritic receptors.	Equivocal results to date; pindolol may not be the ideal drug to test hypothesis
5-HT$_2$ antagonists	5-HT$_2$ antagonists may possess AD effects.	CNS distribution; may regulate DA throughput; important roles in regulating sleep and appetite	Many ADs downregulate 5-HT$_2$s (but not ECS).	Postmortem brain and PET studies are inconclusive; however, PET studies suggest that ADs reduce 5-HT$_2$ binding. Elevated platelet 5-HT$_2$ binding in depression	Agents with 5-HT$_2$ antagonism (e.g., mirtazapine, clozapine) have AD effects; no clinical studies with selective agents
5-HT$_7$ antagonists	5-HT$_7$ agonists may have AD effects and/or ameliorate sleep/circadian disturbances.	CNS distribution; may regulate circadian rhythms; positively linked to cAMP generation	AD and clozapine appear to interact with and/or regulate expression of 5-HT$_7$	None	None
α$_2$ antagonists administered during REM sleep	A very investigational strategy as a rapidly acting AD	α$_2$ antagonists increase firing of LC and release of NE. Enhancing NE function may have AD effects; activating central NE projections during REM sleep may allow released NE to interact with a primed, sensitized postsynaptic environment.	Agents that enhance NE throughput have AD efficacy; sleep deprivation, which has a rapid AD effect, enhances expression of plasticity molecules (e.g., CREB, BDNF) via an NE-dependent mechanism.	Sleep deprivation exerts a rapid AD effect. The LC is quiescent during REM sleep and activated by sleep deprivation.	α$_2$ antagonists (idazoxan, mirtazapine) have been shown to exert AD effects. Use of an α$_2$ antagonist during REM sleep is quite novel; human studies are just getting under way.

CRF antagonists	Enhanced throughput of CRF receptors may mediate some of the signs and symptoms of depression and anxiety; CRF antagonists may be effective ADs and/or anxiolytics.	Regulates NE LC firing; activated by stress; CRF receptors are well placed to regulate many of the neurovegetative symptoms of depression.	Agonists reproduce depression and anxiety-like behaviors in rodents. The orally active CRH antagonist, antalarmin, significantly reduces fear and anxiety responses in nonhuman primates.	HPA axis dysregulation in depression; CSF and postmortem brain studies in depression are supportive.	Positive effects were seen in the initial study; however, the study was stopped because of likely mechanism-unrelated side effects. Several other agents are at various stages of development.
Short-term treatment with GR antagonists	Hypercortisolemia may play an important role in the pathophysiology and/or deleterious long-term consequences of mood disorders.	Hippocampal atrophy mediated in part by hypercortisolemia. (Most studies have concentrated on the hippocampus, but other brain areas may likely show similar changes.) Diabetes, bone mineral density also affected	Injection of a GR antagonist into the dentate gyrus attenuates the acquisition of learned helpless behavior; transgenic and KO mice exhibit some symptoms of anxiety and depression. ADs exert complex effects on GR expression and function.	Abundant data demonstrating HPA axis activation in mood disorders, especially in severely ill patients	Preliminary studies of mifepristone in psychotic depression are very encouraging; larger studies are under way.
NK1 antagonists (substance P receptors)	Enhanced NK1 function in depression; NK1 antagonists may be effective treatments, but data not conclusive	Play important roles in mediating pain (? "psychic pain"); NK1 receptors reduce 5-HT neurotransmission.	Efficacy in animal models of depression; stress regulates re-distribution of NK1 receptors; NK1 KO shows reduced anxiety in certain models	No strong direct supportive evidence	Initial clinical studies positive; subsequent replications failed. Awaiting more definitive studies
NPY receptor agonists	NPY may serve as an endogenous anti-stress, anxiolytic agent. NPY agonists may be efficacious for certain symptoms of depression and anxiety.	May counter many of the deleterious effects of CRF and stress.	Efficacious in animal models of anxiety; NPY KO shows reduced anxiety in certain models. ADs and lithium may increase NPY expression.	CSF NPY may be low in depression. ECT increases CSF NPY-like immunoreactivity	No clinical studies to date

(continued)

TABLE 14–10. Potential Targets for the Development of New Antidepressants and Antibipolar Agents (continued)

Molecule	Hypothesized Involvement in Mood Disorders or Treatment	Function Plausibly Relevant to Mood Disorders	Findings from Animal Models	Direct or Surrogate Human Evidence	Observations from Clinical Treatment Studies
NMDA antagonists	Enhanced throughput of the NMDA receptor may contribute to brain-regional volumetric changes observed in depression; NMDA antagonists may have antidepressant efficacy.	Key regulators of many forms of synaptic plasticity; play an important role in stress-induced hippocampal atrophy and reduction of neurogenesis; implicated in many forms of cell atrophy and death	NMDA antagonists block stress-induced cell atrophy/reduction of neurogenesis; many ADs regulate NMDA receptor subunit expression; NMDA antagonists efficacious in certain animal models of depression	Very indirect—regional volumetric reductions in mood disorders; evidence for glial and neuronal loss/atrophy in mood disorders	Amantadine and especially lamotrigine have antidepressant efficacy; preliminary results suggest that ketamine may have antidepressant efficacy. Studies with other NMDA antagonists are planned.
AMPA Potentiators	AMPA receptors are known to activate MAP kinase cascades and increase plasticity.	Play important roles in neuronal functioning and plasticity	AMPA-potentiating agents have shown efficacy in animal models of depression. An ampakine (CX516) has been shown to produce a marked facilitation of performance in a memory task in rats.	Very indirect—impairment of neuronal plasticity and cellular resilience	No studies yet on mood disorders; preliminary human studies suggest a positive memory encoding effect in certain spheres; beneficial effects seen on measures of attention and memory when added to clozapine in schizophrenia
PDE4 inhibitors	Reduced throughput of cAMP signaling cascade may be involved in depression; enhancement of cAMP signaling may be AD	Enhance cAMP signaling and downstream gene expression, as well as synaptic plasticity and cell survival	PDE inhibitors effective in some models of depression; ADs enhance cAMP-mediated signaling	Postmortem brain studies suggest a potential impairment of cAMP signaling cascade in depression (but not BPD)	Preliminary early clinical studies suggested AD efficacy of rolipram; newer clinical studies with PDE inhibitors as AD adjuncts are under way

MAP kinase phosphatase inhibitors	Enhancement of neurotrophic factor signaling by inhibiting the turn-off reactions may be efficacious in treatment of depression.	MAP kinase signaling cascades are critical mediators of the effects of neurotrophic factors (e.g., BDNF) and play important roles in synaptic and structural plasticity.	ADs and lithium increase BDNF expression; valproate activates the MAP kinase cascade.	Very indirect—regional volumetric reductions in mood disorders; evidence for glial and neuronal loss/atrophy in mood disorders	No clinical studies with specific agents to date
Isozyme selective PKC inhibitors	Enhancement of PKC activity may play a role in the symptomatology of mania; PKC inhibitors may be antimanic.	Play a major role in regulating neuronal firing and neurotransmitter release; may play important roles in psychostimulant-mediated catecholamine release	Lithium and valproate, upon chronic administration, reduce levels of PKC α and ε; certain biochemical and behavioral effects of psychostimulants are attenuated by PKC inhibitors.	A postmortem brain study and human platelet studies suggest activation of PKC isozymes in BPD/mania. Platelet studies also suggest normalization with lithium treatment.	A preliminary study suggests that tamoxifen (an estrogen receptor antagonist and PKC inhibitor) has antimanic efficacy. Larger clinical studies with tamoxifen are under way.
GSK-3 inhibitors, β-catenin upregulators	GSK-3 inhibitors, β-catenin upregulators may have mood-stabilizing effects.	Play important roles in structural plasticity and regulate cell death pathways	Lithium inhibits GSK-3 and upregulates β-catenin; valproate upregulates β-catenin likely via GSK-3 and non-GSK-3 mechanisms; lithium, valproate and lamotrigine protect againt GSK-3 over-expression-induced cell death.	Very indirect—regional volumetric reductions in mood disorders; evidence for glial and neuronal loss/atrophy in mood disorders	Development of CNS-penetrant, selective small molecule GSK-3 inhibitors is currently under way.

(continued)

593

TABLE 14–10. Potential Targets for the Development of New Antidepressants and Antibipolar Agents *(continued)*

Molecule	Hypothesized Involvement in Mood Disorders or Treatment	Function Plausibly Relevant to Mood Disorders	Findings from Animal Models	Direct or Surrogate Human Evidence	Observations from Clinical Treatment Studies
Bcl-2 upregulators	Upregulating Bcl-2 may exert trophic effects and enhance cellular resilience in treatment of mood disorders.	One of the major cell survival signals, and a major downstream effector of neurotrophic factors. Likely plays an important role in neurite outgrowth, neurogenesis, and other forms of neuroplasticity	Lithium and valproate, upon chronic administration, robustly upregulate Bcl-2 levels and exert - neuroprotective effects.	Preliminary postmortem brain studies suggest possible involvement of Bcl-2 in mood disorders; lithium increases gray matter volumes in brain areas of reported atrophy in humans.	Lithium and valproate are effective mood stabilizers; no selective CNS Bcl-2 upregulators currently available. However, pramipexole, in addition to having dopaminergic effects, upregulates bcl-2. Positive antidepressant effects in preliminary studies; larger studies are under way

AD = antidepressant; BDNF = brain-derived neuotrophic factor; BPD = bipolar disorder; CNS = central nervous system; CRF = corticotropin-releasing factor; CRH = corticotropin-releasing hormone; CSF = cerebrospinal fluid; ECS = electroconvulsive shock; ECT = electroconvulsive therapy; GR = glucocorticoid receptor; GSK = glycogen synthase kinase; HPA = hypothalamic–pituitary–adrenal; KO = knockout; LC = locus coeruleus; MAP = mitogen activated protein; NE = norepinephrine; NK = neurokinin; NPY = neuropeptide Y; PET = positron emission tomography; PKC = protein kinase C; REM = rapid eye movement.

Note: See text for references.

Source: Adapted from Nestler and Manji, 2002.

Figure 14–35. The multiple influences on neuroplasticity and cellular resilience in mood disorders. Genetic and neurodevelopmental factors, repeated affective episodes, and illness progression might all contribute to the impairments of cellular resilience, volumetric reductions, and cell death and atrophy observed in mood disorders. Stress and depression likely contribute to impairments of cellular resilience by a variety of mechanisms, including reductions in the levels of BDNF, facilitating glutamatergic transmission via NMDA and non-NMDA receptors, and reducing the cells' energy capacity. Neurotrophic factors such as BDNF enhance cell survival by activating two distinct signaling pathways: the PI$_3$–kinase pathway, and the ERK–MAP kinase pathway. One of the major mechanisms by which BDNF promotes cell survival is by increasing the expression of the major cytoprotective protein, Bcl-2. Bcl-2 attenuates cell death through a variety of mechanisms, including impairment of the release of calcium and cytochrome c, sequestering of proforms of death-inducing caspase enzymes, and enhancement of mitochondrial calcium uptake. The chronic administration of a variety of antidepressants increases the expression of BDNF and its receptor TrkB. Lithium and valproate robustly upregulate the cytoprotective protein Bcl-2 and inhibit GSK-3β, biochemical effects shown to have neuroprotective results. Valproate also activates the ERK–MAP kinase pathway, which may play a major role in producing neurotrophic effects and neurite outgrowth. BAD = pro-apoptotic members of the Bcl-2 family; Bcl-2 and Bcl-x = anti-apoptotic members of the Bcl-2 family; BDNF = brain derived neurotrophic receptor; CREB = cyclic AMP-responsive element-binding protein; GR = glucocorticoid receptor, GSK-3 = glycogen synthase kinase-3; MEK = ERK, components of the ERK-MAP kinase pathway; Ras = Raf; ROS = reactive oxygen species; RSK-2 = ribosomal S-6 kinase; TrkB = tyrosine kinase receptor for BDNF; VPA = valproate. (*Source*: Manji et al., 2001a. Reprinted with permission from Macmillan Publishers, Ltd.)

various mechanisms of synaptic transmission, the molecular mechanisms of receptor and postreceptor signaling, and a finer understanding of the process by which genes code for specific functional proteins that in toto reduce the complexity in gene-to-behavior pathways (Gould and Manji, 2004). Here we synthesize and summarize the major advances pertaining to manic-depressive illness.

The Genetics of Bipolar Disorder

As discussed in Chapter 13, it is clear that we are on the verge of truly identifying susceptibility (and likely protective) genes for bipolar disorder. While the search for predisposing genes had traditionally tended to proceed under the assumption that schizophrenia and bipolar disorder are separate disease entities with different underlying etiologies, emerging findings from many fields of psychiatric research do not fit well with this model (Craddock et al., 2005). Most notably, the pattern of findings emerging from genetic studies shows increasing evidence for an overlap in genetic susceptibility across the traditional classification categories. It is clear that there is not a one-to-one relationship between genes and behaviors so that different combinations of genes (and resultant changes in neurobiology) contribute to any complex behavior (normal or abnormal) (Hasler et al., 2006). It is also critically important to remember that polymorphisms in genes will very likely simply be *associated* with bipolar disorder or recurrent depression; these genes will likely not invariably determine outcome, but only lend a higher probability for the subsequent development of illness. In fact, genes will never code for abnormal behaviors per se, but rather code for proteins that make up cells, forming circuits, that in combination determine facets of both abnormal and normal behavior. These expanding levels of interaction have made the study of psychiatric diseases so difficult. The next task of psychiatric genetic research is to study how and why variations in these genes impart a greater probability to develop manic-depressive illness (to understand pathophysiology) and then to direct therapeutics at that pathophysiology (Gould and Manji, 2004). There is no doubt that knowledge of the genetics and subsequent understanding of their relevant biology will have a tremendous impact on diagnosis, classification, and treatment of psychiatric disease.

An Endophenotype Strategy

It is becoming increasingly clearer that, while the pathways beginning with genes and then expressed through simple biological processes do not necessarily have a single quantifiable endpoint (i.e. behavior), it may be possible to assay the result of aberrant genes through biologically "simpler" approaches (Hasler et al., 2006). The term *endophenotype* is described as an internal, intermediate phenotype (i.e., not obvious to the unaided eye) that fills the gap in the causal chain between genes and distal diseases (Gottesman and Shields, 1973), and therefore may help to resolve questions about etiology. The endophenotype concept assumes that the number of genes involved in the variations of endophenotypes representing more elementary phenomena (as opposed to the behavioral macros found in the DSM) are fewer than those involved in producing the full disease (Gottesman and Gould, 2003).

Will an endophenotype strategy lead to a major payoff? Endophenotypes provide a means for identifying the "upstream" traits underlying clinical phenotypes, as well as the "downstream" biological consequences of genes. The methods available to identify endophenotypes include neuropsychological, cognitive, neurophysiological, neuroanatomical, imaging, and biochemical measures (Hasler et al., 2006). The information revised in this volume suggests that candidate brain function endophenotypes include attention deficits, deficits in verbal learning and memory, cognitive deficits following tryptophan depletion, circadian rhythm instability, and dysmodulation of motivation and reward. Moreover, reduced anterior cingulate volume and early-onset white matter abnormalities represent candidate brain structure endophenotypes. Finally, symptom provocation endophenotypes may be based on recurrent mood disorder patients' sensitivity to sleep deprivation, psychostimulants, and cholinergic drugs (Hasler et al., 2006; see Fig. 14–36). However, it must be acknowledged that there are several potential factors that must be considered. Foremost among these is the fact that none of the suggested endophenotypes have been fully validated. Moreover, while it might seem intuitively obvious that the genetics of these candidate endophenotypes will be simpler than that of manic-depressive illness, this has yet to be clearly established. Thus, these candidate endophenotypes need to be further evaluated with respect to specificity, heritability, temporal stability, and prevalence in unaffected relatives.

Nature and Nurture

In recent years, *epigenetics*—the study of changes to the genome that, unlike mutations, do not alter the DNA sequence—has delineated just how inextricably linked nature and nurture truly are (see Petronis, 2004, for an excellent review). Epigenetics purports to define the molecular mechanisms by which different cells from different tissues of the same organism, despite their DNA sequence identity, exhibit very different cellular phenotypes and perform very different functions. It is presumed that phenotypic and functional differences are the cumulative result of a large number of developmental, environmental, and stochastic events, some of which are mediated through the epigenetic modifications of DNA and chromatin histones. Epigenetic regulation is thus one of the molecular substrates for "cellular memory" that may help us understand how environmental impact results in temporally dissociated, altered behavioral responses.

Do epigenetic factors play a major role in manic-depressive illness? It has been argued that molecular studies of manic-depressive illness would benefit significantly from adding an epigenetic perspective (Petronis, 2004). Thus, epigenetic mechanisms are consistent with various nonmendelian features of manic-depressive illness, such as the relatively high degree of discordance in monozygotic (MZ) twins, the critical age group for susceptibility to the disease, clinical differences in males and females, and fluctuation of the disease course, notably cycling between

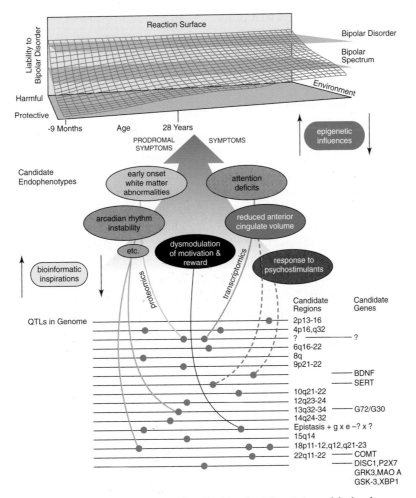

Figure 14–36. Endophenotypes in bipolar disorder. A heuristic model whereby underlying bipolar disorder gene susceptibility loci and implicated genes, modulated by environmental, epigenetic, and stochastic events, predispose to the development of bipolar disorder. Along this lengthy continuum between genes and distal phenotype lie putative bipolar endophenotypes, the identification of which will be useful for studies of the underlying neurobiology and genetics of bipolar disorders, as well as for preclinical investigations, such as the development of animal models. This figure is meant to represent a guide to future studies rather than a definitive portrait of loci, genes, and endophenotypes. QTL = quantitative trait locus. (Copyright 2005 by I.I. Gottesman. *Source*: Hasler et al., 2006. Reprinted with permission from Elsevier.)

phases (Petronis, 2003, 2004). Recent studies have shown that an epigenomic state of a gene can be established through behavioral programming, and it is potentially reversible (Weaver et al., 2004). This line of research is particularly noteworthy since early life stressors (that have been associated with later-life suicide attempts) in bipolar disorder (Leverich et al., 2003) might be amenable to treatment with agents to "undo" the epigenetic changes (e.g., histone deactylase [HDAC] inhibitors) (Zarate et al., 2006a). In this context, recent studies have also suggested that the downregulation of reelin and GAD67 expression in cortical interneurons in schizophrenia and bipolar disorder patients may be mediated by epigenetic hypermethylation of the

respective promoters caused by the selective increase of DNA-methyltransferase 1 in GABAergic neurons (Tremolizzo et al., 2005). In sum, although considerable additional research is needed, our growing appreciation of the molecular mechanisms underlying gene–environment interactions raise the intriguing possibility that environmentally induced neurobiological changes in early life may be amenable to subsequent therapeutic strategies targeting the epigenome (Petronis 2003, 2004).

Cellular Plasticity Cascades

Overall, it should be clear from the information reviewed in this chapter that there are abnormalities in multiple systems and at multiple levels in manic-depressive illness. It is our strong contention that manic-depressive illness arises from abnormalities in cellular plasticity cascades, leading to aberrant information processing in synapses and circuits mediating affective, cognitive, motoric, and neurovegetative function. Thus, manic-depressive illness can be best conceptualized as a disorder of *synapses and circuits*—not "too much/too little" of individual neurotransmitter or neuropeptide systems.

As discussed earlier, cellular signaling cascades form complex networks that allow the cell to receive, process, and respond to information (Bourne and Nicoll, 1993; Bhalla and Iyengar, 1999). These networks facilitate the integration of signals across multiple time scales and the generation of distinct outputs depending on input strength and duration, and regulate intricate feed-forward and feedback loops (Weng et al., 1999). These signaling cascades play a critical role as molecular switches subserving acute and long-term alterations in neuronal information processing.

As we have reviewed already, there is a considerable body of evidence in support of abnormalities in the regulation of signaling as integral to the underlying neurobiology of manic-depressive illness. The pathophysiology of this illness must account for not only the profound changes in mood but also a constellation of neurovegetative features derived from dysfunction in limbic related regions such as the hippocampus, hypothalamus, and brain stem. The highly integrated monoamine and prominent neuropeptide pathways are known to originate and project heavily within these regions of the brain, and it is thus not surprising that abnormalities have been noted in their function across clinical studies. In fact, the contribution of these pathways to the pathophysiology of manic-depressive illness must be reasonably robust, given the variability that might be expected in assessing such dynamic systems under the constraints in experimental design imposed upon such research (Manji and Lenox, 2000b). As we discuss below, the role of cellular signaling cascades offers much explanatory power for understanding the complex neurobiology of manic-depressive illness.

- Signaling cascades regulate the multiple neurotransmitter and neuropeptide systems implicated in manic-depressive illness. While dysfunction within these neurotransmitter and neuropeptide systems is likely to play an important role in mediating some facets of illness pathophysiology, it likely represents the downstream effects of other, more primary abnormalities in cellular signaling cascades. Indeed, even minor variations in ubiquitous regulators of signaling pathways can affect complex functions, yielding detrimental effects on behavior; this is clearly seen in many mouse models, where some genetic

mutations in expressed proteins have little effect on non-CNS functions, but major effects on behavior (Manji et al., 2003a).
- Abnormalities in cellular signaling cascades that regulate diverse physiologic functions likely explain the tremendous comorbidity with a variety of medical conditions (notably cardiovascular disease, diabetes mellitus, obesity, and migraine) and substance abuse. As a corollary, it is worth noting that genetic abnormalities in signaling components are often fully compatible with life, and in many instances, despite the often-ubiquitous expression of the signaling protein, one sees relatively circumscribed clinical manifestations (i.e., the abnormalities are only manifest in some physiologic systems, despite being potentially more widespread). These overt, yet relatively circumscribed, clinical manifestations are believed to ultimately arise from vastly different transcriptomes (all of the transcripts present at a particular time) in different tissues because of tissue-specific expression, haploinsufficiency, genetic imprinting, alternate splicing, varying stoichiometries of the relevant signaling partners in different tissues, and differences in the ability of diverse cell types to compensate for the abnormality (Manji et al., 2003a).
- Signaling pathways are clearly major targets for hormones that have been implicated in the pathophysiology of manic-depressive illness, including gonadal steroids, thyroid hormones, and glucocorticoids.
- Alterations in signaling pathways very likely represent the neurobiological substrates subserving the evolution of the illness over time (e.g., cycle acceleration). Thus, signaling networks play critical roles in cellular memory; cells with different histories, expressing different repertoires of signaling molecules, interacting at different levels, may respond quite differently to the same signal over time. As discussed already, experimental sensitization or kindling models have clearly shown that changes in signaling pathways play important roles in the long-term neuroplastic adaptations observed.
- Alterations in signaling pathways have major effects on circadian rhythms known to be abnormal in manic-depressive illness. It is noteworthy that although this tendency to recur is among the most distinguishing features of manic-depressive illness, in both its bipolar and its highly recurrent unipolar forms, it is poorly described and not well understood. It is noteworthy that studies have begun to uncover the molecular underpinning of circadian cycles (Chang and Reppert 2001). The core clock mechanism appears to involve a transcriptional/translational feedback loop in which gene products are involved in negative feedback of themselves and other genes in the pathway (see Chapter 16). The synchronized multioscillators system offers several advantages; notably,

interactions between neurons not only coordinate the population but decrease cycle-to-cycle variability, allowing behavioral rhythms to be more precise than individual neuronal rhythms (Herzog et al., 2004). A circadian system composed of multiple circadian oscillators can be disadvantageous, however, for the organism when internal desynchrony among circadian pacemakers results from abnormalities in signaling cascades required to provide "fine-tuning" for the system. It is our contention that, along with cyclicity, the switch process is one of the fundamental and defining characteristics of the bipolar disorder subgroup. Thus a greater understanding of the molecular and cellular underpinnings of the switch process could greatly enhance understanding of the neurobiology of the disorder. Unfortunately, the immense practical difficulties inherent in studying medication-free bipolar patients longitudinally have greatly hampered investigators' ability to collect much-needed data on this critical facet of the illness. Nevertheless, important clues have been found, most notably with respect to the catecholaminergic systems and signaling cascades.

- Cellular signal transduction cascades are clearly the targets for our most effective treatments for manic-depressive illness. Indeed, it is likely that the identification of signaling cascades as targets for the actions of lithium and other mood stabilizers has had a profound impact on our understanding of the cellular neurobiology of manic-depressive illness (Manji and Lenox, 2000b; Bezchlibnyk and Young, 2002). While most of our drug development efforts in the past have been aimed at the treatment of the affective states of mania or depression, the unique clinical action of lithium is its ability to prophylactically stabilize the underlying disease process by effectively reducing the frequency and severity of the profound mood cycling in a majority of appropriately selected patients. There is reasonable evidence to suggest that once the disease process has been triggered and clinically manifest, long-term adaptive changes in the central nervous signaling systems predispose an individual to more frequent and severe affective episodes over time. A correction of dysregulated trans-synaptic signaling by mood stabilizers represents a physiological process able to curtail the often wild oscillations in behavioral states associated with manic-depressive illness, especially in its bipolar form. Indeed, regulation of signal transduction within critical regions of the brain by mood stabilizers affects the intracellular signal generated by multiple neurotransmitter systems; these effects undoubtedly represent targets for their therapeutic efficacy, since the behavioral and physiological manifestations of the illness are complex and are likely mediated by a network of interconnected neurotransmitter pathways.

- Abnormalities in cellular plasticity cascades likely also represent the underpinnings of the impairments of structural plasticity seen in morphometric studies of manic-depressive illness. Thus, many of these pathways play critical roles not only in "here-and-now" synaptic plasticity, but also in long-term cell growth and atrophy and cell survival and cell death. Indeed, the atrophic changes observed in multiple cell types (neurons and glia), as well as the reversibility of the changes with treatment, support a role for intracellular plasticity cascades. It is likely that the major defect is in the ability to regulate neuroplastic adaptations to perturbations (both physiological and pathophysiological)—an inability to handle "normal loads" (neurochemical, hormonal, stress-induced, pharmacologically induced, etc.) without failing or invoking compensatory adaptations that overshoot and predispose to oscillations. Indeed, the allostatic load contributes to long-term disease progression (and potentially to cycle acceleration). Many of the very same "plasticity regulators" also play a critical role in cell survival, cell death, and cellular resilience. These observations serve to explain the atrophic (perhaps degenerative) aspect of the illness in some patients, as well as the presence of stigmata normally associated with ischemic/hypoxic insults, such as white matter hyperintensities. (See Figure 14–37 for a depiction of the multiple targets by which neuroplasticity and cellular resilience can be increased in mood disorders.)

In conclusion, since publication of the first edition of this text in 1990, there have truly been tremendous advances in our understanding of the circuits, and especially of the molecular and cellular underpinnings of manic-depressive illness. Through functional brain imaging studies, affective circuits have been identified that mediate the behavioral, cognitive, and somatic manifestations of manic-depressive illness. Key areas of these circuits include the amygdala and related limbic structures, orbital and medial prefrontal cortex, anterior cingulate, medial thalamus, and related regions of the basal ganglia. Imbalance within these circuits, rather than an increase or decrease in any single region of the circuit, seems to predispose to and mediate the expression of manic-depressive illness. Moreover, studies of cellular plasticity cascades in manic-depressive illness are leading to a reconceptualization of the pathophysiology, course, and optimal long-term treatment of the illness. These data suggest that, while manic-depressive illness is clearly not a classic neurodegenerative disease, it is in fact associated with impairments of cellular plasticity and resilience. As a consequence, there is a growing appreciation that optimal long-term treatment will likely be achieved by attempting to prevent the underlying disease progression and its attendant

Figure 14–37. Targets for novel treatments. The functional interactions among monoamine neurotransmitters, glutamate, and neurotrophic signaling cascades, as well as various sites where stress affects these systems are illustrated. Genetic factors and life stress are both likely to contribute to the neurochemical alterations, impairments in cellular resilience, reductions in brain volume, and cell death and atrophy observed in depression. Targets for increasing neuroplasticity and cellular resilience and facilitating new classes of antidepressant medications include the following: (1) Phosphodiesterase inhibitors increase levels of pCREB. (2) MAPK modulators increase the expression of Bcl-2. (3) mGluR II/III receptor agonists modulate the release of excessive levels of glutamate. (4) Drugs such as riluzole and felbamate act on Na^+ channels to attenuate glutamate release. (5) AMPA potentiators upregulate the expression of BDNF. (6) NMDA receptor antagonists such as memantine enhance plasticity and cell survival. (7) Drugs that increase glial release of trophic factors and clear excessive glutamate may have antidepressant properties. (8) CRH antagonists may reverse the anxiogenic and depressogenic effects of extrahypothalamic CRH. (9) Glucocorticoid antagonists may attenuate the deleterious effects of hypocortisolemia. (10) Agents that upregulate Bcl-2 (such as pramipexole) may have antistress and antidepressant actions. α_2-AR = α_2-adrenergic receptor; AC = adenylyl cyclase; AMPAR = α-amino 3-hydroxy-5-methylisoxazole propionate; BDNF = brain-derived neurotrophic factor; CREB = cAMP-responsive element-binding protein; CRH = corticotrophin-releasing hormone; G_i = family of G protein α subunits that includes G_i and G_o; G_q = family of G protein α subunits that includes G_q and G_{11}; Glu = glutamate; GR = glucocorticoid receptor; GSK-3 = glycogen synthase kinase; HDAC = histone deacetylases; MAPK = mitogen-activated protein kinase; mGluR = metabotropic glutamate receptor; NE = norepinephrine; NMDAR = N-methyl-D-aspartate receptor; PKA = protein kinase A; 5-HT = serotonin. (*Source*: Charney and Manji, 2004. Reprinted with permission.)

cellular dysfunction, rather than exclusively focusing on the treatment of signs and symptoms.

There has, unfortunately, been little progress in developing truly novel drugs specifically for the treatment of manic-depressive illness, and most recent additions to the pharmacopeia are brain-penetrant drugs developed for the treatment of epilepsy or schizophrenia. This era may now

be over as there are a number of pharmacologic "plasticity-enhancing" strategies which may be of considerable utility in the treatment of manic-depressive illness. Indeed, these next-generation drugs, in addition to treating the core symptoms of bipolar and/or highly recurrent unipolar disorder, might be able to target other important aspects of the illness. They may, for example, be able to enhance cognition independent of whether mood symptoms improve, prevent, or reverse epigenetic factors that may have long-term negative impact on the course of the illness (e.g., histone deacetylase inhibitors), or reduce certain medical co-morbidities such as diabetes (e.g., GSK inhibitors) (Zarate et al., 2006b).

We are optimistic that the advances outlined here will result in a dramatically different diagnostic system based on etiology, and ultimately in the discovery of new approaches to the prevention and treatment of some of humankind's most devastating and least understood illnesses. This progress holds much promise for developing novel therapeutics for the long-term treatment of severe, refractory mood disorders, and for improving the lives of millions.

NOTES

1. For example, Robbins and Sahakian, 1980; Smith and Helms, 1982; Lerer et al., 1984; Berggren, 1985; Ushijama et al., 1986.

2. Wada et al., 1976; Leviel and Naquet, 1977; Albright and Burnham, 1980; Post et al., 1984c, 1998; Azorin and Tramoni, 1987; Weiss et al., 1990.

3. Wyatt et al., 1971; Louis et al., 1975; Barnes et al., 1983; Koslow et al., 1983; Roy et al., 1985, 1987, 1988; Rudorfer et al., 1985; Veith et al., 1988, 1994; de Villiers et al., 1989. Maas et al., 1987;

4. To begin with, receptors on blood cells are by definition noninnervated, exist in a markedly different environment, and may therefore poorly reflect central, innervated, adrenergic receptors. Another major (often overlooked) consideration when interpreting studies of dynamic receptor regulation in blood cells is that white blood cell counts and the relative proportions of subsets of lymphocytes may vary. Recruitment of cells with different characteristics into the circulation may frequently explain altered receptor function. Precisely such a mechanism appears to be operative in studies demonstrating the seemingly paradoxical increase in lymphocyte beta-adrenergic receptor (βAR) density and responsiveness during short-term isoproterenol infusion, mental arithmetic, and dynamic exercise (procedures that stimulate the sympathetic nervous system) (Maisel et al., 1990; Van Tits et al., 1990). The mechanism appears to be a release of subsets of "fresh" lymphocytes from the spleen into the circulation (Van Tits et al., 1990; Werstiuk et al., 1990). These fresh, activated lymphocytes express enhanced βAR responsiveness, and this probably accounts for the exercise and catecholamine-induced increases in βAR responsiveness.

5. Extein et al., 1979b; Pandey, 1987, 1990; Carstens et al., 1988; Magliozzi et al., 1989.

6. Sarai et al., 1982; Zohar et al., 1983; Cooper et al., 1985; Healy et al., 1985; Mann et al., 1985; Pandey et al., 1985. See Werstiuk et al. (1990) for a critical appraisal of these studies and possible methodological sources of the differences in results (e.g., methods of tissue preparation, types of ligand used, subtypes of patient populations, length of drug-free interval).

7. Extein et al., 1979b; Pandey et al., 1979; Healy et al., 1983; Mann et al., 1985; Klysner et al., 1987; Ebstein et al., 1988; Halper et al., 1988.

8. Matussek et al., 1980; Checkley et al., 1981, 1984, 1985; Charney et al., 1982; Siever et al., 1982; Lechin et al., 1985; Boyer et al., 1986; Uhde et al., 1986; Ansseau et al., 1988; Hoehe et al., 1988.

9. Bunney and Garland-Bunney, 1987; Goodwin and Jamison, 1990; Lenox and Manji, 1998.

10. Murphy et al., 1974; Huey et al., 1981; Goodnick and Meltzer, 1984; G. Goodwin et al., 1986a.

11. Greenspan et al., 1970; Schildkraut 1973, 1974; Beckmann et al., 1975; Murphy et al., 1979; Corona et al., 1982; Linnoila et al., 1983b; Grof et al., 1986; Swann et al., 1987; Goodnick, 1990.

12. Greenspan et al., 1970; Schildkraut, 1973; Beckmann et al., 1975; Bowers and Heninger, 1977.

13. Bond et al., 1972; Jones et al., 1973; Schildkraut et al., 1973; Post et al., 1977; Wehr, 1977.

14. Friedman and Gershon, 1973; Hesketh and Glen, 1978; Ahluwalia and Singhal, 1980; Engel and Berggren. 1980; Ahluwalia et al., 1981; Eroglu et al., 1981; Frances et al., 1981.

15. Fyro et al., 1975; Bowers and Heninger, 1977; Linnoila et al., 1983b; Goodnick and Gershon, 1984; Berrettini et al., 1985b; Swann et al., 1987.

16. Biegon et al., 1987, 1990a,b; Cowen et al., 1987; Arora and Meltzer, 1989a, 1993; Pandey et al., 1990, 1995; Mann et al., 1992; McBride et al., 1994; Hrdina et al., 1995; Sheline et al., 1995.

17. Bunney and Garland, 1983; Bunney and Garland-Bunney, 1987; Price et al., 1990.

18. Collard and Roberts, 1977; Collard, 1978; Ahluwalia and Singhal, 1980; Bunney and Garland, 1983; Shukla, 1985; Treiser et al., 1981.

19. Maggi and Enna, 1980; Treiser and Kellar, 1980; Treiser et al., 1981; Tanimoto et al., 1983; Goodnick and Gershon, 1984; G. Goodwin et al., 1986b; Hotta and Yamawaki, 1988; Godfrey et al., 1989; Mizuta and Segawa, 1989; Newman et al., 1990; Odagaki et al., 1990.

20. Grahame-Smith and Green, 1974; Friedman et al., 1979; Harrison-Read, 1979; G. Goodwin et al., 1986b.

21. G. Goodwin et al., 1986a; Friedman and Wang, 1988; Hotta and Yamawaki, 1988; Wang and Friedman, 1988; Mork and Geisler, 1989; Newman et al., 1990.

22. Fyro et al., 1975; Bowers and Heninger, 1977; Goodnick and Gershon, 1984; Linnoila et al., 1984; Berrettini et al., 1985b; Swann et al., 1987; Goodnick, 1990; Price et al., 1990.

23. Wood and Coppen, 1983; Meltzer and Lowy, 1987; Poirier et al., 1988; Price et al., 1990.

24. Meltzer et al., 1984; Muhlbauer, 1984; Muhlbauer and Muller-Oerlinghausen, 1985; Glue et al., 1986; Cowen et al., 1989; McCance et al., 1989; Price et al., 1989.

25. Gillin et al., 1978; Sitaram et al., 1976, 1978a,b,c, 1979.

26. Lee, 1974; Lingsch and Martin, 1976; Jope et al., 1978, 1980; Rybakowski et al., 1978; Meltzer et al., 1982; Uney et al., 1985; Stoll et al., 1991.

27. Honchar et al., 1983; Jope et al., 1986; Persinger et al., 1988; Hirvonen et al., 1990; Terry et al., 1990; Ormandy and Jope, 1991.

28. Honchar et al., 1983; Jope et al., 1986; Persinger et al., 1988; Hirvonen et al., 1990; Terry et al., 1990; Ormandy and Jope, 1991.

29. In a similar vein, Hong and colleagues (2000) showed that blood levels of reelin were extremely low to undetectable in children afflicted with a variant of lissencephaly. These children had various mutations involving the *RELN* gene and exhibited severe delays in neurologic and cognitive development (Hong et al., 2000). Later, Fatemi and colleagues found deficits in reelin protein in brain and blood of subjects with

autism, another neurodevelopmental disorder characterized by significant cognitive dysfunction in association with a vulnerability to defective reelin inheritance (Fatemi et al., 2001b, 2002; Persico et al., 2001; Fatemi, 2002).

30. Sawaya et al., 1975; Anlezark et al., 1976; Whittle and Turner, 1978; van der Laan et al., 1979; Johannessen, 2000.

31. Witkin, 1993; Li et al., 1997; Tzschentke and Schmidt, 1997; Hotsenpiller et al., 2001; Backstrom and Hyytia, 2003.

32. Several classes of ARPs have been identified, including benzothiadiazides, such as cyclothiazide; pyrrolidones, such as piracetam and aniracetam; and benzoylpiperidines, such as CX-516. Preclinical studies have shown that modulation of AMPA receptors with the piperidine (CX-516) enhances MAPK activation and reduces the extent of synaptic and neuronal degeneration resulting from excitotoxic insults, even when infused after the insult (Bahr et al., 2002). In view of the ability of structurally dissimilar ARPs to increase BDNF expression (Hayashi et al., 1999; Lauterborn et al., 2000; Skolnick et al., 2001), studies investigating the putative efficacy of an ARP (LY392098) in animal models of depression were undertaken. These studies showed that LY392098 produced a reduction in the duration of immobility in the forced swim test similar to that produced by traditional antidepressants, suggesting that ARPs may indeed have utility as novel antidepressants.

33. Several comprehensive texts review the physiology of the HPT axis. See Demeester-Mirkine and Dumont (1980), Ingbar and Braverman (1986), and Martin and Reichlin (1987).

34. Gold and Manji, 2002b; Nemeroff et al., 1985; Hein and Jackson, 1990; Musselman and Nemeroff, 1996; Haggerty et al., 1997.

35. Cho et al., 1979; Cowdry et al., 1983; Bauer et al., 1990; Kusalic, 1992; Oomen et al., 1996.

36. Bartalena et al., 1990; Joffe et al., 1988; Post et al., 1997; Valle et al., 1999.

37. Bauer et al., 1998a,b.

38. Souêtre et al., 1986; Sack et al., 1988; Baumgartner et al., 1990a; Parekh et al., 1998; Orth et al., 2001.

39. For example, Kastin et al., 1972; Prange et al., 1972; Molchan et al., 1991; Rush et al., 1997.

40. Arana et al., 1983; Stokes et al., 1984; Kiriike et al., 1988; Woodside et al., 1989; Swann et al., 1992; Cassidy et al., 1998b.

41. The application of the combined DEX/CRH test consists of the oral administration of 1.5 mg dexamethasone at 11:00 PM the night before an IV bolus administration of 100 µg of human CRH at 3:00 AM. Blood samples for the determination of plasma cortisol and ACTH are then drawn every 15 minutes from 2:00 to 6:00 PM. Recently, a modification of the test has been explored that involves monitoring cortisol levels in saliva, with the intent of making more routine use of the DEX/CRH test (Baghai et al., 2002).

42. This atrophy is observed in the CA3 pyramidal neurons, but not in other hippocampal cell groups (i.e., CA1 pyramidal and dentate gyrus granule neurons). The stress-induced atrophy of CA3 neurons (i.e., decreased number and length of the apical dendritic branches) occurs after 2–3 weeks of exposure to restraint stress or longer-term social stress, and has been observed in rodents and tree shrews (McEwen, 1999a; Sapolsky, 2000a). Atrophy of CA3 pyramidal neurons also occurs upon exposure to high levels of glucocorticoids, suggesting that activation of the HPA axis likely plays a major role in mediating the stress-induced atrophy (Sapolsky 1996, 2000b; McEwen, 1999). The hippocampus has a very high concentration of glutamate and expresses both Type I and Type II corticosteroid receptors, though the latter receptors may be relatively scarce in the hippocampus of primates (Patel et al., 2000; Sanchez et al., 2000) and more abundant in cortical regions. Mineralcorticoid or Type I (MR) receptor activation in the hippocampus (CA1) is associated with reduced calcium currents, whereas activation of glucocorticoid or Type II receptors (GR) causes increased calcium currents and enhanced responses to excitatory amino acids. Very high levels of Type II receptor activation markedly increase calcium currents and lead to greater NMDA receptor throughput that could predispose to neurotoxicity. Indeed, as we discuss in greater detail below, a growing body of data has implicated glutamatergic neurotransmission in stress-induced hippocampal atrophy and death (McEwen, 1999).

43. Using a Golgi-Cox procedure, Wellman (2001) investigated pyramidal neurons in layers II and III of medial prefrontal cortex and quantified dendritic morphology in three dimensions. This study demonstrated a significant redistribution of apical dendrites in corticosterone-treated animals, with the amount of dendritic material proximal to the soma being increased and distal dendritic material being decreased. These findings suggest that stress may produce a significant reorganization of the apical dendritic arbor from medial prefrontal cortex in rats. Most recently, Lyons (2002) demonstrated that 4 years after a brief stressor (intermittent postnatal separations from maternal availability), young adult squirrel monkeys showed significantly larger right ventral medial prefrontal volumes. Neither overall brain volumes nor left prefrontal measures were altered, suggesting selective (rather than nonspecific) effects.

44. CRF$_1$ receptors, which bind CRF with higher affinity than CRF$_2$ receptors, play a major role in regulating ACTH release and have been implicated in animal models of anxiety. Indeed, the central administration of CRF$_1$ antisense oligodeoxynucleotides has been demonstrated to have anxiolytic effects against both CRF and psychological stressors. Although CRF$_2$ receptors appear to act in an antagonistic manner (i.e., CRF$_1$ activates and CRF$_2$ attenuates the stress response), their precise role is still being characterized (Reul and Holsboer, 2002). Interestingly, pretreatment with a CRH antagonist also attenuates the stress-induced increases in MR levels in hippocampus, neocortex, frontal cortex, and amygdala (Gesing et al., 2001). Likewise, rats that underwent a stressor showed increased ACTH and cortisol levels following the administration of an MR antagonist, suggesting that the upregulation of MR in the stressed group was associated with increased inhibitory tone of the HPA axis.

45. Estrogen has been shown to decrease monoamine oxidase (MAO) activity (Klaiber et al., 1971) in human plasma, while progesterone appears to enhance MAO activity (Holzbauer and Youdim, 1973). Although the exact clinical effects in humans are unclear, decreased MAO activity will ultimately increase the levels of monoamine neurotransmitters, an effect generally associated with a positive effect on mood. Preclinical studies indicate that estrogen and other gonadal hormones may facilitate downregulation of 5-HT2 receptors during treatment with antidepressants. Thus, Kendall and colleagues (1982) showed that abrupt withdrawal of estrogen by surgical ovariec-

tomy in rats abolishes antidepressant-induced downregulation of 5-HT2 receptors and that replacement of estrogen (as well as progesterone or testosterone) reverses the effect.

46. Janowsky and colleagues (1979) found that only 2 of 7 manic patients were dramatically calmed, whereas Judd and colleagues (1980) found observable decreases in manic symptoms in 4 of 12 manic patients with the same dose and route of administration. Davis and colleagues (1979) noted some apparent antimanic effects in 4 patients receiving up to 30 mg, but the changes were not sufficiently robust to reach statistical significance. Later, this same group (1980) gave 20 mg subcutaneously to 10 manic patients and reported no improvement in rated mania.

47. In an open trial that included several depressed patients, Kline and Lehmann (1979) noted marked activation in one patient and some improvement in depression in two patients receiving IV p-endorphin. The effect occurred within minutes and lasted for several hours. Angst and colleagues (1979) found that when six depressed patients (four bipolar and two unipolar) received an IV infusion of p-endorphin, all improved in energy, mood, anxiety, and restlessness during the first 20 to 30 minutes, an effect that persisted for 2 hours. Four subsequently relapsed. Three patients switched into mania or hypomania during or soon after the trial, an outcome the authors suggest may have been caused by drug withdrawal, sleep deprivation, or stress.

In a double-blind trial, Gemer and colleagues (1980) also observed significant improvement following IV p-endorphin in 10 depressed patients, who then relapsed the day after the infusion; no hypomania was noted. Similar positive results were observed by Chazot and colleagues (1985) in a randomized placebo-controlled, double-blind trial involving 20 patients hospitalized for major depression (primarily unipolar). Two other double-blind trials were negative—one involving destyrosine y-endorphin (Fink et al., 1981) and the other p-endorphin (Pickar et al., 1981). Extein and colleagues (1979a,b) administered an analog of metenkephalin (FK 33824) to nine medication-free depressed patients (predominantly bipolar) and observed no clinical improvement. In sum, findings of initial open studies (and one double-blind study) suggest that IV p-endorphin or related endogenous opiate substances may improve depression.

48. Terenius' group (1976) initially reported that CSF from manic and depressed patients showed alterations in binding to an opiate receptor preparation. Many of these patients were not studied under medication-free conditions, however, and it is also not clear how many of the depressed patients were bipolar. In a well-controlled study of bipolar illness, Pickar and colleagues (1982a) reported no overall relationship between manic or depressive mood state and total CSF opiate activity as measured by binding in the radioreceptor assay, although all four patients studied in both phases had significantly higher opiate receptor activity during mania than during depression. The opioid peptide precursor proopiomelano-cortin (POMC) is cleaved to form various fragments, including s-endorphin, P-lipotropin, ct-MSH, ACTH, and the N-terminal fragment of POMC (N-POMC). Berrettini and colleagues (1985b, 1987) measured the five fragments in CSF and plasma in 30 normal volunteers and 40 euthymic bipolar patients (15 unmedicated, 25 lithium-treated). None of the five peptides was different in either group of well-state patients compared with controls.

49. Lithium-induced increases in dynorphin were accompanied by an increase in the abundance of prodynorphin mRNA (Sivam et al., 1988), suggesting that the drug's effects on dynorphin levels are at least partially mediated through increased transcription and translation. Acute studies with lithium have demonstrated enhanced release of a number of opioid peptides from hypothalamic slices and have suggested an effect at the inhibitory presynaptic opioid autoreceptor (Burns et al., 1990). Chronic lithium administration did not affect the basal hypothalamic release of any of the opioids, but prevented the naloxone-stimulated release of the peptides in vitro, compatible with lithium-induced autoreceptor subsensitivity (Burns et al., 1990). Lithium is reported to decrease the affinity of opiate receptors in vitro, whereas subchronic lithium administration is reported in some but not all studies to decrease the number of opioid-binding sites in rat forebrain structures (Goodnick and Gershon, 1984). Additional support for effects on the opioidergic system comes from behavioral studies in which lithium produced aversive states in rats that could be blocked by the depletion of central pools of endorphin or by the blockade of opioid receptors. It has also been demonstrated that chronic lithium administration abolishes both the secondary reinforcing effects of morphine and the aversive effects of the opioid antagonist naloxone (Mucha et al., 1985; Blancquaert et al., 1987; Lieblich and Yirmiya, 1987; Shippenberg et al., 1988; Shippenberg and Herz, 1991).

50. When injected with somatostatin intracerebroventricularly, animals exhibit decreased spontaneous activity, increased appetite, decreased slow-wave and REM sleep, and decreased sensitivity to pain. Somatostatin modulates classic neurotransmitters such as NE, serotonin, and DA, and in addition is collocated with neurons containing NE, GABA, or acetylcholine. Several pieces of indirect evidence suggest its potential importance in affective illness. Somatostatin is widely distributed in the CNS, including cortical, limbic, and hypothalamic regions. It exerts inhibitory control over the HPA axis, which, as noted earlier, is often disinhibited in depression and perhaps in some manic states as well. Somatostatin is depleted in temporal cortex and CSF of patients with Alzheimer's disease. It is sometimes reduced in patients with other conditions often accompanied by cognitive impairment, including parkinsonism, multiple sclerosis, and anorexia nervosa. Somatostatin inhibits endocrine responses to a variety of hormones and alters appetite, pain, sleep, and motor activity (Rubinow et al., 1983), all of which are often abnormal in affective illness. It affects a variety of the classic neurotransmitters (NE, 5-HT, DA, GABA, and ACh) and coexists in neurons containing NE, acetylcholine, or GABA, suggesting important regulatory functions in these systems.

51. Clinical evaluations of this hypothesis have used the measurement of CSF vasopressin, plasma vasopressin response to saline infusion challenge, and the behavioral response of depressed patients to a vasopressin analog. A number of studies have found that nonpsychotic bipolar depressed patients had significantly lower levels of vasopressin in CSF than those of manic patients, with normal control levels falling in the middle (Gold et al., 1981b; Gjerris et al., 1985; Sorensen et al., 1985). Gold's group (1984a) also found that vasopressin levels in CSF were significantly correlated with plasma vasopressin responses to hypertonic saline. There ap-

peared to be differences in vasopressin levels across manic and depressive states in the small number of patients receiving hypertonic saline infusion.

These findings suggest that there may be subtle vasopressin changes across manic and depressive mood states that are relevant to alterations in cognitive functioning. However, two studies of euthymic bipolar patients (Berrettini et al., 1982; Berrettini and Post, 1984) found no abnormalities in platelet vasopressin uptake and arginine vasopressin levels in CSF.

As noted, animal research suggests that vasopressin is important in memory processes (Weid, 1975), and several studies have found that administration of vasopressin (or its analogs) to normal volunteers, depressed patients, or amnesic subjects improved some aspects of memory and cognition (Weingartner et al., 1981). Gold and colleagues (1979) report that mood improved in two of seven hospitalized, medication-free depressed patients given l-desamino-8-D-arginine vagopressin (DDAVP); the uniformity of the memory improvement was even more significant. However, Zohar and colleagues (1985) did not find a therapeutic effect of lysine vasopressin on mood in 12 severely depressed, treatment-resistant patients in a double-blind, crossover study.

52. Janowsky and Overstreet, 1995; Maes et al., 1995; Schatzberg and Schildkraut, 1995; Willner 1995; Manji and Potter, 1997; Garlow et al., 1999.

53. Bowden et al., 1997; Manji and Lenox, 2000b; Manji et al., 2000a; Payne et al., 2002.

54. Mathews et al., 1997; Wang et al., 1997; Chen et al., 1999; Warsh et al., 2000.

55. Clearly, caution is necessary when extrapolating from peripheral, accessible tissue in the study of complex CNS disorders. In this context, it is noteworthy that there is a growing body of evidence showing coexpression of abnormal proteins in peripheral cells in several neuropsychiatric disorders (Trottier et al., 1995; Li et al., 1999; Widner et al., 1999), thereby underscoring the potential utility of peripheral cells for such studies. More important for the present discussion, longitudinal studies have previously been undertaken with pharmacological agents known to affect signaling pathways in the brain (most notably lithium), demonstrating effects on several signaling proteins in peripheral cells from humans highly similar to those observed in rodent CNS (Manji et al., 1995a; Manji and Lenox, 1999). Furthermore, at least for some signaling molecules, studies have found a strong correlation between the treatment-induced changes in rodent brain and in platelets obtained from the same rodents (Manji and Lenox, 1999). Together, these results suggest that, with appropriate cautionary measures, peripheral cells can sometimes provide useful information about complex neuropsychiatric disorders.

56. Risby et al., 1991; Mork et al., 1992; Manji et al., 1995b; J. Wang et al., 1999; Manji and Lenox, 2000b.

57. Manji et al., 1995a,b; Stein et al., 1996; Li and El-Mallakh, 2000; Warsh et al., 2000.

58. Jope, 1999; Mork et al., 1992; Wang et al., 1997; Manji et al., 2000a.

59. Furthermore, although some studies have found modest changes in the levels of G protein subunits, the preponderance of the data suggests that the effects of chronic lithium on signal-transducing properties occur in the absence of changes in the levels of G protein subunits per se (Lenox and Manji, 1998). Chronic in vivo lithium treatment has been shown to produce a significant increase in pertussis toxin catalyzed [^{32}P]ADP-ribosylation in rat frontal cortex and human platelets. Since pertussis toxin selectively ADP-ribosylates the undissociated, inactive $\alpha\beta\gamma$ heterotrimeric form of G_i, these results suggest that lithium attenuates G_i function through stabilization of the inactive conformation. These results suggest that removal of the "inhibitory tone" by lithium may be responsible for the elevations in basal AC and the responses to agents activating the stimulatory pathway distal to the receptor.

60. The distinct actions of lithium on the AC system may explain the differing results obtained by investigators using rat membrane preparations and those using slice preparations (Manji et al., 2000a). This possibility led to an investigation of lithium's effects on the AC system in vivo, using microdialysis. These studies found that chronic lithium treatment produced a significant increase in basal and postreceptor-stimulated (cholera toxin or forskolin) AC activity while attenuating the β-adrenergic mediated effect (Masana et al., 1992; Manji et al., 2000a). Interestingly, chronic lithium treatment resulted in an almost absent cAMP response to pertussis toxin, suggesting a lithium-induced attenuation of G_i function. It should be noted, however, that chronic lithium exposure has also been found to increase not only cAMP levels (Wiborg et al., 1999), but also the levels of AC type I and II mRNA and protein levels in frontal cortex (Colin et al., 1991; Jensen et al., 2000). This finding suggests that lithium's complex effects on the system may represent the net effects of direct inhibition of AC, upregulation of AC subtypes, and effects on the stimulatory and inhibitory G proteins.

61. Steketee and Kalivas, 1991; Steketee et al., 1991; Giambalvo, 1992a,b; Gnegy et al., 1993; Steketee, 1993, 1994; Iwata et al., 1997a,b.

62. Lithium has also been shown to have additional potential sites of action in the PI cycle, where it has been reported to inhibit the inositol polyphosphatase that dephosphorylates $I(1,3,4)P_3$ and $I(1,4)P_2$. Because the brain has limited access to inositol other than that derived from recycling of inositol phosphates, the ability of a cell to maintain sufficient supplies of myoinositol can be crucial to the resynthesis of the PIs and the maintenance and efficiency of signaling (Sherman, 1986). Furthermore, because the mode of enzyme inhibition is uncompetitive, lithium's effects have been postulated to be most pronounced in systems undergoing the highest rate of PIP_2 hydrolysis (Berridge et al., 1989; Nahorski et al., 1991, 1992). Furthermore, because several subtypes of adrenergic (e.g., α_1), cholinergic (e.g., m_1, m_3, m_5), serotonergic (e.g., 5-HT$_2$, 5-HT$_1$), and dopaminergic (e.g., D1) receptors are coupled to PIP_2 turnover in the CNS (Mahan et al., 1990; Rana and Hokin, 1990; Vallar et al., 1990; Fisher et al., 1992), this hypothesis offers a plausible explanation for lithium's therapeutic efficacy in treating both poles of manic-depressive disorder by the compensatory stabilization of an inherent biogenic amine imbalance in critical regions of the brain (Manji et al., 1995b).

63. Kendall and Nahorski, 1987; Casebolt and Jope, 1989; Godfrey et al., 1989; Whitworth and Kendall, 1989, discussed in Jope and Williams, 1994; Ellis and Lenox, 1990; Manji and Lenox, 1998.

64. Several lines of evidence suggest that the action of chronic lithium may not be directly manifest in receptor-mediated PI turnover. While investigators have observed that levels of inositol in brain remain reduced in rats receiving chronic lithium (Sherman et al., 1985), it has been difficult to demonstrate that this phenomenon results in reduced resynthesis of PIP_2, which is the substrate for agonist-induced PI turnover. Rather, this observation may be due to the methodological difficulties involved in accurately measuring alterations in a rapidly turning over small signal-related pool of PIP_2 and/or may be explained by recent evidence that resynthesis of inositol phospholipids may also occur through base exchange reactions from other, larger pools of phospholipids, such as phosphatidylcholine (Nishizuka, 1992; Manji and Lenox, 1994). An initial attempt to verify this hypothesis at this level of the PI cycle by examining the effects of lithium on muscarinic-stimulated accumulation of IP_1 in brain slices in the presence of exogenously added inositol were unsuccessful (Kendall and Nahorski, 1987).

Additional support for the critical role of the PI second messenger–generating system in mediating many of lithium's effects comes from numerous biochemical, physiological, and behavioral studies showing that the coadministration of myoinositol attenuates many of the effects of chronic lithium administration (Busa and Gimlich, 1989; Godfrey et al., 1989; Kofman and Belmaker, 1990, 1993; Pontzer and Crews, 1990; Tricklebank et al., 1991; Kofman et al., 1993; Manji et al., 1996). Thus, myoinositol replenishment has been demonstrated to attenuate lithium's effects on agonist-stimulated PI turnover (Godfrey et al., 1989), electrophysiological effects mediated by serotonergic or muscarinic receptors (Pontzer and Crews, 1990), PKC isozymes (Manji et al., 1996), pertussis-catalyzed [32P]ADP-ribosylation (Manji et al., 1996), and various rodent behaviors (Kofman and Belmaker, 1990, 1993; Tricklebank et al., 1991).

65. Since fluoride ion will directly activate G protein–coupled second messenger response, efforts have been made to examine the effect of lithium on NaF-stimulated PI response in brain. Although Godfrey and colleagues (1989) reported a reduction of fluoride-stimulated PI response in cortical membranes of rats treated with lithium for 3 days, no change in response was observed in cortical slices from rats administered lithium for 30 days. More recently, using labeled PI as a substrate (which should bypass any putative inositol depletion), Song and Jope (1992) found an attenuation of PI turnover in response to GTP analogs. Taken together, these results suggest that although chronic lithium administration may affect receptor-mediated phosphoinositide signaling, these effects are unlikely to be due simply to inositol depletion in the CNS (Jope, 1993; Manji and Lenox, 1994; Lenox and Manji, 1995). Through use of a yeast model, it was found that both lithium and valproate perturb regulation of the inositol biosynthetic pathway, albeit through different mechanisms (Murray and Greenberg, 2000; Vaden et al., 2001).

66. Williams and colleagues (2000) demonstrated that lithium, valproate, and carbamazepine all inhibit the collapse of sensory neuron growth cones and increase growth cone area, effects that were reversed by inositol. The authors then used the slime mold dictyostelium, which relies on IP_3 for its development, to identify mutants that confer resistance to the drugs. Null mutations of a gene with unknown intracellular function that encodes prolyl oligopeptidase confer lithium resistance and elevate intracellular levels of IP_3. The authors drew a link between their slime-mold studies and mammals by showing that prolyl oligopeptidase inhibitors abolished the effects of lithium, carbamazepine, and valproate on growth cone collapse and area in mammalian cells. Once again, if further validated in vivo, these observations would add to the body of findings identifying CNS intracellular signaling cascades as targets for mood stabilizers and could ultimately lead to the development of novel, more specific therapies for this devastating illness (Coyle and Manji, 2002).

67. Chen et al., 1994; Watson et al., 1998; Lenox and Hahn, 2000; Manji and Chen, 2000; Manji and Lenox, 2000b.

68. Interest in a putative role for ϖ-3 FA in bipolar disorder has arisen from the following observations: efficacy in models of kindling (antikindling properties in rat models of epilepsy) (Yehuda et al., 1994); incorporation of ϖ-3 FA in the membrane, thereby suppressing the phosphatidylinositol-associated signal transduction pathway (Medini et al., 1990; Sperling et al., 1993); blockade of calcium influx through L-type calcium channels (Pepe et al., 1994); and downregulation/inhibition of various protein kinases (Holian and Nelson, 1992; Slater et al., 1994). Mirnikjoo and colleagues (2001) describe a series of experiments showing that in vitro EPA and DHA significantly reduced the activity of cAMP-dependent PKA, PKC, MAPK, and calcium/calmodulin-dependent protein kinase II (CaMKII), effects not observed with similar fatty acids lacking an ϖ-3 double bound (e.g., arachidic acid). These preclinical observations, the absence of documented drug interaction, the lack of toxicity, and the apparent safety of use in pregnant women and children of ϖ-3 FA have all led to a clinical trial of ϖ-3 FA in bipolar disorder.

69. In an immunohistochemical study of postmortem hippocampus, region-specific reductions in SNAP-25 (an integral component of the SNARE complex) expression were found in both bipolar disorder and schizophrenia (Fatemi et al., 2001a). Likewise, reduced SNAP-25 immunoreactivity was found in Brodman's area 10 of the prefrontal cortex of schizophrenic patients (Young et al., 1998), and reduced SNAP-25 and synaptophysin immunoreactivity in the hippocampal–entorhinal projections of schizophrenic patients (Karson et al., 1999). In a related study, SNAP-25 was found to be elevated in the CSF of schizophrenic patients, and a similar but nonsignificant increase was noted in the small (n=5) number of bipolar patients included (Thompson et al., 1999). A recent study investigating the formation of the SNARE complex in anterior cingulate cortex found that SNAP-25 expression and interaction with syntaxin and synaptobrevin were significantly altered in schizophrenic and depressed suicide victims (Honer et al., 2002). Finally, reduced expression of several isoforms of synapsin was observed in the hippocampus of schizophrenic and bipolar patients (Vawter et al., 2002), and reduced synapsin II mRNA was found in the prefrontal cortex of schizophrenic patients. The authors also showed that chronic lithium or haloperidol has no effect on synapsin expression in rats, a finding confirmed for lithium and extended to valproate (unpublished observations).

70. Two of the primary presynaptic targets of CaMKII are synapsin I and synaptotagmin (Greengard et al., 1993). Synapsin is believed to regulate the movement of vesicles

from the reserve pool to the membrane, and binds tightly to synaptic vesicles, actin, and ATP in a phosphorylation- and Ca^{2+}-dependent manner (Hilfiker et al., 1999a). Synaptotagmin is a secondary constituent of the SNARE complex, which docks vesicles to the presynaptic membrane, and is believed to act as a calcium sensor in calcium-dependent fusion (Hilfiker et al., 1999b). Both of these proteins have been shown to be phosphate enriched following treatment with antidepressants.

71. An additional effect on synapsin was recently noted: Valproate and, to a lesser extent, synapsin are reported to increase the number of synapsin-reactive clusters along neurites in primary neurons. It is unclear what these synapsin clusters represent, but they could be developing synapses or regions of increased cytoskeletal activity or axonal remodeling (a role for synapsins in developmental processes such as neurite outgrowth, branching, and synaptogenesis is hypothesized [Kao et al., 2002]). However, the observed effects on synapsin clustering and phosphorylation (discussed below) are not entirely congruent; increases in synapsin phosphorylation are believed, at least acutely, to cause dispersion of synapsin clusters (Chi et al., 2001; Angers et al., 2002).

72. GSK-3 is a highly conserved enzyme in evolution and is found in two nearly identical isoforms in mammals—α and β (Plyte et al., 1992; Cohen and Frame, 2001; Woodgett, 2001). It was first discovered (and named) on the basis of its ability to phosphorylate and thereby inactivate the enzyme glycogen synthase, an action that leads to a decrease in the synthesis of glycogen. Klein and Melton (1996) discovered that lithium inhibited the action of GSK-3, an effect that occurs through competition with magnesium for a binding site (Ryves and Harwood, 2001). GSK-3 phosphorylates—and thereby inactivates—many targets, including transcription factors and cytoskeletal proteins such as the Alzheimer's protein tau (a previous name for GSK-3 was tau kinase). Inhibition of GSK-3 thus results in the release of this inhibition and activation of multiple cellular targets.

73. GSK-3 is a serine/threonine kinase that is normally highly active in cells and is deactivated by signals originating from numerous signaling pathways (e.g., the Wnt pathway, the PI3 kinase pathway, protein kinase A, and PKC, among many others). It is found in two forms—α and β—that have similar but not always identical biological functions. Cellular targets of GSK-3 are numerous and often depend on the signaling pathway that is acting on it (because of cellular localization and regional sequestration). For example, Wnt pathway inhibition of GSK-3 activates the transcription factor β-catenin, while in the insulin/PI3 kinase signaling pathway, inhibition of GSK-3 results in activation of the enzyme glycogen synthase. Targets of GSK-3 include, among others, transcription factors (β-catenin, CREB, c-Jun), proteins bound to microtubules (tau, MAP1B, kinesin light chain), cell cycle mediators (cyclin D, human ninein), and regulators of metabolism (glycogen synthase, pyruvate dehydrogenase).

Being a component of many signaling pathways with multiple cellular targets from which to choose allows GSK-3 to regulate a diverse array of cellular processes, such as glycogen synthesis, gene transcription, events related to synaptic plasticity, apoptosis, and the circadian cycle. While many of these functions are likely to be critically important to both cellular and organism functioning, at present GSK-3 is the subject of interest primarily as a regulator of apoptosis and cellular resilience. Generally, increased activity of GSK-3 is pro-apoptotic, whereas inhibiting GSK-3 attenuates or prevents apoptosis.

74. In addition to its possible usefulness in the treatment of bipolar disorder, inactivation of GSK-3 has been suggested as a potential therapy for a number of diseases. Diabetes and Alzheimer's disease have received the most attention. Diabetes has drawn interest because GSK-3 phosphorylates and deactivates glycogen synthase (T. Gould et al., 2003, 2004a,b). Alzheimer's disease is a target because of the role GSK-3 plays in both the phosphorylation of tau and the assembly of amyloid-β. Hyperphosphorylation of tau is associated with the formation of neurofibrillary tangles, while accumulation of amyloid-β leads to amyloid plaques. GSK-3 inhibitors may also be useful for the treatment of cardiac ischemic injury, other neurodegenerative disorders, and stroke and other neurotraumatic injuries.

For these reasons, major efforts in industry have focused on the development of selective GSK-3 inhibitors. In 2002 it was reported that more than 45 patents for GSK-3 inhibitors had already been filed. Early-phase clinical trials (likely for Alzheimer's disease or diabetes) of GSK-3 inhibitors will probably be completed in the near future; it is expected that these compounds will also be tested for efficacy in the treatment of bipolar disorder.

75. Steffens and Krishnan, 1998; McDonald et al., 1999; Taylor et al., 1999; Moore et al., 2001; Lenox et al., 2002.

76. Ongur et al., 1998; Rajkowska et al., 1999; Coyle and Schwarcz, 2000; LoTurco, 2000; Rajkowska, 2000; Haydon, 2001; Ullian et al., 2001.

77. Musselman et al., 1998; Steffens and Krishnan, 1998; Doraiswamy et al., 1999; Steffens et al., 1999.

78. BDNF has been shown to potentiate both excitatory and inhibitory transmission, albeit through different mechanisms. BDNF strengthens excitation primarily by augmenting the amplitude of AMPA receptor–mediated miniature excitatory postsynaptic currents (mEPSCs), but enhances inhibition by increasing the frequency of miniature inhibitory postsynaptic currents (mIPSCs) and increasing the size of GABAergic synaptic terminals. Furthermore, full-length TrkB receptor immunoreactivity has been found not only in glutamatergic pyramidal and granule cells but also in some interneuron axon initial segments, axon terminals forming inhibitory-type synapses onto somata and dendritic shafts, and excitatory-type terminals likely to originate extrahippocampally. Together, these results suggest that TkB is contained in some GABAergic interneurons, neuromodulatory (e.g., cholinergic, dopaminergic, and noradrenergic) afferents, and/or glutamatergic afferents.

79. Yuan et al., 2001; Chen et al., 2002; Einat et al., 2003b; Hao et al., 2004.

80. Lawrence et al., 1996; Chen et al., 1997; Merry and Korsmeyer, 1997; Yang and Cortopassi, 1998, and references therein.

81. Volonte and Rukenstein, 1993; D'Mello et al., 1994; Li et al., 1994; Inouye et al., 1995; Pascual and Gonzalez, 1995; Grignon et al., 1996; Alvarez et al., 1999.

82. In a study that may have implications for the treatment of Alzheimer's disease, rats received ibotenic acid lesions of cholinergic basal forebrain nuclei, resulting in a 30–40 percent depletion of both cortical choline acetyltransferase (ChAT) and acetylcholinesterase (AChE) activity (Arendt

et al., 1999). Lithium as well as tetrahydroaminoacridine (THA), given separately either prior to or following the development of the lesion, had small but significant effects on the recovery of cortical ChAT and AChE activity. Intriguingly, when applied in combination, the drugs clearly showed synergistic effects. However, considerable caution is required in the extrapolation of these results to the treatment of humans, since the coadministration of lithium and cholinersterase inhibitors has been shown to be capable of inducing seizures.

After largely regaining my reason, I had another most distinct sensation in the brain. . . . It seemed as though the refreshing breath of some kind Goddess of Wisdom were being blown gently against the surface of my brain. It was a sensation not unlike that produced by a menthol pencil rubbed ever so gently over a fevered brow. So delicate, so crisp and exhilarating was it that words fail me.

—*Clifford Beers (1908, p. 73)*

Converging phenomenological, neuroanatomical, and functional neuroimaging data are yielding insights into the functional neurobiology of affective processing in illness and in health. Affective processing is diverse, as it includes evaluative, experiential, and expressive components that vary in quality and intensity and can occur over differing temporal domains. One approach to these complex phenomena involves subtyping affects by temporal domains, with emotions having the briefest, moods intermediate, and temperaments the most sustained duration. These affects vary in several ways in addition to duration, however (see Table 15–1). Thus, emotions are brief experiences (lasting seconds to minutes) that often are intense, reactive to acute precipitants, and accompanied by autonomic arousal (increased heart rate and blood pressure) and lead to actions. In contrast, moods have longer duration (lasting up to hours in health or months in mood disorders), are somewhat less intense, range from reactive to spontaneous, may be accompanied by more subtle (hypothalamic–pituitary–adrenal axis [HPA] dysregulation) arousal, and tend to yield cognitions. Temperaments, the most sustained (lasting years to decades), are generally the least intense; are largely constitutional, though occasionally modified by persistent experiential factors; usually lack autonomic features; and yield integrative styles of interacting with the environment.

These affects also are related to one another, with different temperaments yielding predispositions to varying moods, which in turn result in tendencies to diverse emotions. Influences can be bidirectional, with repeated emotional experiences yielding particular moods, and chronic moods on occasion resulting in temperamental shifts. Although mood dysregulation is considered central to both bipolar disorder and unipolar major depressive disor-

der (MDD), disturbances in emotion and temperament are also commonly encountered. (Recall that the focus of this book is manic-depressive illness, which includes all *recurrent* mood disorders, both bipolar and unipolar. While some of the imaging literature separates MDD into recurrent and nonrecurrent, most of it does not.) Thus, understanding the neurobiology of bipolar disorder and MDD may be facilitated by appreciating changes in the overlapping cerebral circuits mediating emotion, mood, and temperament. (Unfortunately, in the great majority of the literature relevant to this chapter, recurrent unipolar depression is not identified or analyzed as a distinct group, but represents an unknown and variable portion of the MDD category.)

Recent evidence from functional neuroimaging studies suggests that phylogenetically older anterior paralimbic structures contribute importantly to emotions. Such structures have access to motor circuits, and could thereby provide primitive, perceptually triggered, action-oriented affective processing. More recent overlying prefrontal neocortical elements appear to contribute importantly to moods and could thus provide more refined, complexly (perceptual, mnemonic, cognitive) triggered, cognition-oriented affective processing. Emerging evidence suggests that affective processing involves coordinated activity in basal ganglia–thalamocortical circuits connecting these cortical and subcortical regions.

Neuroanatomical observations dating back to the nineteenth century have suggested that deep midline cerebral structures are important contributors to emotional experiences. Broca (1878) defined the *great limbic lobe* as a midline cortical ring seen in mammals. Papez (1937) suggested corticothalamic mediation of emotion, and MacLean (1952) used the term *limbic system* to describe the limbic cortex and related brainstem structures.

TABLE 15–1. **Temporal Domains and Other Characteristics of Affects**

	Emotions	Moods	Temperaments
Duration	Seconds to minutes	Hours to days Weeks to months[a]	Years to decades
Relative intensity	High	Intermediate	Low
Precipitants	Acute	Variable/absent	Genetic/chronic
Autonomic arousal	Acute, robust	Variable/subtle	Absent/subtle
Products	Actions	Cognitions	Cognitive–affective interactions
Possible neural substrates	Anterior limbic/brain stem	Anterior cortical/anterior limbic	Anterior cortical/anterior limbic/brain stem

[a]In mood disorders.

Source: Reproduced from Ketter et al., 2003, with permission.

Alexander and colleagues (1990) described a series of basal ganglia–thalamocortical circuits, including *limbic* and *lateral orbitofrontal circuits* implicated in affective processes, and *dorsolateral prefrontal circuits* that may contribute to integration of such processes with higher cognitive functions (see Fig. 15–1). Dysfunction in these circuits may yield impaired thalamic gating or modulation of sensory or affective information, which in turn could allow such input to disrupt cognitive and motor processes and thus contribute to the clinical profiles of mood disorders.

Thus, integrative aspects of emotion and mood processing may be related to activity in anterior cortical/anterior paralimbic basal ganglia–thalamocortical circuits. Clinical observations have related damage in such regions to affective changes. For example, the high prevalence of

Figure 15–1. Limbic basal ganglia–thalamocortical circuits. Solid lines indicate positive feedback loops, and dashed lines indicate negative feedback loops. GABA (gamma aminobutyric acid) indicates inhibitory (GABAergic) connections; + glut indicates excitatory (glutamatergic) connections. AM = anterior medial nucleus of thalamus; MDmc = medial dorsal nucleus of thalamus pars magnocellularis; VAmc = ventral anterior nucleus of thalamus pars magnocellularis. (*Source:* Adapted from Alexander et al., 1990, with permission from Elsevier.)

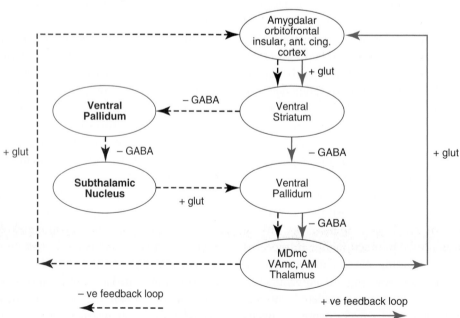

mood disorder symptoms in patients with stroke, Huntington's disease, Parkinson's disease, traumatic brain injury, epilepsy, multiple sclerosis, and brain tumors fueled interest in a provocative but at times controversial literature concerning the neuroanatomy of secondary mood disorders.

Thus, the risk of depression may be greater after anterior compared with posterior and left compared with right strokes, while the risk of mania may be greater after right than after left strokes (Starkstein and Robinson, 1989; Stern and Bachmann, 1991). Such a laterality–valence association has been contested, however (Carson et al., 2000). Basal ganglia strokes may also be associated with secondary depression (Mendez et al., 1989). The profound basal ganglia damage noted in Huntington's and Parkinson's diseases and the high prevalence of mood symptoms in these disorders also support a role for basal ganglia dysfunction in secondary depressions.[1] Left dorsolateral prefrontal and/or left basal ganglia traumatic brain injuries may increase the risk of depression (Federoff et al., 1992), while right temporal basal polar injuries may increase the risk of mania (Jorge et al., 1993). The risk of secondary depression in patients with epilepsy may be greater with left than with right temporal lobe lesions (Altshuler et al., 1990). Temporal (Honer et al., 1987) and left frontal (George et al., 1994) lesions may also increase the risk of depression secondary to multiple sclerosis, although there are discordant data here as well (Moller et al., 1994). Finally, frontal lobe brain tumors may be associated with secondary depression (Direkze et al., 1971; Kanakaratnam and Direkze, 1976).

Primary mood disorders such as bipolar disorder and MDD may be related to the above secondary mood disorders in that similar cerebral circuits are affected by different (more subtle) processes that, although not evident with older technologies such as gross neuropathology and light microscopy, are increasingly being revealed by newer, more sensitive neurochemical, neuropathological, and functional neuroimaging methods. In this chapter, we review neuroimaging studies—first structural, then functional—in bipolar disorder and MDD. In many cases, such studies implicate the expected anterior cortical and anterior paralimbic components of basal ganglia–thalamocortical circuits. In addition, there is increasing evidence of relationships between neuroimaging findings in such regions and important clinical parameters, such as symptoms and treatment response. Emerging data from studies using neurochemically specific radiotracers, now beginning to yield insights into the nature of specific neurochemical changes in such regions, are described in Chapter 14.

STRUCTURAL NEUROIMAGING STUDIES

Computerized Tomography and Magnetic Resonance Imaging

Computed tomography (CT), also known as computer-assisted tomography (CAT), was the first modern neuroimaging method. Computerized analysis of data obtained from sensors detecting ionizing radiation transmitted through tissues yields sets of transaxial (horizontal) slices (tomograms) that reflect cerebral structures. This relatively inexpensive method is limited by the risk of ionizing radiation and limited spatial resolution. Magnetic resonance imaging (MRI) involves assessing paramagnetic (odd atomic number) elements such as hydrogen (^{1}H) in strong magnetic fields by exciting them into a higher-energy state with electromagnetic radiation, and then detecting energy released when these elements relax (return to a lower-energy state). Advantages of MRI over CT/CAT include the absence of ionizing radiation, better spatial resolution, enhanced gray–white matter contrast, less bone artifact, and modifiable acquisition techniques that yield a variety of images. The latter include T_1-weighted images that better reflect neuroanatomy, T_2-weighted images that better reflect neuropathology, diffusion tensor imaging (DTI) that detects white matter pathology, and magnetization transfer imaging (MTI) that reflects white and gray matter integrity. Moreover, magnetic resonance methods can be extended to generate functional brain images (fMRI) and measure cerebral metabolites with magnetic resonance spectroscopy (MRS), a variant of magnetic resonance methodology that allows noninvasive determination of various cerebral chemicals, some of which may be related to affective processing.

Imaging studies need to take into account the influences of age and gender. For example, in healthy volunteers there appear to be regional differences in brain development in childhood and adolescence. Data suggest nonlinear age-related patterns in both the frontal and parietal regions (maximum gray matter volume at 10–12 years, followed by a slight decline) and temporal regions (gray matter volume peak at age 16), but linear increases in the occipital region (Giedd et al., 1999). This nonlinear developmental pattern is also evident with cerebral glucose metabolism (Chugani et al., 1987) and ratios of N-acetylaspartate to choline (Horska et al., 2002). This time course corresponds to that of initial overproduction and subsequent sculpting of excessive neurons, synapses, and dendritic spines in the developing brain. In elderly patients and healthy volunteers, lateral and third ventricle enlargement and cortical sulcal and lateral (Sylvian) fissure prominence increase; in addition, hemispheric, cerebellar, frontal, temporoparietal, parieto-occipital, caudate, putamen, and thalamus size decreases with age.[2] Also, compared with women, men appear to have greater age-related changes (Cowell et al., 1994; Passe et al., 1997; Coffey et al., 1998).

Studies of bipolar and MDD patients compared with one another and with healthy controls have revealed that gender, age, and other parameters can influence the findings of structural neuroimaging. In some reports, for example, increased lateral ventricular enlargement (LVE) is noted in men but not women with bipolar disorder (Andreasen et al., 1990; Swayze et al., 1990). Also, studies suggest that increased subcortical hyperintensities (SCHs) may be seen primarily in older (rather than younger) patients with MDD.[3] Diagnostic subtype may also be important. Hence, some studies note increased LVE (Hauser et al., 2000) and SCHs (Altshuler et al., 1995) in bipolar-I but not bipolar-II patients.

Course of illness can affect findings as well. For example, patients with late-onset MDD may be at greater risk for SCHs than patients with early-onset MDD. Differences related to age at onset among patients with MDD can contribute to our understanding of manic-depressive illness since the more recurrent depressions that are part of the manic-depressive spectrum are very likely to have an early age at onset.[4] Even medication status can influ-ence structural neuroimaging findings, as lithium treatment can increase prefrontal gray matter volume in patients with bipolar disorder (C. Moore et al., 2000) (see Chapter 9).

Although structural neuroimaging methods have proven useful in detecting brain abnormalities in some secondary mood disorders, as well as differences between groups of patients with primary mood disorders and healthy controls, these techniques have lacked the necessary sensitivity or specificity to permit their use as instruments to diagnose primary mood disorders in individual patients. Below we review the findings of such studies in the areas of LVE, cortical sulcal enlargement (CSE), and third ventricular enlargement (TVE); SCHs; frontal, cerebellar, and hippocampal volume decreases; and other structural aspects salient to bipolar disorder and MDD.

Lateral Ventricular Enlargement, Cortical Sulcal Prominence, and Third Ventricular Enlargement

Taken together, 28 CT studies from the 1980s and 1990s[5] and 29 MRI studies since the late 1980s[6] suggest that bipolar and MDD patients compared with healthy controls have increased LVE, CSE, and TVE (see Fig. 15–2). The degree to

Figure 15–2. Lateral ventricular enlargement and subcortical hyperintensities. Left: T_1-weighted SPGR (SPoiled GRASS; 15-degree flip angle) gradient-echo magnetic resonance imaging (MRI) scan showing lateral ventricular enlargement. Right: T_2-weighted (TR 2000; TE 25, 70; slice thickness 2.5 mm) spin-echo axial MRI scan showing subcortical hyperintensities. (*Source:* Ketter and Wang, 2002.)

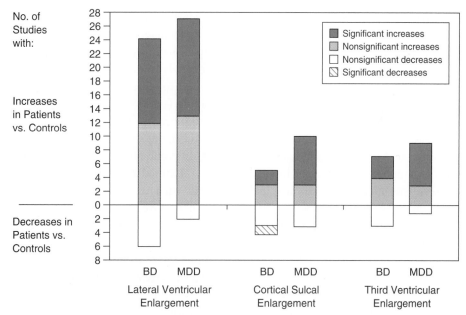

Figure 15–3. Cerebral hypoplasia/atrophy in mood disorders. Summary of 57 controlled studies of cerebral hypoplasia/atrophy in bipolar (BD) and major depressive disorder (MDD) patients compared with healthy controls. Studies with combined diagnostic groups are listed by predominant diagnosis. The graph depicts the number of studies with significant (dark blue) and nonsignificant (light blue) increases (above the horizontal axis), and nonsignificant (white) and significant (striped) decreases (below the horizontal axis) in lateral ventricular enlargement (LVE, left), cortical sulcal enlargement (CSE, middle), and third ventricular enlargement (TVE, right). Although the findings of only about half of the studies were positive, all but a few found at least nonsignificant increases, and only one found a significant decrease. Meta-analyses have confirmed findings of increased LVE and CSE in mood disorders.

which these regionally nonspecific volume deficits reflect hypoplastic developmental problems that precede the onset of affective illness as opposed to atrophic processes related to the progression of mood disorder remains to be established.

Increased LVE has frequently been reported in groups of bipolar and MDD patients compared with healthy controls. Early studies commonly used the ventricular brain ratio (percentage of the whole brain area occupied by the lateral ventricles, in the slice in which the lateral ventricles have their greatest size) as a measure of lateral ventricular size. More recent reports are based on the more accurate approach of calculating ventricular volumes.

LVE in bipolar patients compared with healthy controls has been found to be significantly increased overall in 9 studies,[7] and in male (but not female) (Andreasen et al., 1990), psychotic (but not nonpsychotic) (Woods et al., 1995b), and bipolar-I (but not bipolar-II) (Hauser et al., 2000) patients. LVE has been found to be nonsignificantly increased in bipolar versus healthy subjects in 12 studies[8] and nonsignificantly decreased in 4 studies[9]; 2 reports do not provide the direction of nonsignificant difference (Schlegel and Kretzschmar, 1987; Woods et al., 1995a). Altogether, then, in

bipolar patients compared with controls, LVE was found to be significantly increased in 12 studies, nonsignificantly increased in 14 studies, and indeterminant or nonsignificantly decreased in 6 studies (see Fig. 15–3).

LVE in MDD patients compared with healthy controls has been found to be significantly increased overall in 13 studies,[10] and in nonpsychotic (but not psychotic) patients (Woods et al., 1995b). LVE has been found to be nonsignificantly increased in MDD compared with healthy subjects in 13 studies[11]; 2 reports do not provide the direction of the nonsignificant difference (Schlegel and Kretzschmar, 1987; Greenwald et al., 1997). Thus, in MDD patients compared with controls, LVE was found to be significantly increased in 14 studies, nonsignificantly increased in 13 studies, and indeterminate in 2 studies. In the above summaries, studies with combined diagnostic groups are listed by predominant diagnosis. One additional study found nonsignificant enlargement in mood disorder patients (polarity not specified) (Weinberger et al., 1982).

In summary, about half of the studies reviewed found significantly increased LVE in bipolar and MDD patients compared with controls. It should be noted that limited statistical power related to small sample sizes in individual studies could contribute importantly to negative findings, as all but a few of the above studies found at least nonsignificantly larger ventricles in patients compared with controls, and no study had a significant finding in the opposite direction.

Increased CSE has been reported in bipolar and MDD patients compared with healthy controls. CSE is usually assessed by rating prominence of interhemispheric or Sylvian fissures or frontal or temporal lobe sulci, or by performing volumetric assessment of cortical cerebral spinal fluid (CSF).

CSE in bipolar patients compared with healthy controls has been found to be significantly increased overall in one study (Nasrallah et al., 1982a) and in bipolar patients with (but not without) comorbid substance abuse in another (Lippmann et al., 1985), and significantly decreased in nonpsychotic (but not psychotic) bipolar patients in a study by Woods and colleagues (1995b). CSE has been found to be nonsignificantly increased in bipolar versus healthy subjects in three studies (Dewan et al., 1988a; Iacono et al., 1988; Lim et al., 1999) and nonsignificantly decreased in two studies (Harvey et al., 1994; Dupont et al., 1995b); one report does not provide the direction of the nonsignificant difference (Schlegel and Kretzschmar, 1987).

CSE in MDD patients compared with healthy controls has been found to be significantly increased overall in five studies,[12] in women with endogenous depression (but not in men with endogenous depression or either gender with neurotic depression) (Baumann et al., 1997), and in nonpsychotic (but not psychotic) MDD patients (Woods et al., 1995a). CSE has been found to be nonsignificantly increased in MDD compared with healthy subjects in three studies (Abas et al., 1990; Coffey et al., 1993b; Dupont et al., 1995b), equal in one study (Iacono et al., 1988), and nonsignificantly decreased in one study (Ames et al., 1990); one report does not provide the direction of the nonsignificant difference (Schlegel and Kretzschmar, 1987).

In the above summaries, studies with combined diagnostic groups are listed by predominant diagnosis. One additional study found increased CSE in mood disorder patients (polarity not specified) (Weinberger et al., 1982).

In summary, slightly fewer than half of the studies reviewed found significantly increased CSE in bipolar and MDD patients compared with controls, with the evidence being more robust for MDD patients. Again, limited statistical power related to small sample sizes in individual studies could contribute importantly to negative findings, as most of these studies found at least nonsignificantly increased CSE in patients compared with controls, and only one study had a significant finding in the opposite direction.

Thus, there has been some variability in the findings on LVE and CSE across studies of bipolar and MDD patients compared with controls. Although the direction of change is generally consistent, only about half of the studies reviewed found a statistical significance. Potentially confounding factors that could contribute to such variability include age, nutritional status, comorbid substance abuse, somatic therapies, and heterogeneity (e.g., MDD groups with different ratios of recurrent and nonrecurrent patients). Limited statistical power related to the combination of such confounding influences and small sample sizes may have contributed importantly to the negative findings of individual studies. As noted above, about half of the studies found significantly increased LVE and CSE in bipolar and MDD patients compared with healthy controls. Narrative and "vote counting" reviews (the latter defined as keeping a tally of studies with significant and nonsignificant findings) appear to yield overly conservative conclusions, as these methods unduly emphasize studies finding low statistical power (Hedges and Olkin, 1985). Consideration of the number of studies finding nonsignificant differences in the same direction may appear to offer some additional support but lacks statistical rigor. As described below, meta-analysis methods have proven valuable in confirming structural neuroimaging findings in bipolar disorder and MDD, not only for increased LVE and CSE (Raz and Raz, 1990; Elkis et al., 1995) but also for increased SCHs (Altshuler et al., 1995; Videbech, 1997). Unfortunately, such analyses are currently not available for many neuroimaging findings; in such instances, we consider findings probable if about half of the studies are positive, and no or very few studies have significant findings in the opposite direction.

Raz and Raz (1990) reported on meta-analyses indicating that mood disorder patients compared with controls had increased LVE in 18 studies and increased CSE in 7 studies. The composite sizes for increased LVE and CSE were moderate to small in magnitude (+.55 and +.42, respectively). The corresponding effect sizes for schizophrenia (+.70 and +.35, respectively) did not differ significantly from those for mood disorders.

Elkis and colleagues (1995) reported on meta-analyses likewise indicating that mood disorder patients compared with healthy controls had increased LVE (in 29 studies)[13] and CSE (in 10 studies[14]) (see Table 15–2). The composite effects for increased LVE and CSE were highly significant ($p < .001$), but again moderate to small in magnitude (+.44 and +.42, respectively), and were not systematically related to gender or illness polarity. In addition, the authors noted that schizophrenic patients had greater ventricular enlargement than mood disorder patients. The composite effect size for this finding was highly significant

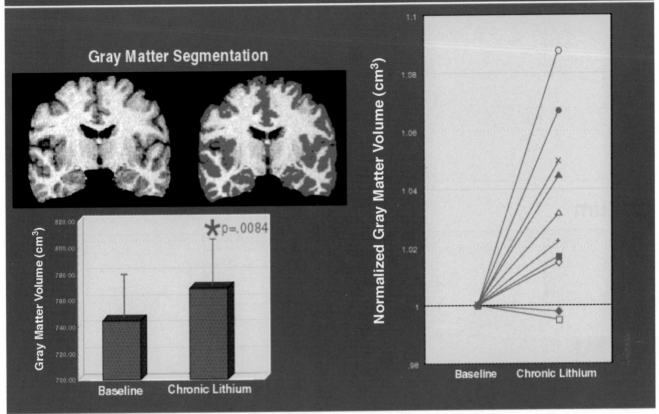

Lithium Increases Gray Matter

Gray Matter Segmentation

Plate 1. Brain gray matter volume is increased following 4 weeks of lithium administration at therapeutic levels in patients with bipolar disorder. Brain tissue volumes were examined by means of high-resolution three-dimensional magnetic resonance imaging (MRI) and validated quantitative brain tissue segmentation methodology to identify and quantify the various components by volume, including total brain white and gray matter content. Measurements were made at baseline (medication-free, after a minimum 14-day washout) and then repeated after 4 weeks of lithium treatment at therapeutic doses. Chronic lithium significantly increases total gray matter content in the human brain of patients with bipolar disorder. No significant changes were observed in brain white matter volume or in quantitative measures of regional cerebral water. (*Source:* Gould, T.D., and Manji, H.K. (2002). Signaling networks in the pathophysiology and treatment of mood disorders. *J Psychosom Res*, 53, 687–697. Reprinted by permission of SAGE Publications, Inc.)

Saline Control

Valproate

Lithium

Bcl-2 Peptide Blocking

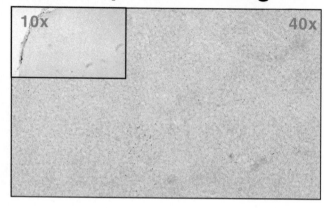

Plate 2. Effects of chronic lithium and valproate treatment on Bcl-2 immunolabeling in frontal cortex. Rats were chronically treated with saline, lithium, or valproate, and immunohistochemistry of Bcl-2 was performed in parallel for each of the groups. Chronic lithium and valproate treatment resulted in a doubling of Bcl-2 levels in FCx. (*Source:* Manji, H.K., Moore, G.J., and Chen, G. (1999). Lithium at 50: Have the neuroprotective effects of this unique cation been overlooked? *Biol Psychiatry*, 46, 929–940. Reprinted with permission.)

Plate 3. Lithium neurogenesis. C57BL/6 mice were treated with lithium for 14 days and then received once-daily bromodeoxyuridine (BrdU) injections for 12 consecutive days while lithium treatment continued. Twenty-four hours after the last injection, the brains were processed for BrdU immunohistochemistry. Cell counts were performed in the hippocampal dentate gyrus at three levels along the dorsoventral axis in all the animals. BrdU-positive cells were counted using unbiased stereological methods. Chronic lithium produced a significant 25 percent increase in BrdU immunolabeling in both right and left dentate gyrus (p <.05). Many BrdU-labeled neurons also stained with NeuN, a neuron-specific marker. (*Source:* Chen, G., Masana, M.I., and Manji, H.K. (2000). Lithium regulates PKC-mediated intracellular cross-talk and gene expression in the CNS in vivo. *Bipolar Disord,* 2, 217–236; Gray, N.A., Zhou, R., Du, J., Moore, G.J., and Manji, H.K. (2003). The use of mood stabilizers as plasticity enhancers in the treatment of neuropsychiatric disorders. *J Clin Psychiatry,* 64(Suppl. 5), 3–17. Reprinted with permission from Blackwell Publishing Ltd.)

Plate 4. Neurotrophic mechanisms in depression. Severe stress causes several changes in hippocampal pyramidal neurons, including a reduction in their dendritic arborizations, and a reduction in brain-derived neurotrophic factor (BDNF) expression (which could be one of the factors mediating the dendritic effects). Antidepressants increase dendritic arborizations and BDNF expression of these hippocampal neurons via growth factor cascades. By these actions, antidepressants may reverse and prevent the actions of stress on the hippocampus and ameliorate certain symptoms of depression. VPA = valproate. (*Source:* Adapted from Nestler, E.J., Barrot, M., DiLeone, R.J., Eisch, A.J., Gold, S.J., and Monteggia, L.M. (2002). Neurobiology of depression. *Neuron*, 34, 13–25. Reprinted with permission from Elsevier.)

Plate 5. Major intracellular signaling pathways regulated by lithium and valproate. Note that these are very rough approximations of the magnitude of effects of the different agents—very few studies have undertaken head-to-head comparisons. Nevertheless, this figure attempts to depict some of the major intracellular signaling pathways involved in neural and behavioral plasticity. Cell surface receptors transduce extracellular signals such as neurotransmitters and neuropeptides into the interior of the cell. Most neurotransmitters and neuropeptides communicate with other cells by activating seven transmembrane-spanning G protein–coupled receptors (GPCRs). As their name implies, GPCRs activate selected G proteins, which are composed of α and β subunits. Two families of proteins turn off the GPCR signal and may therefore represent attractive targets for new medication development. G protein–coupled receptor kinases (GRKs) phosphorylate GPCRs and thereby uncouple them from their respective G proteins. GTPase activating proteins (GAPs, also called RGS, or regulators of G protein–signaling proteins) accelerate the G protein turn-off reaction (an intrinsic GTPase activity). Two major signaling cascades activated by GPCRs are the cyclic adenosine monophosphate (cAMP)–generating second messenger system and the phosphoinositide (PI) system. cAMP activates protein kinase A (PKA), a pathway that has been implicated in the therapeutic effects of antidepressants. Among the potential targets for the development of new antidepressants are certain phosphodiesterases (PDEs). PDEs catalyze the breakdown of cAMP; thus PDE inhibitors would be expected to sustain the cAMP signal, and may represent an antidepressant augmenting strategy. Activation of receptors coupled to PI hydrolysis results in the breakdown of phosphoinositide 4,5-biphosphate (PIP_2) into two second messengers—inositol 4,5-triphosphate (IP_3) and diacylglycerol (DAG). IP_3 mobilizes Ca^{2+} from intracellular stores, whereas DAG is an endogenous activator of protein kinase C (PKC), which is also directly activated by Ca^{2+}. PKC, PKA, and other Ca^{2+}-dependent kinases directly or indirectly activate several important transcription factors, including cAMP-responsive element-binding protein (CREB), cAMP-responsive element modulator (CREM), activating transcription factor 1 (ATF1), c-Fos, c-Jun, Jun-D, and Fos B. Endogenous growth factors such as brain-derived neurotrophic factor (BDNF) use different types of signaling pathways. BDNF binds to and activates its tyrosine kinase receptor (TrkB); this facilitates the recruitment of other proteins (SHC, SOS), which results in the activation of the ERK–MAP kinase cascade (via sequential activation of Ras, Raf, MEK, Erk, and Rsk). In addition to regulating several transcription factors, the ERK–MAP kinase cascade, via Rsk, downregulates BAD, a pro-apoptotic protein. Enhancement of the ERK–MAP kinase cascade may have effects similar to those of endogenous neurotrophic factors; one potential strategy is to use inhibitors of MAP kinase phosphatases (which would inhibit the turn-off reaction) as potential drugs with neurotrophic properties. In addition to using GPCRs, many neurotransmitters (e.g., glutamate and gamma-aminobutyric acid) produce their responses via ligand-gated ion channels. Although these responses are very rapid, they also bring about more stable changes via regulation of gene transcription. One pathway gaining increasing recent attention in adult mammalian neurobiology is the Wnt signaling pathway. The Wnts are a group of glycoproteins active in development but now known to play important roles in the mature brain. Binding of Wnts to the Wnt receptor (WntR) activates an intermediary protein, Dishevelled, which regulates a glycogen synthase kinase (GSK-3β). GSK-3β exerts many cellular effects; it regulates cytoskeletal proteins, including tau, and also plays an important role in determining cell survival and cell death decisions. GSK-3β has recently been identified as a target for lithium's (Lith) actions. GSK-3 also regulates phosphorylation of β-catenin, a protein that when dephosphorylated acts as a transcription factor at LEF (lymphoid enhancer factor) sites. HDACs = histone deacteylases; Rq and Rs = extracellular GPCRs coupled to stimulation or inhibition of adenylyl cyclases (ACs), respectively. Rq/11 = GPCR coupled to activation of phospholipase C (PLC); MARCKS = myristoylated alanine-rich C kinase substrate, a protein associated with several neuroplastic events. VPA = valproate.

Plate 6. Hypofrontality in secondary and primary depression. Transaxial images depicting cerebral metabolic rate (CMR) for glucose in patients with (top row) and without (bottom row) depression. Arrows indicate decreased frontal metabolism in patients with depression secondary to neurological disorders, as well as in those with primary (unipolar) depression. (*Source:* Reproduced with permission from Mayberg, H.S. (1994). Frontal lobe dysfunction in secondary depression. *J Neuropsychiatry Clin Neurosci,* 6(4), 428–442.)

Plate 7. Regional cerebral metabolism (rCM) in moderately to severely depressed unmedicated bipolar patients compared with healthy controls. Z-maps show differences in absolute (top) and normalized (bottom) cerebral metabolism in 17 moderately to severely depressed unmedicated bipolar patients compared with 17 healthy controls. The legend indicates two-tailed p values. Numbers in the upper right corners indicate distances from the intercommissural plane. L = left. Absolute prefrontal and anterior paralimbic cortical metabolic decreases and normalized anterior paralimbic subcortical metabolic increases evident in these images may be state markers for depression in bipolar disorder. Decreased dorsomedial and dorsolateral prefrontal activity has commonly been reported in other studies of bipolar depression. Left ventrolateral structures failed to show the absolute metabolic decreases seen in other prefrontal cortical regions in these moderately to severely depressed bipolar patients (top) or the relative metabolic increases seen in left ventrolateral structures in mildly depressed bipolar patients (Fig. 15–9). (*Source:* Ketter, T.A., Kimbrell, T.A., George, M.S., Dunn, R.T., Speer, A.M., Benson, B.E., Willis, M.W., Danielson, A., Frye, M.A., Herscovitch, P., and Post, R.M. (2001). Effects of mood and subtype on cerebral glucose metabolism in treatment-refractory bipolar disorders. *Biol Psychiatry,* 49(2), 97–109.)

rCMRglu in 16 Mildly Depressed BPs vs 16 Healthy Volunteers
(10 < Ham−D < 18)

Uncorrected 2−tailed p values shown in significant clusters:

Increased / Decreased: <.05 .01 .005 .001 .0005 .0001

Z threshold = 1.96
Cluster probability < .05

Plate 8. Regional cerebral metabolism (rCM) in mildly depressed unmedicated bipolar patients compared with healthy controls. Z-maps show differences in absolute (top) and normalized (bottom) cerebral metabolism in 16 mildly depressed unmedicated bipolar patients compared with 16 healthy controls. The legend indicates two-tailed p values. Numbers in the upper right corners indicate distances from the intercommissural plane. L = left. Increased normalized (but not absolute) metabolism was noted in left inferior, middle, and superior frontal gyri; left insula and left transverse temporal gyrus; left postcentral gyrus; lingular gyrus, cuneus, and hippocampus; and bilateral cerebellum (sparsely). In contrast, decreased normalized (but not absolute) metabolism was noted in right inferior and middle temporal gyri. Ventrolateral metabolic increases have also been reported in depressed unmedicated major depressive disorder patients in the resting state. (*Source:* Ketter, T.A., and Drevets, W.C. (2002). Neuroimaging studies of bipolar depression: Functional neuropathology, treatment effects, and predictors of clinical response. *Clin Neurosci Res*, 2(3-4), 182–192.)

Plate 9. Decreased subgenual prefrontal cortical metabolism in depressed patients with familial major depressive disorder and familial bipolar disorder. Coronal (31 mm anterior to the anterior commissure, or y = 31) and sagittal (3 mm left of midline, or x = −3) sections show negative voxel t values where glucose metabolism was decreased in (7 bipolar and 10 unipolar) familial depressives compared with controls. Decreased activity was accompanied by reduced gray matter volume (Fig. 15–11). A = anterior, L = left, PFC = prefrontal cortex. (*Source:* Drevets, W.C. (2001). Neuroimaging and neuropathological studies of depression: Implications for the cognitive-emotional features of mood disorders. *Curr Opin Neurobiol*, 11(2), 240–249; Drevets, W.C., Price, J.L., Simpson, J.R. Jr., Todd, R.D., Reich, T., Vannier, M., and Raichle, M.E. (1997). Subgenual prefrontal cortex abnormalities in mood disorders. *Nature*, 386(6627), 824–827. Reprinted with permission from Macmillan Publishers Ltd: *Nature.*)

Plate 10. Frontotemporoparietal white matter deficits in schizophrenia and bipolar disorder patients compared with controls. Shown here are white matter deficits in 25 schizophrenia patients versus 52 healthy controls, in red; 37 bipolar disorder patients versus controls, in blue; and both versus controls, in green. Transaxial slices in Talairach orientation are shown with distances in mm from the intercommisural plane. The right side of the brain is depicted by the right side of each slice. (*Source:* Adapted from McDonald, C., Bullmore, E., Sham, P., Chitnis, X., Suckling, J., MacCabe, J., Walshe, M., and Murray, R.M. (2005). Regional volume deviations of brain structure in schizophrenia and psychotic bipolar disorder: computational morphometry study. *Br J Psychiatry.* 186, 369–377. Reprinted with permission from the *British Journal of Psychiatry.*)

Plate 11. The haplotypic structure of the *DAOA* gene. *DAOA*, or D-amino acid oxidase activator (also called G72), has been implicated in bipolar disorder by a number of genetic association studies. It is about 25,000 nucleotides long, and it contains 114 identified single nucleotide polymorphisms (SNPs). This figure shows the location of a portion of those SNPs along the length of the gene. The figure was generated by the software HAPLOVIEW, which identifies the ancestral relationships of the SNPs to each other. Bright red blocks reflect the highest degree of ancestrally related SNPs and have to a large extent persisted over time. Testing just a few key SNPs in the block for association with bipolar disorder can provide almost as much information as testing all of the many SNPs that make up the block.

Plate 12. Gene expression microarray analysis. This is a representative portion of an image generated from a gene expression chip. The chip contains 45,000 25-nucleotide-long segments representing virtually every one of the 20,000–25,000 human genes. RNA was isolated from white blood cells drawn from an invidual with bipolar-I disorder and then placed on the microarray chip. Each dot in the figure reflects the relative abundance of a particular expressed gene in this individual's white blood cells. Dark colors indicate less abundance, while brighter colors reflect higher expression levels. Consistently higher or lower than expected gene expression levels in the tissues of individuals with bipolar disorder could represent an aspect of the disordered biology that leads to illness. (*Source:* From the laboratory of Haiming Chen, Johns Hopkins University.)

Plate 13. Fluorescent in situ hybridization (FISH) image of chromosomes generated from white blood cells carrying *DISCI* reciprocal balanced translocation. A reciprocal balanced translocation refers to a situation in which portions of each of two chromosomes have broken off and rejoined the remaining end of the other chromosome. The exchange of material is even, and this phenomenon can be tolerated, except to the extent that the breakpoints result in the disruption of genes. In this figure, chromosomal DNA has been stained light blue. The long arm of chromosome 1 is labeled in red, and the whole chromosome 11 is labeled in green. For each labeled chromosome, a normal and derived (translocated) form can be seen. The red–green interface on the derived chromosome highlights the physical position of the translocation breakpoints, including the point at which the *DISC1* gene on chromosome 1 is directly disrupted. *DISC1* may play a role in susceptibility to both mood disorders and schizophrenia. (*Source:* From the laboratory of Pat Malloy and Kirsty Millar, University of Edinburgh.)

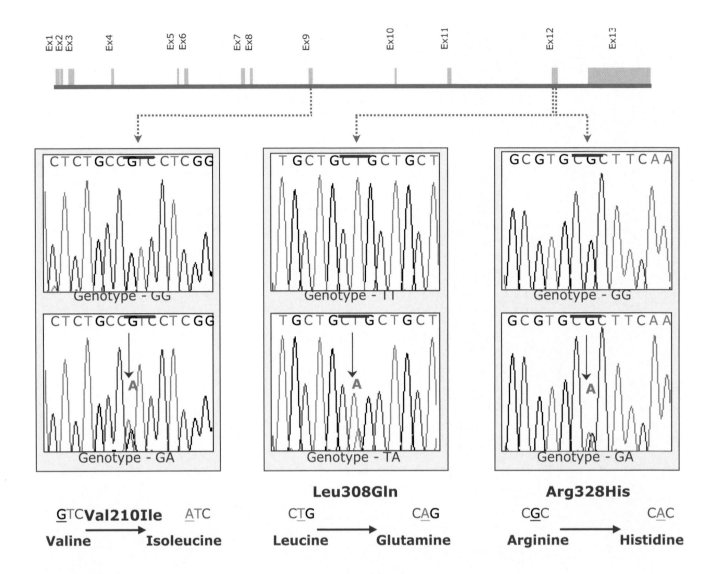

Plate 14. DNA sequencing in the *MLC1* gene reveals three novel missense mutations in inviduals with bipolar disorder. At the top of the figure, the structure of the *MLC1* gene is shown, with its 13 *exons* (Ex), or regions that code for the production of a protein. In the lower portion of the figure, DNA sequencing results are shown for three regions of exons 9 and 12. The four different nucleotides in the DNA chemical alphabet are represented by peaks in four different colors. For each of the three panels, the sequence does not differ between the individual shown in the top half and the other individual shown in the bottom half, except at a single position. The arrow in the lower half of each panel indicates the presence of a rare variation, called a *mutation*, present in each of these individuals. These three mutations are called *missense* because they result in a change in the blueprint by which the gene determines which amino acid will be produced. In the first panel, the standard code indicates the amino acid valine should be produced, but the mutation changes it to isoleucine. The second ordinarily codes for leucine, but the mutated form codes for glutamine. The third changes from arginine to histidine. The resulting altered proteins, acting in brain cells, could influence susceptibility to bipolar disorder. (*Source:* From the laboratory of Ranjana Verma, Institute of Genomics and Integrative Biology, Delhi, India.)

Plate 15. *Torso.* This painting was done during a major depressive episode. (*Source:* La Rue Alegria. Reproduced with permission.)

Plate 16. *To Love and Euphoria.* This painting was done during a manic state. (*Source:* La Rue Alegria. Reproduced with permission.)

Plate 17. *The Gift*. This painting was done after a period of deep depression. The artist was emerging from this depression, and the flowers symbolized a promise of there being something beyond the depression. (*Source:* Meghan Caughey. Reproduced with permission.)

Plate 18. *The Serpent*. "I would lie still. Depression seemed so alive, to thrive on its own like a sleeping serpent in my belly. If I moved and woke it, its overwhelming presence also awakened the voices of the Furies and rekindled the fires of the wound. This malevolent being had a particular hatred of me and seemed without reason to want me to see only despair.

"With it asleep coiled in my abdomen, I would lie immobile or move carefully not to wake it up. For once awake, this beast would unwind and move toward my all too vulnerable throat." (*Source:* Reproduced from The Art of Suicidal Depression by Deenie McKay, with permission.)

TABLE 15–2. Summary of Meta-Analyses of Studies of Ventricular Enlargement and Cortical Sulcal Prominence in Mood Disorders

Hypothesis	No. of Studies	Percent Unipolar	No. of Significant Studies	No. of Nonsignificant Studies	No. of Significant Not Reported	Composite Effect Size	p for Composite Effect Size
More ventricular enlargement in mood disorders than in healthy controls	29	58.4	11	15	3	+.437	.001
More cortical sulcal prominence in mood disorders than in healthy controls	10	58.5	3	5	2	+.421	.001
Less ventricular enlargement in mood disorders than in schizophrenia	11	31.3	0	11	0	−.201	.002
Less cortical sulcal prominence in mood disorders than in schizophrenia	3	—	0	3	0	Insufficient data	

Source: Reproduced from Elkis et al., 1995, with permission.

(p <.002) but small in magnitude (−.2), and was not systematically related to gender or illness polarity. There are too few studies to allow conclusions regarding differences in CSE between mood disorder and schizophrenic patients. Thus, these generalized structural brain abnormalities (increased LVE and CSE) in the former patients may differ less from those in schizophrenic patients than from those in controls, consistent with a continuum model of mood and schizophrenic disorders.[15]

A recent meta-analysis used more robust threshold criteria for inclusion (McDonald et al., 2004). In five studies, bipolar patients compared with controls had a significant (p=.03) 14 percent increase in right lateral ventricular volume, but only a nonsignificant (p=.32) 8 percent increase in left lateral ventricular volume. In six studies, bipolar patients compared with controls tended to have (p=.06) a 17 percent increase in total lateral ventricular volume.

Thus, bipolar and MDD patients appear to have increased LVE and CSE. The clinical significance of these findings remains to be established, however. LVE has received more attention than CSE in this regard. As noted below, there are variable reports on the relationships between LVE and clinical phenomena, and unfortunately meta-analyses regarding such relationships are not yet available.

LVE may increase with age in bipolar patients (Pearlson and Veroff, 1981; Rieder et al., 1983), MDD patients,[16] and healthy subjects.[17] However, negative findings have also been reported in bipolar patients (Pearlson et al., 1984a; Dewan et al., 1988b; Brambilla et al., 2001b), MDD patients,[18] and healthy subjects.[19] Longitudinal studies suggest that LVE may increase with disease duration in patients with mood disorders, perhaps in excess of the increase noted with normal aging (Vita et al., 1988; Woods et al., 1990). In bipolar and MDD patients, LVE has been associated with later or late-life onset in some studies,[20] but not in others.[21]

One study found that multiple-episode bipolar patients compared with both first-episode patients and healthy subjects had larger lateral ventricles, with the degree of enlargement being related to number of prior manic episodes (Strakowski et al., 2002). Another study found that right LVE increased with the number of episodes (Brambilla et al., 2001b). Other studies have reported variable findings on the relationships between LVE and illness chronicity and course,[22] occupational function (Pearlson et al.,1984b; Dewan et al.,1988b), and biological markers (Kellner et al., 1983; Van den Bossche et al., 1991).

LVE was found to be related to psychosis in 31 bipolar-I and 9 bipolar-II patients (Kato et al., 1994b); 66 patients with late-onset depression (Simpson et al., 2001); 22 mood disorder patients (Luchins et al., 1984); and a mixed cohort of 33 MDD, 22 bipolar, and 5 schizoaffective patients (Schlegel and Kretzschmar, 1987). The findings of other studies, however, suggest that LVE may not be related to psychosis in bipolar disorder (Pearlson et al., 1984b; Dewan et al., 1988b; Roy-Byrne et al., 1988), and may (Targum et al., 1983; Rothschild et al., 1989; Shiraishi et al., 1992) or may not (Standish-Barry et al., 1985; Rabins et al., 1991; Hickie et al., 1995) be related to psychosis in MDD patients. LVE may (Kellner et al., 1986) or may not[23] be related to cognitive impairment in bipolar disorder, and may[24] or may not (Andreasen et al., 1990; Simpson et al., 2001) be related to cognitive impairment in MDD patients.

Increased LVE in bipolar (particularly male) compared with MDD patients has been reported (Andreasen et al., 1990; Swayze et al., 1990). Other groups, however, have failed to find this difference (Dolan et al., 1985; Schlegel and Kretzschmar, 1987). Likewise, as noted above, in Elkis and colleagues' (1995) meta-analysis, LVE was not found to be systematically related to polarity or gender. Investigators have also found that LVE generally fails to have a significant association with severity of mood symptoms as assessed by mood rating scales.[25]

Most studies have indicated that LVE is unrelated to dexamethasone suppression status and post-dexamethasone cortisol,[26] although one study noted a trend (Rothschild et al., 1989) and another a significant relationship (Rao et al., 1989). Ventricular enlargement may (Schlegel et al., 1989b) or may not (Dewan et al., 1988b) be related to pre-dexamethasone plasma cortisol, and may (Kellner et al., 1983) or may not (Risch et al., 1992) be related to urinary free cortisol.

Most studies have found that LVE is not related to a history of electroconvulsive therapy (ECT) in bipolar patients[27] or MDD patients (Dolan et al., 1985; Kolbeinsson et al., 1986). Prospectively, ECT did not cause or exacerbate LVE in MDD patients.[28] LVE does not appear to be related to prior treatment with lithium,[29] antidepressants (Dolan et al., 1985; Harvey et al., 1994; Baumann et al., 1997), antipsychotics (Rieder et al., 1983; Dolan et al., 1985; Swayze et al., 1990), or benzodiazepines (Dolan et al., 1985; Swayze et al., 1990), or with alcohol abuse (Rieder et al., 1983; Dolan et al., 1985; Swayze et al., 1990), drug abuse (Swayze et al., 1990), or substance abuse generally (Dewan et al., 1988c; Andreasen et al., 1990). Young and colleagues (1998) found LVE to be associated with poorer response to tricyclic antidepressants, but in other reports, LVE was not shown to be related to response to lithium (Dewan et al., 1988c) or other treatments.

Increased TVE has been reported in bipolar and MDD patients compared with healthy controls. In bipolar versus healthy subjects, TVE was found to be significantly increased in three studies (Dewan et al., 1988; Strakowski et al., 1993; Pearlson et al., 1997), nonsignificantly increased in four studies,[30] and nonsignificantly decreased in two studies (Iacono et al., 1988; Brambilla et al., 2001b); one report does not provide the direction of the nonsignificant difference (Schlegel and Kretzschmar, 1987).

TVE was found to be significantly increased in MDD patients compared with healthy controls in five studies[31] and in women with endogenous depression (but not in men with endogenous or in either gender with neurotic depression) (Baumann et al., 1997), and nonsignificantly increased in three studies (Tanaka et al., 1982; Iacono et al., 1988; Coffey et al., 1993b). One report does not provide the direction of the nonsignificant difference (Greenwald et al., 1997).

Thus, about half of the studies reviewed found significantly increased TVE in bipolar and MDD patients compared with healthy controls, with the evidence being more robust for the MDD patients. Once again, limited statistical power related to small sample sizes in individual studies could contribute importantly to negative findings, as all but a few of these studies found at least nonsignificantly increased TVE in patients, and no study had a significant finding in the opposite direction. A recent meta-analysis using robust threshold criteria for inclusion (McDonald et al., 2004) found that in six studies, bipolar patients compared with controls had a nonsignificant ($p = .35$) 18 percent increase in third ventricular volume.

Because the third ventricle is bounded laterally by the thalamus, TVE is consistent with a decrease in thalamic volume, which in turn supports the hypothesis that basal ganglia–thalamocortical circuit function may be disrupted in bipolar and MDD patients. TVE may (Schlegel and Kretzschmar, 1987) or may not (Dewan et al., 1988a; Brambilla et al., 2001b) be more evident in early-onset bipolar disorder, and may be associated with earlier- (Beats et al., 1991) or later- (Dahabra et al., 1998) onset MDD. There are conflicting data regarding relationships between TVE and dexamethasone suppression status and post-dexamethasone cortisol (Schlegel and Kretzschmar, 1987; Coffey et al., 1993; Mukherjee et al., 1993). TVE and neuropsychological function may not (Dewan et al., 1988) be related in bipolar disorder, and may (Beats et al., 1991) or may not (Dahabra et al., 1998) be related in MDD.

In patients with schizophrenia, LVE appears to be linked to TVE but not to CSE (Raz and Raz, 1990). This finding suggests that in schizophrenia, LVE may represent a subcortical neuropathological process related to third ventricular dilatation, yet independent of CSE. The relationships between these abnormalities in bipolar disorder and MDD remain to be determined. Rieder and colleagues (1983) found that CSE in bipolar patients was correlated

with cerebellar atrophy, but LVE was not correlated with either of these measures. Of interest, in one small study in schizophrenic and depressed patients, those with (but not without) enlarged ventricles and widened Sylvian fissures tended to have lower global metabolism than healthy controls (Kling et al., 1986).

Taken together, the above findings suggest that bipolar and MDD patients have increased LVE and CSE and probably have increased TVE as well. These findings are not anatomically or diagnostically specific, however. Moreover, the clinical significance of these findings needs to be delineated more clearly. Although the currently available data suggest that LVE may be related to age and later- or late-life onset and not to degree of depression or treatment with medications or ECT, there have been variable findings on relationships to illness chronicity, course, and polarity; to psychosis; and to HPA axis dysfunction. Unfortunately, meta-analyses regarding how LVE, CSE, and TVE are related to clinical parameters are currently not available.

Subcortical Hyperintensities

Increased SCHs have been observed in mood disorder patients compared with healthy controls. SCHs are bright areas in deep white, periventricular white, or subcortical gray matter on T2-weighted MRI images. Taken together, 41 studies since 1989 suggest that younger and older bipolar and older MDD patients compared with healthy controls have increased SCHs.[32]

SCHs in bipolar patients were found to be significantly increased overall in 10 studies[33] and in bipolar-I (but not bipolar-II) patients (Altshuler et al., 1995), nonsignificantly increased in 7 studies,[34] and nonsignificantly decreased in 2 studies (Brown et al., 1992; Sassi et al., 2003). With the exception of 2 small pediatric studies (Botteron et al., 1995; Pillai et al., 2002), 1 small elderly adult study (McDonald et al., 1991), and 1 large study involving a broad age range (McDonald et al., 1999), these were studies of nonelderly adult bipolar patients. Altshuler and colleagues (1995) performed a meta-analysis of 8 studies[35] including 198 bipolar patients and 307 controls and found increased frequency of SCHs in the former, with a common odds ratio of 3.3 and 95 percent confidence interval of 1.9–5.6 ($p = .00001$). Videbech (1997) performed an expanded meta-analysis of 10 studies[36] including 296 bipolar patients and 516 controls and found that in all but 1 of these studies (Brown et al., 1992), the odds ratios pointed toward increased frequency of SCHs in the bipolar subjects, with a common odds ratio of 3.3 and 95 percent confidence interval of 2.1–5.1 ($p = .0000001$).

As noted above, SCHs may be more common in bipolar-I but not bipolar-II patients compared with controls (Altshuler et al., 1995), although Krabbendum and colleagues (2000) failed to detect such a difference. In another study, there were no apparent changes in SCHs on repeat scanning 1 year later (Dupont et al., 1990). One study found that 6 of 10 unaffected relatives of patients with bipolar disorder from a loaded pedigree had subcortical gray SCHs (Ahearn et al., 1998).

SCHs in MDD patients were found to be significantly increased overall in 14 studies[37] and in patients with later (over age 50) but not earlier (under age 35) onset (Lesser et al., 1996), nonsignificantly increased in 12 studies,[38] and nonsignificantly decreased in 1 study (Sassi et al., 2003). In contrast to the studies involving bipolar patients noted above, studies involving MDD patients have assessed primarily elderly patients. Videbech (1997) performed a meta-analysis of 7 studies[39] including 254 MDD patients and 511 controls and found that in nearly all of these studies, odds ratios pointed toward increased frequency of SCHs in MDD patients, with a common odds ratio of 3.3 and 95 percent confidence interval of 2.1–4.8 ($p=.00000001$).

Thus, there has been some variability in findings with regard to SCHs across studies of bipolar and MDD patients compared with controls. Although the direction of change has generally been consistent, only slightly more than half of the studies have demonstrated statistical significance.

As with the studies discussed earlier, limited statistical power related to small sample sizes in individual studies could contribute importantly to negative findings, as all but a few of these studies found at least nonsignificantly increased SCHs in patients, and no study had a significant finding in the opposite direction. Indeed, meta-analyses have confirmed increased SCHs in bipolar and MDD patients (Altshuler et al., 1995; Videbech, 1997). This pattern of findings is similar to that for increased LVE and CSE in bipolar and MDD patients noted above. SCHs appear to occur most frequently in the frontal lobe deep white matter in both bipolar patients[40] and MDD patients.[41] This observation does not hold true for all studies, however (Howard et al., 1993; Altshuler et al., 1995).

Deep white matter SCHs have been the subtype studied most frequently and found most consistently to be increased in patients compared with controls. Among 20 studies of bipolar patients, such SCHs were found to be significantly increased in 9 studies,[42] nonsignificantly increased in 8 studies,[43] and equal or nonsignificantly decreased in 3 studies (Brown et al., 1992; Altshuler et al., 1995; Sassi et al., 2003) (see Fig. 15–4). Among 23 studies of MDD patients, deep white matter SCHs were found to be significantly increased in 10 studies,[44] nonsignificantly

Figure 15–4. Subcortical hyperintensities in mood disorders. Summary of 37 controlled studies of subcortical hyperintensities (SCHs) in bipolar (BD) and major depressive disorder (MDD) patients compared with healthy controls. Studies with combined diagnostic groups are shown by predominant diagnosis. The graph depicts the number of studies with significant (dark blue) and nonsignificant (light blue) increases (above the horizontal axis) and nonsignificant (white) decreases and unspecified nonsignificant findings (striped) (below the horizontal axis) in deep white (left), periventricular white (middle), and subcortical gray (right) SCHs. Although only about half of the studies yielded positive findings, all but a few found at least nonsignificant increases, and none found significant decreases. Meta-analyses have confirmed these findings.

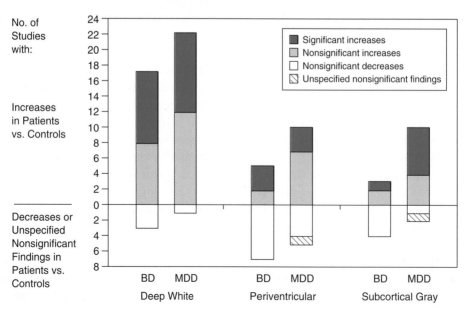

increased in 12 studies,[45] and nonsignificantly decreased in 1 study (Greenwald et al., 1996).

Periventricular SCHs have been assessed less frequently. Among 12 studies of bipolar patients, these SCHS were found to be significantly increased in 3 studies (Altshuler et al., 1995; Woods et al., 1995a; McDonald et al., 1999), nonsignificantly increased in 2 studies (Woods et al., 1995a; Krabbendam et al., 2000), and equal or nonsignificantly decreased in 7 studies.[46] Among 15 studies of MDD patients, periventricular SCHs were found to be significantly increased in 3 studies (Coffey et al., 1990, 1993b; Iidaka et al., 1996), nonsignificantly increased in 7 studies,[47] nonsignificantly decreased in 4 studies,[48] and not significantly different (direction of nonsignificant difference not specified) in 1 study (MacFall et al., 2001).

Subcortical gray matter hyperintensities have been examined least frequently. Among 7 studies of bipolar patients, these SCHs were found to be significantly increased in 1 study (McDonald et al., 1999), nonsignificantly increased in 2 studies (Aylward et al., 1994; Altshuler et al., 1995), and equal or nonsignificantly decreased in 4 studies.[49] In contrast, among 12 studies of MDD patients, subcortical gray matter SCHs were found to be significantly increased in 6 studies,[50] nonsignificantly increased in 4 studies,[51] nonsignificantly decreased in 1 study (Miller et al., 1994), and not significantly different (direction of nonsignificant difference not specified) in 1 study (MacFall et al., 2001).

Thus, SCHs appear to occur in frontal lobes (deep white matter) and in periventricular white matter in nonelderly and elderly bipolar and elderly MDD patients, and in basal ganglia (subcortical gray matter) in elderly MDD patients. The clinical significance of these findings remains to be established, however. As noted below, there are variable reports on the relationships between SCHs and clinical phenomena, and unfortunately meta-analyses in this area are not yet available.

SCHs can occur in patients with other psychiatric and neurological disorders,[52] but lesions in the frontal lobes and basal ganglia may still be related to depressive symptoms. Moreover, SCHs are occasionally observed in clinically healthy individuals in association with ventricular enlargement, cerebral hypometabolism, higher blood pressure, and lower neuropsychological test scores (DeCarli et al., 1995).

SCHs have been reported to increase with age in bipolar patients,[53] MDD patients,[54] heterogeneous psychiatric patients (Deicken et al., 1991; Brown et al., 1992), and healthy volunteers.[55] However, negative findings have also been reported in bipolar patients,[56] MDD patients,[57] and healthy volunteers.[58]

SCHs may be related to hypertension, carotid arteriosclerosis, arteriolar hyalinization, and dilated perivascular spaces.

They have been found to be related to cardiovascular risk factors in MDD patients (Coffey et al., 1989; Lesser et al., 1996; O'Brien et al., 1996), in healthy controls (Coffey et al., 1989; Lesser et al., 1996; O'Brien et al., 1996), and to a lesser extent in bipolar patients (Aylward, et al., 1994). The increased SCHs in bipolar and MDD patients do not, however, appear to be due solely to such risk factors,[59] although Miller and colleagues (1994) failed to find significantly increased SCHs in patients with late-life depression and without such risk factors compared with healthy controls.

Studies have reported variable findings with respect to relationships between SCHs and illness chronicity and course.[60] Among bipolar patients, SCHs may occur in late-onset illness (McDonald et al., 1991) but have also been noted in younger patients (Dupont et al., 1995a,b). Some data (Dupont et al., 1995b) but not all[61] suggest that SCHs may occur preferentially in bipolar patients with later- or late-life onset. Similarly, among MDD patients, some studies[62] but not all[63] indicate that SCHs may occur preferentially in patients with later- or late-life onset.

Among depressed MDD patients, psychosocial stressors have been found to be inversely related to SCHs, suggesting that stress-independent biological factors could be more relevant to these lesions (Fujikawa et al., 1997). Patients with late-onset mania had more or more widespread SCHs than did patients with early-onset mood disorders and late-onset MDD, respectively (Fujikawa et al., 1995), consistent with late-onset mania being a more biologically severe disorder (Fujikawa et al., 1996).

In healthy volunteers, white matter SCHs appear to be related to lower scores on frontal lobe–mediated neuropsychological tests (Boone et al., 1992; DeCarli et al., 1995) and decreased frontal lobe metabolism (DeCarli et al., 1995). SCHs may be related to cognitive impairment in MDD patients,[64] although some studies have failed to detect such a relationship (Zubenko et al., 1990; Dupont et al., 1995b; O'Brien et al., 1996). In bipolar patients, SCHs and cognitive impairment may (Dewan et al., 1988b; Dupont et al., 1990, 1995b) or may not (Swayze et al., 1990; Dahabra et al., 1998; Krabbendam et al., 2000) be related. In elderly individuals (mostly healthy, but some with a history of receiving antidepressants), deep white (but not periventricular) SCHs were found to be associated with depressive symptoms, especially impaired motivation, concentration, and decision making, and this relationship was especially strong in patients carrying the APOE-4 allele (Nebes et al., 2001). Another study of elderly individuals (mostly healthy, but some with a history of depression) found that subcortical and periventricular white matter SCHs were associated with depressive symptoms (de Groot et al., 2000).

SCHs do not appear to be related to severity of depression in bipolar patients (Dupont et al., 1990, 1995a; Altshuler et al., 1995) or MDD patients,[65] although two studies detected such a relationship in the latter patients (MacFall et al., 2001; Murata et al., 2001). SCHs likewise do not appear to be related to psychosis in bipolar patients[66] or MDD patients.[67] SCHs may (Dupont et al., 1990, 1995a) or may not (Altshuler et al., 1995) be related to psychiatric hospitalizations in bipolar patients, and may not be related to psychiatric hospitalizations in MDD patients (Dupont et al., 1995a; Iidaka et al., 1996). SCHs do not appear to be related to dexamethasone suppression status or post-dexamethasone cortisol levels (Rao et al., 1989; Deicken et al., 1991; Coffey et al., 1993b).

SCHs may be more (Sassi et al., 2003) or less (Hickie et al., 1995) common in MDD patients lacking a family history of mood disorders. In contrast, SCHs in bipolar patients have been reported to be unrelated to a family history of mood disorders (Sassi et al., 2003).

Studies have found no relationship between SCHs and prior ECT in either bipolar patients (Swayze et al., 1990; Figiel et al., 1991a) or MDD patients.[68] Prospectively, ECT did not cause or exacerbate SCHs in MDD patients.[69] Basal ganglia lesions may yield patients more susceptible to ECT-induced delirium, however (Figiel et al., 1989b, 1990a,b). Limited evidence suggests that white matter SCHs may predict poorer response to ECT in MDD patients (Coffey et al., 1987; Hickie et al., 1995), perhaps because these SCHs may represent subtle vascular insufficiency (Sackeim, 1996). Other data suggest, however, that SCHs in MDD patients are not related to ECT response (Figiel et al., 1989b).

SCHs do not appear to be related to prior treatment with lithium,[70] carbamazepine (Altshuler et al., 1995), antidepressants (Altshuler et al., 1995), antipsychotics (Dupont et al., 1990; Swayze et al., 1990), or benzodiazepines (Swayze et al., 1990), or to prior alcohol abuse (Swayze et al., 1990), drug abuse (Swayze et al., 1990), or substance abuse generally (Strakowski et al., 1993b). As noted above, earlier-onset MDD patients (who have longer illness duration and greater treatment exposure) compared with later-onset patients may have fewer SCHs, an observation inconsistent with the notion that illness or treatment duration markedly affects these lesions. Moreover, it should be recalled that MDD with an early age at onset is part of the manic-depressive spectrum and as such is genetically different from later-onset MDD (see Chapter 13).

Deep white matter and basal ganglia SCHs may be associated with resistance to antidepressants (Hickie et al., 1995; Simpson et al., 1998). Basal ganglia lesions may increase the risk of antidepressant-induced delirium (Figiel et al., 1989b) and adverse effects on the central nervous system (Fujikawa et al., 1996). After 2 years of naturalistic treatment, MDD patients who had achieved and sustained remission had attenuated increases in white matter SCH volume (11.5 percent) compared with patients who had not achieved or sustained remission (31.6 percent) (Taylor et al., 2003). Less is known about relationships between SCHs and treatment resistance in bipolar patients.

Interpretation of the significance of increased SCHs in bipolar and MDD patients is limited by sparse knowledge of the pathophysiology of these lesions. Emerging data are beginning to address this problem, however. SCHs have been associated with ventricular enlargement in healthy volunteers (DeCarli et al., 1995) and in bipolar (Dupont et al., 1995b) and MDD patients (Coffey et al., 1989; Iidaka et al., 1996), although MDD patients in one study failed to display such a relationship (Dupont et al., 1995b). SCHs have also been associated with CSE in MDD patients (Coffey et al., 1989).

SCHs have been associated with cerebral hypometabolism in healthy volunteers (DeCarli et al., 1995). Elderly patients with depression (who as a group have increased SCHs) commonly have decreased global and regional cerebral blood flow (CBF), which may persist during remission. During hypercapnea challenge, these patients can have diminished CBF responses (decreased vasodilatory reserve), a phenomenon associated with hypertension, late onset, and poor treatment response (Sackeim, 1996). In elderly depressed patients, moreover, periventricular white matter SCHs have been found to be associated with decreased temporal CBF as assessed by single-photon-emission CT using technetium-99m-hexamethylpropyleneamineoxime (99mTc-HMPAO SPECT) (Ebmeier et al., 1998).

SCHs have been found to be associated with altered cerebral metabolite ratios in phosphorous (Sappey-Marinier et al., 1992a) and proton (Sappey-Marinier et al., 1992b) MRS studies of elderly patients, and with decreased N-acetylaspartate (NAA)/creatine (Cr) in elderly MDD patients (Murata et al., 2001).

Diffusion tensor imaging (DTI) is a derivative of MRI that assesses the movement of water in axons. DTI can detect decreases in fractional anisotrophy that are considered indicative of white matter pathology. DTI studies in bipolar patients compared with healthy controls found prefrontal decreased white matter fractional anisotrophy (Adler et al., 2004, 2006) and increased apparent diffusion coefficient (Beyer et al., 2005). In one DTI study, SCHs compared with normal regions displayed increased apparent diffusion coefficients and lower anisotrophy in both elderly depressed patients and controls, suggesting similar pathological changes (Taylor et al., 2001). Also, elderly MDD patients compared with elderly controls had lower right superior frontal gyrus white matter fractional anisotrophy (Taylor et al., 2004). In another DTI study, elderly MDD patients compared with healthy controls showed more robust declines in white matter fractional anisotrophy. In patients but not controls, these declines were related to aging, consistent with emerging data suggesting that late-life depression may be associated with age-related declines in white matter integrity (Choi et al., 2002).

Taken together, the above findings suggest that bipolar and MDD patients have increased SCHs. In individuals without psychiatric disorders and in bipolar and MDD patients, these lesions increase with age. Moreover, in healthy volunteers and MDD patients (and perhaps to a lesser extent in bipolar patients), SCHs appear to be related to cardiovascular risk factors and may thus reflect decreased vascular reserve. There may also be relationships among cerebral regions, diagnosis, and age, as SCHs appear to occur in frontal lobes (deep white matter) in nonelderly and elderly bipolar and elderly MDD patients and in basal ganglia (subcortical gray matter) in elderly MDD patients, consistent with the hypothesis that anterior cortical/anterior paralimbic basal ganglia–thalamocortical circuit function may be disrupted in bipolar and MDD patients. However, the relative paucity of evidence supporting basal ganglia (subcortical gray matter) SCHs in bipolar patients could be due to these lesions being specific to older patients with bipolar disorder (McDonald et al., 1999).

There may be some disassociations between bipolar disorder and MDD in clinical correlates of SCHs. Thus in MDD (perhaps to a greater extent than in bipolar) patients, SCHs may be related to later onset, negative family history, cardiovascular risk factors, cognitive impairment, and treatment resistance. This hypothesis in turn is consistent with there being at least some disassociations between bipolar disorder and MDD in the pathophysiology of SCHs. Importantly, SCHs are not diagnostically specific, and the pathophysiology of these lesions needs to be better understood. Moreover, multiple aspects of the clinical significance of SCHs in bipolar disorder and MDD remain to be established. Although some studies suggest interesting relationships with clinical parameters, there are also multiple negative studies in this regard, and unfortunately, meta-analyses of the clinical relationships are not yet available.

Frontal, Cerebellar, and Hippocampal Volume Decreases

Bipolar and MDD patients compared with healthy controls may have cerebral volume decreases in specific regions. The frontal lobes and cerebellum in bipolar and MDD patients and the hippocampus in MDD patients have been implicated in particular.

Frontal and prefrontal volume decreases appear to occur in mood disorders. A tendency for them to occur in bipolar patients compared with healthy controls was observed in three studies (Coffman et al., 1990; Sax et al., 1999;

Strakowski et al., 1999), but they were not seen in two studies (Strakowski et al., 1993b; Zipursky et al., 1997). A recent meta-analysis using robust threshold criteria for inclusion (McDonald et al., 2004) found that in three studies, bipolar patients and controls had similar left (4 percent smaller, $p = .19$) and right (5 percent smaller, $p = .11$) prefrontal volumes. In MDD patients, these decreases were found to be present in eight studies[71] and absent in only three studies (Pantel et al., 1997; Bremner et al., 2000; Janssen et al., 2004). As noted below, prefrontal CBF and metabolism are commonly decreased in depressed bipolar and MDD patients. Frontal and prefrontal volume decreases may be related to poorer performance on neuropsychological tests (Coffman et al., 1990), such as the continuous performance task (Sax et al., 1999).

Methodological advances (improved scan resolution and gray–white segmentation) have led to emerging data on gray and white matter volumes. Prefrontal gray matter may (Drevets et al., 1997; Lopez-Larson et al., 2002) or may not (Dupont et al., 1995b; Zipursky et al., 1997; Lim et al., 1999) be decreased in bipolar patients compared with healthy controls. Prefrontal gray matter density may also be decreased in bipolar disorder (Lyoo et al., 2004). Findings of a preliminary study suggest that men with bipolar-I disorder (but not men with bipolar-II or women) may be at risk for decreases in left frontal lobe gray matter that tend to correlate with decreases in NAA as assessed by MRS (Dieckmann et al., 2002). One study, however, found that dorsolateral prefrontal cortex, inferior parietal lobule, and superior temporal gyrus gray matter volumes were unchanged in bipolar patients compared with healthy controls (Schlaepfer et al., 1994), and another found that depressed adolescents compared with controls had increased frontal gray matter volumes and decreased frontal white matter volumes (Steingard et al., 2002).

Recently, voxel-based morphometry (VBM) has allowed automated voxel-wise assessments of gray and white matter volumes and densities. Studies to date in patients with bipolar disorder[72] and MDD (Bell-McGinty et al., 2002; Pizzagalli et al., 2004) have had variable findings, perhaps as a result of confounds with respect to age, mood disorder subtype, mood state, prior pharmacotherapy (in view of the putative neurotrophic effects of lithium), current medication status, and methodological variability.

Evidence suggests that gray matter volume is decreased in the prefrontal cortex ventral to the genu of the corpus callosum in both familial bipolar disorder and familial MDD (Drevets et al., 1997), consistent with decreased CBF and metabolism (Drevets et al., 1997) and histopathological changes (Rajkowska, 1997) observed in that region. Gray matter volume decreases in the subgenual portion of the left ventral anterior cingulate cortex in bipolar and MDD patients have been demonstrated by both MRI-based morphometric measures[73] and postmortem neuropathological studies of patients with a family history of bipolar disorder and MDD (Öngür et al., 1998). This reduction in volume was seen in patients with a family history of bipolar disorder (Hirayasu et al., 1999), but was notably not demonstrable in bipolar patients with no family history of mood disorders. The reduction was found early in MDD patients (Botteron et al., 2002) and may follow illness onset, as indicated by preliminary evidence in twins discordant for MDD (Botteron et al., 1999).

Coryell (2005) found decreased volume in a nearby region in patients with psychotic MDD. Kimbrell and colleagues (2002) reported that subgenual anterior cingulate metabolism was inversely correlated with the number of lifetime depressive episodes in MDD patients. Other studies, however, have failed to detect subgenual prefrontal cortical volume decreases in mood disorder patients.[74] A recent meta-analysis using robust threshold criteria for inclusion (McDonald et al., 2004) found that in four studies, bipolar patients compared with controls had nonsignificantly decreased left (20 percent, $p = .31$) and right (6 percent, $p = .36$) subgenual prefrontal volumes. Studies in MDD patients that failed to find a volume decrease in this region, however, found decreased cerebral metabolism in the region in patients with melancholia (Pizzagalli et al., 2004) and decreased gyrus rectus volumes in MDD patients compared with controls (Bremner et al., 2002). Other studies in bipolar patients that failed to detect a volume decrease in this area found more posterior and dorsal cingulate gray matter volume (Lochhead et al., 2004; Nugent et al., 2006) and density (Doris et al., 2004) decreases, as well as decreased left dorsolateral prefrontal cortical gray matter volume in pediatric patients (Dickstein et al., 2005). In addition, MTI demonstrated decreased macromolecular density in the right subgenual anterior cingulate and adjacent white matter (Bruno et al., 2004). Still other studies found that bipolar patients compared with controls had decreased gray matter density in the anterior cingulate close to subgenual prefrontal cortex (Lyoo et al., 2004) and decreased left dorsal anterior cingulate volume (Sassi et al., 2004; Kaur et al., 2005). One study found decreased left cingulate, right medial frontal, and left middle frontal cortical thickness in bipolar patients compared with healthy controls (Lyoo et al., 2006). Ventral prefrontal gray and white matter volumes may decline more rapidly with age in adolescents and young adults with bipolar disorder compared with healthy controls, and rapid cycling may exacerbate and pharmacotherapy may attenuate ventral prefrontal volume deficits (Blumberg et al., 2006). Of interest, decreased orbitofrontal total (Lai et al., 2000) and gray matter (Lacerda et al., 2004; Lavretsky et al., 2004) volumes have been observed in MDD patients.

Although effective treatment with selective serotonin reuptake inhibitors (SSRIs) was not found to alter subgenual prefrontal cortical volume in MDD patients (Drevets et al., 1997), this cortex appeared significantly larger in bipolar patients chronically medicated with lithium or valproate than in bipolar patients who were either unmedicated or medicated with other agents (see Fig. 15–5). These observations are compatible with evidence that chronic administration of these mood stabilizers increases expression of the neuroprotective and neurotrophic proteins in the frontal cortex of experimental animals (Manji et al., 2001). Other investigators, however, have failed to detect subgenual prefrontal cortical volume changes in familial and nonfamilial bipolar and MDD patients (regardless of whether they were taking lithium) compared with healthy controls (Brambilla et al., 2002). One report suggests that, compared with healthy controls, bipolar patients had decreased left anterior cingulate volumes when not medicated but tended to have increased left posterior and right anterior cingulate volumes when taking lithium monotherapy (Sassi et al., 2002b).

Cerebellar volume decreases appear to occur in patients with mood disorders. Compared with healthy controls, such decreases were detected in bipolar patients in six studies[75] but not in four studies,[76] and were detected in MDD patients in two studies (Shah et al., 1992; Escalona et al., 1993) but not in two other studies (Yates et al., 1987; Pillay et al., 1997). In one study, a combined group of bipolar and MDD patients compared with healthy controls tended to have vermian or cerebellar volume decreases (Weinberger et al., 1982). Vermian volume decreases were seen in bipolar patients with (but not without) a history of alcohol abuse (Lippmann et al., 1982). These decreases may tend to be related to number of episodes (DelBello et al., 1999; Brambilla et al., 2001b) and family history of bipolar disorder (Brambilla et al., 2001b), but not to lithium therapy or scores on the Hamilton Rating Scale for Depression (HAM-D) (Brambilla et al., 2001b). In MDD, fluoxetine nonresponders' (but not responders') decreased vermian volumes were found to be associated with higher pretreatment HAM-D scores (Pillay et al., 1997). Cerebellar volume decreases were not related to neuropsychological function in MDD patients, however (Greenwald et al., 1997).

Hippocampal volume decreases have been observed in MDD patients compared with healthy controls. In bipolar patients, however, findings have varied, with hippocampal volumes found to be unchanged in 13 studies,[77] decreased in 3 (Swayze et al., 1992; Noga et al., 2001; Frazier et al., 2005), tending to be decreased in 2 (Strakowski et al., 2002; Blumberg et al., 2003c), and increased in 2 (Kemmerer et al., 1994; Beyer et al., 2004). In a recent meta-analysis

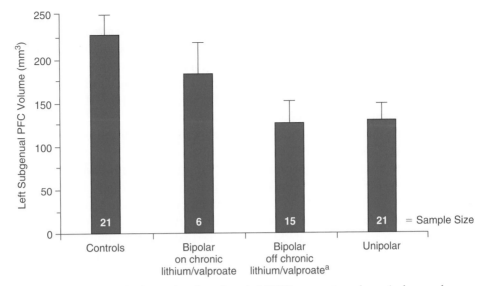

Figure 15–5. Decreased subgenual prefrontal cortical (PFC) gray matter volumes in depressed patients with familial major depressive disorder and familial bipolar disorder. Decreased volumes were accompanied by reductions in cerebral activity (see Fig. 15–11 below). Reduced volumes were not evident, however, in bipolar patients taking chronic lithium or valproate. (*Source:* Adapted from Drevets et al., 2004.)

using robust threshold criteria for inclusion (McDonald et al., 2004), bipolar patients compared with controls were found to have similar left (6 studies, 1 percent larger, $p = .66$), right (6 studies, 1 percent smaller, $p = .60$), and total (8 studies, 1 percent smaller, $p = .24$) hippocampal volumes. One study found that, compared with controls, hippocampal shape anomalies (rounded hippocampus) occurred at a similar rate in familial bipolar disorder, but were more frequent in familial schizophrenia (Connor et al., 2004). Anzalone and colleagues observed that bipolar-I patients compared with healthy controls had right posterior (but not total) hippocampal volume decreases that were related to illness duration. In another study, however, first-episode bipolar patients compared with multiple-episode patients and healthy controls were found to have smaller hippocampal volumes (Strakowski et al., 2002). (One study yielded the curious finding of increased hippocampal volume correlating with poorer neuropsychological function [Ali et al., 2000].) The findings of some studies are consistent with hippocampal volume decreases being more evident on the right (Swayze et al., 1992; Kemmerer et al., 1994; Noga et al., 2001). In one study, however, first-episode affective psychosis patients (polarity not specified) compared with healthy controls showed decreased left (but not right) hippocampal volumes (Velakoulis et al., 1999).

As noted above, there is more consistent evidence of smaller hippocampal volumes in MDD patients. Thus, hippocampal volumes were decreased in 13 studies,[78] tended

to be decreased in 1 study (Steffens et al., 2000), but were unchanged in 5 studies.[79] Indeed, a recent meta-analysis (Campbell et al., 2004) of 12 studies[80] found that a total of 393 MDD patients compared with 303 controls had significantly smaller left and right hippocampal volumes. Significant decreases were more often detected on the left (6 of 12 studies) than on the right (3 of 12 studies). Similarly, another recent meta-analysis (Videbech and Ravnkilde, 2004) of 11 studies[81] found that a total of 351 MDD patients compared with 279 controls had significantly smaller left and right hippocampal volumes. The composite effect sizes for decreased left and right hippocampal volumes were small in magnitude ($-.38$ and $-.32$, respectively). In contrast to observations in bipolar patients, the findings of some studies are consistent with the notion that volume decreases may be more likely for the left hippocampus in MDD patients,[82] although there have been discordant observations (Janssen et al., 2004). In 4 of the 8 studies finding hippocampal volume decreases,[83] these decreases were related to duration of depression, consistent with the notion that chronic hypercortisolemia can lead to progressive hippocampal degeneration. However, there have been discordant observations (Janssen et al., 2004). Another study found that longer total duration of untreated (but not treated) depression was associated with a decrease in hippocampal volume (Sheline et al., 2003), consistent with the hypothesis that reduced adult hippocampal cell proliferation or neurogenesis is involved in the pathophysiology of depression, and that reversal or prevention of decreased neurogenesis may be one way in which antidepressants exert their effects (Malberg, 2004). In a longitudinal study, although no significant hippocampal volume changes were observed in MDD patients or controls between baseline and 1-year follow-up, patients with unremitting illness at follow-up had reduced left and right hippocampal volumes at both baseline and the 1-year follow-up compared with remitting patients, and smaller right hippocampal volumes compared with healthy controls (Frodl et al., 2004). Similarly, in another study, smaller hippocampal volumes were associated with poorer response to antidepressants (Hsieh et al., 2002).

In a study of hippocampal volume, decreases were observed in multiple-episode but not first-episode MDD patients (MacQueen et al., 2003). (MDD with multiple episodes is part of the manic-depressive spectrum.) Another study, however, found hippocampal volume decreases (left-sided gray matter in men and bilateral white matter in men and women) in first-episode MDD patients and failed to detect a relationship between volume decreases and illness duration (Frodl et al., 2002b). Three studies found that greater volume decreases tended to occur with later-onset depression (Steffens et al., 2000; Lloyd et al., 2004; MacMaster and Kusumakar, 2004b), whereas other studies have failed to detect such a relationship (Ashtari et al., 1999; Frodl et al., 2002a).

In some studies, volume decreases were found to be correlated with severity of depression (Ashtari et al., 1999; Vakili et al., 2000), but other investigators have failed to detect such a relationship (Frodl et al., 2002a; MacQueen et al., 2003). One group found hippocampal volume decreases in women with MDD and a history of severe prolonged childhood physical or sexual abuse, but not in MDD patients without such histories. One study found that MDD patients compared with controls had similar hippocampal volumes, but had altered hippocampal shape (Posener et al., 2003). Janssen and colleagues (2004) failed to detect a relationship between hippocampal volumes and subcortical hyperintensities in MDD patients.

MDD patients with the homozygous L/L serotonin transporter genotype were found to have smaller hippocampal gray and white matter volumes than those of controls with this genotype, and significantly smaller hippocampal white matter volumes than those of patients with the L/S or S/S genotype (Frodl et al., 2004). No significant differences were found between patients and controls with the L/S or S/S genotype. The authors suggested that serotonergic influence on neurotrophic factors and excitatory amino acid neurotransmission could account for their findings. Some study findings are consistent with relationships between hippocampal volume loss and poorer cognitive/memory function.[84] For example, Shaw and colleagues (1998) found

that left hippocampal gray matter density was correlated with performance on a verbal memory task.

The above clinical neuroimaging findings of hippocampal volume decreases in MDD, and to a lesser extent in bipolar disorder, are consistent with basic science reports of hippocampal abnormalities in mood disorders.[85] More limited basic science evidence suggests amygdala abnormalities in these disorders (Bowley et al., 2002; Hamidi et al., 2004).

Amygdala findings have been variable in bipolar disorder and MDD. Thus in bipolar disorder, amygdala volumes may be increased,[86] unchanged,[87] tend to be decreased (Chen et al., 2004), or decreased.[88] In a recent meta-analysis using robust threshold criteria for inclusion (McDonald et al., 2004), bipolar patients compared with controls were found to have similar left (four studies, 5 percent larger, $p = .49$), right (four studies, 4 percent larger, $p = .35$), and total (five studies, 1 percent larger, $p = .91$) amygdala volumes. One study in adolescents and young adults found that with increasing age, left amygdala volumes increased in patients but decreased in healthy controls (Chen et al., 2004). These results are consistent with those of most studies including younger populations that have detected amygdala volume decreases in bipolar disorder,[89] although one study involving the very young (mean age 11 years) was negative (Frazier et al., 2005). Blumberg and colleagues (2005) found that decreased amygdala volumes in adolescents and young adults with bipolar disorder persisted 2 years later. Another study found that patients with psychotic (but not nonpsychotic) bipolar disorder compared with those with schizophrenia had increased right amygdala volumes (Strasser et al., 2002). In adults, prior number of episodes may (Altshuler et al., 2000) or may not (Strakowski et al., 1999; Brambilla et al., 2003a) be related to amygdala volume increases. Differences in age, chronicity, and treatment could account for the variation in amygdala volume findings in patients with bipolar disorder.

In MDD, amygdala volumes were found to be unchanged for the entire amygdala[90] and decreased for the entire amygdala (von Gunten et al., 2000) or core nuclei (Sheline et al., 1999), but increased in first-episode (Frodl et al., 2002b) and young female (Lange and Irle, 2004) patients. Thus, Frodl and colleagues (2002c) suggested that amygdala volumes are increased in first-episode but not recurrent MDD patients. A recent meta-analysis (Campbell et al., 2004) of six studies[91] found that a total of 138 MDD patients and 121 controls had statistically similar amygdala volumes. In a longitudinal study, no significant amygdala volume changes were observed in MDD patients or controls between baseline and 1-year follow-up (Frodl et al., 2004).

Amygdala–hippocampal complex volumes appear to be unchanged in bipolar (Swayze et al., 1992) and MDD patients.[92] A recent meta-analysis (Campbell et al., 2004) of four studies[93] found that a total of 126 MDD patients and 165 controls had statistically similar amygdala–hippocampal complex volumes. Thus, although hippocampal volumes appear to be decreased in the latter patients, the absence of decreases or even increases in amygdala volumes could contribute to the lack of difference in amygdala–hippocampal complex volumes.

Temporal lobe findings have been variable in bipolar and MDD patients. Thus in bipolar patients, temporal lobe size was most often found to be unchanged,[94] but in a few studies was found to be decreased (Hauser et al., 1989c; Altshuler et al., 1991) or increased (Harvey et al., 1994; Wilke et al., 2004). A recent meta-analysis using robust threshold criteria for inclusion (McDonald et al., 2004) found that in six studies, bipolar patients compared with controls had similar left (1 percent larger, $p = .63$) and right (1 percent smaller, $p = .55$) temporal lobe volumes. In MDD patients, temporal lobe size has often been found to be unchanged (Coffey et al., 1993b; Pantel et al., 1997; Bremner et al., 2000), but has been reported to tend to be decreased (Kumar et al., 1996, 2000). Decreased left temporal cortical (including hippocampus) gray matter density has been observed in chronic MDD patients (Shah et al., 1998). Later-onset compared with earlier-onset MDD patients had more left medial temporal volume decreases (Greenwald et al., 1997).

In summary, the findings of the above studies suggest that bipolar and MDD patients compared with healthy controls have decreased frontal/prefrontal and cerebellar volumes. In addition, MDD patients appear to have hippocampal volume decreases. To varying degrees, these observations are supported by clinical correlations, but meta-analyses are currently lacking. In contrast, amygdala and temporal lobe volumes have been found to be variable in mood disorders.

Other Structural Neuroimaging Findings

Caudate volumes may be unchanged,[95] decreased (in elderly manic patients) (Bocksberger et al., 1996; Lyoo et al., 2006), or increased (Aylward et al., 1994; Strakowski et al., 1999; Wilke et al., 2004) in bipolar patients; Aylward and colleagues (1994) found increased caudate volumes in men but not women with bipolar disorder. In a study of monozygotic twins with and without bipolar disorder, those with the disorder were found to have increased caudate volumes compared with their normal co-twins. (Noga et al., 2001). A recent meta-analysis using robust threshold criteria for inclusion (McDonald et al., 2004) found that in seven studies, bipolar patients compared with controls had

similar (3 percent larger, $p = .25$) total caudate volumes. Caudate volumes may be decreased in MDD patients (Krishnan et al., 1992, 1993; Greenwald et al., 1997; Parashos et al., 1998) or unchanged.[96] Later-onset compared with earlier-onset MDD patients showed greater left caudate volume decreases (Greenwald et al., 1997).

Compared with controls, putamen volumes were found to be unchanged[97] or increased (in adolescent and first-episode patients and nearly so in multiple-episode patients)[98] in bipolar disorder and unchanged (Pillay et al., 1998; Lenze and Sheline, 1999) or decreased[99] in MDD. In one study that failed to detect caudate and putamen volume differences, anterior and ventral striatal shape differences were seen in drug-naive (but not drug-treated) bipolar patients compared with healthy controls (Lyoo et al., 2006). A recent meta-analysis using robust threshold criteria for inclusion (McDonald et al., 2004) found that in six studies, bipolar patients compared with controls had similar (2 percent larger, $p = .20$) total putamen volumes. A postmortem study found decreased bilateral external pallidum and right putamen volumes in a heterogeneous group of four MDD, two bipolar, and two schizoaffective patients compared with controls (Baumann et al., 1999).

In healthy volunteers, caudate (Jernigan et al., 1991; Krishnan et al., 1992; Murphy et al., 1992) and putamen (Husain et al., 1991) volumes were found to decrease with age; such age-related decreases were also observed in MDD patients (Husain et al., 1991; Krishnan et al., 1992). In another study, age was found to be correlated inversely with left putamen volume in bipolar patients but not healthy controls (Brambilla et al., 2001a), while in geriatric mania patients, putamen volumes failed to be correlated with age but were found to be correlated inversely with age at illness onset (Young et al., 1996). In MDD patients, left putamen volume was observed to decrease with illness duration, while left globus pallidus volume was found to increase with episode number. Illness duration was likewise found to be correlated with putamen volume decreases in bipolar patients (Brambilla et al., 2001a).

Thus basal ganglia volumes have been found to vary in bipolar and MDD patients, with some variability possibly being accounted for by age at illness onset. In contrast, 8 of 15 MRI studies in schizophrenia found enlargement of basal ganglia structures (for a review see Shenton et al., 1997). Medications may yield confounding effects, as typical antipsychotics may result in increased striatal volumes (Chakos et al., 1994).

Thalamic volumes may be unchanged[100] or increased (Dupont et al., 1995b; Strakowski et al., 1999) in bipolar patients. Thus Lochhead and colleagues (2004) reported increased thalamic gray matter density (but not volume) in patients with bipolar disorder, while McIntosh and colleagues (2004) found that bipolar patients compared with controls had decreased thalamic gray matter density. Thalamic volumes may be unchanged,[101] decreased (Dupont et al., 1995b; Kwon et al., 2002), or tend to be increased (Buchsbaum et al., 1997a) in MDD patients. A recent meta-analysis using robust threshold criteria for inclusion (McDonald et al., 2004) found that in five studies, bipolar patients compared with controls had similar (2 percent larger, $p=.54$) total thalamus volumes. Decreased thalamus volumes were seen in MRI studies of schizophrenic patients compared with controls in four of five studies (Shenton et al., 1997) and compared with bipolar patients in the study of McDonald and colleagues (2005).

Pituitary volumes in unipolar patients were found to be unchanged in two studies (Schwartz et al., 1997; Sassi et al., 2001) and increased in two studies (Krishnan et al., 1991; MacMaster and Kusumakar, 2004) (and perhaps are even related to the degree of adrenal escape from dexamethasone suppression; see Axelson et al., 1992). Pituitary volumes were observed to be decreased in patients with bipolar disorder (Sassi et al., 2001) and unchanged with seasonal affective disorder (Schwartz et al., 1997). This variability in findings may be related to differential changes in HPA function within and across disorders.

Corpus callosum size has been reported to be decreased (Coffman et al., 1990; Brambilla et al., 2003b) or unchanged (Hauser et al., 1989b) in bipolar patients, and unchanged[102] or increased in the anterior and posterior subregions in MDD (Wu et al., 1993) and familial MDD patients. One MRI study found that bipolar (but not MDD) patients compared with healthy controls had decreased signal intensity in all subregions of the corpus callosum (Brambilla et al., 2004).

Healthy volunteers have cerebral asymmetry, with right wider than left frontal lobes and left wider than right occipital lobes. In schizophrenia, increased incidence of reversal of this cerebral asymmetry pattern has been reported in some but not other studies. In mood disorder patients, three studies (Weinberger et al., 1982; Tsai et al., 1983; Dewan et al., 1987) found no evidence for and one study (Tanaka et al., 1982) found a trend toward an increased incidence of reversed cerebral asymmetry.

Similar global cerebral volumes have commonly been observed in bipolar[103] and MDD[104] patients compared with healthy controls (see Box 15–1). However, some studies found decreased total cerebral volumes in adolescents with bipolar disorder (Blumberg et al., 2003c; DelBello et al., 2004; Lyoo et al., 2006). Another study found that late-life MDD patients compared with controls had decreased relative (total brain/total intracranial) but similar absolute (total brain) volumes (Kumar et al., 2000). A meta-analysis (Hoge et al., 1999) of seven studies,[105] however, found that

---

BOX 15–1. Structural Neuroimaging Findings in Bipolar and Major Depressive Disorder Patients Compared with Healthy Controls

- Increased lateral ventricular enlargement[a]
- Increased cortical sulcal enlargement[a]
- Increased third ventricular enlargement
- Increased subcortical hyperintensities (younger and older bipolar, older MDD patients)[a]
- Frontal and prefrontal volume decreases
- Cerebellar volume decreases
- Hippocampal volume decreases (in MDD)[a]
- Similar global cerebral volumes[a]

[a]Confirmed with meta-analyses.

---

a total of 160 bipolar patients and 215 controls had similar total cerebral volumes, with a negligible composite effect size of .04 ($p=.56$) and a 95 percent confidence interval of −.17 to .25. A recent meta-analysis using robust threshold criteria for inclusion (McDonald et al., 2004) found that in 11 studies, bipolar patients compared with controls had similar (1 percent smaller, $p=.26$) total cerebral volumes. In 5 studies, bipolar patients compared with controls had similar total gray (1 percent smaller, $p=.71$) and white (1 percent smaller, $p=.66$) matter volumes. In contrast, a meta-analysis of 27 studies revealed decreased total cerebral volumes in schizophrenic patients compared with healthy controls, with a small but significant composite effect size of −.26 ($p <.0001$) and a 95 percent confidence interval of −.35 to −.15 (Ward et al., 1996).

Global cortical gray matter volumes in MDD patients may be unchanged (Dupont et al., 1995b; Pillay et al., 1997), and in bipolar patients may be diffusely decreased (Lim et al., 1999) or unchanged.[106] In the study of Sassi and colleagues (2002b), total gray matter volumes were found to be increased in lithium-treated bipolar patients compared with untreated bipolar patients and healthy controls. Notably, lithium treatment for 4 weeks appeared to increase prefrontal gray matter volume in unmedicated depressed adult bipolar-I patients (Moore et al., 2000b). Cortical white matter volumes in bipolar patients may tend to be decreased (Strakowski et al., 1993b) or unchanged (Lim et al., 1999). In the former study, bipolar patients tended to have decreased global white and unchanged gray matter, and therefore an increased gray/white ratio (Strakowski et al., 1993b).

Thus, the above studies comparing mood disorder patients with healthy controls have yielded variable findings for caudate, putamen, and thalamus volumes, and have generally been negative for whole-brain volumes. Methodological advances allowing segmentation of gray and white matter may enhance the detection of volumetric abnormalities in future studies.

FUNCTIONAL NEUROIMAGING STUDIES

Studies of cerebral activity reflect integrated effects of multiple neurotransmitters and thus have the strength of being able to detect *where* function is altered, even if such alteration is related to actions of multiple neurochemicals on complex networks, such as anterior cortical/anterior paralimbic basal ganglia–thalamocortical circuits. Such studies are limited in their ability to detect *what* function is altered, however. Studies of cerebral activity responses to specific neurochemical challenges can, to a limited extent, address what function is altered, as they reflect the integrated multi-neurotransmitter responses related to alterations in specific neurochemicals.

In contrast, studies of specific cerebral neurochemistry provide data regarding effects on discrete neurochemicals and thus have the strength of being able to detect more specifically *what* function is altered. They may be somewhat limited, however, in their ability to detect *where* function is altered, as they are sensitive only to effects on specific neurochemicals rather than integrated responses related to complex actions of multiple neurochemicals. Also, at least for MRS, poorer spatial resolution (compared with studies of cerebral activity) limits detection of where function is altered.

Clinical studies in mood disorder patients have detected changes in cerebral activity and alterations in specific cerebral neurochemistry in anterior cortical/anterior paralimbic basal ganglia–thalamocortical circuits. Studies of cerebral activity are reviewed in the sections below, followed by a review of studies of specific cerebral neurochemistry using MRS. Studies of specific cerebral neurochemistry using positron emission tomography (PET) and single photon emission computed tomography (SPECT) with specific neurochemical radiotracers are reviewed in Chapter 14.

Studies of cerebral activity include assessments of cerebral metabolic rate for glucose (CMRglu) and CBF. PET with fluorine-18-deoxylglucose (^{18}FDG) assesses CMRglu, and with oxygen-15 water ($H_2^{15}O$) measures CBF. SPECT with ^{99m}Tc-HMPAO, technetium-99m-exametazime (^{99m}Tc-EMZ), and N-isopropyl-p-^{123}I-iodoamphetamine (^{123}IMP) reflects CBF, and with xenon (^{133}Xe) assesses cortical CBF. In addition, fMRI studies yield neurophysiological data considered related to cerebral activity.

CMRglu and CBF generally correlate with one another,[107] although uncoupling can occur with some (Fox and Raichle, 1986; Hallett et al., 1994) but not other (Ginsberg et al., 1988) activation paradigms. Preliminary evidence suggests that global and regional uncoupling of CBF (while performing a passive introspection task) and CMRglu (while performing an auditory continuous performance task) may occur in MDD patients, but not in bipolar patients or healthy volunteers (Dunn et al., 2005). In another study, MDD patients compared with healthy controls were found to have differential left basal ganglia coupling of simultaneously assessed resting CBF and CMRglu (Conca et al., 2000).

CMRglu changes with age. Thus, gray matter CMRglu is low at birth, rises rapidly to adult values by age 2 years, continues to rise to supra-adult values between ages 3 and 12, then declines to adult rates again by the latter part of the second decade (Chugani et al., 1987), similar to the nonlinear developmental patterns seen with gray matter volume (Giedd et al., 1999) and ratios of NAA to choline (Horska et al., 2002). In healthy adults, CMRglu tends to decrease with age,[108] but there is some variability in findings in this regard.[109] Differential regional effects may contribute to such variability. For example, Willis and colleagues (2002) found that in adults, increased age was correlated with decreased global and widespread cortical and increased cerebellar and focal occipital cortical CMRglu.

Although gender has not been found to be related to global CMRglu in most studies,[110] regional differences have been reported. Thus, CMRglu in healthy women compared with men was found to be increased in widespread (Baxter et al., 1987a; Yoshii et al., 1988; Willis et al., 2002) and orbital and medial frontal, caudate, and posterior cingulate regions (Andreason et al., 1994), the thalamus (Murphy et al., 1996), and the cerebellum (Volkow et al., 1997). Compared with men, however, women were observed to have decreased anterior paralimbic (Andreason et al., 1994) and hippocampal (Murphy et al., 1996) or generally similar (Miura et al., 1990) CMRglu. Phase of menstrual cycle may contribute to this variability, as only two studies attempted to control for this parameter (Baxter et al., 1987b; Volkow et al., 1997). Indeed, healthy women during midfollicular phase (lower estradiol and progesterone) were found to have increased thalamic, prefrontal, temporoparietal, and inferior temporal CMRglu, and during midluteal phase (higher estradiol and progesterone) to have increased superior temporal, anterior temporal, occipital, cerebellar, cingulate and anterior insular CMRglu (Reiman et al., 1996).

Cerebral Activity in Affective Processing in Healthy Volunteers

Functional neuroimaging studies in healthy subjects yield important contributions to our understanding of the neural substrates of affective processing. In addition, assessments of regional cerebral function in healthy volunteers provide bases for comparison with mood disorder patients.

For example, activity in anterior compared with posterior cerebral structures is commonly relatively increased (hyperfrontality) in health and relatively decreased (hypofrontality) in depression. Because cerebral function may vary with age and gender, it is important to match patients with healthy controls on these parameters.

The amygdala appears to be important in processing emotional stimuli, especially fear. Amygdala activation was found to be present in 10 studies of emotion evaluation of facial visual stimuli[111] and absent in only 1 (Sprengelmeyer et al., 1998). Anterior cingulate/medial frontal gyrus/basal forebrain was implicated in 7 studies of facial emotion evaluation[112] and not implicated in 3 (Breiter et al., 1996; Morris et al., 1998a; Sprengelmeyer et al., 1998). For both amygdala and anterior cingulate, laterality effects were modest. In spite of considerable variability in paradigms, these studies provide substantial support for amygdala involvement in evaluation of facial emotion, particularly for fearful expressions.

Emerging data indicate that mood disorder patients have attenuated cerebral activation while performing affective processing tasks. For example, these patients compared with healthy controls were found to have attenuated temporal and right insula activation during matching of faces for varied emotions (George et al., 1997a). In another study, adult bipolar patients (about half of whom had mood elevation) compared with healthy controls showed attenuated dorsolateral prefrontal and increased amygdala activation during fearful facial affect recognition (Yurgelun-Todd et al., 2000). In yet another study, manic patients were observed to lack the anterior cingulate and amygdala activation seen in healthy controls during sad facial affect recognition (Lennox et al., 1999). As noted below, the regions showing baseline resting deficits in depressed patients tend to fail to respond in activation studies.

Studies of induction of sadness and happiness have yielded variable findings. Restricting attention to studies using recall of sad events (some of which also used viewing faces), amygdala activation was found to be present in six sadness induction studies[113] but absent in eight.[114] On the other hand, amygdala changes were seen in only two happiness induction studies (Schneider et al., 1995, 1997) and absent in eight.[115] There was a tendency for left-sided amygdala activation to predominate in sadness induction (four left, one bilateral, one right), and left-sided amygdala changes in happiness induction (one left increase, one left decrease). Thus, affective valence appeared to be related more to the presence or absence than to the laterality of activation. Anterior cingulate/medial frontal gyrus changes were seen in eight sadness induction studies[116] but absent in six.[117] These changes were present in only four happiness induction studies[118] and absent in six.[119] Gender may be an

important factor in sadness induction. Three studies (Pardo et al., 1993; George et al., 1996; Schneider et al., 2000) found more widespread activation in women compared with men.

Affect induction can influence cerebral activation during the performance of cognitive tasks. Thus in healthy volunteers, transient sadness induction yielded increased orbitofrontal cortical and decreased rostral medial prefrontal cortical CBF (Baker et al., 1997). Moreover, during transient sadness, subjects had attenuated verbal fluency task–induced left prefrontal, premotor, cingulate, and thalamic activation. The authors noted that the pattern of transient sadness–induced modulation of verbal fluency–induced activations overlapped with resting-state findings of decreased function in these regions in depressed patients.

Pharmacological emotion/mood induction studies have suggested variable cerebral effects across drugs, or even with the same drug across individuals. There are many potential sources of such variability, which may on occasion provide insights into affective processing. In the study of Ketter and colleagues (1996b), for example, acute intravenous procaine yielded robust transient affective experiences ranging from intense euphoria to profound dysphoria. Variability in clinical responses was accompanied by systematic variability in anterior paralimbic responses. That is, in the left amygdala, euphoria occurred with deactivation, and dysphoria was observed with activation.

Physiological and pharmacological induction of affective experiences appears to be accompanied by changes in overlapping anterior paralimbic circuits. Thus, induction of transient sadness or dysphoria by recall of sad events (George et al., 1995b) or by acute intravenous procaine (Ketter et al., 1996b) yielded overlapping anterior paralimbic CBF patterns (see Fig. 15–6).

There are fewer studies of induction of more sustained affective experiences that could perhaps provide more temporally appropriate models of moods. Ketter and colleagues (1996b) found that sustained (30-minute) self-induced sadness yielded decreased metabolism in paralimbic regions that overlapped those where increases were noted with transient sadness induction in other studies. These observations are consistent with the hypothesis that in vulnerable individuals, repeated, prolonged, or intense cerebral activations associated with negative affective experiences may deplete neurochemical substrates, diminishing cerebral metabolism and leading to clinical depression. Similarly, putative hypermetabolism in mania may eventually result in decreased metabolism and postmania depression. Additional functional neuroimaging studies are needed to explore such hypotheses.

Taken together, neuroimaging studies in healthy volunteers suggest that anterior paralimbic structures (especially

Pharmacological
(Procaine-Induced Dysphoria / Euphoria)

Neuropsychological
(Self-Induced Sadness)

A N T E R I O R

P O S T E R I O R

32 Healthy Volunteers
(15 Women, 17 Men)

11 Healthy Volunteers
(All Women)

Figure 15–6. Overlapping limbic regional cerebral blood flow (rCBF) activation with transient induced emotion. Anterior paralimbic activation accompanies both neuropsychologically and pharmacologically induced acute affective changes in healthy volunteers. Images are statistical parametric maps of cerebral blood flow activation in black rendered on the mesial aspect of the left hemisphere. Left: Regions activated during transient self-induced sadness in 11 healthy women (George et al., 1995b). Right: Regions activated during acute intravenous procaine–induced affective symptoms in 32 healthy volunteers (Ketter et al., 1996b).

amygdala and anterior cingulate) contribute importantly to affective processing (particularly fear recognition and transient sadness induction). Emerging data suggest that mood disorder patients compared with healthy controls have differential activation patterns related to affective processing.

Cerebral Activity in Depression

Functional neuroimaging studies have generally implicated anterior cortical and paralimbic changes in cerebral activity in depression, not only in bipolar disorder and MDD, but also in mood disorders secondary to medical and neurological conditions.

Decreased global cerebral activity has been observed in depressed mood disorder patients compared with healthy controls. Thus, global cerebral activity in depressed bipolar patients has commonly been found to be decreased,[120] but has also been found to be unchanged (Rush et al., 1982; Buchsbaum et al., 1984; Cohen et al., 1989) or increased (Buchsbaum et al., 1986). One study found that depressed and mixed-state bipolar patients had lower global CMRglu than manic bipolar patients, euthymic bipolar patients, and depressed MDD patients (Baxter et al., 1985). In depressed MDD patients compared with controls, global activity has commonly been found to be decreased,[121] but has also been observed to be unchanged[122] or increased (Buchsbaum et al., 1986). Thus, a substantial number of studies have detected decreased global cerebral activity in depressed mood disorder patients compared with healthy controls. Findings vary, however, with about half of the

studies detecting decreased and about half similar global cerebral activity in mood disorder patients compared with healthy controls. Of importance, there has been only one report of increased global cerebral activity in depressed mood disorder patients compared with healthy controls (Buchsbaum et al., 1986).

Variability in findings relative to global cerebral activity in depressed mood disorder patients may be related to methodological or demographic differences, or to limited statistical power due to small sample sizes. Moreover, decreased global activity may be more evident in subgroups of depressed patients. Thus, two studies found that global CMRglu was or tended to be decreased in treatment-resistant moderately to severely depressed (but not relatively euthymic) bipolar (Ketter et al., 2001) and MDD (Kimbrell et al., 2002) patients. Global decreases also appeared to be more evident in depressed patients with advanced age and severe depression (Sackeim et al., 1993) or marked weight loss (Delvenne et al., 1997a). Additional factors may contribute to global changes in cerebral activity. For example, in post-thyroidectomy (for thyroid cancer) patients, global CMRglu and CBF were found to be decreased when patients were hypothyroid (with about half also having developed significant depression) after withdrawal of thyroid replacement compared with when they were euthyroid on thyroid replacement (Constant et al., 2001). Moreover, in treatment-resistant mood disorder patients, global CMRglu and CBF were found to be correlated inversely with plasma thyrotropin (Marangell et al., 1997), suggesting that even within the euthyroid range, global cerebral activity decreases with reductions in thyroid function.

Decreased dorsolateral prefrontal activity is the most consistent regional finding in depressed bipolar patients imaged in either the resting condition or while carrying out continuous performance tasks. Thus, studies have commonly detected decreased dorsolateral prefrontal cortical activity, including CMRglu using [18]FDG PET,[123] and CBF using $H_2^{15}O$ PET (Ketter et al., 1996b) or ^{99m}Tc-HMPAO SPECT (Ebert et al., 1993; Ito et al., 1996). Nine of the above studies found bilateral, one found left lateralized (Buchsbaum et al., 1997a), and one found right lateralized (Cohen et al., 1989) decreases, and none found increases in depressed bipolar patients compared with controls. A few studies, however, failed to detect differences between depressed bipolar patients and healthy controls (Cohen et al., 1992; Goyer et al., 1992; Tutus et al., 1998b).

Dorsolateral prefrontal cortical activity has also commonly been found to be decreased in depressed MDD patients compared with healthy controls. These findings include CMRglu assessed with [18]FDG[124] and carbon-11 glucose (^{11}C-glucose) PET (Kishimoto et al., 1987). They also include CBF assessed with oxygen-15 carbon dioxide ($C^{15}O_2$) PET (Bench et al., 1992, 1993; Dolan et al., 1992) and with SPECT employing ^{99m}Tc-HMPAO,[125] ^{99m}Tc-EMZ (Austin et al., 1992; Curran et al., 1993), [123]IMP (O'Connell et al., 1989; Kanaya and Yonekawa, 1990), and gold-195m ([195m]Au)

(Schlegel et al., 1989a). Most of these studies found bilateral decreases, but six found left[126] and three found right (Lesser et al., 1994; Hurwitz et al., 1990; Kimbrell et al., 2002) lateralized decreases. However, slightly fewer than half of the studies in depressed MDD patients compared with healthy controls found similar[127] and three found increased (Buchsbaum et al., 1986; Tutus et al., 1998b; Abou-Saleh et al., 1999) dorsolateral prefrontal activity.

Hypofrontality also has commonly been reported in depression secondary to diverse neurological and medical diseases[128] or other psychiatric disorders.[129] Moreover, return of depressive symptoms induced by depletion of tryptophan (Bremner et al., 1997) and norepinephrine (Bremner et al., 2003) in MDD patients who had responded to SSRIs and desipramine, respectively, was found to be accompanied by decreased dorsolateral prefrontal and orbitofrontal metabolism. Similarly, tryptophan depletion–induced return of depressive symptoms in MDD patients was found to be accompanied by decreased ventral anterior cingulate, orbitofrontal cortex CBF (Smith et al., 1999). Taken together, the above findings suggest the possibility of hypofrontality being a common pathway contributing to depressive symptoms, to some extent independently of illness etiology (primary versus secondary) and subtype (bipolar disorder versus MDD) (see Fig. 15–7).

Anterior cerebral CBF and CMRglu decreases often have been found to be correlated with the severity of primary[130]

Figure 15–7. Hypofrontality in secondary and primary depression. Transaxial images depicting cerebral metabolic rate (CMR) for glucose in patients with (top row) and without (bottom row) depression. Arrows indicate decreased frontal metabolism in patients with depression secondary to neurological disorders, as well as in those with primary (unipolar) depression. (*Source:* Reproduced with permission from Mayberg et al., 1994.)

Figure 15–8. Regional cerebral metabolism in moderately to severely depressed unmedicated bipolar patients compared with healthy controls. Z-maps of differences in absolute (top) and normalized (bottom) cerebral metabolism in 17 moderately to severely depressed unmedicated bipolar patients compared with 17 healthy controls. The legend indicates two-tailed *p* values. Numbers in the upper right corners indicate distances from the intercommissural plane. L = left. Absolute prefrontal and anterior paralimbic cortical metabolic decreases and normalized anterior paralimbic subcortical metabolic increases evident in these images may be state markers for depression in bipolar disorder. Decreased dorsomedial and dorsolateral prefrontal activity has commonly been reported in other studies of bipolar depression. Left (L) ventrolateral structures failed to show the absolute metabolic decreases seen in other prefrontal cortical regions in these moderately to severely depressed bipolar patients (top) or the relative metabolic increases seen in left ventrolateral structures in mildly depressed bipolar patients (Fig. 15–9, bottom). (*Source:* Ketter et al., 2001.)

and secondary[131] depression. Some studies have failed to detect such a relationship, however.[132]

The variability in the above findings may be related in part to differences in affective symptoms. Osuch and colleagues (2000) found depression ratings to be directly correlated with bilateral medial frontal, right anterior cingulate, and right dorsolateral prefrontal globally normalized metabolism. In contrast, anxiety ratings were found to be correlated directly with right parahippocampal and left anterior cingulate and inversely with cerebellum, left fusiform, left superior temporal, left angular gyrus, and left insula globally normalized metabolism. Another study found that parietal operculum, posterior cingulate, left parahippocampus, and ventral thalamus metabolism increased, while bilateral ventrolateral prefrontal cortical metabolism decreased, with degree of depression in MDD patients (Drevets et al., 2002c). In addition, dorsal and posterior cingulate and inferior bank of

superior temporal sulcus metabolism was found to increase with degree of dysfunctional depressive automatic thoughts.

Also of interest, depressed patients with versus those without cognitive impairment were found to have decreased anterior medial prefrontal CBF (Dolan et al., 1992). The degree of cognitive impairment was found to be correlated with the degree of decrease (Dolan et al., 1994). Ketter and colleagues (2001) found that moderately to severely (but not mildly) unmedicated depressed bipolar patients compared with controls carrying out a continuous performance task had decreased absolute prefrontal and anterior paralimbic cortical and increased normalized anterior paralimbic and subcortical metabolism (see Fig. 15–8). Moreover, the degree of depression was found to be correlated negatively with absolute prefrontal and paralimbic cortical and positively with normalized anterior paralimbic subcortical metabolism. This study also found, however, that in mildly (but not moderately to severely) unmedicated depressed bipolar patients compared with healthy controls, relative (i.e., normalized to whole brain) metabolic activity was increased in the left prefrontal cortex, including ventrolateral structures such as the inferior frontal gyrus (see Fig. 15–9)—a finding reported in some studies of unmedicated depressed MDD patients imaged in the resting condition.[133] Of interest, left ventrolateral structures, such as the inferior frontal gyrus in moderately to severely depressed bipolar patients, failed to show the absolute metabolic decreases seen in other prefrontal cortical regions (Fig. 15–8, top) or the relative metabolic increases seen in mildly depressed bipolar patients (Fig. 15–9, bottom). Taken together, these observations are consistent with the view that the topography of cerebral functional changes may be related to the degree of depression in bipolar disorder.

Moderately to severely (but not mildly) depressed bipolar patients compared with healthy controls also were found to have increased normalized metabolism in subcortical paralimbic structures, including ventral striatum, thalamus, and right amygdala (Fig. 15–8, bottom), consistent with a corticolimbic dysregulation model of depression positing that dorsal neocortical hypofunction may lead to ventral paralimbic overactivity or vice versa (Mayberg, 1997; Drevets, 1999, 2000) (see Fig. 15–10). Relative activation of bilateral medioposterior thalamus was also seen, consistent with altered thalamic relay and gating function with respect to communication between subcortical and cortical regions. Drevets and colleagues (1995, 2002c) confirmed the findings of elevated metabolism in the right amygdala and ventral striatum, as well as elevated metabolism in the left amygdala, in depressed bipolar patients relative to healthy controls. Increased ventral striatum and left amygdala metabolism has also been reported in depressed MDD patients meeting criteria for melancholia or familial pure depressive disease.[134]

Another study found decreased CBF (by $H_2^{15}O$ PET) and CMRglu in the prefrontal cortex ventral to the genu of

Figure 15–9. Regional cerebral metabolism in mildly depressed unmedicated bipolar patients compared with healthy controls. Z-maps of differences in absolute (top) and normalized (bottom) cerebral metabolism in 16 mildly depressed unmedicated bipolar patients compared with 16 healthy controls. The legend indicates two-tailed p values. Numbers in the upper right corners indicate distances from the intercommissural plane. L = left. Increased normalized (but not absolute) metabolism was noted in left (L) inferior, middle, and superior frontal gyri; left insula and left transverse temporal gyrus; left postcentral gyrus; lingular gyrus, cuneus, and hippocampus; and bilateral cerebellum (sparsely). In contrast, decreased normalized (but not absolute) metabolism was noted in right inferior and middle temporal gyri. Ventrolateral metabolic increases have also been reported in depressed unmedicated major depressive disorder patients in the resting state. (*Source:* Ketter and Drevets, 2002.)

Figure 15–10. Corticolimbic dysregulation model of depression. Regions with known anatomical connections are grouped into two compartments: dorsal (black) and ventral (gray). Curved black arrows and color-filled regions emphasize inverse correlations between right dorsal prefrontal cortex (dFr 9/46, in black) and subgenual cingulate (Cg 25, in gray) seen with both transient sadness in healthy volunteers (Fr decreases, Cg increases) and mood symptom resolution in depressed patients (Fr increases, Cg decreases). Nonshaded regions are potentially critical to the schematic model. Short black arrows indicate known subcortical pathways. Numbers are Brodmann area designations. Abbreviations, from top to bottom: dFr = dorsolateral prefrontal; inf Par = inferior parietal; dCg = dorsal anterior cingulate; pCg = posterior cingulate; Cg 24a = rostral anterior cingulate; BG = basal ganglia; Th = thalamus; aIns = anterior insula; Hc = hippocampus; Cg25 = subgenual cingulate; Hth = hypothalamus; mb-p = midbrain-pons. (*Source:* Reproduced with permission from Mayberg et al., 1999.)

the corpus callosum (subgenual) in both depressed familial bipolar disorder and depressed familial MDD patients (Drevets et al., 1997) (see Fig. 15–11). Decreased subgenual prefrontal cortical activity was accompanied by reductions in gray matter volume (Drevets et al., 1997; Hirayasu et al., 1999), as noted above (Fig. 15–5). Of interest, Kimbrell and colleagues (2002) reported that subgenual anterior cingulate metabolism was correlated inversely with the number of lifetime depressive episodes in MDD patients. In contrast, Videbech and colleagues (2002) found that nonfamilial depressed MDD patients compared with healthy controls had increased subgenual prefrontal cortical activity.

Drevets (1999) observed that, although baseline subgenual prefrontal cortical CBF and metabolism appeared to be abnormally decreased in PET images during depressive episodes, computer simulations that corrected the PET data for the partial volume effect of reduced gray matter volume suggested that the "actual" metabolic activity in the remaining subgenual prefrontal cortical tissue may be increased in depressive patients relative to controls and decrease to normative levels during effective treatment. This result appears to be compatible with evidence that effective antidepressant pharmacotherapy results in a decrease in metabolic activity in this region in MDD patients[135] and that during

depressive episodes, metabolism shows a positive relationship with depression severity in both depressed bipolar (Ketter et al., 2001) and depressed MDD patients.[136] This mood state dependency of subgenual prefrontal cortical metabolism is also consistent with functional neuroimaging data showing that CBF increases in this region in healthy, nondepressed individuals during sadness induced internally by contemplation of sad thoughts or memories (George et al., 1995b; Damasio et al., 1998; Mayberg et al., 1999).

Variable anterior cingulate/medial prefrontal activity has been noted in other studies of depressed bipolar patients. Some studies of such patients compared with healthy controls have detected decreased anterior cingulate/medial prefrontal metabolism assessed with [18]FDG PET (Buchsbaum et al., 1997a), and CBF assessed with $H_2^{15}O$ PET (Ketter et al., 1996b) and ^{99m}Tc-HMPAO SPECT (Ito et al., 1996). One study detected decreased superior but increased inferior anterior cingulate metabolism in depressed (primarily bipolar-II) patients with summer seasonal affective disorder (Goyer et al., 1992). Others, however, failed to detect differences in anterior cingulate activity in depressed bipolar patients compared with healthy controls.[137] In a study by Ketter and colleagues (2001), anterior cingulate/medial prefrontal metabolism was found to be similar in depressed

Subgenual Prefrontal Hypometabolism in Mood Disorders

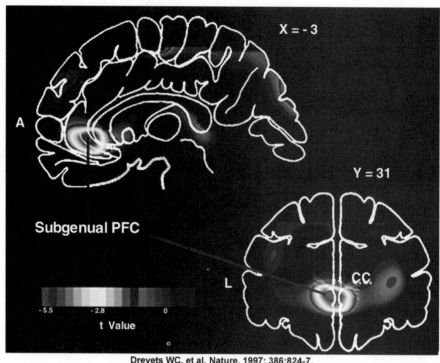

Drevets WC, et al. Nature, 1997; 386:824-7.

Figure 15–11. Decreased subgenual prefrontal cortical metabolism in depressed patients with familial major depressive disorder and familial bipolar disorder. Coronal (31 mm anterior to the anterior commissure, or y=31) and sagittal (3 mm left of midline, or x=−3) sections showing negative voxel *t* values where glucose metabolism was decreased in (7 bipolar and 10 unipolar) familial depressed patients compared with controls. Decreased activity was accompanied by reduced gray matter volume (Fig. 15–5). A=anterior, L=left, PFC=prefrontal cortex. (*Source:* Drevets, 2001; Drevets et al., 1997. Reprinted with permission from Macmillam Publishers Ltd: *Nature*.)

and euthymic bipolar patients and healthy controls, but correlated positively with HAM-D scores in the bipolar patients. Symptoms may be differentially related to anterior cingulate function. Thus in a combined sample of bipolar and MDD patients, HAM-D scores were found to be correlated directly with right anterior cingulate cerebral metabolism and Spielberger Anxiety-State Scale scores with left anterior cingulate cerebral metabolism (Osuch et al., 2000).

There has also been variability in findings on anterior cingulate/medial prefrontal activity in studies of depressed MDD patients. Thus these patients have been reported to have decreased anterior cingulate/medial prefrontal metabolism assessed with [18]FDG PET[138] and CBF assessed with $C^{15}O_2$ (Bench et al., 1992, 1993; Dolan et al., 1992) and $H_2^{15}O$ (Drevets et al., 1997) PET and with ^{99m}Tc-HMPAO[139] and ^{99m}Tc-EMZ (Curran et al., 1993) SPECT. Other studies of depressed MDD patients compared with controls, however, have found unchanged[140] or increased (Drevets et al., 1992; Videbech et al., 2002) anterior cingulate activity. Also, as noted below, subgroups of depressed MDD patients

may have increased anterior cingulate activity related to subsequent response to sleep deprivation[141] or fluoxetine (Mayberg et al., 1997).

Decreased temporal cortical activity has been observed in depressed mood disorder patients compared with healthy controls. Thus several neuroimaging studies in depressed bipolar patients compared with healthy controls have found decreased temporal cortical metabolism with [18]FDG PET (Post et al., 1987; Cohen et al., 1989; Ketter et al., 2001) and CBF assessed with $H_2^{15}O$ PET (Ketter et al., 1996a) and ^{99m}Tc-HMPAO SPECT (Ito et al., 1996). One study detected decreased posterior but increased anterior left temporal cortical metabolism in depressed (primarily bipolar-II) patients with summer seasonal affective disorder (Goyer et al., 1992). Two of the above studies found bilateral (Ketter et al., 1996a, 2001), three found left (Cohen et al., 1989; Goyer et al., 1992; Ito et al., 1996), and one found right (Post et al., 1987) lateralized decreases. Other studies, however, found that depressed bipolar patients compared with healthy controls had increased (Buchsbaum et al., 1997b) or similar[142] temporal cortical activity.

Depressed MDD patients may also have decreased temporal cortical activity. Thus these patients compared with healthy controls were found to have decreased temporal cortical metabolism with [18]FDG[143] and ^{11}C-glucose PET (Kishimoto et al., 1987) and increased CBF with H$_2^{15}$O PET (Drevets et al., 1992) and SPECT employing ^{99m}Tc-HMPAO,[144] ^{99m}Tc-EMZ (Austin et al., 1992; Curran et al., 1993; Edmonstone et al., 1994), [123]IMP (O'Connell et al., 1989; Kanaya and Yonekawa, 1990), and [195m]Au (Schlegel et al., 1989c). Most of the above studies found bilateral decreases, but five found left[145] and three found right (Hurwitz et al., 1990; Drevets et al., 1992; Edmonstone et al., 1994) lateralized decreases. One group noted possible modest lateralized increases in right more than left temporal activity in depressed MDD patients compared with medical controls (Amsterdam and Mozley, 1992), which normalized with recovery (Amsterdam et al., 1995). Other studies by this group, however, failed to detect consistent laterality differences in depressed MDD patients compared with healthy controls (Mozley et al., 1996; Hornig et al., 1997). Kowatch and colleagues (1999) found increased temporal lobe CBF in depressed adolescent MDD patients compared with healthy controls. About half of the studies, however, found that depressed MDD patients and healthy controls had similar temporal cortical activity.[146]

Increased amygdala activity may occur in depressed mood disorder patients compared with healthy controls. Thus in comparison with healthy controls, increased amygdala activity has been noted in depressed bipolar patients through [18]FDG PET (Ketter et al., 2001; Drevets et al., 2002b) and in depressed MDD patients through [18]FDG (Nofzinger et al., 1999; Drevets et al., 2002c) and H$_2^{15}$O PET (Drevets et al., 1992; Videbech et al., 2002) and ^{99m}Tc-HMPAO SPECT (Kowatch et al., 1999). All of the above studies yielded lateralized findings, with four detecting left[147] and two right (Kowatch et al., 1999; Ketter et al., 2001) amygdala activity increases. In one of these studies, left amygdala (but not right amygdala or hippocampus) metabolism was found to be increased in both depressed bipolar and depressed MDD patients, and positively correlated with stressed (PET scan) plasma cortisol levels in both groups (Drevets et al., 2002a). This study also found that in euthymic bipolar patients, left amygdala metabolism was elevated in those patients off but not on mood stabilizers (Drevets et al., 2002c).

In an fMRI study, in a masked (outside of conscious awareness) faces paradigm, depressed MDD patients were found to have exaggerated left (but not right) amygdala activation in response to all faces that was even greater for fearful faces (Sheline et al., 2001). In another study, although depressed MDD patients and controls were found to have similar amygdala CMRglu, negative affect was found to be correlated with right amygdala metabolism in patients (Abercrombie et al., 1998). Depressed MDD patients who later responded to sleep deprivation were found to have baseline increased left amygdala CMRglu in one study (Wu et al., 1992) and right hippocampal–amygdala complex CBF in another (Ebert et al., 1991). Hornig and colleagues (1997) found that treatment-resistant (but not non-treatment-resistant) depressed MDD patients had increased bilateral amygdala–hippocampal CBF. MDD patients who recovered on SSRIs and who had subsequent tryptophan depletion–induced (Bremner et al., 1997) or alpha-methylparatyrosine–induced (Bremner et al., 2003) relapse, but not those who failed to relapse, tended to have increased (laterality not stated) amygdala activity. In other studies, however, amygdala activity was found to be similar in depressed patients and controls.[148]

Compared with healthy controls, depressed MDD patients have shown increased (Ebert et al., 1991; Videbech et al., 2001, 2002), decreased (Saxena et al., 2001), or unchanged (Conca et al., 2000) hippocampal activity.

Decreased basal ganglia activity in MDD patients during depression has been observed in multiple studies. Thus depressed MDD patients compared with healthy controls were found to have decreased basal ganglia metabolism with [18]FDG PET[149] and CBF with H$_2^{15}$O PET (Drevets et al., 1992) and with ^{99m}Tc-HMPAO[150] and ^{99m}Tc-EMZ (Austin et al., 1992; Curran et al., 1993; Edmonstone et al., 1994) SPECT. However, Videbech and colleagues (2002) found increased and most studies found similar[151] basal ganglia activity in depressed MDD patients compared with that in healthy controls.

A few studies have indicated the possibility that depressed bipolar patients have decreased basal ganglia activity. Thus compared with healthy controls, these patients were found to have decreased basal ganglia metabolism with [18]FDG PET (Baxter et al., 1985; Buchsbaum et al., 1986; Cohen et al., 1989) and CBF with H$_2^{15}$O PET (Ketter et al., 1996a). Buchsbaum and colleagues (1997) reported that metabolism in depressed bipolar patients compared with controls was found to be decreased in the left putamen but increased in the entire striatum. In another study, moderately to severely depressed bipolar patients showed relatively increased basal ganglia metabolism compared with mildly depressed and euthymic bipolar patients and healthy controls (Ketter et al., 2001). Other studies, however, failed to detect differences in basal ganglia activity between depressed bipolar patients and healthy controls.[152]

Studies have found both decreased (Baxter et al., 1985; Buchsbaum et al., 1997b) and increased (Ketter et al., 2001) thalamic metabolism assessed with [18]FDG PET in depressed bipolar patients compared with healthy controls. Several other studies have failed to detect differences in thalamic activity in depressed bipolar patients compared with healthy controls.[153]

Depressed MDD patients compared with healthy controls were found to have decreased thalamic metabolism with [18]FDG PET (Hagman et al., 1990; Buchsbaum et al., 1997) and CBF with ^{99m}Tc-HMPAO (Mayberg et al., 1994; Vasile et al., 1996; Kowatch et al., 1999) and SPECT with ^{99m}Tc-EMZ (Austin et al., 1992; Curran et al., 1993). Two studies, however, found increased thalamic activity (Drevets et al., 1992; Saxena et al., 2001) and most found similar[154] thalamic activity in depressed MDD patients compared with healthy controls.

Increased cerebellar activity independent of mood state has been observed in treatment-resistant bipolar patients (Ketter et al., 2001). In another study, however, bipolar patients (mood state not specified) were found to have lower cerebellar blood volume than that of control subjects (Loeber et al., 1999). In the latter study, schizophrenic patients had higher cerebellar blood volume than that of control subjects. Other studies have found similar cerebellar activity in depressed bipolar patients and healthy controls (Baxter et al., 1985; Ebert et al., 1993; Ketter et al., 1996b).

Increased cerebellar activity has also been reported in depressed MDD patients with cognitive impairment (Bench et al., 1992; Dolan et al., 1992) and moderate to severe depression (Videbech et al., 2001, 2002; Kimbrell et al., 2002). However, Kumar and colleagues (1993) found decreased cerebellar metabolism in depressed patients with late-life MDD compared with healthy controls. Other studies found similar cerebellar activity in depressed MDD patients and healthy controls (Baxter et al., 1985; Wu et al., 1992; Biver et al., 1994).

In "activation" studies, mood disorder patients have also manifested altered prefrontal and anterior paralimbic responses compared with healthy controls during diverse conditions (for a more detailed review, see Malhi et al., 2004): affective processing tasks, such as facial emotion recognition (George et al., 1997a; Lennox et al., 1999; Yurgelun-Todd et al., 2000), viewing of emotionally expressive faces,[155] affect-inducing captioned pictures (Malhi et al., 2004), and positive (Mitterschiffthaler et al., 2003) and negative (Davidson et al., 2003; Irwin et al., 2004) affective pictures; self-induced transient sadness[156]; and performance of an emotional version of the Stroop color-word interference test (Malhi et al., 2005). These altered responses also occurred during cognitive tasks, such as the conventional Stroop test (George et al., 1997b; Blumberg et al., 2003a,b; Kromhaus et al., 2006), complex planning (Elliott et al., 1997), planning and guessing with and without feedback (Elliott et al., 1998), word generation,[157] working memory (Adler et al., 2004), visuospatial working memory (Chang

et al., 2004), memory encoding (Bremner et al., 2004), and reaction time and movement velocity scaling, as well as during acute drug challenges with intravenous procaine (Ketter et al., 1993), oral amphetamine (Trivedi et al., 1995), and oral dl-fenfluramine (Mann et al., 1996). In addition, during rapid eye movement (REM) sleep versus waking, depressed MDD patients compared with healthy controls did not show increased anterior paralimbic (including anterior cingulate) metabolism and had decreased gyrus rectus metabolism, but were found to have greater tectal and left hemisphere (sensorimotor and inferior temporal cortex, uncal gyrus–amygdala, and subicular complex) metabolic increases (Nofzinger et al., 1999). Also, during non-REM sleep, depressed MDD patients compared with controls showed increased global and widespread regional (especially posterior cingulate, amygdala, hippocampus, occipital and temporal cortex, and pons) absolute metabolism and decreased prefrontal (especially medio-orbital frontal), anterior cingulate, caudate, and medial thalamus relative metabolism (Ho et al., 1996).

Activation studies may be able to detect cerebral functional differences not apparent with simpler (resting on continuous performance task) behavioral paradigms. For example, although resting and continuous performance task studies have indicated overlapping frontal deficits in schizophrenia and mood disorders, activation studies have demonstrated dissociations. Thus, during the Wisconsin Card Sorting Test, frontal activation was found to be blunted in schizophrenia but preserved in depression (Berman et al., 1993). Similarly, during word generation, frontal activation was blunted in schizophrenic but enhanced in euthymic bipolar patients (Curtis et al., 2001). Moreover, activation studies may detect additional differences between euthymic mood disorder patients and healthy controls. For example, both euthymic bipolar (Krüger et al., 2003) and euthymic MDD (Liotti et al., 2002) patients appear to have altered cerebral activation patterns with transient sadness induction.

Finally, return of depressive symptoms induced by depletion of tryptophan (Bremner et al., 1997) and norepinephrine (Bremner et al., 2003) in MDD patients who had responded to SSRIs and desipramine, respectively, was found to be accompanied by decreased dorsolateral prefrontal and orbitofrontal metabolism. Of interest, increased baseline prefrontal and limbic metabolism predicted vulnerability to such return of depressive symptoms induced by depletion of tryptophan (Bremner et al., 1997) and norepinephrine (Bremner et al., 2003).

In summary, depressed bipolar and MDD patients compared with healthy controls have commonly been found to have decreased global, dorsolateral prefrontal, and temporal cortical activity and increased amygdala activity. The dorsolateral prefrontal finding is the most robust one and is supported by clinical correlations. Basal ganglia but not thalamus activity may also be decreased in depressed MDD patients compared with controls, but there are only sparse variable data for bipolar depression. Mood disorder patients compared with healthy controls have been found to have variable anterior cingulate/medial prefrontal activity, due perhaps in part to heterogeneity related to clinical parameters, such as symptoms and treatment response. Sparse data raise the possibility that cerebellar activity may be increased in at least some mood disorder patients. Although some studies have found lateralized effects, compelling lateralization patterns have not emerged across studies. The above observations from resting or continuous performance task studies have generally been supported by findings from activation studies.

Effects of Mood State and Treatment on Cerebral Activity

Most of the above-mentioned changes in activity in anterior cortical and subcortical components of basal ganglia–thalamocortical circuits appeared to be state related, as they were not evident in euthymic bipolar (Ketter et al., 2001) and MDD (G. Goodwin et al., 1993; Bench et al., 1995) patients. Possible exceptions include the amygdala, where Drevets and colleagues (2002b) observed that metabolism was significantly elevated in a small sample of euthymic bipolar subjects who were not taking mood-stabilizing drugs, relative both to healthy controls and to euthymic bipolar patients taking mood stabilizers. In contrast, amygdala metabolism did not differ between the bipolar subjects taking mood stabilizers and healthy controls. The cerebellum may also show normalized metabolic increases independent of mood state in treatment-resistant bipolar patients compared with healthy controls (Ketter et al., 2001).

Treatment responders compared with their depressed pretreatment baseline often show attenuation (or resolution) of pretreatment cerebral functional abnormalities with various therapies, including mood stabilizers (Ketter et al., 1999), antidepressants,[158] placebo (Mayberg et al., 2002), psychotherapy (Brody et al., 2001b), thyroxine (Bauer et al., 2005), phototherapy (Cohen et al., 1992; Vasile et al., 1997), sleep deprivation,[159] vagus nerve stimulation (Devous et al., 2002), and (nonconvulsive) transcranial magnetic stimulation (TMS) (George et al., 1995c; Pascual-Leone and Pallardó, 1996). Improvements in specific symptoms may be related to normalization of activity in particular components of anterior cortical/anterior paralimbic basal ganglia–thalamocortical circuits (Brody et al., 2001b). There have been some discordant findings, however, such as antidepressants exacerbating baseline abnormalities (Nobler et al., 2000).

One report noted that in MDD patients, recovery from depression was accompanied by metabolism (assessed with [18]FDG PET) increases in neocortical (right dorsolateral prefrontal, inferior parietal) structures and decreases in limbic–paralimbic (subgenual cingulate, anterior insula) regions (Mayberg et al., 1999). That is, baseline abnormalities seen in depression were attenuated or reversed. Of interest, healthy volunteers experiencing transient sadness had the reverse pattern involving the same regions, namely, neocortical increases and limbic decreases in blood flow assessed with $H_2^{15}O$ PET.

In contrast, successful ECT appears to exacerbate decreased anterior cerebral activity (Nobler et al., 1994; Scott et al., 1994; Henry et al., 2001), although other patterns (including normalization) have also been reported (Bonne et al., 1996b; Elizagarate et al., 2001; Mervaala et al., 2001). This apparent divergence could be related to confounding medication effects or to a different mechanism of action of ECT.

Taken together, the above findings suggest that in many instances, differences in cerebral activity in mood disorder patients compared with healthy controls are commonly state related, as they tend to be absent during euthymia and generally attenuate or reverse with successful treatment. Exceptions may occur, however, in specific regions, such as amygdala and cerebellum; in specific subgroups, such as treatment-resistant bipolar patients; and with specific therapies, such as ECT.

Baseline Cerebral Activity Markers of Treatment Response

Comparisons of baseline (pretreatment) cerebral activity in patients who later respond or fail to respond to therapy suggest possible baseline markers of treatment response. Baseline left insular hypermetabolism may be a marker for bipolar patients who are more likely to respond to carbamazepine, while hypometabolism in this region may be related to response to nimodipine (Ketter et al., 1999). Depressed bipolar patients who later respond to valproate may have low baseline rostral anterior cingulate and medial frontal gyrus cerebral glucose metabolism (Ketter et al., 2000). In contrast, depressed MDD patients who later respond to fluoxetine may have high baseline rostral anterior cingulate cerebral glucose metabolism (Mayberg et al., 1997). Thus, complementary baseline differences may be seen in depressed bipolar responders to valproate and depressed MDD responders to fluoxetine. Similarly, depressed MDD patients who later responded to venlafaxine had increased baseline anterior cingulate activation when viewing negative affective pictures (Davidson et al., 2003). Depressed MDD patients who later responded to sertraline had increased baseline gyrus rectus metabolism (Buchsbaum et al., 1997b). In one study of depressed MDD patients compared with healthy controls, however, baseline left middle frontal gyral, bilateral medial prefrontal, and bilateral temporal hypometabolism was seen in those who later responded to venlafaxine or bupropion, whereas baseline cerebellar hypometabolism was evident in those who later failed to respond to these agents (Little et al., 1996). Selectively, compared with control subjects, bupropion responders also had cerebellar hypermetabolism, whereas venlafaxine responders showed bilateral temporal and basal ganglia hypometabolism (Little et al., 2005). Anterior limbic hyperactivity appears to be a baseline marker for MDD patients who obtain antidepressant responses from sleep deprivation.[160]

In MDD patients, degree of treatment resistance was found to be correlated with left orbitofrontal metabolism (Kimbrell et al., 2002). Another study found that medication-free treatment-resistant depression patients had increased hippocampal–amygdalar CBF compared with non-treatment-resistant patients and healthy controls (Hornig et al., 1997). Also, in patients with treatment-resistant mood disorders, widespread (including anterior paralimbic) baseline hypometabolism was found to be associated with better responses to high-frequency (20 Hz) TMS, while baseline hypermetabolism tended to be related to better responses to low-frequency (1 Hz) TMS (Kimbrell et al., 1999). In another study, depressed responders compared with nonresponders to (5 or 20 Hz) TMS had baseline increased inferior frontal lobe CBF (Teneback et al., 1999).

The above studies of baseline markers of treatment response offer preliminary evidence that pretreatment neuroimaging assessments of depressed mood disorder patients may have features that distinguish subsequent responders from nonresponders. Anterior paralimbic (especially anterior cingulate/medial prefrontal) regions may ultimately prove to be of special interest in assessing baseline markers of treatment response. At the same time, it should be noted that the CMRglu and CBF studies reviewed above have important limitations, including small sample sizes, varying methodology, and reliance on measures of cerebral activity rather than assessment of specific neurochemical differences.

Cerebral Activity in Mania, Hypomania, and Rapid Cycling

Because of clinical considerations, there have been relatively few studies of cerebral activity during mania. Thus, only sparse and equivocal data exist regarding changes in global cerebral activity in mania. Kishimoto and colleagues (1987) noted widespread increases in ^{11}C-glucose uptake were noted in three medication-free manic patients

compared with controls. In another study, bipolar patients in mixed (and depressed) states were found to have decreased global CMRglu compared with healthy controls and manic bipolar patients (Baxter et al., 1985). One study found that global cerebral metabolism in medication-free hypomanic or euthymic bipolar patients did not differ from that in healthy controls, but was increased compared with bipolar patients in depressed or mixed states (Schwartz et al., 1987); however, this finding was not replicated by Martinot and colleagues (1990). In other studies, manic patients and controls were observed to lack global differences (Silfverskiöld and Risberg, 1989; Rubin et al., 1995).

There have been variable regional findings in manic patients. Frontal lobe activity was found to be decreased in such patients in four studies.[161] In one of these studies, manic patients were found to have not only decreased resting orbitofrontal CBF but also decreased right rostral prefrontal and right orbital prefrontal CBF activation during word generation (Blumberg et al., 1999). Frontal activity was found to be increased, however, in five studies,[162] with the increased activity occurring in the anterior cingulate or subgenual prefrontal cortex in four of these studies.[163] Baxter and colleagues (1985, 1989) observed an increase in frontal activity in manic compared with depressed bipolar patients. Although lithium withdrawal generally led to decreased anterior cingulate activity, development of mania with lithium withdrawal was found to be associated with increased superior anterior cingulate activity (G. Goodwin et al., 1997).

Temporal lobe activity in mania was found to be decreased in one study (Migliorelli et al., 1993), increased in two studies (O'Connell et al., 1995; Gyulai et al., 1997), and mixed (decreased left amygdala and increased right temporal cortical) in one study (al-Mousawi et al., 1996). Basal ganglia activity was observed to be increased in two studies (Drevets et al., 1995; Blumberg et al., 2000) and increased in about half of patients in another study (O'Connell et al., 1995). Mania ratings were found to be correlated positively with right temporal and caudate CBF by O'Connell and colleagues (1995), but negatively correlated (a trend) with right basotemporal CBF by Migliorelli and colleagues (1993).

Cerebellar blood volume in bipolar-I patients (primarily medicated and in the manic state) compared with controls was found to be similar overall and in patients on lithium or valproate, but decreased in patients on conventional antipsychotics and increased in those on atypical antipsychotics (Loeber et al., 2002). There have also been a few functional neuroimaging studies in patients with mania secondary to medications, alcohol or drug abuse, or general medical conditions. Starkstein and colleagues

(1990) reported right temporal lobe hypometabolism in three patients (two on lithium, one unmedicated) with mania secondary to stroke (Starkstein et al., 1990).

In rapid-cycling bipolar patients, anterior temporal activity may be asymmetric when depressed, manic, or hypomanic but not when euthymic (Gyulai et al., 1997). Global cerebral metabolism (Baxter et al., 1985) and blood flow (Speer et al., 1997) may oscillate as mood state changes.

In summary, the locations of changes noted in neuroimaging studies are consistent with the broad notion that altered anterior cortical/anterior paralimbic basal ganglia–thalamocortical circuit activity may contribute importantly to the pathophysiology of mania. Unfortunately, in contrast with depression, studies of mania have been too sparse and had findings too variable (in terms of the location and direction of changes) to allow more meaningful and specific conclusions. Thus, important issues such as the degree to which the locations and directions of changes in mania compared with depression overlap or are complementary remain to be resolved. For example, the available data are insufficient to determine whether the same regions that have decreased activity in depression have increased activity in mania. Advances in research methodology are needed to make neuroimaging studies in mania more feasible so these issues can be addressed.

Assessment of Specific Cerebral Neurochemistry

Studies of specific cerebral neurochemistry complement studies of cerebral activity in that they can detect more specifically what function is altered, and they are similar in that they can detect where function is altered. Studies using PET and SPECT with specific neurochemical radiotracers to assess specific cerebral neurochemistry are discussed in Chapter 14. Below we review studies using MRS. Clinical MRS studies in patients with mood disorders have begun to detect metabolite alterations in anterior cortical/anterior paralimbic basal ganglia–thalamocortical circuits.

Proton (¹H) Magnetic Resonance Spectroscopy

Proton magnetic resonance spectroscopy (¹H-MRS) allows determination of diverse cerebral metabolites, including NAA, cytosolic choline (Cho) compounds, myoinositol (mI), compounds related to energy metabolism (creatine [Cr], phosphocreatine [PCr]), and amino acids (gamma-aminobutyric acid [GABA], glutamate). Metabolite concentrations may be assessed as absolute or relative (typically compared with Cr) measures.

N-acetylaspartate, an amino acid with putative roles in amino acid metabolism and fatty acid and protein synthesis, is found in mature neurons and may reflect neuronal density and integrity. Although findings vary, evidence is accumulating to support NAA and NAA/Cr changes in

bipolar patients. Thus in bipolar patients compared with healthy controls, NAA or NAA/Cr was found to be decreased in 8 studies,[164] increased in 4 studies,[165] and similar in 11 studies.[166] In contrast, MDD patients and healthy controls were found consistently to have similar NAA and NAA/Cr across 11 studies,[167] while only single studies found decreased caudate NAA/Cr (Vythilingam et al., 2003) and prefrontal NAA/Cr (but not NAA) (Gruber et al., 2003) in MDD patients. In the latter study, decreased prefrontal NAA/Cr in MDD appeared to be related to increased Cr (Gruber et al., 2003).

NAA and NAA/Cr findings in bipolar patients may vary on a regional basis. Thus dorsolateral prefrontal NAA or NAA/Cr in bipolar patients was found to be decreased in three studies (Winsberg et al., 2000; Chang et al., 2001; Sassi et al., 2005) and similar to that of controls in three studies (Bertolino et al., 2003; Michael et al., 2003. While studies found that bipolar patients had decreased medial prefrontal/orbitofrontal NAA (Cecil et al., 2002) and tended to have decreased cerebellar vermis NAA/Cr (Cecil, 2003), multiple other studies found that bipolar patients and controls had similar NAA or NAA/Cr in medial prefrontal (Hamakawa et al., 1999; Frye et al., 2001; Cecil et al., 2003), anterior cingulate,[168] and frontal/prefrontal[169] regions.

In bipolar patients compared with controls, hippocampal NAA (Deicken et al., 2003a) and NAA/Cr (Bertolino et al., 2003) were found to be decreased. In a post hoc analysis of the latter study, bipolar patients compared with those without a history of alcohol abuse had higher hippocampal NAA/Cr (Frye et al., 2000). In another study, however, bipolar patients and healthy controls displayed similar temporal NAA (Moore et al., 2000b). First-episode psychosis patients (46 percent of whom had bipolar disorder) were found to have decreased temporal NAA/Cr (Renshaw et al., 1995). In contrast, euthymic bipolar patients on lithium (but not valproate) showed increased temporal NAA/Cr (T. Silverstone et al., 2003). In a postmortem study, bipolar patients (most of whom had had psychotic symptoms) were found to have decreased superior temporal (but not frontal) cortex NAA, consistent with the notion that temporal lobe NAA deficits may be a common feature of psychotic disorders (Nudmamud et al., 2003).

Bipolar patients compared with controls displayed decreased (Frye et al., 2001), increased (Sharma et al., 1992), or similar[170] basal ganglia NAA/Cr. Medication-free depressed bipolar patients had increased left putamen NAA (Dager et al., 2004). One study found increased NAA (Deicken et al., 2001), but others found similar NAA (Dager et al., 2004) or NAA/Cr (Bertolino et al., 2003) in the thalamus in bipolar patients compared with healthy controls. Parietal and occipital regions have consistently shown similar NAA and NAA/Cr levels in bipolar patients and healthy controls[171] and have commonly been used as control regions. NAA has variable relationships with age.

In bipolar patients, some studies found that dorsolateral prefrontal (Winsberg et al., 2000) and basal ganglia (Kato et al., 1996a; Ohara et al., 1998) NAA/Cr decreased with age, while others found no relationship between age and dorsolateral prefrontal NAA (Brambilla et al., 2005; Sassi et al., 2005), dorsolateral prefrontal NAA/Cr in juveniles (Chang et al., 2001), medial prefrontal NAA (Hamakawa et al., 1999), hippocampal NAA/Cr (Bertolino et al., 2003), or basal ganglia NAA (Hamakawa et al., 1998). In a postmortem study of bipolar patients, superior temporal lobe and frontal NAA were not found to be related to age (Nudmamud et al., 2003). In MDD patients, age was observed to affect caudate NAA/Cr (Vythilingam et al., 2003), but not to be related to anterior cingulate NAA (Pfleiderer et al., 2003) or basal ganglia NAA or NAA/Cr (Hamakawa et al., 1998).

Variable, but most often negative, gender effects have been reported for NAA and NAA/Cr. Hamakawa and colleagues (1998) detected an overall (in euthymic and depressed bipolar and MDD patients and healthy controls) gender effect for left basal ganglia NAA (but not NAA/Cr), but the direction of the effect was not specified. In other studies, however, the same group noted no overall (in euthymic bipolar patients and healthy controls) gender effect on left basal ganglia NAA/Cr (Kato et al., 1996a) and no overall (in euthymic and depressed bipolar patients and healthy controls) gender effect on bilateral medial prefrontal NAA (Hamakawa et al., 1999). In a postmortem study of bipolar patients, superior temporal lobe and frontal NAA were not found to be related to gender (Nudmamud et al., 2003).

NAA/Cr may vary across the menstrual cycle. Thus medial prefrontal (but not occipital) NAA/Cr was found to decline from follicular to luteal phase in women with premenstrual dysphoric disorder (PMDD) by 19 percent and in healthy controls by 16 percent, and there were no statistically significant differences in NAA/Cr between these groups (Rasgon et al., 2001).

Although in one study, bipolar-I patients had bilateral dorsolateral prefrontal NAA/Cr decreases while bipolar-II patients had only unilateral (left) decreases (Winsberg et al., 2000), other researchers found that bipolar-I and -II patients had similar prefrontal (Hamakawa et al., 1999) and basal ganglia (Kato et al., 1996b; Hamakawa et al., 1998) NAA or NAA/Cr. Moreover, one of the latter studies found no basal ganglia NAA differences between bipolar and MDD patients when either depressed or euthymic (Hamakawa et al., 1998).

In bipolar patients, dorsolateral prefrontal NAA/Cr (Winsberg et al., 2000; Chang et al., 2001) and hippocampal NAA showed a tendency to decrease with longer illness duration. However, other studies failed to detect a relationship between duration and dorsolateral prefrontal (Brambilla et al., 2005; Sassi et al., 2005), prefrontal (Hamakawa et al., 1999), basal ganglia (Hamakawa et al., 1998), or thalamus (Deicken et al., 2001) or overall gray or white matter (Dager et al., 2004) NAA or lenticular nucleus NAA/Cr (Ohara et al., 1998). In MDD patients, illness duration was found not to be related to basal ganglia NAA (Hamakawa et al., 1998).

NAA does not appear to vary with mood symptoms. Thus current mood state was not found to be related to NAA or NAA/Cr in prefrontal (Hamakawa et al., 1999; Bertolino et al., 2003), basal ganglia (Hamakawa et al., 1998; Frye et al., 2001), or hippocampal or thalamic (Bertolino et al., 2003) regions in bipolar patients, or in basal ganglia (Hamakawa et al., 1998) in MDD patients. In bipolar patients, HAM-D scores were not found to be related to prefrontal (Hamakawa et al., 1999), basal ganglia (Hamakawa et al., 1998), or overall gray or white matter (Dager et al., 2004) NAA, nor were Young Mania Rating Scale (YMRS) scores found to be related to basal ganglia NAA/Cr (Frye et al., 2001) or to overall gray or white matter NAA (Dager et al., 2004). Similarly, in MDD patients, HAM-D scores were not shown to be related to basal ganglia NAA (Hamakawa et al., 1998). In healthy volunteers, a correlation was not found between the Positive Affect Negative Affect Scale (PANAS), Positive Affect subscale, and left frontal NAA (Jung et al., 2002).

Emerging data suggest possible medication effects on NAA and NAA/Cr. Lithium, in view of its potential neurotrophic effects, is of particular interest. Acute (4-week trial) lithium monotherapy similarly increased prefrontal, temporal, parietal, and occipital NAA in depressed adult bipolar-I patients and healthy controls, but no correlation was found between cerebral NAA and blood lithium concentrations (Moore et al., 2000a). In contrast, in primarily depressed adult bipolar-I and -II patients, lithium for a mean of 3.6 months and valproate for a mean of 1.4 months failed to alter gray or white matter or regional NAA (Friedman et al., 2004). Also, in children and adolescents during manic or mixed episodes, anterior cingulate NAA/Cr showed no change with acute (1-week trial) adjunctive lithium treatment; again, no correlation was found between serum lithium concentrations and brain NAA/Cr (Davanzo et al., 2001). In addition, in adult healthy volunteers, lithium administration for 4 weeks failed to alter dorsolateral prefrontal NAA (Brambilla et al., 2004).

One study found that, compared with healthy controls, euthymic bipolar patients on chronic lithium plus other medications (but not on chronic valproate plus other medications) had increased left temporal NAA/Cr (T. Silverstone et al., 2003). Similarly, bipolar patients taking chronic lithium had increased dorsolateral prefrontal NAA/Cr compared with unmedicated patients and healthy controls (Brambilla et al., 2005). Comparisons of bipolar patients on and not on chronic lithium, however, revealed similar anterior cingulate (Soares et al., 1999) and basal ganglia (Kato et al., 1996b; Ohara et al., 1998a) NAA/Cr and medial prefrontal NAA (Hamakawa et al., 1999); no relationship was found between serum lithium concentrations and basal ganglia or occipital NAA/Cr (Sharma et al., 1992). In euthymic adults with bipolar disorder on chronic lithium, doses were not found to be related to thalamic (Deicken et al., 2001) or hippocampal (Deicken et al., 2003a) NAA.

If lithium increases NAA or NAA/Cr, the presence or absence of chronic lithium could contribute to the variability in NAA and NAA/Cr findings in bipolar patients compared with healthy controls. In studies to date, the percentage of patients taking lithium was lower in studies detecting NAA decreases (N = 27/111, 24 percent)[172] than in those finding no NAA differences (N = 81/189, 43 percent)[173] or those reporting NAA increases (N = 23/65, 35 percent) (Sharma et al., 1992; Deicken et al., 2001; T. Silverstone et al., 2003; Dager et al., 2004). These differences are consistent with the notion that NAA and NAA/Cr increases with chronic lithium therapy could be a confounding factor in detecting putative baseline (unmedicated) decreases in NAA and NAA/Cr in patients with bipolar disorder.

Less is known about the effects of other medications on NAA and NAA/Cr. Bipolar patients taking compared with those not taking chronic anticonvulsants were found to have increased basal ganglia NAA (Hamakawa et al., 1998), but duration of valproate treatment showed an inverse correlation with medial prefrontal NAA (Cecil et al., 2002). Bipolar patients taking compared with those not taking chronic valproate had similar medial prefrontal NAA (Hamakawa et al., 1999), and valproate doses were not found to be related to thalamus (Deicken et al., 2001) or hippocampal (Deicken et al., 2003a) NAA. Patients taking compared with those not taking chronic antipsychotics showed similar medial prefrontal NAA (Hamakawa et al., 1999) and basal ganglia NAA and NAA/Cr (Kato et al., 1996a; Hamakawa et al., 1998). Schizophrenic patients taking atypical antipsychotics compared with those taking typical antipsychotics were found to have higher cingulate NAA (Ende et al., 2000b).

In depressed MDD patients, acute nefazodone (Charles et al., 1994a) and fluoxetine (Sonawalla et al., 1999) did not alter basal ganglia NAA/Cr. The latter study also failed to detect changes when the sample was stratified by patients with sustained response to fluoxetine ("true fluoxetine response") and those with nonresponse or only transient response to the drug ("placebo pattern response/nonresponse") (Sonawalla et al., 1999). Mood disorder patients taking compared with those not taking chronic antidepressants were found to have similar medial prefrontal NAA (Hamakawa et al., 1999) and basal ganglia NAA/Cr (Kato et al., 1996a). In depressed MDD patients, ECT did not alter parietal NAA (Felber et al., 1993), and a course of ECT did not significantly alter bilateral hippocampal NAA (Ende et al., 2000b). These observations are consistent with the notion that ECT may not result in neuronal damage.

There are very few data regarding baseline NAA or NAA/Cr markers of treatment response. In depressed MDD patients, left basal ganglia NAA/Cr was found to be similar in fluoxetine responders and nonresponders (Renshaw et al., 1997) and in those with "true fluoxetine response" and "placebo pattern response/nonresponse" (Sonawalla et al., 1999).

Choline (Cho) is an acetylcholine precursor involved in second-messenger cascades. The "cholinergic–adrenergic" hypothesis of bipolar disorder proposes that depression is related to cholinergic overactivity and adrenergic underactivity, while mania is related to cholinergic underactivity and adrenergic overactivity (Janowsky et al., 1972). In ^{1}H-MRS, the Cho peak represents total cellular Cho stores, the dominant component of which is believed to be from cell membranes (phospholipids) rather than acetylcholine.

Although findings vary, evidence is accumulating to support Cho and Cho/Cr changes in patients with mood disorders. Thus, Cho and Cho/Cr in bipolar patients compared with healthy controls were found to be increased in 5 studies,[174] to tend to be decreased in 3 studies,[175] to be decreased in one cohort but not a second cohort in 1 study (Wu et al., 2004), and to be similar in 17 studies.[176] Cho and Cho/Cr in MDD patients compared with healthy controls were found to be (or to tend to be) increased in 7 studies,[177] decreased in 4 studies,[178] and similar in 3 studies (Auer et al., 2000; Pfleiderer et al., 2003; Smith et al., 2003). Gruber and colleagues (2003) found decreased prefrontal Cho/Cr but not Cho in MDD patients, perhaps related to increased Cr.

Cho and Cho/Cr findings in mood disorder patients may vary on a regional basis. Thus in bipolar patients compared with healthy controls, Cho or Cho/Cr was found to be increased (Soares et al., 1999; C. Moore et al., 2000) or similar[179] in anterior cingulate regions, to tend to be decreased (Cecil et al., 2002) or similar (Hamakawa et al., 1999; Dager et al., 2004) in medial prefrontal regions, and to be decreased (Silverstone et al., 2004; Wu et al., 2004) or similar (Renshaw et al., 1995; Wu et al., 2004) in temporal regions. However, Cho or Cho/Cr in bipolar patients compared with healthy controls was found to be consistently similar in dorsolateral prefrontal,[180] frontal/prefrontal

(Castillo et al., 2000; Amaral et al., 2002; Bertolino et al., 2003), hippocampal (Bertolino et al., 2003; Deicken et al., 2003a), and temporal (Renshaw et al., 1995) regions.

Cho or Cho/Cr in bipolar patients compared with healthy controls was found to be increased,[181] to tend to be increased (Dager et al., 2004), or to be similar (Ohara et al., 1998; Castillo et al., 2000; Bertolino et al., 2003) in basal ganglia, and similar in thalamus (Deicken et al., 2001; Bertolino et al., 2003; Dager et al., 2004). One study found that Cho tended to be increased in bipolar patients compared with controls in left caudate and right putamen, but not in other brain regions or in gray or white matter (Dager et al., 2004). Parietal and occipital regions have consistently shown similar Cho and Cho/Cr in bipolar patients and healthy controls[182] and have commonly been used as control regions.

In MDD patients compared with healthy controls, basal ganglia Cho or Cho/Cr was found to be or to tend to be increased in four studies[183] but decreased in one study (Renshaw et al., 1997). Cho or Cho/Cr in MDD patients compared with healthy controls was observed to be increased in dorsolateral prefrontal (Farchione et al., 2002) and temporal lobe (Mervaala et al., 2000) regions; similar in anterior cingulate (Auer et al., 2000; Pfleiderer et al., 2003) and orbitofrontal (Steingard et al., 2000) regions; and decreased in prefrontal (Gruber et al., 2003), amygdala (Kusumakar et al., 2001), and hippocampal (Ende et al., 2000a) regions. Cho or Cho/Cr in MDD patients was similar to that in healthy controls in thalamus (Vythilingam et al., 2003) and in parietal (Auer et al., 2000) and occipital (Rosenberg et al., 2000) lobes.

In bipolar patients, no age effect was observed on basal ganglia Cho/Cr (Kato et al., 1996b; Hamakawa et al., 1998) or dorsolateral prefrontal (Brambilla et al., 2005) or prefrontal (Hamakawa et al., 1998) Cho. In MDD patients, age was found to be related to thalamic Cho/Cr (Vythilingam et al., 2003), but not orbitofrontal Cho/Cr (Steingard et al., 2000) or prefrontal Cho (Hamakawa et al., 1998).

Data vary regarding the effect of oral Cho administration on cerebral Cho. One group found that in healthy volunteers, acute administration of Cho (choline bitartrate equivalent to 50 mg/kg free Cho) increased basal ganglia Cho/Cr about two-fold by 3 hours, with no significant correlation between brain and serum Cho (Stoll et al., 1995). Another study by the same group showed that acute administration of Cho in older compared with younger healthy volunteers yielded similar (70–80 percent) increases in plasma Cho, but markedly attenuated increases in basal ganglia Cho/Cr, suggesting that uptake of acutely administered Cho may decrease with age (Cohen et al., 1995). Thus it has been proposed that development of cerebral Cho depletion underlies the deteriorating course seen

in some patients with bipolar disorder (Renshaw et al., 1996). These investigators also reported that four patients with rapid-cycling bipolar disorder who responded to 5,000–7,200 mg/day of free Cho added to lithium ± other medications had 30–75 percent increases in basal ganglia Cho/Cr (Stoll et al., 1996). In seven patients with rapid-cycling bipolar disorder, however, Cho ingestion did not alter basal ganglia Cho/Cr after 5 weeks of administration (Demopulos et al., 1997). Also, double-blind choline bitartrate 50 mg/kg/day for 12 weeks in four lithium-treated rapid-cycling bipolar patients failed to alter left basal ganglia Cho/Cr, cerebral lithium, or clinical mood ratings, but decreased left basal ganglia purine/NAA and purine/Cho (Lyoo et al., 2003). The authors commented that decreased purine could reflect decreased adenosine triphosphate (ATP), perhaps reflecting increased ATP consumption with choline. Another group found that acute oral challenge of 50 mg/kg of choline bitartrate did not significantly alter Cho/Cr or Cho in four brain locations (Tan et al., 1998). Still another group found that in young healthy volunteers, both acute (50 mg/kg choline bitartrate single dose) and long-term (lecithin 32 g/day for 4 weeks) administration of Cho failed to alter gray matter, white matter, cerebellum, and thalamus Cho (Dechent et al., 1999b). In a more recent study in 11 healthy young men, oral choline bitartrate to yield 50 mg/kg resulted in increased left putamen Cho/Cr, with a mean peak increase of 6.2 percent approximately 2 hours after ingestion (Babb et al., 2004).

Variable, but most often negative, gender effects have been reported for Cho and Cho/Cr. Studies found no overall (in euthymic and depressed bipolar and MDD patients and healthy controls) gender effect on left basal ganglia Cho and Cho/Cr (Hamakawa et al., 1998), no overall (in euthymic bipolar patients and healthy controls) gender effect on left basal ganglia Cho/Cr (Kato et al., 1996a), and no overall (in euthymic and depressed bipolar patients and healthy controls) gender effect on bilateral medial prefrontal Cho (Hamakawa et al., 1999). In MDD patients, gender was not related to orbitofrontal Cho/Cr (Steingard et al., 2000) or hippocampal Cho (Ende et al., 2000b). Cho/Cr may vary across the menstrual cycle. Thus, occipitoparietal (but not medial prefrontal) Cho/Cr was found to have increased from follicular to luteal phase in women with PMDD by 38 percent and in healthy controls by 13 percent, and there were no statistically significant Cho/Cr differences between these groups (Rasgon et al., 2001).

In one study, bipolar-II patients compared with bipolar-I patients and healthy controls were found to have higher basal ganglia Cho/Cr (Kato et al., 1996a). Later studies by this same group failed to detect bipolar-II versus bipolar-I differences in basal ganglia (Hamakawa et al., 1998) or medial prefrontal (Hamakawa et al., 1999) Cho, but found that depressed bipolar patients had higher basal ganglia Cho than depressed or euthymic MDD patients (Hamakawa et al., 1998). In one report, rapid-cycling compared with non-rapid-cycling bipolar patients showed a tendency to have lower basal ganglia Cho/Cr (Demopulos et al., 1996).

Cho and Cho/Cr do not appear to vary with illness duration in dorsolateral prefrontal (Brambilla et al., 2005), medial prefrontal (Hamakawa et al., 1999), or basal ganglia (Hamakawa et al., 1998; Ohara et al., 1998) regions or overall gray or white matter (Dager et al., 2004) in bipolar patients, or in basal ganglia in MDD patients (Hamakawa et al., 1998).

Cho and Cho/Cr do not appear to have consistent relationships with mood state. As noted above, Hamakawa and colleagues (1998) found that depressed compared with euthymic bipolar patients had higher basal ganglia Cho. In other studies, however, mood state in bipolar patients was not found to be related to Cho or Cho/Cr in medial prefrontal (Hamakawa et al., 1999), dorsolateral prefrontal, anterior cingulate, hippocampal, or thalamic (Bertolino et al., 2003) regions. In bipolar patients, HAM-D scores showed a positive correlation with anterior cingulate Cho/Cr (Moore et al., 2000a), but not with basal ganglia (Hamakawa et al., 1998) or overall gray or white matter (Dager et al., 2004) Cho. In MDD patients, amygdala Cho/Cr displayed a tendency to have a negative correlation with Beck Depression Inventory scores (Kusumakar et al., 2001), while no relationship was observed between HAM-D scores and anterior cingulate (Auer et al., 2000) or basal ganglia (Hamakawa et al., 1998) Cho. In healthy volunteers, however, PANAS Positive Affect subscale scores correlated with left frontal Cho (Jung et al., 2002).

Emerging data suggest possible medication effects on Cho and Cho/Cr. In depressed adult bipolar-I patients, it was found that lithium monotherapy had antidepressant effects and led to decreased prefrontal Cho (Moore et al., 1999). In contrast, in primarily depressed adult bipolar-I and -II patients, lithium for a mean of 3.6 months and valproate for a mean of 1.4 months failed to alter gray or white matter or regional Cho (Friedman et al., 2004). In children and adolescents during manic or mixed episodes, anterior cingulate Cho/Cr did not change with acute (1-week trial) adjunctive lithium treatment and showed no correlation with serum lithium concentrations (Davanzo et al., 2001). Finally, in adult healthy volunteers, lithium administration for 4 weeks failed to alter dorsolateral prefrontal Cho (Brambilla et al., 2004).

Patients taking compared with those not taking chronic lithium were found to have similar basal ganglia Cho/Cr (Lafer et al., 1994; Kato et al., 1996a; Ohara et al., 1998) and Cho (Hamakawa et al., 1998), medial prefrontal Cho (Hamakawa et al., 1999), temporal Cho/Cr (Wu et al., 2004),

and anterior cingulate Cho/Cr (Moore et al., 2000b). Serum lithium concentrations showed no relationship to basal ganglia or occipital Cho/Cr (Sharma et al., 1992).

If lithium alters Cho or Cho/Cr, the presence or absence of chronic lithium treatment could contribute to the variability in Cho and Cho/Cr findings in bipolar patients compared with healthy controls. To date, the percentage of patients taking lithium has been higher in studies finding increases in patients compared with healthy controls (46/84, 55 percent)[184] than in those finding no difference ($N = 97/269$, 36 percent).[185] This difference is consistent with the notion that Cho and Cho/Cr decreases with chronic lithium could be a confounding factor in detecting putative baseline (unmedicated) increases in Cho and Cho/Cr in patients with bipolar disorder.

Less is known about the effects of other medications on Cho and Cho/Cr. Bipolar patients taking compared with those not taking chronic anticonvulsants were found to have similar basal ganglia Cho (Hamakawa et al., 1998), and bipolar patients taking compared with those not taking valproate showed similar anterior cingulate Cho/Cr (C. Moore et al., 2000). Bipolar patients taking chronic antipsychotics compared with those not taking them displayed similar basal ganglia Cho (Hamakawa et al., 1998) and Cho/Cr (Kato et al., 1996b) and medial prefrontal Cho (Hamakawa et al., 1999). Also, in the study of Wu and colleagues (2004), bipolar patients taking lithium had similar temporal Cho/Cr compared with those taking valproate.

By contrast, bipolar patients taking antidepressants compared with those not taking them were found to have higher basal ganglia (Kato et al., 1996b) but not medial prefrontal (Hamakawa et al., 1999) Cho/Cr. In MDD patients, basal ganglia Cho/Cr was found to decrease in patients taking nefazodone (Charles et al., 1994a) and in those with fluoxetine "placebo pattern response/nonresponse" (Sonawalla et al., 1999) but to increase in patients with "true fluoxetine response" (Sonawalla et al., 1999). In MDD patients, depression and physical symptoms induced by SSRI (fluoxetine or paroxetine) discontinuation were observed to be associated with decreased rostral anterior cingulate Cho/Cr (but not NAA/Cr) (Kaufman et al., 2003). In MDD patients, ECT was found to increase hippocampal Cho (Ende et al., 2000b), but not to alter anterior cingulate (Pfleiderer et al., 2003) or parietal (Felber et al., 1993) Cho.

There are very few data on baseline Cho or Cho/Cr markers of treatment response. In depressed MDD patients, pretreatment basal ganglia Cho/Cr was found to be lower in fluoxetine responders than in nonresponders (Renshaw et al., 1997), but similar in patients with "true fluoxetine response" and fluoxetine "placebo pattern response/nonresponse" (Sonawalla et al., 1999).

Myoinositol (mI) is a storage form of six carbon carbohydrate inositol, an agent important in signal transduction that may have antidepressant effects (Levine et al., 1995). Inositol depletion has been proposed as a mechanism of action of lithium (Berridge et al., 1989).

Although findings vary, some evidence suggests that mI and mI/Cr may be altered in patients with mood disorders. Thus, mI and mI/Cr in bipolar patients compared with healthy controls showed a tendency to be increased in five studies,[186] decreased in no studies, and similar in five studies.[187] In MDD patients compared with healthy controls, mI and mI/Cr were found to be (or tend to be) increased in no studies, decreased in two studies (Frey et al., 1998; Gruber et al., 2003), and similar in three studies (Auer et al., 2000; Rosenberg et al., 2000; Vythilingam et al., 2003). One study found decreased prefrontal mI/Cr but not mI in MDD patients, perhaps related to increased Cr (Gruber et al., 2003).

Findings regarding mI and mI/Cr in bipolar patients may vary on a regional basis. Thus in bipolar patients compared with healthy controls, mI or mI/Cr was found to be increased in basal ganglia by Sharma and colleagues (1992), to tend to be increased by Winsberg and colleagues (2000) and Cecil and colleagues (2002), or similar to controls in dorsolateral prefrontal regions by Chang and colleagues (2001), and to tend to be increased in anterior cingulate regions by Davanzo and colleagues (2001, 2003). In multiple other studies, however, bipolar patients and controls were found to have similar mI or mI/Cr in anterior cingulate (Moore et al., 2000a), medial prefrontal (Cecil et al., 2002), frontal and temporal (Silverstone et al., 2002), parietal (Brühn et al., 1993), and occipital (Sharma et al., 1992) regions. One study found that bipolar patients had gray and white matter and regional mI similar to that of controls (Dager et al., 2004).

Two studies found that frontal mI/Cr was decreased in depressed MDD patients compared with age- and gender-matched healthy controls (Frey et al., 1998; Gruber et al., 2003). Multiple other studies, however, found that MDD patients and controls had similar mI or mI/Cr in anterior cingulate (Auer et al., 2000), basal ganglia (Rosenberg et al., 2000; Vythilingam et al., 2003), thalamus (Vythilingam et al., 2003), parietal (Auer et al., 2000), and occipital (Rosenberg et al., 2000) regions.

Oral inositol administration may transiently increase cerebral inositol. By 4 days, 12 g/day mI was found to increase occipital gray (but not parietal white) mI/Cr in healthy volunteers by 20 percent. By 8 days, however, this effect was no longer evident (Moore et al., 1999).

Variable relationships have been noted between mI and age in healthy volunteers. One study found that in depressed MDD patients, right frontal mI/Cr was correlated positively with age (Frey et al., 1998). Variable,

but most often negative, gender effects have been reported for mI and mI/Cr. One study found that in healthy controls (but not in depressed MDD patients), frontal mI/Cr tended to be lower in female than in male subjects (Frey et al., 1998). In contrast to NAA/Cr and Cho/Cr, mI/Cr may not vary across the menstrual cycle (Rasgon et al., 2001), while like these other metabolites, medial prefrontal and occipital mI/Cr was found to be similar in women with PMDD and healthy controls (Rasgon et al., 2001).

There are very few data on relationships between the clinical phenomenology of mood disorders and cerebral mI or mI/Cr. In bipolar patients during manic or mixed states, YMRS scores tended to be correlated positively with prefrontal mI (Cecil et al., 2002). In depressed MDD patients, however, HAM-D scores were not found to be related to anterior cingulate or parietal mI (Auer et al., 2000) or anterior cingulate mI/Cr (Moore et al., 2000b).

Emerging data suggest possible medication effects on mI and mI/Cr in bipolar patients. In view of its ability to inhibit inositol monophosphatase and thus deplete inositol, lithium is of particular interest. In depressed adult bipolar-I patients, lithium monotherapy was found to result in about a 30 percent decrease in prefrontal (but not temporal, parietal, or occipital) mI in patients who were generally still depressed at day 5–7; this decrease persisted until weeks 3–4, at which time patients were generally improved (Moore et al., 1999). The authors proposed that the temporal dissociation between mI decreases and clinical improvement suggests that short-term mI depletion per se is not related to lithium's antidepressant effects. In addition, in children and adolescents during manic or mixed episodes, anterior cingulate mI/Cr was found to decrease with acute (1-week trial) adjunctive lithium therapy in responders (but not in nonresponders), but no correlation was found between cerebral mI/Cr and serum lithium concentrations (Davanzo et al., 2001). Thus short-term mI depletion may be related to lithium's antimanic (rather than antidepressant) effects. In contrast, in adult healthy volunteers, lithium administration for 4 weeks failed to alter dorsolateral prefrontal mI (Brambilla et al., 2004). Also, in adult healthy volunteers, acute (1-week trial) lithium monotherapy was found not to alter temporal mI/Cr (or, as described below, phosphomonoesters, which have a limited inositol phosphate component) (Silverstone et al., 1996, 1999). Moreover, in a more sensitive paradigm in which lithium amplified amphetamine-induced phosphomonoester increases, a similar effect was not detected for mI/Cr (Silverstone et al., 1999). The authors suggested that bipolar patients (but not healthy volunteers) having altered phosphoinositol cycle function that is normalized by lithium may explain the differential effects of lithium on mI/Cr in bipolar patients and healthy volunteers (Silverstone et al., 1999). In contrast, Friedman and colleagues (2004), studying primarily depressed adult bipolar-I and -II patients, found that lithium for a mean of 3.6 months, but not valproate for a mean of 1.4 months, increased gray but not white matter mI.

Compared with healthy controls, euthymic bipolar patients taking chronic lithium showed increased basal ganglia (Sharma et al., 1992), but similar temporal (Silverstone et al., 2002) and occipital (Sharma et al., 1992) mI/Cr and parietal mI (Brühn et al., 1993). No relationship was found between serum lithium concentrations and basal ganglia or occipital mI/Cr (Sharma et al., 1992). Also, bipolar patients taking chronic lithium or valproate compared with healthy controls showed similar anterior cingulate mI/Cr (Moore et al., 2000a). Bipolar patients taking chronic lithium compared with those taking chronic valproate were found to have similar temporal (Silverstone et al., 2002) and anterior cingulate (Moore et al., 2000a) mI/Cr.

If lithium decreases mI or mI/Cr, the presence or absence of chronic lithium could contribute to the variability in mI and mI/Cr findings in bipolar patients compared with healthy controls. In studies conducted to date, the percentage of patients taking lithium was nonsignificantly lower in studies detecting increases in mI and mI/Cr in bipolar patients compared with healthy controls (17/73, 23 percent)[188] than in studies finding no difference (34/100, 34 percent).[189] This nonsignificant difference is consistent with the notion that mI and mI/Cr decreases caused by chronic lithium could be a confounding factor in detecting putative baseline (unmedicated) increases in mI and mI/Cr in patients with bipolar disorder.

There are few data on the potential effects of other medications on mI and mI/Cr. Euthymic bipolar patients taking chronic valproate compared with healthy controls were found to have similar temporal mI and mI/Cr and frontal mI (Silverstone et al., 2002). Depressed bipolar patients taking and not taking antidepressants showed similar anterior cingulate mI/Cr (Moore et al., 2000b) that was also similar to that of healthy controls. Depressed MDD patients taking antidepressants (but not those taking antidepressants) compared with healthy controls, however, displayed decreased frontal mI (Frey et al., 1998).

The MRS *creatine* (Cr or Cr + PCr) peak consists of signals from Cr and PCr. Cr is converted to PCr, which appears to function as an intracellular energy buffer. There are limited data regarding Cr changes in patients with mood disorders. Thus in bipolar patients compared with healthy controls, Cr was found to be increased in one study (Deicken et al., 2001), to be decreased in one study (Deicken et al., 2003a), to tend to be decreased in one study (Sassi

et al., 2005), and to be similar in eight studies.[190] MDD patients and healthy controls have consistently shown similar Cr,[191] with the exception of one report of increased prefrontal Cr in MDD patients (Gruber et al., 2003). The latter finding is noteworthy in that it appeared to drive decreased NAA/Cr, Cho/Cr, and mI/Cr in MDD patients, as absolute NAA, Cho, and mI in patients and healthy controls did not differ (Gruber et al., 2003).

Cr findings in bipolar patients may vary on a regional basis. One group found that bipolar patients compared with healthy controls had decreased hippocampal (Deicken et al., 2003a) and increased thalamic (Deicken et al., 2001) Cr. Another group found that dorsolateral prefrontal Cr tended to be decreased in bipolar disorder (Sassi et al., 2005). Other studies, however, found that bipolar patients and healthy controls had similar Cr in dorsolateral prefrontal (Cecil et al., 2002; Michael et al., 2003; Brambilla et al., 2005), anterior cingulate (Davanzo et al., 2003), medial prefrontal (Hamakawa et al., 1999; Cecil et al., 2002), and basal ganglia (Hamakawa et al., 1998). Dager and colleagues (2004) found that bipolar patients had gray and white matter and regional Cr that was similar to that of controls. MDD patients and healthy controls have consistently shown similar Cr in dorsolateral prefrontal (Farchione et al., 2002), anterior cingulate (Auer et al., 2000; Pfleiderer et al., 2003), hippocampal (Ende et al., 2000a), basal ganglia (Hamakawa et al., 1998; Rosenberg et al., 2000), parietal (Auer et al., 2000), and occipital (Rosenberg et al., 2000).

Cr has shown variable relationships with age. Studies detected no overall age effect (in euthymic and depressed bipolar patients and healthy controls) on medial prefrontal Cr (Hamakawa et al., 1999), no overall age effect (in euthymic bipolar patients) on dorsolateral prefrontal Cr (Sassi et al., 2005), and no overall age effect (in euthymic and depressed bipolar and MDD patients and healthy controls) on basal ganglia Cr (Hamakawa et al., 1998).

Gender effects on Cr have not been extensively reported. Healthy women compared with men were found to have similar Cr in frontal, parietal, occipital, insular (Pouwels and Frahm, 1998), basal ganglia (Charles et al., 1994b), and hippocampal (Ende et al., 2000a). One study (in euthymic and depressed bipolar patients and healthy controls) detected an overall gender effect on right (but not left) medial prefrontal Cr, but the direction of the effect was not specified (Hamakawa et al., 1999). However, another study by the same group (in euthymic and depressed bipolar and MDD patients and healthy controls) found no overall gender effect on left basal ganglia Cr (Hamakawa et al., 1998).

There are limited data on the effect of oral Cr administration on cerebral Cr. In healthy volunteers, Cr 20 g/day for 4 weeks was found to yield increased gray matter, cerebellum, white matter, thalamus, and overall Cr (as well as decreased cerebellum and thalamus NAA and decreased thalamus Cho). Reversal of these changes was detected on repeat scans at least 3 months after Cr had been discontinued (Dechent et al., 1999b). In healthy volunteers, Cr 8 g/day for 5 days was found to result in attenuation of mathematical calculation task–induced mental fatigue and cerebral oxygenated hemoglobin increases (assessed with near infrared spectroscopy, consistent with increased cerebral oxygen utilization) (Watanabe et al., 2002).

Bipolar-II, bipolar-I, and MDD patients showed similar basal ganglia Cr (Hamakawa et al., 1998). Bipolar-II and bipolar-I patients were found to have similar medial prefrontal Cr (Hamakawa et al., 1999).

Cr did not appear to vary with illness duration in dorsolateral prefrontal (Brambilla et al., 2005; Sassi et al., 2005), medial prefrontal (Hamakawa et al., 1999), or basal ganglia (Hamakawa et al., 1998; Ohara et al., 1998) regions in bipolar patients, or in basal ganglia in MDD patients (Hamakawa et al., 1998).

Cr does not appear to have consistent relationships with mood state. Hamakawa and colleagues (1999) found that depressed compared with euthymic bipolar patients had lower medial prefrontal Cr (Hamakawa et al., 1999). In another study by the same group, however, basal ganglia Cr was found to be similar for both bipolar and MDD patients during depression and euthymia (Hamakawa et al., 1998). No relationship was detected between HAM-D scores and basal ganglia Cr in bipolar and MDD patients (Hamakawa et al., 1998), or anterior cingulate or parietal Cr in MDD patients (Auer et al., 2000). In healthy volunteers, no correlation was found between scores on the PANAS Positive Affect subscale and left frontal Cr (Jung et al., 2002).

There are few data regarding treatment effects on Cr. In depressed bipolar-I patients, lithium monotherapy was found to have antidepressant effects by week 3–4, but not to alter prefrontal, temporal, parietal, or occipital Cr at day 5–7 or week 3–4 (Moore et al., 1999). In primarily depressed adult bipolar-I and -II patients, lithium for a mean of 3.6 months and valproate for a mean of 1.4 months failed to alter gray or white matter or regional Cr (Friedman et al., 2004). Also, lithium, valproate, antidepressant, and benzodiazepine therapy was not found to be related to medial prefrontal Cr in bipolar patients (Hamakawa et al., 1999). Bipolar patients taking compared with those not taking antipsychotics showed increased basal ganglia (Hamakawa et al., 1998) but not medial prefrontal (Hamakawa et al., 1999) Cr. MDD patients taking compared with those not taking benzodiazepines displayed increased basal ganglia Cr (Hamakawa et al., 1998). In MDD

patients, ECT was found to modestly increase hippocampal Cr (Ende et al., 2000b), but not to alter anterior cingulate (Pfleiderer et al., 2003) or parietal (Felber et al., 1993) Cr.

Investigators commonly assume that regional Cr is stable enough within individuals and across diagnoses to be used as an internal standard, and thus report other metabolites normalized to Cr.[192] Such a strategy is potentially useful because it increases statistical power by decreasing variability, but it runs the risk of yielding spurious results if Cr varies with time, environmental factors, or diagnosis. As noted above, in healthy volunteers, for example, chronic (4-week) administration of Cr monohydrate 20 g/day was found to increase paramedian parietal gray matter, parieto-occipital white matter, central cerebellum, and thalamus Cr concentrations (Dechent et al., 1999b). In this study, average (across four regions) Cr (but not NAA, Cho, or mI) increased by 8.7 percent, varying between 4.7 percent and 14.6 percent across regions. NAA (but not NAA/Cho and NAA/mI ratios) showed a decrease in cerebellum and thalamus, and Cho (but not Cho/mI ratios) a decrease in thalamus. Hence the confounding influence of referencing metabolites to Cr could be circumvented to some degree by also inspecting results referenced to other metabolites (Mervaala et al., 2000; Steingard et al., 2000; Winsberg et al., 2000).

Some investigators prefer to report metabolite concentrations in absolute units[193]; to report either absolute or normalized concentrations, depending on the study (Kato et al., 1996a; Hamakawa et al., 1998, 1999); or to report both absolute and normalized concentrations.[194] In one such study, it appeared that increased Cr in MDD patients compared with controls drove a finding of decreased NAA/Cr, Cho/Cr, and mI/Cr in MDD, as absolute NAA, Cho, and mI in patients and healthy controls did not differ (Gruber et al., 2003).

Recent advances have allowed MRS assessment of brain GABA and glutamate, which are the main cerebral inhibitory and excitatory amino acid neurotransmitters, respectively. The ability to measure these substances in the brain is of considerable interest because plasma GABA appears to be decreased in bipolar disorder, whereas higher (nearer to normal) levels may predict antimanic (Petty et al., 1996) and possibly even antidepressant (Ketter et al., 2000) responses to the GABAergic agent valproate. Moreover, several new anticonvulsants with GABAergic and/or antiglutamatergic mechanisms appear to have potential roles in the treatment of various symptoms of bipolar disorder (Ketter and Wang, 2003; Ketter et al., 2003)

Emerging data suggest differential cerebral *gamma-aminobutyric acid* changes in depressed MDD and depressed bipolar patients. Thus depressed MDD patients compared with healthy controls were found to have

52 percent lower occipital GABA, but severity of depression (as measured by the HAM-D) showed no correlation with cerebral GABA (Sanacora et al., 1999). Preliminary data from an extension of this work indicate that depressed MDD patients compared with healthy controls and depressed bipolar patients had occipital GABA decreases of 27 percent and 23 percent, respectively, with depressed bipolar patients compared with healthy controls having only a nonsignificant (5 percent) decrease in occipital GABA (Mason et al., 2000). In contrast, euthymic bipolar patients taking GABAergic agents (valproate ± gabapentin) may have occipital and medial prefrontal GABA levels about 50 percent higher than those of healthy controls (Wang et al., 2002).

Gender effects on GABA and GABA/Cr have not been extensively reported. Healthy women and men showed similar orbitofrontal, cingulate, insula, and thalamus GABA/Cr (Grachev and Apkarian, 2000, 2001). Women compared with men, however, showed decreased dorsolateral prefrontal GABA/Cr in young adulthood (ages 19–31) (Grachev and Apkarian, 2000), but not over a more extensive age range (ages 19–52) (Grachev and Apkarian, 2001). In another study involving both depressed MDD patients and healthy controls, women compared with men were found to have increased occipital GABA (Sanacora et al., 1999).

GABA appears to vary across the menstrual cycle. Thus, occipital GABA from follicular to luteal phase was found to decrease by 32 percent in healthy controls, but to increase by 63 percent in women with PMDD (Epperson et al., 2002). Also, PMDD patients compared with healthy controls showed lower follicular phase GABA (Epperson et al., 2002). Occipital GABA was found to be correlated with plasma estradiol and progesterone concentrations negatively in healthy women and positively in those with PMDD (Epperson et al., 2002). Occipital GABA also showed a correlation with plasma allopregnanolone concentrations negatively in healthy women, but not in those with PMDD (Epperson et al., 2002).

In depressed MDD patients, treatment with fluoxetine or citalopram ± yohimbine was found to yield clinical improvement and a 34 percent increase in occipital GABA (Sanacora et al., 2002). Changes in occipital GABA were not correlated with improvement in depression, however. Although no correlation was detected between baseline occipital GABA and clinical improvement, subjects with the lowest and highest baseline occipital GABA showed robust increases or no change in occipital GABA, respectively. In depressed patients, treatment with ECT was found to yield clinical improvement and a 78 percent increase in occipital GABA (Sanacora et al., 2003). No correlation was found, however, between changes in occipital GABA and antidepressant or adverse (memory impairment) effects.

Thus depressed MDD patients may have low baseline cerebral GABA that normalizes with effective SSRI or ECT treatment, while depressed bipolar patients may have near-normal baseline cerebral GABA that rises to supranormal levels with effective treatment with GABAergic agents. It remains to be established whether depressed bipolar patients who obtain antidepressant responses with valproate can be differentiated from those who do not obtain such responses with respect to baseline cerebral levels of the inhibitory neurotransmitter GABA. If so, this or other applications of MRS technology may ultimately have utility in addressing questions about heterogeneity related to diagnosis (such as bipolar disorder versus MDD) and in predicting antidepressant responses to different treatments (such as valproate or SSRIs).

Interpretation of the significance of MRS-assessed cerebral *glutamate* compared with GABA assessments is more complex, as glutamate exists in both metabolic and neurotransmitter pools. In addition, the glutamine and glutamate peaks are overlapping, so that some studies report glutamine/glutamate (Glx) concentrations.

Glx and Glx/Cr in bipolar patients compared with healthy controls have been found to be increased in four studies[195] and similar in one (Davanzo et al., 2001). In MDD patients, they have been found to be decreased in two studies (Auer et al., 2000; Pfleiderer et al., 2003) and increased in one (Rosenberg et al., 2000).

Glx and Glx/Cr findings in patients with mood disorders may vary on a regional basis. Thus in bipolar patients compared with healthy controls, Glx or Glx/Cr was found to be increased in prefrontal (Castillo et al., 2000; Cecil et al., 2002), dorsolateral prefrontal (Michael et al., 2003), and basal ganglia (Castillo et al., 2000) regions, but similar in anterior cingulate (Davanzo et al., 2001) and medial prefrontal (Cecil et al., 2002) regions. One study found that Glx was increased in left insula and tended to be increased in left cingulate (but not in other regions) in bipolar patients compared with controls (Dager et al., 2004). In the latter study, gray (but not white) matter Glx and lactate were increased in bipolar patients compared with controls, consistent with a shift in energy redox state from oxidative phosphorylation toward glycolysis, perhaps reflecting mitochondrial alterations. This study also found that gray and white matter Glx was increased in bipolar-I but not bipolar-II patients. In MDD patients compared with healthy controls, Glx or Glx/Cr was noted to be increased in caudate (Rosenberg et al., 2000), decreased in anterior cingulate (Auer et al., 2000; Pfleiderer et al., 2003), and similar in parietal (Auer et al., 2000) and occipital (Rosenberg et al., 2000) regions.

There are limited data relating Glx or Glx/Cr to clinical parameters. In depressed MDD patients, no relationship was detected between age and anterior cingulate Glx (Pfleiderer et al., 2003). Degree of depression (as measured by the HAM-D) showed no relationship to anterior cingulate or parietal Glx (Auer et al., 2000).

There are also few data relating Glx or Glx/Cr to clinical interventions. In bipolar patients, anterior cingulate Glx/Cr showed no change with acute (1-week) lithium administration and no relationship to plasma lithium concentrations (Davanzo et al., 2001). In primarily depressed adult bipolar-I and -II patients, however, longer-duration lithium (for a mean of 3.6 months) but not valproate (for a mean of 1.4 months) decreased gray but not white matter Glx, suggesting that lithium may attenuate gray matter increases observed by the same investigators in primarily depressed bipolar patients at baseline (Friedman et al., 2004). However, Cecil and colleagues (2002) found an inverse correlation between duration of valproate therapy and prefrontal Glx. In depressed MDD patients, ECT was found to increase anterior cingulate Glx in responders, but not in nonresponders (Pfleiderer et al., 2003).

Euthymic bipolar patients compared with healthy controls showed increased parietal glutamate/Cr (Glu/Cr) (Brühn et al., 1993). On the other hand, depressed MDD patients compared with healthy controls had similar parietal but decreased anterior cingulate Glu (Auer et al., 2000). In the latter study, no relationship was noted between regional Glu and degree of depression (as measured by the HAM-D).

In summary, ^{1}H-MRS studies suggest that patients with mood disorders compared with healthy controls may have metabolite changes in elements of anterior cortical/anterior paralimbic basal ganglia–thalamocortical circuits more than in parietal and occipital regions. Findings may differ to varying degrees with the metabolite considered, region, age, gender, phase of menstrual cycle, diagnosis, illness duration, mood state, and treatment.

Thus about half of the studies of bipolar (but not MDD) patients compared with healthy controls detected NAA or NAA/Cr decreases more than increases, in dorsolateral prefrontal and temporal more than other regions. Lithium may increase NAA or NAA/Cr, confounding efforts to detect putative baseline (unmedicated) NAA and NAA/Cr decreases in bipolar patients.

In about one-fourth of bipolar disorder and one-half of MDD studies, Cho or Cho/Cr tended to be increased compared with that in healthy controls, most often in basal ganglia. In a small number of studies, mI or mI/Cr tended to be increased, compared with that in healthy controls, in about one-half of bipolar and decreased in about one-half of MDD studies. Lithium may decrease mI and mI/Cr in bipolar patients but not in healthy controls, confounding

efforts to detect putative baseline (unmedicated) mI and mI/Cr increases in bipolar patients.

Most of the few Cr studies conducted to date have failed to detect differences between patients with mood disorders and healthy controls, and lithium may not alter Cr in bipolar patients. These negative findings address in a limited fashion concerns that the common method of referencing metabolites to Cr may confound ^{1}H-MRS studies comparing mood disorder patients with healthy controls.

Baseline (unmedicated) occipital GABA may be decreased in depressed MDD but not depressed bipolar patients compared with healthy controls, and increased with SSRIs, ECT, or GABAergic anticonvulsants. Emerging methodology may permit GABA and glutamate assessments in regions with greater relevance to mood disorders, such as anterior cingulate/medial prefrontal cortex.

Phosphorous (^{31}P) Magnetic Resonance Spectroscopy

Phosphorous-31 magnetic resonance spectroscopy (^{31}P-MRS) permits determination of cerebral phospholipids, including phosphomonoesters (PMEs), phosphodiesters (PDEs), inorganic phosphate, high-energy phosphates, and related compounds such as PCr, as well as intracellular pH. PMEs consist of phosphoethanolamine, phosphocholine, phosphoserine, and sugar phosphates such as inositol-1-monophosphate, while PDEs consist of glycerophosphocholine, glycerophosphoethanolamine, and mobile phospholipids. PMEs and PDEs include cell membrane precursors and degradation products, respectively, and are of interest in view of relationships to intracellular signaling and membrane phospholipid changes proposed in bipolar disorder. PMEs may to a limited extent reflect inositol-1-monophosphate concentrations, which account for about 10 percent of the PME signal (Gyulai et al., 1984), but use of PMEs to indicate inositol monophosphate has been criticized (Agam and Shimon, 2000).

Decreased prefrontal phosphomonoesters have been observed in euthymic bipolar patients in clinical research. Studies have most consistently detected PME changes in bipolar-I patients. Thus, euthymic bipolar-I patients appear to have decreased prefrontal PMEs consistent with abnormal membrane phospholipid metabolism, which in turn may reflect changes in signal transduction putatively related to the pathophysiology of bipolar disorder (Manji and Lenox, 2000). Kato and colleagues reported on a series of ^{31}P-MRS studies in primarily medicated bipolar patients. In these studies, prefrontal PMEs in euthymic bipolar-I patients compared with healthy controls were found to be significantly decreased in four studies (Kato et al., 1992b, 1993a, 1994a,b) and nonsignificantly decreased in a fifth study (Kato et al., 1991). No correlation was detected between

PMEs and brain lithium concentrations (Kato et al., 1993a). In addition, Deicken and colleagues found that euthymic medication-free bipolar-I patients had decreased PMEs compared with controls in bilateral prefrontal (Deicken et al., 1995a) and temporal (Deicken et al., 1995b) regions. Prefrontal PMEs in euthymic bipolar-I patients were also found to be significantly decreased compared with depressed bipolar-I patients (Kato et al., 1992a, 1994b), manic bipolar-I patients (Kato et al., 1991, 1993b), and euthymic MDD patients (Kato et al., 1992a). Prefrontal PMEs in manic bipolar-I patients compared with healthy controls were found to be significantly increased in one study (Kato et al., 1991) and nonsignificantly increased in another (Kato et al., 1993a). Depressed bipolar-I and depressed MDD patients showed similar prefrontal PMEs (Kato et al., 1992b).

Studies in bipolar-II patients or mixed samples of bipolar-I and -II patients have detected PME changes less consistently. Thus, euthymic bipolar-II patients were found to have prefrontal PMEs that did not differ significantly from those of healthy controls (Kato et al., 1994b,c) or across mood states (Kato et al., 1994c). Depressed and hypomanic bipolar-II patients compared with healthy controls, by contrast, showed increased prefrontal PMEs (Kato et al., 1994c). In studies of combined groups of primarily medicated bipolar-I and -II patients, prefrontal PMEs in euthymic bipolar patients compared with healthy controls were found to be nonsignificantly decreased in one study (Kato et al., 1994b) and nonsignificantly increased in another (Kato et al., 1995a), compared with depressed bipolar patients were found to be nonsignificantly decreased (Kato et al., 1995a), and compared with manic bipolar patients were found to be nonsignificantly increased (Kato et al., 1995b). Medication-free euthymic bipolar patients compared with healthy controls showed nonsignificantly increased PMEs (Kato et al., 1998). Similar occipital PMEs were detected in euthymic bipolar patients and healthy controls (Murashita et al., 2000). One study found that prefrontal PMEs in depressed bipolar patients were (significantly on the left and nonsignificantly on the right) increased compared with those of healthy controls and nonsignificantly increased compared with those of manic bipolar patients, and in manic patients were not significantly different from those of healthy controls (Kato et al., 1995a). Also, euthymic bipolar patients taking chronic lithium or valproate showed similar left temporal PMEs compared with healthy controls (Silverstone et al., 2002).

Prefrontal PMEs were found to decrease with age in euthymic bipolar patients but not in healthy controls, consistent with an illness progression effect, but the decrease was not clearly related to onset or duration of illness, psychosis, duration of lithium therapy, or LVE (Kato et al., 1994b).

Considering studies including both bipolar-I and -II patients, Yildiz and colleagues (2001b) reported on meta-analysis of eight ^{31}P-MRS studies involving 139 bipolar patients and 189 controls[196] that confirmed the finding of decreased prefrontal PMEs in euthymic bipolar patients. Thus across six studies, a total of 100 euthymic bipolar patients compared with 130 controls showed lower prefrontal[197] or temporal (Deicken et al., 1995a) PMEs ($p = .014$). Likewise, across three studies, a total of 39 euthymic bipolar patients compared with 34 depressed bipolar patients had lower prefrontal PMEs ($p = .0005$) (Kato et al., 1992a, 1994a, 1995b). In other PME comparisons, no significant differences were detected between manic and euthymic bipolar patients (Kato et al., 1991, 1993b, 1995b),[198] between depressed bipolar patients and controls, or between manic bipolar patients and controls. Yildiz and colleagues (2001b) thus concluded that the data suggest trait-dependent PME changes in bipolar disorder, but that there have been too few studies to permit a definitive assessment of state-dependent alterations. Of interest, prefrontal PME decreases have consistently been reported in schizophrenic patients (Pettegrew et al., 1991; Kato et al., 1995b).

There have been a few studies of PMEs in MDD patients, with varying results. Depressed MDD patients were found to have basal ganglia (Moore et al., 1997) and prefrontal (Kato et al., 1992b) PMEs similar to those of healthy controls, with the latter study also not detecting differences in euthymic MDD patients compared with depressed MDD patients or with healthy controls. In contrast, another study found that depressed MDD patients had increased prefrontal PMEs compared with those of healthy controls, but that PMEs were correlated inversely with degree of depression (Volz et al., 1998).

Because lithium inhibits inositol monophosphatase (Hallcher and Sherman, 1980), investigators have assessed its effects on PMEs, which have a limited (about 10 percent) inositol phosphate component (Gyulai et al., 1984). If lithium proved to increase PMEs, this could be related to its inhibiting the conversion of inositol-1-phosphate to inositol. Technical limitations and potential differences between the effects of lithium in patients and healthy controls may have contributed to the varied findings on this issue. In schizophrenic patients, acute lithium was found to have no overall effect on PMEs, but to tend to result in complementary biphasic longitudinal changes in the first 2 weeks of therapy in both responders and nonresponders (Keshavan et al., 1992). In six manic bipolar patients, however, lithium failed to alter prefrontal PMEs significantly (Kato et al., 1993a). In healthy volunteers, lithium administration for 1 week failed to alter left temporal PMEs significantly (Silverstone et al., 1996, 1999), but in a more sensitive paradigm, the drug was found to amplify amphetamine-induced PME increases (Silverstone et al., 1999). Also in healthy volunteers, a study with enhanced sensitivity derived from using proton decoupling and a large (620 cc) voxel centered on the superior corpus callosum detected increased PMEs after 7 and 14 days of lithium (Yildiz et al., 2001a). Euthymic bipolar patients taking chronic lithium compared with those taking chronic valproate showed similar temporal PMEs (Silverstone et al., 2002).

Findings for *phosphodiesters* (PDEs), in contrast to those for PMEs, are variable in bipolar patients. Thus euthymic bipolar-I patients compared with healthy controls showed similar prefrontal (Kato et al., 1992b, 1993b) and bilateral temporal PDEs (Deicken et al., 1995b) but increased bilateral prefrontal (Deicken et al., 1995a) PDEs. In a combined sample of medication-free euthymic bipolar-I and -II patients, prefrontal PDEs were found to be correlated with SCHs, but patients and healthy controls showed similar PDEs (Kato et al., 1998). One study found occipital PDEs in euthymic bipolar patients and healthy controls to be similar (Murashita et al., 2000). In a meta-analysis of four studies, Yildiz and colleagues (2001b) found that a total of 51 euthymic bipolar patients compared with 57 controls had statistically similar prefrontal (Kato et al., 1992b, 1993b; Deicken, et al., 1995b) and temporal (Deicken et al., 1995a) PDEs ($p = .597$). Other PDE comparisons across mood states and diagnoses were also negative.

Inorganic phosphate (Pi) contains PO^- and PO_4^{2-} and is seen in multiple metabolic pathways. There is little evidence of Pi changes in bipolar disorder, however. Thus medication-free euthymic bipolar-I patients and healthy controls were found to have similar bilateral prefrontal (Deicken et al., 1995a) and temporal (Deicken et al., 1995b) Pi. Also, prefrontal Pi was found to be similar to that of healthy controls in bipolar-I patients, independent of mood state (Kato et al., 1992b, 1993b), and in a combined sample of medication-free euthymic bipolar-I and -II patients (Kato et al., 1998). Likewise, similar occipital Pi was detected in euthymic bipolar patients and healthy controls (Murashita et al., 2000).

There is also little evidence of changes in *high-energy phosphates* in bipolar disorder. Thus prefrontal high-energy phosphates were found to be similar in bipolar-I patients and healthy controls, independent of mood state (Kato et al., 1992b, 1993a), and beta-adenosine triphosphate (beta-ATP) was found to be similar to that of healthy controls in medication-free euthymic bipolar-I patients in bilateral prefrontal (Deicken et al., 1995a) and temporal (Deicken et al., 1995b) regions. Also, a combined sample of medication-free euthymic bipolar-I and -II patients showed prefrontal beta-ATP similar to that of healthy controls (Kato et al., 1998). In contrast, depressed MDD patients compared with healthy controls showed decreased beta-ATP and total nucleotide triphosphates in basal ganglia (Moore et al., 1997) and bilateral prefrontal regions (Volz et al., 1998). Of interest, decreased left basal ganglia beta-ATP has also been reported in schizophrenic patients (Deicken et al., 1995a).

Phosphocreatine is considered a high-energy phosphate buffer. Early work demonstrated decreased prefrontal PCr in bipolar-II patients (independent of mood state) compared with healthy controls (Kato et al., 1994c), but failed to detect such differences in bipolar-I patients (Kato et al., 1992b, 1993b) (aside from a decrease in severe compared with mild depression [Kato et al., 1992a]) and MDD patients (independent of mood state) (Kato et al., 1992a). The investigators suggested that decreased prefrontal PCr in bipolar-II patients may be related to decreased Cr or Cr phosphokinase activity, increased intracellular magnesium, or mitochondrial dysfunction (Kato et al., 1994c). Simultaneous consideration of prefrontal PCr and PMEs appears to allow for some discrimination between euthymic bipolar-II (low PCr) and bipolar-I (low PMEs) patients (see Fig. 15–12) (Kato et al., 1994c).

Later work revealed decreased left prefrontal PCr in depressed bipolar-I patients (correlated with degree of depression) and right prefrontal PCr in manic and euthymic bipolar-I patients (Kato et al., 1995a). Euthymic medication-free bipolar-I patients and healthy controls showed similar bilateral prefrontal and temporal lobe PCr (Deicken et al., 1995a,b). A combined sample of medication-free euthymic bipolar-I and -II patients also displayed prefrontal PCr similar to that of healthy controls (Kato et al., 1998). Euthymic medicated bipolar-I patients were found to have resting and post–photic stimulation occipital PCr similar to that of healthy controls, while lithium-resistant (but not lithium-responsive) patients showed decreased PCr for 12 minutes after photic stimulation (Murashita et al., 2000). The investigators suggested that this observation is consistent with mitochondrial dysfunction in lithium-resistant bipolar-I patients.

Some *intracellular pH* differences have been detected in bipolar disorder, perhaps reflecting altered sodium–hydrogen ion transport. Thus prefrontal intracellular pH was found to be decreased in euthymic bipolar-I patients compared with depressed (Kato et al., 1992b) and manic (Kato et al., 1993b) bipolar-I patients and healthy controls (Kato et al., 1992b, 1993b). Prefrontal intracellular pH was also found to be decreased in combined samples of euthymic bipolar-I and -II patients compared with healthy controls (Kato et al., 1994b, 1998); correlated positively with duration of lithium therapy, but not with age, illness onset, or illness duration (Kato et al., 1994b); and related to SCHs (Kato et al., 1998). On the other hand, intracellular pH was observed to be similar to that of healthy controls in

Figure 15–12. Low prefrontal phosphocreatine in euthymic bipolar-II (BP-II) patients and low phosphomonoesters in euthymic bipolar-I (BP-I) patients. Prefrontal phosphocreatine levels are shown on the vertical axis, and phosphomonoester levels on the horizontal axis. Euthymic bipolar-I patients (squares) have significantly lower phosphomonoesters and nonsignificantly higher phosphocreatine compared with euthymic bipolar-II patients (circles). These relationships allow correct classification of 18/21 patients as bipolar-I (above the diagonal line) and bipolar-II (below the broken line). HC = healthy controls. [a] p <.05 versus BP-I, healthy controls; [b] p <.01 versus BP-II, healthy controls. (*Source:* Reproduced with permission from Kato et al., 1994b.)

medication-free euthymic bipolar-I patients in bilateral prefrontal (Deicken et al., 1995a) and temporal (Deicken et al., 1995b) regions, in bipolar-II patients independent of mood state in prefrontal regions (Kato et al., 1994b), and in a combined sample of euthymic bipolar-I and -II patients in the occipital lobe (Murashita et al., 2000).

In summary, ^{31}P-MRS studies suggest that euthymic bipolar-I patients have decreased prefrontal PMEs consistent with abnormal membrane phospholipid metabolism, which in turn could reflect altered signal transduction. Prefrontal PMEs in euthymic bipolar-I patients are also significantly decreased compared with those in depressed bipolar-I, manic bipolar-I, and euthymic MDD patients. Studies in bipolar-II patients and in mixed samples of bipolar-I and -II patients have detected PME changes less consistently. Nevertheless, meta-analyses of studies including both bipolar-I and -II patients confirm decreased prefrontal PMEs in euthymic bipolar patients compared with healthy controls and depressed bipolar patients. In contrast, data on PMEs in MDD patients are sparse and variable. Some data suggest that lithium may increase PMEs, but other findings fail to support this hypothesis, perhaps because of methodological and sampling differences. PDEs, in contrast to PMEs, do not appear to be systematically altered in bipolar patients. There is some evidence of pH

and PCr differences, but little evidence of Pi or high-energy phosphate changes in bipolar patients.

Lithium Magnetic Resonance Spectroscopy

Brain lithium concentrations determined by lithium-MRS are about half those seen in serum and tend to be correlated with serum lithium concentrations.[199] Brain/serum lithium ratios may be lower in children and adolescents than adults, suggesting that younger patients may require higher serum lithium levels than adults to achieve similar brain lithium concentrations (Moore et al., 2002). Brain (prefrontal) lithium may correlate better with serum than with red blood cell lithium levels (Kato et al., 1993). When serum lithium concentrations are restricted to therapeutic range, however, brain lithium levels can vary markedly and may be correlated only modestly with serum lithium (Sachs et al., 1995). Patients taking alternate-day compared with daily lithium therapy with similar mean 12-hour trough serum lithium levels were found to have similar brain lithium concentrations (Jensen et al., 1996). Patients taking lithium in a single bedtime dose compared with twice daily also showed similar brain lithium concentrations, but increased brain/serum lithium ratios (Soares et al., 2001). MDD and schizophrenic patients taking short-term (4–8 weeks) and long-term (over 6 months) lithium therapy

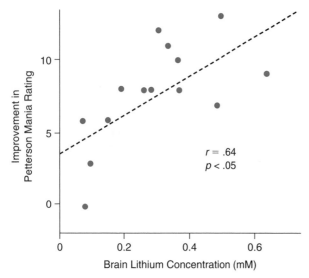

Figure 15–13. Correlation between cerebral lithium concentrations and antimanic responses. Change in Petterson Mania Rating Scale (PMRS) scores are shown on the vertical axis and brain lithium levels on the horizontal axis. The correlation coefficient is .64 ($p < .05$). The regression is shown as a dotted line. (*Source:* Reproduced with permission from Kato et al., 1994c.)

may have similar whole-brain/serum lithium ratios, but whole-brain lithium may be better correlated with serum lithium in long-term than in short-term treatment (Riedl et al., 1997). Relationships between mood and brain lithium concentrations remain to be established, as brain lithium has been reported to be higher when patients are both manic (Kato et al., 1992) and euthymic (Sachs et al., 1995).

Brain lithium concentrations may need to be at least .2 millimoles per liter (mmol/l) for adequate therapeutic effects (Gyulai et al., 1991; Kato et al., 1994a). Hand tremor may be related more closely to brain than to serum lithium levels (Kato et al., 1996b), as subtherapeutic prefrontal lithium levels (less than .2 mmol/l) were observed in 25 percent of patients without and only 7 percent of patients with hand tremor. Thus in patients with inadequate responses and no hand tremor, an increase in lithium dosage should be considered because of the possibility of subtherapeutic cerebral lithium levels, even if serum lithium levels appear to be within the therapeutic range.

Antimanic responses may correlate with brain (prefrontal) lithium level (Fig. 15–13) and brain/serum lithium ratio, but not serum lithium level or lithium dose/weight (Kato et al., 1994a). This observation raises the possibility that some patients may be resistant to lithium because of insufficient central nervous system lithium entry or retention, despite having therapeutic serum lithium levels.

In summary, lithium-MRS studies indicate that cerebral lithium concentrations are about half those seen in serum, tend to be correlated with serum lithium concentrations, and may be related to lithium's therapeutic and adverse effects. In

contrast, there are relatively few data regarding relationships between mood state and cerebral lithium concentrations.

CONCLUSIONS

Structural Neuroimaging

To date, structural neuroimaging cannot be used to diagnose bipolar disorder or MDD. For example, despite there being mean differences in structural parameters between groups of mood disorder patients and groups of healthy controls, the ranges overlap so that the groups are not discretely separated. Moreover, the abnormalities seen in groups of mood disorder patients compared with groups of healthy controls are nonspecific, as they can occur in other psychiatric disorders, such as schizophrenia. For example, compared with healthy controls, both schizophrenic and bipolar patients had frontal, temporoparietal, and corpus callosum white matter volume decreases, while volumes in these areas were statistically similar in the two patient groups (McDonald et al., 2005). However, the deficits in schizophrenia may be more severe and widespread than those seen in bipolar disorder. Thus, schizophrenic patients had anterior paralimbic thalamorcortical (amygdala, hippocampus, insula, caudate, thalamus, lateral prefrontal and temporal cortex) gray matter volume decreases compared with both bipolar patients and healthy controls, whereas the latter two groups had statistically similar volumes in these regions (McDonald et al., 2005). This pattern of findings was also evident in first-degree relatives of patients with schizophrenia and bipolar disorder (McDonald et al., 2004). In a similar fashion, another group found that, compared with healthy controls, anterior thalamic gray matter density was decreased in both schizophrenic and bipolar patients and their relatives, with schizophrenia but not bipolar disorder also being associated with decreased middle prefrontal gyrus and dorsomedial thalamus gray matter density (McIntosh et al., 2004). Moreover, this group found that, compared with healthy controls, anterior limb of internal capsule white matter density was decreased in both schizophrenic and bipolar patients, with schizophrenia but not bipolar disorder also being associated with decreased corpus callosum and frontal subgyral white matter density (McIntosh et al., 2005).

Structural neuroimaging can be used to diagnose general medical conditions associated with secondary mood disorders. Primary (bipolar disorder and MDD) and secondary (due to substance abuse or general medical conditions) mood disorders may represent extremes of a continuum, bracketing intermediate mood syndromes with varying ratios of primary to secondary components. For example, it has been suggested that SCHs may contribute to the development of depression in at least some patients (Alexopoulos et al., 1997; Krishnan et al., 1997; Steffens and Krishnan, 1998). Thus, these structural brain changes suggestive of mild cerebrovascular insufficiency not severe enough to merit a diagnosis of depression secondary to stroke may contribute to mood symptoms, treatment resistance, and poor prognosis in late-life or late-onset depression.

Further along the continuum, frank vascular lesions in basal ganglia–thalamocortical circuits may lead to secondary mood disorders. Thus, vascular subtypes of mania and depression have been proposed, with criteria including clinical and/or neuroimaging evidence of cerebrovascular disease (history of stroke, transient ischemic attacks, focal neurological signs, SCHs) or neuropsychological impairment (decreased cognitive processing quality or speed) (Steffens and Krishnan, 1998). Proposed supporting features include onset of or change in affective symptoms after age 50, marked anhedonia, psychomotor retardation, marked impairment in basic activities of daily living, and lack of family history of mood disorders.

Methodological advances—including new methods of image acquisition, such as DTI, and new image processing techniques, such as the ability to segment images into gray and white matter—promise to advance structural neuroimaging studies. Limited statistical power related to clinical heterogeneity and small sample sizes in individual studies needs to be addressed, however. This problem is particularly salient with respect to understanding the clinical correlates of structural imaging abnormalities in mood disorder patients. Large collaborative studies and/or standardized designs that facilitate meta-analyses may help surmount this problem.

Functional Neuroimaging

Taken together, the functional neuroimaging literature reviewed above suggests that elements of anterior cortical/anterior paralimbic basal ganglia–thalamocortical circuits may contribute importantly to affective processing in health, and can have altered function in bipolar and MDD patients (see Box 15–2).

The cerebral activity studies reviewed here have important limitations, including small sample sizes, varying methodology, and reliance on measures of patterns of activity across cerebral structures rather than assessment of specific neurochemical differences. Their findings need to be combined with emerging data from studies of specific cerebral neurochemistry using specific neurochemical radiotracers (reviewed in Chapter 14) and MRS (described above) to yield more comprehensive understanding of the nature of the neurobiology of mood disorders.

Methodological advances in MRS studies are beginning to allow in vivo assessment of specific cerebral

---

BOX 15–2. **Functional Neuroimaging Findings in Depressed Bipolar and Major Depressive Disorder Patients Compared with Healthy Controls**

- Decreased global cerebral activity (in older, more depressed patients)
- Decreased dorsolateral prefrontal activity
- Decreased temporal cortical activity
- Decreased basal ganglia activity (in MDD)
- Variable anterior cingulate and medial prefrontal activity
- Increased amygdala activity
- Decreased prefrontal phosphomonoesters (in *euthymic* bipolar patients versus healthy controls and depressed bipolar patients)[a]

[a]Confirmed with meta-analysis.

---

neurochemistry that is less invasive (no ionizing radiation) and more generally available (no need for an on-site cyclotron, radiochemistry team, or PET scanner) than PET techniques using specific neurochemical radiotracers. MRS studies are limited, however, by relatively poor spatial resolution, and by the ability to assess only a small and in some cases inadequately characterized group of metabolites.

Studies of specific cerebral neurochemistry share important limitations with those of cerebral activity, such as small sample sizes and varying methodology. Technical advances, including new methods of image acquisition (such as MRS sequences to detect GABA and glutamate with enhanced spatial and temporal resolution), promise to advance functional neuroimaging studies. As with structural neuroimaging studies, however, limited statistical power related to clinical heterogeneity and small sample sizes in individual studies remains problematic. Also as with structural neuroimaging studies, large collaborative studies and/or standardized designs that facilitate meta-analyses may help address these difficulties.

Future Directions

Despite providing substantial contributions to our understanding of which cerebral structures mediate affective processing in health and mood disorders, neuroimaging has not yet realized its potential to be a clinically relevant tool in the diagnosis and treatment of major mood disorders. Technological innovations to enhance spatial and temporal resolution, decrease or eliminate exposure to ionizing radiation, increase neurochemical specificity, increase availability, and decrease expense are needed if research is to further advance our knowledge of the neuroanatomical and neurochemical substrates of these disorders. As these technological innovations unfold, it becomes even more important that we put considerably more effort into improved methods for diagnosis and clinical evaluation, including an agreed-upon standard for distinguishing the more recurrent forms of MDD that fall within Kraepelin's concept of manic-depressive illness. More careful differentiation between state and trait is also needed, as are consensus protocols for assessing the multiple sources of variance in these measures. Given the great promise and expense of these technologies, we can afford to do no less. While it remains to be seen whether such advances will ultimately yield clinical applications to facilitate diagnosis and target treatments more effectively in patients with mood disorders, it is clear that this potential will not be realized unless we invest more effort in standardizing the clinical characterization of the patients we study.

NOTES

1. Mindham, 1970; Caine and Shoulson, 1983; Folstein and Folstein, 1983; Horn, 1974.
2. Lisanby et al., 1993; Passe et al., 1997; Coffey et al., 1998; Parashos et al., 1998; Kumar et al., 1999.
3. Figiel et al., 1991b; Lesser et al., 1991; Fujikawa et al., 1993; Howard et al., 1993; Krishnan et al., 1993; Hickie et al., 1995; O'Brien et al., 1996; Salloway et al., 1996.
4. Figiel et al., 1991a; Lesser et al., 1991; Fujikawa et al., 1993; Howard et al., 1993; Krishnan et al., 1993; Hickie et al., 1995; O'Brien et al., 1996; Salloway et al., 1996; Dahabra et al., 1998.
5. Jacoby and Levy, 1980; Pearlson and Veroff, 1981; Hazama et al., 1982; Nasrallah et al., 1982b; Tanaka et al., 1982; Kellner et al., 1983; Scott et al., 1983; Targum et al., 1983; Luchins et al., 1984; Pearlson et al., 1984a, 1989; Shima et al., 1984; Dolan et al., 1985, 1986; Lippmann et al., 1985; Kolbeinsson et al., 1986; Schlegel and Kretzschmar, 1987; Iacono et al., 1988; Rossi et al., 1989; Abas et al., 1990; Ames, et al., 1990; Beats et al., 1991; Van den Bossche et al., 1991; Lauer et al., 1992; Raz, 1993; Wurthmann et al., 1995; Baumann et al., 1997.
6. Besson et al., 1987; Dupont et al., 1987, 1995b; Dewan et al., 1988b; Johnstone et al., 1989; Andreasen et al., 1990; Swayze et al., 1990; Figiel et al., 1991a; Lewine et al., 1991; McDonald et al., 1991; Rabins et al., 1991; Coffey et al., 1993b; Strakowski et al., 1993b, 1999; Harvey et al., 1994; Kato et al., 1994b; Botteron et al., 1995; Woods et al., 1995b; Iidaka et al., 1996; Greenwald et al., 1997; Pearlson et al., 1997; Zipursky et al., 1997; Pantel et al., 1998; Roy et al., 1998; Lim et al., 1999; Hauser et al., 2000; Brambilla et al., 2001b.
7. Pearlson and Veroff, 1981; Nasrallah et al., 1982b; Pearlson et al., 1984b; Lippmann et al., 1985; Figiel et al., 1991b; Raz, 1993; Kato et al., 1994b; Zipursky et al., 1997; Strakowski et al., 1999.
8. Kellner et al., 1983; Besson et al., 1987; Dewan et al., 1988c; Johnstone et al., 1989; Swayze et al., 1990; McDonald et al., 1991; Strakowski et al., 1993b; Harvey et al., 1994; Botteron et al., 1995; Dupont et al., 1995b; Roy et al., 1998; Lim et al., 1999.
9. Dupont et al., 1987; Iacono et al., 1988; Lewine et al., 1991; Brambilla et al., 2001a.
10. Scott et al., 1983; Targum et al., 1983; Luchins et al., 1984; Shima et al., 1984; Dolan et al., 1985; Kolbeinsson et al., 1986; Pearlson et al., 1989; Ames et al., 1990; Rabins et al., 1991; Lauer et al., 1992; Wurthmann et al., 1995; Pantel et al., 1998.
11. Jacoby and Levy, 1980; Tanaka et al., 1982; Iacono et al., 1988; Rossi et al., 1989; Abas et al., 1990; Andreasen et al., 1990; Beats et al., 1991; Lewine et al., 1991; Van den Bossche et al., 1991; Coffey et al., 1993b; Dupont et al., 1995b; Iidaka et al., 1996; Baumann et al., 1997.
12. Tanaka et al., 1982; Dolan et al., 1986; Kolbeinsson et al., 1986; Rabins et al., 1991; Wurthmann et al., 1995.
13. Jacoby and Levy, 1980; Pearlson and Veroff, 1981; Nasrallah et al., 1982a; Weinberger et al., 1982; Kellner et al., 1983; Scott et al., 1983; Targum et al., 1983; Luchins et al., 1984; Pearlson et al., 1984a, 1989; Shima et al., 1984; Dolan et al., 1985; Kolbeinsson et al., 1986; Besson et al., 1987; Schlegel and Kretzschmar, 1987; Dewan et al., 1988c; Iacono et al., 1988; Johnstone et al., 1989; Rossi et al., 1989; Abas et al., 1990; Andreasen et al., 1990; Swayze et al., 1990; Beats et al., 1991; Rabins et al., 1991; Van den Bossche et al., 1991; Lauer et al., 1992; Coffey et al., 2001; Raz, 1993; Strakowski et al., 1993b.
14. Nasrallah et al., 1982b; Tanaka et al., 1982; Weinberger et al., 1982; Dolan et al., 1986; Kolbeinsson et al., 1986; Dewan et al., 1988c; Iacono et al., 1988; Abas et al., 1990; Rabins et al., 1991; Coffey et al., 1993b.
15. Raz and Raz, 1990; Jeste et al., 1988; Elkis et al., 1995; Ketter et al., 2004.
16. Shima et al., 1984; Dolan et al., 1985; Rossi et al., 1987; Beats et al., 1991; Alexopoulos et al., 1992; Coffey et al., 1993b; Iidaka et al., 1996; Wurthmann et al., 1995.
17. Shima et al., 1984; Dolan et al., 1985; Pearlson et al., 1989; Jernigan et al., 1990; Coffey et al., 1992; Murphy et al., 1992; Pfefferbaum et al., 1994; Botteron et al., 1995.
18. Pearlson et al., 1989; Rossi et al., 1989; Baumann et al., 1997; Dahabra et al., 1998.
19. Pearlson et al., 1984a; Rossi et al., 1987, 1989; Baumann et al., 1997; Brambilla et al., 2001a.
20. Jacoby and Levy, 1980; Shima et al., 1984; Rossi et al., 1987; Alexopoulos et al., 1992; Dahabra et al., 1998; Simpson et al., 2001.
21. Pearlson et al., 1984b; Dolan et al., 1985; Dewan et al., 1988c; Rossi et al., 1989; Harvey et al., 1994; Brambilla et al., 2001b.
22. Jacoby et al., 1981; Nasrallah et al., 1984; Pearlson et al., 1984a; Shima et al., 1984; Dolan et al., 1985; Kolbeinsson et al., 1986; Roy-Byrne et al., 1988; Johnstone et al., 1989; Beats et al., 1991.
23. Nasrallah et al., 1984; Pearlson et al., 1984a; Dahabra et al., 1998; Dewan et al., 1988b; Andreasen et al., 1990.
24. Pearlson et al., 1989; Rothschild et al., 1989; Abas et al., 1990; Greenwald et al., 1997.
25. Luchins et al., 1984; Schlegel et al., 1989c; Van den Bossche et al., 1991; Brambilla et al., 2001b.
26. Targum et al., 1983; Standish-Barry et al., 1985; Schlegel and Kretzschmar, 1987; Dewan et al., 1988c; Schlegel et al., 1989b; Van den Bossche et al., 1991; Coffey et al., 1993a; Mukherjee et al., 1993.
27. Rieder et al., 1983; Nasrallah et al., 1984; Pearlson et al., 1984b; Andreasen et al., 1990; Swayze et al., 1990; Harvey et al., 1994.
28. Coffey et al., 1987, 1988a, 1991; Figiel et al., 1989b; Pande et al., 1990.

29. Pearlson et al., 1984b; Dolan et al., 1985; Johnstone et al., 1986; Swayze et al., 1990; Harvey et al., 1994; Brambilla et al., 2001a.

30. Botteron et al., 1995; Roy et al., 1998; Lim et al., 1999; Strakowski et al., 1999.

31. Schlegel and Kretzschmar, 1987; Beats et al., 1991; Rabins et al., 1991; Wurthmann et al., 1995; Iidaka et al., 1996.

32. Figiel et al., 1989b, 1991b; Dupont et al., 1990, 1995a,b; Coffey et al., 1990, 1993a; Swayze et al., 1990; Zubenko et al., 1990; Beats et al., 1991; Lesser et al., 1991, 1996; McDonald et al., 1991, 1999; Rabins et al., 1991; Brown et al., 1992; Guze and Szuba, 1992; Howard et al., 1993; Krishnan et al., 1993; Strakowski et al., 1993a; Aylward et al., 1994; Miller et al., 1994; Altshuler et al., 1995; Botteron et al., 1995; Lewine et al., 1995; Woods et al., 1995a,b; Greenwald et al., 1996; Iidaka et al., 1996; O'Brien et al., 1996; Persaud et al., 1998; Lenze et al., 1999; Krabbendam et al., 2000; Kumar et al., 2000; MacFall et al., 2001; Losfescu et al., 2002; Pillai et al., 2002; Sassi et al., 2003; T. Silverstone et al., 2003; Videbech and Ravnkilde, 2004.

33. Dupont et al., 1990, 1995a,b; Swayze et al., 1990; Figiel et al., 1991a; McDonald et al., 1991, 1999; Aylward et al., 1994; Woods et al., 1995; Pillai et al., 2002.

34. Strakowski et al., 1993; Botteron et al., 1995; Lewine et al., 1995; Woods et al., 1995; Persaud et al., 1997; Krabbendam et al., 2000; P. Silverstone et al., 2003.

35. Swayze et al., 1990; Dupont et al., 1990; Figiel et al., 1991b; McDonald et al., 1991; Brown et al., 1992; Strakowski et al., 1993b; Aylward et al., 1994; Altshuler et al., 1995.

36. Swayze et al., 1990; Figiel et al., 1991a; McDonald et al., 1991; Brown et al., 1992; Strakowski et al., 1993a; Aylward et al., 1994; Altshuler et al., 1995; Dupont et al., 1995b; Lewine et al., 1995; Woods et al., 1995.

37. Figiel et al., 1989b; Coffey et al., 1990, 1993; Zubenko et al., 1990; Beats et al., 1991; Lesser et al., 1991; Rabins et al., 1991; Brown et al., 1992; Krishnan et al., 1993; Greenwald et al., 1996; Iidaka et al., 1996; O'Brien et al., 1996; Kumar et al., 2000; MacFall et al., 2001.

38. Guze and Szuba, 1992; Howard et al., 1993; Miller et al., 1994; Dupont et al., 1995a,b; Lewine et al., 1995; Woods et al., 1995; Greenwald et al., 1998; Lenze et al., 1999; Losfescu et al., 2002; T. Silverstone et al., 2003; Videbech and Ravnkilde, 2004.

39. Zubenko et al., 1990; Lesser et al., 1991; Brown et al., 1992; Krishnan et al., 1993; Dupont et al., 1995a; Lewine et al., 1995; O'Brien et al., 1996.

40. Dupont et al., 1990, 1995b; Aylward et al., 1994; Krabbendam et al., 2000.

41. Krishnan et al., 1988, 1993; Figiel et al., 1991a; Guze and Szuba, 1992; Dupont et al., 1995a; Iidaka et al., 1996; O'Brien et al., 1996; Greenwald et al., 1998; MacFall et al., 2001.

42. Dupont et al., 1990, 1995a,b; Figiel et al., 1991b; McDonald et al., 1991, 1999; Aylward et al., 1994; Woods et al., 1995a; Pillai et al., 2002.

43. Swayze et al., 1990; Strakowski et al., 1993a; Botteron et al., 1995; Lewine et al., 1995; Woods et al., 1995b; Persaud et al., 1997; Krabbendam et al., 2000; T. Silverstone et al., 2003.

44. Figiel et al., 1989b; Coffey et al., 1990; Zubenko et al., 1990; Lesser et al., 1991, 1996; Rabins et al., 1991; Brown et al., 1992; Krishnan et al., 1993; O'Brien et al., 1996; MacFall et al., 2001; Sassi et al., 2003.

45. Coffey et al., 1993a; Howard et al., 1993; Miller et al., 1994; Dupont et al., 1995a,b; Lewine et al., 1995; Woods et al., 1995b; Iidaka et al., 1996; Greenwald et al., 1998; Lenze et al., 1999; Brambilla et al., 2003a; T. Silverstone et al., 2003.

46. Swayze et al., 1990; McDonald et al., 1991; Brown et al., 1992; Botteron et al., 1995; Persaud et al., 1997; Sassi et al., 2003; P. Silverstone et al., 2003.

47. Rabins et al., 1991; Howard et al., 1993; Woods et al., 1995b; Greenwald et al., 1996; O'Brien et al., 1996; Lenze et al., 1999; P. Silverstone et al., 2003.

48. Beats et al., 1991; Brown et al., 1992; Miller et al., 1994; Sassi et al., 2003.

49. Figiel et al., 1991b; McDonald et al., 1991; Botteron et al., 1995; Sassi et al., 2003.

50. Figiel et al., 1989a; Coffey et al., 1990; Beats et al., 1991; Rabins et al., 1991; Greenwald et al., 1996; Iidaka et al., 1996.

51. Coffey et al., 1993b; Greenwald et al., 1998; Lenze et al., 1999; Sassi et al., 2003.

52. Swayze et al., 1990; Deicken et al., 1991; Brown et al., 1992; Woods et al., 1995b; O'Brien et al., 1996.

53. Brown et al., 1992; Strakowski et al., 1993a; Aylward et al., 1994; Altshuler et al., 1995; Woods et al., 1995b.

54. Dewan et al., 1988c; Krishnan et al., 1988; Coffey et al., 1989; Figiel et al., 1989a; Rabins et al., 1991; Brown et al., 1992; Guze and Szuba, 1992; Miller et al., 1994; Dupont et al., 1995a,b; Hickie et al., 1995; O'Brien et al., 1996; Greenwald et al., 1997; Lenze et al., 1999.

55. Jernigan et al., 1990; Zubenko et al., 1990; Deicken et al., 1991; Coffey et al., 1992; Guze and Szuba, 1992; Howard et al., 1995; O'Brien et al., 1996.

56. Dupont et al., 1990, 1995a,b; Figiel et al., 1991a.

57. Zubenko et al., 1990; Beats et al., 1991; Krishnan et al., 1993; Iidaka et al., 1996; Dahabra et al., 1998.

58. Rabins et al., 1991; Brown et al., 1992; Krishnan et al., 1993; Dupont et al., 1995a,b; Woods et al., 1995a.

59. Coffey et al., 1989; Krishnan et al., 1993; Altshuler et al., 1995; O'Brien et al., 1996; McDonald et al., 1999.

60. Dupont et al., 1990, 1995a,b, 1987; Altshuler et al., 1995; O'Brien et al., 1996; Moore et al., 2001; Sassi et al., 2003.

61. Dupont et al., 1990, 1995a; Figiel et al., 1991b; McDonald et al., 1999.

62. Figiel et al., 1991b; Lesser et al., 1991, 1996; Fujikawa et al., 1993; Howard et al., 1993; Krishnan et al., 1993; Hickie et al., 1995; O'Brien et al., 1996; Salloway et al., 1996; Dahabra et al., 1998.

63. Zubenko et al., 1990; Churchill et al., 1991; Rabins, et al., 1991; Miller et al., 1994; Dupont et al., 1995a,b; Greenwald et al., 1996; Iidaka et al., 1996; Dahabra et al., 1998.

64. Lesser et al., 1991, 1996; Hickie et al., 1995, 1997; Salloway et al., 1996; Jenkins et al., 1998; Kramer-Ginsberg et al., 1999.

65. Coffey et al., 1989; Dupont et al., 1995a; Lesser et al., 1996; O'brien et al., 1996.

66. Dupont et al., 1987, 1990; Figiel et al., 1991a; Altshuler et al., 1995; Krabbendam et al., 2000.

67. Coffey et al., 1989; Rabins et al., 1991; Hickie et al., 1995; O'Brien et al., 1996.

68. Coffey et al., 1988b, 1989, 1991; Hickie et al., 1995; O'Brien et al., 1996.

69. Coffey et al., 1987, 1991; Figiel et al., 1989b; Pande et al., 1990.

70. Dewan et al., 1988c; Swayze et al., 1990; Figiel et al., 1991b; Altshuler et al., 1995; Dupont et al., 1995b.

71. Krishnan et al., 1992; Coffey et al., 2001; Kumar et al., 1996, 1997, 1998, 2000; Parashos et al., 1998; Lavretsky et al., 2004.

72. Adler et al., 2005; Bruno et al., 2004; Doris et al., 2004; Lochhead et al., 2004; Lyoo et al., 2004; McDonald et al., 2004, 2005; McIntosh et al., 2004, 2005, 2006; Wilke et al., 2004; Dickstein et al., 2005; Nugent et al., 2006.

73. Drevets et al., 1997; Hirayasu et al., 1999; Sharma et al., 2003; Wilke et al., 2004.

74. Brambilla et al., 2002; Bremner et al., 2002; Kegeles et al., 2003; Bruno et al., 2004; Doris et al., 2004; Pizzagalli et al., 2004; Lochhead et al., 2004; Dickstein et al., 2005; McDonald et al., 2005; Sanches et al., 2005; Nugent et al., 2006.

75. Heath et al., 1982; Lippmann et al., 1982; Nasrallah et al., 1981, 1982b; DelBello et al., 1999; Strakowski et al., 2002.

76. Yates et al., 1987; Dewan et al., 1988c; Coffman et al., 1990; Brambilla et al., 2001.

77. Hauser et al., 1989a, 2000; Pearlson et al., 1997; Altshuler et al., 1998, 2000; Sax et al., 1999; Strakowski et al., 1999; Brambilla et al., 2003b; Chen et al., 2004; Chang et al., 2005; Dickstein et al., 2005; McDonald et al., 2005; Nugent et al., 2006.

78. Sheline et al., 1996, 1999; Bremner et al., 2000; Mervaala et al., 2000; Bell-McGinty et al., 2002; Colla et al., 2002; Frodl et al., 2002a; Vythilingam et al., 2002; MacQueen et al., 2003; Janssen et al., 2004; Lange and Irle, 2004; Lloyd et al., 2004; MacMaster and Kusumakar, 2004a.

79. Ashtari et al., 1999; Vakili et al., 2000; von Gunten et al., 2000; Rusch et al., 2001; Posener et al., 2003.

80. Ashtari et al., 1999; Sheline et al., 1999; Bremner et al., 2000; Mervaala et al., 2000; Steffens et al., 2000; Vakili et al., 2000; von Gunten et al., 2000; Rusch et al., 2001; Frodl et al., 2002b; Vythilingam et al., 2002; MacQueen et al., 2003; Posener et al., 2003.

81. Ashtari et al., 1999; Bremner et al., 2000; Mervaala et al., 2000; Steffens et al., 2000; Vakili et al., 2000; von Gunten et al., 2000; Frodl et al., 2002b; MacQueen et al., 2003; Posener et al., 2003; Rusch et al., 2001; Sheline et al., 2003.

82. Bremner et al., 2000; Mervaala et al., 2000; Steffens et al., 2000; von Gunten et al., 2000; Vythilingam et al., 2002; Frodl et al., 2002; MacMaster and Kusumaker, 2004.

83. Sheline et al., 1996, 1999; Colla et al., 2002; MacQueen et al., 2003.

84. Shah et al., 1998; Ashtari et al., 1999; Sheline et al., 1999; von Gunten et al., 2000.

85. Benes et al., 1998; Vawter et al., 1998, 1999, 2002; Dowlatshahi et al., 2000; Eastwood and Harrison, 2000; Fatemi et al., 2000, 2001; Rosoklija et al., 2000; Law and Deakin, 2001; Webster et al., 2001; Heckers et al., 2002; Dean et al., 2003.

86. Altshuler et al., 1998, 2000; Strakowski et al., 1999; Brambilla et al., 2003a.

87. Swayze et al., 1992; Strakowski et al., 2002; Frazier et al., 2005; McDonald et al., 2005; Nugent et al., 2006.

88. Pearlson et al., 1997; Blumberg et al., 2003c; Chen et al., 2004; DelBello et al., 2004; Chang et al., 2005; Dickstein et al., 2005.

89. Blumberg et al. 2003c; Chen et al., 2004; DelBello et al., 2004; Chang et al., 2005; Dickstein et al., 2005.

90. Sheline et al., 1999; Mervaala et al., 2000; Frodl et al., 2003, 2004.

91. Sheline et al., 1998, 1999; Bremner et al., 2000; Mervaala et al., 2000; von Gunten et al., 2000; Frodl et al., 2002b.

92. Axelson et al., 1993; Coffey et al., 1993a; Pantel et al., 1997; Ashtari et al., 1999.

93. Axelson et al., 1993; Coffey et al., 1993b; Pantel et al., 1997; Ashtari et al., 1999.

94. Johnstone et al., 1989; Swayze et al., 1992; Pearlson et al., 1997; Altshuler et al., 1998, 2000; Roy et al., 1998; Hauser et al., 2000; Brambilla et al., 2003a; Chen et al., 2004.

95. Swayze et al., 1992; Strakowski et al., 1993b, 2002; Dupont et al., 1995b; Sax et al., 1999; Brambilla et al., 2001a; Chang et al., 2005; Sanches et al., 2005.

96. Dupont et al., 1995b; Pillay et al., 1998; Lenze and Sheline, 1999; Bremner et al., 2000.

97. Swayze et al., 1992; Aylward et al., 1994; Brambilla et al., 2001; Sanches et al., 2005; Lyoo et al., 2006.

98. Strakowski et al., 2002; DelBello et al., 2004; Wilke et al., 2004.

99. Husain et al., 1991; Krishnan et al., 1992, 1993; Parashos et al., 1998.

100. Strakowski et al., 1993a, 2000, 2002; Buchsbaum et al., 1997b; Sax et al., 1999; Caetano et al., 2001; Lochhead et al., 2004; Chang et al., 2005; Frazier et al., 2005; McDonald et al., 2005.

101. Krishnan et al., 1993; Parashos et al., 1998; Caetano et al., 2001.

102. Husain et al., 1991; Lammers et al., 1991; Parashos et al., 1998.

103. Hauser et al., 1989a ; Strakowski et al., 1993b; Aylward et al., 1994; Harvey et al., 1994; Schlaepfer et al., 1994; Dupont et al., 1995b; Ohaeri et al., 1995; Zipursky et al., 1997; Sax et al., 1999; Wilke et al., 2004; Chang et al., 2005; Nugent et al., 2006.

104. Husain et al., 1991; Krishnan et al., 1992; Axelson et al., 1993; Coffey et al., 1993a; Dupont et al., 1995b; Sheline et al., 1996; Kumar et al., 1997, 1998; Pillay et al., 1997; Ashtari et al., 1999; Bremner et al., 2000; MacQueen et al., 2003.

105. Hauser et al., 1989b; Strakowski et al., 1993a; Aylward et al., 1994; Schlaepfer et al., 1994; Dupont et al., 1995b; Ohaeri et al., 1995; Zipursky et al., 1997.

106. Strakowski et al., 1993a; Harvey et al., 1994; Schlaepfer et al., 1994; Dupont et al., 1995b; Pearlson et al., 1997; Zipursky et al., 1997.

107. Raichle et al., 1976; Baron et al., 1982, 1984; Lebrun-Grandie et al., 1983; Fox and Raichle, 1986; Ginsberg et al., 1988.

108. Kuhl et al., 1982; Schlageter et al., 1987; Yoshii et al., 1988; Moeller et al., 1996; Murphy et al., 1996; Petit-Taboue et al., 1998; Willis et al., 2002.

109. de Leon et al., 1983, 1987; Kushner et al., 1987; Salmon et al., 1991; Wang et al., 1994; Ernst et al., 1998.

110. Baxter et al., 1987b; Yoshii et al., 1988; Miura et al., 1990; Andreason et al., 1994; Gur et al., 1995; Murphy et al., 1996; Volkow et al., 1997; Willis et al., 2002.

111. George et al., 1993; Breiter et al., 1996; Morris et al., 1996, 1998a,b; Phillips et al., 1997, 1998; Whalen et al., 1998; Baird et al., 1999; Blair et al., 1999.

112. George et al., 1993; Morris et al., 1996, 1998a; Phillips et al., 1997, 1998; Whalen et al., 1998; Blair et al., 1999.

113. Grodd et al., 1995; Schneider et al., 1995, 1997, 1998, 2000; Damasio et al., 1998.

114. Pardo et al., 1993; George et al., 1995b, 1996; Gemar et al., 1996; Lane et al., 1997; Damasio et al., 1999; Mayberg et al., 1999; Liotti et al., 2000.

115. George et al., 1995b, 1996; Grodd et al., 1995; Lane et al., 1997; Damasio et al., 1998, 1999; Schneider et al., 1998, 2000.

116. George et al., 1995a, 1996; Gemar et al., 1996; Lane et al., 1997; Schneider et al., 1997; Damasio et al., 1999; Mayberg et al., 1999; Liotti et al., 2000.

117. Pardo et al., 1993; Grodd et al., 1995; Schneider et al., 1995, 1998, 2000; Damasio et al., 1998.

118. George et al., 1996; Lane et al., 1997; Schneider et al., 1997; Damasio et al., 1999.

119. George et al., 1995c; Grodd et al., 1995; Schneider et al., 1995, 1998, 2000; Damasio et al., 1998.

120. Baxter et al., 1985; Martinot et al., 1990; Cohen et al., 1992; Goyer et al., 1992; Ketter et al., 2001.

121. Rush et al., 1982; Raichle et al., 1985; Kishimoto et al., 1987; Schlegel et al., 1989c; O'Connell et al., 1989; Kanaya and Yonekawa, 1990; Sackeim et al., 1990, 1993; Upadhyaya et al., 1990; Kumar et al., 1993; Lesser et al., 1994; Mayberg et al., 1994; Delvenne et al., 1997a.

122. Gur et al., 1984; Baxter et al., 1985; Kuhl et al., 1985; Reischies et al., 1989; Silfverskiöld and Risberg, 1989; Hagman et al., 1990; Bench et al., 1992, 1993; Berman et al., 1993; Maes et al., 1993; Murphy et al., 1993; Biver et al., 1994; Rubin et al., 1995; Delvenne et al., 1997b; Kimbrell et al., 2002.

123. Buchsbaum et al., 1984, 1986, 1997a; Baxter et al., 1985, 1989; Cohen et al., 1989; Martinot et al., 1990; Ketter et al., 2001.

124. Baxter et al., 1989; Hurwitz et al., 1990; Kumar et al., 1993; Biver et al., 1994; al-Mousawi et al., 1996; Delvenne et al., 1997a; Nofzinger et al., 1999; Kimbrell et al., 2002.

125. Ebert et al., 1991; Lesser et al., 1994; Mayberg et al., 1994; Ito et al., 1996; Vasile et al., 1996; Awata et al., 1998; Galynker et al., 1998; Tutus et al., 1998b; Navarro et al., 2001.

126. Ebert et al., 1991; Bench et al., 1992, 1993; Biver et al., 1994; Tutus et al., 1998b; Nofzinger et al., 1999.

127. Baxter et al., 1985; Kuhl et al., 1985; Kling et al., 1986; Hagman et al., 1990; Upadhyaya et al., 1990; Drevets et al., 1992; Maes et al., 1993; Philpot et al., 1993; Edmonstone et al., 1994; Bonne et al., 1996b; Mozley et al., 1996; Buchsbaum et al., 1997a; Delvenne et al., 1997b; Hornig et al., 1997; Wu et al., 1999; MacHale et al., 2000; Saxena et al., 2001; Videbech et al., 2001, 2002.

128. Stroke (Mayberg et al., 1991; Grasso et al., 1994); epilepsy (Bromfield et al., 1992); Parkinson's (Mayberg et al., 1990; Ring et al., 1994), Huntington's (Mayberg et al., 1992), and Alzheimer's (Hirono et al., 1998) diseases; acquired immunodeficiency syndrome (Renshaw et al., 1992); and postherpetic encephalitis (Caparros-Lefebvre et al., 1996).

129. Obsessive–compulsive disorder (Baxter et al., 1989), bulimia (Hagman et al., 1990; Andreason et al., 1992), and cocaine abuse (Volkow et al., 1991).

130. Baxter et al., 1989; O'Connell et al., 1989, 1995; Schlegel et al., 1989c; Kanaya and Yonekawa, 1990; Kumar et al., 1991; Austin et al., 1992; Drevets et al., 1992; Cohen et al., 1992; Yazici et al., 1992; Bench et al., 1993; Bonne et al., 1996b; Iidaka et al., 1997; Ketter et al., 2001; Kimbrell et al., 2002.

131. Baxter et al., 1989; Mayberg et al., 1990; Volkow et al., 1991; Andreason et al., 1992; Grasso et al., 1994; Hirono et al., 1998.

132. Maes et al., 1993; Philpot et al., 1993; Thomas et al., 1993; Lesser et al., 1994; Mayberg et al., 1994; Vasile et al., 1996.

133. Baxter et al., 1987a; Cohen et al., 1992; Drevets et al., 1992; Biver et al., 1994.

134. Drevets and Raichle, 1992; Drevets et al., 1992, 2002c; Wilson et al., 2002.

135. Buchsbaum et al., 1997a; Mayberg et al., 1999; Drevets et al., 2002a,b,d.

136. Buchsbaum et al., 1986; Cohen et al., 1989; Drevets et al., 2002a,b.

137. Baxter et al., 1985; Cohen et al., 1992; Ebert et al., 1993; Ketter et al., 2001.

138. Hagman et al., 1990; Hurwitz et al., 1990; Kumar et al., 1993; Drevets et al., 1997; Mayberg et al., 1997; Nofzinger et al., 1999.

139. Mayberg et al., 1994; Ito et al., 1996; Awata et al., 1998; Galynker et al., 1998.

140. Baxter et al., 1985; Kuhl et al., 1985; Austin et al., 1992; Biver et al., 1994; Edmonstone et al., 1994; Bonne et al., 1996a; al-Mousawi et al., 1996; Mozley et al., 1996; Vasile et al., 1996; Buchsbaum et al., 1997b; Hornig et al., 1997; MacHale et al., 2000; Navarro et al., 2001; Saxena et al., 2001; Videbech et al., 2001; Kimbrell et al., 2002.

141. Ebert et al., 1991, 1994; Wu et al., 1992, 1999; Holthoff et al., 1999.

142. Baxter et al., 1985; Buchsbaum et al., 1986; Martinot et al., 1990; Cohen et al., 1992; Ebert et al., 1993; Tutus et al., 1998a.

143. Hurwitz et al., 1990; Kumar et al., 1993; Nofzinger et al., 1999; Conca et al., 2000; Kimbrell et al., 2002.

144. Yazici et al., 1992; Philpot et al., 1993; Lesser et al., 1994; Mayberg et al., 1994; Bonne et al., 1996b; Ito et al., 1996; Vasile et al., 1996; Awata et al., 1998; Conca et al., 2000.

145. Philpot et al., 1993; Bonne et al., 1996a; Ito et al., 1996; Nofzinger et al., 1999; Conca et al., 2000.

146. Baxter et al., 1985; Kuhl et al., 1985; Buchsbaum et al., 1986, 1997; Kling et al., 1986; Hagman et al., 1990; Upadhyaya et al., 1990; Bench et al., 1992, 1993; Dolan et al., 1992; Maes et al., 1993; Biver et al., 1994; al- Mousawi et al., 1996; Mozley et al., 1996; Delvenne et al., 1997b; Hornig et al., 1997; Tutus et al., 1998a,b; Abou-Saleh et al., 1999; MacHale et al., 2000; Navarro et al., 2001; Videbech et al., 2001.

147. Drevets et al., 1992, 2002d; Nofzinger et al., 1999; Videbech et al., 2002.

148. Bench et al., 1992, 1993; Dolan et al., 1992; Biver et al., 1994; Mayberg et al., 1997; Saxena et al., 2001.

149. Baxter et al., 1985; Buchsbaum et al., 1986; Hagman et al., 1990; Hurwitz et al., 1990; Kumar et al., 1993; Delvenne et al., 1997a; Wu et al., 1999; Conca et al., 2000.

150. Mayberg et al., 1994; Vasile et al., 1996; Awata et al., 1998; Kowatch et al., 1999; Conca et al., 2000; MacHale et al., 2000.

151. Kuhl et al., 1985; Kling et al., 1986; O'Connell et al., 1989; Kanaya and Yonekawa, 1990; Bench et al., 1992, 1993; Dolan et al., 1992; Wu et al., 1992; Philpot et al., 1993; Biver et al., 1994; Bonne et al., 1996b; Mozley et al., 1996; Delvenne et al., 1997a; Hornig et al., 1997; Navarro et al., 2001; Saxena et al., 2001; Videbech et al., 2001; Kimbrell et al., 2002.

152. Martinot et al., 1990; Cohen et al., 1992; Goyer et al., 1992; Ebert et al., 1993.

153. Cohen et al., 1992; Goyer et al., 1992; Ebert et al., 1993; Ketter et al., 1996b.

154. Baxter et al., 1985; Kuhl et al., 1985; Kling et al., 1986; Hurwitz et al., 1990; Kanaya and Yonekawa, 1990; Bench et al., 1992, 1993; Dolan et al., 1992; Wu et al., 1992; Kumar et al., 1993; Biver et al., 1994; Edmonstone et al., 1994; Bonne et al., 1996b; Mozley et al., 1996; Delvenne et al., 1997a; Hornig et al., 1997; Awata et al., 1998; MacHale et al., 2000; Navarro et al., 2001; Videbech et al., 2001; Kimbrell et al., 2002.

155. Drevets et al., 2001; Sheline et al., 2001; Thomas et al., 2001; Lawrence et al., 2004; Blumberg et al., 2005.

156. George et al., 1995b; Mayberg et al., 1999; Liotti et al., 2002; Krüger, 2003, 2006.

157. Matsuo et al., 2000, 2002; Curtis et al., 2001; de Asis et al., 2001.

158. Baxter et al., 1989; Kanaya and Yonekawa, 1990; Drevets and Raichle, 1992; G. Goodwin et al., 1993; Bench et al., 1995; Buchsbaum et al., 1997b; Tutus et al., 1998a,b; Smith et al., 1999; Mayberg et al., 2000; Brody et al., 2001a; Kennedy et al., 2001; Nofzinger et al., 2001; Sheline et al., 2001; Drevets et al., 2002a,d.

159. Ebert et al., 1991; Wu et al., 1992, 1999; Volk et al., 1997; Holthoff et al., 1999; Smith et al., 1999.

160. Ebert et al., 1991, 1994; Wu et al., 1992, 1999; Holthoff et al., 1999.

161. O'Connell et al., 1995; Rubin et al., 1995; al-Mousawi et al., 1996; Blumberg et al., 1999.

162. Drevets et al., 1995, 1997; G. Goodwin et al., 1997; Blumberg et al., 2000.

163. Drevets et al., 1995, 1997; G. Goodwin et al., 1997; Blumberg et al., 2000.

164. Renshaw et al., 1995; Winsberg et al., 2000; Chang et al., 2001; Frye et al., 2001; Cecil et al., 2002; Bertolino et al., 2003; Deicken et al., 2003a; Sassi et al., 2005.

165. Sharma et al., 1992; Deicken et al., 2001; P. Silverstone et al., 2003; Dager et al., 2004.

166. Stoll et al., 1992; Kato et al., 1996a; Hamakawa et al., 1998, 1999; Ohara et al., 1998; Soares et al., 1999; Castillo et al., 2000; Moore et al., 2000a; Davanzo et al., 2001; Amaral et al., 2002; Michael et al., 2003.

167. Charles et al., 1994b; Renshaw et al., 1997; Hamakawa et al., 1998; Auer et al., 2000; Ende et al., 2000b; Mervaala et al., 2000; Rosenberg et al., 2000; Steingard et al., 2000; Kusumakar et al., 2001; Farchione et al., 2002; Pfleiderer et al., 2003.

168. Soares et al., 1999; Davanzo et al., 2001; Amaral et al., 2002; Bertolino et al., 2003; Dager et al., 2004.

169. Castillo et al., 2000; Moore et al., 2000b; Amaral et al., 2002; Bertolino et al., 2003; Dager et al., 2004.

170. Kato et al., 1996b; Hamakawa et al., 1998; Ohara et al., 1998; Bertolino et al., 2003.

171. Sharma et al., 1992; Stoll et al., 1992; Moore et al., 2000b; Frye et al., 2001; Bertolino et al., 2003.

172. Renshaw et al., 1995; Winsberg et al., 2000; Frye et al., 2001; Cecil et al., 2002; Bertolino et al., 2003; Deicken et al., 2003a; Sassi et al., 2005.

173. Stoll et al., 1992; Kato et al., 1996a; Hamakawa et al., 1998, 1999; Ohara et al., 1998; Castillo et al., 2000; Moore et al., 2000a; Davanzo et al., 2001; Amaral et al., 2002; Michael et al., 2003; Brambilla et al., 2005.

174. Lafer et al., 1994; Kato et al., 1996a; Hamakawa et al., 1998; Moore et al., 2000a; Sharma et al., 1992.

175. Demopulos et al., 1996; Cecil et al., 2002; Silverstone et al., 2004.

176. Stoll et al., 1992; Brühn et al., 1993; Renshaw et al., 1995; Ohara et al., 1998; Hamakawa et al., 1999; Castillo et al., 2000; Winsberg et al., 2000; Chang et al., 2001; Davanzo et al., 2001, 2003; Deicken et al., 2001, 2003a; Amaral et al., 2002; Bertolino et al., 2003; Michael et al., 2003; Brambilla et al., 2005; Sassi et al., 2005.

177. Charles et al., 1994b; Hamakawa et al., 1998; Mervaala et al., 2000; Rosenberg et al., 2000; Steingard et al., 2000; Farchione et al., 2002; Vythilingam et al., 2003.

178. Renshaw et al., 1997; Ende et al., 2000b; Kusumakar et al., 2001; Gruber et al., 2003.

179. Davanzo et al., 2001 2003; Amaral et al., 2002; Bertolino et al., 2003.

180. Chang et al., 2001; Winsberg et al., 2001; Cecil et al., 2002; Bertolino et al., 2003; Michael et al., 2003; Brambilla et al., 2005; Sassi et al., 2005.

181. Sharma et al., 1992; Lafer et al., 1994; Kato et al., 1996b; Hamakawa et al., 1998.

182. Sharma et al., 1992; Stoll et al., 1992; Brühn et al., 1993; Bertolino et al., 2003.

183. Charles et al., 1994a; Hamakawa et al., 1998; Rosenberg et al., 2000; Vythilingam et al., 2003.

184. Sharma et al., 1992; Lafer et al., 1994; Kato et al., 1996b; Hamakawa et al., 1998; Soares et al., 1999; C. Moore et al., 2000.

185. Stoll et al., 1992; Brühn et al., 1993; Renshaw et al., 1995; Ohara et al., 1998; Hamakawa et al., 1999; Castillo et al., 2000; Winsberg et al., 2000; Davanzo et al., 2001, 2003; Deicken et al., 2001, 2003a; Amaral et al., 2002; Bertolino et al., 2003; Chang et al., 2003; Michael et al., 2003; Dager et al., 2004; Wu et al., 2004; Brambilla et al., 2005; Sassi et al., 2005.

186. Sharma et al., 1992; Winsberg et al., 2000; Davanzo et al., 2001, 2003; Cecil et al., 2002.

187. Brühn et al., 1993; Moore et al., 2000a; Chang et al., 2001; Silverstone et al., 2002; Dager et al., 2004.

188. Sharma et al., 1992; Winsberg et al., 2000; Davanzo et al., 2001, 2003; Cecil et al., 2002.

189. Brühn et al., 1993; Moore et al., 2000a; Chang et al., 2001; Silverstone et al., 2002; Dager et al., 2004.

190. Hamakawa et al., 1998, 1999; Cecil et al., 2002; Davanzo et al., 2003; Michael et al., 2003; Dager et al., 2004; Wu et al., 2004; Brambilla et al., 2005.

191. Hamakawa et al., 1998; Auer et al., 2000; Ende et al., 2000b; Rosenberg et al., 2000; Farchione et al., 2002; Pfleiderer et al., 2003.

192. Sharma et al., 1992; Charles et al., 1994a; Renshaw et al., 1995, 1997; Steingard et al., 2000; Winsberg et al., 2000; Castillo et al., 2000; Mervaala et al., 2000; Moore et al., 2000b; Chang et al., 2001; Davanzo et al., 2001; Amaral et al., 2002.

193. Dechent et al., 1999b; Moore et al., 1999a,b; Auer et al., 2000; Deicken et al., 2001, 2003a,b; Cecil et al., 2002.

194. Brühn et al., 1993; Davanzo et al., 2003; Gruber et al., 2003; Wu et al., 2004.

195. Castillo et al., 2000; Cecil et al., 2002; Michael et al., 2003; Dager et al., 2004.

196. Kato et al., 1991, 1992b, 1993b, 1994b,c, 1995; Deicken et al., 1995a,b.

197. Kato et al., 1991, 1992a, 1994b, 1995a; Deicken et al., 1995b.

198. Although two studies found that euthymic compared with manic bipolar-I patients had decreased PMEs (Kato et al., 1991, 1993b) one study with both bipolar-I and -II patients failed to replicate this finding (Kato et al., 1995b).

199. Renshaw and Wicklund, 1988; Komoroski et al., 1990, 1993; Gyulai et al., 1991; Kato et al., 1992a, 1993a, 1994a, 1996b; Gonzalez et al., 1993; Kushnir et al., 1993; Plenge et al., 1994; Sachs et al., 1995; Jensen et al., 1996; Riedl et al., 1997; Soares et al., 2001; Moore et al., 2002.

For our body is like a clock; if one wheel be amiss, all the rest are disordered, the whole fabric
suffers: with such admirable art and harmony is a man composed.

—*Robert Burton*, The Anatomy of Melancholy *(1621, p. 171)*

As surely as the sun rises in the morning and bears hibernate in the winter, human functioning heeds its own innate rhythms. Body temperature rises and falls in oscillations, as do hormone secretions, cell division, heart rate, urine flow, allergic reactions, motoric activity, even mathematical finesse—and, most obvious of all, the need for sleep. Mood also fluctuates, waxing and waning, although the regularity of mood cycles is not synchronized with the clock as precisely as is the case with other biological rhythms. Indeed, abnormalities of biological rhythms have been proposed to represent endophenotypes or markers of manic-depressive illness (perhaps particularly the bipolar subgroup), presumably being present not only in patients but also in some relatives without manifest mood disorder. Sleep disruption is closely associated with recurrent affective illness. Sleep loss is a major symptom as well as a trigger of manic episodes, and when applied clinically (sleep deprivation) is one of the most effective antidepressant interventions[1]—certainly the fastest acting. In addition to the diurnal, or circadian, rhythms associated with sleep, the observation that the seasons of the year influence the expression of mood disorders is as old as the classical descriptions of manic-depressive illness itself.

In this chapter we review the literature on circadian rhythms, sleep disturbances, and their relationship to affective illness. We also review the less extensive body of work on the relationship between seasonal rhythms and mood disorders. We begin by reviewing the physiology of circadian rhythms and of sleep. Next we look at the relationship between sleep and affective disorders, and that between disturbances of circadian rhythms and manic-depressive illness. We then examine the literature on experimental alterations of sleep and other biological rhythms as treatments for affective illness. Finally, we review what is

known about the relationship between seasonal rhythms and affective disorders.

PHYSIOLOGY OF CIRCADIAN RHYTHMS

As the earth rotates through its 24-hour cycle, a world of light alternates with a world of darkness. To enhance survival and conserve energy, animals have adapted their activity patterns to a diurnal, nocturnal, or crepuscular[2] existence, retreating at other times to a relatively protected environment where they rest and sleep. Such circadian rhythms are approximately 24-hour oscillations or alternations of biological processes that are observed in a broad spectrum of organisms. Although these rhythms are generated endogenously by internal clocks, they do not function in isolation from their surroundings; rather, they are synchronized with temporal variations of the environment by external cues, especially the light–dark cycle. Circadian rhythmicity allows organisms not only to respond to but also to anticipate regular changes in the environment, aligning their physiological and behavioral capabilities to best fit environmental demands.

A clock entrained to the natural environment has a 24-hour period, while a free-running (non-24-hour) circadian clock (in constant dark or dim–light conditions) has a slightly different period, with marked variability among species and individuals. In humans, for example, the period is slightly longer than 24 hours, while in most rodents it is slightly less. The components of a circadian system include the clock itself, which generates the biological rhythm; input pathways that transmit environmental cues to the clock; and output pathways that transmit the clock's rhythms to the rest of the organism, influencing a large number of endocrinologic, biochemical, and electrophysiological processes.

The Master Circadian Clock

Molecular analysis reveals that the master circadian clock is located in the *suprachiasmatic nuclei* (SCN), which are small, paired clusters of cells situated in the anterior hypothalamus. The SCN receive input from the retina for adjustment to the light–dark cycle and have extensive modulatory innervation from serotonergic neurons in a part of the midbrain called the *raphe*. The first indication that the master clock is located in the SCN came from ablation studies in rodents. Stephan (1983) and then Kafka and colleagues (1985) demonstrated that ablation of the SCN in rats abolishes circadian rhythms of drinking activity. Conversely, cultures of an SCN cell line that exhibit robust circadian metabolic rhythms (Earnest et al., 1999) can restore circadian rhythms of locomotor activity when transplanted into the third ventricle of SCN-lesioned rats without circadian rhythms. Thus, this cell line is sufficient to generate and drive circadian rhythmicity at the level of the whole organism. Such behavioral rescue is not trivial, since circadian rhythms in vivo are not restored by other cell lines, such as fibroblasts, that may show oscillatory properties.[3] Is the clock function a result of the interactions of SCN neurons, i.e., a result of the neuronal network, or is it an intrinsic function of each neuronal cell? The latter possibility appears more likely at this point, based on the work of Welsh and colleagues (1995).[4]

In recent years, several genes representing components of the mammalian clock have been identified, among them *clock, cry,* and *per*[5]; evidence linking certain clock genes to bipolar disorder is reviewed later. How are these clock genes linked to rhythms of electrical activity in the SCN? These genes and their products are involved in interacting positive and negative feedback loops in transcription (transforming chemical information from DNA to messenger RNA [mRNA]) and translation (transforming chemical information from mRNA to proteins) of clock genes.[6] It is from these feedback loops (which span 24 hours) that self-sustained circadian oscillations arise. The electrical activity of the clock is an output, not a necessary constituent of the clock because the clock's time-keeping function continues even if the electrical output is silenced with anesthetic agents (Reppert and Weaver, 2001). The electrical activity of the SCN is the result of activation of a related set of genes called *clock-controlled genes* (CCGs). CCGs are rhythmically regulated by the clock but are not part of the clock per se because their products are not essential to its functioning.[7]

To function effectively, the SCN must synchronize their approximately 20,000 neurons for a coordinated output. It appears that gamma-aminobutyric acid (GABA), the principal neurotransmitter in the SCN (and involved in the action of some of the medications used in treating bipolar

disorder), is essential for this synchronization (Liu and Reppert, 2000), although other neurotransmitters, including neuropeptides, may also be involved.[8] In mammals, including humans, visual stimuli are required for entrainment of physiological and behavioral rhythms to the light–dark cycle (Yamazaki et al., 1999; Rugier et al., 2003).[9] The major pathway is the retinohypothalamic tract (RHT). Its major neurotransmitter is glutamate, with additional modulation from substance P (Hamada et al., 1999) and pituitary adenylate cyclase activating peptide (Chen et al., 1999).[10] In addition, abundant terminals of serotonergic neurons from the raphe modulate the activity of the SCN.

Along with neurotransmitters (the "wiring"), neurohumoral modulatory factors reach the SCN. The most important of these is melatonin, which modulates phase shifts by binding to specific melatonin receptors; melatonin also reduces the firing of SCN neurons (Liu et al., 1997a).[11]

The output pathways (and neurohumoral mediators) from the SCN are not completely understood (Reppert and Weaver, 2001). GABA-containing axonal terminals from the SCN to the paraventricular nuclei regulate melatonin synthesis in the pineal gland (Kalsbeek et al., 1996) and thus participate in the circadian and seasonal rhythms of melatonin.[12]

The timing of several rhythms is identical in diurnal and nocturnal species relative to the day–night cycle. For example, electrical activity of the SCN and vasopressin levels in the cerebrospinal fluid are higher during the daytime, while melatonin is produced at night in all species regardless of whether they are active during the day or night. On the other hand, important physiological rhythms, such as body temperature and hypothalamic–pituitary–adrenal activity, are linked predominantly with the day–night rest–activity rhythm.

Circadian Rhythms in Humans

Evidence that human circadian rhythms are endogenous came from experiments in which people lived for weeks or months in caves, underground bunkers, or windowless, sound-proof apartments, isolated from external time cues (Chouvet et al., 1974; Siffre, 1975; Wever, 1979). Under these conditions, circadian rhythms ran according to their own intrinsic period, which, as noted above, is usually slower (i.e., longer) than one cycle every 24 hours in humans.[13] Experimental results indicate that external time cues synchronize circadian rhythms not only with the day–night cycle but also with one another. When entrained by "zeitgebers" (see endnote 13), homeostatic mechanisms ensure that the various rhythms maintain distinct phase relationships to the environment and to one another. In humans, for instance, the temperature minimum nearly always occurs

diff. circ. rhythms

during the last third of the night, just before dawn. Internally, circadian rhythms that are normally synchronized with each other can dissociate when one becomes disentrained from the zeitgeber. The temperature rhythm of a night shift worker, for example, may continue to be entrained to the day–night cycle but become dissociated from the sleep–wake cycle when the worker sleeps during the day. Or consider what would happen under free-running conditions (i.e., in the absence of zeitgebers). The two cycles, each following their own intrinsic periodicity, would go in and out of phase with each other (see Fig. 16–1). This internal desynchronization can create what has been called a *beat phenomenon* (such as when two peaks periodically coincide), analogous to the audible beat produced by two tuning forks of slightly different frequencies (Halberg, 1968; Kripke et al., 1978).

Proper functioning of the human circadian system depends on continuous sensory input from the environment. This feature may be particularly relevant to understanding circadian disturbances in manic-depressive illness. Equally important, behavior regulates biological rhythms by exposing a person to or shielding him or her from the entraining zeitgebers—that is, behavior serves a gating function. The depressive patient who hides under the covers is certainly less likely to be exposed to light and other zeitgebers than is the manic patient who races through the day and sleeps little at night.

The normal phase relationships between circadian oscillators and their overt rhythms can be temporarily disturbed during rapid transmeridian travel and shift work, as well as in experimental laboratory conditioning. As demonstrated in isolation experiments, the oscillators may spontaneously dissociate and oscillate with unequal periods when humans are deprived of external time cues. The

timing of circadian rhythms relative to the day–night cycle and to one another is homeostatically controlled and reflects in part the period of the intrinsic rhythm of the driving oscillators. Such a system may be altered by disease and treatment interventions. Alterations can occur in the intrinsic periods of the oscillators, in the coupling between oscillators, or between the oscillators and the external day–night cycle. Such changes may affect the phase position of circadian rhythms entrained to the day–night cycle and even their capacity to be entrained at all (Aschoff, 1981a,b).

An essential concept for understanding how light or other zeitgebers synchronize or desynchronize internal and external rhythms is the phase response curve (PRC). In short, light during midday has minimal if any phase-shifting effects, while light in the late afternoon and evening delays circadian rhythms, and late night–early morning light advances them. (It is important to note that the terms *midday, afternoon, evening, night,* and *morning* refer to internal time.[14]) In contrast to light, melatonin and behavioral arousal have a PRC that is distinct from, and even somewhat complementary to, that of light (Duncan et al., 1996). Thus, melatonin phase advances the rest–activity rhythm when administered between internal midday and early night, while producing a phase delay when administered between late night and midday. Given that the circadian period in humans is slightly longer than 24 hours, the synchronization of the circadian system in normal individuals occurs through daily phase advances.[15]

Biological Day and Night, Biological Dusk and Dawn

The circadian pacemaker imposes daily variation on the activity of human neuroendocrine systems. Similar to the changes in environmental light that define day, night, and twighlight, these changes exhibit waveforms characterized by distinct diurnal and nocturnal periods with relatively short transitions between them (corresponding to a biological dusk and a biological dawn). In humans, for example, periods characterized by absence of melatonin secretion, low prolactin secretion, falling cortisol levels, decreasing theta activity in the electroencephalogram (EEG), and decreasing propensity to rapid eye movement (REM) (biological day) all alternate with nocturnal periods of active melatonin secretion, high prolactin secretion, rising levels of cortisol, increasing theta activity, and increasing propensity to REM sleep (biological night). In response to light, the circadian pacemaker synchronizes biological day and night so that their timing and duration are appropriately matched with the timing and duration of the external day and night.[16,17] These processes are summarized in Figure 16–2.

Figure 16–1. The beat phenomenon. This hypothetical model shows two circadian rhythms. Oscillator A is synchronized to the day–night cycle and always peaks during the day. Oscillator B free-runs slightly faster than one cycle per 24 hours and therefore goes out of phase with A. When A and B are in phase, their ratio is stable, but when they are out of phase, the ratio of B to A may become very high. This ratio indicates the cyclic beat phenomenon that occurs every few days. (*Source*: Adapted from Halberg, 1968, and Kripke et al., 1978.)

Biological Dawn entrained to dawn	Biological Dusk entrained to dusk	Biological Dusk entrained to dawn
BIOLOGICAL DAY No melatonin secretion Increasing core body temperature Decreasing sleepiness Decreasing waking EEG theta activity Decreasing REM sleep propensity Decreasing cortisol levels Wakefulness		**BIOLOGICAL NIGHT** Melatonin secretion Decreasing core body temperature Increasing sleepiness Increasing waking EEG theta activity Increasing REM sleep propensity Increasing cortisol levels Sleep

(handwritten note: ← natural tendency)

Figure 16–2. Temporal organization of the human circadian timing system. Profiles of a number of circadian rhythms in humans exhibit distinct diurnal and nocturnal states with abrupt switch-like transitions between them. These states and transitions can be conceptualized as a biological day and night and a biological dawn and dusk. They are generated within the organism and mirror or anticipate features of the solar day to which they correspond and with which they are synchronized. EEG = electroencephalogram; REM = rapid eye movement. (*Source*: Wehr et al., 2001b. Reprinted with permission from Blackwell Publishing, Ltd.)

(handwritten note: What's fon of REM sleep?)

PHYSIOLOGY OF SLEEP

Sleep is a distinct behavioral and physiological state, as defined by EEG and behavioral characteristics. In preparation for sleep, animals seek a protected environment, assume a characteristic sleep posture, and pass briefly through a drowsy state before falling asleep. Despite intense research, the function of sleep remains unknown. Nevertheless, it is well known that sleep serves a vital function, this despite its evolutionary disadvantages, such as increased vulnerability to predators. Mammals totally sleep deprived for 2–3 weeks die, as they would if deprived of food for a similar duration.[18]

Stages of Sleep

The discrete stages of sleep are marked by variations in EEG patterns, eye movements, and muscle tone. By convention, human sleep is divided into two major phases that alternate throughout the night: a REM phase and a non-REM (NREM) phase. On falling asleep, healthy adults go into NREM sleep, the period of rest and energy conservation, when the brain literally cools while respiration, blood pressure, heart rate, and other physiological processes slow down, eyes are still or move only slowly, and muscles are relaxed but not flaccid. This first phase comprises four stages of progressively deeper sleep. On EEG recordings, the frequency of electrical waves decreases steadily from stage 1 to stage 4, while the amplitude—the energy discharged at each impulse—increases (see Fig. 16–3). Stages 3 and 4 consist of predominant slow and ample delta waves (slow-wave sleep), the result of highly synchronized brain activity.

Following the NREM phase is REM sleep, marked by intense mental activity, vivid dreaming, and rapid and diffuse cerebral metabolism. Blood flow and most neuronal firing rates, and probably brain temperature, are higher than during either NREM or awake states, while, paradoxically, the large muscles are virtually paralyzed. Bursts of REM occur, pulse and blood pressure rise and fall, and respiration becomes irregular. EEG activity shows a sawtooth pattern, low in amplitude (voltage) and variable in frequency, similar to stage 1 NREM sleep (the brief transition period between wakefulness and sleep). Dement and Kleitman (1957) observed that in normal individuals, the distribution of REM sleep during the night was skewed, with more occurring toward the end of the night than at the beginning.

In the normal sleep of a young adult, the first period of NREM sleep (through all four stages) is followed, after an average of about 90 minutes, by a 15- to 20-minute period of REM sleep. Slow-wave sleep (stages 3 and 4, part of the NREM phase) predominates during the first part of the night, whereas REM sleep periods become progressively longer and are most concentrated in the hours before waking. While an internal self-sustaining circadian pacemaker appears to govern the propensity for REM sleep, homeostatic processes determine other sleep patterns, such as the amount of slow-wave sleep, which turns out to be proportional to the length of time the person has been awake prior to sleep.

Advances in understanding of the neurophysiological basis of the sleep EEG (Steriade, 1994; Amzica and Steriade, 1998), in conjunction with quantitative EEG analysis (Borbely et al., 1989; Aeschbach and Borbely, 1993; Achermann and Borbely, 1998), have confirmed that the EEG is influenced by prior and ongoing individual experience. In addition, there is evidence that genetic factors contribute to sleep regulation and abnormalities (for reviews of animal research, see Franken et al., 1999; Toth, 2001). For example, EEG parameters of recovery sleep after sleep deprivation in mice are strain-specific. These differences have been linked to a locus on chromosome 5 near one of the clock genes and may reflect differences in circadian timing of sleep.[19] Sleep alterations in knockout mice[20] are another means of evaluating genetic contributions to sleep.[21]

Neural Substrates for Sleep

A pandemic of encephalitis letargica, a presumed viral infection, swept much of the globe during World War I, causing severe daytime sleepiness in most affected individuals. A group of individuals had the opposite problem, however—a prolonged state of insomnia. A Viennese neurologist, Baron von Economo (1930), reported that the increased sleepiness was due to injury of the posterior hypothalamus and rostral midbrain, while the severe insomnia resulted from lesions of the preoptic area and basal forebrain. On the basis of this observation, von Economo postulated that a region in the anterior hypothalamus contains sleep-promoting neurons, while a region in the posterior hypothalamus contains wakefulness-promoting neurons. Lesioning studies in animals proved his predictions correct, and

the pathways responsible for the hypothalamic regulation of wakefulness have now begun to be understood (Saper et al., 2001).[22]

During REM sleep, cholinergic neurons in the caudal midbrain and rostral forebrain fire at their maximum, while the serotonergic, noradrenergic, and catecholaminergic pathways are at their minimum. These monoaminergic neurons inhibit the cholinergic REM-promoting neurons and thus terminate REM sleep.[23] NREM sleep is associated with hypersynchrony of thalamocortical rhythms, with an active inhibition of the arousal centers.[24] Conversely, when activated, these neurons abort sleep and induce wakefulness.[25] The brain structures involved in the control of NREM sleep are also involved in thermoregulation. As noted, lowering of the set point for body temperature occurs in NREM sleep. Thus, lesions that result in disruption of NREM sleep also disrupt thermoregulation. Of clinical importance, heating the body promotes NREM sleep. For example, as part of sleep hygiene, a warm bath before going to bed is recommended for patients with insomnia. In contrast to NREM sleep, more highly discrete brain areas are involved in the regulation of REM sleep. Neurons in the pontine tegmentum (the pedunculopontine tegmental nucleus and lateral dorsal tegmental nucleus) are active during REM sleep and waking and inactive during NREM sleep. Drugs that boost acetylcholine levels to these areas activate REM sleep, while

Figure 16–3. Normal sleep: electroencephalogram (EEG) patterns, distribution of non–rapid eye movement (NREM) and REM periods. EMG = electromyography; EOG = electro-oculogram. (*Source*: Hobson and Steriade, 1986.)

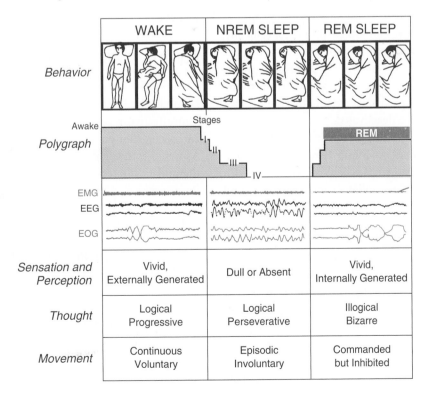

blockers of muscarinic receptors suppress REM sleep. Noradrenergic neurons in the locus ceruleus and serotonergic neurons of the dorsal raphe are active during waking, less active during NREM sleep, and inactive during REM sleep. These neurons inhibit the cholinergic neurons of the pontine tegmentum to terminate REM sleep. A less-than-active serotonergic or noradrenergic system (perhaps in depression) may result in disinhibition of REM sleep. While these discrete pontine structures are involved in REM sleep initiation, other neurons, such as those in the lateral hypothalamus, the amygdala, and other limbic structures, are involved in the maintenance of REM sleep.

In addition to GABA, histamine, acetylcholine, serotonin, norepinephrine, and orexin/hypocretin (described briefly above and in the associated notes), other neurotransmitters have an important role. For example, dopaminergic neurons promote wakefulness. In addition, cholecystokinin, prostaglandins, interleukin-1, and adenosine have a modulatory role. Adenosine in particular has been implicated in mediating the homeostatic mechanisms of sleep. Caffeine increases alertness by blocking adenosine receptors, which are widespread in the brain. Receptors on the cholinergic neurons of the basal forebrain appear to regulate adenosine's effect on sleep.[26]

Functional Neuroimaging of Sleep

Positron emission tomography (PET) studies have used either O15 water (for blood flow) or deoxyglucose-F18 (FDG) (for cerebral metabolism), each having its advantages and disadvantages.[27] PET studies have shown that global cerebral metabolism is similar in REM sleep and wakefulness, but regional blood flow differs. Specifically, several limbic structures, such as the cingulate gyrus, are more active during REM than waking conditions, while areas of high-order association, such as the orbitofrontal cortex, the dorsolateral prefrontal cortex, and the inferior parietal lobe, tend to be deactivated.[28] In contrast, slow-wave sleep is characterized by deactivation in the brain stem, thalamus, and basal forebrain (Braun et al., 1997). Compared with NREM, REM sleep is associated with higher metabolic rates in midline frontal, cingular, and dorsolateral prefrontal regions (Buchsbaum et al., 2001).

The Two-Process Model of Sleep

The timing and duration of sleep and wakefulness are the result of the interaction of circadian rhythms paced by the SCN (process c) and a sleep–wake-dependent ("homeostatic") process (process s). Process c represents a circadian variation in sleep propensity that can be understood as fluctuating thresholds for falling asleep and waking up, while process s tracks the increase in sleep pressure during waking and a corresponding decrease during sleep (Borbely, 1982; Borbely

and Wirz-Justice, 1982). This two-process model attempts to account for the compensatory role played by the SCN with respect to process s. For example, as sleep appetite increases throughout the day, the SCN drives a signal of increased alertness to avoid a mandatory cessation of activity (a "wake maintenance zone"). This phenomenon can be conceptualized as an increase in the threshold for falling asleep, and sleep latency at this time is prolonged. Furthermore, as sleep appetite decreases toward early morning, the threshold for being asleep is lowered (a "sleep maintenance zone").[29]

Physiology of Sleep Duration

In patients with bipolar disorder, reduction of sleep duration can trigger mania. But how long do we need to sleep? Sleep duration and amount of sleep needed differ somewhat among individuals; genetic factors may play a role in determining sleep duration in humans (Partinen et al., 1983; Webb and Campbell, 1983), as well as in rodents (Franken et al., 1999; Tafti et al., 1999; Huber et al., 2000). In experimental conditions consisting of imposed rest and long artificial nights for up to 15 weeks, healthy volunteers slept almost 11 hours during their first night, interpreted as the result of "paying" the sleep debt that had accumulated from daily life before the study began. Thereafter, subjects slept progressively less on subsequent nights until reaching an average steady-state duration of 8.25 hours in the fourth week (with very little individual variation) (Wehr et al., 1991, 1993). Sleeping less than one needs results in metabolic and endocrine alterations, such as lower glucose tolerance, lower thyrotropin concentration, and elevated cortisol and sympathetic nervous system activity (Spiegel et al., 1999).[30,31]

SLEEP IN AFFECTIVE DISORDERS

Clinical and research evidence provides tantalizing leads for understanding the connection between sleep and recurrent affective illness. Switches from depression to mania can occur after patients miss a night of sleep, for example. As noted earlier, sleep depriving a patient with depression therapeutically often results in a striking albeit temporary improvement in mood (see also Chapter 19); resuming sleep, even for a short nap, can often cause the patient to sink back into depression.

Time Course of Sleep Abnormalities in Affective Disorders

Polysomnographic abnormalities in affective disorders may be present long before the clinical onset of the disorder and continue to persist indefinitely (thus representing a "vulnerability" or "trait"). Alternatively, the abnormality may appear only with a disordered mood state; if it persists for a long time after mood has normalized, it may represent a "scar" marker, while if it is present only during the mood episode, it is a "state" marker. Thus some researchers have found persistent REM sleep abnormalities after depressed patients have achieved remission (Rush et al., 1986; Steiger et al., 1989, 1993a,b,c). For example, in 78 unmedicated depressed patients, Thase and colleagues (1998) found that certain sleep abnormalities (sleep efficiency, REM density) were to some degree reversible with remission, while others were independent of mood state. In contrast, other researchers have found that persistent REM sleep abnormalities have a tendency to normalize after mood state has normalized,[32] even to nearly complete restoration of normal sleep in remitted depressed patients (Knowles et al., 1986).

Several studies have found shortened REM latencies in healthy relatives of depressed patients (Giles et al., 1987a,b, 1988, 1989). Gillin's group (Gillin et al., 1982; Jones and Berney, 1987) hypothesized that because euthymic individuals with a family history of affective illness have an increased response to arecholine and because relatives with affective illness have an increased REM response to arecholine relative to those without affective illness, cholinergic supersensitivity may be a vulnerability marker for affective illness. This hypothesis was confirmed by Schreiber and colleagues (1992), who found that subjects with a positive family history but negative personal history for affective illness had more frequent sleep-onset REM periods with cholinergic stimulation than did healthy controls.

Of particular relevance to the notion that recurrence is central to manic-depressive illness, some polysomnographic sleep abnormalities appear to reflect a vulnerability to recurrence of depression. Thus Thase and colleagues (1995) found more frequent REM sleep abnormalities in patients with recurrent depression than in those experiencing a single episode. Similarly, Buysse and colleagues (1997) observed that sleep abnormalities predicted future recurrence in patients with recurrent major depression. More recently, Perlman and colleagues (2006) found that a persistent sleep deficit after recovery (at least partially) from a mood episode in bipolar patients predicted depressive symptoms during a 6-month follow-up period. (Manic/hypomanic symptoms could have been undercounted because if they were brief, they were likely to have been missed in the once-a-month assessments.)

Some methodological issues tend to complicate interpretation of the state versus trait literature. These issues include variable or imprecise definitions of relapse and recurrence, an overly short interval from mood normalization to the sleep study, and uncontrolled medication effects. For example, when patients were medication-free for several years rather than for several weeks or months, sleep was more likely to normalize (Riemann and Berger, 1989; Buysse et al., 1997; Riemann et al., 2001).

Sleep in the Bipolar Subgroup

As noted above, sleep loss is often a precursor and/or precipitant of hypomania or mania in bipolar patients.[33] As we emphasized in the first edition of this text, maintaining stable sleep–wake cycles is of central importance to the maintenance of stability in bipolar illness, a point subsequently confirmed empirically (Brown et al., 1996; Frank et al., 1997). During episodes of depression, bipolar patients often report sleeping too much, although, as noted above, this hypersomnia appears predominantly in bipolar depression of mild to moderate severity. Hypersomnia is one of the symptoms of an "atypical depression syndrome," which overlaps with many cases of bipolar depression (other symptoms being overeating, increased appetite, and weight gain). These atypical features tend to be associated with a lower incidence of the type of polysomnographic abnormalities reported in classic melancholic depression. Of relevance here is the finding that no REM sleep disinhibition or decrease in slow-wave sleep has been found[34] in patients with winter depression or seasonal affective disorder (SAD) (which is characterized by atypical features). Moreover, Schwartz and colleagues (2000) reported that patients with SAD, compared with controls, actually had significantly longer NREM episodes and more slow-wave sleep during NREM periods.

Sleep during Mania/Hypomania

Just as sleep loss can trigger mania in bipolar patients, reduction in sleep is a good predictor of hypomania or mania the next day in rapid-cycling bipolar patients (Leibenluft et al., 1996a). This 1-day latency is similar to observations of sleep loss triggering or intensifying mania (Wehr et al., 1987; Barbini et al., 1996) and is consistent with the recent report of Bauer and colleagues (2006), who collected longitudinal self-ratings of mood and sleep in 59 bipolar outpatients undergoing routine treatment. They found for many patients an inverse relationship between a change in sleep and a subsequent change in mood, with a usual lag period of 1 day.

But what do we know about sleep during manic/hypomanic episodes? Obviously this is a difficult question to research, especially in mania. Van Sweden (1986) studied two unmedicated severely manic patients who had been hospitalized after 2 and 3 weeks of mania. He found that, contrary to the common assumption that manic patients are unable to sleep, the EEGs of both patients showed stage 2 sleep within seconds of closing their eyes. In a study of eight unmedicated manic men, Linkowski and colleagues (1986) found that REM latency, as well as the percentage of time spent in any stage of sleep, was no different than in age-matched normal men, although the patients took longer to fall asleep and spent less time asleep. In a slightly larger study, however, Hudson and colleagues (1988) found shorter REM latencies and higher REM densities in nine unmedicated manic patients relative to normal controls. Thus, the patients showed hypersomnia and sleep continuity disturbances very similar to those seen in bipolar depression, although to a lesser degree. Unlike patients with major depression, however, the manic patients in the Hudson group's study did not have disturbances in delta sleep (stages 3 and 4).

In a patient with rapid cycling, Gann and colleagues (1993) found that very short REM latencies, including sleep-onset REM periods, followed depressive days, and after hypomanic days, REM latency was prolonged but still shorter than normal. Feldman-Naim and colleagues (1997) described a diurnal variation in the direction of mood switch in rapid-cycling bipolar disorder. They observed an "up-switch" from depression to hypomania/mania during the daytime and a "downswitch" at night. For the great majority of bipolar patients, however, most switches into mania occur overnight (Bunney et al., 1972a,b).

Circadian abnormalities, discussed in more detail later, may underlie some sleep–wake abnormalities in patients with bipolar disorder. For example, 48- or 72-hour rhythms have been observed in rapid-cycling patients when they shift from depression to mania (Wehr et al., 1982; Mizukawa et al., 1991). This phenomenon is similar to that seen in healthy volunteers under conditions in which external time cues have been eliminated (Weitzman, 1982; Wever, 1983). Other chronobiological abnormalities in a manic state include phase advances in the nadir of the cortisol rhythms relative to the time of sleep onset, as found by Linkowski and colleagues (1994) in eight unmedicated patients in a manic state. It is possible that a phase advance of the circadian rhythms in mania is the consequence rather than the cause of sleep abnormalities, and may also reflect a previously reported supersensitivity to light (Lewy et al., 1985; Eagles, 1994). A more recent report confirmed the original finding only partially (Nurnberger et al., 2000). A plausible hypothesis is that, given the brevity of sleep in mania, such patients are exposed to bright light very early in the morning, so that under conditions of supersensitivity to light, rhythms may shift to a more advanced position.

What can be learned from bipolar patients with regard to state–trait abnormalities? Knowles and colleagues (1986) studied 10 remitted bipolar depressed patients for 5 nights. Although the patients reported more frequent arousals, no significant differences in EEG sleep parameters relative to age-matched controls were observed. Similar findings were reported by Jones and colleagues (2005). On the other hand, Harvey and colleagues (2005) showed that euthymic bipolar patients have impaired sleep efficiency, along with higher-than-normal levels of anxiety about having poor-quality sleep, and Millar and colleagues

(2004) found that sleep duration and nighttime wakening were more variable in remitted bipolar patients compared with controls. Furthermore, Sitaram and colleagues (1982) found increased density and percentage of REM among bipolar patients in the well state compared with normal controls. More striking, however, was their finding that when infused with arecholine (an acetylcholine agonist that can produce a shortened REM latency), the recovered bipolar patients in the well state were more sensitive to its effects on REM latency than were the normal controls (see the discussion of cholinergic sensitivity below).

Sleep in Major Depression

Lenox and colleagues (2002) and Gould and Manji (2002a,b) proposed that circadian disturbances and disinhibition of REM sleep (such as a greater shortening of REM latency with cholinergic agents) may represent endophenotypes for recurrent unipolar depression, whereas a hypomanic or manic response to sleep deprivation may represent an endophenotype for bipolar disorder. Both unipolar and bipolar manic-depressive patients can, of course, have sleep disorders unrelated to their illness, such as sleep apnea, which may disrupt sleep and result secondarily in mood instability. In such cases, consultation with a sleep specialist may bring dramatic improvement to an occasional, apparently treatment-resistant situation while also improving overall functioning.

Initial efforts to distinguish recurrent unipolar depression from bipolar depression on the basis of sleep characteristics have been confounded by issues of overall severity and comorbid anxiety. Thus for the sake of clarity, our discussion here focuses on depression in general; where adequate data exist, we distinguish between the recurrent unipolar and bipolar forms.

In general, sleep and depression appear to be inversely related. Thus some impairment of sleep quality is reported by more than 90 percent of depressed patients (Tsuno et al., 2005), while approximately 25 percent of patients complaining of chronic insomnia suffer from major depression (Vollrath et al., 1989). Breslau and colleagues (1996) reported a relative risk of 4.0 for new onset of major depression among individuals with a history of insomnia. Insomnia also appears to be a prominent risk factor for developing major depression in the future (Pfaffenberger et al., 1994; Chang et al., 1997). Further longitudinal studies will be necessary, however, to distinguish between insomnia as a true predictor of depression and as a subclinical or prodromal symptom of depression. Conversely, timely treatment of insomnia can reduce the likelihood of a major mood episode (Weissman et al., 1997).

What is the nature of the sleep disorder in major depression? Patients with the endogenous or melancholic form of depression tend to report global insomnia, that is, some difficulty falling asleep, frequent nocturnal awakenings, and early-morning awakenings. In contrast, hypersomnia is encountered more frequently among bipolar patients who are moderately depressed (Detre et al., 1972; Thase et al., 1989) and in patients with SAD (Rosenthal et al., 1984). Sleep abnormalities in depression have been characterized by polygraphic EEG recordings (so-called polysomnographic studies), pioneered by Snyder at the National Institute of Mental Health (NIMH) and by Kupfer's group (Kupfer and Foster, 1972; Foster et al., 1976). Kupfer's group found a decreased REM latency in depression (a shortening of the interval between sleep onset and the occurrence of the first REM period), typically accompanied by a reduction in slow-wave sleep. In addition, they found greater frequency of eye movements during REM sleep, a characteristic referred to as increased REM density. The early hypothesis that decreased REM latency may be a biological marker for primary melancholic rather than secondary depression (Kupfer, 1976; Kupfer et al., 1976) has not been confirmed by more recent studies. Rather, the phenomenon has been reported in nonmelancholic and secondary depression, in other psychiatric disorders, and even in normal aging (Benca et al., 1992; Riemann et al., 2001).

Medication Effects on Sleep in Depression

Almost all antidepressants suppress REM sleep (Sitaram et al., 1978b), an effect once considered a possible mechanism of their antidepressant activity. It is now clear, however, that suppression of REM sleep is not necessary for an antidepressant effect (Riemann et al., 2001), as some antidepressants, such as nefazodone (Sharpley et al., 1992) and bupropion (Nofzinger et al., 1995), appear to enhance rather than decrease REM sleep. There is disagreement over the time course of REM suppression, with one group reporting that it attenuated over the first 3–5 weeks of treatment (Berger et al., 1986; Riemann and Berger, 1990) and another that it persisted beyond 1 year (Kupfer et al., 1994; Reynolds et al., 1997).

Mood stabilizers have a smaller and more variable impact on REM sleep and may exert their influence mainly by increasing slow-wave sleep. Such effects have been described for lithium (Friston et al., 1989) and carbamazepine (Yang et al., 1989). Valproate decreases REM and increases slow-wave sleep (Harding et al., 1985), whereas lamotrigine and gabapentin increase rather than decrease REM sleep in patients with seizure disorders (Placidi et al., 2000a,b,c). Electroconvulsive therapy (ECT) decreases REM latency in depressed patients, and the antidepressant response is poorer in patients who continue to have sleep-onset REM periods after ECT (Grunhaus et al., 1997).

Cholinergic Sensitivity in Patients with Manic-Depressive Illness

As noted in the first edition of this text and earlier, cholinergic–adrenergic balance has been considered important for sleep regulation. According to this hypothesis as first proposed in 1972 (Janowsky et al., 1972), mania is related to decreased and depression to increased cholinergic activity. This hypothesis, although overly inclusive, did generate some useful research. Thus a cholinergic agonist such as arecholine, administered during sleep, was found to hasten the occurrence of REM sleep.[35] This finding may be related to the observation in patients with recurrent affective illness that REM latency is shorter than normal, although there are conflicting results as to whether this reflects a state or trait.[36]

CIRCADIAN RHYTHM DISTURBANCES IN MANIC-DEPRESSIVE ILLNESS

Many patients with manic-depressive illness, both the bipolar and recurrent unipolar forms, lead productive lives and work late hours, work in shifts, or are engaged in transmeridian travel. In addition to the intrinsic dysregulation of sleep–wake cycles and biological rhythms in such patients, these environmental challenges strain a fragile system, especially for bipolar patients. Because of the major potential of the sleep–wake cycle to disrupt mood stability in these patients, we introduce this section with a recommendation that both clinicians and patients be aware of these risks. The psychiatrist treating individuals who work nights or travel across meridians should either be well versed and current in the principles of treating abnormalities of circadian phase, jet lag, or shift work–related complaints, or consult with or refer to colleagues who are.

As outlined in the first edition of this volume, early clinical studies of circadian rhythms in depression carried out in England in the 1950s and 1960s were inspired by Lewis and Lobban's (1957) discovery that placing a subject on unusual schedules during the Arctic summer altered the relative timing of his or her various circadian rhythms. The English clinical studies (e.g., Lobban et al., 1963; Palmai and Blackwell, 1965) were designed to explore whether early-morning awakening in depressed individuals is related to an analogous but pathological internal phase disturbance. Early studies of circadian rhythms sometimes showed dramatic phase disturbances in depressive patients, but no consensus emerged about the significance and pattern of these changes. That situation appears to be changing.

Until the 1970s, normal circadian physiology remained largely unexplored, so that no context was available in which to place findings on depression. Investigative groups studying circadian rhythms were distant from one another, their studies widely separated in time. An initial fruitful period in the development of methodologies encompassing interactions between sleep and circadian systems in the clinical domain was followed by a period of relative stagnation (possible contributing factors are discussed later) and contradictory results. Given its complexity and cost, the gold standard, forced desynchrony,[37] has not been employed in this more recent work, so that some important questions about the physiology involved remain obscure. Simpler methods, such as constant routine,[38] raise ethical and clinical questions, as they usually involve loss of at least one night of sleep. Yet during this period of relative inactivity in the physiological realm, progress has been made in unraveling some of the molecular mechanisms underlying sleep and the circadian clock. Before discussing specific models of alterations in the timing of daily circadian rhythms and then possible homeostatic mechanisms, it is important to place circadian rhythm disturbances in a broader context. Figure 16–4 illustrates a hypothesized relationship among genetic vulnerability, stress, circadian rhythm disturbances, neurotransmitter–neuroendocrine immune dysregulation, and the symptoms of manic-depressive illness. The link between circadian rhythm disturbances and clinical symptoms (perhaps through neurotransmitter–neuroendocrine intermediaries) is, in our opinion, likely to be a closed loop, with rhythmic disturbances producing symptoms that reinforce or exacerbate abnormal rhythmic processes—or vice versa, the arrows of causation going in both directions. Also, we agree with those who have speculated that, with respect to affective disorders, the circadian biological clock provides an intriguing link between biological and psychosocial perspectives (Wehr and Goodwin 1983a; Ehlers et al., 1988, 1993).

Desynchrony and the Free-Running Hypothesis

As discussed earlier, circadian rhythms are synchronized with external zeitgebers (the most important being the light–dark cycle) and with each other. It is possible that recurrent affective illness is analogous to jet lag, with certain biological rhythms being desynchronized relative to sleep–wake cycles and to each other. Among the first hypotheses regarding abnormalities in the biological rhythms of depressed individuals was Georgi's (1947) suggestion that the rhythms are out of synchrony. Georgi proposed that the patient's own circadian rhythms are desynchronized either with one another (internal phase disorder) or with the entraining day–night cycle (external phase disorder). Later, Halberg (1968) formulated a more specific desynchronization hypothesis. He suggested that some circadian rhythms in affectively ill patients (particularly those with rapid cycles) may not be entrained to the 24-hour day–night cycle but free run, gradually going in and out of phase with other circadian rhythms that remain synchronized with the day–night cycle. According to Halberg, such phase disturbances leading to affective episodes (perhaps analogous to the "beat" phenomenon mentioned earlier) would occur periodically every few days or weeks. In support of Halberg's hypothesis, Kripke and colleagues (1978; Kripke, 1983) found that five of seven rapid-cycling bipolar patients had some circadian rhythms that appeared to free run with periods shorter than the 24-hour day–night cycle. Wehr's group (1985b) studied four patients (three bipolar, one unipolar) under free-running (isolation) conditions. One bipolar patient experienced an abnormally short intrinsic period, as predicted by the hypothesis of a fast circadian pacemaker. Unlike

Figure 16–4. Hypothesized relationship among genetic vulnerability, stress, circadian rhythm disturbances, neurotransmitter–neuroendocrine immune dysregulation, and the symptoms of manic-depressive illness.

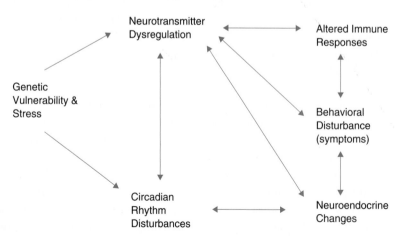

Kripke's and Wehr's groups, Pflug and colleagues (1983) failed to detect free-running circadian rhythms in patients living on normal schedules, that is, entrained to the environment. Follow-up studies on these initial observations are lacking.

The behavioral consequences of living under conditions without zeitgebers are not well understood; anecdotal accounts suggest that mood disturbances may occur (Kripke, 1983). In contrast, the few manic-depressive patients studied in isolation have, if anything, shown amelioration of depression. Thus, one of the three bipolar patients studied by Wehr and colleagues (1985b) switched into mania, and the unipolar patient improved. As proposed by Wehr and Goodwin (1983c) and Kripke (1983), stable depression may occur in patients in whom an overly fast, intrinsic pacemaker rhythm causes circadian rhythms to become abnormally but stably advanced relative to the day–night cycle. Cyclic depression, by contrast, may result from an overly fast rhythm that escapes from entrainment and free runs, advancing repeatedly through 360 degrees relative to the day–night cycle.

The possibility of free-running circadian rhythms has far-reaching implications for research on manic-depressive illness. Not only could such a mechanism drive the dramatic cyclicity observed in some bipolar and highly recurrent unipolar patients through the beat phenomenon (Wehr and Wirz-Justice, 1982), but it could also result in epiphenomena that are misinterpreted as biological correlates of changes in the mood cycle. If, for example, a biological variable is sampled at a fixed time of day, its level appears to change cyclically as the rhythm goes in and out of phase with the sampling time, even if its mean 24-hour level never changes.

Findings of longitudinal studies with hamsters indicate that some antidepressant drugs can slow certain intrinsic rhythms of circadian oscillators, and lead to lengthening of the sleep–wake cycle and a temporary escape from the primary mode of entrainment (Wehr and Wirz-Justice, 1982). Clinically, this drug effect may lead to the frequently recurring escapes and double-length (48-hour) sleep–wake cycles found naturalistically to be associated with switches into mania (Wehr et al., 1979, 1982). Most of these patients experienced 48-hour sleep–wake cycles at the beginning of each manic phase.[39] Based on carefully timed sleep deprivation experiments in patients with rapid cycles, Wehr and colleagues concluded that the insomnia associated with these 48-hour cycles probably helps trigger switches into mania or exacerbates switches that have just begun. Thus, a drug-induced slowing of the intrinsic rhythm of circadian oscillators, leading to more frequent escapes from the primary mode of entrainment, may be one mechanism underlying drug-induced rapid manic-depressive cycles. Studies using constant routine and forced desynchrony procedures

would be necessary to follow up on these initial studies, but have been precluded by ongoing obstacles, including the inherent difficulties and risks of these procedures, ethical considerations, and costs and funding priorities.

Abnormalities of Phase Position: The Phase-Advance Hypothesis

Briefly, this hypothesis is based on a desynchrony between the sleep–wake cycle, which stays in a normal or phase-delayed position, and other circadian rhythms, which tend to occupy a phase-advanced position. Just as jet lag (which is a mismatch between imposed sleep–wake rhythms at the destination and circadian rhythms, which tend to remain closer to the place of origin) manifests with fatigue, mood changes, and physical malaise, so, too, the desynchrony represents a perpetuating factor in individuals predisposed to depression.

In his original formulation of the desynchronization hypothesis, Georgi (1947) linked depression to a phase disturbance.[40] One initial explanation of circadian phase abnormality was shortened REM latency, a characteristic of some affectively ill patients discussed earlier. The link between the patterns of REM sleep and nonsleep circadian processes was made in 1964 by Maron and colleagues. The following year, in one of the first EEG studies of sleep in depressed patients, Gresham and colleagues (1965) found that the normal pattern of REM sleep was altered. Depressive patients had more REM sleep than controls in the first third of the night and less REM sleep in the last third of the night. Most subsequent EEG sleep studies of depression have been variations on this theme. All the changes in the temporal distribution of REM sleep in depressed patients[41] may result from a phase advance of the circadian rhythm governing the propensity for REM sleep. If the rhythm were advanced, its maximum, instead of occurring near dawn, would occur nearer to the beginning of sleep (Papoušek, 1975; Lewy et al., 1981; Wehr and Goodwin, 1981).

In addition to REM propensity, the circadian rhythms studied most extensively among nonseasonal depressed patients are those of temperature and plasma cortisol. In 1981, Wehr and Goodwin reviewed all of the studies in which the circadian pattern of a biological or physiological variable in depressed patients had been considered. They concluded that in the majority of studies, the phase position among the depressed patients (as reflected in the peak, nadir, or both) was variably advanced, generally occurring 1 to 4 hours earlier than in control subjects. In a review of the literature on circadian rhythms in nonseasonal depression, Souêtre (1990) found 80 studies involving a total of 1,061 patients and focusing on various measures, including cortisol, temperature, thyroid-stimulating hormone (TSH), melatonin, various neurotransmitter markers, heart rate, and motor activity. Taken together, the results of these studies suggest that phase-advanced rhythms are quite common, although there is considerable variability among individuals and studies. It is of interest that reports of a phase delay have been strikingly less frequent than would be expected by chance. One might conclude that circadian rhythms tend to be abnormal or unstable in affective illness, with a bias toward assuming a phase-advanced position some of the time (see the review of Duncan et al., 1996). In mania, Linkowski and colleagues (1994) showed an early timing of the nadir of cortisol.

In circadian phase interpretation, age must be controlled, since circadian abnormalities associated with aging have been reported. These abnormalities consist mainly of a phase advance of sleep and delay of temperature and melatonin rhythms compared with normal sleep (Duffy et al., 1998, 2002; Dijk et al., 2000). Other important variables are diagnostic: whether patients are unipolar or bipolar, and whether the disorder is cyclic (that is, highly recurrent) or relatively noncyclic. Thus Linkowski and colleagues (1985a,b) found a significant phase advance in the cortisol nadir among unipolar patients, but only a trend among bipolar patients.

One clinical antidepressant treatment that appears to support the phase-advance hypothesis (described in more detail later) is a sleep schedule manipulation that advances the time of morning wakening, producing a temporary antidepressant response in a significant proportion of patients with nonseasonal depression.[42] Figure 16–5 illustrates how depriving patients of sleep in the second half of the night or advancing their sleep might help synchronize the abnormally advanced rhythm of REM sleep, temperature, and cortisol with the oscillator controlling sleep and wakefulness. By advancing sleep (or eliminating its second half), the abnormal phase relationship in the second half of the night would be corrected.

Figure 16–5. Hypothesized correction of an abnormally advanced oscillator by partial sleep deprivation or phase-advance treatment. (*Source:* Wehr and Wirz-Justice, 1981.)

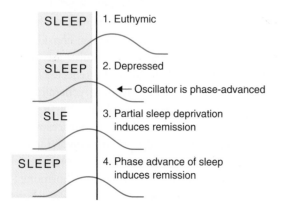

It would be consistent with the phase-advance hypothesis for the antidepressant effect of light to be observed with evening administration (delaying cortisol, melatonin, and temperature rhythms and thus realigning them with the sleep–wake rhythm), coupled with a worsening of depression with morning light (which should further advance circadian rhythms). However, it has been found that the timing of light administration in nonseasonal depression is unimportant to its effect (Yamada et al., 1995; Kripke, 1998; Wirz-Justice et al., 1999a) and further, that morning light, rather than being detrimental, is as effective as evening light (Yamada et al., 1995). Light therapy is discussed in more detail later in the chapter.

Riemann and colleagues (1996) compared an experimentally advanced (from 5 PM to 12 AM) sleep period with a normal (from 11 PM to 6 AM) sleep period in patients who had responded to total sleep deprivation. Two-thirds of subjects in the latter group relapsed after one night of sleep, while two-thirds of subjects in the former group did not. Thus phase advance of the sleep–wake cycle can prolong the antidepressant effect of sleep deprivation.[43] In a subsequent study, Riemann and colleagues (1999) compared the ability of sleep phase advance and sleep phase delay to preserve the antidepressant effects of total sleep deprivation. They hypothesized that sleep phase advance would be more effective in preventing relapse in responders to the treatment. Among their original sample of 54 depressed patients, 77.2 percent were found to be responders to total sleep deprivation and were randomized to either the phase-advance or phase-delay experimental condition. After 7 days, 75 percent of the sleep phase–advance patients were still stabilized, compared with only 40 percent of the sleep phase–delay patients. (See also the later section on therapeutic sleep deprivation.)

Phase Instability: Evidence from Longitudinal Studies of Temperature and REM Propensity

As reviewed in the first edition of this text, findings of a few longitudinal case studies suggest a dramatic correspondence between changes in the circadian temperature rhythm and manic-depressive cycling. In two cases (Pflug et al., 1976, 1981; Wehr and Wirz-Justice, 1982), the temperature rhythm was advanced by several hours during the switch into depression. In two other cases (Pflug et al., 1981), temperature rhythms were advanced, then later delayed during the course of depressive episodes. In three cases (Kripke et al., 1978), temperature rhythms were advanced continually through all phases of the manic-depressive cycle. Only one study monitored both sleep EEG and temperature in the same patient (Wehr and Wirz-Justice, 1982). In that study, before the patient switched into depression, advances occurred in the phase position of the temperature rhythm that were accompanied by advances in the temporal distribution of REM sleep within the sleep period. Although not inconsistent with a circadian rhythm, phase-advance model of depression, these data suggest that in cycling patients, the circadian phase position may be more related to the stage of the episode than to the state of depression or mania per se. Studying 65 inpatients with "various mental disorders" (half with major depression), Tsujimoto and colleagues (1990) found that 24-hour body temperature rhythm varied more widely in depressed and manic patients than in normal controls or schizophrenic patients.

Apparent instability of phase position may also characterize depression in noncycling patients. In studies of mixed groups of unipolar and bipolar depressed patients, Wehr and Goodwin (1983c) and Kripke (1983) found a bimodal distribution in the time of the temperature minimum, with many of the patients experiencing both modes (early and late) when sampled on different days. Thus there may be, on the one hand, a certain phase instability inherent to depression, perhaps reflecting poor entrainment by environmental zeitgebers, and, on the other hand, a phase instability linked to shifting phases of bipolar illness. Since the stability of a circadian system is positively correlated with amplitude (Aschoff and Wever, 1980; Wever, 1980), we next consider the amplitude of circadian rhythms in affective disorders.

Amplitude of Circadian Rhythms: The Temperature Dysregulation Hypothesis

As reviewed by Duncan (1996), an elevated nocturnal temperature is frequently reported in depressed patients, while increased diurnal temperature and a blunted circadian amplitude are sometimes noted. Schulz and Lund (1985, pp. 70–71) hypothesized that alterations in the timing of REM sleep could be explained by a "flattening of the arousal cycle. . . . [I]ndicators of this hypothetical arousal cycle are measures of subjective sleepiness and body core temperature." The authors based this hypothesis on their earlier finding (Schulz and Lund, 1983) that subjects with sleep-onset REM periods (perhaps reflecting phase-advanced REM) had significantly reduced amplitude of the circadian temperature curve (peak-to-trough difference) compared with those without such periods. The findings of research on the amplitude of the temperature rhythm in depressed patients are inconsistent, perhaps reflecting differences in the populations of "depressed" patients studied. Thus elevated nocturnal temperature is reported by some authors, whereas blunting of or no change in the temperature rhythm is noted by others.[44]

A variety of antidepressant treatments, including tricyclic antidepressants, ECT, bright light, sleep deprivation, and phase-advance treatment, have been reported to increase

circadian amplitudes of temperature, cortisol, or TSH in patients. More recently, experimentally lengthening the duration of the dark period has been shown to increase the amplitude of circadian rhythms and been proposed as one of the plausible theoretical premises for the application of extended rest and darkness in the treatment of rapid-cycling bipolar illness (Wehr et al., 1998), as described in more detail below.

If relatively low-amplitude rhythms were somehow intrinsic to recurrent depression or bipolar illness, one would expect such rhythms to be more vulnerable to perturbation by internal or external influences, since the stability of a circadian system is positively correlated with amplitude (Aschoff and Wever, 1980; Wever, 1980). Not only do the frequency and timing of environmental zeitgebers vary considerably under normal conditions, but the dramatic behavioral shifts associated with manic-depressive illness (especially the bipolar subgroup) also multiply this variability. Thus, blunted amplitudes associated with affective disorder would be expected to be associated with phase instability. For example, using actigraphic recordings, Jones and colleagues (2005) have demonstrated that bipolar patients, even in recovery, have less stable and more variable circadian activity patterns than normal controls. This decreased stability/increased variability in activity patterns has recently been reported among individuals deemed to be at risk for bipolar disorder as defined by a threshold score on the Hypomanic Personality Scale (Meyer and Maier 2006).

One explanation for decreased circadian amplitude is poor entrainment by external zeitgebers (Aschoff and Wever, 1981), as observed in normal individuals isolated from time cues under free-running conditions. Such reduced or irregular entrainment—initially the consequence of depression (due, e.g., to loss of social zeitgebers during withdrawal)—could then feed the depression through the resulting disturbance in rhythms (Ehlers et al., 1988).

In this context, it is necessary to consider a paradox. Lewy and colleagues (1981, 1985) found that, compared with normal controls, bipolar (but apparently not unipolar) patients (Cummings et al., 1989; Lam et al., 1990) are supersensitive to light, as reflected by a lower threshold required to reduce nighttime plasma melatonin levels; moreover, this supersensitivity appears to be state independent. However in a subsequent study of euthymic bipolar patients subjected to a 500 lux light between 2 AM and 4 AM on one night and left in the dark for a comparable time period on another night, no group-level differences in melatonin suppression were found among the bipolar group, the unipolar group, and controls (Nurnberger et al., 2000). While the hypothesis that bipolar patients have an increased sensitivity to light was not confirmed, abnormalities in melatonin secretion were found in the bipolar-I subgroup.[45]

If increased sensitivity to light is a trait marker of at least some bipolar patients, how can one posit decreased entrainment of zeitgebers? First, although light is indeed important to entrainment, it is hardly the only influence, since activity and temperature are important as well. Second, one could view the increased sensitivity to light as compensatory, that is, an attempt to offset the reduced entrainment due to either the compromising of other zeitgebers (e.g., activity) by the illness or an intrinsic defect in the clock mechanism. The latter possibility is particularly interesting in light of evidence that monkeys with lesions in the SCN can compensate by becoming more sensitive to certain zeitgebers (Van Cauter and Turek, 1986). The inverse relationship is also possible: that the phase instability is primary, producing the appearance of low amplitude when individual data are averaged for a group. We might refer to this as a smearing effect. In the extreme, if individuals' phase positions were randomly distributed along the time axis, the group mean would exhibit no circadian rhythm. If the group-average pattern were simply smeared by interindividual variability, the average amplitude for the group would appear to be decreased (Wehr and Goodwin, 1983c).

The preceding discussion is relevant only to phase instability. What about the apparent tendency for this instability in phase position to express itself as a phase advance? One situation that might produce both instability and a bias toward advance would be a clock with an intrinsic period length of about 24 hours—faster than the normal period of the rest–activity cycle in humans when measured under free-running conditions, which, as noted earlier, is longer than 24 hours in the majority of individuals. Findings of basic research on the factors that determine circadian phase position under conditions of entrainment (Pittendrigh and Daan, 1976; Wever, 1979) indicate that the faster the intrinsic period of the pacemaker or clock, the earlier its phase position relative to the entraining schedule—that is, it is relatively phase advanced. Furthermore, if the intrinsic period of the clock is just fast enough so that it happens to coincide with the external day–night cycle (i.e., 24 hours), it might be expected to wobble, that is, to be unstable. This is the case because under normal conditions, the intrinsic period is slower than 24 hours, a discrepancy that produces constant tension in the system: the 24-hour environmental light–dark cycle continuously pulls backward the intrinsic 25-hour clock. This constant tug of the environment on the internal circadian mechanisms would be expected to provide stability. Under conditions in which the intrinsic period of the clock is very close to the external day–night cycle, little or no tug or tension exists, and the clock is free to wobble. This mechanism would link the

evidence of a faster-than-normal clock in some patients with the findings of phase instability and the tendency toward advance.

As discussed in the first edition of this text, another possible explanation for phase advance is an increased sensitivity to zeitgebers. Given that in humans the intrinsic period of the circadian pacemaker is slower than that of the day–night cycle, environmental zeitgebers tend to pull the pacemaker closer to 24 hours, and a pacemaker that is more sensitive to zeitgebers might be expected to assume a relatively more advanced phase position (Wever, 1979). Relevant to this observation is the finding just noted—that in some studies, bipolar patients apparently have an increased sensitivity to light, which appears to be independent of the state of illness.[46] It is important to mention, however, that melatonin suppression by light is not equivalent to phase shifting by light, and future phase-shifting experiments are needed to sort this out. Obviously, the many gaps and even some apparent contradictions in the circadian literature preclude a complete synthesis. Clinical heterogeneity is a major confounding variable and may well explain apparent contradictions.

Throughout this discussion, we have referred, explicitly or implicitly, to the concept of a closed loop involving the circadian system and the phenomenology (and biochemistry) of depressive and manic episodes. We return to this subject here because it remains the most significant conceptual challenge in interpreting the circadian literature. Until we have more data from manic-depressive patients studied under forced desynchrony, we will be unable to answer the question of whether a disturbance in the function of the circadian clock is primary, and therefore driving the symptoms, or is itself simply a physiological symptom secondary to the large shifts in mood, sleep, and behavior that characterize the illness. This possibility deserves further consideration in light of evidence showing that behavioral arousal may feed back directly to the circadian pacemaker's behavior (Mrosovsky, 1988).

Mood Stabilizers and Circadian Rhythms

As reviewed in Chapter 20, lithium is effective in reducing cycling in bipolar as well as highly recurrent unipolar depression. This reduction in cycling is not immediate, nor is it immediately lost upon discontinuation of treatment. On the other hand, patients who are abruptly discontinued from lithium are at an elevated risk for increased cycling and shifting into hypomania/mania.

Lithium modifies the period and phase of circadian rhythms in species ranging from unicellular organisms to insects, mice, and humans (Klemfuss, 1992; Healy and Waterhouse, 1995; Klemfuss and Kripke, 1995). These effects, which might be considered analogous to the effects of lithium on mood cycling, are achieved with clinically meaningful doses and do not occur immediately after initiation of the drug—as with its clinical effects, there is a lag. Most consistently, lithium lengthens the free-running circadian period across species, from single cells to whole organisms.[47] Also, there have been some reports of period-lengthening effects in normal volunteers under free-running conditions,[48] as well as phase-delayed rhythms in humans living on a 24-hour schedule (Kupfer et al., 1970; Mendels and Chernik, 1973; Kripke, 1983), which may reflect a lengthening of the period of the circadian oscillator.[49]

How do mood stabilizers affect the previously discussed increased sensitivity of melatonin secretion to light in some bipolar patients? In the original studies, the increased sensitivity was reported to be greatest in patients who were medication free for at least 5 weeks, while in those taking lithium, the sensitivity was not different from that of healthy controls (Nurnberger et al., 2000). This finding is consistent with lithium's reduction of the melatonin-suppressive effect of light in healthy volunteers (Hallam et al., 2005a). Valproate has also been reported recently to reduce melatonin suppression by light in healthy volunteers (Hallam et al., 2005b). The potent mood-stabilizing effects of both lithium and valproate could, at the very least, be partially explained by their chronobiological effects, as inhibition of suppression of melatonin by light could result in an altered circadian period (specifically, a prolonged period) and thus changes in alignment between sleep–wake and biological day–night.

Clock Genes and Bipolar Disorder

As noted briefly above, certain clock genes have been associated with circadian rhythm sleep disorders[50]; examples are *PER3* (Ebisawa et al., 2001; Archer et al., 2003; Pereira et al., 2005) and *CSNK1* (Takano et al., 2004) in delayed sleep-phase syndrome, and the *PER2* gene in familial advanced sleep-phase syndrome (Toh et al., 2001). Recently, linkage to and association with bipolar disorder have been examined for 10 circadian genes (*ARNTL, CLOCK, CRY2, CSNK1, DBP, GSK3β, NPAS2, PER1, PER2,* and *PER3* (Nievergelt et al., 2005). Linkage analysis in 52 affected families revealed suggestive evidence for linkage to *CSNK1*, but this was not confirmed in an association study of 185 parent–proband triads. Through single-gene permutation tests, haplotypes in *ARNTL* and *PER3* were found to be significantly associated with bipolar disorder, the strongest association being with *PER3*. Because, as noted above, *PER3* has also been associated with circadian rhythm sleep disorder, this may represent an underlying mechanism for circadian abnormalities in bipolar disorder, as well as

overlapping features between delayed sleep disorders and bipolar disorder (Nievergelt et al., 2005). Ultimately, as Bunney and Bunney (2000) hypothesized, the circadian rhythm abnormalities in major depression and SAD may be due to altered clock genes, and genetic knowledge and technology may now be advanced enough to enable exploration of this hypothesis directly in patients. Similarly, the discovery of melanopsin[51] as an important molecule in circadian photo-transmission is very recent, and clinical applications of this discovery can now be anticipated. (See the Web site for this volume for further information on genetic contributions to abnormalities of sleep.)

Other (Noncircadian) Mechanisms of Sleep Disturbance in Affective Disorders

The previously discussed cholinergic–aminergic hypothesis postulates that increased REM latency is secondary to increased activity of a REM excitatory cholinergic mechanism. This increased activity is accompanied by decreased activity in REM inhibitory aminergic mechanisms (including serotonin-containing raphe neurons, norepinephrine-containing neurons of the locus ceruleus, and histamine-containing neurons of the mammilary body).

Also as discussed earlier, the two-process model posits that the onset and maintenance of sleep are regulated by the interaction of process s, which represents a need for NREM sleep (measurable with delta power in sleep EEG), and process c, which reflects the circadian variation in the threshold for the onset of sleep (van den Hoofdakker and Beersma, 1985). The antidepressant effect of sleep deprivation may result from increased sleep pressure (process s) during prolonged wakefulness. In the future, it may be of interest to measure sleep pressure using theta waves in the waking EEG (Aeschbach et al., 1999) rather than delta waves during sleep.

EXPERIMENTAL ALTERATIONS OF SLEEP AND OTHER BIOLOGICAL RHYTHMS IN AFFECTIVE ILLNESS

One important clinical advantage of the circadian and sleep therapies listed in Table 16–1 is their shorter time lag compared with drugs or psychotherapy (Wirz-Justice et al., 2005). Box 16–1 presents the recommendations of the Committee on Chronotherapeutics in Affective Disorders of the International Society for Affective Disorders with regard to such therapies.

Despite their advantages, the current research effort on chronobiological interventions is less than what might be expected from the richness of the early findings in the field. Commenting on the relative lack of research interest even

TABLE 16–1. **Circadian and Sleep Therapies for Major Depression**

Therapy	Therapeutic Latency	Response Duration
Total sleep deprivation (TSD)	Hours	~1 day
Partial sleep deprivation (PSD) (2nd half of the night)	Hours	~1 day
Repeated TSD or PSD	Hours	Days/weeks
Repeated TSD or PSD with antidepressants	Hours	Weeks/months
Phase advance of the sleep–wake cycle	~3 days	1–2 weeks
TSD followed by sleep phase advance	Hours	1–2 weeks
Single or repeated TSD or PSD followed by light therapy	Hours	Weeks
Single or repeated TSD or PSD followed by phase advance and light therapy	Hours	Weeks
Single or repeated TSD or PSD combined with lithium, pindolol, or SSRIs	Hours	Months
Light therapy (winter seasonal MDD)	Days	Weeks/months
Light therapy (nonseasonal MDD)	Weeks	Weeks/months
Light therapy with SSRIs (nonseasonal MDD)	1–2 weeks	Weeks/months
Dark or rest therapy (for rapid cycling or mania)	Days	Throughout maintenance of treatment

MDD = major depressive disorder; SSRI = selective serotonin reuptake inhibitor.
Source: Wirz-Justice et al., 2005. Reprinted with permission from Cambridge University Press.

in the most dramatically effective of such interventions—sleep deprivation—Wirz-Justice (2005) wrote:

> In our opinion, two factors may be responsible for the current lack of interest [in sleep deprivation]. First, considerable relapses were frequently observed after recovery sleep. Second, the dominance of pharmacology and neurochemistry in research on pathogenesis and therapy of psychiatric disorders may be responsible. It is difficult to obtain funding for non-pharmacological and non-neurochemical clinical research (the same is true for another efficacious antidepressant modality, light treatment). Nevertheless, the rapidity and the magnitude of the clinical changes brought about by [sleep deprivation] and sleep still remain highly intriguing and may provide clues for understanding the pathophysiology of depression. In fact, it is surprising that no pharmaceutical company has focused on this model in the search for that

much-needed rapid-acting antidepressant; don't clinicians want a drug that works within a day?

Therapeutic Sleep Deprivation

After observing the effects of sleep on severely depressed patients, clinicians have from time to time concluded independently that sleep itself exacerbates depression. Ostenfeld (1986) reported that this clinical observation was one of several that led him to try iatrogenic asomnia to treat a manic-depressive patient in 1954 at a time when ECT was the only available treatment known to be effective. Since then, investigators using sleep deprivation and many other experimental manipulations of sleep have produced a body of evidence suggesting that the dramatic changes in the timing and duration of sleep during manic and depressive episodes are not mere epiphenomena.

It is now well established that total sleep deprivation (Pflug and Tölle, 1971) and, in some studies, even partial sleep deprivation in the second half of the night (Schilgen and Tölle, 1980) can induce temporary remissions in depressed unipolar and bipolar patients.[52] In their meta-analysis, Wu and Bunney (1990) reported that 50–60 percent of patients showed a temporary improvement in mood following total sleep deprivation, with 80 percent sinking back into depression after one night of sleep. Indeed, as noted earlier, even a nap has been found to result in relapse of depressed mood in 50 percent of patients (Wiegand et al., 1987), with morning naps being more detrimental than those in the afternoon (Weigand et al., 1993). This rapid loss of efficacy may help explain why interest in sleep deprivation in the United States has lagged behind that in Europe despite the treatment's established therapeutic

value. Wehr and Sack (1988, p. 208) emphasized the importance of sleep deprivation studies:

> The single most important argument that sleep is an important factor in mental illness is the observation that sleep deprivation rapidly induces remissions in the majority of depressed patients, and induces mania in bipolar patients, and that recovery sleep after sleep deprivation rapidly induces depression in the majority of patients who have responded to sleep deprivation.

Are there differences between unipolar and bipolar patients in the efficacy and safety of response to sleep deprivation? From the occasionally dramatic mania-inducing effect of losing one night of sleep, one might presume a more intense effect in bipolar patients. Indeed, Barbini and colleagues (1998) reported that bipolar patients had a greater response than unipolar depressed patients to three cycles of total sleep deprivation and, contrary to some expectations, that no unipolar patient switched to bipolar during the treatment. It is not known, however, what proportion of the unipolar group had the more recurrent forms of unipolar depression (which in some patients may be associated with a diathesis for bipolar disorder). Another intriguing observation of this study is that subjective ratings of mood (on visual analogue scales) improved only in the bipolar group.

A large study of 206 bipolar depressed patients who underwent three nights of sleep deprivation alternated with three nights of sleep (Colombo et al., 1999) found that the risk of switch into mania was 4.85 percent and into hypomania was 5.83 percent (the rate of antidepressant response was not reported). Initial estimates suggested a risk of one in four bipolar patients, but these estimates were based on a small population of patients with a history of rapid cycling, a subgroup especially vulnerable to mood switches.

In general, there is a feed-forward relationship between sleep deprivation and mania in bipolar patients (the mania maintaining insomnia and arousal) (Wehr et al., 1987), in contrast to a feedback relationship between sleep deprivation and fatigue (causing sleepiness) in nonbipolar depressed patients. Lenox and colleagues (2002) hypothesized the response to sleep deprivation to be a genetically heritable condition and possibly an endophenotype of bipolar illness (Lenox et al., 2002).

Predictors of response to sleep deprivation include diurnal variation in mood, with spontaneous improvement in mood occurring in the afternoon and evening hours (Reinink et al., 1990); increased diurnal variation in mood independent of the direction (Reinink et al., 1993); decreased REM latency (Riemann et al., 1991), which normalizes after sleep deprivation (Duncan et al., 1980; Riemann and Berger, 1990); and "endogenous" rather than "reactive" or "neurotic" features of depression (Wu and Bunney, 1990). Gender, age, previous hospitalizations, severity of depression, and duration of depressive episodes do not predict response to sleep deprivation (Kuhs and Tölle, 1991). The less tired (Bouhuys et al., 1995) and more aroused a patient is prior to sleep deprivation (Van Den Burg et al., 1992), the better is his or her response to the treatment. As noted earlier, some but not all studies have found a greater response in bipolar than in unipolar patients, but the clinical features just reviewed are generally not controlled for in these comparisons.

If neither placebo nor gross confounding factors account for the effects of sleep deprivation, could the explanation be as simple as the fatigue disinhibiting brain sites that modulate the expression of depressive affect or inhibiting centers that mediate depressive affect? In fact, this is the essence of a hypothesis that the influence of some subcortical areas having both an alerting and a depressogenic effect is decreased in parallel with the fatigue induced by sleep deprivation (Van Den Berg et al., 1992; Bouhuys et al., 1995).

As to the question of what underlying neuroanatomical structures are involved in the effects of sleep deprivation, brain imaging studies have indicated that increased activity is found in the orbitofrontal cortex and anterior cingulate prior to sleep deprivation in patients who respond to the treatment, but not in nonresponders,[53] and that improvement in mood parallels a decrease in blood flow in these areas.[54] Mayberg and colleagues (1997) found that the ventral anterior cingulate cortex was activated in association with an antidepressant response to total sleep deprivation.[55] The anterior cingulate cortex appears to play a major role in affective regulation and cognition (Devinsky et al., 1995) and in depression (Drevets et al., 1997; Drevets, 1999).

Earlier in our discussion of the regulation of sleep, we briefly considered some of the mechanisms that may underlie the antidepressant effect of sleep deprivation. First, could it simply be a placebo effect? While this possibility cannot be ruled out, it appears unlikely given that the usual expectations of the patient being deprived of sleep tend to be negative (van den Hoofdakker, 1997).[56] Numerous factors, such as light exposure, body posture, and motor activity, are confounded with sleep deprivation, but they do not appear to be major contributors to its antidepressant effect (van den Hoofdakker, 1997).

Regarding molecular mechanisms, the cholinergic hypothesis of sleep discussed earlier appears to offer an attractive explanation of the effects of sleep deprivation because the cingulate receives cholinergic projections from the basal forebrain; however, there are as yet no direct data on cholinergic mechanisms in sleep deprivation. Data do exist that suggest the involvement of both serotonergic and dopaminergic pathways in the effects of sleep deprivation.

Implicating serotonin, Benedetti and colleagues (1999b) reported better mood amelioration with sleep deprivation in subjects with the long variant of 5-HTT-linked polymorphisms, associated with increased density of the 5-HT transporter. Moreover, sleep deprivation increases brain serotonin turnover in rats (Asikainen et al., 1997) and increases firing in the serotonergic neurons in the raphe (Gardner et al., 1997). In bipolar patients, pindolol, a 5-HT_{1A} autoreceptor blocker (which blocks the receptor that puts the break on the release of serotonin, thereby enhancing serotonin release) was found to increase the antidepressant response to sleep deprivation and decrease the tendency to relapse after the procedure (Smeraldi et al., 1999). It appears that the role of serotonin in the effects of sleep deprivation is complex, and some of the data are conflicting. In one study, for example, sleep deprivation in rats resulted in reduced rather than increased serotonin and 5-HIAA in the frontal cortex (Borbely et al., 1980). And not only did Neumeister and colleagues (1998a,b,c) fail to find a hypothesized blocking of the effects of sleep deprivation with tryptophan depletion (which decreases brain serotonin), but they also noted that tryptophan depletion could actually block relapses back into depression.

Gerner and colleagues (1979) reported increased concentrations of homovallic acid (HVA), a metabolite of dopamine, in the cerebrospinal fluid of responders to sleep deprivation, but not in nonresponders (Gerner et al., 1979). Related to this finding is that of Ebert and colleagues (1994): compared with nonresponders, responders had significantly greater displacement of a ligand for the D2 receptor after sleep deprivation, a result suggesting dopamine receptor activation. Rigidity, bradykinesia, and gait disorder improve in patients with Parkinson's disease after therapeutic sleep deprivation (Demet et al., 1999), which could also reflect enhanced dopamine function (alternatively, it could reflect an anticholinergic effect of sleep deprivation). However, other studies have failed to find an association between sleep deprivation and dopamine enhancement. For example, Benedetti and colleagues (1996) reported that a dopamine receptor agonist (stimulant) blocks rather than enhances the effects of sleep deprivation. Thus the involvement of dopamine receptor regulation in the clinical effects of sleep deprivation is probably complex. Can sleep deprivation be considered analogous to the effect of an antidepressant drug? Given the rapidity of onset as well as the transient nature of the antidepressant effect of sleep deprivation compared with the lag and the more sustained response seen with antidepressants, a more reasonable pharmacological analogy might be with psychostimulants, whose effect on dopamine (enhancing release from presynaptic stores) is both immediate and relatively short-lived (Ebert and Berger, 1998).[57]

It has been speculated that the therapeutic effect of sleep deprivation does not depend on the loss of sleep per se but is associated with not being asleep in the second half of the night. Thus Sack and colleagues (1988) compared the effects of an equivalent amount of sleep loss (4 hours) in either the first or second half of the night. Improvement was associated only with the latter. Because REM sleep is distributed predominantly in the second half of the night, this finding led to speculation that sleep deprivation may act by suppressing REM sleep.[58] Indeed, Vogel and colleagues (1980) deprived patients of REM sleep with selective nocturnal awakenings over a 3-week period and found that a 50 percent reduction in REM sleep had a significant antidepressant effect. However, REM deprivation alone cannot account for the immediate effects of sleep deprivation, since it usually requires several weeks to produce an antidepressant effect.

Combinations of sleep deprivation and other treatment options have been attempted to either extend the duration of mood improvement gained through sleep deprivation alone or augment or hasten the effect of the other treatments. For example, total sleep deprivation was found to hasten the effect of fluoxetine in treating major depression (Benedetti et al., 1997). Another treatment with antidepressant effects—bright light (but not dim light), discussed in more detail later—was used to maintain the beneficial effects of sleep deprivation in patients with major depression (Neumeister et al., 1996). In this context, it is of interest that response to sleep deprivation predicts response to light therapy in both seasonal and nonseasonal depression (Fritzsche

et al., 2001). In bipolar depressed patients, Colombo and colleagues (2000) found that light treatment in combination with lithium maintained the improvement in self-reported mood achieved with total sleep deprivation.[59] This finding is consistent with that of Smeraldi and colleagues (1999) that lithium successfully stabilized the antidepressant effect of sleep deprivation for 3 months in 13 of 20 bipolar patients (versus a stable antidepressant effect of sleep deprivation in only 2 of 20 patients not on lithium) (Smeraldi et al., 1999).

An obvious question is whether sleep deprivation in bipolar patients will precipitate mania or hypomania or increase mood cycling. Although the Committee on Chronotherapeutics of the International Society for Affective Disorders concluded that the rates of switch into mania or hypomania are similar to those associated with the newer antidepressants (Colombo et al., 1999; Wirz-Justice et al., 2005), we would recommend caution in the use of this treatment for bipolar-I patients, especially those with a history of rapid cycling (or an otherwise unstable course) and/or a history of psychotic mania. And, of course, sleep deprivation should not be undertaken unless and until the patient is on a mood stabilizer—the same recommendation we make with respect to the initiation of antidepressants.

As noted earlier, in addition to sleep deprivation, advancing the entire sleep period by 4–6 hours (sleep phase advance) has been shown to produce antidepressant effects, further suggesting that the effects of sleep deprivation may depend less on the amount of sleep than on its timing. These relationships are illustrated in Figure 16–6. In contrast with sleep deprivation, the improvement seen

Figure 16–6. Relationship between the timing of sleep and the antidepressant effect of sleep deprivation. (*Source*: Wehr and Goodwin, 1981.)

than SD.

with ongoing sleep phase advance is more stable. One possible explanation for the efficacy of sleep phase advance is a realignment of the sleep–wake cycle with other circadian endogenous rhythms, such as cortisol and temperature, which tend to occupy a phase-advanced position in major depression.

Initiating sleep phase advance (Sack et al., 1985) in the evening following total sleep deprivation (as it is easier to fall asleep at 5 PM after a night without sleep) maintains the antidepressant effect of sleep deprivation in a proportion comparable to that of treatment with antidepressant medication.[60] Benedetti and colleagues (2001a) observed that, compared with unmedicated patients, those taking lithium showed greater improvement with a combination of total sleep deprivation and sleep phase advance. The authors explained their results as a double action to realign sleep–wake with other biological rhythms, the sleep phase advance bringing sleep earlier and lithium delaying the metabolic rhythms.

Extended Rest–Dark Period as a Treatment for Rapid Cycling

Given the above-noted vulnerability of bipolar patients to sleep deprivation and their apparently increased sensitivity to light (Wehr et al., 1993; Wehr, 1996), the modern use of artificial light into the nighttime may be detrimental for bipolar patients as it may modify the duration and timing of sleep, thus altering circadian rhythms. Wehr and colleagues (1998) attempted to stabilize a bipolar patient who was rapidly cycling despite being on mood stabilizers by depriving him of light for 14 hours (keeping him in the dark from 8 PM to 6 AM) each night for several weeks. His highly unstable mood and sleep cycles were stabilized (Wehr et al., 1998).[61] Another group reported on a treatment-resistant rapidly cycling bipolar patient in whom extended darkness and bedrest for 10 hours resulted in immediate mood stabilization, initially in the depressed range and then, following the addition of midday light treatment, in the euthymic range (Wirz-Justice and van den Hoofdakker, 1999; Wirz-Justice et al., 1999a,b).[62]

Interpersonal and Social Rhythm Therapy

Frank and colleagues (2000) built on the intimate relationships among mood, the circadian system, and the sleep–wake cycle, as described in the first edition of this text, to design interpersonal and social rhythm therapy (IPSRT). The central concept of IPSRT is that a manic switch is often preceded by a disruptive social event, such as death and bereavement, which may entail a combination of psychosocial challenge, threat or loss, and sleep deprivation (Wehr and Goodwin, 1983b; Malkoff-Schwartz et al., 1998; Ashman et al., 1999).[63] IPSRT is discussed in Chapter 22.

SEASONAL RHYTHMS AND RECURRENT AFFECTIVE DISORDERS

> Melancholy occurs in autumn whereas mania in summer.
> —*Posidonius, fourth century*

> Repeatedly I saw in these cases moodiness set in autumn and pass over in spring, "when the sap shoots in the trees," to excitement, corresponding in a certain sense to the emotional changes which come over even healthy individuals at the changes of the seasons.
> —*Emil Kraepelin, 1921, p. 139*

> [T]he gloom of the Arctic night sets in, and although the Eskimos spent their time telling stories and legends and tried hard to amuse us, I could notice a depression among ourselves, as well as among the people . . . that reached its climax at Christmas . . . we were all very blue.
> —*Frederick A. Cook, M.D, Surgeon to the Peary Arctic Expedition, 1894*

The clinical lore surrounding affective disorders has alluded to their seasonal nature since ancient times. Seasonal trends emerge in the epidemiology of populations of patients, and seasonal patterns become evident in the course of manic-depressive illness in individual patients. Onsets of episodes tend to cluster in the spring and fall, especially among those prone to annual recurrences. As Wehr and Rosenthal (1989) pointed out, these patterns imply that environmental changes can both cause and ameliorate episodes of affective illness.

Nineteenth-century psychiatrists, unlike those of today, had the opportunity to observe the course of untreated manic-depressive illness for long periods (see Chapter 1). Several leading psychiatrists of the era[64] recorded many cases in which the pattern of recurrence was seasonal. In one pattern, depressions began in spring and summer. In another, the onset of depression occurred in fall or winter, while mania or hypomania appeared in the summer. These patterns also emerge in longitudinal data published by Baastrup and Schou (1967) in their now-classic lithium studies and by Kukopulos and Reginaldi (1973). Analysis of the frequency distribution of the cycle lengths of episodes drawn from a longitudinal study of 105 bipolar patients (Zis and Goodwin, 1979) shows a very large peak at 12 months, with smaller peaks at subsequent multiples of 12 (see Fig. 16–7). Although reporting bias may account for some of these findings, it is probably not sufficient to explain the magnitude of the seasonal effect.

Slater (1938) was the first to apply systematic statistical analysis to the study of seasonal patterns among manic-depressive patients. He noted that for each patient, recurrences were significantly more likely to occur at the same

Figure 16–7. Seasonal variation in the length of the photoperiod and in its rate of change: relationship to seasonal peaks in depression, mania, and suicide. (*Source*: Zis and Goodwin, 1979.)

time of the year than at random; that is, variability in the month of onset for any one patient was less than half the variability among patients. The study of seasonality did not resurface in the literature for nearly half a century. In the early 1980s, Goodwin's group at NIMH (Rosenthal et al., 1985) identified a specific syndrome—winter depression, one form of SAD—which since that time has been investigated extensively in the United States, Europe, Great Britain, Australia, and South America. In 1984, Rosenthal and colleagues studied recurrent winter depressions, often with summer hypomania, and published the original criteria for SAD.

Wehr and Rosenthal (1989) attributed the long hiatus in psychiatric interest in seasonality to changing fashions in theory—from the ancient humoral theories emphasizing seasonal influences to contemporary theories stressing internal psychological and biological processes. Another possible reason for the neglect may be that modern life had so shielded psychiatric observers from environmental influences that they no longer considered seasonal patterns, which in addition had become obscured by modern treatments. The authors also noted that both psychiatrists and patients may have been inclined to see episodes of affective illness as linear rather than cyclical, a shift in thinking about time that may be general in modern culture.

Physiological Mechanisms Involved in Seasonality in Mammals

Seasons are the result of the combined action of the tilted axis of the earth and its movement around the sun, which cause changes in the duration of day (photoperiod) and night (scotoperiod) with a period of 1 year. The magnitude of photoperiodic changes, as well as climatic seasonal changes (temperature, humidity, skycover, and rainfall), is directly related to latitude. Numerous species experience marked seasonal changes in physiology and behavior. Many have developed specialized neuronal circuits that detect, store, anticipate, and respond to changes in day length. Photoperiodic organisms use both absolute measures of day length and direction of day-length change to regulate their seasonal changes (see Goldman's [2001] review of mammalian photoperiodic systems). There are variations in photoperiodic responses among species, among breeding populations within species, and among individuals within single breeding populations (Goldman, 2001). This point is particularly important for understanding SAD, as individual humans differ markedly with regard to seasonality.

The SCN are not only the master circadian pacemaker (as discussed earlier) but also the central neuronal structure involved in seasonal responses (Moore, 1996a,b). Destruction of the SCN abolishes photoperiodic responses (Schwartz et al., 2001b). SCN neurons have a higher firing rate during the daytime and less intense firing during the night, with sharp transitions around dusk and dawn, a pattern that persists in hypothalamic slices and dissociated cell cultures under constant conditions (Schwartz et al., 2001b). To understand seasonality, it is important to know that the duration of diurnal firing under constant conditions reflects the day length to which the animal has previously been exposed—shorter when the previous daylength was shorter, longer when it was longer (Mrugala et al., 2000). This suggests that the SCN cells "remember" the previous photoperiod to which they have been exposed (Jac et al., 2000a,b). Photoperiod-induced changes in melatonin secretion, as well as in SCN firing rate and other output markers of SCN activity, are ultimately determined by temporally sequenced gene expression (Hastings et al., 2001).

Pittendrigh and Daan (1976) proposed that the mammalian pacemaker consists of a morning "oscillator" (M) locking on to dawn and an evening oscillator (E) locking on to "dusk," and that these two oscillators may be used to measure day length and adjust seasonal timing (Schwartz et al., 2001a,b). Information on day length reaches the SCN via the retinohypothalamic tract, and it modifies the duration of firing of the SCN neurons. The axons of the SCN neurons inhibit the firing of the paraventricular neurons in the hypothalamus. If uninhibited, the paraventricular neurons stimulate (via a multisynaptic pathway) the secretion of melatonin by the pineal glad.[65] Thus SCN firing ultimately results in inhibition of melatonin secretion. The duration of day length is encoded in the duration of increased SCN firing and then in the duration of time without melatonin secretion. Therefore, seasonal information starts with clock information and is then transformed into hormonal information—the duration of melatonin secretion—which in turn conveys seasonal information to other hypothalamic hormonal systems and to other organs and tissues (Malpaux et al., 1998; Morgan et al., 1999).

To what degree have these mechanisms persisted in humans? Wehr (2001) discussed this topic in detail in his review of photoperiodism in humans and other primates. He reported that neuroanatomical and physiological elements that mediate seasonality in mammals (described above) are preserved in humans. Human reproduction is not seasonal in the sense of being confined to a distinct period of the year as it is in many other mammals, including some other primates. However, it has been shown that human reproduction has a distinct seasonal variation.[66] This variation has both cultural and biological components (perhaps reflecting evolutionary forces), which would tend to shut off reproduction at certain times of the year, especially in females (Davis and Levitan, 2005).

Some humans manifest changes with season that are similar to those seen in photoperiodic mammals (animals that show marked changes in behavior in response to changes in day length, both under naturalistic conditions and in the laboratory). For example, during the late fall/winter months, some individuals become passive and less assertive, sleep more, eat more, gain weight, and have decreased interest in sex; opposite changes occur in summer (Wehr and Rosenthal, 1989; Lam and Levitt, 1999). (A summer form of SAD has also been described, as discussed further below [Wehr et al., 2001a,b]. Because the literature on summer SAD is so limited, our future references to SAD refer to the winter form unless otherwise noted.) These seasonal changes are distinct but mild in 10–20 percent of the adult U.S. population and are not associated with major depressive episodes. In 1–4 percent of the U.S. population, however, pathological changes in mood and related changes in energy, sleep, and appetite are associated with SAD. Seasonal major depression accounts for 11 percent of all major depression (Levitt et al., 2000).

Seasonality in Manic-Depressive Illness

Although there is clearly some overlap with SAD, seasonality in manic-depressive illness deserves a separate discussion. Many sources of variance confound the collection of data on seasonality in bipolar or recurrent unipolar disorder. For example, although hospital admission dates may be meaningful markers for the onset of manic episodes, they are unlikely to reflect the true onset of depressive or hypomanic episodes. In fact, hospitalizations for depression are more likely to reflect the eventual severe or suicidal phase of an evolving depressive episode than its onset. Moreover, voluntary admissions and hospital schedules (rotation of physician staff or holidays) may affect data on seasonal patterns, and diagnostic criteria vary from hospital to hospital. Despite these methodological problems, however, the consistency of findings in seasonality studies of both affective episodes and suicide is noteworthy (Eastwood and Peter, 1988). Two broad peaks are evident in the seasonal incidence of major depressive episodes: a substantial spring peak and a smaller autumn peak. This pattern tends to parallel the seasonal pattern for suicide: to date, 23 of 27 studies have reported a suicide peak in spring,[67] while many studies have also identified a suicide peak in early fall (see Chapter 8). The evidence gains further weight from the fact that virtually all the studies were carried out after the widespread use of lithium had begun, which may have dampened the natural pattern of seasonal variability. Changes in light conditions are most rapid in spring and fall, and it may be that patients with recurrent affective disorders are more susceptible to rapid changes in the photoperiod.[68,69]

While most of the earlier studies of the seasonal incidence of depression did not differentiate bipolar and unipolar patients, some more contemporary studies, taken together, suggest that a spring peak is predominant in unipolar depression, while bipolar depression is more likely to show a (smaller) fall/winter peak.[70] A recent study of 958 consecutively admitted patients with major depression (Sato et al., 2006) found that those with "depressive mixed states" (see Chapter 1) showed a seasonal pattern similar to that of the bipolar group and different from that of the unipolar patients without such states, which is consistent with the hypothesis that these states are part of the bipolar spectrum. While the above studies employed *clinical* samples, Shin and colleagues (2005) recently confirmed the high rate of seasonality in bipolar patients compared with patients with major depression or normal controls in a large *community* sample.

Although the data on mania are somewhat more limited and therefore a bit less compelling, peak incidences tend to occur in the summer months (Takei et al., 1992). Analyzing hospital admissions, Cassidy and Carrol (2002) found that admissions for pure mania were more frequent in spring (when photoperiod increases rapidly), which coincided with the peak for total admissions for mania. However, the peak for mixed episodes was in late summer, when photoperiod starts decreasing more rapidly, and the ambient temperature is still high. Myers and Davies (1978) and Carney and colleagues (1988) showed significant correlations between admissions for mania and total monthly hours of sunshine and average monthly day length, but not environmental temperature. Peck (1990) found that rates of mania were related to hours of sunlight in the preceding month. In England, by contrast, increased relapse of mania was not observed in any particular season, a finding that may relate to the extensive cloud cover over that country (Hunt et al., 1992; Silverstone et al., 1995).

Figure 16–8 displays these spring and fall peaks in major depression and suicide and also includes SAD, which is characterized predominantly by regularly recurring atypical depressions in winter, sometimes with hypomania in summer. The light–dark cycle shown in the figure is the principal seasonal variable of interest. Note that the overall length of the photoperiod has two extremes—longest in summer and shortest in winter—whereas the rate of change in the ratio of light to dark has two peaks—one in late winter/early spring, the other in late summer/early fall. Thus if manic-depressive patients were abnormally sensitive to seasonal light changes, this could be reflected in either opposite behavioral patterns at the two extremes (winter and summer) or behavioral disturbances in early spring or early fall, reflecting the period of rapidly increasing and rapidly decreasing light, respectively.

Moving beyond variations in photoperiod, Postolache and colleagues (2005a) hypothesized that cytokine released during seasonal inflammatory disorders may trigger decompensation/exacerbation of mood disorders in

Figure 16–8. Frequency distribution of cycle lengths among bipolar patients, showing 12-month peaks. BP-I = bipolar-I; BP-II = bipolar-II. (*Source*: Zis and Goodwin, 1979.)

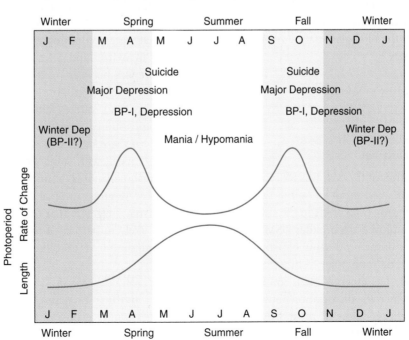

vulnerable individuals. In a U.S.-wide epidemiological study, women showed at least a doubling of the rate of suicide during periods of high tree pollen counts (tree pollen has a massive peak in spring), after adjustment for environmental light (Postolache et al., 2005b). Consistent with a possible effect of allergens in exacerbating spring-time depression and triggering suicide in women, preliminary research found increased gene expression of cytokines to be involved in allergic reactions in the orbital cortex of female victims of suicide (Tonelli et al., 2005). Recently, moreover, in female Brown Norway rats, sensitization to tree pollen produced anxiety- and depression-like behavioral changes and activation of molecular and cellular mediators of allergy within the brain (Tonelli and Postolache 2006).

In one study on twins discordant for bipolar-I disorder in Finland, the twins with the disorder reported greater seasonality of mood and sleep length and a greater positive response to sunny days compared with their healthy co-twins (Hakkarainen et al., 2003). It is important to note that morningness–eveningness did not differ between bipolar patients and controls, an observation that argues against a circadian phase change difference underlying the greater seasonality of mood in the bipolar twins.

Diagnostic Criteria for Seasonal Affective Disorder

As noted earlier, Rosenthal and colleagues (1984) first published criteria for diagnosing SAD. By 1987, criteria for a seasonal pattern of mood disorders had been incorporated into the *Diagnostic and Statistical Manual* (DSM)-III-R. Table 16–2 compares the original criteria of Rosenthal and colleagues with the broader criteria of DSM-IV, which encompass other seasonal patterns. We consider the Rosenthal criteria to be superior to the DSM-IV criteria because they better reflect both the biological nature of the disorder and its clinical course.[71]

Epidemiological Studies of Seasonal Affective Disorder

Relationship between Seasonal Affective Disorder and Bipolar Disorder

At the time the first edition of this text was written, the literature indicated that on average, about half of those with SAD were bipolar, primarily bipolar-II. In the subsequent literature, which has employed the broader DSM-IV definition of SAD, estimates of the proportion of patients with SAD who also meet criteria for bipolar disorder have been lower, but no consensus has emerged. It is important to consider the extent to which the dissociation between SAD and bipolar disorder reflects nature. If most SAD is not a variant of bipolar disorder, attempts to integrate circadian

studies of SAD with those of bipolar disorder will be misleading.

Ethnicity

According to a review by Magnusson (2000), the prevalence of SAD (diagnosed using criteria based on the Seasonal Pattern Assessment Questionnaire) across 20 retrospective studies varied from 0 to 9.7 percent. Winter SAD was found to be more prevalent than summer SAD in all but four studies—three in China and Japan (Ozaki et al., 1995a; Han et al., 2000a) and a fourth in the tropics (Morrisey et al., 1996). It may be that a specific ethnic factor, genetic or environmental, protects those of Asian ethnicity from winter SAD and makes these individuals more vulnerable to summer SAD.[72] Given the size of the Chinese population, summer SAD is not a small problem at the global level.

Latitude and Weather

Initial studies using the Seasonal Pattern Assessment Questionnaire found an effect of latitude, with winter SAD being more prevalent at higher latitudes, a finding consistent with the hypothesis that the disorder is caused by reduced light in the winter. Of three studies that examined the effect of latitude in Scandinavia, however, only one found such an effect; a latitude effect was observed in Japan, but not in Italy or Australia (Magnusson, 2000). Studies using DSM-IV criteria instead of the Seasonal Pattern Assessment Questionnaire applied to large populations found no latitude effect (Blazer et al., 1998, reviewed by Magnusson, 2000). A possible explanation may be that latitude is only a small predictor of how much sunlight people will actually receive, since meteorological conditions such as cloud cover may have an effect. Wacker and colleagues (1992), however, found no difference in the prevalence of SAD between regions that were predominantly sunny and those that were overcast in Switzerland. Similarly, a study in Iceland found no differences between those who worked outdoors and those who worked indoors (Magnusson and Stefansson, 1993). As with all studies failing to find a difference, however, the possibility of type II error (false negative) must be assessed for these studies. In sum, the literature on weather effects is mixed, with some studies reporting correlations with sunshine and/or temperature and others not (reviewed by Magnusson et al., 2000).[73] What these mixed findings may suggest (other than type II error) is that SAD is more likely to be related to the direction of changes in day length than to its absolute value (Wehr et al., 2001a,b).

Acclimatization

Is SAD a dysfunctional response, or is it adaptive? Over time, does longer exposure to a higher latitude result in more drastic and consolidated behavioral changes, or do

TABLE 16–2. **Criteria for Seasonal Affective Disorder and Seasonal Pattern**

Seasonal Affective Disorder (Rosenthal et al., 1984)	Seasonal Pattern (DSM-IV, 1994)
1. Recurrent fall–winter depressions	1. Regular temporal relationship between onset of episode of affective disorder and a particular 60-day period of the year.
2. No seasonally varying psychosocial variables that might account for the recurrent depressions	2. Do not include cases in which there is an obvious effect of seasonally related psychosocial stressors (e.g., regularly being unemployed every winter).
3. Regularly occurring nondepressed periods in the spring and summer	3. Full remissions (or a change from depression to hypomania or mania) during a characteristic time of year (e.g., depression disappears in the spring).
4. At least two of the depressions occurred during consecutive years	4. In the last 2 years, two major depressive episodes have occurred that demonstrate the temporal seasonal relationships described in previous points, and no nonseasonal major depressive episodes have occurred during the same period.
5. At least one of the depressions met Research Diagnostic Criteria (Spitzer et al., 1978a) for major depression	5. The corresponding criterion is implicit here, as "seasonal pattern" is provided as a modifier of other DSM-IV diagnoses: bipolar disorder or recurrent major depression.
6. No other Axis I psychopathology	6. Seasonal episodes of mood disturbance substantially outnumbered nonseasonal episodes.

seasonal responses habituate and decrease over time? The bulk of the data support the latter conclusion.[74]

Syndromal versus Subsyndromal Seasonal Affective Disorder and the Dual-Vulnerability Hypothesis

The term *subsyndromal SAD* has two definitions. The first is based on cross-sectional epidemiological studies using a seasonality questionnaire (the Seasonal Pattern Assessment Questionnaire), which defines the syndrome according to a global seasonality score above a certain cutoff point reflecting the severity of the "problems" related to seasonal changes in mood (Kasper et al., 1989b). The second definition is based on clinical interviews, and characterizes subsyndromal SAD as reflecting winter depressive episodes that are significant but do not meet the full DSM criteria for a major depressive episode (Kasper et al., 1989a).

There are two views on the difference between SAD and subsyndromal SAD. The classic one is that the difference is mainly quantitative (Blehar and Lewy, 1990), that is, that SAD represents the extreme of a seasonality dimension (Blehar and Lewy, 1990; Avery et al., 1998). Consistent with this view is the fact that the distribution of seasonality scores in the general population is continuous (Kasper et al., 1989b; Jang et al., 1997a,b). Others postulate separate factors for seasonality and for depression, and suggest that when this dual vulnerability obtains, SAD results (Lam et al., 2001c). The trigger for the seasonal vulnerability is said to be a decrease in photoperiod, while possible triggers for depression include a seasonal loss of energy and drive with an attendant compromised ability to meet societal demands. Depending on the relative degree of loading on these two factors, different categories emerge. For example, loading on seasonality with little or no loading on depression would be expected to result in subsyndromal SAD (which consists mainly of vegetative symptoms, such as increased appetite, weight gain, fatigue, and hypersomnia). If the degree of loading on both factors is similar, the full syndrome of SAD might be expected.[75] If one has loading on depression with little or no loading on seasonality, a nonseasonal major depression would be expected. This dual-vulnerability hypothesis was initially proposed by Young and colleagues (1991) and further developed by Lam and colleagues (2001a,b,c). Light treatment was known to be effective for both subsyndromal SAD and SAD (Kasper et al., 1989a; Norden and Avery, 1993). Subsequently, however, Lam and colleagues (2001c) showed that subsyndromal SAD (more loading on seasonality than on depression) appears to be more responsive to the treatment. On the other hand, a meta-analysis by Kripke and colleagues (1997) found that the antidepressant effect of light treatment in nonseasonal depression is equivalent to that seen in seasonal depression.[76]

Pathophysiology of Seasonal Affective Disorder

There are three levels (presumably interrelated) at which one can address the pathophysiology of SAD: genetic factors, neurotransmitter dysfunction, and chronobiological dysregulation. In addition, one must look at associations between SAD and both sensitivity to light and other, nonlight factors. Here we look briefly at each of these associations. An excellent, balanced review of SAD pathophysiology is that of Lam and colleagues (2000). A more detailed review of genetic and neurobiological (including chronobiological) associations in SAD, along with discussion of sensitivity to both light and nonlight factors in SAD, is provided on the Web site for this volume.

Genetic Factors

A large study involving 4,639 adult twins pairs from Australia found that genetic factors accounted for 29 percent of the variance in seasonality (Madden et al., 1996). The heritability of seasonality was associated with a preponderance of the vegetative symptoms of depression, such as increased appetite, weight gain, and increased sleep, which are also good predictors of response to light therapy (Lam et al., 1993; Sher et al., 2001). This latter association also provides circumstantial support for a dual-vulnerability model, as seasonality in appetite, weight, and sleep is associated with loading on vulnerability for seasonality as opposed to dysphoria and anhedonia, which result from loading on vulnerability for depression. Another twin study involving 339 twin pairs (Jang et al., 1997b) found a more substantial genetic contribution than that found in the study by Madden and colleagues (1996). The authors also reported that heritability accounted for more variance in seasonality in men (69 percent) than in women (45 percent). Linkage studies have reported genetic associations between SAD and the serotonin 5-HT$_{2A}$ promoter polymorphism—1438G/A (Enoch et al., 1999)—as well as the 218C allele of tryptophan hydroxylase (Levitan et al., 1999a,b). An association between seasonality as a trait and the short allele

of the serotonin transporter promoter gene has also been reported (Postolache et al., 1998; Rosenthal et al., 1998). Replications in larger samples are awaited.

Neurotransmitter Dysfunction

It is important to note that the subjects for the studies discussed below were patients with SAD. Therefore, the degree to which the study findings are related to seasonality in manic-depressive illness, either bipolar or recurrent depression, is unknown (see the earlier discussion of the overlap between SAD and bipolar disorder).

Serotonin. Certain indirect measures of serotonin activity, such as levels of precursors and metabolites, fluctuate markedly with the seasons. For example, plasma L-tryptophan, the precursor of serotonin, is at its highest levels in spring, declining in late (Wirz-Justice and Richter, 1979) or early (Wirz-Justice et al., 1979; Swade and Coppen, 1980) fall. In a recent study of 101 healthy men in which serotonin metabolites in the jugular vein were measured, turnover of serotonin by the brain was found to be lowest in winter ($p = .013$). In addition, the rate of production of serotonin by the brain was correlated positively with the level of ambient light, and the strongest correlation was with the day of testing (i.e., the relationship was not particularly lagged) (Lambert et al., 2002). Results of animal studies indicate that serotonin content in the hypothalamus shows a marked seasonal variation, with a minimum in the winter (Carlsson et al., 1980). The major metabolite of serotonin, 5-HIAA, measured in the cerebrospinal fluid, has its trough in springtime, which may reflect low serotonergic activity during winter (Brewerton et al., 1988). Neumeister and colleagues (2001) reported reduced serotonin transporter availability in the hypothalamic/thalamic area in winter compared with summer in healthy subjects.

Because dietary carbohydrates enhance serotonin synthesis and transmission through increased tryptophan uptake into the brain (Fernstorm and Wurtman, 1971), the observation that patients with SAD feel activated following high-carbohydrate meals whereas normal controls feel more sedated (Rosenthal et al., 1989) may suggest altered serotonin metabolism in SAD. Several studies have shown that treatment with tryptophan can improve mood in patients with SAD to a degree similar to that achieved with light treatment (Ghadirian et al., 1998; McGrath et al., 1990). Tryptophan may also augment light treatment, one study finding that it converted 9 of 14 patients from nonresponders to responders (Lam et al., 1997).

The hypothesis that SAD may involve serotonin has also been examined using tryptophan depletion, by which central serotonin synthesis can be reduced. Tryptophan depletion results in a relapse of depressive symptoms in SAD patients who formerly responded to light treatment in winter, as shown in three different studies (Lam et al., 1996; Neumeister et al., 1997, 1998a). Tryptophan depletion in summer resulted in relapse in one study (Neumeister et al., 1998a) but not in another (Lam and Levitan, 1996). The association of tryptophan depletion with depressive relapse is not specific to seasonal depression, also being seen in nonseasonal cases (Bremner et al., 1997), which suggests that the phenomenon is related more to depression than to seasonality per se. Preliminary data suggest that D-fenfluramine, a serotonin-releasing agent, may benefit SAD patients (O'Rourke et al., 1987). Selective serotonin reuptake inhibitors (SSRIs) are also effective in the treatment of SAD, as reported for fluoxetine (Lam et al., 1995) and sertraline (Moscovitch et al., 1995). When added to light treatment, citalopram improves the efficacy of the treatment in the long run, but not in the short run (Thorell et al., 1999).

One serotonergic finding appears to be specific to SAD. Whereas patients with nonseasonal major depression do not show altered hormonal or abnormal behavioral responses to the 5-HT$_{2C}$ agonist m-chlorophenylpiperazine (m-CPP) (Anand et al., 1994), patients with SAD show blunted hormonal responses and experience "activation euphoria"—a consistent finding in both uncontrolled (Joseph-Vanderpool et al., 1993; Jacobsen et al., 1994; Garcia-Borreguero et al., 1995) and controlled (Schwartz et al., 1997; Levitan et al., 1998) studies. These changes are normalized after successful light therapy, suggesting that the response to m-CPP is a state marker in SAD.

In conclusion, there is convincing evidence that serotonergic dysfunction plays a role in SAD. Some of these abnormalities, involving either 5-HT$_{2C}$ or 5-HT$_7$, may be specific to the state of winter depression rather than being associated with depression in general.

Dopamine. There is some evidence, mostly indirect, suggesting dopamine involvement in SAD. Low resting prolactin levels independent of season have been reported in SAD patients (suggesting a trait marker), a finding interpreted as reflecting upregulation of D2 receptors secondary to reduced presynaptic dopamine (Depue et al., 1989, 1990). Another presumed indicator of altered dopamine function is blunted thermoregulatory heat loss in the winter in patients with SAD compared with normal controls (Arbisi et al., 1989, 1994), which is reversed by successful light treatment. A more direct test of the dopamine hypothesis failed when a double-blind, placebo-controlled trial of L-dopa/carbidopa yielded negative results (Oren et al., 1994b). On the other hand, the antidepressant bupropion,[77] whose mechanism of action is thought to involve enhanced dopamine (and norepinephrine) function, was found to be effective in one placebo-controlled study of SAD (Modell

et al., 2005). Perhaps also consistent with dopamine involvement in SAD, findings of a recent study indicate that adults with residual attention deficit disorder may have high seasonality scores (Levitan et al., 1999a).

Norepinephrine. An inverse relationship between depression scores in patients with SAD and levels of norepinephrine metabolites in cerebral spiral fluid has been reported (Rudorfer et al., 1993). Results of other studies, however, suggest a lower plasma norepinephrine concentration in untreated SAD patients relative to controls and in untreated versus light-treated conditions (Schwartz et al., 1997). Also after light treatment, plasma norepinephrine levels (Skwerer et al., 1988), as well as norepinephrine turnover, were found to increase (Anderson et al., 1992); both of these findings are consistent with the effectiveness of bupropion, as cited above.

Neumeister and colleagues (1998c) subjected SAD patients to both tryptophan and catecholamine depletion[78] (i.e., both dopamine and norepinephrine) and sham depletion with an active placebo (benztropine). A temporary relapse in depressive symptoms resulted from both interventions, leading the authors to conclude that catecholamines, not just serotonin, are involved in the effect of light treatment on SAD.

Chronobiological Dysregulation

There are two hypotheses regarding dysregulation of seasonal rhythms in patients with SAD. The first is based on a different duration (specifically, the duration of melatonin secretion) of the internal night between winter and summer. The second is based on a shift of the phase of the circadian rhythms.

Melatonin Duration Hypothesis. According to this hypothesis, inspired by the animal literature, a longer internal night in patients with SAD matches a longer external night in winter, and this winter–summer difference in the duration of the internal (biological) night is what drives seasonal changes in behavior. This hypothesis found additional support in initial findings of an increased prevalence of SAD with a more northern latitude characterized by more drastic changes in photoperiod, although these findings were not confirmed in studies in clinical populations (reviewed by Magnusson, 2000). A consequence of this hypothesis was the administration of light in early morning (6 AM to 9 AM) and late afternoon (4 PM to 7 PM), designed to reduce the duration of winter darkness to a level similar to that in the summer.

Because in many mammals the photoperiod signal is encoded in the duration of melatonin secretion and because light suppresses melatonin secretion, it was hypothesized that light in the morning and evening reduces the duration of melatonin secretion, bringing it to summer levels. However, suppression of melatonin secretion is not sufficient to produce an antidepressant effect (Wehr et al., 1986). Specifically, more drastic suppression, as with atenolol, a long-acting beta-blocker, did not result in improvement (Rosenthal et al., 1988). On the other hand, a short-acting beta-blocker administered in early morning resulted in maintenance of improvement in SAD patients (Schlager, 1994). A problem in the study, however, was that propranonol was administered at a time when it may have been too late to suppress the melatonin secretion in most patients, so that the study may not represent a valid test for the melatonin duration hypothesis.

A strong argument against the melatonin duration hypothesis is the effectiveness of a late-afternoon dose of melatonin (Lewy et al., 1998, 2006).[79] According to the theory, the presence of melatonin in the blood for an increased duration would make patients more depressed. The findings of two other studies are also inconsistent with the melatonin duration hypothesis. Winton and colleagues (1989) measured melatonin profiles in SAD patients receiving two schedules of combined morning and evening light treatment. Although both treatments resulted in an equivalent shortening of melatonin secretion, the antidepressant effect was greater in the treatment group with more exposure to light. Wehr and colleagues (1986) found that two regimens of light treatment were equally effective even though only one of them was expected to shorten the photoperiod. This study cannot be considered conclusive, however, because melatonin profiles were not obtained, sample sizes were small, and patients were exposed to room lighting from 7 AM to 11 PM, which could have diminished the contrast between the two conditions.

Interest in the melatonin duration hypothesis was revived after Wehr's group (Wehr, 1991a,b; Wehr et al., 1991, 1993) showed that in humans, as previously described in rodents, the duration of nocturnal melatonin secretion reflects the extent of light exposure in the immediately preceding photoperiod. Because no changes in normal volunteers were found between winter and summer, it was suggested that artificial light suppresses melatonin and thus the hormone's response to changes in photoperiod (Wehr et al., 1995). Young and colleagues (1991, 1997) found that photoperiod may be related to the onset of vegetative symptoms in SAD, symptoms that, according to the dual-vulnerability hypothesis, are an expression of seasonality more than of depression per se. Wehr and colleagues (2001a,b) found that SAD patients, but not controls, had a winter–summer difference in the duration of active melatonin secretion. This study showed for the first time that patients with SAD generate a signal of change in season similar to that used by nonhuman mammals to regulate seasonal behavior.

Circadian Phase-Shift Hypothesis. As previously described in the section on physiology of circadian rhythms, light is a potent synchronizer and shifter of these rhythms. Building on the phase-advance hypothesis of nonseasonal depression (Kripke et al., 1978; Wehr et al., 1979), Lewy and colleagues (2003, 2006) and Burgess and colleagues (2004) suggested that a phase shift in circadian rhythms is conducive to SAD. In short, the theory posits that for most SAD patients, the internal clock is phase delayed relative to the external day–night cycle. (On the other hand, Murray and colleagues [2006] could not confirm this at a statistically significant level, although trends in their data were consistent with the phase-shift hypothesis.)

An elaboration of the phase-shift hypothesis is the hypothesized misalignment between the sleep–wake cycle and other biological rhythms (such as cortisol and melatonin secretion and body temperature) and the notion that light will realign these rhythms (Lewy et al., 1987; Lewy and Sack, 1989). According to this theory, evening light should further delay the internal clock and thus be less antidepressant than morning light. Another study (Sack et al., 1990) did indeed find delayed melatonin rhythms, consistent with the phase-shift hypothesis. The authors also found that morning light resulted in a phase advance.

A subsequent study by Terman and colleagues (2001) found no relationship between dim-light melatonin onset (DLMO), a marker of circadian phase, and severity of depression; between baseline DLMO and treatment response; or between post–light treatment DLMO and depression rating (but a type II error cannot be ruled out). Moreover, after evening light, patients with larger delays were not more depressed than those with smaller delays. In support of the phase-shift hypothesis, however, the authors found a correlation between the magnitude of the phase advance to morning light and improvement in depression scores (consistent with the findings of Lewy et al., 1987b, 1998; Sack et al., 1990).

Another strength of the Terman et al. (2001) study is that it addressed the phase-angle difference between sleep and other circadian rhythms as involved in SAD (rather than the phase shift alone), requiring that the correction in phase angle by light treatment be involved in the antidepressant response (Lewy and Sack, 1988). However, Terman and colleagues (2001) found that changes in phase-angle difference between sleep onset and melatonin onset did not predict response to treatment. In fact, morning light increased the gap between sleep and melatonin onset, having a greater phase-advancing effect on melatonin rhythms than on the sleep–wake cycle. The authors wrote, "one would conclude that phase advance is neither necessary nor sufficient for the therapeutic effect" (Terman et al., 2001). The ideal scheduling for light treatment, according to the authors, would be based on circadian time and not sleep time, and would commence 8.5 hours after melatonin onset.

The phase-shift hypothesis in SAD has received significant support from the reported improvement in depression resulting from melatonin administered in the late afternoon, at a time when it results in a phase advance (Lewy et al., 1998, 2006). Moreover, the antidepressant effect of melatonin administration was found to be correlated with normalizing circadian alignment (Lewy et al., 2006). Other support for the phase-shift hypothesis in SAD comes from constant routine studies. Because waveforms of circadian rhythms are distorted by such factors as sleep, activity, natural and artificial light exposure, and feeding, constant routine (as compared with forced desynchrony) is a relatively simple and reliable way to unmask circadian rhythms. In short, subjects are studied for 36 hours, awake in dim light and with no time cues. In constant routine conditions, patients with SAD showed phase-delayed DLMO, core temperature, and cortisol rhythm, with these abnormalities being corrected by light treatment (Avery et al., 1993; Dahl et al., 1993). Again, however, the improvement in depression was not related to the degree of phase advance.

Results of other studies, however, fail to support a phase-shift hypothesis and the phase-advance mechanism of action of light. A number of studies did not find circadian markers (body temperature, cortisol, prolactin, thyrotropin) to be phase delayed in SAD patients (Rosenthal et al., 1990; Eastman et al., 1993; Oren et al., 1996). Many tests of the phase-shift hypothesis have assessed the antidepressant response of different timings of bright light administration. To support the phase-delay hypothesis, according to the previously described phase response curve, morning light would have to improve and evening light to worsen depression. It is true that morning light is a more potent antidepressant than evening light, as shown by direct comparisons (Lewy et al., 1998; Terman et al., 1998) and by most meta-analyses (Terman et al., 1989a; Thomson et al., 1999; Vitaterna et al., 1999). However, some studies have found evening light to be as effective as morning light (Wirz-Justice et al., 1993a,b) or nearly so (Eastman et al., 1998). Most important, even as evening light was less effective than morning light, it was more effective than placebo and certainly not detrimental, as the phase-shift theory would predict. However, the large placebo component of light that varies among subjects and studies would mitigate depressant effects of shifting the clock in the wrong direction.

Several factors may account for the somewhat conflicting results of the various circadian studies addressing SAD (reviewed by Lam and Levitan, 2000). These include small sample sizes; selection of patients not always representative of the entire SAD group (e.g., including only hypersomnic patients, excluding patients with severe phase abnormality);

and masking of effects of environmental factors, sleep, activity, and social cues. Light administered at a constant external clock time may vary greatly according to individual circadian time, by up to several hours. Thus the magnitude of a phase shift will vary considerably among individuals. According to Terman and colleagues (2001), the ideal timing of light treatment is related to a circadian marker and not to clock time. However, Terman appears to have assumed that all SAD patients are phase delayed, whereas Lewy and colleagues (2006) recently confirmed that a subgroup of patients are phase advanced and should be treated with evening bright light and/or morning low-dose melatonin administration. Lewy also cautioned against overshifting across the therapeutic window (DLMO = 6 hours before midsleep).

Seasonal Affective Disorder Patients and Sensitivity to Light

A parsimonious explanation of SAD might be that light exposure in winter compared with that in summer is significantly lower in patients with SAD relative to controls. This explanation does not hold, however, as similar light exposures have been reported in normal controls and in SAD (Oren et al., 1994a) or subsyndromal SAD (Guillemette et al., 1998) patients. If light exposure does not differ between SAD patients and controls, perhaps differences in sensitivity to light may explain the behavioral differences between individuals with and without SAD. Experiments with albino rats have shown that the retina of these animals adapts to variations in ambient light, with increased sensitivity in dim light (Schremser and Williams, 1995a,b), a phenomenon termed *photostasis*. This phenomenon is believed to have evolved for adaptation to seasonal changes in illuminance (Penn and Williams, 1986). Both a hyperphotostatic (increased sensitivity) (Beersma, 1990) and a hypophotostatic (decreased sensitivity) (Reme et al., 1990) adjustment to light have been proposed as potential etiologies for SAD (although there is no evidence that photostasis exists in humans).

Measuring retinal sensitivity indirectly with an electrooculogram (EOG), Ozaki and colleagues (1995b) found a higher sensitivity in winter than in summer in normal subjects (interpreted as a compensatory mechanism triggered by a decrease in natural sunlight), whereas in SAD patients, retinal sensitivity remained constant across the two seasons. With a more accurate technique, the electroretinogram (ERG), Lam and colleagues (1992a) found lower-than-normal amplitudes (using a mixed cone–rod response) in females with SAD and higher-than-normal amplitudes in males with SAD compared with matched controls (Lam et al., 1992a). In another study, Hebert and colleagues (2002), opting to use a stimulus for the rod system exclusively (because photostasis was described for that system), with subsyndromal SAD patients (who are less likely to have been exposed to light treatment) as subjects, found lower sensitivities to light in these patients, with a positive correlation between their global seasonality scores and a winter decrease in rod sensitivity (Hebert et al., 2002).

It is far from clear whether alterations in sensitivity to light are contributory to SAD, a consequence of neurotransmitter dysregulation in the central nervous system, or a consequence of aberrant behaviors of SAD patients. If neurotransmitter dysfunction were the cause, one would expect that light treatment, correcting the dysfunction, would normalize the patients' retinal sensitivity. However, the persistence of those abnormalities after light therapy (Ozaki et al., 1993) argues against that alternative. Finally, higher cone sensitivity (and rod adaptation) was found in SAD patients in winter than in controls in a study using self-reported dim-light detection (Terman and Terman, 1999).

Factors Other Than Light

Light treatment, although effective, does not completely shift patients with SAD from a winter to a summer state (Postolache et al., 1988). Consequently, factors other than light may be involved in seasonal changes in behavior. Two studies found a correlation between SAD symptoms and atmospheric temperature (Molin et al., 1996; Okawa et al., 1996). This finding is consistent with the animal literature showing that low ambient temperature accelerates short-day responses in seasonal animals (Larkin et al., 2001).

Findings of other studies on seasonal behavior in animals suggest that olfaction could be involved in seasonality (Nelson and Zucker, 1981; Nelson, 1990; Schilling and Perret, 1993). Postolache and colleagues (2002d) hypothesized that patients with SAD would differ from normal controls with regard to olfactory acuity. They compared olfactory detection thresholds in patients and normal controls in both winter and summer and found that patients with SAD had an ability to detect odors greatly exceeding that of the controls. The difference was statistically significant across seasons, although there was a trend for it to be more apparent in the summer.

CONCLUSIONS

Sleep reflects a critical phase of a core circadian rhythm in humans, and thus our coverage of sleep and biological rhythms belongs in the same chapter. Sleep disturbances are central to the pathophysiology of manic-depressive illness; they are not only a key symptom of both mania and depression, but also the earliest indication of major

switches in mood state. Moreover, a manipulation of sleep—sleep deprivation—while the fastest-acting antidepressant known, can all too readily switch bipolar patients into mania. And because the clinical course of manic-depressive illness, particularly the bipolar subgroup, is cyclic, the illness is itself an abnormal rhythm. Yet despite centuries-old observations of seasonal and circadian patterns of symptoms in manic-depressive illness, the physiology of these rhythms has been explored systematically only in the last two or three decades. Further, since the publication of the first edition of this text in 1990, new research on the physiology of rhythms in manic-depressive illness has been sparse, while pharmacological and basic neurobiological research has flourished. Although such physiological research is painstaking and time-consuming, it is all the more necessary today because of rapid advances in understanding the molecular biology and genetics of the circadian clock. Without a sophisticated understanding of the phenomenology and physiology of the specific rhythmic disturbances in manic-depressive patients, the full potential of the new genetic and molecular discoveries in the field will not be realized.

Heritability of circadian disturbances has been demonstrated in both humans and animals.[80] An important focus for future research would be the prevalence of these disturbances in patients with manic-depressive illness versus normal controls, as well as the prevalence of affective illness in subjects with familial circadian disturbances. The integrity of clock genes in patients with manic-depressive illness is another potentially fruitful subject for research, as is the relationship between central and peripheral oscillators, especially the amplitude, phase, synchronization, and stability of molecular rhythms in patients with bipolar and highly recurrent unipolar disorders.

Research on the melatonin receptor agonists (one, ramelteon, recently approved by the U.S. Food and Drug Administration for treatment of insomnia) represents an advance in chronobiology. Having a greater affinity for melatonin receptors and a more favorable and predictable pharmacokinetic profile, as well as lacking contaminants, the melatonin receptor agonists might be used for synchronization and shifting in placebo-control paradigms.[81] Continuing work in this area is a priority for future research on the relationship between sleep and circadian rhythms and manic-depressive illness.

NOTES

1. In the United States, however, sleep deprivation remains little known and seldom used, perhaps because of its loss of efficacy after even a short nap and a society that has become increasingly concerned about the consequences of sleep loss.

2. Active at and around dawn or dusk.

3. Earnest and colleagues (1999) noted that the difference between an oscillator and a pacemaker is the ability to orchestrate and direct rhythmicity in other cells, resulting in behavioral changes at the organismic level. A diffusible substance from these SCN cells is able to induce and is also necessary to maintain rhythmicity in cocultured fibroblasts (Allen et al., 2001).

4. Welsh and colleagues (1995) showed that a spontaneous action potential could be recorded from individual SCN cells weeks after they had been dispersed and cultured. When the same method was used with SCN neurons from *tau* mutant hamsters (Liu et al., 1997b) and *clock* mutant mice (Herzog et al., 1998), which have altered circadian cycle lengths, it was shown that alterations in cycle length are present in the electric potential of individual cells. Moreover, variation in sensitivity to circadian phase-shifting agents is a property not only of the SCN but also of individual cells (Liu and Reppert, 2000). Thus as the clock was identified inside each cell, its molecular components were not merely supportive elements of the clock; rather, they made up the clock itself.

5. *Clock* was the first gene cloned in mammals. In heterozygous mutant mice with the *clock* mutation, the circadian period is abnormally long. In homozygous *clock* mutants, complete arhythmicity follows after the animals are placed in constant darkness (Vitaterna et al., 1994).

The products of *Cryptochrome* genes (*mcry1* and *mcry2*), the mCRY proteins, are the negative regulators in the clock. The identification of *cry* as a clock gene in mammals came as a surprise, given that the cryptochromes function as circadian blue-light photoreceptors in plants and insects. The importance of *mcry* to the clock was demonstrated using targeted deletions: deletion of *mcry1* alone lengthens circadian period, deletion of *mcry2* alone lengthens circadian period, and deletion of both results in complete arhythmicity in constant darkness (van der Horst et al., 1999; Vitaterna et al., 1999). Three mammalian *period* genes have been identified: *per1, per2,* and *per3*. Although these genes were identified by homology with *Drosophila per*, the functions of the mammalian *per* appear to be very different from those of its insect counterpart. While the *Drosophila per* has an autoinhibitory effect, *mPER* proteins in mammals have little effect on the negative regulation of the clock; on the contrary, *mPER2* appears to have a positive regulatory function (Zheng et al., 1999). The role of *mPER1* and *mPER2* is not yet known.

A putative mammalian *timeless* gene has been identified (Zylka et al., 1998). While in *Drosophila*, the *tim* gene is essential for the entrainment of the clock to light, its function is unclear in mammals, as its SCN levels are not rhythmic and not altered by light pulses (Field et al., 2000). *Mtim* may be more related to the newly discovered insect gene *Timeout* and may have a developmental rather than a circadian role in mammals (Benna et al., 2000). The *cry* genes assumed in mammals the role of *tim* genes in insects.

6. See Shearman and colleagues (2000a). For recent reviews, see Reppert and Weaver (2001) and Herzog and Schwartz (2002).

7. An example is vasopressin prepropressophysin protein, which is highly rhythmic in the SCN and augments the SCN's electrical firing.

8. Because some of the medications used in treating bipolar patients are GABAergic, it is important to note that GABA may have a different effect on SCN neurons during subjective daytime—when in fact it appears to be excitatory—than at night, when it may be inhibitory as in the rest of the central nervous system (Wagner et al., 1997). In isolated neurons, GABA remains characteristically inhibitory, with inhibition causing phase shifts (Liu and Reppert, 2000). Many medications used for bipolar disorder enhance GABA activity, and thus may consolidate circadian rhythms through an increased excitatory role during the daytime and inhibitory role at night.

9. Despite one report that extraocular light may shift melatonin rhythms in humans (Campbell and Murphy, 1998), melatonin secretion cannot be suppressed by light in blindfolded or bilaterally enucleated subjects (Czeisler et al., 1995; Lockley et al., 1998). Moreover, only free-running (non-24-hour) cycles have been observed in bilaterally enucleated individuals (Lockley et al., 1998; Skene et al., 1999).

10. Two additional indirect pathways have been described. The first originates from the same retinal cells whose axons compose the RHT, but instead of projecting to the SCN, synapses in the intergeniculate leaflet of the lateral geniculate nucleus; then a geniculohypothalamic tract, most likely using GABA, neuropeptide Y, and enkephalin as neuromodulators, projects to the same neurons in the SCN where the retinohypothalamic tract projects. The second detour from the retina to the SCN, through the raphe nuclei, imparts a large serotonergic innervation to the SCN. These alternative pathways may play a role in nonphotic phase shifts—significantly in manic-depressive illness—including phase shifts caused by behavioral arousal (Mistlberger and Holmes, 2000).

11. Illumination of the retina induces release of glutamate at the level of the SCN. Remarkably, however, what happens after that depends on the subjective time (internal, biological, circadian) at which the stimulus is applied, similar to the behavioral effects of light. In the late night, light or, in vitro, glutamate receptor activation induces phase advances; glutamate stimulates nitric oxide production, increases cyclic guanosine monophosphate (cGMP), activates cGMP-dependent protein kinase, and phosphorylates cyclic adenosine monophosphate (cAMP)- response element binding protein (CREB) (Ding et al., 1997, 1998). In contrast, during early night, light-induced glutamate release acts via N-methyl-D-aspartate receptors, with release of calcium, activation of several kinases, phosphorylation of CREB, and induction of gene expression. Light or glutamate receptor activation can phosphorylate CREB only during the zone of sensitivity in the biological night or, in cardiology terms, the "vulnerable" period. That ability is absent during the subjective daytime, which is a refractory period for phase shift.

12. These efferents work by turning off a stimulatory signal from the paraventricular nucleus to the pineal via multisynaptic pathways.

13. It had been reported that the period of the free-running body temperature rhythm ranged from 24.2 to 25.1 hours (Campbell et al., 1993; Middleton et al., 1996). However, a number of factors may affect the generalizability of these findings, including knowledge of the time of day, activity, and exposure to ordinary room light. In a "forced desynchrony" protocol (Czeisler et al., 1999) involving a "28-hour day," with bedtime scheduled to occur 4 hours later each day for more than 3 weeks under constant low light, the average circadian period was 24.18 hours, in contrast with the previously reported

period of 24.7 hours (Campbell et al., 1993). Thus the duration of the circadian period in humans is longer than 24 hours, but only slightly. In normal everyday life, the intrinsic human circadian period adjusts to 24 hours to synchronize with the environment as a result of periodic factors that serve as 24-hour time cues, or "zeitgebers." Light is probably the principal zeitgeber.

14. For example, the PRC to light in a subject who is flown to a geographic location with a 12-hour difference from the point of departure (e.g., 2 PM is equivalent to 2 AM) will accord with the time of origin rather than that of destination.

15. Prior to the cloning of the *clock* genes, the retina was considered the only structure other than the SCN to contain a circadian clock. With the cloning of these genes, it became apparent that the *clock* genes are widely expressed, both in the brain and in many peripheral tissues, and that they oscillate independently in these tissues (Reppert and Weaver, 2001).

16. The rhythms of cortisol and sleep onset are delayed approximately 1 to 3 hours as compared with melatonin, temperature, prolactin, EEG theta waves, and REM sleep propensity rhythms (Wehr et al., 2001a).

17. In the Pittendrigh and Daan (1976) model of the rodent circadian system and in the elaboration of that model by Illnerova and Vanecek (1982), it is proposed that the circadian pacemaker consists of two component oscillators. One is entrained to dusk and controls an evening bout of locomotor activity and the onset of melatonin secretion in nocturnal rodents. The other is entrained to dawn and controls a morning bout of locomotor activity and the offset of melatonin secretion. Separate entrainment of the oscillators to dawn and dusk makes it possible for the pacemaker to adjust the duration of nocturnal periods of activity and melatonin secretion to conform to seasonal changes in night length. As applied to humans, the dusk- and dawn-entrained components of the complex circadian pacemaker could be considered to control evening and morning transitions in melatonin secretion, core body temperature, sleepiness, EEG theta activity, sleep propensity, REM sleep propensity, cortisol secretion, and sleep–awake state. The pacemaker also adjusts the timing of these transitions in response to seasonal changes in day length.

18. A major argument that sleep is vital for survival comes from marine mammals, which must be awake constantly to surface for air. Instead of being permanently alert, they sleep with one cerebral hemisphere at a time.

19. With regard to REM sleep distribution in mice, associations were found with loci on chromosomes 2, 17, and 19 (Tafti et al., 1999).

20. Knockout mice—those missing a single gene that has been knocked out—are used in biomedical research.

21. Induced mutations in serotonin receptors, somnogenic cytokines (such as interleukin 1β and tumor necrosis factor α), and the prion protein gene, implicated in the human condition of fatal familial insomnia (Chapman et al., 1996), result in alterations of sleep (for a review and a note of caution in interpreting these data, see Toth, 2001).

22. Transections of the brain stem at the midpons or below do not reduce wakefulness, while transections at or above a midcollicular level cause an acute loss of wakefulness. The tissue at the rostral pontin–caudal midbrain interface is thus essential for maintaining wakefulness. One set of neurons is located in a group of nuclei that have been identified as the pedunculopontine and laterodorsal tegmental nuclei (PPT–LDT). These neurons project to the thalamus, intralaminar nuclei, thalamic relay nuclei, and reticular nucleus of the thalamus. The cholinergic input from these neurons to the thalamus has a major role in regulating thalamocortical transmission.

There is another group of neurons, also situated in the midbrain and pons, that ascend toward the hypothalamus and not the thalamus, among them neurons from the noradrenergic locus ceruleus and dorsal and median raphe nucleus. Their axons run through the lateral hypothalamus, where they are joined by cholinergic axons from basal forebrain cholinergic neurons and histaminergic axons from the tuberomamillary nucleus of the hypothalamus. These axons project diffusely to the cerebral hemispheres.

The PPT–LDT cholinergic neurons fire rapidly during wakefulness and even more so during REM sleep (REM-on neurons), and are inhibited during NREM sleep. The monoaminergic nuclei (raphe, ceruleus, and tuberomammilary), by contrast, are almost silent during REM sleep (REM-off neurons), while firing actively during wakefulness and slowing down during NREM sleep.

23. Just as there are ascendant axons, there are also important descendent axons that have an important role in the switch between sleep and wakefulness. One source of these fibers is the ventrolateral preoptic nucleus (VLPO), located in the anterior hypothalamus. The VLPO neurons innervate the tuberomammilary, raphe, and serotonin neurons, and their terminals contain GABA and galanin and have an inhibitory nature. The VLPO neurons fire twice as fast during sleep as during wakefulness, and twice as fast during sleep preceded by sleep deprivation as during sleep not preceded by sleep deprivation.

The VLPO appears to contain subregions specific to REM versus NREM regulation. Specifically, more peripheral areas of the VLPO inhibit the monoaminergic neurons and stimulate the PPT–LDT neurons to produce REM sleep.

The VLPO has a reciprocal inhibiting relationship with the monoaminergic neurons. During sleep, the VLPO's rapid firing inhibits the monoamine neurons and thus disinhibits its own firing. During wakefulness, the monoamine neurons' firing inhibits the VLPO and thus disinhibits their own firing. The overall large influences of the circadian and homeostatic processes may shift the relative balance of mutual inhibition; the pattern of firing and inhibition is reversed rapidly toward a new steady state. This is called a "flip-flop mechanism," intended to maintain the stability of sleep and wakefulness in the face of transient fluctuations in the input to the SCN and to avoid intermediate states and frequent fluctuations in behavioral states (Saper et al., 2001).

Other important descending fibers that have a similar flip-flop stabilizing role are the axons of the hypocretin-orexin-containing neurons in the lateral hypothalamus, which innervate and stimulate all the components of the ascending arousal system. Orexin-containing neurons stabilize and promote wakefulness and decrease both REM and NREM sleep.

24. Specifically, cells in the preoptic anterior hypothalamic nucleus (POAH) send GABAergic projections to reduce the activity of the histaminergic neurons in the tuberomamillary nucleus of the posterior hypothalamus.

25. In the absence of alerting stimuli from the tuberomamillary nucleus and the ascending reticular activating system

(cholinergic neurons located in the pons in the vicinity of the midbrain), higher-frequency firing oscillations disappear, and synchronous firing of thalamocortical neurons occurs. This phenomenon is responsible for the slowing and increased amplitude of the NREM EEG.

26. The contributions of hypocretin/orexin to sleep regulation represent some of the most novel findings on sleep regulation and dysregulation, as well as one of the most fascinating examples of recent scientific history.

27. For a review see Buchsbaum and colleagues (2001). The FDG PET allows for a more "naturalistic" setting (i.e., the patient sleeps in bed, not in the scanner). In addition, the spatial resolution is better with FDG; however, the temporal resolution is better with O15 water (this being important for events that follow in succession).

28. Maquet and colleagues (1996) reported an activation of amygdala during REM sleep that is potentially responsible for the affective components of dreams. Nofzinger and colleagues (1997, 2000) noted widespread activation during REM sleep, encompassing midline limbic and paralimbic structures. They suggested that one function of REM is to integrate neocortical activity with that of limbic motivational and regulatory centers (Buchsbaum et al., 2001).

29. EEG changes observed during sleep were instrumental in crystalizing the two-process model, with delta waves representing the accumulation of process s. Conversely, in the waking EEG, theta waves reflect both the wake-dependent homeostatic process and the circadian process and are related to sleepiness, while high-frequency alpha waves have little wake-dependent variation but significant circadian variation and are related to alertness.

30. Because these changes are related to cardiovascular morbidity and mortality, having a sleep debt may decrease longevity (see, however, Kripke and colleagues' [2002] counterargument). We suggest that sleep debt is best defined in relative terms. Thus a long sleeper needing to sleep 10 hours a night and sleeping 8 would accumulate 2 hours of sleep debt daily, while a short sleeper needing and sleeping 6 hours daily would accumulate no sleep debt.

Besides reporting less sleepiness on the Stanford Sleepiness Scale during extended wakefulness—congruent with EEG data suggesting a higher tolerance in long sleepers to sleep pressure as compared with short sleepers (Aeschbach et al., 2001a)—long sleepers have a longer biological night (see below) than that of short sleepers (Aeschbach et al., 2003).

31. As previously discussed, the two-process model posits that the timing and duration of sleep have two determinants: the SCN (the internal, subjective clock time) and a sleep–wake-dependent process, which can be understood as the time since one was awake or asleep (Dijk et al., 1992). Monk and colleagues (1992), using a constant routine protocol, found that mood in normal subjects also reaches its lowest values around body temperature minimum. Totterdell and colleagues (1994) confirmed through sleep displacement studies that the timing of sleep significantly influences mood. In these studies, prior duration of wakefulness and endogenous rhythms were shown to be confounded. Bolvin and colleagues (1977) were the first to use a forced desynchrony to study circadian and homeostatic influences on mood in normal subjects. They found that mood was related to the interaction between the internal clock and the time awake; the

influence of the former exceeded that of the latter. Not only how long but also when one sleeps and when one stays awake influence one's mood (see below), as well as cognitive and psychomotor functioning.

32. Hauri et al., 1974; Schultz and Trojan, 1979; Schulz et al., 1979; Cartwright, 1983; Buysse et al., 1997.

33. Wehr, 1989, 1991a, 1992a,b; Hudson et al., 1992; Barbini et al., 1996; Benedetti et al., 1996.

34. Rosenthal et al., 1989; Partonen and Lonnqvist, 1993; Partonen et al., 1993b; Anderson et al., 1994; Brunner et al., 1996.

35. Sitaram et al., 1976, 1978b; Gillin et al., 1978.

36. Gillin et al., 1979a; Sitaram et al., 1980, 1982; Berger et al., 1989; Nurnberger et al., 1989.

37. Forced desynchrony is the current gold standard in chronbiological research. It separates the sleep–wake cycle from the circadian rhythm without changing the ratio between sleep and wakefulness and without depriving patients of sleep. The principle is that while the circadian pacemaker is able to alter the duration of internal night or day to match changes in photoperiod or scotoperiod that would occur naturally, it is unable to match drastically reduced or extended periods of imposed light–dark and rest–activity cycles. Consequently, while subjects sleep and are awake on these very short (e.g., 20 hours) or very long (28- to 30-hour) days, the SCN continues to "pace" with a period of approximately 24 hours. The intent behind the procedure is to have the subjects sleep and be awake at different circadian periods, while the ratio of 33 percent sleep duration to 66 percent wakefulness duration is maintained.

38. Constant routine is an experimental procedure designed to eliminate the confounding influence of sleep. It is used to establish circadian markers, such as temperature minimum, onset and offset of melatonin secretion, cortisol and prolactin rhythms, rhythms in subjective sleepiness, cognitive and psychomotor performance rhythms, and electroencelographic circadian parameters (e.g., EEG theta and alpha rhythms and REM sleep propensity). It consists of prolonged wakefulness of 30–50 hours, often of 40 hours, enforced by a technician present in the room, with dim light and with the patient in a semirecumbent position. Food and water are distributed throughout day and night, at equal short intervals. If patients are used, their medications must be divided into q2 hour doses. The effects of process s, a consequence of the time-awake interval, are eliminated using mathematical models before process c is analyzed by fitting a cosine function. The major limitation of constant routine in mood research is that it modifies the studied phenomenon. As discussed earlier, sleep deprivation improves mood in patients with depression, and in bipolar patients may precipitate mania. Thus, the patient's mood state is expected to change as the procedure progresses. Moreover, several assumptions may not hold up to severe scrutiny. First, the cosine function assumes that studied parameters change as a continuous undulation rather than discontinuous alternation (see below). Second, processes s and c are assumed to have an additive interaction, whereas it is possible that at times synergistic or less-than-additive interactions are possible. Nevertheless, there is no procedure as good as constant routine for determining important markers for the timing of light interventions, such as circadian temperature minimum. Validation work is needed to find models that can eliminate the need for extended wakefulness in patients with affective illness, especially bipolar patients.

39. Wehr's group (Wehr and Wirz-Justice, 1982; Wehr et al., 1982) found that most patients who had rapid (1- to 6-week) manic-depressive cycles experienced one or more double-length (48-hour) sleep–wake cycles at the onset of each manic phase of their mood cycle. Upon switching from the depressed to the manic phase, they often had alternate nights of total insomnia. Conceivably, these recurring escapes of the sleep–wake cycle from its primary (1:1) mode to its secondary (1:2) mode of coupling to the day–night cycle result from its driving oscillator having an overly long intrinsic period. Because the sleep–wake oscillator is weak, its oscillations remain relatively well coordinated with the day–night cycle and other circadian rhythms. Thus, the dissociation of its oscillations is expressed only in the periodic 24-hour phase jumps associated with double-length sleep–wake cycles. In free-running circadian rhythm experiments in which all external time cues have been eliminated, normal individuals sometimes experience similar 48-hour sleep–wake cycles (Wever, 1979, 1983; Wehr and Wirz-Justice, 1982; Wehr et al., 1982; Weitzman, 1982). Thus, 48-hour sleep–wake cycles in manic patients may resemble the behavior of normal sleep-regulating mechanisms under free-running conditions, perhaps associated with uncoupling of oscillators that are normally linked.

40. According to Georgi (1947, p. 1267), "In the true endogenous depressive we see a shift in the 24-hour rhythm, a phase shift, that can express itself from a slight phase shift to a complete reversal—the night becomes day. Anyone knowing the material would look for the CNS origin in the midbrain, where the entire vegetative nervous system is controlled by a central clock whose rhythmicity . . . regulates and balances the biological system."

41. The literature on circadian rhythms in depression has focused on nonseasonal depression. Seasonal (winter) depression (described later in the chapter) may involve a circadian phase delay.

42. Wehr et al., 1979; Sack et al., 1985; Souêtre et al., 1985; Vollmann and Berger, 1993; Berger et al., 1997; Albert et al., 1998; Riemann et al., 1999.

43. Contrary to expectations, REM latency was not different between the two groups, and the REM density was decreased to a greater degree in the "normal" sleep period group. It is thus unlikely that phase advance combined with sleep deprivation acts by reducing REM disinhibition.

44. von Zerssen et al., 1985; Souêtre et al., 1988, 1989; Nagayama et al., 1992; Dietzel and Ciullo, 1996.

45. These abnormalities included a trend to increased dark-adjusted melatonin suppression compared with matched controls, significantly lower baseline melatonin levels and nadir levels on the light night, a trend to greater amplitude of variation in melatonin secretion compared with matched controls on the dark night, and significantly later peak time (Nurnberger et al., 2000).

46. This increased sensitivity is also present in offspring of bipolar patients more commonly than in healthy controls (Nurnberger et al., 1988), making it a candidate for an endophenotype for bipolar disorder.

47. Kavaliers and Ralph, 1981; Welsh and Moore-Ede, 1990; Klemfuss and Kripke, 1995; Kripke, 1995; Abe et al., 2000.

48. Johnsson et al., 1979, 1980, 1983; Klemfuss, 1992.

49. As described in Chapter 14, the enzyme glycogen synthase kinase 3-beta (GSK-3β) appears to be a target of lithium action (Phiel and Klein, 2001). GSK is a highly conserved enzyme in evolution (Plyte et al., 1992; Cohen and Frame, 2001; Woodgett, 2001). The basic amino acid sequence and substrate specificity are common among species from unicellular organisms to Drosophila and humans. Of possible relevance to the circadian actions of lithium, GSK-3β has a Drosophila ortologue called SHAGGY, which happens to phosphorylate the timeless protein, a component of the Drosophila molecular clock mechanism (Martinek et al., 2001).
Overexpression of SHAGGY results in shortening of the free-running circadian period, while a decrease in SHAGGY activity has the opposite effect of increasing the free-running circadian period (Martinek et al., 2001). Given the participation of GSK-3β in the circadian clock of Drosophila and the well-known effects of lithium in inhibiting GSK-3β while prolonging the circadian period, Gould and Manji (2002a) have raised the possibility that GSK-3β represents a putative cellular mechanism for altering circadian physiology in very diverse organisms, from unicellular to complex (Klemfuss, 1992), and represents a molecular target for the circadian action of lithium.

50. Sleep disruption leading to excessive sleepiness or insomnia that is due to a mismatch between the sleep–wake schedule required by a person's environment and his or her circadian sleep–wake pattern.

51. Provencio et al., 1998, 2000, 2002; Gooley et al., 2001; Barinaga, 2002; Berson et al., 2002; Hannibal et al., 2002; Hattar et al., 2002.

52. For reviews, see Gillin, 1983; Brown, 1984; Wehr, 1990; Leibenluft and Wehr, 1992; Wirz-Justice and van den Hoofdakker, 1999; Riemann et al., 2001.

53. Ebert et al., 1991, 1994; Wu et al., 1992; Volk et al., 1997.

54. Wu et al., 1992, 1999, 2001; Leonhardt et al., 1994; Smith et al., 1999.

55. This concept was confirmed and advanced using a new technology called low-resolution electromagnetic tomography (LORETA), which computes the three-dimensional intracerebral distributions of current density for specific EEG frequency bands. Pizzagalli and colleagues (2001) reported that increased EEG theta activity in the anterior cingulate during the pretreatment period predicted antidepressant response to nortriptyline. In that study, pretreatment theta activity in the medial frontal region extending to the anterior cingulate gyrus correlated positively with percent improvement in depression after treatment. Of interest, it was only the theta band activity in the pretreatment condition that correlated with depression in the study by Pizzagalli and colleagues (2001), because theta activity in the waking EEG reflects accumulation of both process s and process c (Aeschbach et al., 1999). Moreover, the rostral anterior cingulate may be an important generator for theta activity in the human brain (Asada et al., 1999; Ishii et al., 1999). In the future, it would be interesting to correlate response to sleep deprivation with midfrontal theta wave dynamics and cingulate activity using neuroimaging.

56. It is possible, however, that after an initial dramatic response, a particular patient would respond even better to sleep deprivation in the future, given that an expectation factor may add to any biological effect.

57. Payne and colleagues (2002) suggested that sleep deprivation may act by imposing a temporal coincidence on normally

dissociated events (maintaining the activity of noradrenergic neurons of the locus ceruleus at a time when tissues innervated by the locus ceruleus show the highest sensitivity).

58. It is only during REM sleep, and not during NREM sleep or wakefulness, that neurons in the locus ceruleus, the main source of noradrenergic stimulation of the brain, are inactive and noradrenergic receptors have their highest sensitivity (Siegel and Rogawski, 1988). Thus the hypothesis that REM sleep deprivation is the mechanism of action of sleep deprivation implicates noradrenergic mechanisms.

59. In this study, adding both lithium and light treatment to total sleep deprivation did not result in further improvement, suggesting a ceiling effect.

60. Vollmann and Berger, 1993; Berger et al., 1997; Albert et al., 1998; Riemann et al., 1999.

61. In fact, the periods with greatest mood instability were those when his circadian rhythms in sleep, melatonin, and rectal temperature appeared to lose their entrainment to the 24-hour sleep–wake cycle and free run around the clock with a period longer than 24 hours. The therapeutic premise was to increase the number of hours available for sleep, overriding sleep deprivation–induced mania. Because animal research showed that a reduction in scotoperiod (duration of darkness) may decrease the ability of the circadian pacemaker to reset the response to light (Goldman and Eliott, 1988), a therapeutic increase in scotoperiod would result in increased amplitude of biological rhythms and thus decreased ability of the circadian pacemaker to synchronize downstream rhythms with the light–dark cycle.

62. The authors chose to use midday light on the basis of the preliminary observations of Leibenluft and colleagues (1995)—who followed 13 patients with rapid-cycling bipolar disorder on light therapy for 3 months—that morning light could result in increased cycling and hypomania; that evening light was largely ineffective; and that midday light, thought initially to be a placebo intervention, appeared to be the most effective (indeed, it has since been interpreted as a stabilizing, entraining stimulus for a process underlying hypomania). Kusumi and colleagues (1994) found a similar effect with morning administration of light combined with vitamin B12, without increased cycling or hypomania. Unfortunately, to our knowledge, no controlled study has followed up on these observations.

63. The purpose of IPSRT is on the one hand to regulate circadian rhythms and sleep–wake cycles (with a major intended impact on hypomania, mania, and cycling) and on the other hand to address losses, stresses, and interpersonal tensions and difficulties (with a major intended impact on depression). An example of how the social domain can interact with the circadian domain is a new baby's disrupting parents' sleep at night. Besides resulting in sleep deprivation and thus possibly in a manic switch, such disruption may expose the circadian system to light at a time of increased potential for large switches (around temperature minimum). These switches may result in depression or inadequate social functioning (e.g., falling asleep or feeling sleepy in the late afternoon in the case of phase advance) and may further contribute to deterioration of the sleep–wake cycle (inability to fall asleep and to wake up in the case of phase delay).

While the interpersonal component of the therapy focuses on four "traditional" aspects of treatment—grief, role disputes, role transitions, and interpersonal deficits—the circadian and sleep–wake component focuses on the disruption of social zeitgebers (e.g., personal relationships and social demands and tasks) that entrain biological rhythms and the occurrence of zeitstörers (time disrupters) that may be physical (e.g., exposure to light as in transmeridian travel), chemical (e.g., medications), or psychosocial (e.g., a new baby or work deadlines). Monk and colleagues (1990) designed the Social Rhythm Metric (SRM) that is used in IPSRT. The patient and therapist review the first 3–4 weeks of SRM measures to find rhythms that are particularly unstable, such as variation in the time of going to bed from day to day or from weekday to weekend days. The therapist encourages stabilization of such social rhythms, searching for rhythm disrupters, especially ongoing environmental stressors, and making recommendations for life changes to enhance protection of circadian rhythms and the sleep–wake cycle. A slightly more regular day job, even if less lucrative, is highly desirable for some patients. Difficulty may arise with certain patients (analogous to medication nonadherence; see Chapter 24) as a very stable lifestyle may appear unappealing, and some patients may mourn their lost hypomanias. The therapist works toward achieving a healthy balance between stability and spontaneity. Another area of focus is the anticipation of changes in routines with changes in one's social climate (e.g., breakup with a partner, divorce or separation, death of a spouse, leaving for college), resulting in the loss of social zeitgebers.

An analogy with alcohol may be appropriate. Many individuals can use small amounts of alcohol intermittently with no apparent detrimental effect, but there is some consensus that a recommendation for its intermittent use is not okay for alcoholics. Similarly, while some degree of instability in social rhythms is likely okay for a majority of individuals, it is highly detrimental for bipolar patients. Even in recovered individuals, craving persists. Just as alcoholics may continue to crave alcohol, bipolar patients may continue to crave the roller coaster, the spontaneity of living, and hypomania. Ongoing therapy (e.g., Alcoholics Anonymous for the alcoholic, the preventive phase of IPRST for the bipolar patient) helps reduce the risk of relapse.

64. Baillarger, 1854; Griesinger, 1867; Falret, 1890; Kraepelin, 1921.

65. The enzyme responsible for the conversion of serotonin to melatonin is pineal N-acetyltranspherase.

66. Two peaks have been identified in human conceptions—one in fall and one in spring. Usually the spring peak is dominant, although a shift toward the fall peak has been noted in the United States over the last several decades. Seasonal variation in conception has decreased in amplitude over the last 100–200 years, possibly as a result of the advent of artificial lighting and indoor temperature control. An alternative explanation is changes in nutrition. In female rats, for example, ad libitum feeding renders the pituitary–ovarian axis insensitive to melatonin, while restricted feeding sensitizes it to the effects of melatonin (Wilamowska et al., 1992). Since subsistence-level feeding may have been prevalent in earlier periods of human history (Wehr, 2001), it may have contributed to greater seasonality of reproduction. (For further support see *Journal of Biological Rhythms*, June 2004.)

67. Among them Petridou and colleagues (2002) in the United States, Rasanen and colleagues (2002b) in Finland, Morken

and colleagues (2002) in Norway, van Houwelingen and Beersma (2001a,b) in the Netherlands, and C. Cantor and colleagues (2000) in Australia.

68. Increased levels of potentially depressogenic interleukins have been found in bipolar patients with SAD (Leu et al., 2001), as well as in patients with bipolar disorder in general (Tsai et al., 2001). Nelson (2004), who brought immunology to the forefront of seasonality, suggested that immune functions are activated during winter to enhance survival in the "bottleneck" created by high-energy thermoregulatory demands at a time of reduced availability of nutrients. While preparing to defend the body from infections, the immune cells communicate via cytokines to the brain and the rest of the body that a behavioral inhibition may be necessary to conserve energy.

69. Studies aimed at distinguishing effects of depression and seasonality may produce more consistent results if SAD patients are compared not with controls but with patients experiencing nonseasonal recurrent depression. According to the vulnerability hypothesis, one could also compare subsyndromal SAD patients with normal controls.

The melatonin hypothesis could be further tested with improved designs involving either administration of light at a time when it would suppress early-morning versus later melatonin secretion or pharmacologic manipulations. Antidepressant interventions might include a bedtime delayed-release preparation of propranonol or selective melatonin receptor antagonists. On the other hand, loss of the antidepressant effect of light or the induction of a winter state during summer may result from appropriately timed administration of melatonin, a melatonin receptor agonist, or a serotonin receptor antagonist (5-HT_{1B} receptors mediate the inhibitory effect of the serotonergic system on retinohypothalamic axons).

An important contribution to our understanding of seasonality in humans, as well as to optimal treatment of SAD, may result from examining the potential role in seasonality of factors other than light, such as other physical, chemical, and biological factors, as well as interventions such as immunological, olfactory, and temperature manipulations in addition to light treatment. Also valuable would be research on melanopsin-based photoreception in patients with SAD versus controls and on retinal sensitivity to the narrow spectrum that would have maximum effect on melatonin suppression and shifting. The most important directions for future research may involve focusing at the molecular level to explore the underlying mechanisms of heterogeneity in seasonality, such as mutations in clock genes or genes that code for melatonin receptors, as well as the numeric and topographic distribution of those receptors in individuals with versus without seasonal changes in mood, level of energy, sleepiness and sleep, weight and appetite, and interest in socialization and sex.

70. Wehr and colleagues (1987) also hypothethized that summer SAD may involve a specific abnormality in thermoregulation that increases the individual's sensitivity to heat.

71. For example, the DSM-IV criterion of two major depressive episodes occurring in the last 2 years is rarely fulfilled because approximately half of SAD patients do not become depressed each winter and, most important, because many SAD patients today treat themselves with light before experiencing a full-blown episode of major depression, thereby aborting the episode.

72. One study showed that aborigines from Northern Scandinavia have less variation in mood than other Scandinavians (Saarijarvi et al., 1997). SAD is less common in the Icelandic population (which has lived in virtual isolation during the past 1,000 years) (Magnusson and Stefansson, 1993) and its descendants in Canada (Magnusson and Axelsson, 1993) than on the eastern coast of the United States (Magnusson, 2000). This difference may be due to environmental factors—most likely "portable" environmental factors associated with lifestyle, such as diet or activity schedule, rather than "fixed" environmental factors, such as climate—or to genetic factors.

73. Young and colleagues (1997) hypothesized that weather may explain the year-to-year variation in the onset of depressive symptoms in SAD. After careful adjustment for photoperiod, however, they found no significant effect of weather on the onset of depressive symptoms in SAD.

74. In a recent study by Postolache's group (Yousuffi et al., 2003), African college students living in the Washington, D.C., metropolitan area for at least 3 years reported more problems with changes in season than their African American colleagues, a finding consistent with a habituation hypothesis. Results of only one study, however, support the sensitization hypothesis: Murase and colleagues (1995) reported increased prevalence of winter-type SAD in long-staying as compared with short-staying Japanese residents of Sweden. In contrast, Murase and colleagues (1995) reported increased prevalence of winter-type SAD in long-staying as compared with short-staying Japanese residents of Sweden.

75. If the loading on seasonality exceeds that on depression, one would expect SAD with full remission in the summer; on the other hand, if the loading on depression exceeds that on SAD, summer remissions would be incomplete.

76. The term "hypophyseal insufficiency associated with lack of light" (first used by Marx, a German physiologist, in 1946) represents the first scientific description of SAD. Marx also hypothesized that light affected patients' behavior via the retino-hypothalamic tract, which he termed "the hypothalamic root of the optic nerve."

Animal seasonal rhythms provided the analogies and the impetus for SAD research. In photoperiodic animals, seasonal changes they experience are mediated by the duration of melatonin secretion. The report of Lewy and colleagues (1980) that melatonin is suppressed by bright light in humans was followed somewhat logically and somewhat serendipitously by the description of the first SAD patient and his treatment with light (Lewy et al., 1982), and then a more complete description of the syndrome and a preliminary evaluation of light treatment (Rosenthal et al., 1984). Light treatment was proven effective in a double-blind, placebo-controlled paradigm (Eastman et al., 1998; Terman et al., 1998). Wehr and colleagues (2001b) showed that patients with SAD, and not matched controls, have a longer duration of active melatonin secretion in winter than in summer, similar to changes in melatonin duration in animals. Individual variability is high in humans, but even in species with more drastic and uniform behavioral changes in response to photoperiodic changes than those experienced by humans, some individual animals do not respond at all to changes in photoperiod (Puchalski and Lynch, 1986; Gorman and Zucker, 1997).

77. Bupropion was used prophylactically to prevent the onset of winter depression in SAD.

78. Administration of the tyrosine hydroxlase inhibitor alpha-methyl-paratyrosine was used to deplete catecholamines.

79. Rather than describing phase position relative to external time, describing it relative to wake–sleep time may be more clinically relevant. Thus in a recent study (Lewy et al., 2006), the duration of the interval between melatonin onset and sleep onset (the melatonin–sleep interval, or MSI) predicted depression scores in patients with SAD. The ideal MSI is 2 hours; the more MSI deviated in either direction from 2 hours, the higher were the depression scores. Moreover, with specifically timed administration of physiological doses of melatonin, changes in depression scores were correlated with the movement toward or away from the 2-hour standard. Thus defining phase advance as MSIs greater than 2 hours and phase delay as MSIs less than 2 hours (rather than relative to astronomical time) may help guide treatment, that is, the use of timed administration of melatonin and/or light to shift abnormal phase positions.

80. Jones et al., 1999; Lowrey et al., 2000; Allada et al., 2001; Toh et al., 2001.

81. In fact, agomelatine, another melatonin receptor agonist with additional $5-HT_{2C}$ receptor antagonist properties, was shown in 711 depressed patients to be effective and well tolerated, with a higher efficacy than placebo and a faster response than paroxetine (Loo et al., 2002). In addition, agomelatine, in contrast to paroxetine, was not associated with a discontinuation syndrome (Montgomery et al., 2004).

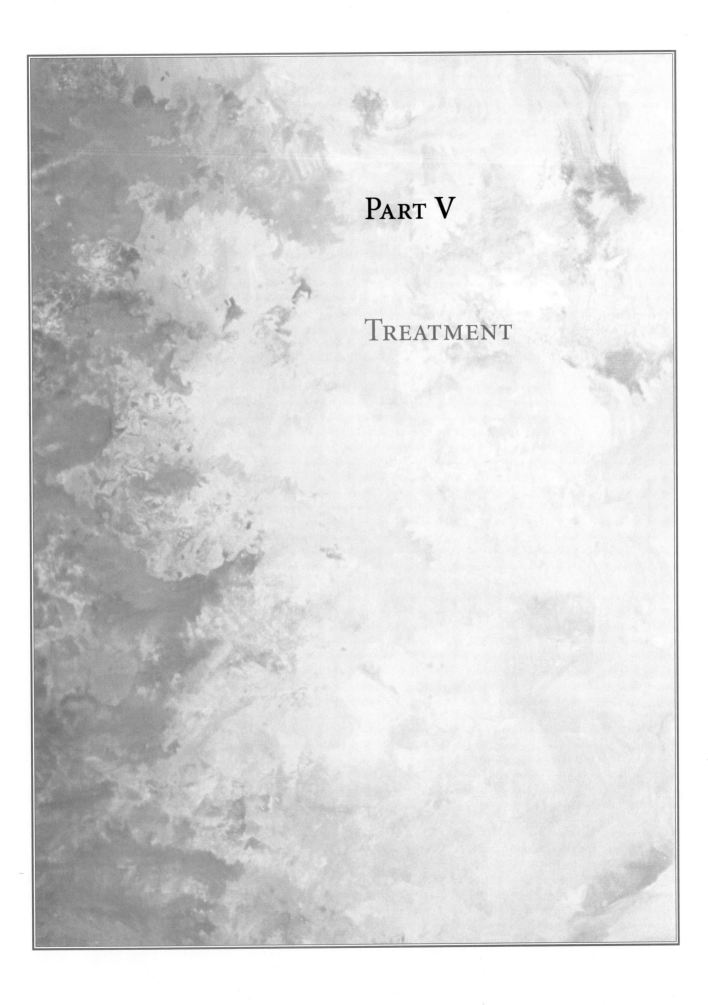

Part V

Treatment

17 Fundamentals of Treatment

Of all our conversations, I remember most vividly [Robert Lowell's] words about the new drug, lithium carbonate, which had such good results and gave him reason to believe he was cured: "It's terrible, Bob, to think that all I've suffered, and all the suffering I've caused, might have arisen from the lack of a little salt in my brain."

—*Robert Giroux, 1967*

Until the middle of the twentieth century, manic-depressive illness had remained intractable, frustrating the best efforts of clinical practitioners and their forebears to treat it. This long history ended abruptly with the discovery of lithium's therapeutic benefits. The impact of the discovery of lithium has been profound and long-lasting (Goodwin and Ghaemi, 1999; Bauer et al., 2006). Not only did it reaffirm psychiatry as a medical specialty in an era when the ideology behind "the myth of mental illness" and "mental illness as a normal response to a crazy world" was in ascendancy (particularly in the United States and the United Kingdom), but the fact that lithium's effects were specific to a particular diagnosis reinforced the importance of nosology at a time when many in the mental health field were deriding the very concept of a diagnosis as "labeling." The benefits of lithium established beyond rational dispute that a major mental illness did indeed have a strong biological component with which a chemical treatment was obviously interacting; this, in turn, initiated what has become a sea change in the public's perception of the mentally ill and of mental health professionals.[1] In an ironic turn of events, moreover, the psychopharmacology revolution set in motion by lithium eventually mobilized a renaissance in the psychotherapy of manic-depressive patients. Substantially freed of the severe disruptions of mania and the profound withdrawals of depression, patients and therapists could sustain their focus on the many psychological issues related to the illness, and also confront basic developmental tasks. Most important, lithium has saved the lives of hundreds of thousands of patients and immeasurably changed for the better the course and outcome of manic-depressive illness for millions more.

For the research community and, more broadly, the mental health community, lithium and the psychopharmacology revolution it launched can be said to have led to the development of today's formal diagnostic systems, the *Diagnostic Statistical Manual* (DSM)-IV and the *International Classification of Diseases* (ICD)-10. Because the early psychopharmacology researchers required reliable diagnoses to define their study populations, the Research Diagnostic Criteria were developed and subsequently became the basis for today's diagnostic systems. Moreover, lithium and the drugs that followed gave substantial impetus to modern neuroscience. Prior to the discovery of the clinical effects of lithium, the phenothiazines, and the antidepressants, basic and clinical scientists focused largely on neuroanatomy. Efforts to understand how these new drugs were exerting their powerful and often specific effects required a shift from a predominantly structural to a functional neuroscience focused on neurotransmitters, neuromodulators, receptors, and, more recently, mechanisms of postsynaptic signal transduction and gene induction. Today, of course, the cutting edge of neuroscience reflects the integration of functional and anatomical approaches. Here, too, the mechanisms of action of lithium continue to be a major emphasis (see Chapter 14).

THE HUMAN AND ECONOMIC COSTS OF MANIC-DEPRESSIVE ILLNESS

We have chosen here to discuss the impact of manic-depressive illness (its human and economic costs) first, followed by a brief review of "real-world" patterns of medication use and their effectiveness. In reality these issues are intertwined: contemporary data on the impact of the illness involve patient populations receiving various levels of treatment, from none to high-quality combinations of medications and psychotherapy delivered by specialists. The literature on the impact of manic-depressive illness and the application and effectiveness of treatments has focused on the bipolar subgroup; while there is a robust literature on depressive disorders, to our knowledge recurrent depression has not been analyzed separately in these studies.

The impact of bipolar disorder on individual lives starts with its usual age at onset—adolescence and the twenties—precisely the time when individuals must navigate the critical developmental transition from childhood to adulthood (Calabrese et al., 2003; Post, 2005). In Chapter 4 we review the evidence suggesting that earlier ages at onset are associated with a less favorable course of illness. The extent to which interference with developmental processes (including interrupted educational and career trajectories) accounts for this association is not clear. What is clear is that in the aggregate, bipolar illness is associated with major functional impairment, include physical disability. Indeed, the World Health Organization (WHO) has estimated that bipolar disorder is the sixth-leading cause of disability for those in the age range most associated with the onset of the disorder—15 to 44 (Murray and Lopez, 1996). The WHO data and results of other epidemiological surveys related to the disability associated with bipolar disorder are reviewed in Chapter 5. A relationship between early age at onset and disability is suggested by the striking finding of Gillberg and colleagues (1993) that 89 percent of adolescents with bipolar disorder were receiving full disability benefits in the United States by age 30 despite treatment (primarily lithium).

As reviewed in Chapter 4, among patients receiving treatment in the community (see below), considerable functional impairment often persists even in the face of full symptomatic or syndromal recovery.[2] For example, Dion and colleagues (1988) found that while 80 percent of their bipolar patients hospitalized for mania were symptom-free or only mildly symptomatic 6 months after discharge, only 43 percent were employed, and only 21 percent were working at their pre-illness level. Employment status was better following a first hospital admission: 64 percent of such patients were employed versus only 33 percent of those with previous admissions.[3] Conus and colleagues (2006) examined symptomatic and functional outcomes following a first episode of psychotic mania in a catchment area sample, that is, a sample broadly representative of the community. They found that at 1 year, while 90 percent of the patients had achieved syndromal recovery, 61 percent had failed to return to their previous level of functioning. Predictors of functional outcome were substance abuse, earlier age at onset, and a family history of affective disorder. Particularly striking was the impact of substance abuse: patients with this comorbidity were 19 times less likely to return to their previous level of functioning.[4] In addition, the families of recovered euthymic

bipolar patients can still experience considerable caregiver burden (Reinares et al., 2006).

It is the extent of depressive, not manic, symptoms that predicts[5] poor functional outcome during follow-up (Bauer et al., 2001; Judd et al., 2005; Altshuler et al., 2006); it is also depressive morbidity that explains why bipolar disorder compared with unipolar depression is associated with more than twice the number of days lost from work according to the U.S. National Comorbidity Survey (Kessler et al., 2006). In the three chapters that follow, we note the imbalance between the impressive number of medications developed for the treatment of mania and the paucity of agents developed for the treatment of bipolar or highly recurrent unipolar depression. Given that depressive symptoms are primarily responsible for the burden of illness, any continuation of this imbalance is unacceptable. It should be noted that in the Bauer and colleagues (2001) Veterans Health Administration study, clinical status (primarily the extent of depression) predicted only about half of the variance in functional outcome, the remainder being associated with individual patient factors, such as the ability to engage in treatment and to manage life tasks despite the illness.

Functional impairment and disability associated with bipolar disorder incur considerable financial costs—for the patient, the family, and society at large. Estimates of such costs vary according to the assumptions used. One of the most widely cited figures is that of Wyatt and Henter (1995), who estimated the direct and indirect costs of bipolar disorder in the United States at $45 billion, 84 percent of which comprised indirect costs, such as lost productivity, unemployment compensation, disability payments, and law enforcement. More recently, Begley and colleagues (2001) estimated the lifetime cost for new cases of bipolar disorder in the United States during 1998 at $24 billion, with a lifetime cost per case of up to $625,000 for those with chronic, treatment-resistant symptoms. Yearly cost estimates globally range from $12,000 to $18,000 per patient, 80 percent of which consists of indirect costs (Kleinman et al., 2003; Dardennes et al., 2006). The very high ratio of indirect to direct costs suggests it should be possible to demonstrate that clinically effective treatments can be cost-effective as well (Chisholm et al., 2005). Perhaps especially relevant to policy makers today is the increased cost of medical care among bipolar patients (Kupfer, 2006; McIntyre et al., 2006; Gardner et al., 2006), which exceeds that for diabetes (Simon and Unutzer, 1999). More effective treatments would be expected to reduce these medical costs. And since mental health care generally accounts for only 6 to 7 percent of total health care costs, it has been argued that cutting back on psychiatric care for bipolar patients in an attempt to reduce health care costs is penny wise and pound foolish (Hyman et al., 2006).

"REAL-WORLD" PHARMACOTHERAPY AND ITS EFFECTIVENESS

In the three chapters that follow, we review the *efficacy* of various drugs in treating mania and depression and in preventing recurrences; the knowledge base for these chapters comes almost entirely from controlled studies of single drugs, and substantially from patients not only without comorbidities but also well enough to give informed consent for research. To understand this growing knowledge base in a larger context, it is useful first to understand the reality of how medications are actually being used in the community and how *effective* they are, that is, how well they work under circumstances in which the "average" patient has both physical and psychiatric comorbidities and is taking more than one drug. Obviously, patterns of use and effectiveness are inexorably intertwined with the illness's human and economic costs as discussed above. While available treatments could allow many manic-depressive patients to lead relatively normal lives—lives less painfully interrupted by illness and less often ended prematurely by suicide—the reality falls far short of meeting this modest expectation. One has only to recall the naturalistic follow-up studies of the modern era (see Chapter 4), during which contemporary treatments have been available, to find support for this conclusion. Myriad interrelated factors contribute to this therapeutic shortfall, including long delays in seeking and receiving treatment and differences in health care delivery systems, in patients' attitudes toward treatment, in clinicians' skills and training, in the availability of family and social supports, in comorbid conditions, and so on. Before briefly examining some of these factors (many of which are also covered in the individual treatment chapters that follow), we must restate the fundamental reality emphasized in the first edition of this text: we simply do not yet have an adequate understanding of the illness in all of its various forms and complexities, including its interactions with *individual differences* that is, differences in environment and in the patient's character and psychological and physical resilience. By thus citing the limits of our knowledge, we in no way intend to diminish the very substantial progress that has been made since the first edition was published. On the contrary, it is most encouraging that this progress has occurred on virtually all fronts, not the least of which is the development of new pharmacological and psychosocial treatments, as described in the following chapters.

In their recent review of epidemiological studies from around the world, Schaffer and colleagues (2006) concluded that anywhere from one-fourth to nearly two-thirds of individuals with bipolar disorder have never sought any sort of treatment for a mental disorder. For those who do seek

treatment, there is often a lengthy delay (approximately 10 years) before a correct diagnosis is made and appropriate pharmacotherapy initiated.[6] This delay contributes substantially to worse long-term outcomes and to reduced effectiveness of treatments once they are started.[7,8] More often than not, delay in the initiation of appropriate treatment means inappropriate treatment rather than simply the absence of treatment. This is the case because about half of bipolar patients are initially diagnosed as unipolar and treated with antidepressants (Ghaemi et al., 2000; Blanco et al., 2002; Perlis et al., 2006). As discussed in Chapter 19, such inappropriate treatment can have major negative consequences for the illness, including increased costs of care (Li et al., 2002; Matza et al., 2005). Whatever factors contribute to the absence of appropriate treatment in an individual patient, results of studies in nonacademic community settings indicate that half or more of all bipolar patients are not taking a mood stabilizer (see, e.g., Lim et al., 2001; Wang et al., 2005; Schaffer et al., 2006).

What does the literature tell us about the effectiveness of contemporary pharmacotherapy? It is difficult to develop an estimate of effectiveness for the "average" bipolar patient. Most studies are from academic centers, which on the one hand are likely to deliver high-quality care, but on the other are dealing with the kinds of patients who tend to end up in tertiary referral centers, that is, those with more severe and treatment-resistant illness. For example, 2-year data from the largest treatment study of bipolar disorder ever undertaken—the National Institute of Mental Health's (NIMH) Systematic Treatment Enhancement Program for Bipolar Disorder (STEP-BD) (involving academic centers) (Perlis et al., 2006)—indicate that the "best treatment available" was associated with full remission in just over half of the bipolar patients, and that nearly half of the recovered patients relapsed at least once during the 2-year study (see Chapter 20). Similarly, a Stanley Foundation Bipolar Network academic center follow-up study (Levine et al., 2000) found that fewer than half of the patients were able to live independently or be employed, and more than half made at least one suicide attempt during the study. Results from another academic tertiary referral center (Gitlin et al., 1995) are similar: 73 percent of bipolar patients receiving "aggressive maintenance treatment" relapsed during the 5-year follow-up period, and two-thirds of those who relapsed did so more than once.

Combining the studies reviewed in this and the previous section (as well as in Chapter 4) reveals a picture suggesting that, with respect to syndromal recovery, treatment effectiveness in community samples is better than that in referral centers, but with respect to functional recovery, results in neither setting are encouraging. Perhaps functional disabilities derive substantially from the psychological and social scars of having had episodes, rather than primarily from the severity of symptoms during episodes. It is perhaps for this reason that pharmacological treatments appear to be more effective against syndromes and symptoms than against dysfunction and disability. Obviously, the importance of psychosocial rehabilitation can hardly be overstated.

STRUCTURE AND RATIONALE OF THE TREATMENT CHAPTERS

This part of the book departs from earlier parts in its emphasis on the application of accumulated knowledge to the pragmatic business of treating individual patients. As one medical sociologist and historian has observed, "While the aim of all sciences is the maximum of generality, that of medicine ought always to be action aimed at the maximum welfare of the individual" (Wightman, 1971, p. 14). It is this principle that has guided the writing of these chapters. The chapters that follow address practical therapeutic choices faced by the clinician and summarize the clinical research on the efficacy and effectiveness of available treatments. Application of the medication strategies outlined in the next three chapters requires a psychiatrist skilled in psychopharmacology, but not necessarily a highly specialized background in manic-depressive illness. However, consultation may be necessary in some situations, such as when the diagnosis is uncertain, when the decision to hospitalize is difficult, when the response to initial treatment is poor, when the patient fails to adhere to a prescribed regimen, or, especially, when there is a danger of suicide. Although bipolar illness remains the primary focus in these chapters, highly recurrent unipolar illness and its management are considered, especially in our discussions of prophylactic treatment.

We have chosen a somewhat unconventional organization for these chapters, with clinical recommendations preceding the evidence that supports them. There are two reasons for this choice. First, our treatment recommendations represent more than a distillation of research findings. They are drawn from our reading of the literature and, we believe, represent the essential core of the evidence. Where we find the literature to be incomplete or equivocal, we supplement it with the seasoned judgments of our colleagues and opinions based on our own clinical experience. Our second reason for organizing these chapters as we did is our belief that the formal literature has more meaning when framed by clinical treatment issues. Although future research certainly will alter and supplement any of our specific recommendations, it is our hope that the fundamental principles outlined here will have lasting value for the clinical care of patients with manic-depressive illness.

Following this chapter (which includes a review of the basic pharmacology of the major classes of drugs used in treating manic-depressive illness) are three chapters devoted to medical treatment of adults, including medication, electroconvulsive therapy, novel central nervous system (CNS) stimulation techniques, and manipulation of sleep and light. The treatment of manic episodes is covered in Chapter 18 and that of depressive episodes in Chapter 19. Long-term prophylactic treatment is discussed in Chapter 20, as is the issue of side effects, which in our experience becomes most salient during prophylactic treatment. Chapter 21 focuses on the special issue of adherence to medical treatments, while Chapter 22 deals with psychotherapy and related issues. Chapter 23 addresses the pharmacological and psychological treatment of children and adolescents. Chapters 24 and 25, respectively, are focused on two special and important populations: those with comorbid conditions and those at risk for suicide. The presence of comorbid conditions, both psychiatric and medical, is increasingly recognized as a complicating and limiting factor in the treatment of manic-depressive illness; successful management of the illness depends on the clinician's ability to recognize and treat these comorbid conditions, especially anxiety and substance abuse/dependence. Finally, far too many manic-depressive patients kill themselves, and clinicians must be astute not only in assessing suicide potential but also in knowing how to manage it, both pharmacologically and psychologically.

Stages of Treatment

In reading this section, it is important to keep in mind the natural course of manic-depressive illness, described in Chapter 4. Although many treatments can alter acute symptoms dramatically, the nature and logic of planning treatment should be shaped by respect for the course of the illness: its inherently, insidiously recurrent nature, as well as its tendency to worsen over time. Throughout these chapters, we use several terms to describe stages of medical and psychotherapeutic treatment that are linked conceptually to aspects of the illness's natural course:

- *Acute treatment* is treatment administered during the period from the beginning of a manic or depressive episode to a clinical response—ideally, remission. This phase usually lasts from 6 to 12 weeks.
- *Continuation treatment* is the ongoing treatment of a depressive or manic episode from the point of clinical response to the point at which spontaneous recovery would be expected to occur in untreated patients. Although overt clinical symptoms of illness may remit within a few weeks, an underlying "tail" of vulnerability can remain for some time. The duration of continuation

treatment is determined by the natural course of the illness. In nonrecurrent unipolar patients, antidepressants are usually recommended for a period of 9 to 12 months after remission, but the natural course of bipolar disorder suggests a somewhat shorter continuation phase after a depressive episode—approximately 6 months. While the natural course of mania would suggest a continuation phase of about 4 months, clinically it can be longer, involving the management of a postmania depression or a sometimes protracted period of mood instability dominated by dysphoria as the patient attempts to repair the external and internal damage wrought by the manic episode.

- *Maintenance treatment* is intended to prevent or attenuate future mood episodes in patients with bipolar or recurrent unipolar illness, and it is used somewhat more selectively than are acute and continuation treatment. A word of clarification is in order, however. Although commonly used, the term *maintenance treatment* is less precise than *long-term prophylactic treatment*, or *prophylaxis*, in referring to the effects of treatment on the long-term course of manic-depressive illness. The concept of maintenance overlaps both the continuation and prophylactic phases of treatment, whereas prophylactic effects range from prevention of future episodes to attenuation of their frequency, duration and/or severity. Thus while we use the common term *maintenance treatment* throughout the volume, particularly in Chapter 20, we intend it to refer specifically to prophylaxis.

General Clinical Considerations

Psychiatric Evaluation and Diagnosis

Evaluation of the patient before treatment is the most important stage in managing the illness. As extensively as the patient's clinical condition permits, the evaluation should cover the pattern and duration of symptoms, exposure to possibly stressful life events, suicide potential, substance abuse, and personal and family history. If at all possible, the patient's spouse or a close family member should participate; clinicians evaluating depressed patients without the participation of a family member will miss prior manic (and especially hypomanic) episodes half of the time. Screening instruments can help, but a form of the screening questions for the family member to fill out should be employed as well, since the patient's response to such questions depends on (1) the individual's memory of manic/hypomanic behaviors and feelings, and (2) sufficient insight to realize the states were not normal. Also, the presence of family members serves as an opportunity for the clinician to assess their attitudes about such issues as medications and hospitalization. The situation provides an occasion as well for

evaluating the family's ability and willingness to participate further in treatment and follow-up. This ongoing involvement can be especially helpful in the early detection of prodromal symptoms (Jackson et al., 2003), such as decreased sleep; detection of prodromal signs has been shown to prolong time to manic relapse and improve social functioning significantly (Perry et al., 1999).

Differential diagnosis, discussed fully in Chapter 3, often involves:

- Patients who are in a hyperactive psychotic state and whose personal or family history is not available. In these cases, acute schizophrenia and organic and drug-induced psychoses must be ruled out.
- Patients with mild manic-like symptoms. Normal elevated mood must be differentiated from clinical hypomania.
- Patients with severe depressive symptoms whose history is unknown. The most important alternative diagnosis to consider is unipolar depression. Schizophrenia and schizoaffective illness, drug-induced states, and dementia also must be ruled out.
- Patients with moderate depressive symptoms. Major depressive illness, either unipolar or bipolar, must be distinguished from milder forms. Manic-depressive illness (bipolar or highly recurrent unipolar) should be considered whenever recurrent, discrete episodes are present.

Medical Evaluation

The medical evaluation preceding treatment, like the psychiatric evaluation, should be shaped by the clinical situation. When lithium treatment is being considered, emphasis must be given to thyroid and renal function; for carbamazepine and valproate, hepatic and hematopoetic function, and for valproate, gonadal hormone function in females; for lamotrigine, prior sensitivity to rashes; and for some atypical antipsychotics, risk factors for weight gain, metabolic syndrome, and diabetes. Since pretreatment medical evaluation is most critical for long-term treatment, specific recommendations for laboratory tests are discussed in Chapter 20. Finally, clinicians often discover previously undiagnosed medical problems in the course of their routine pretreatment evaluations. This potential dividend provides a further reason to exercise care in the initial phase of treatment.

The Therapeutic Alliance in Drug Treatment

Chapters 21 and 22 deal extensively with the relationship between psychotherapy and medication. Here we pause briefly to underscore a fundamental truth in psychopharmacology: to achieve its full potential, any drug should be given in the context of a solid and positive clinician–patient relationship. Unfortunately, a working therapeutic alliance is not always achieved in the context of a busy practice, especially given the constraints imposed by managed care.[9] Today most formal psychotherapy is the responsibility of nonmedical mental health professionals. The challenge is how to ensure coordination between the psychopharmacologist and the psychotherapist given that there is no reimbursement for the time professionals devote to coordinating care. Since the psychotherapist spends more time with the patient, he or she is generally in a better position to know more about side effects and quality-of-life issues. The importance of coordination of care was recently demonstrated by Simon and colleagues (2005, 2006), who randomized 441 bipolar patients in a staff model health maintenance organization (HMO) to treatment as usual or to a multicomponent intervention (initially described by Bauer et al., 2001). The latter intervention involved case monitoring by nurses, structured group psychoeducation, and monthly telephone monitoring of mood and adherence, followed by feedback to the treating professionals and facilitation of needed follow-up care, including outreach and crisis intervention. The coordinated care group had significantly fewer manic symptoms and time spent manic. While the incremental mental health cost of the intervention was $1,251, one would expect that extra cost to be offset by a decrease in the high cost of medical care associated with bipolar disorder. Unfortunately, medical care costs were not reported, but on the basis of earlier studies, it appears reasonable to assume that cost savings associated with the reduction in frequency and severity of mania achieved would more than offset this modest incremental direct cost of mental health care. In a concurrent 3-year trial involving bipolar patients in 11 Veterans Affairs hospitals (who were generally sicker and more frequently hospitalized than the HMO patients in the above study), Bauer and colleagues (2006a,b) randomized 306 subjects to a similar collaborative care program or to usual care. Their results were strikingly similar to those achieved in the HMO population: there was a significant 6.2-week reduction in time spent in an affective episode (primarily manic), as well as improvements in social role functioning and quality-of-life measures. The intervention was slightly and nonsignificantly less costly than usual care, with increases in outpatient costs being more than offset by reductions in inpatient costs, both psychiatric and medical-surgical.

There is no substitute for clinical experience in applying the general principles listed in Box 17–1 and research knowledge to the treatment of manic-depressive illness with drugs. One cannot predict with complete certainty that a given patient will tolerate and benefit from a particular drug, nor can one predict the safest and most effective dose. Experimentation and adjustment are required when treatment

---

BOX 17–1. Some General Principles for the Management of Manic-Depressive Illness

- Include a family member in the initial evaluation and (on occasion and where appropriate) in the ongoing evaluation of treatment.
- Use a life chart to record the patient's history and to monitor the course of the illness.
- Aim for "balanced effectiveness"; that is, give equal weight to a drug's tolerability, efficacy, and safety. Among agents with evidence of efficacy, it is generally better to start with the most tolerable one. The side effects of most concern to patients are weight gain, neurocognitive impairment, and sedation.
- Treat breakthrough symptoms, substance abuse, comorbid anxiety and side effects vigorously. Bipolar-II patients may be more sensitive to side effects than bipolar-I patients.
- Focus psychotherapy on adherence, psychoeducation, and circadian integrity.
- Watch for suicidal behavior and persistent suicidal ideation, especially if the patient has a specific plan.
- If antidepressants are needed for the acute treatment of bipolar depression, include a mood stabilizer. Do not maintain antidepressants in bipolar patients unless attempts to taper off repeatedly fail; watch for early signs of a hypomanic/manic switch and/or increased cycling.
- When mood stabilizer monotherapy proves inadequate, use combinations in modest doses. Lithium may interact synergistically with some anticonvulsants.

---

begins, and the patient should be advised accordingly. The patient is most likely to cooperate if the clinician approaches drug treatment as an investigative undertaking—one depending on active collaboration. Controlled double-blind studies of antidepressant drugs not infrequently have shown success rates below those reported in some open trials. Some of this difference certainly can be attributed to the positive expectations of the clinicians in the open trials, but much of it is probably due to better adherence and the positive and reinforcing effects of the therapeutic alliance.

Clinicians are in the best position to help a depressed or manic patient when they convey an attitude of serious concern for the individual's suffering, while at the same time communicating confidence in their own ability and measured optimism about the ultimate outcome of treatment. It is important not to oversell a treatment. If the first approach fails without the patient's having been advised about the possibility of failure, not only is the patient's trust eroded, but the clinician can feel defeated and discredited—feelings that, in turn, may be subtly conveyed back to the patient. When both clinician and patient view a treatment as an experiment, even a poor response can be seen as an important piece of new information that can contribute substantially to the rational choice of subsequent treatments. Patients who are prescribed drugs should be told that if they fail to respond to one class of drugs, they may, by that very fact, be more likely to respond to an alternative class.

The Role of Lifestyle Changes in Optimizing Treatment

Another key component of treatment is education of the patient about the importance of regular exercise and a good diet. The patient should be made aware of studies supporting an antidepressant effect of vigorous aerobic exercise, as well as evidence that exercise, when done roughly at the same time every day, helps synchronize the circadian clock (which tends to be less stable in manic-depressive illness, particularly the bipolar subgroup; see Chapter 16). Equally important is a good diet, particularly one in which simple carbohydrates are kept to a minimum. It is helpful to explain how bipolar patients tend to have a pattern of reactive hypoglycemia, in which simple carbohydrates in the morning can produce an excessive increase in blood sugar, followed by an excessive decrease; this reactive hypoglycemia is associated with symptoms patients assume are related to their mood disorder or medication, such as feeling tired, "fuzzy-headed," or irritable. To relieve these symptoms, patients often ingest more carbohydrates (in effect "chasing" their blood sugar throughout the day), and in the process take in many additional calories. The fact that a number of the medications patients take can cause both carbohydrate craving and weight gain further supports the importance of diet and exercise in the comprehensive management of manic-depressive illness.

The clinician should also be familiar with the benefits of stress reduction techniques, such as meditation and yoga, and be able to make referrals to professionals who understand the application of these techniques to patients taking medication for mood disorders. For many patients, moreover, religious faith is not only an important part of their identity but also a source of considerable support and comfort. The clinician should be alert for clues to and always be respectful of the patient's religious or spiritual life (Griffith and Griffith, 2002; Josephson and Peteet, 2004).

To optimize recovery and reintegration, self-help groups can be invaluable. All clinicians should be familiar with the principal support groups in their area (either patient-run, such as local chapters of the Depression and Bipolar Support Alliance [DBSA], or family-focused, such as the National Alliance for the Mentally Ill [NAMI]), and be prepared to direct their patients to those groups. Given the importance of such groups to patients' recovery, we encourage clinicians to support them, not only financially but also through direct participation, such as by giving talks at local meetings or volunteering as a consultant.

Finally, there is perhaps nothing more important to the stability of the bipolar patient than good sleep management. Indeed, disturbances of sleep/circadian rhythms are so central to the pathophysiology of recurrent mood disorders that we have devoted a separate chapter to the topic. As noted above, regularity of the circadian clock is especially critical to the bipolar patient. This means a stable sleep cycle. Patients with difficulty falling asleep should be educated about the importance of having a quiet, low-stimulation environment to prepare for sleep. For example, they should avoid going to sleep with the television on and avoid arguments late at night, avoid the use of stimulants such as coffee and caffeine-based cola beverages, and for most patients, it is best not to read oneself to sleep especially if it involves a computer screen. When reading in bed use a dim (25 watt) bulb. Patients should also be made aware of the importance of avoiding alcohol just before bed; while it may help with the onset of sleep, it will make the patient more likely to awaken later. For most patients, 8 hours of sleep is optimal; less than that over time produces chronic sleep deprivation, with symptoms that can be misread as depression or, when irritability predominates, as a mild mixed state. "How are you sleeping?" is therefore a question that should be part of every clinical contact. The clinician should obtain a detailed description of when sleep onset is occurring, how often and for how long the patient awakens during the night, when the patient arises, and what if any naps are taken during the day.

Summary

Competent and compassionate treatment assumes a thorough knowledge of the diagnosis, clinical description, and natural course of manic-depressive illness. In addition, it assumes an understanding of the pharmacological and psychotherapeutic options available and the lifestyle changes that can optimize treatment, as well as the ability to establish a good therapeutic relationship and a willingness to communicate clearly with patients, their families, and the other professionals involved in patient care. The healing role of the clinician and the potentially life-saving influence of competent and compassionate psychotherapy are too often overlooked in an era of increasingly sophisticated psychopharmacology. The extraordinarily important role of the therapeutic relationship in treatment and recovery was described thus by Morag Coate (1964, p. 214) in *Beyond All Reason*:

> Because the doctors cared, and because one of them still believed in me when I believed in nothing, I have survived

to tell the tale. It is not only the doctors who perform hazardous operations or give life-saving drugs in obvious emergencies who hold the scales at times between life and death. To sit quietly in a consulting room and talk to someone would not appear to the general public as a heroic or dramatic thing to do. In medicine there are many different ways of saving lives. This is one of them.

UNDERSTANDING AND INTERPRETING THE TREATMENT RESEARCH LITERATURE

We now turn to the key methodological and conceptual issues one must understand to properly interpret the treatment research literature. While an extensive review of the principles of study design and analysis is beyond the scope of this discussion, we examine some common issues that arise in treatment research. Our focus is on bipolar disorder, although the principles delineated apply as well to recurrent unipolar disorder.

Observational (Naturalistic) Studies

Historically, new ideas and hypotheses have been born in the course of direct clinical observation. Unlike controlled studies, naturalistic studies, at their best, capture the richness and complexity of the seasoned clinician's observations of individual patients. Indeed, the observations of Kraepelin, the father of the study of manic-depressive illness, are continually rediscovered today. To quote Jonathan Himmelhoch (2003), himself a clinical investigator having wide direct experience with manic-depressive patients whose own novel observations have stood the test of time, "anecdotes that break new ground because of the careful clinical observation behind them have far greater sensitivity than can be produced by any instrument." We could not agree more. It has generally been assumed that observational studies report larger effects of a treatment than do randomized controlled trials. In an analysis of 136 reports on 19 various treatments in medicine, however, Benson and Hartz (2000) found little evidence to support this assumption.

On the other hand, with respect to the kind of observational study that compares groups of patients receiving different treatments, definitive conclusions are impossible because the treatments are not administered randomly; that is, the patients are treated by clinicians with particular drugs for certain reasons. This individual decision making means that confounding factors—those other than the one thought to be at issue—could explain the result observed. For example, an observational study of antidepressant discontinuation in bipolar disorder (Altshuler et al., 2003) found that after initial response to a mood stabilizer plus an antidepressant, those patients whose psychiatrist decided to keep them on the combination stayed well longer than those whose psychiatrist decided the antidepressant should be stopped. Since the nonrandom nature of the treatment choices was not noted in the study's abstract, many readers concluded that the results obtained demonstrated better outcomes with long-term continuation of antidepressants in bipolar patients.

To assess possible confounding bias, readers must put themselves in the place of the treating clinicians: Why would one stop antidepressant use after recovery from an acute episode? There is a literature suggesting that antidepressants can indeed cause mixed states or worsen rapid cycling in patients with bipolar disorder. Thus if a patient had rapid-cycling illness, some clinicians would be inclined to stop the antidepressant after recovery from an acute episode. This might also be the case if a patient had a history of antidepressant-induced mania that was common or severe. Likewise, some clinicians would be less likely to continue antidepressant use in a patient with bipolar-I disorder than in one with bipolar-II disorder. In other words, in such a study we do not know how many patients did worse because they were taken off the antidepressant and how many were taken off the drug because they were doing (or might do) worse. In trying to interpret an observational study, then, it is necessary to know as much as possible about the characteristics of those who were treated one way versus the other. This information is often provided in an initial table of demographic and clinical characteristics so readers can see whether there are any differences, which then might be confounders. A common mistake is for researchers to compare two groups, note a p value above .05, and then conclude that there is "no difference" and thus no confounding effect. However, this use of p values is generally inappropriate, as discussed further below, because such comparisons are usually not the primary purpose of the study (which might be focused on antidepressant outcome, not age or gender differences between groups). Usually, such studies are underpowered to detect many clinical and demographic differences, and thus p-value comparisons are irrelevant.

Levels of Evidence and the Evidence-Based Medicine Movement

A key feature of the evidence-based medicine movement is the concept of levels of evidence (see Box 17–2). Ideally, levels of evidence should guide researchers in making consistent and justified comparisons of different studies and their findings, and enable clinicians to evaluate the validity of the research literature.

It must be borne in mind that each level of evidence has its own strengths and weaknesses, so it cannot be assumed (as those not well versed in the realities of clinical

BOX **17–2.**   **Levels of Evidence**

Level I: Double-blind randomized trials (parallel-group or
            on–off designs)

   Ia: Placebo-controlled monotherapy

   Ib: Non-placebo-controlled comparison trials, or placebo-
            controlled add-on therapy trials

Level II: Open randomized trials

Level III: Naturalistic studies

   IIIa: Nonrandomized controlled studies (with a comparison
            group)

   IIIb: Large nonrandomized, uncontrolled studies (N > 100)

   IIIc: Medium-sized nonrandomized, uncontrolled studies
            (100 > N > 50)

Level IV: Small naturalistic studies (nonrandomized, uncontrolled)
            (50 > N > 10)

Level V: Case series (N < 10), case reports (N = 1), expert opinion

Source: Adapted from Gray (2002). Revised in accordance with evidence regarding the validity of naturalistic studies derived from the medical literature and with types of studies frequently published in the psychiatric literature.

trials often do) that a "higher" level always trumps a "lower" one. Consider one major problem that plagues contemporary level I randomized controlled trials in bipolar disorder—the ethical difficulty of enrolling (and maintaining) very ill patients in a trial in which some will be randomized to placebo, especially if the duration of the trial is long (Vieta and Carne, 2005). Thus when a level I trial leads to the conclusion that a given treatment has not been shown to be effective, and that conclusion conflicts with much of the existing expert clinical opinion, it is wise to consider the limited generalizability of that trial's database before dismissing the opinion of those with extensive clinical experience, including experience with the sickest patients. Many other selection factors operate (intentionally or unintentionally) to limit the generalizability of level I trials.[10] Ideally, of course, the results of double-blind, placebo-controlled studies will be more valid than those of studies at the other, less rigorous levels. In reality, however, open randomized and large observational studies of bipolar disorder can be as accurate as level I studies while having the advantage of being more generalizable (Benson and Hartz, 2000).

In summary, the theory behind evidence-based medicine is not unreasonable. The problems it raises arise from the way it is applied—by the architects of guidelines, third-party payers, health care planners, and regulatory authorities, many of whom tend to overvalue level I research by minimizing its difficulties while nearly dismissing other levels of evidence, particularly if the evidence is based only on a consensus among experienced clinicians.

The Bias against Off–On, On–Off (Mirror-Image) and Crossover Designs, Even When Placebo Controlled

The seminal observation of lithium's prophylactic effect was a within-patient comparison of episode frequency before and while taking lithium. As described in Chapter 20, the result of this much-criticized study was later confirmed by multiple level I studies. As Post and colleagues (2000) pointed out, the inherent variability and heterogeneity of individual bipolar patients can all too easily undermine the parallel-group randomized controlled trial, which, because this design is perceived to be virtually required by regulatory agencies, is the staple of industry-supported clinical trials, as well as of university institutional review boards. Crossover designs (which mirror good clinical practice) are especially suited to addressing options for those resistant to an initial monotherapy, who unfortunately represent a majority of bipolar patients. The relative strengths and limitations of the traditional parallel-group randomized controlled trial and the off–on, on–off design are outlined in Tables 17–1 and 17–2, respectively.

Challenges in Interpreting Level I Studies

A number of challenges arise in the interpretation of level 1 studies. First, *the use and misuse of p values is a major error in treatment studies.* False positive results occur when too many p value–based comparisons are made (type I or multiple-comparison error). The extent of this problem is often not adequately recognized. The basic idea can be understood by considering certain facts about probability. Suppose we are willing to accept a p value of .05, meaning that assuming the null hypothesis is true, the observed difference is likely to occur by chance 5 percent of the time. The chance of inaccurately accepting a positive finding (rejecting the null hypothesis) would be 5 percent for 1 comparison, about 10 percent for 2 comparisons, 22 percent for 5 comparisons, and 40 percent for 10 comparisons. This means that if in a randomized controlled trial, the primary analysis is negative but one of four secondary analyses is positive with $p = .05$, that p value actually reflects an unacceptably high (22 percent) probability of a chance positive finding. One option would be to apply a correction for multiple comparisons, such as the Bonferroni correction, which would require that the p value be maintained at .05 overall by being divided by the number of comparisons made. Thus for 5 comparisons, the acceptable p value would be .05/5, or .01. The other approach would be simply to accept the finding, but to give less and less interpretive weight to a positive result as more and more analyses were performed.

This is the main reason why, when a randomized controlled trial is designed, researchers should choose one or

TABLE 17–1. **Strengths and Limitations of Traditional Parallel-Group Randomized Controlled Trials in Bipolar Illness**

Strengths	Limitations
• Usually requires for approval by regulatory agencies • Standard in the literature	• Cumbersome, inflexible for initial phases of drug discovery • Dose schedule usually predetermined • Confounds assessment of individual and placebo response • Requires large sample sizes, typically from many centers, increasing variance • Subject to type II errors • Placebo exposure (often lengthy) required • Homogeneous populations required, but strict entry criteria limit generalizability given that the illness is characteristically pleomorphic • Very costly and difficult to manage

Source: Adapted from Post et al., 2003.

a few primary outcome measures for which the study should be properly powered (a level of .80 or .90 [power=1–type II error] is a standard convention). Usually there is a main efficacy outcome measure, with one or two secondary efficacy or side-effect outcome measures. An efficacy effect or side effect to be tested can be established either a priori (which is always the case for primary and secondary outcomes) or post hoc (after the fact, which should be viewed as exploratory but not confirmatory of any hypothesis). For example, in a randomized controlled trial of olanzapine added to standard mood stabilizers (divalproex or lithium) for prevention of mood episodes in bipolar disorder (see Chapter 20), results were reported as positive, with the group taking combined olanzapine and mood stabilizer doing better than those taking mood stabilizer alone. However, this positive finding was a secondary outcome.

TABLE 17–2. **Strengths and Limitations of Off–On, On–Off Designs**

Strengths	Limitations
• Flexible, suitable for pilot studies • Dose exploration easy • Smaller sample sizes possible • Not prone to type II error • Cost-effective • Patient serves as own control • Trial length can be individualized • Length of placebo periods is reduced • Response can be confirmed in individuals • All patients available for biological measures and response predictors • Adaptable for heterogeneous groups; broader entry criteria feasible • Amenable to drug combination studies • Causality of side effects can be established and confirmed	• Traditionally not accepted • No consensus on statistical approaches or on trial length • "Off" periods still pose risk of illness exacerbation • Carryover effects may obscure results • Number of such "sample of 1" studies sufficient to demonstrate generalizable results is uncertain

Source: Adapted from Post et al., 2003.

The primary outcome was time to a new mood episode, and on this outcome, there was no difference. Among a number of secondary outcomes, there was one—defined as time to decreased ratings of mania or depression—on which the olanzapine plus mood stabilizer group did better ($p = .023$). To give the researchers the benefit of the doubt, let us assume that there were only two secondary analyses. Under these conditions, the apparent p value of .023 would represent a true likelihood above the .05 cutoff for statistical significance. Furthermore, even if valid, the outcome is generalizable only to the group of patients experiencing full acute remission with olanzapine, and the benefit was not in prevention of new episodes per se but in somewhat reduced symptomatic burden.

Second, *in presenting descriptive results (as opposed to testing hypotheses), effect-estimate statistics are generally more appropriate than t tests, since the latter can often be misleading* (increased likelihood of being falsely positive with multiple comparisons or falsely negative with underpowered comparisons). Effect-size estimates are calculated with 95 percent confidence intervals (CIs). If the CIs do not cross the null (i.e., the ratio of the numbers being compared is 1), the comparison will be statistically significant in hypothesis-testing terms. For example, in an analysis of the first 500 participants in the NIMH STEP-BD program, Ghaemi and colleagues (2006) examined medications used at baseline and reported that 43 percent of those with a history of psychosis were taking an antipsychotic, compared with only 20 percent of those without such a history; given a relative risk of 2.2 with a 95 percent CI of 1.65–2.93, one can assume that this difference is likely to be real.

A common situation in which t tests can lead to false negative results is comparison of rates of side effects with an active drug versus placebo. For example, in studies of atypical antipsychotics, rates of extrapyramidal syndrome (EPS) for most of these drugs have been reported as not significantly different from those for placebo by t test. However, these efficacy studies are not powered to detect such a difference. It is not uncommon for the risk of EPS to be three- or four-fold higher than that with placebo, but the sample size required to detect this observed difference statistically (i.e., using significance hypothesis-testing procedures) would be over 1,000. Thus absence of evidence is not evidence of absence.

Third, *if a study appears valid, the generalizability of the results should always be assessed.* After overcoming the limitations of confounding bias and chance, a reader might conclude that the results of a study are valid. The final step (noted above in our discussion of the limitations of level I studies) is to assess the generalizability of these valid results. Here the question is, given that these results are correct, to whom do they apply? One must search the methods

section of a study carefully to answer this question, usually by looking for the inclusion and exclusion criteria employed. This issue is especially relevant to maintenance studies of bipolar disorder (which may or may not represent demonstrations of true prophylaxis).

Even when samples are described as meeting diagnostic criteria, one must question whether they are truly representative with respect to treatment response. This issue is particularly relevant when one is comparing a new treatment with an older, established one. An old adage in medicine states, "the longer a successful treatment is available, the more difficult it becomes for researchers to show that it still works." Let us assume, for example, that one is comparing a new putative mood stabilizer with lithium; it is unlikely that those patients in the community who are doing well on lithium would be interested in participating in a trial of a new drug, particularly if there were a chance that they would end up taking placebo, and their clinicians might consider it unethical to refer them. Indeed, in the initial placebo-controlled trial comparing lithium and divalproex in treating acute mania, the sample included quite a few prior lithium nonresponders. Thus in interpreting the literature, it is useful to remember that new drugs tend to have some advantage over older ones simply because of this referral bias.

Another generalizability issue in maintenance research derives from the fact that there are two basic study designs: prophylaxis and relapse prevention. In the prophylaxis design, any patient who is euthymic, regardless of how that person got well, is eligible to be randomized to drug versus placebo or a comparator. In the relapse prevention design, only those patients who respond acutely to the drug being studied are eligible to enter the maintenance phase, when they are randomized to remain on the drug or be switched (usually abruptly) to placebo and/or an active comparator. For example, the 6-month relapse prevention study of aripiprazole versus placebo started with manic or mixed patients being given the drug open label (see Chapter 20); 37 percent of the original group both tolerated the drug and met response criteria, and it was they who were then randomized to placebo or continued on aripiprazole. Obviously, the 6-month results can be generalized only to the minority who responded acutely. Thus results from a prophylactic design are generalizable, whereas those from a relapse prevention trial are not.

A further problem with the relapse prevention design is that it introduces the possibility of a withdrawal syndrome. Consider the maintenance study of olanzapine versus placebo (see Chapter 20), in which all patients who entered the placebo-controlled phase of the study had to have already responded to open-label olanzapine for acute mania (49 percent of them had). In that study, the placebo relapse rate was very high, and for 75 percent of the patients the relapse occurred in the first 1–2 months after initiation of the study, which may represent withdrawal relapse after recent acute efficacy. Such results really reflect continuation-phase efficacy, not maintenance-phase or prophylactic efficacy, which, as noted above, is generally defined as starting 6 months to a year or longer after resolution of the acute episode.

Still another generalizability issue emerges from studies of combination therapy, often a comparison of an atypical antipsychotic plus a standard mood stabilizer with mood stabilizer monotherapy in treatment of acute mania (see the review by Zarate and Quiroz, 2003). Such studies tend routinely to show benefit with combination treatment, yet it is important to note that the patients in almost all these studies must fail to respond initially to mood stabilizer monotherapy. Indeed, the few studies of combination therapy that have started with "fresh" patients have tended to show no difference between monotherapy and combined therapy.

Fourth, *meta-analysis is an observational study, and thus cannot be accepted at face value.* Meta-analysis represents an observational study of studies; in other words, one combines the results of many different studies into one summary measure. The "apples and oranges" dilemma is, to some extent, unavoidable in that clinicians and researchers must attempt to pull different studies together into some useful summary of the state of the literature on a topic. There are different ways to go about this, with meta-analysis perhaps being the most useful, but all such reviews have their limitations.[11] Meta-analysis weights studies by their samples sizes, but in addition, it corrects for the variability of the data (some studies have smaller standard deviations, and thus their results are more precise and reliable). The problem still remains that studies differ from each other; this problem of heterogeneity introduces confounding bias when the actual results are combined. One option is to exclude certain confounding factors. For instance, a meta-analysis may include only women, so that gender is not a confounder, or may be limited to the elderly, thus excluding confounding by younger age. Often, meta-analyses are limited to randomized controlled trials, as in the Cochrane Collaboration, the idea being that patient samples will be less heterogeneous in the highly controlled setting of such trials than in observational studies. Nonetheless, given that meta-analysis itself is an observational study, it is important to realize that the benefits of randomization are lost. Often readers may not be aware of this, and thus it may appear that a meta-analysis of 10 randomized controlled trials is more meaningful than each trial alone. However, each large, well-conducted randomized controlled trial is basically free of confounding bias, which is never the case

for meta-analysis. The most meaningful conclusions can be reached when both the individual randomized controlled trials and the overall meta-analysis point in the same direction.

Another way to handle the confounding bias of meta-analysis, just as in single observational studies, is to use stratification or regression models, often called *meta-regression.* For instance, if 10 randomized controlled trials exist, but 5 used a crossover design and 5 a parallel design, one could create a regression model that could be used to obtain the relative risk of benefit with drug versus placebo, corrected for the variables of crossover and parallel design. Meta-regression methods are relatively new.

Besides the "apples and oranges" problem, meta-analysis has the publication bias, or "file-drawer," problem: the published literature may not be a valid reflection of the reality of research on a topic because positive studies are published more often than negative ones. This occurs for various reasons. Editors may be more inclined to reject negative studies given the limits of publication space. Researchers may be less inclined to put effort into writing and revising manuscripts on negative studies given the relative lack of interest engendered by such reports. And, perhaps most important for treatment studies in bipolar disorder, pharmaceutical companies that conduct randomized controlled trials have a strong economic motivation not to publish negative studies of their drugs. If they did so, their competitors would likely seize upon those negative findings to malign the drugs, and the cost of preparing and producing such manuscripts would likely be difficult to justify to the top management of a publicly owned for-profit company. One possible approach to addressing this problem is to create a data registry in which all randomized controlled trials on a topic would be registered. If studies were not published, managers of the registry would obtain the actual data from negative studies and store them for systematic reviews and meta-analyses. This solution is limited, however, by its dependence on voluntary cooperation; in the case of the pharmaceutical industry, most companies refuse to provide such negative data. The patent and privacy laws in the United States protect companies on this issue, leaving definitive scientific reviews of evidence difficult to accomplish.

The potential impact of the bias toward positive findings in the publication of industry-supported studies appears to be reflected in two recent reviews. Heres and colleagues (2006) examined industry-supported studies of atypical antipsychotics and found that in 90 percent of the studies, the outcome was favorable to the sponsor's drug. This phenomenon can be reflected in contradictory findings about the same drug studied by two different sponsors. An example is the comparison of divalproex and olanzapine in treating acute mania, in which the results of the Lilly-sponsored study (Tohen et al., 2002) favored that company's drug (olanzapine), while in the Abbott-sponsored study (Zajecka et al., 2002), the risk/benefit analysis favored that company's drug (divalproex) (see Chapter 18). In a similar vein, Perlis (2005) compared randomized controlled trials in which the author(s) reported a financial conflict of interest and trials without such potential conflicts; the former were 4.9 times more likely to report positive results. Related to these observations is the proliferation of papers with "executive authors," in which data derived from large trials conducted by a pharmaceutical company are analyzed "in house." A manuscript is drafted by medical writers working for the company, and one or more academic opinion leaders (who may or may not have been involved as investigators when the data were initially collected) are recruited to serve as lead authors. Obviously, reviewing data already selected by company scientists and analyzed by company statisticians is not the same as selecting and analyzing one's own data de novo.

Fifth, *intent-to-treat analyses are more valid than completer analyses*. In general, in randomized controlled trials, intent-to-treat analyses are considered more valid than completer analyses because they preserve randomization. What this means is that randomization equalizes all potential confounding factors for the entire sample at the beginning of the study. If that entire sample is analyzed at the end of the study, there should be no confounding bias. However, if some of that sample is not analyzed at the end of the study (as in completer analysis, which does not include dropouts before the end of the study), one cannot be sure that the two groups are still equal at the end of the study on all potential confounding factors. If some patients drop out of one treatment arm because of less efficacy or more side effects, these nonrandom dropouts will bias the ultimate results of the study in a completer analysis. Thus in general, an intent-to-treat approach is used. From the study design perspective, this approach is called *intent to treat* because the researchers intend to treat all the patients for the entire duration of the study, regardless of whether they remain in the study until the very end. From the statistical analysis perspective, this approach is called the *last observation carried forward* because it comes down to taking the last data point available for the patient and pretending that it occurred at the very end of the study. The problem with this approach is that it assumes the last outcome for the patient in the study would have remained the same until the study's end, that is, that the patient would not have gotten any better or any worse. This is less of a problem in a short-term than in a maintenance study. Nonetheless, it is important to realize that there are assumptions built into both this and completer analyses and that no approach fully removes all possibility of bias. The presence of some potential for bias in even the best-crafted randomized controlled trial means one can never be completely certain that the results of any such trial are valid. Thus replication with multiple randomized controlled trials is necessary to get closer to establishing causation.

Finally, *in survival analysis, one always needs to know the sample size at each time point; if there are many dropouts, the survival curve may be misleading.* Survival analysis, a statistical method commonly used in maintenance studies of bipolar or highly recurrent unipolar disorder, measures the time until an event, as opposed to simply counting the frequency of an event. The reason this approach is so prevalent is that it provides more information, and thus more statistical power, than simply assessing the number of patients who respond. In a long-term study, for instance, if one patient relapsed at 1 month and another at 1 year, both would be counted simply as patients who relapsed. Survival analysis makes it possible to take into account that one person relapsed after a much longer period of staying well compared with the other person. One can use a regression model, called *Cox regression*, for survival outcomes to provide an effect size called a *hazard ratio*, which is the survival equivalent of risk ratios or odds ratios for other outcomes.

The primary problems with survival analysis are sample size and dropouts. Sample size decreases with time in a survival analysis. This is expected because patients drop out for a variety of reasons, such as illness relapse, side effects, or having achieved the end point of the study. In general, a survival analysis is most valid for the earlier portions of the curve, where there is a larger number of patients. Thus, a treatment may appear to show a major effect after 6 months, but the sample at that point could be 10 patients in each arm, as opposed to 100 in each arm at 1 month. The results would not be statistically significant, and the effect size would not be meaningful because of the high variability of such small numbers. Nonetheless, researchers continue to rely on survival analysis, mainly because there are no other options at this time. Again, this situation highlights the need to recognize the statistical issues involved, as well as to exercise a good deal of caution in interpreting the results of even the best randomized controlled trials.

The main statistical issue is that since dropouts are unavoidably nonrandom, a survival analysis is more valid if there are few dropouts "lost to follow-up" (i.e., where one has no idea why the patient has left the study). Statisticians have tended to designate a ballpark figure of 20 percent lost to follow-up as tolerable overall so as to maintain reasonable confidence in the validity of a survival analysis.[12] In fact, the dropout rates in maintenance studies of bipolar disorder tend to be in the 50–80 percent range, which hampers the ability to be certain of the validity of survival analysis in bipolar research. Researchers resign themselves to the fact that this population is highly nonadherent and thus difficult to study. For example, the problem of differential dropouts can be illustrated by a study comparing olanzapine and divalproex in treating bipolar disorder (see Chapter 20). Data on weight gain have been presented in a survival analysis with up to 1-year follow-up. The survival curves appear to show that olanzapine is associated with much more weight gain than divalproex in the first few months, but by 1 year, the rates of weight gain appear to converge. Although not obvious from the survival curves, by 1 year about 85 percent of the sample had dropped out, with many of the dropouts in the olanzapine arm being due to weight gain. Thus, the apparent decline in weight gain with olanzapine could reflect the fact that those who gained weight discontinued the agent earlier in follow-up.

In the above discussion, we have attempted to alert the reader to some of the methodological complexities one encounters in reading the treatment literature relevant to manic-depressive illness. The importance of emphasizing these issues in this volume is underscored by a recent methodological examination of published studies on the treatment of bipolar disorder (Soldani et al., 2005). The authors reported that of the 100 papers randomly selected from the five psychiatric journals with the highest impact ratings, only 19 percent were randomized; most of the rest were small, nonrandomized case series, relying primarily on contrasts between baseline and end point without a control group. Of the 100 papers, 53 made no reference to study design or statistical methods.

Even when considering level I randomized controlled trials, however, we emphasize the need for caution when interpreting their results—whether they indicate a difference between drug and placebo (or between two drugs) or fail to show a difference, especially when this finding is based on nonsignificant p values in the absence of effect-size estimation. The best bulwark against erroneous conclusions remains the requirement for multiple independent replications.

TREATMENT GUIDELINES AND ALGORITHMS FOR BIPOLAR DISORDER

Given the substantial increase in treatment options since the first edition of this text was published, the clinician faces what might appear to be a bewildering array of choices. Thus guidelines and algorithms have understandably been welcomed by many busy clinicians. As long as guidelines remain *advisory* to the clinician, they can be helpful to both the professional and the patient. We become concerned when they are used by managers of care and third-party payors in an effort to enhance the cost-effectiveness of care by reducing the number of treatment options. This has already happened to those patients in Texas whose treatment is funded by the state. If the tendency to make guidelines coercive continues to grow, both quality and innovation will be threatened (G. Goodwin, 2003a). Since guidelines are, by definition, yesterday's practice of medicine, they inevitably begin going out of date even before they are published.

In their review, Fountoulakis and colleagues (2005) identified a total of 27 guidelines for the treatment of bipolar disorder published since 1994. Table 17–3 lists, in reverse chronological order, the major guidelines for the treatment of adults that have been published since 2002 from North America, Europe, Australia/New Zealand, and the World Federation of Societies of Biological Psychiatry. (Guidelines for the treatment of children and adolescents with bipolar disorder are reviewed in Chapter 23.) Direct comparisons of even the more recent guidelines are limited by the reality that each was developed in its own time frame. Obviously, the more recent guidelines are the most relevant, but even they can quickly become obsolete as new findings emerge from the research literature. Nevertheless, it is useful to examine the existing guidelines to highlight those general approaches for which there is broad consensus, and to take note of important cross-national differences.

The process by which guidelines are developed also differs in ways that may affect the recommendations made. In general, the process begins with a committee of experts who undertake an evaluation of the existing treatment research literature, ranking studies according to the levels of evidence outlined in Box 17–2. Because of the inherently limited generalizability of controlled trials, as discussed above (see also Box 17–3), guideline developers have, to varying degrees, attempted to incorporate expert opinion, thus allowing observational studies and clinical experience to fill in some of the gaps left by controlled studies, such as combined medications, the treatment of comorbid conditions, and drug–psychotherapy interactions. Developers of the Expert Consensus Guidelines in the United States (Keck et al., 2004) have assessed expert opinion most systematically, using a statistical analysis of the answers given independently by 47 experts in bipolar disorder to a series of specific questions about what they would do in particular circumstances. This approach avoids the problem associated with conclusions arising from the deliberations of a committee—that the strongly held opinions of a few members may carry more weight, given that the committee's task is to reach agreement.

TABLE 17–3. **Recent Treatment Guidelines**

Algorithm	Year of Publication	Reference
American Psychiatric Association Guidelines	2002	Hirschfeld et al., 2002
World Federation of Societies of Biological Psychiatry Guidelines	2002, 2003, 2004	Grunze et al., 2002, 2003, 2004
British Association for Psychopharmacology Guidelines	2003	G. Goodwin et al., 2003
Guidelines from the Danish Psychiatric Association	2003	Licht et al., 2003
Expert Consensus Guidelines (U.S.)	2004	Keck et al., 2004
Texas Medication Algorithm	2005	Suppes et al., 2005
Canadian Network for Mood and Anxiety Treatments Algorithm	2005	Yatham et al., 2005

The various guidelines differ in their level of specificity and coverage. Some, for example, such as the Texas Medication Algorithm (Suppes et al., 2005), the British Association for Psychopharmacology Guidelines (G. Goodwin, 2003b), and the World Federation of Societies of Biological Psychiatry Guidelines (Grunze et al., 2002, 2003, 2004), offer no advice on the treatment of bipolar-II patients, citing the virtual absence of level I studies, and most guidelines fail to address comorbid conditions for the same reason. As might be expected of an evolving process, the three most recent sets of guidelines—the Texas Medication Algorithm, the Canadian Network for Mood and Anxiety Treatments Algorithm (Yatham et al., 2005), and the Expert Consensus Guidelines (all of which happen to be North American in origin)—are the most comprehensive and up to date. The Canadian guidelines present the most thorough review of the literature; they also do a better job than the others of covering assessment issues, bipolar-II, mixed states, and older patients while placing relatively less emphasis on the risk/benefit ratio of different treatment options. The Texas Medication Algorithm also presents an impressive review of the literature and, in its introduction, is clear about the difference between continuation treatment and true prophylaxis. In the specific recommendations included as "maintenance" treatment, however, are two atypicals for which the bulk of the drug–placebo difference occurred in the first few months after recovery from an acute manic episode, that is, in the continuation phase of treatment.

There are two principal differences between the North American and European guidelines. First, the Europeans place more emphasis on lithium treatment and less on valproate; in North America, the pharmaceutical industry plays a larger role, and as a result there is a great deal more exposure to the newer income-generating, patent-protected drugs, such as divalproex (valproate), and relatively less exposure to such drugs as lithium and carbamazepine (Lieberman et al., 2006; see also Box 17–4). In some European countries, antidepressants are considered first-line treatment for bipolar depression (as long as an antimanic mood stabilizer is used concurrently), whereas the North American guidelines emphasize mood stabilizers for the acute treatment of depression while acknowledging the need for adjunctive antidepressants in more severe cases. For example, the Texas Medication Algorithm considers antidepressants fourth-line treatment after mood stabilizers and combinations thereof.[13] Another difference between the North American and European guidelines lies in recommendations for when to initiate maintenance treatment: in the North America guidelines, its initiation is clearly recommended after the first manic episode; the European guidelines recommend that maintenance treatment begin after the second manic episode, but can be "considered" after the first if that episode is severe enough (Vestergaard, 2004).

BOX 17–3.   Understanding Treatment Guidelines for Bipolar Disorder

- Most guidelines are based primarily on randomized, placebo-controlled trials (RCTs), and are thus affected by the limited generalizability of such trials. For example:
  - In placebo-controlled trials, the sickest patients are under-represented because of ethical concerns about exposing them to placebo, particularly over an extended period of time.
  - Most large RCTs are of monotherapy, whereas most bipolar patients are taking combined medications.
  - Patients with comborbid conditions are excluded from most RCTs, yet most bipolar patients have comorbid diagnoses.
- The level of agreement across guidelines varies with the proportion of RCTs focused on particular states. These differences are especially pronounced between European and North American guidelines.
  - Because the majority of RCT's have been of treatments for acute mania, there is a high level of agreement across those guidelines.
  - Prophylactic treatment has been addressed by an intermediate number of RCT; accordingly, the level of agreement across those guidelines is intermediate.
  - Bipolar depression has been the subject of the fewest RCTs, and therefore the level of agreement across those guidelines is lowest.
- Guidelines follow classification systems (primarily the *Diagnostic and Statistical Manual* [DSM]-IV), and thus are affected by the limitations of those systems (see the text and Chapters 1 and 3 for discussion of these limitations).

While we refer in the chapters that follow to recommendations from various guidelines as they apply to specific treatment situations, we must pause to note that to date, there is scant evidence that guidelines are having much effect on clinical practice in the community. For example, a recent analysis of prescriptions in the community for 7,760 bipolar patients (Baldessarini et al., 2006) found that half received antidepressants, while only a quarter were prescribed a mood stabilizer.[14] Turning to psychiatric settings, a survey of prescribing patterns for 1,864 bipolar-I patients in more than 100 psychiatric inpatient units in the United States (Lim et al., 2001) found that in the treatment of manic or bipolar depressed patients without psychosis, guidelines were followed only 16–17 percent of the time (the percentages were higher for those with psychosis, but still only 38 and 31 percent for mania and depression, respectively). A 1999 survey revealed that one in six psychia-

---

BOX 17–4.   Changing U.S. Prescribing Patterns for Mood Stabilizers

In the United States between the mid-1990s and the turn of the century, a fairly marked shift occurred from lithium to valproate (principally divalproex) for the treatment of bipolar disorder, a trend not seen in most of the rest of the world (Fenn et al., 1996; Goodwin, 1999; Goodwin and Ghaemi, 1999; Blanco et al., 2002). There are many possible explanations for this change. One reason suggested is the intense marketing of divalproex to psychiatrists that occurred during the mid- to late 1990s. Given that divalproex has generated at least 20 times more sales revenue than lithium, it is no surprise that American psychiatrists have had far greater exposure to it through marketing and Abbott Laboratories–supported continuing medical education programs (Goodwin et al., 2003b; Lieberman et al., 2006). In our opinion, a clinician cannot be considered even minimally competent to treat patients with bipolar disorder unless he or she knows how to use lithium.

---

trists was not even aware that guidelines existed (Jaffe and Yager, 1999), and almost half had not read the guidelines for bipolar disorder. Consistent with these findings are those of Blanco and colleagues (2002), who analyzed data on psychiatrists from the National Ambulatory Medical Care Survey for the years 1992 to 1999. Over one-third of bipolar patients did not receive a mood stabilizer, whereas antidepressant use was "common": 45 percent of office visits were associated with such a prescription, and for half of these visits there was no accompanying prescription for a mood stabilizer. Unfortunately, this apparent underuse of mood stabilizers accompanied by the apparent overuse of antidepressants was no different when data for the early and late 1990s were compared.

Not surprisingly, the correspondence between guidelines and practice is better in academic settings and in staff model HMOs (where almost all bipolar patients are pharmacologically treated by psychiatrists, and adherence to guidelines tends to be tracked). Two large U.S. datasets reflecting "real-world" open treatment as provided by psychiatrists associated with academic centers (which provide largely tertiary care) are those of the Stanley Foundation Bipolar Network and the NIMH STEP-BD program. An analysis of 457 bipolar-I patients who participated in a Stanley center voluntary registry revealed that 82 percent were taking a mood stabilizer upon entry into the registry (Levine et al., 2000); most were receiving combined treatment involving more than one mood stabilizer. Thus among the 50 percent of the total group taking lithium and the 40 percent taking valproate, only 18 percent and 10 percent, respectively, received the mood stabilizer as monotherapy. Similarly, in an analysis of medications received just prior to the entry of the first 500 patients into the STEP-BD program (73.6 percent of whom were bipolar-I), Ghaemi and colleagues (2006) found that 72 percent were taking mood stabilizers, but only 11 percent as monotherapy. In another tertiary care setting (the NIMH Intramural Program), it was observed that the proportion of patients receiving combined medications increased sharply from the mid-1970s to the mid-1990s; the proportion of discharged bipolar patients taking three or more medications rose from 3 to 44 percent. By contrast, in two staff model HMOs (Kaiser Northern California and Group Health of Puget Sound) providing primary care psychiatry (whose guidelines for bipolar disorder reserve combined therapy for those who fail monotherapy), only 11.5 percent of patients were treated with more than one mood stabilizer (Hunkeler et al., 1995).

While the largely tertiary-care populations involved in the STEP-BD program and the Stanley centers reflected recent North American guidelines with respect to the central role of mood stabilizers in bipolar disorder, there was less correspondence with guidelines for the adjunctive use of antidepressants: 57 percent of the Stanley patients (including 55 patients not on a mood stabilizer) and 41 percent of the STEP-BD patients were taking antidepressants. The Stanley data reflected treatment patterns in the mid-1990s, whereas the STEP-BD data were collected later, in 1998 and 1999. It is possible that this difference in time frame is relevant to the modest differences reported in antidepressant use, given that the first U.S. guidelines cautioning about the use of antidepressants in bipolar disorder were published in 1994 (American Psychiatric Association, 1994) and 1996 (Frances et al., 1996). While it might be argued that the relatively high rate of antidepressant use is related to the presence of sicker patients in tertiary care settings, antidepressant use was also common in the two HMO primary psychiatric care settings referred to above: 75 percent of patients had received at least one such prescription. The primary care (HMO) data were collected from 1994 to 2001, a period that includes some time prior to the publication of the above-mentioned guidelines.

It is of interest that even though the 2003 British guidelines include antidepressants as a first-line option, the Maudsley Bipolar Project (Frangou et al., 2002) and a survey conducted in northeast England (Lloyd et al., 2003) found that only 14 and 23 percent, respectively, of bipolar patients were taking an antidepressant, whereas in both surveys the use of mood stabilizers was similar to that in the United States.

In conclusion, although there are differences among guidelines (primarily cross-national in nature), they agree on the centrality of mood stabilizers in the management of bipolar disorder and on the inappropriateness of antidepressant monotherapy. Further, all three of the most recent guidelines, to varying degrees, express caution about the use of antidepressants even when combined with a mood stabilizer. Thus far, the impact of guidelines on practice in the United States has not been obvious in the data on prescription patterns; no doubt this is due, at least in part, to the fact that prescription data are derived from all physicians, not just psychiatrists. Finally, it must be noted that guidelines are organized according to current diagnostic schema; that is, there are separate guidelines for bipolar disorder and major depression, but none for the highly recurrent unipolar group, which in effect falls between the cracks.

MEDICATIONS USED TO TREAT MANIC-DEPRESSIVE ILLNESS

Here we review the basic pharmacology of the medications used for acute, continuation, and maintenance treatment of manic-depressive illness. Clinical detail on the use of these agents, including additional findings concerning dosage and drug interactions, is presented in the chapters that follow. Since side effects and adverse events are most salient during maintenance treatment, they are covered in Chapter 20, while information on the use and side effects of the various medications related specifically to children and adolescents is presented in Chapter 23.

Lithium

Although the mechanism of lithium's action in acute treatment of mania and depression and in prophylactic therapy for bipolar disorder is unknown, several productive theories are being tested (see Chapters 18, 19, and 20, respectively, and Chapter 14). The standard oral formulation is the carbonate salt of lithium, whereas the liquid formulation uses the citrate or chloride salt. The U.S. Food and Drug Administration (FDA) has approved lithium carbonate for both the treatment of manic episodes and maintenance treatment of bipolar disorder.

Lithium carbonate is readily absorbed throughout the gastrointestinal tract. There are preparations that delay absorption somewhat (Eskalith CR, Camcolit, Priadel, and Lithobid) and to some extent reduce the peaks and valleys of serum lithium levels throughout the day. The principal advantage of these preparations is a lower frequency of initial gastrointestinal side effects, which may enhance adherence. These preparations also appear to have less of an effect on urinary osmolarity, which would be consistent with a reduced long-term impact on renal function (although this has not yet been studied directly) (Vestergaard and Schou, 1987). Lithium is excreted primarily in urine; renal excretion is rapid under normal circumstances. The drug is passed into the glomerular filtrate and is indistinguishable from sodium in the proximal tubule, where both are reabsorbed. It is reabsorbed to a much lesser extent in the loop of Henle and is not reabsorbed at all in the distal tubule.

The half-life of lithium is initially about 12 hours, but reaches approximately 24 hours once steady-state serum levels have developed at about 5 days. The conventional trough serum lithium level occurring 12 hours after the last dose is the standard level for measurement. The dose/blood-level ratio is influenced by the individual's clinical state (manic or depressed), gender, age, weight (especially muscle mass), salt intake, extent of sweating, intrinsic renal clearance capacity for lithium, and use of other medications. A relatively higher dose/blood-level ratio is associated with being manic, younger, male, and heavier and having a higher salt intake. Although controlled studies are lacking, results of open trials suggest that therapeutic blood levels for children and adults are about the same.

To predict dosage requirements, some investigators recommend a test dose of lithium, followed 24 hours later by a plasma-level determination (Cooper and Simpson, 1976; Fava et al., 1984; Perry et al., 1984). Although this technique probably can be applied reliably when the mood state is stable, its practical value in treating acute mania is limited. Errors in the predicted dose may, for example, be due to changes in patients' sleep and activity, which cause changes in glomerular filtration rate (Perry et al., 1984). In addition, use of this method necessitates a 24-hour delay in treatment.

Because the proximal tubule reabsorbs lithium as it does sodium, it is essential for the patient to maintain normal salt and adequate fluid intake to prevent the development of lithium intoxication. Although decreased tolerance to lithium has been reported to ensue from protracted sweating, the only test of this effect in a small number of healthy long-distance runners did not find a tendency toward increased lithium levels following vigorous exercise. Nonetheless, some caution is warranted. The risk of elevation of serum lithium levels as a result of diarrhea and vomiting is undeniable. Should these conditions occur, supplemental fluid and salt should be administered, and lithium therapy may need to be stopped temporarily until fluid and salt balance can be restored.

The gap between therapeutic and toxic levels of lithium is narrow. Thus the frequency of serum monitoring of lithium should be proportional to the risks associated with particular patient profiles. When there is reason to believe that lithium levels may be fluctuating—because of erratic adherence, a sudden change in clinical state (e.g., a switch from mania into depression),[15] the presence of medical conditions that could affect renal function, concurrent medications, individual sensitivity to the effects of lithium, a low-salt diet, or excessive sweating—and whenever there is clinical suspicion of impending toxicity, serum-level monitoring must be more frequent (Goodwin and Goldstein, 2003). Serum lithium levels should be obtained whenever there is a change in dosage and at least every 6 months in stable patients. Elderly and frail patients should be tested more often.[16]

Anticonvulsants

Valproate

Valproate is a gamma-aminobutyric acid (GABA)-enhancing anticonvulsant approved by the FDA for the treatment of epilepsy and acute mania and for migraine prophylaxis. Preparations include capsules, elixir, rectal forms, and, most recently, an intravenous (IV) formulation; none of these forms appears to offer any particular advantage for treatment of bipolar disorder. Nor has the rapid oral loading protocol that most patients tolerate (McElroy et al., 1998) been shown to result in a faster onset of antimanic action compared with slower titration protocols. The level of gastrointestinal irritation is dramatically reduced with the sodium divalproex formulation of valproate, which has largely replaced the original formulation. Still, indigestion and nausea, along with sedation, are the most common side effects.

Valproate inhibits the enzymes that metabolize several other drugs, including, most notably, lamotrigine. The therapeutic range of this and other psychotropic drugs is difficult to define precisely, but it would appear that levels above 70 and below 120 milligrams per milliliter (mg/ml) are as close to optimal as is practical for most patients (Ellenor and Dishmon, 1995).

Carbamazepine

Carbamazepine, a tricyclic compound that is classified as an iminostilbene derivative, has been shown to be effective in the treatment of mania. Results of trials comparing its prophylactic effect with that of lithium suggest that it probably has maintenance efficacy, but it has never been submitted to the FDA for this indication.

Carbamazepine[17] is reported to be absorbed slowly and erratically from the gastrointestinal tract. After chronic use, the time to peak plasma concentrations is several hours following ingestion (Pugh and Garnet, 1991). Carbamazepine is lipophilic; therefore, no parenteral forms have been developed, and different brands of the drug cannot be assumed to produce the same blood levels. Bioavailability can be estimated at about 80 percent (Ketter et al., 1999). Although carbamazepine undergoes only modest first-pass metabolism, it is extensively metabolized in the liver. Approximately 75 percent of the drug is protein bound. Carbamazepine can induce its own metabolism such that over time, dose increments may be needed. The drug can also impact the metabolism of some other agents, most notably inducing lamotrigine metabolism such that the dose of the latter may need to be increased when the two drugs are used in combination.

Oxcarbazepine

Oxcarbazepine is a chemical derivative of carbamazepine with a similar structure and antiepileptic profile. It is rapidly and extensively converted to the 10-hydroxy metabolite, suggesting that it may be an easier drug to administer than carbamazepine, with fewer drug interactions, and easier to tolerate with less neurotoxicity. Oxcarbazepine's most common side effects are tiredness, headache, dizziness, and ataxia. Also, it has been reported to cause allergic reactions and hypoatremia, although less frequently than carbamazepine. It is also associated with a lack of effects on the hematopoietic system. Large controlled studies of its efficacy in bipolar patients is lacking.

Lamotrigine

Lamotrigine is a phenyltriazine structure; controlled trials have demonstrated its maintenance efficacy against depression in bipolar patients, for which it has an FDA indication. It is probably also effective in the acute treatment of bipolar depression. Lamotrigine inhibits the release of glutamate, which may be the basis for its anticonvulsant activity, but neither this nor the basis for its putative antidepressant action is known. It is readily absorbed in the gut and is only about 50 percent bound to plasma proteins; about 90 percent is metabolized to inactive metabolites in the liver, while 10 percent is excreted unchanged. Its half-life is about 24 hours. Birth control medications can decrease plasma levels of lamotrigine, but the converse is not true.

Gabapentin

Gabapentin is structurally related to GABA but does not bind to the GABA receptor as a GABA analogue, as was originally believed when the drug was developed in the early 1970s. It does enhance GABA function in some indirect manner. What role, if any, the drug has in the management of bipolar patients is unclear, especially after it failed to separate from placebo in controlled trials of treatment of mania. It has looked somewhat more promising as an adjunctive agent based on the results of uncontrolled studies. Gabapentin is readily absorbed, is not protein bound, is not

metabolized, and is excreted almost exclusively in its original form by the kidney. Thus it has a very short half-life of about 6 hours, indicating the need to give it in multiple daily doses. Because there is no known relationship between blood level and therapeutic response for the drug, there is no indication for therapeutic monitoring, and perhaps most difficult, a wide range of possible therapeutic doses exists (600–4500 mg/day). From a kinetic point of view, the drug would be advantageous in patients with liver function problems or those taking other drugs that affect hepatic metabolism, but there would be a corresponding need for caution in patients with impaired or unstable renal function.

Topiramate

Topiramate is described as a fructopyranose. It is an antiepileptic agent thought to increase GABA activity and to inhibit excitatory glutamate receptor activation. It is readily absorbed and largely unmetabolized, and about 70 percent is excreted in free unchanged form by the kidney; about 15 percent is protein bound. It has a serum half-life of about 21 hours. Phenytoin and carbamazepine lower its serum levels and its half-life, while topiramate can increase serum levels of those two anticonvulsants. In several controlled trials with manic patients it has not been better than placebo.

Tiagabine

Tiagabine is a nipecotic acid derivative whose mechanism of action in epilepsy is thought to be related to GABA action. There is little evidence, controlled or otherwise, for its utility in treating bipolar disorder. It is rapidly absorbed, with peak serum levels occurring within 1 hour of a first dose. It is predominantly protein bound in serum. Almost all of tiagabine is metabolized in the liver; however, other routes are also known to play some role. The mean half-life of the drug is 8 hours, but is decreased by carbamazepine and other enzyme inducers.

Antidepressants

Monoamine Oxidase Inhibitors

Monoamine oxidase inhibitors (MAOIs) inhibit enzymes responsible for the neuronal breakdown of catcholamine and idoleamine neurotransmitters. The original MAOIs were irreversible inhibitors of both types of monoamine oxidase enzyme, A and B, which are found primarily on the outer membrane of mitochondria. In the past decade, both reversible MAO-A inhibitors and a selective MAO-B inhibitor in patch form have been developed, adding the potential for greater specificity and safety to the profile of this group of antidepressants.

MAOIs are absorbed quickly when administered orally. Peak MAO inhibition occurs within several days following the initial low dose, which is then gradually increased based on therapeutic effects and tolerability of side effects. Tranylcypromine is administered 10 mg/day; phenelzine can be given at a higher dosage of 15 mg/day. Effects of these drugs are often not observed for 2–4 weeks. Sometimes, amounts as high as 90 mg are required for an adequate response and reduction in depressive symptoms. MAOIs should be discontinued gradually, as sudden withdrawal can result in delirium and agitation.

Tricyclics

Tricyclic antidepressants—the first widely studied agents to treat depression successfully—putatively act by inhibiting the norepinephrine and serotonin uptake in nerve endings. Imipramine was the first tricyclic used and remains the most thoroughly studied (Kuhn, 1957). Amitriptyline, clomipramine, desipramine, doxepin, nortriptyline, protriptyline, and trimipramine are other widely available tricyclic preparations.

Tricyclic antidepressants are absorbed quickly and almost completely by the small bowel. Peak plasma concentrations usually occur within 2–3 hours of ingestion. The half-lives of tricyclic antidepressants are relatively long and variable, ranging from 6 to 198 hours. Protriptyline, for example, has a half-life of 80 hours. Tricyclic antidepressants are highly lipophilic and bind strongly to plasma proteins in the heart and to brain tissue.

Plasma levels have been correlated with both therapeutic (Ziegler et al., 1978) and toxic (Spiker and Pugh, 1976) effects. Wide variation in plasma levels is due largely to genetic differences in the hepatic enzymes responsible for the drugs' metabolism. Sampling should be performed 1 week following administration to ensure a steady-state level, and 10–12 hours following the last dose to ensure complete absorption and distribution. The therapeutic ranges suggested in the literature are 50–140 nanograms per milliliter (ng/ml) for nortriptyline and 110–180 ng/ml for all other tricyclic antidepressants (except protriptyline).

Selective Serotonin Reuptake Inhibitors

Selective serotonin reuptake inhibitors (SSRIs) block 5-HT reuptake from synaptic clefts, making more of this neurotransmitter available at postsynaptic receptors. Their popularity, particularly outside of psychiatry, is due primarily to their having fewer side effects, far less potential for lethal overdose, and drug interactions compared with the older antidepressants, as well as a reduced requirement for medical testing (e.g., electrocardiogram) prior to their use and the elimination of plasma monitoring. The absorption of SSRIs is generally efficient, although results of one study suggest that the concentration of sertraline in plasma is 32 percent higher when taken with food. The metabolism of SSRIs is influenced by age, disease, gender, environmental agents, and type and amount of drug administered.

The specific SSRI dosage varies depending on the particular drug. The simplest regimens, for citalopram, fluoxetine, and paroxetine, are 20 mg/day from the initial day of treatment. Sertraline and fluvoxamine are usually titrated upward until a clinical effect is achieved. Most SSRIs have elimination half-lives ranging from 15 to 26 hours. However, norfluoxetine, the active metabolite of fluoxetine, has a half-life of 7–9 days. Because of this longer half-life, the usual 2-week "wash-out" period recommended when switching an SSRI to an MAOI should be extended (usually to 5 weeks) when a patient is being switched from fluoxetine to an MAOI.

Bupropion, Selective Norepinephrine Reuptake Inhibitors, and Other Antidepressants

Bupropion is a weak blocker of the neuronal uptake of serotonin and norepinephrine, but it does increase norepinephrine turnover by other mechanisms; it also inhibits the neuronal reuptake of dopamine to some extent. In humans, following oral administration of bupropion, peak plasma bupropion concentrations are usually achieved within 2 hours, followed by a biphasic decline. The terminal phase has a mean half-life of 14 hours, with a range of 8 to 24 hours. The distribution phase has a mean half-life of 3 to 4 hours. The mean elimination half-life (±standard deviation [SD]) of bupropion after chronic dosing is 21 (±9) hours, and steady-state plasma concentrations of the drug are reached within 8 days. Plasma bupropion concentrations are dose-proportional following single doses of 100 to 250 mg; however, it is not known whether the proportionality between dose and plasma level is maintained in chronic use.

Venlafaxine and its major metabolite, O-desmethylvenlafaxine (ODV), are potent inhibitors of neuronal serotonin and norepinephrine reuptake and weak inhibitors of dopamine reuptake. Venlafaxine is well absorbed, with peak plasma concentrations occurring approximately 2 hours after dosing. The drug is extensively metabolized, with peak plasma levels occurring approximately 4 hours after dosing. The mean elimination half-lives for venlafaxine and its active metabolite are 5 (±2) and 11 (±2) hours, respectively.

Duloxetine is a balanced selective serotonin and norepinephrine reuptake inhibitor. It appears to be fairly well absorbed after oral doses; peak plasma levels occur in 6–10 hours (dose-dependent). The drug is extensively metabolized in the liver to active metabolites; most of an oral dose is excreted in the urine, only a small amount of which is unchanged. An elimination half-life of 11–16 hours has been reported.

Reboxetine is a novel selective norepinephrine reuptake inhibitor that is well absorbed after oral administration. Its absolute bioavailability is 94.5 percent, and maximal concentrations are generally achieved within 2 to 4 hours. Food affects the rate but not the extent of absorption. The mean half-life of the drug (approximately 12 hours) is consistent with the recommendation to administer it twice daily.

Nefazodone exerts dual effects on serotonergic neurotransmission through blockade of 5-HT$_2$ receptors and inhibition of serotonin reuptake. These two properties combine to increase serotonergic neurotransmission through other serotonin receptors, such as the 5-HT$_{1A}$ receptor. Nefazadone is rapidly and completely absorbed but is subject to extensive metabolism, so that its absolute bioavailability is low—about 20 percent—and variable. Peak plasma concentrations occur at about 1 hour, and the drug's half-life is 2–4 hours.

Typical Antipsychotics

In 1952, the first conventional antipsychotic, chlorpromazine, was found to be therapeutic for schizophrenia, an effect thought to be related to its blockade of dopamine D2 receptors. Since that time, a multitude of new antipsychotic drugs have been introduced. These drugs are categorized into five distinctive classes: phenothiazines, butyrophenones, dibenzoxazepines, thioxantheses, and dihydroindolones. All typical antipsychotics act equally to relieve psychotic symptoms, such as hallucinations, delusions, and thought disorders.

All antipsychotics are well absorbed; however, oral administration can result in less predictability in absorption, and food and antacids can affect absorption by the gastrointestinal tract. Most antipsychotics peak at approximately 3 hours following oral administration, but peak plasma levels can occur within 30 minutes or after up to 5 hours. Steady-state blood levels are reached within 3 to 5 days. Metabolism occurs mainly in the liver, but also in the intestinal wall. The bioavailability of most of the antipsychotics is relatively high, but for some is considerably lower. Haloperidol tablets, for example, have an average bioavailability of only 60 percent. The elimination half-life of typical antipsychotics can range from 1.5 hours to 26 days.[18]

Atypical Antipsychotics

Following oral administration of atypical antipsychotics, the gastrointestinal system absorbs the drug rapidly and almost completely. Food appears to have no effect on the rate and extent of absorption of these agents with the exception of ziprasidone, which is absorbed to a lesser extent on an empty stomach. Peak plasma concentrations for the original compound usually occur between 1 and 6 hours. A steady-state level can be achieved within 5 to 6 days. It has been found that atypical antipsychotics have a very high bioavailability and protein binding. The elimination half-lives for all atypical antipsychotics range from 3 to 27 hours.

Benzodiazepines

Although benzodiazepines are now prescribed for a wide range of indications, they were introduced in the 1970s as powerful and rapid-acting antianxiety or hypnotic drugs. These drugs bind benzodiazepine receptors, which allosterically modulate GABA receptors, the most ubiquitous inhibitory neurotransmitter in the brain. In bipolar disorder, the high-potency benzodiazepines (clonazepam and lorazepam) are used either for their sedative properties (for example, to abort an emerging hypomanic/manic episode by aiding sleep) or as treatments for comorbid anxiety symptoms.

Following oral administration, lorazepam is absorbed rapidly and completely, whereas clonazepam is absorbed more slowly. Peak serum levels for lorazepam occur within 1–2 hours, whereas clonazepam requires several hours. All benzodiazepines exhibit first-order kinetics over the therapeutic dosage range, with metabolism occurring in the liver; they all bind to plasma proteins at levels of 70 percent or higher. Lorazepam has a relatively short half-life of 10–20 hours, whereas that of clonazepam is 18–50 hours.

NOTES

1. Indirectly, lithium also made possible the birth of the first patient-run support/advocacy group, the National Depressive and Manic Depressive Association (now the Depressive and Bipolar Support Alliance [DBSA]), by helping many patients function well enough to form and run an effective national organization.
2. Tohen et al., 1990, 1992, 2000, 2006; Coryell et al., 1993; Strakowsky et al., 1998, 2000.
3. In a recent survey in Norway, bipolar patients were more than three times as likely as controls to be unemployed and three times as likely to be on disability, despite the fact that the patients enjoyed a significantly higher educational level than that of the controls (Schoyen et al., 2006).
4. Earlier studies, largely from academic health centers, while noting the expected relationship between substance abuse and symptomatic and/or syndromal outcome, did not find such a relationship with functional outcome (reviewed in Bauer et al., 2001). The difference between these studies and that of Conus and colleagues (2006) may reflect the fact that patients in tertiary referral academic centers are generally sicker, with both high rates of substance abuse and poor functional outcome, making it more difficult to demonstrate a relationship.

5. The word *predicts* is used here in the statistical sense, reflecting an association between two variables without implying the direction of causality.

6. See, e.g., Lish et al., 1994; Ghaemi et al., 2002; Goldberg and Ernst, 2002; Hirschfield et al., 2003.

7. Not surprisingly, the bulk of the data establishing this relationship comes from studies of lithium.

8. Prien et al., 1974; Abou-Saleh and Coppen, 1986; Gelenberg et al., 1989; O'Connell et al., 1991; Winokur et al., 1993; Lish et al., 1994; Baldessarini et al., 1999; Franchini et al., 1999; Swann et al., 1999.

9. One managed care problem that is rarely addressed is the practice of pharmacy benefit managers allowing patients to obtain only 30 days of a prescription at one time; this practice substantially increases the likelihood of patients missing medications and thus going through periods of withdrawal.

10. See, for example, Calabrese and Rapport, 1999; Baldessarini et al., 2000; Post et al., 2000; Rush et al., 2000; Licht et al., 2002; Rothwell et al., 2005.

11. The least acceptable approach to a review of the literature is the classic "selective" review, in which the reviewer selects those articles that agree with his or her opinion and ignores those that do not. In this approach, any opinion can be supported by selectively choosing among studies in the literature. Unfortunately, most reviews of the literature on bipolar disorder fall into this category. The opposite of the selective review is the systematic review. In this approach, some effort is made, usually with computerized searching, to identify all studies on a topic. Once all studies have been identified (ideally including some that may not have been published), the question is how these studies can be compared.

  The simplest approach to reviewing a literature is the "box score" method: How many studies were positive and how many negative? The problem with this approach is that it fails to take into account the quality of the various studies (i.e., sample sizes, randomized or not, control of bias, adequacy of statistical testing for chance). The next-most rigorous approach is a pooled analysis. Unlike the "box score," this approach corrects for sample size, but nothing else. Other features of studies are not assessed, such as bias in design, randomization or not, and so on. Sometimes, those features can be controlled by inclusion criteria that might, for instance, limit a pooled analysis to randomized studies.

12. Sometimes a sensitivity analysis can be done, where one assumes a best-case scenario (all dropouts remain well) and a worst-case scenario (all dropouts relapse) to see whether the conclusions change. Nonetheless, a high percentage of dropouts means one cannot be certain whether results are valid.

13. The Texas Medication Algorithm does include the olanzapine–fluoxetine combination (OFC) as one third-line option, given that it was approved by the U.S. Food and Drug Administration for bipolar depression based on adequate data from randomized controlled trials. However, when comparing treatment options, it is important to note that OFC is not a drug—it is two drugs marketed as a single pill. Scientifically, it should be compared with other combinations of two drugs.

14. It should be noted that these data include all prescriptions, not just those written by psychiatrists.

15. In the lithium treatment of acute mania, the patient's clinical state is one of the factors affecting the dose/blood-level ratio. Some patients when manic retain lithium in body pools outside the plasma, possibly in bone (Greenspan et al., 1968; Almy and Taylor, 1973). In practice, more lithium may be needed to achieve a given blood level during mania than during euthymia or depression (Goodwin et al., 1969; Serry, 1969; Kukopulos et al., 1985).

16. When renal concentrating ability is substantially impaired or the patient excretes in excess of 4 liters of urine per 24 hours, careful monitoring (by the patient and the physician) of fluid balance is required to avoid dehydration and lithium intoxication (Vestergaard and Shou, 1987). Although renal concentrating ability usually improves if lithium is discontinued, the improvement can be quite delayed and incomplete if the impairment has been long-standing. Lithium discontinuation studies indicate that increases in 24-hour urine output remain the same or decrease only slightly after lithium is discontinued.

17. More sedation and ataxia occur with rapidly rising levels of carbamazepine than with most other modern anticonvulsants, and as a consequence, titration often needs to be slowed, especially when multiple drugs are being used together. Most of these cases have occurred in the elderly and within the first 4 months of treatment.

18. Serious side effects are associated with the typical antipsychotics. Common central nervous system side effects involve altered thermoregulation, extrapyramidal syndrome, neuroleptic malignant syndrome, and tardive dyskinesia. Orthostatic hypotension is also observed. Erectile dysfunction, blurred vision, constipation, and urinary retention are common anticholinergic effects. Cardiovascular effects include electrocardiogram changes, tachycardia, and torsade de pointes. Changes in the endocrine system, including amenorrhea and galactorrhea, occur as well. Occasionally the hematological system can be involved, with agranulocytosis and leucopenia occurring. Liver enzyme elevations are sometimes seen early in treatment; they usually resolve even with continued treatment, but can cause bilirubin with cholestatic jaundice to occur. Other pertinent side effects include allergic reactions and skin photosensitivity and all immune-mediated agranulyctopenia. Sedation and weight gain are observed as well. So-called low-potency antipsychotics cause more sedation and vascular side effects (orthostasis), whereas the more potent drugs are more commonly associated with extrapyramidal syndrome. The greatest concern arises for extrapyramidal syndrome, the potentially fatal neuroleptic malignant syndrome, and potentially irreversible tardive dyskinesia. These severe side effects have led to a recent trend toward the use of atypical antipsychotics, especially for patients newly diagnosed.

18 Medical Treatment of Hypomania, Mania, and Mixed States

[Robert Lowell] showed me the bottle of lithium capsules. Another medical gift from Copenhagen. Had I heard what his trouble was? "Salt deficiency." This had been the first year in eighteen he hadn't had an [manic] attack. There'd been fourteen or fifteen of them in the past eighteen years. Frightful humiliation and waste. . . . His face seemed smoother, the weight of distress–attacks and anticipation both gone.

—*Richard Stern (cited in Hamilton, 1982, p. 370)*

Despite the availability of many effective pharmacological agents for treating mania and hypomania, the management of both states is often challenging. Unlike the depressed patient, who usually seeks out treatment, the manic patient—and especially, perhaps, the hypomanic patient—often resists treatment. Moreover, the physician treating the first manic episode in a previously untreated patient must engage the patient's cooperation in treatment, simultaneously educate family and friends about the illness, and coordinate efforts with hospital staff and even law enforcement agencies. In many ways, the pharmacological treatment of the manic patient, the main focus of this chapter, may be the easiest part of the clinical work performed by the physician.

This chapter addresses hypomanic, manic, and mixed affective states, the latter usually characterized by a combination of the dysphoric mood of depression and the pressured agitation of mania; the management of mixed states resembles that of mania much more than that of bipolar depression (see Chapter 19). Note that this chapter focuses on medical treatment during the acute and continuation stages of these conditions, as defined in Chapter 17. Long-term maintenance (prophylactic) treatment is covered in Chapter 20, while psychotherapeutic treatment is discussed in Chapter 22. Two important related topics—medication adherence and psychotherapy—are addressed in Chapters 21 and 22, respectively. Note also that many of the drugs discussed here for acute and continuation treatment of hypomania, mania, and mixed states are used as well for patients with acute bipolar depression and for maintenance treatment, and are therefore discussed in Chapters 19 and 20 as well. The reader interested in a detailed review of the drugs themselves, including their functioning and their side effects, should refer to those chapters.

The chapter begins with a discussion of clinical management, emphasizing proven and/or widely accepted approaches to treatment. We then review the literature supporting these approaches, as well as newer and less proven but nevertheless promising interventions that may become more standard in the future. All of the drugs mentioned in the first section of the chapter are discussed in detail in the second.

CLINICAL MANAGEMENT

A patient in the throes of a manic or mixed episode can be intensely agitated, uncooperative, psychotic, aggressive, and quite dangerous. By the time the clinician is contacted, both patient and family may be confused and distraught, and the clinician may have little time to ponder available choices. Ideal treatment involves both persuasion and medication, but is the patient persuadable, and which drug is best for this patient in this situation? To what degree is there a danger to staff, accompanying family, or the patient in the manic or mixed state? Should the selected drug be offered orally, or will parenteral administration be quicker and more effective? Each decision calls for balancing the high-risk manic agitation against the consequences of intervention—a medication's potency against its side effects, for example, or the patient's safety against the risks and responsibilities of forced medication and possible involuntary hospitalization. Our recommendations for the selection of appropriate treatments for particular patients are presented later in the chapter.

This section addresses the key aspects of clinical management of hypomania, mania, and mixed states. Discussed in turn are evaluation of the manic, mixed-state, and hypomanic patient; hospitalization; general considerations involved in medical treatment; clinical features that modify medication management; medication dosages and therapeutic monitoring; hypomanic symptoms; and general psychological issues related to the medical treatment of mania. Detailed discussion of special considerations in treating children and adolescents is presented in Chapter 23, and of issues involving drugs and pregnancy in Chapter 20.

Evaluation of the Manic, Mixed-State, and Hypomanic Patient

By definition, the manic or mixed-state patient is highly agitated and not easily amenable to examination. It is critical, then, to obtain the patient's history from family, friends, coworkers, law enforcement officers, or whoever may be available to give information about the course of illness and development of symptoms. A history of prior manic or depressive episodes will, of course, be very helpful in making a diagnosis, but mania should be suspected in any disorganized patient with marked psychomotor agitation (see also the discussion of diagnosis in Chapter 3). A differential diagnosis will include schizophrenia, drug-induced states, and delirium from metabolic or other medical causes, but because the emergent treatment of all these conditions is generally similar, behavioral management of the potentially dangerous patient will usually take priority over the subtleties of the usual psychiatric diagnostic process. Nevertheless, a mental status examination assessing such symptoms as euphoric or irritable mood, pressured speech, and grandiose themes should be performed when feasible. Although the usual structured cognitive examination may not be possible, it is important to rule out delirium by means of questions addressing orientation and awareness of surroundings.[1]

Laboratory testing is extremely important in evaluating the agitated psychiatric patient. Even if the history obtained clearly suggests a diagnosis of mania, the patient's psychiatric condition can be exacerbated by and the clinical picture confused by drug use or medical conditions. The patient's condition may also be affected by nonadherence to treatment for concurrent medical conditions, such as diabetes and hypertension. Manic patients will frequently be dehydrated and may be at risk for rhabdomyolysis, or they may present with simultaneous alcohol or drug intoxication or withdrawal (see Chapter 7). Testing for electrolyte abnormalities, hypo- and hyperglycemia, liver and renal dysfunction, and illicit drug use is thus an essential part of the initial evaluation.

The hypomanic patient will show less psychomotor agitation than the manic patient and can often be examined in greater detail. These patients may be less than forthcoming during the exam, however, and quite unreliable when it comes to giving a medical or psychiatric history. Indeed, hypomanic patients may actively withhold information or even prevaricate regarding symptoms and behavior if they believe doing so is necessary to avoid hospital confinement. Furthermore, mental status examination of hypomanic patients, who may evidence little more than slightly pressured speech and infectious high spirits, can belie the dangerousness of their situation. Such patients will be more likely than disorganized, agitated manic patients to enter into ruinous business deals or sexual indiscretions. Again, information from other individuals is vital for treatment planning.

Hospitalization

Patients exhibiting severe mania will need to be hospitalized, often involuntarily. When manic symptoms are still in the mild to moderate range, judging the need for and the timing of hospitalization is more difficult. In deciding whether to hospitalize a patient, the clinician must keep in mind that mild mania can progress rapidly and unexpectedly to more severe forms. The medical, social, occupational, and legal risks of such extreme behavior must be weighed against the financial, social, and personal consequences of hospitalization.

The uncomfortable affect of the mixed state, together with its disinhibition paranoia, and behavioral activation, can be an especially dangerous combination. Such patients are at very high risk of self-harm, sometimes higher than that for patients with pure major depression (see Chapter 8). A history of serious suicide attempts, as well as of previous hospitalizations, further increases the risk of suicide. Expressions of desperation or hopelessness in a manic patient indicate the need for immediate hospitalization.

The interpretation of commitment laws and the details of the commitment process vary considerably from community to community, even within the same state. Therefore, familiarity with local commitment laws is indispensable for the clinician involved in the treatment of manic, mixed-state, or hypomanic patients. Many states require that the clinician have first-person knowledge of disturbed behavior or suicidality before a psychiatric patient is hospitalized involuntarily—knowledge sometimes not available to the clinician who is at the receiving end of a phone call from a desperate family member. The clinician may have to spend considerable time educating family members about the steps necessary to initiate involuntary commitment of their loved one. Family members may resist taking on this responsibility, regarding it as a betrayal of their relative; some may worry about future physical or psychological reprisals. First-hand knowledge of the commitment process will enable the clinician to provide the necessary guidance and support. Advance directives, executed when the patient was euthymic, can be of help (see Chapter 22).

Safety issues will frequently inform the decision whether to hospitalize the manic patient, and here the choice is often more clear-cut. Patients showing severe behavioral dyscontrol and marked psychomotor agitation will obviously need to be hospitalized. In the case of the hypomanic patient, such overt evidence of poor impulse control, potential suicidality, or imminent violence may be absent. The decision-making process then shifts from focusing on the patient's current condition to assessing the probability that this condition will deteriorate, as well as the likelihood of being able to intervene quickly should that occur. Several questions arise: How insightful is the patient about his or her condition? Has the patient shown a willingness to seek more intensive treatment in the past when asked to do so by family or physician? Is there a complicating substance abuse problem? Do patient and family have quick and easy access to the clinician, day and night if necessary? The availability and competence of the patient's community support system—family members, a reliable and available therapist or case manager, and law enforcement officials who are informed and experienced in the care of psychiatric patients—also come into play.

Medical Treatment: General Considerations

Treatment goals for management of the manic or mixed-state patient include emergency management to allow for safe care in a standard inpatient setting; initial behavioral stabilization; mood stabilization; and, finally, transition to maintenance treatment.

Emergency Management

In general, the sooner an agitated manic patient can be effectively medicated, the better. A medication that is easy to use, safe, and rapidly calming is the ideal. Haloperidol given intramuscularly (IM) is the most widely used emergency treatment for acute mania (although other high-potency typical antipsychotics, such as fluphenazine, are just as effective and slightly less likely to cause extrapyramidal syndrome [EPS]).[2] Three of the atypicals—olanzapine, ziprasidone, and risperidone (a depot preparation)—are now available in parenteral form. IM ziprasidone, 2–10 mg, was shown in one study to offer a short-term advantage over IM haloperidol for acute agitation and to be associated with less EPS (Brook et al., 2000). IM clonazepam (.5–1.0 mg) and IM lorazepam (1–2 mg) have also been used for short-term treatment of agitated manic states; however, they are not as effective as the high-potency antipsychotics in calming most manic patients. For example, IM olanzapine has been shown to be superior to IM lorazepam for the treatment of acute manic agitation (Meehan et al., 2001). Nevertheless, benzodiazapines can be highly effective and provide some welcome drowsiness for patients in a mixed manic state with a moderate degree of agitation; they also are less likely to leave the patient as dysphoric as some feel after receiving antipsychotics. On the other hand, the short-term risk of disinhibition with benzodiazepines is a hazard in the already hyperactive patient, although it is uncommon after a single dose.

Initial Behavioral Stabilization

The treatments of choice in the first days of dealing with moderately severe to severe mania vary by institution and locale. Many American centers begin with valproate and/or lithium or with a typical antipsychotic, the latter remaining the most common choice for combination treatment (Chou et al., 1996; Keck et al., 1996; Tohen et al., 2001), although use of atypicals is increasing (Letmaier et al., 2006). By contrast, many centers outside the United States continue to use the typical antipsychotics as first-choice agents (Letmaier et al., 2004), either alone or in combination with lithium, valproate, or carbamazepine. Both the more sedating atypical antipsychotics, such as clozapine, olanzapine, and quetiapine, and those that tend to be less sedating—risperidone, aripiprazole, and ziprasidone—are gaining in popularity, and controlled data support their effectiveness as monotherapy or for use in combination treatments to stabilize the manic patient. In applying these controlled data on the new atypicals to clinical situations involving severe psychotic mania, however, it is important to realize that the ethics of placebo-controlled trials mean the sickest patients are less likely to be included.

The primary caution with antipsychotic combinations (especially the typical antipsychotics) relates to side effects, such as weight gain and metabolic syndrome, EPS, effects involving dopaminergic systems, and antipsychotic malignant syndrome. Moreover, concurrent administration of multiple medications makes it difficult for the clinician to determine which side effects and which beneficial effects are due to which drug. Despite substantial evidence supporting the efficacy of atypical antipsychotic monotherapy for acute mania, a sizable fraction of patients do not fully recover when these drugs are used alone, ultimately necessitating a typical antipsychotic and/or the addition of lithium or an anticonvulsant. Furthermore, because manic patients are prone to rapid shifts in mood and behavior during the early phases of recovery, those taking lithium or an anticonvulsant alone will frequently require high-potency antipsychotics or benzodiazepine medications on an as-needed basis during the first week or so of treatment. Combination therapies therefore predominate in treatment for acute mania, despite the paucity of clinical studies specifically assessing their use. More detail about individual drugs (doses, blood levels, and the like) is provided below.

If a patient fails to improve or manic behavior escalates despite the use of antipsychotics, lithium, and/or anticonvulsants, electroconvulsive therapy (ECT) is a valuable alternative. Both a randomized controlled trial (Small et al., 1988) and a large retrospective study (Black et al., 1987) found that ECT compares favorably with lithium for the treatment of acute mania or mixed states.[3] ECT may also be especially useful for women in the first trimester of pregnancy, when it is preferable to avoid medications, and for those in mixed states with a high risk of suicide. Obtaining informed consent for ECT, however, can be quite difficult with acutely manic or mixed patients. Some clinical investigators believe bilateral electrode placement may be necessary to obtain the full antimanic effect of ECT (Milstein et al., 1987), whereas others find no difference between unilateral and bilateral placement (Black et al., 1987). If ECT is used, lithium dosage should be reduced or discontinued because of the risk of delirium (Rudorfer et al., 1987). Rapid transcranial magnetic stimulation (rTMS) may turn out to be a useful alternative to ECT in some patients.

In acutely manic patients who do not respond to or cannot tolerate lithium, valproate, carbamazepine, or antipsychotics, the question arises of whether newer anticonvulsants may be adequate alternatives. Topiramate had been of interest because of its potential to produce weight loss, but controlled data have failed to demonstrate its antimanic efficacy. Oxcarbazepine has also been of interest because of its relatively more benign side-effect profile, especially the fact that it lacks the hematopoietic effects of the parent compound. Yet while some open studies have found it to be helpful (perhaps especially in patients with milder manic symptoms), there have been no adequately controlled studies establishing its efficacy as monotherapy. Gabapentin has shown no antimanic efficacy in controlled trials, although its sedative or anxiolytic properties may be useful when it is combined with an antimanic agent. Phenytoin and levetiracetam appear to show some antimanic activity as adjuncts, but controlled monotherapy data are still lacking.

Mood Stabilization

The likelihood that manic symptoms will resolve rapidly or slowly often becomes apparent within the first 4 to 5 days of inpatient care. While the occasional extremely agitated and delusional patient will remain calm for days after a single IM injection of antipsychotic medication, other patients will remain manic to the point of requiring seclusion and physical restraint for a week or more despite receiving high-dose antipsychotics combined with an anticonvulsant and lithium. Most patients' response to treatment falls somewhere between these extremes, and the length of time to recovery cannot be predicted accurately.

When patients accept short-term medical management, they often do so without really understanding or accepting their diagnosis and its implications, especially in the initial stages of their recovery. With clinical improvement, however, many manic patients will develop at least partial insight into the full consequences of uncontrolled mania and sign on to the treatment plan. At this point, the physician will be able to have more meaningful though still limited discussion of the advantages and disadvantages of the various treatment options with the patient. When the patient recovers the capacity to exercise sufficient judgment, it becomes possible for patient and physician to collaborate on a plan for continued acute treatment and a strategy for remission maintenance. Day hospital is often an ideal setting for manic patients who are partially recovered and cooperative to attain adequate control of their symptoms and improved insight and judgment. When dealing with hypomanic patients in particular, it can be helpful to point out that hypomania, albeit more than pleasant at the moment, usually can be thought of as the beginning of the next depression.

Continuation Treatment and the Transition to Maintenance Therapy

Even with aggressive pharmacotherapy, severely ill manic patients can take 4 weeks or longer to attain a stable affective state with sufficient insight to permit outpatient care. With careful monitoring of the therapeutic benefits as well as the side effects of treatment, titration of the lithium, anticonvulsant, or antipsychotic dose into the therapeutic range (using blood levels where appropriate), along with a gradual decrease in the dose of any typical antipsychotic medication, can be substantially accomplished within 1–2 weeks of initiation of treatment. By the third week, some patients can be maintained on lithium, an anticonvulsant, or an atypical antipsychotic alone. Recovering manic patients should not be discharged to day hospital or outpatient care unless they are well enough to make an informed and reliable commitment to medication adherence (see Chapter 21) and regular office or clinic visits; in addition, it is helpful to enlist family members whose involvement can increase the likelihood that the treatment plan will be followed.

The danger of discharge without sufficient improvement and insight is not merely a theoretical concern. Patients who appear to be improving over the short term can rapidly relapse into manic symptoms if they do not adhere to treatment; even if they do adhere, they may cycle into the depressed phase of the illness. Moreover, many patients with bipolar disorder are at substantial risk for suicidal behavior, regardless of the polarity of the acute episode (see Chapter 8).[4] Rucci and colleagues (2002) found that an intensive treatment program, which included closely monitoring treatment adherence and tracking down patients who missed appointments, virtually eliminated suicide attempts in bipolar patients in the period following an acute manic episode.

Clinical Features That Modify Medication Management

Extreme Hyperactivity

Extreme hyperactivity poses substantial direct and indirect risks to manic patients; these include dehydration, cardiovascular stress, and the medically necessitated physical restraint and seclusion often associated with intense agitation. It should not be forgotten that many manic patients died of exhaustion before the advent of modern treatments (see Fig. 18–1). Typical antipsychotics are the most rapidly effective agents in controlling this set of symptoms; in these situations, they are often combined with lithium, an anticonvulsant, or an atypical antipsychotic.

Psychotic Symptoms

Approximately 50 percent of inpatient manic patients suffer from delusions, usually grandiose or paranoid in nature. Formal thought disorder and auditory hallucinations, although less common, also occur relatively frequently (see Chapter 2). Antipsychotics (both typical and atypical) are quite effective in treating these symptoms.

Euphoric versus Mixed Mania

Prior to the availability of anticonvulsants and atypical antipsychotics, a combination of lithium and typical antipsychotics was generally used for the acute treatment of mixed

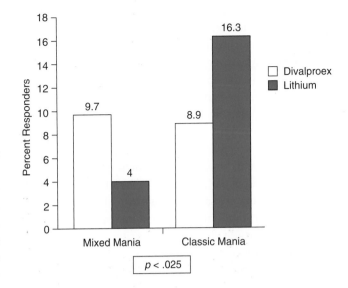

Figure 18–2. Percent response to divalproex and lithium in classic vs. mixed mania. (*Source*: Adapted from Bowden et al., 1994. Reprinted with permission.)

states. Some studies have shown lithium to be more effective in typical manic states than in dysphoric/mixed or rapid-cycling acute states, whereas valproate is particularly effective in mixed or acute rapid-cycling states (Juckel et al., 2000). Two separate analyses of the original divalproex registration trial showed divalproex monotherapy to be superior to lithium monotherapy for the treatment of manic states in patients with elevated depression scales and in those with multiple previous episodes. However, this is confounded by the high number of prior lithium failures in the sample. Carbamazepine may be superior to lithium for mixed states (Emilien et al., 1996).

It is important to note that in the divalproex registration trial, lithium was more effective than divalproex among patients with the "classic" manic features of euphoria and grandiosity (see Fig. 18–2). This trial is also noteworthy for finding that prior good response to lithium predicted a good response during subsequent manic episodes and a poorer response to anticonvulsants—an argument for using lithium in some patients with mixed states despite the apparent superiority of valproate in treating such states. Olanzapine, either as monotherapy or adjunctively, has been shown to be as effective in mixed mania as in pure mania. There are similar data for other atypical antipsychotics, suggesting a class effect. However, each atypical is unique in its clinical profile, and many patients do poorly on one but very well on another.

Rapid-Cycling Bipolar Disorder

A history of rapid cycling, usually defined as four or more affective episodes within 1 year, has implications for the

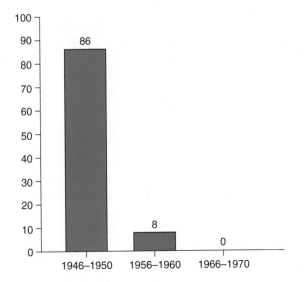

Figure 18–1. Deaths from psychotic exhaustion. Mortality statistics for psychotic exhaustion, Royal Park Hospital, for the years 1946–1950, 1956–1960, 1966–1970. (*Source*: Cade, 1978.)

treatment of acute mania in that it makes sense to start medications in the short term that have proven beneficial for this subgroup of patients in the longer term. Early studies of lithium prophylaxis suggested that patients with a history of at least four affective episodes in 1 year were disproportionately overrepresented among those who failed to experience a prophylactic effect from lithium (Dunner and Fieve, 1974). However, a more recent naturalistic study of rapid-cycling and non-rapid-cycling patients found that lithium was equally effective in both groups (Baldessarini et al., 2000), a finding that may, in part, be related to the relatively conservative use of antidepressants in this particular group of patients. Another important consideration is that in the Dunner and Fieve study, the minimum criterion for treatment failure was a single new episode, whereas Baldessarini and colleagues examined the overall reduction in morbidity associated with lithium treatment in the two groups of patients; clinically, the latter is a more relevant measure. Indeed, Dunner (2000) himself advocated starting lithium acutely in patients with a history of rapid cycling and only adding an anticonvulsant later if needed. Likewise, McElroy and Keck (2000), based on their review of the literature, recommended that manic or mixed-state patients with a history of rapid cycling be started on lithium, reserving adjunctive valproate for those who fail to respond to lithium. However, contemporary North American guidelines recommend that rapid-cycling patients be started on an anticonvulsant acutely (valproate is recommended most frequently; see Sachs et al., 2000), with the option of adding lithium later depending on the response to the anticonvulsant. This recommendation may be modified in light of the recent carefully controlled trial of Calabrese and colleagues (2005) showing that lithium and divalproex monotherapy had equivalent (poor) maintenance efficacy in rapid-cycling patients who had been stabilized on the combination (see Chapter 20).

Rapid cycling has also been shown to predict an acute antimanic effect for carbamazepine (Post et al., 1986a), although results of other studies indicate that this effect does not translate into prophylaxis against mania in patients with a history of rapid cycling (Denicoff et al., 1997). In the initial studies that established olanzapine as an antimanic agent, it was equally effective among rapid and nonrapid cyclers (Tohen et al., 2004), and this appears to be true for other atypicals as well. Furthermore, among patients with a history of rapid cycling who are nonresponders to lithium or anticonvulsants, the addition of atypical antipsychotics has been shown to be effective for the treatment of acute mania (Sanger et al., 2003), although the data do not support giving an atypical to all patients with a history of rapid cycling in the absence of other indications.

Medication Dosages and Therapeutic Monitoring

Lithium

Lithium's antimanic effects correlate more closely with serum levels than with dosage. Early studies of its efficacy in mania indicate that its antimanic (as well as its prophylactic) serum level is positively correlated with blood levels. Results of several monotherapy studies suggest that levels below .8 milliequivalents per liter (mEq/l) are not as effective as those above this level. Although there is an upper limit of therapeutic benefit in serum lithium level, this limit appears to be set by toxicity rather than by loss of therapeutic benefit. Prien and Caffey's (1976) systematic search of their controlled trial data established .9 mEq/l as the lower limit for antimanic efficacy and 1.4 mEq/l as the limit above which additional benefit could not be demonstrated because of high rates of toxicity. It is important to note that when lithium is administered to an acutely manic patient, it is generally necessary to adjust the dose downward as the mania begins to subside in order to maintain the blood level in a reasonable range. As detailed in the first edition, the ratio of dose to plasma level is higher in mania than in euthymia or depression. The mechanism by which lithium excretion appears to be enhanced during manic states is unknown, but probably involves changes in aldosterone levels. Following resolution of the acute mania (that is, when shifting to the continuation phase of treatment), the blood level should gradually be reduced, if possible, to the .6–.8 mEq/l range (see Chapter 20).

Anticonvulsants

As with lithium, the therapeutic benefit of anticonvulsants in mania appears to correlate with serum levels rather than with dosage. Thus studies of valproate suggest that levels above 45 micrograms per milliliter (µg/ml) are necessary for antimanic efficacy (Bowden et al., 1996) and that side effects become increasingly problematic at levels above 125 µg/ml.

Oral medication loading strategies have been devised for speeding up the onset of the antimanic action of anticonvulsants. For valproate, the strategy is to dose at 30 milligrams per kilogram (mg/kg) of body weight for days 1 and 2 of therapy, followed by 20 mg/kg on days 3–10 (Hirschfeld et al., 1999). In one double-blind study, valproate loading was shown to be at least as rapid in reducing manic symptoms as treatment with haloperidol (McElroy et al., 1996), and in a pooled analysis of randomized, double-blind studies, the loading strategy was found to be more rapidly effective than standard-titration valproate and equivalent to olanzapine (Hirschfeld et al., 2003). Intravenous loading has also been reported to be rapidly effective and may be an option for some patients (Grunze et al., 1999a).

Serum carbamazepine levels of 8–12 mEq/ml appear to be optimal for the treatment of mania (Post et al., 1986a). Although oxcarbazepine has been studied in Europe since the early 1980s, its optimal dose and therapeutic serum level have not been established for the treatment of bipolar disorder. A dose that is 1.5 times that of carbamazepine (oxcarbazepine dose of 600–1200 mg/day) is recommended for epilepsy (Dam, 1994), and clinical experience suggests this ratio is probably appropriate for mania as well.

Typical Antipsychotic Agents

Although clinicians have frequently used larger oral doses of antipsychotics for acute mania than for schizophrenia, results of controlled studies suggest that lower doses are effective for mania as well. Haloperidol remains widely used at doses ranging from 2 mg/day up to as high as 50 mg/day (25 mg orally every 12 hours).[5] Chlorpromazine, thioridazine, and other low-potency antipsychotic agents are now used rarely because of high rates of orthostatic hypotension and extrapyramidal side effects.[6]

Atypical Antipsychotic Agents

A major change in the treatment of mania since 1990, especially in the United States, has been the emergence of atypical antipsychotics as effective antimanic agents. Olanzapine, risperidone, quetiapine, ziprasidone, and aripiprazole have received the approval of the U.S. Food and Drug Administration (FDA) as antimanic agents, and as of this writing, the European regulatory agency has approved olanzapine, risperidone, and quetiapine. In the United States, olanzapine, quetiapine, and clozapine have largely replaced chlorpromazine and thioridazine as the favored *sedating* antipsychotics. However, it is worth noting that these new drugs are not always an adequate replacement for the typical agents, especially in cases of more severe mania and when rapid control of psychosis and hyperactivity are required, such as in an emergency room setting. As Licht and colleagues (1997) pointed out, placebo-controlled trials of atypicals have, of necessity, tended to involve more moderately ill patients in order to obtain ethically acceptable informed consent.

Olanzapine is usually begun at oral doses of 2.5–5 mg every 6 hours for treatment of mania, titrated up to 20 mg/day (although some studies suggest 2.5–5 mg/day may work as well). Quetiapine is dosed on the basis of height, weight, and clinical response, but not blood levels; the usual starting dose is 100 mg/day, with a target dose ranging from 400 to 800 mg/day and averaging 600 mg/day. Clozapine is begun at 25–50 mg every 6 hours and titrated up to 1,000 mg/day.

Use of the less sedating oral antipsychotics risperidone, aripiprazole, and ziprasidone is also increasing. Risperidone is started at 1 mg every 6–8 hours and usually does not exceed 6–10 mg/day. Aripiprazole doses of 30 mg/day are generally recommended, with an option to decrease this dose to 15 mg/day if tolerability is a problem. Oral ziprasidone is started at 40 mg twice daily (BID) with food, increased to 60 or 80 mg BID on the second day, then adjusted in the range of 40–80 mg BID. The IM dose in acute psychotic states is usually about 10–20 mg every 4 hours, up to 40 mg/day.

It has been suggested that there may be clinically important differences among the various atypical antipsychotics in the initial onset of antimanic effects (Keck, 2005). However, such a conclusion is premature given the design differences among the various registration trials for these drugs. For the risperidone and ziprasidone trials, the first ratings were obtained at 1 or 2 days, for aripiprazole at 4 days, and for olanzapine at 7 days. The impression that ziprasidone and risperidone have a more rapid onset of action than the other drugs is probably an artifact of these design differences.

Benzodiazepines

High-potency benzodiazepines, including lorazepam and clonazepam, have been shown to have short-term benefits in the treatment of acute manic agitated states, especially in emergency room settings. IM or oral doses of 1–2 mg up to every 2 hours are most common (Lenox et al., 1992). Adjunctive oral benzodiazepines can also be useful, such as in the management of the initial activation sometimes seen with ziprasidone or aripiprazole.

Hypomanic Symptoms

Hypomanic symptoms need not always be treated aggressively, as they will often resolve with watchful waiting. However, repeated episodes of hypomania can be indicators of more general mood instability that should lead the clinician to reassess the adequacy of the maintenance strategy (see Chapter 20). The threshold for treating hypomanic symptoms in a particular patient depends on diagnostic considerations: the threshold should be lower in patients with a history of similar symptoms evolving into full-blown mania (i.e., bipolar-I disorder) than in those whose hypomanic episodes have never progressed to mania (i.e., bipolar-II). Hypomania with depressive features (dysphoric hypomania) is not uncommon (see Chapters 1 and 2), and this makes it more likely that pharmacological intervention will be sought and needed.

The decision regarding treatment can often be difficult, however; patients early in the course of illness whose diagnosis is less than clear and those who are unreliable present obvious challenges. It is important to remember that patients with mild hypomania can be disinhibited enough to suffer substantial interpersonal, professional, or financial or legal adverse consequences from a period of even mildly elevated mood. Approaches thought to be useful for the treatment of mania have generally been extrapolated to the treatment of hypomania, as there is a paucity of clinical research data specifically on the treatment of hypomania. Finally, it is reasonable to consider the possibility that treatment of hypomania may reduce the likelihood and/or severity of subsequent depressive episodes. Indeed, as noted earlier, it can be useful to point out that a period of hypomania is often the beginning of the next depression when dealing with a hypomanic patient reluctant to be treated.

An evaluation for possible etiological factors is an initial step in deciding how to proceed. Iatrogenic causes should be investigated, specifically the recent addition to the patient's regimen of a medication, such as an antidepressant, that may precipitate hypomanic symptoms (see Chapter 19). Numerous over-the-counter preparations—including nutritional supplements such as St. Johns Wort (Nierenberg et al., 1999), dehydroepiandrosterone (DHEA) (Dean, 2000), and others—have been reported to be associated with hypomanic symptoms. Patients not infrequently supplement their prescribed medications with such preparations without informing their physicians because they fear disapproval or do not realize the potential for adverse effects. Surreptitious substance abuse is another important and all-too-common factor, as is sleep deprivation.

Lowering the dose of or discontinuing such potentially mania-inducing agents is a sensible first step in addressing hypomanic symptoms. Thereafter, a reasonable initial intervention is to optimize whatever antimanic treatment the patient is already receiving. Dosage increases need to be guided by serum drug levels when possible, while the implications for long-term management should be considered before another agent is added. The addition of an anticonvulsant to lithium or vice versa may be indicated if the current hypomanic episode is one of many and appears to signify a pattern of inadequate maintenance treatment. The addition of an atypical antipsychotic agent is frequently recommended for the short-term control of hypomanic symptoms, especially given the fairly rapid onset of benefit, which may be due to immediate improvement in sleep. Vieta and colleagues (2001) examined this strategy in an open study of 44 patients with bipolar-II disorder. In the 34 patients who completed the study, the Young Mania Rating Scale (YMRS) score dropped from a mean of 22.1 to 3.1 (essentially asymptomatic) within 2 weeks when risperidone was added to various other medications being taken, including lithium, anticonvulsants, and combinations.

Benzodiazepines also have a place in the treatment of hypomanic symptoms. The temporary use of adjunctive clonazepam often can abort the beginning of a hypomanic episode by stabilizing sleep, although systematic data on this strategy are lacking.

Figure 18–3 outlines our recommended approach to the treatment of acute mania/ hypomania.

Psychological Issues Related to Medical Treatment of Mania

Many manic or mixed-state patients in acute care will undergo treatment without real insight into their condition. Although each situation is unique, some general guidelines can be offered to the clinician working with acutely manic patients whose judgment is substantially impaired.

The most extreme situation is when the patient is dangerous but will not or cannot give informed consent for treatment. In most states, commitment to a hospital is sufficient legal grounds for emergency medication against the patient's wishes, but not for routine medication, which often requires a separate administrative review. In more moderate circumstances, the patient is intermittently agreeable to treatment, or is consistently agreeable to some medication interventions but not to others. In such cases, establishing a few firm, non-negotiable limits very calmly and without rhetorical flourish or rancor can minimize a confrontation in the acute care situation.[7] Once a degree of cooperation has been achieved, it is important to begin educating manic patients about diagnosis and treatment to the extent that they are able to comprehend these matters, while gradually negotiating a path toward a full commitment to maintenance therapy. (These issues are explored in detail in Chapter 22.) As noted in Chapter 17, the most effective approaches involve the integration of drugs and psychotherapy.

Although family members are often no more able than the treating clinician to win a manic patient's cooperation, they are in a position to strengthen the patient's resolve *against* treatment if they do not understand the disorder and the rationale for the treatment. Families can easily become frightened by the intrinsically imprecise nature of pharmacological treatment of mania; they may worry that the patient taking multiple medications is being overmedicated and become concerned about the quality of care. It is important to inform family members about the sedative effects of medications and the extent to which such effects may be unavoidable (or even welcomed). Warning family members about likely side effects (such as periods of oversedation) and options for their management will reassure them and help gain their trust in and collaboration with the treatment process.

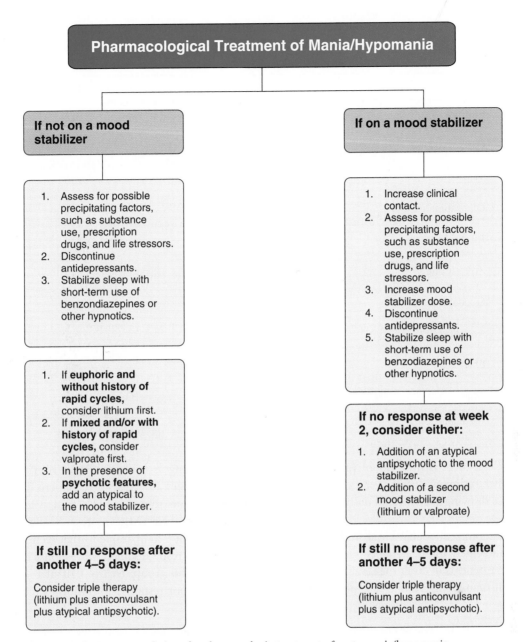

Figure 18–3. Recommendations for pharmacologic treatment of acute mania/hypomania.

REVIEW OF THE LITERATURE

In this section we review the literature on the various medications used to treat hypomania, mania, and mixed states: lithium, anticonvulsants, typical and atypical antipsychotics, and benzodiazepines. Other treatments, including ECT, TMS, calcium channel blockers, omega-3 fatty acids, and cholinergic agents, are discussed as well. Results of randomized, double-blind monotherapy trials for each of the major pharmacological agents are summarized in Table 18–1 and Figure 18–4, while results of non-placebo-controlled trials and placebo-controlled add-on trials are summarized in Table 18–2.

Lithium

Earlier controlled studies of lithium clearly established its superiority to placebo in treating acute mania. Studies conducted since 1990 were designed to compare newer medications with lithium as the reference antimanic agent (e.g., Bowden et al., 1994).

As detailed in the first edition of this volume, early placebo-controlled studies[8] established lithium as an effective, although not rapidly acting, treatment of choice for mania.[9] Many of these studies varied as to dosage, serum levels, and rapidity of dosage titration, making it difficult to establish the precise time to onset of lithium's antimanic

TABLE 18–1. Summary of Randomized, Double-Blind, Placebo-Controlled Monotherapy Trials That Have Demonstrated Acute Antimanic Efficacy

Drug	No. of Studies	Sample Size[a]
Lithium	5	358
Carbamazepine	4	600
Valproate	2	215
Olanzapine	2	254
Risperidone	2	549
Ziprasidone	2	412
Quetiapine	2	386
Aripiprazole	2	534
Phenytoin	1	27
Totals	20	2,137

[a]Combined drug and placebo groups.

action. Nonetheless, there is little doubt that lithium is as effective as other antimanic agents over a 3-week period, with some studies showing a more rapid onset of action (as little as 10 days).

The largest randomized, double-blind study of lithium versus placebo in acutely manic patients was actually designed to study the benefits of divalproex (valproate) for the treatment of acute mania, with lithium- and placebo-treated groups serving as controls (Bowden et al., 1994; Swann et al., 1997, 2002). In this study, 49 percent of the lithium-treated patients responded (i.e., had at least a 50 percent reduction in their YMRS scores) during the 3-week trial period (efficacy comparable to that seen for the valproate group). This result doubled the response rate of 25 percent in the placebo group. Nearly half of the patients had a history of poor response to lithium, which predicted the

Figure 18–4. Response rates for acute mania monotherapy. Mg/d = milligrams/day. (*Source*: Bowden et al., 2005.)

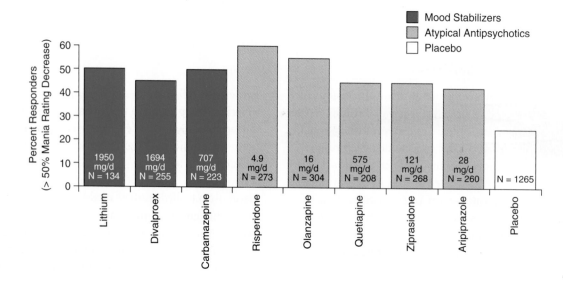

TABLE 18–2. **Drugs Demonstrating Acute Antimanic Efficacy in Non-Placebo-Controlled Comparison Trials or in Placebo-Controlled Add-On Trials**

Drug	No. of Studies	Sample Size	Findings
Lithium	16	775	Equivalent to typical antipsychotics or valproate
Carbamazepine	5	230	Equivalent to typical antipsychotics
Valproate	6	620	Equivalent to lithium or typical antipsychotics
Oxcarbazepine	2	72	Equivalent to both lithium and haloperidol
Phenytoin	1	39	Modest additional benefit when added to haloperidol among partial responders
Clozapine	1	27	Open-labeled monotherapy benefit or equivalent to chlorpromazine
Chlorpromazine	8	521	More effective than or equivalent to lithium
Haloperidol	9	901	Equivalent to lithium and atypical antipsychotics
Clozapine	4	115	Open-labeled monotherapy benefit or additional benefit when added to mood stabilizers
Risperidone	6	463	Equivalent to lithium; more effective than placebo as adjunct among non- or partial responders to lithium or anticonvulsants
Olanzapine	6	1,539	Equivalent to haloperidol, lithium, and valproate; more effective than placebo as adjunct among non- or partial responders to lithium or valproate
Quetiapine	5	440	More effective than placebo as adjunct among non- or partial responders to lithium and valproate
Electroconvulsive therapy (ECT)	2	64	Equivalent to lithium; ECT + chlorpromazepine more effective than ECT alone
Totals	65	5,246	

Note: Many of the individual studies comparing two active drugs without a placebo control lack sufficient statistical power to make it possible to evaluate whether the observed absence of a difference actually means equivalence.

differential response seen in this trial. Thus among the prior lithium responders who received lithium in this trial, there was a 15-point mean reduction in YMRS scores (a 60 percent improvement), compared with only a 1-point mean improvement in the previously nonresponsive group (Bowden et al., 1994). Among the prior lithium responders randomized to valproate, by contrast, there was only a 27 percent improvement, compared with the 60 percent improvement with lithium.

In another analysis of the data from this study, Swann and colleagues (1997) found evidence of some pharmacological specificity in that patients with mixed manic-depressive symptoms had a better response to valproate than to lithium, while those with typical manic symptoms did better on lithium (Bowden et al., 1995; see Fig. 18–2). Still another analysis of the same dataset, illustrated in Figure 18–5, revealed that manic patients with more than 10 prior affective episodes (of any polarity) also had a poorer response with lithium than with valproate (Swann et al., 1999). (Details of the findings on the efficacy of valproate are discussed below.)

A 12-week trial designed to evaluate quetiapine in acute mania included 98 patients on lithium as an active control

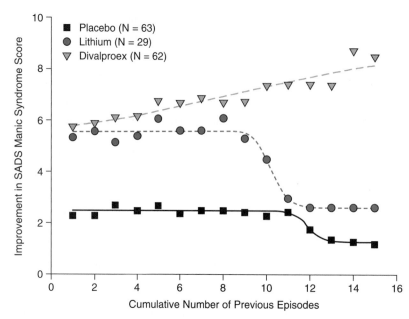

Figure 18–5. Number of prior episodes as a predictor of acute antimanic response to lithium or divalproex. SADS = Schedule for Affective Disorders and Schizophrenia. (*Source*: Swann et al., 1999. Reprinted with permission from the *American Journal of Psychiatry*, copyright 1999, American Psychiatric Association.)

(mean serum lithium .77 mEq/l). The response rate among the latter patients (defined as a decrease in YMRS scores of 50 percent or more) was 53 percent—identical to the response rate among the 107 patients on quetiapine and significantly better than that among the placebo group (27 percent). Discontinuation because of adverse events was infrequent with both drugs (lithium 6.1 percent, quetiapine 6.5 percent) (Bowden et al., 2005).

The response rates to lithium in the relatively recent studies of valproate and quetiapine are somewhat lower than the rates found in earlier studies. While this difference may relate in part to the evolution of research methodologies, another explanation (noted in Chapter 17) is (unintentional) referral bias. It is an old adage in medicine that the longer a successful treatment is available to clinicians, the more difficult it becomes for investigators to show that it still works. The reasons for this are straightforward. Among the bipolar patients referred to research centers for the evaluation of a new drug, those who are already doing well on lithium would tend to be underrepresented. Neither the patients nor their physicians have much of an incentive for participation in a trial of a new agent in which they have a chance to end up taking placebo. We also refer the reader to Box 17–4 in Chapter 17, which reviews the shift in prescribing patterns in the United States away from lithium and toward valproate, and suggests a possible nonmedical explanation for part of this shift.

There has been one trial of rapid administration (loading doses) of lithium to treat acute mania, aimed at assessing the potential to reduce the delay in the drug's onset of action (Keck et al., 2001b). In this trial, 15 manic and mixed-state patients were treated with 20 mg/day of lithium given in two doses. Concomitant lorazepam up to 4 mg/day through day 6 and up to 2 mg/day through day 8 was also allowed during the study. All patients achieved lithium levels above .6 mEq/l after 1 day of treatment. Two could not tolerate the rapid titration and stopped—one because of tachycardia and the other because of tremor, fatigue, and diarrhea—and one subject did not adhere to the regimen. Among the remaining 12 subjects, 7 were well enough to be discharged before the 10-day trial was completed. The mean YMRS score for these subjects was 11. Overall, 9 of 15 patients had achieved a greater than 50 percent reduction in YMRS scores by day 10 (by definition they were "responders").

As noted in Chapter 14, one hypothesis for the therapeutic action of lithium in mania is its inhibition of inositol monophosphatase, which by reducing brain inositol levels decreases the ability of neurons to generate certain second messengers. In a recent pilot open study, Shaldubina and colleagues (2006) evaluated the effect of an inositol-deficient diet on the clinical efficacy of lithium in a mixed group of 15 bipolar patients. Seven of these patients were in a manic episode that had not responded to lithium, and the remainder were lithium- or valproate-resistant rapid cyclers. Ten of the patients evidenced a substantial reduction in symptom severity, beginning in the first 1–2 weeks of treatment; of the 5 who did not respond, 3 did not adhere to the diet. A controlled replication of this intriguing observation is awaited.

Anticonvulsants

The use of anticonvulsant agents for the treatment of bipolar disorder was a watershed event for psychiatry in the late twentieth century. The clear effectiveness of some anticonvulsants for patients who do not respond well to or cannot tolerate lithium has made these drugs a welcome addition to the armamentarium. Controlled trials have shown both valproate and carbamazepine (including the new extended-release formulations of each) to be more effective than placebo and, as noted above, as effective as lithium for treatment of acute mania.[10] Moreover, a series of small non-placebo-controlled studies has found that oxcarbazepine, the 10-keto metabolite of carbamazepine, appears to have antimanic action similar to that of its parent compound, but requiring a higher dose. It has also become clear that not all anticonvulsants are effective antimanic agents. Thus while several case reports and open studies had suggested that topiramate might be effective for the treatment of acute mania, controlled studies have failed to show its efficacy as monotherapy for this state. Results of open studies suggest its usefulness as an adjunct, but these results need to be confirmed with placebo-controlled studies. There are also a few case reports of apparent precipitation of manic symptoms with topiramate.[11] One controlled study supports the efficacy of phenytoin as an adjunct, while monotherapy studies of gabapentin and the gamma-aminobutyric acid (GABA) analogue tiagabine have shown no apparent benefit in manic patients. Results of open studies suggest some efficacy for levetiracetam in treating acute mania, but there are as yet no controlled data. Other, newer anticonvulsants that have not been assessed in systematic studies of bipolar patients include losigamone, progabide, and vigabatrin.

Carbamazepine

Starting in the 1970s, a number of studies showed carbamazepine to be superior to placebo, although not necessarily equivalent to lithium, in the short-term treatment of mania.[12,13] Okuma and colleagues (1990) conducted a double-blind, placebo-controlled study of manic patients who were undergoing treatment with antipsychotics without substantial benefit. Half of the 105 patients were given 400–1200 mg/day of carbamazepine, and the other half were given lithium in amounts sufficient to establish relatively low mean serum levels of .46; all the patients continued on haloperidol. The final assessment revealed moderate to marked improvement in both groups of patients.[14] Since no group was assigned to continue antipsychotics alone, however, it remains unclear how much of the improvement seen was due to the adjunctive mood stabilizers versus the antipsychotics themselves. Small and colleagues (1991) conducted an 8-week double-blind comparison of carbamazepine and lithium in 52 hospitalized acutely manic patients. They found that the two drugs were equally effective in reducing manic symptoms (as judged by YMRS scores),[15] a conclusion supported by a later meta-analysis (Emilien et al., 1996).

Post and colleagues (1987) studied carbamazepine for the treatment of mania and concluded that rapid-cycling illness was a predictor of the drug's efficacy in treating acute mania. Subsequent investigators reported, however, that many patients with rapid cycling did not have good control of mania symptoms over the long term on carbamazepine monotherapy. For example, Denicoff and colleagues (1997) found that fewer than 20 percent of patients with rapid-cycling illness remained in remission during a 1-year study of the drug. More recently, however, two large multicenter double-blind, placebo-controlled trials of the extended-release formulation of carbamazepine showed its superiority over placebo for the acute treatment of mania or mixed states (Weisler et al., 2004, 2005). On the basis of these two trials,[16] extended-release carbamazepine has been approved by the FDA for the acute treatment of mania/mixed states.

In one of the few available studies of combinations of anticonvulsants, a retrospective chart review revealed that 12 bipolar manic patients but none of 4 schizoaffective manic patients did well with a combination of valproate and carbamazepine (Tohen et al., 1994). Small and colleagues (1995) conducted an 8-week inpatient trial of carbamazepine plus lithium compared with haloperidol plus lithium in manic patients. About half of the original 60 patients dropped out of the study during the 2-week placebo washout phase, primarily because of worsening mania. Among the 33 remaining patients, 17 treated with carbamazepine plus lithium and 16 with haloperidol plus lithium showed comparable levels of improvement. However, more of the latter patients left the study prematurely because of side effects. Conversely, more of the former patients terminated the protocol because of nonadherence; this group also needed more "rescue" medications for aggressive, uncooperative behavior in the first week of therapy.

Valproate

The French psychiatrist Lambert first reported a possible role for valproate in the treatment of bipolar disorder in the course of its first clinical trials in patients with epilepsy in the 1960s (Lambert et al., 1966). Many years later, Calabrese and Delucchi (1990) found that the drug appeared to have marked effects in treating mania, mixed states, and cycling. They also noted that most patients (63 percent) with a good response to the drug had failed to improve on lithium or carbamazepine (or both). The most striking results were seen in patients with mixed mania; for the group as a whole there was minimal evidence of any benefit during the depressive phases of illness.[17] Calabrese and colleagues (1992) later suggested that the subgroup of patients for whom valproate had shown some antidepressant effect were likely to have experienced an antimanic effect as well.

Muller-Oerlinghausen and colleagues (2000) reported on a double-blind, placebo-controlled study in which valproate was added to the medications used more commonly to treat acute mania in European centers—typical antipsychotics. A total of 136 patients taking haloperidol and/or perazine or some other antipsychotic received either valproate at a fixed dose of 20 mg/kg or placebo. The patients receiving valproate experienced a more rapid remission of symptoms and required progressively lower doses of the antipsychotic relative to patients in the placebo group. (It is not clear whether the sample was all "fresh" patients or included any non- or partial responders to antipsychotic monotherapy.) Studies of the reverse—an adjunctive antipsychotic among patients not responding adequately to lithium or anticonvulsant—are reviewed in the section on antipsychotics below.

Randomized, placebo-controlled studies have compared valproate with placebo and with lithium. In the first such study (Pope et al., 1991), 17 patients were randomized to divalproex and 19 to placebo. The divalproex-treated patients showed a median improvement in YMRS scores of 54 percent, versus only 5 percent for the placebo group ($p = .003$). Similar benefit was seen on the Global Assessment of Social Scale (GAS) and the Brief Psychiatric Rating Scale (BPRS). A significant problem with this and several other studies of mania is that the completion rate for the 3-week study was only 24 percent in the divalproex group and 21 percent in the placebo group.

In the largest placebo-controlled study of acute mania conducted to date (referred to above in our review of lithium studies), 179 patients with acute mania were treated with either divalproex, lithium, or placebo for 21 days (Bowden et al., 1994) (as in the Pope et al. [1991] study, a large number of patients failed to complete this study). About half of the patients in the divalproex- and lithium-treated groups but only one-fourth of the patients in the placebo-treated group showed marked improvement. While the authors concluded that the efficacy of divalproex appeared to be independent of prior responsiveness to lithium, in fact the drug showed only a 27 percent response rate among prior lithium responders (compared with a 60 percent response rate with lithium) while having greater effi-

cacy among prior lithium nonresponders. As noted above, in a later analysis of this study, Swann and colleagues (1999) found that a history of many previous episodes (but not rapid cycling or mixed states) predicted a poor response to lithium and placebo but not to valproate.

An earlier double-blind study comparing lithium and divalproex in the treatment of acute mania found that high pretreatment depression scores (i.e., mixed-mood symptoms) predicted a favorable response to divalproex but not to lithium, although lithium had a slightly higher efficacy rate overall, with a trend toward better efficacy in patients with classic euphoric mania (Freeman et al., 1992). Several subsequent analyses have supported the preferential use of divalproex for irritable–dysphoric, mixed, and rapid-cycling states (Bowden et al., 1994; Swann et al., 2002), while lithium has shown some advantage for patients with "classic" euphoric/grandiose mania (see Fig. 18–2), although the apparent advantage of lithium in this group is not reflected in the various North American treatment guidelines. It has been suggested that manic patients treated with valproate have shorter hospital stays and lower associated costs than patients treated with lithium. One retrospective study examining this issue reported a 40 percent reduction in length of stay for patients on divalproex monotherapy compared with those on lithium monotherapy (Frye et al., 1996); however, another, similar study found no such advantage (Dalkilic et al., 2000).

Recently, high-dose intravenous valproate (20 mg/kg over 30 minutes) was evaluated in seven acute manic patients, with no benefit noted. The authors speculated that the antimanic effect of anticonvulsants requires changes in cell signaling systems over time (Phrolov et al., 2004). The new extended-release form of divalproex, which allows once-a-day dosing was recently approved by the FDA for the acute treatment of mania after it was shown to be superior to placebo in a 3-week randomized, parallel-group, multicenter study (Bowden et al., 2006).

Oxcarbazepine

Oxcarbazepine is one of two major products of the microsomal metabolism of carbamazepine. It is nearly devoid of hematological side effects, and, compared with carbamazepine causes fewer allergic skin reactions, and appears to be much less active as a hepatic enzyme inducer (i.e., causes less autoinduction). It is, however, a significant contributor to the occasional gastrointestinal, teratogenic, endocrine, and central nervous system toxicity seen with carbamazepine. Hyponatremia is the one adverse effect that may occur more frequently with this drug than with the parent compound (see the recent review by Ketter, 2005).

Several 2-week open clinical trials conducted in Germany in the 1980s indicated that relatively high doses of oxcarbazepine had an effect equivalent to that of haloperidol (mean dose of 42 mg/day) in acutely manic patients; the oxcarbazepine was very well tolerated compared with the high-dose haloperidol regimen. Two randomized comparisons, one with valproate (Emrich et al., 1985) and one with lithium (Emrich, 1990), found that oxcarbazepine had comparable efficacy over 2 weeks, with roughly similar side-effect profiles; however, the absence of a placebo group in these studies renders their conclusions tentative. A more recent study of oxcarbazepine for treatment of mania using an on–off design had a high dropout rate that likewise makes its results difficult to interpret (Hummel et al., 2002). Nevertheless, some of these mild to moderately manic patients had a greater than 50 percent reduction in their YMRS scores, suggesting that further studies should be done to assess this agent for antimanic efficacy. A comparative study in which 23 of 42 patients with mania being treated with valproate were switched to oxcarbazepine found comparable reductions in the Clinician Administered Rating Scale for Mania (CARS-M) at 10 weeks. More of the patients who continued on valproate had a significant weight gain compared with those who switched to oxcarbazepine (Hellewell, 2002).

Given that oxcarbazepine appears to have a relatively benign side-effect profile, it has been the subject of considerable clinical interest, and some open studies have suggested its usefulness as an adjunct (Benedetti et al., 2004). To date, however, a single adequately powered placebo-controlled study of its efficacy as monotherapy in treating mania is still lacking.

Topiramate

There have been several single-case reports and open studies indicating the apparent benefits of topiramate in the treatment of mania.[18,19] McElroy and colleagues (2000) treated more than 50 bipolar patients with topiramate in addition to other medications in an open design as part of the Stanley Foundation Bipolar Network studies. In patients with manic symptoms (N=30), the mean YMRS score was 10 at the start of the study, indicating relatively mild manic symptoms. At 10 weeks, the reduction in score was statistically significant, albeit of questionable clinical salience given the long duration of antimanic treatment and the relatively mild symptoms at the outset. The patients lost an average of 2.4 pounds in 4 weeks and remained stable in weight over 10 weeks.[20] However, in a recent randomized placebo controlled trial of topiramate in bipolar patients experiencing a manic/mixed episode while on lithium or valproate, the addition of topiramate (400 mg) was no more effective than placebo (Chengappa et al., 2006).

Given its failure to separate from placebo in five large randomized controlled trials (Powers et al., 2004; Kushner

et al., 2006; Chengappa et al., 2006), one cannot recommend topiramate monotherapy for the treatment of mania in adults, and indeed none of the guidelines do so. There is, however, some evidence suggestive of a beneficial effect in adolescents (see Chapter 23), although this controlled trial was unfortunately terminated early by the manufacturer after the failure of the adult trials (DelBello et al., 2005). Yet, unlike many other anticonvulsants, topiramate does not cause weight gain and actually causes weight loss in many patients. In light of this advantageous side-effect profile, it is unfortunate that the controlled attempts to demonstrate the drug's efficacy in treating adult mania failed. We can hope that the somewhat encouraging results with adolescents will spur further work in this age group, given how problematic weight gain can be in the young bipolar patient. Moreover, the drug has also shown promise as an adjunctive agent, making randomized, double-blind adjunctive trials another potentially valuable area for future work.

Lamotrigine

Lamotrigine is an anticonvulsant with sodium channel blocking activity similar to that of carbamazepine and phenytoin. Case reports and open studies have suggested some efficacy for this drug in treating mania,[21] but this finding was not confirmed in controlled studies. A small (30 subjects) 4-week randomized controlled trial compared lamotrigine with lithium for treatment of hospitalized manic patients (Ichim et al., 2000). Patients in the lithium group received a fixed dose of 800 mg/day, achieving an average plasma level of .743 millimoles per liter (mmol/l) arguably not an adequate lithium dose for mania. The lithium and lamotrigine groups shared similarly reduced YMRS scores, but the absence of a placebo group renders the results of this underpowered study inconclusive. Other controlled studies in patients with mania/mixed states and hypomania found no significant difference between lamotrigine and placebo (Anand et al., 1999; Frye et al., 2000). An open study of patients with a history of rapid cycling found lamotrigine to be helpful in some rapid-cycling patients with mania, but not in those with the most severe manic symptoms (Bowden et al., 1999).

Gabapentin

A number of case reports and uncontrolled studies of gabapentin in patients with manic and mixed states have suggested a beneficial effect when the drug is used adjunctively.[22] On the other hand, Pande and colleagues (2000) found that gabapentin was less effective than placebo as an adjunctive agent for treating mania in patients taking lithium, valproate, or both, while Frye and colleagues (2000) found that it was no different from placebo in refractory bipolar disorder. There have also been a number of reports of mania associated with the initiation of gabapentin (Short and Cooke, 1995; Ghaemi et al., 1998).

Other Anticonvulsants

Tiagabine is a GABA uptake inhibitor used for the adjunctive treatment of partial complex seizures. One open study of patients with bipolar disorder treated with this agent indicated a possible benefit (Schaffer et al., 2002). In another open study, however, fewer than one-quarter of 13 treatment-refractory patients with bipolar disorder appeared to be helped by adjunctive tiagabine (Suppes et al., 2002). In a third study, none of 8 acutely manic patients appeared to benefit from tiagabine as either monotherapy or an adjunctive agent (Grunze et al., 1999b).

Some case reports and small open studies have indicated beneficial responses in manic patients treated with zonisamide (Kanba et al., 1994; Berigan, 2002), a drug associated with weight loss in obese bipolar patients. In an open-label trial of adjunctive zonisamide, investigators in the Stanley Network (McElroy et al., 2005) noted significant improvements in YMRS and CGI scores among 34 manic or mixed patients who had not responded to conventional treatment ($p < .001$); 14 of the 34 patients were "much" or "very much" improved after 8 weeks of treatment. In an open study, adjunctive zonisamide (300–600 mg/day) at bedtime was associated with significant weight loss in obese euthymic bipolar patients on maintenance medication (Yang et al., 2003).

Other open studies have noted antimanic and/or mood-stabilizing effects associated with levetiracetam.[23,24] A 6-week open-label, add-on study of mexiletine (an antiarrhythmic drug with anticonvulsant properties) in "treatment-resistant" bipolar patients found that four of the five patients with manic or mixed states in the study had a "full" response and the remaining patient a "partial" response as measured by a derived scale that estimated symptom burden (Schaffer and Levitt, 2005).

Surprisingly little work has been done on one of the oldest anticonvulsants—phenytoin—in the treatment of bipolar disorder. Mishory and colleagues (2000) in Israel reported on 39 patients in whom they examined the antimanic efficacy of phenytoin given with haloperidol in a double-blind, placebo-controlled study. Significantly more improvement was observed in the manic patients who received phenytoin and haloperidol than in those who received placebo and haloperidol.

Typical Antipsychotics

As reviewed extensively in the first edition of this volume, from the 1960s through the early 1990s, typical antipsychotics, particularly haloperidol, were unchallenged as the fastest-acting treatment for acute manic agitation. They were generally considered the treatment of choice for acute mania, and this practice was reasonably well supported by the literature of the time (Prien et al., 1972; Shopsin et al., 1975; Garfinkel et al., 1980). These studies found that antipsychotics and lithium were equally effective after 3 weeks, but that antipsychotics had a more rapid onset of antimanic action in highly active, acutely manic patients. While American studies were limited to the use of chlorpromazine and haloperidol, European studies often included zuclopenthixol and flupenthixol as well. As Schatzberg and Nemeroff (1998) concluded, "All of the traditional antipsychotic drugs are effective in reducing manic excitement. In comparison with lithium, valproic acid, and carbamazepine, antipsychotic drugs often have a more rapid onset of action." Today, despite the relative deemphasis on typical antipsychotics in the U.S. Expert Consensus Guidelines and other recent treatment algorithms/guidelines, these agents continue to be widely used in Europe and the United States in the treatment of hospitalized manic patients.

Haloperidol, although by no means the first choice of all clinicians for treatment of acute mania, is still frequently used for this purpose, perhaps more in Europe than in the United States. A small double-blind, prospective study compared the efficacy of three different doses of haloperidol for acute mania (10, 30, and 80 mg/day) over a 6-week period and found no advantage for doses over 10 mg/day (Riflan et al., 1994). By contrast, another double-blind study compared haloperidol at doses of 5 and 25 mg/day for 21 days and found the higher dose to be more effective. Adding lithium enhanced the antimanic effect of the lower but not the higher dose (Chou et al., 1999). Typical antipsychotic medications frequently are combined with lithium in acute treatment of mania, and these combinations have been the focus of controlled studies (Small et al., 1995; Sachs et al., 2002). To our knowledge, however, there has been only one well-designed double-blind study of manic patients not selected for prior poor response to lithium, which demonstrated the superiority of such combinations over lithium monotherapy (Garfinkel et al., 1980).[25]

In more recent studies, typical antipsychotics have been compared with atypical agents for the treatment of manic states.[26] Barbini and colleagues (1997) compared chlorpromazine (mean dose 3.10 mg/day) with clozapine (166 mg/day) and found a more rapid onset of antimanic action at 2 weeks in the clozapine-treated group. However, the two groups were comparable by 4 weeks of treatment. A comparison of haloperidol and olanzapine monotherapy for the treatment of acute mania found comparable symptomatic improvement with the two agents, but concluded that patients taking olanzapine had an enhanced return to normal functioning at 12 weeks as measured by scores on the Health-Related Quality of Life questionnaire and self-report work status (Shi et al., 2002). In a large randomized, double-blind comparison of olanzapine (n=234) with haloperidol (n= 219), Tohen and colleagues (2003b) found that the proportions remitting were comparable, which is in line with the conclusion of a recent Cochrane database systematic review (Cipriani et al., 2006). Similar results were found in large double-blind, randomized comparisons of risperidone with haloperidol (Smulevich et al., 2005) and quetiapine with haloperidol (McIntyre et al., 2005).[27]

To our knowledge, there has been only one controlled study in which an atypical showed superior efficacy to a typical. This was a large randomized, double-blind comparison of aripiprazole (15–30 mg/day) and haloperidol (10 to 15 mg/day) (Vieta et al., 2005).[28] The advantage of the atypical agents over the typicals is generally believed to depend on their greater tolerability. On the basis of median YMRS scores at entry, studies of atypicals in acute mania were comparing typical and atypical antipsychotics in moderately manic subjects. It is possible that a comparison in a naturalistic setting involving more severely manic patients would show some advantage for the typical agent. However, in a chart review of 106 consecutively admitted manic inpatients in a routine clinical setting, Letmaier and colleagues (2006) found more improvement at 2 weeks (and less EPS) in those treated with an atypical versus a typical, even though the two groups had comparable severity on admission as measured by the CGI scale.

Atypical Antipsychotics

As noted above, during the past decade the treatment of mania has been significantly altered by the introduction of atypical antipsychotics, especially in North America. The more favorable side-effect profile of these drugs, particularly the lower incidence of extrapyramidal symptoms (at least as compared with haloperidol in controlled monotherapy trials in schizophrenia), was a significant factor prompting research into their efficacy for patients with bipolar disorder. It soon became apparent, however, that these agents also have effects on mood more specific than those of the typical antipsychotics, with antimanic and possibly some antidepressant and maintenance efficacy in bipolar patients (including those with mixed states; see Suppes et al., 1992; Benabarre et al., 2001) not shared to the same extent by their predecessor compounds.

Table 18–3 summarizes key findings from the literature on the efficacy of the various atypicals. Essentially, the controlled data indicate equivalent antimanic efficacy for each of these drugs, whether studied as monotherapy (Perlis et al., 2006a) or in combination with lithium or valproate. It is important to note that the studies of atypicals as adjunctive agents all started with patients who had already failed to have a satisfactory response to lithium or an anticonvulsant. Differences in the drugs' tolerability profiles, as outlined briefly in the table, can affect the choice of treatment, but these differences become more important in maintenance treatment and are thus emphasized in Chapter 20.

Among the atypical antipsychotics, olanzapine and risperidone have been studied most extensively. Initially, case reports and open studies suggested that these two agents had antimanic effects, but some patients appeared to experience a worsening of manic symptoms. However, this reported worsening was not supported by subsequent controlled studies: a post hoc analysis of the results of two placebo-controlled trials of olanzapine in treatment of acute mania (Tohen et al., 1999, 2000) found that a worsening of mania occurred in 38 percent of placebo- and 21 percent of olanzapine-treated patients (Chengappa et al., 2003). Although these results do not eliminate the possibility that the atypical antipsychotics can cause a worsening of mania, they do not support the idea either.

Clozapine

Clozapine has been studied for treatment of mania only in open studies, presumably because of its side-effect profile (including sedation, hypotension, and hematological dyscrasias). In the earliest such study, Muller and Heipertz (1977) found that about half of 52 patients with mania responded quickly to clozapine treatment. Nearly 20 years later, investigators at the McLean Hospital reported a small case series of treatment-resistant bipolar patients who improved substantially on clozapine, especially in manic, mixed, and rapid-cycling states (Zarate et al., 1995). Calabrese and colleagues (1996) reported on an open trial of clozapine monotherapy in 10 bipolar and 15 schizoaffective patients who had failed to either tolerate or respond to lithium.[29] All but 3 of the patients completed the 13-week trial, and 18 (72 percent) showed marked improvement on the YMRS and BPRS. It was clear that the bipolar patients experienced more improvement than the schizoaffective patients, and those with rapid cycling did not respond to clozapine as well as the other patients.

An open prospective clozapine trial involving 22 psychotic manic patients who had failed other therapies found that the 14 patients who completed at least 10 weeks of the trial had a better than 50 percent improvement on the YMRS and BPRS and a 39 percent improvement on the CGI (Green et al., 2000). Barbini and colleagues (1997) found clozapine to be as effective as but more rapidly acting than chlorpromazine in a group of 27 manic patients. Suppes and colleagues (1999) compared clozapine adjunctive therapy with treatment as usual in bipolar and schizoaffective patients with a history of mania. Although their study was conducted primarily to assess outcome at 1 year, they also observed that 65 percent of the clozapine-treated patients showed at least 30 percent improvement by 3 months.[30]

TABLE 18–3. **Efficacy and Side-Effect Profiles of Various Atypical Antipsychotics for Treatment of Mania**

Agent	Efficacy Summary	Side-Effect Profiles
Clozapine	Effective as adjunctive agent in open trials among non- or partial responders to lithium or anticonvulsants. Effective as monotherapy in open studies.	Sedating; weight gain +++; dyslipidemia ++; prolactin elevation +/0; hypotension common; risk of blood dyscrasias necessitates frequent white blood count determinations
Olanzapine	Effective in adjunctive trials among non- or partial responders to lithium or anticonvulsants. Monotherapy superior to placebo and comparable to lithium and valproate in randomized, double-blind trials.	Sedating; weight gain +++; dislipidemia +++; prolactin elevation +/0; dose-related extrapyramidal syndrome (EPS) +; parenteral form rapidly effective
Risperidone	Efficacy as adjunctive agent in open and randomized, double-blind trials among non- or partial responders to lithium or anticonvulsants. Monotherapy superior to placebo in two randomized, double-blind trials; as effective as lithium or haloperidol monotherapy in randomized, double-blind trials among non- or partial responders to those drugs.	Less sedating; weight gain ++; dyslipidemia +; prolactin elevation +++; dose-related EPS ++
Quetiapine	Efficacy as adjunctive agent in open trials and one randomized, double-blind trial among non- or partial responders to lithium or anticonvulsants. Monotherapy superior to placebo in two randomized, double-blind trials.	Sedating; weight gain ++; dyslipidemia +; prolactin elevation 0; dose-related EPS +/0
Ziprasidone	Monotherapy superior to placebo in two randomized, double-blind trials	Sedating at high doses; weight gain +/0; dyslipidemia +/0; prolactin elevation +/0; dose-related EPS +; parenteral form rapidly effective
Aripiprazole	Monotherapy superior to placebo in two randomized, double-blind trials	Less sedating; weight gain +/0; dyslipidemia +/0; prolactin elevation 0; dose-related EPS +

The studies of adjunctive atypicals were conducted in patients who had failed to respond adequately to lithium or an anticonvulsant and cannot be generalized beyond that population. Number of plus signs indicates severity of side effects. For individual literature references see the text.

Olanzapine

This atypical agent has been shown to be superior to placebo in several randomized, double-blind comparisons in acutely manic patients. In the first of these studies, olanzapine at a dose of 5–20 mg/day resulted in substantially greater improvement over that seen in placebo-treated subjects in a 3-week study (Tohen et al., 1999). The olanzapine-treated patients' response rate (defined as a reduction in YMRS score) was 48 percent, compared with 24 percent for the placebo-treated group. The difference favoring olanzapine was not apparent, however, until the third week of the study. Even though twice as many patients responded to olanzapine as to placebo, it is sobering to consider that at 3 weeks, fewer than half of the patients on the atypical met response criteria, an observation that can also be made about acute mania trials with other atypical antipsychotics.

There was no significant EPS in the olanzapine-treated subjects, but several had transient elevation of liver enzymes, and the olanzapine-treated group gained an average of 3 pounds during the 3-week study. A second randomized, placebo-controlled study yielded similar results, except that the difference in efficacy between olanzapine and placebo appeared after only 1 week of treatment and was sustained throughout the remainder of the trial (Tohen et al., 2000).[31] The olanzapine-treated subjects with mixed mania experienced improvement in depressed mood that was statistically superior to that among the placebo group. It is also worth noting that in both studies, the improvement rate for the olanzapine-treated manic subjects was equivalent for those with nonpsychotic and psychotic mania; similar findings have been reported with other atypical agents.

Taken together, these findings support the conclusion that the effect of the atypicals in treating mania is truly antimanic, rather than nonspecifically antipsychotic or sedative (Baker et al., 2003b). Along the same lines, Baldessarini and colleagues (2003) found olanzapine response to be independent of number of prior episodes, rapid cycling, and lifetime substance abuse.[32] It is likely that such findings represent a class effect for the atypicals rather than being unique to olanzapine.

In addition to the comparisons of typical and atypical antipsychotics discussed above, a number of studies have compared olanzapine with other mood stabilizers. In a randomized, double-blind comparison of lithium and olanzapine monotherapy, impressive improvements were seen in manic symptoms for both agents over the 4 weeks of the study. All but one of the four scales employed[33] showed equivalent, dramatic improvement; the fourth[34] indicated greater improvement among the olanzapine-treated patients. Mean lithium level was only .74 mg/L, however, which almost certainly favored the olanzapine treatment regimen (Berk et al., 1999).

In a 3-week randomized, double-blind study comparing olanzapine (5–20 mg/day, mean dose 17.4 mg/day) with divalproex (500–2,500 mg/day, mean dose 1,401 mg/day, achieving a mean blood level of 82 mg/ml) for the treatment of acute manic or mixed episodes in 248 patients, Tohen and colleagues (2002) demonstrated a slight but significant advantage for olanzapine over divalproex as measured by the percentage of patients achieving a greater than 50 percent decrease in YMRS score, by the percentage achieving remission as defined by a YMRS score of 12 or lower, and by the mean reduction in score among the two groups. A 44-week double-blind extension of this study found that only after 15 weeks of treatment was the efficacy of valproate comparable to that of olanzapine (Tohen et al., 2003b). Zajecka and colleagues (2002), by contrast, found that olanzapine and valproate had comparable efficacy in a 12-week randomized, double-blind study involving 120 patients with acute mania. The difference between the results of these two studies appears to be explained by dose: compared with the Lilly-funded Tohen et al. study, the Abbott-funded Zajecka et al. study used a lower dose of olanzapine (mean daily doses were 14.7 mg) and a higher dose of valproate (2,115 mg/day). In both studies, patients in the olanzapine group experienced significantly more side effects, especially somnolence and weight gain, than those in the valproate group. Finally, Baker and colleagues (2004) found that, for those with mixed states not responding adequately to a mood stabilizer, adjunctive olanzapine produced significantly more improvement in scores on the Hamilton Rating Scale for Depression (HAM-D) compared with the mood stabilizer alone.[35]

Some case reports (primarily from the schizophrenia literature) have suggested that olanzapine might occasionally exacerbate mania. This question was examined systematically by Baker and colleagues (2003a), who pooled the results of two large randomized, placebo-controlled studies of manic patients. Among the 254 patients in these studies, manic exacerbations were significantly more frequent in the placebo group (38 versus 22 percent). However, patients in controlled trials are less likely to have some of the risk factors (such as substance abuse) associated with switching, and they have just experienced a spontaneous manic episode to qualify for the trial.[36]

To our knowledge, there has been only one comparative study of the IM formulation of olanzapine, in which it was compared with IM lorazepam and placebo as a sedating agent in acutely agitated manic patients in a randomized trial (Meehan et al., 2001). The investigators found that 10 mg of olanzapine was superior to 2 mg of lorazepam or placebo at 2 hours and remained superior to placebo in reducing manic agitation at 24 hours. Olanzapine had no more side effects than lorazepam during the acute period.

Risperidone

In open studies of manic patients, Tohen and colleagues (1996) found a 50 percent or greater reduction in manic symptoms in 10 of 12 patients when risperidone was added to lithium. Keck and colleagues (1995) studied a mixed group of patients treated with risperidone, noting that all 9 bipolar patients with mania showed moderate to marked improvement when the drug was added to a mood-stabilizing regimen consisting of lithium, valproate, or carbamazepine. Ghaemi and Sachs (1997) found that 9 of 14 bipolar patients, most with mania or mixed states, responded well to the addition of risperidone in small doses, averaging under 3 mg/day. In contrast to some early reports of antidepressant activity (Hillert et al., 1992) and even aggravation of manic symptoms (Dwight et al., 1994), Ghaemi and Sachs saw no evidence of worsening of mixed or manic symptoms, a finding consistent with those of the controlled studies described below.

Three large randomized, double-blind trials have demonstrated the superiority of risperidone over placebo in the treatment of mania/mixed states (Vieta et al., 2003; Hirschfeld et al., 2004; Khanna et al., 2005); these studies constitute the database for FDA registration of this drug as an antimanic agent. The largest of the three (Khanna et al., 2005) was conducted in India, where 144 hospitalized manic or mixed patients were randomized to placebo and 146 to a flexible dose of risperidone (1–6 mg/day) for 3 weeks; at end point, a clinical response (50 percent or greater decrease in YMRS scores) was observed in 73 percent of the risperidone patients versus 36 percent of the placebo patients ($p < .001$). The major side effect was EPS (primarily mild), in 35 percent of risperidone-treated patients versus

6 percent of placebo-treated patients. The authors noted that their patients' manias were, on average, substantially more severe than those of patients participating in controlled trials elsewhere.[37] This was reflected in the unusually large mean change in YMRS scores (−23.2). In the other large study, Hirschfeld and colleagues (1999) randomized 134 manic patients to risperidone (mean modal dose 4.1 mg/day) and 125 to placebo, also for 3 weeks. Again, improvement in mania (YMRS score) was significantly greater in the risperidone group, with separation from placebo evident as early as 3 days; 43 percent of those randomized to risperidone met response criteria at 3 weeks, versus 24 percent in the placebo group. Remission rates (decline in YMRS score ≤12) were 38 percent for risperidone versus 20 percent for placebo. The most common adverse event was somnolence; while EPS rating scale scores were significantly higher in the active treatment group in all three studies, these symptoms were generally mild.

A randomized, double-blind study of risperidone in combination with lithium, carbamazepine, or valproate showed a significantly more rapid decline in YMRS scores for patients taking risperidone in addition to their other medication. The mean modal dose in this study was 4 mg/day (Yatham et al., 2003). In another prospective double-blind, placebo-controlled trial of risperidone as adjunctive treatment for mania (added to lithium or valproate, to which the patients were not responding adequately), Sachs and colleagues (2002) noted more improvement in YMRS scores with risperidone than with placebo at the end of weeks 1, 2, and 3.[38] Similar findings were reported by Yatham and colleagues (2004), who randomly added risperidone (n=75) or placebo (n=75) to lithium or valproate, noting significantly more reduction in mania (YMRS scores) with the combined treatment.

What about comparisons of risperidone and other antimanic agents? In a randomized, double-blind trial of risperidone monotherapy, 45 manic patients took risperidone 6 mg/day, haloperidol 10 mg/day, or lithium 800–1,200 mg/day in a 3-week trial.[39] There were no differences in treatment outcomes among the three groups, all of which showed a mean improvement of about 50–60 percent on the YMRS, as well as substantial improvements on general psychopathology and functioning scales (Segal et al., 1998). The fact that lithium and risperidone showed similar efficacy in this monotherapy study appears at first glance to be at odds with the results of controlled studies reviewed above in which adjunctive risperidone was superior to lithium (or valproate). But each of these adjunctive studies started with patients already on a mood stabilizer *to which they had not had an adequate response*. As discussed in Chapter 17, such designs, which characterize most studies of adjunctive atypicals in treating mania, select for

poor responders to a mood stabilizer. In a recent randomized double-blind comparison, risperidone and olanzapine had equivalent antimanic efficacy; olanzapine was associated with a greater reduction in depressive symptoms but more weight gain (Perlis et al., 2006b).

Quetiapine

Several case reports (Dunayevich and Strakowski, 2000) and retrospective case series[40] suggest a useful role for the atypical antipsychotic quetiapine when used as adjunctive treatment for mania and/or mixed states.

Two large international multicenter randomized, double-blind, placebo-controlled trials evaluated the efficacy of quetiapine monotherapy (400–800 mg/day) in hospitalized manic patients. In one (Bowden et al., 2005), 302 patients were randomized to quetiapine (n=107), lithium (n=98), or placebo (n=95). At 3 weeks the decrease in YRMS scores was significantly greater ($p < .001$) for both drugs compared with placebo; the extent of the improvement was virtually identical for the two drugs. The other study (McIntyre et al., 2005) was of the same size and design, except that the active comparator was haloperidol; results were similar as well, except that at 3 weeks, the effect of haloperidol was slightly more robust than that of quetiapine. In both studies, quetiapine had a significantly greater effect than placebo on depression ratings (see Chapter 19). On the basis of these two studies, quetiapine (Seroquel) received FDA approval for treatment of "acute mania associated with bipolar disorder." Somnolence, dry mouth, and postural hypotension were the principal side effects differentiating quetiapine from placebo.

Two large randomized, placebo-controlled trials (Sachs et al., 2004; Yatham et al., 2004) examined the efficacy of adjunctive quetiapine in 402 hospitalized manic patients who were still substantially symptomatic (YMRS scores ≥ 20) after a minimum of 7 days of lithium or divalproex. In both studies, the combined treatment was significantly better than the mood stabilizer alone. As noted above regarding adjunctive olanzapine and risperidone, it is important to note that patients entered these studies after at best a partial response to a week or more on the mood stabilizers alone; thus the generalizability of the study findings is limited.

Ziprasidone

The neuropharmacology of this atypical is of interest because its effects include monoamine reuptake inhibition, which might suggest efficacy in depression. Also, ziprasidone stands with aripiprazole (see below) as one of only two atypicals producing little or no weight gain.

Keck and colleagues (2003a) conducted a multisite randomized, double-blind, placebo-controlled study involving 210 inpatients in a manic or mixed state. They assigned 140 of the patients to ziprasidone monotherapy at a dosage of 80–160 mg/day and 70 to placebo. The patients were also allowed to receive lorazepam or temazepam. Ziprasidone was found to be significantly superior to placebo at 2, 4, 7, 14, and 21 days as measured by the YMRS and from day 4 on according to the CGI scale. The main side effects were somnolence (37 percent with ziprasidone versus 13 percent with placebo) and dizziness (22 percent with ziprasidone versus 10 percent with placebo). These results were subsequently replicated in a 21-day randomized, double-blind, placebo-controlled trial (Potkin et al., 2005) involving 202 manic patients (137 on ziprasidone, 65 on placebo); again, separation from placebo was achieved at day 2. The results of the two studies taken together show approximately linear dose–response relationships. Ziprasidone was not effective for mania at the 40 mg/day dose, whereas 160 mg/day appeared to be substantially more effective than the lower doses. Combined analysis of the two trials indicates that, as with other atypicals, the antimanic efficacy of ziprasidone was similar among those with and without mixed states or psychotic features.

The combination of ziprasidone and lithium versus lithium alone was evaluated in 198 manic patients in a 21-day randomized, double-blind, placebo-controlled trial (99 patients on ziprasidone plus open lithium, 99 on placebo plus open lithium). The group with adjunctive ziprasidone had greater mean decreases in YMRS scores, but the difference achieved significance only at day 4, suggesting that the combination of lithium and ziprasidone may accelerate response (Weisler et al., 2004). Compared with lithium monotherapy, the addition of ziprasidone was associated with more extrapyramidal symptoms, somnolence, dizziness, agitation, and discontinuation due to adverse events (8 versus 4 percent).

An IM form of ziprasidone at 10 mg was found to be very rapidly acting in a group of patients described as psychotic—in fact, more so than haloperidol (at 2.5–10 mg IM) or placebo (Brook et al., 2000). The efficacy of IM ziprasidone in psychotic manic, mixed, or schizoaffective patients was evaluated in a subgroup analysis of two randomized, double-blind studies (Daniel et al., 2004). Doses of 10–20 mg/day (up to 80 mg/day) were compared with a very low "control" dose (2–8 mg/day). There was a significantly higher response rate in the high-dose group (80 percent) than in the low-dose control group (18 percent). The FDA has approved oral ziprasidone for treatment of mania.

Aripiprazole

This atypical antipsychotic (now available as orally disintegrating tablets) has a pharmacodynamic profile that distinguishes it from other antipsychotics by virtue of its being a partial agonist rather than an antagonist at dopamine D2 receptors. Keck and colleagues (2003a) conducted a 3-week double-blind, placebo-controlled study of aripiprazole for the treatment of mania in 262 hospitalized patients. They found a 40 percent response rate (defined as a decrease of 50 percent or more in YMRS scores) compared with 19 percent for placebo. These findings were subsequently replicated in a second multisite 3-week study involving 272 manic patients (135 on aripiprazole, 137 on placebo). On the basis of the results of these two large studies, the FDA has approved aripiprazole for the treatment of acute mania/mixed states.

How does this agent compare with haloperidol? Vieta and colleagues (2005) addressed this question in a large double-blind comparison in which 347 manic/mixed-state patients were randomized 1:1. The first 3 weeks of treatment was completed by 76.6 percent of the aripiprazole group but only 55.2 percent of the haloperidol group; by 12 weeks these percentages were 50.9 and 29.1, respectively. At week 12, significantly more patients in the aripiprazole group met response criteria of 50 percent or greater improvement (49.7 versus 28.4 percent). The high dropout rate in the haloperidol group was due at least in part to low tolerability, which can be attributed largely to the protocol's not allowing anticholinergic medication to deal with EPS. The authors also noted another factor limiting the generalizability of the comparison: the limited dose range allowed for haloperidol.

Amisulpiride

In a trial in schizophrenic patients, this selective, dose-dependant D2–D3 antagonist appeared to be more effective against affective symptoms than haloperidol or risperidone (Peuskens et al., 2002). This finding led to a preliminary open prospective 6-week study in 20 patients meeting DSM-IV criteria for mania (Vieta et al., 2005). Among the 14 patients who completed the study, a significant improvement was seen in mania ratings, as was a significant albeit less robust effect on depression ratings. The principal side effect was sedation; 10 percent of the subjects experienced EPS.

Zotepine

This first-generation atypical antipsychotic, which, like ziprasidone, inhibits reuptake of monoamines, has been studied in two small open-label trials. Harada and Otsuki (1986) reported beneficial effects in the majority of their 16 moderately manic patients, most of whom were already on lithium. More recently, Amann and Grunze (2005) evaluated zotepine somewhat more formally as monotherapy in a group of more severely manic patients. Nine of the 12 patients met response criteria (a 50 percent reduction YMRS scores), and 5 of them achieved this improvement within 4 days. There have as yet been no randomized, placebo-controlled trials.

Benzodiazepines

In the 1980s, the potential value of two high-potency benzodiazepines—clonazepam and lorazepam—for the treatment of mania was noted. Previously, it had been hoped that these agents might become alternatives to the antipsychotics that would not share their tendency to cause tardive dyskinesia. Results of early open studies suggested that efficacy and speed of onset were similar for high-potency benzodiazepines and antipsychotics, and that the benzodiazepines could be used as short-term antimanic agents for patients who had not taken lithium long enough for it to have an antimanic effect (Modell et al., 1985).

Edwards and colleagues (1991) compared clonazepam with placebo in 40 manic patients, with additional doses of chlorpromazine being given to patients in either group as needed. The clonazepam-treated group showed greater improvement on the YMRS and had a trend toward requiring fewer doses of chlorpromazine. In a crossover study comparing clonazepam with lithium in acutely manic patients, Chouinard and colleagues (1983) found the former to be more effective in reducing manic symptoms. However, the length of the study was only 10 days, with patients receiving either drug for only 5 days before switching to the other. Thus the study findings are probably better seen as reflecting the sedating effect of clonazepam and the known lag time in lithium's antimanic effect than a superior antimanic effect for clonazepam. Also of note, patients in both groups were able to receive haloperidol as needed, further casting doubt on any claim to antimanic efficacy for the benzodiazepine.

Lenox and colleagues (1992) compared lorazepam and haloperidol as adjuncts to lithium in a double-blind study involving 20 hospitalized patients. They found no significant difference between the two drugs in length of time to response. More patients in the haloperidol group dropped out because of side effects, and more patients in the lorazepam group dropped out because of lack of efficacy. Gouliaev and colleagues (1996) obtained similar results comparing clonazepam with the antipsychotic zuclopenthixol. A comparably designed study of clonazepam versus haloperidol found that the haloperidol-treated patients responded more quickly, probably reflecting that drug's more rapid onset of action (Chouinard et al., 1993). Bradwejn and colleagues (1990) found lorazepam to be superior to clonazepam in a double-blind study involving 24 acutely manic patients, a finding that in retrospect also probably reflects differences in pharmacodynamics between the two agents. On the other hand, a recent meta-analysis of the controlled studies concluded that while clonazepam is effective for the treatment of mania, the evidence for lorazepam is not as conclusive (Curtin and Schultz, 2004).

Early on in research on the use of benzodiazepines to treat acute mania, it became apparent that the antimanic effect of these agents is short-lived. Aronson and colleagues (1989) reported on a study of clonazepam monotherapy that was terminated after all five patients treated with the drug for mania relapsed within weeks. It gradually became clear that the apparent antimanic effects of benzodiazepines are more likely due to their acute sedating effect than to a more specific effect on manic symptoms, and that their appropriate role in the treatment of mania is as adjunctive agents for rapid sedation of agitated patients and stabilization of sleep. Finally, the possibility must be considered that some manic patients may experience further disinhibition with these agents.

Electroconvulsive Therapy

Although it is clear from clinical experience that ECT is an effective and rapidly acting treatment for mania (Fink, 2006), there have been only a handful of controlled prospective studies to support this conclusion. This is a reflection, perhaps, of four factors. First, given the efficacy and wide range of available pharmaceutical agents, few patients receive ECT for mania. Second, the effect is often so dramatic as to make controlled study appear unnecessary. Third, it is difficult to justify and maintain blinded conditions with sham ECT for such a controlled trial in acutely manic patients. Finally, unlike drug treatments, ECT requires written informed consent (Fink, 2006), which can be difficult to obtain, particularly from more severely ill patients for whom ECT may well have an advantage over medication.

Given this lack of data, it is difficult to say how ECT is best used for treating mania. The optimal electrode placement and number of treatments also remain unclear. For example, some have suggested that mania might be expected to respond more favorably to right-sided placement and depression more to left-sided placement. In one study of seven manic patients, however, right unilateral ECT was not effective (Milstein et al., 1987).

Although systematic and controlled studies are lacking, an excellent review of the published experience with lithium by Mukherjee and colleagues (1994) suggested that about 80 percent of manic patients treated with ECT showed marked improvement or full recovery. On the other hand, an analysis of manic and schizoaffective manic patients receiving ECT (Winokur et al., 1990) confirmed the earlier observation (Winokur and Kadrmas, 1989) that these patients had more subsequent hospital admissions for mania than those not receiving ECT, although the ensuing total number of episodes of mania and depression did not differ between ECT- and non-ECT-treated patients. The authors concluded that this finding probably reflects some difference in the patients selected to receive ECT rather than medication alone, although they could not rule out the possibility that ECT might have had an adverse effect on the severity of subsequent manic episodes.

Zarate and colleagues (1997) studied a series of seven bipolar patients who were given ECT while continuing on anticonvulsants (valproate or carbamazepine), including two who were receiving ECT for mania. They found that the combined use of ECT and anticonvulsants was safe and appeared to be effective. Seizure duration was slightly shorter with unilateral (but not bilateral) ECT despite the use of a more powerful electrical stimulus with unilateral ECT in patients on valproate or carbamazepine.[41] Ciapparelli and colleagues (2001) evaluated the effectiveness of ECT for patients with mixed states and reported dramatic reductions in depression scores. The effect of maintaining ECT in mania is discussed in Chapter 20.

Rapid Transcranial Magnetic Stimulation

There have been two studies of the use of rTMS for the treatment of mania. Grisaru and colleagues (1998) evaluated the efficacy of right-sided versus left-sided rTMS in 16 hospitalized patients with mania taking various medications and found that the former produced more improvement in manic symptoms than the latter (which in fact appeared to worsen manic symptoms, leading to premature termination of the study). Since left-sided rTMS treatments have been shown to be more effective for the treatment of depression in most (though not all) studies, these results suggest a lateralized control of mood in the brain, a finding supported by experiments evaluating the results of right-sided versus left-sided rTMS on mood in normal volunteer subjects (Pascual-Leone and Catala, 1996).

Michael and Erfurth (2004) administered right-sided prefrontal rTMS treatments to nine patients hospitalized with mania. Eight of the patients were on various medications, while one received rTMS as monotherapy. All nine patients had "sustained reduction of manic symptoms."

As is true for the treatment of depression with rTMS, clinical data on the use of rTMS to treat mania are scant and preliminary but encouraging. They suggest that rTMS may turn out to be a valuable addition to the therapeutic options available for the treatment of mania.

Other Treatments

Calcium Channel Blockers

The use of calcitonin, verapamil, and diltiazem for treatment of mania was proposed in the early 1980s, but few controlled data were brought forth to support this recommendation.[42] Subsequent controlled studies have shown mixed results. Two parallel studies compared verapamil with lithium. In one (Garza-Trevino et al., 1992), no difference was seen between the two agents over a 4-week period. In the other (Walton et al., 1996), lithium was found to be superior to verapamil. Janicak and colleagues (1998) found no benefit from verapamil compared with placebo in a 3-week double-blind study.

Post and colleagues (2000) studied the L-type calcium channel blocker nimodipine in patients with ultrarapid (ultradian) bipolar illness (patients who cycle several times in a 24-hour period). They noted marked improvement in some patients (Pazzaglia et al., 1998), including one whose mood again destabilized when verapamil was substituted for nimodipine.

Magnesium sulfate, used in a variety of clinical contexts, including treatment of cardiac arrhythmias, exerts at least some of its pharmacological effects through competitive antagonism with calcium at cellular calcium channels. Heiden and colleagues (1999) added intravenous magnesium sulphate to the drug regimens of 10 patients with severe, treatment-resistant manic agitation and noted a marked improvement in 7.

Levy and Janicak (2000) reviewed these and other studies of calcium channel antagonists and concluded that there is at best quite limited support for their efficacy. Because of their lack of demonstrated superiority over other agents, the calcium channel blocking agents have been relatively neglected in the clinical research literature. Thus their role in the treatment of acute mania remains to be determined.

Tamoxifen

This nonsteroidal antiestrogen is widely used in the treatment and relapse prevention of estrogen-dependent cancers, particularly of the breast. Because it is also a potent inhibitor of phosphokinase C, which is thought to be involved in the mechanism of action of mood stabilizers (see Chapter 14), it has been used experimentally for treating mania and found to be effective in a small series of patients (Manji and Chen, 2002).

Omega-3 Fatty Acids

Although there has been interest in these compounds for the treatment of bipolar disorder, reports and trials have been limited to bipolar depression and possible uses in prophylaxis (see Chapters 19 and 20). There has been at least one report of possible induction of hypomania in a patient using over-the-counter fish oil preparations (Kinrys, 2000). What if any benefit these substances may have for manic patients is as yet unknown.

Cholinergic Agents

Reports on the use of cholinergic agents, such as pilocarpine, for the treatment of mood states appeared as early as the late nineteenth century. Severe side effects limited the use of these older agents, but new agents developed for the treatment of Alzheimer's disease have a much more favorable side-effect profile. Burt and colleagues (1999) reported on a small open case study of the use of the cholinesterase inhibitor donepezil in patients with treatment-resistant bipolar disorder. Of the 11 patients in the study, 10 were in a manic, hypomanic, or mixed state. Of these, 6 were very much improved by the end of 2 weeks. However, in a subsequent double-blind, placebo-controlled trial of adjunctive donepezil in 11 manic patients, Eden Evins and colleagues (2006) were unable to demonstrate efficacy. Cases of mania evidently precipitated by donepezil have been reported as well (Benazzi, 1998).

CONCLUSIONS

The discovery of the antimanic effects of lithium launched the psychopharmacology revolution in psychiatry, and today lithium remains one of the most documented choices for the treatment of euphoric nonpsychotic mania or hypomania. Beyond lithium, however, our armamentarium has been considerably enriched by anticonvulsants and atypical antipsychotics. In comparison with the treatment of bipolar depression or maintenance treatment, the clinician enjoys the choice of a wide range of drugs that have been shown to be effective in treating acute mania and/or mixed states. Indeed, in the United States alone there are nine FDA-approved agents for mania. Recall, however, that in the placebo-controlled literature, "response" means an improvement of 50 percent or better, and that even with this modest definition of improvement, the response rates from monotherapy studies average around 50 percent. Thus most manic patients will ultimately require a combination of medications, although when possible, it is generally advisable to evaluate monotherapies first. Given that a drug or drug combination initiated for mania or hypomania will likely be carried forward into the continuation phase of treatment (not to be confused with true maintenance or prophylactic treatment; see Chapter 17), both efficacy and tolerability must be considered from the outset. For the acute management of more severely ill patients, the older typical antipsychotics still have a role, while for the patient with moderate to moderately severe symptoms, the atypical antipsychotics represent an important addition to the armamentarium.

The manic patient presents multiple clinical challenges beyond the issue of choice of medication, such as dealing with law enforcement and deciding when to hospitalize involuntarily, how best to involve the family, and how to enhance adherence to the treatment regimen. For those patients whose manic episodes are heralded by a hypomanic period (the "hypomanic alert"), the clinician may have an opportunity to prevent escalation through the aggressive use of drugs to restore normal sleep. An ongoing relationship with the family is the best way for the clinician to be assured of being alerted in time.

NOTES

1. Delirious mania—a syndrome of the acute onset of the insomnia, excitement, grandiosity, emotional lability, and psychotic symptoms characteristic of mania, accompanied by the disorientation and altered consciousness characteristic of delirium—is fortunately now rare. See Chapter 2 and Fink (1999) for a review.
2. IM droperidol had also been widely used for emergency sedation until concerns about cardiac arrhythmia and reports of sudden death led to its virtual elimination from the armamentarium in the late 1990s. More detailed analyses have cast some doubt on the wisdom of abandoning this highly effective agent so quickly (Chase and Biros, 2002).
3. To our knowledge there have been no studies comparing ECT with atypical antipsychotics in the treatment of mania.
4. For example, a Finnish study of bipolar patients who committed suicide found that about 1 in 10 were in or had recently recovered from a period of psychotic mania at the time of their death (Isometsa et al., 1994).
5. However, in a randomized study, Rifkin and colleagues (1994) compared three doses of haloperidol for mania (10, 30, and 80 mg/day) and found no difference among the three doses. They concluded that more than 10 mg/day offers no additional advantage in treating mania.
6. Adapted from the first edition of this text: Comparisons of lithium and neuroleptics have been limited largely to chlorpromazine. The largest such study, the Veterans Affairs (VA)–National Institute of Mental Health (NIMH) study (Prien et al., 1972), warrants extensive discussion because of its size—255 newly admitted manic and schizoaffective patients in 18 VA hospitals—and its unusual findings. Patients were differentiated not only by diagnosis but also by activity level: "highly active" or "mildly active." Among the highly active patients who completed the 3-week treatment trials, both the lithium-treated and the chlorpromazine-treated groups improved significantly on a wide range of symptoms. However, 38 percent of the lithium-treated patients dropped out, compared with only 8 percent of those treated with chlorpromazine, in part reflecting more side effects attributable to lithium in this group since the dose was pushed in an effort to control the hyperactivity. Both drugs produced significant improvement in the mildly active patients who completed the study, but in this group severe side effects were more frequent among the chlorpromazine-treated patients. The investigators concluded that chlorpromazine was superior to lithium in the initial treatment of the highly active patients. The neuroleptic not only reduced motor activity, excitement, grandiosity, hostility, and psychotic disorganization, but also sharply decreased the patients' need for ward supervision in the first week. By the end of 3 weeks, however, the two drugs were equivalent. Among the mildly active patients, there were fewer dropouts related to lithium than to chlorpromazine, primarily because lithium did not make them feel as "sluggish and

fatigued." Neither discharge rates nor overall improvement rates were reported in this study. In other studies, however, discharge rates and clinical evaluations have favored lithium over neuroleptics, thus underscoring the ultimate advantage of lithium. The dropout rate in the VA-NIMH study may reflect limitations in clinical management more than inherent limitations of the drugs in question.

Diagnosis is also a critical issue. Prien and colleagues did not specify how the differential diagnosis was made between the manic phase of manic-depressive illness and schizoaffective psychosis. Other investigators might have diagnosed their highly active patients as schizoaffective or "atypical." Although some studies have suggested that such patients do not respond as well to lithium as the more typical manic-depressive patients do (reviewed by Goodwin and Ebert, 1973), other investigators have failed to find any difference in lithium response between the groups (reviewed by Goodnick and Meltzer, 1984). This discrepancy is probably more apparent than real. Goodnick and Meltzer (1984) have shown that, compared with manic patients, schizoaffective manic patients require more than twice as long to achieve a full antimanic response to lithium alone (9 weeks versus the 4 weeks for manic patients). Many of the reports of relatively poor lithium response rates among schizoaffective manic patients involve trials of 4 weeks or less. Again, from a practical point of view, this means that schizoaffective manic patients are likely to require other medications in addition to lithium for the acute treatment of mania. Finally, it is important to recall that even though the antipsychotics had been the established treatment for acute mania, and lithium's introduction was clouded (particularly in the United States) by reports of deaths associated with its initial use as a salt substitute, lithium nevertheless became the preferred treatment for most acutely manic patients.

7. As an example of such limit setting, consider the following: "I am doing my best to appreciate your reasoning and wishes. I understand that you disagree with me, but I have decided that for now this is what must happen. We must give you x mg of olanzapine now and three times a day over the next 3 days to get to a therapeutic range."

8. Schou et al., 1954; Maggs, 1963; Goodwin et al., 1969; Stokes et al., 1971.

9. A delay of 7–10 days in the onset of lithium action includes the 5–6 days it usually takes to establish a steady-state level.

10. Post et al., 1986a; Small et al., 1991; Bowden et al., 1994, 2006; Weisler et al., 2004, 2005.

11. Ichim et al., 2000, Lessig et al., 2001; Jochum et al., 2002; Margolese et al., 2003.

12. Ballenger and Post, 1980; Okuma et al., 1981; Desai et al., 1987; Lerer et al., 1987.

13. As noted in the first edition, in a number of these early studies the carbamazepine-treated patients were also on lithium.

14. The average carbamazepine level was 7.3 μg/ml, while the average lithium level was .46 mEq/l. In this study, both medications were used at doses that resulted in relatively low serum levels, and they had approximately the same efficacy.

15. The mean YMRS scores at the end of the 8-week study period (17/60) were the same in both groups but were nevertheless fairly high. The authors noted that although the two agents were equally effective, neither was sufficiently effective to be recommended as monotherapy for treatment of severe manic

states. They suggested that combination treatment would be needed for most acutely manic patients. At the same time, they noted that most of the patients in their study had a prior history of failing a lithium trial.

16. The registration trials for extended-release carbamazepine were undertaken after encouraging results were obtained in a 6-month open-label evaluation by Ketter and colleagues (2004).

17. In this study, 63 percent of the subjects also remained on lithium therapy throughout the study period.

18. Marcotte, 1998; Normann et al., 1999; Calabrese et al., 2001; Letmaier et al., 2001; Pecuch and Erfurth, 2001; Bozikas et al., 2002.

19. An open study of 14 patients with mania (9 of whom took topiramate as monotherapy) found the drug to be helpful in 62 percent of the subjects (Bozikas et al., 2002). Calabrese and colleagues (2001) treated 10 manic patients with topiramate as monotherapy in an open trial over a period of up to 4 weeks. The subjects' mean YMRS score dropped from 32 to 22; however, only 3 of 10 patients had a decline in score of 50 percent or more, while 5 had a decline of less than 20 percent. Marcotte (1998) reviewed the charts of 44 patients treated for bipolar-I manic or mixed or bipolar-II disorder with an average of 200 mg/day of topiramate in addition to "existing therapy" for an average of 16 weeks. Moderate to marked improvement was experienced by 23 (52 percent) of the patients, while 5 patients (11 percent) were rated as worse; 1 patient became delirious. No weight gain (or loss) was reported in the group.

20. Chengappa and colleagues (1999) used topiramate in another open-label study of 12 manic, 1 hypomanic, 5 mixed, and 6 rapid-cycling patients also taking other medications. The mean YMRS score declined from 30 to 18 in 3 weeks and to 12 by 5 weeks. In this study, patients lost an average of 6 pounds at 3 weeks and 9 pounds at 5 weeks. Grunze and colleagues (2001) gave topiramate to 11 acutely manic patients who were taking other medications, including lithium, valproate, carbamazepine, haloperidol, and lorazepam. After 10 days of receiving topiramate, 7 of the patients had positive responses that deteriorated when the drug was discontinued. When the topiramate was reinstituted, 8 of the 9 patients who completed the study experienced a 50 percent or greater decrease in their YMRS score.

21. In an open study, lamotrigine was given either as monotherapy or in addition to other agents to patients experiencing acute mood episodes of bipolar disorder (Calabrese et al., 1999). Of the 31 patients with manic, hypomanic, or mixed states, 33 percent were "very much improved" on the CGI scale at the end of 48 weeks. Of the total group of 75 patients, 8 experienced a worsening of or the onset of manic symptoms that required hospitalization. A study of lamotrigine as a prophylactic agent in rapid-cycling bipolar disorder (Calabrese et al., 2000) had a preliminary open phase that included 66 patients with mania or hypomania. After being treated with lamotrigine for 6 weeks, about half of these patients had experienced sufficient remission of their symptoms to enter the next phase of the study.

22. Bennett et al., 1997; McElroy et al., 1997; Stanton et al., 1997; Erfurth et al., 1998; Altshuler et al., 1999; Cabras et al., 1999; Hatzimanolis et al., 1999; Perugi et al., 1999; Sokolski et al., 1999; Ghaemi and Goodwin, 2001.

23. Goldberg and Burdick, 2002; Braunig and Kruger, 2003; Grunze et al., 2003; Bersani, 2004.

24. In Grunze and colleagues' (2003) open-label study, the efficacy of levetiracetam added to haloperidol was examined in 10 acutely manic patients in an on–off–on study design. There was an improvement in mean YMRS scores during the first on phase of the study, a worsening during the off phase, and then another improvement during the second on phase.

25. The single comparison study of zuclopenthixol for treatment of acute mania was limited by its design. The study compared the combination of zuclopenthixol and clonazepam with that of lithium and clonazepam in 28 hospitalized patients with acute mania. The two combinations were found to be of similar efficacy (Gouliaev et al., 1996).

26. Miller and colleagues performed a retrospective chart review of 204 patients with acute mania admitted to a university hospital over a 30-month period, comparing typical and atypical antipsychotic medications as add-ons to mood-stabilizing medications. In this naturalistic study, patients taking atypical antipsychotic medications showed greater clinical improvement and fewer side effects than those treated with typical antipsychotic medications, but the clinicians may have tended to use the typical agents in the sicker patients (Miller et al., 2001).

27. Sachs and colleagues (2002) reported on a comparative trial of risperidone (mean dose 4 mg/day) or haloperidol (mean dose 6 mg/day) versus placebo as adjunctive treatment for patients taking either lithium or valproate for acute mania. Similar degrees of improvement on the YMRS were seen with both. In a nonrandomized observational study, Gonzalez-Pinto and colleagues (2001) evaluated the relative efficacy of adjunctive olanzapine versus an adjunctive typical antipsychotic in the treatment of 45 hospitalized patients with mixed states already on a mood stabilizer; those treated with olanzapine showed significantly more improvement in depressive symptoms compared with those taking the typical antipsychotics. In the one randomized comparison of olanzapine and haloperidol as monotherapy in treating mania, Tohen and colleagues (2003b) evaluated 453 patients and found that approximately 50 percent in each group met remission criteria (low scores on both mania and depression scales) after 6 weeks of treatment. During an additional 6 weeks of followup, relapses into depression occurred more rapidly with haloperidol than with olanzapine, and in a secondary analysis, those without psychotic features ("pure" mania) did better on olanzapine than haloperidol. As might be expected, olanzapine was associated with more weight gain, while haloperidol produced more EPS.

28. The absence of a placebo group in this aripiprazole–haloperidol comparison limits interpretation of the results.

29. Most patients had also had poor responses to carbamazepine or valproate. All 25 subjects had experienced at least one episode of mania in the 24 months prior to the trial. The mean number of hospitalizations was 15.

30. A chart review study of bipolar-I patients treated with adjunctive clozapine, risperidone, and olanzapine found no difference in efficacy among the groups (Guille et al., 2000). Olanzapine caused the greatest weight gain, although olanzapine plus lithium was associated with less weight gain than olanzapine plus valproate.

31. However, there was an even higher placebo response rate in this series—43 percent, compared with the 25 percent rate in the earlier study.

32. A secondary analysis of the first placebo-controlled trial (Tohen et al., 1999) by Baker and colleagues (2002) indicated that the efficacy of olanzapine in acute mania was independent of whether the patient had previously failed to respond to lithium or valproate.

33. Brief Psychiatric Rating Scale, Clinical Global Impression for Bipolar Disorder scale identifying manic, hypomanic, depressive, or mixed symptoms.

34. Simpson-Angus Scale.

35. Generalizability is quite limited for studies in which the new agent is added to ongoing treatment to which the patient is not yet responding since this is, in effect, selecting for non- or partial response to the original agent, in this case lithium or valproate.

36. The Baker et al. (2002) data could also be interpreted as suggesting that olanzapine was superior to placebo in preventing early relapses into mania after acute treatment of the episode.

37. This difference may relate to the fact that in India, families can give consent for participation in treatment research when the validity of a patient's consent is compromised by the illness.

38. In this study, there was also a haloperidol-treated group. It is interesting that three placebo- and three haloperidol-treated subjects on lithium or valproate became manic, but none of the risperidone-treated patients did.

39. In Segal and colleagues' (1998) study, mean serum lithium levels were .53, .62, and .72 mmol/l at the end of weeks 1, 2, and 3, respectively.

40. Ghaemi and Katzow, 1999; Zarate et al., 2000; Chisholm et al., 2001; Sajatovic et al., 2001.

41. Coexisting lamotrigine does not appear to require any increase in the electrical stimulus.

42. Giannini et al., 1984; Dose et al., 1986; Dubovsky et al., 1986; Barton and Gitlin, 1987.

Medical Treatment of Depression

Monsieur le Docteur, since you are quite aware of what in me is capable of being attacked (and healed by drugs). . . . I hope you have the know–how to give me the quantity of subtle liquids, of specious agents, of mental morphine which will uplift my abasement, balance what is crumbling, reunite what is separated, recompose what is destroyed.

—*Antonin Artaud (1924, pp. 27–28)*

The treatment options for recurrent depression, especially bipolar depression, have finally begun to expand over the last few years. In the first edition of this volume, a treatment algorithm for bipolar depression listed only four interventions, or classes of interventions, by name: lithium, the tricyclic and monoamine oxidase inhibitor (MAOI) antidepressants, and electroconvulsive therapy (ECT) (although fluoxetine and bupropion were discussed in the text). Since then, entirely new classes of medications have been introduced and shown to benefit patients with bipolar depression.[1]

Medical treatments for bipolar depression are also being explored. Entirely new classes of medications have been introduced and shown to benefit patients with bipolar depression. An expanded clinical literature now informs the use of thyroid hormones for depression, and research continues into the relevance of adrenal agents. The use of sleep deprivation and phototherapy to augment pharmaceutical treatments has proven beneficial. New techniques for electrical stimulation of the central nervous system are being studied, while nonprescription pharmaceuticals, such as St. John's wort, and dietary supplements, including those containing omega-3 fatty acids, have been the subject of intense interest in the lay press. Finally, our continued, strong belief in the importance of psychotherapeutic treatments is reflected in their being the subject of a separate chapter.

Despite the newly available medical interventions, however, the successful treatment of bipolar depression remains a challenge for the clinician. Many options for the treatment of mania (discussed in the previous chapter) have been established by randomized, placebo-controlled trials, as reflected in the large number of antimanic agents approved by the U.S. Food and Drug Administration (FDA). Research on the treatment of bipolar depression has been minimal in comparison with that on mania, or especially that on unipolar depression. Reflecting this paucity of data, as of this writing only two agents are FDA approved for treatment of bipolar depression—the atypical antipsychotic quetiapine and the combination of olanzapine and fluoxetine. Even long-term maintenance treatment (see Chapter 20) has been the subject of more controlled studies than have been conducted for the acute treatment of bipolar depression. Moreover, although the few available controlled studies are weighted toward bipolar-I patients, some do include bipolar-II patients, but usually without separately analyzing the results for these two very different groups. Thus the treatment of bipolar-II depression remains woefully understudied, despite the disorder's being at least as common as bipolar-I disorder.

Patients with bipolar depression often respond more slowly[2] and less completely to pharmacotherapeutic interventions than patients who have manic or mixed symptoms, and some clinical studies suggest that they are substantially less likely to experience full remission of their symptoms (Hlastala et al., 1997; Calabrese, 2005). A 2001 survey of patients being treated for bipolar-II disorder, for example, found that despite treatment, nearly half had suffered residual depressive symptoms of at least 2 years' duration (Benazzi, 2001), findings very similar to the recent analysis of the Systematic Treatment Enhancement Program for Bipolar Disorder (STEP-BD) data (Perlis et al., 2006). Likewise, in the follow-up phase of the National Institute of Mental Health (NIMH) Collaborative Program on the Psychobiology of Depression-Clinical Studies (Judd et al., 2003), 67 percent of those receiving routine treatment available in the community continued to have substantial depressive morbidity.

This chapter begins with a discussion of the clinical management of depressed patients, addressing the evaluation and treatment planning process and providing an overview of proven and widely accepted treatment approaches. We review the literature supporting these approaches, and then survey less proven but nevertheless promising interventions that may become more commonplace in the future. All of the drugs mentioned in the first section of the chapter are discussed in detail in the second.

Before proceeding, a note on the scope of the discussion is in order. As mentioned in Chapter 1, our discussion of depression encompasses both bipolar and highly recurrent unipolar major depression; however, given the paucity of studies of acute treatment of recurrent depression per se, our emphasis is primarily on bipolar depression. Moreover, as discussed in Chapter 17, we conceptualize treatment of manic-depressive illness in three stages—acute, continuation, and long-term maintenance. This chapter, like the preceding one, focuses on acute treatment; Chapter 20 focuses on maintenance treatment. The continuation stage is not so easily apportioned to a single chapter. Relapses into a major depressive syndrome from a state of euthymia, postmanic depressions, and breakthrough minor depressive symptoms are categories whose boundaries in real-life treatment situations can be unclear. Therefore, while the management of severe major depressive episodes, which can represent a medical emergency, is an important focus of this chapter, approaches to breakthrough or residual symptoms, particularly the former, are also addressed here, as well as in Chapter 20.

CLINICAL MANAGEMENT

This section addresses the key aspects of the clinical management of depression. Discussed in turn are the evaluation of the depressed patient, hospitalization, general considerations involved in medical treatment, and selection of a treatment approach. Our recommendations for the selection of appropriate treatments for particular patients are presented later in the chapter. Detailed discussion of special considerations in treating bipolar children and adolescents is presented in Chapter 23, and issues involving side effects of psychiatric medications and their use in pregnancy are addressed in Chapter 20.

Evaluation of the Depressed Patient

Diagnosing bipolar depression can be difficult, and the importance of taking a comprehensive history and performing a careful mental status examination as the foundation for treatment of the depressed patient cannot be overemphasized. Often the evaluating psychiatrist is not the first mental health professional, the first physician, or even the first psychiatrist to see the patient. Patients may previously have been told, erroneously, that they suffer from another psychiatric disorder, such as unipolar depression or, less commonly, schizoaffective disorder, schizophrenia, or a personality or substance abuse disorder. The clinician should neither accept such prior diagnoses at face value nor dismiss them out of hand, but rather use them as a starting point for fuller consideration of the clinical picture, as well as a means of engaging the patient and family in a discussion of history and symptoms.

The patient should be told that the inclusion of family members or a close friend in at least part of the diagnostic interview is routine and expected. Doing so is especially important in diagnosing a depressive syndrome potentially associated with bipolar disorder. As discussed in Chapters 3 and 21, patients often lack insight into the problems associated with hypomanic or even manic episodes, and therefore may not report the salient details, even with careful questioning; the more objective perspective of an outside observer is generally necessary. In conducting the diagnostic interview, the clinician should be sure to address the following matters:

- **Course-of-illness** questions should inquire into mood cycling—over the course of a day (diurnal mood variations), month (premenstrual exacerbations), and year (seasonal affective disorder [SAD]). Mood symptoms in the postpartum (puerperal) period or exacerbation of affective symptoms following antidepressant treatment should also be addressed specifically. The use of a life chart (as described in Chapter 11) is highly recommended for recording these important course variables.
- It is imperative to take a comprehensive survey of the patient's **use of alcohol and other intoxicating substances** (see Chapter 7); the clinician should ask specifically about a family history of alcoholism or drug abuse. Substance abuse is often viewed by patients as not being a "psychiatric" problem. Surreptitious substance abuse is frequently an illness-sustaining factor responsible for refractory depressive symptoms, antidepressant-related switches, and/or cycling, medication nonadherence, and an apparent lack of response to adequate treatment. Therefore, questioning family members and previous providers about substance use and abuse may be the only way to obtain this history accurately. Practitioners should have a low threshold for obtaining urine toxicology screens and hepatic transaminase determinations if there is any suspicion in this regard.
- Patients, when asked about their **treatment history**, may present an extensive list of medications that they report have been ineffective for them in the past. Frequently such lack of benefit can be attributed to inadequate medication trials. Thus it is essential to request details on adherence, the dosing and duration of these past medication

trials, and results of blood-level determinations for appropriate agents; records from past providers should be obtained whenever possible. Reports of side effects should be treated with empathy but some skepticism and elucidated in as much detail as possible. Patients may experience a variety of minor somatic symptoms more accurately attributable to depression than to a medication, or more closely related to a total side-effect burden associated with multiple medications than to a single agent. The clinician should also ask about a history of a decreased need for sleep, abnormal increases in energy, euphoria and/or irritability, suicidal thinking or behavior, or other signs of psychomotor activation in response to treatments for depression, as these symptoms may indicate an underlying bipolar diathesis.

- In taking the **family psychiatric history**, the clinician should focus not only on the diagnosis of family members but also on their response to particular treatments. Although the field of pharmacogenetics is still in its infancy, it is possible that, given the clear genetic mechanisms at work in the etiology of mood disorders, a patient will have a favorable response to an agent that successfully treated a similarly ill family member. Clinical experience suggests that this is not uncommonly the case.

Hospitalization

The first treatment decision the clinician must make is whether a depressed patient can safely be treated on an outpatient basis. More than two-thirds of completed suicides by persons with bipolar disorder occur during a major depressive episode (Isometsa et al., 1994) (see Chapter 8). The patient expressing fear of acting on suicidal urges clearly needs to be considered for hospitalization, but the decision is often less than clear-cut, depending, for example, on whether there is a previous history of serious suicide attempts, whether the patient expresses hopelessness, whether the patient has a history of impulsiveness and/or violence, and whether the patient has access to lethal means and/or lives alone. Comorbid substance abuse substantially increases the suicide risk; thus the threshold for hospitalizing the depressed patient who is actively abusing drugs or alcohol should be lower than that for a patient who is not.

The patient with severe psychomotor retardation should usually be hospitalized. Even if the close support of family members is available to these patients, their nutritional status and ability to comply with treatment recommendations are poor, and their illness can decompensate quickly into an acutely life-threatening condition. The risk of suicide may actually rise as these patients begin to emerge from their depression. Under some circumstances, a patient may need to be placed under one-to-one observation, or suicide watch (see Chapter 8). Energy level and volition often increase well before mood state improves; thus patients who literally have been too depressed to harm themselves may quite suddenly become much more likely to kill themselves.

Hospitalization offers many opportunities for monitoring of both symptoms and medication adherence that are not available in the course of outpatient treatment. Diurnal variations in mood, brief hypomanic periods, mixed affective symptoms, and symptoms of withdrawal from surreptitiously abused drugs are just some of the complicating factors that may become apparent only during hospitalization. Side effects can be identified and managed more quickly, and hospitalized patients can be educated and supported in tolerating the temporary discomforts often experienced with new medications. The clinician should also consider hospitalizing a depressed patient for ECT early in the process of planning treatment, not as a last resort. We discuss factors favoring ECT as a first-line treatment in a later section.

Day-hospital programs and hospital-based intensive outpatient programs can sometimes achieve the goals of inpatient treatment. Such programs are much less disruptive to the patient's personal and family life than hospitalization, while also incurring substantially lower financial costs.

Medical Treatment: General Considerations

Patients presenting to the psychiatrist with symptoms of bipolar depression vary tremendously in the severity of their symptoms, the complexity of their course of illness, and their previous treatment history. Nevertheless, some general considerations will serve the clinician well in almost all instances:

- **Adequacy of medication trials.** The benefits of pharmaceutical interventions for depression may take several weeks to become apparent, and patients may continue to improve for months after starting on a new medication. Once the presumed therapeutic dose range has been reached, futher dosage increases should generally occur at intervals of not less than 2 weeks. Improvement in response to medications does not always follow a smooth pattern, so it is important for patients to be ready to experience a "sawtooth"-like pattern (see Figure 22-1 in Chapter 22).[3] Symptoms should not be declared refractory to a particular agent unless the patient has taken it at the maximum recommended dosage or, if serum determinations are available, at the top of the therapeutic range, for at least 4 weeks.
- **Mood cycles and fluctuations.** Some mood fluctuations in patients being treated for bipolar disorder reflect cyclic or phasic changes associated with the illness that will normalize with time and do not necessarily require pharmaceutical intervention. Many patients will, for example,

have brief depressive periods following periods of mania or hypomania. Being too quick to intervene during these periods can result in prescribing unnecessary and sometimes ultimately destabilizing antidepressants or other agents. Watchful waiting, along with psychotherapeutic and psychoeducational support, is often the better approach. Nonpharmaceutical adjunctive treatments, such as phototherapy, sleep deprivation, and exercise, can be helpful as well.

· **Breakthrough depressions in patients on maintenance mood stabilizers.** This is the most common situation in which the clinician encounters bipolar depression. The first consideration should be optimization of the mood stabilizer regimen. As reviewed in the first edition of this volume (and now incorporated into several of the treatment guidelines for bipolar depression), a temporary increase in the patient's lithium level (to above .8 milliequivalents per liter [mEq/l]) can often abort a breakthrough episode, and there is reason to think that such a strategy may be effective with other mood stabilizers as well. While we emphasize watchful waiting above, in some situations attention to prodromal or subsyndromal symptoms may allow an intervention that can prevent an episode from progressing at a time when it may be more rapidly responsive to intervention. In our experience, cognitive symptoms, such as diminished concentration and indecisiveness, are the most frequent prodromes; this observation is consistent with that of Keitner and colleagues (1996). Subtle mood and psychomotor changes are also common (see the reviews of Jackson et al., 2003, and Marangell, 2004).

· **Assessment of progress.** Recovery from bipolar depression can be slow and characterized by starts and stops. Therefore, frequent assessment (weekly during the initial stages of treatment and at least every 2 weeks as long as there are significant residual symptoms) is essential. Family members should be encouraged to attend follow-up appointments to report their impressions. Patients can also be encouraged to keep a journal or mood chart[4] and bring the results to appointments. In addition, the clinician should consider using an objective rating scale to record assessments of improvement. The Montgomery-Asberg Depression Rating Scale (MADRS) (Montgomery and Asberg, 1979) is more sensitive to symptom change in bipolar depression than the more frequently used Hamilton Rating Scale for Depression (HAM-D) because it focuses more on core depressive symptoms than on anxiety, insomnia, and somatic symptoms (Montgomery and Asberg, 2001). A self-administered version of the MADRS is also available. (See also Chapter 11.)

· **Rational combined pharmacotherapy and irrational polypharmacy.** Although rational combined pharma-

cotherapy (the use of several pharmaceutical agents to treat a single condition) is often necessary in treating bipolar depression, the risk of irrational or haphazard combinations (polypharmacy) looms large. Patients, family members, and, increasingly, reviewers for insurance companies insist that "something" be done to provide quicker symptom relief or discharge from the hospital, and multiple medications are added in the mistaken belief that more aggressive treatment will achieve this end. Several adjunctive medications for insomnia, anxiety, or agitation may be initiated during a period of exacerbated symptoms, and can result in such problems as oversedation and fatigue that can mimic depressive symptoms. These problems, in turn, can result in the use of even more medications. The preferable strategy is to recognize that improvement from medications used to treat depression requires time.

· **Switches and cycle acceleration associated with antidepressants.** Perhaps the most important issue regarding the risk/benefit assessment associated with combining agents is the addition of an antidepressant to a mood stabilizer; because of its importance, this issue is discussed extensively in the present chapter. In addition to the possibility of acute manic switches associated with antidepressants, we have chosen to include coverage here of the potential for long-term induction of cycles (destabilization) by these agents because it is a key consideration in planning the acute treatment of depression, especially with bipolar patients.

· **Comorbidities.** Attention to complicating comorbid conditions that may be illness-sustaining is vital (see Chapters 7 and 24). Substance abuse, anxiety and eating disorders, and thyroid dysfunction are perhaps the most important and commonly overlooked of these conditions, but alertness to any coexisting systemic, neurological, or endocrinologic illness in a patient and close collaboration with all treating practitioners are essential.

· **Highly recurrent unipolar depression.** As discussed in Chapter 1, a substantial subset of unipolar patients share certain important features with bipolar patients: a high frequency of recurrence (cycle lengths averaging 2 years or less), a family history of mania, and an early age at onset (teens and twenties). Indeed, recurrent unipolar depression was part of Kraepelin's original construct of manic-depressive illness. While there is a paucity of treatment studies focused on this group, it is probably wise to keep in mind the principles outlined here for the management of bipolar depression, particularly the cautions about sustained antidepressant monotherapy and the importance of considering the use of mood stabilizers, especially those with robust effects against depression.

Selection of a Treatment Approach

As outlined in Chapter 17, there are many published guidelines, algorithms, and consensus statements on the treatment of bipolar depression. Though the details vary, most recommend using mood stabilizers—lithium and/or the activating anticonvulsant lamotrigine—as the foundation for treatment, and adding other agents as needed to enhance an incomplete antidepressant effect or provide symptomatic treatment for insomnia, anxiety, or agitation. For many treatment decision points, however, research data are insufficient to provide confidence in recommending one approach over another. The specific pharmacological approach for an individual patient must be based on an assessment of family history, past and present symptoms, course of illness, past treatment responses, appearance and tolerance of side effects, and adherence issues.[5] As noted above, the focus of the great majority of the literature has been on bipolar-I depression; treatment of bipolar-II depression has, unfortunately, been very inadequately studied. What information is available is addressed later in our review of the literature. Our recommendations for the treatment of bipolar-I and -II depression are presented in Figures 19–1a and 19–1b, respectively.

Lithium

Given data demonstrating the apparent ability of long-term treatment with lithium to protect patients with bipolar disorder against suicidal behavior (see Chapter 25), one can argue that lithium should be included in the regimen for many if not most bipolar patients. Lithium remains a strong choice for monotherapy for bipolar-I depression in patients presenting with no previous treatment history. Indeed, the practice guidelines of the American Psychiatric Association (APA) (2002) for the treatment of patients with bipolar disorder recommend lithium as an initial treatment for bipolar depression of mild to moderate severity. The most recent guidelines—the Texas Algorithm (Suppes et al., 2005)—recommends as a first step for bipolar depressed patients already taking lithium that the lithium level be increased to above 0.8 mEq/l.

A typical clinical scenario is the patient presenting with depressive symptoms who, on closer questioning of both patient and family member(s), is found to have experienced previous episodes of clear hypomania (or even mania) that did not come to clinical attention or were not properly diagnosed and treated. Patients with such a history will often resist the idea of having bipolar disorder rather than just "depression" and may recoil at the mention of lithium, a medication they may associate with severe mental illness. Thus, before some patients will agree to take lithium, they must be educated about its well-demonstrated, albeit often

modest, antidepressant effects and its prophylactic efficacy in treating recurrent mood disorders. It can also be helpful to point out that the side-effect profile described in reference publications, such as the *Physicians' Desk Reference*, is based on studies that are now more than three decades old in which substantially higher doses of lithium were used.

Another common clinical situation is the patient already taking an antidepressant prescribed by another physician who comes to the psychiatrist with refractory or residual depressive symptoms, and from whom a history of previously undetected hypomanic symptoms is elicited for the first time. While there is solid evidence supporting the use of lithium to augment an antidepressant (as discussed below), many patients with bipolar depression will get well and stay well on lithium alone. Should the clinician recommend discontinuing the antidepressant when such a patient recovers after starting lithium? Or (as discussed below) should the antidepressant be gradually replaced by lamotrigine, a stabilizer with antidepressant effects that appear to be more robust than those of lithium? To answer these questions, the clinician must engage the patient and family members as partners in treatment decisions. How important is taking only one medication for this patient? What is this patient's risk of self-destructive behavior upon becoming depressed? Is there a history suggesting that an antidepressant may be destabilizing for this patient (a history of mixed symptoms, rapid cycling, or substance abuse)? Is there a supportive family member who will help monitor symptoms and adherence? Can the patient afford to pay for the medication (in this case lamotrigine)?

As noted in the first edition of this volume, lithium's antidepressant effects may not become noticeable for up to 3 to 5 weeks, a lag time that can be somewhat longer than that experienced with antidepressants; some patients, however, respond within the first week or two. The original studies on lithium monotherapy for bipolar depression recommended doses that would achieve serum levels of up to 1.2 mEq/l, considerably higher than the levels now recommended for maintenance treatment. While it appears that higher levels are more effective in treating acute depressive symptoms, they are associated with more side effects and problems with adherence (Gelenberg et al., 1989; see also Chapter 21). Often, however, achieving these levels for a relatively short period of time can produce an antidepressant response, after which the dose can be lowered.

Some have suggested that rapid cycling (defined as at least four episodes of mania or depression within 12 months) predicts poorer acute antidepressant response to lithium, especially as compared with response to the anticonvulsant agents (see, e.g., Bowden, 2001). Although this work has examined primarily efficacy in preventing relapse, it has been extended to the treatment of acute depression, and

a

Treatment of Bipolar-I Depression

If not on a mood stabilizer

1. Evaluate thyroid function, and supplement as necessary.
2. Start lamotrigine combined with lithium or valproate.
   a. For severe depression, consider electroconvulsive therapy (ECT) or an antidepressant plus an antimanic mood stabilizer.
   b. For psychotic depression, add an atypical.
   c. If the patient has seasonal depression, use adjunctive bright light in the morning.

stabilizer w̄ antidep. effects.

If no response at week 4:
Add quetiapine.

If no response at week 6:
Consider olanzapine plus fluoxetine as an alternative to quetiapine.

If no response at week 8:
Discontinue olanzapine plus fluoxetine and add bupropion or a selective serotonin reuptake inhibitor (SSRI), depending on symptom pattern,[a] while maximizing the antimanic mood stabilizer.

If no response at week 10:
Consider ECT or an alternative antidepressant, such as a monoamine oxidase inhibitor (MAOI) (preferably), a tricyclic; pramipexole, or a stimulant and/or sleep deprivation.

If on lithium or valproate

1. Assess for possible precipitating factors, such as substance use, prescription drugs, or life stressors.
2. Evaluate thyroid functioning; supplement if necessary.
3. If on lithium, increase dose.
4. Add lamotrigine.

If no response at week 4:
Add quetiapine, and consider thyroid augmentation.

If no response at week 6:
Consider olanzapine plus fluoxetine as an alternative to quetiapine.

If no response at week 8:
Discontinue olanzapine plus fluoxetine and add bupropion or SSRI, depending on symptom pattern,[a] while maximizing the antimanic mood stabilizer.

If no response at week 10:
Consider ECT or an alternative antidepressant, such as an MAOI (preferably), a tricyclic, pramipexole, or a stimulant and/or sleep deprivation.

Figure 19–1. *a*: Recommendations for treatment of bipolar-I depression. Bupropion is preferred for psychomotor retardation/slowing; SSRIs are preferred for irritability or comorbid anxiety, panic, or obsessive-compulsive disorder. *b*: Recommendations for treatment of bipolar-II depression. Note: There have been very few controlled studies focusing on bipolar-II depression; therefore, any recommendations for treating this condition must be considered more tentative than those for treating bipolar-I.

b

Treatment of Bipolar-II Depression

If not on a mood stabilizer

1. Start lamotrigine.
   a. For severe depression, consider electroconvulsive therapy (ECT) or an antidepressant plus an antimanic mood stabilizer.
   b. For psychotic depression, add an atypical antipsychotic to lamotrigine.
   c. If the patient has seasonal depression, use adjunctive bright light in the morning.
   d. For persistent irritability, consider adjunctive valproate.

If no response at week 4:

Consider a second-generation antidepressant plus an antimanic mood stabilizer or quetiapine.

If no response at week 6:

Consider other combinations (quetiapine plus lamotrigine, lithium plus lamotrigine, olanzapine plus fluoxetine, monoamine oxidase inhibitor [MAOI] plus antimanic mood stabilizer).

If on a mood stabilizer

1. Increase clinical contact.
2. Assess for possible precipitating factors, such as substance use, prescription drugs, or life stressors.
3. Evaluate thyroid functioning; supplement as necessary.
4. If on lithium, increase dose.
5. Add lamotrigine.

If no response at week 4:

Consider a second-generation antidepressant plus an antimanic mood stabilizer or quetiapine.

If no response at week 8:

Consider other combinations (quetiapine plus lamotrigine, lithium plus lamotrigine, olanzapine plus fluoxetine, MAOI plus antimanic mood stabilizer).

Figure 19–1. *(continued)*

some guidelines recommend using valproate as first-line monotherapy for depressed patients with a history of rapid cycling (see, e.g., Sachs et al., 2000). However, a meta-analysis of studies of efficacy in rapid-cycling and non-rapid-cycling bipolar patients concluded that anticonvulsants have not been shown to be more effective than lithium in preventing relapse (Baldessarini et al., 2002). As suggested by the maintenance study of Calabrese and colleagues (1999b, 2005), neither lithium nor valproate is very effective against the depressive phase in rapid-cycling patients.

Because of lithium's relatively low therapeutic index, it is important to hold a detailed discussion with patients regarding certain precautions before they start taking the drug. Patients should be advised, for example, to take care not to become dehydrated in hot weather. Patients should also let the treating clinician know if they are taking prescription drugs from other physicians (especially thiazide diuretics) or over-the-counter preparations, especially those containing nonsteroidal anti-inflammatory drugs (NSAIDs), so their lithium blood levels can be checked. Issues also arise regarding the use of lithium during pregnancy. Potentially suicidal patients should have their access to possibly dangerous quantities of lithium limited. All of these medical issues are discussed in more detail in Chapter 20.

Anticonvulsants

For patients who remain depressed on lithium, recommendations regarding the choice of an adjunctive agent were based in the past on whether the patient had a history of symptoms associated with a more complex and brittle bipolar disorder, usually thought to be indicated by a history of rapid cycling or mixed episodes. The literature supporting the efficacy of certain anticonvulsants in the treatment of mixed states and rapid cycling supports the adjunctive use of these agents in patients with such a history who experience lithium-resistant bipolar depression, as do studies indicating synergistic or at least additive effects of lithium and valproate at both the clinical (Young et al., 2000) and cellular levels (see Manji et al., 2001; see also Chapter 14). Some patients with bipolar depression will respond to valproate monotherapy; compared with lithium, however, there is less data supporting valproate as a first-line agent for depression. However, when a bipolar depressed patient is suffering from comorbid anxiety, valproate or carbamazepine may be a reasonable first-line choice. (See also our review of the literature below.)

Lamotrigine is different from the other anticonvulsants (such as valproate or carbamazepine) in that the evidence indicates it to be effective in treating the core symptoms of bipolar depression, and unlike traditional antidepressants, it is much less likely to be associated with a switch into mania (although switches into hypomania have been reported). Indeed, lamotrigine has joined lithium as a first-line agent for bipolar depression. In the Texas Algorithm (Suppes et al., 2005), for patients not already taking lithium, lamotrigine is the first-line recommendation for bipolar depression (together with an adjunctive antimanic agent for bipolar-I patients). Because of the slow titration schedule required to minimize the risk of a serious rash, there is some concern that the acute antidepressant effect of the drug may not be rapid enough for some clinical situations. While this may well be true for severe depression, for many patients at least partial antidepressant effects can begin at doses as low as 50 mg; indeed, as noted in the review of the literature below, 50 mg of lamotrigine was found to be superior to placebo, a dose that can be reached in the third week of administration. Patients who are going to respond completely usually do so at doses between 100 and 200 mg/day, but some (who may be rapid metabolizers) fail to respond until higher doses, up to 400 mg/day.[6] For bipolar-II depression, lamotrigine can be used as monotherapy, while for bipolar-I depression, it is generally best combined with another stabilizer that works more effectively in the prevention of mania. The British guidelines (G. Goodwin et al., 2004) specify that lamotrigine monotherapy for bipolar-I depression may be appropriate "where depressive symptoms are less severe."

The antidepressant efficacy of gabapentin monotherapy is not well supported by the research literature (see below), but gabapentin can be useful as an adjunctive agent in the presence of comorbid anxiety and/or insomnia. For this latter use, its short half-life is an advantage because the drug is not likely to be associated with daytime sedation. Topiramate is another anticonvulsant without controlled data to support its use as monotherapy for bipolar depression, but it may be useful as an adjunctive agent because of its ability to produce weight loss.[7] Likewise, there is a paucity of controlled data for oxcarbazepine, whose main advantage is its low incidence of drug interactions and more benign side-effect profile (compared with carbamazepine).

Antidepressants

Analysis of U.S. prescribing patterns in the 1990s indicates that approximately half of all visits to a psychiatrist by bipolar patients involved the administration of an antidepressant, often in the absence of a mood stabilizer (Blanco et al., 2002; Baldessarini et al., 2006). While such practice is, in our view, clearly inappropriate, adding an antidepressant to a mood stabilizer can be justified in some circumstances. By and large, the North American treatment guidelines suggest that antidepressant monotherapy is not appropriate for bipolar depression (especially bipolar-I depression) and that even in combination with a mood stabilizer, antidepressants should be reserved for more severe cases of depression.[8] It should be noted that some European experts believe the North American guidelines are too negative with regard to antidepressants. At any rate, earlier reluctance (especially in the United States) to recommend antidepressants for patients with bipolar disorder because of concerns about precipitating manic symptoms has been attenuating somewhat in the face of evidence (albeit limited) that, compared with the tricyclics, the newer antidepressants (in the presence of a mood stabilizer) are less likely to be associated with acute switching into manic/hypomanic episodes (Gijsman et al., 2004). With regard to long-term cycle induction, however, the newer agents may be no safer than the older ones (Ghaemi et al., 2004).

Given the reality that most patients with bipolar disorder experience substantially more morbidity from depressive than from manic/hypomanic symptoms, antidepressants continue to have some role in the treatment of bipolar depression, perhaps especially for the bipolar-II patient. In our view, however, antidepressants should generally be reserved for patients who are severely depressed or those for whom a combination of two mood stabilizers (including lamotrigine) or a combination of a mood stabilizer and quetiapine has failed. Our conclusion, which is similar to the recommendation of the Texas Algorithm (see below) was reinforced by the finding of the Stanley Foundation Bipolar Network that only 15 percent of 549 bipolar patients (65 percent bipolar-I) taking mood stabilizers whose breakthrough depression was treated with an adjunctive antidepressant remained in remission for a minimum of 2 months (Altshuler et al., 2003).

Because maintenance antidepressants have been implicated in mood destabilization, gradually discontinuing these agents is often the first step in eventually achieving mood stability. Indeed, in the first edition of this text we recommended that antidepressants be gradually withdrawn shortly after the antidepressant response in patients with bipolar-I disorder and maintained only in those who repeatedly relapse after antidepressant discontinuation, which in our experience are about 15 to 20 percent of bipolar depressed patients (Ghaemi and Goodwin, 2001b).

This recommendation has been called into question by the results of three open, nonrandomized studies (two retrospective, one prospective) that examined 1-year outcomes in patients with bipolar depression (approximately two-thirds bipolar-I) who had been treated with one of the newer antidepressants added to a mood stabilizer. Each of these studies found that, compared with those kept on their antidepressant for the full year of observation, those whose antidepressant was discontinued were significantly more likely to relapse into depression, whereas the risk of manic relapse was not related to the duration of antidepressant treatment (Altshuler et al., 2001a, 2003; Joffe et al., 2005).[9] However, the patients in these studies were not randomized, nor were the studies controlled for a host of potentially confounding variables (Goldberg and Ghaemi, 2005). For example, the question remains open as to why the treating psychiatrists chose to keep some patients on the antidepressant (presumably the more stable patients) while withdrawing it from others (presumably those whose course may have been destabilized by the antidepressant, as demonstrated in several studies). In other words, it is not possible to know how many patients in these studies did worse because they were taken off antidepressants and how many were taken off because they were doing worse.[10]

It is also important to note that an earlier randomized study (i.e., without the confounds just discussed) found that antidepressant (tricyclic) discontinuation in bipolar-I patients maintained on lithium plus placebo did not result in more depressive episodes over 2 years compared with those maintained on lithium plus imipramine (Prien et al., 1984). A later randomized clinical trial by the same group compared lithium, imipramine, and a combination of the two (Prien et al., 1988). The authors analyzed a subgroup of 25 patients with dysphoric mania and found that imipramine (alone or in combination with lithium) was associated with higher recurrence at up to 2 years of follow-up compared

with lithium alone. Of relevance to the newer second-generation antidepressants, a recent randomized study within the NIMH STEP-BD program (detailed in our review of the literature below) found that over 1-year follow-up of bipolar patients who had responded to a mood stabilizer–antidepressant combination, the adjunctive antidepressant was not associated with a better outcome compared with the mood stabilizer alone.

Ghaemi and Goodwin (2005) applied the technique of decision analysis to all of the available literature addressing the role of antidepressants in bipolar-I disorder (the analysis was weighted toward the newer agents, as well as toward randomized controlled trials, and involved conservative assumptions). They concluded that the available literature supports mood stabilizer monotherapy or a mood stabilizer plus short-term use of an antidepressant, but does not support long-term use of an antidepressant, even with a mood stabilizer.

Among second-generation agents, the APA and Expert Consensus guidelines recommend bupropion or paroxetine, whose use for treating bipolar depression has been supported by the results of randomized, placebo-controlled studies. Ultimately, however, the clinician must tailor this decision to the particular patient, based on such factors as symptom pattern, individual or family history of response to a particular agent, and side-effect profile. For example, when psychomotor retardation/decreased energy and lack of motivation are the most prominent features of the depression, bupropion, with its activating profile, is preferred; when comorbid anxiety, panic, or obsessive-compulsive symptoms predominate, a selective serotonin reuptake inhibitor (SSRI) is likely to be the best choice. A moderate amount of crossover data is available to support such choices. On the basis of studies covered in our review of the literature, as well as our clinical experience, the following conclusions and recommendations are particularly relevant:

- Tricyclics are problematic for the treatment of bipolar depression with regard to both stabilization and efficacy. For a contrary view see Moller and Grunze (2000), as well as a detailed critique of that paper[11] (Ghaemi et al., 2003a).
- The MAOIs remain underutilized for treating bipolar depression (Himmelhoch et al., 1991; Balon et al., 1999). Although they are well documented to be effective for that purpose and uniquely effective for some patients who fail to benefit from any other agent, many psychiatrists never prescribe them because of misapprehensions about side effects and required diet. Many published diets are overly restrictive, however, being based on case report data on drug reactions that are of questionable validity

given that such reports focus on negative outcomes (see Walker et al., 1996). Moreover, selegiline, a MAOI now available in patch form, is reported to have a low incidence of all tyrimine-related reactions. MAOIs may be particularly helpful for patients with more severe depressive symptoms with atypical features as defined in the *Diagnostic and Statistical Manual* (DSM)-IV—anergia, psychomotor retardation, and reverse vegetative signs (hypersomnia and hyperphagia)—although patients without these features can benefit as well. Guidelines for the use of MAOIs (e.g., after mood stabilizers have failed) are the same as for other antidepressants.

- Second-generation antidepressants such as bupropion and the SSRIs have largely replaced the older drugs. In addition to being somewhat less likely than tricyclics to precipitate a switch (with the exception of venlafaxine), although perhaps not less likely to be associated with cycle induction, they have a more favorable side-effect profile than the older drugs.

- Antidepressant monotherapy is contraindicated in bipolar-I depression; for bipolar-II depression, we advise caution in using antidepressant monotherapy until more data are available.

- When bipolar-I depression is treated with an adjunctive antidepressant (including the second-generation agents), an effort should be made to taper and discontinue the drug shortly after remission (or maximal response) has been achieved. For bipolar-II disorder, the risk/benefit ratio of maintenance antidepressants has not been established.

- Restoring and/or maintaining the integrity of sleep is an important consideration in choosing an antidepressant for the bipolar patient. Other things being equal, bupropion has an advantage over SSRIs in that it preserves normal sleep architecture when given early in the day (which may be why it is apparently less likely than an SSRI to be associated with a switch into mania/hypomania).

Box 19–1 outlines our conclusions about the role of antidepressants in treating bipolar disorder.

Given the differential response of individuals with major depression to different agents, tapering and switching is a reasonable strategy when a patient does not respond to one antidepressant. Most guidelines recommend switching to an antidepressant in a class different from the failed agent, for example (as noted above), to bupropion in a patient showing no response to an SSRI (see Fava, 2000, for a discussion of switching strategies with a focus on avoiding discontinuation syndromes). Differential responses to different drugs in the same class have certainly been demonstrated, however; for example, some (unipolar) depressed

---

BOX 19–1.   The Role of Antidepressants in Treating Bipolar Disorder

- The efficacy of maintenance antidepressants in treating bipolar disorder is not established.
- Cycling and/or switches while on antidepressants have been demonstrated in three randomized, placebo-controlled studies.
- Antidepressant monotherapy is not recommended for bipolar-I disorder; data are insufficient to support a recommendation for bipolar-II.
- Antidepressants (with a mood stabilizer) should generally be reserved for severe bipolar depression, or cases in which adjunctive mood stabilizers have failed.
- When antidepressants are used, they should be tapered and discontinued after recovery from depression; they should be maintained only in those who repeatedly relapse soon after discontinuation.

Source: Adapted from Ghaemi et al., 2003.

---

patients not responding to sertraline have been shown to benefit from fluoxetine (Thase et al., 1997).

Antipsychotics

Some patients with bipolar depression will benefit from antipsychotic medications. These agents are certainly indicated for patients with depression complicated by delusions and hallucinations. The agitation and extreme dysphoria and distress associated with severe depression can be significantly ameliorated with antipsychotics as well. And given in the evening, these agents can be especially helpful in stabilizing sleep.

The newer, atypical antipsychotics have positive effects on mood while also being somewhat less prone to cause acute or delayed extrapyramidal symptoms; thus they are clearly preferred over the older agents. Indeed, given the ability of some of these drugs to improve mood, even when the clinical picture does not include psychotic features, they may be preferable to benzodiazepines in patients with severe insomnia or extreme anxiety with physical restlessness and agitation. It should be noted that the doses of these agents useful in treating depression are often lower than those needed to treat schizophrenia or manic states. The atypicals are 5-hydroxytryptamine(2) (5-HT$_2$) receptor antagonists at low doses, and it has been suggested that as a result, they may have an antidepressant effect through serotonergic mechanisms at these doses.

Olanzapine has been studied extensively in bipolar disorder. In addition to its clear antimanic action, there is evidence of a modest antidepressant effect, even in monotherapy (Tohen et al., 2003a), although the size of this effect is small and derives almost entirely from the drug's beneficial effect on insomnia, anxiety, and irritability. When olanzapine is combined with fluoxetine (Tohen et al., 2003b) or other antidepressants (Thase, 2002), the effect is more robust. Recently, another atypical, quetiapine, was found to have a robust antidepressant effect, including some effect on core depressive symptoms, in two large randomized, placebo-controlled studies of bipolar patients; indeed, quetiapine is the first drug to have attained an FDA indication for bipolar depression (see our review of the literature below).

There have been reports of olanzapine and other atypical antipsychotic medications causing hypomanic and manic symptoms in patients with bipolar disorder. Two critical reviews by the same group (Aubry et al., 2000; Rachid et al., 2004) evaluated published case reports covering a total of 60 patients and concluded that for more than half of these patients, a causative role for an atypical antipsychotic was "highly suggestive." On the other hand, an analysis of 129 patients participating in controlled trials of olanzapine found a significantly higher switch rate in the placebo group than in those taking the drug (Baker et al., 2003). It should be noted, however, that patients participating in controlled trials are less likely than nonparticipants to have some of the risk factors (such as substance abuse) associated with switching. Also, because the participants had to have just experienced a spontaneous manic episode to qualify for the trial, their situation was different from that of the bipolar patient being treated for depression.[12]

Although the risk of causing extrapyramidal symptoms is likely lower with the atypical than with the typical antipsychotics (see Chapter 20), some, though not all, of the former have metabolic side effects, including increased serum lipids, triglycerides, and glucose (Osser et al., 1999). Weight gain associated with the use of some of these medications is well documented,[13] and cases of new-onset diabetes mellitus have been reported (Wirshing et al., 1998). Monitoring of weight is therefore essential when certain of these medications are prescribed, as is the usual attention to the serum lipids that are important to cardiac health (see Chapter 20 for details on the individual drugs).

Complex Regimens

Many bipolar patients with refractory depressive symptoms will need to take lithium as well as an anticonvulsant, such as lamotrigine, and clinical experience has shown that a few will need to take lithium and more than one anticonvulsant, an atypical antipsychotic, and an antidepressant as well. The clinician must be sure to approach such complex regimens cautiously. Optimizing of dosages (using serum drug-level determinations when possible) or simply watchful waiting for full benefit to be achieved from the addition of an agent may be all that is necessary. The

clinical utility of the latter strategy cannot be overemphasized; increased mood instability from adding an antidepressant can take many months to become apparent, and even then it is easily missed by clinicians not employing a life chart methodology (see Chapter 11).

Thyroid Augmentation

Attention to the thyroid status of the depressed bipolar patient is essential. Determination of thyroid-stimulating hormone (TSH) and free thyroxine (fT_4) by dialysis should be part of the assessment of patients with depression at the first sign of resistant symptoms. Correction of thyroid deficiencies is obviously important, but patients with "normal" thyroid determinations may benefit from adjunctive treatment with thyroid hormone as well (see our review of the literature below). In the next chapter, we review studies indicating that lower mean thyroid indices (albeit in the "normal range") are associated with incomplete recovery from bipolar depression. Psychiatrists should thus be familiar with thyroid physiology, know the signs and symptoms of hyper- and hypothyroidism, and, most important, understand the concept of subclinical hypothyroidism.

Recommendations as to which depressed patients to treat with adjunctive thyroid hormone and at what point can be difficult to make. Female patients, those with rapid-cycling disorders, and those with levels of TSH above the 50th percentile of normal and with fT_4 below the 50th percentile have shown particular benefit from thyroid augmentation. Given that about 50 percent of patients with treatment-resistant depression benefit from augmenting antidepressant medication with triiodothyronine (T_3), a low-risk intervention, it would be reasonable to recommend adding T_3 to an antidepressant sooner rather than later, perhaps even after concluding that the patient has not benefited from the second or even the first antidepressant added to lithium and anticonvulsant(s). For long-term management of bipolar patients, it is appropriate to shift gradually to T_4 (see Chapter 20).

Sleep Deprivation and Phototherapy

Sleep deprivation has clearly been demonstrated to benefit depressed patients and can bring about rapid and dramatic relief in those with bipolar depression. While the antidepressant benefits of sleep deprivation can be short-lived, they can be prolonged by lithium and antidepressant medications, as detailed later in our review of the literature. Even if the actual antidepressant effects of sleep deprivation are short-lived, there is an important psychological effect whose implications can be more lasting: the hopeless feeling that one will never recover is clearly challenged by the dramatic, albeit temporary, improvement. Patients can thus be helped to realize that they still have the capacity to feel well; the remaining challenge is to sustain this feeling.

In the first edition of this text, we suggested that partial sleep deprivation (during the second half of the night) was probably as effective as total sleep deprivation, noting that the former was easier for patients. However, results of recent research appear to indicate that total sleep deprivation is indeed the most effective technique (Giedke et al., 2003). Although somewhat difficult to achieve in the outpatient setting, it can easily be accomplished in the hospital with the support and direction of nursing staff. Patients should be kept awake for 36 hours (all night and the following day) and then allowed a night of recovery sleep. Several published efficacy studies recommend a series of three sleep-deprived nights alternating with recovery-sleep nights, although even one night of sleep deprivation is sufficient for some sensitive patients to benefit. For certain patients, however, partial sleep deprivation may be effective, and for outpatients it is not unreasonable to try this approach first and then move on to total sleep deprivation if necessary.

Sleep deprivation can be a highly effective technique for accelerating the response to a new medication for a depressive episode, and can also provide relief for minor breakthrough depressive symptoms without necessitating a change in the patient's medication regimen. Some, though not all, studies have found a greater response in bipolar than in unipolar patients, but the clinical features that predict response are generally not controlled for in these comparisons. Switches into mania/hypomania have been reported following sleep deprivation, so clinicians are well advised to employ the treatment only in patients on mood stabilizers. In addition to the clinical correlates of the treatment's effectiveness, studies relevant to its mechanism of action are reviewed in Chapter 16.

Phototherapy is another low-risk treatment for depression that is accomplished even more easily than sleep deprivation.[14] The most obvious situation requiring this treatment is when the depressive phase is occurring during the winter months, a pattern not uncommon among bipolar patients. However, phototherapy can also be helpful at other times of the year, probably because of its nonspecific activating effects (it can be especially effective against daytime somnolence that can be associated with mood stabilizers) and its ability to help synchronize the circadian cycle, thereby contributing to the stabilization of sleep.

Despite over a decade of research, the precise timing of light exposure necessary to derive its maximum benefit for winter depression has not been definitively established, although most experts recommend first thing in the morning. Certainly early-morning exposure is required for normalizing a phase-delay sleep disorder in which the patient gets to sleep late and then finds it difficult to get up in the morning.

No advantage of broad-spectrum light over bright white light has been demonstrated.[15] Current recommendations are for at least 30 minutes of exposure to 5,000–10,000 lux at a distance of 18 to 24 inches. All patients with a seasonal pattern to their mood symptoms, as well as those with phase-shifted sleep patterns, should probably invest in their own phototherapy light box, as should all psychiatric inpatient units. It should be noted that occasional switches into hypomania and mania have been reported to be associated with phototherapy.

Electroconvulsive Therapy

In our opinion, it is unfortunate that ECT is often relegated to last-resort status in treatment guidelines and protocols. We believe the clinician should not hesitate to recommend ECT to severely ill patients as a first-line treatment. For the delusional or suicidal patient—indeed, for any depressed patient who is so ill that only the most reliably and rapidly effective treatments should be considered—ECT is the clearly superior alternative. ECT should also be offered to patients with treatment-resistant depression who have a history of adverse reactions to antidepressants (increased cycling, induced mania or agitation) whenever their symptoms threaten to become chronic or begin to have a significant negative impact on family or on occupational or academic functioning.

Depression in elderly patients is especially responsive to ECT. Since older patients often need to be started on lower doses of medications and their dosages titrated up more slowly than is the case for younger patients, ECT is frequently the most rapidly effective treatment for severe depression in this population.

It is important to remember that the antidepressant effect of a standard course of ECT is generally temporary, and that patients who are not started on medication at the conclusion of their course of treatment are likely to relapse. For a discussion of maintenance ECT, see Chapter 20.

Alternative Treatments

A variety of alternative treatments have been claimed to benefit some patients with bipolar depression. These include novel antidepressant combinations, stimulant medications, dopamine agonists, the "wakefulness" agent modafinil, nutritional supplements (including omega-3-fatty acids), and others. (See our review of the literature for details.) It is appropriate here to comment on one especially important form of "alternative" treatment—regular exercise (see Chapter 17). Not only has regular vigorous aerobic exercise been shown to have an antidepressant effect in numerous studies, but when at least some exercise is done at approximately the same time every day and not too close to the time for sleep, it can help stabilize circadian rhythms and enhance the integrity of the sleep cycle (see Chapter 16). The positive psychological impact of successfully pursuing a treatment whose benefits derive entirely from the patient's own efforts is difficult to overstate.

REVIEW OF THE LITERATURE

This section presents a detailed review of the evidence regarding the treatments surveyed above. We review in turn the literature on lithium, anticonvulsants, antidepressants, antipsychotics, ECT, novel central nervous system stimulation techniques, dopamine agonists, psychostimulants, hormonal agents, sleep deprivation, phototherapy, and nutritional supplements. Results of randomized, double-blind monotherapy trials for each of the major pharmacological agents are summarized in Table 19–1, while results of randomized, non-placebo-controlled monotherapy trials and placebo-controlled add-on trials are summarized in Table 19–2.

Lithium

Several early reports on lithium's efficacy in treating mania suggested that it lacked significant antidepressant effects (Cade, 1978). Subsequent studies, however, demonstrated its effectiveness in preventing depressive relapses in patients with recurrent major depression (see, e.g., Baastrup and Schou, 1967; Baastrup et al., 1970). By the early 1980s, several studies, focused on patients hospitalized for depression, had found that lithium was superior to placebo (see Table 19–3, as well as the review by Zornberg and Pope, 1993). Several of these studies suggested that lithium was more likely to be effective in patients with bipolar than unipolar depression (especially less recurrent forms) and that the time to therapeutic response was longer than was typically reported for tricyclic antidepressants—on the order of 3 to as long as 8 weeks. In several double-blind studies comparing lithium with tricyclics, lithium was found to be as effective as amitriptyline, desipramine, and imipramine

TABLE 19–1. **Randomized, Double-Blind, Placebo-Controlled Monotherapy Trials Demonstrating Acute Antidepressant Efficacy of Various Drugs**

Drug	No. of Studies	Sample Size[a]	Findings
Lithium	10	179	Moderate effect size
Carbamazepine	3	30	Small effect size
Lamotrigine	3	432	Moderate to large effect size
Olanzapine	1	833	Small effect size; primarily improves insomnia, anxiety, and anorexia
Valproate	3	89	Moderate effect size; trend ($p=.1$) in one study; significant separation from placebo by random regression analysis in the other
Imipramine	5	638	Effect size similar to that of lithium
Desipramine	1	12	Effect size similar to that of lithium
Flouxetine	3	255	Methodological problems, but probably equivalent to tricyclic antidepressants in efficacy and rate of switch into mania
Meclobemide	2	537	Low mania switch rate[b]
Total	31	3,005	

[a]Combined drug and placebo groups.
[b]Bipolar-II patients
Source: Adopted from Ghaemi and Hsu, 2005.

TABLE 19–2. Drugs Demonstrating Acute Antidepressant Efficacy in Randomized, Non-Placebo-Controlled Comparison Trials or in Placebo-Controlled Add-On Trials

Drug	No. of Studies	Sample Size	Findings
Lithium	2	144	Equivalent to imipramine and to paroxetine
Valproate	1	27	Valproate and lithium equivalent to paroxetine + lithium or valproate
Topiramate	1	36	Equivalent to bupropion when added to lithium
Risperidone	1	22	May speed onset of response when added to paroxetine
Bupropion	3	99	Equivalent to desipramine, with lower switch rate
Imipramine	3	191	Equivalent to lithium, with higher switch rate
Desipramine	1	15	Equivalent to bupropion when added to lithium, with higher switch rate
Tranylcypromine	1	56	More effective than imipramine when added to lithium; acute switch rates equivalent to those with imipramine
Pramipexole	2	43	More effective than placebo when added to lithium; low switch rate

Source: Adapted from Ghaemi and Hsu, 2005.

TABLE 19–3. Lithium Treatment in Patients Hospitalized for Depression: Results of Placebo-Controlled Studies

Study	Sample Size	Patient Characteristics	Results
Goodwin et al., 1969	18	13 with bipolar depression, 5 with "noncyclic depression"	10 of 13 bipolar patients showed some response, versus only 2 of 5 "noncyclic" depressed patients
Stokes et al., 1971	18	Manic-depressive	Lithium trial lasted only 10 days, showed a nonsignificant trend toward response
Goodwin et al., 1972	52	Primary affective disorder—40 bipolar (-I or -II), 12 unipolar	32 of 40 bipolar patients responded, versus 4 of 12 unipolar patients ($p<.05$)
Noyes et al., 1974	22	Manic-depressive, depressed with "endogenous features"—6 bipolar, 16 unipolar	6 of 6 bipolar patients responded, versus 7 of 16 unipolar patients ($p<.05$)
Johnson, 1974	10	Endogenous depression with recurrent histories	5 showed "marked improvement"
Baron et al., 1975	23	Primary affective disorder (Feighner criteria)—9 bipolar (-I and -II), 14 unipolar	7 of 9 bipolar patients responded, versus 3 of 14 unipolar patients ($p<.05$)

Note: Response rates (complete and partial) for all studies combined are bipolar, 64/81 = 79%; unipolar, 20/55 = 36%.

in treating mixed groups of bipolar and unipolar depressed patients (see Table 19–4). One of these studies (Watanabe et al., 1975) found lithium to be equally effective in bipolar and unipolar depressed patients.

These earlier studies have been criticized on a number of methodological grounds, including the on–off nature of some of the designs (perhaps confounding the placebo period with lithium withdrawal symptoms) and the modest number of subjects, increasing the risk of type II (false negative) errors (Bhagwagar and G. Goodwin, 2002). In the understudied area of treatments for bipolar depression, however, methodological limitations are by no means confined to lithium. Thus two reviews of treatment options for bipolar depression (Yatham et al., 2003; Ghaemi and Hsu, 2005) concluded that lithium comes closest to meeting those authors' criteria for a first-line treatment for bipolar depression (that is, the treatment should be efficacious in treating bipolar depressive symptoms, should be effective in preventing further depressive and/or manic episodes, and should not be associated with manic switching or increased cycling).

There has been only one randomized, double-blind clinical trial comparing lithium monotherapy for acute bipolar depression with the use of second-generation antidepressants (Nemeroff et al., 2001). In a secondary analysis, these investigators found that at blood levels of .8 mEq/l or above, lithium alone was as effective as lithium plus either paroxetine or imipramine. Since many of the patients in the study had previously failed to respond to lithium, it is reasonable to assume that these results likely understate the effectiveness of lithium in a more representative group of patients with bipolar depression.

Numerous studies have shown that the addition of lithium to antidepressant therapy results in remission of symptoms that have not improved or have been ameliorated only partially with antidepressants alone. This has been shown to be true for patients with both bipolar and unipolar depression and for lithium added to tricyclics, MAOIs, SSRIs, and other newer antidepressants. These studies are reviewed here because of their possible relevance to the antidepressant effects of lithium.[16] Table 19–5 summarizes three meta-analyses of lithium augmentation of antidepressants, primarily tricyclics.

One of the first of these studies (De Montigny et al., 1981) found that eight of eight unipolar depressed patients who had failed to respond to 3 weeks of various tricyclic antidepressants experienced notable relief from their symptoms with lithium. This effect was observed in all these patients within 48 hours of starting lithium, although this rapid improvement was not always seen in subsequent studies. Numerous open and blind studies have shown lithium to be an effective augmentation agent for the tricyclics in about 50 percent of patients to whom it is given (Joffe et al., 1993). Lithium added to MAOIs was shown to be an effective strategy in several case reports and small open trials in the 1970s.[17]

TABLE 19–4. Lithium Treatment of Patients Hospitalized for Depression: Results of Double-Blind Comparisons with Tricyclic Antidepressants

Study	Sample	Design	Results
Fieve et al., 1968	21 bipolar	Imipramine comparison	Significantly more improvement on imipramine; lithium had "mild" antidepressant effects
Mendels et al., 1972	12 bipolar and 12 unipolar	Desipramine comparison	Lithium as effective as desipramine
Watanabe et al., 1975	45 mixed	Imipramine comparison	Lithium as effective as imipramine
Worrall et al., 1979	29 bipolar and unipolar	Imipramine comparison with elimination of initial placebo responders	All 14 patients on lithium improved, but not until second week; patients on imipramine who improved did so during first week; response was significantly more uniform on lithium
Khan, 1981	30 recurrent unipolar	Amitriptyline comparison	Lithium as effective as amitriptyline
Arieli and Lepkifker, 1981	33 bipolar	Clomipramine comparison	Lithium as effective as clomipramine
Linder et al., 1989	22	Clomipramine comparison	Lithium as effective as clomipramine
Total sample size	276	Conclusion: 6 of 7 studies found lithium equivalent to the antidepressant.	

Note: Most of these relatively small studies were underpowered to detect modest differences between active treatments.

TABLE 19–5. **Lithium Augmentation of Antidepressants: Results of Three Meta-Analyses**

Analysis	Studies Analyzed	Patients	Conclusions	Odds Ratio (CI)
Austin et al., 1991	5 double-blind, placebo-controlled studies in which patients with treatment-resistant depression took lithium and had a serum lithium level ≥.4 mEq/L	99	Response rate of approximately 40%	6.85 (2.27–20.00)
Bauer and Döpfmer, 1999	9 double-blind, placebo-controlled studies in which patients took 250–1,200 mg of lithium daily; lithium levels reported for 5 studies (serum levels of .5–1.1 mEq/L)	234	Response rate of 50%	3.89 (2.14–7.08)
Bauer and Döpfmer, 1999 (strict criteria)	3 double-blind, placebo-controlled studies in which patients took at least 800 mg/day of lithium or had serum lithium level ≥.5 m Eq/L for at least 2 weeks	110	Response rate of 27% during lithium treatment tripled compared with placebo	3.31 (1.46–7.53)

CI = confidence interval.

Some, though not all, studies of lithium augmentation of SSRIs have also shown positive results.[18] Successful lithium augmentation of venlafaxine-refractory depression has been reported in open trials.[19] Lithium augmentation of mirtazapine has been identified as an effective strategy in case reports (Moustgaard, 2000). However, a double-blind comparison indicated that this strategy may be less effective than a lithium–imipramine combination (Bruijn et al., 1998).

One of the meta-analyses listed in Table 19–3, encompassing studies of lithium augmentation of various (mainly tricyclic) antidepressants (including five studies that were placebo-controlled), concluded that the odds of remaining ill were cut in half by the addition of lithium (Austin et al., 1991). A more rigorous analysis examined only the three double-blind, placebo-controlled studies (totaling 110 patients) in which lithium was administered at a dosage of at least 800 mg/day for a minimum of 2 weeks (or a serum lithium level of at least .5 mEq/l was achieved) (Bauer and Döpfmer, 2000). The authors reported a response rate 27 percent higher in patients who received lithium than in those receiving placebo. When the authors incorporated into the analysis an additional 234 patients who had taken lower doses of lithium or had participated in studies in which the results were gathered after less than 2 weeks on lithium, the overall response rate was approximately 50 percent. These results suggest that lower lithium doses (600–800 mg/day) may be sufficient to achieve successful antidepressant augmentation, at least in some depressed patients. The study also indicates that patients whose symptoms have not responded to lithium augmentation within 12 days are unlikely to respond to a longer trial of the drug. Finally, an-

other placebo-controlled study found that patients were more likely to respond to lithium augmentation of either fluoxetine or lofepramine (a tricyclic similar to imipramine) if they had serum lithium levels of at least .4 mEq/l (Katona et al., 1995).

Surveys of practicing psychiatrists have indicated that lithium augmentation in treating refractory depression is, despite its proven efficacy, probably underutilized. A 1996 survey found that 39 percent of responding U.S. psychiatrists and only 12 percent of U.K. psychiatrists would add lithium as their next step in treating a patient with refractory major depression who had shown no improvement after taking 150 mg of amitriptyline for 6 weeks (Shergill and Katona, 1997).

Finally, an extensive body of literature has established that lithium dramatically reduces the risk of suicide (see Chapter 25). For up-to-date analyses of the antidepressant effects of lithium as monotherapy and as augmentation for traditional antidepressants, see the reviews by Davis and colleagues (1999) and Bauer and colleagues (2006).

Anticonvulsants

Reports of the antidepressant effects of anticonvulsant medications have appeared in the clinical literature for several decades, resulting in the incorporation of these agents into several algorithms for the treatment of bipolar disorder, including bipolar depression. Unfortunately, however, there have been few controlled studies of the use of anticonvulsants as antidepressants to inform their use in depressed bipolar patients. An exception is a growing literature on the antidepressant uses of lamotrigine, an agent that appears to be effective in treating bipolar depression.

Valproate

Results of case reports and open studies suggest that valproate has antidepressant properties in some patients.[20] An open study of 33 unipolar depressed outpatients (some of whom had not responded to previous antidepressant treatment) found a 54 percent response rate (Davis et al., 1996). However, in a review of four open studies of 195 acutely depressed patients with bipolar (-I or -II not designated) or schizoaffective diagnoses, only 30 percent had an antidepressant response to valproate (McElroy and Keck, 1993). With regard to the three controlled studies of the efficacy of valproate as an antidepressant, the results are modest. In one study, Sachs and colleagues (2004) found a 45 percent response rate for valproate compared with 27 percent for placebo, but with only 45 subjects, this difference failed to reach statistical significance ($p < .3$).[21] On the other hand, a relatively small 8-week study of 25 outpatients by Davis and colleagues (2005) was able to show a 43 percent decrease in HAM-D scores with valproate compared with 27 percent with placebo, which was statistically significant in a random regression analysis. As might be expected with a gamma-aminobutyric acid (GABA)ergic anticonvulsant, the effect on anxiety was greater than that on depression. Finally, in a recent randomized double-blind study of 19 bipolar depressed patients (mostly type I) (Dunn et al., 2006), valproate was found to be superior to placebo. Analysis of individual MADRS items, the primary outcome, demonstrated some benefit in treating core mood symptoms. The effect size in this study was larger than that in the previous studies.

With regard to bipolar-II depression, there has been one small open study of valproate in 11 medication-naïve patients, 82 percent of whom responded (as measured by a 50 percent decrease in HAM-D scores) (Winsberg et al., 2001). As in Sachs and colleagues' (2004) study, the effect of valproate nearly reached statistical significance among the bipolar-II subgroup. In a recent review of the literature, Bowden, the investigator associated most prominently with the evaluation of valproate in treating bipolar disorder, and his colleagues (2006) concluded that "the acute effectiveness of valproate in depression is modest." It has been suggested that response to valproate may be predicted by failure to respond to lithium and vice versa. That is, lithium-responsive and valproate-responsive depressed patients may represent distinct clinical subgroups (Bowden et al., 1994; Ghaemi and Goodwin, 2001b).

There are even fewer controlled data on the commonly used strategy of combining valproate and lithium. A double-blind study of 27 patients with bipolar-I or -II disorder who had experienced major depression while taking either lithium or valproate compared the antidepressant response to the SSRI paroxetine with that to a second mood stabilizer (valproate was added if the patient had become depressed on lithium, and vice versa). Significant and comparable improvement in depression scores was seen among the SSRI and adjunctive mood stabilizer groups after 6 weeks of treatment (Young et al., 2000). These results can be interpreted as supporting the suggestion that, with respect to lithium and valproate, patients who do not respond to one will benefit from the other; the results may also suggest a synergistic effect of the two agents. It should be noted that in this study, more patients in the mood stabilizer group than in the SSRI group developed drug intolerance, perhaps reflecting the side-effect burden when full doses of these agents are used simultaneously.[22] We await a controlled study of drug combinations in which less-than-full doses of each drug are used. Such a study would provide a more accurate test of both clinical practice and the laboratory-based conclusion that lithium and valproate (and perhaps other anticonvulsants) can act synergistically.

Carbamazepine and Oxcarbazepine

There have been six relatively small randomized, placebo-controlled trials of carbamazepine in the treatment of depression, with an average response rate of 44 percent (Post et al., 1996). Three of these trials involved a total of 30 bipolar patients, and in one of these studies carbamazepine was combined with lithium; again the antidepressant effect can be described as modest (Ghaemi and Hsu, 2005). The findings of these controlled studies are consistent with those of the open study of Dilsaver and colleagues (1996).

Oxcarbazepine is a 10-keto analog of carbamazepine that has a clinical profile similar to that of an anticonvulsant but a somewhat more benign side-effect profile and fewer drug interactions than the parent compound. Although there have as yet been no randomized controlled trials of this agent in treating bipolar depression, results of two open studies indicate that it may have some antidepressant effect (Berv et al., 2002; Ghaemi et al., 2002).

Lamotrigine

Lamotrigine differs from the GABAergic anticonvulsants (carbamazepine and valproate) by virtue of its modulating effects on glutaminergic transmission, which appear to contribute to its activating profile. Antidepressant efficacy was reported in the early 1990s in case reports and small open case series.[23]

There have been three positive randomized, placebo-controlled trials of lamotrigine monotherapy—two with a crossover design and one a large industry-supported study with a parallel-group design. In the two placebo-controlled crossover studies, lamotrigine was found to be significantly more effective than placebo or gabapentin in treating refractory depressed patients. The first study involved 31 bipolar patients at NIMH (Frye et al., 2000); the second (Obrocea et al., 2002) involved 35 bipolar and 10 unipolar patients who underwent randomized successive 6-week trials with lamotrigine, gabapentin, and placebo separated by 1 week. In the latter trial, the responders to lamotrigine were more likely to have a bipolar diagnosis and to be male (Obrocea et al., 2002).

The large parallel-group study revealed clear antidepressant efficacy (Calabrese et al., 1999b). In this study, 195 depressed outpatients received either 50 or 200 mg/day of lamotrigine or placebo for 7 weeks. Because of the gradual dosing necessary with lamotrigine to minimize the risk of serious rash, both lamotrigine groups took the same dose of medication for the first 3 weeks of the study (i.e., up to 50 mg); both showed improvement over the placebo group within this time—response rates of 48 and 54 percent, respectively, compared with the placebo rate of 29 percent. On the other hand, there have been two unpublished adequately powered double-blind, randomized, placebo-controlled trials involving patients with bipolar depression in which lamotrigine failed to separate from placebo (Goldsmith et al., 2003; Gao and Calabrese, 2005). The lamotrigine response rates across all 5 studies were remarkably consistent; what differentiated the two failed trials was higher placebo response rates. Indeed, in an analysis of the pooled data from all three of these parallel-group trials, involving 291 patients treated with lamotrigine and 282 with placebo, the drug was found to be significantly better than placebo for those MADRS items that reflect core symptoms of depression—apparent and reported sadness, lassitude, and inability to feel; pessimistic thoughts nearly achieved statistical significance (Gao and Calabrese, 2005; Hirschfeld et al., 2005).

Taken together, results of the above five studies are quite suggestive of an acute antidepressant effect of lamotrigine. The drug was very well tolerated in all five studies, with transient headache being the only side effect that differentiated it from placebo.

A 9-week placebo-controlled, double-blind study involving 40 patients with acute bipolar or unipolar major depression compared the antidepressant efficacy of a combination of lamotrigine and paroxetine with that of paroxetine alone (Normann et al., 2002). Although HAM-D scores did not differ between the two groups at the end of the study, the patients who took the combination reported improvement in several depressive symptoms significantly

sooner than patients on paroxetine alone; the numbers were not sufficient for a separate analysis of the bipolar subgroup. In a recent randomized double-blind comparison of adjunctive lamotrigine versus citalopram in bipolar depression, the mean reduction in MADRS scores was virtually identical in the 2 groups (Schaffer et al., 2006). Finally, a randomized[24] comparison of adjunctive lamotrigine versus risperidone or inositol in 66 treatment-resistant bipolar depressed patients (documented failure to respond to a mood stabilizer and at least one antidepressant) enrolled in the NIMH STEP-BD program (Nierenberg et al., 2006), lamotrigine was associated with the numerically highest rate of recovery (sustained for at least 8 weeks); post hoc analyses of "relevant continuous outcomes" indicated that adjunctive lamotrigine is superior to risperidone or inositol for treatment-resistant bipolar depression.

Can lamotrigine precipitate or exacerbate manic symptoms, as is seen with antidepressants? There have been a few case reports of switches in bipolar patients on lamotrigine, which may be related to relatively rapid titration and higher doses (Raskin et al., 2006) and/or combination with a high dose of an antidepressant (Margolese et al., 2003). Unfortunately, many published studies on the drug's efficacy have not addressed this issue specifically, often incorporating the development of mania or hypomania into analyses of "adverse effects." In the pooled analysis of the three large randomized, placebo-controlled studies cited above, switch rates for lamotrigine and placebo did not differ. Further, in an analysis of pooled data on 827 patients taking lamotrigine and 685 taking placebo in eight controlled studies lasting from 3 weeks to 18 months, the risk of developing manic, hypomanic, or mixed symptoms with lamotrigine was comparable to that associated with placebo, as well as to that among subjects taking lithium (Bowden et al., 2003; G. Goodwin et al., 2004).[25] It should be noted, however, that these studies were not sufficiently powered to rule out an increase in manic switches (Ghaemi et al., 2003b).[26] Finally, there is an interesting recent report of the simultaneous use of lamotrigine and ECT (Penland and Ostroff, 2006) noting that the combination was well tolerated and that, importantly, lamotrigine had a minimal effect on standard ECT parameters, unlike most other anticonvulsants.

Riluzole

This drug is related to lamotrigine by virtue of its effects on glutamatergic transmission; it is FDA-approved for the treatment of amyotrophic lateral sclerosis. In an 8-week open-label study of riluzole in 14 treatment-resistant bipolar depressed patients, Zarate and colleagues (2005) found significant antidepressant effects across a wide range of items on the MADRS. There were no switches into hypomania or mania. It is of interest that three of the four patients who had previously failed to respond to lamotrigine responded to riluzole. While these open data are preliminary, they are consistent with the results of a recent trial of riluzole in patients with treatment-resistant unipolar depression (Zarate et al., 2004).

Topiramate

Interest in the possibility that the novel anticonvulsant topirimate may provide some benefit in bipolar depression has been heightened by its ability to reduce weight. Several case reports and open studies in fact do suggest that the drug may have some effect in treating bipolar depression, especially in the 100–200 milligrams per deciliter (mg/dl) range (Marcotte, 1998; Ghaemi et al., 2001). In an open trial, topiramate was given to 45 bipolar-I and 18 bipolar-II patients who were suffering from a major depressive episode and had not benefited from or were intolerant of two mood stabilizers. Although nearly a third of these patients dropped out of the study because of side effects or lack of efficacy, 42 percent had an essentially complete antidepressant response within 4 weeks (HAM-D scores below 7), and another 27 percent had a partial antidepressant response (HAM-D scores between 8 and 12) (Hussain and Chaudhry, 1999).

McIntyre and colleagues (2002) found that topiramate compared favorably with bupropion as an adjunctive treatment in depressed bipolar-I and -II patients who had not improved despite 2 weeks of treatment with either lithium (13 patients) or valproate (23 patients). In this randomized, single-blind study (blind rater), the addition of either topiramate or bupropion resulted in a reduction in HAM-D scores of at least 50 percent in about half of the patients, and about a quarter of both groups had scores below 7.[27] As is typically the case with new agents, an assessment of the safety and efficacy of topiramate must rely on sometimes conflicting case reports and small open studies in complex, often treatment-refractory patients who are frequently taking other medications as well. Although results thus far are encouraging, further research and clinical experience will be required before the role of this agent in the treatment of bipolar depression becomes clear.

Other Anticonvulsants

Data on the efficacy of other anticonvulsants in treating bipolar depression are quite preliminary. To our knowledge there has been only one double-blind, randomized clinical trial involving gabapentin as monotherapy, and it had negative results.[28] Gabapentin has, however, been reported to be useful as an adjunctive agent (primarily for its anxiolytic and sedative properties) in several open studies of bipolar depression.[29]

Clinical data are limited on the use of tiagabine for treating bipolar disorder. A series of three refractory bipolar patients with mixed but predominantly depressive symptoms benefited from tiagabine added to other agents, including valproate, carbamazepine, and antidepressants (Kaufman, 1998). Clearly, however, it is difficult to draw conclusions from such a small sample size.

Another anticonvulsant with mechanisms of action that overlap both the GABAergic and antiglutamatergic agents is zonisamide; the ability of this agent to reduce weight is of obvious interest to clinicians managing bipolar patients.[30] Since the initial open study noting some benefit of this agent in treating mania (Kanba et al., 1994), there have been several reports on its use in treating depression. Baldassano and colleagues (2004) reviewed the charts of 12 patients with bipolar depression (-I and -II), finding 6 that met their response criteria based on a change in scores on the Clinical Global Impressions (CGI) scale. Anand and colleagues (2005) found open-label adjunctive zonisamide effective in 5 of 10 bipolar depressed patients who had not tolerated or were resistant to their existing treatment.[31] A similar open adjunctive trial in 22 bipolar depressed patients not responding to at least one "standard" mood stabilizer also found a significant decrease in mean bipolar depression severity scores on the CGI scale ($p < .001$); however, only 32 percent of the subjects completed the 8-week trial and were classified as responders (McElroy et al., 2005). Recently, Ghaemi and colleagues (2006) conducted an open prospective study of adjunctive zonisamide (mean dose 222 mg) in 20 depressed bipolar patients (bipolar-I, -II, and -not otherwise specified [NOS]); while the observed antidepressant effect was relatively robust (a mean 8 point decrease in MADRS ratings, $p < .001$), half of the patients terminated because of side effects, principally nausea/vomiting, cognitive dysfunction, and sedation. Obviously, controlled data (especially monotherapy data) on zonisamide are needed.

Antidepressants

Tricyclics and Monoamine Oxidase Inhibitors

The existing literature on the efficacy of tricyclic antidepressants is dominated by studies in patients with unipolar depression. The consensus of this literature is quite clear: tricyclics have been more effective than placebo in more than two-thirds of controlled trials, with an overall efficacy rate in the treatment of major depression ranging from 50 to 85 percent and averaging 65 to 70 percent. The data on bipolar depression are much thinner, however. Indeed, in a recent Cochrane analysis it was noted that bipolar patients (that is, bipolar patients recognized and treated as such) represent only 1 percent of all depressed patients in randomized, placebo-controlled clinical trials (Gijsman et al., 2004).

In the first edition of this text, after analyzing 77 studies involving 3,226 patients, we concluded that the clinical literature provided almost no information about the relative efficacy of this group of drugs in treating bipolar versus unipolar depression. Small studies suggesting that bipolar depression was tricyclic-resistant had occasionally appeared (e.g., Kupfer and Spiker, 1981). Uniformly, however, these studies had not set out to compare medication efficacy in bipolar and unipolar depressed patients. Rather, "bipolarity" or a history of mania was reported as one of several predictors of antidepressant nonresponse in drug efficacy studies or course-of-illness investigations. Yet the results of a large retrospective study intended to answer the question of the efficacy of tricyclics in treating bipolar versus unipolar depression (Moller et al., 2001) indicate that this may not be the case. In this naturalistic chart review, the treatment of 2,032 consecutive patients admitted for a major depressive episode between 1980 and 1992 was assessed to determine whether there was a difference in antidepressant efficacy between bipolar and unipolar patients as measured by several outcome scales. Almost all these patients were prescribed tricyclic (or "tetracyclic") antidepressants; no difference in drug efficacy was found between the bipolar and unipolar patients. However, this observational study did not attempt to control for confounding variables.

Two recent but conflicting meta-analyses bear on this question. The first is the Cochrane meta-analysis of five acute (4–10 weeks duration) randomized, parallel-group, double-blind, controlled trials (Gijsman et al., 2004) in which a traditional unimodal antidepressant (n = 213) was compared with placebo (n = 449); 75 percent of these bipolar depressed patients were on a concomitant atypical antipsychotic (the majority) or a mood stabilizer. Relevant to our discussion here, only two of the trials involved a tricyclic. Compared with those on placebo, the antidepressant-treated patients were 1.96 times more likely to respond and 1.4 times more likely to achieve remission. The overall effect size was judged to be comparable to what has been published for unipolar depression and for lamotrigine in bipolar depression. The tricyclics were somewhat less effective than the newer antidepressants (risk ratio [RR] = .84), but this difference did not achieve statistical significance.

As with meta-analyses in general (discussed in Chapter 17), considerable care is in order when interpreting these conclusions. The results are substantially driven by one very

large study (456 patients) in which olanzapine alone (the "placebo" condition) was compared with olanzapine plus a nontricyclic antidepressant—fluoxetine (Tohen et al., 2003a). Whether an antidepressant effect of fluoxetine plus olanzapine should be the principal basis for a generalization about the effectiveness of antidepressants in bipolar patients on a mood stabilizer is questionable at best. One study included in the Cochrane analysis (Nemeroff et al., 2001) directly addressed the question at hand—whether combinations of an antidepressant and a mood stabilizer are more effective than standard mood stabilizers alone. In that study, 117 patients, all on lithium, were randomized to placebo, imipramine, or paroxetine; among those with lithium levels adequate for an antidepressant effect (.8 mEq/l or above), no added advantage was associated with either antidepressant. Unfortunately, in the meta-analysis this study was overwhelmed by the much larger study of fluoxetine plus olanzapine. Another recent meta-analysis (Ghaemi et al., 2003b) examined nine studies of long-term prophylactic use of antidepressants, including but not limited to tricyclics (with follow-up periods of 6 months or longer), and concluded that there is no overall benefit with use of an adjunctive antidepressant.[32] The discrepancy between these two meta-analyses likely relates to the fact that one focused on acute studies and the other on long-term studies.

MAOIs have been claimed to be particularly effective in treating bipolar depression. Starting in the early 1970s, a group of investigators at the Western Psychiatric Institute in Pittsburgh published a series of studies on the use of tranylcypromine in patients with bipolar depression, alone and in combination with lithium. Following several reports of MAOI efficacy in open studies of depressed patients who had not benefited from lithium or lithium plus a tricyclic, Himmelhoch and colleagues (1991) carried out a double-blind study on 56 patients with "anergic" bipolar-I or -II depression, comparing the efficacy of tranylcypromine and imipramine monotherapy. "Anergic" depression was defined as a syndrome similar to DSM's "atypical features," including psychomotor retardation and "reverse vegetative signs" (i.e., hypersomnia and hyperphagia). The response rate (defined as "moderate" or "marked" improvement on the CGI scale) in the tranylcypromine group during the "acute treatment" phase of this study (4 weeks) was 81 percent, double that of the imipramine group. A year later, the same investigators reported on a double-blind crossover study of depressed bipolar patients taking either imipramine or tranylcypromine: 9 of 12 patients who crossed over from imipramine to tranylcypromine responded, compared with only 1 of 4 patients crossing over from tranylcypromine to imipramine (Thase et al., 1992).

Moclobemide is a reversible inhibitor of monoamine oxidase A (MAO-A) approved for the treatment of depression in many countries throughout the world, but not in the United States. In a randomized, double-blind, multicenter study of bipolar depressed patients, most of whom were on a mood stabilizer,[33] Silverstone (2001) found no significant difference between moclobemide (n = 81) and imipramine (n = 75) with respect to changes in HAM-D and MADRS scores, although there were nonsignificant trends favoring the tricyclic. Switches into mania were observed in 3.7 percent of those on moclobemide versus 11 percent of those on imipramine. The fact that MAOIs were only slightly (and nonsignificantly) better than tricyclics in the analysis of Gijsman and colleagues (2004) may be due to the inclusion of this moclobemide study (the largest one in the analysis): moclobemide is generally thought to be less effective than other MAOIs, and in the Silverstone study tended to be less effective than imipramine (as perhaps also reflected in the lower mania switch rate).

Bodkin and Amsterdam (2002) conducted a double-blind, placebo-controlled study of 177 unipolar depressed outpatients in which transdermal selegiline was found to be effective and well tolerated. This MAOI is more specific to the isoenzyme monoamine oxidase B (MAO-B) at low doses and is less active in inhibiting MAO-A, the isoenzyme that predominates in intestinal epithelium and whose inhibition necessitates a low-tyramine diet. This specificity is unfortunately lost at the higher oral doses required to treat depression; in this study, however, a comparatively low dose (20 mg/day) delivered by a transdermal patch was effective. Although patients in this study kept to a low-tyramine diet, the study raises the possibility that MAOI therapy without (or with less stringent) dietary restrictions may be possible by means of a transdermal drug delivery system.[34] The selegiline patch was recently approved by the FDA.

Second-Generation Antidepressants

Selective Serotonin Reuptake Inhibitors. As is true of the tricyclics, SSRIs have clearly been shown to be effective in the acute treatment of unipolar depression. However, this general conclusion may be more applicable to the mainstream unipolar depressed patient without frequent recurrences. Thus it is interesting that in the recent report from the "real-world" NIMH Sequenced Treatment Alternatives to Relieve Depression (STAR*D) trial of the antidepressant citalopram, only 28 percent of patients with fairly recurrent forms of unipolar depression (average of six prior episodes) achieved remission (Trivedi et al., 2006).

Compared with unipolar depression in general, data on the efficacy of SSRIs in the acute treatment of bipolar depression are more limited (see Table 19–6). Kupfer and colleagues (2001) conducted an 8-week open study of citalopram added to lithium, valproate, carbamazepine, or a combination of these agents in 33 patients with bipolar-I or -II depression. They found that 64 percent experienced a reduction in depressive symptoms (Kupfer et al., 2001).[35]

The largest controlled study of the acute antidepressant effect of an SSRI in bipolar disorder, noted above in our discussion of tricyclics, involved comparing fluoxetine plus olanzapine with olanzapine alone; there was no fluoxetine-alone group. While there is no question that this combination is effective—indeed, it was given an FDA indication for the treatment of bipolar depression—one cannot use these results to assess the efficacy of SSRIs themselves in treating bipolar depression.

A 6-week double-blind study of 89 patients with bipolar depression (-I or -II not specified) found response rates for fluoxetine, imipramine, and placebo of 86 percent, 57 percent, and 38 percent, respectively (Cohn et al., 1989). The results are difficult to interpret, however, because about half of the study participants were also taking lithium, and a disproportionate number of those patients were in the fluoxetine group.[36] In the largest and best-designed study comparing the efficacy of paroxetine and imipramine in bipolar depressed patients (mentioned previously), Nemeroff and colleagues (2001) compared each antidepressant with placebo over 10 weeks under double-blind conditions in 117 patients who were also taking lithium (some were taking valproate or carbamazepine as well). No significant differences in efficacy among the three groups were found. In a post hoc analysis, the groups were stratified according to their lithium levels. It was found that imipramine and paroxetine were superior to placebo (and equivalent to each other), but only in patients with lower lithium levels (less than .8 mEq/l). Thus lithium was as effective as the two antidepressants when given at doses that achieved levels of .8 mEq/l or greater.

There has been considerable interest in using second-generation antidepressants to treat bipolar-II depression (see Box 19–2). Several studies of SSRI monotherapy for this indication are available. In a post hoc analysis of pooled data from randomized clinical trials involving patients with unipolar depression (in which some bipolar-II patients were included), Amsterdam and colleagues (1998) noted that the efficacy of fluoxetine in 89 bipolar-II patients was comparable to its efficacy in matched and unmatched unipolar depressed patients.

Bupropion. This drug, which enhances both noradrenergic and dopaminergic transmission through different mechanisms, may have unique advantages in the treatment

TABLE 19–6. Studies of Selective Serotonin Reuptake Inhibitors in Treating Bipolar Depression

Study	Sample	Design	Results
Cohn et al., 1989	89 bipolar (-I or -II not specified)	6-week double-blind comparison of fluoxetine, imipramine, and placebo; results confounded because more of the fluoxetine patients were also taking lithium	86% of fluoxetine-treated patients improved, compared with 57% of imipramine- and 38% of placebo-treated patients.
Simpson and DePaulo, 1991	16 bipolar-II	Open case series of fluoxetine monotherapy in patients refractory to other treatment (including tricyclics, MAOIs, and/or lithium); patients treated 13.6 ± 5.2 months	15/16 patients showed some benefit; 10/13 taking fluoxetine for at least 10 months had a good to very good response.
Young et al., 2000	11 bipolar-I, 16 bipolar-II	6-week double-blind, randomized study comparing the addition of paroxetine or a mood stabilizer to the regimen of patients already taking a mood stabilizer	Both treatments were effective in improving depressive symptoms; however, the mood stabilizer add-on group had a significantly lower completion rate (related to more side effects).
Kupfer et al., 2001	30 bipolar-I, 15 bipolar-II	8-week open-label add-on study	33 patients completed the study, 21 of whom were considered responders (64%).
Nemeroff et al., 2001	117 bipolar (-I or -II not specified)	10-week double-blind, placebo-controlled study comparing paroxetine, imipramine, and placebo; patients also took lithium or anticonvulsants	Both paroxetine and imipramine were superior to placebo only in patients with subtherapeutic lithium levels.
Ghaemi et al., 2004	78 patients (41 bipolar, 37 unipolar); 63% of bipolar patients were bipolar-I	228 trials as adjunct; naturalistic with systematic diagnostic criteria and assessment of response	Nonresponse was 60% more likely in the bipolar group; loss of response was 3.4 times more likely in the bipolar group.

Note: In evaluating this literature, it is important to be aware of the observation by Sachs and colleagues (2003) that there is no systematic method for correcting for improved depression scores that occur as part of a switch into mania. For example, about a quarter of the impressive response rates reported in some studies of tranylcypromine and imipramine monotherapy represent subjects who became manic during the study.

Source: Adapted from Ghaemi and Hsu, 2005.

of bipolar depression. Many experts believe it is at least as efficacious as SSRIs and tricyclics for the treatment of bipolar depression while having a significantly more benign side-effect profile, causing neither the heavy anticholinergic side effects of the tricyclics nor the problems of sexual dysfunction and long-term weight gain common with the SSRIs. Moreover, as an activating agent, it may have some advantage in the majority of bipolar patients whose depression involves primarily psychomotor retardation. In addition, results of two randomized trials suggest bupropion may be less likely to provoke a switch into mania than either a tricyclic or venlafaxine (see below).

In an open prospective study of adjunctive bupropion, 8 of 13 patients with complex, refractory bipolar disorder

taking a variety of other agents, including some who were taking other antidepressants, had a greater than 50 percent reduction in their MADRS scores (Erfurth et al., 2002). A prospective 8-week double-blind study compared bupropion and desipramine in 15 depressed bipolar patients also taking lithium, valproate, or carbamazepine (Sachs et al., 1994).[37] About two-thirds of all the patients had at least a 50 percent reduction in their HAM-D scores, with comparable efficacy being observed for the two antidepressants. The most comprehensive comparison of adjunctive bupropion with other second-generation antidepressants is the randomized, double-blind Stanley Foundation Bipolar Network study (Post et al., 2006), in which 174 bipolar patients experiencing a breakthrough depression were randomized

BOX 19–2. Treatment of Bipolar-II Depression

While numerous studies have examined the clinical characteristics and epidemiology of bipolar-II disorder, relatively few have focused on treatments specifically for bipolar-II depression. Because patients with bipolar-II disorder have more frequent episodes of depression than bipolar-I patients and may be at higher risk for suicide, research into the treatment of bipolar-II depression deserves urgent attention.

Bipolar-II patients have been included in efficacy studies of lithium, anticonvulsants, antidepressants, and other agents. All too often, however, bipolar-II patients are not separated out in the discussion of results. Nevertheless, a survey of the literature leads to the conclusion that available treatments for bipolar-I depression are also effective for the treatment of bipolar-II depression (see MacQueen and Young, 2001, for a discussion of efficacy studies).

A number of studies of the use of the sedating anticonvulsants (such as valproate or carbamazepine) in treating bipolar-II disorder suggest that these agents are quite useful in treating the impulsiveness, irritability, and dysphoric moods often seen in these patients, symptoms that, while not classic, may lead to more self-harming behavior and psychosocial disability. Results of several preliminary studies suggest that valproate may be modestly effective in treating bipolar-II patients. In a small open study of divalproex monotherapy in 19 bipolar-II depressed outpatients, nearly two-thirds of the subjects showed a greater than 50 percent reduction in HAM-D scores after 12 weeks (Winsberg et al., 2001). There have been two double-blind, placebo-controlled studies. The first investigated the effects of valproate as monotherapy in 30 patients with bipolar-II disorder who also met criteria in the *Diagnostic and Statistical Manual* (DSM)-IV for borderline personality disorder. The valproate group experienced a significant reduction in dysphoric symptoms, such as irritability and anger. There was also a nonsignificant trend toward reduction of depressive symptoms, though this finding may be explained by the fact that patients with active major depression had been excluded from the study (Frankenburg and Zanarini, 2002). The second controlled study, conducted by Sachs and colleagues (2001), failed to show a significant advantage over placebo for the overall group, but did identify a trend favoring valproate over placebo in the bipolar-II subgroup.

Lamotrigine may be effective in patients with bipolar-II depression, but there have been no placebo-controlled studies or head-to-head comparisons with lithium or other anticonvulsants.

Any number of studies of antidepressants for the treatment of bipolar depression have included bipolar-II patients. For example, bipolar-II patients have been included in studies of the use of selective serotonin reuptake inhibitors (SSRIs) for treating bipolar disorder (see Table 19–6). As with lithium and the anticonvulsants, however, the data are insufficient to conclude that any particular agent is especially superior for treating bipolar-II depression. The key issue here is whether the risk of switch and/or destabilization is lower among bipolar-II than among bipolar-I patients. While recent data suggest that this might be the case, there is still no consensus and we still recommend that if antidepressants are used in treating bipolar-II depression, they be combined with a mood stabilizer.

---

to adjunctive bupropion, sertraline, or venlafaxine (see Fig. 19–2). The three drugs showed modest efficacy overall, with about one-third of the patients achieving remission; however, on the outcome of most importance to the clinician—remission without a switch into mania/hypomania (see below)—on average an uncomplicated remission was achieved by only 25 percent of the patients. With regard to the drugs individually, bupropion performed best (38 percent), compared with sertraline (27 percent) and venlafaxine (just 18 percent). In other words, with respect to the most desirable outcome, bupropion was twice as good as venlafaxine (RR for bupropion versus venlafaxine = 2.13 [95 percent confidence interval (CI) 1.15–3.94]).

Serotonin/Norepinephrine Reuptake Inhibitors (SNRIs). Venlafaxine has garnered significant interest because of its "dual reuptake" effects—acting as both a serotonin and noradrenergic reuptake inhibitor. Some data suggest that venlafaxine has a more rapid onset of therapeutic action and results in higher remission rates than SSRIs in patients with unipolar depression (Thase et al., 2001). However, these differences have not been demonstrated as yet in the few studies on bipolar patients. Amsterdam and Garcia-Espana (2000) reported on a nonrandomized study of venlafaxine monotherapy for 15 bipolar-II and 17 unipolar patients being treated for major depression. About two-thirds of the patients in both groups had a reduction in HAM-D and MADRS scores of 50 percent or greater. A 6-week single-blind (blind rater) study of 60 patients with bipolar-I or -II major depression taking lithium or anticonvulsants found equal response rates (about half the patients) in those taking venlafaxine and paroxetine, with no significant difference in the bipolar-I and -II patients (Vieta et al., 2002). With regard to the proportion who responded without a switch, however, paroxetine outperformed venlafaxine. This result is consistent with the Stanley Foundation Bipolar Network results noted above (Post et al., 2006), and both reports suggest that venlafaxine

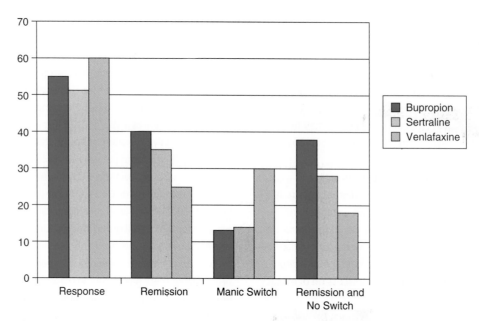

Figure 19–2. Outcomes for patients taking bupropion, sertraline, and venlafaxine. Note: Response and remission rates based on Inventory of Depressive Symptomatology (IDS) criteria only; mania switch and remission/no switch rates based on Young Mania Rating Scale or Clinical Global Impressions-Bipolar criteria. (*Source*: Post et al., 2006. Reproduced with permission.)

may be more like tricyclics, with a less favorable ratio of responses to switches compared with other second-generation antidepressants, especially bupropion.

Results of several open studies of the use of nefazodone in treating bipolar depression have not been encouraging. El-Mallakh (1999) found only transient improvement over a period of 8 weeks in 5 outpatients who took nefazodone with other medications. In another open trial, Goldberg and colleagues (2002) noted that about two-thirds of 13 patients who took nefazodone in addition to lithium, anticonvulsants, and antipsychotics had a 50 percent reduction in HAM-D scores during the course of the study, but that half of these patients experienced some relapse of depressive symptoms by the eighth week.

The new SNRI duloxetine was approved by the FDA for the treatment of major depression in 2004 on the basis of several large placebo-controlled trials involving more than 1,400 patients (Detke et al., 2002; Goldstein et al., 2002; Nemeroff et al., 2002). To our knowledge, studies of this agent focused on bipolar depression have not yet been published.

Selective Noradrenergic Reuptake Inhibitors. Reboxetine is a norepinephrine reuptake inhibitor with a structure distinct from that of the tricyclics. Although it is comparable in norepinephrine reuptake inhibition potency to the tricyclics, its selectivity for noradrenergic reuptake inhibition can be compared with that of the SSRIs in inhibiting serotonin reuptake. Reboxetine has thus been referred to as the first selective norepinephrine reuptake inhibitor, and

as such represents the first of what may become a new class of antidepressants (Wong et al., 2000). Reboxetine has been shown to be superior to placebo in treating unipolar depression and comparable to tricyclics and fluoxetine (Berzewski et al., 1997; Versiani et al., 1999; Schatzberg, 2000). To date, there have been no published studies of its use in treating bipolar depression, although three cases of probable reboxetine-induced mania in bipolar patients have been reported (Vieta et al., 2001).

Long-Term Efficacy of Antidepressants in Bipolar Disorder

As noted earlier, we chose to introduce the issue of the long-term effects of antidepressants (both benefits and risks) in this chapter because they are important considerations in the choice of a treatment for acute depression. With regard to highly recurrent unipolar depression, insufficient data are available to estimate a risk–benefit ratio, so our focus here is on bipolar depression.

In a university clinic, Ghaemi and colleagues (2004) found that, over periods of observation that averaged appoximately 1 year, there was a 51.3 percent nonresponse rate among 41 bipolar depressed patients, compared with only a 31.6 percent nonresponse rate among 37 unipolar patients. In addition, loss of response during treatment occurred 3.4 times more often among the bipolar than the unipolar patients. These results are in the same range as those of the Stanley Foundation Bipolar Network study: Post and colleagues (2003) found that while about 50 percent of their bipolar-I patients given a second-generation antidepressant in addition to a mood stabilizer were "much" or "very much" improved (as measured by the CGI scale), only 19 percent were able to complete the intended 1 year of continued antidepressant use. In a similar vein, Sachs and colleagues (2003) reported preliminary outcomes for the first 1,000 subjects enrolled in the NIMH STEP-BD program. During the first year of follow-up, 181 subjects experienced the new onset of at least one episode of major depression, and 50 of these patients experienced multiple depressive episodes[38]; no statistically significant advantage was associated with the adjunctive use of second-generation antidepressants.[39] Finally, a recent randomized study within the NIMH STEP-BD program (mentioned briefly in the section on clinical management) evaluated 69 bipolar patients who had recovered from a depressive episode on a combination of a second-generation antidepressant and a mood stabilizer (Ghaemi et al., 2006). After being stable for 2 months, the patients were openly randomized to continue with the combined treatment or the mood stabilizer alone (that is, antidepressants were tapered and discontinued); after adjusting for other clinical variables,[40] antidepressant continuation did not result in lower overall mood morbidity at 1-year follow-up compared with mood stabilizer alone.[41] Note that these results are quite different from those of the three nonrandomized studies reviewed in the section on clinical management that have, unfortunately, been interpreted by some as indicating that bipolar patients who have responded acutely to antidepressants should be continued on them. Clearly only a minority of bipolar patients do well when kept on antidepressants plus mood stabilizers, but the results of observational studies do not provide clinicians with a basis for judging which of their patients might be expected to do so.

The reader will note that scattered throughout our review of the literature are studies of the effectiveness of various agents in "treatment-resistant depression." The importance of such studies is underscored by evidence that resistance to standard antidepressants is one of the characteristics that may make the condition of a given patient more likely to be part of the bipolar spectrum (see Chapter 1). For example, Sharma and colleagues (2005) studied 61 patients with major depression who had failed to respond to two adequate antidepressant trials, two-thirds of whom had initially been diagnosed as unipolar. Upon careful diagnostic reevaluation in the course of 1-year follow-up, only 21 percent were still diagnosed as unipolar, with 79 percent now meeting criteria for bipolar disorder, primarily bipolar-II. Rybakowski and colleagues (2005) reported on a cohort of 447 unipolar depressed patients, 106 of whom met criteria for bipolar spectrum disorder; those with bipolar spectrum features were twice as likely as the "pure" unipolar patients to have

a history of treatment-resistant depression (30 versus 15 percent). Approaching this relationship from a different direction, Hantouche and colleagues (2005) evaluated the lifetime treatment history of 256 patients diagnosed as having unipolar major depression and found that those whose antidepressant had been augmented by a mood stabilizer (implying antidepressant resistance) had higher scores on a hypomania checklist and were more likely to have cyclothymic temperaments. However, not all studies have found a relationship between bipolar features and antidepressant resistance in unipolar patients (personal communication, D.J. Smith, October 14, 2005, University of Edinburgh).

Switches and Cycle Acceleration Following the Initiation of Antidepressants

Switches. In the first paper describing the antidepressant effects of imipramine, Kuhn (1958, p. 463) observed that "if [a patient's] depressions are easily and frequently replaced by manic-like phases or actual manic states, the reaction [to imipramine] is less favorable. . . .[T]he tendency arises for the depression to switch over into a manic phase." This observation is not limited to imipramine. Angst (1985) conducted an intriguing retrospective study of patients admitted to the Burghoelzli Psychiatric Hospital with a mood disorder between 1920 and 1982 (see Fig. 19–3). His findings indicate that the incidence of depressed patients experiencing manic symptoms increased with the development of medical treatments for depression (ECT and medications).[42]

In the ensuing decades, this "switch" phenomenon has been reported for every class of antidepressant, for many other classes of psychotropics, for medications used to treat nonpsychiatric conditions, for nonpharmocological

Figure 19–3. Switch rate of hospitalized depressed patients (unipolar or bipolar). Note: Only one episode per patient was considered. (*Source*: Angst, 1985.)

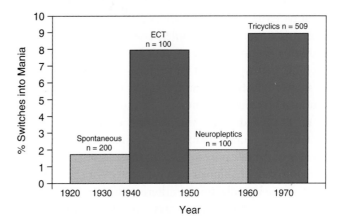

interventions (ECT, phototherapy, sleep deprivation), and even for herbal preparations.[43] In our above discussion of the efficacy of antidepressants in bipolar patients, we briefly noted reports of switching.[44] Table 19–7 builds on our considerable coverage of this issue in the first edition by summarizing recent studies of mania/hypomania following the initiation of antidepressants. Similarly, reports have appeared since the 1960s that in some bipolar patients, an antidepressant medication can be associated with increased mood cycling (see below). It has been posited that these agents can hasten the onset of new mood episodes in patients, accelerating the rhythm of their cycles and destabilizing mood.

If anything, the question of possible antidepressant-related worsening of bipolar illness has taken on more urgency since the first edition was published as a result of the enormous increase in prescriptions for antidepressants that has followed from the continuing introduction of new, easier-to-use agents into the market. Thus since 1990 there has been more than an eight-fold increase in prescriptions within the SSRI class alone (Grunebaum et al., 2004). Because the bulk of this increased prescribing is by nonpsychiatric physicians, there is an increased risk of undiagnosed bipolar patients being on antidepressants without a mood stabilizer.

A variety of methods have been used in an attempt to quantify how frequently switches occur, to assess whether drug-related and spontaneous switches differ,[45] to identify which agents are more likely to cause switching, and to alert clinicians to risk factors that may make particular patients more vulnerable. A number of factors have conspired to make this work quite difficult: (1) the inherent cycling pattern of the disorder makes it challenging to separate spontaneous from drug-induced changes in symptoms and course of illness; (2) the diagnostic categories for bipolar disorder are empirically derived and may not validly differentiate patients according to the undoubtedly complex and heterogeneous neurobiological underpinnings that may determine how they respond and react to pharmacological interventions; and (3) changes in treatment patterns over the years, especially the increasing use of multiple agents and complex treatment regimens, make gathering groups of patients with a similar treatment history increasingly difficult for the long-term studies needed to answer questions about the effects of specific pharmaceuticals on course of illness.

First, what do we know about the frequency of the switching phenomenon in patients on antidepressants? Estimates of the rate of switching into manic, mixed, and hypomanic states in bipolar patients treated with antidepressants range broadly among different studies (10 to nearly 70 percent, with the higher rates generally associated with

the tricyclics), a variability no doubt associated with the confounding factors just noted, especially patient selection and methods used to ascertain and score occurrences of mania/hypomania (Ghaemi et al., 2003c; Goldberg and Truman, 2003; Goldberg and Ghaemi, 2005).[46] As an example, one of the largest studies to date (Altshuler et al., 1995) used a retrospective life chart method to analyze the temporal association between tricyclic and MAOI antidepressants and the course of illness of 51 patients hospitalized with an episode of bipolar disorder. Manic or hypomanic episodes were categorized as likely to have been antidepressant related on the basis of such criteria as an episode occurring within 8 weeks of initiation of the drug or a change in illness pattern (the episode would have been "unexpected" given the prior course of the patient's illness). The authors concluded that one-third of the patients experienced an antidepressant-induced mania and that one-fourth experienced cycle acceleration at some time during the course of their illness. Of the switches that occurred, 75 percent were in bipolar-I patients and 25 percent in bipolar-II; half of the patients experienced rapid cycling (having had four or more mood episodes in the year prior to the study), and all were lithium refractory. Some patients were taking lithium at the time of the switch or cycle acceleration, and others were not. Given this heterogeneous group of ill patients, generalizing of these rates of adverse effects to other patient groups and the total group of patients with bipolar disorder is not possible.

Results of prospective studies that have specifically set out to identify manic episodes following the initiation of antidepressants indicate that approximately one-quarter of patients with bipolar disorder experience mania or hypomania within weeks to months of first taking these drugs (most studies set the criterion at 2 months; see Table 19–7). Some have suggested that patients with bipolar-I disorder are more likely than those with bipolar-II to experience a switch, but to our knowledge, these two populations have never been compared prospectively in the same study.

Switch rates calculated from clinical trials of antidepressants in bipolar depression (see Tables 19–8a and 19–8b) tend to be lower than those reported from naturalistic studies. For one thing, controlled trials tend to screen out patients who are at a higher risk of switching, such as those with substance abuse histories (Goldberg and Whiteside, 2002; Manwani et al., 2006). In addition, as Sachs (2005) has pointed out, given the ethical constraints associated with randomized, double-blind trials, antidepressants would hardly be continued if there were any signs of incipient mania. Patients showing evidence of abnormal mood elevation are typically removed from the study

TABLE 19–7. Observational Studies Since the First Edition (1990) Focused on the Emergence of Mania/Hypomania Following Initiation of Antidepressants

Study	Sample	Study Design	Results
Altshuler et al., 1995	38 bipolar-I, 13 bipolar-II	Lifetime life chart review of consecutive patients admitted to a clinical research ward	35% had a manic episode "likely" due to heterocyclic antidepressants, 21% due to MAOIs
Benazzi, 1997	103 unipolar, 8 bipolar-I, 92 bipolar-II	3–6 month prospective, naturalistic treatment of private-practice patients	Manic/hypomanic switch occurred in 25% of bipolar-I, 17.3% of bipolar-II, and 5.8% of unipolar patients; unipolar patients who switched resembled bipolar-I patients in age at onset and "atypical" features
Boerlin et al., 1998	29 bipolar-I (79 "episodes")	2-month prospective, naturalistic study in which patients taking antidepressant alone were compared with patients taking antidepressant and lithium or anticonvulsant	28% of patients had mania/hypomania, but in only 10% was it "severely disruptive"; there was no significant difference between patients taking antidepressant and those taking antidepressant plus lithium or anticonvulsant; switch rates were lower for SSRIs vs. tricyclics or MAOIs
Bottlender et al., 1998	158 bipolar depression	Retrospective study of medical records	25% of patients had switched to a maniform (mania and hypomania) state during the treatment period in the hospital; among that group, the phenomenon occurred in 23 patients (15%) as a hypomania and in 16 patients (10%) as a mania
Ghaemi et al., 2000	85 bipolar or unipolar	Retrospective study of medical records	55% of bipolar patients taking antidepressants developed hypomania or mania; 23% developed new or worsening rapid-cycling course
Henry et al., 2001	31 bipolar-I, 13 bipolar-II (95 "treatment phases")	6-week prospective, naturalistic study comparing patients who switched with those who did not; 90% of patients were on an SSRI, 10% on a tricyclic	27% of patients switched; there was no difference between rates in bipolar-I and -II patients or between antidepressants and ECT; lithium was more protective than anticonvulsants
Goldberg and Whiteside, 2002	53 bipolar (-I or -II not specified)		39.6% switched into mania or hypomania; no apparent impact of concomitant mood stabilizers
Joffe et al., 2002	51 bipolar-I, 18 bipolar-II (113 "trials")	1-year prospective, naturalistic study comparing SSRIs (including venlafaxine) with bupropion; all patients taking lithium or anticonvulsant	12.4% of patients developed mania; bipolar-I > bipolar-II; there was no difference between rates in the two drug classes

(continued)

TABLE 19–7. Observational Studies Since the First Edition (1990) Focused on the Emergence of Mania/Hypomania Following Initiation of Antidepressants *(continued)*

Study	Sample	Study Design	Results
Post et al., 2003	127 bipolar patients on lithium and/or valproate given an adjunctive secondary antidepressant for depression; 42% reported a history of rapid cycling	Assessed using National Institute of Mental Health life chart methodology for 1 year; 10-week prospective study with 1-year continuation phase; randomized to bupropion, sertraline, or venlafaxine; nonresponders rerandomized	Half responded (=<50% improvement) to acute antidepressant treatment, but half of responders switched into hypomania/mania (with some dysfunction) in either the acute or the continuation phase
Serritti et al., 2003	297 bipolar-I, 119 bipolar-II	Retrospective case–control study with interviews, medical records, and life charts	43% of switchers were bipolar-I vs. 19% of switchers who were bipolar-II ($p < .0001$); switchers were 5.8 times more likely to have history of rapid cycles; 3 times fewer switches occurred with antidepressant + mood stabilizer vs. antidepressant alone (51% vs. 17%); depression–mania–interval (DMI) pattern more frequent among switchers ($p < .0002$)
Ghaemi et al., 2004	41 bipolar depression, 37 unipolar depression	Analysis of clinical records for outcomes of antidepressant trials	Switches into mania were not observed in any unipolar patient, but occurred in 84.2% of bipolar patients not taking any antimanic agent, vs. 31.6% taking at least one antimanic agent; compared with tricyclics, newer antidepressants were not associated with lower rates of cycle acceleration

and their response reported as an adverse event, "manic reaction," but not as an episode of mania or hypomania.

In most studies comparing apparent antidepressant-related switch rates in bipolar patients with and without mood stabilizers, those on mood stabilizers have been found less likely to switch.[47] Thus in those studies in which all patients were taking lithium or anticonvulsants, the rate of switching was roughly half that reported in studies of patients treated with antidepressants in the absence of a mood stabilizer. The protective effect of mood stabilizers (especially atypical antipsychotics) is illustrated by the recent Cochrane meta-analysis of five randomized trials of short-term treatment for bipolar depression, comparing antidepressants and placebo (Gijsman et al., 2004). In this study, 84 percent of the patients were on a "mood stabilizer," primarily (77 percent) olanzapine. The switch rates were low in both the antidepressant plus "mood stabilizer" and "mood stabilizer" alone groups.[48]

A number of studies have addressed potential risk factors for drug-related switching. One such factor is gender. In a randomized, double-blind, 3-year prospective comparison of lithium versus lithium plus imipramine, Quitkin and colleagues (1981) noted 2.5 times more switches in the combined-treatment group, but this differential was significant only among females, a finding similar to that of Yaldez and Sachs for antidepressant-related cycling (see below). In an observational study, by contrast, Goldberg and Whiteside (2002) found no difference in the gender ratio of bipolar patients who switched on antidepressants versus those who did not.

Another factor examined is episode sequence. Koukopoulos and colleagues (1980) noted that the episode sequence mania–depression–interval (MDI) was less likely to be associated with switching than the depression–mania–interval (DMI) sequence, a conclusion presumably related to his observation that the MDI pattern was associated with longer,

TABLE 19–8A. Reported Rates of Emergent Mania in Association with Antidepressants in Randomized Studies of Bipolar Depression

Study	Medication	Sample Size	Study Duration	Mean Dose	Switch Rate	Comments
Cohn et al., 1989 (95)	Fluoxetine	30	3–6 weeks	62 mg/day	0.0%	Concurrent lithium in 23% taking fluoxetine, 17% taking imipramine, 20% taking placebo; 16% of imipramine or placebo nonresponders who then took fluoxetine became hypomanic within 1 month during unblinded extension
	Imipramine	30	3–6 weeks	62 mg/day	7.0%	
	Placebo	29	3–6 weeks	N/A	3.0%	
Himmelhoch et al., 1991 (71)	Tranylcypromine	16	6 weeks	37 mg/day	21.0%	No concomitant mood stabilizers used
	Imipramine	16	6 weeks	246 mg/day	25.0%	
Thase et al., 1992 (91)	Tranylcypromine	12	4–12 weeks	39 mg/day	17.0%	Double-blind crossover of study of nonresponders from a prior tranylcypromine study
	Imipramine	4	4–12 weeks	246 mg/day	25.0%	
Sachs et al., 1994 (75)	Bupropion	9	8-week acute	358 mg/day	11.0%	Cotherapy with lithium, valproate, or carbamazepine
	Desipramine	10	1-year continuation	140 mg/day	50%	
Young et al., 2000 (78)	Paroxetine	11	6 weeks	36 mg/day	0.0%	All subjects initially took lithium or valproate; study drug was then added
	Lithium or valproate	16	6 weeks	Lithium 1,300 mg/day Valproate 1,200 mg/day	6.3%	
Nemeroff et al., 2001 (77)	Paroxetine	35	10 weeks	33 mg/day	0.0%	All patients on lithium; switch rate significantly lower on paroxetine vs. imipramine, but two of the three imipramine patients who developed mania and the 1 placebo patient who developed mania were in subtherapeutic serum lithium level group
	Imipramine	39	10 weeks	167 mg/day	7.7%	
	Placebo	43	10 weeks	N/A	2.3%	
Silverstone, 2001 (81)	Moclobemide	78	8 weeks	450–750 mg/day	3.7%	"Switch" defined as Young Mania Rating Scale score >10
	Imipramine	78	8 weeks	150–250 mg/day	11.0%	
Vieta et al., 2002 (92)	Paroxetine	30	6 weeks	32 mg/day	3.0%	Open-label randomized; paroxetine and venlafaxine both effective and safe in treatment of depressive breakthrough episodes in bipolar disorder; there was a suggestion of a slightly higher risk for switch to mania or hypomania with venlafaxine
	Venlafaxine	30	6 weeks	79 mg/day	13.0%	

N/A = not available.

TABLE 19–8B. Reported Rates of Emergent Mania in Association with Antidepressants in Nonrandomized Studies of Bipolar Depression

Study	Medication	Sample Size	Study Duration	Mean Dose	Switch Rate (%)	Comments
Fogelson et al., 1992 (65)	Bupropion	11	6 weeks	286 mg/day	54.5	Coexisting lithium and carbamazepine or valproate in 5 of 6 patients who switched
Baldassano et al., 1995 (64)	Paroxetine	20	8 weeks	23 mg/day	5.9	1 patient on lithium + carbamazepine developed hypomania
Kupfer et al., 2001 (93,94)	Citalopram	45	8-week acute, then 16-week continuation	34.5 mg/day	6.7	All subjects on lithium, valproate, or carbamazepine
Erfurth et al., 2002 (90)	Bupropion	13	4 weeks	286 mg/day	0.0	Bupropion added to diverse combination therapies in a treatment-refractory group

more stable depressions. More recently, Serretti and colleagues (2003) conducted a retrospective case–control study of 169 bipolar patients who switched while taking an antidepressant versus 247 who did not (matched for age and gender); they also found switches more likely with the DMI pattern. On the other hand, MacQueen and colleagues (2002) presented detailed life-chart data for 42 bipolar depressed patients indicating that those whose depression was preceded by a manic/hypomanic episode (presumably the MDI pattern) were more likely to have an antidepressant-related switch than those whose depression was preceded by a period of euthymia. Given the design and size of these studies, it appears fair to conclude that the weight of the literature suggests switching is more likely to be associated with the DMI pattern. A third factor studied is comorbid substance abuse. Goldberg and Whiteside (2002) found that switch risk was associated with a history of substance abuse and/or multiple previous antidepressant exposures.

What about the relative risk in bipolar-I versus bipolar-II? By far the majority of the data on switching has come from studies of bipolar-I patients, although some of the studies reviewed above included both bipolar-I and -II patients. Two studies (Joffe et al., 2002; Serretti et al., 2003) noted more switching in bipolar-I than in bipolar-II, while two found no difference (Henry and Demotes-Mainard, 2003; Bauer et al., 2005). The resolution of this question has been advanced considerably by two sets of data from the Stanley Network—one concerning acute treatment (Altshuler et al., 2006) and the other focused on long-term follow-up (Leverich et al., 2004). Both reveal that, compared with bipolar-I patients, those with bipolar-II have a lower switch rate, and when they do switch, it is into hypomania.

Finally, as might be expected, Sato and colleagues (2004) found that bipolar patients with depressive mixed states (see Chapters 1 and 2) are more likely to switch when antidepressants are added to mood stabilizers than are bipolar patients with "pure" depression. Related findings come from an analysis of the NIMH STEP-BD database (Goldberg et al., 2004), which found that among bipolar patients with depressive mixed states, antidepressants worsened manic symptoms without improving depressive ones. In a recent comparison of switchers and nonswitchers among bipolar patients on antidepressants in the Stanley Network, Frye and colleagues (2006) found three specific manic-like symptoms during depression that were associated with a switch—more motor activity, more talkative, and showing new interests; increased sexual activity just missed significance. The results of these last three studies are important for the clinician to keep in mind because such "depressive mixed states" are often confused with agitated depression; the specificity of the individual symptom predictors in Frye and colleagues' study should prove especially useful to the clinician.

Do antidepressant-related switches differ from spontaneous ones? In a prospective study of consecutive admissions, Tamada and colleagues (2004) compared 12 patients on mood stabilizers who switched within 12 weeks of starting an antidepressant and 12 patients with spontaneous mania. Those who switched while taking an antidepressant had been ill longer with more previous episodes, had a higher prevalence of subclinical hypothyroidism, and had a history of more previous antidepressant-related switches. In the largest observational study comparing spontaneous and antidepressant-related switches, Akiskal and colleagues (2003) evaluated 493 consecutive patients with DSM-IV major depression (196 were bipolar-II or bipolar-NOS; bipolar-I patients were excluded). Spontaneous hypomania was experienced by 29 percent of the entire cohort; an additional 10.5 percent were hypomanic only while on antidepressants. The latter group had experienced significantly more psychotic features, greater suicide risk, a more chronic course with more previous hospitalizations, and more previous treatment with mood stabilizers, and were less responsive to lithium. Finally, in an interesting retrospective case–control study of 56 bipolar depressed patients on an antidepressant, Mundo and colleagues (2001) found that those with the short allele of the promoter region of the serotonin transporter gene experienced twice as many switches as those without that allele.[49]

In summary, the most consistently reported predictors of antidepressant-related switching among patients with bipolar-I disorder are a history of multiple acute episodes (particularly those with a course characterized by the DMI sequence), exposure to multiple antidepressant trials, a history of previous antidepressant-related switches, a history of substance abuse, and isolated manic-like symptoms ("depressive mixed states"). Risk among patients with bipolar-II disorder is also associated with substance abuse and perhaps with psychotic features, but appears to differ from bipolar-I risk by its association with a more chronic course. In light of the two recent Stanley Network studies, it now appears likely that the relative risk is greater in bipolar-I than in bipolar-II, but more data are needed to settle this point, particularly with respect to long-term destabilization. For comprehensive reviews of clinical and demographic predictors of antidepressant-related switching, see Goldberg and Truman (2003) and Visser and Van der Mast (2005).

Related to switching is the phenomenon of conversion from a unipolar to a bipolar diagnosis, which bears on the question of which patients with unipolar depression might be vulnerable to an antidepressant-related switch. Examining the relationship between the likelihood of such a conversion and premorbid personality characteristics, Akiskal and colleagues (1995) followed 559 patients with major depressive disorders for up to 11 years.[50] They reported a "temperamental triad" of mood lability, energy/activity,

and "daydreaming" as being predictive of the conversion from unipolar to bipolar-II, but not to bipolar-I. This triad was associated with early age at first depression, chronicity, and a high rate of substance abuse. The association between early age at onset of unipolar depression and subsequent switch to a bipolar diagnosis has been noted in several studies.[51] In the Akiskal et al. (1995) study just described, switching from unipolar to bipolar-I was associated with psychotic features when the patient was depressed, a finding that agrees with those of Kovacs (1996), Coryell and colleagues (1995), and Goldberg and Whiteside (2002).

Are there differences among the antidepressants in their propensity to precipitate switching? Among the older drugs there was some indication that, compared with MAOIs, tricyclics were associated with switches that occurred more rapidly and led to more severe dysphoric manias (Himmelhoch et al., 1991). The most important question today is whether the newer, second-generation drugs are associated with a lower prevalence of switching. Peet (1994) assessed manic symptoms in unipolar depressed patients taking part in clinical trials (some bipolar-II patients participated since DSM-IIIR did not include that condition under bipolar illness) who were taking SSRI versus tricyclic antidepressants. To do so, he performed a post hoc analysis of data from randomized clinical trials of fluoxetine, fluvoxamine, paroxetine, and sertraline and comparison groups treated with tricyclics or placebo. He found switch rates below 1 percent in all the unipolar groups. The switch rate in the bipolar group taking an SSRI was not significantly different from that in the placebo group—about 4 percent—and was significantly lower than an 11 percent switch rate reported in the studies involving tricyclics. The relative position of the newer versus older drugs in this study is probably more valid than the absolute percentages because the database of clinical trials Peet examined reflected the result of vigorous efforts to screen out patients with mania/hypomania or even with risk factors for switching, such as a history of substance abuse. Also, as noted above, the ethical requirements of randomized controlled trials mean that patients with any sign or symptom suggesting the possibility of mania are very likely to be dropped from the study, resulting in the undercounting of manic switches. Therefore, it is not surprising that Peet's post hoc analysis yielded results differing from those of some observational studies, including the work of Altschuler and colleagues (1995) and Ghaemi and colleagues (2004). For example, the latter study found that 49 percent of bipolar depressed patients switched within 2 months of starting a second-generation antidepressant (primarily SSRIs); most of these patients were also on a mood stabilizer.

In a study comparing desipramine and bupropion, Sachs

and colleagues (1994) found a switch rate in the tricyclic group five times higher than that in the bupropion group over a 1-year follow-up period (50 percent [5/10] versus 11 percent [1/9]). The authors therefore speculated that bupropion might be especially safe with respect to switching. Consistent with this speculation is the observation of Erfurth and colleagues (2002), who reported no switches with bupropion in a 4-week study of 13 bipolar patients on a mood stabilizer. However, the results of one nonrandomized study employing a much higher dose of the old immediate-release (IR) formulation (450 versus 200 mg) are at odds with the purported low incidence of mania following the initiation of bupropion. Fogelson and colleagues (1992) found that 6 of 11 bipolar patients taking lithium or an anticonvulsant developed hypomanic or manic symptoms when 450 mg of IR bupropion was added. However, 10 of these 11 patients had previously cycled into mania when prescribed an antidepressant, suggesting that this may have been a particularly vulnerable group, not representative of the larger population of patients with bipolar disorder. Also relevant here is the report of Goren and Levin (2000) on the case of a bipolar patient who did not develop manic symptoms until his dose of bupropion was raised to 600 mg/day. The authors reviewed several other case reports of manic symptoms associated with bupropion and concluded that the risk of inducing manic symptoms increases significantly in patients taking more than 450 mg/day.[52]

What about venlafaxine? In our earlier review of efficacy studies, we cited the work of Vieta and colleagues (2002), who compared venlafaxine and paroxetine in bipolar depressed patients on a mood stabilizer. The rate of development of manic symptoms was four times higher in the venlafaxine group (13 versus 3 percent), a rate similar to that reported for tricyclics in other studies.[53] This result is consistent with that of a 10-week study from the Stanley Network (Post et al., 2003) (previously mentioned in our review of efficacy) in which 174 bipolar patients (73 percent bipolar-I) experiencing a breakthrough depression on lithium, valproate, or a combination of the two were randomized under double-blind conditions to bupropion, sertraline, or venlafaxine. While response and remission rates were similar with all three antidepressants, there were significantly more switches into mania/hypomania[54] with venlafaxine (29.2 percent) than with sertraline (8.6 percent) or bupropion (9.8 percent). If venlafaxine resembles the tricyclics in its tendency to precipitate manic symptoms, this may be due to its dual reuptake inhibition, both serotoninergic and noradrenergic. However, in a short-term (6-week) study of venlafaxine monotherapy in 17 bipolar-II patients, Amsterdam (1998) observed no switches into mania.

Cycle Acceleration. In addition to the issue of acute switches following the initiation of antidepressants, antidepressants may be associated with increased cycling over the longer course of bipolar disorder. While maintenance treatment is the subject of the next chapter, we discuss here the effect of antidepressants on the long-term course of the illness since this is a key consideration in planning the acute treatment of bipolar depression. Indeed, compared with the issue of acute switching, of which most clinicians are well aware, we consider it even more important to emphasize the potentially damaging effects of cycle acceleration because it is a phenomenon so easily missed by clinicians who do not use life charting. Moreover, formal studies addressing cycle acceleration involve methodological challenges. As far back as 1965, the German literature reported that tricyclic antidepressants may cause destabilization, increasing the frequency of recurrences after the acute treatment of a depressive episode (Arnold and Krysprin-Exner, 1965; Till and Vuckovic, 1970). Furthermore, the very first report of an antidepressant (the MAOI iproniazid) cited rapid cycling following initiation of the drug (Crane, 1956). In the first edition of this text we reviewed a number of case reports, retrospective reviews, and uncontrolled prospective studies, as well as the placebo-controlled studies of Wehr and Goodwin (1979b) and Quitkin and colleagues (1981) (see below), all of which involved tricyclics (with some MAOIs included in the naturalistic studies). Taken together, the results of these studies were consistent with the conclusion reached by earlier observers, as were the more contemporary findings of Altshuler and colleagues (1995) (cited above in our discussion of acute switches). The latter authors studied 51 hospitalized bipolar-I patients retrospectively using life charting; 25 percent of the subjects experienced cycle acceleration while on tricyclics or MAOIs. Similar studies finding no such association have also been conducted (for a review see Altshuler et al., 1995). Nonetheless, the best data available—from both a small and a larger randomized clinical trial (see below)—indicate that cycle acceleration following the initiation of tricyclics does occur.

One factor that may contribute to the mixed results in the literature is that antidepressant-related cycling may be relatively gender specific, with females being more vulnerable. This confound was suggested by Yildiz and Sachs (2003), who found that among 129 bipolar patients, the association between subsequent cycling and prior antidepressant use held only for females. This finding is reminiscent of an earlier report by Quitkin and colleagues (1981), discussed above in the section on antidepressant-related switching.

Much of the literature examining the issue of increased cycling in bipolar disorder in apparent association with tricyclics or MAOIs has approached the question by attempting to identify episodes of rapid cycling that are temporally related to initiation of the antidepressant. A large observational study of patients with bipolar disorder conducted by Coryell and colleagues (1992) found no association between periods of antidepressant use and rapid cycling. In this study, 919 patients were followed for at least 1 and up to 5 years, with semiannual evaluations; patients' treatment was monitored but not controlled by the study. Nearly 1 in 5 patients experienced a period of rapid cycling; after controlling statistically for episodes of major depression, the authors found that treatment with tricyclics or MAOIs "did not seem to anticipate rapid cycling" (p. 129). Rather, the authors suggested that an episode of major depression heralding a period of rapid cycling is a feature of the natural history of the illness, and that any association between antidepressant treatment and rapid cycling is thus an epiphenomenon. However, this conclusion appears to be overstated since the patients were not randomized to receive or not receive antidepressants, and it is impossible to know why clinicians chose to use or not use the drugs for some patients or at certain times.

In the first edition we made a similar point about the influential study of Lewis and Winokur (1982), who opened the debate when they reported no increase in switching or cycling among a group of bipolar patients receiving acute and continuation treatment with tricyclics chosen by the physician. The interpretation of their finding is quite problematic, however, in view of the high switch rate among the untreated controls (41 percent) and the variety of uncontrolled factors that could lead to such a high rate among patients whose physicians chose not to administer antidepressants. The negative conclusion from this study was reinforced by Angst (1985), who, when reanalyzing his data on admission patterns from 1920 to 1982 (see Fig. 19–3), inexplicably combined the ECT-era data (with their expected high switch rates) with the data from the presomatic treatment era and concluded that switch rates did not increase after the introduction of tricyclics. In sum, controlled studies examining the course of bipolar disorder over the longer term have consistently identified patients in whom there appears to be a clear relationship between tricyclic antidepressants and acceleration of the illness cycle (see Table 19–9).

Wehr and Goodwin (1979a) presented data on a small group of patients closely followed prospectively over a period of years at NIMH in a placebo-controlled clinical trial. These patients entered and exited a series of double-blind studies in which they took lithium plus placebo or lithium plus tricyclics for periods of up to a year, thus serving as their own controls. When the length of the cycle (onset of mania to onset of mania) was compared for periods on and off antidepressants, a striking shortening of cycle became evident during periods of antidepressant therapy. Moreover, cycling slowed again when the antidepressant was stopped. Lithium provided no protection against cycling in these patients.

In a subsequent and larger controlled clinical trial, Wehr and colleagues (1988) found a similar temporal relationship between antidepressant treatment and shortening of the mood cycle in about half of a group of 51 patients with rapid-cycling bipolar disorder on lithium (see Table 19–9). The inability of a mood stabilizer to prevent tricyclic-related

TABLE 19–9. Randomized, Placebo-Controlled Studies of Antidepressant-Related Long-Term Mood Destabilization of Bipolar Illness

Study	Sample Size	Mean Duration of Follow-up (Months)	Treatments	Results
Wehr and Goodwin, 1979a	5	27	Lithium + desipramine vs. lithium + placebo	4 times more rapid cycling in lithium + desipramine treatment vs. lithium + placebo treatment alone
Quitkin et al., 1981	75	19	Lithium + imipramine vs. lithium + placebo	2.4 times more manic episodes in lithium + imipramine group vs. lithium + placebo group
Wehr et al., 1988	51	59	Lithium + tricyclics vs. lithium + placebo	33% higher rapid-cycling rate with lithium + tricyclics vs. lithium + placebo

Note: Long-term mood destabilization in these studies is limited to cycle acceleration, defined as two or more DSM-IV affective episodes during antidepressant treatment versus similar exposure times immediately before antidepressant treatment. The Quitkin and colleagues (1981) finding was a post hoc finding. Other randomized controlled trials with tricyclics failed to find evidence of worsened course in post hoc analyses. The Wehr and Goodwin (1979) and Wehr and colleagues (1988) studies were the only studies designed to assess prospectively the issue of antidepressant-induced mood destabilization, and they both found evidence for this association.

Source: Ghaemi et al., 2003b. Reprinted with permission.

cycling was also noted in the randomized, double-blind, parallel-group comparison of lithium plus placebo versus lithium plus imipramine discussed earlier; over the 3 years of this prospective study, there were 2.4 times more manic episodes in the lithium plus tricyclic group than in those taking lithium plus placebo (Quitkin et al., 1981) (see Fig. 19–4). These placebo-controlled prospective trials represent the best data available for establishing that tricyclic-related cycle acceleration does indeed occur. The answer to the question of how frequently it occurs must come from larger naturalistic studies. As noted earlier, Altshuler and colleagues (1995) reported cycle acceleration occurring in about a quarter of recently hospitalized bipolar patients when their course of illness was studied retrospectively. Other observational studies have likewise reported frequent tricyclic-related cycle acceleration (for example, Koukopoulos et al., 1980).

What about the effects of the second-generation antidepressants on cycle length? Joffe and colleagues (2002) addressed this question in a prospective, open, naturalistic study of SSRIs and bupropion. They examined 113 individual antidepressant trials involving 69 bipolar-I and -II patients, identifying cycle shortening using the life-charting method developed by Post and colleagues (1986); patients were followed for at least 1 year. In 6 of the individual trials (7.8 percent), patients showed acceleration in their cycling. Of these 6 patient trials, 5 involved bipolar-I disorder, and all 5 were SSRI trials; all the patients were taking lithium or anticonvulsant medication or a combination thereof in addition to the antidepressant.

In two other naturalistic studies (Ghaemi et al., 2000, 2004) rates of antidepressant-related cycle acceleration were

23 and 25.6 percent, respectively, figures higher than those reported by Joffe and colleagues (2002) but very similar to data from the Stanley Network. In a year-long evaluation of the treatment of bipolar depression with adjunctive antidepressants, 39 percent of patients experienced at least one switch during the continuation phase, suggesting cycle acceleration (Post et al., 2003; Altshuler et al., 2006). In a subsequent analysis of the Stanley Network trial of the use of newer antidepressants for breakthrough depression in patients maintained on lithium, valproate, or a combination of the two (Post et al., 2006), 49–53 percent of patients met criteria for response, but switching and/or cycle acceleration (overall rate of 21 percent) was twice as likely among responders. As discussed earlier, bupropion had the most favorable ratio of response to switch/cycle acceleration, while venlafaxine had the least favorable. In a preliminary analysis of the STEP-BD data, Sachs and colleagues (2003) found that while depressive morbidity did not differ between bipolar patients given a second-generation antidepressant with a mood stabilizer and those given a mood stabilizer alone, the antidepressant-treated patients experienced 60 percent more manic episodes. Sachs and colleagues (2004) coined the term "roughening" to describe destabilization involving mood lability of an amplitude that does not reach criteria for an episode of depression or mania, but there have not yet been quantitative studies of this phenomenon. Here it is worth recalling the STEP-BD study described earlier (Filkowski et al., 2006; Ghaemi et al., 2006), in which bipolar patients randomized to antidepressant continuation did no better (in terms of overall mood morbidity over 1 year) than those on a mood stabilizer alone, and in fact experienced more rapid relapse and more manic episodes, albeit fewer full depressive episodes.[55]

In another independent examination of data from STEP-BD, Goldberg and Truman (2003) found that a switch into mania/hypomania was observed in 19.5 percent of 1,250 antidepressant trials within 3 months of initiation of the antidepressant. These antidepressant "switchers" were more likely to switch again if reexposed to another antidepressant of the same class. By contrast, a recent naturalistic prospective study of 80 bipolar-I and -II patients, 47 of whom were taking antidepressants (92 percent were second-generation drugs), found no more switches or cycling in those on antidepressants (Bauer et al., 2005). The incidence of switching and rapid cycling did not differentiate bipolar-I from -II. It is important to note that 89 percent of those taking antidepressants were also taking at least one mood stabilizer. Of interest, patients on antidepressants in this naturalistic setting reported more depression than those not on antidepressants. Of course, as we observed previously, it is impossible in a naturalistic study of this kind to know what factors may have influenced the decisions of

Figure 19–4. Inability of mood stabilizer to prevent antidepressant-related cycling during a 3-year randomized double-blind prospective study. Note: Average relapse time was 7–19 months, reflecting cycle induction rather than acute switching. (*Source*: Quitkin et al., 1981.)

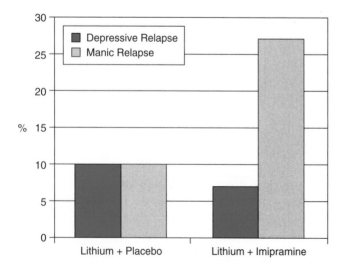

individual clinicians to use or not use antidepressants in a particular patient (confounding by indication).

Although not absolutely conclusive, results of the available studies indicate that at least some patients with bipolar disorder experience an acceleration of their illness during periods of treatment with antidepressants and that for many if not most patients, this effect is reversible when the antidepressants are stopped (Wehr and Goodwin, 1979b; Wehr et al., 1988). As is apparently the case with the induction of mania and hypomania by antidepressants, cycle acceleration may be more common in bipolar-I than in bipolar-II patients, although this has not been established by comparative controlled trials. Rates associated with SSRIs may not be lower than those associated with tricyclics or MAOIs, and results of one study suggest that the risk may actually be higher (Goldberg and Truman, 2003). In contrast to switches, the risk of cycle acceleration may not be reduced by simultaneous treatment with lithium or anticonvulsant medications, although further research on this critical question is clearly needed.

It is often assumed that cycle induction must involve manic or hypomanic symptoms. But in patients taking a combination of an antidepressant and an effective antimanic mood stabilizer, the mood stabilizer may well prevent the manic symptoms, so that the underlying cycle is evidenced only by an increased frequency of depressive episodes. Finally, a frequently observed phenomenon that may reflect cycle induction is the development of tolerance to an antidepressant; that is, rather than being viewed as a loss of the effect of the antidepressant, tolerance can just as easily be thought of as the medication's ongoing effect—driving the cycle and bringing the next natural episode closer. Thus in a previously mentioned observational study of 40 bipolar and 38 unipolar patients (Ghaemi et al., 2003c), loss of effectiveness after response was noted in 57 percent of the bipolar patients but only 18 percent of the unipolar patients. Consistent with this observation are the findings of Sharma and colleagues (2005), who studied clinical characteristics of 61 depressed patients initially referred as unipolar with a history of loss of response to at least two antidepressants. On follow-up and reevaluation, 80 percent of these patients were found to have DSM-IV bipolar disorder or met criteria for bipolar spectrum disorder by the criteria of Ghaemi and colleagues (2002).

Antipsychotics

Prior to the introduction of the newer atypical antipsychotic agents, the literature on the use of antipsychotic medications in the depressed phase of bipolar disorder was quite sparse. In one open study, flupenthixol decanoate was given to 30 lithium-intolerant periodic and cyclic depressive patients, some of whom had a history of mania, and was found to have a "prophylactic effect . . . similar to the effect of lithium salts" (Kielholz et al., 1979, p. 307). Consistent with this finding, several retrospective studies have reported depressive relapse in patients with bipolar disorder after discontinuation of typical antipsychotics (see, e.g., Hendrick et al., 1994). On the other hand, as noted in the previous chapter, the treatment of mania with typical antipsychotics alone was not infrequently followed by a postmania depressive episode.

The use of atypical antipsychotics in the treatment of depression has drawn increasing interest. In case reports and open studies, these agents appear to have beneficial effects when added to SSRI and MAOI antidepressants (for a review see Thase, 2002). A randomized, double-blind clinical trial found an olanzapine–fluoxetine combination to be superior to either agent alone in nonpsychotic treatment-resistant depressed patients (Dube et al., 2002).

With regard to bipolar depression, in the largest randomized clinical trial ever conducted in this population (n = 833), olanzapine monotherapy was found to be superior to placebo. The effect size was quite modest, however, and the bulk of the improved rating items related to sleep and appetite rather than to core mood symptoms. On the other hand, combination of olanzapine and fluoxetine (included in the Cochrane analysis discussed above) was found to be substantially superior to placebo and to olanzapine alone (Tohen et al., 2002), with an effect size equivalent to that for lamotrigine and, like lamotrigine, producing improvement in core depressive symptoms (Williamson et al., 2006). During the 8-week duration of the study, the switch rate was low and comparable in all three groups, and it stayed low (5.9 percent) throughout a subsequent 24-week open-label extension study (Corya et al., 2006). A fixed-dose olanzapine–fluoxetine combination (OFC-Symbyax) has been approved by the FDA as a treatment for bipolar depression. Recently, OFC was compared head to head with lamotrigine in a 7-week randomized double-blind trial in 410 bipolar-I depressed patients. While there was no significant difference in response rates,[56] time to response showed an advantage for OFC, as did the extent of reduction in MADRS ratings and CGI severity scores. However, there were significantly more side effects with OFC (somnolence and sedation, increased appetite, weight gain, dry mouth, and tremor), as well as higher levels of triglycerides and cholesterol. Indeed, the seriousness of the weight gain and metabolic problems associated with some atypicals (especially olanzapine and OFC) has to be taken into account when assessing the risk/benefit ratio of these drugs; this point is made in the most recent set of guidelines for the treatment of bipolar depression, the Texas Algorithm (Suppes et al., 2005).

Evidence for the efficacy of another atypical—quetiapine—in the treatment of depressive symptoms in a variety of psychotic and mood disorders (including bipolar disorder, rapid-cycling bipolar disorder, and adolescent mania) has been reported in several open-label studies.[57] More recently, two large randomized, placebo-controlled trials revealed robust antidepressant effects for quetiapine in bipolar patients. These 8-week multisite studies involved a total of 506 bipolar depressed patients (339 on quetiapine and 167 on placebo; two-thirds bipolar-I, one-third bipolar-II) (Calebrese et al., 2005). The first study found a 58 percent response rate (greater than 50 percent decrease in MADRS scores) compared with 36 percent for placebo; the rate for remission (decline in MADRS scores of less than 12) was 53 percent for quetiapine versus 28 percent for placebo. The core depressive items on the MADRS scale[58] showed significant separation from placebo ($p < .001$). Onset of action was rapid, with separation from placebo at the end of week 1; both doses of quetiapine—300 and 600 mg —were roughly equivalent in efficacy, but side effects (dry mouth, sedation/somnolence, dizziness, constipation) were more common at the higher dose. The effect size with the 300 mg dose was equivalent to that achieved with the olanzapine–fluoxetine combination (OFC), and at 600 mg it exceeded the latter results. However, the magnitude of the quetiapine effect was substantially reduced when the items related to insomnia and anxiety were removed from the analysis. Similar results were obtained in the replication study (Hirschfeld et al., 2006), and the FDA has now approved quetiapine for the treatment of bipolar depression.

It is important to note that studies of DSM-IV-defined bipolar depression (such as the above quetiapine studies) can include patients with up to three manic-like symptoms (because of the strict DSM-IV definition for a mixed episode, that is, meeting full criteria for both mania and depression). Whether these "depressive mixed-state" patients may respond preferentially to antipsychotics has not yet been reported, but the possibility should be assessed. Most formal studies of antipsychotics in mixed states per se use the DSM-IV criteria and therefore involve dysphoric mania rather than depressive mixed episodes, but such data may still have relevance to the evaluation of these agents as possible antidepressants. For example, Gonzalez-Pinto and colleagues (2001) compared two groups of patients with dysphoric mania, all of whom were treated with either valproate or lithium but also took either typical antipsychotics (haloperidol and/or levomepromazine) or an atypical (olanzapine). Patients treated with the adjunctive atypical had statistically significant reductions in HAM-D scores (as well as Young Mania Rating Scale scores) compared with those who took the typical antipsychotic.

Other atypical antipsychotics, including clozapine, risperidone, ziprasidone, aripiprazole, and amisulpride (which is available in Europe but as of this writing not in the United States), have, to varying degrees, been shown to be effective in ameliorating depressive symptoms in patients with schizophrenia, and for some of these drugs, when used adjunctively, there is evidence of efficacy in treatment-resistant depression. Some are now undergoing testing in bipolar depression. Whether monotherapy with some atypical antipsychotic agents will turn out to be sufficiently robust to achieve remission in the majority of patients with bipolar depression remains an open question.

Electroconvulsive Therapy

There is an extensive literature on the use of ECT in the treatment of major depression (see Fink, 2001, for a review, and Abrams, 1997, for a comprehensive discussion). Approximately 50 years after the introduction of ECT, Janicak and colleagues (1985) conducted a careful meta-analysis of 25 studies selected for their rigorous methodology, which together included more than 1,200 patients. These studies variously compared ECT with simulated ECT, placebo, tricyclics, and MAOIs and found indisputable evidence of the superiority of ECT over all these other treatments for severe depression. Most of these studies included patients with both unipolar and bipolar illness. This conclusion was reinforced by the most recent and most extensive meta-analysis comparing ECT with pharmacotherapy, conducted by the UK ECT Review Group (2003). Examining 18 trials (1,144 patients), they found that ECT was significantly better than antidepressant medication. As noted earlier, ECT has been shown to be a safe and especially effective treatment for elderly patients, including the very elderly (Salzman et al., 2002); it has also proven to be safe in pregnant patients (Miller, 1994) and even those with intracranial mass lesions (Zwil et al., 1990). Indeed, one can find reports of ECT having been administered to patients safely and successfully regardless of almost any imaginable medical or psychiatric complication.

There is a modest amount of data on the use of ECT specifically to treat bipolar depressed patients. Zornberg and Pope (1993) reviewed nine studies of the use of ECT in 723 such patients. Of the seven trials comparing ECT with antidepressant agents, five found it be more effective. ECT appears to be equally effective for unipolar and bipolar depressed patients. Daly and colleagues (2001) compared the response rates and rapidity of response to ECT in 228 patients with unipolar and bipolar-I and -II depression who were participating in three different protocols. There was no difference in efficacy rates[59] among the diagnostic groups, although the bipolar patients who responded to ECT needed fewer treatments than the unipolar responders.

Grunhaus and colleagues (2002) also found no unipolar–bipolar differences.

It appears that clinically significant ECT-induced mania is rare. Given that ECT is a highly effective treatment for mania, this is perhaps not surprising. Nevertheless, there have been a number of case reports of mania and hypomania following ECT (see, e.g., Serby, 2001), and one case series found that about a third of 57 patients with depression (unipolar or bipolar not specified) treated with ECT had hypomanic symptoms following their course of treatment (Koukopoulos et al., 1980). In another retrospective chart review study, however, the switch rate into mania or hypomania in hospitalized bipolar patients who had received ECT did not differ from that in bipolar patients who had not received the therapy (Angst et al., 1992). The evidence for cycle induction or acceleration caused by ECT per se is even less convincing, especially since most patients who receive ECT are treated with antidepressants either during or following the therapy (see Koukopoulos et al., 1980).

Novel Central Nervous System Stimulation Techniques

Transcranial Magnetic Stimulation

Transcranial magnetic stimulation (TMS) takes advantage of a principle of electromagnetism first demonstrated in 1831 by the British physicist Michael Faraday: one can induce an electrical current in a conductor by bringing a changing magnetic field in close proximity to it. In TMS, an apparatus that develops a rapidly changing magnetic field is applied to the scalp (hence the more common name for the technique—rapid transcranial magnetic stimulation, or rTMS) to induce a small current in underlying neural tissue (see Daskalakis et al., 2002, for a review). Unlike ECT, rTMS does not produce a seizure[60] or even alteration of consciousness, and thus can be carried out without anesthesia on individuals with only the most minimal discomfort from scalp tingling and the noise generated by the apparatus. The technique has been used for neurophysiological studies and is increasingly being used as a treatment for depression and other psychiatric conditions.

Because sham rTMS is easily performed, it has been possible to carry out placebo-controlled studies of the treatment. In a comprehensive review and meta-analysis of 23 randomized controlled studies of rTMS in treating depression, Burt and colleagues (2002) noted that the effect was highly significant statistically, and the average effect size was substantial, raging from .67 to .79. This is essentially the same conclusion reached in an earlier meta-analysis of 12 studies by Holtzheimer and colleagues (2001).[61]

As with other new interventions for treating depression, the literature on rTMS is evolving. The current lack of consistency regarding the size of the effect across studies may be due to differences in technique (right- versus left-side stimulation, for example) and overselection of treatment-resistant patients for some studies, as well as other factors. The ultimate role of rTMS in the treatment of mood disorders is far from clear, but the results of controlled studies thus far are encouraging. There have been two small studies involving patients with bipolar depression. In the first, Dolberg and colleagues (2002) randomized 20 patients to TMS or sham TMS (5 sessions per week); by the end of the second week, the TMS group showed a greater reduction in HAM-D ($p < .05$) and BPRS ($p < .01$) scores compared with the sham group. In a subsequent study of bipolar depression (Nahas et al., 2003), left prefrontal TMS showed only a nonsignificant trend to outperform the sham condition, but there were too few subjects (N = 23) to rule out a type II error.

Other types of magnetic stimulation may turn out to be helpful in the treatment of bipolar depression. Rohan and colleagues (2004) investigated the antidepressant effects of exposure to magnetic stimulation less intense than that of the rTMS technique, spurred by the serendipitous observation of mood improvement in subjects with bipolar depression who had volunteered for a neuroimaging study of bipolar disorder. Echo-plantar magnetic resonance spectroscopic imaging (EP-MRSI) is a neuroimaging technique that also employs oscillating magnetic fields, but the magnetic force generated is weaker and more generalized than that in rTMS. Significant differences in mood improvement were observed in subjects who received actual EP-MRSI compared with those receiving sham EP-MRSI (Rohan et al., 2004).

Vagus Nerve Stimulation

Zabara (1988) first demonstrated that experimental seizures in dogs could be ameliorated by electrical stimulation of the vagus nerve (cranial nerve X), and in 1988, the first vagus nerve stimulator was implanted in a human patient to treat epilepsy. The sensory connections of the vagus project to many brain regions, including the locus coeruleus and other regions implicated in the regulation of mood. After antidepressant effects were reported in patients who had received a vagus stimulator, interest developed in vagus nerve stimulation (VNS) as a treatment for depression, and the first VNS device was implanted in a patient to treat depression in 1998. In VNS, a programmable electrical pulse generator (much like a cardiac pacemaker) is implanted subcutaneously in the chest wall, and a lead is connected to the left vagus nerve near the carotid artery in the neck. (For reviews of VNS, see George et al., 2000, and Krahl et al., 2004.)

Rush and colleagues (2000) conducted an open multicenter study of 21 unipolar, 4 bipolar-I, and 5 bipolar-II patients with treatment-resistant major depressive episodes. They found that 40 percent achieved at least a 50 percent reduction in symptoms (as measured by the HAM-D and MADRS) after 10 weeks of VNS. Analysis of the efficacy of VNS in this group, expanded by the addition of another 29 patients (for a total of 59, including 6 bipolar-I and 10 bipolar-II subjects), found similar results—a 31 percent response rate with a 15 percent remission rate (Rush et al., 2005)—but those with the most treatment resistance (having failed 7 or more antidepressant trials) did not benefit (Sackeim et al., 2001). In a 1-year follow-up of those completing 3 months of acute treatment, the benefits of VNS were sustained, and there was some indication of additional benefit, with a significantly increased proportion of these patients achieving remission from their symptoms— 29 percent versus 17 percent in the original 10-week study (Marangell et al., 2002). In a subsequent 2-year follow-up of the same cohort, Nahas and colleagues (2005) confirmed that the response rate at 1 year surpassed that at 3 months (31 percent versus 44 percent), with the additional improvement persisting at 2 years (42 percent response rate). The same collaborative group (George et al., 2005) compared the 1-year results of Marangell and colleagues (2002) with those achieved in a separate study of patients with treatment-resistant depression receiving similar treatment as usual (TAU); the patients in this 1-year observational study of TAU had baseline clinical characteristics and demographics that were statistically comparable to those of the patients in the VNS study. VNS plus TAU was superior to TAU alone as assessed by monthly improvement in the self-rated Inventory of Depressive Symptomatology (IDS-SR) across 12 months ($p <.001$) or by response rates (last observation carried forward [LOCF] analysis of changes in HAM-D scores): 27 percent for TAU plus VNS versus 13 percent for TAU alone ($p < .01$); post hoc analysis revealed no unipolar–bipolar difference in response to VNS.

In the largest controlled study of acute VNS to date, Rush and colleagues (2005) randomized 235 patients with treatment-resistant depression[62] to VNS or sham VNS for 10 weeks. While the primary outcome variable—response as measured by a 50 percent decline in HAM-D score (LOCF analysis)—did not show a significant difference between VNS (15.2 percent response rate) and sham treatment (10 percent response), a secondary outcome—IDS-SR—did (17 percent versus 7.3 percent response rate, $p = .032$, by LOCF analysis). Thus it appears that VNS, especially when evaluated over 1 year or more, is somewhat more effective than TAU for a very difficult-to-treat group of patients, many of whom have bipolar or recurrent unipolar depression. A VNS device has been approved by the U.S. FDA for just such patients and is now marketed by Cyberonics.

Dopamine Agonist Agents

The role of dopaminergic agents in the treatment of mood disorders is evolving, and preliminary data are encouraging. Several currently available antidepressants (bupropion, sertraline, and venlafaxine) inhibit presynaptic dopamine reuptake to varying degrees. One selective dopamine reuptake inhibitor, nomifensine, was marketed as an effective antidepressant for about 10 years in Europe and more briefly in the United States before being withdrawn because of associated hemolytic anemia.

Bromocriptine, a dopamine agonist used in the treatment of Parkinson's disease, has been reported to be an effective antidepressant in several small studies comparing it with tricyclic antidepressants in patients with major depressive disorder (see Perugi et al., 2001, for a review). The drug has never gained wide acceptance as an antidepressant, however, perhaps because it lacks clear superiority over available agents and is associated with a substantial side-effect burden. Pergolide, a dopamine agonist 20 to 30 times more potent than bromocriptine, has been used to augment antidepressant treatment of major depression in both unipolar and bipolar patients. In one open study, 11 of 20 refractory depressed patients experienced improvement when pergolide was added to either a tricyclic or MAOI. Transient hypomanic symptoms in some patients responded to lowering the dose of the drug (Bouckoms and Mangini, 1993).

The antidepressant effects of pramipexole, another potent dopamine agonist that has been used to treat Parkinson's disease, have also been investigated in both unipolar and bipolar patients. A number of case reports and open studies indicate those effects to be significant, especially when the drug is combined with other agents. In one of these open trials, a related compound, ropinirole, showed similar results. In a retrospective evaluation of 32 unipolar and bipolar patients treated with pramipexole for depression for an average of 6 months, there was only one case of transient hypomania (Sporn et al., 2000). And in the first double-blind, randomized clinical trial of pramipexole in treating bipolar depression, Goldberg and colleagues (2004) found it to be significantly superior to placebo and reported a mania/hypomania switch rate of 7 percent. A second randomized, placebo-controlled study involving 21 patients with bipolar-II disorder found a 60 percent response rate (greater than 50 percent decrease in MADRS score) for pramipexole compared with 9 percent for placebo; 1 patient developed hypomania, compared with 2 in the placebo group (Zarate et al., 2004). Ironically, there are more data from randomized, double-blind, placebo-controlled trials for the efficacy and safety of pramipexole in bipolar depression than for all but one standard antidepressant (paroxetine), yet the other standard antidepressants are used much more extensively than pramipexole.

Psychostimulants

The use of amphetamine drugs and related compounds, such as methylphenidate, in the treatment of symptoms of depression has a long history. These agents have been used alone, as well as in conjunction with antidepressant and other psychotropic agents, for several decades in the treatment of mood disorders, and a large but often rather confusing body of literature is frequently cited in support of these uses. The verdict on stimulants as the sole agents for treating major depression is, however, quite clear. In a review of the literature on the use of stimulants as monotherapy for the treatment of primary depressive disorders, Satel and Nelson (1989, p. 248) concluded that these agents "demonstrated no significant advantage over placebo in the treatment of primary depression." Nevertheless, a large body of literature supports the use of stimulants to treat depressive symptoms for patients with debilitating medical conditions in which fatigue and lethargy are prominent features, such as acquired immunodeficiency syndrome (AIDS) (Wagner and Rabkin, 2000), as well as for those who experience the opiate-related fatigue and somnolence that occur in the palliative care of patients with cancer) (see Rozans et al., 2002, for a review). Whether the improvement seen in these patients can be called an antidepressant effect or simply the amelioration of primarily somatic depressive symptoms seen in seriously ill patients is a matter of debate, however. The lack of significant and sustained efficacy in patients who have more uncomplicated depression would appear to argue for the latter conclusion.

Several case reports and open series support the use of stimulants as an augmentation strategy in patients with major depression who have only a poor or incomplete response to antidepressant medications. Stoll and colleagues (1996), for example, reported on five patients who cited robust symptom reduction when methylphenidate was added to SSRI antidepressants. The literature on the use of stimulant medications in treating bipolar depression is very limited, however, perhaps in part because of clinicians' reluctance to report their experiences treating patients with a controlled substance. A retrospective chart review of eight adolescent bipolar patients (both bipolar-I and -II) treated consecutively with adjunctive stimulants for comorbid attention-deficit hyperactivity disorder (ADHD) indicated moderate symptomatic improvement and substantial functional improvement, with no evidence of switching or abuse (Carlson et al., 2004). Still, a number of case reports suggest that stimulants can induce manic and hypomanic states (see Lake et al., 1983, for a review), and this work is often cited as a reason to avoid the use of these drugs in bipolar patients. In one open case series, when methylphenidate was added to an existing mood stabilizer in 15 bipolar patients experiencing a breakthrough depression, a 56 percent mean reduction in MADRS scores was observed over the next 3 weeks. However, 20 percent of the patients dropped out because of hypomania or anxiety/agitation (El-Mallakh, 2000). This issue is an important one in planning the treatment of children or adolescents with bipolar disorder because of the comorbidity of bipolar disorder and ADHD in these age groups and because of suggestive evidence that stimulants may hasten the onset of bipolar disorder in children (see Chapter 23).

Modafinil is a novel psychostimulant that has less dopaminergic activity and appears to have less abuse potential than older stimulant medications. In a retrospective case series of seven patients who took modafinil as an adjunct to antidepressant medication, three patients with bipolar depression achieved full or partial remission (Menza et al., 2000). A subsequent prospective trial (DeBattista et al., 2004) indicated that among 33 patients whose major depression had been only partially responsive to 4 weeks of antidepressant use, there was a rapid and significant improvement in both fatigue and overall depressive symptoms for the group as a whole ($p < .0001$). This was followed by a large (N=314), multicenter, 8-week randomized, placebo-controlled study of adjunctive modafinil (200 mg) among partial responders to SSRIs with persistent fatigue/sleepiness (Fava et al., 2005); compared with placebo, modafinil was associated with significantly more improvement on the CGI scale. To our knowledge, there has been only one controlled study of adjunctive modafinil in bipolar depression (Frye et al., 2005). Among the 41 patients randomized to modafinil (100–200 mg/day), there were significantly more responders than among the 44 placebo patients ($p = .038$), with no difference in manic switches. The absence of switches was also noted in a retrospective chart review of 39 bipolar patients who received modafinil at some point during their treatment (Nasr et al., 2006). However, we should note that two cases of manic-like symptoms have been reported among patients taking this drug (Ranjan and Chandra, 2005).

Hormonal Agents

Hypothalamic–Pituitary–Thyroid Axis

There is a substantial literature on the use of thyroid hormones in the treatment of mood disorders, as well as on the interrelationships between mood disorders and abnormalities of the hypothalamic–pituitary–thyroid axis. A higher-than-expected prevalence of clinical and subclinical hypothyroidism, elevations of circulating antithyroid antibodies, and levels of fT_4 significantly lower than those of controls have all been reported in patients with bipolar disorder.[63]

The early reports of Gjessing (1938) (from the prelithium era) that hypermetabolic doses of thyroid hormone could stabilize periodic catatonia (now thought to be related to bipolar disorder) represented the first suggestion that thyroid enhancement could affect behavioral or mood stability. Since then, virtually all of the data on the subject have related to adjunctive use of thyroid hormone, generally T_3 in acute depression and T_4 in maintenance treatment.

Results of open and placebo-controlled studies conducted over several decades support the adjunctive use of T_3 for patients unresponsive to antidepressants alone. The positive results of the first controlled study of this combination treatment (Goodwin et al., 1982) were confirmed by most subsequent studies, as indicated by a meta-analysis (Aronson et al., 1996) that examined eight studies involving a total of nearly 300 patients with depression refractory to tricyclic antidepressants whose treatment was augmented with T_3. The authors concluded that this strategy effectively doubled the response rate compared with that of control groups, but also cautioned that the various studies were uneven in quality and, although encouraging, could not be considered definitive. In another analysis of this literature, Joffe (1992) concluded that the addition of T_3 was an effective augmentation strategy in 55–60 percent of tricyclic-refractory depressed patients. Reports of successful augmentation of SSRIs (Joffe, 1992; Abraham et al., 2006) and MAOIs (Joffe, 1988) have appeared as well.

Another treatment strategy involving thyroid hormone is the use of T_3 to accelerate the response of depressive symptoms to antidepressant medications. A meta-analysis of this literature by Altshuler and colleagues (2001b) included six placebo-controlled studies in which "relatively untreated" depressed patients (unipolar or bipolar not specified)—that is, patients who had not been selected for refractory depressive symptoms—were started on T_3 along with amitriptyline or imipramine. It was found that patients who started on 20–25 micrograms (μg) of T_3 along with a tricyclic experienced a statistically significant acceleration of their treatment response compared with those who did not receive the thyroid hormone. It was also found that the effect size of this intervention increased as the proportion of female patients in the studies increased.

It has been proposed that the augmentation effect of T_3 on antidepressant treatment is the result of an interaction between thyroid hormone and serotonergic neurotransmitter systems. This hypothesis is based on various findings—for example, that administration of T_3 to animals results in increased cortical serotonin concentration and reduced sensitivity of auto-inhibitory 5-hydroxytryptamine (1A) (5-HT_{1A}) receptors in the raphe area (see Bauer et al., 2002).

It has also been postulated that the benefits of thyroid hormones in treating depression derive from their effect on subtle thyroid dysfunction that might be clinically insignificant in persons who are not depressed. Cole and colleagues (2002) examined the relationship between pretreatment thyroid hormone levels and time to treatment response in 65 depressed bipolar-I patients and found a significant association between lower-normal fT_4 index (FTI) and higher-normal TSH levels. Patients with FTI values above the mean and TSH values below the mean experienced remission of their symptoms an average of 4 months sooner than other patients in this group. The authors concluded that nearly two-thirds of bipolar patients may have a thyroid profile that, although technically in the normal range, is nevertheless inadequate for an optimal treatment response. They cited these results in support of the hypothesis that the low-normal thyroid functioning seen in some patients represents an inadequate homeostatic response to the stress of a depressive episode. Similar results come from a recent chart review of 135 bipolar-I patients on maintenance medication (primarily lithium), which revealed that the 36 percent with chemical evidence of hypothyroidism, compared with those without such evidence, spent significantly longer in acute treatment and had significantly higher HAM-D scores during maintenance treatment (Fagiolini et al., 2006).

The use of supraphysiological thyroid hormones in the treatment of bipolar disorder has also been the subject of considerable interest, primarily for patients with rapid-cycling mood episodes, but also for depressed patients (Bauer and Whybrow, 1986, 1990; Whybrow, 1994). After noticing what appeared to be a more rapid response of depressive symptoms to high-dose T_4 in treatment-resistant, non-rapid-cycling bipolar patients, Bauer and colleagues (1998) conducted an open trial of a high-dose T_4 augmentation strategy. In this study, 17 patients with major depression (12 with bipolar depression) who were taking various combinations of antidepressants, lithium, and anticonvulsants were started on T_4, with the dose gradually being raised to 500 mg/day, double the usual maximum recommended dose for the treatment of hypothyroidism. Of the 17 patients, 10 experienced remission (defined as a greater than 50 percent reduction in HAM-D scores, with a final score of less than 9) within 12 weeks of starting on high-dose T_4. In open-trial investigations of high-dose T_4 treatment by this same group, approximately 50 percent of patients with treatment-resistant depression of a mean duration of more than 15 months experienced remission (defined as above) (Rudas et al., 1999). Patients with nonrapid but nevertheless "intractable" bipolar cycling experienced a significant reduction in the number of mood episodes when T_4 was added to other treatments.

Although the importance of normal thyroid functioning for the regulation of mood appears clear, the mechanisms by which thyroid function, dysfunction, and manipulation affect mood are unclear, and apparent contradictions abound. It is well known, for example, that depression can be a symptom of both hyperthyroidism and hypothyroidism. The administration of thyroid hormones, sometimes in supraphysiologic doses, to some depressed patients is effective in treating depression. Yet increased levels of T_4 are consistently reported in association with major depression, and a reduction of circulating T_4 (free and/or total) is seen after successful treatment with ECT, antidepressants, and bright light, as well as after cognitive psychotherapy (see Bauer et al., 1998).

Whether the addition of thyroid hormones to other treatments for depression corrects a subtle thyroid dysfunction in some patients, sensitizes a target cortical system important to mood regulation through manipulation of monoamine mechanisms, or works by some other as yet unknown mechanism remains to be elucidated. (These issues are also discussed in Chapter 20.)

Hypothalamic–Pituitary–Adrenal Axis

Abnormalities in the functioning of the hypothalamic–pituitary–adrenal (HPA) axis have been reported in association with mood disorders for several decades (see Chapter 14). Elevated plasma cortisol levels in depressed patients were first reported in the 1950s. Subsequent investigations have demonstrated in depressed patients elevated cortisol levels in the urine and cerebrospinal fluid, enlarged pituitary and adrenal glands, and a loss of the normal circadian rhythm of cortisol secretion by the adrenal gland (as demonstrated by a positive dexamethasone-suppression test). This HPA overactivity is thought to be caused by oversecretion of corticotropin-releasing hormone (CRH) by the hypothalamus, possibly in response to a dysfunction of glucocorticoid receptors in patients with mood disorders.[64] Chronically high levels of circulating glucocorticoids have been implicated in the mood symptoms and cognitive impairment seen in depressed patients.

Cortisol-lowering agents have been used to treat unipolar and bipolar depressed patients, with mixed results. Ketoconazole has been the most frequently investigated cortisol-lowering drug, but aminoglutethimide and metyrapone have been used as well. Case reports and small open series in unipolar and bipolar depressed patients have shown encouraging results, with some patients experiencing dramatic and long-lasting symptom remission (see Brown et al., 2001, for a review). One small placebo-controlled study found significant reductions in HAM-D scores in nine patients with major depression (unipolar or bipolar not specified) treated with ketoconazol monotherapy for 4 weeks compared with patients given placebo, but only in those patients who were hypercortisolemic prior to participating in the study (Wolkowitz et al., 1999a). Another placebo-controlled study found no advantage of ketoconazol over placebo (Malison et al., 1999).

Substantial risks of hepatotoxicity and hypoadrenalism have limited the investigation and routine clinical use of cortisol-lowering agents. Nevertheless, because of the striking and consistent findings of glucocorticoid abnormalities in patients with mood disorders, interest in the HPA axis as a therapeutic target remains high. Substantial work on corticotropin-releasing factor (CRF) antagonists is ongoing (see Holsboer, 2001), and the glucocorticoid receptor antagonist mifepristone (RU-486) has been investigated as well (see Wolkowitz and Reus, 1999, for a review of the use of various antiglucocorticoid agents).

Dehydroepiandrosterone (DHEA) is a steroid compound secreted by the adrenal gland that, along with its sulfate-ester metabolite (DHEA-S), is one of the most abundant circulating adrenal hormones. DHEA and DHEA-S are precursors to testosterone and estrogen and have been proposed to have a broad range of effects on mood. DHEA levels progressively decrease after age 30, and treatment with supplemental DHEA has been reported to increase the sense of well-being in aging men and women. DHEA acts as an antiglucocorticoid and has been shown in animal studies to counteract deleterious neuronal effects of cortisol. Young and colleagues (2002) found an elevated cortisol/DHEA ratio in 39 drug-free unipolar depressed patients compared with 41 healthy comparison subjects. In a small double-blind study, DHEA either alone or with an antidepressant effected a greater than 50 percent decrease in HAM-D scores in about half of depressed patients and none of those receiving placebo. This study included two bipolar-II depressed patients, but the authors did not report which group they were assigned to or whether they were responders (Wolkowitz et al., 1999b).

DHEA is widely available in vitamin stores and supermarkets in the United States as a dietary supplement and is promoted as an antiaging compound that enhances mood, immune functioning, and even libido. Younger persons, especially young men, also take DHEA because of its reported effect of increasing muscle mass. There have been several case reports of mania in individuals with bipolar disorder (Dean, 2000), as well as in those with no previous psychiatric history (Kline and Jaggers, 1999), who started taking DHEA. Decisions on its use in men over 50 should take into account a possible increase in the risk of prostate cancer related to any elevation of androgen levels.

While the potent effects of various glucocorticoids in producing or exacerbating affective syndromes have been clearly demonstrated, elucidation of the mechanisms of these effects remains speculative. The rational therapeutic use of pharmaceutical manipulation of the HPA axis to ameliorate mood disorder symptoms has thus far proven an elusive goal.

Hypothalamic–Pituitary–Gonadal Axis

As with the other endocrine systems discussed above and in Chapter 14, clinical research and epidemiological data clearly indicate that the physiology of the hypothalamic–pituitary–gonadal (HPG) endocrine axis is important in mood disorders. The increased prevalence of depressive illness in women and the striking vulnerability of women with bipolar disorder to manic episodes during the postpartum (puerperal) period are but two examples of the probable influence of this system on mood. The mechanisms of these influences are, however, even more obscure than in the case of other endocrine systems. HPG abnormalities in patients with mood disorders have yet to be convincingly demonstrated, in either women (for an overview see Young and Korszun, 2002) or men (see Schweiger et al., 1999).

There is some evidence that depressive symptoms in women who also have low serum estrogen levels can be ameliorated by the administration of estrogen. Several open studies have demonstrated the benefits of estrogen therapy in women with postpartum depression. Ahokas and colleagues (2001) found that the administration of ß17-estradiol reduced MADRS scores from a mean of over 40 to 11 in 23 postpartum women who had abnormally low serum estrogen levels. The authors found similar results in 10 women with postpartum psychosis also having abnormally low estrogen levels (Ahokas et al., 2000). Although these studies did not include women diagnosed with bipolar disorder, their findings may have some relevance to the treatment of bipolar depression, given the high risk of developing mania during this period for women with bipolar disorder.

The addition of estrogen did not improve the response of premenopausal depressed women to imipramine in several early studies (see, e.g., Shapira et al., 1985). Results of more recent studies in perimenopausal and postmenopausal women, however, support the efficacy of physiologic doses of estrogen in treating a variety of depressive disorders. The largest study to date was a double-blind, placebo-controlled study conducted by Soares and colleagues (2001) in which 50 women received transdermal ß17-estradiol for 12 weeks as monotherapy for major depression, minor depression, or dysthymia. More than 68 percent of the patients experienced remission as measured by scores of less than 10 on the MADRS, compared with 20 percent of the patients who received placebo.

Although there have to our knowledge been no studies on the treatment of bipolar depressed women with estrogen preparations, results of the above studies suggest a possible role for the hormone in bipolar women with low serum estrogen levels. The risk of malignancies and other serious complications of estrogen replacement therapy, however, makes estimating the risk/benefit ratio of such a strategy difficult, particularly since the Women's Health Initiative Study (National Institutes of Health, 1991) did not include data on depression.

Testosterone replacement has been reported to help alleviate depressive symptoms in men with low testosterone levels. In an open study conducted by Seidman and Rabkin (1998), five men with low testosterone levels and SSRI-resistant major depression experienced complete remission of depression (mean score of 4 on the HAM-D) after 8 weeks of taking testosterone in addition to the SSRI (Seidman and Rabkin, 1998). As with estrogen, long-term side effects of testosterone treatment are not known, including whether there is an increased risk of prostate cancer, and the relevance of this finding to the treatment of bipolar disorder is far from clear.

Sleep Deprivation

Since first being described in the 1970s, the antidepressant effect of sleep deprivation has been replicated in numerous studies involving various diagnostic groups: unipolar as well as bipolar depression, depression with psychotic features, premenstrual dysphoria, depression associated with dementia, and even negative symptoms of schizophrenia (for a review see Wirz-Justice and van den Hoofdakker, 1999, and Wu and Bunney, 1990). Indeed, nearly two-thirds of depressed patients will experience an improvement in mood after sleep deprivation. Unfortunately, about 80 percent of such (unmedicated) patients experience a relapse into depressed mood after their next night's sleep (Wu and Bunney, 1990). Indeed, even a brief nap has been found to result in relapse of depressed mood in 50 percent of patients (Wiegand et al., 1987), with morning naps being more detrimental than those in the afternoon (Weigand et al., 1993). Repeated sleep deprivation has been evaluated as a stategy for maintaining the initial antidepressant effect, and studies alternating 3 nights of total sleep deprivation (three cycles of 36 hours of wakefulness) with 3 nights of sleep (Benedetti et al., 1996; Barbini et al., 1998; Colombo et al., 2000) have found some sustained benefit.

There is some evidence that patients with bipolar depression respond better than unipolar depressed patients to sleep deprivation. In a carefully designed study, Barbini and colleagues (1998) compared the response to sleep deprivation in patients with bipolar-I depression, bipolar-II depression, a first episode of major depression, and "unipolarity" (defined as having had three or more previous major depressive episodes and no family history of bipolar disorder in first-degree relatives). No patients had taken lithium or antipsychotics in the 6 months before sleep deprivation, and none had taken antidepressants in the week prior to the study. After three cycles of total sleep deprivation (no sleep on nights 1, 3, and 5 of the study and ad lib sleep on nights 2, 4, and 6), both groups of bipolar patients had significantly larger decreases in HAM-D scores compared with the unipolar patients. The bipolar patients also reported significantly more improvement in their perceived mood than did the unipolar patients, as measured by a visual analog scale. Although the numbers of patients in this study were small, the results are striking and confirm the findings of several (though not all) earlier studies hampered by methodological problems.

Pharmacotherapy has been demonstrated to prevent rapid relapse into depression following sleep deprivation in a significant proportion of patients. Benedetti and colleagues (1999) found that hospitalized depressed patients with bipolar-I disorder who had responded to three cycles of total sleep deprivation were more likely to continue to be in remission 10 days after the last sleepless night if they had been taking lithium for at least 6 months (14 of 20 patients) prior to the sleep deprivation cycles, compared with patients not treated with lithium (2 of 20 patients).[65] In subsequent studies of bipolar depressed patients also on lithium, this same group (Benedetti et al., 2001a,b, 2005) found that the beneficial effect of sleep deprivation could be extended by 3 days of subsequent phase advance (in which the patient both goes to sleep and wakes up about 4 hours earlier than normal), a result in agreement with those of others (see e.g., Berger et al., 1997; Riemann et al., 2002) and a strategy suggested in the first edition of this text. In other studies of pharmacological enhancement, Smeraldi and colleagues (1999, 2003) found that mood benefits were sustained 4 days after sleep deprivation when depressed bipolar-I patients were given pindolol, an antagonist of the presynaptic serotonin receptor (which therefore increases serotonin release in the central nervous system). In addition, pindolol significantly improved the overall efficacy of sleep deprivation, suggesting that the effect may involve serotonergic mechanisms.

The rate of switch into mania and hypomania after sleep deprivation appears to be at least comparable to that associated with the SSRIs and other newer antidepressants. In an open series of 206 bipolar depressed patients treated with three cycles of total sleep deprivation either alone or in combination with other medications, Colombo and colleagues (1999) observed that about 5 percent of the patients developed manic and 6 percent hypomanic symptoms. However, some patients may be more vulnerable than these data suggest. In the NIMH study reviewed in the first edition (Wehr et al., 1982), nine rapidly cycling patients in a depressed phase were asked to simulate a 48-hour sleep–wake cycle by remaining awake for 40 hours; eight switched out of depression, and seven were rated as manic or hypomanic. For further discussion of sleep deprivation and phase advance, see Chapter 16.

Phototherapy

A seasonal pattern of symptoms is common among mood disorder patients (see Chapter 16). A retrospective analysis of the records of more than 1,500 patients with affective disorders entering outpatient treatment in Italy found that about 10 percent had a seasonal pattern of symptoms. Of these patients, about half had a unipolar and half a bipolar affective disorder, with bipolar-I diagnoses outnumbering bipolar-II about three to two in the group (Faedda et al., 1993). In the first edition of this text, we reviewed 11 studies of SAD, reporting that the proportion of patients who met criteria for bipolar disorder (-I or -II) ranged from 8 to 90 percent, a degree of variation that may reflect both regional differences in seasonal extremes and variation in diagnostic criteria. Our weighted average of the 11 studies in the first edition (45 percent) is higher than that of the Faedda data, as well as that of other more recent studies. This difference may reflect some broadening of the diagnostic criteria for SAD since the syndrome was first described by Goodwin's group at NIMH (Rosenthal et al., 1984).

Since the first description of the improvement of symptoms of SAD in response to bright light (Rosenthal et al., 1984), there have been numerous studies of phototherapy in depressed patients. An early meta-analysis of trials involving a total of 332 patients found improvement rates of 67 percent in mildly depressed patients and 40 percent in patients with "moderate to severe depression" (Terman et al., 1989); maximum improvement was correlated with exposure to at least 2,500 lux for 2 hours a day. Morning light exposure appears to be more effective than evening (Lewy et al., 1998). More recently, shorter exposure to higher-intensity light has been demonstrated to have equal benefit.[66]

While these open studies have demonstrated the benefits of monotherapy with bright light in depressed patients, the results of attempts at placebo-controlled studies have been much more mixed, perhaps because these studies have been hampered by methodological problems. The studies have varied in the timing and intensity of light exposure, and designing true placebo-controlled studies has been challenging. A study comparing light exposure of 6,000 lux for 1.5 hours a day in the morning or evening with "sham negative ion generators" in 96 patients with SAD found a statistically significant difference between morning light and the sham condition in the number of patients achieving complete or nearly complete remission (61 versus 32 percent).[67] When the mean change in depression ratings was measured in this study, however, there was no difference in efficacy between bright light and placebo (Eastman et al., 1998). A similar study comparing bright light with an active negative ion generator found no difference in the two treatments (Terman et al., 1998).

Although earlier work emphasized the benefits of phototherapy in patients with disorders displaying a seasonal component, the treatment appears to help those without a seasonal symptom pattern as well (Kripke, 1998; Tuunainen et al., 2004; Golden et al., 2005). As with other treatments effective in depression, there have been case reports associating light therapy with switches into mania/hypomania, and a meta-analysis of 20 controlled studies of light therapy in nonseasonal depression (from the Cochrane database) found a 4.9-fold increase in risk for hypomania associated with the treatment (Tuunainen et al., 2004). As with sleep deprivation, the combination of phototherapy and pharmacotherapy appears to be the most useful strategy. Results of several European studies indicate a possible synergistic effect of the two treatments (see, e.g., Colombo et al., 2000; Benedetti et al., 2003; and the review of Kripke, 1998). For a more comprehensive discussion of SAD and the antidepressant effect of bright light, see Chapter 16.

Nutritional Supplements

Various herbal preparations and other nutritional supplements reported to help individuals with mood disorders have received extensive publicity in the lay press. Often touted as "natural" and therefore supposedly superior to synthetic pharmaceuticals, nutritional preparations have fervent adherents and equally fervent critics (a rather striking exception is the tendency to overlook lithium as a natural substance). Frequently, neither group is well informed about the scientific literature, or lack thereof, that supports their use. Patients will frequently ask about nutritional supplements, and the clinician should have some familiarity with them and be comfortable in making suggestions regarding their use (for an overview, see Wong et al., 1998a; Desai and Grossberg, 2003).

St. John's Wort

The medicinal use of St. John's wort (*Hypericum perforatum*) dates to ancient times and is recommended in the medical texts of Pliny and Hippocrates, as well as in Burton's seventeenth-century classic *The Anatomy of Melancholy*. Contemporary use of hypericum extract has been as an antidepressant, with hypericin being the putative active ingredient. Hypericum extract shows affinity for the several neurotransmitter receptors, and serotonin reuptake inhibition and monoamine oxidase inhibition have been proposed as its mechanisms of action (reviewed by Wong et al., 1998a). Hypericum's side-effect profile is generally quite benign, but clinically significant interactions with warfarin, human immunodeficiency virus (HIV) proteases, theophyllin, digoxin, and pharmaceuticals metabolized by the cytochrome P450 system have been reported (Henderson et al., 2002). Hypericum has also been noted to be associated with the onset of hypomania.

Early studies of hypericum extracts as antidepressants were hampered by variability in the extracts used, subtherapeutic doses of comparison drugs, and heterogeneity of patients. Subsequent controlled studies have led to conflicting conclusions about efficacy and resulted in intense controversy in both the scientific and lay press. Although several placebo-controlled studies from Europe have demonstrated superior efficacy for hypericum compared with placebo (see Kasper and Dienel, 2002, for a meta-analysis), two large studies from the United States have not (Shelton et al., 2001; Hypericum Depression Trial Study Group, 2002). Shelton and colleagues' study assigned 340 outpatients with major depression to three groups treated with either hypericum, sertraline, or placebo. No difference in efficacy was found among any of the groups as measured by the HAM-D. Sertraline but not hypericum was more effective than placebo in bringing about improvement as measured by the CGI scale. Hypericum extracts have not been studied as a treatment for bipolar patients, although there have been case reports of manic symptoms thought to have been caused by their use (Nierenberg et al., 1999).

Hypericum extract continues to be widely recommended in Europe for the treatment of depression. Enthusiasm for its use has waned in the United States, however, perhaps as a result of increasing concern about significant drug interactions in the face of its equivocal efficacy for treating depression.

Omega-3 Fatty Acids

Docosahexaenoic acid (DHA), ethyl-eicosapentaenoate (EPA), and linoleic acid are naturally occurring fatty acids abundant in brain tissue and the retina that cannot be synthesized by the body (hence the term *essential* fatty acids). Dietary intake is thus the only source of these substances, which are found in significant amounts in cold-water fish and such plant oils as canola, soybean, and flaxseed oils.

Omega-3 fatty acids are thought to play important roles in cell membrane fluidity and neuronal signal transduction. Epidemiological studies have indicated that a diet rich in omega-3 fatty acids is protective against coronary and cerebrovascular disease (Djousse et al., 2001), and it has been suggested that omega-3 fatty acids have anti-inflammatory effects and may even inhibit tumor growth (Tevar et al.,

2002). It has also been suggested that differences in diet, specifically fish consumption, may underlie epidemiological differences in rates of depression among various populations (such as certain Asian and Western populations) and explain the increasing incidence of depression in contemporary societies (Hibbeln et al., 1998; Mischoulon and Fava, 2000; Hibbeln, 2002; Freeman et al., 2006). These data have led to intense interest in supplemental omega-3 fatty acids as treatment for mood disorders (reviewed by Parker et al., 2006 and Freeman et al., 2006).

Stoll and colleagues (1999) reported that fish oil capsules containing omega-3 fatty acids were superior to placebo (olive oil capsules) in preventing relapse over a 4-month period in 30 patients with bipolar disorder otherwise receiving (and resistant to) "usual" treatment.[68] In this study, very high doses of fish oil capsules were used (over 9 grams/day of the combination of EPA and DHA), but later studies have generally used much lower doses. In a subsequent study of bipolar patients with depressive symtoms and functional impairment, Osher and colleagues (2005) reported that the open-label addition of 1.5–2.0 grams of EPA was associated with 50 percent or greater improvement in 8 of 10 patients who were followed for at least 1 month. More recently, Frangou and Lewis (2006) conducted a study involving 75 moderately depressed bipolar patients not responding to 8 weeks of conventional treatment. The patients were randomized under double-blind conditions to adjunctive placebo (n = 26) or EPA at either 1 gram (n = 24) or 2 grams (n = 25) over 12 weeks. There was significantly more improvement in the EPA-treated groups than in the placebo group, while the two doses of EPA were equivalent.

There have been somewhat more studies focusing on major depression. In a placebo-controlled study of 20 unipolar patients who were experiencing major depressive symptoms despite 4 months of treatment with antidepressants (mainly SSRIs), the addition of 2 grams/day of EPA, DHA, or both resulted in a more than 50 percent reduction in HAM-D scores, compared with a 10 percent reduction among patients taking placebo (Nemets et al., 2002). Likewise, in a double-blind, placebo-controlled trial of adjunctive combined EPA/DHA, Su and colleagues (2003) found a significantly greater reduction in HAM-D scores in the omega-3 group.

There have been fewer studies of omega-3 fatty acids as monotherapy. In a double-blind, placebo-controlled study of DHA, 36 patients with major depressive disorder showed no significant difference compared with placebo (Marangell et al., 2003). On the other hand, in a study of EPA monotherapy in patients with unipolar depression, Peet and Horrobin (2002) found 1 gram/day more effective than placebo; however, there was no effect at higher doses (4 and 9 grams). Their positive findings at lower doses of EPA are

similar to those of Zanarini and Frankenburg (2003) in an 8-week study of 30 borderline personality disorder patients. The negative results of Peet and Horrobin at higher doses are similar to those of the Stanley Foundation Bipolar Network study (Keck et al., 2006), in which EPA monotherapy at 6 grams/day over 4 months was no more effective than placebo in 59 patients with bipolar depression and 62 with rapid cycling.

In summary, results of four controlled studies of *adjunctive* omega-3 fatty acids have been positive—two involving bipolar patients and two unipolar patients—but experience with these compounds as *monotherapy* has been, at best, mixed. Since these supplements have essentially no side effects, many clinicians are routinely recommending them for their patients in addition to standard treatment, although more systematic study is still needed.

Inositol

About 1 gram/day of inositol, a precursor of the phosphatidyl inositol second messenger system, is present in a normal diet. There have been reports of reduced inositol in the cerebrospinal fluid (CSF) of patients with unipolar and bipolar depression (Coupland et al., 2005), as well as in the frontal cortex of bipolar patients (Shimon et al., 1997), and one of the proposed mechanisms of action of mood stabilizers involves stabilization of inositol signaling. Orally administered inositol has been shown to increase CSF levels in humans substantially, and at doses of 6–20 g/day has been associated with improvement in unipolar and bipolar depression (Levine et al., 1995; Chengappa et al., 2000). Recently, Edens and colleagues (2006) reported that among 17 bipolar patients allready on lithium or valproate, compared with those on placebo, there was a trend for more subjects on inositol to show improvement in depressive symptoms; this was the case especially in those with high baseline levels of anger and hostility.

S-Adenosylmethionine

S-adenosylmethionine (SAMe) is formed in the body when methionine, one of the essential amino acids, is activated by adenosine triphosphate (ATP) in a reaction catalyzed by methionine adenosyltransferase. SAMe serves as a methyl donor in numerous important transmethylation reactions, including deoxyribonucleic acid (DNA) methylation reactions involved in gene regulation, as well as the catalysis of proteins, phospholipids, and neurogenic amines, including norepinephrine, dopamine, and serotonin (see Lieber and Packer, 2002, for an introduction to this compound). SAMe has been a prescription antidepressant in some parts of Europe for several decades, where it has often been administered parenterally, and it was released for sale in the United States as an (oral) over-the-counter nutritional supplement in 1998. In addition to its purported benefits in treating affective disorders, SAMe has been reported to benefit individuals with osteoarthritis and cirrhosis, perhaps through its antioxidant effects.

Bressa (1994) published a meta-analysis of clinical studies using SAMe either orally or parenterally in doses ranging from 45 mg /day intravenously to 1,600 mg/day orally to treat depressed patients. These studies were hampered by small numbers of patients, variations in route and dosing of SAMe, and short duration (several as short as 7 days and most 14–21 days). Nevertheless, Bressa concluded that SAMe's antidepressant efficacy was significantly superior to that of placebo and comparable to that of tricyclic antidepressants.[69] An earlier open study of 9 patients who were given intravenous SAMe at a dose of 100–200 mg/day for major depressive symptoms included 6 patients with bipolar disorder (Lipinski et al., 1984). Two of these patients developed manic symptoms within days of starting SAMe. A more recent open study of the adjunctive use of this compound (Alpert et al., 2004) noted a 50 percent response rate and a 43 percent remission rate among 45 patients with major depression showing no more than a partial response to an SSRI or venlafaxine.

SAMe appears to have a benign side-effect profile, with only mild gastrointestinal discomfort commonly reported. It has been recommended that individuals taking SAMe supplement its use with a multivitamin that contains folic acid and vitamins B12 and B6 to avoid increases in homocysteine levels.[70] This methyl donor appears to be a promising compound that has been curiously neglected in studies of antidepressants, probably because of questions about whether meaningful amounts reach the brain after oral administration. More study is clearly needed before SAMe can confidently be recommended to patients with depressive disorders, and it should probably be avoided by individuals with bipolar disorder, certainly in the absence of a mood stabilizer.

Botanicals and Vitamin and/or Mineral Supplements

Botanical preparations often recommended by herbalists for symptomatic treatment of insomnia and anxiety include chamomile, kava, lemon balm, skullcap, and valerian. These preparations contain a variety of flavonoids, pyrones, and fatty acids, and several have been shown to provide symptomatic relief of more minor psychiatric symptoms with a very low incidence of side effects (see Wong et al., 1998b, for a more extended discussion).

There has long been interest in treating psychiatric disorders with vitamins and minerals, an endeavor known variously as *nutritional* or *orthomolecular psychiatry*. During the

revival of interest in alternative medicine that occurred in the late 1990s, a preparation of vitamins, minerals, amino acids, and various botanicals (including gingko biloba and germanium sesquioxide), manufactured under the brand name "E.M. Power +," was developed by family members of bipolar patients specifically for the treatment of bipolar disorder. An open study found that 11 patients with bipolar disorder taking other standard medications experienced a 50 percent reduction of symptoms over a period of 6 months when this preparation was added to their other medications (Kaplan et al., 2001). Another nutritional supplement proported to have mood-stabilizing properties is Equilib, but as yet no systematic trials of this supplement have been published. Reports from uncontrolled trials that chromium was associated with substantial improvement in treatment-resistant mood disorders (see, for example, McLeod and Golden, 2000) led to a placebo-controlled trial in 15 patients with major depressive disorder, atypical type (as noted earlier, atypical depression is often antidepressant resistant and overlaps considerably with bipolar depression) (Davidson et al., 2003). This group found that 70 percent of the chromium-treated patients met response criteria compared with none in the placebo group ($p < .02$).

CONCLUSIONS

Even though depression accounts for the preponderance of the morbidity in bipolar disorder, research on bipolar depression has until very recently been minimal compared with that on the acute treatment of mania or the treatment of unipolar depression. As an illustration of this imbalance, one has only to note that every drug developed for the treatment of bipolar disorder—with one recent exception (lamotrigine)—has been introduced as an antimanic agent. Furthermore, we believe the tacit assumption that the antidepressant drugs developed for unipolar depression will show the same risk/benefit ratio for bipolar depression can now be challenged, primarily by data on switch rates and increased cycling among patients taking antidepressants; while such data are not yet conclusive, they are highly suggestive.

The relatively recent findings on the antidepressant effects of the anticonvulsant lamotrigine, the atypical antipsychotic quetiapine, and the combination of olanzapine plus fluoxetine have significantly enlarged the armamentarium for dealing with bipolar depression and clearly represent good news. The bad news, however, is that even with these agents, most patients do not achieve remission. Thus for the majority of patients with bipolar depression, a combination of medications will still be required, a situation that only highlights the unfortunate reality that virtually all of the available controlled data are on monotherapy.[71]

NOTES

1. These new medications include the anticonvulsant lamotrigine and the atypical antipsychotic quetiapine. In addition, the combination of olanzapine and fluoxetine, marketed as a single pill, has been shown to be efficacious in treating bipolar depression.

2. A rapid response to an antidepressant may presage a subsequent manic switch.

3. The "mini relapses" associated with drug-related recovery from a depressive episode can be very discouraging to the patient until they are explained as evidence that the drug is beginning to work.

4. An excellent patient-generated mood chart with instructions on its use can be downloaded from the Web site of the Harvard Bipolar Research Program at <http://www.manic-depressive.org/moodchart.html>, as can the mood chart of the National Institute of Mental Health (NIMH). See the further discussion in Chapter 22.

5. In addition to the literature review that forms the second part of this chapter, these recommendations are drawn from Sachs et al., 2000; Grunze, et al., 2002; and Thase et al., 2003.

6. In the positive parallel-group controlled trial, the 400 mg arm was not statistically different from the 200 mg arm, but these represent averages.

7. The fact that topiramate has been reported to produce depressive symptoms in some patients (*Physicians' Desk Reference*, 2006) should be kept in mind.

8. It has also been suggested that this combination may be called for when a more rapid antidepressant response is needed, but there are no controlled data to support this suggestion.

9. Altshuler and colleagues (2001a) found that over two-thirds of bipolar patients treated with an antidepressant had a relapse of depression within a year of discontinuing the drug, versus less than a third of those who continued it. The incidence of manic relapse was the same in both groups. However, treatments were not randomly assigned, and it appears likely that the patients taken off their antidepressant were doing poorly, including cycling. Further, of the original sample exposed to antidepressants, only 15 percent remained well on antidepressants for up to 1 year, despite continuation. The others either did not respond, became manic, or had other adverse reactions. Thus it is not clear that there are grounds for generalizing these results to more than a minority of bipolar patients.

10. In response to a letter to the editor about potential confounds in the Altshuler et al. study, the authors noted that no subjects with a history of rapid cycling were included among those remaining on an antidepressant during the 1-year observational study; that is, no rapid-cycling patients remained well on long-term antidepressants.

11. For example, Moller and Grunze (2000) cited naturalistic data supporting antidepressant effectiveness in bipolar depression, but not similarly naturalistic data supporting the opposite conclusion.

12. Baker and colleagues' (2003) data could be interpreted as suggesting that olanzapine was superior to placebo in preventing early relapses into mania after acute treatment of the episode.

13. Clozapine appears to pose the highest risk of causing weight gain, followed by olanzapine and quetiapine. There is a lower risk with risperidone and sertindole. Ziprasidone and aripiprazole do not appear to cause weight gain (McAskill et al., 1998; Taylor and McAskill, 2000).

14. Common side effects include headache, eyestrain, jitteriness, and insomnia. It has been suggested that prolonged exposure to full-spectrum light in the absence of a mechanism to screen out ultraviolet wavelengths (which most light boxes have) poses a risk for the development of cataracts and skin cancer. There have also been case reports of the induction of manic symptoms by phototherapy (Terman and Terman, 1999).

15. Although there is now at least one marketed product that employs blue light, almost all efficacy and safety studies have used bright white light.

16. While it may be intuitively appealing to expect that depressed bipolar patients will respond better than unipolar patients to lithium augmentation, this notion has never been studied. A related question—whether a favorable response to lithium augmentation in bipolar patients is simply a response to lithium rather than to the combination of agents—also remains unanswered (see Austin et al., 1991; Ernst and Goldberg, 2002).

17. One study examined the lithium–MAOI combination in patients who had not responded to lithium added to other antidepressants. In this open trial, 12 patients who had not responded to 2 weeks of lithium augmentation of a non-MAOI antidepressant (either desipramine, bupropion, or the experimental drug adinazolam) took the MAOI tranylcypromine with lithium instead (Price et al., 1985). All 12 patients experienced significant improvement in their depression, including two patients with bipolar-II depression who were discharged from the hospital either "much" or "very much" improved.

18. A double-blind, placebo-controlled study involving bipolar and unipolar depressed patients found that 6 of 10 patients refractory to treatment with citalopram alone had a greater than 50 percent reduction in HAM-D scores when lithium was added, whereas only 2 of 14 patients taking citalopram and placebo experienced a similar reduction in symptoms (Baumann et al., 1996). On the other hand, Fava and colleagues (1994) randomized depressed patients refractory to 20 mg of fluoxetine to three groups: an increased dose of fluoxetine (40–60 mg) and augmentation with either lithium or desmethylimipramine (DMI); the 40–60 mg fluoxetine group did significantly better than either augmented group, leading the authors to the conclusion that high-dose fluoxetine is the most effective treatment for partial responders to previous treatment.

19. In a study conducted by Hoencamp and colleagues (2000), 23 patients who had a less than 50 percent reduction in their initial HAM-D scores despite 7 weeks of treatment with 225 mg/day of venlafaxine were given a dose of lithium sufficient to maintain serum levels of .6–1.0 mEq/L. After 7 weeks of this combination treatment, 35 percent of the subjects had a HAM-D score reduction of at least 50 percent. Likewise, Walter and colleagues (1998) found that two adolescents with major depression experienced a rapid improvement in their symptoms when lithium was added to venlafaxine.

20. Some studies purporting to investigate the effect of pharmaceuticals on bipolar "depression" actually focused on the reduction of depressive symptoms in patients in a mixed

affective state, a common finding for a number of anticonvulsants. Unless otherwise noted, the studies of efficacy in bipolar depression detailed here involved patients without mixed symptoms.

21. Given that there were only 45 subjects, this failure to find a difference between valproate and placebo may well reflect a type II error (false negative); such data might be analyzed more meaningfully by using odds ratios with confidence intervals, as suggested by Ghaemi and Hsu (in press). In this study, response to valproate occurred 50 percent more often than response to placebo.

22. Given the evidence suggesting that lithium and valproate (and perhaps other anticonvulsants) may act synergistically on postsynaptic signal transduction, studies of these agents used simultaneously at less than full doses are needed.

23. Kusumakar and Yatham, 1997; Sporn and Sachs, 1997; Calabrese et al., 1999a; Suppes et al., 1999.

24. Patients were randomly assigned to receive one of the three treatments—lamotrigine, risperidone, or inositol. Since many patients had previously taken at least one of these three medications, they could be randomized to two of the three or only one of two, a strategy referred to as "equipoise randomization."

25. See our later discussion of the possibility of underestimating the risk of manic switches when examining data from controlled studies.

26. In an analysis of all controlled studies to date (Ghaemi, personal communication, 2006), the combined frequency of mania, hypomania, or mixed states was 3.7 for lamotrigine-treated patients versus 2.5 for placebo (risk ratio 1.45; 95 percent confidence interval [CI] .62–3.41). To properly evaluate whether this 45 percent difference is real would require a sample size of over 1,000, nearly three times the sample available from the controlled studies. For further discussion of this point, see Chapter 17.

27. On the other hand, Klufas and Thompson (2001) reported on three patients with bipolar disorder taking a variety of other medications who became profoundly depressed shortly after being prescribed topiramate for mild symptoms of irritability, agitation, or depression, a state that remitted within days of discontinuation of the drug. It should also be noted that induction of mania has been reported with topiramate (Schlatter et al., 2001).

28. As noted above, Frye and colleagues (2000) compared gabapentin monotherapy with lamotrigine monotherapy and placebo in 31 patients suffering from refractory bipolar depression (11 bipolar-I and 14 bipolar-II) or unipolar depression (6 patients) using a crossover design. Gabapentin was no more effective than placebo in treating either manic or depressive symptoms.

29. See, for example, Young et al., 1997; Ghaemi et al., 1998; Altshuler et al., 1999; Ghaemi and Goodwin, 2001a.

30. Patients with sensitivity to sulfa compounds should probably not take zonisamide.

31. Of the 8 subjects who completed the 8-week study, 5 had a greater than 50 percent reduction in HAM-D scores and were "much improved" on the Clinical Global Impressions of Improvement (CGI-I) scale.

32. The conclusion of Ghaemi and colleagues is consistent with results of an earlier retrospective chart review that found no difference in the length of the depressive episode among bipolar patients on mood stabilizers and those on mood stabilizers plus antidepressants (Frankle et al., 2002).

33. Fifty-nine percent of those treated with moclobemide were on lithium or an anticonvulsant, compared with 64 percent of those treated with imipramine.

34. Several selective reversible MAO-A inhibitors have been reported to be effective in studies on depression. None are available in the United States. Brofaromine is discussed by Waldmeier (1993) and moclobemide by Waldmeier (1993) and Kennedy (1997).

35. The open design of the Kupfer et al. study was intended to minimize barriers to enrollment in treatment studies: the use of placebo and the need to accept randomization. Surprisingly, however, not only did the study fall far short of its recruitment target, but only 21 of the 45 (47 percent) enrolled subjects met the acute response criteria, and only 31.1 percent achieved sustained remission.

36. Another problem with the study by Cohn and colleagues (1989) was that the imipramine group was titrated up to a target dose of 300 mg, which induced many dropouts due to intolerance, distorting the efficacy comparison with the more tolerable fluoxetine.

37. Three patients who had no response to one agent after 8 weeks made a blind switch to the other agent, for a total of 19 acute treatment trials (10 bupropion and 9 desipramine). No attempt was made to classify the patients as bipolar-I or -II.

38. A standardized clinical monitoring form is used in STEP-BD to collect prospective assessments of symptom severity and assigns a clinical status based on DSM-IV criteria at every follow-up visit.

39. A subsequent report on 349 bipolar depressed patients with concomitant manic or hypomanic symptoms (mixed-state patients) from the STEP-BD program (Goldberg et al., 2004) noted that, while time to recovery was not altered by the addition of an antidepressant to a mood stabilizer, those with a higher level of manic symptoms at baseline experienced more severe manic symptoms later when on the antidepressant–mood stabilizer combination.

40. Patient expectations were one of the variables included in the regression analysis because the study was not blinded.

41. Also, it appeared that antidepressant continuation led to more rapid relapse into a full mood episode, although less frequently a depressive one.

42. Angst actually concluded in this later paper that his data did not support "treatment-induced switching." He suggested that the apparent increase in switching since the introduction of medical treatments for depression was due to an increase in the diagnosis of bipolar disorder in the later decades of the study.

43. A comprehensive listing of references on agents reported to induce manic states, dating from the 1960s through the mid-1990s, can be found in Moller and Grunze (2000).

44. See the studies of Fogelson et al. (1992), Sachs et al. (1994), Amsterdam and Garcia-Espana (2000), Goren and Levin (2000), Nemeroff et al. (2001), Vieta et al. (2001), Erfurth et al. (2002), and Peet (2004).

45. For example, Stoll and colleagues (1994) retrospectively matched the charts of 49 patients who met their criteria for an antidepressant-related switch to 49 patients with spontaneous mania and reported that the antidepressant-related episodes were shorter and less severe.

46. For example, studies of outpatients that do not include family members as sources of information will certainly underestimate the occurrences of mania/hypomania.

47. See, for example, Prien (1984), Bottlender et al. (1998), Serretti et al. (2003), and Mundo et al. (2006); not all studies agree, however (see, for example, Goldberg and Whiteside, 2002).

48. In this meta-analysis, however, important issues of heterogeneity were not explored. In two studies comparing use of an antidepressant without a mood stabilizer and no treatment (placebo only), no mania was observed in any patients—an oddity, if true, since it would suggest that even spontaneous mania did not occur while those patients were studied or that perhaps manic symptoms were not adequately assessed. Another study preferentially prescribed lithium more in the antidepressant group (Cohn et al., 1989), providing possibly unequal protection against mania. While the olanzapine/fluoxetine data suggest no evidence of switch while using antipsychotics, it is noteworthy that in our reanalysis of the lithium plus paroxetine (or imipramine) study, there was a three-fold higher manic switch rate with imipramine versus placebo (relative risk 3.14), with asymmetrically positively skewed confidence intervals (.34, 29.0). As discussed earlier, these studies were not powered to assess antidepressant-induced mania, and thus lack of a finding is liable to be due to type II (false negative) error. It is more effective to use descriptive statistics as above, which suggest some likelihood of a higher manic switch risk at least with tricyclics compared with placebo. Taken together with the results of other studies reviewed showing higher switch rates with tricylics than with other antidepressants, this heterogeneity suggests that one cannot rule out antidepressant switch. Thus, apparent agreement among studies masks major conflict between the results of the only adequately designed study using the most proven mood stabilizer, lithium, and the results of the remaining studies (which used either no mood stabilizer or less proven agents).

49. Unfortunately, Mundo and colleagues' (2001) nonrandomized study did not analyze important potential differences between the two groups, such as treatment duration and use of mood stabilizers.

50. The patients were from the NIMH Collaborative Program on the Psychobiology of Depression-Clinical Studies and had initially sought treatment at one of five university centers, 80 percent of which was inpatient treatment. During prospective follow-up, they received routine care in the community.

51. Rao and Nammalvar, 1977; Coryell et al., 1995; Hantouche et al., 1998; Geller et al., 2001.

52. Of course, at these levels the dose of bupropion must be divided, and with half of it given in the late afternoon, the likelihood of sleep disruption may increase. This in turn may increase the risk of switch.

53. This difference did not achieve statistical significance by t test. Since this study was not powered to rule out mania, the finding is more appropriately evaluated as relative risk ratio with confidence intervals (RR 4.00; 95 percent CI .47–33.7).

54. Defined as an increase of 2 on the 7-point CGI scale for mania. Using the CGI, the mean switch rate for all three drugs was 21 percent, whereas by the more stringent requirement of a Young Mania Rating Scale score of 13 or above, the mean was only 9 percent.

55. Overall mood morbidity, which was the primary outcome of this study, relates to the roughening concept. *Mood morbidity* is defined as meeting any number of DSM-IV mood episode criteria for mania or depression, thus capturing subsyndromal and chronic outcomes, which have been shown to constitute the major morbidity of bipolar illness. Further, overall mood morbidity represents a more sensitive outcome measure than relapse into a full mood episode.

56. Response was defined as a 50 percent or greater reduction in MADRS scores.

57. Zarate et al., 2000; Sajatovic et al., 2001, 2002; DelBello et al., 2002; Vieta et al., 2002; Ghaemi et al., 2003c; Post et al., 2003; Suppes et al., 2004.

58. Sadness, lassitude, inability to feel, pessimistic thoughts, suicidal thoughts.

59. This study did not attempt to determine an overall efficacy rate for ECT in treating unipolar or bipolar depression, and the treatment techniques in the three protocols differed in electrode placement and stimulus strength. A 1986 retrospective review of the naturalistic treatment with ECT of about 400 patients with unipolar and bipolar depression at a university medical center found that about 70 percent of patients in both groups showed marked improvement with the treatment (Black et al., 1986).

60. Seizures can be induced at high levels of stimulation, and rTMS has, in fact, been proposed as an alternative seizure-induction strategy to the direct application of electrical current used in ECT (Lisanby et al., 2001a).

61. For example, in a double-blind controlled study involving 70 depressed patients, Klein and colleagues (1999) demonstrated that right prefrontal rTMS led to a greater than 50 percent reduction in HAM-D scores after 2 weeks (compared with only 25 percent with sham treatment), whereas Lisanby and colleagues (2001b) and others found only a small effect. In a study of 20 bipolar patients, Dolberg and colleagues (2002) reported a significant but only modestly robust effect. However, in interpreting these data it is important to be aware that studies of TMS involve patients who have failed conventional treatments.

62. The patients in both the VNS and sham treatment groups continued to receive their usual treatment.

63. For an overview of the psychoneuroendocrinology of mood disorders and thyroid physiology, see Frye et al. (1999) and Bauer et al. (2002, 2003).

64. For an overview of HPA physiology with special reference to mood disorders, see McQuade and Young (2000).

65. These results are similar to those of the study by Szuba and colleagues (1994).

66. An excellent review of the details of the technique is found in Daskalakis et al. (2002).

67. Measured by a 50 percent decrease in scores on the Structured Interview Guide for the Hamilton-Seasonal Affective Disorder (SIGH-SAD) (the 21-item HAM-D plus 8 additional items concerning common SAD symptoms, such as hypersomnia and increased appetite), as well as a score at the end of the study of 8 or lower.

68. This 4-month relapse prevention study is not clearly either an acute trial or a maintenance trial, so it is reviewed both here and in the next chapter. The benefit of the omega-3 fatty acids appeared to be related primarily to an antidepressant effect; however, the definition of improvement was vague, rendering problematic a definitive interpretation of these results.

69. An Italian group carried out two double-blind comparison studies of SAMe and imipramine (Delle Chiaie et al., 2002). Unipolar depressed patients who met the DSM-IV diagnostic criteria for major depression without psychosis received 150 mg/day of imipramine and either SAMe 400 mg/day given intramuscularly (in a 4-week study) or 1,600 mg/day taken orally (in a 6-week study). In these studies, patients in both SAMe groups had decreases in mean HAM-D and MADRS scores that were not significantly different from those of patients given imipramine. The percentage of responders in the SAMe groups (defined as a greater than 50 percent decrease in HAM-D score) was not significantly different from that in the imipramine group.

70. High homocysteine levels have been thought to contribute to atherosclerosis.

71. The focus of the pharmaceutical industry on monotherapy trials no doubt reflects its perception that regulatory agencies strongly prefer such trials. This strong preference, however, has historically applied selectively to psychiatric drugs.

20 | Maintenance Medical Treatment

Art is long, life short, opportunity fleeting, experiment dangerous, judgment difficult, nor is it sufficient that the physician should attend to his work, but it is necessary also that the patient and those around him should do theirs.

—*Hippocrates (cited in Whitwell, 1936, p. 61)*

Preventing new episodes of manic-depressive illness has been an ambition of clinical investigators since the inherently recurrent nature of the illness was first recognized. In the middle of the twentieth century, the pursuit led many clinicians to treat their patients with intensive psychotherapy, but with little success. Maintenance electroconvulsive therapy (ECT) appeared to be effective for some patients, but it was pharmacology that enabled the realization of this long-standing ambition. The development of lithium as an effective prophylactic treatment for manic-depressive illness was one of the most important advances in modern psychiatry, and it fundamentally altered both the prognosis for patients and the concepts of the disorder. While the earlier trials of lithium prophylaxis were for manic-depressive illness (they encompassed both bipolar and recurrent unipolar disorders), the contemporary literature focuses on the bipolar form.

In the first edition of this text, the terms "maintenance" and "prophylactic" were both used to indicate prevention of *a new episode,* and the maintenance phase of treatment (for non–rapid-cycling bipolar patients) was defined as beginning only after 6 to 12 months had passed since an acute episode. Anything short of 6 months was considered continuation treatment of the acute episode.[1] However, the meaning of these classic concepts has become somewhat obscured in recent years because of the proliferation of "relapse prevention" trials in which (1) the length of the trial is less than 1 year, or (2) even when the length of the trial is adequate, the critical period during which most of the drug–placebo differences can be demonstrated is in the range of 2 or 3 months—in effect, the period *of relapse* after withdrawal of the active drug to which the patient had responded acutely. We took note of these methodological issues in Chapter 17 and do so again in

our subsequent review of the literature when we consider how to interpret relapse prevention data for individual drugs. We do not consider studies whose entire period of observation is less than 6 months to be "maintenance" or "prophylactic" studies, so they are not reviewed in this chapter.

A related issue is how to define "mood stabilizer," a question to which we devoted a great deal of attention in the first edition of this text. The U.S. Food and Drug Administration (FDA) has not defined the term, nor is there yet consensus on the issue among researchers. The strictest definition requires that an agent demonstrate efficacy in the acute treatment of both mania and depression, as well as the ability to prevent future episodes of both (Goodwin and Jamison, 1990; Calabrese and Rapport, 1999; Bauer and Mitchner, 2004). As proposed later in our review of the literature, lithium comes closest to meeting that definition. A somewhat less stringent definition, suggested by Ghaemi (2001), requires a drug to be efficacious in two of three phases of treatment of the illness (acute mania, acute depression, and prophylaxis of mania and/or depression), one of which must be prophylaxis; lithium, lamotrigine (and possibly valproate) fits this definition. The least stringent definition, suggested by Bowden (1998) and Sachs (1996), requires an agent to demonstrate efficacy against only one phase of the illness as long as it does not worsen any other phase, including increasing the frequency of episodes. The atypical antipsychotics as a class fit that definition. Our view is that a demonstration of *prophylactic* efficacy (that is, the prevention of new episodes) should be fundamental to the definition of a mood stabilizer, and that including drugs in this category simply on the basis of acute efficacy against depression and/or mania renders the term so broad as to be essentially meaningless.

As reviewed by Bech (2006) in an essay written in tribute to Mogens Schou, the use of lithium in "endogenous affective disorder" was first recommended by Frederick Lange in 1893 and subsequently by his brother Carl Lange in 1897 (reviewed more extensively by Schioldann [2001] in an excellent commemorative tribute to Carl Lange). After the rediscovery of lithium by Cade half a century later (for the acute treatment of mania), lithium prophylaxis in manic-depressive illness was first described by Noack and Trautner (1951), who observed that the drug appeared to prevent additional manic episodes in patients in whom it had alleviated acute mania. Shortly thereafter, Schou and colleagues (1954) provided the first case report demonstrating the benefits of lithium for treating both manic and depressive episodes. The 10 to 12 episodes a year that their patient had experienced before treatment were markedly attenuated in duration and severity after 2 years of taking lithium continuously. In the above-mentioned essay, Bech (2006) reminds us of some important history:

> The term "mood normalizer" for lithium (Cade, 1949) was originally introduced by Mogens Schou in 1963, with reference to Baastrup's findings regarding long-term therapy of lithium and its high recurrence prevention of both manic and depressive episodes in bipolar patients. In the 1950s, clinicians used the term "mood stabilizer" to refer to a combination of amphetamine and a barbiturate to treat patients with neurotic instability, but not patients with bipolar disorders. By "mood-normalizer" Schou meant a compound acting specifically on a disease process rather than on a symptom level (Schou, 1963). During long-term therapy with lithium in bipolar disorder, Schou and Baastrup saw a normalisation of the abnormal mood swings, while normal emotions seemed not to be affected in any way, as they were when the combination of amphetamine and barbiturate was used. Now, fourty [sic] years later, the definition of a "mood stabilizer" has changed to exactly what Schou had called "mood-normalizer", i.e. a drug with prophylactic properties in regard to mania and depression, and in this sense lithium still is the only drug that meets the criterion.

In the first section of this chapter, we provide practical clinical guidelines for the long-term maintenance treatment of manic-depressive illness, focusing on the bipolar form. These guidelines cover the complex issues of the selection of medications, the management of side effects, and the problem of breakthrough episodes. The second section examines the relevant research literature, emphasizing studies of treatment efficacy, predictors of response, and the important issue of the effects of long-term treatment on other organ systems.

CLINICAL MANAGEMENT

In this section we discuss key aspects of clinical management for maintenance treatment of manic-depressive illness. Following an overview of the issues involved, we address, in turn, embarking on maintenance treatment, selecting medications, treating the elderly patient, treating pregnant and breastfeeding women, and dealing with breakthrough episodes. Note that issues of maintenance treatment for children and adolescents are addressed separately in Chapter 23.

Overview

Manic-depressive illness, especially the bipolar-I form, is the prototypical diagnostic indication for maintenance treatment. When to commence maintenance therapy and whether it is ever reasonable to stop are currently matters of only modest controversy.[2] As detailed in Chapter 4, mood disorders are often highly recurrent illnesses, frequently characterized by residual symptoms and substantial risk of chronicity (this appears to be especially true of illness characterized by more prominent depressive symptomatology). One 5-year prospective follow-up study found that nearly 90 percent of 172 individuals with bipolar-I disorder experienced a relapse of illness within 5 years after their recovery from an acute mood episode (Keller et al., 1993). Many of these patients had been actively in treatment throughout the period since recovery (see also Keller et al., 1992). In a recent prospective study of 1,469 bipolar patients participating in the National Institute of Mental Health's (NIMH) Systematic Treatment Enhancement Program for Bipolar Disorder (STEP-BD) (Perlis et al., 2006), 58 percent achieved recovery, but nearly half of these patients (49 percent) had a recurrence of illness during the follow-up period of up to 2 years. Recurrence was associated with the persistence of residual symptoms after treatment of the acute episode.[3]

The substantial morbidity (including medical morbidity) and significant mortality associated with recurrences of bipolar disorder, the financial burden resulting from the decreased productivity of affected persons and associated health care costs, and the toll in human misery (including substance abuse, violence, and suicide) all argue for making every possible effort to prevent new episodes. Patients who have had a manic episode and a major depressive episode—thus all patients with bipolar-I disorder—are at high risk of relapse throughout their lives; barring contraindications, long-term maintenance therapy is indicated for all such patients. We agree with the recommendations of the various North American treatment guidelines that long-term prophylactic treatment should generally begin after the first manic episode; in most of the European guidelines, prophylaxis is recommended after the second episode of mania, but it can be "considered" after the first manic episode if that episode is severe enough (Vestergaard, 2004). At the same time, it is important to note that treatment decisions must be made in context of individual patients and their diagnoses. In clinical situations, moreover, a significant amount of time, often several months, is usually required to determine whether an individual can tolerate a particular long-term maintenance medication at a dose that is likely to be helpful. And it takes at least a year, and more often 2 to 3 years, to develop a clear picture of how effective the treatment is in preventing recurrence. When evaluating treatment times of less than 1 year, it is difficult to distinguish prevention of relapse back into the acute episode from true prophylaxis (prevention of a new episode). Thus decisions about prophylactic medications must be made and reconsidered over periods of many years.

Long-term maintenance is also indicated for bipolar-II patients, primarily because of the toll of depressive morbidity (Judd et al., 2005) and the availability of new mood stabilizers that can reduce the likelihood of new depressive episodes in a significant percentage of bipolar patients. Bipolar-II disorder differs from bipolar-I in several ways that suggest a modification of the usual maintenance recommendations for the latter. The defining characteristic that differentiates bipolar-II from bipolar-I is, of course, the absence of full-blown manic episodes. For example, the risk of manic switch is lower, which may make antidepressants safer than they are in bipolar-I patients. The importance of maintenance treatment for bipolar-II is underlined by the finding that individuals with the disorder have more frequent mood episodes and are ill a greater percentage of time than those with bipolar-I disorder (Tondo et al., 1998; Judd et al., 2005). There are suggestions that patients with bipolar-II disorder are at greater risk of suicide as well; this may increase the importance of lithium prophylaxis in these patients (see Chapter 25), the clear benefits of which for bipolar-II patients have repeatedly been demonstrated in studies extending back several decades (Suppes and Dennehy, 2002). Fewer data are available on anticonvulsant medications in treating bipolar-II disorder. The increased cycling seen in patients with the disorder suggests that valproate may have a role, although its antidepressant efficacy (like that of lithium) has been shown to be modest at best in patients with rapid cycling (Calabrese and Delucchi, 1990; Calabrese et al., 2005). Valproate may be useful in treating the impulsiveness, irritability, and dysphoric moods often seen in bipolar-II patients, features that may be associated with more self-harming behavior and psychosocial disability.

Lamotrigine's demonstrated maintenance effect against depression in bipolar disorder suggests an important role for this agent in the treatment of patients with bipolar-II. In contrast to bipolar-I patients, for whom it is recommended that lamotrigine be coadministered with an agent such as lithium or valproate that can protect more completely against mania/hypomania (i.e., "from above" [Ketter and Calabrese, 2002]), lamotrigine monotherapy is generally appropriate for the bipolar-II patient, for whom the risk of a manic switch is lower. Also, as noted later in our review of the literature, lamotrigine is the only mood stabilizer with any evidence of a prophylactic effect as monotherapy for rapid cycling, and this effect was seen (in a secondary analysis of one study) only among the bipolar-II subgroup. Studies demonstrating the clear benefits of lithium and some of the anticonvulsants in preventing relapses in bipolar-II patients also reveal the shortcomings of these agents: they delay but rarely eliminate further mood episodes in studies of sufficient length. Patients in these studies not infrequently suffer from relapses, usually with depressive symptoms, despite taking lithium and the anticonvulsants carbamazepine and valproate. Thus the new data on lamotrigine are especially encouraging. By "stabilizing from below" (i.e., reducing or preventing depression), this agent may obviate the need for adjunctive antidepressants, which pose some risk of switching and cycle induction even in bipolar-II patients; before the availability of lamotrigine, maintenance antidepressants were widely used in treating bipolar-II disorder (even as monotherapy), given the substantial morbidity associated with its frequent depressive phases (see the discussion of switching and cycle acceleration in Chapter 19).

At the same time, lamotrigine, even in combination with another stabilizer, is not always effective in treating or preventing bipolar-II depression. Therefore, antidepressants will continue to play a role in treatment for some patients. Whether patients with bipolar-II are at lower risk of antidepressant-induced mood destabilization than bipolar-I patients is still something of an open question, and, as noted earlier, there are clearly some bipolar-II patients for whom antidepressant treatment is not without risk (Suppes and Dennehy, 2002). Of the 28 bipolar-II depressed patients who completed a 26-week study of fluoxetine monotherapy, only 1 developed hypomanic symptoms, but the dropout rate was nearly 90 percent. Although the numbers are small, this 1 patient represented 3.6 percent of those who completed the study; moreover, among the large number of dropouts, it is not known how many were due to mania (Amsterdam et al., 1998). A number of studies of the use of antidepressants for the acute treatment of bipolar depression have included bipolar-II patients (see Chapter 19), but the data are insufficient to conclude that any particular antidepressant is superior in preventing depression in patients with bipolar-II disorder.

With regard to maintenance treatment of recurrent unipolar depression, contemporary U.S. guidelines recommend antidepressants. However, it is important to realize that this recommendation is based on studies in which "recurrent" represents patients with as few as two episodes (the minimum *Diagnostic and Statistical Manual* [DSM]-IV definition). It has been estimated that as many as half of patients with DSM-IV recurrent unipolar depression will experience a relapse despite maintaining a full dose of the antidepressant to which they have responded acutely (Byrne and Rothschild, 1998). This phenomenon is variously referred to as "poop out," "tachyphylaxis," or "tolerance." All of these terms imply that the relapse represents a loss of the drug's therapeutic effect, a phenomenon for which many explanations have been advanced (Fava, 2003; Solomon et al., 2005). Yet rarely is the possibility considered that in some patients, the phenomenon may reflect the *ongoing efficacy* of the antidepressant, bringing the next depression on sooner by accelerating the natural cycle of the more recurrent forms of unipolar depression (Goodwin, 1989).[4] In this regard, it is interesting that in the recent report from the "real-world" NIMH Sequenced Treatment Alternatives to Relieve Depression (STAR*D) trial of the antidepressant citalopram, only 28 percent of patients with fairly recurrent forms of unipolar depression (average of six prior episodes) achieved remission (Trivedi et al., 2006).

With regard to the use of mood stabilizers for prevention of recurrent unipolar depression, as reviewed in the first edition of this text and more recently in two meta-analyses (Souza et al., 1990; Davis et al., 1999), substantial evidence indicates that lithium is highly efficacious in the prevention of recurrent unipolar depression. Most of this evidence has involved patients with frequent recurrences, often as frequent as those experienced by the typical bipolar patient. Thus in their careful analysis, Davis and colleagues (1999) noted that most of the earlier maintenance studies of unipolar patients had involved subjects with two to three episodes during the 2 years before the study, a frequency well within the range of that of the typical bipolar patient. For highly recurrent unipolar patients, recommended lithium monotherapy levels are in the same range as those for bipolar-II (.4 to .6 mEq/l). While some of the patients in these earlier studies might today be considered as falling within the "bipolar spectrum," the size of the effect (which is as large as that in all of the lithium studies of bipolar disorder taken together) and the remarkable consistency across studies argue against misdiagnosis as an adequate explanation for these findings. To our knowledge, there have been no studies of other putative mood stabilizers in the prevention of recurrent unipolar depression.

Embarking on Maintenance Treatment

Patients recovering from an episode of mania will usually be taking lithium and/or an anticonvulsant and/or an atypical antipsychotics. Patients recovering from an episode of depression may be taking an antidepressant in addition to lithium and/or an anticonvulsant. Since many patients can be protected against recurrences of their illness with lithium or an anticonvulsant alone, adjunctive medications often can be gradually tapered off and discontinued. However, substantial numbers of patients with bipolar disorder will need to take a combination of medications to remain well.

For the recently manic patient, standard practice, reflected in published guidelines and consensus statements from North America, is to continue the medication or medications found to be effective during the acute phase of illness.[5] While this practice is appropriate for managing the period immediately after resolution of the acute episode (the continuation phase of treatment), it is certainly not the best approach to true prophylaxis. Unfortunately, the North American guidelines do not distinguish adequately between true prophylaxis and continuation treatment. Simply because a drug has antimanic properties (and if continued, will protect against relapse back into mania in the months after the acute episode), one cannot assume that it will be effective in the prevention of new episodes in the future, particularly depressive episodes. While this assumption may be true (to some extent) for lithium, it is not well supported by the data with respect to all the other antimanic agents. Indeed, a recent post hoc analysis of the combined data from two 18-month randomized comparisons of lithium, lamotrigine, and placebo that focused on the period between 6 and 18 months (i.e., beyond the continuation phase) demonstrated that for the patients maintained on placebo, 84 to 86 percent of recurrences were to an episode whose polarity was *opposite* of that of the index episode (Calabrese et al., 2006; Goodwin and Calabrese [in preparation]). Box 20–1 outlines some issues involved in understanding what "maintenance" treatment means as the term is used today and provides a perspective on contemporary maintenance treatment guidelines, the evidence base for which is heavily weighted by trials involving relapse prevention after acute response, primarily antimanic response (see also Chapter 17).

Perhaps the most valuable and necessary resources for successful maintenance treatment of bipolar disorder are ones that, especially in the United States, are available in ever-decreasing supply: adequate time for assessment (in terms of both duration and frequency of appointments), and continuity of care over a period of months and years that allows the physician to become familiar with the rhythms and permutations of the patient's illness and the individually unique signs of relapse. Evaluation of patients on a weekly basis during the initial stages of recovery from an acute episode and at least every 2 weeks thereafter as long as significant residual symptoms remain is necessary for an accurate assessment of continued recovery. Patients can be

---

BOX 20–1.   Understanding Maintenance Treatment Guidelines

- Classically, three phases of treatment have been distinguished:
  - *Acute*: control of acute symptoms
  - *Continuation*: ongoing control of the acute episode (the length of this phase is proportional to the natural history of episodes)
  - *Maintenance* or *prophylactic*: prevention or attenuation of new episodes
- Because the natural history of bipolar disorder is for it to recur, on average, every 16–18 months, true prophylaxis cannot be evaluated in 6 or 12 mo.
- Contemporary relapse prevention designs that have generated U.S. Food and Drug Administration (FDA) "maintenance" indications show drug–placebo differences primarily in the continuation phase.
- Some guidelines recommend different maintenance treatments depending on whether the most recent episode was a mania or depression. However, this recommendation appears to be based on two studies* of drug–placebo differences in the first few months after an acute episode; later relapses (which were more likely to be new episodes) were of the opposite polarity 85 percent of the time.

---

*The two studies were of maintenance lamotrigine versus placebo—one with patients who had recently been depressed and the other with those who had recently been manic or hypomanic.

---

encouraged to keep a journal and a mood chart[6] and to bring the results to appointments. Family members should always be encouraged to attend follow-up appointments with some regularity to report their impressions.

Selecting Medications

Clinical decision making is the art of making prudent choices based on insufficient information. Controlled data have not yet caught up with the realities and exigencies of clinical practice in the treatment of bipolar disorder (including, among other things, individual differences, comorbidities, and combined medications), especially in the area of long-term prophylactic treatment. Clearly, lithium is the most proven agent for the prevention of affective episodes, followed by lamotrigine, both of which have generated FDA "maintenance" indications; valproate may be effective in long-term prevention, but this conclusion is based on secondary analysis of one controlled trial, insufficient to support an FDA indication. In the North American guidelines (with the notable exception of those for the Veterans Health Administration), lithium and valproate are nonetheless given equal rank as first-line maintenance treatments. However, other guidelines around the world still rank lithium ahead of valproate, a position in line with

the most recent (and rigorous) Cochrane review of controlled studies of valproate, which concluded that "at present, the observed shift of prescribing practice [from lithium] to valproic acid is not based on reliable evidence of efficacy" (Macritchie et al., 2001). Olanzapine and aripiprazole have also been approved by the FDA for "maintenance" treatment of bipolar disorder (although, as discussed later, the evidence for atypicals is focused less on long-term prophylaxis and more on prevention of relapse into mania shortly after recovery from a manic episode, which is more properly referred to as continuation treatment). Finally, substantial data, primarily European, support use of the non–FDA-approved anticonvulsant carbamazepine. Other agents and combinations clearly have a role as well, as discussed in detail later in this chapter. A medication regimen for an individual patient will be based on diagnosis, the relative preponderance and severity of manic versus depressive symptoms, responses of the patient and family members to particular agents, comorbid conditions, cost, and drug allergies and sensitivities.

The 2006 prescription data for bipolar disorder in the United States show that lithium is the most prescribed agent, followed closely by lamotrigine, then divalproex, then quetiapine. In 2001, divalproex was the most prescribed, followed closely by lithium. For 2006, carbamazepine and oxcarbazepine combined had less than half the market share achieved individually by lithium, lamotrigine, or divalproex. The most dramatic change in U.S. prescription patterns from 2001 to 2006 is the sharp increases in market share for lamotrigine and quetiapine, accompanied by comparable decreases in divalproex and lithium. The European market for medications for bipolar disorder is somewhat different. Lithium remains the market leader with a share almost identical to that in the United States; valproate and valpromide combined are second, followed by olanzapine, then lamotrigine, then carbamazepine. Between 2001 and 2006, lithium's market share in Europe declined by 24 percent, while carbemazepine's share dropped by 48 percent and valproate's share doubled. It should be noted that these data reflect all uses of the drugs in bipolar patients, including both acute and maintenance treatment.

It is important to bear in mind that some fluctuations of mood in patients being treated for bipolar disorder reflect cyclic or phasic changes of the illness that will normalize with time and do not necessarily call for additional pharmaceutical intervention. Patients may have brief depressive periods following a period of mania or transient episodes of mild hypomania following recovery from depression. Experienced clinicians know that being too quick to intervene during these periods can result in the prescription of unnecessary additional medications that may ultimately be destabilizing in the case of antidepressants or oversedating in the case of anticonvulsants and antipsychotics. During the maintenance phase of treatment, mood *stability* should be a treatment goal comparable with that of euthymia. At times, interventions designed to further one of these goals may require restraint in interventions addressing the other.

The decision as to when and how quickly to attempt tapering off and discontinuing a medication that may have been used for an acute episode must always be an individualized one as well. The patient's previous course of illness, demonstrated response to and requirement for particular medications, and willingness to accept the risks of ongoing medication treatment versus the risk and consequences of relapse will offer important guidance. Likewise, although the best available research data indicate that lithium should be the mainstay in the treatment of bipolar disorder in most circumstances, an individual patient's inability to tolerate lithium therapy, as well as breakthrough or residual symptoms, may dictate the selection of alternative or adjunctive agents. That said, it is beyond regrettable that many young psychiatrists in the United States have never really learned the science and art of lithium treatment, and that they excuse their ignorance by convincing themselves that lithium has been surpassed by more effective medications or that it is too difficult to use—a self-fulfilling prophesy. It is our belief that clinicians who are unable or unwilling to include the skillful use of lithium in their armamentarium should not be considered competent to treat bipolar disorder.

There are, of course, many patients who legitimately need and benefit from alternatives or adjuncts to lithium, and fortunately, controlled data and clinical experience are increasingly available to guide the clinician in identifying those agents. Emerging data suggest that lamotrigine may be especially helpful for the prevention of depressive episodes, and valproate and carbamazepine for the prevention of manic episodes. As noted earlier, the role of the atypical antipsychotics, such as olanzapine and aripiprazole, in the long-term prevention of new manic episodes is less clear. Although these two drugs have "maintenance" indications from the FDA, results of existing studies are probably best interpreted as demonstrating their prevention of relapse back into the acute manic episode (continuation treatment), leaving open the question of whether they can prevent future new episodes, especially of depression (that is, whether they are true prophylactic agents).

The full range of available clinical data will be necessary in making decisions for individual patients, many of whom inevitably resemble the subjects that are excluded from or drop out of controlled studies because of severe and/or complex illness or inability to tolerate particular agents. For example, the data on the ability of lamotrigine to prevent depressive relapses, taken together with the more ambiguous data on this agent's mania-preventing effects, might argue for its being added to rather than substituted for lithium in a patient with bipolar-I disorder who experiences breakthrough depressive symptoms on lithium alone. On the other hand, the addition of an antidepressant rather than lamotrigine makes sense for a patient with bipolar-II disorder who has similar symptoms but a history of developing a severe rash when taking an antibiotic. For the bipolar-I patient whose history suggests a high risk of manic recurrences and who is developing renal complications while taking lithium, valproate, carbamazepine, or an atypical antipsychotic might be used as a substitute for lithium (accompanied by the latter's *gradual* withdrawal) rather than as an adjunctive agent.

In each of the above situations, there are reasons not to pursue the particular course of action described, and it is quite possible to justify other approaches. In the absence of definitive data, the clinician has little choice but to craft each patient's treatment plan gradually based on a careful assessment of target symptoms over time and on the patient's response to treatment—always with an eye to the development of medication intolerances and side effects. It is well to keep in mind that the great majority of the time, the next new episode following a mania is a depression and vice versa (see our later review of the literature).

Below we review in turn the use of lithium, valproate, carbamazepine/oxcarbazepine, lamotrigine, other anticonvulsants, and the atypical antipsychotics for maintenance treatment of manic-depressive illness, with an emphasis on the bipolar subgroup. The pretreatment evaluation and ongoing monitoring recommended for maintenance mood stabilizers are outlined in Table 20–1; similar recommendations for maintenance atypical antipsychotics are outlined in Table 20–2.

Lithium

Some debate continues regarding optimal serum lithium levels for maintenance monotherapy of recurrent affective disorders, particularly the bipolar subgroup. How to balance the greater efficacy and increased side-effect burden with increasing serum levels is a clinical decision that must be individualized for each patient (Luby and Singareddy, 2003). Gelenberg and colleagues (1989) compared the ability of "standard" (.8 to 1.0 mEq/l) and lower (.4 to .6 mEq/l) levels to prevent recurrences among bipolar-I patients. Although the higher levels were associated with superior protection against relapse, they were also associated with greater dropout rates due to side effects. A major problem with this study, however, is that the findings actually reflect the effect of lowering the lithium level from the

Agent	Therapeutic Range (blood level)	Monitoring	Other Considerations
Lithium	0.6–0.8 mEq/l for bipolar-I; lower for bipolar-II, highly recurrent unipolar, and adjunctive use (0.4–0.6 mEq/l)	• Serum lithium level: 6-mo intervals in euthymic patients. Consider more frequent determinations in the elderly or medically ill or in special circumstances, such as need to check postoperative status or compliance. • Serum creatinine: 6- to 12-mo intervals (more frequent in elderly or medically ill patients). • Urine volume (24-hr output) if history of substantial polyuria is obtained. • TSH free triiodothyronine (T_3), T_4 by dialysis, thyroid peroxidase antibodies at 12-mo intervals. Consider ultrasound thyroid scan after 1–2 yr of treatment.	• Monitor weight; intervene at >5 lb (focus on carbohydrate control and exercise). • Tremor generally responds to low-dosage beta-blockers. • Once-a-day dosing is best for most patients. • Slow/extended-release preparations are associated with fewer side effects. • Office-based lithium assay technology markedly increases convenience for both patient and clinician.
Carbamazepine	4–12 µg/ml	• Pregnancy test (HCG) • Hepatic profile. • Complete blood count (CBC), including platelets every 2 wk for 2 mo, then quarterly. • Electrolytes, especially sodium.	• Induces metabolism of many agents, including itself. • Higher doses of oral birth control agents recommended. • Monitor weight; intervene at >5 lb.
Valproate	45–125 µg/ml (median = 84)	• Pregnancy test (serum HCG). • Hepatic profile, amylase, and electrolytes periodically.	• Regular monitoring of reproductive history (menstrual cycle, galactor-rhea, and hirsutism) recom-especially for younger women. • Monitor weight; intervene at >5 lb.
Lamotrigine	Not determined	• Assessment for rash, especially during first 12 wk. • Pretreatment antigen screen can reduce background rate of benign rash (see text).	• Severe dermatological reactions are rare with gradual titration (≈ 1/5,000). • Plasma level is doubled by valproate and decreased by carbamazepine but not oxcarbazepine.

(continued)

TABLE 20–1. **Pretreatment Evaluation and Ongoing Monitoring for Maintenance Mood Stabilizers** *(continued)*

Agent	Therapeutic Range (blood level)	Monitoring	Other Considerations
Oxycarbazepine	Not determined	• Pregnancy test (serum, HCG).	• Less induction than carbamazepine. • Higher dosage of oral contraceptive required.

Notes: General pretreatment evaluation for mood stabilizers encompasses medical history focusing on renal, endocrine, cardiac, hepatic, hematopoietic, and nervous systems; catalog of present and past drug use, including prescriptions, over-the-counter drugs, illicit drugs, caffeine, nicotine, and alcohol; baseline blood pressure, complete blood count (CBC), electrolytes, hepatic profile, creatinine, thyroxine (T_4), thyroid-stimulating hormone (TSH), and urinalysis; and pregnancy test (serum human chorionic gonadotrophine [HCG]) where appropriate. Only lithium and lamotrigine have been approved by the U.S. Food and Drug Administration for maintenance use.

Source: Adapted with permission from Bowden et al., 2000b.

standard to the low level, which may have been associated with a lithium withdrawal effect (Perlis et al., 2002). Another limitation of the study is that it did not include a group with levels in the key range of .6 to .8 mEq/l. A finer-grained analysis was provided by Maj and colleagues (1986), who randomized 80 consecutive bipolar patients to one of four different plasma levels: .3–.45, .46–.6, .61–.75, and .76–.9 mEq/l. All but the group with the lowest level showed a significant reduction in affective episodes and overall morbidity.

Recommended serum levels have trended downward over the decades since lithium was first introduced, with most experts now recommending a compromise between the levels studied by Gelenberg and colleagues (1989) and Maj and colleagues (1986). Akiskal (2000) recommended a rather broad range of .3 to .8 mEq/l in his chapter on mood disorders in the *Merck Manual*. Schou (2001), the father of modern maintenance lithium therapy, narrowed this range a bit to .5 to .8 mEq/l, while Maj and colleagues (1986) concluded that beyond .8 mEq/l, negative outweigh positive effects. It may be that most studies have failed to show a relationship between lithium levels within the generally accepted range of .5 to 1.0 mEq/l and clinical response (see, e.g., Vestergaard et al., 1998) because the potentially greater efficacy at higher levels is offset by more problems with adherence (G. Goodwin and Geddes, 2003). The guidelines of the American Psychiatric Association (2002) note that .6 to .8 mEq/l is the range commonly chosen by bipolar-I patients and their psychiatrists for lithium monotherapy, while .4 to .6 mEq/l is recommended for adjunctive lithium therapy for bipolar-I or monotherapy for bipolar-II or highly recurrent unipolar depression (Goodwin and Goldstein, 2003).[7] An interesting recent paper (Severus et al., 2005) reviewed the lithium-level data from both earlier and more recent studies (in the latter, lithium was included as an active "control" in trials of new putative mood stabilizers). The conclusion of this paper was that relatively lower levels are optimal for prevention of

depression (as we noted in the first edition of this text), whereas relatively higher levels may be best for prevention of mania, yielding an optimal range of .5 to .8 mEq/l for overall stabilization.

Serum lithium levels should be obtained whenever there has been a change in dosage and at least every 6 months in stable patients. Recently, obtaining lithium levels has become significantly easier for both patient and physician with the development of a reliable office-based instant blood test that can be accomplished as part of the patient's regular visits to the psychiatrist (Glazer et al., 2004). The instant feedback provided by this technology has obvious advantages for clinical management, particularly in addressing issues related to adherence.[8] Elderly and medically frail patients should, of course, be tested more often (treatment of the elderly is discussed in greater detail later in this chapter). Most of lithium's side effects correlate with serum levels and can often be ameliorated by changing the dosage schedule or using sustained-release preparations (which result in lower peak levels). Gastrointestinal symptoms are not uncommon but are generally transient.[9] Polydipsia and polyuria, as well as edema that occurs early on, often resolve with time and can be managed with low doses of loop diuretics or potassium-sparing diuretics, such as amiloride; patients who develop polyuria only after months or years should be evaluated for nephrogenic diabetes insipidus (see the later discussion). Diuretics, especially thiazide diuretics, may alter lithium excretion, and serum lithium levels must be closely monitored in these patients to avoid toxicity.[10]

Side effects associated with lithium treatment, with particular reference to long-term effects, are shown in Table 20–3; they include weight gain, some cognitive dulling and fine hand tremor (both dose-related), dermatological problems, nephropathy in a very small number of patients, nephrogenic diabetes insipidus, and thyroid-suppressing effects. The latter effects may be temporary in some patients, but in others may proceed to clinical or subclinical

TABLE 20–2. Pretreatment Evaluation and Ongoing Monitoring for Maintenance Atypical Antipsychotics

Agent	Monitoring	Other Considerations
Clozapine	• Blood pressure at 3 mo, then annually; weight (and BMI) every month for the first 3 mo, then quarterly. • Waist measurement annually; fasting plasma glucose at 3 mo, then annually. • Fasting lipid profile at 3 mo, then annually. • CBC with differential weekly for 6 mo, then every other week for the next 6 mo, then monthly.	• Early anticholinergic effects and postural hypotension are common. Baseline electrocardiogram (ECG) needed. • May need to discontinue if substantial weight gain in the first 2 wk.
Risperidone	• Blood pressure at 3 mo, then annually. • Weight (and BMI) every month for the first 3 mo, then quarterly. • Waist measurement annually. • Fasting plasma glucose at 3 mo, then annually. • Fasting lipid profile at 3 mo, then annually.	• EPS at higher doses (>6 mg/day) in monotherapy studies; may be more frequent with combined treatment and/or comorbidities in clinical settings. • Some anticholinergic effects; some postural hypotension. • Available in depot formulation (every 2 wk).
Olanzapine	• Blood pressure at 3 mo, then annually. • Weight (and BMI) every month for the first 3 mo, then quarterly. • Waist measurement annually. • Fasting plasma glucose at 3 mo, then annually. • Fasting lipid profile at 3 mo, then annually.	• Early anticholinergic effects and postural hypotension are common. • Some EPS seen in clinical settings. • May need to discontinue if substantial weight gain in the first 2 wk. • Available in intramuscular (IM) formulation.
Quetiapine	• Blood pressure at 3 mo, then annually. • Weight (and BMI) every month for the first 3 mo, then quarterly. • Waist measurement annually; fasting plasma glucose at 3 mo, then annually. • Fasting lipid profile at 3 mo, then annually.	• Anticholinergic effects and postural hypotension are common. • Some EPS seen in clinical settings.

(continued)

TABLE 20–2. **Pretreatment Evaluation and Ongoing Monitoring for Maintenance Atypical Antipsychotics** *(continued)*

Agent	Monitoring	Other Considerations
Ziprasidone	• Blood pressure at 3 mo, then annually. • Weight (and BMI) at baseline, then annually.	• Activation and insomnia at lower doses; sedation at higher doses. • Administer with food to ensure absorption. • Some anticholinergic effects. • No consensus on utility of pretreatment ECG, but we believe it is unnecessary in the absence of pretreatment cardiac pathology. • Available in intramuscular (IM) formulation.
Aripiprazole	• Blood pressure at 3 mo, then annually. • Weight (and BMI) at baseline, then annually.	• Some anticholinergic effects. • Some EPS in community settings. • Some initial activation. • Available as oral liquid.

Notes: General pretreatment evaluation for atypical antipsychotics: medical history focusing on endocrine, cardiac, hepatic, hematopoietic, and nervous systems; catalog of present and past drug use, including prescriptions, over-the-counter drugs, illicit drugs, caffeine, nicotine, and alcohol; baseline blood pressure, complete blood count (CBC), electrolytes, hepatic profile, creatinine, thyroxine (T_4), thyroid-stimulating hormone (TSH), urinalysis; pregnancy test (serum human chorionic gonadotrophine [HCG]) where appropriate. In addition (for clozapine, olanzapine, risperidone, and quetiapine), weight (and body mass index [BMI]), waist measurement, personal/family history of weight problems and/or diabetes, fasting plasma glucose, and fasting lipid profile. Olanzapine and aripiprazole are FDA-approved for relapse prevention. Data derived primarily from controlled monotherapy trials with little or no comorbidity. Prevalence of extrapyramidal syndrome (EPS) with use of atypical antipsychotics in bipolar patients appears to be considerably higher among those treated in the community (Ghaemi et al., 2006).

Source: Reprinted with permission.

hypothyroidism (which of course should be treated early with replacement thyroid hormones). Indeed, thyroid supplements may enhance stability and help reduce some side effects in bipolar patients in whom formal hypothyroidism is not present (Bauer and Whybrow, 2001; Goodwin and Goldstein, 2003). We recommend starting at .025 mg of thyroxine (T_4), increased by .025 mg every 3 to 4 weeks until the free T_4 level is in the upper quartile of the normal range or until side effects ensue (such as, overactivation, tachycardia, tremor, or changes in body temperature regulation), at which point the dosage can be decreased. Unfortunately, some of the published guidelines for maintenance treatment do not even mention thyroid supplementation.

Weight gain is not uncommon with lithium use, and the mechanisms of this weight gain remain unexplained.[11] Approximately one-quarter to one-half of patients taking lithium experience a 5 to 10 percent weight gain (Perselow et al., 1980; Fagiolini et al., 2002). Excessive weight gain, in addition to its inherent deleterious effects, is a common reason for nonadherence to lithium use (see Chapter 21). Temporary fluid retention can be expected to result in a gain of 2 to 3 pounds; however, the clinician should act aggressively to prevent a gain of more than 5 pounds. Increased serum leptin levels have been detected in lithium-treated bipolar patients (Atmaca et al., 2002) but not in healthy volunteers taking lithium (Baptista et al., 2000). Diet (especially the control of simple carbohydrates), exercise, and perhaps correction of reduced thyroid function may be helpful in managing lithium-induced weight gain.[12] There are also reports of reduction of lithium-induced weight gain with the adjunctive use of topiramate (Chengappa et al., 2002; Nemeroff, 2003), but the additive effects of the two drugs on cognitive function often limit the usefulness of this combination.

Cognitive dulling, with complaints of poor concentration, impaired memory, and mental slowing, is known to be

TABLE 20–3. Principal Adverse Effects of Drugs Used as Monotherapy at Recommended Doses for Maintenance Treatment

Drug	Neurocognitive Impairment	Sedation	Weight Gain	Other (see also Table 20–2)
Lithium	++	0 / +	++	Gastrointestinal (initially), thyroid, renal (nephrogenic diabetes insipidus), tremor, dermatological
Carbamazepine	+ / ++	+	+	Hematological, rash, diplopia, ataxia, drug interactions
Oxycarbazepine	+	+	+ / 0	Rash, drug interaction with oral contraceptives, diplopia
Valproate	+ / ++	+ / ++	++	Tremor, hair loss, hepatic and reproductive changes including polycystic ovary syndrome, pancreatitis (rare)
Lamotrigine	0	0	0	Rash, transient headache
Clozapine	?[a]	++	+++	Aplastic anemia (monitor for), orthostatic hypotension, anticholinergic effects, hyperlipidemia and metabolic syndrome
Olanzapine	?[a]	++	+++	Hyperlipidemia, metabolic syndrome
Risperidone	?[a]	++	+	Hyperprolactinemia, extrapyramidal syndrome, hyperlipidemia (low risk), metabolic syndrome
Quetiapine	?[a]	++	++	Hyperlipidemia
Ziprasidone	0	0	0	Some QTc prolongation, but its clinical significance is questionable; initial (low-dose) activation/agitation
Aripiprazole	[a]	0/+	0	Activation/anxiety initially in some patients

[a]To varying degrees, atypical antipsychotics cause sedation, which some may regard as a neurocognitive side effect.
EPS = extrapyramidal syndrome; PCOS = polycystic ovary syndrome.

caused by lithium; this problem generally responds to reducing the dosage, shifting the entire dose to bedtime,[13] and/or enhancing thyroid function. Fine tremor is another dose-related side effect. Tremor sometimes subsides spontaneously after several weeks of treatment, and it can be worsened by coadministered medications such as selective serotonin reuptake inhibitors (SSRIs) and bupropion; it generally responds to treatment with beta-blockers. Dermatological problems associated with lithium use include acne and, occasionally, hair loss, problems that are usually minor. Acne responds to local treatment and antibiotics; isotretinoin should be used with caution because of the possible risk of exacerbating suicidality. Lithium can exacerbate preexisting psoriasis so severely as to preclude its use, although some patients with psoriasis will respond to the agents usually effective for the condition (Tsankov et al., 2000).[14] Lithium has also been associated with a variety of benign electrocardiogram (ECG) changes, but significant cardiac conduction changes or arrhythmias are very uncommon (Steckler, 1994).

As the long-term effects of lithium on the kidney have become clearer, earlier concerns about its nephrotoxicity have eased significantly.[15] While the risk of reduced glomerular function with lithium appears to be very low, a small number of patients appear to develop glomerular and tubulointerstitial nephropathy[16] that can progress to renal insufficiency and be irreversible if not detected early enough. It appears that in this small group of vulnerable patients, lithium interacts with other medical conditions (e.g., hypertension) or familial or environmental problems to cause progressive renal failure. In a review of such cases, the reversibility of renal insufficiency after discontinuation of lithium appeared to be associated with serum creatinine levels lower than 2.5 mg/dl, further highlighting the need for monitoring of renal function in patients taking lithium. Creatinine clearance determinations are no longer recommended for routine monitoring; obtaining serum creatinine determinations every 3 to 12 months, depending on such factors as age and general medical conditions, is reasonable. Patients who have serum creatinine levels consistently greater than 1.6 mg/dl (or whose level is 25 percent or more above the pretreatment baseline) should be referred for medical evaluation, which should start with a creatinine clearance determination. The more common lithium-associated renal problem is nephrogenic diabetes insipidus (reflected in "creeping creatinine"), seen in about 20 percent of those taking lithium for 15 to 20 years or longer (Lepkifker et al., 2004),[17] which is caused by lithium-induced reductions in the capacity of the distal tubules to reabsorb electrolytes. This condition is accompanied by a mild but significant decrease in urine-concentrating ability,[18] which has been demonstrated in most (though not all) longitudinal studies of lithium's effects on the kidney. It appears that this effect is due to a lithium-induced interference with the sensitivity of the distal tubule to antidiuretic hormone. Earlier cross-sectional studies suggested a correlation between duration of lithium treatment and decreased maximum urine osmolality. More recent longitudinal studies have not found a progressive decrease over time, however, suggesting that there is a decrease in urine-concentrating ability during the first few years of lithium treatment and little or no further progression in ensuing decades. Results of lithium discontinuation studies indicate that increases in 24-hour urine output remain the same or decrease only slightly (at least in the short term) after the drug is discontinued. Patients should be asked about polyuria and a 24-hour urine volume measurement obtained if polyuria is suspected.[19] Reducing polyuria can be especially important when nocturia is significant enough to interfere with sleep since sleep disruption can destabilize the illness.

All the studies of lithium's renal effects have involved standard immediate-release lithium. There are some data to suggest that slow- or extended-release preparations have significantly less impact on urinary osmolality (Miller et al., 1985) and might therefore be expected to have a more benign renal profile. There have as yet been no long-term studies of slow- or extended-release preparations to permit direct evaluation of this hypothesis, however.

Results of two relatively recent studies appear to suggest that serious long-term effects of lithium use on renal functioning may not be rare (Markowitz et al., 2000; Bendz et al., 2001). However, these studies involved a small sample of lithium users within a much larger sample of patients with renal deficiencies, and in one study (Markowitz et al., 2000), the proportion of lithium users within the sample was the same as that within the general population, a finding not consistent with a lithium effect. Kallner and colleagues (2000) studied nearly 500 patients treated with lithium for up to 30 years and found no deaths related to chronic renal insufficiency. Likewise, to our knowledge no clinical studies have found an increase in end-stage renal disease that could be attributed to lithium use in the absence of other risk factors.

Lithium decreases thyroid hormone release and may interfere with other steps in the synthesis of thyroid hormones, and has been reported to inhibit the conversion of T_4 to triiodothyronine (T_3) in the periphery and neurons (reviewed by Kleiner et al., 1999). Patients may respond to these thyroid-suppressing effects with a rise in thyroid-stimulating hormone (TSH) that is usually temporary. Some patients on lithium therapy, however, progress to clinical or subclinical hypothyroidism. Bocchetta and colleagues (2001) reported on the thyroid function of patients followed in an Italian lithium clinic for more than 10 years and concluded that patients are at increased risk of developing clinical or subclinical hypothyroidism during the first few years of lithium therapy, with rates declining to near those of the general population thereafter.[20] Their 10-year follow-up study of 150 patients who had already been taking lithium for various lengths of time when they entered the study found that the incidence of new-onset hypothyroidism, goiter, and thyroid autoimmunity did not differ from that reported for the general community (Bocchetta et al., 2001). This study found that women and individuals with thyroid autoimmunity were at highest risk of developing hypothyroidism while taking lithium. The authors recommended testing for baseline thyroid function at the start of lithium therapy; determination of TSH, free T_3, free T_4, and thyroid peroxidase antibodies (TPO Abs), as well as ultrasonic scanning of the thyroid, after 1 or 2 years of lithium treatment; annual TSH determinations thereafter; and TPO Abs and thyroid ultrasound scans at 2- to 3-year intervals. Regarding autoimmune thyroiditis itself, a large study by the Stanley Foundation Bipolar Network (Kupka et al., 2002) found that the prevalence of TPO Abs was significantly higher among 226 bipolar patients than among 3,190 psychiatric patients of any diagnosis or 252 community controls; while the frequency of TPO Abs was not associated with lithium exposure, hypothyroidism was. Kleiner and colleagues (1999) suggested that both TPO Abs and antithyroidglobulin be determined for patients at the beginning of lithium therapy to identify those at greater risk for developing hypothyroidism. They recommended TSH determinations as the most sensitive and therefore only needed test to monitor patients for lithium-induced thyroid dysfunction. They recommended that TSH be measured every 3 months during the first year of lithium therapy and semiannually to annually thereafter (Kleiner et al., 1999).[21]

Treatment of Lithium Toxicity

Prevention is the most important principle in managing lithium toxicity or intoxication. By detecting early signs and adjusting dosages, the problem can be averted. The most sensitive indicator of incipient lithium toxicity is the central nervous system (CNS) perhaps particularly the cerebellum. Patients must be alerted in advance to CNS symptoms, and each encounter with the patient should include some assessment of CNS functioning. The agitation and restlessness of early lithium intoxication are similar to symptoms of mixed affective states, and distinguishing between the two phenomena can be difficult.

If the intoxication is so severe that lithium withdrawal is not sufficient, the patient should be admitted to a hospital and cared for by a specialist in the treatment of poisoning. The first of several methods used to treat lithium poisoning is the vigorous application of general supportive measures appropriate in any CNS poisoning. Obviously, kidney function should be preserved by maintaining blood pressure and replacing fluids and salt, but if it falters, hemodialysis is necessary. Although most patients recover after deliberately or accidentally overdosing on lithium, some are left with a persistent neurological or renal defect, and a few die. Because of these severe complications, the possibility of lithium intoxication should never be taken lightly. Patients with preexisting vulnerabilities, particularly in kidney or CNS function, plainly require more careful monitoring. Further information about lithium intoxication and treatment guidelines for managing it are available on our Web site.

Valproate

Compared with lithium, there are fewer data on effective levels of valproate for maintenance treatment; at this point it appears reasonable to use the levels published in the large, multisite 1-year maintenance trial conducted by Bowden and colleagues (2000a) (see Table 20–1). Side effects become increasingly problematic at levels greater than 125 µg/ml. Dose-related side effects of valproate (see Table 20–3) include neurocognitive dysfunction and weight gain, as well as nausea, vomiting, and other gastrointestinal complaints, such as abdominal pain and heartburn. If possible, the drug should be started gradually to avoid these gastrointestinal symptoms, and a temporary reduction in dose can often alleviate them. Sedation is a common side effect, so it is best to take most if not all of the daily dose at bedtime. Indeed, given the importance of maintaining sleep stability in bipolar patients, this particular side effect can be turned into an advantage. Tremor is not uncommon; indeed, in the 1-year comparison of lithium, valproate, and placebo carried out by Bowden and colleagues (2000b), both drugs produced tremor at the same rate, sedation and hair loss were significantly greater with valproate, and weight gain showed a trend to be more frequent with valproate than with lithium. There are reports that adjunctive topiramate can reduce valproate-induced weight gain (McElroy et al., 2000; Chengappa et al., 2002), but as with lithium, additive cognitive side effects limit the usefulness of this combination for many patients. Transient minor elevations in hepatic transaminases are common when treatment with valproate is initiated and usually subside over time. Valproate can cause severe hepatotoxicity, but the risk to adults appears to be very low; most fatalities have occurred within 4 months after initiation of therapy. Careful monitoring of liver function is recommended when valproate is first administered as the hepatotoxicity is reversible in some cases if the drug is withdrawn. Similarly, rare cases of hemorrhagic pancreatitis have been reported that appear to be related to initiation of the drug or dosage increase in susceptible individuals. Delay of diagnosis has been implicated as a factor contributing to these rare cases, and patients should be warned about the symptoms and potential severity of pancreatitis. Another observed idiosyncratic response with valproate is thrombocytopenia, although documented cases of abnormal bleeding are lacking.

Some though not all reports of women treated for epilepsy have linked valproate with a high rate of gynecological problems, including menstrual irregularities, polycystic ovary syndrome (PCOS), and androgenization.[22] A recent large, multicenter study of epileptic patients compared valproate ($n=225$) and lamotrigine ($n=222$)[23] and found significantly more PCOS symptoms among the valproate-treated patients (54 versus 38 percent; $p<.01$). Although it has been suggested that women taking valproate for psychiatric conditions have less risk of these reproductive abnormalities, two small studies of bipolar patients taking valproate obtained results similar to those of the Isojarvi study of epileptic patients (O'Donovan et al., 2002; McIntyre et al., 2003). More important, a recent NIMH STEP-BD study of 230 bipolar women aged 18 to 45[24] found 7.5 *times* more PCOS (10.5 versus 1.4 percent, $p<.002$) in the 12 months following initiation of valproate compared with women who had initiated a variety of other mood stabilizers (Joffe et al., 2006). Obviously, regular monitoring of reproductive function in female patients taking valproate is needed, with questions being raised during visits regarding menstrual disorders, fertility, weight gain, hirsutism, and galactorrhea. Table 20–1 summarizes the monitoring that should be performed when valproate and the other anticonvulsants (discussed in the following sections) are used for maintenance treatment of bipolar disorder.

Carbamazepine/Oxcarbazepine

A therapeutic range for carbamazepine in the maintenance treatment of bipolar disorder has not been determined by studies correlating serum levels with clinical efficacy (see Table 20–1). In clinical trials, however, levels comparable to those used to treat epilepsy have typically been attained (Post et al., 1986, 1987). Carbamazepine has the ability to induce the hepatic microsomal enzymes responsible for its own metabolism, and considerable dosage adjustments may be necessary during the first weeks of therapy. In several studies of epileptic patients or volunteers on dosage regimens exceeding 1 month, the clearance of carbamazepine increased two-fold over initial treatment. Carbamazepine also decreases the clearance of other drugs, including valproate and benzodiazepines, and increases the metabolism of lamotrigine, ethinylestradiol, and progesterone. Contraceptive failure can occur with oral contraceptives containing less than 50 μg of ethinylestradiol (see Crawford, 2002).

The most common dose-related adverse effects of carbamazepine are diplopia and ataxia. Other dose-related complaints include mild gastrointestinal upset, unsteadiness, cognitive slowing, and, at much higher doses, drowsiness.[25] Hyponatremia and water intoxication have occasionally occurred and may be dose-related (see Table 20–3). Idiosyncratic blood dyscrasias, including fatal cases of aplastic anemia and agranulocytosis, are the most serious concern with carbamazepine.[26] Periodic blood counts are recommended to monitor for these effects of the drug, along with educating the patient on the signs and symptoms of these reactions. A retrospective study of 977 psychiatric inpatients taking carbamazepine found a 2.1 percent incidence of moderate to severe leucopenia, occurring mainly within the first few weeks, with none of the cases progressing to life-threatening illness (Tohen et al., 1995). A mild and persistent leukopenia is seen in some patients and is not necessarily an indication to stop treatment. There have been a few reports of hepatic failure in patients taking carbamazepine. A complete blood count with platelet count and liver function tests should be performed on patients starting carbamazepine every 2 weeks during the first month of treatment, at least every 3 weeks for the next few months, and then every 2 to 3 thereafter. Patients should be instructed regarding the signs and symptoms of hematological and hepatic reactions.

Other blood dyscrasias, including thrombocytopenia and hemolytic anemia, can also occur. Because of this risk, hematological monitoring is required before carbamazepine is initiated and fortnightly for the first few months

of treatment. If the white blood cell count falls to less than 3,000 cells/mm[3] or the neutrophil count to less than 1,000/mm[3], the carbamazepine should be reduced or stopped while further monitoring takes place (Sobotka et al., 1990). It may take 2 weeks or longer for white blood counts to return to normal after the drug is discontinued. Clinically, apparent hepatitis is uncommon, but transient elevation of the liver enzymes is not. Benign rashes are quite common (up to 15 percent) in carbamazepine-treated patients. Dermatological hypersensitivity, including Stevens-Johnson syndrome and the sometimes fatal toxic epidermal necrolysis, is a serious though rare idiosyncratic reaction to carbamazepine (Table 20–4).

Although controlled data on the efficacy of oxcarbazepine in treating bipolar disorder are still scant, it has at least one advantage over carbamazepine—aplastic anemia and agranulocytosis have not been associated with its use (Chen et al., 1999). Effective doses of oxcarbazepine are a third to a half higher, but unlike carbamazepine, oxcarbazepine does not induce its own hepatic metabolism, obviating the need for dosage adjustment after the initial treatment period. Moreover, oxcarbazepine is a much weaker inducer of the cytochrome P450 system and is not as highly bound to serum proteins, so it has fewer interactions with other protein-bound drugs, such as phenytoin and warfarin; also, it does not affect the metabolism of lamotrigine or valproate. As with carbamazepine, however, plasma levels of estrogen and progesterone tend to be reduced by oxcarbazepine, so only high-dose contraceptives should be used, to counteract this effect (see Ahmed and Anderson, 2001). To our knowledge there have been no studies examining the relationship between plasma levels of oxcarbazepine and clinical efficacy in treating bipolar disorder. The most common side effects of oxcarbazepine are dizziness, sedation, and blurred vision. Rashes also occur, and although they are seen less commonly than with carbamazepine, 25 to 30 percent of

TABLE 20–4. Estimated Risk of Stevens-Johnson Syndrome and Toxic Epidermal Necrolysis among Anticonvulsants

Anticonvulsant	Risk per 10,000 New Users
Phenytoin	8.3
Phenobarbital	8.1
Lamotrigine	2.5
Carbamazepine	1.4
Valproate	0.4

Source: The German Rash Registry, Mockenhaupt et al., 2005.

patients with hypersensitivity to carbamazepine are also hypersensitive to oxcarbazepine.

Lamotrigine

Clinical trials of lamotrigine for acute and maintenance treatment of bipolar disorder have employed doses ranging from 50 to 400 mg/day, and a target daily dose of 200 mg/day for maintenance treatment appears to be reasonable (Calabrese et al., 1999a; Bowden, 2003b). Adjunctive use of an anticonvulsant drug that induces hepatic microsomal enzymes (e.g., carbamazepine, phenobarbital, phenytoin, primidone) increases the clearance of lamotrigine; conversely, valproate interferes with the metabolism of lamotrigine, approximately doubling its half-life. Although serum levels of lamotrigine are routinely available, a therapeutic range for the treatment of bipolar disorder has not been determined.

As noted in Table 20–3, lamotrigine has a very favorable side-effect profile, with transient headache and dizziness being the most common complaints. In contrast to lithium and valproate, when lamotrigine is used as monotherapy at recommended doses, it does not appear to be associated with neurocognitive side effects (Lieberman and Goodwin, 2004) and unlike lithium and valproate and most of the atypical antipsychotics, it does not cause sedation or weight gain (Sachs et al., 2006). Indeed, it has been associated with weight loss in obese bipolar patients (body mass index greater than 30 kg/m^2 [Bowden et al., 2006]).

Of particular concern with lamotrigine, however, are reports of severe dermatological reactions associated with rapid initial upward titration of the dose, including Stevens-Johnson syndrome and toxic epidermal necrolysis. Serious rash may be more common in younger patients, and lamotrigine therefore is not approved for use in patients under age 16.[27] Based on results of clinical trials in bipolar patients, the incidence of serious rash has been estimated to be 1 in 1,200 (the current FDA labeling), but this estimate was derived by counting all patients who had a rash of any sort in whom the drug was discontinued and the patient was hospitalized. In reality, the drug was typically discontinued for any rash, and the hospitalizations were not necessarily related to rash. Indeed, among 2,624 patients in the clinical trials, only 1 was hospitalized for a rash, and that patient's dose had reached 100 mg by the end of the second week (data on file, GlaxoSmithKline). The most reliable rash data come from the German rash registry, which estimates the risk of serious rash to be about 1 in 5,000 lamotrigine exposures among patients being treated for epilepsy. Since almost all of these data are based on the use of the drug by neurologists, even this estimate is probably too high when applied to the more gradual titration employed in the treatment of bipolar disorder. Because benign rashes are not uncommon with this drug (about 2 to 5 percent greater frequency than with placebo), it is important to be able to distinguish them[28] from those rare cases in which a rash may signal the development of Stevens-Johnson syndrome or toxic epidermal necrolysis.

Figure 20–1 provides a decision-making flowchart for dealing with rash in patients taking lamotrigine. Dangerous rashes typically are confluent (covering virtually all of the skin) and/or involve the facial or genital area given the proximity of each to mucous membranes; also, dangerous rashes are almost always accompanied by systemic symptoms such as fever, elevated white blood cell count, and flu-like symptoms. It is of interest to note that in the German registry, a number of other drugs, including some anticonvulsants, rank ahead of lamotrigine in the frequency with which they are associated with serious rashes (see Table 20–4). Kanner and Frey (2000) reported that valproate can be added to lamotrigine safely if the dose of the latter is lowered by 50 percent after the start of valproate therapy. These findings suggest that rash resulting from the combination of the two drugs is not due to a pharmacodynamic interaction, but to a pharmacokinetic one in which a sudden increase in lamotrigine levels occurs in the presence of valproate. Finally, there have been a few case reports of agranulocytosis among patients taking lamotrigine (de Camargo and Bode, 1999; Solvason, 2000), but a causal relationship has not been established.

Other Anticonvulsants

No therapeutic ranges have been established for gabapentin, tiagabine, or topiramate. These agents generally have favorable side-effect profiles, with the exception of the dulling cognitive effects of topiramate. Thus no routine therapeutic monitoring is presently recommended for patients taking these agents.

Atypical Antipsychotics

Typical antipsychotic medications have been used mainly as adjunctive agents in the acute phases of bipolar disorder, especially for manic states (see Chapter 18), and they still form the mainstay of acute treatment for mania in many European centers. Given the risk of tardive dyskinesia with the typical antipsychotics,[29] they have usually been viewed as having only a temporary role in the treatment of bipolar disorder, with discontinuation recommended as soon as symptoms stabilize. Because they were for a long time the only psychotropics available as long-acting depot agents,[30] they have been used, when effective, in a small number of patients who have failed to adhere to oral medication regimens (Littlejohn et al., 1994).

Figure 20–1. Lamotrigine Rash Decision-Making Flowchart. CBC = complete blood count; LFT = liver function test. (*Source*: Calabrese et al., 2002. Reprinted with permission.)

While the atypical antipsychotics are generally considered safer than the typicals because they are less likely to cause extrapyramidal syndrome (EPS), the relatively low EPS rates found in large multicenter registration trials may be misleading because they reflect monotherapy in patients without psychiatric or medical comorbidities and are based on data from the randomized phase, which are limited to patients who have already demonstrated that they can tolerate the drug. A recent study conducted in a "real-world" setting (reflecting combined treatment of patients often with comorbid disorders) found rates of EPS that exceeded 60 percent, principally akethesia (Ghaemi et al., 2006).[31] Furthermore, Leucht and colleagues (2003) noted that most of the controlled trials comparing EPS rates in patients taking typical versus atypical antipsychotics have used the high-potency agent haloperidol (which is associated with a high rate of EPS) as the comparator. In their meta-analysis of 31 studies comparing atypical antipsychotics with lower-potency typical antipsychotics such as chlorpromazine (median of mean doses = 440 mg/day),[32] only clozapine (15 studies) was associated with significantly less EPS, while the lower frequency seen with olanzapine (4 studies) was of borderline significance ($p = .07$), and the rates for zotepine (6 studies) were similar to those for the low-potency typicals. We should note, however, that for quetiapine, ziprasidone, aripiprazole, amisulpride, and sertindole, the data were insufficient to draw conclusions.[33]

Perhaps the feature that most distinguishes the atypical antipsychotics from their older cousins is that they are more effective as thymoleptic agents; that is, they appear to have a more specific ameliorative effect on mood, including depressive symptoms. The use of these agents to treat breakthrough hypomanic/manic/mixed and depressive symptoms is discussed in Chapters 18 and 19, respectively. Their use as monotherapy for maintenance treatment of bipolar disorder is still being evaluated in controlled trials, but positive results have been obtained with olanzapine and aripiprazole in studies of relatively short-term relapse prevention (see the later discussion), specifically relapse into mania among those who recently had a full antimanic response to the atypical. These results have led to FDA approval of these two agents as "maintenance treatment" for relapse prevention, primarily manic relapse, and suggest an ongoing role for their use in patients with illness characterized by more frequent and treatment-resistant manic symptoms, either in combination with lithium and/or an anticonvulsant or perhaps as a sole agent. As of this writing, the only atypical antipsychotic available in depot form is risperidone. As more such formulations become available, a much greater role for the atypicals can be anticipated for patients who are nonadherent, even partially or episodically, to treatment with lithium or anticonvulsants.

Our recommendations for pretreatment evaluation and ongoing monitoring for maintenance atypical antipsychotics are outlined in Table 20–2. Most are administered initially in low dosages and titrated upward based on clinical response and tolerance of side effects. Typically, clozapine is begun at 12.5 mg/day and increased in 25 mg increments as tolerated. Final effective doses for clozapine range from 300 to 800 mg/day. It is crucial for patients to take the prescribed clozapine daily as syncope is not uncommon in those who miss several doses and then restart it at the therapeutic dose previously achieved through titration. Laboratory monitoring of white blood cell count should be carried out for patients taking clozapine to detect agranulocytosis. The usual initiating dose of olanzapine is 2.5 to 5 mg/day. For risperidone, the initial dose is usually 1 mg, with the effective dose ranging from 2 to 6 mg/day for most patients. Quetiapine is begun at doses of 25 to 50 mg, with usual effective doses ranging from 150 to 750 mg/day. Ziprasidone is usually started at 40–80 mg BID with food,[34] while for aripiprazole the starting dose is 5–15 mg. When possible, atypical antipsychotics should be tapered slowly to reduce the likelihood of withdrawal symptoms.

Because bipolar disorder itself has been associated with obesity, as well as an elevated risk of diabetes and related metabolic disturbances (see Chapter 7), it becomes critical to understand the potential contribution of the atypical antipsychotics to these problems. Soon after the introduction of clozapine in the mid-1970s, excessive weight gain was reported in many patients taking certain atypical antipsychotics, especially clozapine and olanzapine. Although weight gain in the short term is often modest, several studies have shown that it can continue for many months. Table 20–3 shows the weight gain risks of the various atypical antipsychotics. Clozapine and olanzapine are associated with the highest risk; risperidone and quetiapine are intermediate; and ziprasidone, aripiprazole, and amisulpride pose the lowest risk (there is also no evidence associating these latter three drugs with adverse metabolic effects). In a 5-year study of weight changes associated with clozapine, the gain did not level off until 46 months after treatment was initiated (Henderson et al., 2000). Thus the potential for significant weight gain in patients receiving long-term treatment with some atypical antipsychotic medications is substantial. Furthermore, the weight gain associated with these drugs most commonly results in central or abdominal obesity, a pattern thought to pose more health risks, particularly cardiovascular risk, than generalized obesity. These risks also include dyslipidemia and insulin resistance, which along with abdominal obesity, constitute the "metabolic syndrome," associated with an increased risk of type 2 diabetes mellitus, coronary artery disease, and other conditions.[35] Although the risk of diabetes with these drugs appears to be of the same rank order as that of weight gain, weight gain alone may not fully explain all of the metabolic effects (Newcomer et al., 2002).

The primary mechanism for the weight gain associated with some atypical antipsychotics appears to be a centrally mediated increase in appetite, although it has also been suggested that atypical antipsychotics alter the regulation of leptin, a polypeptide synthesized in adipose tissue and thought to be involved in insulin sensitivity and regulation of adiposity. A direct effect of these agents on glucose uptake by target cells has also been proposed (for excellent reviews see Baptista et al., 2002; Newcomer 2006). The effects of the drug probably interact with genetic predispositions to pancreatic and glucose dysfunction, putting some individuals at higher risk than others for the development of diabetes (Guo et al., 2006).[36] Psychiatrists should take these risks into account when selecting antipsychotic agents, and when possible prescribe those agents less likely to cause weight gain in already obese patients and those with diabetes or a family history of the disease. Body weight, blood glucose, and serum lipid levels should be monitored at the beginning of treatment and regularly thereafter in patients taking atypical antipsychotics for maintenance treatment; obviously, the drugs with the greatest potential to cause weight gain require the closest monitoring. It is especially important to monitor weight closely during the first few weeks of therapy since it has been shown that a gain of 2 kg (4.4 lb) or more during the first 3 weeks of olanzapine administration is a reasonably accurate predictor of substantial subsequent weight gain (Lipkovich et al., 2006). Clinicians should discuss with patients symptoms that could reflect emerging diabetes, such as excessive thirst and urination, fatigue, frequent infections, and blurred vision. Nutritional counseling for patients taking these agents is important, emphasizing portion-size control, low-fat and low-carbohydrate foods, and regular exercise.

Several small studies of the pharmacological treatment of antipsychotic-related obesity with fenfluramine and other appetite-suppressing agents have yielded results that can be characterized as modest at best (Allison, 2001). On the other hand, a recent double-blind, randomized, placebo-controlled trial of adjunctive amantadine in patients who had gained at least 5 lb while taking olanzapine found that, compared with placebo, amantadine plus olanzapine was associated with no further weight gain (Graham et al., 2005). In another encouraging report, Vieta and colleagues (2004) found that the combination of olanzapine and topiramate over 12 months appeared to prevent the weight gain that would have been expected with olanzapine.[37] Finally, orlistat, a lipase inhibitor that is not active in the CNS, may also have some potential for the treatment of medication-induced weight gain. However, while orlistat has a very benign side-effect profile, its use in psychiatric patients has not been systematically investigated.[38]

Several drugs, including lithium, valproate, carbamazepine, and SSRI antidepressants, have been known to increase the therapeutic effects of atypical antipsychotics when administered concurrently.[39] Other drugs, including fluoxetine, paroxetine, quinidine, and tricyclic compounds, can inhibit the metabolism of atypical antipsychotics. Bupropion and almost all antipsychotics, including the atypicals, can lower the seizure threshold, and this possibility should be considered before combined use of these agents is initiated.

Treating the Elderly

Modifications of recommendations for the maintenance treatment of bipolar disorder when treating the elderly address primarily the increased sensitivity of these patients to adverse effects and toxicity associated with the usual agents. There are no data suggesting differences in the efficacy of various agents in older patients, although this issue has not been investigated directly with controlled studies. In their prospective study of 166 bipolar and recurrent unipolar outpatients, Murray and colleagues (1983) found no age-related decrease in lithium efficacy. They did note that manic symptoms grew increasingly prevalent and severe with age, a trend they interpreted as reflecting the natural course of the illness. It has been suggested that lower serum lithium levels are effective in the elderly, although this observation has been based on retrospective literature reviews rather than controlled data (Van Gerpen et al., 1999). However, lower levels are clearly associated with fewer adverse effects, an important consideration in this population. Further, some experienced clinicians believe, and we agree, that "stability can beget stability"; accordingly, we recommend that clinicians consider discussing with some patients a gradual and modest reduction in dose after years of stability have been achieved.

A number of case reports and open studies indicate that valproate is safe in the elderly, although no controlled studies addressing its prophylactic efficacy in this population are available. A retrospective chart review involving 72 long-term nursing facility patients over age 55 taking lithium or valproate for bipolar disorder, dementia, or both found that lithium was associated with more adverse medication-related effects and concluded that valproate was a safer treatment, at least in this very fragile population. However, the bulk of the lithium-related adverse effects appeared to reflect poor management in that they were associated with "toxicity and/or dehydration," including blood levels in excess of 1.2 mEq/l (Conney and Kaston, 1999). Furthermore, a recent study comparing patients in their 70s who were taking comparable doses of lithium and valproate (Shulman et al., 2005) found that the two drugs were quite similar in their impact on neuropsychological functioning (Fig. 20–2).

Lamotrigine may have an advantage in this population because of its impressive tolerability; particularly important in older patients is the absence of cognitive impairment and sedation. Sajatovic and colleagues (2005) analyzed the data for 98 bipolar subjects over the age of 55 who were part of two large 18-month studies comparing lamotrigine, lithium, and placebo (G. Goodwin et al., 2004) and found lamotrigine to be significantly better than placebo in preventing depressive relapses (and lithium significantly better than

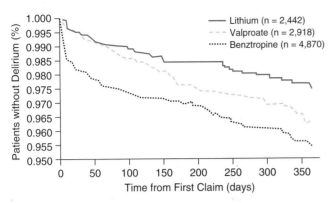

Figure 20–2. Kaplan-Meier survival curves for incidence of delirium in new users of lithium, valproate, or benztropine among older adults. (*Source*: Shulman et al., 2005. Reprinted with permission.)

placebo in preventing manic/hypomanic relapses); there were significantly fewer side effects with lamotrigine than with lithium. When using antipsychotics in this population, agents with a low risk of postural hypotension (such as ziprasidone and aripiprazole) should be considered.

Treating Pregnant Women

Maintenance treatment for women during their childbearing years involves the art of balancing competing priorities. A healthy pregnancy and postpartum (puerperal) period and, of course, a healthy baby, as well as continued remission from symptoms of bipolar disorder, are no longer regarded as being mutually exclusive. In balancing the risks (Table 20–5) and benefits of continuing some medication during at least a portion of the pregnancy (Altshuler et al., 1996; Warner, 2000; Chaudron and Pies, 2003; Gentile, 2006), it must be remembered that bipolar episodes themselves pose a risk to the fetus or newborn[40] (Box 20–2). Table 20–6 presents a more detailed review of the FDA categories of drug safety during pregnancy.

It has been suggested that pregnancy exerts a protective effect against the recurrence of mood symptoms in women with "classic" bipolar disorder, as characterized primarily by complete recovery between episodes (Grof et al., 2000). However, this suggestion is not supported by the results of studies of unselected bipolar patients, largely in U.S. tertiary care academic centers (Viguera et al., 2002). Whether pregnancy is or is not "protective" in some patients, the postpartum (puerperal) period is clearly a time of greatly increased risk for relapse, especially into mania and psychosis, rates of which are estimated at 50 to 75 percent, respectively.[41]

Several large studies have documented that postpartum (puerperal) episodes in patients with manic-depressive illness cluster in families (Dean et al, 1989; Jones and Craddock, 2001; Forty et al, 2006). In the one study that focused only on bipolar women (Jones and Craddock, 2001) those with a family history of postpartum psychosis were more than six times more likely to have a postpartum episode than those without such a family history. Given the magnitude of this difference in risk, it is prudent to consider family history when advising women of the risks of being off medication during pregnancy and/or when considering adjunctive treatments aimed at preventing postpartum episodes. (See, for example, Sharma et al, 2006).

For several decades, lithium was considered quite teratogenic and thus virtually contraindicated during pregnancy because of an increased incidence of major cardiac defects, notably Ebstein's anomaly. More recent data, based on consecutive series rather than case registries, have substantially reduced the risk estimates for Ebstein's anomaly to a range of 1 in 1,000 to 1 in 2,000 live births (Jacobson et al., 1992; Cohen et al., 1994). Nevertheless, a gradual reduction of the lithium dose for women who wish to become pregnant can be considered, at least for the first trimester. If the patient's episodes have been seasonal in the past (seen most commonly with manic/hypomanic episodes in the spring or summer), the pregnancy might be timed so that there will be a relatively safe period for temporary lithium withdrawal. The tapering off should be done slowly, over at least several weeks, because abrupt discontinuation of lithium substantially increases the risk of suicide and relapse, particularly manic relapse. Restarting lithium after the first trimester does not appear to increase the risk of teratogenicity. It is advisable to restart the drug well before parturition so as to minimize the risk of postpartum mania, psychosis, and depression (Stewart et al., 1991; Austin, 1992). It is important to keep in mind that the maximum therapeutic and prophylactic effect of lithium may take many months, even years, to achieve, and there is no guarantee that restarting the drug in the second trimester will recapture the prior level of protective efficacy, which is essential during the high-risk postpartum period. There have been reports of neonatal lithium toxicity in infants exposed to lithium during labor and delivery, but this appears to be rare as long as the lithium level is lowered to .3 mEq/l or less for a day or two before parturition (Newport et al., 2005). On the other hand, discontinuing lithium altogether clearly puts the mother at substantial risk of relapse (especially into mania, which itself, as noted above, puts the baby at risk) and should be avoided if at all possible.[42] For some patients whose history suggests a high risk of relapse when off lithium even for a few months (or who evidence breakthrough symptoms when the tapering is undertaken), the drug should be continued even through the first trimester.

A variety of malformations have been linked to treatment with valproate (Thisted and Ebbesen, 1993) and carbamazepine (Kallen, 1994) during pregnancy. These two

TABLE 20–5. Fetal and Neonatal Risks Associated with Drugs Used for Maintenance Treatment

Drug	Fetal Risks
Lithium	• Ebstein's cardiac malformation (risk much lower than earlier estimates, now .05–.1% (1 in 1,000 to 1 in 2,000) • Neonatal hypothyroidism, nephrogenic diabetes insipidis, polyhydramnios (rare) • Secreted in breast milk at one-half maternal plasma concentration • FDA Pregnancy Category C (see Table 20–6) based on old data
Carbamazepine and oxcarbazepine	• Spina bifida (approximately 1–2% risk), dysmorphic facies • Secreted in breast milk • FDA Pregnancy Category D
Valproate	• Spina bifida (approximately 3–5% risk) • Structural defects in heart and limb, dysmorphic facies • Secreted in breast milk • FDA Pregnancy Category D
Typical antipsychotics	• Teratogenic risk low, but limited data available • Secreted in breast milk • FDA Pregnancy Category C, except clozapine (Category B) • Phenothiazines—not yet categorized
Atypical antipsychotics	• Teratogenic Risk unknown • Secreted in breast milk • FDA Pregnancy Category C
Benzodiazepines	• Possible cleft palate, cleft lip • Secreted in breast milk • FDA Pregnancy Category D
Lamotrigine	• Increase in nonsyndromic cleft palate or cleft lip associated with first-trimester exposure in the North American Antiepileptic Drug (AED) Registry, but not in four other registries • Secreted in breast milk • Risks of major defects may increase with concomitant use of valproate • FDA Pregnancy Category C
Other anticonvulsants	• Unknown teratogenic risks for gabapentin, oxcarbazepine, topiramate • Secreted in breast milk • FDA Pregnancy Category C
Antidepressants	• Selective serotonin reuptake inhibitors (SSRIs) and tricyclic antidepressants thus far not associated with major fetal anomalies • Infants exposed to SSRIs in utero may experience respiratory distress, irritability, and feeding problems • Infants exposed to tricyclics in utero may experience transient withdrawal effects • Secreted in breast milk • FDA Pregnancy Category C[a]

[a]Applies to most SSRIs, including fluoxetine; some tricyclic medications are in Category D.

Source: Adapted from Viguera et al., 2002; Lamotrigine Pregnancy Registry; Nonacs and Cohen, 2003. Reprinted with permission.

BOX 20–2.   Increased Risks to Fetus and Newborn during an Affective Episode

- Stress, including release of stress-related hormones
- Alcohol and drug use (including nicotine)
- Poor nutrition
- Sexually transmitted diseases
- Risk to newborn from postpartum mania, depression, and psychosis
- Maternal suicide
- Physical violence
- Impaired maternal care of infant

drugs are much more dangerous to the fetus than lithium, causing a variety of major and minor congenital defects, most notably neural tube defects such as spina bifida. Because of teratogenicity and the increased risk of reproductive abnormalities, some guidelines now recommend that alternatives to valproate be used for mood stabilization in women of childbearing age; we agree. Information regarding the teratogenicity of the newer anticonvulsants gabapentin, oxcarbazepine, and topiramate is sparse, and until proven otherwise, they should probably be considered higher-risk agents.[43] Initial reports on lamotrigine monotherapy during the first trimester were reassuring: among 596 first-trimester exposures to lamotrigine monotherapy or combined therapy excluding valproate, the incidence of anomalies was 2.9 percent, consistent with the risk in the general population (Cunnington and Tennis, 2005). However, recent analysis of the ongoing North American Antiepileptic Drug (AED) Pregnancy Registry noted 5 cases of isolated nonsyndromic cleft palate or cleft lip out of 564 first trimester monotherapy exposures (.89 percent)—higher than the rates in general population registries (which range from .037 to .22 percent). However, an increased risk of cleft lip or palate has not been observed in a number of other international registries. Three recent studies (reviewed by Gentile, 2006) noted a 60 to 65 percent decrease in plasma lamotrigine levels in the third trimester compared with prepregnancy levels.

Relative to lithium and most anticonvulsants, the typical neuroleptics pose a low risk of teratogenicity, and apparently this is true of the newer atypical agents as well (Ernst and Goldberg, 2002; McKenna et al., 2005), although pregnancy appears to increase the risk of metabolic syndrome in women treated with olanzapine (reviewed by Gentile, 2006). Both first- and second-generation antidepressants are also generally considered low-risk during pregnancy, although this view is at odds with package insert labeling for various drugs.[44]

Treating Breastfeeding Women

While data on the impact on the fetus of psychoactive drug use by pregnant women are sparse, they are even more so when it comes to the question of how these drugs might affect newborns who are breastfed.

Compared with most other drugs used in the maintenance treatment of manic-depressive illness, a relatively high percentage of maternal lithium—ranging from 24 to

TABLE 20–6.   U.S. Food and Drug Administration (FDA) Categories of Drug Safety during Pregnancy

Category	Description
A	Adequate, controlled human studies have demonstrated no fetal risks; these drugs are the safest.
B	Animal studies show no risk to the fetus and no controlled human studies have been conducted, or animal studies show a risk to the fetus but well controlled human studies do not.
C	No adequate animal or human studies have been conducted, or adverse fetal effects have been shown in animals but inadequate human data are available.
D	Evidence of human fetal risk exists, but benefits may outweigh risks in certain situations (e.g., life-threatening conditions or serious diseases for which safer drugs cannot be used or are ineffective).

Notes: These categories can be quite misleading because they are, by and large, based on data available at the time of the drug's initial approval. Typically, once a drug is off patent, new data are not submitted to the FDA. For example, newer data indicate that lithium (Category D) is safer than either carbamazepine (Category D) or valproate (Category C). Adequate human data for valproate were not available at the time it was approved, and newer data indicate a substantial risk of spina bifida with the drug.

72 percent—is found in breast milk (Chaudron and Jefferson, 2000). Because of this and a handful of case reports of adverse effects, the American Academy of Pediatrics (AAP) recommends that if lithium is administered to a breastfeeding woman, it should be done with caution and with careful monitoring of the infant, especially for lethargy and hypotonia (see the review by Ernst and Goldberg, 2002).[45]

Chaudron and Jefferson (2000) and the AAP consider use of anticonvulsants to be compatible with breastfeeding. The concentration of valproate in breast milk is low, representing less than 10 percent of maternal levels. For carbamazepine, a higher percentage of the drug's maternal blood level gets into breast milk than is the case with valproate, and there are at least nine case reports of adverse effects of carbamazepine in breastfed babies (Ernst and Goldberg, 2002). There are fewer data on lamotrigine in breast milk (and very little of this is monotherapy data), but because the amount found in breast milk represents a relatively high proportion of maternal levels (estimated at 60 percent), caution is advised (Ernst and Goldberg, 2002; data on file, GlaxoSmithKline).

Few or no data exist on the penetration of the atypical antipsychotics, as a group, into breast milk; however, use of these agents is generally considered compatible with breastfeeding, perhaps because of older (albeit still limited) evidence that a low proportion of the mother's dose of typical antipsychotics enters breast milk.

A prospective, controlled study of mothers exposed throughout pregnancy to either tricyclic antidepressants ($n = 46$) or fluoxetine ($n = 40$) (half of whom breastfed their babies) compared with 36 mothers who were not exposed to antidepressants (Nulman et al., 2002) found no adverse effect of drug exposure on the children's global intelligence quotient (IQ), language development, or behavior when they were tested between ages 15 and 71 months. In contrast, IQ and language development were significantly and adversely affected by uncontrolled depressive symptoms in the mothers. Further discussion of the risk/benefit calculation for the use of psychotropic drugs in pregnancy and breastfeeding can be found in two recent reviews (Gentile, 2004, 2006; Malone et al., 2004).

Dealing with Breakthrough Symptoms

The appearance of hypomanic/manic or (especially) depressive symptoms during the course of maintenance treatment of bipolar disorder is so common as to appear almost inevitable. The clinician who has treated a particular patient for years will likely know how to react (or not react) to breakthrough symptoms in that patient, but more often the decision is a difficult one. A young person who is early in the course of illness presents an obvious challenge; the patient whose adherence to treatment recommendations is difficult

to judge is another. The first step in addressing breakthrough symptoms is to assess their etiology. Possible reasons for such symptoms in previously stable patients include the following:

- *Nonadherence to recommended treatment*—Nonadherence can be both intentional and unintentional. It may be due, for example, to the patient's reducing the dosage of a medication to alleviate side effects, misunderstanding instructions, or forgetting doses; in a study of patients referred for lithium prophylaxis and followed prospectively for 2 years, ongoing substance abuse emerged as the best predictor of nonadherence (Aagaard and Vestergaard, 1990). Regular laboratory monitoring is important not only because of the medical issues involved, but also because it reinforces for the patient the clinician's understanding that the proper dose of medication is important to treatment. As suggested earlier, the use of long-acting depot medications (haloperidol, fluphenazine, risperidone) is an option for patients in whom regular adherence to oral medications is consistently problematic. Family members are excellent resources for evaluating the possibility of nonadherence in the patient with unexplained worsening of symptoms. Treatment adherence is discussed in detail in Chapter 21.

- *Psychosocial stressors*—It is important to differentiate between mood symptoms that represent recurrence of illness and those that represent normal reactions to circumstances. That having been said, drawing this distinction can be a fiendishly difficult task. The appearance of mild depressive symptoms is not uncommon in the context of a personal setback and may respond to reassurance and support; thus it is important for the clinician to convey interest in and a willingness to discuss the patient's personal issues. On the other hand, a period of psychosocial stress can precipitate an episode of illness, and neither the patient nor the physician should be too complacent about symptoms that appear to be explained by circumstances. At the very least, more frequent contact with the patient will be required to monitor the symptoms and intervene promptly if more aggressive treatment is indicated. Often the mechanism by which psychosocial stress destabilizes the illness is sleep loss, so careful monitoring of sleep is as essential as the clinician's willingness to address the problem pharmacologically. Brief supportive psychotherapy, with referral to a competent psychotherapist if necessary, is an intervention easily undertaken by all psychiatrists caring for patients with mood disorders (see Chapter 22). Indeed, as noted throughout this volume, it is our belief that manic-depressive illness is best managed by a combination of pharmacological and psychotherapeutic treatment.

- *Destabilizing factors*—These may include substance abuse; antidepressants; medications with psychotropic effects prescribed by other physicians, such as steroids or interferon; or endogenous factors, such as the onset of thyroid abnormalities. The symptomatic patient may not be the best source of information on these factors, an observation that reinforces the need to develop collaborative relationships with family members and other professionals involved in the patient's care.

- *True relapse*—Only after other possibilities have been ruled out should the clinician contemplate changes in medication to address breakthrough symptoms. Even then, questions will remain. How aggressively should the symptoms be treated? The severity of the immediate symptoms will naturally inform this decision, as will consideration of the course of the patient's illness. Have mild symptoms progressed to severe illness previously, and if so, how quickly? Can this breakthrough episode be related to previous ones in a way that suggests a specific intervention? (For example, if depressive symptoms recur in winter months, supplemental phototherapy may be helpful.) Once the decision has been made to treat breakthrough symptoms, a reasonable first step is to maximize the effectiveness of the patient's current medication regimen. Therapeutic monitoring is crucial in determining whether dosages can be increased safely. Dosages of agents with dose-related efficacy should generally be maximized before the addition of new agents is considered. As noted previously, the trigger for or earliest indication of a breakthrough manic or hypomanic episode often is decreased sleep. Thus the early, short-term use of sedative hypnotics may be able to abort an emerging episode before it escalates. Agents useful for this purpose include benzodiazepines, zolpidem, eszopiclone, ramelton, gabapentin and some other sedative anticonvulsants, and some atypical antipsychotics.

Approaches to managing breakthrough manic/hypomanic and depressive symptoms are discussed in Chapters 18 and 19. Here we only emphasize that there are almost no controlled data to guide the clinician in choosing a particular combination regimen for an individual patient. Medication combinations are clearly effective for many patients. Goodwin and Goldstein (2003), for example, reviewed data on several medications, such as valproate, that may work synergistically with lithium (allowing reduced dosages of each drug), potentially enhancing maintenance treatment by increasing the ratio of therapeutic to side effects. Another frequently used combination is lithium plus lamotrigine, combining a stabilizer that works best "from above" (lithium) with one that works best "from below" (lamotrigine) (Ketter and Calabrese, 2002). When using combinations, however, downward dosage adjustment should generally be attempted (which is feasible for both of the combinations just mentioned) since combinations of two or more drugs at full monotherapy doses increase the risk of side effects and nonadherence.

REVIEW OF THE LITERATURE

In this section, we provide a detailed review of the literature on the medications discussed above for maintenance treatment of manic-depressive illness: lithium, valproate, carbamazepine/oxcarbazepine, lamotrigine, other anticonvulsants (for which the data on efficacy are sparse), and the antipsychotics. We also review the literature on combination maintenance treatments and on other agents and approaches, including maintenance ECT, thyroid hormones, calcium channel blockers, nutritional supplements, and extended bed rest and darkness. Maintenance treatment for children and adolescents is discussed in Chapter 23.

Lithium

In the introduction to this chapter, we noted the pioneering work of the Lange brothers, as well as that of Cade and Noack and Trautner. But the first major systematic study of lithium's prophylactic efficacy in manic-depressive illness occurred through the collaboration of Baastrup and Schou (1967). They analyzed the results of a retrospective study initiated at the Psychiatric Hospital in Glostrup, Denmark, involving all patients with recurrent affective disorders admitted from 1960 through 1966 (a total of 88 patients). Those selected for analysis had an episode frequency ranging from two or more episodes in a year to one episode per year for at least 2 years before lithium administration. All had taken lithium for at least 1 year.

The study's results were striking. Following the initiation of lithium, episodes (defined as rehospitalization) had become clearly less frequent among 83 (94 percent) of the 88 patients. The magnitude of the effect is suggested by the fact patients were ill on average 13 weeks a year before starting lithium, compared with less than 2 weeks a year while taking lithium—an almost seven-fold reduction. The frequencies of manic and depressive episodes were affected equally; however, lithium's ability to prevent rehospitalization for depression, not always evident initially, appeared to improve with time. In this sample, lithium was equally effective in patients with bipolar and recurrent unipolar depression[46] (see the review below of lithium studies in this group) but was less so in schizoaffective patients (Baastrup and Schou, 1967). In a follow-up study, Angst and colleagues (1970) obtained similar results.

Baastrup and Schou's 1967 report, a medical landmark, stimulated many trials of the use of lithium in the prophylactic management of manic-depressive illness. By 1972, more than 60 clinical studies comparing the course of the illness before and while taking the drug had been published. Virtually all showed decreases in the frequency, duration, and severity of episodes; those studies that distinguished between manic and depressive episodes found that lithium reduced both.

By this time, most clinicians who had studied lithium's effects on recurrent affective illness were favorably impressed. Skeptics such as Blackwell and Shepherd (1968), however, noted that patients selected for a trial because of a history of relatively frequent episodes might be expected to experience a decreased frequency of episodes during the study period as part of the natural course of the illness, reflecting a regression toward the mean rather than a drug effect. But the assumption underlying this view—that the natural course of manic-depressive illness is random—was contradicted by data indicating a strong tendency for the average frequency of manic-depressive episodes to be non-random and to increase with time (see Chapter 4). Three independent studies (Laurell and Ottosson, 1968; Isaksson et al., 1969; Angst et al., 1997) examined the natural course of manic-depressive illness in patients with 2-year histories of frequent episodes—the kind of patients selected for the trials just discussed. Patients in all three studies were found to be at high risk for subsequent episodes in the next 2 years if they remained off lithium. Blackwell and Shepherd (1968) had also noted that in the absence of double-blind procedures, observer bias or patient expectation may have accounted for the favorable results obtained. Clinicians highly familiar with the illness knew, however, that full-blown mania (and probably also severe depression) is unlikely to respond meaningfully to psychological suggestion alone.

In the remainder of this section, we review in turn the results of placebo-controlled studies of the prophylactic efficacy of lithium conducted before 1980, the renewed controversies that arose during the mid-1980s regarding the drug's effectiveness and results of contemporary studies in which lithium served as an active comparator in maintenance trials of new agents, lithium's relative prophylactic efficacy in treating mania and depression, its effect on normal mood, the issues of withdrawal and rebound, clinical features that may predict the drug's prophylactic effectiveness, its prophylactic efficacy in bipolar-II disorder, and finally the surprisingly robust literature supporting its prophylactic efficacy in recurrent unipolar depression. Finally, we should note that maintenance lithium can prolong life, not only by dramatically reducing the likelihood of suicide, but also by reducing the elevated cardiovascular mortality associated with manic-depressive illness (Ahrens et al., 1995) (see Chapter 7). The relationship between lithium and the risk of suicide in patients with recurrent affective disorders is reviewed in Chapter 25.

Results of Placebo-Controlled Studies Prior to 1980

The first substantial response to Blackwell and Shepard's (1968) criticism came when the Danish group undertook a study in which female patients were given lithium in a clinic setting and stabilized on the drug for at least 1 year, then continued on either lithium or placebo under double-blind conditions (Baastrup et al., 1970). Although the results of this study were even better than those of the open studies discussed previously, the study was also widely criticized. One criticism was that limiting the trial to patients who had been successfully stabilized on lithium for a year prior to the study introduced a bias in favor of lithium responsiveness (a problem, discussed later, that continues to plague contemporary studies using relapse prevention designs). Another criticism was the possibility that abrupt cessation of lithium made the placebo group relapse more quickly than would otherwise have been the case (a criticism that clearly deserves consideration; see below). A subsequent study in England by Coppen and colleagues (1971) also involved prior lithium responders, but the period of stabilization on lithium prior to randomization was only 6 weeks, which is perhaps why the findings of this investigation helped increased acceptance of lithium in Europe.

The major study influencing the acceptance of lithium prophylaxis in the United States was that of Prien and colleagues (1974), a collaborative effort of the Veterans Health Administration and NIMH.[47] This study, which formed the principal basis for the FDA's 1974 decision to approve the marketing of lithium, was initiated at a time when the drug was poorly accepted in the United States, largely because of unfortunate experiences with toxicity when it was being used as a salt substitute.

For most observers, the positive randomized, placebo-controlled, parallel-group studies of Baastrup and colleagues (1970), Melia (1970), Coppen and colleagues (1971), Stallone and colleagues (1973), and Prien and colleagues (1974) (summarized in Fig. 20–3) essentially laid to rest reservations based on the results of the earlier mirror-image studies.[48] However, there was still the question of whether patients selected for and maintained on lithium become "dependent" on it; if so, they would be more likely to relapse when taken off the drug. Three studies examined this question directly. Schou and colleagues (1970), Grof and colleagues (1970), and Sashidharan and McGuire (1983) all compared patients' relapse rates during lithium withdrawal with those before lithium treatment and found no difference in either frequency or severity. These results appear to differ from those of more contemporary studies in which the frequency of relapse during the first year after abrupt lithium withdrawal appears to have exceeded

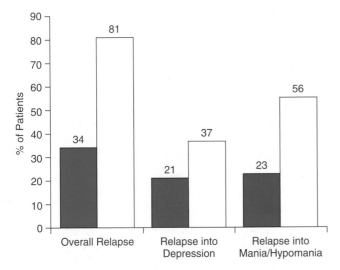

Figure 20–3. Results of double-blind lithium versus placebo maintenance trials conducted in the 1970s. Blue bars = lithium treatment (*n* = 251); white bars = placebo treatment (*n* = 263). (*Source*: Gyulai et al., 2003. Reprinted with permission.)

baseline recurrence rates (see the later discussion of the work of Suppes and colleagues [1991]). Perhaps the best explanation for this discrepancy is that offered by Grof and colleagues (1994) and Grof and Alda (2000)—that the earlier studies were of classic Kraepelinian manic-depressive illness with free intervals and without the mood-incongruent psychotic features allowed by contemporary diagnostic systems. It is also worth noting that in a more recent analysis of the older randomized, placebo-controlled studies, Keck and colleagues (2000) noted that the likelihood of relapse on placebo was not related to whether the lithium withdrawal occurred in newly treated patients or after a long period of stabilization on the drug.

Renewed Controversies and Results of Contemporary Studies Using Lithium as a Comparator

From the mid- to late 1980s until recently, despite the apparently definitive study results reported above, the clinical effectiveness of lithium was again called into question by a series of reviews proposing that there had been a steady decrease in the drug's effectiveness in the treatment of bipolar disorder since the studies of the 1970s had been conducted (Dickson and Kendell, 1986; Markar and Mander, 1989). It was suggested that the earlier studies had led to an overly optimistic view of the benefits of lithium, and that the drug's inadequacies were becoming apparent with wider and longer-term use.

Coryell and colleagues (1997) published a naturalistic (nonrandomized) study of the course of illness of 181 patients with bipolar-I disorder who were followed semiannually for 5 years, comparing the course of 139 patients who were taking lithium with that of 42 patients who were not.

Lithium showed a clear prophylactic effect against the return of symptoms only during the first 32 weeks of treatment following an episode of mania or depression; during weeks 33 through 96, there appeared to be no relationship between lithium treatment and relapse. The authors questioned the necessity of longer-term lithium prophylaxis for patients who have had 8 months or more of euthymia, suggesting that lithium discontinuation studies be performed to elucidate the issue. They also speculated that patient selection bias in treatment decisions may have reduced the size of the lithium treatment effect, and that only a minority of patients with bipolar disorder are at risk of relapse over the longer term and thus require continuous treatment. Kleindienst and colleagues (1999) reanalyzed these data using a complex mathematical model assuming that lithium's efficacy is not transient and, most important, that some patients are at high risk of relapse and others at lower risk. They were thereby able to generate survival curves virtually identical to those of Coryell and colleagues (1997). They concluded that individuals at low risk for relapse would inevitably predominate in the later months of a nonrandomized naturalistic study, thus accounting for the very small treatment effect observed for that period.

Maj and colleagues (1996) reported on 65 patients with bipolar disorder who had remained well on lithium for 5 years and who were followed for another 5 years during which they remained adherent to treatment. During the 5 years of follow-up, 12.7 percent of these stable patients experienced at least two episodes despite good adherence. These "late nonresponders" had experienced a significantly higher number of previous affective episodes and hospitalizations and a significantly longer duration of illness. The authors argued that these factors indicate a more severe illness that will eventually overwhelm the prophylactic efficacy of lithium, a conclusion they suggested is supported by their review of previous studies.

It is not surprising that the notion that the intrinsic inadequacies of lithium as a prophylactic treatment for bipolar disorder emerged at a time when alternatives to lithium were becoming available. Overlooked in most of these reviews was the inherent selection bias that arises once a treatment has become established in the community: those who tend to respond to the treatment are likely to remain in the care of practitioners, while those who are less responsive become overrepresented in samples available to investigators, who usually work in referral centers. Indeed, a recent naturalistic comparison of lithium and valproate among 201 bipolar-I patients followed for 1 year after hospitalization (Revicki et al., 2005) found that the two treatments were equally effective for those patients who stayed in treatment.[49] Nevertheless, it is likely that certain secular trends (such as increased substance abuse and much greater use of antidepressants) have resulted in more lithium-resistant cases (at least in some countries) compared with a decade or two ago.

Baldessarini and Tondo (2000) addressed these issues in a review of the 24 open and controlled long-term lithium trials published between 1970 and 1996 (most of which were from outside the United States). They found that subjects in more recent studies (1982–1996) actually had lower recurrence rates than those in earlier ones (1970–1981). They also found that pretreatment recurrence rates did not differ in earlier as opposed to later studies, suggesting the absence of secular factors that had been hypothesized to worsen the illness in more recent decades. Moreover, and importantly, recurrence rates were not significantly different in open versus blinded trials of lithium, a point also made by Davis and colleagues (1999). In another analysis of 28 studies comparing the recurrence risk with and without lithium treatment, the same authors addressed the concern that earlier studies had exaggerated lithium–placebo differences by including patients who had been withdrawn from lithium before randomization to placebo (Baldessarini et al., 2002). They showed that the reduction in recurrence attributable to lithium was the same in the half of the studies that involved prior lithium withdrawal as in the half that did not, which challenged the notion that lithium "dependence" skewed the data on its prophylactic effects. Furthermore, among the 11 "gold standard" blinded, randomized, placebo-controlled, parallel-group studies, the average reduction in recurrence risk associated with lithium was 3.6-fold. In a meta-analysis of the five randomized, placebo-controlled trials that met the requirements of the Cochrane database,[50] Geddes and colleagues (2004) concluded that lithium was clearly effective, reducing overall relapses to 65 percent of the frequency observed with placebo.

Critics had also charged that lithium's *efficacy* in treating bipolar disorder (its proven ability to treat the illness successfully in research studies) was much better than its *effectiveness* (its ability to treat the broad range of patients with bipolar disorder successfully under real-life clinical conditions).[51] To address this question, Baldessarini and Tondo (2000) also retrospectively analyzed the illness course of 360 patients treated with lithium over a period of 30 years at an Italian mood disorder clinic. Patients had been in treatment for at least 1 year and for a mean of about 5 years. These patients apparently adhered to lithium treatment and had no complicating substance abuse diagnoses, but were otherwise not selected by clinical factors; they included bipolar-I and -II patients, as well as patients with rapid cycling, some with predominantly mixed states, and some with psychotic features. Again, the authors found no cohort effect and no evidence of any decrease in lithium's effectiveness for these patients over time (see Tondo et al., 2001, for a detailed analysis). A slight increase in the numbers of patients with mixed and psychotic illness was offset by a decrease over time in the numbers of patients with rapid cycling.

It is worth noting that these data are from a large lithium clinic in Italy where the use of antidepressants is minimal. In our opinion, some of the reported decline in lithium's effectiveness in the United States is real; that is, it cannot be attributed to either referral bias or changes in the nature of maintenance studies. Some possible reasons for this decreased effectiveness (including the sharp increase in the use of antidepressants) are discussed below.

In three relatively recent large randomized controlled trials, lithium was compared with placebo for prophylaxis in bipolar-I disorder. In these studies, which were designed to evaluate the prophylactic efficacy of valproate and lamotrigine, those two agents were compared with lithium and with placebo. The valproate trial (Bowden et al., 2000a) is the only long-term trial not to have shown statistical superiority of lithium over placebo in a maintenance protocol (valproate was also not superior to placebo). The authors suggested several possible reasons for this surprising finding: the number of lithium-treated subjects entered into the study was small (half the number treated with valproate); there were many dropouts in the lithium group (67 percent, a rate perhaps related to the high doses of lithium used); and the study duration (1 year) was shorter than that of studies showing clear differences between lithium and placebo (2 years). Perhaps the overriding issue was this: because the primary outcome variable was relapse, there were ethical concerns about including very sick patients in the trial; with mild to moderately ill patients, it is likely that the placebo did too well. In Chapter 17 we review design issues relevant to studies of maintenance treatment for bipolar disorder.

In the two studies of lamotrigine versus lithium versus placebo, lithium was shown to be superior to placebo in preventing recurrence of mood episodes over 18 months in patients with bipolar-I disorder who had recently been manic or hypomanic (Calabrese et al., 2003) or depressed (Bowden et al., 2003b). The demonstrated efficacy of lithium in these two studies is all the more remarkable given that the sample was partially enriched with lamotrigine responders, and there is some evidence that lithium and lamotrigine responses represent different clinical profiles (Passmore et al., 2003). In both studies, lithium was found to be more effective in preventing mania than depression; in a combined analysis of both studies (G. Goodwin et al., 2004), however, lithium showed a trend toward superiority over placebo against depression ($p = .12$) (lamotrigine was also more effective than placebo, as discussed later). The authors noted that this was "the first study in which lithium differentiated from placebo using modern survival analytic methods and arguably provides some of the strongest evidence available for the efficacy of lithium in maintenance treatment of bipolar disorder" (Bowden et al., 2003b, p. 398).

In these two multicenter trials, lithium was included as an active control to assess "assay sensitivity"—that is, the ability of the trial to reveal differences between active drug and placebo. The size of the lithium effect was not as large as that seen in the earlier lithium studies reviewed above. In a careful comparison of the older and newer lithium literature, Deshauer and colleagues (2005) analyzed nine randomized, placebo-controlled trials involving 1,432 patients. They noted that the older studies tended to start with patients who were already taking lithium, whereas in the two recent studies in which lithium separated from placebo, the patients had already been stabilized, at least briefly, on lamotrigine. With regard to the size of the lithium effect, there was an 11-fold difference between the older, "lithium-enriched" and the newer, "lamotrigine-enriched" studies.[52]

In a 5-year prospective naturalistic study of more than 400 bipolar-I patients in the lithium clinic at the University of Naples, Maj and colleagues (1998) noted that about 25 percent of these patients had no relapses while taking lithium, about 40 percent had at least one relapse, but nearly 33 percent had stopped taking lithium (often because they felt well and saw no need for further treatment). A 2-year prospective study from New Zealand yielded similar results (Silverstone et al., 1998). A retrospective analysis of 76 patients attending a lithium clinic found that nonadherent patients were less accepting of the need for lithium prophylaxis, less convinced of its efficacy, and less likely to believe they had a serious illness (Schumann et al., 1999).

Several factors led to the above reappraisal of lithium's central role in the prophylactic treatment of manic-depressive illness (with the contemporary studies focusing on the bipolar form) and of the previously held view of lithium as the "gold standard" of treatment for the illness:

- Changes in the nature of the randomized controlled trials, including referral bias, as discussed above.
- The emergence of "effectiveness" in addition to "efficacy" studies, which included among their outcome variables differences due to patients' adherence to treatment, clinicians' adherence to good prescription practices, and toxicity, as well as blood-level monitoring. That is, real-world experience will not, on average, match the practice standards that obtain in controlled efficacy studies.
- Changes in the apparent nature of bipolar disorder in recent years:
  - Expansion at the lower end of severity with the new category of bipolar-II, perhaps bringing more Axis II comorbidity into the picture

  - The inclusion of more psychotic features in the diagnostic criteria for mania, especially in the United States
  - Lower age at onset
  - Increased comorbidity with substance abuse (the rates of which vary across countries)
  - Substantially increased use of antidepressants
  The latter three factors are associated with "atypical" features of bipolar disorder (e.g., rapid cycling, mixed states, psychotic features) that may respond better to some of the newer drugs, such as anticonvulsants (lamotrigine, valproate, carbamazepine) and the atypical antipsychotics, than to lithium (Bowden et al., 1994; Goodwin and Goldstein, 2003).
- The development of potential alternatives to lithium maintenance (especially anticonvulsants and the newer atypical antipsychotics), which remain under patent protection and thus can support substantially more marketing and sponsored educational events for psychiatrists than is the case for lithium—the perennial "low earning orphan" drug.

Nonetheless, contemporary reviews and meta-analyses of older data, as well as new data generated during investigations of more recently introduced agents, support the conclusion that reports of the demise of lithium's central role in the treatment of manic-depressive illness, including bipolar disorder, were, indeed, premature.

Lithium's Relative Prophylactic Efficacy in Treating Mania and Depression

Some earlier reviewers, primarily Americans, appeared to assume that lithium is better at preventing mania than depression, a position perhaps influenced by then-prevailing biological theories postulating that mania and depression are opposite states. Conversely, many European investigators and clinicians apparently expected that both phases would respond equally since both were viewed as intrinsic aspects of the same illness. Few of the important early European studies distinguished manic from depressive episodes in reporting relapse frequencies. In their landmark study, Baastrup and Schou (1967) did not specifically analyze the differential effects of lithium on mania and depression. As noted earlier, however, inspection of their individual case histories indicates equivalent prevention of manic and depressive episodes (defined as a period in which symptoms were sufficiently pronounced to require hospitalization or supervision in the home). The authors also noted that "very many of the patients suffered during these non-psychotic intervals from phases with slight to moderate depressive or, less often, hypomanic symptoms" (Baastrup and Schou, 1967, p. 90).

Three studies using balanced mirror-image pretreatment and on-lithium periods, careful selection of patients, and quantitative rating instruments attempted to answer directly the question of lithium's relative efficacy in preventing depression versus mania. In one of these studies (Holinger and Wolpert, 1979), a similar decrease in manic and depressive episodes was observed among patients taking lithium. The other two studies (Poole et al., 1978; Rybakowski et al., 1980) actually found better prophylaxis against depression than mania.

Of eight double-blind, placebo-controlled studies conducted in the 1970s to address this question, two found a greater effect in preventing mania or hypomania than depression (Cundall et al., 1972; Dunner et al., 1976), two had indeterminate results (Stallone et al., 1973; Fieve et al., 1976), and four found lithium to be equally effective in preventing both types of episodes.[53] More recent retrospective studies have also failed to demonstrate significant differences in lithium's effectiveness against manic and depressive symptoms (Berghofer et al., 1996; Tondo et al., 1998). In two more recent randomized, placebo-controlled maintenance trials involving lithium and lamotrigine (discussed earlier), lithium was found to be more effective in preventing mania than depression, but recall that this was a population partially enriched with lamotrigine responders. In the Cochrane meta-analysis cited earlier, Geddes and colleagues (2004) found the effect of lithium to be somewhat more robust for mania than for depression (relative risk .62 and .72, respectively), but this result may be due to the fact that two of the five trials included in the analysis involved the partially lamotrigine-enriched samples.

As is clear from a detailed analysis of the controlled studies conducted to date, there is little support for the notion that lithium is substantially more effective in the prevention of mania than of major episodes of depression. However, mild depressive symptoms do appear to be noted more frequently than mild hypomanic symptoms among patients taking maintenance lithium. In an early study, Jamison and colleagues (1979) found that physicians were more likely than patients to report lithium's being less effective against depression than mania. In interpreting this finding, however, one should remember that patients are probably less likely to report hypomanic than depressive symptoms.

Lithium's Effect on Normal Mood

Lithium's effect on nonpathological mood states has intrigued researchers for many decades. Schou and colleagues (1968), for example, took lithium at therapeutic doses for several weeks and reported feelings of indifference, decreased initiative, and a sense of being "separated from [the] environment by a glass wall" (Schou et al., 1968, p. 93). The issue has significant therapeutic implications: an agent that prevents abnormal mood episodes at the cost of blunting or even deadening normal mood variability may be quite undesirable for many patients.

Several researchers have compared mood states and day-to-day mood variation in normal subjects and euthymic bipolar patients taking lithium. Folstein and colleagues (1982) reported the results of two such studies, in which they found that bipolar subjects had mean mood ratings similar to those of controls but less day-to-day mood variation as measured by visual analog mood scales (DePaulo et al., 1982; Folstein et al., 1982). Although these results were consistent with a mood-constricting effect of lithium, the authors cautioned that it may not be valid to compare the mood ratings of bipolar subjects, who have experienced major depressions and manias, with those of control subjects, who have not. Two crossover comparison studies of lithium and placebo were conducted to assess whether lithium attenuates mood fluctuations to the same extent in bipolar patients and controls. Both studies showed no difference in mood variation related to lithium use in those without a history of mood disorders, suggesting that lithium does not have a significant effect on normal mood (Calil et al., 1990; Barton et al., 1993). As more putative mood stabilizers appear, it will be important to evaluate their effects on normal mood fluctuations as well.

Lithium Withdrawal and Rebound

Lithium withdrawal delirium or nonspecific agitation was suggested by a few case reports (DePaulo et al., 1982; King and Hullin, 1983) but was never strongly supported by subsequent studies. More attention has been focused on the issue of whether rapid (as opposed to gradual) cessation of lithium in patients with bipolar disorder actively promotes rapid relapse, particularly into mania. This question is important clinically for obvious reasons, but as alluded to earlier, it also is salient to the interpretation of results of lithium studies in which rapid cessation of the drug is part of the protocol. Suppes and colleagues (1991) performed a meta-analysis of 14 studies involving 257 bipolar-I patients and found that more than half of new episodes (which were primarily mania) occurred within 3 months after stopping lithium[54]; the number of relapses was 28-fold higher than that seen when the patients were taking lithium, suggesting that the withdrawal-related relapses represented more than just a return of the illness. Coming to a different conclusion, Davis and colleagues (1999) performed an exhaustive meta-analysis of 19 randomized controlled studies of prophylactic lithium in "recurrent affective illness" (including both bipolar and unipolar disorders), calculating the frequency of relapses before, during, and after lithium use in the reviewed studies. They assumed for their analysis that if a lithium-cessation rebound existed as a withdrawal phenomenon, it should be seen in the first several days after abrupt cessation, a time course consistent with the pharmacodynamics of lithium. In fact, most relapses occurred 3 to 9 months after cessation, suggesting to the authors that there was little support for the concept of relapses related primarily to lithium withdrawal as opposed to return of the illness in the absence of an effective medication. The difference in the conclusions reached by Davis and colleagues and Suppes and colleagues is probably due to the fact that the former group included in their analysis the substantial literature on lithium in recurrent unipolar depression, in which lithium withdrawal relapse has not been demonstrated (not surprising given that the majority of withdrawal relapses in bipolar patients are into mania).

Baldessarini and colleagues (1996, 1997, 1999a) addressed this issue by analyzing a clinical population rather than research subjects, pooling data from 227 patients with bipolar disorder (136 bipolar-I, 91 bipolar-II) in whom lithium had been discontinued for various reasons in the course of their treatment at a university-affiliated mood disorders clinic. They divided patients into "abrupt" (1–14 days) and "gradual" (15–30 days) discontinuation groups and performed a survival analysis to identify recurrences of mania or depression (by DSM-IV criteria). They found that time to 50 percent risk for any illness recurrence was four times shorter in the abrupt-discontinuation than in the gradual-discontinuation group. Rapid discontinuation of lithium resulted in a 50 percent risk of mania at 2 months and a 50 percent risk of depression at 6 months, compared with 10 months for mania and 17 months for depression in the gradual-discontinuation group. Bipolar-I patients fell ill more rapidly than bipolar-II patients in both groups. Patients who discontinued abruptly were most likely to fall ill during the first year after lithium discontinuation, primarily in the first 10 weeks; relapse rates returned thereafter to those experienced by untreated bipolar subjects.[55] Although it is not clear that this phenomenon should be called lithium "rebound" or lithium "withdrawal," rapid discontinuation of lithium in bipolar patients is clearly associated with increased relapses and an increased risk of suicide (see Chapters 8 and 19) during the first few months. These data suggest, moreover, that this phenomenon represents something distinct from simple loss of the benefits of lithium in patients with bipolar disorder, although its mechanism remains obscure.

It has also been reported that a subgroup of bipolar patients (perhaps 15 to 20 percent) who abruptly discontinue lithium become refractory to the drug when it is restarted (see Post et al., 1992; Maj et al., 1995). Other studies, however, have found that lithium is neither more nor less effective following a period of cessation in bipolar patients (see Tondo et al., 1997; Coryell et al., 1998). G. Goodwin (1994) suggested that the phenomenon of relapse after abrupt withdrawal of lithium should be taken into account in treatment planning. Based on the data in the above-noted analysis of Suppes and colleagues (1991), he recommended that lithium not be started unless the patient is committed to taking it for at least 2 years, advice that found its way into the treatment recommendations of the International Exchange on Bipolar Disorder (Bowden et al., 2000b).

A related issue is whether a longer latency in initiating preventative treatment for bipolar disorder is associated with worse outcomes. The "kindling" hypothesis would predict that patients who start prophylactic treatment early in the course of their illness will have a lower risk of relapse and better treatment response. Although earlier studies of this question yielded contradictory answers, two relatively recent large studies appear to have settled the matter. Baldessarini and colleagues (2003) studied 450 bipolar patients (two-thirds bipolar-I, one-third bipolar-II), 86 percent of whom were maintained on lithium essentially as monotherapy. While longer treatment latency did not predict greater morbidity during treatment, *pretreatment* morbidity was associated with shorter treatment latencies; that is, the sicker patients entered treatment earlier, resulting in a larger relative reduction in morbidity with earlier treatment. The second study, this one prospective, followed 147 bipolar patients receiving maintenance therapy over an average of 7 years (Baethge et al., 2003) and, like the work of Baldessarini and colleagues (2003), used a multivariate approach. This study, too, found no relationship between treatment latency and subsequent response to treatment. Both groups of authors pointed out that studies finding the opposite (i.e., that prompt initiation of maintenance treatment ameliorates the course of illness) did not control for illness severity prior to prophylaxis. Although there are certainly many arguments for the prompt initiation of prophylaxis in bipolar disorder, favorable modification of the future course of illness would not appear to be one of them. Nevertheless, the results of these studies clearly indicate, as the authors concluded, that it is never too late to start maintenance therapy.

Predictors of Lithium's Prophylactic Efficacy

It has generally been thought that patients with typical euphoric manias and a clearly episodic course of illness with well intervals (Duffy et al., 2002; Passmore et al., 2003) have an especially good prophylactic response to lithium monotherapy, while those with dysphoric or mixed manias (Goldberg et al., 1998) are less likely to have a favorable long-term response. As noted in the first edition of this text, the relationship between episode frequency and lithium response was first evaluated in a placebo-controlled study by Dunner and Fieve (1974), who found that bipolar patients with rapid cycles (four or more episodes per year) were more likely to relapse while taking lithium than those without rapid cycles. Table 20–7 reviews the major studies

TABLE 20–7. Results of Studies Evaluating Maintenance Lithium and/or Anticonvulsants in Rapid-Cycling Illness

Study	Sample	Design	Conclusion
Dunner and Fieve, 1974	55 BP NS	Naturalistic prospective cohort study of patients taking lithium over 6–66 mo	Patients with >4 episodes/year were disproportionately represented among 27 of 56 patients with prophylaxis failure.
Dunner et al., 1977	390 BP NS	Retrospective chart review	Most patients treated with lithium had fewer and less severe mood episodes while taking lithium.
Okuma, 1993	215 BP NS	Retrospective chart review	Rapid-cycling patients had poorer outcomes than non–rapid-cycling counterparts, whether taking lithium or carbamazepine.
Maj et al., 1998	402 BP NS	Prospective study of lithium therapy in a cohort of patients with BP	Rapid cycling absent in BP patients deemed good responders to lithium, but observed in 26% of those with poor response. Rapid cycling predicted poor outcome independently of treatment.
Bowden et al., 1999	75 BP NS	Add-on study of lamotrigine in patients with refractory BP (60 patients received add-on therapy; 15 received monotherapy)	Lamotrigine was generally effective and well tolerated.
Baldessarini et al., 2000	218 BP-I, 142 BP-II	Naturalistic prospective cohort study of patients taking lithium over an average of 13.3 yr	Lithium was equally effective in patients with and without a history of rapid cycling in delaying relapse and decreasing total time ill. Rapid-cycling patients, however, experienced more relapses.
Baldessarini et al., 2000	360 BP NS	Naturalistic, prospective; patients with BP-I or -II monitored on average for more than 13 yr	Similar morbidity was observed while both rapid-cycling and non-rapid-cycling patients were taking lithium, arguing against the idea that lithium is less effective in rapid-cycling BP.
Calabrese et al., 2000	225 BP-I, 98 BP-II	Randomized study of lamotrigine added to current regimen of euthymic or ill patients; other agents then tapered off	Adding lamotrigine resulted in remission or continued wellness in about half of patients, and the remission was sustained after other agents were tapered over 4–8 wk.
Swann et al., 2000	372 BP NS	Stabilized BP patients randomized to divalproex, lithium, or placebo	Although response to lithium decreased in patients with increased numbers of past depressive or manic episodes, only one subject randomized to lithium had rapid-cycling BP.
Kupka et al., 2003	3,709 BP NS	Meta-analysis of 20 studies that made direct comparisons between rapid-cycling and non–rapid-cycling BP	59% of all lithium-treated rapid cyclers achieved at least 50% improvement. A significant association between current rapid cycling and hypothyroidism was noted.
Tondo et al., 2003	317 BP NS	Meta-analysis	Overall, rapid cycling was associated with lower effectiveness of all treatments evaluated; not specific to lithium.

(continued)

TABLE 20–7. **Results of Studies Evaluating Maintenance Lithium and/or Anticonvulsants in Rapid-Cycling Illness** (continued)

Study	Sample	Design	Conclusion
Calabrese et al., 2005	24 BP-I, 36 BP-II	Patients first stabilized on lithium + valproate for up to 6 mo, then randomized to monotherapy with one of the two drugs gradually withdrawn and placebo substituted; then followed for 20 mo	Relapse into any mood episode occurred in 56% of patients taking lithium vs. 50% of those taking valproate. Time to relapse not specified.

BP = bipolar disorder; BP NS = bipolar-I or bipolar-II not specified.

that have evaluated this question. It has been suggested that the finding that rapid-cycling patients do poorly on maintenance lithium may simply mean such patients are more severely affected and as such are more difficult to treat; they may have a likelihood of improvement on lithium equal to that of non–rapid-cycling patients, but the improvement often is not sufficient to bring them into or sustain them in remission. Tondo and colleagues (2001) found that about two-thirds of their patients with bipolar disorder, including those with illness features often thought to predict less lithium responsiveness, experienced a reduction in frequency of episodes, as well as in total time ill, of at least 50 percent when observed over at least 1 year of lithium treatment. This same group (Tondo et al., 2003) conducted a meta-analysis of comparative studies of mood stabilizers in rapid-cycling versus non-rapid-cycling patients (16 studies; 905 rapid-cycling and 951 non-rapid-cycling patients), and found that lithium was superior to anticonvulsants among the latter and equivalent to valproate among the former patients.[56] The most definitive comparison of lithium versus divalproex in rapid-cycling patients (Calabrese et al., 2005), discussed later in the section on valproate, likewise found that the two drugs were not significantly different. As noted earlier, the use of antidepressants may also play a role in the relative treatment resistance of rapid-cycling patients. For example, there have been several reports of more favorable lithium results in the absence of (or with minimal use of) antidepressants (Kukopulos et al., 1980; Wehr et al., 1988; Baldessarini et al., 2000). In fact, the only intervention shown in a double-blind, placebo-controlled design to be effective in rapid-cycling bipolar-I disorder is discontinuation of antidepressants (Wehr et al., 1988).

There is evidence that mood-incongruent psychotic features predict a more lithium-resistant illness, although it appears clear that such patients can nevertheless derive substantial benefit from lithium prophylaxis. For example, Maj and colleagues (2002) followed patients with mood-incongruent psychotic features for 5 years and compared the course of their illness with that of a control group of patients with no such history. They found that the former patients were more likely to have stopped taking lithium at the 5-year point (78 versus 57 percent), and although about half of them had experienced at least a 50 percent reduction in time spent in the hospital, as a group they did not fare as well as those without psychotic features, 80 percent of whom had a comparable decrease in hospitalization time. In a randomized controlled trial that compared lithium and carbamazepine for prevention of mood episodes in bipolar patients with mood-incongruent features, the two agents were found to be equally effective (Greil et al., 1997).

Recently, Kleindienst and colleagues (2005) made a substantial contribution to the response-predictor literature. They found nearly 2,000 papers on lithium response predictors written from 1966 through 2003, 43 of which met their criteria for analysis.[57] Seven of the studies were randomized controlled trials, 10 involved a prospective cohort design, and 26 were retrospective case–control studies. Because of substantial heterogeneity in the effect sizes of different studies and the well-known publication bias in favor of positive studies, the authors applied a highly conservative "fail safe" procedure to increase the likelihood that a predictor reported in several studies was real: they added two large (N=1,000) hypothetical studies with zero correlation; if a particular predictor was still statistically significant after this maneuver, it was considered likely to be real. Among the 42 possible response predictors, this conservative analysis could identify only 5 for which there was enough agreement across studies to consider them likely predictors. The two predictors of good lithium response were the mania–depression–interval (MDI) course pattern and an age at onset in the intermediate range. Predictors of poor lithium response were a large number of previous hospitalizations, the course pattern of depression–mania–interval (DMI), and continuous cycling. Given that the effect sizes for any one predictor are, at best, moderate, the authors suggested that

TABLE 20–8. Clinical Characteristics Likely to be Associated with Differential Maintenance Response to Lithium versus Anticonvulsants

LITHIUM		VALPROATE, CARBAMAZEPINE, LAMOTRIGINE	
Good	Poor	Good	Poor
Family history of bipolar disorder	Negative family history for bipolar disorder	Negative family history for bipolar disorder	
Course variables:		Course variables:	
Intermediate age at onset	Earlier age at onset		
Mania–depression–interval course sequence	Depression–mania–interval course sequence		
Fewer previous hospitalizations and/or episodes	More previous hospitalizations and/or episodes	Multiple previous episodes (valproate)	
Non-rapid-cycling	Rapid-cycling[a]	Non-rapid-cycling; rapid-cycling bipolar-II (lamotrigine)	Rapid cycling (valproate)
Full remissions between episodes	Chronic course with comorbid substance abuse and anxiety	Chronic course with comorbid substance abuse and anxiety (lamotrigine)	

[a]May not apply in the absence of antidepressant use; see text for details.

the application of clinical predictors should be based on many variables (Table 20–8). Some of the clinical characteristics previously identified in individual studies that did not hold up in this meta-analysis are rapid cycling,[58] duration of illness, nature of the index episode, type of mania (euphoric-grandiose versus mixed), and bipolar-I versus bipolar-II.[59] The authors noted that in general, past history was better than the current clinical picture at predicting prophylactic lithium response.

Lithium's Prophylactic Efficacy in Bipolar-II

Table 20–9 outlines the limited literature on the efficacy of maintenance treatments for bipolar-II disorder. With regard to lithium, we know of only one adequately powered study that directly compared its prophylactic efficacy for bipolar-I and bipolar-II disorder. This open prospective study of bipolar patients on lithium maintenance for an average of 6.35 years, which included 129 patients with bipolar-II disorder, found that the latter patients had interepisode intervals nearly six-fold longer than those of the bipolar-I patients and were twice as likely to have no new mood episodes after lithium was initiated (Tondo et al., 1998). With regard to the relative efficacy of lithium against hypomania and depression in bipolar-II patients, one small study (Dunner et al.,

1976) found that the effect of lithium versus placebo was significant for depression but not for hypomania, a result reminiscent of some, but not all, of the mirror-image studies described previously.

Lithium's Prophylactic Efficacy in Recurrent Unipolar Depression

Many contemporary observers, particularly in the United States, will be surprised to learn that there are substantially more data on lithium's prophylactic efficacy in recurrent unipolar depression (primarily cases with recurrence frequencies in the bipolar range) than in bipolar-II disorder. Indeed, there are more data on lithium as maintenance treatment for recurrent unipolar depression than there are for all of the anticonvulsants and atypical antipsychotics combined as maintenance treatments for bipolar-I disorder (Davis et al., 1999).

In their extensive and careful meta-analysis, Davis and colleagues (1999) summarized nine randomized, blinded, placebo-controlled trials involving a total of 229 patients with recurrent unipolar depression. They found that relapse rates (primarily rehospitalization) averaged 75 percent for placebo versus 36 percent for lithium—virtually the same difference noted for similar studies of bipolar dis-

TABLE 20–9. **Results of Studies of Maintenance Treatment with Lithium for Bipolar-II Disorder**

Study	Sample Size	Duration	Drugs Studied	Results
Dunner et al., 1976	26	33 mo	Lithium vs. placebo	Effect of lithium greater than that of placebo for depression; not significant for hypomania (limited statistical power).
Fieve et al., 1976	18	48 mo	Lithium vs. placebo	Effect of lithium greater than that of placebo for prevention of depression.
Kane et al., 1982	22	24 mo	Lithium, imipramine, lithium + imipramine	Effect of lithium nonsignificant for bipolar-II (limited statistical power).
Tondo et al., 1998	129	75 mo (6.3 yr)	Lithium vs. placebo	Effect of lithium greater for bipolar-II than for bipolar-I.
Greil and Kleindienst, 1999	57	30 mo	Lithium vs. carbamazepine	No difference (limited statistical power).

Note: Studies with an observation period of 6 mo or less are not considered "maintenance" and are not included here.
Source: Adapted from Suppes and Dennehy (2002).

order. Moreover, the lithium effect in these most rigorous designs was the same as that observed in the many placebo-controlled trials that involved lithium withdrawal, as well as in the numerous matched case–control and mirror-image trials, a point made by Baldessarini and colleagues (1996) with reference to trials in bipolar disorder.

Valproate

Although valproate is clearly an effective antimanic agent, its role in maintenance therapy is less clear than that of lithium. As early as the 1970s, Lambert and colleagues (1971) reported preliminary evidence of a long-term benefit of the drug in treating bipolar disorder. In the United States, much of the initial interest in what was then, for psychiatry, a new agent was focused on its potential usefulness in patients who were not doing well on lithium, principally rapid cyclers. Calabrese and colleagues (1993) reviewed six open trials that assessed the efficacy of valproate in the maintenance treatment of 124 rapid-cycling bipolar patients; the two largest of these studies, comprising 101 patients, found that both valproate and lithium had marked antimanic but poor antidepressant effect.[60] Denicoff and colleagues (1997a), studying 18 rapid-cycling patients, found that only 6 of 18 responded to valproate, and all but one of the responders were also taking lithium (the question of the efficacy of valproate in combination with lithium is discussed later in the section on combined treatments). Indeed, in their review, Calabrese and colleagues (2001) concluded that rapid cyclers have a relatively poor response to all treatments for bipolar disorder, especially monotherapies. In the most careful and

comprehensive comparison of divalproex versus lithium for rapid-cycling bipolar disorder ever conducted, Calabrese and colleagues (2005) followed 60 rapid cyclers who had been stabilized for up to 6 months on a combination of lithium plus divalproex and were then randomized to have lithium or divalproex gradually tapered off with placebo substitution. During the monotherapy phase, which lasted 20 months, no significant differences were seen in relapse rates between divalproex- and lithium-treated subjects (50 versus 56 percent),[61] although there was a nonsignificant trend for the divalproex group to have a longer time to intervention. Studies of valproate and rapid-cycling disorder are included in Table 20–7.

With regard to maintenance valproate in non-rapid-cycling bipolar patients, a naturalistic study with a mean duration of follow-up of nearly 2 years (90 weeks) found that in a setting of minimal antidepressant use, divalproex was equivalent to lithium overall; lithium nonresponders did well on divalproex (50 percent by the Clinical Global Impressions-Bipolar [CGI-BP] scale) and vice versa (44 percent) (Ghaemi and Goodwin, 2001). Prevention of depressive relapses was noted with both agents, but divalproex was superior to lithium in reducing scores on the Hamilton Rating Scale for Depression (HAM-D) ($p < .003$).[62]

By far the most extensive and well-controlled evaluation of the maintenance efficacy of valproate is the parallel-design, randomized comparison of divalproex, lithium, and placebo for the maintenance treatment of bipolar disorder undertaken by Bowden and colleagues (2000a); indeed, it represents one of the largest studies of the prophylaxis of bipolar disorder to date.[63] The primary or planned analysis was a comparison of survival curves (i.e., time to first relapse) in the divalproex-, lithium-, and placebo-treated patients. This analysis found no significant difference among the three treatment groups. In secondary analysis, however, divalproex emerged as superior to placebo in having a lower rate of discontinuation for a recurrent mood episode, a finding consistent with that of a subsequent reanalysis of the data by a Cochrane Review group. The Cochrane reviewers concluded, however, that the results were difficult to generalize because "the inclusion of a placebo-treated group led to the inclusion of a less severely ill group of patients than is generally found in clinical practice" (Macritchie et al., 2002, p. 140). Here the reviewers were referring to the previously mentioned ethical constraints on a placebo-controlled study in which the end point is relapse.

In another secondary analysis, Bowden and colleagues (2000a) suggested less worsening of depressive symptoms during divalproex compared with lithium therapy, yet the high dropout rate in the lithium group (perhaps related to the high blood levels maintained) renders these comparisons problematic. It should also be recalled (as we review in Chapter 17) that secondary analyses are hypothesis generating, not hypothesis testing. Bowden and colleagues (2000a) suggested further that, compared with lithium, subjects treated with divalproex had symptom-free intervals of longer duration. A subsequent secondary analysis of this same database (Gyulai et al., 2003) found that among the patients given a "rescue" SSRI for breakthrough depressive symptoms, a lower percentage of those taking divalproex compared with placebo discontinued early because of depression. These authors also noted that those who had been given divalproex in the open period relapsed into depression later on divalproex than on lithium. But an advantage for divalproex in the maintenance phase might be expected among patients who were selected by their clinicians as being likely to respond to divalproex in the acute open phase. In a subsequent analysis of this maintenance treatment database, Bowden and colleagues (2005) examined the relationship between the symptom pattern during the acute manic phase and the subsequent response to maintenance treatment with either divalproex or lithium. They found that those patients whose manic episode had been dysphoric were more sensitive to the side effects of both lithium and divalproex during the maintenance trial. Regarding maintenance efficacy in the dysphoric group, the two drugs were equivalent. Among those patients who had been euphoric during their mania, more depressive symptoms (primarily motoric slowing) and more premature discontinuations were associated with lithium than with divalproex, although, as noted earlier, this finding might be explained by the high doses of lithium employed in this study.

With regard to valproate as maintenance treatment for bipolar-II disorder, we know of no controlled studies of pure bipolar-II patients that has directly addressed this question. However, in a double-blind, placebo-controlled study of 30 patients with bipolar-II disorder who also met DSM-IV criteria for borderline personality disorder, the divalproex group showed a significant reduction in dysphoric effects, such as irritability and anger (Frankenburg and Zanarini, 2002), but the drug did not separate from placebo in the prevention of depressive relapses.

Carbamazepine/Oxcarbazepine

Carbamazepine, initially used to treat a wide range of seizure disorders and various paroxysmal pain syndromes, was tried in manic-depressive (primarily bipolar) patients because it had stabilized the moods of some patients with convulsive disorders and because it counteracted kindling in laboratory animals. Much of the early work on carbamazepine in treating bipolar disorder was done in Japan during a time when lithium was unavailable for treatment of the disorder in that country because of regulatory issues, making identification of alternative treatments an urgent need. Okuma and colleagues (1973) found a prophylactic effect in 14 of their 27 bipolar patients in an open study, which they followed up with a 1-year placebo-controlled prophylactic trial in 22 bipolar patients (Okuma et al., 1981). Six of the 10 carbamazepine-treated patients, compared with 2 of the 9 taking placebo, had no affective recurrences during the trial, a result that tends to indicate a prophylactic effect. In what was actually the first double-blind trial, Ballenger and Post (1980) noted a prophylactic effect in 13 bipolar patients (many of whom had rapid-cycling illness or had failed to respond to lithium) maintained on carbamazepine for up to 4 months.[64] Kishimoto and colleagues (1983) suggested that responders to carbamazepine prophylaxis are likely to be those with onset of illness before age 20 and with frequent illness episodes, a conclusion similar to the analysis of the divalproex data by Swann and colleagues (1999). Additional studies that appeared through the 1980s suggested that carbamazepine is useful for the prophylactic management of bipolar patients who respond poorly to lithium (Placidi et al., 1986; Watkins et al., 1987). In the ensuing decades, five published controlled studies compared carbamazepine with lithium for the treatment of acute mania or depression.[65] Although these cannot be viewed as straightforward studies of prophylaxis of recurrences, they support some prophylactic benefit for carbamazepine.

There have been several prospective, parallel, randomized, double-blind trials comparing carbamazepine with lithium as a prophylactic agent in treating bipolar disorder. Coxhead and colleagues (1992) carried out such a study of 31 stable bipolar patients, 16 of whom were switched from lithium to carbamazepine, and found no difference in relapses, which had occurred in 50 percent of both groups by the end of the 12-month study. All relapses in the carbamazepine group had occurred within 2 months of switching, while only 3 of the 8 relapsing lithium-treated patients had relapsed at 2 months. The remaining 5 had relapsed between 2 and 6 months after the start of the trial. This study was too small for formal statistical analysis. Denicoff and colleagues (1997b) entered 52 bipolar patients into a randomized crossover 3-year trial comparing the efficacy of lithium, carbamazepine, and the combination (for 1 year each) in preventing recurrences.[66] The combination was significantly superior to either drug alone in preventing recurrent manic episodes and was also more effective in previously rapid-cycling patients.[67,68]

Greil and colleagues (1997) conducted a larger comparative trial of carbamazepine versus lithium over 2.5 years in 144 bipolar patients (Fig. 20–4).[69] Survival curves for rates of full relapse and rehospitalization showed trends favoring lithium, but the differences were not statistically significant. When relapse was defined by the need for other psychotropic medications and/or symptoms of depression or mania, however, the advantage for lithium achieved statistical significance ($p = .03$). When the curve was calculated using treatments and/or need for additional medication and/or dropouts due to side effects, lithium's advantage was even greater (35 percent [26/74] versus 51 percent [36/70]; $p = .007$). A placebo control group was not used for ethical reasons, given earlier studies showing lithium's advantage over placebo in bipolar disorder.

Figure 20–4. Survival curve for maintenance patients taking carbamazepine ($n = 70$) or lithium ($n = 74$), based on intention-to-treat analysis. Lithium showed a clear superiority ($p = .007$) when dropouts for hospitalization, symptom recurrence, need for additional medication, or intolerable side effects were considered. (*Source*: Greil et al., 1997. Reprinted with permission.)

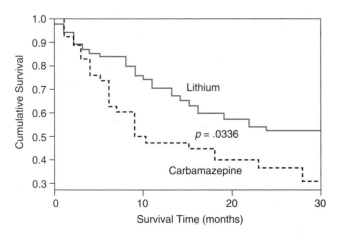

Subsequent analyses by these authors found that lithium's prophylactic benefit was particularly strong for "classical bipolar cases" (bipolar-I patients with no mood-incongruent delusions) (lithium>carbamazepine, $p < .01$), while carbamazepine was slightly (but not significantly) more efficacious than lithium for "nonclassical" bipolar disorder, a category including patients with mixed states. The authors also concluded that for the group as a whole, lithium's prophylactic effect was superior to that of carbamazepine when assessed by global measures of outcome (likelihood of remaining in treatment, rehospitalization, and residual symptomatology not requiring hospitalization) (Kleindienst and Greil, 2002).

With regard to carbamazepine in bipolar-II disorder, a 2-year randomized open trial of 57 patients with bipolar-II or bipolar-not otherwise specified (NOS) disorder was conducted, in which no significant differences were found between carbamazepine and lithium in preventing recurrence of symptoms (Greil and Kleindienst, 1999). However, the study was underpowered for establishing the absence of a difference.

To date there have been no controlled prophylaxis trials of oxcarbazepine. In one small study (Ghaemi et al., 2002)—a retrospective analysis of 13 subjects treated with the drug (either adjunctively or as monotherapy) for bipolar disorder—2 patients (16 percent) showed moderate improvement and 6 (46 percent) mild improvement during a period of 1–24 weeks. Unfortunately, 7 (54 percent) of the 13 patients stopped the medication because of side effects. Munoz (2002) reported on 28 patients with acute symptoms who were able to reduce the mean number of other medications taken over 12 weeks. Nasr and Caspar (2002) found that 28 patients with bipolar disorder who took oxcarbazepine for 9 months had significant improvement in severity of illness; bipolar-II patients appeared to benefit the most. Clearly, further study of oxcarbazepine for maintenance treatment of bipolar disorder is needed.

Lamotrigine

Lamotrigine has now been studied in a number of open and controlled trials as a maintenance treatment for bipolar disorder. Open add-on trials lasting several weeks to several months showed similar encouraging results in bipolar-I and -II subjects (Sporn and Sachs, 1997; Calabrese et al., 1999a; Suppes et al., 1999a).[70]

Two large randomized, placebo-controlled, double-blind studies of lamotrigine for maintenance treatment of bipolar-I disorder have been completed, both comparing it with lithium and placebo. The first involved 175 patients who had recently been manic/hypomanic (Bowden et al., 2003a), while the second involved 349 patients who had recently

TABLE 20–10.   Drugs Demonstrating Maintenance Prophylactic Efficacy versus Placebo in Randomized, Double-Blind Trials

Drug	No. of Studies	Sample Size	Findings
Lithium	17	1,551	About half of the studies involved abrupt lithium withdrawal before randomization, but lithium–placebo differences were similar in studies with and without abrupt withdrawal.
Carbamazepine	2	32	The carbamazepine–placebo difference was modest.
Lamotrigine	2	645	Superiority to placebo was due primarily to prevention of depressive episodes, while for the comparator, lithium, it was due primarily to the drug's effect against mania/hypomania.
Lamotrigine (in rapid cycling)	1	182	In secondary analysis, lamotrigine was found to be superior to placebo among the bipolar-II subgroup.
Divalproex	1	372	The primary outcome variable did not separate divalproex from placebo, but divalproex did separate in some secondary analyses.
Fluoxetine	1	10	Possible benefit was found in the bipolar-II subgroup in retrospective post hoc analysis of a unipolar cohort.
Olanzapine	1	361	Compared with placebo, olanzapine delayed relapse in bipolar-I patients who responded to open-label acute treatment with olanzapine for a manic or mixed episode. This was a 1-year trial, but 75% of placebo relapses occurred in the first 2 mo.
Aripiprazole	1	567	Time to relapse of manic symptoms was significantly longer, and there were fewer total manic relapses with aripiprazole treatment than with placebo. This was a 6-mo trial.
Total	26	3,720	

Source: Adapted from Ghaemi and Hsu, 2005.

been depressed (Bowden et al., 2003b) (Fig. 20–5). Patients entered these studies in an open phase of up to 16 weeks during which lamotrigine was slowly titrated up while other psychotropics were gradually withdrawn. Patients who met criteria for stabilization on lamotrigine plus the medication that was gradually withdrawn (they were taking lamotrigine alone for at least 1 week) were then randomized to receive either lamotrigine, lithium (to achieve serum levels of .8–1.1 mEq/l), or placebo. The partially enriched sample that was randomized represented about half

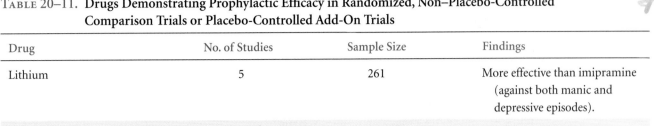

Table 20–11. Drugs Demonstrating Prophylactic Efficacy in Randomized, Non–Placebo-Controlled Comparison Trials or Placebo-Controlled Add-On Trials

Drug	No. of Studies	Sample Size	Findings
Lithium	5	261	More effective than imipramine (against both manic and depressive episodes).
Valproate	1	251	Equivalent to olanzapine.
Carbamazepine	2	64	Slightly less effective than lithium in study of mostly "typical" patients; slightly more effective than lithium in study of "atypical" patients.
Oxcarbazepine	1	15	Equivalent to lithium, but study underpowered.
Flupenthixol	2	53	Equivalent to placebo when added to lithium, but study underpowered.
Olanzapine	3	778	Equivalent to lithium or valproate; more effective than placebo when added to lithium or valproate among nonresponders or partial responders.
Clozapine	1	38	Clozapine plus treatment as usual (TAU) more effective in prevention of mania than TAU among nonresponders to two mood stabilizers.
Imipramine	2	192	Equivalent to placebo when added to lithium; significantly more manic episodes over 3 yr in one study with careful monitoring of lithium levels.
Omega-3 Fatty Acids	1	30	Somewhat more effective than placebo when added to standard mood stabilizers in a rapid-cycling sample.
Total	18	1,682	

Source: Adapted from Ghaemi and Hsu, 2005.

of the approximately 1,300 patients who initially met the study's screening criteria. Time until the need for intervention for breakthrough symptoms was the primary end point in both studies. In the study of recently manic/hypomanic patients, both lamotrigine and lithium were found to be superior to placebo in delaying the need for intervention for any mood episode (about 50 percent of patients in both treatment groups needed some additional treatment, compared with more than 80 percent of the placebo group). When the measure of any early discontinuation from the study was used as an end point, both active drugs were still statistically superior to placebo, but the difference

Figure 20–5. Comparison of lithium or lamotrigine with placebo for the prevention of mood episodes. Shown are Kaplan-Meier survival curves for time to intervention for any mood episode (e.g., need for additional medication) in 171 patients with bipolar disorder. (*Source:* Bowden et al., 2003b, p. 392. Reprinted with permission.)

was less impressive. With respect to time to intervention for any episode and survival in the study, essentially the same results were obtained with the recently depressed patients. In both studies considered independently, lamotrigine (but not lithium) was superior to placebo in delaying or decreasing the likelihood of interventions for depressive symptoms, while lithium (but not lamotrigine) was superior in delaying or decreasing the likelihood of interventions for manic/hypomanic symptoms.

However, a combined analysis of both datasets (employing appropriate statistical adjustments) showed that lamotrigine was significantly superior to placebo not only for depressive episodes, but also for manic episodes, although lithium was significantly better than lamotrigine for prevention of mania. As noted earlier in our discussion of lithium, there was only a trend for lithium to be superior to placebo in delaying time to relapse for depression, but it should be recalled that this sample was partially enriched with lamotrigine responders, who may represent a somewhat different clinical profile from that of lithium responders (see the later discussion). The fact that lithium works best "from above" while lamotrigine works best "from below" implies that in the maintenance treatment of bipolar-I disorder, the two drugs should be combined. However, given that lamotrigine apparently has a modest prophylactic effect against mania, it should be possible when using the drug for prevention of depression in a bipolar-I patient to use lower doses of an adjunctive stabilizer, such as lithium or valproate, "from above," thereby reducing the overall side-effect load and preserving one of lamotrigine's major advantages—its impressive

tolerability (especially lack of weight gain and neurocognitive side effects).

The data from these two studies have been interpreted as supporting the conclusion that the polarity of the acute episode predicts the polarity of relapse in the maintenance phase. However, a subsequent analysis by Calabrese and colleagues (2006) found that when the early relapses (those occurring in the first 3 to 6 months) are not considered, both lamotrigine and lithium continue to separate robustly from placebo, suggesting that they are preventing new episodes (recurrences) rather than just relapses. In addition, a separate analysis of the 6 to 18 month data among those randomized to placebo (Goodwin and Calabrese, in preparation) showed that these late relapses (recurrences) were much more likely to be into the *opposite* phase; that is, following an index mania, 85 percent of the late relapses were into depression and vice versa for index depressive episodes.[71] This new analysis brings these clinical trial data into line with results of studies of the natural course of the illness described in Chapter 4 (manic episodes tend to follow depressive ones and vice versa). What is perhaps most important about this new analysis is that it effectively undermines the all too common recommendation (which unfortunately has found its way into some treatment guidelines) that whatever works for the acute episode should simply be continued as the foundation for long-term maintenance treatment.

Lamotrigine's ability to stabilize mood over time has been reported in rapid-cycling patients as well.[72] In the first double-blind, placebo-controlled trial of any agent for rapid-cycling bipolar-I and -II disorder, a prospective 26-week study of lamotrigine, the drug showed a small but not significant advantage over placebo in time to additional intervention for symptoms in the entire sample, but in a post hoc analysis of the bipolar-II group, it was found to be superior to placebo (Calabrese et al., 2000)[73] (see the discussion of bipolar-II that follows). This stands as the first placebo-controlled maintenance study with rapid-cycling bipolar patients. In a 1-year open trial of lamotrigine versus lithium in 14 rapid-cycling bipolar patients, those taking lamotrigine were much more likely to have fewer than four affective episodes during the year of the study (Walden et al., 2000). The authors acknowledged that, as in the earlier lithium–divalproex comparisons, their protocol favored inclusion of prior lithium-nonresponsive patients, which obviously could bias any comparisons with lithium.

Passmore and colleagues (2003) compared several clinical and family history characteristics of 21 patients with bipolar disorder—14 classified as responders to lamotrigine and 7 as responders to lithium. They found that the lamotrigine responders tended to have more chronic symptoms, rapid cycling, and comorbid panic disorder and substance abuse and to have larger numbers of family members with schizoaffective disorder, major depression, and panic disorder. They suggested that lamotrigine may be especially helpful for patients with these clinical characteristics. An overall impression of lamotrigine's effectiveness in a clinical setting can be gleaned from recently reported STEP-BD data from Stanford University in the United States (Champion et al., 2006). Among 201 trials with a mean duration of 432 days, lamotrigine was continued throughout in 64 percent of the trials (32 percent as monotherapy, 42 percent with an additional drug).[74] Six percent of patients discontinued lamotrigine because of lack of efficacy. There were no serious rashes, but 3 percent discontinued the drug because of a benign rash.

Other Anticonvulsants

Emerging but not definitive maintenance data exist for several other anticonvulsants. Some of these agents were studied in the past with ambiguous results as to their efficacy; several others are being actively studied as of this writing.

Gabapentin

Although some evidence supports an anxiolytic and sedative effect of gabapentin, no evidence from controlled trials supports its benefit as monotherapy in maintenance treatment of bipolar disorder. Trials of gabapentin versus lamotrigine and placebo at NIMH provided no evidence that gabapentin's benefit exceeded that of placebo (Frye et al., 2000). This result, coupled with the drug's failure as an antimanic agent (Pande et al., 2000), has discouraged

pursuit of its use in prophylaxis for bipolar disorder. A few open reports and one recent controlled study do suggest acute antimanic and antidepressive effects of *adjunctive* gabapentin. For example, in a study of 23 patients with bipolar disorder (Altshuler et al., 1999), 19 patients were taking two or more medications in addition to gabapentin. Thus although most did recover during the study period, it is impossible to assess critically the role, if any, played by gabapentin. Knoll and colleagues (1998) reported similar results for 12 treatment-resistant patients taking multiple medications and followed for up to 60 weeks. In the only controlled maintenance trial of gabapentin in bipolar disorder, Vieta and colleagues (2006) randomly assigned 25 euthymic bipolar-I and -II patients already taking lithium, carbamazepine, or valproate (or any combination of these, but excluding antidepressants and antipsychotics) to receive either adjunctive gabapentin or placebo under double-blind conditions. This trial is notable for its use of a true prophylactic design rather than one based simply on relapse prevention following acute response (see Chapter 17). Compared with those taking placebo, the gabapentin group showed significantly more change on the CGI-BP, Modified long-term outcome scale ($p < .005$); that is, the blinded clinician raters perceived more overall improvement among those taking adjunctive gabapentin.

Tiagabine

To date there have been no controlled studies of tiagabine in bipolar disorder (Young et al., 2006). As noted in Chapter 18, the drug did not have obvious antimanic benefit in an early study of eight acutely manic inpatients for whom other treatments had failed (Grunze et al., 1999). However, Schaffer and Schaffer (1999) reported on two patients with recurrent manic, mixed, and to some extent depressive relapses who appeared to improve over 3 and 5 months, respectively, when tiagabine was added to their medication regimen. A later study conducted by the same authors (Schaffer et al., 2002) assessed tiagabine as an adjunctive treatment for patients with refractory bipolar disorder and found that 8 of 22 patients (36 percent) were "much" or "very much" improved on the CGI scale after 6 months of taking tiagabine.[75]

Topiramate

Topiramate has been used to treat acute phases of bipolar disorder, and the results reported have been equivocal at best (see Chapters 18 and 19). Results of several open reports on slightly longer-term use of the drug are also inconclusive. Nevertheless, topiramate is a fairly common component of the pharmacotherapy of bipolar disorder, given its ability to reduce appetite and weight. Yet for many patients it can be a challenge to find a dose that produces positive effects without causing unacceptable neurocognitive side effects.[76] Marcotte (1998) reviewed the charts of 44 patients treated for bipolar-I manic or mixed states or bipolar-II disorder with an average of 200 mg/day of topiramate in addition to existing therapy for an average of 16 weeks. Of these patients, 23 (52 percent) were rated as showing moderate to marked improvement, and 5 (11 percent) were rated as worse; 1 patient became delirious.

McIntyre and colleagues (2002) reported on 109 outpatients with bipolar-I and -II disorder with chronic mood instability in whom topiramate was added to lithium, valproate, or both for 16 weeks. Although more than one-third (39) of the patients dropped out of the study because of adverse events or insufficient response, about two-thirds of those remaining showed reductions of 50 percent or more in their Young Mania Rating Scale (YMRS) or Montgomery-Asberg depression scores at the end of the 16 weeks. Vieta and colleagues (2002) conducted a 6-month open-label add-on trial of topiramate in 34 subjects with treatment-resistant bipolar spectrum disorders (schizoaffective disorder-bipolar type, bipolar-I, bipolar-II, and bipolar-NOS). More than half of the patients (who had refractory manic, depressive, or mixed symptoms) could be classified as responders based on reductions in YMRS, HAM-D, and CGI scores (Vieta et al., 2002). The same group reported comparable results in a similarly designed 12-week study involving 16 subjects with bipolar-II disorder (Vieta et al., 2003).

In sum, topiramate's efficacy for the maintenance treatment of bipolar disorder is far from clear. Indeed, as reviewed in Chapter 18, it has not yet been possible to demonstrate the drug's antimanic effects acutely. Clearly, then, more data will be required before this agent can be recommended with any confidence, even for adjunctive use.

Phenytoin

Mishory and colleagues (2003) studied 23 subjects with bipolar-I or schizoaffective disorder taking a variety of other medications in a double-blind, placebo-controlled, crossover study of add-on phenytoin, with a 6-month observation period for each phase. During a total of 30 observation periods in these subjects, 3 relapsed while taking phenytoin and 9 while taking placebo. These results suggest that phenytoin may be helpful in prophylaxis, but more controlled studies clearly are needed.

Antipsychotics

Until fairly recently, there had been few studies of antipsychotic medications for the long-term treatment of bipolar disorder except in combination with other agents. In the mid-1990s, however, the development of the atypical antipsychotics led to a resurgence of interest in antipsychotics for maintenance treatment of bipolar disorder. Actually, the

first evaluation of an antipsychotic as maintenance treatment for manic-depressive illness predated the atypical drugs by nearly 20 years. In an early open study whose coauthors included Schou and Baastrup, the typical antipsychotic flupenthixol was given to 93 patients with manic-depressive illness (bipolar disorder or recurrent unipolar depression) who had experienced a poor response to or were unable to tolerate lithium (Ahlfors et al., 1981). The patients experienced a significant decrease in manic episodes but an excessive number of depressive episodes compared with when they were taking lithium alone. Overall, the antipsychotic was considered a suitable substitute for lithium therapy only for those patients who failed to respond to lithium or who would not or could not take it. A second study, with a randomized, double-blind, crossover design, failed to show any benefit of flupenthixol (Esparon et al., 1986).

During the mid-1990s, the first atypical antipsychotic, clozapine, was the subject of case reports and open series reporting that it was helpful as an adjunctive treatment in patients with bipolar disorder (Banov et al., 1994; Zarate et al., 1995). Ciapparelli and colleagues (2000) retrospectively reviewed the naturalistic use of clozapine in 91 patients with treatment-refractory symptoms of schizophrenia, bipolar disorder with psychotic features, or schizoaffective disorder and found that those with mood disorders showed significantly greater improvement than those with schizophrenia. In a randomized study of adjunctive clozapine versus treatment as usual in 38 patients over a period of 1 year, the clozapine-treated group showed significant improvement on scales for global functioning, psychotic symptoms, and mania, but not on those for depression (Suppes et al., 1999b).[77]

There have been preliminary but promising reports as well on the efficacy of risperidone for maintenance treatment of bipolar disorder. Ghaemi and Sachs (1997) prospectively assessed the outcome of openly adding risperidone to the medication regimen of 12 outpatients with bipolar-I disorder who suffered breakthrough episodes despite adequate maintenance medication (lithium, divalproex, or carbamazepine, or a combination of these).[78] Four patients discontinued medication—two because of lack of efficacy and two because of side effects. Among the remaining eight patients, four experienced an improvement of 10 to 25 points in Global Assessment of Functioning scores and were rated much better on the CGI-Improvement scale. Although one patient suffered a major depressive recurrence (at week 22), none experienced worsening of mania. A more recent continuation study of adjunctive risperidone, while somewhat larger, was limited by the brevity of the follow-up period— just 10 weeks. Among 48 bipolar patients who completed the 10 weeks of treatment after an acute manic episode, those who received a mood stabilizer plus risperidone showed significantly more improvement in mania and depression ratings than those who were taking a mood stabilizer plus placebo (Bowden et al., 2004). The recent availability of a long-acting (about 2 weeks) form of injectable risperidone (Respiridol Consta in the United States) expands the options for dealing with adherence problems.

The atypical antipsychotic that has been studied most extensively as a maintenance treatment for bipolar disorder is olanzapine. Several open studies of the adjunctive use of this atypical agent have showed encouraging efficacy in reducing breakthrough symptoms and preventing relapses in patients whose illness was difficult to control (Narendran et al., 2001; Vieta et al., 2001b). These findings led to interest in the use of this agent as monotherapy for the maintenance treatment of bipolar disorder, first investigated in the continuation phase of a placebo-controlled study of the drug for treatment of acute mania (Sanger et al., 2001). In this study, 113 patients who had responded acutely in the open-label extension and remained well on olanzapine during the 3-week placebo-controlled phase continued into a 49-week open-label phase. The investigators had the option of adding lithium or fluoxetine for residual or breakthrough symptoms and did so for nearly two-thirds of the patients. Like many longer-term studies of patients with bipolar disorder, this study had a high dropout rate (over 60 percent). Nevertheless, the 41 percent of patients who received olanzapine monotherapy recovered and remained well over a period of 1 year. Somnolence and weight gain and complaints of "depression" were the most frequently reported side effects.

Tohen and colleagues reported on three separate double-blind studies of olanzapine for relapse prevention after successful treatment of a manic or mixed episode with olanzapine—one comparing olanzapine with lithium in 431 patients (Tohen et al., 2002), one comparing it with divalproex in 248 patients (Tohen et al., 2003), and one comparing it with placebo in 361 patients (Tohen et al., 2006). In the olanzapine versus lithium study, patients were entered into the maintenance phase if they both tolerated and had a complete antimanic response to the open-label combination of olanzapine plus lithium (representing 33 percent of the initial population); they were then randomized to have one of the drugs discontinued abruptly and followed for up to 52 weeks. The group that remained on olanzapine had a significantly lower rate of relapse back into mania (28.0 versus 14.3 percent) than the group that remained on lithium, while relapses into depression were nearly identical in the two groups. This international collaborative study, which included many sites with considerable experience in the use of lithium, represents the first large-scale demonstration of any drug's surpassing lithium in the prevention of relapse back into mania. In a subsequent post hoc analysis, Ketter and colleagues (2006) examined treatment response in relation to the number of previous manic episodes. For those with two prior episodes (early-stage illness), olanzapine was significantly better than lithium in preventing relapse into mania, while for those with either three to five (intermediate-stage illness) or more than five (later-stage illness) prior episodes, there was no significant difference between the two treatments, although the intermediate-stage group showed a trend favoring olanzapine. The authors concluded that olanzapine maintenance after acute recovery from a manic episode may be particularly effective early in the course of the illness.

The 47-week randomized study of olanzapine versus divalproex started with the acute double-blind treatment of manic or mixed patients, the results of which are reviewed in Chapter 18.[79] Responders then entered a 44-week double-blind extension, in which they remained on the drug to which they had responded acutely (flexibly dosed olanzapine or divalproex[80]). The mean improvement in YMRS scores was significantly greater for the olanzapine group, and the median time to symptomatic remission of mania was shorter for olanzapine. On the other hand, the overall rate of bipolar relapse, including relapse into depression, did not differ, and adverse effects (including somnolence, dry mouth, weight gain, and akathisia) were significantly more frequent among the olanzapine-treated patients. The high dropout rates for both olanzapine- and divalproex-treated patients (84 percent overall) limit the interpretation of these results, especially for a study with no placebo group.[81] A subsequent post hoc analysis of these 47-week data (Suppes et al., 2005) examined differential treatment response as a function of the presence or absence of rapid cycling; the advantage of olanzapine in mean improvement in mania ratings was seen only in the non-rapid-cycling patients.

The study of olanzapine versus placebo (Tohen et al., 2006) started with bipolar patients whose manic/mixed episode had responded to and tolerated olanzapine (representing 49 percent of the initial group); after being well for a period of 1 to 4 weeks, the patients were randomized to either continue olanzapine or be assigned to placebo (that is, they were abruptly withdrawn from olanzapine). Compared with the placebo group, the olanzapine continuation group was significantly less likely to relapse back into mania (hazard ratio 3.9) or (to a lesser extent) into depression (hazard ratio 2.1).[82] The ability of olanzapine to prevent relapse was independent of psychotic features during mania or a history of rapid cycling. Perhaps the most important issue in evaluating this study as evidence of a "maintenance" effect is the fact that the bulk of the drug–placebo difference was evident in the first 2 months, suggesting that a withdrawal effect contributed substantially to the results (Fig. 20–6). The authors addressed this possibility by

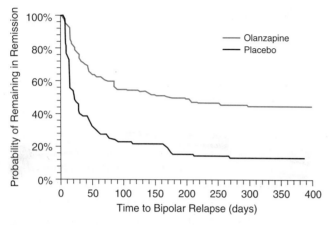

Figure 20–6. Time to relapse into mania or depression with olanzapine versus placebo. (*Source*: Tohen et al., 2003. Reprinted with permission.)

pointing to two post hoc analyses.[83] However, those analyses did not address the fundamental issue—that most of the drug–placebo difference occurred within the first 2 months, a period of time we believe is too short to allow evaluation of whether olanzapine prevents the occurrence of new episodes. Although the FDA has approved olanzapine for "maintenance" treatment,[84] studies of the drug's long term *prophylactic* efficacy are still needed. The reader is referred to Chapter 17 for a discussion of maintenance designs and their meaning.

The most recent evaluation of an atypical antipsychotic for use beyond the acute episode involved aripiprazole. Following stabilization of an acute manic/mixed episode with open-label aripiprazole for a minimum of 6 weeks, 567 bipolar-I patients (37 percent of those who entered the open phase)[85] were randomized to continue the drug for up to 6 months or to have it withdrawn abruptly and replaced by placebo (Keck et al., 2006). The majority of relapses were into mania—hardly surprising for patients who had recently recovered from a manic episode. Time to relapse into manic symptoms was significantly longer and fewer total manic relapses occurred with aripiprazole treatment than with placebo. Relapses into depression were low in both groups and were virtually identical. The only adverse effects that were more common (by t test) in the aripiprazole group were anxiety and nervousness, while sedation and somnolence were actually less frequent with aripiprazole than with placebo (McQuade et al., 2004). As with the olanzapine studies, however, this study was underpowered to detect differences in side effects, and under these circumstances, a simple t test can be quite misleading.[86] As with the olanzapine studies, moreover, both the efficacy and side-effect results can be generalized only to those who tolerate and respond acutely to aripiprazole. Relative to the olanzapine–placebo comparison, this study's results are less confounded by withdrawal effects because it employed a longer open-label stabilization period (minimum of 6 weeks) before randomization and because the aripiprazole–placebo difference continued to widen throughout the 6 months. Nevertheless, a randomized phase lasting a maximum of only 6 months is too short to permit evaluation of true prophylactic effects; longer studies of aripiprazole are awaited. Table 20–12 summarizes the strength of the evidence from the controlled monotherapy maintenance studies reviewed above.

TABLE 20–12. Strength of the Evidence for Efficacy of Mood Stabilizers from Placebo-Controlled Monotherapy Studies

Drug	Depression	Mania	True Prophylaxis[a] (prevent recurrence)	Continuation/"Maintenance" (FDA) (prevent relapses)
Lithium	++	+++	++++	++++
Valproate	+	+++	+ ?	+ ?
Carbamazepine	+/−	+++	+	?
Lamotrigine	++	—	+++	+++
Olanzapine	+	+++	+ ?	+
Aripiprazole	No data	+++	No data	+
Quetiapine	++	+++	No data	No data

[a]Prophylaxis is defined based on data from placebo-controlled studies demonstrating efficacy during the maintenance phase (>6 mo after the acute phase).

Note: The + signs indicate the strength of the data, not the size of the effect.

Combination Maintenance Treatments for Bipolar Disorder

Retrospective and open-label studies of the use of combinations of psychotropic agents for maintenance treatment of bipolar disorder are too numerous to review individually. Some of these studies involved as few as 5 to 15 patients, and many lasted less than 1 year. As with the treatment of acute depression and mania with combinations of drugs, the literature offers scant empirical information to guide the clinician in the choice of agents for complex regimens. (The reasons for the paucity of controlled studies of combination treatments are discussed in Chapter 17.) Most studies of combination treatments start with a group of patients who are not responding or are inadequately responding to a monotherapy; this limits the generalizability of the results. Another problem with this literature is that almost exclusively, full doses of each drug are used, whereas in clinical practice, additive effects are generally taken into account so that lower doses of each drug are used. Further, when there is some suggestion from studies of mechanism of action that two drugs may act synergistically, combining lower doses of two drugs with different side-effect profiles can result in a higher ratio of therapeutic to side effects (Goodwin, 2003). Finally, because of the higher side-effect burden of combination treatments, dropout rates from such studies are high, making statistical comparisons somewhat problematic.

Lithium and Anticonvulsants

Freeman and Stoll (1998) provided a comprehensive review summarizing the large and inconclusive compilation of uncontrolled studies of combinations of lithium and anticonvulsants, noting that the "interactions of such combinations are sometimes complex, often very useful, and potentially dangerous." They suggested that the combinations are safe, with that of lithium and valproate probably having the best overall profile of safety and efficacy given the limitations of the published data on combination treatments. They suggested further that this combination may be especially useful for patients with rapid cycles and mixed states.[87] It has also been suggested that the combination of lithium and carbamazepine is particularly effective (Kishimoto, 1992). Bocchetta and colleagues (1997) reported on 22 patients with bipolar or schizoaffective disorder, followed for up to 13 years, whose cumulative affective morbidity was markedly reduced when carbamazepine was added to lithium.

With regard to controlled studies of the lithium plus anticonvulsant combination, in our earlier review of carbamazepine we mentioned the randomized, placebo-controlled study of Denicoff and colleagues (1997b), which included a crossover design and which found that combination to be superior to either drug alone, particularly among patients with a history of rapid cycles. In a further study of 24 patients who had failed to respond to lithium plus carbamazepine, this same group found that 59 percent did respond to lithium plus valproate; 3 of the 7 who failed to respond to lithium plus valproate did respond to the triple combination of lithium plus valproate plus carbamazepine. Another small randomized study (Solomon et al., 1997) found fewer relapses among bipolar patients taking the combination of lithium plus valproate compared with lithium plus placebo, but the former combination was associated with more side effects.

Recently, considerable experience has been gained with the combination of lithium and lamotrigine (see, e.g., Ghaemi et al., 2006), which, as noted previously, is an especially advantageous combination for maintenance treatment of bipolar-I patients, combining prevention "from below" with that "from above." Because lithium has no drug–drug interactions with lamotrigine, in these circumstances it has an advantage over valproate (which inhibits the metabolism of lamotrigine). Also, as noted earlier, lamotrigine has some modest mania-preventing capacity of its own, so its use should enable lower doses of the antimanic agent (lithium, another anticonvulsant, or an atypical antipsychotic) when treating bipolar-I patients, thus reducing the overall side-effect burden (Goodwin and Goldstein, 2003).[88]

Combinations with Antidepressants

Despite the frequency with which antidepressants are prescribed for patients already taking medications for bipolar disorder, a 2001 review by Ghaemi and colleagues (2001a) concluded that the use of antidepressants on a long-term basis in patients with bipolar disorder has been "extraordinarily understudied." Indeed, surveys indicate that twice as many prescriptions are written for antidepressants as for mood stabilizers for bipolar patients (Garza-Trevino et al., 1992; Ghaemi et al., 2001b; Baldessarini et al., 2006). Thus in a naturalistic study of outpatients with affective disorders, Ghaemi and colleagues (2000) found that only 33 percent of the bipolar subset had ever received mood stabilizers alone, while 78 percent had been prescribed antidepressants at some time. Additionally, mania or hypomania was observed after the initiation of antidepressants in 55 percent of the bipolar patients, and 23 percent experienced rapid cycling or cycle acceleration. In the largest study to date, Baldessarini and colleagues (2006) analyzed initial prescriptions for 7,760 bipolar patients in the United States and found that half of them were for an antidepressant, while only 24.6 percent were for a mood stabilizer.

Seven long-term studies have involved combinations of lithium and antidepressants.[89] These studies (summarized in Table 20–13) were of varying design and allow few conclusions about the efficacy or safety of these combinations.

TABLE 20–13. Blind, Controlled Trials of Long-Term Antidepressant Treatment in Bipolar Disorder[a]

Study	Diagnoses (Sample Size)	Design	Duration (mo)	Outcome Assessed	Results
Prien et al., 1973b	BP-I (44)	Lithium vs. imipramine vs. placebo	Up to 24	Hospitalized or new treatment	Efficacy: lithium >imipramine = placebo
Wehr and Goodwin, 1979	BP-I (5)	Lithium carbonate vs. lithium carbonate + desipramine	27 (mean)	Nurse ratings	Efficacy: lithium + desipramine >lithium (?); switch and cycling rate: lithium + desipramine ≫lithium
Quitkin et al., 1981	BP-I (75)	Lithium vs. lithium + imipramine	19 (mean)	RDC episodes	Efficacy: lithium = imipramine; mania: imipramine >lithium (women)
Kane et al., 1982	BP-II (27), UP (22)	Lithium vs. imipramine vs. lithium + imipramine vs. placebo	11 (mean)	RDC episodes	Efficacy: lithium >placebo; imipramine = placebo
Prien et al., 1984	BP-I (117), UP (150)	Lithium vs. lithium + imipramine vs. imipramine	Up to 24	RDC episodes	Efficacy: lithium = lithium + imipramine; imipramine more manic switches
Sachs et al., 1994	BP-I (15) (19 treatment trials)	Bupropion vs. desipramine	Up to 12	DSM-III-R episodes	Efficacy: lithium + bupropion = lithium + desipramine; mania: desipramine >bupropion
Amsterdam et al., 1998	BP-II (80), matched UP (79), unmatched UP controls (661)	Fluoxetine vs. placebo	Up to 14	DSM-III-R episodes	Efficacy: fluoxetine similar in BP-II and UP; switch rate: BP >UP
Parker et al., 2006	BP-II (10) (4-day duration for hypomania not required; no previous treatment with antidepressant or mood stabilizer)	Escitalopram vs. placebo, followed by crossover	9 (3-mo baseline, 3-mo SSRI or placebo, 3-mo placebo or SSRI)	Various self-ratings daily, monthly HAM-D and YMRS	Compared with placebo, a significant reduction in depression severity and days spent depressed or high; no worsening of course

[a]See the companion Web site for an updated version of this table.

Note: Efficacy results related to BP depressive symptoms unless otherwise stated.

BP = bipolar disorder; DSM-III-R = *Diagnostic and Statistical Manual*, 3rd edition, revised; HAM-D = Hamilton Rating Scale for Depression; RDC = Research Diagnostic Criteria; SSRI = selective serotonin reuptake inhibitors; UP = unipolar depression; YRMS = Young Mania Rating Scale.

Source. Adapted from Ghaemi et al., 2001a.

None of these studies showed an advantage of imipramine over lithium for preventing depression, but their results do point to the risk of hypomanic and manic switches in bipolar patients taking imipramine. The table also includes three studies involving second-generation antidepressants. (See Chapter 19 for a more extensive discussion of both the acute and long-term efficacy of antidepressants in bipolar disorder and the relationship between antidepressants and switching and/or illness destabilization.)

Combinations with Antipsychotic Medications

Many patients discharged from the hospital after having been treated for mania are taking antipsychotic medications and continue to do so for weeks or months thereafter. Clinical variables associated with being treated with antipsychotics for at least 6 months after discharge from the hospital include being male, having multiple manic episodes with severe symptoms, and failing to adhere to the treatment regimen (Keck et al., 1996; Frangou et al., 2002). Results of studies involving the older (typical) antipsychotic medications have been rendered less relevant with the emergence of the newer, atypical agents and their putative lower risk of EPS and tardive dyskinesia.[90] The potentially serious risk of significant weight gain was noted earlier.

Results of several relatively long-term studies of atypical antipsychotics added to lithium or anticonvulsants are now available. In the preceding section on the atypical antipsychotics, we discussed the randomized study of Suppes and colleagues (1999b), which showed that adjunctive clozapine was associated with significant clinical improvement, but the improvement did not include depressive symptoms. An Italian study of 60 patients with schizoaffective disorder or bipolar disorder with psychotic features found significant improvement on the CGI-Severity of Illness scale that extended over a 24-month period after clozapine was added to their regimen (Ciapparelli et al., 2000). Chang and colleagues (2006) found that, among 51 treatment-refractory bipolar patients given adjunctive clozapine and followed for at least 6 months, 90 percent experienced a reduction in the number and duration of hospitalizations ($p<.01$); significant reductions were noted in hospitalizations for both manic and depressive but not mixed episodes. Two similar studies by Vieta and colleagues used adjunctive risperidone for 6 months in more than 400 patients with schizoaffective or psychotic bipolar disorder (Vieta et al., 2001a) and olanzapine for 43 weeks in 23 patients with bipolar-I or -II disorder (Vieta et al., 2001b); comparable results were obtained in the two studies.

Tohen and colleagues (2004) compared the efficacy of olanzapine added to lithium or valproate with that of the mood stabilizer alone for the prevention of mood episodes in an 18-month randomized, double-blind study of bipolar-I subjects. Participants in a previous study of the treatment of acute manic or mixed episodes who had a prior documented failure to respond to either lithium or valproate were given an open-label combination of olanzapine plus one of the two mood stabilizers for 6 weeks. Those who achieved remission were randomized under double-blind conditions to either continued use of the combination or abrupt withdrawal of olanzapine with continuation of the mood stabilizer plus placebo. The time to relapse into a manic, mixed, or depressive episode according to DSM-IV criteria did not differ between the two groups. However, a secondary analysis revealed that the time to development of a "symptomatic relapse" (defined as a YMRS or HAM-D-21 score of 15 or greater) was significantly shorter for the mood stabilizer monotherapy group.[91] At the same time, the apparent symptomatic advantage of adjunctive olanzapine must be balanced against the 10-fold higher incidence of weight gain associated with its use as compared with lithium or valproate alone (20 versus 2 percent). There was no significant difference in the polarity of the relapses with and without the adjunctive olanzapine. As we noted earlier when presenting the results of the monotherapy study of olanzapine versus placebo, most of the difference in symptomatic relapse occurred during the first 2 months (which is part of the continuation phase of treatment), suggesting that withdrawal effects played a role.

Other Agents and Approaches

Additional approaches to the maintenance treatment of bipolar disorder have been examined in the literature. These include the use of maintenance ECT, thyroid hormones, calcium channel blockers, psychostimulants such as methylphenidate, nutritional supplements, and extended bed rest and darkness.

Maintenance Electroconvulsive Therapy

A number of case reports and open series have addressed maintenance ECT for the prevention of mood episodes in patients with various disorders, including affective disorders, schizophrenia, and Parkinson's disease. These reports have uniformly described patients with intractable symptoms poorly controlled with medications who have benefited from ECT given on a schedule ranging from weekly to monthly, or even less often (for reviews see Abrams, 1990; Andrade and Kurinji, 2002; Vaidya et al., 2003). Petrides and colleagues (1994) reported on the institutional experience of continuation and maintenance ECT for patients with affective disorders between 1985 and 1991, including 1-year follow-up data for 21 patients; they cited a reduction in relapse rate compared with rates before the start of the ECT program. Vanelle and colleagues (1994) reviewed the records of 22 patients who received approximately monthly ECT treatments for intractable, recurrent unipolar and bipolar mood disorders, some for up to 2 years, including many with rapid cycles. They reported a substantial reduction in the time these patients spent hospitalized (7 percent) compared with the previous year (44 percent). Recently, a very favorable response to maintenance ECT was reported for two bipolar patients whose treatment-resistant recurrences were predominantly manic (Nascimento et al., 2006; Sienaert and Peuskens, 2006).

As the results of these studies indicate, maintenance ECT is considered an appropriate choice for patients who consistently relapse when attempts are made to stop ECT and maintain remission with medications, and it has been incorporated into some of the international guidelines for maintenance treatment, such as those of the World Federation of Societies of Biological Psychiatry (Grunze et al., 2002). As new pharmacological approaches become available, it may be possible to reduce the number of patients for whom maintenance ECT is necessary. Rhodes (2000) described the case of a woman who had to stop taking lithium because she developed renal insufficiency while taking it, and who was able to stay reasonably well without it (although with considerable residual depressive symptoms) only by receiving an ECT treatment every 4 to 6 weeks. After starting on lamotrigine, she experienced complete remission and was able to stop ECT. Her recovery had lasted 34 months at the time of the report.

Newer techniques involving electrical stimulation of the CNS (transcranial magnetic stimulation and vagus nerve stimulation) have been examined only in short-term studies focused on the relief of acute symptoms (see Chapter 19). How beneficial these techniques may be for prophylaxis remains to be demonstrated.

Thyroid Hormones

Thyroid indices in the "normal" range do not necessarily indicate sufficiently robust thyroid functioning for some patients with bipolar disorder to remain well. Cole and colleagues (2002) examined the relationship between pretreatment thyroid hormone levels and time to treatment response in 65 depressed bipolar-I patients and found a significant association between delayed response to treatment and lower-normal free thyroxin index (FTI) and higher-normal TSH levels. They concluded that nearly two-thirds of bipolar patients may have a thyroid profile that, although technically in the normal range, is nevertheless inadequate for an optimal treatment response. Related findings were published by Frye and colleagues (1999), who found that among bipolar patients with free T_4 in the

"normal" range, those below the median were more depressed, had poorer antidepressant responses to lithium or carbamazepine, and had more mood instability regardless of their mood stabilizer status.

Substantial numbers of patients with bipolar disorder have a blunted TSH response to thyrotropin-releasing hormone (Hendrick et al., 1998), and under these circumstances, the absence of a TSH elevation may be misleading. Psychiatrists should be familiar with thyroid physiology, especially the concept of subclinical hypothyroidism, and become comfortable with the assessment and therapeutics of thyroid replacement for their patients taking lithium. T_4 supplementation is an effective strategy for managing hypothyroidism associated with lithium therapy (Kusalic, 1992; Kirov et al., 2005).

Supraphysiological doses of T_4 have been reported to increase the efficacy of pharmacological treatments for affective disorders. A prospective open-label study of 21 patients included 13 patients with bipolar disorder who had failed two previous prophylactic trials. These 13 patients took a mean dose of 378 µg of T_4 along with their other medications and were followed for a mean of about a year. They showed improvement on the CGI-BP, as well as having fewer relapses and spending less time in the hospital compared with the period before starting treatment (Bauer et al., 2002).[92] Baumgartner (2000) reviewed eight open trials of the use of supraphysiological doses of T_4 involving a total of 78 patients, and concluded that the T_4 benefited approximately 50 percent of patients who were entirely resistant to all other antidepressant and prophylactic treatments. Further detail on the use of thyroid hormones in treating bipolar disorder is provided in Chapter 19.

Calcium Channel Blockers

Interest in the use of calcium channel blockers for the treatment of mania has extended to maintenance treatment. Pazzaglia and colleagues (1993) reported on the results of the first double-blind, placebo-controlled study of the calcium channel blocker nimodipine in 12 patients with treatment-resistant "ultra-ultra-rapid-cycling" bipolar disorder in a placebo–nimodipine–placebo design. Of the 9 patients completing the study, 5 were classified as responders, with 1 bipolar-II subject showing a complete response. The results with these 9 subjects were included in a subsequent analysis of 30 treatment-resistant patients with affective disorder (23 bipolar-I or -II) who were receiving nimodipine monotherapy and were studied over periods of approximately 6 months; 10 patients showed a moderate or marked response. Fourteen of the 20 patients who did not respond to nimodipine had carbamazepine added to their regimen in a blinded fashion (Pazzaglia et al., 1998), and 4 of them responded to the carbamazepine augmentation.

Because verapamil, another calcium channel blocker, is relatively safe during pregnancy, it has been cited as a substitute for lithium or anticonvulsants in women with bipolar disorder who become pregnant (see Goodnick, 1993; Wisner et al., 2002).[93] In addition to the need for safer alternatives during pregnancy, there is a need for better treatments for unstable, rapid-cycling illness. These factors underline the need for more work on the calcium channel blockers as prophylactic treatment for bipolar disorder.

Psychostimulants

Our major discussion of the role of psychostimulants in the maintenance treatment of manic-depressive illness is in Chapter 23, dealing with the treatment of children and adolescents. As noted in Chapter 19, the literature on the use of these agents in the treatment of depressive symptoms in adults is scant, no doubt in part because of their status as controlled substances. We could find only one published report on the long-term use of a psychostimulant (methylphenidate) in bipolar patients: a chart review of 16 patients taking adjunctive methylphenidate for an average of 14 months (Lydon and El-Mallakh, 2006). Most patients reported various kinds of improvement following the addition of the stimulant to their ongoing treatment, including better concentration and less depressed mood; the most common side effects were mild irritability and/or agitation. There were no manic/hypomanic switches and no apparent abuse of the stimulant or other substances. Obviously, controlled studies of this treatment are needed.

Nutritional Supplements

Because nutritional supplements cannot be patented, there is no large industrial base of support for research on these compounds. Nevertheless, it is important for clinicians to be as educated as possible in this area, in which patients regularly have many questions.

There now have been a number of reports on the use of nutritional supplements in the treatment of mood disorders. As discussed in Chapter 19, clinical research thus far, while not definitive, has yielded some encouraging results (along with some negative findings) about the addition of omega-3 fatty acids to the armamentarium of treatments for affective disorders. The exploration of the therapeutic potential of these compounds grew out of epidemiological observations that linked high levels of fish oil with relatively low rates of depression and bipolar disorder (see Chapter 5). Many clinicians are now routinely recommending fish oil for their patients to supplement the established mood stabilizers. A number of case reports and an open case series in adults with bipolar disorder (Kaplan et al., 2001) and in a group of children with a variety of mood and behavioral problems, three with bipolar disorder (Kaplan et al., 2004), demonstrated

significant improvement in mood stability in these subjects over a period of months. Controlled studies of the use of micronutrients (the collective term for minerals and vitamins) are ongoing (see Popper, 2001). Assistance in sorting out the various levels of "information" in this area can be obtained from the Alternative Medicine Foundation (http://www.amfoundation.org [accessed September 14, 2006]), the *PDR for Herbal Medicines* (3rd edition) (Gruenwald et al., 2004), and http://www.quackwatch.com (accessed September 14, 2006).

Extended Bed Rest and Darkness

In Chapter 19, we discuss the potential effectiveness of sleep deprivation, sleep phase manipulation, and light therapy in treating depression. Given that each of these techniques has also been shown to carry some risk of triggering mania, Wehr and colleagues (1998) explored what might be called the opposite of sleep deprivation and light in the management of a patient with treatment-resistant rapid-cycling bipolar disorder.[94] Over a period of several years, the patient's clinical state was assessed with twice-daily self-ratings, once-weekly observer ratings, and continuous activity recordings with a wrist monitor; sleep was assessed periodically with polygraph recordings. The results were striking: compared with the unstable sleep and mood the patient experienced on his "normal" schedule, extended bed rest and darkness (14 hours a day) were associated with stabilization and normalization of both sleep and mood.

CONCLUSIONS

Because manic-depressive illness, particularly the bipolar form, is a chronic, episodic illness involving substantial functional impairment, long-term prevention of new episodes and enhancement of interepisode functioning should be the core first principles of clinical management. Unfortunately, the priority that should be accorded maintenance treatment is not reflected in the amount and quality of available controlled data. Virtually every drug on the market for bipolar disorder has been introduced as an antimanic agent. While it is common clinical practice simply to continue an effective antimanic agent as maintenance treatment, this approach, with the exception of lithium and lamotrigine, is not based on solid evidence of true *prophylactic* efficacy—meaning the ability to prevent new episodes. Obtaining such data will require that the field, the regulatory agencies, and the pharmaceutical industry move beyond contemporary relapse prevention designs.

Clearly, today's major unmet need is for more effective and more tolerable agents for the prevention of depressive episodes in bipolar patients and in those with highly recurrent unipolar depression. Given that (1) there is no convincing evidence that long-term antidepressants are effective in the prevention of bipolar-I depression, while (2) the results of three placebo-controlled studies indicate that at least some antidepressants can be associated with destabilization of the disorder, this class of drugs cannot be recommended for routine long-term use, at least for the bipolar-I patient. Fortunately, emerging evidence suggests that certain mood stabilizers, such as lithium and lamotrigine, and potential mood stabilizers, such as quetiapine, have some efficacy in preventing depressive relapses without destabilizing bipolar illness (see Table 20–12).

Given the limited efficacy of single agents for many patients, combined treatment is more or less standard for the majority of patients. But here we face a paradox: virtually all of the large randomized, placebo-controlled trials have been of monotherapy, even though such treatment is the exception in the real world of clinical practice, while the amount of controlled data to inform the use of medication combinations is comparatively limited. Moreover, much of the existing data on combination treatments is of limited relevance to clinical practice because the data are based on full monotherapy doses of each drug; as might be expected, the result is more side effects, which can offset any enhanced effectiveness by causing decreased adherence. Recent attempts to close the gap between clinical practice and research, under the auspices of the Stanley Foundation Bipolar Network and the NIMH STEP-BD program, clearly represent important efforts in the right direction.

NOTES

1. This classic distinction between continuation and maintenance derived from consideration of the natural history of the disease. For noncyclic unipolar depression, there was a clear consensus that the continuation phase comprised the first year after the episode, and anything beyond that was considered maintenance or prophylactic treatment (Frank et al., 1991). For the average bipolar patient, an untreated depressive episode would be expected to last about 6 months, with a manic episode lasting 3 to 6 months; hence the shorter continuation phase for bipolar treatment.

2. Coryell and colleagues (1997) speculated that lithium may protect against relapse in the period immediately following an episode of illness, but not against recurrence of illness months later. They also questioned the necessity of longer-term lithium prophylaxis for patients who have had 8 months or more of euthymia and suggested that lithium discontinuation studies be performed to elucidate the issue. This argument, however, has been rebutted by several other groups (see the section on "Renewed Controversies" in our later review of the literature).

3. Moreover, the tendency of the illness to accelerate in some patients as they age, with episodes occurring more frequently and lasting longer, has been noted since Kraepelin's descriptions of the disorder more than a century ago.

4. If the natural sequence of recurrent unipolar illness goes from depression to recovery and then eventually to the next episode, treatments that accelerate recovery of the index depression could also accelerate the onset of the next episode.

5. This practice is based on findings from some large contemporary "maintenance" trials that the polarity of the acute episode predicts the polarity of relapses; apparently, however, this prediction holds only for relapses within the first few months after the acute episode (i.e., in the continuation phase) (Joseph Calabrese, personal communication, March 2004).

6. An excellent patient-generated mood chart with instructions for its use can be downloaded from the Harvard Bipolar Research Program at http://www.manicdepressive.org/moodchart.html (accessed September 14, 2006).

7. For a review of the literature on lithium levels, see Hopkins and Gelenberg (2000). Lithium levels should generally be obtained 12 hours after the last dose. With slow- or sustained-release preparations, the 12-hour level will be about 15 to 20 percent higher than that seen with the immediate-release preparations.

8. The fact that the charge for this simple and rapid procedure will be reimbursed by insurance companies should increase its acceptance by practitioners.

9. Slow- or controlled-release formulations are not generally associated with gastric symptoms, but some patients taking these formulations may initially experience more diarrhea.

10. The clinical features and treatment of lithium toxicity (lithium poisoning) were outlined in the first edition of this text and have recently been described by Eyer and colleagues (2006), based on an analysis of 22 cases of lithium overdose. Most patients received hemodialysis (the treatment of choice); loop diuretics did not enhance lithium clearance, contrary to what would have been expected from animal studies.

11. It is thought that the effect of lithium on carbohydrate metabolism, including a mild anti-insulin effect, plays a role in weight gain, and therefore carbohydrate restriction is recommended.

12. Goodwin and Goldstein (2003) suggested the following measures to help control lithium-induced weight gain. Lifestyle measures include regular exercise, restriction of sugary fluids, and avoidance of simple carbohydrates, especially early in the day since they can induce mild hypoglycemia and thus increased caloric intake as patients "chase" their blood sugar throughout the day. Medical and pharmacological measures include supplementing T_4 if necessary, avoiding concurrent medication with an additive weight gain effect (olanzapine, clozapine, quetiapine, conventional antipsychotics, valproate, gabapentin, some selective serotonin reuptake inhibitors [SSRIs]), and consulting with a primary care physician about other options if weight gain exceeds 5 lb despite preventative measures.

13. However, some patients will experience lithium-related activation and insomnia when the full dose is taken at bedtime.

14. A recent randomized, double-blind, placebo-controlled crossover study by Allan and colleagues (2004) found that inositol supplements reduce psoriasis associated with lithium treatment, but not that in patients not taking lithium.

15. For an excellent review of lithium's renal effects, see Gitlin (1999).

16. For a detailed discussion of the renal pathology associated with progressive renal insufficiency due to lithium, see Markowitz et al., 2000.

17. In the retrospective study by Lepkifker and colleagues (2004), covering durations of lithium therapy ranging from 4 to 30 years, nephrogenic diabetes insipidus was associated with longer durations of lithium treatment, past episodes of lithium intoxication, and medical illnesses or treatments that could affect renal function. Others have found the renal effects of lithium to be associated with the cumulative amount of the drug ingested over the years (Presne et al., 2003).

18. If renal concentrating ability is substantially impaired or the patient excretes more than 4 liters of urine per 24 hours, careful monitoring (by patient and physician) of fluid balance is required to avoid dehydration and lithium intoxication (Vestergaard and Schou, 1987). Although the renal concentrating ability usually improves if lithium is discontinued, the improvement can be quite delayed and incomplete if the impairment has been long-standing. Lithium discontinuation studies indicate that increases in 24-hour urine output remain the same or decrease only slightly after lithium is discontinued.

19. A 24-hour urine volume greater than 3 liters is generally considered clinically significant polyuria. Estimates of the condition's frequency range from 15 to 40 percent; it has been reported that concomitant use of other unspecified psychotropic drugs is associated with reduced urinary concentrating ability and increased urinary volume (Bendz et al., 1983). More recently, Movig and colleagues (2003) found that, compared with lithium monotherapy, coadministration of SSRIs is associated with four times more polyuria, perhaps related to hyponatremia (Movig et al., 2002). Nonpsychotropic drugs that can decrease urinary concentrating ability (and increase urine volume) include thiazide diuretics, nonsteroidal anti-inflammatory drugs (NSAIDs), and angiotensin-converting enzyme (ACE) inhibitors. Although there is not yet a full consensus on the relationship between renal function and frequency of lithium dosing, most of the evidence supports the assertion we made in the first edition of this text, that once-a-day dosing is associated with a lower frequency of renal problems (see Plenge et al., 1982; Bowen et al., 1991; Gitlin, 1999).

20. A retrospective chart review study of 718 British patients also concluded that the risk of developing hypothyroidism is greatest during the first 2 years of lithium therapy (Johnston and Eagles, 1999).

21. Because some patients with an affective disorder have hypothalamic dysfunction reflected in a failure to mount a normal TSH response to infused thyroid-releasing hormone (TRH), a normal TSH level may not always be a reliable indicator of the integrity of thyroid function.

22. Isojarvi et al., 1993; Bauer et al., 2000; Ernst and Goldberg, 2002; Joffe et al., 2003.

23. In the GlaxoSmithKline study, the lamotrigine and valproate were used either as monotherapy or adjunctively; the period of observation was up to 1 year.

24. Funded jointly by NIMH and Abbott Laboratories.

25. More sedation and ataxia occur with rapidly rising levels of carbamazepine than with most other modern anticonvulsants; as a consequence, titration often needs to be slowed, especially when multiple drugs are being used together.

26. The occurrence of these complications is rare, at a rate of about 1 in 20,000 patients. Most of these cases have been in the elderly and within the first 4 months of treatment.

27. In a retrospective case review at five epilepsy centers in England, Wong and colleagues (1999) found that higher starting doses, a rapid titration (increase) of the dose of lamotrigine, and the combined use of lamotrigine with valproate (which increases the half-life of lamotrigine, resulting in higher serum levels) were associated with the greatest risk of serious rashes requiring hospitalization. Gradual dose titration is therefore recommended by the manufacturer for patients starting lamotrigine, with an extremely slow titration recommended for those who are taking valproate (starting at 25 mg every other day for 2 weeks).

28. Ketter and colleagues (2005) have developed "antigen precautions" for consideration prior to the initiation of lamotrigine; using this approach, they have been able to reduce rates of benign rash substantially.

29. Serious side effects are associated with typical antipsychotics. Common CNS side effects involve altered thermoregulation, extrapyramidal syndrome (EPS), neuroleptic malignant syndrome, and tardive dyskinesia. Orthostatic hypotension is also observed. Erectile dysfunction, blurred vision, constipation, and urinary retention are common anticholinergic effects. Cardiovascular effects include ECG changes, tachycardia, and torsade de pointes. Changes in the endocrine system, including amenorrhea and galactorrhea, occur as well. Occasionally, the hematological system is involved, with agranulocytosis and leucopenia occurring. Liver enzyme elevations are sometimes seen early in treatment; they usually resolve even with continued treatment, but can cause release of bilirubin with cholestatic jaundice. Other pertinent side effects include allergic reactions and skin photosensitivity and all immune-mediated agranulocytopenias. Sedation and weight gain are observed as well. So-called low-potency antipsychotics cause more sedation and vascular side effects (orthostasis), whereas the more-potent drugs are more commonly associated with EPS. The greatest concern arises for EPS, the potentially fatal neuroleptic malignant syndrome, and for potentially irreversible tardive dyskinesia.

30. Risperidone is now available in a long-acting depot form.

31. Risk of EPS was assessed using the Abnormal Involuntary Movement Scale, Barnes Akathisia Rating Scale, and Simpson-Angus Scale. Mean duration of treatment was 25.5 weeks, and 61 percent of the patients were female. The EPS rate found in this study—63 percent—is somewhat higher than that reported in similar studies of patients with schizophrenia, consistent with earlier findings that bipolar patients are more sensitive to antipsychotic-induced EPS (Goodwin and Jamison, 1990).

32. Leucht and colleagues (2003) referred to meta-analyses by Baldessarini (1988) and Bollini and colleagues (1994), which concluded that no additional efficacy is achieved in the treatment of schizophrenia when doses of chlorpromazine or its equivalent exceed 500 to 600 mg/day.

33. Also relevant are the findings of the recent NIMH Clinical Antipsychotic Trials in Intervention Effectiveness (CATIE) (Dettling and Anghelescu, 2006), comparing a typical antipsychotic with several different atypicals in "real-world" settings. No differences in rates of EPS were noted between the typical agent, perphenazine, and the atypicals.

34. Ziprasidone is the one atypical antipsychotic in which the "start low, go slow" approach is not recommended because at low doses its activating effects, predominate.

35. In a recent cross-sectional study of 171 bipolar-I and schizoaffective patients in a clinic, almost half met the National Cholesterol Education Program criteria for abdominal obesity, and 30 percent met criteria for metabolic syndrome. Most patients were taking more than one medication, 29 percent were taking one of the atypicals associated with weight gain, and 44 percent were taking lithium (Fagiolini et al., 2005). Among 367 patients taking atypicals, the presence of the metabolic syndrome (in 37 percent of the patients) was associated with a two-fold increase in the risk of coronary events (angina, myocardial infarction, and sudden cardiac death) (Correll et al., 2006).

36. Guo and colleagues (2006) used a large managed-care database to conduct a retrospective, population-based case–control study of the relative risk of diabetes among bipolar patients treated with various atypicals. After controlling for age, gender, other drugs, and psychiatric and medical comorbidities, they found significant risk ratios for clozapine (7.0), risperidone (3.4), olanzapine (3.2), and quetiapine (1.8).

37. Adjunctive topiramate has also been reported to control olanzapine-induced weight gain in schizophrenic patients (Levy et al., 2002).

38. For a review of management options for the weight gain associated with antipsychotics, see Birt (2003) and Keck and McElroy (2003).

39. When low doses of some atypical antipsychotics are added to mood stabilizers, enhanced cognitive organization is sometimes observed.

40. Applaby et al., 1998; Ernst and Goldberg, 2002; Newport et al., 2002; Bonari et al., 2004; Spinelli, 2004; Yonkers et al., 2004; Eberhard-Gran et al., 2005.

41. Austin, 1992; Viguera et al., 2000; Wisner et al., 2004; Jones and Craddock, 2005.

42. For a more comprehensive discussion of these issues, see Viguera et al. (2002).

43. Anticonvulsants such as valproate can be used for a few weeks before parturition and in the postpartum period. However, the effectiveness of valproate for the prevention of postpartum episodes has been called into question by a study failing to find any benefit (Wisner et al., 2004).

44. See Stewart (2000) for a discussion.

45. On the other hand, Moretti and colleagues (2003) followed 11 babies who were breastfed while their mothers were taking lithium and found that for half of the mothers, the calculated dose the infant received via breast milk averaged only about 10 percent of the mother's weight-adjusted dose; more important, no overt adverse effects were observed among the 11 infants. Accordingly, some experts suggest that the benefits of breastfeeding probably outweigh the risk posed by lithium (see, e.g., Chaudron and Jefferson, 2000).

46. The recurrent unipolar group in this study may have included some patients who today would be diagnosed as having bipolar spectrum disorder.

47. The study of Prien and colleagues (1974) also included some patients already taking lithium, so the question of a bias toward lithium is relevant.

48. Although mirror-image studies are frequently criticized, in their meta-analysis of the literature, Davis and colleagues (1999) showed convincingly that the efficacy suggested by the results of such studies is of the same magnitude as that reported in randomized, placebo-controlled trials.

49. Compared with the lithium-treated patients, however, those on valproate were less likely to discontinue treatment for adverse effects or lack of efficacy (12 versus 23 percent). Adherence to either treatment was associated with better functional outcome and more than three-fold lower total medical care costs.

50. Studies were excluded if randomization to placebo involved abrupt withdrawal of lithium after the patient had been stable on the drug for a long time.

51. Dickson and Kendell, 1986; Markar and Mander, 1989; Harrow et al., 1990; Licht et al., 2001.

52. These authors noted that "diagnostic drift" is also a factor contributing to a smaller lithium effect size in contemporary studies, although it has a much smaller impact than the enrichment differences. Specifically, the older literature used diagnostic criteria, such as the Research Diagnostic Criteria (RDC), that excluded psychotic features, whereas contemporary studies use the much broader DSM-IV diagnostic criteria, which include psychosis and other "atypical" features.

53. Baastrup et al., 1970; Coppen et al., 1973; Prien et al., 1973a,b.

54. Subsequently this research group (Faedda et al., 1993; Baldessarini et al., 1997) and others (G. Goodwin et al., 1997; Cavanagh et al., 2004), using more refined analyses, further developed the research base, confirming that rapid discontinuation carries substantially more risk and that most relapse events occur within a few months of withdrawal.

55. This result can explain why the previously mentioned analysis of the efficacy literature by Baldessarini and colleagues (1999b) found that *long-term* lithium effectiveness was no different in trials with and without the placebo group's having been withdrawn from lithium.

56. There was a trend for both lithium and valproate to be superior to carbamazepine among rapid-cycling patients.

57. Kleindienst and colleagues (2005) applied the following criteria for inclusion in their review of predictors of response: (1) the observation period lasted at least 6 months; (2) lithium was the primary prophylactic agent, or the lithium group was analyzed separately; (3) at least one clinical response "predictor" was evaluated in a quantitative manner; and (4) the study was focused on a bipolar sample or analyzed a bipolar subgroup separately.

58. The related phenomenon of "continuous cycling" did predict a relatively poor response to lithium.

59. Other variables that appeared to predict poor lithium response, but in a small number of studies that failed to pass the "fail safe" test, were comorbid personality disorder and mood-incongruent psychotic features. Longer treatment latency had also been reported to be associated with decreased lithium response, but as noted earlier, Baldessarini and colleagues (2003) and Baethge and colleagues (2003) have pointed out that this relationship can best be explained by the fact that the sickest patients receive treatment earlier; given that such patients have the most pathology, the treatment effect appears larger. Kleindienst and colleagues (2005) suggested that the potential predictors identified in their review should each undergo this same kind of detailed analysis.

60. In a small retrospective chart review, Ghaemi and Goodwin (2005) found that the maintenance effectiveness of lithium and valproate was equivalent (54 versus 53 percent responders, respectively).

61. This lack of difference between lithium and valproate in rapid-cycling patients was also found in the meta-analysis of Tondo and colleagues (2003).

62. HAM-D ratings are weighted toward items that might be expected to respond favorably to divalproex, such as anxiety and insomnia.

63. A 2-year randomized trial comparing lithium monotherapy, valproate monotherapy, and a combination of the two in patients with a history of mania studied in "real-world" settings is currently under way in the United Kingdom (Geddes et al., 2002). An attempt is being made to recruit more than 1,000 subjects for this study.

64. In most of the patients, carbamazepine was added to lithium, and so this evaluation is, in reality, an assessment of adjunctive carbamazepine.

65. Okuma et al., 1976; Ballenger and Post, 1978; Placidi et al., 1986; Watkins et al., 1987; Luznat et al., 1988.

66. In this study, 29 (69 percent) of 42 patients completed the year on lithium, 12 (34 percent) of 35 patients completed the year on carbamazepine, and 22 (76 percent) of 29 patients completed the year on the combination. The proportion of patients with moderate to marked improvement was 33 percent for lithium alone, 31 for carbamazepine alone, and 55 for the combination.

67. The authors pointed out that a large fraction of the patients had previously received lithium alone, carbamazepine alone, and/or a combination of the two. Thus, the results of the study must be seen in the context that these patients were not naïve to the study drugs and had, for the most part, responded poorly to them in the past.

68. A small double-blind trial of carbamazepine versus lithium for treatment of bipolar disorder was carried out by Hartong and colleagues (2003). In this study, 12 (27 percent) of 44 patients assigned to lithium had recurrences during treatment, compared with 21 (14 percent) of 150 patients assigned to carbamazepine.

69. The mean serum carbamazepine level was 6.4 μg/ml, and the average serum lithium level was .63 mEq/l.

70. In the Calabrese et al. (1999b) open study, conducted over 48 weeks, lamotrigine was added to the currently used maintenance treatment in 60 bipolar-I and -II patients and was used as monotherapy for another 15 patients. Fifty percent (48) of the patients had depressive symptoms at the onset of the trial, while 40 percent (31) were experiencing hypomanic, manic, or mixed symptoms. The majority of patients showed significant improvement in ratings on depression and mania scales, although several developed manic symptoms, perhaps not unexpected in this preliminary study involving patients with complex illnesses and taking a variety of other medications (more than one in most cases), including antidepressants, lithium, valproate, carbamazepine, and antipsychotics.

71. Thus among those patients on placebo, later recurrences after an index depression were 6 times more likely to be a mania/hypomania than another depression; conversely, for those whose index episode had been mania/hypomania, later recurrences were 6 times more likely to be a depression than another mania/hypomania. In other words, overall, 85 percent of the recurrences were of the opposite polarity.

72. Walden and colleagues (1996) reported on a patient with lithium-resistant rapid-cycling bipolar disorder who improved within days when lamotrigine was added to valproate monotherapy; the improvement was sustained for more than a year.

73. However, for the entire group there was a small but significant advantage of lamotrigine over placebo when treatment dropout was considered, an event the authors suggested may often be a sign of relapse.

74. Of the adjunctive agents used, 21 percent were for anxiety/insomnia, 19 percent for depression, and 12 percent for mood elevation.

75. Doses ranged from 1 to 8 mg/day. Thirteen patients did not improve but also did not tolerate the side effects of tiagabine at higher doses; the remaining patient did not adhere to the regimen. A German group reported that tiagabine at doses of 20 mg/day and higher was not useful because of severe complications encountered at this dose range (Carta et al., 2002). Further evaluation of tiagabine at lower doses is needed for full assessment of its utility.

76. There have been scattered reports suggesting that agents used in the treatment of dementia may be helpful in managing neurocognitive side effects of psychoactive medications. Thus Jacobsen and Comas-Diaz (1999) found the cholinesterase inhibitor donepezil to be helpful for memory loss associated with a variety of psychotropic agents, while Burt and colleagues (1999) reported that it improved mood scores in treatment-resistant bipolar disorder. More recently, Schrauwen and Ghaemi (2006) reported that the new cholinesterase inhibitor/nicotinic receptor agonist galantamine was effective in reducing cognitive impairment in two of four medicated bipolar patients.

77. In a subsequent comparison of adjunctive clozapine over 1 year in rapid-cycling versus non–rapid-cycling bipolar-I patients, Suppes and colleagues (2004) found that the latter group evidenced greater improvement.

78. Patients were rated prospectively on the CGI and Global Assessment of Functioning scales for a mean of 6 months and took a mean dose of 2.75 mg/day of risperidone (range 1–4.5 mg/day).

79. Although there was some controversy about the dosing of the acute mania study (conducted by the manufacturer of olanzapine)—that the Depakote dose, while following the *PDR* (3rd edition), was not as high as subsequent studies had indicated it should be for optimal response in acute mania (Allen et al., 2006)—the 47-week double-blind continuation study used flexible doses based on clinical response and side effects.

80. The only adjunctive drug allowed was lorazepam, up to a maximum of 2 mg/day.

81. The 84 percent dropout rate could be interpreted as meaning that neither drug was particularly effective, but without a placebo group, one cannot know.

82. This study employed HAM-D ratings to evaluate the impact of olanzapine on depression. Since the HAM-D scale was developed to assess unipolar depressed patients, it is not considered as good as other rating systems (e.g., the Montgomery-Asberg scale) for the assessment of bipolar depression. In particular, because the HAM-D places much emphasis on such items as insomnia and anxiety, it would be expected that an atypical antipsychotic could reduce ratings on this scale without having a significant effect on core depressive symptoms.

83. These analyses indicate (1) that time in remission before randomization (1, 2, 3, or 4 weeks) was not associated with risk of relapse, and (2) that the drug–placebo differences were similar (and both were significant) among those who remained in remission in the double-blind phase for a minimum of 2 weeks compared with the smaller group who

remained in remission for a minimum of 8 weeks (half of those originally randomized to olanzapine and one-fourth of those randomized to placebo).

84. FDA indications do not use the terms "prophylaxis" or "mood stabilizer"; "maintenance" is a much broader term encompassing both the classic concept of continuation treatment and prophylaxis. Since giving maintenance indications to olanzapine and aripiprazole, the FDA has revised its guidelines and recommendations. Future maintenance indications should be based on studies in which there has been at least a 6-month period of stabilization before randomization into the maintenance phase.

85. Apparently only 37 percent of those who entered into the open-label phase both tolerated and responded to aripiprazole. And because the dropout rate during the randomized phase was 58 percent, it would appear that only 21.5 percent of the original sample were still stable after 6 months of treatment.

86. For example, compared with patients taking placebo, those taking aripiprazole were 13 times more likely to have clinically significant weight gain and 6 times more likely to have EPS.

87. Baethge and colleagues (2005) offered an up-to-date review of the lithium plus carbamazepine combination in a post hoc analysis of their own long-term data on 46 bipolar-I patients—data that generally reflect the literature by showing both substantial benefit and increased adverse effects.

88. For other excellent reviews of combination mood stabilizers, see Pies (2000) and Zarate and Quiroz (2003).

89. Prien et al., 1973a; Wehr and Goodwin, 1979; Quitkin et al., 1981; Sachs et al., 1994; Post et al., 2001.

90. The conclusion that atypical antipsychotics pose a negligible risk of tardive dyskinesia is based in part on extrapolating the low rates of EPS reported from randomized controlled trials.

However, it should be remembered that these trials involved patients with a single diagnosis who received a single drug. In real-world settings, rates of EPS are not negligible, with one recent report estimating that more than half of the bipolar patients taking atypical antipsychotics were positive for EPS by rating-scale criteria (Ghaemi et al., 2006).

91. See note 82 on the limitation of the HAM-D scale for evaluating bipolar depression.

92. Earlier, Bauer and Whybrow (1990) treated 11 refractory rapid-cycling bipolar patients with high-dose adjunctive levothyroxine; 10 showed a "clear-cut" response of depressive symptoms, and 5 of the 7 patients with manic symptoms experienced a decrease in these symptoms while taking T_4. In all but one of the responsive patients, "supranormal" levels of circulating T_4 were required for the clinical response.

93. Goodnick (1993) described the cases of three women who took verapamil during pregnancy; two had become manic at the beginning of pregnancy, one taking no medication and one having discontinued carbamazepine. The other patient was in remission from mood symptoms on lithium when she discovered she was pregnant; she stopped the lithium and started verapamil. All three women had a good response. The two patients with mania had a good acute response to verapamil, and all three remained well during pregnancy while taking the drug. Wisner and colleagues (2002) reported on nine women with bipolar-I and -II disorder who took verapamil for 2 to 14 months (two patients took the drug as monotherapy). Six of these nine women remained well while taking verapamil.

94. While a single case report would not ordinarily merit this much coverage in a text such as this, the innovative nature of this study deserves our attention.

21 Medication Adherence

The endless questioning finally ended. My psychiatrist looked at me; there was no uncertainty in his voice. "Manic-depressive illness." I admired his bluntness. I wished him locusts on his lands and a pox upon his house. Silent, unbelievable rage. I smiled pleasantly. He smiled back. The war had just begun.

—*Patient with manic-depressive illness*[1]

Many patients with mood disorders appear to have little or no difficulty with taking potent daily medications for an indeterminate period. They do not appear to be unduly concerned about potential or actual side effects, nor do they struggle with the existential issues that might reasonably be raised when a person is required to take powerful mind- and mood-altering drugs. For whatever reason—perhaps temperament or past experience—they do not protest or disobey their physicians' orders; instead, they are grateful for the medications and appreciative of the doctors who prescribe them. Often such patients state that lithium, other mood stabilizers, or antidepressants have rescued them from chaos, despair, hospitalization, or suicide. These patients are an interesting, although inadequately studied, group. Certainly they are a source of gratification to their physicians.

For every patient who follows the treatment course, however, there is at least one who does not—one who resists, protests, objects, takes too little, takes too much, or takes none at all. The perspective of one such patient, more common than most clinicians perhaps appreciate, is presented in Box 21–1.

This chapter deals with medication adherence among patients with the bipolar form of manic-depressive illness, a topic that merits a separate chapter for several reasons:

- The consequences of medication nonadherence are profound and can be life-threatening, clinically equivalent to those of untreated or inadequately treated manic-depressive illness. Nonadherence commonly precipitates the recurrence and intensification of affective episodes that may in turn result in personal anguish, conjugal failure, chaos in other family and interpersonal relationships, alcohol and drug abuse, financial crises, psychiatric hospitalization, suicide, and violence. A recent study

of bipolar juvenile offenders, for example, found that the number of felonies and misdemeanors committed among those off medication was 4.8 times higher than among those on medication (Dailey et al., 2005). This point may be obvious, but it is frequently ignored. Unlike nonresponsiveness to treatment, however, nonadherence is potentially reversible and can be changed through experience, education, learning, and psychotherapy. Such interventions are discussed later in this chapter and in Chapter 22.

- Lithium, anticonvulsants, and antipsychotic medications are prescribed on an exceptionally long-term or lifelong basis. For this reason, unique challenges arise for the patient, the physician, and other clinicians involved in the treatment program.

- Medication nonadherence is a frustrating, common, and perplexing clinical problem, and yet far less discussion and training are devoted to this matter than to the intricacies of prescribing medication effectively.

- Poor adherence is almost certainly the single most important factor in poor treatment response.

- Failure to consider nonadherence may bias research findings in clinical studies related to the outcomes of medication treatment. Frank and colleagues (1985, p. 42) stressed that investigators "have an obligation to account for nonadherent patients in their analyses" by specifying how many and which patients fail to comply (patient, history of illness, and therapist variables) and accounting for dropouts and discontinuation in their statistical evaluations of outcome. Such accounting is rarely undertaken and seldom adequate.

In this chapter, we first discuss approaches to clinical management of medication adherence. We then review

BOX 21–1.   **Rules for the Gracious Acceptance of Lithium Into Your Life**

1. Clear out the medicine cabinet before guests arrive for dinner or new lovers stay the night.
2. Remember to put the lithium back into the cabinet the next day.
3. Don't be too embarrassed by your lack of coordination or your inability to do well the sports you once did with ease.
4. Learn to laugh about spilling coffee, having the palsied signature of an 80-year-old, and being unable to put on cufflinks in less than 10 minutes.
5. Smile when people joke about how they think they "need to be on lithium."
6. Nod intelligently, and with conviction, when your physician explains to you the many advantages of lithium in leveling out the chaos in your life.
7. Be patient when waiting for this leveling off. Very patient. Reread the Book of Job. Continue being patient. Contemplate the similarity between the phrases "being patient" and "being a patient."
8. Try not to let the fact that you can't read without effort annoy you. Be philosophical. Even if you could read, you probably wouldn't remember most of it anyway.
9. Accommodate to a certain lack of enthusiasm and bounce you once had. Try not to think about all the wild nights you once had. Probably best not to have had those nights anyway.
10. Always keep in perspective how much better you are. Everyone else certainly points it out often enough, and, annoyingly enough, it's probably true.
11. Be appreciative. Don't even consider stopping your lithium.
12. When you do stop, get manic, get depressed, expect to hear two basic themes from your family, friends, and healers:
    • But you were doing so much better. I just don't understand it.
    • I told you this would happen.
13. Restock your medicine cabinet.

Source: Jamison, 1995.

the key findings of the literature on nonadherence, particularly among bipolar patients. Before proceeding, however, we must note two issues of terminology. First, the term *compliance* has been roundly criticized as having a paternalistic connotation, suggesting a doctor–patient relationship not typical of current practice. Many believe that the term *adherence* reflects more accurately the complex processes of collaboration and mutual decision making involved. Therefore, we use the latter term in this chapter. Second, most of the research and clinical discussion concerning the problem of medication adherence has

focused on lithium, as opposed to other mood stabilizers. Consequently, much of this chapter addresses lithium in particular; however, the discussion is relatively generalizable to other medications, with exceptions being noted as they arise.

CLINICAL MANAGEMENT

As discussed in earlier chapters, both clinician and patient face a number of challenges in maintaining an effective treatment regimen. From the patient's point of view, many daunting issues arise concerning the meaning of the illness, attitudes and expectations about the role of medication, the supportive resources available, and the consequences of adherence or nonadherence. These issues are complex, involving both rational and irrational, conscious and nonconscious processes. Moreover, adherence is a dynamic phenomenon, changing over time.

The clinician's task is critical, as well as difficult, with respect to the goal of treatment adherence, and it encompasses multiple potential roles: a teacher providing clear, complete, and accurate information; a skilled therapist allowing for an open, safe, accepting discussion of the patient's concerns, beliefs, and expectations; a skilled psychopharmacologist knowledgeable about options, dosages, side effects, and drug interactions; an advocate/facilitator informing significant others and enlisting their positive participation in treatment; and a scientist maintaining knowledge and skills concerning effective treatment practices in the context of rapidly expanding research on the etiology and course of illness. Among the inherent obstacles to the effective management of adherence are several noted briefly in the following sections; suggestions for addressing these issues and facilitating adherence are also provided. Chapters 18, 19, 20, and 22 elaborate in greater detail some of these considerations in psychopharmacology and psychotherapy.

Clinician Attitudes

Patients who fail to follow their therapists' suggestions have in the past been perceived as motivated by pathological processes and nefarious personal traits, labeled "resistant," and thereby in some measure blamed for the failure of their treatment. Yet nonadherence rarely involves only the patient's pathological or irrational side; the truth is far more complex. The clinician plays a vital role in creating a collaborative, honest, and supportive environment in which to raise issues concerning treatment adherence with the patient.

Clinicians, of course, experience frustration, impatience, and even anger when patients discontinue medication or fail to follow the prescribed regimen—particularly when the stakes are high and involve personally devastating consequences to the patient. But even more subtle processes may undermine the effectiveness of the treatment collaboration. Clinicians may not take enough time to elicit information about adherence, attitudes, or side effects. They may focus excessively on medical side effects to the relative neglect of other effects that patients may find more distressing, such as cognitive changes and blunted enthusiasm and diminished energy.

Physicians are relatively poor judges of adherence and may assume that patients are fully adherent when they are not (Blackwell, 1980; World Health Organization, 2003; Osterberg and Blaschke, 2005). It is important to question patients about adherence directly and frequently. When discussing the issue of adherence, it is also important to do so in a nonjudgmental way, making an admission of nonadherence socially acceptable, for example, by asking: "Many people have trouble taking all their pills. Do you have trouble taking all of yours?"

Also critical are the attitudes of treating clinicians toward mood-stabilizing and other medications. In general, clinicians who are ambivalent about the paramount role of biological factors in the causation and treatment of affective disorders tend to convey that ambivalence to their patients and may thereby contribute to nonadherence. Results of a study by Cochran and Gitlin (1988) underscore the importance of the role of the patient's psychiatrist in ensuring adherence. Their findings suggest that the more strongly the psychiatrist believes in the treatment regimen, the more likely the patient is to take the medication as prescribed.

While it is increasingly uncommon for bipolar patients to encounter clinicians who are reluctant to acknowledge the biological basis of the disorder, the opposite problem may be encountered and can also be detrimental to patients' attitudes. Clinicians with an extreme biological bias may oversell the efficacy of medication, for instance, and thereby pave the way for the patient's disillusionment when relapses occur. Or they may underestimate the role of psychological factors in the illness and its treatment, underutilize psychotherapy, and overlook "subjective" symptoms, such as emotional dulling or memory disturbance, that many patients find troublesome. Excessively narrow clinical perspectives that unduly emphasize the biology of the disorder may undermine patients' own views of the complex nature of their problem; medication adherence may be discouraged if patients experience a sense of futility and are led to believe that only medication can help them.

Suggestions for Facilitating Adherence to Medication

A brief list of practical suggestions for all clinicians who treat bipolar patients is presented in Box 21–2. Schou (1997),

---

BOX 21–2. Practical Suggestions for Maximizing Medication Adherence

Assessment and Education

- Educate the patient and family members about the course of the illness and the benefits of treatment.
- Teach monitoring and recognition of early symptoms of mania and depression.
- Assess adherence history and potential risk factors for nonadherence.
- Include family members, and inform them about the illness, its treatment, and the risks of no treatment.
- Encourage patients and family members to read about bipolar illness and its treatment; encourage them to question what you are doing and why you are doing it.

Medication and Treatment Alliance Issues

- Create a collaborative relationship, facilitating the patient's role in dosage/treatment decisions as appropriate.
- Minimize the number of daily doses, and discuss techniques for facilitating regular use of the medication (including pillboxes), as well as management of multiple medications.
- Involve family members as appropriate.
- Provide oral and written information about side effects.
- Elicit and respond to concerns about and treat side effects.

Monitoring of Adherence

- Initiate an open discussion of adherence issues; provide enough time for assessing and discussing patients' concerns.
- Inquire about and discuss adherence frequently.
- Obtain regular blood levels of medications as appropriate.
- Encourage support and monitoring by significant others as appropriate.

Adjunctive Treatments

- Recommend, as appropriate, psychotherapeutic treatment for adherence issues specifically, or for bipolar disorder generally.
- Encourage participation in self-help groups.

---

along with many other researchers and clinicians, emphasized the importance of patient education. He recommended that patients and their families be given instruction booklets concerning the benefits and costs of using and not using medications, as well as the costs of interrupting or discontinuing treatment. He noted that constructing life charts of the course of illness may help patients understand the recurrent nature of the disorder and how the risk of recurrence is magnified by nonadherence. Advocacy of such patient and family education is reflected in many psychoeducation programs, increasingly sophisticated psychotherapeutic techniques, and the development of a wide network of self-help organizations and support groups (see Chapter 22).

Enlisting the support of family members is important. Not only do relatives need to be educated about the facts of bipolar disorder and its course and treatment, but they can also play a unique role in facilitating adherence by conveying their attitudes about the need for regular medication, providing encouragement and reinforcement for adherence, and facilitating regular routines that include medication consumption.

Several investigators have suggested that, given the magnitude of the problem of nonadherence and the need for close patient monitoring, specialty clinics may be advisable to address adherence issues (e.g., Gitlin and Jamison, 1984; Goldberg et al., 1996; Schou, 1997). Such clinics may be best equipped to follow practice guidelines carefully, monitor adherence closely, and deal with unique patient clinical profiles and side effects through the use of multiple therapeutic agents and psychotherapy. The development of easier monitoring methods (for example, a new 2-minute, office-based test for serum lithium levels) may also have an impact on adherence (Glazer et al., 2004).

Adjunctive Psychotherapy and Self-Help Alliances

As we emphasize in Chapter 22, psychotherapy often helps bipolar patients deal with a variety of issues. A number of specialized psychotherapeutic treatments have been developed for bipolar patients to supplement medication regimens, and a major component of these treatments relates to the management of adherence issues. Cognitive-behavioral approaches, family-based treatments, and interpersonal psychotherapy, for example, have been tested and are continuing to be evaluated in more extensive trials. Research presented in Chapter 22 indicates that such interventions improve clinical and functional outcomes. Some of the studies have specifically included a treatment adherence component, and their findings indicate that psychotherapeutic interventions may facilitate adherence to medication.

Self-help groups, such as those organized by the Depression and Bipolar Support Alliance and the National Alliance on Mental Illness, are beneficial as well to many patients and their families. The increasing use of the Internet to facilitate self-help and chatroom discussions may prove to be beneficial in encouraging the sustained use of medications and in providing educational materials that can make patients informed consumers, aware of their illness and their treatment options. Caution must be exercised, however, in that the accuracy of information provided on the Internet is highly variable. A list of Web sites and other sources of information about bipolar illness, including self-help groups, is given in the Resources section at the end of this volume.

REVIEW OF THE LITERATURE

This section begins with a discussion of definitional and measurement issues related to adherence. Next we present findings on rates of nonadherence among bipolar patients. We then discuss two key questions commonly addressed in research on this subject: What are the reasons for nonadherence that can be articulated by patients, and what are the empirical correlates of nonadherence? Finally, we present an overview of the effectiveness of psychotherapy in facilitating adherence, a topic developed more fully in Chapter 22.

Before proceeding, it is important to note that nonadherence to medication regimens is not at all unique to bipolar disorder, although the latter has certain distinctive characteristics that will be discussed. Overall, as Young and colleagues (1999) pointed out, rates of adherence in general medical practice are about 50 percent, and various studies have found a range of 15 to 85 percent for common medical illnesses.[2] These rates are consistent with estimates of the World Health Organization (2003) that adherence among patients with chronic diseases in developed countries averages only 50 percent. Nonadherence is especially common in outpatients and in those with chronic relapsing disorders, such as diabetes and hypertension. Blackwell (1973) found, for example, that adherence is lowest when the condition is prolonged and requires prophylactic treatment and when the consequences of discontinuation are not immediate. Even in situations in which the fear of fatal consequences is high and the period of treatment is short, adherence is not ensured. Rates of adherence to antibiotic prophylaxis during the highly publicized 2001 anthrax threat, for example, ranged from only 31 to 64 percent (Brookmeyer et al., 2003).

Table 21–1 shows the factors associated with adherence and nonadherence in general medical patients. Factors that appear to predict adherence include chronicity of illness, number of symptoms experienced, extent of disability, health beliefs of the patient (perceived seriousness of illness and perceived efficacy of treatment), and social supports. Aspects of the treatment regimen—such as complexity, number and cost of medications, and route and ease of administration—are also predictive, as are aspects of the health care delivery system (convenience of the clinical setting, continuity of care, and extent of supervision by others). Demographic variables, such as age (except in its extremes), gender, intelligence, and education level, are not generally predictive of adherence. The relationship of personality variables and medication side effects to general medical adherence is uncertain, although these factors appear to be more relevant to adherence to mood-stabilizing drugs (Aagaard and Vestergaard, 1990; Colom et al., 2000).

TABLE 21–1. **Factors Associated with General Medical Adherence**

Factor	Predictive of Adherence	Predictive of Nonadherence	Not Predictive	Unclear
Disease				
Chronicity of illness	■			
Amount of time asymptomatic		■		
Severity of disease				
As a general factor			■	
Number of symptoms experienced	■			
Extent of disability	■			
Type of illness—psychiatric		■		
Patient				
Demographics				
Age (except extremes)			■	
Sex			■	
Intelligence			■	
Education level			■	
Personality and attitudes				■
Personality				
Health beliefs				
Seriousness of illness	■			
Perceived efficacy of treatment	■			
Social supports				
Living alone		■		
Unstable/nonsupportive family		■		
Treatment				
Treatment regimen				
Complexity of regimen		■		
Number and cost of medications		■		
Oral administration	■			
Safety caps		■		
Frequency of dosage				■
Side effects of medication				■
Health care delivery				
Clear information	■			
Counseling	■			
Reminding strategies	■			
Convenience of clinical setting	■			
Continuity of care	■			
Extent of supervision by others	■			

Source: Based on data in Haynes et al., 1979, 2003; Blackwell, 1980; McDonald et al., 2002; World Health Organization, 2003; DiMatteo, 2004; Osterberg and Blaschke, 2004.

A great deal of research on nonadherence among psychiatric patients has focused on schizophrenia and has yielded findings of considerable relevance to bipolar disorder. Young and colleagues (1999) reviewed 29 studies of nonadherence to antipsychotic oral medications, conducted between 1986 and 1997. They found a median nonadherence rate of 46 percent, with a range of 5 to 85 percent. Fenton and colleagues (1997) reviewed empirical correlates and predictors of nonadherence among schizophrenic patients; their findings are summarized in Box 21–3. Consistent with these

---

BOX 21–3. Empirical Correlates of Nonadherence in Patients with Schizophrenia

Patient-related factors

Greater severity of illness, grandiosity, or both
Lack of insight into the illness
Substance abuse comorbidity

Medication-related factors

Medication side effects, especially dysphoric ones
Subtherapeutic or excessively high dosages

Environmental factors

Inadequate support or supervision
Practical barriers, such as lack of money or transportation

Clinician-related factors

Poor therapeutic alliance

Source: Adapted from Fenton et al., 1997. Used with permission.

---

findings, Young and colleagues (1999) noted important shifts of emphasis in the treatment of schizophrenia, supporting the significance to adherence of a strong therapeutic alliance and patient insight. A recent study of 228 patients hospitalized with schizophrenia, for example, found that patients' relationships with staff and the prescribing physician were predictive of attitudes toward treatment (Day et al., 2005). Perkins and colleagues (2006) conducted a 2-year prospective study of 254 patients recovering from a first episode of schizophrenia or schizophreniform or schizoaffective disorder. They found that patient beliefs about the benefits of medication and the need for treatment, as well as the perceived negative aspects of the antipsychotic medications (haloperidol or olanzapine), were predictive of medication nonadherence. Nearly one-half of the patients were nonadherent by the end of the first year of treatment; those who received olanzapine were significantly more likely to be adherent than those receiving haloperidol.

A meta-analysis of adherence rates for antidepressant treatments (Pampallona et al., 2002) showed high rates of nonadherence (approximately one-third). The authors suggested that adjunctive treatments, such as psychotherapy, that address issues relevant to taking medication may enhance adherence—although they identified no one such intervention as being uniformly effective. We revisit these themes in a later section.

Definitional and Measurement Issues

What is meant by treatment adherence? Various definitions exist, and different studies operationalize the concept in different ways, often as a percentage of time during which physician directions are followed as prescribed. According to Boyd and colleagues (1974a, p. 326), medication nonadherence is "the failure to comply (intentional or accidental) with the physician's directions (expressed or implied) in the self-administration of any medication." Blackwell (1976, 1980, 1982) specified how nonadherence can occur through four types of errors: (1) omission, where the patient either fails to fill the prescription at all or, once having filled it, fails to take the drug; (2) dosage, taking too much or too little; (3) timing, including failure to follow directions about when to take the drug or for how long, or when to change levels; and (4) purpose or commission (taking the drug for the wrong reason). One study of nonpsychiatric patients (Boyd et al., 1974a,b) found the most common medication errors to be mistimed dosages (56 percent of prescriptions), premature termination of the drug (45 percent), and deliberate skipping of dosages (35 percent).

Patterns of nonadherence to mood stabilizers may also vary over time and from patient to patient. Some patients refuse to take the medication at all; some adhere to a given medication but titrate their own dose instead of following the physician-prescribed schedule; and some alternate between total and partial adherence. *Full adherence* refers to the practice of patients who take medication in the manner prescribed and for the period of time specified by their physicians. This pattern is relatively uncommon; most patients who are considered adherent only approximate full adherence. A pattern of *late adherence* is often observed—initial resistance to medication, followed by recurrences of affective illness and subsequent hospitalizations. There may then be a sudden shift toward adherence as patients begin to recognize the relationship between stopping the medication and recurrence of their illness. In *intermittent adherence,* probably the most common pattern, patients adhere for a period of time (usually days to months) and then stop taking the medication (or start taking it in a manner not prescribed) against medical advice. After a recurrence of their illness, they begin taking the medication again. Before more consistent adherence is achieved, these patients stop and start the medication, take it in subtherapeutic dosages, and experience recurrences of illness. This pattern, however, varies greatly from patient to patient. The most extreme pattern is, of course, *total nonadherence,* which every physician encounters at some time and which is the focus of most of the research in this area. It may also be noted that "behavioral nonadherence" may involve issues apart from pharmacological nonadherence: failure to keep appointments; failure to divulge important information on symptoms; and a lack of willingness to follow suggestions, such as getting regular sleep (Colom and Vieta, 2002).

The most commonly employed methods for measuring adherence include review of chart notes, patient self-reports, records of unkept appointments and unfilled prescriptions, blood and urine levels of the drug in question, spousal estimates of the patient's drug-taking behavior, physician assessments of such behavior, pill counts, and measures of illness outcome (the latter assuming a direct relationship between medication adherence and exacerbation or recurrence of illness). All of these measures of medication adherence pose substantial problems of reliability and validity. Physician ratings of adherence generally agree poorly with other sources, and it has been noted that patient self-reports of adherence are far less potentially valid than those of nonadherence (e.g., Young et al., 1999). A recent study found that self-reported adherence levels and actual plasma levels of mood stabilizers were inconsistent predictors of outcome (rehospitalization); the investigators suggested that self-reported adherence may be a proxy measure for additional health-enhancing behaviors and may therefore be predictive of better outcomes (Scott and Pope, 2002b).

Rates of Nonadherence among Bipolar Patients

The first reported instance of lithium nonadherence in a bipolar patient was the first patient treated with the drug. Years after recounting the initial dramatic success of lithium, Cade (1978, p. 13) described the subsequent course of events:

> It was with a sense of the most abject disappointment that I readmitted him to hospital 6 months later as manic as ever but took some consolation from his brother who informed me that Bill had become overconfident about having been well for so many months, had become lackadaisical about taking his medication and finally ceased taking it about 6 weeks before.

Of the thousands of articles written about lithium and other mood stabilizers, remarkably few deal in a substantive way with nonadherence—the primary clinical problem associated with these treatments. This lack of research is extraordinary given the extent of the clinical problem posed by patients who refuse to take medications as prescribed. There is little information about how many patients stop taking mood stabilizers against medical advice; for what reasons they do so, for how long, and at what point in their therapeutic regimen or mood cycles; and whether there are gender and age differences in reasons for nonadherence or incomplete adherence. Little systematic research has been done on patients' perceptions of the positive and negative consequences of taking medications regularly and the effect of these perceptions on actual patterns of use. There is even less information on the use of frequently prescribed combination treatments.

Despite its paucity, the research on rates of medication nonadherence in bipolar patients, summarized in Table 21–2, clearly establishes the magnitude of the problem. In a recent review of 25 studies of medication adherence published between 1976 and 2003, Perlick and colleagues (2004b) calculated the median rate of nonadherence in bipolar patients to be 42 percent. Studies based on multiple medications have reported similar figures. Keck and colleagues (1997), in a study of 140 bipolar manic patients, found an overall adherence rate of 49 percent during a 1-year follow-up, with 31 percent of patients being totally nonadherent. The authors reported 59 percent adherence among those receiving lithium and 48 percent among those receiving divalproex; adherence was only 11 percent for those receiving carbamazepine monotherapy. Of particular note, there was 100 percent adherence to the combination of lithium and divalproex; the sample size of this subgroup was not reported, however, and the authors observed that patients were not randomly assigned, so that self-selection may have affected adherence. (Nonetheless, it is of interest that a recent 18-month comparison of lithium or divalproex plus placebo or olanzapine found that the dropout rate was higher for patients on monotherapy [90 percent] than for those on combination therapy [69 percent] [Tohen et al., 2004]. Likewise, a recent study of 184 bipolar patients found that adherence was higher in patients who were taking a greater number of different medications [Sajatovic et al., 2006a]).

Weiss and colleagues (1998) obtained bipolar patients' retrospective recall of rates of adherence to their medications since first prescribed. About 60 percent of patients reported having adhered to the various medications "more than two-thirds of the time." However, full adherence was reported by 50 percent for divalproex and by only 21 percent for lithium. According to the authors, these figures may reflect in part longer histories with lithium, and hence more opportunity for nonadherence, than was the case for the more recently prescribed divalproex. All of the patients were also substance abusers, and it may be that divalproex is better accepted among that subgroup. By far the largest study of adherence was undertaken utilizing the Veterans Affairs National Psychosis Registry (Sajatovic et al., 2006b). Approximately 45 percent of the 73,964 bipolar patients (n = 32,993) were prescribed antipsychotic medications; as a group they were younger and more often had comorbid substance abuse or post-traumatic stress disorder than those bipolar patients who had not been prescribed antipsychotics. Approximately half (52 percent) of those prescribed antipsychotics were fully adherent; 21 percent were partially adherent, and 27 percent were nonadherent.

Another way to view the issue of nonadherence is to track the number of days of continuous use. Johnson and

TABLE 21–2. **Rates of Nonadherence to Mood Stabilizers and Antipsychotic Medications (Percentage)**

Study	Lithium	Divalproex	Carbamazepine	Antipsychotics
Angst et al., 1970	18[a]			
Van Putten, 1975	20–30			
Bech et al., 1976	24			
Jamison et al., 1979	47			
Cochran, 1982	52			
Connelly et al., 1982	25			
Kucera-Bozarth et al., 1982	52			
Vestergaard and Amdisen, 1983	23[a]			
Danion et al., 1987	53			
Cochran and Gitlin, 1988	46			
Maarbjerg et al., 1988	23[a]			
Lenzi et al., 1989	51		38	
Aagaard and Vestergaard, 1990	42[b]			
Mukherjee et al., 1993	30			
Keck et al., 1997	41	52	89	
Weiss et al., 1998	79[c]	50		
Bonin, 1999	37			
Schumann et al., 1999	55[d]			
Colom et al., 2000	39[b]			
Svarstad et al., 2001	33[e]			
Pope and Scott, 2003	46			
Kleindienst and Greil, 2004	14		18	
Sajatovic et al., 2006b				48[f]
Gonzalez-Pinto et al., 2006	22			

[a]Within the first 6 months of treatment.
[b]Within 2 years.
[c]Lifetime rate.
[d]Discontinued at least once in 6 yr follow-up. Half of 76 lithium patients were bipolar. No differences between diagnostic groups.
[e]Any prescribed mood stabilizer.
[f]Partially adherent, 21 percent; nonadherent, 27 percent.

McFarland (1996) studied records of a large number of lithium users in a health maintenance organization. They determined that the median period of continuous lithium use was 65 days in a 6-year observation period.

Whether one looks at rates of nonadherence or days of use, the above figures indicate that, across diverse medications, populations, and facilities, a lack of adherence to medication regimens is a substantial problem for patients with bipolar disorder. The consequences of this nonadherence appear obvious but bear emphasis: patients who discontinue medication or use it incompletely or inappropriately greatly increase their risk for relapse and recurrence of episodes, as well as suicide (e.g., Suppes et al., 1991). Results of several studies underscore earlier findings in this regard. For instance, Marken and colleagues (1992) cited nonadherence—along with substance abuse and stressful life events—as a key factor precipitating rehospitalization among their inpatient sample (see also Johnson and McFarland, 1996).

From the reverse perspective, Keck and colleagues (1998) found that full adherence was associated with significantly better syndromic recovery during a 1-year follow-up. Likewise, Tsai and colleagues (2001) found that full medication adherence was the strongest predictor of good clinical outcome over a 15-year period among a sample of Taiwanese bipolar patients. Another study, unique for its use of serum lithium levels to monitor adherence, revealed that poor lithium adherence was the strongest predictor of more episodes per year over the follow-up period among a large sample of Indian bipolar patients (Kulhara et al., 1999). And Silverstone and colleagues (1998), having compiled follow-up data on several samples in the United Kingdom and New Zealand, found that 94 percent of patients who totally discontinued lithium became manic, usually within a few weeks; these patients accounted for a sizable portion (44 percent) of those who experienced recurrences over a 2-year course. Although the authors pointed out, as have many others, that the recurrence rate is high even when medication adherence is good, it is clear that nonadherence is a potent determinant of significantly poorer clinical course. Chapters 8 and 25 further underscore the various clinical costs and suspected biological consequences of both sudden discontinuation and intermittent use of mood stabilizers.

Reasons for Nonadherence

Why do patients in general, and individuals with bipolar disorder specifically, not follow their prescribed medication regimen? The common but seemingly irrational failure to take steps prescribed to prevent unwanted medical and psychiatric consequences has been studied from several perspectives, the most important of these being the clinical and the empirical/descriptive. From the clinical perspective, anecdotal and impressionistic information about medications from both patients and practitioners has led to a number of widely held assumptions, which serve as the basis for questionnaires and interviews. The empirical/descriptive approach, adopted largely in medical and psychiatric studies of adherence, typically involves examining variables in four domains: medication-related, patient-related, environmental, and clinician-related. Finally, although less common, theories based in social psychology and behavioral medicine have been proposed. An example is the Health Belief Model, which emphasizes complex interactions among variables, including a mental calculus of attitudes about the costs and benefits of adherence in relation to personal goals and resources.

While all of these research perspectives contribute important information, they also remind us that each investigator's approach may encompass some but not all of the important factors. Moreover, the various factors likely interact in highly complex ways for different individuals. And some of the most important variables may be exceptionally difficult to measure. These include beliefs, expectations, personal predictions, and subjective weighing of costs and benefits—all cognitive operations that may be distorted by mood and judgment.

Clinical Reports of Reasons for Nonadherence

Several anecdotal reports on lithium nonadherence have been published, along with proposed explanations for the phenomenon. In an early study, Polatin and Fieve (1971) emphasized that patients often attribute decreases in creativity and productivity to lithium. They also stressed the role of denial in chronic, serious illness. Fitzgerald (1972) speculated that refusal to take lithium stems from intolerance of reality-based depressions, preference for a hypomanic way of life, or provocation from a spouse or other family member who also misses the patient's hypomanic episodes. Van Putten (1975), in addition to stressing the preference for hypomania, noted the importance of side effects and lithium-induced dysphoria, characterized by a driveless, anhedonic condition. Like Schou and colleagues (1970), he suggested that depressive relapses, as well as a tendency to feel well and to see no further need for medication, are significant variables in lithium refusal. Grof and colleagues (1970) reported that the majority of their patients who stopped lithium of their own accord had been free of relapse and felt no motivation to continue. Van Putten and Jamison (1980) likened the clinical situation to that of penicillin prophylaxis in rheumatic fever, where adherence is positively related to the individual's estimate of the likelihood of having another attack; many bipolar patients in the early stages of their illness are not convinced that a relapse is probable. Schou and Baastrup (1973) cited several reasons for lithium nonadherence: decreased energy, enthusiasm, or sexuality; increased marital difficulties; and a common perception that life is flatter and less colorful than before lithium treatment began. Some of these complaints no doubt result from direct effects of lithium on the illness, such as dampening or eliminating periods of hypomania, and some are due to side effects. Kerry (1978) suggested that the social stigma associated with manic-depressive psychosis may lead to rejection of lithium, the most concrete symbol of the illness. After several decades of work with patients taking lithium, Schou (1997, p. 361) summarized the factors that he and other researchers believe are involved in lithium nonadherence as follows:

> Non-adherence is a complex phenomenon and may have a number of causes. Patients may be inadequately instructed or negligent, they may stop taking lithium because it is not as effective as they had expected it to be, or they may stop taking the drug because it is so effective that there are no further recurrences and they think that they no longer need medication. Patients may stop taking lithium because of side-effects, because they dislike having their mood regulated by a drug, or as a result of anti-drug pressure by the media or the patients' immediate environment.
>
> Patients may also stop lithium because they miss the exhilaration and excess energy experienced during previous hypomanias. If, despite lithium maintenance treatment, patients develop a slight manic recurrence, they may feel unusually well, "on top of the world," and in no need of further lithium. They may then discontinue the treatment, with the result that the impending mania develops into a full-blown one. . . .

It is also clear that attitudes toward medication and adherence may change over time. Cochran (1982), while conducting a brief intervention focused on adherence among bipolar patients, noted that during treatment of nonadherence, patients often followed a pattern in their ability and willingness to articulate their attitudes toward lithium. Initially, they discussed their appreciation of the drug and expressed little ambivalence. By the third session, however, they frequently spoke of extreme ambivalence about lithium and expressed considerable concern about future adherence. Cochran observed that patient concerns centered on the following issues:

- Personal control—frustrations with the "medical model," which patients perceived as focused more on symptoms than on personal gains, and insufficient emphasis on the establishment of alternative means of control, such as changes in diet or reduction in stress.
- Changes in life brought about by successful lithium treatment—missing of highs and the impact of stabilization on relationships.
- Lack of predictability in the course of the illness, possible breakthrough episodes, and length of time on lithium and discomfort about having to be passive in light of possible impending episodes.
- Issues concerning lithium, such as its safety, mechanism of action, side effects, and efficacy.

These issues, observed by most clinicians who have treated bipolar patients, are discussed in greater detail later in this chapter.

Empirical Studies of Reasons for Nonadherence

It is important to note that a "reason" for adherence or nonadherence may not be the same as a "cause." Patients may vary in their ability to articulate or identify their beliefs or theories about why they take (or fail to take) medication as prescribed. Moreover, while information based on consciously held perceptions is vitally important, it may be limited by awareness, influenced by cognitive and emotional factors, and shaped by beliefs that are subject to inaccuracies of various kinds.

In one of the first systematic explorations of the earlier clinical reports of beliefs described previously, Jamison and colleagues (1979) pursued two obvious sources of information and experience about taking medication for bipolar illness: the attitudes of patients (47 lithium patients from the Affective Disorders Clinic at the University of California, Los Angeles [UCLA]) and, independently, the attitudes of clinicians well experienced in the use of lithium (50 physicians, each of whom had treated at least 50 patients with lithium). Nearly one-half of the patients reported having stopped taking lithium at some time against medical advice, and 34 percent of those patients said they had stopped more than once. Of those who reported not having stopped, more than 90 percent stated that they had never considered doing so. These findings raise the possibility that patients tend to divide into two distinct subgroups with regard to adherence—a distribution perhaps more bimodal than continuous in nature.

The results of this study and others investigating reasons for and predictors of nonadherence are summarized in Table 21–3 (see also the later discussion on empirical correlates of nonadherence). The UCLA study revealed no significant demographic (gender, age, education, or income) differences between those who discontinued lithium and those who continued. It is interesting that the adherent and nonadherent groups had equally positive beliefs about the effectiveness of the drug in preventing recurrences of mania and, to a somewhat lesser extent, depression. Both groups also indicated that fear of depression was a stronger motivation for adherence to lithium than fear of mania.

Table 21–4 lists, in order of importance, the reasons for nonadherence cited by the entire patient sample in the UCLA study, by the group that reported nonadherence, and by the clinicians. (When patients reported that they had always complied, they were asked to give reasons that might cause them not to comply.) From the nonadherent

TABLE 21–3. Correlates of Medication Adherence: Data-Based Studies

Study	Sample Size	CORRELATES OF	
		Adherence	Nonadherence
Bech et al., 1976	74 (49 BP)[a]		Side effects; lack of efficacy
Jamison et al., 1979	47 (38 BP)		Disliked the idea of moods being controlled by medication; missed highs; felt depressed
Connelly et al., 1982	48 (40 BP)	Male; perception of continuity of care	Elevated mood; not married
Kucera-Bozarth et al., 1982	37 BP		Lower SES; not married; higher external locus of control score
Frank et al., 1985	216 BP	History of good adherence; higher education	Not married; younger
Danion et al., 1987	73 (36 BP)		Lower cognitive functioning; personality disorder
Cochran and Gitlin, 1988	48 BP		Lack of knowledge about medication; concerns about stigma; side effects
Maarbjerg et al., 1988	133 (61 BP)		Early age at illness onset; greater number of prior hospitalizations; personality disorder; substance abuse
Lenzi et al., 1989	67[a] (53 BP)	Social support; unpleasant psychotic experience	Grandiosity; living alone; manic phase; somatic concerns
Aagaard and Vestergaard, 1990	133 (61 BP)		Substance abuse; personality disorder; greater number of hospitalizations
Miklowitz, 1992	23 BP	Mood-congruent psychosis; better social functioning	
Mukherjee et al., 1993	114 BP	Male; Caucasian	Older age; shorter duration of illness
Keck et al., 1997	140 BP		Substance abuse; denial; side effects
Weiss et al., 1998	44 BP		Substance abuse; side effects; denial
Bonin, 1999	149 BP		Younger; male; less perception of treatment efficacy
Schumann et al., 1999	76 (38 BP)		Resistance to long-term treatment; side effects
Colom et al., 2000	200 BP		Personality disorder; schizotypal symptoms; fewer episodes but more hospitalizations
Greenhouse et al., 2000	32 BP	Acceptance of illness; good coping and low-denial strategies	
Scott and Pope, 2002a	98 (78 BP)		Denial; history of nonadherence

(continued)

TABLE 21–3. Correlates of Medication Adherence: Data-Based Studies *(continued)*

Study	Sample Size	CORRELATES OF Adherence	CORRELATES OF Nonadherence
Stratigos et al., 2002	111 BP		Disliked the idea of moods being controlled by medication; felt well, saw no need for medication; felt illness more related to life events than biologically based
Pope and Scott, 2003	72 (61 BP)		Disliked the idea of moods being controlled by medication; disliked the idea of having a chronic illness; felt depressed
Kleindienst and Greil, 2004	171 BP	Higher age; greater trust in medication and physician[b]	
Perlick et al., 2004b	101 BP[c]		Greater perceived family burden; emotional overinvolvement of caregiver
Sajatovic et al., 2006a	184 BP	Greater number of medications	Current substance abuse
Sajatovic et al., 2006b	32,993 BP[d]		Younger age; minority ethnicity; substance abuse; homelessness

Note: Most earlier studies focused primarily on lithium treatment; more recent studies have included anticonvulsants and antipsychotic medications.

BP=bipolar; SES=socioeconomic status.

[a]35 patients on lithium, 32 on carbamazepine, all female.
[b]For lithium but not carbamazepine patients.
[c]101 patients matched with identified caregivers.
[d]Prescribed antipsychotic medications.

TABLE 21–4. Rank Ordering of General Reasons for Nonadherence: UCLA Study

Rank Order	Total Patient Sample (*n*=47)	Patients Who Reported Discontinuing Lithium Treatment (*n*=22)	Independent Clinician Sample (*n*=50)
1	Bothered by idea that moods are controlled by medication	Bothered by idea that moods are controlled by medication	Felt well; saw no need for lithium
2	Felt depressed	Missed highs	Missed highs
3	Bothered by idea of chronic illness	Felt depressed	Bothered by idea of chronic illness
4	Felt less attractive to spouse	Bothered by idea of chronic illness	Felt less creative
5	Felt well; saw no need for lithium	Felt well; saw no need for lithium	Felt less productive
6	Hassle to take medication	Hassle to take medication	Bothered by idea that moods are controlled by medication
7	Missed highs	Felt less attractive to friends	Hassle to take medication
8	Felt less creative	Felt less creative	Felt less attractive to friends
9	Felt less productive	Felt less productive	Felt depressed
10	Felt less attractive to friends	Felt less attractive to spouse	Felt less attractive to spouse

Source: Adapted from Jamison et al., 1979.

patients' perspective, the four most important reasons for nonadherence were as follows:

- They disliked the idea of medication controlling their moods.
- They missed their highs.
- They felt depressed.
- They disliked the idea of having a chronic illness, symbolized by the necessity for lithium therapy.

Patient and clinician perceptions occasionally diverged, and when they did, the differences were significant. Patients were much more bothered than clinicians believed them to be by having medication control their moods. Those patients who reported discontinuing lithium were more likely than clinicians to report that feeling depressed was a significant factor. Although both clinicians and discontinuers ranked missing highs as particularly important in nonadherence, discontinuers were less likely to state that decreases in productivity and creativity were important in their decision to discontinue. This finding contrasts with prevailing notions about reasons for nonadherence and suggests that many patients do not necessarily equate highs with creativity or productivity. From the clinicians' point of view, the three most important reasons for lithium nonadherence were as follows:

- The patient felt well and saw no need to continue the medication. (Nearly two-thirds of physicians thought that lithium nonadherence was "somewhat" or "very"

related to patients' acting out their denial of a serious lifelong illness.)
- The patient missed the highs of hypomania and/or mania.
- The patient was bothered by the idea of having a chronic illness.

More than 20 years after the UCLA study, Pope and Scott (2003) attempted to replicate it using a British sample of 72 patients and 41 psychiatrists (Fig. 21–1). They concluded that the reasons patients gave for medication nonadherence had "hardly altered since Jamison et al.'s (1979) original study" (p. 291). They also found, as the UCLA investigation had, that physicians' perceptions of reasons for nonadherence remained at variance with those of patients. Psychiatrists, for example, believed that patients stopped taking their medication because they missed their highs, which is certainly true for many patients, but most patients were more concerned about feeling depressed while medicated. Psychiatrists also failed to recognize the importance to patients of having to deal with a chronic illness, as well as having their moods controlled by medication. Psychological issues of control were paramount in a study of bipolar patients conducted by Stratigos and colleagues (2002), as well as in an extensive European study of patient attitudes (Morselli et al., 2003). By far the most important concern patients cited was "feeling dependent" on taking medication; next in importance was their perception that taking medication was tantamount to "slavery."

Figure 21–1. Primary reasons for stopping medication identified by clinicians ($n=41$) and by previously nonadherent (PNAD, $n=33$) and adherent (AD, $n=37$) patient groups. (*Source*: Pope and Scott, 2003. Reprinted with permission from Elsevier.)

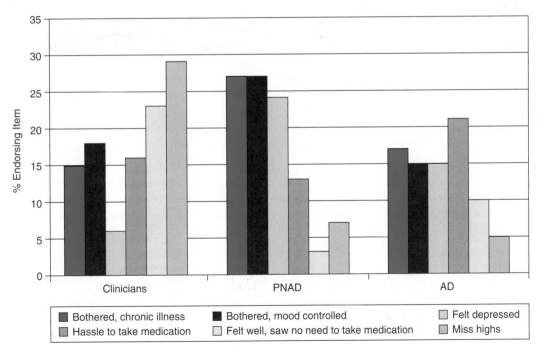

Additional studies have attempted to understand patients' subjective reasons for nonadherence or to predict adherence over time. Some studies have tested versions of a "health belief" model in which patients' perceptions of the severity of their illness and beliefs about the benefits of medication, about themselves, and about control over their illness combine to predict adherence. For instance, Cochran and Gitlin (1988) assessed various attitudes and beliefs among a later sample from the UCLA Affective Disorders Clinic and tested a complex social psychological model of adherence. For the most part, their results confirmed the model, indicating that attitudes about lithium and its effects can predict adherence. An important finding was patients' belief that if their psychiatrist and their friends and family had positive views of the treatment and its effects—and if they themselves were motivated to meet the psychiatrist's and others' expectations—adherence was more likely. The investigators noted that relevant relationships, including the patient–physician relationship, may be important sources of adherence-related attitudes.

Keck and colleagues (1997) assessed patients' reasons for nonadherence to their medication regimen (various mood stabilizers and combinations of drugs) using a questionnaire derived from previous studies of reasons for nonadherence. In their sample of 140 hospitalized manic patients followed for a 1-year period, they found that only 31 percent were totally adherent. The most commonly cited reasons for total or partial nonadherence were denial of illness or poor insight (63 percent); side effects (27 percent); belief that they had recovered from the illness (11 percent); and others, including practical considerations such as the cost of medication.

Schumann and colleagues (1999) reported on a 6-year retrospective study of reasons for nonadherence among 76 patients in two clinics in Vienna and Berlin; 50 percent of the patients were bipolar, with the remainder being unipolar or schizoaffective. Although results were not reported by diagnostic group, the investigators indicated that diagnosis was not significantly associated with adherence or reasons cited for discontinuation of medication. They found that 54 percent of the patients had discontinued treatment at least once during the 6-year period. The most commonly cited reason was "resistance against long-term treatment." Comparisons of adherent and nonadherent patients revealed significant differences on three attitude items: resistance to prophylaxis, denial of the effectiveness of lithium, and denial of the severity of illness.

Greenhouse and colleagues (2000) specifically tested the role of cognitive acceptance or denial of illness in predicting self-reported adherence during a 1-week period. Acceptance and denial were defined by items on a coping questionnaire—for example, "I've been accepting the reality of the fact that it [diagnosis of bipolar-I disorder] has

happened" and "I've been saying to myself, 'this isn't real.'" The authors found that with lower acceptance and higher denial, medication adherence scores declined sharply. Noting that the correlations between acceptance and denial were only moderate, they argued that both processes may contribute separately to medication adherence. Adams and Scott (2000) found that patients' beliefs about the benefits of treatment and the severity of their illness contributed substantially to the prediction of adherence. They also observed that believing health is controlled by external rather than internal factors enhanced adherence.

In a prospective study of the relationship between illness concepts and medication adherence, Kleindienst and Greil (2004) randomly assigned 171 bipolar patients to either lithium or carbamazepine treatment. Illness concepts—trust in medication, trust in the treating physician, and absence of negative treatment expectations—were predictive of adherence to lithium but not to carbamazepine.

Side Effects: A Complex Issue

Several studies, especially those based on primarily lithium-treated patients, have found that side effects are often cited in subjective reports of reasons for nonadherence (e.g., Weiss et al., 1998; Scott and Pope, 2002a). In the prospective study of Kleindienst and Greil (2004), however, neither the number nor the severity of side effects was related to adherence in patients taking lithium or carbamazepine.

Side effects are a complex issue for several reasons. The side effects of a medication may be real, but their importance to patients may be highly subjective in ways unrelated to their frequency or to the perceptions of others, and they may or may not be related to adherence. For example, Gitlin and colleagues (1989) found that the most common side effects of lithium—thirst and polyuria—were far less bothersome to patients than weight gain and cognitive effects. The total number of side effects was related to nonadherence only slightly and nonsignificantly; specific side effects (especially tremor and mental slowness) were associated most strongly (although only moderately) with actual nonadherence. Further, patients indicated that weight gain was the major side effect *potentially* bothersome enough to cause them to stop lithium. Thus the role of side effects in actual medication nonadherence is somewhat ambiguous.

Jamison and colleagues (1979) found further that clinicians may misperceive the role of side effects; the clinicians in their study viewed side effects as more important in nonadherence than did patients who had discontinued lithium treatment. Clinicians may also attribute some "side effects" to mood episodes rather than to medication. Such tendencies may reflect a reluctance to acknowledge certain negative effects, such as cognitive changes, or they may accurately characterize illness factors that patients attribute to their medication. Not only may mood symptoms be misperceived as medication side effects, but mood symptoms—especially depression—may affect the degree to which patients experience and are bothered by somatic side effects (e.g., Abou-Saleh and Coppen, 1983). Indeed, it is likely that personality and interpersonal–environmental characteristics influence patients' perceptions and tolerance of medication side effects.

Side effects, therefore, represent both real deterrents to medication adherence and psychological issues that may play a complex role in adherence. There are some indications that different mood stabilizers may have fewer or differing side effects, resulting in varying levels of adherence to the prophylactic regimen, but significant differences have not been convincingly documented. One study of adherence to antipsychotic medication among a sample of outpatient veterans (most diagnosed with schizophrenia) is suggestive. The investigators found significantly better rates of adherence to atypical than to typical antipsychotic medications, as measured by prescription refills (Dolder et al., 2002). Yet while better adherence was found for the medications with fewer side effects at 6-month follow-up, no differences were seen at 12 months. A recent large study of claims data for antipsychotic treatment in more than 15,000 commercially insured bipolar patients found greater adherence for individuals taking atypical rather than typical antipsychotics (Gianfrancesco et al., 2006). British researchers, however, found significantly lower adherence to atypical antipsychotics than to lithium (Horne et al., 2006).

Greater availability of medical resources to treat adverse side effects may enhance acceptance of long-term medication. Certainly, education about side effects is essential. A recent British study found that more than 60 percent of the 223 patients surveyed were dissatisfied with the information they received about side effects from their physicians (Bowskill et al., 2006). It must be emphasized, however, that subjective and psychological factors also play an important role in patients' reactions to side effects. In their prospective study of adherence in bipolar patients, for example, Kleindienst and Greil (2004) demonstrated that concepts patients hold about their illness strongly influence the subjective impairment caused by medication. Chapters 18 through 20 address side effects and their management in greater detail.

Empirical Correlates of Nonadherence

In addition to the reasons for nonadherence that can be articulated by patients, further information is available from studies of empirical correlates of nonadherence. Table 21–3, presented earlier, summarizes studies of adherence among bipolar patients. Most of these studies focused on lithium and examined a variety of demographic and clinical factors,

using diverse measures of adherence and populations from a range of clinical settings. These studies were characterized by numerous methodological and conceptual shortcomings, including the use of predominantly small sample sizes, which precludes subgroup comparisons and limits generalizability; a relative absence of theoretical or predictive models to guide the analyses; and failure to evaluate complex interactions among variables and changes in medication use over time. Nevertheless, these studies serve as useful first steps toward understanding adherence issues.

Patient-Related Factors

As noted earlier, few demographic variables (age, gender, income, education) appear to predict adherence to lithium or other medications reliably, an observation consistent with results of medication adherence studies in general (see Table 21–1). Among the exceptions to this rule are findings that being married is associated with better adherence and that living alone is associated with poorer adherence[3]; less consistently, adherence increases with age.[4]

Clinical features are also inconsistently associated with adherence, with the exception of a constellation of variables related to elevated mood. As discussed earlier, Jamison and colleagues (1979) found that missing of highs was one of the few factors significantly differentiating adherent from nonadherent patients (see Table 21–4). Likewise, Connelly and colleagues (1982) observed that nonadherence was associated with elevated mood. Lenzi and colleagues (1989) found that grandiosity was significantly associated with nonadherence, while Rosen and Mukherjee (unpublished data) noted that nonadherence was associated with a history of grandiose delusions. Similarly, a study of patients with bipolar-I disorder showed lithium adherence to be less likely among those who experienced recurrent manic episodes (without evidence for clinical depression) than among those who experienced both disabling depressive and manic episodes (Lenzi et al., 1989).

Miklowitz (1992) found that among manic patients, those with more severe psychotic symptoms (and schizoaffective-manic patients generally) were more nonadherent. Other illness factors, such as polarity of episodes, severity, family history, diagnostic subtype, and frequency of affective episodes, are ambiguously or inconsistently related to adherence. Nonetheless, it might be predicted that number of years ill, in complex interaction with age and clinical history, would affect adherence. Clinical experience suggests that younger patients tend to be less accepting of their diagnosis and prognosis, and their attitudes change with experience and the consequences of the illness over time.

The role of mania, and perhaps psychosis in particular, may be especially relevant to the patient's level of insight, awareness, and acceptance of illness. Ghaemi (1997) reviewed studies examining insight (awareness that one has a mental disorder or that one is exhibiting symptoms of psychopathology) among patients with severe psychopathology and its correlation with clinical features. In general, he found that lack of insight is just as prevalent in patients with mania as in those with schizophrenia. Yen and colleagues (2004) found that poorer insight in bipolar illness is more likely in males and in patients with a shorter duration of illness and a history of psychosis. It is also related to the nature of the clinical episodes experienced by patients (see Chapter 22). Patients who experience pure mania show less insight than those who have predominantly mixed states (Cassidy et al., 2001; Dell'Osso et al., 2002); depressed patients show greater insight than manic patients[5]; and bipolar-II patients appear to show less insight than bipolar-I patients (Pallanti et al., 1999). Ghaemi (1997) found no studies examining the role of insight in medication adherence among bipolar patients; however, results of studies previously mentioned concerning patients' beliefs that they are not ill, or no longer ill, clearly reflect a similar concept. Research in the field of schizophrenia has demonstrated a strong association between lack of insight and nonadherence (e.g., Fenton et al., 1997; Young et al., 1999), and further studies of the meaning, correlates, and consequences of lack of insight among bipolar patients are needed. Treatment for bipolar illness often results in improved insight,[6] but the effect of this on adherence has not been adequately studied.

Two further patient characteristics warrant consideration in the context of adherence. The first is substance abuse, which is increasingly recognized as a common and complicating feature of the course of bipolar disorder (see Chapter 7). It may play a particularly pernicious role in poor adherence to medication, as several studies have now reported.[7]

A second salient patient characteristic is one that has rarely been examined: personality disorders that may interact with clinical and attitudinal variables to affect adherence. One large study of 200 bipolar-I and -II patients found that personality disorders assessed by the Structured Clinical Interview for the *Diagnostic and Statistical Manual* (DSM) (SCID) II were strongly associated with medication nonadherence (Colom et al., 2000), as did an earlier, considerably smaller study (Danion et al., 1987) and a Danish one (Aagaard and Vestergaard, 1990). On the other hand, another study, which did not report details on the method used for assessing personality disorders, did not find such an association (Schumann et al., 1999), nor did a recent prospective study of 171 bipolar patients conducted in Germany (Kleindienst and Greil, 2004). It might be speculated that the relatively poor clinical course associated with many forms of personality disorder (see Chapter

10) involves medication nonadherence as a key mechanism of the effects of personality pathology. Personality pathology is highly likely to contribute not only to behavioral problems, such as poor perseverance and inadequate environmental supports, but also to increased substance abuse and maladaptive understanding of the illness, its consequences, and the role of medication. However, patients with personality pathology may also respond more poorly to medication and thus perceive less benefit from adhering to their treatment regimen.

In their comprehensive review of 25 studies of medication adherence in bipolar patients, Perlick and colleagues (2004b) concluded that the most consistent risk factors for nonadherence are comorbid substance abuse, comorbid personality disorder, being single or living alone, having limited insight or knowledge about bipolar illness, and difficulties with side effects (especially cognitive changes, weight gain, lethargy, and problems with tremor and coordination). For an important subgroup, manic symptoms and missing highs are also important. Less clearly related are gender, number of affective episodes, and age.

Environmental Factors

Supportive resources and practical matters have been identified as key contributors to medication adherence in patients with schizophrenia, but have been studied far less often in the context of bipolar disorder. Many studies have found that living alone or being single is predictive of nonadherence in bipolar patients[8]; in a related finding, Lenzi and colleagues (1989) noted that adherence was associated with degree of social support (see also Tables 21–1 and 21–3). The existence of positive relationships doubtless affects adherence in both direct and indirect ways, and such issues deserve considerably more investigation. Also, of course, marriage and adherence may both be associated with positive personal attributes and a relatively better clinical course. Obviously, too, if supportive relationships help facilitate medication adherence, psychotherapy may be an important source of support and may influence adherence directly as well as indirectly (see Chapter 22).

Environmental factors also include the occurrence of chronic and episodic stressors and the extent to which such experiences may undermine efforts to adhere to medication. To date, only one study has directly investigated the potential effect of life events on symptomatology through the mechanism of changes in adherence. Johnson and colleagues (1998) examined this model among a sample of 67 bipolar-I patients over a 1-year period but found no such effect; instead, they found that both adherence and life events affected symptomatology independently and directly.

Other issues concerning practical matters—in particular, medication costs and treatment affordability and availability—are obviously important but have not been adequately studied.

Clinician-Related Factors

The therapeutic alliance has rarely been studied in the context of bipolar patients' adherence to medication, although its importance has been well documented in studies of schizophrenia (see, e.g., the review by Fenton et al., 1997). As noted previously, Cochran and Gitlin (1988) tested a complex model of attitudes associated with adherence and found that patients' perceptions of physicians' attitudes about lithium were important to the patients' own attitudes, although that study did not examine the quality of the therapeutic relationship. Yet it appears probable that the clinician's role is critical, extending well beyond the mechanics of appropriate prescribing (Frank and Frank, 1991; Slavney, 2005).

Medication-Related Factors

Patients' perceptions of both the efficacy and the side effects of the medications they take, or do not take, are clearly important. The relationship between perceived efficacy of medication and adherence is complex and little studied. Two studies (Jamison et al., 1979; Connelly et al., 1982) found no association between adherence and patients' evaluation of medication efficacy, but two others found to the contrary (Bech, 1982; Bonin, 1999). Adherence, as we have seen, is complexly affected by individual differences in perception and toleration of side effects. Several studies have found that nonadherence is associated with the severity or number of subjective concerns about side effects.[9] Other investigators, however, have not found this association.[10]

Certain intrinsic features associated with the pharmacological treatment of bipolar patients may result in exceedingly difficult clinical situations that clinicians must work to overcome. These intrinsic qualities of lithium and the other medications used to treat bipolar illness are listed below with respect to lithium; their generalizability to other medications is apparent, although incomplete.

- Lithium (unlike analgesics, neuroleptics, or benzodiazepines) has a long-delayed therapeutic action: 5 to 7 days for an antimanic effect, usually much longer for an antidepressant effect.
- Patients are expected to stay on the drug for an indeterminate time, much of it in a more or less normal clinical state, with no immediate felt need for the drug.
- If a patient stops the medication, the negative consequences of nonadherence (recurrence of mania and/or depression) are often delayed. Rarely is there an immediate negative effect.

- The cessation of lithium, on the other hand, is often accompanied by relatively immediate positive experiences, either because of the disappearance of side effects or because of breakthrough hypomania (often a contributing factor to lithium nonadherence in the first place).
- The initiation of lithium treatment often is associated with unpleasant events in the patient's memory (e.g., psychosis, hospitalization, violence, agitation).
- If lithium is first prescribed for a manic episode, the natural history of the illness predicts that the patient is at significant risk for a postmanic depression, which further associates the onset of lithium treatment with unpleasant psychological and physical experiences.

Compounding these difficulties, lithium has no known intrinsic reinforcing qualities, either immediate or delayed.

Psychotherapy and Medication Adherence

We cannot emphasize enough the importance of psychotherapy for patients who have bipolar illness, especially those to whom medication adherence does not come easily. We review specific psychotherapeutic interventions, as well as their impact on recurrence of illness and adherence, in Chapter 22. Sajatovic and colleagues (2004) recently summarized clinical trials that specifically examined interventions designed to enhance medication adherence; we reproduce their summary here (Table 21–5) and discuss the details of the psychotherapeutic techniques and specific psychotherapy studies in Chapter 22. Several clinical trials have been completed since the review of Sajatovic and colleagues. Two found no significant difference in medication adherence between the treatment and comparison groups (Ball et al., 2006; Scott et al., 2006); two found increased adherence in the treatment groups (Miklowitz et al., 2003; Lam et al., 2005). These studies are discussed in Chapter 22.

CONCLUSIONS

Many clinicians, having once diagnosed bipolar illness and prescribed an effective medication, tend to assume that the difficult part is over. On the contrary, in the words of one patient, "the war has just begun." Nonadherence to the use of lithium and other medications is costly not only to bipolar patients, but also to those who know them, and to society as a whole.

Research on the factors involved in nonadherence among bipolar patients is relatively sparse, but much information exists in research conducted on related illnesses, such as schizophrenia. One set of factors includes patient variables such as attitudes about the illness and the role of medication, as well as reactions to side effects. The role of the patient's insight into the disorder may be crucial, with

TABLE 21–5. Summary of Studies of Interventions to Enhance Treatment Adherence among Patients with Bipolar Disorder

Study	Design	Intervention	Participants	Outcome	Comments
Shakir et al., 1979	Mirror design	Weekly interpersonal group psychotherapy	$N = 15$; bipolar-I = 12, bipolar-II = 3	Lithium levels; pretreatment = .53 mEq/l; post-treatment = .94 mEq/l	Average duration of group treatment was 51 wk; mean number of participants per session was 8.2
Cochran, 1984	Randomized controlled trial	Weekly modified cognitive-behavioral intervention for 6 wk	$N = 28$; 14 to intervention, 14 to usual care	Significantly enhanced adherence immediately after intervention and at 6 mo	Patients who received the intervention stopped lithium less often and were hospitalized less often
Van Gent and Zwart, 1991	Randomized controlled trial	Five theme-oriented groups for partners of patients with bipolar disorder	$N = 26$ partners of patients; 14 to intervention, 12 to control group	Nonadherence did not differ between groups	Group support was of benefit to partners; partners in both groups reported increased well-being
Harvey and Peet, 1991	Randomized controlled trial	Videotaped lecture on lithium, handout, and home visit	$N = 59$; 29 to educational group, 30 controls	Intervention group had fewer missed lithium doses ($p < .07$)	Improved adherence was associated with improved attitudes toward lithium[a]
Clarkin et al., 1998	Randomized controlled trial	Manual-driven marital therapy (25 sessions)	$N = 42$; 19 to intervention, 23 to usual care	Mean level of medication adherence was higher in the intervention group ($p = .008$)	Patients receiving marital therapy had better overall functioning but were not less symptomatic
Perry et al., 1999	Randomized controlled trial	Individual teaching of early symptom recognition (7 to 12 sessions)	$N = 69$; 34 to intervention, 35 to control group	No difference in adherence between groups	Experimental treatment was effective in reducing relapse to mania but not to depression

866

Study	Design	Intervention	Sample	Adherence findings	Other findings
Weiss et al., 2000	Controlled trial, sequential block enrollment	Weekly integrated group therapy (12–20 sessions)	N=45; 21 to intervention, 24 to control conditions; all participants had dual diagnoses[b]	No difference in adherence between groups	Improvements in substance dependence and mania but not depression for intervention group
Miklowitz et al., 2000	Randomized controlled trial	Manual-driven family-focused psychoeducational treatment; 21 sessions over 9 mo	N=101; 28 to family treatment, 51 to control group; 22 terminated early	No main effect of psychosocial treatment on predicting medication adherence	Over 12 mo, family therapy provided greater prophylaxis against relapse to mood disorder, particularly depression
Lam et al., 2000	Randomized controlled trial	Cognitive-behavioral therapy, 12–20 sessions within 6 mo (mean=16.3 sessions)	N=25; 13 to intervention, 12 to control group	Therapy group showed significantly better adherence over 12 mo ($p<.05$)[c]	Patients in the therapy group had significantly fewer bipolar episodes and fewer hospitalizations
Colom et al., 2003	Randomized controlled trial	Psychoeducational group program, 21 sessions, 90 min each	N=120 euthymic bipolar-I and -II patients; 60 to intervention, 60 to control group	At 2 yr follow-up, intervention patients had higher lithium levels ($p=.03$)	Group psychoeducation significantly reduced the number of patients who had relapses, the number of recurrences per patient, and hospitalizations
Lam et al., 2003	Randomized controlled trial	Individual manual-driven cognitive therapy	N=103; 51 to intervention, 52 to control group	Significantly greater adherence in treatment group ($p=.02$ for self-report; $p=.06$ for serum levels)	Cognitive therapy reduced relapse, improved social functioning

[a] As measured by the Lithium Attitudes Questionnaire.
[b] Bipolar disorder and substance dependence.
[c] As measured by the Medication Compliance Questionnaire.
Source: Sajatovic et al., 2004. Reprinted with permission from *Psychiatric Services.* Copyright 2004, American Psychiatric Association.

factors that reduce such insight (e.g., mania, being young or at an early stage of the illness, comorbid substance abuse) contributing to nonadherence. Other important factors in adherence involve the clinician–patient relationship and the patient's environment, including the extent of supportive relationships with others. Further research on adherence among bipolar patients is needed to further our understanding of issues that may be unique to this population.

Clinicians wishing to increase medication adherence can take several steps: minimize medication levels to the extent possible; minimize and treat aggressively any side effects; track the patient's adherence; examine their own, as well as the patient's, concerns about long-term medication maintenance; educate patients and their families about bipolar illness and the role of medication in attenuating its course; and, when indicated, actively encourage adjunctive psychotherapy.

NOTES

1. This description and others by "a patient with manic-depressive illness" were written by one of the authors, Kay R. Jamison. Some were modified slightly and incorporated into her memoir, *An Unquiet Mind* (New York: Alfred A. Knopf, 1995).

2. See Mazullo and Lasagna, 1972; Haynes et al., 1979; Becker and Maiman, 1980; Docherty and Fiester, 1985; Fenton et al., 1997.

3. Connelly et al., 1982; Kucera-Bozarth et al., 1982; Frank et al., 1985; Lenzi et al., 1989; Aagaard and Vestergaard, 1990; Bonin, 1999; Perlick et al., 2004b; Gonzalez-Pinto et al., 2006.

4. Frank et al., 1985; Greenhouse et al., 2000; Perlick et al., 2004a; Rosen and Mukherjee, unpublished.

5. Amador et al., 1994; Michalakeas et al., 1994; Ghaemi et al., 1995; Peralta and Cuesta, 1998; Dell'Osso et al., 2000; Pini et al., 2001; Dell'Osso et al., 2002.

6. Michalakeas et al., 1994; Fennig et al., 1995; Peralta and Cuesta, 1998; Yen et al., 2003.

7. Danion et al., 1987; Maarbjerg et al., 1988; Aagaard and Vestergaard, 1990; Keck et al., 1997; Colom et al., 2000; Gonzalez-Pinto et al., 2006; Sajatovic et al., 2006a,b.

8. Connelly et al., 1982; Kucera-Bozarth et al., 1982; Frank et al., 1985; Lenzi et al., 1989; Aagaard and Vestergaard, 1990; Bonin, 1999.

9. Bech et al., 1976; Frank et al., 1985; Gitlin et al., 1989; Weiss et al., 1998; Scott and Pope, 2002a.

10. Connelly et al., 1982; Danion et al., 1987; Lenzi et al., 1989; Kleindienst and Greil, 2004.

22 Psychotherapy

At this point in my life, I cannot imagine leading a normal life without both taking lithium and being in psychotherapy. Lithium prevents my seductive but disastrous highs, diminishes my depressions, clears out the wool and webbing from my disordered thinking, slows me down, gentles me out, keeps me from ruining my career and relationships, keeps me out of a hospital, alive, and makes psychotherapy possible. But, ineffably, psychotherapy heals. It makes some sense of the confusion, reins in the terrifying thoughts and feelings, returns some control and hope and possibility of learning from it all. Pills cannot, do not, ease one back into reality; they only bring one back headlong, careening, and faster than can be endured at times. Psychotherapy is a sanctuary; it is a battleground; it is a place I have been psychotic, neurotic, elated, confused and despairing beyond belief. But, always, it is where I have believed—or have learned to believe—that I might someday be able to contend with all of this.

No pill can help me deal with the problem of not wanting to take pills; likewise, no amount of analysis alone can prevent my manias and depressions. I need both. It is an odd thing owing life to pills, one's own quirks and tenacities, and this unique, strange and ultimately profound relationship called psychotherapy.

—Patient with manic-depressive illness[1]

Manic-depressive illness is, by any measure, gravely serious—complex in its origins, diverse in its expression, unpredictable in its course, severe in its recurrences, and too often fatal in its outcome. Yet in the bipolar subgroup milder forms of the disorder may, in some individuals, enhance productivity, creativity, and sociability (see Chapters 10 and 12). Severe mania and depression are debilitating, but mild hypomania is a state that is often sought. Moods are such an essential part of the substance of life, of individuality and identity, that distinguishing normal moods from mild and moderate expressions of the illness is an exacting task for patients. Given such complexity, it is clearly unrealistic to expect treatment to proceed smoothly simply because effective medications are available.

Psychological support for the treatment of bipolar patients ranges from a few minutes with the prescribing physician to combined use of psychoeducation and individual, family, and group psychotherapy. Most commonly, a general psychiatrist or psychopharmacologist provides support for patients who are taking mood stabilizers, usually within a limited time frame of 20 to 30 minutes every few weeks. Although psychotherapeutic work per se may not take place in such a context, the physician can create an emotionally supportive atmosphere, be aware of and focus on the general psychological issues involved in taking a mood stabilizer and having a mood disorder, and encourage patients to express their concerns. Creating and maintaining such an atmosphere is essential to good clinical care.

The practice guidelines of the American Psychiatric Association (2002) for managing bipolar disorder recommend that clinicians (1) perform a diagnostic evaluation, (2) evaluate the patient's safety and determine a treatment, (3) establish and maintain the therapeutic alliance, (4) monitor treatment response, (5) provide education to the patient and family, (6) enhance treatment adherence, (7) promote awareness of stressors and regular patterns of activities and sleep, (8) work with the patient to anticipate and address early signs of relapse, and (9) evaluate functional impairments. A therapeutic relationship of this kind not only increases the likelihood of medication adherence, but also makes it more likely that the patient will be referred for formal psychotherapy should the need arise. Formal, structured psychotherapy best follows control of acute episodes. Unfortunately, many physicians do not provide this type of therapeutic relationship, nor do they make the necessary referrals to qualified psychotherapists.

Indeed, the very efficacy of mood stabilizers and other medications may lead clinicians to minimize the value of psychotherapy or their own role in the treatment of bipolar illness. In 1990, a consensus conference of the National Institute of Mental Health (NIMH) identified as the most underdeveloped area in the treatment of bipolar illness the use of adjunctive psychosocial therapies to alleviate the behavioral and social adjustment problems associated with the disorder (Prien and Potter, 1990). Likewise, Vasile and colleagues (1987) found that psychiatrists and mental health professionals often de-emphasize psychotherapy in the treatment of affectively ill patients. Patients themselves, by contrast, often find psychotherapy a potent adjunct to mood stabilizers. In the one study in which patients and therapists were actually asked about the value of psychotherapy in the treatment of bipolar illness, twice as many patients as physicians thought psychotherapy was helpful to them in remaining adherent to medication (Jamison et al., 1979). These findings are consistent with those of a survey of a national depression and bipolar support group completed two decades later (Goodale and Lewis, 1999).

While medication is the central treatment for bipolar disorder—in both the acute and maintenance phases—psychotherapy is a particularly important adjunct to medication in maintenance treatment. This is true for several reasons.

First, problems that typically accompany bipolar illness invite psychotherapeutic intervention. The personal, interpersonal, and social consequences of the disorder, which are usually severe, can include suicide, violence, alcoholism, drug abuse, unemployment, divorce, parental neglect, and hospitalization. Although biological variables predominate in the etiology, the primary manifestations of bipolar illness are behavioral and psychological, with profound changes in perception, attitudes, personality, mood, and cognition. Psychotherapeutic interventions can be of unique value to patients undergoing such devastating changes in the way they perceive themselves and are perceived by others, providing the needed monitoring of mood and life changes. Indeed, some of the newer psychotherapies focus on monitoring these changes as a way of preventing recurrences. The psychosocial consequences of bipolar disorder—such as loss of employment or a significant decline in employment status, alcohol or other substance abuse, alienation from loved ones, and frequent marital and other interpersonal disputes—are also precipitants of recurrences of the disorder. Such life events, often the subject matter of psychotherapy sessions (Coryell et al., 1993; Goldberg et al., 1995), may trigger manic or depressive episodes through, for example, disruption of circadian rhythms, loss of sleep, or distorted cognitions (Wehr et al., 1987a; Frank et al., 1994; Miklowitz et al., 1996). In helping to alleviate the stress-related precipitants of manic and depressive episodes, psychotherapy may temper the progression of the natural course of the illness (Post et al., 1986).

Second, suicide tends to occur early in the illness (see Chapters 8 and 25), when patients have the least support

and information and are most likely not to adhere to medication. Indeed, nonadherence to lithium or other mood stabilizers becomes a major theme in the therapy of many patients (Jamison et al., 1979; Jamison, 1995; Keck et al., 1997) (see Chapter 21). Confusion often arises because the illness itself, as well as its pharmacological treatments, can affect cognition, perception, mood, and behavior. Psychotherapeutic sessions frequently involve concerns about being on medication. For example, the effectiveness of medication in ameliorating the illness is not always welcome because it deprives some patients of energy and much-sought-after highs and can burden them with bothersome side effects. Moreover, some patients (at least 10 to 15 percent) have a poor response to mood stabilizers (Goldberg and Harrow, 1999), which may be due in part to nonadherence. Close monitoring of adherence is therefore important, especially because discontinuation of medication may lead to recurrences of mania and/or depression and increased risk of suicide.

Third, there are times when clinicians treat bipolar patients who are not taking medication, such as those who refuse it, those who have medical contraindications or need surgery, and women who stop taking medication during their pregnancies. In such cases, psychotherapy may have to serve as the sole treatment, providing critical support and monitoring. Psychotherapy, in conjunction with medication or electroconvulsive therapy (ECT), may also be the treatment of choice for acutely suicidal patients or for breakthrough depressions in patients prone to antidepressant-induced cycling.

The emphasis in this chapter is on psychotherapeutic interventions for patients maintained on mood stabilizers. The first section focuses on psychotherapeutic issues of importance in the clinical management of bipolar illness. These issues are relevant to all aspects of clinical management, whether the patient is being seen for medications only (the most common clinical situation) or for medications in conjunction with formal psychotherapy—individual, group, or family—or with involvement in a self-help group. The discussion encompasses new developments in psychotherapeutic practices, as well as educational and informational resources, including books, self-help groups, and websites. Some psychotherapies have been modified for bipolar patients and described in manuals for testing in clinical trials; a number of such trials are either completed or ongoing. The literature on these psychotherapies and their efficacy is reviewed in the second section of the chapter, with a focus on treatment modalities combining psychotherapy and mood stabilizers. Psychotherapeutic techniques per se, however, are not discussed in detail, in part because we assume a basic knowledge of the principles and practice of psychotherapy and in part because no one type of psychotherapy has been demonstrated to be *uniquely* effective in this patient population. The lack of psychotherapeutic specificity in the discussion here reflects the reality of clinical practice, namely, the predominance of pharmacological treatments for bipolar disorder and the relatively recent emphasis on psychological interventions. However, we wish to reemphasize our belief that formal psychotherapy is beneficial to many, if not most, bipolar patients and is unquestionably essential for many others, especially those who are suicidal or unwilling to take medication in the manner prescribed. The limitations of even the most beneficial medications are increasingly apparent to clinicians treating affective illness. It may be hoped that ongoing and future research efforts will determine the specific nature of the most effective psychological interventions.

CLINICAL MANAGEMENT

We begin this section by summarizing the historical context for the psychotherapeutic treatment of bipolar disorder. We then review key issues that arise during such treatment. The section ends with discussion of important aspects of psychotherapeutic treatment of bipolar illness, including mood charting, patient education, family education and family therapy, and the self-help programs of national and local support associations.

Historical Context

Clinical pragmatism, buttressed by biological assumptions about etiology, long ago determined the dominance of medical therapies in the treatment of bipolar illness. Thus physicians, ancient and modern, have for the most part sought cures for mania and melancholia not through talking and listening, but through direct actions of control: mineral baths, bloodletting, herbs, chains, vapors, bromides, opiates, warm waters, cold waters, and physical and chemical restraints.[2]

Psychotherapy, as generally conceptualized, is a set of formal psychological procedures or exercises that are followed by a therapist and patient and that are designed to relieve symptoms, improve function, or produce insight. These procedures, discussed at length later in the chapter, are derived from a particular theory of psychological development or change.[3]

Even the pioneers of psychotherapy, the psychoanalysts, tended to perceive patients suffering from bipolar illness as not very good candidates for psychotherapeutic treatment. Fromm-Reichmann (1949) characterized them as lacking in "complexity and subtlety"; Abraham (1911) as "impatient, envious, exploitive, and with dominating possessiveness"; and Rado (1928) as continually involved in a "raging orgy of self-torture." Bipolar patients generally were

compared with schizophrenic patients and found to lack introspection and to be too dependent and "clinging" (Fromm-Reichmann, 1949), disconcertingly capable of finding vulnerable spots in the therapist (Fromm-Reichmann, 1949; Janowsky et al., 1970), and prone to eliciting strong feelings of countertransference in the analyst (English, 1949; Rosenfeld, 1963). Despite these perceived difficulties, many leading analysts from the prepharmacotherapy era sustained a dedicated commitment to the psychoanalytic treatment of bipolar illness. Thus in 1911, Abraham noted:

> Psycho-analysis, which has hitherto enabled us to overcome this obstacle [depression interfering with the development of transference], seems to me for this reason to be the only rational therapy for manic-depressive psychoses. (Abraham, 1927, pp. 153–154)

Nevertheless, before lithium was available, enthusiasm for treating bipolar illness was limited—and understandably so. One can imagine the frustration of attempting to treat a hypomanic or manic patient in psychotherapy. Getting such a patient into the office and keeping him there would have been difficult enough; engaging in a meaningful therapeutic endeavor could only have been daunting. Likewise, any clinician can appreciate the different kind of frustration involved in treating a profoundly depressed patient. The high spontaneous remission rate characteristic of bipolar illness no doubt encouraged therapists in some cases to attribute clinical changes to their therapeutic interventions; conversely, when no change or a relapse occurred, therapists tended to assume responsibility as well or to blame the patient.

The psychoanalysts and early psychotherapists provided a source of clinically descriptive information, virtually all of it from unmedicated patients. This material is all the more significant because present medical ethics strongly discourage the psychotherapeutic treatment of unmedicated patients with bipolar illness. The psychoanalytic school is also important because it has had a profound effect on clinical thinking about bipolar illness. Not only most psychotherapists, but also many who contributed to the early biological and pharmacological literature, have been deeply influenced by psychoanalytic conceptions of the illness.

Psychotherapeutic Issues

The competent and compassionate psychotherapy of bipolar illness is predicated on a solid knowledge of the disorder. Kraepelin's injunction to his turn-of-the-century medical students remains compelling: "It is one of the physician's most important duties to make himself, as far as possible, acquainted with the nature and phenomena of insanity" (Kraepelin, 1904, p. 3). A solid knowledge of bipolar disorder encompasses phenomenology, the natural history of the illness (including its recurrent nature, problematic course, high mortality rate, and seasonal patterns), biological aspects (including medication responses in mania and depression), biological theories of etiology, and mechanisms of action of the drugs used for treatment. Therapists with a good scientific grasp of the psychological phenomenology of the illness, as well as the biological, will be more therapeutically competent. They will also be more likely to avoid the biological determinism that is common in therapists who are well grounded in biological theories but poorly trained in psychological studies such as personality theory and development, neuropsychology, and social psychology.

The psychotherapy of bipolar illness requires considerable flexibility in style and technique. Flexibility is necessary because of the patient's changing moods, thinking, and behavior, as well as fluctuating levels of therapeutic dependency intrinsic to the illness. Fluctuations in functioning that occur within as well as between episodes of the illness pose a serious challenge to therapists, who must adjust their treatment options, strategies, and attitudes to meet the demands of the individual patient and the specific phase of the illness. In the therapeutic relationship, a long-lead approach is often useful to maximize the patient's awareness of and sense of control over his or her behavior. It is important not to attempt to control the patient unduly and not to allow medications to become the focus of a power struggle; various psychoeducational treatments have been developed and tested for this purpose (see the later discussion). A thin line exists between too much and too little therapeutic control: too much may lead to increased dependency, maladaptive rebellion, decreased self-esteem, or nonadherence; too little may lead to feelings of insecurity, an unnecessarily tenuous hold on reality, and feelings of abandonment. The patient may see signs of caring in the therapist's firm, consistent orders for routine medication levels or tests of thyroid, liver, and kidney functioning but engage in unnecessary power struggles and refuse to comply with medication regimens when the therapist places undue emphasis on precise medication patterns (e.g., not allowing for some degree of self-titration).

Because bipolar disorder has a long-term course with highly variable manifestations, therapeutic alliance and support play a central role in treatment. The alliance is the product of good rapport, combined with knowledge about the course of the individual patient's illness. Collaborative aspects of management through self-ratings, chartings, and patient and family education (using films, lectures, books, or handouts), discussed later in the chapter, are integral to good clinical care. The therapist must also be able to use hospitalization, when appropriate, as an occasionally necessary adjunct to outpatient care and must not regard it as an indication of failure in the therapeutic endeavor.

In the remainder of this section, we review issues that commonly arise in the psychotherapeutic treatment of bipolar illness: anger, denial, and ambivalence surrounding both the illness and its treatment; disappointment and frustration attendant to less-than-complete treatment success; losses associated with medication; fears of recurrence; the problem of learning to discriminate normal from abnormal moods; the need to deal with developmental tasks of late adolescence and early adulthood; concerns about family and other relationships; concerns about genetics; and clinician attitudes and expectations. First, however, we discuss patients' perspectives on some of the major psychological issues of importance in psychotherapy.

Perspectives of Patients

The following description of the bipolar form of manic-depressive illness was written by a patient who, by age 30, had been through two violently psychotic, ecstatic manic episodes, countless expansive and euphoric hypomanias, occasional mixed states, several lengthy and incapacitating suicidal depressions, and a nearly lethal suicide attempt:

> There is a particular kind of pain, elation, loneliness, and terror involved in this kind of madness. When you're high it's tremendous. The ideas and feelings are fast and frequent like shooting stars and you follow them until you find better and brighter ones. Shyness goes, the right words and gestures are suddenly there, the power to seduce and captivate others a felt certainty. There are interests found in uninteresting people. . . . Feelings of ease, intensity, power, well-being, financial omnipotence, and euphoria now pervade one's marrow. But, somewhere, this changes. The fast ideas are far too fast and there are far too many; overwhelming confusion replaces clarity. Memory goes. Humor and absorption on friends' faces are replaced by fear and concern. Everything previously moving with the grain is now against—you are irritable, angry, frightened, uncontrollable, and enmeshed totally in the blackest caves of the mind. You never knew those caves were there. It will never end. Madness carves its own reality.
>
> It goes on and on and finally there are only others' recollections of your behavior—your bizarre, frenetic, aimless behaviors—for mania has at least some grace in partially obliterating memories. What then, after the medications, psychiatrist, despair, depression, and overdose? All those incredible feelings to sort through. Who is being too polite to say what? Who knows what? What did I do? Why? And

most hauntingly, when will it happen again? Then, too, are the annoyances—medicine to take, resent, forget, take, resent, and forget, but always to take. Credit cards revoked, bounced checks to cover, explanations due at work, apologies to make, intermittent memories (what *did* I do?), friendships gone or drained, a ruined marriage. And always, when will it happen again? Which of my feelings are real? Which of the me's is me? The wild, impulsive, chaotic, energetic, and crazy one? Or the shy, withdrawn, desperate, suicidal, doomed, and tired one? Probably a bit of both, hopefully much that is neither. Virginia Woolf, in her dives and climbs, said it all: "How far do our feelings take their colour from the dive underground? I mean, what is the reality of any feeling?" (Patient with manic-depressive illness[1])

Alluded to here are many of the fears and worries common to most individuals with bipolar illness: the frightening, tumultuous, and extremely damaging aspects (to self and others) of mania and depression; the powerful effects of the illness on subsequent functioning and ongoing and potential relationships, as well as general expectations of the future; the inherent unpredictability of the course of the disease; and the pervasive fear, often terror, of recurrence. Practical consequences of mania and depression usually include, among others, the alienation of friends, lovers, and family members; the inability to move forward or naturally in a career; and major financial problems stemming from overspending, ill-considered investments, substantial and often uninsurable medical expenses, and legal difficulties. Alcohol and substance abuse are common (see Chapter 8). Additionally, many individuals who have bipolar illness find it difficult to adjust to the idea of having a serious, chronic, and life-threatening illness, one that generally requires lifelong maintenance medication, with side effects, for its control. Consequential features pervade this illness, including a fundamental, if usually transitory, inability to perceive reality with accuracy and to judge a course of action with prudence. Once an acute episode is over, the person is left with palpably shaken self-confidence. For a considerable period after a manic or depressive episode, many patients continue to question their judgment, their ability to assess situations, and their capacity to understand their relationships with other people.

Etiological assumptions about the disorder deeply affect the highly individualized experience of bipolar illness. Despite the compelling arguments for its biological origins—and despite the potential of such arguments to alleviate the associated guilt and stigma—patients often find these explanations intuitively unpersuasive, especially in the early stages of illness. Thus although some patients come to believe that profound depression is biologically rooted, others interpret it as a character problem or a spiritual crisis, and

still others as psychological in origin. Hypomania is often perceived as highly intoxicating, powerful, productive, and desirable; patients have difficulty thinking of it as a sickness or as part of the same illness as depression and mania.

In the following sections, we review common themes that appear repeatedly in patients' descriptions of their illness: they are fearful of recurrence; they are concerned about transmitting it to their offspring; they feel shame and humiliation; they suffer the havoc wrought by each episode on their relationships with others; they confront disturbing psychological, financial, and social issues during recovery; and they reflect on the long-term meaning of the illness in their lives.

Fears that the illness will return are common, and a profound mistrust of the future often forms the crux of patients' concerns about work and personal relationships. A physician hospitalized several times for mania described his fears of recurrence (especially of mania), as well as the damaging effects of his illness on his career, thus (Anonymous, *Lancet*, 1984, p. 1268):

Two years is a long time out of professional medical circulation—things forgotten, things not learned or heard of, but the most daunting problem is the prospect of further episodes of mania. The depression if it occurs is a more private feature of the syndrome. Mania is very public and is accompanied by a multitude of embarrassing excesses and, not infrequently, scandals.

Questions remain: will there be further episodes; how frequently; and will they be as debilitating? No-one can offer guarantees or even reliable answers yet. Meanwhile what about my capacity to work, earn a living, to occupy myself, and fulfill my responsibilities? The qualities for a doctor are vastly different from those of a poet. A hospital consultant is nothing if not reliable. My unreliability is already manifest.

Another typical concern derives from the heritable component of bipolar illness and recurrent depression. Many patients, having grown up in an environment of mental illness and/or extreme mood swings, express fear that they will end up like the affected parent, especially if that parent has been severely disabled, repeatedly hospitalized, violent, or alcoholic. The fear is even greater if the parent died by suicide. The daughter of a woman with bipolar disorder described her fear of inheriting the illness and her difficulty in establishing an independent identity (Anthony, 1975, p. 292):

Ever since I was small, I have been told that I was just like my mother. I was named after her, and very soon I took to thinking that I was going to be committed when I was 21, like she was. . . . I was sure that they were going to come and haul me away. . . . I felt that the only way I could separate my thoughts and feelings from her would be for her to die, and I often hated her and wished for her death, especially when she was manic.

Often, too, patients (and their spouses) agonize over the possibility of passing on the illness to children. Playwright and producer Joshua Logan wrote about this fear in describing a conversation with his first wife (Logan, 1976, p. 153):

> I asked her if she wanted to have children with me.
> She said no.
> I asked why, but she refused to answer. . . . She would
>   never have children by me, and that
> I should know why. I looked at her blankly, and she added:
> "I have no wish to bring insane children into this world."

Individuals who suffer from bipolar illness experience acute shame and humiliation for many reasons, including psychosis and resulting bizarre and inappropriate behavior or violence, financial irregularities, and sexual indiscretions, to name but a few. In the words of one patient, "No one who has not had the experience can realize the mortification of having been insane" (Reiss, 1910). Another patient (Graves, 1942) wrote:

> While the intoxication of mania lasts, I for one have no disposition to embrace death. After the intoxication is over, my chief emotional reaction is shame and disgust with myself, and a wonder that my fear of death could be so wonderfully and idiotically twisted. That the facing of humiliation, despair, or deprivation should produce a desire for death is quite natural.

In portions of two letters to T. S. Eliot, Robert Lowell (cited in I. Hamilton, 1982, pp. 286, 307) described his embarrassment following two different manic episodes:

> [June 1961] The whole business has been very bruising, and it is fierce facing the pain I have caused, and humiliating [to] think that it has all happened before and that control and self-knowledge come so slowly, if at all.
>
> [March 1964] I want to apologize for plaguing you with so many telephone calls last November and December. When the "enthusiasm" is coming on me it is accompanied by a feverish reaching to my friends. After it's over I wince and wither.

The widely varying reactions of others to a person who has bipolar illness include anger, concern, withdrawal, unrealistically high or low expectations, rejection, and denial of the illness.[4] Robert Lowell (1977) wrote of the isolation, pain, and misunderstanding experienced during one of his hospitalizations for mania:

> At visiting hours, you could experience
> my sickness only as desertion. . . .

> Dr. Berners compliments you again,
> "A model guest . . . we would welcome
> Robert back to Northampton any time,
> the place suits him . . . he is so strong."
> I am on the wrong end of a dividing train—
> it is my failure with our fragility.

John Custance (1952, p. 115), a British writer and former naval intelligence officer who suffered from severe, psychotic manias and depressions, described the denial of others after his release from a psychiatric hospital. He also depicted his own denial and the gradual sealing-over process so characteristic of the recuperation period:

> But once I get out of a Mental Hospital all this changes. I find myself in a totally different "atmosphere". I cannot, however hard I try, get even my most intimate relatives and friends to understand or take any interest in what may or may not have happened to me during my "madness". Gradually the vividness of my memory fades; like my relatives, I try to put the whole experience out of my mind, and in fact it does to a certain extent disappear into "lower levels of my Unconscious". Then I find myself genuinely wondering whether these memories so far as they are conscious at all, are not "delusions", "hallucinations," as "unreal" as the actual technical hallucination I know I have had and have described earlier.

A different kind of denial, a "conspiracy of silence," was described by Norman Endler (1982, pp. 148–149), a Canadian psychologist writing about his hypomania and depression and their effects on those around him:

> In April 1977, when I first started getting depressed, not only did I deny it to myself but so did my friends and colleagues. My secretary and administrative assistant, as indicated earlier, asked me what was wrong. My gradual withdrawal from interaction, my lack of cheerfulness, and my quietness were interpreted by them as anger at something done wrong. After about four weeks my wife insisted that I should see a doctor. My children said nothing to me. My colleagues at York said nothing to me, and the professionals (psychiatrists, psychologists, and social workers) in the Department of Psychiatry, Toronto East General Hospital, said nothing to me. I'm sure that some, if not most of them, must have noticed that something was wrong with me. (If they had not, they shouldn't be working in the mental health field.)
> Why did my colleagues participate in an unintended "conspiracy of silence"? There are a number of factors to consider. First, suppose they commented on my depression and they were wrong. Suppose I wasn't really depressed but only very tired. This would have been most embarrassing for them. Second, some people do not like

to interfere or intrude in the lives of others. Third, suppose it were true that I was depressed. How could they handle it without embarrassing me? The fact that I was chairman might have been another factor. Because the "show" was running smoothly, there was no need to question the chief executive officer. My guess is that my friends didn't say anything because they probably couldn't believe that it was true. . . . when I was hypomanic, none of my colleagues confronted me. Here, again, they were following the social norm of not interfering. Because I had previously been depressed, they probably perceived it as a recuperative period and gave me the benefit of the doubt.

The postpsychotic or recovery phase is an important but seldom-discussed aspect of bipolar illness. The transition from disturbed to normal thinking and feeling and the adjustment to the interpersonal, medical, professional, and financial consequences of mania and depression are usually slow, exhausting, frustrating, and partially futile experiences for patients.

Virginia Woolf (1910), writing from a hospital where she was confined for mania (letter to Vanessa Bell, July 28, 1910), described the slowness and subtlety of psychological recovery: "I have been out in the garden for 2 hours; and feel quite normal. I feel my brains, like a pear, to see if its [sic] ripe; it will be exquisite by September." She also described the gradual return from depression to normality: "I think the blood has really been getting into my brain at last: It is the oddest feeling, as though a dead part of me were coming to life."

The recovery period typically is filled with anxiety about things done, or left undone, during the preceding mania or depression, fears about the future, and concerns about the completeness of recovery. Uncertainty about the future, as well as confusion about the origins and meaning of the illness, was expressed by Joshua Logan (1976, p. 178):

Still, none of that shook off the dreariness of having an illness that didn't seem like one, of not knowing how or when I'd be rid of it, of not knowing even why it had happened to me, of having iron bars on the windows—even though those bars were fashioned like curlicued decorative devices. Was I ever, ever, going to get out? And if I did—what would I do? Where would I go?

Inevitable ruminations about behavior when ill, especially when manic, are part of the recovery phase (Lowell, cited in I. Hamilton, 1982, p. 218):

I've been out of my *excitement* for over a month, I think, now, and am in good spirits, though I don't feel any rush of eloquence to talk about the past. It's like recovering from some physical injury, such as a broken leg or

jaundice, yet there's no disclaiming these outbursts—they are part of my character—me at moments. . . . The whole business was sincere enough, but a stupid pathological mirage, a magical orange grove in a nightmare. I feel like a son of a bitch.

Lowell, born into an old-line Boston family where "Lowells talk only to Cabots and Cabots talk only to God," wrote poignantly of his fall from "pedigreed tulip to weed" in his painful recovery (Lowell, 1959, p. 84):

Recuperating, I neither spin nor toil.
Three stories down below,
a choreman tends our coffin's length of soil,
and seven horizontal tulips blow.
Just twelve months ago,
these flowers were pedigreed
imported Dutchmen; now no one need
distinguish them from weed.
Bushed by the late spring snow,
they cannot meet
another year's snowballing enervation.

I keep no rank nor station.
Cured, I am frizzled, stale and small.

Anger, Denial, and Ambivalence

History bears witness to the tendency of some people to resist with passion when cornered by fate—to, in the words of Dylan Thomas, "rage against the dying of the light." Others submit more readily to what may or may not have been inevitable. Such different reactions are understandable in individuals who face an uncertain future because of bipolar illness. Some patients resist for years, irate at their diagnosis, their treatment, and their physicians. Others accept the illness and its treatment with remarkable equanimity. Most fall between the two extremes.

Bipolar disorder can push patients to the limits of their resources. It is a complicated and frustrating illness, seemingly impossible to sort through. It takes a heavy emotional toll on family members and friends, the repercussions of which place further psychological stress on the patient. The illness often seems within the patient's control, but usually it is not. It frequently carries with it a psychotic diagnosis and an uncertain course, and almost always a lifetime sentence of medication. Especially when not treated early and aggressively, it is costly in loss of self-esteem, disrupted relationships, secondary alcoholism and drug abuse, violence, economic chaos, hospitalizations, lost jobs, years consumed by illness, and suicide.

Contending with such a reality understandably rouses patients to anger, which can be seen as natural and, up to a point, highly adaptive. Anger is useful because it drives patients to question assumptions and to refuse to accept the unacceptable. At the same time, it often leads patients to reject irrationally an effective treatment or to direct their wrath—at times legitimately, but more often not—at the clinicians who treat the disease. Moreover, determining the extent to which anger is a symptom of the disorder can be difficult.

Bipolar patients also use denial to cope with their illness. Even in the presence of severe and obvious pathology, they deny the disorder's severity, the odds of its recurring, its consequences, and at times its very existence. Like anger, denial is a normal response to the unpleasant, the painful, the unpredictable, and the destructive in life. Not to deny some aspects of a serious disease such as bipolar illness would be unusual, even troubling. Denial clearly is an essential part of healing, allowing slow assimilation of otherwise overwhelming thoughts and feelings. Too much denial, however, can be dangerous.

Not surprisingly, patients' level of insight into their illness varies depending upon the predominant nature of their clinical episodes. Patients who experience pure mania generally show less insight than those who have mixed states (Dell'Osso et al., 2000, 2002; Cassidy, 2001), although Cassidy and colleagues (1998) had failed to find this difference in an earlier study. Depressed patients usually show greater insight than manic patients[5]; those with bipolar-II disorder appear to show less insight than those with bipolar-I (Pallanti et al., 1999). Poorer insight is also related to the presence of psychotic features (Yen, 2003), as well as residual subsyndromal manic symptoms (Dell'Osso, 2002; Yen, 2003). Although not well studied, there is evidence that impaired insight persists during remission for many patients (Varga et al., 2006); recent research on patients with schizophrenia suggests that neurocognitive deficits, which persist during remission, play a significant role in impaired insight (Aleman et al., 2006).

Symptoms of bipolar illness contribute to the process of denial. Patients' judgment is often suspended during episodes of acute mania, to the point that they become incapable of recognizing the destructiveness of their behavior (Jamison, 1995; McAlpin and Goodnick, 1998). Likewise, cognitive and other memory impairments during depression often are pronounced, producing problems of recollection even without denial. Repression, psychological distance, and the need to adapt to the realities of life frequently cause memories of depression to pale over time. The severity and nature of manic episodes similarly are frequently minimized or forgotten. This can be due to the relatively clearer perception of earlier, milder, and more enjoyable stages of mania; amnesia resulting from the cognitive fragmentation characteristic of manic psychosis; repression; and the sheer volume of thoughts, perceptions, behaviors, and feelings that occur during mania

and make storage of memories or good recall unlikely. Denial often leads to medication nonadherence, an issue discussed in detail in Chapter 21.

The treatment of denial, although not always successful, frequently becomes easier as time passes and the illness reappears too often to be disowned, even unconsciously. Denial can be dealt with effectively in psychotherapy by exploring the meaning and consequences of the illness for the patient. Ongoing education about the natural history of the illness, with emphasis on its high relapse rate, undercuts the process of denial as well, as do straightforward and informed discussions of the risks and benefits of medication.

Ambivalence is another common reaction among patients with bipolar disorder, especially when caused by the incongruence between the behavioral expression of the illness and its biological treatment. As a disorder of mood and behavior, bipolar illness has symptoms and consequences that are largely psychological and interpersonal in nature. At the same time, effective mood stabilizers can result in relatively rapid improvement. The treatment response is obvious and gratifying to the clinician, if not the patient, and lends credence to a strongly biological treatment program. This belief is further encouraged by the demonstrated inability of psychotherapy alone to relieve or prevent bipolar episodes. Also encouraging a biological focus is the fact that treatment with mood stabilizers is imbued with a medical ambiance and embedded in a highly structured medical regimen: the physician orders laboratory tests of serum levels of mood stabilizers, as well as kidney, liver, and thyroid functioning, and asks specific medical questions about side effects, usually somatic rather than cognitive in nature. This understandable focus of physicians on the medical aspects of bipolar illness often stands in a point–counterpoint relationship to the perspective of patients, who are likely to be more focused on the psychological aspects of their illness and its treatment. These disparate perspectives can easily lead to a quite arbitrary split between the biological and the psychological.

Conceptualizing bipolar illness as fundamentally a medical disorder has many advantages for the patient. It can decrease stigma, result in effective and specific treatment, and minimize unwarranted family and individual responsibility for the emergence of the illness. At the same time, however, it can discourage discussion of significant life issues and problems involved in adjusting to the illness and its consequences. An overly medical approach can also mean that psychological concerns about taking medication may be ignored. Furthermore, taking medication can create its own stigma because society and patients themselves often disparage the continuing need for psychiatric drugs.

Biological assumptions about the illness can also make it more difficult for patients to feel a sense of personal control.

Many, for example, maintain the belief that if only they changed their work, exercise, or dietary habits; if only they conducted their love affairs in a different way; if only they heeded more stringently the counsel of their priests, therapists, and consciences—in other words, if only they behaved as they think they should—they would be able to prevent recurrences of manic and depressive episodes. When treatment with mood stabilizers has beneficial results, some patients continue to believe that they ought to have been able to handle things without the medication. Some may attribute their improvement to a combination of their own efforts and the efficacy of the medication. Others believe the medication alone made the difference, and they had little or no control over the illness. Psychotherapy can help clarify the ambivalence that inevitably results from such beliefs, underscore the patient's role in the medication regimen, and identify psychological issues that are important and amenable to the patient's control. There is also evidence that psychotherapy can help the patient change irregular sleep habits and deal with family conflicts, as well as teach the patient to monitor mood, cognitive, behavioral, and sleep changes for incipient relapses or recurrences.

Disappointment and Frustration

Expecting the treatment of bipolar illness to proceed in a straightforward manner is likely to create problems. For many patients, mood stabilizers are an uncertain treatment imposed upon an uncertain illness, a problematic treatment for a problematic disease. For many, life before medication can be likened to a kite on a string in exceedingly unpredictable winds. Mood stabilizers allow some control over the winds, but often it is not complete, and therein lies much of the disappointment and frustration. Clinicians and patients frequently define successful control very differently. The clinician looks at certain types of evidence—fewer or no hospitalizations or little or no need for adjunctive mood stabilizers, antipsychotics, and antidepressants—and finds drugs to be effective. The patient who continues to experience disruptive and upsetting mood swings is likely to interpret the same evidence in much more equivocal terms. In essence, physicians focus more often on the successes of medication, that is, the contrasts with untreated illness. Patients, while living with those successes, live with the failures and disappointments of medication as well. The improvements achieved tend to be forgotten, and with time, the seriousness of the illness is denied. Day-to-day discontents then emerge as the compelling factor in feelings about medication. In the words of one P. G. Wodehouse character (Wodehouse, 1975), "I could see that, if not actually disgruntled, he was far from being gruntled." Bipolar patients on medication are often far from being gruntled.

The resentment patients feel at their partial cure is, in some respects, proportional to the severity of the illness and concomitant hope. Unrealistic expectations of medications and of physicians not only derive from the fragile hopes of patients, but also are rooted in the exaggerated claims of some pharmaceutical manufacturers and physicians. Paradoxically, the very existence of mood stabilizers as effective treatments has given rise to a new generation of patients with a new set of expectations. When lithium was first used in Scandinavian clinical trials, there was no alternative, and patients were generally "grateful for a treatment that revolutionized their lives" (M. Schou, personal communication). The availability and efficacy of a variety of mood stabilizers have made them a part of the pharmaceutical establishment, which in turn has created an inevitable groundswell of expanded expectations, disappointments, and criticism.

Perceived Losses Associated with Medication

The subtle and powerful clinician–patient alliance that is possible in pharmacotherapy is predicated on a thorough understanding of not only the benefits of the medications to the patient, but also the realistic and unrealistic fantasies of loss that many patients experience during treatment. These fantasies often focus on missing the highs of bipolar illness and cannot be adequately understood through the simplistic view that the patient is shortsighted, self-destructive, or escapist. Effective therapy with bipolar patients—whether it involves using drugs alone or in combination with psychotherapy—must address the reality of the patient's positive perceptions of the illness, as well as the altered states of perception induced by its occasional elevated-mood, high-energy phases (Jamison et al., 1979, 1980).

Patients may experience many different kinds of losses, realistic and otherwise, as a result of taking a mood stabilizer. These losses and their relationship to medication nonadherence are discussed in detail in Chapter 21. Here we present an overview of the psychotherapeutic issues involved.

Realistic losses are those undesirable changes brought about by medication. They can include decreased energy level, loss of euphoric states, increased need for sleep, decreased productivity and creativity, less interpersonal verve, and diminished sexuality. One patient described the subtle effects of lithium thus:

> People expect that you will welcome being "normal," be appreciative of lithium, doctors, and modern science, and take in stride having normal energy and sleep. But if you are used to sleeping only 5 hours a night and now sleep 8, are used to staying up all night for days and weeks in

a row and now cannot, it is a very real adjustment to blend into a formal schedule which, while comfortable to many, is new, restrictive, seemingly less productive, and for sure less fun. People say, when I complain of being less lively, less energetic, "Well, now you're just like the rest of us," meaning, among other things, to be reassuring. What they don't realize is that I compare myself with my former self, not with others. Not only that, I always compare my current self with the best I have been, which is when I have been hypomanic. When I am my present "normal" self, I am far removed from when I have been my liveliest, most productive, most intense, most outgoing and effervescent. In short, for myself, I am a hard act to follow. (Patient with manic-depressive illness[1])

The results of a study of bipolar patients in remission suggest that many patients feel their illness makes positive contributions to their lives in one or more important ways (Jamison et al., 1980). A substantial majority of the patients in this study perceived pronounced short- and long-term positive effects from their bipolar illness in addition to whatever disabling and dysphoric symptoms they may have experienced. Most patients reported increased sensitivity, sexual intensity, productivity, creativity, and social ease. Men and women varied considerably in what they regarded as the most enjoyable and important changes when hypomanic: for men it was increased social ease, whereas for women, increases in sexual intensity, productivity, and social ease were rated equally important.

In a recent, related study, Culver and colleagues at Stanford (2006) assessed benefit finding in 57 euthymic bipolar patients (42 percent bipolar-I, 46 percent bipolar-II, 12 percent bipolar–not otherwise specified [NOS]). They found that these patients commonly identified benefits associated with their affective illness; most frequently, they endorsed the beliefs that bipolar illness "made me more understanding of others who have problems"; "increased my self-awareness"; "helped me become a stronger person, more able to cope effectively with future life challenges"; "led me to be more accepting of things"; "taught me how to adjust to things I cannot change"; and "led me to want to help others." Benefit finding correlated significantly with the more effective use of coping skills.

Such attributions are important for several reasons. From a behavioral perspective, it is essential to realize the meaning, nature, and value of positive behavioral and mood changes (as well as negative ones) for an individual patient. Such euphoric states serve for some patients as powerful addictive states, providing significant benefits on the one hand and posing the risk of severe emotional and pragmatic problems on the other. The sense of loss that occurs when medication eliminates those states, if unaddressed,

may hinder the patient's adjustment to treatment. Moreover, the side effects of a medication can be difficult to separate from the medication's effect on hypomanic symptoms; they are also sometimes indistinguishable from symptoms of inadequately treated depressive episodes.

Treatment management under such circumstances is not straightforward. For example, adherence to a mood stabilizer regimen, which at best has a tenuous and delayed relationship to alleviation of the dysphoric features of bipolar illness, competes with behavior maintained by a highly positive and intermittent reinforcement schedule—an exceedingly difficult behavior pattern to modify. It is in some ways analogous to a drug self-administration paradigm in which a highly pleasurable and relatively rapid state can be obtained. For some patients, hypomania or even mania itself may represent, in effect, an endogenous stimulant addiction. Clinical experience suggests that patients may attempt to induce mania by discontinuing medication not just when they are depressed, but also when they face problematic decisions and life events. Because the negative consequences of such behavior are delayed, it is not always clear to the patient that the benefits of medication outweigh its costs. Thus the clinician must be aware of the positive features of mood swings to better understand and thereby treat the bipolar patient.

Other realistic losses include cognitive, perceptual, physical, emotional, or social changes that result from the side effects of medications, as well as negative social consequences, such as self-labeling or social stigma (Jamison, 2006). Among the more significant side effects from a psychotherapeutic point of view, described further in Chapters 20 and 21, are those detailed in early papers by Schou and Baastrup (1973) and Schou (1980): decreased energy, enthusiasm, and sexuality (all of which can be a factor in increased marital problems); curbing of activities; and the common perception that life is flatter and less colorful. Cognitive dulling and weight gain are also important—indeed, more important to many patients (Gitlin et al., 1989; Perlick et al., 2004). Moreover, the need to adhere to a regimented lifestyle, underscored by frequent monitoring of medical and psychiatric status, may trigger the patient's feelings of being controlled and hopeless (Jamison, 1995; McAlpin and Goodnick, 1998).

Unrealistic losses include circumstances in which medication and psychotherapy come to symbolize the patient's personal failures. In addition to experiencing the normal difficulties of adjusting to the need for treatment, patients occasionally project their other life failures, thwarted ambitions, and personal and professional inadequacies onto medication, which can thereby become the psychological scapegoat and represent a rationalization for other failures that predate the onset of the illness.

Fears of Recurrence

The worst fear for most bipolar patients is recurrence of the illness. Many patients maintain a deep and fatalistic pessimism, however entwined with denial and optimism, about again becoming manic or depressed. In a poem from *Day by Day*, Robert Lowell (1977, p. 31) wrote, "if we see a light at the end of the tunnel, / it's the light of an oncoming train." This is a sentiment to which many of Lowell's fellow sufferers can relate only too well. Some patients become preoccupied with such fears of recurrence and are almost illness-phobic. They become unduly self-protective and hyperalert for signs of an impending episode. These concerns are often reflected in the process of learning to differentiate normal from abnormal moods and states (see the later discussion). A perceived decreasing tolerance for affective episodes is a concern that is usually secondary to the stress of the illness and to the large amount of psychological energy consumed by earlier bouts. Patients, often with good cause, fear that their families and friends will grow ever more intolerant with each new recurrence. Bipolar illness also takes a severe toll on other relationships, professional activities, finances, and patients' ability to handle the emotional stress of their affective episodes. Thus Lowell wrote, "but the breakage can go on repeating once too often" (1977, p. 113). Likewise, in his autobiography, Joshua Logan (1976, p. 338) described a certain weariness after yet another manic attack: "I was only forty-five years old, but I felt exhausted by this last experience, hollowed out, as though I were a live fish disemboweled."

Learning to Discriminate Moods

Problems with learning to discriminate normal from abnormal moods are common throughout the psychotherapy of bipolar patients. Because of the experience of their illness and the intensity of their emotional responses, many patients fear that a normal depressive reaction will deepen into a major episode and that a state of well-being will escalate into hypomania or mania. Many common emotions range across several mood states, spanning euthymia, depression, and hypomania. For example, irritability and anger can be a part of normal human existence, or can be symptoms of both depression and mania. Tiredness, sadness, and lethargy can be due to normal circumstances, medical causes, or clinical depression. Feeling good, being productive and enthusiastic, and working hard can be either normal or pathognomonic of hypomania.[6] These overlapping emotions can be confusing and arouse anxiety in many patients, who may then question their own judgment and, as discussed previously, become unduly concerned about recurrences of their affective illness. Occasionally, patients become conservative or excessively conforming (Benson, 1976).

The need to help patients discriminate normal from abnormal affect is common in psychotherapy. Patients must learn to live within a narrower range of emotions, yet master the skill of using those emotions with greater subtlety and discretion. Closely related to the discrimination of moods is the slow, steady process involved in patients' learning to disentangle what is normal personality from what the illness has superimposed upon it—turbulence, impulsiveness, lack of predictability, and depression. Patients whose premorbid temperament has been predominantly depressive may have unrealistic expectations about how much change can be brought about by medication. Likewise, those with an underlying exuberant temperament may have to become more finely tuned to discerning normal from pathological enthusiasms (Jamison, 2004).

Dealing with Developmental Tasks

Developmental tasks previously overshadowed by bipolar illness often become issues for patients in remission. Ironically, the illness can act as a protection against many of the slings and arrows of fortune encountered in normal life. Because late adolescence and early adulthood are the highest-risk periods for the onset of the illness, many of the developmental tasks of these periods—separation from parents and family, development of close personal relationships, romantic involvements, hurts and rejections, childbearing and childrearing, and career development—are impaired or postponed. (Conversely, these developmental transitions or crises can also precipitate the occurrence of episodes.) Once the illness is under control, patients often must deal with these problems, as well as those of a more general, existential nature, within the therapeutic relationship.

Concerns about Family and Other Relationships

Concerns about the effects of bipolar illness on family and other relationships can be profound. Patients report feeling guilty about things done while manic and those left undone while depressed. The most frequently voiced concerns center on the interpersonal consequences of the illness, effects felt strongly by family members, spouses, and friends. Unmarried patients are often unclear about when and what to tell people they are dating about their illness. Similar concerns arise in relationships with employers and coworkers. Psychotherapy can help encourage patients to suspend major personal decisions during episodes and to manage family and work crises associated with the illness. Interpersonal aspects of bipolar illness are covered more fully in Chapter 10.

Concerns about Genetics

Many patients worry about possible transmission of bipolar disorder to their children. They tend to overidentify with any close family member who has the illness, particularly a parent. Occasionally, they feel guilty about receiving effective treatments that were not available to an afflicted parent. This latter phenomenon, although not common, is particularly striking in those patients whose parents committed suicide or were hospitalized for a long time. Similar guilt is sometimes seen in patients successfully treated with medication whose siblings or parents have refused treatment.

Recent advances in locating specific genetic variations involved in bipolar illness (see Chapter 13) are likely to increase such concerns, as well as the desire for information. Indeed, study results indicate a strong desire for counseling about prenatal susceptibility (Smith et al., 1996; Trippitelli et al., 1998; Jones et al., 2002). Trippitelli and colleagues (1998) at Johns Hopkins studied knowledge and attitudes among 90 bipolar patients and their spouses with regard to the possibility of inheriting bipolar disorder, genetic testing, and decisions about childbearing. Most said they would agree to take a test for bipolar disorder if it were available, but that knowing they or their spouse had a gene or genes for bipolar illness would not change their decision to marry or to have children. Most also said they would not consider abortion if they discovered the fetus had the gene(s) for bipolar disorder. In research conducted at the University of California, San Francisco (Smith et al., 1996), both bipolar patients and psychiatry residents stated that they would be much more likely to consider terminating a pregnancy if the fetus's bipolar illness were hypothesized to have a severe clinical course than if it were not; the residents were more likely to endorse abortion. As of this writing, these issues are still academic. As more precise information on the genetic etiology and risk of bipolar disorder emerges, such concerns will become more prominent in the psychotherapeutic management of the illness. Issues associated with genetic counseling for bipolar patients are discussed in Chapter 13.

Clinician Attitudes and Expectations

As noted earlier, many psychoanalysts who worked in the prelithium era found it frustrating to treat bipolar patients. The psychoanalytic literature addressed countertransference issues extensively and described in some detail the anger analysts felt toward patients for their seeming inconstancy and lack of insight (or desire for insight):

> The extraverted, apparently unsubtle, manic depressive is a threat. . . . in several ways: In the first place, communicative efforts are a strain because of the lack of response. Secondly, the so-called healthy extraverted approach to reality is likely to fill the more sensitive, introspective person [the psychoanalyst] with self-doubts as to the possibility that he makes mountains out of molehills, reads meanings

> in where none were meant, and so forth. . . . Thirdly, the therapist tends to dislike this sort of person and to think of him as "shallow." And, finally, the patient's difficulty in recognizing or discussing his or another's feelings or meanings throws the therapist into a situation of helplessness, since these things are the coin in which he deals. (Cohen et al., 1954, p. 131)

English (1949, p. 126) stated succinctly what others have said at great length: "The manic-depressive rejects you because he seems to be unsure that he needs you at all."

Although many aspects of therapeutic work with bipolar patients have changed radically as a result of effective mood stabilizers, patients continue to elicit strong feelings from some therapists. One clinical team put it thus:

> . . . bipolar patients, with their alienating behavior, incessant demands, opaqueness, and difficulty in adhering to medication regimens, are generally viewed as difficult to treat, providing a therapist with a sense of unease and minimal gratification. (Davenport et al., 1979, p. 33)

Other therapists who work with bipolar patients are frustrated by the inconsistencies patients display in their behavior and attitudes toward self, therapist, therapy, and medication during different mood states. Unstable moods can result in fluctuating levels of intimacy and trust within the therapeutic relationship, both from patient to therapist and from therapist to patient. The patient who appears at a session in an angry and irritable state may produce a reaction in the therapist, whose feelings may then persist longer than the patient's fleeting mood. Or the therapist may make a suggestion at one session, find the patient feeling better at the next, and attribute the improved mood to the suggestion—only to discover the patient is depressed again at the next session. If the therapist fails to understand that fluctuating mood is not a reliable signal, but rather is intrinsic to the illness, such situations can lead to a misperception of the role of therapy.

Anger and frustration can also be engendered in the therapist when the patient rejects an effective treatment. This situation may arise when the therapist fails to comprehend what the illness means to the patient or the patient fails to understand, usually through processes of denial, the consequences of rejecting such a treatment regimen. Greenson (1967) emphasized that the therapist should have a broad and rich background for empathy. A breadth of imagination is particularly relevant and useful to the therapist dealing with manic patients, whose emotions and ideas often are not from the same experiential base as that of the therapist (see Chapter 2). In addition to having the kind of personal background advocated by Greenson, a therapist can reduce feelings of being excluded from and not understanding the patient's experience by having a solid grounding in the phenomenology of the illness.

Patients who stop their medication, or take it only fitfully and become ill again, can be an enormous source of frustration to their clinicians (see Chapter 21). The therapist often experiences anger and feelings of helplessness when the patient's denial leads to medication nonadherence and results in rehospitalization for manic or depressive episodes, suicide attempts, or exacerbation of hostile and aggressive behaviors. Even when the patient is adherent, feelings of inadequacy and failure can develop when the illness recurs (see the earlier discussion). Indeed, such feelings may be commonplace when therapists treat patients who are depressed, suicidal, or hypomanic (Fromm-Reichmann, 1949; Janowsky et al., 1970). Hypomanic and manic patients regularly show special sensitivity to vulnerabilities in the therapist, and this tuning in to the "jugular" is at the core of many therapists' acute and intense feelings of anger. Although such a pattern of interaction is most likely to occur during hypomania and mania, it is not uncommon during the depressive phase, when the patient's levels of paranoia, irritability, and hopelessness have increased. Patients under such circumstances are often exquisitely aware of feelings of frustration, annoyance, and impotence in the therapist. The anger and hopelessness a patient expresses at such times can have a significant impact on the already vulnerable therapist. Therapists, of course, must recognize their own attitudes and feelings and cope with them effectively to minimize repercussions for the patient.

Yet another potential problem with clinicians' reactions to their patients centers on misinterpretation of resistance in bipolar patients. We have already discussed such patients' difficulties in differentiating normal from pathological mood states and their fears of recurrence. Therapists occasionally assume that a patient's depression is a reaction to a particular environmental, interpersonal, or therapeutic event. The therapist's tendency to link depression to external events can be problematic. Even when depressions are not really endogenous, the patient is often frightened by the similarity between such thoughts and feelings and those experienced earlier in severe major depressive episodes. Therapists need to take a delicate approach in helping the patient differentiate various types of feelings, while at the same time recognizing when they themselves may have overlooked recurrence or to see psychological causality when little exists.

Problems can also develop when the therapist "acts out" through the patient. The therapist is in an unusual position to influence the patient by unwittingly encouraging both medication nonadherence and the behaviors linked to affective states. The special appeal of hypomania is particularly relevant here. The seductive aspects of that state are often impossible to ignore. Guilt over depriving the patient of a special state may occur when the patient proclaims that he misses the highs of the disorder. Moods are contagious, and occasionally the loss of a patient's hypomania results in a corresponding, albeit lesser, loss reaction in the therapist. A few therapists may also romanticize "madness." This romanticization can range from a tendency to overvalue the positive aspects of bipolar illness and minimize the negative, painful ones to a conviction that psychopharmacological interventions are oppressive or contraindicated. The consequences of such romanticization are usually catastrophic.

Mood Charting

Before turning to a discussion of psychotherapy, we examine the role of other components of psychological care: mood charting, patient and family education, and self-help groups. Mood charting by patients can provide invaluable information about seasonal and premenstrual patterns of moods; psychological, environmental, and biological correlates of mood swings; and response to treatment, including possible worsening of the illness (e.g., increased cycling induced by antidepressant therapy; see Chapter 19).

Administration of a visual analogue scale is straightforward, requiring little time on the part of the patient (see Chapter 13 for further discussion). The patient is given sheets of paper, each with a 100 mm line, anchored by 1 ("worst I've ever felt") on the left or the bottom and 100 ("best I've ever felt") on the right or the top. The patient is then asked to put a mark across the line at the point most representative of his overall mood (or whatever other variable, such as energy or anxiety level, is being assessed) for the day. To control for diurnal variations in mood and behavior, ratings should be recorded at approximately the same time of day or evening. Significant life events and additional medications required are noted on the rating sheet. After completion, the dated form is set aside to avoid influence from earlier ratings. The results can then be graphed, with time plotted along the horizontal axis and mood ratings, from 1 to 100, along the vertical. In some instances, patients can do their own graphing.

Two other instruments have been developed for mood charting: the retrospective Life-Chart Method (LCM-r) (Leverich and Post, 1993) and the NIMH prospective Life-Chart Method (NIMH LCM-p) (Denicoff et al., 1997). The two follow the same guidelines but differ in the unit of measure—LCM-r is monthly, whereas LCM-p is daily. For LCM-p, patients are given a computer-readable form to take home once a month, with instructions to rate their mood and functioning each day, morning and evening. Self-ratings of mood are plotted along a 100 mm line with 25 points corresponding to a continuum from most depressed ever, to balanced (middle), to most manic ever. Functional impairment is rated as none, mild, moderate, or severe.

A third method of tracking mood fluctuations as they relate to daily social and circadian rhythms is the Social Rhythm Metric (Monk et al., 1991; Frank et al., 2000). This chart, completed by the patient at the end of each day, is used to assess 17 daily activities (e.g., waking up, first communication with another person, morning beverage, afternoon nap) as to the time of the day they occurred, whether they involved other people, and how stimulating they were. This daily mood rating can help the patient understand the relationship among changes in a regular schedule, stimulation induced by daily routines, and mood fluctuations. Using the results of this charting, the therapist collaborates with the patient to find realistic ways of stabilizing these daily rhythms. This charting method has been incorporated into interpersonal psychotherapy for bipolar patients, described later.

Mood ratings can be useful not only in identifying patterns of mood and treatment response, but also in giving patients a sense of control, instilling a sense of collaboration, and underscoring the importance of systematic observation. They also provide a relatively objective basis for persuading patients when treatment regimens require modification. At the beginning of treatment, other patients' charts may be used as examples of various patterns of mood fluctuation to illustrate the use of daily mood ratings in diagnostic and treatment decisions. Figure 22–1 portrays one such pattern, in which the time course and efficacy of antidepressant medications are demonstrated in a woman with bipolar-II disorder. The essential point for the patient to note is that there is an uneven, sawtooth nature to the recovery pattern. Predicting occasional serious relapses on the way to remission is important in minimizing serious, potentially lethal discouragement in a high-risk (i.e., transitional) period. It also alerts patients to the potential danger of transitional and mixed states, which should be reported to the clinician.

Patient Education

"Am I manic-depressive?" "We don't use that term, but I would guess from the record that you are bipolar." "Which is a nice way of saying that yes, I'm manic-depressive? . . . that I'm lucky as all get-out to be a complete nut because we real bats get much more help from lithium than simple neurotics can—" "I've never heard it put just that way, but there is some truth in it." (Sloan Wilson, describing a conversation with his psychiatrist, 1976, p. 436)

Most affective disorder clinics and some practitioners routinely provide formal and informal education to patients and families through lectures, books, articles, pamphlets, discussion groups, videotapes, and ongoing communication between clinician and patient. Although this is the ideal scenario, it is not the prevailing one. Patients often express resentment at how little information they receive about bipolar illness and its treatment. Yet clinicians, in whatever setting, have an ethical and clinical obligation to engage patients in a continuing process of education, which clearly is integral to informed consent. Patients vary considerably in their ability to assimilate information about their medications and illness, and they need to participate actively in the treatment process. Too often a physician becomes a unilateral advocate of maintenance medication, and the result frequently is an adversarial rather than a collaborative relationship.

Figure 22–1. Course of recovery in a female patient with bipolar-II disorder treated with antidepressant medications.

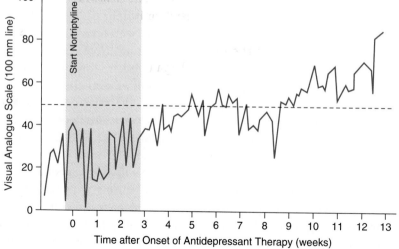

The collaborative nature of the patient–clinician relationship is central to effective treatment. Not only must patients be taught about the natural course and symptoms of bipolar illness, but they should also be actively encouraged to question their clinicians about diagnosis and treatment, to discuss their concerns about undue delays in achieving the desired results, and to seek second opinions when appropriate. If the treating physician or psychotherapist disparages second opinions or consultations, patients should be encouraged to challenge this view and obtain the consultation anyway.

In the course of patient education, the chronic and highly recurrent nature of bipolar illness should be emphasized and reemphasized to the patient. Charts illustrating the relapse rate and worsening course of the untreated illness (e.g., Fig. 22–2) and the dramatic effect of a mood stabilizer can highlight these points for patients, as well as their families (Fig. 22–3). Patients should be encouraged to read about the illness and its treatment (suggested reading is listed in the appendix to this volume), including the potential neuroprotective effects brought about by lithium and other mood stabilizers (see color plates 1–4 and Chapter 14). They should also be given specific information about their medications and potential risks and side effects. The safety and efficacy of various treatments and the risks of no treatment should be outlined. Special attention should be paid to discussing the potential dangers of antidepressant use in bipolar patients, such as induction of mania or mixed states, worsening of the natural course of the illness (i.e., shortening of the cycle length), and severe agitation (see Chapter 19). Patients prescribed lithium should be advised that sudden discontinuance may substantially increase the risk of relapse and suicide (see Chapter 25). Education and informed consent do not end with a discussion of risks and benefits and the distribution of fact sheets, however. Ongoing talks between patient and clinician are essential, perhaps supplemented with lectures and/or videotapes.

Patients need to be alerted to the symptoms of impending episodes and, with the therapist's assistance, encouraged to identify their own individual prodromal patterns. These patterns have been studied extensively.[7] Changes in sleep patterns are particularly important because they precede, exacerbate, and accompany mania, and because mania may be precipitated by sleep loss. As discussed in Chapter 16, environmental factors leading to insomnia (e.g., anxiety, excitement, grief), as well as other circumstances (e.g., hormonal changes, travel, drugs), can lead to mania through sleep deprivation. Wehr and Goodwin (1987) advised warning bipolar patients that a single night of unexplainable sleep loss should be taken as an early warning of possible impending mania. They further

suggested counseling patients to avoid situations likely to disrupt sleep and advised clinicians to consider prescribing hypnotics to prevent significant sleep loss. Factors leading to sleep reduction and their relationship to the precipitation of mania are illustrated in Figure 22–4. This illustration can be used in educating patients about the necessity of maintaining adequate levels of sleep. The importance of regularizing circadian rhythms by establishing patterns in meals, exercise, and other activities should also be stressed to patients.

Education regarding the impact of the disorder on interpersonal relations, employment, position in the community, and general health should also be provided. Patients often need guidance in dealing with the consequences of risky, illegal, or embarrassing behaviors that occur during mania, and in handling professional, family, or financial responsibilities during either depression or mania. For patients who experience significant employment difficulties as a result of the illness, the therapist can be helpful in recommending and exercising career counseling or vocational rehabilitation options.

A large amount of educational material on bipolar disorder can be found on the Internet. This material includes information on symptomatology, treatment options, support for patients and families, and referral sources; websites of discussion/advocacy groups; and reading matter. The quality of these materials varies enormously. Reliable sources include the NIMH, the Depression and Bipolar Support Alliance (DBSA; known until 2002 as the National Depressive and Manic-Depressive Association), the National Alliance on Mental Illness (NAMI), the National Foundation for Depressive Illness (NAFDI), and the National Mental Health Association (NMHA). In addition, Internet chatrooms provide bipolar patients and their families with a forum for the exchange of information and support, although some patients may find the information overwhelming and confusing. The appendix at the end of this volume includes various Internet sites and chatrooms relevant to bipolar disorder.

Finally, the ability to exercise informed consent, even for the well-educated patient, may be compromised when the patient is manic or depressed. In some states and countries, patients who know when rational and in a normal mood that they wish to have electroconvulsive therapy or be hospitalized when depressed (or manic) but that they are unlikely to consent in the midst of an episode can draw up "Odysseus" agreements (Joshi, 2003; Keefe and Pinals, 2004; Srebnik et al., 2005). Swanson and colleagues (2006) have shown that a 2-hour structured facilitation session, conducted by trained research assistants, is an effective way to help patients complete advanced directives so that they contain useful information about the patient's

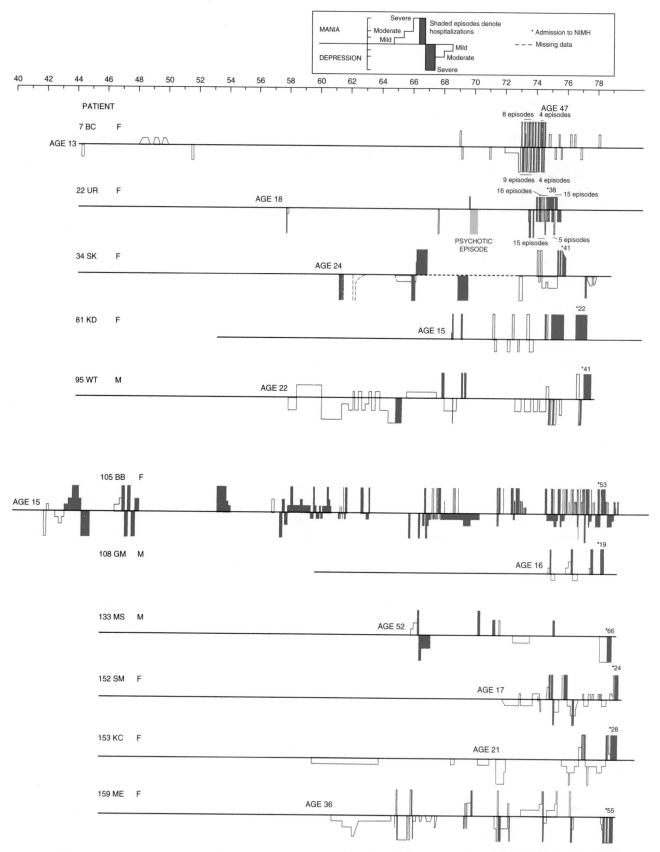

Figure 22–2. Life course of manic and depressive episodes in bipolar affective illness. Patterns of recurrent affective illness are illustrated in individual bipolar-I patients (those hospitalized for a manic episode). Manias are plotted above the line and depressions below. Hospitalizations are shaded, and dotted lines indicate uncertain or missing data. Note that most patients show a course of increased severity or frequency of affective episodes over time. NIMH = National Institute of Mental Health. (*Source*: Squillace et al., 1984.)

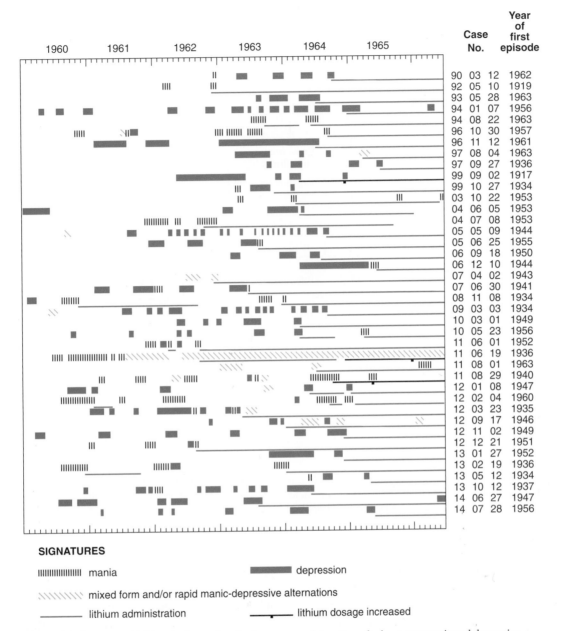

Figure 22–3. Effect of lithium in decreasing the frequency and duration of subsequent manic and depressive episodes. The patient records are arranged according to age; the first two digits of each case number indicate the year of birth. In the second column is shown the year when the first manic or depressive episode appeared. The diagram shows, for each patient, all psychotic episodes that occurred between January 1, 1960, and July 1, 1966. (*Source*: Baastrup and Schou, 1967.)

preferences for treatment. Derived from the same principle as that used by Odysseus when he sought protection from seduction by the Sirens, such agreements allow patients to consent in advance to certain treatments. General guidelines for drawing up advance directives are given in Box 22–1.

Family Education and Family Therapy

Family members and close friends often find that the educational information provided to patients is useful to them as well. Families are, of course, in a unique position to observe the behavior and moods of bipolar patients. Education about the illness can increase family members' awareness and acceptance of the patient's condition and underscore their role in encouraging the patient to take prescribed medications and live sensibly. Waiting for symptom-free intervals between episodes to discuss the meaning and nature of bipolar illness allows for education and collaborative decision making in a less emotionally charged and more cognitively astute atmosphere.

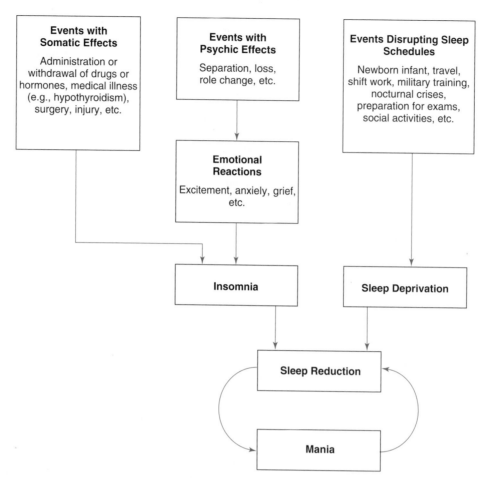

Figure 22–4. Diagram of the hypothesis of sleep reduction as the final common pathway of diverse factors thought to precipitate mania. (*Source*: Adapted from Wehr et al., 1987b. Reproduced with permission from the American Psychiatric Association.)

In addition to being educated about the illness and medications, family members should be informed about the importance of recognizing the early signs and symptoms of hypomanic, manic, and depressive episodes. Changes in sleep patterns, sexual and financial behavior, mood (expansiveness or undue enthusiasm, volatility, pessimism and hopelessness), and judgment, as well as involvement in excessive numbers of projects, are all highly characteristic of impending affective episodes. As noted earlier, such prodromes, as well as others more subtle or idiosyncratic (e.g., increased religious or political interest, avoidance of eye contact), can escape the patient's attention. These changes often are first noted by family members, who therefore can play a crucial role in early intervention, although Highet and colleagues (2005) found that many family members who care for patients with depression are able to recognize prodromal symptoms only in hindsight. In a comprehensive review of studies of early symptom identification by patients, Jackson and colleagues (2003) found that a median of 82 percent of patients could identify early symptoms of bipolar depression, such as changes in mood (48 percent) and psychomo-

tor symptoms (41 percent); prodromal sleep changes were far less easily identified (24 percent), however. The opposite was true for the prodromal symptoms of mania: the great majority of patients (77 percent) could identify sleep disturbance as an early symptom of mania, compared with 47 percent for psychomotor symptoms, 43 percent for changes in mood, and 34 percent for psychomotor changes. Overall, the prodromes of mania were of longer duration and easier to identify than those of bipolar depression.

If possible, strategies for contacting the clinician should be determined between patient and family during times when the patient is euthymic. To the extent feasible, general contingency plans and agreements should be formulated in advance to cover possible emergencies (e.g., suicidal thinking and behavior), hospitalization plans for mania or depression, and financial protection for patient and family during hypomanic and manic episodes.

The "relapse drill" is a roadmap to guide the family's plans and actions should mania or depression recur (Marlatt and Gordon, 1985; Miklowitz and Goldstein, 1997). During the drill, the therapist identifies the prodromal

BOX 22–1.   Advance Directives for Patients with Bipolar Illness

The Depression and Bipolar Support Alliance (2004) provides the following guidance on the use of advance directives:

> One way to put self-knowledge and self-advocacy into practice is to create an advance directive—a written document outlining the treatment the patient would like to receive if his illness renders him incapable of making decisions. In your advance directive, you might choose to give another person the authority to make decisions about your treatment for you.
>
> Advance directives for mental health are a relatively new development, and a few legal precedents are in place. Each U.S. state has a different set of laws governing the use and enforcement of advance directives. You may want to consult a qualified disability law attorney to be sure your advance directive is enforceable.

Using an advance directive may:
- Ease stress on you and your loved ones.
- Help you avoid treatment you know is not helpful.
- Help you get the right treatment when you need it most.

> You must be mentally competent at the time you make your advance directive. Binding advance directives are usually signed by at least one witness and one physician who can verify that you are in good mental health at the time you write it. State what treatment you want, where and by whom, and under what circumstances. Your instructions may include:

- Emergency contact information for all of your health care providers.
- Medications (and dosages) that help you.
- Medications that have unpleasant side effects or do not help you.
- Treatments, such as electroconvulsive therapy, that you do or do not wish to be given.
- The facility or hospital where you prefer to be treated.
- Family members and friends who are authorized to make decisions about your treatment according to your written preferences.
- What you would like your loved ones to do if your symptoms cause you to be a danger to yourself or others.
- Things people can say or do to calm you or convince you to accept treatment.
- Warning signs that you may be in crisis.

> You may also want to add instructions for legal professionals on how to assist you if you break the law and get arrested while you are ill.
>
> Review your advance directive with your loved ones and health care providers. Give each of them an up-to-date copy. Check your advance directive periodically to be sure it still reflects your needs.
>
> Having an advance directive does not guarantee your treatment will go smoothly. However, creating advance directives can be a beneficial addition to treatment. The entire process can be empowering. It can help you strengthen relationships with your health care providers and loved ones.

Note: This information is not meant to take the place of consultation with a qualified legal professional.

---

symptoms of mania, hypomania, and depression and helps the patient and family develop plans for contacting the treatment team, dealing with practical problems that result from the relapse (e.g., parenting, financial arrangements), handling work and social responsibilities, and deciding when hospitalization is necessary and how to proceed. Realistic plans should be made with other adults (relatives or friends) who can support the patient's family during a crisis. The therapist can also formulate a mutually acceptable plan for helping the patient adhere to a medication regimen if he or she tends to skip doses.

Potential problems involving the violation of clinician–patient confidentiality are substantial and need to be discussed openly with both patients and their families. Szmukler and Bloch (1997) recommended that clinicians consider overriding the patient's refusal to involve family members only if harm (to the patient or family members) is probable and could be serious, if no acceptable alternatives are available, if the patient's decision-making ability is impaired, or if excluding the family could result in greater restrictions on the patient's rights and freedom. Whenever possible, however, patients should be strongly encouraged to involve their families in at least the early stages of treatment. (There are, of course, obvious if infrequent exceptions to this general guideline.)

Finally, family therapy, when indicated, can be a useful adjunct to treatment. Many issues arise in treating families with one or more members who suffer from bipolar illness (see Chapter 10). Specific studies involving family interventions are reviewed later in this chapter.

National and Local Support Associations

Both bipolar patients and their families can participate in excellent self-help groups, many of which operate under the auspices of DBSA. There are now approximately 1,000 such groups in the United States. The stated purpose of DBSA is "to provide personal support and direct service to persons with clinical depression or manic depression and their families; to educate the public concerning the nature and management of these treatable medical disorders; and to promote related research." The importance of educating both the public and health professionals about early symptoms of bipolar disorder is underlined by DBSA's survey of members, in which half of bipolar respondents reported not having received any treatment during the first 5 years after the onset of symptoms (Lish et al., 1994).

Services provided by chapters of DBSA and other advocacy and support organizations, such as NAMI, include educational programs for patients, their family members, and the general public; self-help support groups for patients and families; determination of medication levels; Alcoholics Anonymous meetings; telephone hotlines for emergencies; newsletters; summaries of relevant research findings; employment counseling; and referrals to clinicians with expertise in treating bipolar and depressive illness. DBSA and NAMI work in collaboration, not in competition, with clinicians.

A survey of 2,049 members of DBSA support groups in 190 U.S. cities was conducted in three waves between 1997 and 1998. Among the survey respondents, 59 percent reported having bipolar disorder. The substantial majority (71 percent) of these respondents reported that psychotherapy was an essential part of their treatment. So, too, was participation in support groups. More than half (58 percent) of those who had experienced difficulty in adhering to treatment reported a significant improvement in adherence between the initial and follow-up surveys. The longer the patient had attended a support group, the lower was the chance of discontinuing medication against medical advice. Even those who had attended a DBSA group for less than a year reported a significant reduction in barriers to adherence (e.g., "problems in relationship with the doctor," "missing medication doses"). In addition, respondents who had attended a group for longer than a year reported significantly lower hospitalization rates. Although there is no clear cause–effect relationship between group attendance and better outcomes (members with more severe symptoms or functional impairment may be more likely to drop out of the groups), members cited the support, education, and advocacy of DBSA groups as important factors in dealing successfully with bipolar disorder and depression (Goodale and Lewis, 1999).

Although most major cities now have a branch of DBSA or a similar organization, 57 percent of respondents to a 1997–1998 survey of DBSA members reported not learning of the group's existence until more than a year after their diagnosis (Goodale and Lewis, 1999). Patients and their families should be encouraged to seek support from their local DBSA, NAMI, or other such group. If there is no local branch of DBSA or NAMI, the organizations' national offices can be contacted for information about the nearest group (contact information is given in the appendix to this volume).

REVIEW OF THE LITERATURE

We have emphasized our belief that psychotherapy is important, often essential, in the treatment of bipolar illness, and have discussed a number of issues that can complicate overall clinical management and are the targets of such therapy. Until recently, however, scientific data from controlled clinical trials on the efficacy of psychotherapy in treating bipolar illness were nearly nonexistent.

At one time, the diversity of psychotherapeutic approaches discouraged research on psychotherapy for any disorder. Each psychotherapist was considered impenetrably unique, as was each patient, and there was little way to know what the therapist was actually doing in the office with a given patient. Psychotherapy was regarded as an art form that could not be addressed by science.

Over the past two decades, that view has changed. Methods have been developed or adapted for the testing of psychotherapeutic approaches, including the use of clinical trials, random assignment, and outcome measures that tap the areas of change one might expect as a result of psychotherapy. Most important among these new tools have been psychotherapy manuals that outline accepted procedures, provide technical specifications with scripts for intervention, and offer guidelines on what should be covered during treatment (Hibbs et al., 1997; Weissman et al., 2000). Such manuals can make psychotherapy a relatively uniform and therefore testable treatment. Audiotaping or videotaping of ongoing psychotherapy sessions provides an objective record of adherence to and delivery of the treatment set forth in a manual, and has been incorporated into numerous trials of psychotherapy for major depression and other disorders. Although bipolar patients have usually been excluded from these trials, possibly because medication has been viewed as the fundamental treatment for the disorder, this situation has begun to change.

The new psychotherapeutic approaches now being tested for treatment of bipolar disorder are different from the open-ended psychoanalytic approaches of the 1940s and 1950s, which focused on early-childhood experiences, transference, and dreams. Modern approaches are designed to be used as adjuncts to medication. They include attention to making a precise diagnosis; a psychoeducation component, with emphasis on medication adherence; monitoring of symptoms through symptom checklists; a focus on current problems; regulation of daily routine through life charts; and efforts to improve current relationships to prevent relapse and build ways of coping with the consequences of the illness in work and family contexts. Bipolar disorder is viewed not as a character flaw, but as a chronic illness that requires varying levels of intervention over a lifetime. The norm is to employ psychotherapy as needed, rather than as an intensive treatment over many years. The family is an important ally, not an adversary, in the treatment. The emphasis is on the transactions between patients and their significant others, rather than the relationship between patient and therapist. The goal is not only gaining insight, but also learning to cope with having a chronic, usually devastating, and potentially lethal illness.

Not all of the new approaches have all these features. For example, some focus only on education, whereas others emphasize interpersonal and family relationships and use group or family modalities. The more comprehensive treatments—cognitive-behavioral therapy (CBT), interpersonal and social rhythm therapy (IPSRT), family-focused treatment (FFT), and the Life Goals Program—emphasize the achievement of functional goals through skills training and reduction of interpersonal conflict with significant others. These approaches include protocols for relapse prevention (the action plans in CBT and the Life Goals Program, the symptom monitoring and management plan for IPSRT, the relapse drill for FFT).

The new psychotherapeutic approaches appear to be consistent with the clinical reality of bipolar disorder. Whether they make a difference in altering patterns of relapse, however, cannot be known without further results from controlled clinical trials.

Tables 22–1 through 22–5 provide details of the interventions, study designs, results, and clinical observations of the clinical trials of various psychotherapeutic approaches conducted or ongoing as of this writing. It is obvious from these summaries that the samples have been relatively small, that many studies need to be replicated, and that only a few modalities have been tested. Tables 22–1 through 22–4 describe efficacy studies, and Table 22–5 ongoing effectiveness studies. The latter studies are designed to test psychotherapy in actual clinical practice among large, heterogeneous samples of bipolar patients. Such studies were recently initiated to compensate for the paucity of data on the psychotherapeutic management of bipolar illness. The following subsections review the most salient features and findings of studies addressing psychoeducation, CBT, IPSRT, and family/couples therapy (including FFT), as well as ongoing effectiveness studies.

Psychoeducation

Psychoeducation for bipolar disorder focuses on education about the illness, including symptoms (prodromal and during the episode), treatment options, and the importance of sleep regulation and adherence to medication. An essential component of almost every new psychotherapy for bipolar disorder, it has also been tested as a specific method. Its purpose is to encourage the active and informed involvement of patient and family in the treatment process, following an "alliance, not adherence" philosophy (Frank et al., 1995; Toprac et al., 2000; Berk et al., 2004). In a recent survey, 500 British and American psychiatrists cited the education of patients as one of their most important clinical priorities (Roy and Williams, 2005). A Brazilian study of 106 bipolar patients found that level of knowledge about treatment, in this case lithium, was directly related to treatment adherence (Rosa et al., in press).

Psychoeducation deals with two of the most predominant problems in the management of bipolar disorder: nonadherence to medication and relapse despite adherence. Nearly one-half of patients with bipolar illness fail to adhere to their treatment (see Chapter 21); however, even highly adherent patients can suffer relapses (Keck et al., 1998). As discussed earlier, psychoeducation can help prevent relapses by teaching patients to recognize prodromal signs and symptoms and notify their treatment team and relatives. A summary of the results of studies examining the effect of psychoeducation and psychotherapy on medication adherence is presented in Table 21–5 in Chapter 21.

Various approaches to psychoeducation were employed in the studies listed in Table 22–1, including lectures; videotapes; group discussion; and fact sheets on symptoms, their management, and medication. Sometimes only the patient was included and sometimes key relatives, in individual or group settings. The length of the intervention varied from 2 to 6 weeks; all of the studies included follow-up at periods of 3 to 18 months. Outcomes ranged from improving knowledge and understanding and medication adherence to reducing rates of relapse. (Clinical trials of psychoeducation using CBT techniques are included in Table 22–2 and discussed in that section.)

In general, the results of these studies were modest. Some demonstrated significantly increased knowledge about the illness. Results varied regarding improvement in adherence to medication, and in some cases revealed improvement in relatives' attitudes. The one study that assessed impact on clinical status found no effect of brief psychoeducation on relapse rate.

The most comprehensive psychoeducation program, the Patient and Family Education Program, was developed by the Texas Medication Algorithm Project (Toprac et al., 1998, 2000). The aim was to develop medication algorithms for the treatment of individuals with bipolar disorder, depression, or schizophrenia and to test the clinical and cost-effectiveness of these algorithm-driven treatments

TABLE 22–1. Clinical Trials of Brief Psychoeducation in the Treatment of Bipolar Patients

Study	Intervention	Study Design	Results	Clinical Observations
Haas et al., 1988	Inpatient family psychoeducation to increase acceptance and knowledge of BP in families (average 6 weekly sessions).	Families of BP patients randomized to psychoeducation plus standard hospital care ($n = 12$) or standard inpatient care alone ($n = 8$). Follow-up at 6 and 18 mo.	At 6 and 18 mo, female patients with BP who received the treatment had significantly better role functioning than female BP patients in the control group.	Family attitudes toward treatment improved in the psychoeducation group compared with the controls.
Peet and Harvey, 1991	Group psychoeducation involving a videotaped lecture on lithium action and side effects, followed by a home visit (2 sessions).	BP patients in remission randomly assigned to group psychoeducation ($n = 30$) or a wait-list control group ($n = 30$). Follow-up at 6 mo. Blood levels and tablet omission monitored to determine adherence.	At termination and follow-up, knowledge about lithium had increased significantly in the psychoeducation group. Improvement in medication adherence was significantly associated with improvement in knowledge about lithium.	Even short video psychoeducation increased knowledge about and adherence to lithium. Clinical status not assessed.
Van Gent and Zwart, 1991	Group psychoeducation with partners of BP patients (5 sessions). Focus on symptoms of the disorder, functioning, medication action, side effects, and hereditary factors.	Partners of BP outpatients randomly assigned to psychoeducation ($n = 14$) or no intervention ($n = 12$). Follow-up at 6 mo (partners) or 12 mo (patients).	Partners' knowledge about the illness, mood stabilizers, and coping strategies had increased significantly at termination and 6 mo. No difference in medication adherence was seen at 12 mo.	Clinical status not assessed.

Honig et al., 1997	Multifamily group psychoeducation (6 biweekly sessions). Focus on symptoms of BP, coping strategies, patient support and advocacy.	BP patient and a key relative assigned on a first-come, first-served basis to the psychoeducation group (n=29) or a wait-list control group (n=23). Follow-up at 3 mo.	No significant difference in relapse and medication adherence was observed in the two groups. Significantly more relatives in the psychoeducation group changed from high to low expressed emotion.	Even a brief intervention can result in changes in levels of expressed emotion in families.
Suppes et al., 2000	Psychoeducation as part of patient care in the Texas Medication Algorithm Project for BP, depressive, and schizophrenic patients.	Outpatient (n=44) and inpatient (n=25) BP patients received psychoeducation and algorithm-driven treatment. A large controlled trial is under way.	Both inpatient and outpatient groups experienced significant symptom improvement. Improvement in social functioning was significant for the inpatient group.	
Miller et al., 2004	Multifamily psychoeducational group therapy (6 sessions) or family therapy (average of 12 sessions), plus standardized pharmacotherapy.	BP-I patients randomly assigned to pharmacotherapy alone (n=29), family therapy plus pharmacotherapy (n=33), or group therapy plus pharmacotherapy (n=30).	No differences were found among groups in rates of recovery or time to recovery.	No measures of psychosocial functioning or recurrence of illness were used. The study involved a relatively small number of therapy sessions. The patient population may have been particularly refractory.

Note: Clinical trials of psychoeducation using cognitive-behavioral therapy are reviewed in Table 22–2. BP=bipolar disorder.

TABLE 22–2. Clinical Trials of Cognitive-Behavioral Therapy for Patients with Bipolar Disorder

Study	Intervention	Study Design	Results	Clinical Observations
Cochran, 1984	Individual CBT for BP outpatients to enhance medication adherence compared with standard clinic care (6 weekly sessions). Targeted cognition and behavior that affect adherence based on Beck's model.	BP patients randomized to CBT ($n=14$) or standard clinical care ($n=14$). Follow-up at 3 and 6 mo.	The CBT group showed significantly greater adherence to medication at baseline and 6 mo follow-up (but not at 3 mo follow-up). Physician and independent evaluator reports showed improved adherence, whereas self- and informant reports did not. Although the two groups did not differ significantly in affective episodes, the CBT group had significantly fewer hospitalizations.	A brief intervention appeared to improve adherence to medication. The positive results disappeared at the 3 mo follow-up and reappeared at 6 mo, indicating the importance of long-term follow-up.
Hirschfeld-Becker et al., 1998	Group CBT (11 weekly sessions). Treatment included psychoeducation, cognitive approaches to depressive and manic behavior, preventive mood hygiene, medication adherence, problem solving around suicidality, and stress and conflict management.	BP patients randomly assigned to group CBT and medication ($n=15$) or medication only ($n=15$). Follow-up at 3 mo.	The CBT group had significantly longer periods of euthymia and significantly fewer new episodes than controls at both termination and follow-up.	A longer follow-up and a larger number of patients are needed to determine long-term efficacy.
Perry et al., 1999	Individual CBT psychoeducation for relapse prevention (7–12 sessions). Focus on early identification of relapse symptoms and a plan for seeking treatment.	BP patients with a history of relapse in the previous year but euthymic at baseline randomly assigned to psychoeducation combined with treatment as usual (TAU) ($n=34$) or TAU only ($n=35$). Follow-up at 6, 12, and 18 mo.	The psychoeducation group had significantly fewer manic relapses over 18 mo but no difference in the number of depressive relapses (in fact, the number slightly increased). Social functioning improved significantly. Adherence to mood stabilizers as indicated by blood levels did not differ.	This relatively short intervention resulted in a significant reduction of manic but not depressive episodes over a long follow-up period (18 mo).
Weiss et al., 2000	Group CBT for relapse prevention (12 or 20 weekly sessions) for patients with comorbid bipolar and substance-abuse disorders.	Euthymic BP (-I and -II) patients with substance abuse dependence within the past 30 days and taking a mood stabilizer enrolled in	The CBT group had significantly lower Addiction Severity Index scores and more months of abstinence from	Age was nonrandomly distributed. After controlling for age differences, reduction of mania symptoms in the

	Intervention	Method	Results	Comments
	In addition to psychoeducation and support, groups focused on identifying and coping with triggers, recognizing prodromal symptoms, and dealing with setbacks.	sequential blocks: BP patients ($n=21$) in group CBT in addition to any other psychosocial treatment compared with BP patients ($n=24$) who received assessment only. Both groups were assessed for mood, substance abuse, and medication adherence before, during, and after treatment monthly. Follow-up at 3 mo.	both drugs and alcohol. No significant differences in mood episodes or hospitalizations were seen.	CBT group no longer reached significance. At baseline, the therapy group had significantly more severe alcohol problems than controls, making results difficult to interpret. This is the only psychotherapy thus far for comorbid bipolar and substance-abuse disorders.
Lam et al., 2000	Individual CBT for relapse prevention (12 to 20 weekly sessions over 6 mo). Psychoeducation, CBT skills for coping with prodromal and residual symptoms. Emphasis on the importance of routine and sleep regulation.	Euthymic BP-I patients taking regular prophylatic medication with a history of recurrence. Random assignment to CBT plus TAU ($n=13$) or TAU only ($n=12$). Monthly mood and medication adherence ratings. Follow-up at 6 mo.	The CBT group had significantly fewer hypomanic episodes and a lower total number of episodes than the control group at follow-up. They also showed significantly fewer fluctuations in symptoms and higher medication adherence at termination and follow-up. They were significantly less depressed and hopeless at follow-up and showed significantly better social functioning and self-control behavior. Significantly fewer neuroleptics were prescribed in the CBT group.	Raters were not blinded to patients' status. CBT showed the best results at the end of follow-up, suggesting gains even after therapy had been completed.
Scott et al., 2001	Individual CBT (25 weekly sessions) focused on managing symptoms, altering dysfunctional thoughts and attitudes, managing barriers to adherence, and preventing relapses.	BP outpatients randomly assigned to CBT ($n=21$) or a 6 mo wait-list control group ($n=21$), followed by CBT. Medication prescribed by the preexisting treating physician. Follow-up at 6 and 12 mo.	The CBT group showed significant reductions in symptomatology and functioning at termination and follow-up (with a non-significant trend toward symptom increase at follow-up). Depressive symptoms were significantly reduced, and there was a trend toward fewer manic symptoms (self-rated manic	The authors suggest the need for a more extensive course of maintenance given the slight deterioration in symptomatology after termination.

(continued)

TABLE 22–2. Clinical Trials of Cognitive-Behavioral Therapy for Patients with Bipolar Disorder (continued)

Study	Intervention	Study Design	Results	Clinical Observations
			activation was significantly reduced). Hospitalization rates were also significantly reduced in the CBT group.	
Colom et al., 2003a	Group CBT psychoeducation for relapse prevention (21 sessions, 8–12 BP patients in each group). Focus on illness awareness, early identification of relapse symptoms, treatment adherence, and a plan for seeking treatment.	Euthymic BP (-I and -II) patients randomly assigned to psychoeducation group combined with medication ($n=60$) or unstructured group combined with medication ($n=60$). Follow-up every 2 mo up to 28 mo.	The psychoeducation group had significantly fewer manic, hypomanic, and depressive relapses, as well as fewer and shorter hospitalizations, relative to the control group at termination and follow-up.	This is the only psychoeducation clinical trial that resulted in a significant reduction of manic as well as depressive relapses over a long follow-up period (28 mo).
Colom et al., 2003b	Group CBT psychoeducation for relapse prevention in adherent patients using the same treatment program as above.	Euthymic BP-I patients, adherent to medication, randomly assigned to psychoeducation combined with TAU ($n=25$) or TAU only ($n=25$). Follow-up every month up to 28 mo.	The psychoeducation group had significantly fewer overall recurrences and depressive episodes than the control group at termination and follow-up.	Because the patients were already adherent to medication, the positive results of psychoeducation seen in this study suggest that its therapeutic mechanisms extend beyond adherence enhancement.
Lam et al., 2003	Individual cognitive therapy (12–18 sessions during first 6 mo, 2 booster sessions during second 6 mo). Focus on preventing relapse, promoting social functioning, and monitoring mood and illness prodromes.	BP patients randomly assigned to cognitive therapy plus mood stabilizer ($n=51$) or control group ($n=52$), which received mood stabilizer plus regular psychiatric care. Monthly follow-up for 12 mo.	The cognitive therapy group had significantly fewer bipolar episodes, hospitalizations, and days affectively ill. They coped better with manic prodromes at 12 mo, and their medication adherence was better, although not significantly so.	It was more difficult to teach patients to monitor depressive than manic prodromes. There was no assessment of sleep routines or control for medication prescribed.
Lam et al., 2005b	18 mo follow-up of Lam et al. (2003) study.	Continuation of Lam et al. (2003) study design.	Over 30 mo, the cognitive therapy group had significantly better outcomes in terms of time to relapse. The effect of relapse prevention was seen primarily in the first year. Medication adherence was significantly higher in the cognitive therapy group.	The cognitive therapy group spent 110 fewer days in bipolar episodes (out of a total of 900 possible days) over the entire 30 mo and 54 fewer days (out of 450 possible days) for the last 8 mo. Booster sessions or maintenance therapy may be a helpful addition to treatment programs.

Ball et al., 2006	Individual cognitive therapy sessions (18–20) focusing on education, identification of early warning signs, establishment of stable routines, identification and modification of cognitions, and expression of emotions.	BP patients randomly allocated to a 6 mo trial of cognitive therapy plus mood-stabilizing medications ($n=25$) or medication TAU ($n=27$).	The cognitive therapy group had less severe depression scores, less dysfunctional attitudes, and a trend toward a longer time to depressive relapse. At 12 mo follow-up, the cognitive therapy group showed a trend toward lower mania scores and improved behavior control.	The study was the first to use emotive techniques systematically. The sample size was small, and the number of dependent variables was large. A single therapist administered the cognitive therapy, and there was poor adherence with blood testing in both groups. There was no significant difference between the groups in self-reported medication adherence. Clinical benefits diminished after the cognitive therapy was completed, suggesting that maintenance treatment or booster sessions may be advisable.
Scott et al., 2006	20 sessions of CBT, weekly until week 15 and then in reduced frequency until week 26. Two booster sessions offered (at weeks 32 and 38).	BP patients randomly assigned to CBT plus TAU ($n=127$) or TAU (medication plus occasional clinical contact) ($n=126$). Patients assessed every 8 weeks for 18 mo.	No significant differences between groups were observed in recurrence rates or medication adherence. CBT appeared to be more effective in those with a history of fewer episodes.	Interpretation of the findings is problematic because of heterogeneity of the patient population: 32% were in acute episodes, the remainder euthymic; 31% had a history of 6 or fewer episodes, 25% a history of 30 or more. Many (40%) of the CBT patients did not receive the entire treatment sequence; 16% of patients in both groups were not taking mood stabilizers.

CBT = cognitive-behavioral therapy; BP = bipolar disorder.

TABLE 22–3. Clinical Trials of Interpersonal and Social Rhythm Therapy for Patients with Bipolar Disorder

Study	Intervention	Study Design	Results	Clinical Observations
Frank, et al., 1999; Frank, 2000	Individual IPSRT plus behavioral strategies to help regulate patients' daily routines. Administered weekly in the acute phase until stabilization, biweekly for 12 wk during the preventive phase, monthly for 2 yr. Frequency increased in case of a new episode.	BP patients, acutely ill, randomly assigned to medication plus IPSRT (n=45) or medication plus clinical status and symptom review treatment (CSSRT), matching the frequency of IPSRT and including psychoeducation and treatment adherence training (n=45). After stabilization, patients were reassigned to either IPSRT or CSSRT for the preventive phase.	Preliminary results: patients in the IPSRT group had significantly more regular routines than those in the comparison condition. There was no significant difference in recovery time from manic and depressive episodes between the two conditions. IPSRT was associated with significantly longer periods of euthymia than the comparison condition. No such difference was found for manic/mixed versus euthymic states.	Changing treatment modality (whether IPSRT or the control treatment) was associated with significantly faster recurrence and worse symptomatology, suggesting the importance of stability in the treatment of BP.
Frank et al., 2005	Acute and maintenance IPSRT, acute and maintenance intensive clinical management (ICM), acute IPSRT followed by maintenance ICM, or acute ICM followed by maintenance IPSRT.	Acutely ill BP patients (n=175) randomly assigned to one of the four treatment strategies; 2 yr preventive maintenance phase.	No difference was found among treatment strategies in time to stabilization. Patients assigned to IPSRT in the acute treatment phase survived longer without a new affective episode.	Medically healthy married patients without comorbid anxiety disorders benefited most from treatment.

BP = bipolar disorder; IPSRT = Interpersonal and Social Rhythm Therapy.

TABLE 22–4. Clinical Trials of Family/Couples Therapy for Patients with Bipolar Disorder

Study	Intervention	Study Design	Results	Clinical Observations
Miller et al., 1991	Family group therapy (8–12 sessions) initiated during hospitalization and continued for 18 wk after discharge.	BP patients randomly assigned to standard treatment alone ($n=7$) or combined with family group therapy ($n=7$). Follow-up at 2 yr.	Significantly fewer hospitalizations and relapses had occurred in the family therapy group at 2 yr follow-up.	Although the number of patients was small, the significant results are promising.
Clarkin et al., 1998	Marital therapy with BP patient (either married or living with a partner for >6 mo); 25 sessions over 11 mo.	Euthymic BP patients randomly assigned to medication and marital therapy ($n=19$) or medication only ($n=23$). No follow-up.	At termination, medication adherence and overall functioning were significantly better for the psychotherapy group. There was no difference in symptomatology between the two groups.	The authors argued that aggressive treatment delivered earlier in the marriage could have been more successful.
Miklowitz et al., 2000	FFT including extensive family psychoeducation on BP, communication skills, and family problem solving; 21 sessions over 9 mo.	BP patients recruited during or immediately after an episode, randomized to either FFT for 9 mo ($n=31$) or standard psychiatric care ($n=70$). Follow-up at 3 mo intervals for 1 yr.	The FFT group experienced significantly fewer depressive relapses and longer interepisode intervals than the comparison group. The FFT group also showed an overall decrease in depressive but not in manic symptoms.	The effects of FFT were independent of medication adherence, although higher adherence in both groups was associated with greater stabilization of manic symptoms. FFT was associated with a more positive nonverbal interactional style, which partially mediated a more favorable outcome. BP patients from families with high expressed emotion showed the most dramatic symptom reduction.
Miklowitz et al., 2003	FFT as described above, 21 sessions, compared with crisis management (CM), 2 sessions. Both groups received pharmacotherapy.	BP patients randomized to FFT ($n=31$) plus pharmacotherapy or CM ($n=70$) plus pharmacotherapy. Follow-up at 3–6 mo intervals for 2 yr.	The FFT group experienced fewer relapses, longer survival intervals, greater reduction in mood symptomatology, and better treatment adherence.	FFT involved more extensive therapist contact. There was a lack of control over patients' medical regimens.
Rea et al., 2003	FFT as described above (21 sessions) or individual therapy focused on support, problem solving, and education (21 sessions).	BP patients randomly assigned to FFT ($n=28$) or individual therapy ($n=25$). Assessments at 3 mo intervals for 1 yr period of active treatment and follow-up at 1 yr after treatment.	The FFT group was much less likely to be rehospitalized or to have illness relapses during the 2 yr study period. Both groups showed high levels of medication adherence (no significant difference between groups).	The effect of FFT was strongest after completion of the treatment protocol. Patients with poor premorbid status were protected from relapse by FFT but not by individual therapy.

BP = bipolar disorder; FFT = Family-Focused Treatment.

897

TABLE 22–5. Effectiveness Studies Involving Psychotherapy for Patients with Bipolar Disorder

Study	Intervention	Study Design	Results	Clinical Observations
Sachs et al., ongoing	Systematic Treatment Enhancement Program for Bipolar Disorder (STEP-BD). Clinical trials of interpersonal and social rhythm therapy (IPSRT), family-focused therapy (FFT), cognitive-behavioral therapy (CBT), or collaborative care (the control condition, psychoeducation) as adjunct to medication.	A multisite randomized effectiveness study. BP patients (n=5,000) to be recruited in 17 centers.	Not yet available.	Not yet available.
Callahan and Bauer, 1999	Life Goals Program: group psychotherapy with psychoeducation for relapse prevention (5 weekly sessions); individual behavioral treatment with social/educational goals.	Initial open trial with bipolar patients (n=29) at two Veterans Affairs (VA) Hospital sites.	69% of patients completed psychoeducation and showed increased knowledge of BP; 70% of these patients reached behavioral goals. Multisite open trial is ongoing.	The program is currently being evaluated against VA treatment as usual in a 12-site randomized controlled clinical trial.
Simon et al., 2005	An effectiveness trial of the Life Goals Program plus monthly telephone monitoring by nurses at a health maintenance organization.	BP patients (n=441). Clinical/functional status assessed every 3 mo for 12 mo.	Patients in the intervention group had significantly lower mania ratings and spent one-third less time in hypomanic or manic episodes. Mean depression ratings did not differ between the groups.	Those who completed five or more group sessions had better clinical outcomes but also had less severe symptoms at baseline. It is difficult to separate the effects of greater attention and support from those of specific intervention components.

BP = bipolar disorder.

compared with treatment as usual. The study cited in Table 22–1 tested only feasibility; a trial of this program is currently under way (Suppes et al., 2001). The psychoeducation in this approach has unique features. The program was developed mainly by a committee of members of patient advocacy and support groups, working in collaboration with clinicians. The educational material used during the acute phase of treatment is introduced by the physician and followed up by staff responding to patients' questions. When patients are less symptomatic, more complex material is presented to help with symptom recognition and to explore barriers to adherence to treatment (including side effects). Apart from individual meetings with the clinical team, patients and their families have the option to participate in group meetings that may include videotape presentations and consumer discussions (Toprac et al., 2000). The results of the ongoing trial, which includes a comprehensive consumer-guided educational program and large sample sizes, will provide important information about the effectiveness of this approach.

Cognitive-Behavioral Therapy

CBT, developed by Beck and colleagues (1979), is currently the most widely used and tested psychotherapeutic approach for which a manual has been created. It was originally developed for major depression but has been adapted and tested for numerous other conditions, including bipolar disorder. The underlying assumption is that depression-prone individuals possess negative self-schemata (beliefs), labeled the "cognitive triad." Specifically, depressed patients have negative views of themselves as worthless, inadequate, unlovable, deficient; of their environments as overwhelming, filled with obstacles and failure; and of their futures as hopeless, as though no effort will change the course of their lives. There have been far fewer studies of cognitive style in bipolar disorder than in major depression. The results of those that have been conducted suggest that cognitive styles in both mood disorders are similarly fragile and that negative self-esteem is a robust predictor of depressive and manic relapses (Scott et al., 2000; Scott and Pope, 2003; Jones et al., 2005). In administering CBT, the therapist is active and directive and, applying principles of logic and the scientific method, facilitates a rational approach to thinking with regard to the patient's current life circumstances. The patient's thoughts and assumptions are treated as hypotheses that can be tested to verify their accuracy.

To foster a spirit of collaborative empiricism, CBT therapists typically begin treatment by educating patients about their disorder. When a new technique is introduced, the therapist begins by presenting its rationale. In educating patients, the therapist builds the therapeutic alliance. To maximize rapid response to treatment, emphasis is placed on homework outside of therapy sessions. By the end of each session, therapist and patient agree on at least one assignment the patient can complete to either test beliefs or build skills. Cognitive therapy focuses on understanding how patients interpret events in their lives. The therapy is based on the premise that if distorted thoughts and images can be changed, the accompanying negative emotional states and behaviors will change as well. In this cognitive model of emotion, affect and behavior are seen for the most part as mediated by cognition.

The CBT adaptation for bipolar disorder is based on the observation that stressful life events can interact with negative cognitive styles to precipitate manic and depressive symptomatology in individuals with the disorder (Alloy et al., 1999). Various studies (Hollon et al., 1986; Alloy et al., 1999) led to the somewhat surprising finding that many persons with bipolar illness exhibit cognitive styles as negative as those associated with unipolar mood disorders, suggesting that similar psychological processes may predispose to both manic and depressive episodes or that the underlying disorders may result in similar cognitive manifestations.

Antimanic cognitive techniques include early identification of manic thoughts, cognitive restructuring geared to realistic interpretation of events, and evaluation of plans before taking action. Behavioral techniques focus on coping with sleep disturbance and on increasing medication adherence (when the chance of discontinuation is high), such as by associating the taking of medication with certain daily routines. Also employed are methods of reducing risk-taking behavior, such as giving credit cards to a relative or friend permanently or at the first sign of a relapse to control spending, and the imparting of skills needed to prioritize and decrease the number and intensity of activities (Bauer et al., 1991; Basco and Rush, 1995; Scott, 1996). Cognitive and behavioral interventions during depressive phases include teaching behavior activation techniques to end the lethargy cycle (such as an increase in pleasant activities or assignment of tasks to reduce workload) and techniques for countering negative thoughts.

More than 10 efficacy trials of CBT in treating bipolar disorder have been completed (see Table 22–2). In addition, CBT is included in NIMH's ongoing Systematic Treatment Enhancement Program for Bipolar Disorder (STEP-BD) (discussed later). The CBT interventions studied were generally similar, but differed in the degree of structure of the manuals employed, as well as in the emphasis placed on cognitive or behavioral interventions and psychoeducation. Several studies used a group format (Hirschfeld-Becker et al., 1998; Weiss et al., 2000; Colom et al., 2003a,b). In most of the studies, CBT was conducted primarily on euthymic bipolar patients and was compared with treatment as usual. The length of the interventions varied from 6 to 25 sessions.

The results of these studies suggest that CBT may be a particularly useful adjunct to medication for relapse prevention, and may result in increased medication adherence and fewer relapses (both manic and depressive). In one study, cognitive dysfunctional attitudes remained unaffected despite symptomatic relief by the end of the treatment (Zaretsky et al., 1999), and in another, the positive effects of CBT were greater by the end of follow-up (Lam et al., 2000), indicating that CBT for bipolar patients may need to extend over time. Other investigations also have found that "booster" psychotherapy may be necessary to maximize outcome (Scott et al., 2001; Ball et al., 2006). Results of a recent study by Lam and colleagues (2005a) suggest that the combination of cognitive therapy and mood stabilizers is superior to mood stabilizers alone with regard to not only clinical outcome, but also cost-effectiveness. The cost of adding cognitive therapy to a medication-only regimen was offset by reduced costs for other services, such as inpatient or community core programs. The most recent randomized control study of CBT (Scott et al., 2006) is the only study to show no significant differences between the CBT and treatment as usual groups, but its results are difficult to interpret. The results may be due to the heterogeneity of the patient population (one-third were in acute episodes, and there was wide variability in affective histories). Moreover, many CBT patients did not complete all of their treatment sessions, and nearly one of every five patients was not taking a mood stabilizer (see Lam, 2006, for a detailed critique of the study's methodology).

Several of the studies (Cochran, 1984; Perry et al., 1999; Colom et al., 2003a,b) used CBT techniques for psychoeducation to assist patients in changing their attitudes about adherence and in solving problems related to relapse prevention (see Box 22–2 for the content of the Barcelona Psychoeducative Program). Results of these studies showed significant changes in the clinical status of the patients or their number of hospitalizations as a result of extensive psychoeducation. In Cochran's (1984) six-session intervention, significantly fewer hospitalizations occurred in the CBT group (although no difference in mood episodes was found). The study by Perry and colleagues (1999) showed a reduction in manic relapses, whereas Colom and colleagues (2003a), who conducted the longest psychoeducational intervention, found a reduction in both manic and depressive relapses; thus it may take a longer intervention to help patients learn how to avoid depressive relapses. In addition, the study of Colom and colleagues (2003b)—a group psychoeducation study with adherent bipolar patients—sheds light on the possible mechanisms of action of psychoeducation: that it exerts its effect not

---

BOX 22–2. Contents of the Barcelona Psychoeducation Program

1. Introduction
2. What is bipolar illness?
3. Causal and triggering factors
4. Symptoms (I): Mania and hypomania
5. Symptoms (II): Depression and mixed episodes
6. Course and outcome
7. Treatment (I): Mood stabilizers
8. Treatment (II): Antimanic agents
9. Treatment (III): Antidepressants
10. Serum levels: Lithium, carbamazepine, and valproate
11. Pregnancy and genetic counseling
12. Psychopharmacology vs. alternative therapies
13. Risks associated with treatment withdrawal
14. Alcohol and street drugs: Risks in bipolar illness
15. Early detection of manic and hypomanic episodes
16. Early detection of depressive and mixed episodes
17. What to do when a new phase is detected
18. Lifestyle regularity
19. Stress management techniques
20. Problem-solving techniques
21. Final session

Source: Colom and Vieta, 2006. John Wiley & Sons. Reproduced with permission.

---

only through increased adherence (since the participants in that study were already adherent), but also through assistance provided to the patient in recognizing and managing the prodromal symptoms of a relapse. In a subanalysis of their data, Colom and colleagues (2005) found that mean serum lithium levels were higher and more stable in patients who had received psychoeducation than in those who had not (Colom et al., 2005). An individual treatment manual based on the CBT model of this study has been developed and is currently being tested in STEP-BD. This manual has optional sections that can be used to address comorbid disorders often associated with bipolar disorder (see Chapter 7).

Interpersonal and Social Rhythm Therapy

Interpersonal psychotherapy is a time-limited psychotherapy, specified in a manual, that was developed for major depression and has been modified for other disorders and tested in numerous clinical trials (Klerman et al., 1984; Weissman et al., 2000). It makes no assumption about the cause of illness, but makes use of the connection between onset of symptoms and current interpersonal problems. The approach deals with current rather than past relationships and the immediate social context of the illness. It attempts to intervene in symptom formation and social dysfunction and not in personality. The initial phase includes a systematic diagnostic evaluation, psychoeducation, a review of medication, and an examination of current relationships and changes proximal to the emergence of symptoms. At least one of four problems (grief, interpersonal disputes, role transitions, role deficits) becomes the focus of treatment.

Frank and colleagues (1994) adapted interpersonal psychotherapy for bipolar disorder by adding a behavioral component to regulate patients' social rhythms and termed their approach IPSRT. The importance of regulating such rhythms had been demonstrated earlier in research conducted at NIMH (Wehr et al., 1987a,b). The focus of the method is on disruptions in interpersonal relationships that precede the onset of recurrence of an episode (manic or depressive). The four problem areas of interpersonal psychotherapy are also considered potential triggers of episodes in this adaptation. In IPSRT, grief includes not only grief for the death of a loved one, but also the mourning frequently experienced by bipolar patients over the loss of a healthy self that used to function productively (see Jamison and Goodwin, 1983; Jamison, 1991, 1995). Frank and colleagues (1994) argued that if this issue is not addressed, it may manifest itself in medication nonadherence and other self-destructive behavior. Interpersonal disputes are common among bipolar patients, especially in the manic phase, when angry and impulsive outbursts may alienate and frighten loved ones. Role transitions or life changes—such as starting a new job; relocating; having a new baby; experiencing the death of a spouse, family member, or close friend; or undergoing a divorce—may disrupt a routine that has provided a sense of familiarity and predictability, and may also disturb patients' sleep–wake cycle and daily rhythms. Interpersonal deficits are prominent in bipolar patients, as the damage and turmoil that follow manic episodes lead some patients to reduce their involvement in social relationships and work.

As noted earlier, major interpersonal disruptions may precipitate a manic or depressive episode. Based on findings from earlier research carried out by Wehr and colleagues (1987a,b) at NIMH, IPSRT postulates that the link between the patient's biological vulnerability and interpersonal events lies in the interplay between zeitgebers (events that stabilize the biological clock) and zeitstorers (events that disrupt the biological clock) (see Chapter 16). Thus, the mediating mechanism that may lead to an episode is disruption of the patient's circadian rhythms and daily routines (Wehr et al., 1987a; Ehlers et al., 1988; Frank et al., 1994). Early in the treatment, the therapist introduces the Social Rhythm Metric to chart the regularity and stimulation of 17 daily activities (e.g., getting out of bed, having the first meal), as well as the patient's mood at the end of each day. This procedure is intended to help the patient become more aware of the patterns of change in daily rhythms and life events and their relationship to mood.

IPSRT is conducted in four phases:

- In the initial phase, the therapist takes a thorough history of previous episodes and their interpersonal context; provides psychoeducation on bipolar disorder; introduces the Social Rhythm Metric, focusing on the most recent episode; and identifies the patient's main interpersonal problem area(s). The therapist is looking for evidence of disruption of daily rhythms that preceded episodes and educating the patient about the impact of rhythm dysregulation on mood.
- In the second phase, therapist and patient work toward regulating the patient's routine, as well as resolving the interpersonal problem areas relevant to episodes.
- The goal of the third phase is for the patient to become more independent and proficient in the use of IPSRT to address the links among events, biology, and mood.
- Termination is the fourth phase, with particular emphasis on enhancing the patient's independent functioning and developing strategies for relapse prevention.

Frank and colleagues conducted an efficacy study of IPSRT (Frank et al., 1999, 2000), comparing it with clinical status and symptom review treatment, a form of intensive clinical management (see Table 22–3). All patients also received medication. Preliminary results for 90 patients who participated in the preventive phase showed significantly more regular social/circadian rhythms in the IPSRT than in the comparison group. There was no significant difference in the number of episodes (manic or depressive) between the two conditions. However, IPSRT was associated with significantly longer periods of euthymia relative to the comparison group, which experienced more depressive symptoms over time. There was no difference between the two conditions in the proportion of manic/mixed and euthymic states over time (Frank et al., 2000). Preliminary findings also indicated that patients assigned during the preventive phase to a treatment different from that received during the acute phase (regardless of what that treatment was) were at higher risk for relapse, suggesting that stability in treatment delivery can be a regulating factor for bipolar patients (Frank et al., 1999). IPSRT is also being tested in the NIMH STEP-BD study (see the later discussion).

In a study of 175 acutely ill bipolar patients, Frank and colleagues (2005) compared two psychosocial interventions, IPSRT and intensive clinical management (ICM), in a randomized controlled trial involving four treatment strategies: acute and maintenance IPSRT, acute and maintenance ICM, acute IPSRT followed by maintenance ICM, and acute ICM followed by maintenance IPSRT. During the 2-year preventive maintenance phase, they found no difference among the treatment strategies in time to survival. Those who had been assigned to IPSRT during the acute treatment phase survived longer without a new affective episode. As might be expected, the participants in the IPSRT group showed more regularity of social rhythms at the end of the acute treatment phase. Moreover, medically healthy patients without comorbid anxiety disorders derived greater benefit from treatment.

Family/Couples Therapy

Because bipolar disorder takes a considerable toll on marriage and family life, early psychotherapy studies focused on families and couples (see Chapter 10). It has been found that families with high levels of expressed emotion toward the patient, characterized by hostility, rejection, and overinvolvement, are associated with higher rates of relapse (Fallon et al., 1984; Miklowitz et al., 2004). Patients' sensitivity to such criticism is also predictive of poorer outcomes (Miklowitz et al., 2005). In an adaptation of behavioral family management methods tested with schizophrenic patients (Fallon et al., 1984), FFT was developed for bipolar patients recently treated for an acute episode as inpatients or outpatients (Miklowitz and Goldstein, 1990). Family attitudes, communication, and problem-solving style are the targets of treatment. FFT, lasting 9 months and usually delivered in 21 sessions, has five stages:

- In the "joining phase," the therapist introduces the protocol to the family.
- The initial assessment phase focuses on evaluation of levels of expressed emotion in the family and on the quality of communication and problem-solving styles.
- Family psychoeducation consists of 7 sessions during which information on bipolar disorder is introduced, including the patient's particular patterns of onset for both manic and depressive episodes, symptom course, and suicidal ideation. A central component of family psychoeducation is the relapse drill discussed previously. The therapist also explores patient and family attitudes toward medication and emphasizes the importance of adherence, including regular monitoring of blood levels. A vulnerability–stress model is adopted, and the therapist identifies risk and protective factors that affect relapses. In this context, the entire family is encouraged to promote a regular, predictable, and low-stress environment.
- Communication enhancement training, lasting about 7 sessions, teaches family members skills of listening actively, expressing positive and negative feelings in an accepting and nonintrusive manner, and making nonjudgmental requests for change.

- Problem-solving techniques are addressed in about 5 sessions, in which participants learn to define problems, evaluate each option, and implement solutions. The family, with the help of the therapist, resolves problems concerning medication adherence, living arrangements, and resumption of previous social and occupational roles (Miklowitz and Goldstein, 1997).

There have been five efficacy trials of family/couples therapy with bipolar patients (see Table 22–4), which have varied in the number of participants (14–101) and length of follow-up period (from none to 2 years). A study conducted by Miller and colleagues (1991) had a very small sample and, despite the high probability of type II error, yielded significant results with regard to relapse prevention over 2 years. Clarkin and colleagues (1998) failed to show significant symptomatic change, but they did not conduct a follow-up evaluation and may have missed the delayed effect present in other studies. The largest efficacy studies conducted thus far (Miklowitz et al., 2000; Rea et al., 2003) showed that FFT led to a significant reduction in depressive relapses and symptomatology as compared with clinical management or individual therapy. The results of these studies suggest that therapy with some family involvement may be efficacious for bipolar patients, with a selective effect for depressive symptomatology. However, the variability in the treatments used in these studies limits conclusions about a specific type of family treatment. FFT is also included in STEP-BD (discussed later).

Psychotherapy for Children and Adolescents

Interest in the early presentation of bipolar disorder in children and adolescents has been growing (see Chapter 6). Since there are still so many unknowns regarding the early signs, diagnostic criteria, and comorbid conditions of pediatric bipolar disorder, it is no surprise that there are only a few tested mood stabilizers for this population and no proven psychotherapeutic approaches (Pavuluri et al., 2002).

Fristad and colleagues (1998) described a manual-driven, adjunctive, multifamily group treatment approach for youths aged 8 to 12 with bipolar and depressive disorders. This method includes psychoeducation about the disorders and the role of medications, training in communication skills to improve interactions between parents and children, stress management, and development of coping strategies. In a later study, Fridstad and colleagues (2002) showed that multifamily psychoeducation groups were characterized by increased knowledge about bipolar disorder and treatment options, better skills for dealing with the bipolar child, more active attitudes toward mobilizing resources to benefit the child, and an increased sense of support compared with a wait-list control group.

Miklowitz and colleagues developed a manual for adolescents aged 13 to 17 with bipolar-I disorder. This manual, an adaptation of the FFT model for bipolar adults, is designed to make the approach appropriate for this age group and to address clinical issues specific to juvenile bipolar disorder. In an open trial of 20 bipolar adolescents (mean age 14.8 years; standard deviation=1.6), this adapted approach was associated with improvements in depression and mania symptoms, as well as in behavioral problems (Miklowitz et al., 2004).

Greene (2001) developed a collaborative problem-solving model that focuses on parents' assistance to their children. This approach helps parents avoid engaging their children when the children are in the midst of a rage attack. Only after an attack subsides can the parent encourage collaborative problem solving. The approach is controversial since the model emphasizes no consequences for the rage behavior or associated actions.

Pavuluri and colleagues (2002) developed a treatment program that involves parent-and-child sessions for 8- to 12-year-olds with bipolar disorder, termed Child- and Family-Focused Cognitive-Behavioral Therapy. Central to this approach is building the youth's self-esteem and helping all involved parties understand that pediatric bipolar disorder is a neuropsychiatric problem of affect dysregulation, rather than willful misbehavior. Over 12 sessions, parents are trained as coaches while engaging in parallel therapy to address their own affect regulation in dealing with their children, restructure their thoughts regarding their effectiveness as parents, and learn to resolve conflicts with their children through empathy. Both parents and children are instructed in the use of "RAINBOW":

- R=the importance of a routine (including sleep hygiene).
- A=affect regulation/anger control (including knowledge about the disorder, medication, and life charts).
- I="I can do it" (positive self-statements).
- N=no negative thoughts (restructuring negative thinking)/living in the "now."
- B=be a good friend/balanced lifestyle (also for parents).
- O="Oh, how can 'we' solve it?" (letting the rages pass, interpersonal and situational problem solving).
- W=ways to ask for and get support.

The child's school receives a work folder documenting what has been accomplished in the individual sessions. In addition, a teleconference is held with school staff members to educate them in the use of the RAINBOW program. A preliminary investigation of 34 patients with pediatric bipolar disorder (mean age 11.3 years, standard deviation=3.1) found that the RAINBOW child- and family-focused intervention resulted in significant reductions in severity of symptoms of aggression, mania, psychosis, depression, and sleep disturbance (Pavuluri et al., 2004).

Finally, an interpersonal psychotherapy–based preventive intervention for adolescent children of bipolar mothers is under way at New York State Psychiatric Institute (Verdeli, 2004). Seven adolescents whose mothers are receiving treatment for bipolar-I disorder and who themselves have subsyndromal bipolar symptomatology and/or mild functional impairment attend sessions of family psychoeducation about the mother's disorder and also receive individual interpersonal psychotherapy–based counseling (12 sessions). The intervention aims to (1) educate the adolescents and their parents/caretakers about bipolar disorder; (2) help the family make realistic plans in the event of the mother's relapse; (3) help the adolescents deal more adaptively with stressful interpersonal situations (including the mother's disorder); and (4) when necessary, help the adolescents regulate their circadian rhythms, social stimulation, and daily habits.

Ongoing Effectiveness Studies

The multisite STEP-BD effectiveness study being conducted by Sachs and colleagues should provide more definitive data on the relative value of the various psychotherapeutic approaches discussed here (see Table 22–5). This trial will be carried out over the next 5 to 8 years in 17 treatment centers and will include 5,000 bipolar patients. Data will be obtained on the effectiveness of CBT, IPSRT, and FFT in combination with pharmacotherapy treatment algorithms. Collaborative care, the control condition, is patient-directed in that the patients watch a psychoeducational videotape on bipolar disorder and receive a self-help workbook. The psychotherapeutic treatments are expected to improve remission of symptoms from acute depression, maintain treatment gains after recovery, and improve medication adherence. The large sample and the inclusion of psychotherapeutic approaches developed and/or adapted for bipolar disorder make this an important study. Early results suggest that intensive psychotherapy may be most helpful for those patients with the more severe forms of bipolar illness, whereas briefer treatment may be adequate for those who are less ill (Miklowitz et al., 2006).

The Life Goals Program encompasses a five-session psychoeducation phase followed by an individual behavioral treatment to improve functional status by working toward interpersonal/occupational goals identified by the patient (Callahan and Bauer, 1999). This program has been tested in an open trial in two Veterans Affairs (VA) sites with 29 bipolar patients, 70 percent of whom achieved their behavioral goal during the second phase of the study. Likewise, a 12-month effectiveness study based on the Life Goals Program, involving 441 patients at health maintenance organization centers in Seattle, found that patients in the intervention group spent one-third less time in manic or hypomanic episodes (Simon et al., 2005). In an open study of 45 bipolar patients, Swiss researchers found that the great majority of those who completed the initial phases of the Life Goals Program were very satisfied with the information received and reported subjective improvements in mood stability, relapse prevention strategies, and methods of coping with relapse (de Andrés et al., 2006). The Life Goals Program is currently being compared against treatment as usual in 12 VA hospitals in a multisite randomized controlled trial.

In general, effectiveness studies are not initiated until there is evidence of a treatment's efficacy in homogeneous samples under the controlled conditions of an efficacy study. The push to conduct these large effectiveness studies reflects the relative paucity of data on the psychotherapeutic management of bipolar patients and the urgent need to close this gap.

Meta-analyses of Psychological Treatments

Scott and Gutierrez (2004), studied the overall efficacy of psychotherapeutic interventions for bipolar illness by conducting meta-analyses of randomized controlled trials of psychological therapies added to standard psychiatric treatment versus medication and standard psychiatric treatment alone. Most although not all of the psychological therapies used cognitive-behavioral techniques. Only studies that reported relapse rates during the treatment phase and a follow-up period of at least 6 months were included in the analysis. The analysis results, shown in Figure 22–5, clearly demonstrate that psychological interventions are effective in reducing the risk of bipolar relapse, although it is not clear which specific approaches are most efficacious. There is without doubt sufficient evidence to support the use of psychological treatments to improve the course and outcome of bipolar illness.

CONCLUSIONS

Both clinical experience and emerging evidence suggest that bipolar illness is treated most effectively with a combination of mood stabilizers or other medications and psychotherapy. Drug treatment, which is primary, frees most patients from the severe disruptions of manic and depressive episodes. Psychotherapy can then help patients come to terms with the repercussions of past episodes and comprehend the practical and existential implications of having bipolar illness. When medications are administered in an emotionally supportive atmosphere, patients are more likely to express their concerns, physicians are better able to assess the need for psychotherapeutic interventions, and medication adherence is enhanced. Moreover, educating patients and their families is essential because it aids them in recognizing symptoms of emerging episodes. It is also essential to informed consent for treatment, which is imperative for both clinical and legal reasons. Charting of moods appears to be useful to provide an objective record of patterns of mood and treatment response and to give patients a sense of control and collaboration in their treatment.

Although not all patients need psychotherapy, most may benefit from one of its many forms—individual, group, or family. Participation in a self-help group can supplement or, on occasion, supplant formal psychotherapy. Which option

Figure 22–5. Odds ratios of relapse in randomized controlled trials of psychological treatments for bipolar disorder. (*Source*: Scott and Gutierrez, 2004. Reproduced with permission from Blackwell Publishing, Ltd.)

Early, smaller trials

Study	Sample Size		Effect	p-value
Cochran, 1984	28		0.12	0.02
Lam et al., 2000	23		0.02	0.00
Perry et al., 1999	68		0.59	0.34
Scott et al., 2001	42		0.38	0.17
Fixed combined (4)	161		0.28	0.00
Random combined (4)	161		0.22	0.01

0.01   0.1   1   10   100

Favors Psychotherapy

Recent, large-scale trials

Study	Sample Size		Effect	p-value
Colom et al., 2003a	120		0.41	0.02
Lam et al., 2003	96		0.26	0.00
Miklowitz et al., 2000	101		0.46	0.08
Fixed combined (3)	317		0.37	0.00
Random combined (3)	317		0.37	0.00

0.01   0.1   1   10   100

Favors Psychotherapy

is most appropriate can usually be determined by the psychiatrist or psychopharmacologist who supervises the patient's medications. No one psychotherapeutic approach, even among the newer techniques, has been shown to be uniformly superior for bipolar patients. The therapist must be guided by knowledge of the illness itself and its manifestation in the individual patient. In style and technique, the therapist must remain flexible to adjust to the patient's fluctuating moods, cognition, and behavior. The therapist must be especially alert to the emotions commonly engendered in clinicians who work with bipolar patients.

Psychotherapeutic issues are dictated by the character of the illness. Although reactions vary widely, patients typically feel angry, confused, and ambivalent about both the illness and its treatment. They may deny the existence of the illness, its severity, or its consequences; such denial may cause them to stop taking their medication. When treatment is not completely successful, patients are understandably disappointed and frustrated. Patients also may be disturbed at losing the energy and vitality that accompany mania. They fear recurrences. They have difficulty discriminating normal from abnormal moods. And they are concerned about relationships and the possibility of transmitting a genetic illness to their children.

During the 1970s and 1980s, research in psychotherapy for bipolar patients was characterized by small open trials, without the guidance of treatment manuals or attention to therapists' adherence to the treatment. Functional and symptomatic outcomes were not systematically assessed, and treatment randomization was rare. The empirical evidence for the efficacy or effectiveness of psychotherapy for bipolar disorder remains limited for adults and is virtually nonexistent for children and adolescents. In the 1990s, a number of randomized clinical trials of the efficacy of various psychotherapeutic approaches set the stage for multisite effectiveness trials now under way. Psychotherapy manuals, independent evaluators blinded to the treatment being given, and expanded outcome measures (including symptoms, social functioning, cost-effectiveness, and medication

adherence) are now the recognized tools for testing the new approaches. Of course, the demonstrable efficacy of manual-driven psychotherapeutic interventions does not rule out the efficacy of other, as yet untested types of psychotherapy.

Clinically, psychotherapy aimed at patient and family education and/or management of the consequences and environmental triggers of the illness makes sense, but there is still a gap between clinical wisdom and evidence. The results of ongoing trials should provide the strong base of empirical evidence that is needed to fill this gap.

NOTES

1. This passage, as well as others by "a patient with manic-depressive illness," was written by one of the authors, Kay R. Jamison. Some were modified slightly and incorporated into her memoir, *An Unquiet Mind* (Jamison, 1995).

2. For obvious reasons, psychotherapy has never been as integral or comfortable a part of the treatment of bipolar illness as it has been of unipolar illness. Clearly, the psychotic disorders and their empirically derived remedies long predate psychological treatments. Both history and necessity have embedded bipolar illness in medicine, much more so than other psychiatric disorders. Unipolar depressions, on the other hand, have had an easier alliance with psychotherapy, partly because they generally constitute a wider spectrum of psychopathology that shows a range of milder syndromes with prominent psychological factors. Because the concept of *depression* encompasses a relatively normal spectrum of emotions and feeling, it has traditionally stimulated counsel from priests, physicians, and friends.

3. For a more comprehensive discussion of the nature and methods of psychotherapy, see Jerome Frank's classic book, *Persuasion and Healing* (1961), and Phillip Slavney's *Psychotherapy* (2005).

4. Many of these reactions are discussed further in Chapter 10.

5. Ghaemi, 1995; Peralta and Cuesta, 1998; Dell'Osso et al., 2000, 2002; Pini et al., 2001.

6. G. Goodwin (2002) has described many of the difficulties that arise from attempts to establish clear boundaries between the manic states.

7. Molnar et al., 1988; Smith and Tarrier, 1992; Basco and Rush, 1996; Lam and Wong, 1997; Perry et al., 1999.

23 Treatment of Children and Adolescents

The prognosis of insanity in children must of course be very variable. . . . Judicious management, which is the most essential condition of amendment, is very difficult to obtain.

—D. H. Tuke (1892, p. 204)

Research on treatment in the field of child and adolescent psychiatry has been roughly a generation behind that in adult psychiatry. Several reasons explain this lag, such as the power and persistence of the analytic model in child psychiatry, concerns about pharmacological therapies interfering with a child's normal development, and ethical dilemmas in conducting pediatric clinical trials. Most important, diagnostic criteria for adults were not developed with children in mind, and children of different ages pose a variety of assessment challenges not encountered with adults. Because of these difficulties, there is a lack of consensus on what constitutes affective disorder, especially mania, in children (see Chapter 6).

Despite these barriers, however, research on treatment of manic-depressive illness in children and adolescents (virtually all of it focused on the bipolar subgroup) has been accelerating, spurred by a number of forces. These include incentives introduced by the U.S. Food and Drug Administration (FDA) in 1997 to stimulate industry-sponsored trials; research initiatives by the National Institute of Mental Health (NIMH); and, more recently, the activism of organizations such as the Depression and Bipolar Support Alliance (DBSA) and the Child and Adolescent Bipolar Foundation (CABF) in providing on-line support, destigmatization, and public education, especially their efforts to raise parents' awareness of the urgent need for more research.

We begin this chapter with a discussion of the unique diagnostic and other challenges posed by affective (especially bipolar) disorders in children and adolescents (sometimes referred to collectively here as youths or pediatric populations). We then turn to clinical management, presenting our recommendations for treatment, as well as for preven-

tion in at-risk youths. Next we review the literature supporting our recommendations for acute and maintenance pharmacological treatment, focusing on bipolar disorder (while there is essentially no literature on recurrent unipolar depression per se in this age group, we do discuss prepubertal depression and the frequency with which it evolves into bipolar disorder). In this section we also examine the literature on the offspring of adults with bipolar disorder, on psychiatric and medical adverse events, and on the use of electroconvulsive therapy (ECT) and psychotherapy in pediatric patients.

CHALLENGES POSED BY EARLY-ONSET BIPOLAR DISORDER

Diagnosis

"Classic" bipolar disorder is a recurrent condition in which mood and activity level are either significantly increased (hypomania and mania) or decreased (depression), with a return to premorbid levels of functioning between episodes. Our understanding of manic-depressive illness, especially the bipolar form, has emerged largely from the vast clinical experience of psychiatrists, such as Kraepelin, in recognizing the syndromal similarities among hundreds of patients over the course of time. By contrast, our understanding of the illness in youths, more specifically the bipolar subgroup, did not emerge from many years of intense study of the patients treated by child psychiatrists. Rather, it began with attempts to find in pediatric populations equivalents of what Kraepelin and others appeared to be describing (see Glovinsky, 2002; Carlson, et al., 2005). When early clinicians tried to do so, they found that classic Kraepelinian manic-depressive illness did indeed exist in youths, but occurred mainly in adolescents. Anthony and Scott (1960) explored the question of classic "manic-depressive psychosis," strictly defined, in preadolescents in a literature review and found it to be uncommon in this population, generally beginning to emerge with any frequency at about age 11 (see Chapter 6 for a comprehensive discussion).

When the bipolar form of manic-depressive illness was misdiagnosed in adolescents, it was because the psychosis in mania and depression was often very severe and was misattributed to schizophrenia (see, e.g., Carlson and Strober, 1978). In preadolescents, the diagnostic conundrum has been separating mania from a variety of behavioral disorders in children in which activation, short attention span, and irritability co-occur chronically. The essential question becomes whether the frequent and brief episodes of intense mood volatility and irritability that are being called "prepubertal mania" or "juvenile bipolar disorder" represent the same illness as that in adults (McClellan, 2005). The further one diverges from the description of bipolar disorder as it has been conceptualized for the past century, the more difficult it becomes to extrapolate those findings to children. At this point, it is unclear to what extent these children will evolve into adults with bipolar disorder as defined by the *Diagnostic and Statistical Manual* (DSM)-IV, let alone the classic form with clearly delineated episodes and good intermorbid functioning (Biederman et al., 1998; Geller et al., 2004). Thus when people say bipolar disorder is much more common in children than heretofore believed, this statement is reflecting, at least in part, the broadening of the concept of the disorder.

Classic bipolar disorder is, at best, uncommon in children; however, the results of large retrospective studies of adult bipolar patients would appear to be at odds with this conclusion. In their recent review, Post and Kowatch (2006) cited retrospective data from two relatively large samples of adults with DSM-IV bipolar disorder—those of the Systematic Treatment Enhancement Program for Bipolar Disorder (STEP-BD) and the Bipolar Collaborative Network (BCN; formerly the Stanley Foundation Bipolar Network). In STEP-BD, 28 percent of adult bipolar patients reported their age at onset as younger than 13; in the BCN, 15 percent did so. Post and Kowatch also cited another finding from the BCN data: that the earlier the age at onset, the longer was the delay to first treatment (16.8 years for childhood onset, 11.3 years for adolescent onset, and 4.6 years for adult onset) and the worse the long-term outcome. In citing these data, however, the authors implicitly acknowledged the limitations of retrospective data: "The field is in agreement that prospective assessment and follow-up of large cohorts of children need to be conducted in order to better define initial diagnostic subgroups and their ultimate

trajectories into classic bipolar illness . . ." (p. 115). We certainly agree. We also agree that there are many children with markedly labile mood and episodic behavioral dyscontrol who appear to need and benefit from the mood stabilizers used in the treatment of adolescents and adults with bipolar disorder. But the relationship between these serious and very real syndromes in children and adolescent and adult bipolar disorder has not yet been clarified (see the discussion later in this chapter and in Chapter 6).

Furthermore, although DSM-III-R and -IV have been used to diagnose bipolar disorder in children as well as adolescents and adults, there is little uniformity in how these criteria are operationalized for children. Leibenluft and colleagues (2003) proposed an approach that requires strict adherence to criteria for mania in adults for a "narrow phenotype," as opposed to an "intermediate phenotype" (based on the DSM-IV criterion for mania but with a duration of less than 4 days) and a "broad phenotype" (encompassing severe mood dysregulation that many believe characterizes what is being called "juvenile mania"). This approach, inherently inclusive, strikes us as quite sensible.

Geller and colleagues (2002a) have reoperationalized several of the DSM criteria (most notably euphoria and grandiosity) to make them what the authors believe to be developmentally appropriate for children. Not everyone agrees with this reformulation, however (Harrington and Myatt, 2003). In a recent cross-national study (United States and United Kingdom) of five cases of children with mood symptoms in whom bipolar disorder might have been a diagnostic consideration, disagreement on diagnosis occurred in three of the five cases. The reason for this appears to be differing interpretations of specific symptoms. DSM's reliance on symptom counts (used in the United States) may result in a conceptualization that differs from the gestalt of bipolar disorder as described in the *International Classification of Diseases* (ICD)-10, used in the United Kingdom. Specifically, in a preadolescent patient with classic mania, agreement was close (96.4 percent of U.S. and 88.9 percent of U.K. physicians made a manic diagnosis). In the prepubertal child with both attention-deficit hyperactivity disorder (ADHD) and manic-like symptoms, however, 86.2 percent of U.S. child psychiatrists diagnosed mania, in contrast to only 31.1 percent of their U.K. colleagues (Dubicka et al., 2005).

Other Challenges

Beyond diagnosis, other unique challenges posed by early-onset bipolar disorder ultimately have an impact on treatment. First, most clinical trials include only adolescents, or include mixed samples that are not large enough to permit separate analysis of children and adolescents. By our rough estimate, fewer than one-third of clinical trials discussed later in our review of the literature involved solely children. That means most of our knowledge bears on adolescents rather than children. If childhood-onset bipolar disorder is a fundamentally distinct disorder, it is questionable at best to extrapolate treatments from adolescents to children. Further, even clinical trials of adolescents can be difficult to interpret because they often fail to distinguish the age at onset of the disorder, whether in childhood or adolescence. Some trials are of inpatients, some of outpatients. Inpatient trials more closely approximate adult "acute mania" studies. Outpatient trials usually address bipolar spectrum disorders or include subjects whose generally lower levels of severity allow them to be seen only monthly. These trials are reviewed later in the chapter.

Second, because Axis I–based structured interviews are used to assess bipolar disorder in most studies, developmental disorders, as well as conditions such as mild autism that used to be Axis II and that may occur in nearly two-thirds of bipolar children and adolescents (Towbin et al., 2005), are overlooked. Moreover, the presence of such children in a clinical sample may affect treatment response since adverse events are higher in these children (Carlson, 2005; Carlson and Mick, 2003).

Third, bipolar patients in whom the disorder started in childhood have more complicated developmental histories than those whose disorder started in adolescence or early adulthood (Carlson and Meyer, 2006). In an adult who has had many years to establish baseline functioning, recognizing the onset of something new and different is relatively easy. On the other hand, a child who enters kindergarten at age 5 and becomes disruptive may be manifesting the onset of bipolar disorder, suffering from an altogether different disorder, or simply having serious trouble adjusting to the academic and social demands of school.

Fourth, bipolar disorder in children almost never occurs without some other comorbidity (see Chapter 6). When manic symptoms are superimposed on or coexist with other kinds of psychopathology (e.g., ADHD, conduct disorder, anxiety disorder), episodes become more difficult to distinguish and to treat. Moreover, the meaning of comorbidity is unresolved. The hope in the field has been that the underlying comorbidity is actually a manifestation of bipolar disorder and with adequate treatment will resolve. Although this may turn out to be true once better treatments have been identified, the current armamentarium does not sufficiently treat underlying comorbidities. That is, a child with mania in addition to ADHD or conduct disorder usually continues to have the latter two conditions, although ratings of hyperactivity may improve with antimanic treatments. It appears that early onset and comorbidity interact and may change both the course of bipolar illness and its response to treatment. Two studies have found that the duration of the index

episode increases with younger age at onset (Carlson et al., 2002; Geller et al., 2004), and underlying comorbidity appears to predict poorer functional outcome (Carlson et al., 2002). There are also data suggesting that the presence of ADHD worsens response to lithium (Strober et al., 1988, 1998; Kafantaris et al., 1998).

Although the percentage of males and comorbid ADHD diagnoses both appear to decline with increasing age at onset of bipolar disorder, a history of ADHD can still be ascertained in 10 to 20 percent of patients with adult-onset bipolar illness (Carlson et al., 2000). Moreover, adult-onset bipolar patients with comorbid substance abuse may well have had externalizing disorders (conduct disorder and ADHD) as children and adolescents (Carlson et al., 1999). This externalizing disorder comorbidity likely complicates treatment response as well. Finally, anxiety disorders co-occur with bipolar disorder at high rates in youth and adults. Several selective serotonin reuptake inhibitors (SSRIs) (fluoxetine, fluvoxamine, clomipramine) have established efficacy for treating anxiety disorders, including obsessive-compulsive disorder, in children and adolescents (Reinblatt and Walkup, 2005). However, the same risks that complicate the use of SSRIs for treatment of bipolar depression (see the later discussion) obtain here as well.

Fifth, early onset of bipolar disorder is associated with increased genetic loading (see Chapters 6 and 13). The level of complexity of bipolar disorder may be heritable as well, and this, too, has an impact on treatment. For instance, there is suggestive evidence that parental response to medication may select a more homogeneous group of bipolar subjects (Duffy et al., 1998) and that offspring of lithium-responding bipolar parents have a milder condition[1] than offspring of bipolar adults with comorbid conditions (Biederman et al., 2000b).

Finally, severe emotional and behavioral lability in children and adolescents is significantly impairing but may be nonspecific. Several longitudinal studies have identified "bipolar symptoms" in children that did not evolve into bipolar disorder later on (e.g., Johnson et al., 1999; Lewinsohn et al., 2000; Hazell et al., 2003), although mood symptoms (depression and anxiety) did persist. While children with these "bipolar" symptoms certainly need treatment and may well respond to mood stabilizers, this fact alone does not clarify the relationship between these states and classic bipolar disorder.

CLINICAL MANAGEMENT

Overview

The American Academy of Child and Adolescent Psychiatry (AACAP) has developed practice parameters, the most recent of which were published in 1997 and are being up-dated as of this writing. In the interim, given the immediate need to have something more current available for treatment of the manic, depressive, and maintenance phases of bipolar disorder in pediatric populations, a consensus conference was convened in July 2003, initiated and supported by the CABF. Experts in child and adolescent bipolar disorder summarized recommendations for the field based on inter-pretation of existing information (Kowatch et al., 2005). Our treatment recommendations, which follow, integrate our own views with those consensus recommendations.

Adequate assessment of bipolar disorder in a child or adolescent takes several hours and may require multiple visits (Youngstrom et al., 2004). The assessment should in-clude interviews with parent(s) and child, as well as infor-mation gathered from other observers of the child (e.g., teachers). The information thus obtained should encom-pass not only symptoms of mania and depression, but also symptoms of other psychiatric disorders that may be con-fused with or co-occur with bipolar disorder. Standard-ized rating scales and interviews are often useful adjuncts. Evidence of psychiatric disorders in the youth's immediate family is essential not only because it can provide impor-tant genetic information, but also because such evidence can bring into focus issues that need to be addressed in psychotherapy. A developmental history, including ascer-tainment of social, academic, and family functioning, is necessary as well. Psychoeducational testing is often ex-tremely helpful in formulating a treatment plan for school. Decisions regarding the impairment produced by mood symptoms can be addressed by the "FIND" approach (Kowatch et al., 2005), encompassing *f*requency (symp-toms occur most days during the week), *i*ntensity (extreme disturbance caused in two or more settings), *n*umber (symptoms occur three or four times a day), and *d*uration (symptoms occur a total of 4 or more hours a day, not nec-essarily contiguous). The information obtained should in-clude whether the predominant mood is mania or depres-sion and whether there are comorbidities in addition to the mood disorder. If there has been a positive response to medication treatment (or lack thereof), it is important to know the details, such as the dose and the length of the trial. It is equally important to determine what adverse ef-fects may have occurred.

After assessment, psychoeducation of the patient and family members is important, and it should accomplish the following:

- The education of all concerned about the nature of the disorder(s) being treated (not only what is known about child, adolescent, and adult bipolar disorder, but also the comorbidities that may exist).

- Clarification of the advantages, limitations, and risks of medications, as well as the consequences of not using them:
  - Discuss the importance of following the exact pre-scription and of keeping medications secure.
  - Anticipate that a number of different medications may be used, so as to spare the patient multiple blood draws, and cover all bases by establishing a baseline: complete blood count (CBC), platelets, fasting blood sugar, liver and renal functioning, cholesterol, lipids, and thyroid functioning (specifically thyroid-stimulating hormone [TSH] and free thyroxine [T_4] by direct measure).
  - Obtain baseline ratings for the major symptoms being addressed (e.g., aggression/irritability, psychosis, hy-peractivity, inattention, anxiety, depression, shifts in mood/behavior) to make it possible to track and quan-tify any response or worsening.
  - Establish the priority of drugs for trial, and inform other members of the treatment team, patient, and family. The fact that a parent says "we've tried that" may not mean that an adequate trial has taken place.
  - Tell parents to allow each dose adequate time to work.
- Address any aspects of the disorder and its treatment that have an impact on the family and functioning in school. This can involve cognitive-behavioral therapy for the child, training of the parent(s), neuropsychological test-ing, and academic intervention; it can also include treat-ing any family members with psychiatric disorders that have an impact on parent–child functioning.

It is important to remember that any comorbidities war-rant their own psychoeducational focus. If ADHD coexists with bipolar disorder, for example, the clinician must ex-plore with patient and parent(s) all of the comorbidities that can occur with ADHD, including learning, language, and motor coordination problems. These latter comorbidi-ties are likely to require an individual educational plan that accommodates them, such as smaller classrooms with higher teacher/pupil ratios. Depending on the severity of the ma-nia, depression, or comorbidity, the child may also need a day program, periods of hospitalization, or even long-term residential treatment.

Children/adolescents and their parents need to under-stand the complexities of the conditions involved; the im-portance of adherence to treatment; and the need to stabi-lize the environment, aspects of which may be exacerbating the disorder. Information sources for parents are noted in the appendix at the end of this volume.

The reality that early-onset bipolar disorder is genetic means other family members with whom the child lives may need treatment for their own mood disorders. This observa-tion is especially important for the patient's caregiver. Care of a bipolar child is, to say the least, challenging. A depressed or manic parent afflicted with the dysfunctions that can accompany the condition poses additional management problems.

A candid discussion of medication risks is also necessary. If side effects of a particular medication are minimal and treatment efficacy is clear, it obviously makes sense to continue treatment. If adverse events appear to be worse than the condition being treated, the medication should be slowly discontinued or a lower dose administered. The decision to try another, similar medication or the same medication at a lower dose must be made on a case-by-case basis. The reason it is necessary to establish a clear baseline of symptoms and functional impairment is to be able to make such decisions with greater confidence. With respect to treatment for ADHD and/or antidepressant use, it remains prudent (1) to warn parents about hypomania/mania and nonspecific activation/agitation (including suicidal or other self-harm behaviors) as potential side effects of antidepressants, and activation/agitation as a side effect of stimulants; (2) to obtain as part of the family history information on any medication responses and intolerances; and (3) to provide careful follow-up (see the discussion later in this chapter).

It is unclear whether the absence of a classic presentation of bipolar disorder in prepubertal children hinders response to medication, or whether there are developmental differences that influence the medication response of young children, or both. Until this question can be answered, we believe the confidence one has in extrapolating treatment data from adults to children should be directly proportional to how closely the child's history and presentation correspond to a pattern of clear episodes of mania, depression, and euthymia. The following is an overview of treatment choices for the various phases of bipolar disorder:

- *Mania/hypomania/mixed episodes*—Given that the evidence base is rapidly changing, an evidence-based approach (see Chapter 17) requires the clinician to monitor closely the results of published studies. As of this writing, lithium,[2] divalproex, and atypical antipsychotics are supported as monotherapies and, when monotherapy is inadequate, in combination.
- *Mania and ADHD*—Mania is treated first, followed by treatment for ADHD if symptoms have not remitted. There is no consensus on cases in which the differential diagnosis is unclear. We advise discussing with parents the risks and benefits of using atypical antipsychotics or mood stabilizers first versus starting with treatment for ADHD (see the later discussion). There are many more years of experience with stimulant medication than with atypical antipsychotics or mood stabilizers. If the patient

becomes more irritable or aggressive with ADHD treatment, however, it makes most sense to switch to an atypical or a mood stabilizer, than retrying the ADHD treatment.
- *Bipolar depression*—One open trial of lithium monotherapy for hospitalized adolescents with bipolar depression found a reduction in depressive symptoms, although most of this amelioration occurred during the hospitalization. There has also been a positive open trial using lamotrigine alone or with other medication in adolescents. No placebo-controlled or otherwise randomized data exist, however. Thus for adolescents with clear bipolar depression, it may make sense to apply the findings from the literature on adult bipolar depression, which increasingly advocates the use of lamotrigine or quetiapine. The long-term use of quetiapine may be problematic, however, given the dramatic increase in obesity among adolescents, especially in the United States. This caution applies as well, of course, to some of the other atypicals, especially olanzapine and the olanzapine–fluoxetine combination.
- *First episode of depression with a bipolar family history*—This is another thorny issue on which there is no clear consensus, and for which it is necessary to have a discussion with family members of the risks and benefits of alternatives (Carlson, 2005a). In a young person at risk for a bipolar course, the clinician must weigh the risk that an antidepressant may precipitate mania or hypomania, versus the risk that a mood stabilizer alone may not alleviate the depression, versus the risk of using two drugs, one of which may not be needed. Adult data cited in Chapter 19 suggest that the beginning of an antidepressant response to lamotrigine is often evident by 3 weeks, which may help in the decision-making process. Regarding the use of traditional antidepressants to treat early-onset depression, there is as yet no consensus in child psychiatry on the importance of trying a mood stabilizer first or even on the need to combine the antidepressant with a mood stabilizer. We have seen young people destabilized by antidepressants, as well as others kept on mood stabilizers alone in the face of persistent depression. Regarding some mood stabilizers, moreover, it should be noted that children and adolescents may balk at taking medication at all if blood must be drawn or if there is a possibility of weight gain. Thus the clarity of a history suggestive of a bipolar diathesis (including a clear history of bipolar disorder in first-degree relatives), the reliability of parent observation and the patient's adherence to treatment, and family preference should all be carefully weighed in the decision-making process.
- *Maintenance*—Results of the few extant maintenance studies suggest that even with good medical follow-up,

young people with bipolar disorder have higher relapse rates than adults. It is unclear whether this is because children have higher rates of rapid cycling (and therefore are comparable to rapid-cycling adults) and/or because the higher rates of illicit drug use common in young people increase relapse; erratic sleep patterns or other factors may contribute as well. Both the available data and clinical experience suggest, however, that if remission is achieved on a particular regimen, that regimen should be continued as long as possible, and at least until the patient has navigated his or her most important developmental, academic, and social milestones.

In the following sections, we present in greater detail our recommendations for acute treatment of mania/hypomania, mania/ADHD, and bipolar depression in children and adolescents; maintenance and psychosocial treatments in these populations; and prevention in at-risk youths.

Mania/Hypomania

How one initiates treatment for bipolar disorder in children and adolescents depends on whether the patient is acutely manic or hypomanic. Evidence is best for adolescents with mania, for whom randomized, double-blind, controlled trials of atypical antipsychotics have shown clear efficacy, as have large open trials of lithium. In smaller samples of children and adolescents with mania, hypomania, and bipolar disorder-not otherwise specified (NOS) and/or those at risk for bipolar disorder, there are placebo-controlled data on lithium, which is the only antimanic medication approved by the FDA for adolescents. Lithium's approval was "grandfathered" from the FDA's requirement for efficacy and safety data specifically on children and adolescents. Data from open studies exist for anticonvulsants and atypicals.

The guidelines of Kowatch and colleagues (2005) (described earlier) include two treatment algorithms for use when the mania presents with versus without psychosis. Here again, what follows is an integration of our own recommendations with these guidelines. When a child or adolescent presents with manic or mixed symptoms without psychosis, monotherapy is generally preferred initially, for reasons of safety. Treatment can be initiated with lithium, a sedating anticonvulsant (the most data exist for valproate),[3] or an atypical antipsychotic (such as olanzapine, quetiapine, or risperidone, for which the most data are available), while keeping in mind the adolescent's vulnerability to weight gain. If the clinical response is only partial, a drug of a different class should be used adjunctively (adding an atypical to a mood stabilizer or vice versa), with appropriate dose adjustments to minimize additive side effects. If there is no response to the initial monotherapy, we recommend switching to a drug of a different class (from lithium to an anticonvul-

sant, or from lithium or an anticonvulsant to an atypical). If the second agent fails to produce a satisfactory response, the evidence supports combined therapy (see the literature review below).

If the manic or mixed syndrome presents with psychotic features and/or prominent symptoms of severe agitation and aggression, we recommend that treatment be initiated with a combination of a mood stabilizer and an atypical antipsychotic. Based on data for adults, when a partial response is encountered under these circumstances, we recommend that a second mood stabilizer be added (for a total of three medications—an anticonvulsant, plus lithium, plus an atypical).

In the case of nonresponse (or intolerance) to the initial mood stabilizer/atypical combination, we recommend switching to an alternative mood stabilizer (lithium for anticonvulsant nonresponse/intolerance and vice versa). If there is still no response at this point, we recommend use of an alternative atypical agent or mood stabilizer.

For children and adolescents who have not responded to combination treatment involving three medications, we recommend clozapine. Haloperidol has also been used as an adjunctive treatment in several trials (Kafantaris et al., 2001). ECT is recommended for adolescents only, but for treatment refractory children with severe delusional depression, it may be justified (see the literature review below). Finally, although hospitalization is not a psychiatric medication, clinical experience suggests that some children and adolescents need the structure, decreased stimulation, or removal from stress that this intervention provides.

Differentiating Mania from ADHD

As noted earlier, it can be difficult to distinguish manic symptoms from those of severe ADHD in young people, particularly in the absence of clear *episodes* of mania. This is especially so in children, in whom mania tends to be chronic rather than episodic and is often comorbid with oppositional defiant disorder, a condition whose associated irritability and affective aggression are often indistinguishable from similar symptoms encountered in mania. Frequently, the classic manic symptoms of euphoria and grandiosity are not present. When they are, euphoria can be difficult to distinguish from the "class clown" antics of a child with ADHD, and grandiosity requires sufficient cognitive and linguistic maturity to understand the concept. Other symptoms of mania and ADHD overlap as well, such as talkativeness, hyperactivity–psychomotor agitation, and distractibility (Harrington and Myatt, 2003; Carlson et al., 2005). Although the specific criteria for ADHD appear to be different from those for mania (see Chapter 3), the overlap is heightened when ADHD-associated symptoms such as temper outbursts and mood lability are present (DSM-IV Text Revision [TR] p. 88).

The overlap between ADHD and mania raises three therapeutic questions. First, when both conditions occur, which should be treated first? Second, if it is unclear whether one is dealing with mania or severe ADHD and oppositional defiant disorder, which should be treated first? Third, if a child has an adverse response to a stimulant or atomoxetine, is that reaction suggestive of bipolar disorder? Some issues are clearer than others. When one is treating both mania and ADHD, results of clinical trials support treating the mania first, then proceeding with treatment for ADHD. Two small, systematic trials (Carlson et al., 1992; Scheffer et al., 2005) have examined combined treatment with a mood stabilizer and a stimulant. Neither found worsening of manic symptoms or significant side effects.

Atypical antipsychotics also appear to decrease rates of hyperactivity/impulsivity as measured by ADHD rating scales, although it is unclear whether this represents a nonspecific sedating effect. Teacher ratings and other measures of academic impact, which are traditionally part of efficacy studies in ADHD, have not been obtained. The implication of studies involving atypicals is that they can improve ADHD behavior through their ability to enhance cognitive organization, but this effect has not been studied formally. Clinically, it appears that additional specific ADHD treatment is often necessary.

When it is not clear whether the clinical picture reflects mania or ADHD with oppositional defiant disorder (or when a positive family history of mania indicates a risk for the development of bipolar disorder), we believe the clinician should talk with family members to advise them of the various alternatives and their risks. While there is concern that ADHD treatments may hasten the onset of bipolar disorder in children with ADHD and some manic symptoms (DelBello et al., 2001; Soutullo et al., 2002), more definitive data are needed on this critical question.

There are two important treatment issues—efficacy and adverse events. With regard to efficacy, in outpatient children who clearly have ADHD and also display some mood lability (which some call manic symptoms), limited data suggest that both the ADHD and "manic" symptoms not uncommonly show a robust response to stimulants immediately, as well as over the next 14 months (Galanter et al., 2003). Moreover, the majority of inpatient children with ADHD and manic symptoms studied systematically by Carlson and Kelly (1998) improved with and could tolerate stimulants, though stimulants alone clearly were inadequate to treat severely disruptive children with multiple comorbidities.

In contrast to its effectiveness in treating mania, the available data indicate that lithium is ineffective for the treatment of ADHD and mood lability (Greenhill et al., 1973; DeLong and Aldershof, 1987; Carlson et al., 1992a).

Moreover, even if lithium provides some benefit in treating aggression (see Steiner et al., 2003 and Table 23–1), it must be administered for at least 1 month to achieve this effect. Data on the use of anticonvulsants to treat ADHD are lacking, although there is some evidence of their efficacy in the treatment of affective aggression (see Table 23–1). Of interest, risperidone appears to be effective in treating both irritability and ADHD symptoms in cognitively impaired, irritable, aggressive children (Aman et al., 2002); added to stimulant medication, it produces significantly better control than stimulants alone in these patients.

With regard to adverse events, some children do not tolerate stimulants (or atomoxetine). Given its clinical importance, the paucity of data on this issue is surprising. Children who develop rebound on stimulant medication (i.e., a worsening of behavior as the medication wears off) (Carlson and Kelly, 2003) do not appear to have higher rates of bipolar disorder than of other disorders, although more data are needed. In a follow-back study of children with minimal brain dysfunction/hyperkinesis who were reinterviewed in young adulthood, there was no evidence that treatment response differed in those with childhood manic symptoms or that treatment triggered the onset of bipolar disorder in childhood or young adulthood (Carlson et al., 2000). Follow-up studies of children with ADHD who were treated with stimulants (Mannuzza et al., 1998) have not shown increased rates of bipolar disorder compared with controls—which would be expected if 16 to 20 percent of children with ADHD were misdiagnosed as having mania, as has been reported in some clinics (Wozniak et al., 1995; Biederman et al., 1996, 1998). In addition, there is suggestive evidence that young children, especially those with ADHD (L.L. Greenhill, personal communication, 2006), as well as those with pervasive developmental disorder, may be more sensitive to behavioral toxicity in general, including mood and behavioral instability (Carlson and Mick, 2003; Carlson et al., 2005). In other words, young people with bipolar disorder may well worsen on stimulants, but not everyone whose behavior worsens on stimulants has bipolar disorder. Although it is prudent to discontinue a medication that worsens a child's behavior, data are as yet inadequate to support the conclusion that acute behavioral toxicity predicts the development of a subsequent bipolar course.

In summary, then, for a child whose dominant symptoms clearly reflect ADHD (as distinct from a mood disorder), we recommend treatment with a stimulant first. If the child's behavior clearly becomes worse, either on the medication or after it wears off, addition of a mood stabilizer or an atypical antipsychotic is advised. It should be noted that adjunctive atypicals cannot be recommended for long-term maintenance treatment in the same way that

TABLE 23–1. Controlled Studies of Aggression Lasting at Least 4 Weeks

Study	Sample Size	Age (yr)	Diagnosis	Medication	Duration	Measures	Outcome[a]
Lithium							
Campbell et al., 1984	61	9	CD/aggression (inpatient)	Lithium compared with haloperidol	6 wk	CPRS	Lithium and haloperidol both better than placebo
Campbell et al., 1995	50	9	CD/aggression (inpatient)	Lithium	1 mo	CPRS	Lithium better than placebo
Malone et al., 2000	40	12.5	CD	Lithium	6 wk	CGI, OAS	Lithium better than placebo
Divalproex							
Donovan et al., 2000	20	10–18	CD, ODD	Divalproex	12 wk	OAS, SCL 90	Divalproex better than placebo
Steiner et al., 2003	58 males	16	CD	Divalproex low vs. high dose	8 wk	CGI severity, CGI improvement	53% responders with high dose vs. 8% with low dose
Risperidone							
Findling et al., 2000	20	6–14	CD	Risperidone	10 wk	Rating of Aggression against People and Property Scale	Risperidone better than placebo
Buitelaar et al., 2001	38	Adolescent (IQs 36–84)	Disruptive behavior disorders	Risperidone	6 wk	CGI Severity Overt Aggression Scale-Modified Aberrant Behavior Checklist	Risperidone better than placebo overall and on hyperactivity scales
Aman et al., 2002	118	5–12 (IQs 36–84)	Disruptive behavior disorders	Risperidone	6 wk	Nisonger Child Behavior Rating	46.2% change relative to baseline on risperidone vs. 18% on placebo

a"Better than" indicates a statistically significant difference at the $p < .05$ level or better.

CD = conduct disorder; CGI = Clinical Global Impressions scale; CPRS = Comprehensive Psychopathological Rating Scale; IQ = intelligence quotient; OAS = Overt Aggression Scale; ODD = oppositional defiant disorder; SCL = symptom checklist.

one would recommend mood stabilizers for youths with clear bipolar disorder.

Bipolar Depression

In young people, as in adults, there have been far more attempts to study treatment response in mania than in bipolar depression. The few studies in which lithium or adjunctive lithium was administered to depressed prepubertal children or adolescents with or without predictors of future bipolarity have demonstrated little or no efficacy. While further studies under controlled conditions are needed, recommendations for adults with bipolar depression appear to be relevant to pediatric populations, at least to adolescents. On the other hand, antidepressant responses in children do not necessarily mirror those in adults (placebo responses are more frequent, and drug responses may differ), so direct extrapolation becomes more tenuous.[4]

Emerging data on adults with bipolar depression suggest that mood stabilizers, such as lamotrigine, can stabilize primarily against depression (that is, "from below"; see Chapter 20), apparently without destabilizing the illness. In adults, bupropion is often cited as having advantages for the treatment of bipolar depression since it appears to have a lower switch rate (perhaps because it has little or no disruptive effect on sleep when given early in the day) and a favorable clinical profile for most bipolar patients (especially those with psychomotor retardation). Bupropion also has the most benign side-effect profile of any antidepressant. For this reason, it may be especially suitable for young patients, who tend to be more sensitive than adults to side effects. Thus in the absence of data, but based on clinical experience (including that with adults), the consensus panel (Kowatch et al., 2005) recommended using bupropion or an SSRI adjunctively with a mood stabilizer when treating bipolar depression in youths.

More problematic is treatment of depression when future bipolarity is uncertain. In adolescents, bipolar illness commonly starts with depression rather than mania, a fact that is troubling clinically because of the risk of precipitating a manic episode in a vulnerable patient by using antidepressants. This concern escalates in the case of a seriously depressed young person with a history of bipolar disorder in first-degree relatives. As with ADHD and mania, scant controlled data exist on which to base advice on the treatment of early-onset depression when the possibility of converting to a bipolar course is uncertain. Results of follow-up studies of clinical samples of children and adolescents with depression indicate that on average, 20 percent subsequently develop bipolar disorder, with a range of 6 percent (Weissman et al., 1999a) to 48.6 percent (Geller et al., 2001)[5] (see Chapter 6). Thus the clinician using an antidepressant

without a mood stabilizer to treat young people with serious depression (or even dysthymia) must be mindful of the risk that they will develop bipolar disorder or at least mood/behavioral instability (sometimes referred to as "roughening"). Although the odds ratio for subsequent bipolar disorder in offspring of bipolar parents is higher than that for unipolar depression, this differential is influenced by the fact that rates of mania in the general population are much lower than those of depressive disorder.[6] In fact, more offspring of bipolar parents develop depression than bipolar disorder (LaPalme al., 1997; Meyer et al., 2004), although clearly the lengthy age range of risk for developing mania makes this statistic an unstable one.

The clinician, then, must weigh the modest but important risk of patients' becoming bipolar against the greater likelihood of their having a nonbipolar depression (although the possibility of antidepressants inducing unipolar cycling, as has been suggested for adults with recurrent unipolar depression, should be kept in mind). For children and adolescents at risk for the development of bipolar disorder or destabilization, there are two questions embedded in the treatment dilemma. The first is whether to use an antidepressant even with a concomitant mood stabilizer. The second is how to understand psychiatric adverse events that may occur as a result of antidepressant exposure including manic symptoms (drug-induced mania), activation/disinhibition (which may be different from mania), long-term cycle induction, and suicidal behavior. Unfortunately, assessment of these events has not been well operationalized in medication studies in children and adolescents (Carlson, 2005).

To summarize some treatment implications for early-onset depression, a trial of lamotrigine may make sense when there is a strong suggestion of a bipolar diathesis. Other choices are combinations of an antidepressant with an antimanic mood stabilizer or with an atypical antipsychotic, although it has not been established that such agents protect against antidepressant-related mania and/or destabilization in pediatric populations (Baumer et al., 2006). If the parents and/or the child are especially concerned about the use of a mood stabilizer or antipsychotic, antidepressant medication alone may sometimes be used, provided that the child does not have both a bipolar first-degree relative and evidence of subthreshold bipolarity, and provided that there is adequate discussion of the risks and benefits involved, and that the child is monitored carefully.

Maintenance Treatment

Maintenance trials are generally undertaken after definitive acute studies have been conducted. Since data from acute trials of treatment of bipolar children and adolescents are just beginning to emerge, it is not surprising that information on maintenance treatment in these populations is sparse. The one study designed to test lithium or valproate as maintenance monotherapy in children and adolescents who had been stabilized on the combination failed to establish the superiority of either drug. As discussed later, the relapse rate to mania was high with both medications (Findling et al., 2005).

Despite the lack of data on the efficacy of maintenance treatment, the consensus panel observed that, given the high lifetime recurrence rates for untreated bipolar disorder, medication should be recommended for the long term for patients with well-documented bipolar disorder (Kowatch et al., 2005). We would add that the foundation of maintenance treatment should be a mood stabilizer. Moreover, patients and families should be educated about both the high rate of relapse in young people and the especially noxious contribution of illicit drugs. When the prospect of lifetime medication appears overwhelming, we encourage patients to continue drug therapy until they have completed high school, college, or trade school or are beyond an anticipated major life stressor (e.g., starting a new job, getting married). If the patient and/or family insists on discontinuing medication, this should be undertaken very gradually and at a time when it will have the least impact on life, and ongoing monitoring and social support will be available to provide for prompt referral should an episode occur. The recommendation that any discontinuation be undertaken very gradually is based on evidence of an increased likelihood of mania (Suppes et al., 1991) and of severe suicide attempts among adults following after rapid versus gradual discontinuation of lithium (Baldessarini et al., 1999). In cases where the diagnosis is less clear, the decision on medication continuation should be based on how successful the treatment is in mitigating symptoms. Continuation of medications providing marginal benefit in the face of high rates of adverse events is not recommended.

Based on results of clinical trials in adults, the consensus panel supported the efficacy of lithium, lamotrigine, and olanzapine as maintenance treatments for youths (Kowatch et al., 2005). The advantage of lamotrigine is its benign side-effect profile, noted earlier. Agents with high side-effect profiles, particularly weight gain (e.g., olanzapine, valproate, and lithium) and neurocognitive impairment (e.g., lithium and valproate), are more likely to lead to poor adherence (and, in the case of weight gain, to medical complications).

When the diagnosis of bipolar disorder is more tenuous, the presence of baseline ratings of irritability/mood instability, depression, and executive dysfunction (all of which can occur in children with ADHD), along with periodic reassessment of those ratings, will help determine how effective mood stabilizer treatment is and therefore how vigorously

to maintain it. Obviously, the less robust the treatment response, the more reason there is to discontinue medications associated with significant adverse events. Recommendations for the use of antipsychotics to treat aggression in children and adolescents have been discussed by Schur and colleagues (2003) and Pappadapulos and colleagues (2003).

It is premature to draw conclusions about the clinical or pharmacological significance of apparent drug-related "activation" in young people because the data on this issue are so limited. How specifically to address the issue depends on what the symptoms are, how severe they are, and how effective the medication is. Choices obviously range from stopping the drug, to lowering the dose and/or changing the dosing schedule, to adding another medication that mitigates the unwanted symptoms. Before any medication is initiated, families should always be warned about the potential for psychiatric adverse events, with particular caution being exercised for young children; those with developmental disabilities; and those with preexisting problems involving severe emotional dysregulation, such as ADHD and bipolar disorder.

Psychosocial Treatments

Psychosocial treatments have an important complementary role to play in the treatment of bipolar disorder in young people. The reasons for this include (1) the impact of the disorder on overall functioning in school and within the family, (2) the high rates of comorbidity and treatment nonadherence in these patients (one study, for example, found nonadherence rates of 31 percent, even over a short, 6-week trial [Kowatch et al., 2000]), and (3) higher-than-normal rates of family psychopathology (see Chapter 22). Research supports the importance of both psychoeducation and approaches aimed at reducing "expressed emotion" within the family (i.e., destructive criticism that sometimes characterizes families with mental illness).

There are a number of common themes in three promising family therapy treatments developed for children (Fristad et al., 2003; Pavuluri et al., 2004a) and adolescents (Miklowitz et al., 2004). The underpinnings consist of psychoeducation and problem solving within a cognitive-behavioral framework. The premise of the former is that if parents are given information about the biology of bipolar disorder, they will be less likely to blame each other and/or their children, allowing a greater focus on positive solutions. Additionally, by educating families about aspects of the disorder that are worsened by environmental stresses (disordered routine, decreased sleep, harsh criticism, parental fighting and inconsistency) and by helping families develop constructive ways of solving problems, many aspects of the illness can be brought under more effective control.

Prevention in At-Risk Youth

Do early intervention and treatment ameliorate the course of bipolar disorder? The potential for preventive intervention has been raised by the emerging hypothesis that bipolar disorder is a progressive neurobiological process (see Chapter 14). However, clinical research has not yet reached the point of testing pharmacological and/or psychological therapies for their preventive potential. One first step would be to develop a reliable means of identifying children and adolescents in the prodromal phases of bipolar disorder. In the meantime, two trials involving children of adults with bipolar-I and -II disorder have been completed. One small, open trial conducted by Chang and colleagues (2003) showed promise for the use of valproate in children who were experiencing mood and behavior difficulties, but not yet bipolar disorder. In the other trial, Findling and colleagues (2001) failed to demonstrate the efficacy of valproate, although improvement was suggested in children whose parents both had bipolar disorder. While this is a vitally important issue, it is not possible as yet to recommend evidence-based, specific clinical management strategies beyond those that would be recommended for children with known psychopathology in a population not "at risk."

REVIEW OF THE LITERATURE

In this section we review the literature behind the clinical management strategies recommended above. Our focus, by virtue of the nature of the available evidence, is on clinical trials of pharmacological treatments for acute mania—lithium, anticonvulsants, and atypical antipsychotics—as well as drug combinations; we also touch briefly on the efficacy of these treatments for aggression in pediatric populations. We then discuss in turn the findings of the literature on treatment of bipolar depression, maintenance treatment, offspring of adults with bipolar disorder, psychiatric adverse events, medical adverse events, ECT, and psychotherapies.

Treatment of Acute Mania

As discussed previously, the overall evidence base for treating pediatric bipolar disorder in general and acute mania in particular is sparse when compared with the extensive database from studies of adults, as reviewed in Chapter 18. There have been a few placebo-controlled studies of lithium involving a small number of children or adolescents, most of whom had conditions other than acute mania (see the later discussion). Five industry-sponsored clinical trials of medications for children and/or adolescents with acute mania have been completed: topiramate versus placebo

(DelBello et al., 2006); quetiapine versus divalproex (DelBello et al., 2006), oxcarbazepine versus placebo (Wagner et al., 2006), olanzapine versus placebo (Tohen et al., 2006), and divalproex-extended release (ER) versus placebo (data on file, Abbott Laboratories, December 2006). The largest lithium studies have been open trials, some involving hospitalized adolescents with acute mania (Kafantaris et al., 2004) and some involving outpatient children and adolescents with mania/hypomania or bipolar-NOS or children considered at risk for developing bipolar disorder. Placebo-controlled trials of other atypical antipsychotics (risperidone, aripiprazole, ziprasidone) and anticonvulsants (valproate) approved for adults are ongoing as of this writing. There have also been open and discontinuation studies. As noted earlier, there has been one controlled trial of maintenance therapy (Findling et al., 2005).

Table 23–2 summarizes the currently available information for children and adolescents on drugs used to treat mania in adults, organized by the level of evidence. As noted in the table, safety data are available for several other medications (anticonvulsants) because they are approved for the treatment of convulsive disorders in youths. Placebo-controlled trials in mania have not yet established efficacy for any of the anticonvulsants or the atypical antipsychotics; hence they have not been approved by the FDA for this purpose. The FDA has requested that drug sponsors conduct more clinical trials in youths, and NIMH is also supporting treatment trials. Although the following summary reflects considerable advances since the first edition of this text was published, the evidence base, including placebo-controlled trials, is expected to grow considerably over the next decade. In addition to the traditional randomized, placebo-controlled designs, there is a need for more practical, "clinician-friendly" trials (see Chapter 17), such as crossover and randomized open comparative studies that can assess differences in tolerability (and perhaps even efficacy) (Post and Kowatch, 2006). As Post and colleagues pointed out (2002), such designs are more likely to be accepted by parents, especially when very young children are involved.

Lithium

Early Lithium Trials. The earliest studies of lithium in young people were case reports involving episodic illness. Annell (1969) noted: "We began using lithium at the Department of Child and Youth Psychiatry in Uppsala in 1965 . . . for older adolescents and for typical manic conditions; but as time went on, we began giving it to younger patients and for conditions other than typical mania. All . . . had severe mental complaints and all showed sudden changes in their conditions during the course of the year." The 12 youths on whom Annell reported were aged 9 to 18,

TABLE 23–2. **Summary of Evidence for Drugs Used to Treat Mania in Children and Adolescents**

Drug	Status as Treatment for Bipolar Disorder
Lithium	U.S. Food and Drug Administration (FDA) approved for treatment of mania in adults and in youths aged 12 and above. Placebo-controlled trials in samples that included some children and adolescents with acute mania, but acute mania was not specifically studied; results mixed. Otherwise, open and discontinuation trials with mostly positive results.
Divalproex	FDA approved for treatment of mania in adults. Safety data in youths because of approval for treatment of seizures. For mania in children and adolescents, positive open trials, discontinuation trials, add-on trial, and randomized comparator trials. The one placebo-controlled trial (divalproex-extended release [ER]) was negative.
Carbamazepine	Off label in adults and children. Safety data in youths because of approval as anticonvulsant in children and adolescents. For mania, open randomized trial and case reports in children and adolescents with positive results.
Topiramate	Off label in adults and children. Some safety data because of approval for partial-onset seizures in children aged 2–16 years. For mania, one placebo-controlled trial in children and adolescents aged 6–17 years; inconclusive results because underpowered.
Oxcarbazepine	Off label in adults and children. Some safety data in youths because of approval as adjunctive treatment for partial complex seizures in youths aged 4–16 years. For mania, case reports.
Risperidone	FDA approved for mania in adults. Chart review series, positive open trials, positive add-on trial, placebo-controlled trials in children with irritable aggression associated with conduct disorder and autism, ongoing industry-sponsored randomized controlled trial for youths aged 10–17 years.
Olanzapine	FDA approved for mania in adults. In children and adolescents, 10 positive open trials and case reports. Randomized controlled trial found olanzapine significantly better than placebo.
Quetiapine	FDA approved in adults for treatment of mania. In adolescents, positive add-on study and randomized comparison with divalproex; ongoing randomized controlled trial for youths aged 10–17 years.
Ziprasidone	FDA approved in adults for treatment of mania. In children and adolescents, chart reviews and small case series. Randomized controlled trial under way in youths aged 10–17 years.
Aripiprazole	FDA approved in adults for treatment of mania. In children and adolescents, chart reviews. Randomized controlled trial under way for youths aged 10–17 years.
Clozapine	FDA approved only for treatment-resistant schizophrenia in adults. Off label for mania in adults. In children and adolescents, case series.
Lamotrigine	FDA approved for maintenance treatment of adults with bipolar-I disorder to delay time to occurrence of mood episodes (depression, mania, hypomania, mixed states). Safety data in youths because approved for patients aged 2 and older with simple or complex partial seizures. For bipolar disorder, chart review and one positive open study for bipolar depression in adolescents.
Symbyax (combined olanzapine and fluoxetine)	FDA approved for treatment of bipolar depression in adults. No studies of bipolar depression in children and adolescents, although fluoxetine is FDA approved for treatment of major depression in children and adolescents.

although onset had occurred at ages as young as 7.5 years; 25 percent of the sample (*n*=3) were younger than age 12. Of the 11 youths for whom follow-up data were available, 7 responded very positively; the responders consisted of both children and adolescents. Only 2 responders showed typical mania (dominated by euphoria and grandiosity), but all had experienced the clearly demarcated onset of a condition distinctly different from their premorbid state.

Most had family members with manic-depressive illness. Not long thereafter, a much wider net was cast to find subjects with psychopathological conditions and a positive family history who might be responsive to lithium.

In an early summary of the possible effectiveness of lithium in young people, most cases were not even considered bipolar disorder in today's terminology. Reviewing the extant case reports and studies, Youngerman and Canino

(1978) found 211 cases; of these, there was sufficient information for only 46 to allow tentative conclusions about the reasons lithium was used. Twenty-two patients were children: 2 had "manic-depressive illness," 2 had an "atypical mood disorder," 8 were hyperkinetic, and 10 had autism/childhood schizophrenia. Twenty-four of the 46 were adolescents: 9 had "manic-depressive illness," 13 had "atypical mood disorder," and 2 had hyperkinesis. Thus, there were very few studies of children or even adolescents who could be considered bipolar. Even placebo-controlled trials had heterogeneous subjects and few with classic bipolar disorder. Samples encompassed youths with a variety of psychotic-like and developmental disorders (Gram and Rafaelsen, 1972), hyperkinesis and equivocal stimulant response (Dyson and Barcai, 1970; Greenhill et al., 1973), and autism and schizophrenia (Campbell et al., 1972), as well as offspring of lithium-responding parents (McKnew et al., 1981).

Several observations can be made about these early studies of lithium in youths: (1) the rarity of classic bipolar disorder in children compared with adolescents; (2) the early interest in trying to find a symptom constellation, especially in younger children, that would be lithium responsive; and (3) the poor treatment response in these subjects, which may have deterred clinicians from conducting more studies. Early studies in adults, whose samples appeared equally heterogeneous, showed higher response rates. These results with adults were promising enough to encourage not just further investigation, but a whole revolution in treatment. The fact that the response rates were highest in adults with what is considered classic manic-depressive illness (bipolar disorder and recurrent unipolar depression) may explain why young people, whose presentation is less likely to be classic, were less likely to respond.

Placebo-controlled lithium trials that occurred prior to the first edition of this volume are summarized in Table 23–3. Those occurring since the first edition are listed in Table 23–4.

Lithium Treatment for Mania in Hospitalized Adolescents.

Although lithium has been used in young people for more than 40 years, there have been no published randomized, double-blind, placebo-controlled studies of adolescents meeting DSM-IV criteria for acute mania. One placebo-controlled discontinuation study has been conducted (Kafantaris et al., 2004), and other studies are in progress. The largest open trial (Kafantaris et al., 2003) involved 100 adolescents initially hospitalized for mania and treated with lithium over 4 weeks; 55 percent were responders, as defined by a 50 percent reduction in scores on the Young Mania Rating Scale (YMRS). If the psychotic or aggressive manic adolescents received an adjunctive antipsychotic, the response rate improved to 65 percent. Of interest, 40 of

the responders to open lithium monotherapy were subsequently randomized under double-blind conditions to placebo or continued lithium and followed for 2 weeks (Kafantaris et al., 2004); both groups relapsed at about the same rate—52.6 percent of those on lithium and 61.9 percent of those on placebo. The adolescents who relapsed on lithium in the blind phase were subsequently restabilized on lithium under open conditions (V. Kafantaris, personal communication, 2006). It is likely that in the double-blind phase, the investigators tended to withdraw patients on blind lithium from the trial prematurely if they were showing even mild breakthrough symptoms (perhaps assuming that any given patient might be on placebo), and thus these lithium patients were scored as relapses even though they went on to respond to open lithium.

In an open study of manic adolescents, the response rate to lithium (defined as a 33 percent reduction in YMRS scores and a Clinical Global Impressions [CGI] rating of 1 or 2) was 53.5 percent; the presence of prior ADHD made no difference in the likelihood of responding to the drug (Kafantaris et al., 1998). On the other hand, psychotic features were associated with a significantly lower response rate. Subsequently, the same group treated 42 hospitalized manic adolescents with both lithium and antipsychotic medication. Ultimately, of 28 adolescents who completed at least 4 weeks of treatment, only 14 were judged clinically stable enough to discontinue their antipsychotic medication. Of these 14, only 8 maintained their response on lithium monotherapy for an additional 4 weeks (sustained responders). The other 6 experienced a clinically significant exacerbation of symptoms on lithium monotherapy and resumed treatment with their adjunctive antipsychotic (Kafantaris et al., 2001).

There have been two systematic case series of hospitalized manic adolescents. Strober and colleagues (1988, 1998) found response rates of 67 to 80 percent in adolescents with classic mania, while response rates in manic adolescents with a prior history of ADHD were lower (33 to 40 percent). An 18-month naturalistic follow-up study of adolescents who had discontinued lithium (because of nonadherence) after inpatient stabilization revealed that 90 percent had relapsed, compared with only 37.5 percent of those who had remained on lithium (Strober et al., 1990). Whether this result reflects the effectiveness of lithium or simply the difference between adherent and nonadherent youngsters cannot be determined for this nonrandomized study.

Lithium Treatment for Mania in Hospitalized Children.

There have been two clinical trials of lithium in hospitalized children with mania or manic-like symptoms. In the first, 11 patients with bipolar-NOS were treated with lithium and tested by a trained rater, teachers, and nursing staff at baseline, 4 weeks, and 8 weeks (7 of these children also

TABLE 23–3. Early Placebo-Controlled Trials of Lithium in Children and Adolescents with a Variety of Conditions

Study	Sample	Psychopathology Addressed	Methodology	Results	Comments
Gram and Rafaelsen, 1972	$N=18$; ages 8–22 yr; 13 males, 5 females; pupils at a special school in Denmark	"Psychosis or pronounced psychotic traits"; 7 with autism/pervasive developmental disorder, 2 "borderline," 2 psychosis, 1 personality disorder, 1 speech and language disorder	2 groups: lithium for 6 mo, then placebo, and vice versa; parent/teacher ratings on 11 items: hyper- or hypoactivity, elevated or depressed mood, anxiety, obsessive behavior or stereotypies, speech disturbances, aggression to others/self, concentration, school performance	8 unchanged; 1 best on placebo, 9 best on lithium, 7 worsened when lithium stopped; significant improvement by chi square $p<.001$; "no patient became totally free of symptoms"; symptoms improving included aggression, depressed/elevated mood, speech disturbances and stereotypies in school	In current nosology, these youths had autism or psychotic spectrum disorders; none were bipolar, but mood component was important anyway; response rate 50%, meaning improvement but not cure
Campbell et al., 1972	$N=10$; ages 3–6 yr; inpatients	Severely disturbed preschoolers; developmental quotient <60 in 50%; mostly autistic/pervasive developmental disorder; 2 "hyperkinetic," 1 "organic" with "withdrawing reaction"	Children matched on hyperactivity and hypoactivity; lithium compared with carbamazepine; 7–10 wk for each drug, 4 wk drug free before the crossover; lithium levels .25–1.19 mEq/L; carbamazepine about 90 mg	Using global improvement: lithium—1 with marked, 4 with slight, 5 with no improvement and 1 worse; carbamazepine—3 with marked, 6 with slight (1 received thiothixine), 1 with no change; $p=$ not significant (ns); lithium may have improved explosiveness, aggressiveness, hyperactivity, psychotic speech	"Margin between toxic and optimal" doses small; improvement did not outweigh toxicity; a very difficult population to treat, however
Greenhill et al., 1973	$N=9$; ages 7–14 yr; hospitalized for study at National Institute of Mental Health, then outpatient for 6 wk	Hyperactive children unresponsive to stimulant medication by parent history; 2 "unsocialized aggressive," 5 hyperactive–immature–inadequate labile type, 2 no diagnosis stated but looked equally labile and hyperactive by case report	Conners rating scale by nurses/teachers; "blind" psychiatrist-made global ratings; 2 stages: (1) 1 wk single-blind placebo, dextroamphetamine, lithium; (2) randomly alternating 3-wk trials of each condition; children seen at home, school, outpatient department visits	On dextroamphetamine: 3 improved, 3 slightly improved, 3 worse (including one delusional); on lithium, 5 worse, 1 no change, 1 dropout, 2 markedly improved (with deterioration after lithium was stopped), but improvement not sustained over the next 3 mo; Conners scale failed to detect differences	No attempt to call these youths bipolar, but addressed whether very hyperactive youths with a history of poor stimulant response would improve on lithium; they did not

Study	Sample	Diagnosis/Characteristics	Design	Results	Comments
DeLong, 1978	$N=12$, although only 4 were placebo controlled; ages 4–14 yr; outpatient	Disruptive, nonpsychotic behavior problems, rages/aggression, or cyclical behavior patterns	Open trial involving 12 children; all improved by parent ratings; 4 who had been stable for 9–21 mo had a placebo crossover	All 4 deteriorated on placebo and improved when lithium was resumed	A discontinuation study of children who had already improved
McKnew et al., 1981	$N=6$; ages 9–12 yr; outpatient	Offspring of lithium-responding parents: 2 with bipolar-II, 2 unipolar (1 mother, 1 grandmother), 2 with bipolar-I (1 mother, 1 father); parents all comorbid; children: 2 with bipolar mixed, 3 with attention-deficit hyperactivity disorder (ADHD) and mood problems, 1 with recurrent major depressive disorder (MDD)	Double-blind crossover design; 16–18 wk with 2 placebo periods; seen weekly; rated on the Child Psychiatric Rating Scale and Children's Affective Rating Scale; Clinical Global Impressions (CGI) ratings using information from both parent and child	2 children with bipolar disorder definitely improved; 2 children improved on some ratings by some raters (i.e., equivocal response); 2 children, including 1 with ADHD and cyclothymia and 1 with recurrent MDD, did not improve	Very small, very heterogeneous sample; it did not appear that parent mood or response status predicted anything in this small sample

TABLE 23–4. Contemporary Placebo-Controlled Trials of Lithium in Children and Adolescents

Study	Sample	Psychopathology Addressed	Methodology	Results	Comments
Carlson et al., 1992a	$N=11$; ages 5 yr 11 mo to 12 yr 10 mo; inpatient	K-SADS ADHD/ODD; severe aggression; bipolar symptoms; YMRS scores 15–35 in 10 children, 1 child with YMRS score of 12 had "episodic ADHD"; inadequate response to stimulant or severe rebound or depression	11 children completed an 8-wk trial of lithium, with ratings by staff and teachers at baseline, 4 wk, and 8 wk; 7 children treated with methylphenidate (MPH) alone and with adjunctive lithium and MPH, with a placebo discontinuation phase at the end of the study	Lithium alone produced modest changes in YMRS and CDRS-R scores, but no relapse off lithium; adjunctive MPH appeared to act synergistically with lithium by nurses' ratings of inattention, but lithium blocked MPH improvements on computerized laboratory measures	It was not possible to discriminate milieu response from lithium response because children did not relapse when lithium was stopped; over-all response modest compared with the psychopathology of the children
Geller et al., 1998	$N=25$; ages 12–18 yr; outpatient	Teenagers with any kind of substance abuse and comorbid bipolar-I, bipolar-II, or major depressive disorder with risk for developing bipolar disorder; specific mood state not mentioned	Diagnosis by K-SADS; CGI score improvement >65 was outcome measure; randomized trial, 6 wk, 4 wk on lithium; "interpersonal therapy" in both groups	21 subjects completed; 6/10 lithium group responded (60%) vs. 1/12 (9.3%) on placebo ($p=.046$); no measures of mood outcome	Although this is always cited as a double-blind, placebo-controlled study of lithium in bipolar disorder, it did not address the treatment of pure bipolar disorder per se
Kafantaris et al., 2004	$N=40$; ages 12–18 yr; initially inpatient	Met criteria for current manic episode; YMRS score >16	Open trial of lithium or lithium + antipsychotic for 4 wk, then lithium alone; 19 randomized to take lithium, 21 to placebo after a 3 day tapering off period	YMRS scores dropped from a mean of 25.62 (7.37) to 8.53 (5.53), CGI scores from 4.95 (.85) to 2.68 (.89) during open phase; 52.6% on lithium and 61.9% on placebo got "worse or very much worse"; no difference (i.e., no protection) with lithium	Discharge could have complicated findings; ethical concerns may have necessitated a quick stop to the study; or lithium may not work well in hospitalized teens

ADHD=attention-deficit hyperactivity disorder; CDRS-R=Children's Depression Rating Scale-Revised; CGI=Clinical Global Impressions scale; K-SADS=Kiddie Schedule for Affective Disorders and Schizophrenia; ODD=oppositional defiant disorder; YMRS=Young Mania Rating Scale.

received adjunctive methylphenidate [MPH] between their first and second lithium testing periods, during which they received no medication, as well as placebo at the end of the study). Patients, nursing staff, and raters were blinded to the medication condition (Carlson et al., 1992b). Results were mixed. Improvement in YMRS scores at 4 weeks was not sustained at 8 weeks, while scores on the Children's Depression Rating Scale-Revised (CDRS-R) (depression) improved by 8 weeks relative to scores at 4 weeks (Poznanski et al., 1984). Greater improvement was seen in teachers' ratings of self-control (Teacher Self Control Rating Scale [Humphrey, 1982]) than in nurses' ratings at both 4 and 8 weeks. Since most improvement did not reverse when lithium was discontinued, nonspecific improvement due to hospitalization was believed to account for some of the improvement observed. The sample size was limited because of the advent of managed care (Carlson et al., 1992a). The second trial of lithium was open and involved 10 prepubertal children identified as acutely manic and psychotic. All showed a "positive clinical response" to the drug (Varanka et al., 1988).

Lithium Treatment for Mania in Outpatient Settings. An old but large *case series* of lithium-treated children and adolescents was reported by two research neurologists who collected data on 196 such patients over the course of 10 years. DeLong and Aldershof (1987) divided their outpatient sample into those with clear mood disorder and those with other disorders with manic-like symptoms. They determined response based on whether patients were continued on the drug over a 10-month period. The duration of follow-up was highly variable but appeared to average about 3.5 years. Two-thirds (39/59) of the "classic" bipolar youths remitted on lithium, and one-third of those who remitted remained well after lithium was stopped. Lesser responses were seen in youths with unipolar depression (5/29, 17 percent), ADHD with affective symptoms (3/8, 38 percent, with 5 considered "worsened"), and explosive/aggressive behavior (5/9, 56 percent). The children with ADHD and affective symptoms all discontinued lithium without further problems. A modest percentage (5/21, 29 percent) of rageful, autistic/developmentally or neurologically impaired young people improved, but at the expense of high rates of serious side effects.

Formal outpatient *trials* of bipolar children and adolescents are more common than inpatient trials, but the samples are somewhat more heterogeneous, both diagnostically and by age. Here we review only those trials that used a systematic assessment for diagnosis and had a large enough sample size to allow interpretation of treatment response. A 6-month open trial of either lithium or valproate in combination with risperidone was conducted by Pavuluri and

colleagues (2004b). The study included 37 subjects aged 5 to 18 with mania or mixed episodes of bipolar disorder. Using three outcome measures (YMRS, CGI-Bipolar [CGI-BP], and CDRS-R), the researchers found lithium in combination with risperidone to be as effective as valproate plus risperidone. Both combination therapies were well tolerated. In a double-blind, placebo-controlled study, Geller and colleagues (1998a) administered lithium over 6 weeks to 11 substance-abusing adolescents with various bipolar diagnoses (bipolar-I, bipolar-II, and major depressive disorder with "bipolar predictors"). Response was defined as a score of 65 or higher on the Children's Global Assessment Scale (Shaffer et al., 1983) (at study entry, the average score was 38). The response rate was higher in lithium-treated adolescents than in those receiving placebo.

Anticonvulsants

Several controlled and uncontrolled trials of valproate and other anticonvulsants have been conducted in various inpatient or outpatient populations (see Tables 23–5 and 23–6). A number of open studies and chart reviews of valproate had results encouraging enough to stimulate controlled trials in outpatients.[7] The numbers studied were small, however, and the studies suffered from the usual methodological problems (see Table 23–5).

There have been several positive open-label trials with a reasonable sample size in which children and adolescents were treated with divalproex alone or in combination with other medications (see Table 23–6). One was a trial of divalproex in 40 children and adolescents, 61 percent of whom improved (>50 percent decline in YMRS score) over the 8 to 10 weeks of initial stabilization. However, the study had been designed as a discontinuation trial and was hampered by the fact that 23 of 40 subjects had to discontinue prior to randomization because of poor efficacy, inability to discontinue concomitant lithium or haloperidol as required, nonadherence, or refusal to continue in the study once stable (Wagner et al., 2002). Pavuluri and colleagues (2005) reported the results of an open trial of divalproex in 34 children and adolescents with mania or mixed mania. They found that 73.5 percent responded (≥50 percent decline from baseline YMRS score and ≤40 score on CDRS-R), and 52.9 percent remitted.

A randomized, open-label, 8-week trial compared the benefits of lithium, divalproex, and carbamazepine in 42 outpatient youths aged 8 to 18 (Kowatch et al., 2000). Twenty of the subjects had bipolar-I and 22 bipolar-II; 71 percent had comorbid ADHD, among other comorbidities. Forty-six percent of subjects responded to divalproex, 42 percent to lithium, and 34 percent to carbamazepine, with response defined as a 50 percent reduction in YMRS score and designation as improved or very much improved on

TABLE 23–5. Open Acute Trials of Divalproex in Children and Adolescents with Manic or Mixed States

Author	Sample and Type of Study	Diagnosis, Measures, and Duration of Trial/Study	Other Medications Taken	Doses and Levels	Response and Adverse Events
West et al., 1994	$N = 11$; ages 12–17 yr; open add-on trial; mean age 14.5; 9 M, 2 F; inpatients accrued over 10 mo	DSM-III-R bipolar mixed state or mania diagnosed by SCID, mean YMRS score 19; 63.4% comorbid ADHD; duration: valproate treatment over 6–26 days	Haloperidol—63.4%, perphenazine—36.4%, thioridazine—9%, lithium—45.5%; divalproex added to these medications	Dose range 500–2,000 mg/day, mean 1068 mg; valproate levels 38–91 µg/ml	Mild improvement—18.2%, moderate improvement—54.5%, marked improvement—27.3%; sedation in 2 cases
Papatheodorou et al., 1995	$N = 15$ (13 finished); ages 12–20 yr, mean age 17.3; 13 F, 2 M; open trial inpatient, then outpatient	Bipolar mixed state or mania diagnosed by K-SADS, Blackburn Mania Scale, MMRS, BPRS, GAS, CGI	Only Practice Research Network (PRN) chlorpromazine allowed	Dose range 750–2,000 mg/day; mean 1,423 mg; mean blood level 64.2 µg/ml	MMRS drop: 69.54 → 18.08; BPRS drop: 36.31 → 12.0; CGI impairment drop: 5.4 → 2.4; GAS increase: 30.0 → 55.0; valproate side-effect scale drop: 11.8 → 5.5 (subjects felt better, reported fewer side effects); adverse events: 1 transient liver enzyme elevation; 1 developed hypothyroidism (thyroid stimulating hormone 3.80–7.26 IU/l)
Deltito et al., 1998	$N = 36$, 20 manic or bipolar mixed episode; ages 13–18 yr, mean age 15.6; no gender noted; inpatient chart review	Chart data recorded systematically; comorbidity not described	Milieu treatment on ward; duration of stay not described; PRNs allowed; specifics not described	Dose range 700–900 mg/day; levels not reported	For those with mania or mixed states, overall changes reported: 66–70% change in mania, 79% change in depression, 83–87% change in aggression, 70–74% change in mood fluctuation

ADHD = attention-deficit hyperactivity disorder; BPRS = Brief Psychiatric-Rating Scale; CGI = Clinical Global Impressions scale; DSM-III-R = *Diagnostic and Statistical Manual*, 3rd edition, revised; F = female; GAS = Global Assessment Scale; K-SADS = Kiddie Schedule for Affective Disorders and Schizophrenia; M = male; MMRS = Modified Mania Rating Scale; SCID = Structured Clinical Interview for DSM; YMRS = Young Mania Rating Scale.

TABLE 23–6. Controlled Acute Trials of Divalproex in Children and Adolescents with Manic or Mixed States

Study	Sample and Type of Study	Diagnosis, Measures, and Duration of Trial/Study	Other Medications Taken	Doses and Levels	Response and Adverse Events
Kowatch et al., 2000	n = 42 in open comparison of lithium, carbamazepine, divalproex; n = 15 received divalproex as outpatients	Mania or hypomania diagnosed by K-SADS, YMRS, CGI; 71% comorbid for ADHD, 38% for ODD	Chlorpromazine PRN allowed; 3 subjects needed it	20 mg/kg/day at start, aiming at blood levels 85–110 µg/L; final average divalproex level 82.8 µg/l	YMRS change from baseline to endpoint 14.53; effect size 1.63; 46% had both a ≥50% change in YMRS and CGI ≤2; side effects: nausea (20%) and sedation (20%)
DelBello et al., 2006	N = 30; ages 12–18 yr, mean age 14.3; 16 M, 14 F; open treatment with divalproex; 15 subjects each simultaneously randomized to quetiapine or placebo; inpatient 7–14 days	Mania or mixed state diagnosed by Washington University (WASH-U) K-SADS, YMRS, PANSS-P, CDRS, CGAS; 60% ADHD, 47% psychosis; duration: 6 wk	PRN drugs allowed; 4 subjects needed 1 dose of lorazepam; 1 subject required 3 doses	20 mg/kg/day, adjusted for levels of 80–130 µg/l; valproate level 114 µg/l; by 7 day	73% completed 6-wk trial; if the divalproex + placebo subjects are considered the divalproex response group, 53% showed a ≥50% response from baseline on the YMRS; average YMRS scores dropped from about 30 to about 15 (from graphs); significant improvement noted in CDRS, PANSS-P, and CGAS, but scores not given
Wagner et al., 2002	N = 40; ages 7–19 yr, mean age 12.1; 25 M, 15 F; discontinuation trial that was basically an open trial (only 17 made it to randomization, and 14 of those stopped prematurely); inpatient, outpatient	Mania, hypomania, mixed state diagnosed by K-SADS, Mania Scale (Endicott and Spitzer, 1978), BPRS, CGI severity; 23% had ADHD	PRN drugs allowed; rates of significant use of other medication: lorazepam—18%, haloperidol—20%, lithium—10%, stimulant—15%	Dose last day: 813 mg/day; mean—17.5 mg/kg; valproate level—8.34 µg/l	23 patients discontinued before randomization: 15% ineffective, 15% did not meet randomization criteria, 15% could not tolerate medication, 15% nonadherent; using last observation carried forward (LOCF) in 36 cases, 22/26 (61%) showed >50% improvement on CGI; effect size 1.12 for mania scale change from baseline; side effects: headache, nausea, vomiting, diarrhea, somnolence
Findling et al., 2003a	N = 90; ages 5–17 yr, mean age 10.9; bipolar-I or -II with episode within past 3 mo (95% bipolar-I; 81.1% manic or mixed); open trial	Mania or mixed state diagnosed by K-SADS Present and Lifetime Version (PL) or K-SADS Epidemiologic Version (E), YMRS, CDRS, CGI, CGAS; 71% comorbid disruptive behavior disorder; 66.6% ADHD; duration: 20 wk	Other medications ever during study: stimulants—58.9%, atypicals—21.1%, alpha-adrenergic agents—24.4%	End of study: divalproex dose 862.5 (397.5) mg/day, level: 79.8 (25.9) µg/ml; lithium: 923.3 (380.2) mg/day, level: .9 (.3) mmol/l	48 nonremitters: 19 discontinued for nonadherence, 3 were hospitalized, 15 were discontinued for medication intolerance, 7 had continued psychosis, 4 had continued mood symptoms; 42 remitted: 46.7% defined by CDRS <40, YMRS <12.5, CGAS ≥51; rating scale changes: CDRS 31.7 (14) → 21 (7.9), YMRS 21.8 (8.2) → 5.7 (8.5), CGI severity 4.1 (.9) → 2.3 (1.3), CGAS 50 (7.2) → 65.2 (12.9)

(continued)

925

TABLE 23–6. Controlled Acute Trials of Divalproex in Children and Adolescents with Manic or Mixed States *(continued)*

Study	Sample and Type of Study	Diagnosis, Measures, and Duration of Trial/Study	Other Medications Taken	Doses and Levels	Response and Adverse Events
Findling et al., 2005	*N*=60; ages 5–18 yr, mean age 10.7; 91.7% bipolar-I, 50% rapid cycling; subjects were remitted with prior treatment with lithium+divalproex; randomized double-blind to lithium+placebo or divalproex+placebo; maintenance trial	Mania or mixed state diagnosed by K-SADS PL or K-SADS E, YMRS, CDRS, CGI, CGAS; ADHD 63.3% ODD/conduct disorder 30%; most subjects from prior study; duration: 76 wk	Stimulant use 58.3%	End of study blood levels: lithium 0.84 (0.30) mmol/L divalproex 75.3 (29.4) µg/ml	Only 10% completed 76-wk trial: 56.7% exited because of relapse into mania/hypomania, 6.7% because of relapse into depression, 26.6% for other reasons (eg., nonadherence, side effects); time to relapse for mood reasons: lithium—114 days (standard error [SE] 57.4 days), divalproex—112 days (SE 56 days); time to discontinuation for any reason: lithium—91 days (SE 30 days), divalproex—56 days (SE 19.9 days); no significant difference between lithium and divalproex; young age predicted relapse into mania; no other predictors
Pavuluri et al., 2005	*N*=34; ages 5–18 yr, mean age 12.1 (3.7); open trial of divalproex; visits monthly	Mania or mixed state diagnosed by WASH-U K-SADS, YMRS, CDRS, CGI-BP, Children's Global Assessment of Functioning Scale (CGAS); 76.5% ADHD, 55.9% ODD; duration: 6 mo	Other medications in study: methylphenidate (MPH) 38.2%; risperidone at some point 50%	Final dose: mean 950 (±355) mg/day; level 109 (±33) µg/ml	Response (≥50% change from baseline on YMRS; ≤40 on CDRS): 73.5%; remission (response + CGI-BP improvement ≤2; CGAS ≥51): 52.9%; mean change from baseline: YMRS—19.8 points, CDRS—27.4 points
Abbott Laboratories (data on file, Dec. 2006)	*N*=150; ages 10–17; randomized DB to placebo or divalproex-ER	DSM-IV-TR mania or mixed state diagnosed by WASH-U KSADS; minimum YMRS score 20 on entry; assessed by CGAS, CGI, CDRS-R; duration: 4 wk	Full information not yet available	Initial dose 15 mg/kg/day, titrated to maximum of 35 mg/kg/day (plasma levels of 80–125 mcg/ml)	No significant drug–placebo differences in YMRS scores or secondary outcome measures

ADHD=attention-deficit hyperactivity disorder; BPRS=Brief Psychiatric Rating Scale; CDRS=Child Depression Rating Scale; CGAS=Children's Global Assessment Scale; CGI=Clinical Global Impressions; DB=double blind; DSM-IV-TR = *Diagnostic and Statistical Manual*, 4th edition, text revised; ER = extended release; K-SADS=Kiddie-Schedule for Affective Disorders and Schizophrenia; ODD=Oppositional Defiance Disorder; PANSS-P=Positive and Negative Syndrome Scale; PRN=Practice Research Network; TR=text revised; YMRS=Young Mania Rating Scale.

the Clinical Global Impressions-Improvement (CGI) scale. The sample sizes in these studies were too small to permit comparison of responses by diagnostic subtype or age.

In the first randomized, double-blind, placebo-controlled trial of an anticonvulsant in treating pediatric bipolar disorder—a large multicenter study of oxcarbazepine as treatment for bipolar-I mania/mixed states[8]—Wagner and colleagues (2006) failed to find a significant difference between drug and placebo on the primary outcome measure, change in YMRS score over 6 weeks (drug=10.9, placebo=9.8). There was a trend for more of the oxcarbazepine patients to respond (at least 50 percent improvement in YMRS score): 42 percent of those on the drug versus 26 percent of those on placebo. The oxcarbazepine response rate, nearly identical in children (43 percent) and adolescents (41 percent), was very similar to the response rates reported from open trials of lithium, valproate, and carbamazepine in bipolar children and adolescents (Kowatch et al., 2000). Nineteen percent of the oxcarbazepine patients discontinued because of side effects (primarily dizziness, somnolence, diplopia, and fatigue), compared with 4 percent of those receiving placebo. Recently, 150 DSM-IV manic or mixed-state patients ages 10 to 17 (minimum YMRS score at entry: 20) were randomized to divalproex-ER or placebo for 4 weeks; there were no significant differences in the primary or secondary end points. The drug was generally well tolerated, although there was a significant increase in mean plasma ammonium levels (2.1 versus 18.6), which in 1 patient was associated with disorientation requiring hospitalization, data on file, Abbott Laboratories (December 2006).

The less-than-impressive performance of mood stabilizers as monotherapy prompted a variety of other trials of combined medications. In a subsequent study, for instance, Kowatch and colleagues (2003) randomized 35 outpatient child and adolescent bipolar-I and -II subjects into a continuation phase of treatment, which had been initiated with mood stabilizer monotherapy (lithium, carbamazepine, or divalproex). For the nearly half of the patients (17 of 35) who had not responded acutely to monotherapy, other medications were added. Twelve improved on a second mood stabilizer, antipsychotic, or antidepressant, while 12 needed stimulant medication as well.

With regard to other anticonvulsants, there have been scattered case reports and the one open randomized trial that included carbamazepine, described earlier. In addition, there have been seven case reports of young adolescents cited in three studies (Hsu and Starzynski, 1986; Woolston, 1999; Craven and Murphy, 2000). All but one of the seven responded to carbamazepine. The anticonvulsant gabapentin has not been studied specifically for treating acute mania in youths, although there is one published case report on its utility (Soutullo et al., 1998). A placebo-controlled study of topiramate involving 56 manic and mixed-state adolescents was recently undertaken simultaneously with a trial involving manic adults as part of a registration study, but was halted because of a lack of antimanic efficacy in the adults. There was some suggestion of a positive treatment effect of the drug in the adolescents, however (DelBello et al., 2005). The mean total reduction in YMRS scores was twice as large for those adolescents treated with topiramate ($n=29$) as for those receiving placebo ($n=27$), but given the small number of subjects, this difference did not reach statistical significance. At the final visit, however, 34.5 percent of the topiramate-treated subjects versus 22.2 percent of the placebo-treated subjects had improved either much or very much on the CGI-I scale relative to baseline ($df=1$, $p=.310$).

Atypical Antipsychotics

Until recently, the available database on atypical antipsychotics as treatment for bipolar disorder in children and adolescents included only chart reviews for risperidone (Frazier et al., 1999), olanzapine (Soutullo et al., 1999; Chang and Ketter, 2000), quetiapine (Schaller and Behar, 1999), and clozapine (Fuchs, 1994; Masi et al., 2002; Kant et al., 2004). However, the status of atypicals in the treatment of child and adolescent bipolar disorder is evolving (Findling and McNamara, 2004). The strong incentive for the pharmaceutical industry to conduct trials to determine the safety and efficacy of the drugs in children and adolescents has been a major impetus for the emergence of a controlled database on their use in treating bipolar disorder in these populations. To this end, multicenter placebo-controlled studies are now under way within the broad framework espoused by the consensus conference discussed earlier (Carlson et al., 2003).

An 8-week open trial of olanzapine was conducted among outpatient children and adolescents aged 5 to 15, 61 percent of whom improved (Frazier et al., 2001). The definition of improvement in this study was problematic, however, requiring only a 30 percent decline in YMRS score or a CGI score of 3 or greater. Biederman and colleagues (2005a) conducted an 8-week open trial of risperidone as monotherapy among 30 youths with mania, mixed mania, and hypomania. Stimulants were used as needed. The authors reported a 70 percent response rate (CGI scores improved or very much improved). Other symptoms of psychopathology were also responsive. Data on clozapine are limited to a chart review that found decreases in mania, depression, and aggression ratings in 10 adolescents with mania/mixed episodes in residential treatment for whom other treatments had failed (Masi et al., 2002). With regard to aripiprazole, data from retrospective chart reviews suggest that it may be effective and well tolerated in children and adolescents with bipolar disorder (Barzman et al., 2004; Biederman et al., 2005b). In a case series of three youths not responding to traditional mood stabilizers, some symptom alleviation was observed after a switch to ziprasidone monotherapy (Barnett, 2004).

A recent study of mania/mixed episodes in 50 hospitalized adolescents compared quetiapine (400–600 mg/dl) against divalproex (blood levels 80–120 mg/dl) in a randomized, double-blind design (DelBello et al., 2006). *Within* each treatment group, a statistically significant improvement in YMRS scores was seen from baseline to endpoint.[9] There was no statistically significant difference in YMRS scores *between* the two groups over the 28 days of the study (F[1,48]=1.0, p=.3, Cohen's d=.28]). Measures of depression and psychosis also improved significantly with both medications. Over a 4-week period, 72 percent of those treated with quetiapine and 40 percent of those receiving divalproex had an end-point YMRS score of 2 or less, a statistically and clinically significant change. The slopes of recovery indicated that adolescents randomized to quetiapine improved more quickly than those receiving divalproex. Other than higher rates of sedation in the quetiapine-treated youths (60 percent versus 36 percent with divalproex), there were no differences in side effects, although it should be noted that, as in virtually all comparative clinical trials, the study was not powered to detect smaller side-effect differences.[10]

The first study to emerge as a result of FDA approval of an atypical antipsychotic for treatment of adult acute mania was one involving olanzapine in adolescents aged 13 to 17 (undertaken before the inclusion age was lowered to 10). Preliminary findings of this study are encouraging (Tohen et al., 2006). This 3-week double-blind, placebo-controlled, multisite study included 107 olanzapine-treated and 54 placebo-treated adolescents given doses that ranged from 2.5 to 20 mg/day (average 8 to 10 mg/day). The retention rate was reasonable (79 percent for those receiving active medication), and the response rate (50 percent decline in YMRS scores and CGI severity<3) was 44.8 percent with olanzapine versus 18.5 percent with placebo (p=.002); remission rates were 35 percent with olanzapine and 11 percent with placebo (p=.001). Ratings of aggression (on the Overt Aggression Scale of Yudofsky) and ADHD symptoms were significantly better with the medication, suggesting an overall calming effect and a decrease in activation.

Finally, regarding other medications with potential utility in treating mania, there have been case reports on the utility of verapamil (Kastner and Friedman, 1992), nimodipine (Davanzo et al., 1999), lecithin (Schreier, 1982), and melatonin (Robertson and Tanguay, 1997).

Drug Combinations

In an open trial of combined medications, 90 bipolar-I and -II children and adolescents who had not responded to either lithium or valproate were treated with a combination of both (Findling et al., 2003). Using a strict definition of remission (YMRS score<12.5, with a mean score of 21.8 entering the study), 42 of the subjects (46.7 percent) remitted. It is of note that this remission rate is in the same range as "response" rates in the monotherapy trials, which require only 50 percent improvement. The dropout rate due to side effects or nonadherence was high, but if the subjects could tolerate the combination of medications, they appeared to improve substantially. It would be interesting to know whether a combination of less-than-full monotherapy doses of lithium and valproate (given the evidence that their postsynaptic mechanisms show some synergism and their side-effect profiles are somewhat different) would produce a more favorable ratio of benefit to side effects.

In a small placebo-controlled crossover study of seven inpatients with mixed manic symptoms and ADHD, Carlson and colleagues (1992b) found that measures of inattention and overactivity showed greater improvement with lithium and MPH than with MPH alone. Scheffer and colleagues (2005) examined 40 children and adolescents with bipolar mania treated openly with valproate and then randomized to added placebo or added dextroamphetamine (Adderall). The added stimulant led to greater improvement on the YMRS compared with the added placebo (i.e., valproate alone), and also was effective for the ADHD symptoms. The study did not find worsening of manic symptoms or significant side effects. In another study of combined treatment, Pavuluri and colleagues (2004b) examined the combination of risperidone (up to 3 mg/day) and either lithium or divalproex in a 6-month, nonrandomized open trial. The study included 37 subjects aged 5 to 18 with mania or mixed episodes.[11] Based on three outcome measures (YMRS, CGI-BP, and CDRS-R), divalproex in combination with risperidone was found to be as effective and as well tolerated as the combination of lithium and risperidone.

Finally, as part of a double-blind, placebo-controlled study of adjunctive quetiapine, DelBello and colleagues (2002) randomized 30 hospitalized adolescents with mania or mixed episodes to divalproex plus placebo or divalproex plus quetiapine. There was a significant decline (p<.01) in YMRS scores with divalproex plus placebo (i.e., divalproex alone) and significant additional improvement with quetiapine. The response rate (improved or very much improved on the CGI or 50 percent decline in YMRS scores) was 53 percent for divalproex. Adding quetiapine (versus adding placebo) raised the response rate an additional 15 percent, a statistically significant difference.

Treatment of Aggression

Although a thorough discussion of the treatment of aggression and conduct disorder is beyond the scope of this chapter, it is important to state that most of the medications approved for the treatment of acute mania in adults have also demonstrated some efficacy in treating affective aggression in pediatric populations (see Table 23–1). Ironically, far more children with aggression and conduct disorder than with mania have been studied using lithium under controlled conditions (Campbell et al., 1984, 1995; Malone et al., 2000). One randomized trial of divalproex found that a higher dose was better than a lower dose for treating conduct disorder (Steiner et al., 2003).

Antipsychotics have also proven effective in randomized, placebo-controlled trials involving more than 500 children with aggression associated with either conduct disorder/ADHD[12] or autism/pervasive developmental disorder (McCracken et al., 2002). For example, with a responder defined as a subject with an end-point rating of much or very much improved on the CGI scale, the percentage of responders in one study (Aman et al., 2002) was 53.8 percent for the risperidone group and 7.9 percent for the placebo group, a significant difference.

One problem with these studies is that outcome measures of irritability/aggression (Aman et al., 1985, 1996) include behaviors elevated in mania: temper tantrums; irritability; depressed mood; demanding behavior; crying over minor annoyances; rapid mood changes; deliberately hurting oneself; arguing; explosive behavior; being easily angered; getting into physical fights; and talking back to teachers, parents, or other adults (Biederman et al., 1995; Carlson et al., 1998; Mick et al., 2003). In trials involving bipolar children and adolescents in which both aggression and mania have been measured directly,[13] the decline in aggression has been similar to the decline in "mania" scores.

Treatment of Bipolar Depression

As of this writing, no large, placebo-controlled clinical trials of medications for pediatric bipolar depression (including antidepressants) have been published or are currently under way. There has been one 6-week open trial of lithium involving 28 hospitalized bipolar adolescents. This study demonstrated a significant reduction in depressive symptoms (Patel et al., 2006), with 48 percent of the patients showing a greater than 50 percent reduction in CDRS-R scores (Poznanski et al., 1984) relative to baseline, although the baseline scores were so high that in fact only 30 percent met response criteria after 6 weeks (decline in CDRS-R scores <28 and CGI improvement <2). Interpretation of the apparent treatment response is complicated by the fact that there was no placebo control (depression has a notoriously high placebo response in youths); moreover, the major improvement in mood symptoms took place within the first 2 weeks of treatment, during which 82 percent of the adolescents remained hospitalized. Indeed, 6 weeks is a brief time frame for measuring antidepressant response.

Current understanding of lamotrigine treatment in youth began with a study by Kusumakar and Yatham (1997) that included 7 adolescents among a sample of bipolar adults and found an improvement in scores on depression rating scales. Carandang and colleagues (2003) reported on a case series of lamotrigine (both as monotherapy and as an adjunct) in 9 adolescents with refractory depressive disorders, 6 of whom were bipolar. In this series, 8 of the 9 patients responded well (mean dose 142 mg/day), as determined by achieving a score of 1 or 2 on the CGI-BP scale. Finally, Chang and colleagues (2006) recently completed a study using up to 150 mg/day of lamotrigine over 8 weeks in youths aged 12 to 18. Remarkably, of 19 subjects, 16 (84 percent) were considered responders by virtue of achieving a score of 1 or 2 on the CGI-I-BP. Remission was achieved in 11 of 19 (58 percent) of the subjects.[14]

Quetiapine is another promising agent for adults with bipolar depression (see Chapter 19). A controlled study examining this treatment option is currently in progress.

Maintenance Treatment

The question of how long a child or adolescent with bipolar disorder should be treated is clearly important. Insofar as youths have a condition in which clear episodes of mania, depression, and euthymia are occurring, one can probably extrapolate from adult monotherapy studies. In broader pediatric "bipolar" populations, however, the limited data currently available suggest that maintenance with single mood stabilizers generally does not provide adequate coverage. For instance, using subjects from their sample of children and adolescents stabilized on combined lithium and valproate (and adding other subjects to form a sample size of 60), Findling and colleagues (2005) conducted a maintenance trial in which those patients who had responded to combined lithium and divalproex were randomized to monotherapy. The study hypothesis, based on an adult trial (Calabrese et al., 2005), was that divalproex would be superior to lithium as maintenance monotherapy in patients with rapid cycling (50 percent of the subjects). Outpatients ranging in age from 5 to 17 were first openly stabilized on combined lithium and divalproex for 20 weeks and then randomized under double-blind conditions to have one of the mood stabilizers withdrawn while continuing on the other. Relapses were frequent and rapid over the next 3 to 4 months, with only 10 of the 60 subjects completing the trial. Moreover, neither drug was found to be superior. Interpretation of the study results is limited by the lack of a placebo control, and especially by the confound represented by the withdrawal effect (Findling et al., 2005).

In addition to this one controlled study, there have been some naturalistic studies of medication continuation. For instance, in a study of adolescents hospitalized with "classic" bipolar disorder who were treated with lithium and then followed for 18 months, those who discontinued lithium had a high rate of relapse compared with those who maintained the treatment (92 versus 37 percent) (Strober et al., 1990). Finally, in a naturalistic 4-year follow-up study contrasting bipolar patients first hospitalized in adolescence with those first hospitalized after age 30, the proportion remaining on maintenance medication through the follow-up was similar in the two groups (55 percent of the youths versus 59 percent of the adults) (Carlson et al., 1999). In the adolescent-onset group, however, those who remained on maintenance medication had a relapse rate of 67 percent, similar to the 70 percent among those who stopped treatment. As might be expected, comorbid behavior disorders and substance abuse in the adolescents complicated both medication adherence and relapse. Cessation of substance abuse was associated with fewer episodes and greater functional improvement at the 4-year point in this follow-up.

Offspring of Adults Treated for Bipolar Disorder

Using a family history of lithium response as the basis for trying medication in children with a variety of psychiatric symptoms, Dyson and Barcai (1970) studied two children with "hyperkinesis" who had a parent considered to be a lithium responder. One child responded to both dextroamphetamine and lithium; the second responded to lithium alone. McKnew and colleagues (1981) attempted to replicate this study with a slightly larger sample ($N=6$) of symptomatic offspring of lithium-responding parents or grandparents, but without success (see Table 23–3).

There have been two more contemporary studies examining the use of divalproex in children and adolescents believed to be at risk for bipolar disorder by virtue of their family history. In one open 12-week trial, 24 children with "mood symptoms" whose parents had bipolar disorder improved globally (Chang et al., 2003). In another study, 53 children or adolescents (aged 5 to 17) with a bipolar parent who themselves had mood symptoms not sufficient to meet criteria for mania or depression were randomized to divalproex or placebo. Median time until a mood event for those randomized to placebo (196 days, standard error [SE] ±117.6 days) was not significantly different from the mean survival time among the youths randomized to divalproex (148 days, SE ±137.1 days). Among those with more bipolar disorder among first-degree relatives, however, the mood stabilizer was significantly superior to placebo (Findling et al., 2003a).

Finally, there have been two recent studies of quetiapine by the same group involving the non–bipolar-I offspring of a bipolar-I parent. In one, a 12-week open study of quetiapine monotherapy (mean dose 447 mg/day) in 25 adolescents with major depression, the score on the CDRS-R was reduced from 40 to 29 ($p<.0001$) (Barzman et al., 2006). In the other study, 20 adolescents with dysthymia, major depression, depressive disorder-NOS, cyclothymia, bipolar-II disorder, or bipolar-NOS were treated in a single-blind fashion (blind rater) with quetiapine (300 to 600 mg/day) for 84 days. Mean YMRS scores declined from 18 to 8 at end point ($p<.0001$), and CDRS-R scores fell from 38 to 27 ($p<.0006$) (Strakowski et al., 2006). The most common side effects were sedation (65 percent), dry mouth (40 percent) and headache (40 percent).

Psychiatric Adverse Events

The diagnostic and treatment implications of activation associated with medications (which may manifest as symptoms of mania) complicate clinical decision making in general and that for patients with bipolar disorder in particular. As detailed in Chapter 19, the frequency of manic symptoms in adults with bipolar depression within 2 months of initiation of a second-generation antidepressant is about 20 percent.[15] Rates can vary widely, depending on rating criteria, cohort characteristics, duration of treatment with the antidepressant, possibly the type of antidepressant used, and whether a mood stabilizer is used concurrently (Post et al., 2003). Results of studies in adults appear to suggest that rapid-cycling bipolar patients are especially vulnerable to destabilization (Ghaemi et al., 2003; Post et al., 2003; Altshuler et al., 2003). This finding is relevant to pediatric bipolar patients, among whom the percentage with a rapid-cycling course ranges from 19 percent (Faraone et al., 1997) to 83 percent (Tillman et al., 2003), depending on the study.

There are as yet no prospective studies evaluating the frequency with which antidepressant-induced switching or cycle induction occurs. Biederman and colleagues (2000a) used multivariate analysis to examine 50 charts of child and adolescent outpatients with bipolar depression treated with SSRIs plus a mood stabilizer and found a three-fold increase in the relative risk (RR) for destabilizing the condition (RR=3.0, 95 percent confidence interval [CI]=1.2–7.8; $p=.02$). However, it should be noted that there was a greater likelihood of improving the condition (RR=6.7, 95 percent CI=1.9–23.6; $p=.003$). Although mood stabilizers (primarily lithium and valproate) ameliorated manic symptoms, they did not prevent the antidepressant-related increase in cycling as reflected by more episodes of bipolar depression. Another chart review involving 82 children with a modified diagnosis of bipolar disorder found that 58 percent developed treatment-emergent mania shortly after receiving mood-elevating agents (Faedda et al., 2004). Baumer and colleagues (2006) recently published the first study to assess, by direct semistructured interview of both parent and offspring, antidepressant-related mania in adolescents and children who not only are at risk for bipolar disorder (i.e., at least one parent with a *Diagnostic and Statistical Manual* (DSM)-IV bipolar-I or -II diagnosis as determined by the Structured Clinical Interview for DSM [SCID-I]), but who also meet criteria for bipolar-I or -II disorder according to the Kiddie Schedule for Affective Disorders and Schizophrenia (K-SADS) or subsyndromal bipolar disorder (ADHD symptoms with a YMRS score of 12 or more or CDRS-R score of 30 or more). They reported that, in agreement with the findings of Faedda and colleagues (2004), 50 percent of the subjects experienced an antidepressant-related mania as reflected in YMRS ratings and in accordance with DSM-IV criteria (except that only 1 day of symptoms was required because most subjects stopped the antidepressant with 1 to 4 days of the onset of mania).

It has been estimated that psychotically depressed, hospitalized adolescents who became hypomanic on a tricyclic antidepressant had at least a 20 percent chance of developing a bipolar course (Strober and Carlson, 1982; Akiskal et al., 1985). DelBello and colleagues (2003) attempted to replicate this in a sample of 157 adolescents and adults who were hospitalized with psychotic depression and followed for a relatively short time (up to 2 years); they found that only 13 percent developed DSM-IV mania or hypomania (which, of interest, was independent of age at onset). However, 13 percent is probably an underestimate in light of the finding of Baumer and colleagues (2006), noted previously, that the antidepressant is generally discontinued as soon as manic/hypomanic symptoms appear, and thus not all of the episodes would have met DSM-IV durational criteria (at least 1 week for mania and 4 days for hypomania).

Rates of agitation/activation in short-term trials of seven antidepressant drugs used to treat children and adolescents were recently summarized by Cheung and colleagues (2005). They reported the relative risk of treatment-emergent agitation or hostility to be modest but significant (RR=1.79, 95 percent CI=1.16–2.76). In the Treatment of Adolescent Depression study (March et al., 2004), the rate of agitation/anxiety/irritability in fluoxetine-treated subjects was 5.5 percent, compared with 3.57 percent in those treated with placebo. The rate of mania/hypomania was 2.3 percent versus 1.7 percent for placebo over the 12-week trial; these drug–placebo differences become more sig-

nificant given that bipolar youths were specifically excluded.[16]

In longer-term studies, follow-up data on prepubertal depressed children do not suggest that tricyclic antidepressants precipitate mania in early-onset *nonbipolar* depressed children (Craney and Geller, 2003). Nor does that suggestion emerge from a meta-analysis of 13 clinical trials of tricyclics involving more than 500 young people (from which bipolar youths were excluded) (Hazell et al., 2002). However, in interpreting this literature, it is important to recall the point made earlier that because DSM-IV mania requires at least 1 week of symptoms (2 weeks in the study of Geller and colleagues [2002]), cases in which the mania was ameliorated by immediate antidepressant discontinuation would not be counted.

The most interesting study of young people and their response to antidepressants examined a large insurance database involving "real-world" patients and treatments. This study found that children and adolescents had higher rates of administration of mood stabilizers 3 months or longer after being treated with antidepressants compared with adults. Along with the use of mood stabilizers was an accompanying diagnosis of bipolar disorder. Although it is possible that the diagnosis was made to justify the change in treatment, the vulnerability of young people to psychiatric adverse events is sobering. Comparing rates of "conversion" in those unexposed versus exposed to antidepressants, the study reported the following: for children aged 10 to 14, 3.1 versus 12.7 percent; aged 15 to 19, 4.8 versus 10.9 percent; aged 20 to 24, 4.3 versus 7.6 percent (Martin et al., 2004). At a minimum, these data suggest that young people are particularly vulnerable to psychiatric adverse events that trigger the clinician's choice to use a mood stabilizer.[17] Unfortunately, the study did not explore whether antidepressants were stopped and/or the change in treatment approach was continued and led to improved outcomes. That is, had it been possible to follow the sample longitudinally, one could have seen whether mood stabilizer treatment continued and whether the frequency of visits declined.

The question of antidepressant-induced "suicidal behavior" has been a contentious and confused topic, perhaps primarily because the term "suicidal behavior" has had no clear definition, and its relationship to actual suicide or serious attempts is tenuous at best (see the detailed discussion in Chapter 25). In 24 pediatric trials of antidepressants, the FDA (2004) found an increased risk for suicidal behavior (overall RR=1.78, 95 percent CI=1.14–2.77): about 2 percent with placebo versus about 4 percent in SSRI-treated subjects (there were no actual suicides). These rates are, in fact, similar to those for activation/agitation. Unfortunately, the relationship of suicidal behavior to agitation was not examined as a primary outcome measure. Even if it had been, agitation and activation were measured in such inconsistent ways

(Carlson and Mick, 2003) that conclusions would have been impossible. The Columbia Reclassification Project, requested by the FDA to reexamine data from industry-sponsored trials of antidepressant treatment in youths, has substantiated the small but significant "signal" of increased suicidal behavior compared with placebo with short-term use of antidepressants in these patients. However, bipolar subjects are excluded from the FDA database, and results of the few studies of bipolar youths indicate that the frequency of antidepressant-related suicidality is considerably higher: 14 percent in the study of Faedda and colleagues (2004) and 25.5 percent in the study of Baumer and colleagues (2006). Although these findings have not translated into an increased risk for actual suicide, it is prudent to monitor young people closely, especially those with or at risk for bipolar disorder, when starting these medications. Information for parents and clinicians on this issue is provided at http://www.parentsmedguide.org (accessed September 19, 2006).

Medical Adverse Events

Adverse events associated with medications in adults are described in Chapters 17 and 20, and all of these findings are applicable to children and adolescents. Several additional concerns need to be emphasized, however, as reviewed by Correll and Carlson (2006):

- *Lithium and thyroid suppression*—Lithium's thyroid suppression effect is well known. In a brief, 4-week study of adolescents conducted by Kafantaris and colleagues (2003), lithium produced only minor, transient elevations in serum TSH, which corrected spontaneously. In a study in which lithium was administered along with divalproex, however, a significant number (24 percent) of patients developed serum TSH levels greater than 10 mU/l (Gracious et al., 2004) within only 20 weeks. This much larger thyroid impact suggests a synergistic effect of valproate and lithium such that extra caution should be exercised in thyroid monitoring for young people receiving the combination.
- *Valproate and polycystic ovaries*—Polycystic ovary syndrome (PCOS)—chronic anovulation and hyperandrogenism with or without actual polycystic ovaries—is associated with oligomenorrhea, hirsutism, and acne. Given that menstrual irregularities are common in adolescents, it is important to obtain a baseline menstrual history when evaluating the impact of valproate. See Chapter 20 for a review of two recent large studies of bipolar adults, whose results indicate a very substantial divalproex-related increase in PCOS and menstrual irregularities compared with other mood stabilizers. These findings are especially important to the management of adolescents, considered to be most vulnerable to this adverse effect.

- *Atypical antipsychotics and prolactin*—As reviewed in Chapter 14, dopamine-2 (D2) receptor antagonism is associated with elevated prolactin, as dopamine blocks the release of prolactin. The affinity of atypical antipsychotics for this receptor and thus their likelihood of causing hyperprolactinemia can be summarized as follows: risperidone >olanzapine >ziprasidone >quetiapine >clozapine >aripiprazole. Postpubertal children and adolescents may be more susceptible than adults to drug-induced prolactin elevations (Wudarsky et al., 1999). However, a rise in prolactin does not necessarily translate into a clinical problem. Moreover, the rise in prolactin appears to be relatively transient (Findling et al., 2003b), so it is unnecessary to measure prolactin levels routinely. Prolactin levels should be measured if, after initiation of an atypical, amenorrhea or oligomenorrhea develops in an adolescent who previously had regular menses. The clinical manifestations of hyperprolactinemia in adolescents include breast enlargement/engorgement and/or galactorrhea, failure to enter or progress through puberty, and the development of hirsutism.
- *Weight gain associated with atypical antipsychotics, lithium, and divalproex*—This is a concern for patients of all ages, and as detailed in Chapter 20, combinations of these drugs are likely to increase the risk. Some of the atypical antipsychotics have an especially significant tendency to promote weight gain, particularly in patients who have not had prior exposure to psychotropic medication (Correll et al., 2005), as is the case for young people. This point is relevant because the occurrence of the metabolic syndrome in young people predicts development of atherosclerosis and vascular disease early in adulthood, while obesity during adolescence predicts later coronary artery disease and colorectal cancer even more strongly than obesity during adulthood. Data on adults (Allison et al., 1999; American Diabetes Association, 2004; Casey, 2004) and from an ongoing large-scale naturalistic study involving children and adolescents (Correll et al., 2005) suggest the following rank order among the atypicals in terms of ability to promote weight gain and development of the metabolic syndrome: clozapine = olanzapine >> risperidone >> quetiapine > ziprasidone > /= aripiprazole. In addition, the prospect of weight gain is likely to affect medication adherence, particularly among adolescents, for whom appearance is especially important.
- *Lamotrigine and Stevens-Johnson syndrome*—This potentially lethal condition is quite uncommon in young people with appropriate dosing—according to the German rash registry, 1 in 1,700 for those under age 16 versus 1 in 10,000 in adults (most of the youths in the registry were being treated for epilepsy with multiple rash-producing

drugs).[18] It is important for the clinician to follow carefully the gradual upward titration schedule outlined in Chapter 20.

Summary of Pharmacological Studies of Bipolar Disorder

Numerous problems beset pharmacological studies of bipolar disorder in young people. The relative rarity of DSM-IV bipolar disorder in prepubertal children limits the number of subjects available for systematic trials. Moreover, from the earliest studies, there has been a great deal of heterogeneity in the subjects involved; this has been the case even in studies involving only adolescents. And although more recent studies have used structured interviews and rating scales such as the YMRS, the high prevalence of comorbidities across studies makes their results too heterogeneous to be compared meaningfully. Comorbid conditions may well affect the action of mood-stabilizing medications as well. In the case of placebo-controlled studies, the study duration and the severity of symptoms among subjects are limited by ethical constraints. Outpatient studies suffer from major problems with adherence, interfering stressors, family crises, and high dropout rates (Carlson et al., 2003). Inpatient studies are expensive and, some would suggest, not as generalizable.

Despite the difficulties faced by placebo-controlled studies, treatment research in pediatric bipolar disorder is moving forward at an accelerating pace. Whereas just a short while ago there were few agents and little agreement among experts, today there are many agents and many more areas of consensus. We are encouraged by the number and scope of controlled studies currently under way. While we await their results, we must note that in the many areas in which placebo-controlled data are inadequate, experts are still able to reach substantial agreement on recommendations by drawing on results of open studies and clinical experience. Thus today, clinicians, patients, and families enjoy an expanded array of options, many of them supported by extensive observations in the "real world" of clinical practice.

Electroconvulsive Therapy

The body of knowledge on the use of ECT in young people has grown to the point that a practice parameter has been developed to provide advice to child and adolescent psychiatrists (Ghaziuddin et al., 2004). Several reviews have summarized the literature on ECT, including its successful use in treating mania in bipolar adolescents (at least those without comorbid personality disorder) (Rey and Walter, 1997; Walter et al., 1999; Walter and Rey, 2003). There have

been no controlled studies, but these reviews have identified 60 reports (63 percent of which were case studies) describing the use of ECT in 396 patients. Rates of improvement across studies were 63 percent for depression, 80 percent for mania, 80 percent for catatonia (which is often related to bipolar disorder), and 42 percent for schizophrenia. One study evaluated adolescents about 5 years after they had undergone ECT. Compared with carefully matched psychiatric controls, 11 adolescents given ECT for psychotic depression or mania were similar in school and social functioning. Bipolar disorder was the most common follow-up diagnosis, however, suggesting that for some, the antidepressant effectiveness of the procedure was accompanied by a switch into mania (Taieb et al., 2002). The only data on prepubertal children come from a report on 2 successfully treated patients with refractory mania (Hill et al., 1997) and 1 with severe depression with catatonic features (Russell et al., 2002).

Psychotherapy

Fristad and colleagues (1998) used a manual-driven, adjunctive, multiple-family group treatment approach for children aged 8 to 12 with bipolar and depressive disorders. This method includes psychoeducation about the disorder and the role of medications, training in communication skills to improve interactions between parents and children, stress management, and development of coping strategies. In a randomized controlled trial, this same group (Fristad et al., 2002) showed that multifamily psychoeducation was associated with increased knowledge about bipolar disorder and treatment options, better skills in dealing with the bipolar child, more active attitudes toward mobilizing resources to benefit the child, and an increased sense of support compared with a wait-list control group.

Miklowitz and colleagues (2000, 2004) developed a manual for adolescents aged 13 to 17 years with bipolar-I disorder. This manual is an adaptation of the family-focused therapy model for bipolar adults, designed to make it appropriate for this age group and to address clinical issues specific to juvenile bipolar disorder. In an open, 1 year observational study of 20 bipolar adolescents, the approach, in combination with mood stabilizers, moderately improved symptoms of depression and mania and behavior problems (Miklowitz et al., 2004). Greene and colleagues (Greene et al., 2003; Greene and Ablon, 2005) developed a "collaborative problem-solving" model that focuses on parents' assistance to their children. Parents are encouraged to avoid engaging their children until after a rage attack subsides, at which point collaborative problem solving can be encouraged. This approach is controversial, however, since the model emphasizes no consequences for the rage behavior or associated actions. Pavuluri and colleagues (2004a) developed a treatment program that involves parent-and-child sessions for 8- to 12-year-olds with bipolar disorder, termed child- and family-focused cognitive-behavioral therapy, described in detail in Chapter 22.

CONCLUSIONS

A serious psychiatric condition such as bipolar disorder that begins in childhood or adolescence does more than interfere with the patient's life: it also interferes with development. Thus it is encouraging that information on the treatment of bipolar disorder in children and adolescents, while still lagging behind that for adults, is improving. In the not-too-distant future, ongoing research is expected to resolve the dilemma of how to diagnose children (younger than age 12) more accurately and how to distinguish bipolar disorder in this population from a host of common comorbidities, including ADHD. Once consensus exists on how to classify children, more advanced treatment strategies for this age group can be pursued in clinical trials. In the meantime, most of our knowledge about treatment for children comes from open studies and clinical experience, combined with what is known from controlled studies of adolescents.

Although the evidence base is far from strong, this chapter provides clinical guidance on the use of medical and psychotherapeutic treatments for both children and adolescents. As of this writing, a number of clinical and industry-sponsored trials have just been launched, and their results can be expected to greatly increase the current knowledge base.

To summarize our treatment recommendations, mania should be treated with lithium, an anticonvulsant, and/or an atypical antipsychotic, depending on the clinical presentation. One common and perplexing question is how to treat a youngster whose symptoms of bipolar disorder may actually be symptoms of ADHD, or one who has ADHD comorbid with bipolar disorder. When a diagnosis of mania is clear, a mood stabilizer should be prescribed first, followed by treatment for the ADHD. When a mania diagnosis is less clear, we believe the ADHD should be addressed; if the child becomes more irritable, an atypical antipsychotic may be used and the ADHD readdressed as needed. With regard to a first depression in youths with a clear positive family history of mania in first-degree relatives, lamotrigine should be offered initially; if there is a family history of lithium response, lithium may be preferred over lamotrigine. An antidepressant can be added later if the response to the mood stabilizer is inadequate. If the clinical situation makes it appear unwise to wait, however, the antidepressant can be started simultaneously with the mood stabilizer. If the family or child resists a mood stabilizer or is simply unhappy with taking two medications, an antidepressant may be initiated alone, but only if the patient can be monitored very carefully for any signs of incipient mania or mixed state.

With regard to maintenance therapy for bipolar disorder, treatment guidelines in adults extrapolated to young people suggest the use of lithium or lamotrigine. The jury is still out as to whether olanzapine and aripiprazole, which have FDA "maintenance" indications, will prove to prevent new episodes (a prophylactic effect) as opposed to simply being effective continuation treatments following an acute antimanic response.

Psychosocial approaches are a vital component of treatment. They can improve social, academic, and family functioning, as well as promote adherence to pharmacological therapies. Evidence-based psychosocial therapies include psychoeducation and family therapy to help families devise constructive ways of problem solving.

NOTES

1. Duffy et al., 1998; Egeland et al., 2000, 2003; Shaw et al., 2005.
2. For the acute treatment of mania in children and adolescents, side-effect considerations appear similar to those in adults, although some investigators have noted fewer side effects in children (see McClellan and Werry, 1997). Lithium has a shorter half-life in children because of their more efficient renal physiology and, therefore will reach steady-state levels more quickly. Children may be more susceptible to the cognitive dulling seen in adults at higher serum levels (Silva et al., 1992).
3. The issue of a possible effect of valproate on female reproductive function is important for girls and young women who are taking the drug. Regular monitoring of reproductive function in female patients taking valproate is recommended, including questioning patients during visits regarding menstrual disorders, fertility, weight gain, hirsutism, and galactorrhea.
4. Compared with adult trials, ethical constraints make it more difficult to get seriously ill children admitted to trials with placebo controls. Therefore, placebo responses are often high, which can obscure an active drug effect.
5. The Geller and colleagues (1999) data emerged from a tricyclic antidepressant trial that found no relationship between antidepressant use and the development of subsequent bipolar disorder.
6. Odds and odds ratios are based on comparison of rates of bipolar disorder in the offspring of adults with the disorder versus another sample, usually a population sample. Rates of bipolar disorder are just over 1 percent, and of depression are nearly 10 percent. Thus if rates of disorder in bipolar offspring are 5 percent for bipolar disorder and 20 percent for unipolar depression, more have unipolar depression. But the rate of bipolar disorder is 5 times higher than that in the general population, whereas the rate of unipolar depression is only 2 times higher.
7. West et al., 1994, Papatheodorou et al., 1995; Deltito et al., 1998.
8. Oxcarbazepine is a 10-keto analogue of carbamazepine that apparently is without the parent compound's hematopoietic problems.

9. For quetiapine, the baseline mean was 35 (standard deviation [SD] = 8), and the end-point mean was 12 (SD = 11). For divalproex, the baseline mean was 36 (SD = 7), and the end-point mean was 17 (SD = 11).

10. Other potentially relevant information on quetiapine comes from an open safety trial in 10 adolescents with "chronic or intermittent psychosis" (i.e., not specified as bipolar) who were subsequently followed for 88 weeks (McConville et al., 2000). Doses of 300 to 800 mg/day were used, reportedly with minimal side effects.

11. As opposed to most studies of combined medications, these subjects were not selected on the basis of nonresponse to monotherapy.

12. Findling et al., 2000; Aman et al., 2002; Snyder et al., 2002; Turgay et al., 2002.

13. Frazier et al., 1999; ACNP, 2005; Biederman et al., 2005a.

14. The starting dose was 25 mg/day (12.5 mg in three subjects also taking valproate) for 2 weeks, 50 mg for 2 weeks, then 100 mg, 125 mg, and 150 mg, with a final mean dose of 132 mg/day. No rashes developed (Chang et al., 2006).

15. Clearly, if 20 percent of bipolar adults destabilize on antidepressants, 80 percent do not, as is suggested by other studies (Maj et al., 2002; Altshuler et al., 2003; Gijsman et al., 2004; Joffe et al., 2005; Carlson et al., 2006).

16. We can only assume that if some early-onset depressive patients are going to become bipolar but have not yet manifested mania, some will inadvertently be included in these trials.

17. The possibility that clinicians treating young versus older people are quicker to use mood stabilizers if they perceive that certain side effects are occurring cannot be ruled out.

18. The safety profiles of the anticonvulsants are well characterized for children and adolescents taking these agents for epilepsy. Younger patients may be at greater risk of rare idiosyncratic hepatic and dermatological reactions, as these problems have generally been reported more frequently in children than in adolescents and adults. The manufacturers of lamotrigine do not recommend its use in patients younger than age 16 years, except for special antiepilepsy indications, because of the apparently higher incidence of toxic epidermal necrolysis in the young.

Two months of intense self–analysis–dream interpretation etc. Remarried. . . . Wife left me because of drinking. . . . Many barbiturates and tranquilizers . . . Many hospitalizations. . . . Severe memory loss, memory distortions. DT's. . . . Quart of whisky a day for months in Dublin working hard on a long poem. Dry 4 months 2 years ago. Wife hiding bottles, myself hiding bottles.

—*John Berryman (cited in Haffenden, 1982, pp. 374–375)*

For most of the medical and psychiatric conditions that are comorbid with manic-depressive illness, a combination of psychosocial approaches and medication is optimal. Few controlled trials of pharmacotherapy have been conducted, however, despite the high prevalence of comorbidity in patients with manic-depressive illness, especially the bipolar subgroup. Most clinical trials aim for a "pure" presentation of the disorder being studied and therefore exclude patients with comorbid conditions. As a result, it is difficult to select treatment based on demonstrated efficacy in a specific comorbid population. Instead, the focus has tended to be on identifying treatment for the comorbid condition that will not destabilize the mood disorder.

Mood stabilizers that have been shown to be effective in noncomorbid bipolar patients are an obvious first choice for the treatment of comorbid illnesses because they can contribute to the stabilization of both conditions simultaneously. If additional agents are required, the first consideration is that they should not exacerbate depression, mania, or cycling. Thus the risk of the comorbid illness must be weighed against the risk of the adjunctive treatment. In practice, this type of risk assessment is difficult given the paucity of controlled studies available to guide the clinician. A realistic approach is to rely on clinical judgment and knowledge of a patient's unique presentation while conducting regular assessments of the patient's response to a given treatment. Such ongoing assessment will enable the clinician to detect any destabilization of the mood disorder in response to the treatment for the comorbid condition so that alternative treatment strategies can be pursued.

In this chapter, we review in turn what is known about the treatment of the following comorbid conditions commonly seen in patients with manic-depressive illness: substance abuse, anxiety disorders (panic disorder, social anxiety disorder, obsessive-compulsive disorder, and post-traumatic stress disorder), eating and personality disorders, and general medical disorders (cardiovascular disease, obesity, and thyroid dysfunction). Since the management of comorbid ADHD involves primarily children and adolescents, it is covered in Chapter 23.

SUBSTANCE ABUSE

The first step in the treatment of any disorder is to conduct a comprehensive assessment. For patients with substance abuse comorbidity, an initial assessment must include an evaluation of the effects of the substance(s) on the patient's affective stability. Differentiating mood changes brought about by affective illness from those brought about by alcohol or drug abuse can be a subtle and complex process.

In some cases, simple coincidence accounts for the coexistence of two disorders in the same individual, whereas in others, the alcohol and drug abuse may reflect genetically influenced behavioral traits that overlap the mood and addictive disorders (such as stimulus seeking and poor impulse control). Alternatively, the substance abuse may simply reflect an attempt at self-treatment of depression, mania, or especially mixed states.

Just as affective illness can mask substance abuse, the reverse is also true. Accurate diagnosis of both disorders is vital because it is the basis for important treatment decisions. For example, it is unnecessary and unwise to prescribe mood stabilizers or antidepressants for transient mood symptoms secondary to substance abuse that will spontaneously remit with abstinence. Many investigators (e.g., Schuckit, 1983; Driessen et al., 2001) have noted that with primary alcoholism and an apparent secondary affective disorder, affective symptoms usually remit within 2 to

4 weeks after cessation of alcohol use. Treating only substance abuse in the presence of an independent affective illness, on the other hand, risks persistence of the problems associated with mood disorders.

Adequate assessment of a patient with possible diagnoses of bipolar or recurrent unipolar disorder and substance abuse requires systematic inquiry using standardized diagnostic criteria. Family histories of affective and substance abuse problems, as well as a detailed chronicling of symptom onset, also are important. Such histories aid in teasing out the more probable or primary diagnosis; moreover, they assist the clinician in identifying and counseling the manic-depressive patient who has a family history of alcoholism, a history that makes the patient more liable to become an alcoholic (Morrison, 1975). It is also important to differentiate between adolescent-onset affective disorders and early-onset alcoholism, which, like the bipolar form of manic-depressive illness, can be associated with aggressive and impulsive behavior. Indeed, early-onset alcoholism tends to be associated with a high degree of comorbidity. For example, Famularo and colleagues (1985) diagnosed bipolar illness in 7 of 10 cases of alcohol abuse developing before the age of 13. Driessen and colleagues (1998) studied a sample of 250 hospitalized alcohol-dependent patients and found that the majority of late-onset subjects were either not comorbid at all or had Axis I comorbidity only. Early-onset alcohol dependence, on the other hand, was preferentially associated with personality disorders. Gender differences also play a role. Goldstein and colleagues (2006), in a large-scale study of data from the 2001–2002 National Epidemiologic Survey on Alcohol and Related Conditions, found that among those with comorbid bipolar-I and alcohol abuse disorders, the former was more likely to go untreated among males and the latter more likely to go untreated among females.

In addition to a comprehensive diagnostic interview, a urine screen for drugs is important, as indicated by the finding of Estroff and colleagues (1985, p. 38) that there existed "little relationship between patients' self-reported patterns of drug abuse . . . and the results of the urine analysis." On the other hand, another study that evaluated patients seeking treatment specifically for drug problems found that self-reports of drug use were generally reliable (Brown et al., 1992), as reflected in the .65 reliability coefficient (kappa) between self-report and urinalysis results for most of the substances studied.

As with comorbid conditions in general, there is a paucity of data on how best to treat patients with comorbid mood and substance abuse disorders. Unfortunately, alcohol and drug abuse disorders are among the most common exclusionary criteria for patients entering clinical trials. At the same time, studies of substance abusers generally exclude patients with co-occurring psychiatric disorders. Clinicians must therefore rely primarily on their clinical acumen in addition to the sparse empirically derived data when determining which treatments are best for patients with co-occurring bipolar and substance abuse disorders.

Treatment for the two disorders can be structured in a number of different ways: selective treatment of only one of the comorbid conditions, sequential treatment of first one and then the other, parallel treatment of each, and integrated treatment of the two together. It is important to note that no pharmacological treatment for substance abuse has been shown to be effective in the absence of psychosocial therapy. Therefore, any strategy that involves treatment of the substance abuse disorder must have a psychosocial component, which should include Alcoholics Anonymous (AA), Narcotics Anonymous (NA), or their equivalent.

Because it is easy for one of the two diagnoses to be missed (usually the substance abuse), selective treatment of only one of the two conditions is common. In such cases, favorable outcomes and long-term stabilization are unlikely. Because substance abuse triggers and exacerbates bipolar and recurrent unipolar disorders (and vice versa), such an approach is analogous to the partial treatment of an infection; the untreated pathology reactivates the morbid process. In a minority of cases, it is conceivable that effective treatment of the mood disorder will attenuate the substance abuse disorder such that the patient is able to recover from the latter without professional intervention. Nevertheless, treatment of only the mood disorder results in significant numbers of patients being labeled incorrectly as treatment resistant. These patients, especially the bipolar subgroup, fail to stabilize despite multiple trials of mood stabilizers not because of some factor intrinsic to their mood disorder, but as the consequence of an unrecognized or inadequately treated comorbid substance abuse disorder.

When co-occurring illnesses are diagnosed accurately, some patients may receive treatment first for one and then for the other. Such sequential treatment may be the result of factors within the system of care. Some mental health clinics are unable to treat patients with active substance abuse problems, while some substance abuse programs require that co-occurring psychiatric disorders be stabilized prior to enrollment. Although it is not ideal, sequential treatment can be effective for some patients. Because the two illnesses interact in harmful ways, stabilization of one can facilitate improvement in the other, making remission more likely.

Parallel treatment involves addressing both disorders concurrently but independently. Thus comorbid bipolar disorder is approached in the same way as the disorder without co-occurring substance abuse. Such an approach, however, fails to address the ways in which the two illnesses interact. Therefore, the best approach is an integrated one that takes the comorbid substance abuse into account in choosing a treatment for the affective disorder. The interactions between the disorders are considered in selecting both pharmacological and psychosocial treatments. Specialized programs that offer integrated treatment are rare, however, and for many patients, accessing such treatment is not possible. Integrated treatment is discussed in more detail below in the section on psychosocial therapies.

Most psychiatrists are familiar with the large body of evidence supporting the efficacy of available treatments for recurrent depression and bipolar disorder. There tends to be widespread pessimism, however, about the long-term efficacy of treatments for substance abuse disorders. There are a number of reasons for this unfounded pessimism. For example, clinicians may initially be exposed to the most seriously ill substance abuse patients, many of whom are seen in emergency rooms. These patients demonstrate poor adherence to treatment recommendations, have very limited support networks, and often show little motivation for change. Clinicians may come to view these intractable cases as typical of substance abuse disorders. Substance abuse in patients with good prognoses, on the other hand, may not be recognized because the pathology is more subtle. Such patients may be employed and have homes, and their substance abuse may not be diagnosed unless a clinician specifically inquires about it with both the patient and the family. Clinicians who believe that substance abuse disorders do not respond to treatment may neglect to ask patients and family members about them, fail to identify the most treatable individuals, and consequently develop only limited experience with those who successfully overcome their addictions.

Inappropriate measurements of efficacy also contribute to the belief that substance abuse treatment does not work. For patients with substance dependence, full abstinence is the long-term goal; achieving this goal is a gradual process, however, and improvement may occur only incrementally. Judging a treatment based on its ability to achieve this long-term goal rapidly can be misleading. Thus it is useful to think of substance abuse as a chronic relapsing illness, similar to diabetes or hypertension, for which it is not clinically meaningful to expect that treatment will lead in the short term to an asymptomatic state. In this respect, substance abuse and psychiatric disorders differ: many treatments commonly used in psychiatry demonstrate efficacy over a period of weeks to months, whereas substance abuse treatments may take months to years to be fully effective.

Despite the belief that substance abuse does not respond well to treatment, a study of 51 patients with comorbid bipolar disorder and substance abuse found that the treatment for the addiction was more successful than the treatment for the mood disorder. Over the course of 3 years, symptoms of bipolar disorder improved only modestly, whereas 61 percent of the subjects were in full remission from their substance abuse disorder at the end of the study period (Drake et al., 2004). Successful treatment of the substance abuse in this study was associated with greater rates of independent living, employment, social contacts with non–substance abusers, and overall quality of life. Indeed, measuring psychosocial functioning is the most appropriate way to evaluate a behavioral intervention.

Before taking a more detailed look at pharmacological and psychosocial treatments for comorbid manic-depressive illness and substance abuse, we wish to reemphasize that although comparatively little is known about the most effective ways to treat these patients, recovery is unlikely unless both illnesses are addressed. Recognition of the substance abuse problem is the essential first step, and lack of recognition is a common obstacle to effective treatment. Substance-abusing patients with comorbid mood disorders are more difficult to treat, and long-term abstinence may take longer to achieve. Nevertheless, the extensive literature demonstrating that noncomorbid substance abuse disorder can be managed successfully with currently available treatments suggests the possibility, or even the likelihood, of good outcomes for appropriately treated manic-depressive patients as well.

Pharmacological Treatment

Although pharmacological treatment in the absence of psychosocial intervention is not an adequate treatment for substance abuse, effective medication can contribute to a positive outcome. This strategy may also allow the clinician to reduce the total number of drugs a patient must take, which may increase treatment adherence. Table 24–1 presents the results of open-label and placebo-controlled trials of mood stabilizers in patients with affective disorders and comorbid substance abuse (Levin and Hennessy, 2004).

Bipolar disorder in the presence of a comorbid substance abuse disorder may not respond well to lithium. A retrospective review of the medical records of 204 bipolar-I inpatients found that patients with substance abuse histories who received divalproex or carbamazepine remitted during hospitalization more often than did those who received lithium as the sole mood stabilizer (Goldberg et al., 1999). Additionally, an assessment of 44 patients using a structured interview found that dually diagnosed patients were more likely to be adherent to valproate than to lithium (Weiss et al., 1998). It may be that patients who are good lithium responders, that is, those with predominantly euphoric, or "classic" manias, may be less likely to use alcohol and drugs

TABLE 24–1. Open-Label and Placebo-Controlled Trials of Mood Stabilizers in Mood Disorders (Primarily Bipolar) with Comorbid Substance Abuse

Study	Substance (Sample Size)	Affective Disorder Diagnosed (Diagnostic Criteria)	Type of Trial/Setting	Medication/ Duration (weeks)	Concurrent Therapy	Affective Disorder Outcomes[a]	Drug Craving[a]	Drug Use[a]
Gawin and Kleber, 1984	Cocaine (16)	4 cyclothymia, 3 dysthymia, 2 major depressive disorder (MDD), 7 no diagnosis (Diagnostic and Statistical Manual, 3rd edition [DSM-III])	Open-label/ outpatient	Lithium[b]/12	Weekly individual and group therapy	Not assessed	↓ for 3-year lithium-treated cyclothymic patients only; measured by a 20-point analog scale	Self-reported ↓ for lithium-treated cyclothymic patients only; urine drug screen (UDS) collected every 3 to 6 weeks during the trial
Nunes et al., 1990	Cocaine (10)	Hypomania or cyclothymia (DSM-III, revised [DSM-III-R])	Open-label/ outpatient	Lithium/12	Drug counselor weekly	Improved hypomania in 5 patients as assessed by General Behavior Inventory (GBI)	↓ in 5 patients as assessed by Cocaine Craving Scale	3 patients cocaine-free for 3 weeks, as assessed by weekly UDS; of these, one achieved sustained abstinence
Brady et al., 1995	Alcohol, cocaine, or multiple substances (9)	Bipolar-I disorder (DSM-III-R)	Open-label/started medication inpatient, then followed outpatient	Valproate/24	None	↓ Hamilton Depression Scale (HAM-D) and Young Mania Rating Scale (YMRS)	Not assessed	↓ in days and amounts of substance used as assessed by Time-Line Followback (TLFB); UDS collected every other month

Study	Substance abuse (n)	Psychiatric diagnosis	Design/setting	Medication/duration (weeks)	Psychosocial treatment	Psychiatric outcome		Substance use outcome
Geller et al., 1998	Alcohol (7); marijuana (2); alcohol and marijuana (14); inhalant (1); alcohol, inhalant, and cough syrup (1) (total of 25 adolescents)	Bipolar-I or -II disorder, or MDD with bipolar predictors (DSM-III-R)	Placebo-controlled/outpatient	Lithium or placebo/6 (13 lithium treated, 12 placebo treated)	Weekly interpersonal therapy modified for families	↑Children's Global Assessment Scale (CGAS)[c]	Not assessed	Percentage of positive UDS significantly decreased in the lithium group compared with the placebo group[c]; UDS collected weekly
Calabrese et al., 2001	Alcohol, marijuana, and/or cocaine (56)	Rapid-cycling bipolar-I or -II disorder (DSM, 4th edition, [DSM-IV])	Open-label/Outpatient	Lithium + divalproex/24	12-step–based intensive outpatient chemical dependency program	↓ HAM-D, ↑ YMRS, ↑ Global Assessment Scale (GAS) after 4 weeks of treatment; statistical/clinical significance not reported	Not assessed	14 patients met DSM-IV criteria for full remission of alcohol or drug abuse disorder after 6 months; no UDS
Brady et al., 2002	Cocaine (139: 57 with affective disorder [AD[d]], 82 with no affective disorder [NAD[d]])	Lifetime diagnosis of bipolar-I or -II disorder, MDD, cyclothymia, dysthymia, or NAD (DSM-III-R)	Placebo-controlled/outpatient	Carbamazepine (CBZ) or placebo/12 (AD: 30 CBZ,[d] 27 placebo; NAD: 42CBZ,[d] 40 placebo)	Non-study-related, outpatient substance abuse treatment	Not significant (NS) ↓ HAM-D and Beck Depression Index (BDI)[c] but not YMRS for the CBZ/AD group	↓ for the entire sample, assessed by a 10-point Likert-type rating scale	Compared with other three groups, CBZ/AD group had NS trend toward ↓ percentage of positive UDS and significantly longer time to first cocaine use, as assessed by TLFB and Cocaine Use Inventory[c]; UDS collected weekly

(continued)

TABLE 24–1. Open-Label and Placebo-Controlled Trials of Mood Stabilizers in Mood Disorders (Primarily Bipolar) with Comorbid Substance Abuse (continued)

Study	Substance (Sample Size)	Affective Disorder Diagnosed (Diagnostic Criteria)	Type of Trial/Setting	Medication/ Duration (weeks)	Concurrent Therapy	Affective Disorder Outcomes[a]	Drug Craving[a]	Drug Use[a]
Brown et al., 2002	Cocaine (17)	Bipolar-I or -II disorder (DSM-IV)	Open-label/ outpatient	Adjunctive quetiapine (12)	Non-study-related[a]	↓ HAM-D, YMRS, and Brief Psychiatric Rating Scale[c] (BPRS)	↓ as assessed by Cocaine Craving Questionnaire (CCQ)[c]	NS ↓ days of cocaine use, money spent on cocaine; slight increase in positive UDS[c]
Brown et al., 2003	Cocaine (30)	Bipolar-I, -II, or not otherwise specified (NOS) (DSM-IV)	Open-label/ outpatient	Lamotrigine, adjunctive or monotherapy/ 12	24 patients in non-study-related substance abuse treatment	↓ HAM-D and YMRS, BPRS[d]	↓ as assessed by CCQ[c]	NS ↓ days of use, money spent on cocaine; no change in positive UDS[c]; UDS collected weekly

Note: ↑ = increased; ↓ = decreased.
[a]Results are statistically or clinically significant unless otherwise noted by "NS."
[b]Subgroup of 3 cyclothymic, 1 dysthymic, and 2 with no diagnosis received lithium. Others received desipramine (6) or psychotherapy only (4).
[c]Intent-to-treat and computer analyses.
[d]Six patients were involved in substance abuse treatment, and 11 were not.
Source: Reprinted from Levin and Hennessy, 2004, with permission from the Society of Biological Psychiatry.

to self-medicate than those who have predominantly mixed states (and may therefore be more likely to respond to anticonvulsants).

As summarized in Table 24–1, only a few double-blind, placebo-controlled trials have included a substantial number of substance-abusing patients with affective illness (primarily bipolar disorder). A recent 24-week controlled study followed 59 patients with comorbid bipolar-I disorder and alcohol dependence who had been randomized in a double-blind fashion to receive either valproate or placebo in addition to standard therapy with lithium (Salloum et al., 2005). Patients who received valproate had significantly fewer heavy drinking days. Valproate plus lithium therapy also significantly prolonged the time to relapse to sustained heavy drinking—to an average of 93 days, compared with an average of 62 days for those taking lithium alone. Supporting the specific benefit of the anticonvulsant, higher valproate serum concentrations correlated with improved alcohol abuse outcomes. There were no statistically significant differences in mood symptoms between the two groups, reflecting the mood-stabilizing efficacy of lithium in both. This finding suggests that the reduced drinking observed in the valproate group was not simply the result of a more stable mood, and that a separate mechanism played a role in reducing alcohol intake.

Valproate enhances gamma-aminobutyric acid (GABA), which may be affected in substance abuse disorders. GABA neurons projecting to the nucleus accumbans, the reward center of the brain where addictive drugs have their effects, diminish the release of dopamine and may attenuate the reinforcing properties of these substances. Although the antimanic efficacy of valproate is well established, data on its use in patients with substance abuse disorders are limited. In one open-label study, the efficacy of valproate for acute detoxification of noncomorbid alcohol-dependent subjects was demonstrated. Valproate reduced the symptoms of withdrawal more rapidly and consistently than benzodiazepines (the current standard of care), and valproate-treated patients were abstinent at 6-week follow-up (Longo et al., 2002). Valproate is an attractive option in this population because, unlike benzodiazepines, it does not have abuse potential.

While the anticonvulsants carbamazepine and topiramate have not been examined in bipolar patients with comorbid alcohol abuse, both have been shown to have a place in the treatment of alcohol dependence. Carbamazepine has been used successfully to treat acute alcohol detoxification. In a study of 100 noncomorbid outpatients, carbamazepine was more effective than placebo in reducing symptoms of alcohol withdrawal, and patients taking it experienced a more rapid improvement in their ability to work (Bjorkqvist et al., 1976). In another study, carbamazepine was shown to work more rapidly than a benzodiazepine in reducing symptoms of alcohol withdrawal (Malcolm et al., 2002). Carbamazepine was also found to be as effective as oxazepam—the standard of care in detoxification units—in a double-blind study, and by one measure it was superior. Subjects taking oxazepam showed an increase in global psychological distress from day 3 to day 7, whereas those taking carbamazepine exhibited a decline (Malcolm et al., 1989). After day 7, there was no difference between the two treatments.

Actively abusing patients generally require detoxification as a precursor to sobriety. However, detoxification is not a treatment for the underlying abuse disorder because by itself, it does not address the central issue of managing long-term craving and relapse. A 12-month study of carbamazepine provided evidence of its potential usefulness in preventing relapse. This double-blind, placebo-controlled study of 29 noncomorbid adult alcoholics found that carbamazepine decreased the number of drinks per drinking day and delayed the time to first episode of heavy drinking (Mueller et al., 1997).

Similarly, a double-blind, placebo-controlled trial of topiramate found a robust effect on the core symptoms of alcohol dependence. In this study, 150 subjects were treated over a period of 12 weeks with either placebo or an average of 300 mg/day of topiramate. Subjects receiving topiramate had fewer drinks per day, fewer heavy drinking days, and more days abstinent (Johnson et al., 2003). In another study, topiramate significantly reduced both alcohol consumption and craving in alcohol-dependent subjects (Johnson et al., 2003). On the other hand, while open-label studies have shown promising results for topiramate in the treatment of mania in noncomorbid patients with bipolar disorder, controlled trials have failed to confirm its antimanic efficacy (see Chapter 18).

Lamotrigine, an anticonvulsant with antiglutamatergic properties, is an effective mood stabilizer, especially against depression; that is, it stabilizes "from below" (see Chapter 19). We could find only one study of lamotrigine involving bipolar patients with comorbid alcohol dependence, that of Rubio and colleagues (2006). They gave open-label lamotrigine to 28 patients (21 bipolar-I, 7 bipolar-II, as diagnosed by the Structured Clinical Interview for DSM [SCID]) and assessed weekly changes in scores on the Hamilton Rating Scale for Depression (HAM-D), the Young Mania Rating Scale (YMRS), the Brief Psychiatric Rating Scale (BPRS), and a self-rated craving scale, as well as change in a biochemical indirect measure of alcohol consumption, carbohydrate-deficient transferrin (CDT). Significant improvement was noted in scores on all three mood scales ($p < .01$) and in both craving and consumption (as reflected in CDT) ($p < .001$).

Unlike mood stabilizers, other drugs that are effective in the treatment of substance abuse disorders may carry a risk of destabilizing a comorbid manic-depressive patient. For example, naltrexone has demonstrated efficacy in preventing relapse in noncomorbid alcohol dependence. However, some studies (Hollister et al., 1981; Latt et al., 2002), though not all (Chick et al., 2000), have raised the question of whether naltrexone causes depression when used to treat alcohol dependence, possibly by blocking the positive mood effects associated with opioid peptides. Two cases reported by Sonne and Brady (2000) illustrate the potential problems bipolar patients can experience when given naltrexone for comorbid alcohol dependence. Both patients experienced severe adverse effects after taking a single dose of naltrexone and refused to continue the medication. One experienced dysphoria. Both were hypomanic at the time of naltrexone administration, and the authors noted that mania may be associated with the production of higher levels of endogenous opiates (Olson et al., 1996), which would make individuals in this state exquisitely sensitive to the actions of an opiate antagonist.

Disulfiram may also be problematic in some comorbid patients. Under normal conditions, the prospect of the aversive alcohol–disulfiram reaction would discourage alcohol use. However, manic patients experiencing impaired judgment and impulsivity may not adequately appreciate the serious consequences of drinking while taking this drug.

Acamprosate is the most recently approved treatment in the United States for the maintenance of abstinence from alcohol. Unlike naltrexone, acamprosate does not reduce the reward associated with alcohol consumption, nor does it cause an aversive reaction as does disulfiram. Indeed, the mechanism of action of acamprosate in the treatment of alcohol dependence is not well understood. It is thought, however, that acamprosate affects both GABA and glutamate activity. Animal studies suggest it restores the normal balance between neuronal excitation and inhibition that is altered in chronic alcohol abuse (Berton et al., 1998). A large multicenter trial comparing acamprosate and placebo in 455 alcohol-dependent adults found that the mean cumulative duration of abstinence was significantly greater in the acamprosate group (139 versus 104 days). At the end of the 1-year study, 41 (18.3 percent) of the acamprosate-treated patients and 16 (7.1 percent) of the placebo-treated patients had been continuously abstinent (Whitworth et al., 1996). None of the patients in the study had comorbid mood disorders, however. Similar results were reported by Sass and colleagues (1996), who found that over a period of 48 weeks, acamprosate-treated patients (with no comorbid mood disorder) were abstinent 62 percent of the days, compared with 45 percent for patients taking placebo.

Acamprosate is well tolerated; diarrhea was the most common side effect reported by Whitworth and colleagues (1996). Potentially relevant to the treatment of comorbid patients, however, are results of clinical trials showing an elevated risk of suicidality among acamprosate-treated patients compared with those taking placebo. Completed suicides were similar in the two groups: 3 (.13 percent) of 2,272 acamprosate-treated and 2 (.10 percent) of 1,962 placebo-treated patients (.10 percent). However, suicidal events, including attempts and ideation, occurred in 2.4 percent of patients who received acamprosate for at least a year, compared with 0.8 percent of those who received placebo. The clinical relevance of these numbers is not yet fully understood, however, and it is essential to weigh the long-term risks of the untreated illness against the potential risks of this demonstrably effective medication.

Cocaine abuse and dependence are also common among patients with bipolar disorder, in part because of the drug's short-term antidepressant effect and in part because it extends and heightens hypomanic periods. As with alcohol abuse, the antimanic anticonvulsant medications may be useful in the treatment of cocaine abuse. In one study of a group of adults with cocaine dependence, some of whom also had a major affective disorder, there was a trend toward fewer cocaine-positive urine tests for those taking carbamazepine compared with those taking placebo (Brady et al., 2002). More than half of the patients in this study did not have a concurrent mood disorder, however, and among these "pure" cocaine abusers, carbamazepine had no effect on cocaine use compared with placebo. The benefit, therefore, may have been mediated by carbamazepine's mood-stabilizing capability rather than by an effect on cocaine craving per se. This finding supports the possibility that comorbid patients who receive treatment for bipolar disorder alone may be better able to reduce their substance abuse. This finding also is consistent with the observation that periods of abnormal mood tend to be associated with increased drug use.

Open-label lamotrigine was found to produce a statistically significant improvement in mood and a significant reduction in drug craving (but not a reduction in drug use) in a group of 30 bipolar patients with comorbid cocaine dependence (Brown et al., 2003). In a subsequent extension of this study involving an additional 32 cocaine-dependent bipolar patients, Brown and colleagues (2006) replicated their initial findings of improved mood and reduced craving, and in addition were able to document a significant reduction in cocaine use, as reflected in money spent on the drug. In another group of such patients, reductions in craving and improvement in mood were reported with open-label quetiapine (Brown et al., 2002).

Psychosocial Treatment

The most widely known and used psychosocial program for alcoholism, AA, has more than 1 million members participating in more than 30,000 groups that convene in at least 70 different countries. Determining the program's efficacy and delineating the types of individuals for whom it is most beneficial are difficult in anonymous, self-help group settings, however. As Ogborne and Glaser (1985) pointed out, it remains unclear (1) what proportion of any population of problem drinkers would either accept or benefit from a referral to AA; (2) whether benefits derived from involvement with AA are greater than those gained from other substance abuse treatment programs; and (3) whether involvement with AA can have any detrimental effects on some of those who participate. A meta-analysis of the literature on AA found that the correlation between participation and drinking outcomes was more positive among outpatient than inpatient samples; better-designed studies were more likely to report positive psychosocial outcomes related to AA attendance. In general, however, studies of AA have lacked sufficient statistical power to detect relationships of interest (Tonigan et al., 1996).

While there is a paucity of well-controlled studies, our clinical experience supports the widely held belief that AA benefits many individuals at little or no cost to themselves or to society. The program apparently derives much of its success from the continuous support, hope, and help provided by peers; from exposure to successfully abstinent alcoholics; from the substitution of other AA members for former drinking companions; and from increased self-regard gained through helping others in like circumstances (Vaillant, 1978). On the other hand, not all alcoholics are attracted to or able to tolerate AA's self-examining approach or religious underpinnings. Of particular relevance to manic-depressive patients with drinking problems is the opposition expressed by some AA members to the use of "chemicals" other than alcohol, including mood-stabilizing medications. Yet AA neither endorses nor prohibits the use of psychiatric medications by its members. The pamphlet *AA: Medications and Other Drugs*, published by the AA General Service Conference, clearly distinguishes necessary and important prescription medications from self-administered drugs.

To assess systematically the attitudes of AA members toward the use of medications, 277 AA members were surveyed anonymously. They were asked about their attitudes toward the use of alcohol relapse prevention medication and their experiences with any psychotropic medications while in AA. Nearly a third (29 percent) reported personally experiencing some pressure to stop taking a medication (of any type); however, 69 percent of these individuals continued taking the medication. Only 12 percent of respondents said they would tell another member to stop taking medication (Rychtarik et al., 2000).

Double Trouble in Recovery (DTR) is a 12-step self-help program specifically designed for persons with chronic mental illness and a comorbid substance abuse disorder. The program was started in 1989 and currently has more than 200 groups in the United States. DTR specifically supports both abstinence from intoxicating substances and adherence to psychiatric medication regimens. Indeed, a 1-year prospective longitudinal study of 310 participants in the program found that consistent attendance at DTR meetings was associated with better adherence to medication regimens (Magura et al., 2002). Although the study was not randomized, this relationship persisted after controlling for baseline variables that were independently associated with adherence (living in supported housing, having fewer stressful life events, and having a lower severity of psychiatric symptoms). A fifth of the patients in the study had bipolar disorder, a fifth had unipolar depression, and about half had schizophrenia.

More recently, 129 stabilized outpatients meeting *Diagnostic and Statistical Manual* (DSM) criteria for drug dependence (cocaine, heroin, or cannabis) and serious mental illness (55 percent affective disorders, polarity not specified) were randomly assigned to 6 months of Behavioral Treatment for Substance Abuse in Severe and Persistent Mental Illness (BTSAS) or to a manualized control condition, Supportive Treatment for Addiction Recovery (STAR) (Bellack et al., 2006). BTSAS entails a social learning intervention, including motivational interviewing, social skills training, and a urinalysis contingency. Participants were taught how to refuse drugs, engage in alternative social activities, and develop non-drug-using social contacts. The STAR program consisted of support groups, some education, and checking of urine samples, but with no systematic feedback. The BTSAS program was significantly more effective than STAR in terms of attendance at treatment sessions, clean urine test results, and survival in treatment. BTSAS participants reported a significant increase in general life satisfaction, were less likely than STAR participants to be hospitalized, and were less likely to be arrested.

Group therapy has been shown to be effective for treatment of both bipolar disorder and substance abuse disorders; however, few structured group therapies have been developed to address comorbid substance abuse and bipolar disorder simultaneously. An exception is Integrated Group Therapy (IGT), a manualized relapse prevention therapy that achieves an integrated approach by addressing topics that are relevant to both disorders and by highlighting common aspects of recovery from, and relapse to, each disorder (Weiss et al., 1999, 2007). A 6-month, nonrandomized pilot study found that, compared with patients who did not receive group therapy, those who received IGT had significantly better outcomes on the Addiction Severity Index drug composite score, spent more months abstinent, and were more likely to achieve at least two consecutive abstinent months. The nonrandom design of this study did not make it possible to compare the efficacy of IGT and other forms of group therapy, however. A more recent, randomized study of 62 patients found that those receiving IGT had significantly less substance abuse (Weiss et al., 2007).

In contrast to the benefits of the manualized IGT, unstructured therapy does not appear to be helpful, and it may actually be harmful, for substance-abusing patients. Weiss and colleagues (2000) followed 24 patients receiving unstructured psychosocial treatment after hospital discharge. It was found that psychotherapy and AA attendance decreased over time among the study subjects, and the focus of patients' psychotherapy gradually became more general, so that decreasing emphasis was placed on their specific disorders. During this period, there was a trend toward more frequent drug use, while the patients' mood symptoms did not change significantly.

ANXIETY DISORDERS

Panic Disorder

Uncomplicated panic disorder is generally treated pharmacologically with selective serotonin reuptake inhibitors (SSRIs) or high-potency benzodiazepines. While the use of SSRIs in unipolar depression is relatively straightforward, in bipolar patients the risk of switches into mania/hypomania/mixed states and the risk of long-term destabilization must be taken into account (see Chapter 19 for a full discussion of these critical issues). The risk of switch/destabilization with antidepressants may be increased by substance abuse comorbidity. For example, in a sample of 48 bipolar patients, 20 of whom had comorbid substance abuse, the probability of having a history of an antidepressant-induced mania was seven times greater among the comorbid patients. Overall, 60 percent of the bipolar patients with comorbid substance abuse had become manic when given an antidepressant (Goldberg and Whiteside, 2002). Although comorbid panic disorder represents a case in which an SSRI may well be needed, it is critical to first optimize mood stabilization. Indeed, as noted later, some mood stabilizers themselves have been shown to have therapeutic effects in panic disorder that could obviate the need for an SSRI.

Benzodiazepines, which are also effective in panic disorder, are frequently used during acute mania. Although they may not possess inherent mood-stabilizing properties, they can be highly effective in helping to normalize sleep, which

is a central objective in the treatment of mania. Apart from some reports of alprazolam-induced mania (Goodman and Charney, 1987), benzodiazepines do not appear to destabilize bipolar disorder. Given the high prevalence of substance abuse disorders in this population, however, benzodiazepines must be used cautiously because of their potential for abuse.

The frequency with which panic disorder occurs comorbidly with bipolar disorder may reflect a common underlying etiology (see Chapter 7). Use of a mood stabilizer to treat both illnesses simultaneously can be an advantageous strategy. Unfortunately, lithium, for which there is the largest database demonstrating efficacy in bipolar disorder, has not been the subject of controlled studies in anxiety disorders. There are more data on antipanic/anxiolytic effects among the anticonvulsants. For example, valproate has been reported to have some beneficial effects in the treatment of panic disorder, possibly due to GABA agonism (Keck et al., 1993). An open-label study of the efficacy of valproate in rapid-cycling bipolar disorder found that 95 percent of patients with comorbid panic disorder reported improvement in their panic symptoms when taking the drug. On the other hand, a related anticonvulsant, carbamazepine, was not found to be effective in a small trial of 14 patients with noncomorbid panic disorder. Only one patient experienced marked and sustained clinical improvement on the drug, while 50 percent actually experienced an increase in panic attacks (Uhde et al., 1988). A double-blind, placebo-controlled study of gabapentin in 103 patients with panic disorder (Pande et al., 2000) found it to be no different than placebo. However, a post hoc analysis did reveal that gabapentin was superior to placebo among the most severely ill patients. With respect to bipolar disorder, placebo-controlled trials have failed to demonstrate efficacy in mania (Pande et al., 1999). Pregabalin, a novel anticonvulsant that binds to a subunit of certain calcium channels, is approved as an add-on in the treatment of partial seizures. It has been found to be effective in controlled trials of generalized anxiety disorder,[1] with a side-effect profile that is generally more favorable than that of comparators such as benzodiazepines or SSRIs. In a recent placebo-controlled, head-to-head comparison of pregabalin with venlafaxine in treating generalized anxiety disorder, only pregabalin achieved significant efficacy, as early as the first week, on all a priori primary and secondary efficacy measures (Montgomery et al., 2006). Pregabalin, 400 mg, was better tolerated than venlafaxine, as reflected in significantly fewer dropouts due to side effects. These results (if replicated), together with evidence that among the second-generation antidepressants, velafaxine is associated with the highest risk of manic switch (Leverich et al., 2006), underscore the importance of evaluating the efficacy of pregabalin in the treatment of comorbid anxiety disorders in bipolar patients.

Atypical antipsychotics are playing an increasingly important role in the treatment of bipolar disorder. All have significant effects on the serotonin system; in contrast to the SSRIs, however, this effect consists of direct stimulation or inhibition of presynaptic and postsynaptic serotonin receptors. Results of some studies suggest that certain of these agents, as well as the typical antipsychotics, including trifluoperazine (Mendels et al., 1986), may have anxiolytic properties in general (Wilner et al., 2002; Gao et al., 2006) as well as in bipolar patients (Hirschfeld et al., 2006). To our knowledge, however, there have been no controlled trials of atypical antipsychotics in the treatment of panic disorder per se, so their utility for this purpose remains speculative.

For optimal results, psychotherapeutic interventions should generally be part of the comprehensive management of comorbid panic disorders. Cognitive-behavioral therapy has been shown to be effective in treating many anxiety disorders and is considered a first-line treatment.

Social Anxiety Disorder

Little is known about the pharmacological treatment of comorbid social anxiety disorder. Monoamine oxidase inhibitors (MAOIs) and serotonergic agents such as SSRIs are effective for noncomorbid social anxiety disorder, but as noted earlier, these medications can destabilize bipolar disorder. Although gabapentin has not been shown to be effective in bipolar disorder, one double-blind trial showed positive results in 69 patients with noncomorbid social anxiety disorder (Pande et al., 1999). Presumably, gabapentin would be less likely than antidepressants to cause destabilization in patients with comorbid social anxiety disorder. The role of some of the atypical antipsychotics in reducing anxiety symptoms in bipolar disorder has already been noted. As with the other comorbid anxiety disorders, cognitive-behavioral therapy should generally be part of the management strategy.

Obsessive-Compulsive Disorder

Serotonergic antidepressants are the most frequently used treatment for obsessive-compulsive disorder (OCD); benzodiazepines (Hollander et al., 2003) and antidepressants without serotonergic activity (Vulink et al., 2005) are not effective for patients with this disorder. The use of antidepressants carries risks for these patients, however. A study of 263 patients with OCD who had not been diagnosed with bipolar disorder nevertheless found that 13 percent had experienced a hypomanic episode, and that many of the hypomanias occurred after treatment with an antidepressant (Lensi et al., 1996). Only 1.5 percent had experienced full manias, a finding consistent with data showing that most patients with comorbid OCD and bipolar disorder have the bipolar-II type (Perugi et al., 1997).

As noted earlier, mood stabilizers such as lithium and the atypical antipsychotics have some degree of serotonergic activity, but the evidence supporting their efficacy in treating OCD is mixed. The findings of two controlled studies of lithium augmentation of SSRIs in the treatment of refractory OCD without comorbid bipolar disorder were negative (McDougle et al., 1991; Pigott et al., 1991). On the other hand, randomized, double-blind, placebo-controlled trials of atypical antipsychotics (risperidone and quetiapine) have shown some efficacy when these drugs are taken adjunctively by OCD patients resistant to SSRIs (McDougle et al., 2000; Denys et al., 2004).

Among patients with OCD, the degree of insight into the irrationality of obsessions varies along a spectrum. In the most severe cases, the degree of insight is low, and many such patients have psychotic delusions. These patients also tend to have less favorable responses to standard antidepressant treatment (Solyom et al., 1985). Antipsychotic augmentation of SSRIs has been studied in resistant cases of OCD, with mixed results. A small open-label study of risperidone augmentation showed beneficial effects (Saxena et al., 1996), but in a case series of six patients, risperidone actually exacerbated OCD symptoms while successfully treating psychotic symptoms (Alevizos et al., 2002). Antagonism of postsynaptic serotonin receptors is a hypothesized explanation for this detrimental effect. A double-blind study of olanzapine augmentation in patients nonresponsive to fluoxetine likewise did not show a positive effect (Shapira et al., 2004).

The treatment studies described above all evaluated patients with noncomorbid OCD. Evidence suggests, however, that comorbid OCD is different in important ways and may respond differently to treatment (see Chapter 7). Some data suggest that that the co-occurrence of OCD and bipolar disorder reflects variability in the expression of a single morbid process that is responsible for both the mood and anxiety disorders (Strakowski et al., 1998). This hypothesis would suggest that a focus on mood stabilization is the most effective way to address a comorbid patient's OCD symptoms.

A naturalistic study of 38 inpatients with comorbid bipolar disorder and OCD found that drug treatment with clomipramine and, to a lesser extent, with SSRIs was associated with hypomanic switches in these patients, especially those not treated concomitantly with mood stabilizers (Perugi et al., 2002). A combination of multiple mood stabilizers was necessary in 16 of the patients (42.1 percent), and a combination of mood stabilizers with atypical antipsychotics was required in 4 cases (10.5 percent). Overall, OCD–bipolar patients tended to show a less positive outcome with respect to both mood symptoms and general functioning (Perugi et al., 2002).

Post-Traumatic Stress Disorder

No controlled studies have specifically evaluated treatment for the comorbidity of bipolar disorder and post-traumatic stress disorder (PTSD). Because of the greater severity of pathology seen with this comorbidity compared with PTSD alone, effective treatments for noncomorbid PTSD may not work as well when used with bipolar patients. Nevertheless, there is substantial interaction between the two illnesses, whereby the symptoms of one can destabilize the other: abnormal mood states can decrease resilience and increase the risk of developing PTSD in response to a traumatic experience; conversely, both acute and chronic overarousal associated with PTSD can exacerbate mood states by increasing stress and interfering with sleep. Given this interaction, improvement of either disorder has the potential to reduce the symptoms of the other.

There is good evidence for the efficacy of both pharmacotherapy and psychotherapy in patients with noncomorbid PTSD. In particular, an international consensus group has identified SSRIs as an appropriate medication for PTSD because of the large database of randomized controlled trials supporting their efficacy (Ballenger et al., 2004). As with other anxiety disorders, however, the risks associated with PTSD must be carefully weighed against the risks of antidepressant treatment in patients with bipolar disorder, and other alternatives considered. It appears appropriate to attempt other strategies first, such as optimizing mood stabilizers.

With one exception, there are no data from controlled trials on any of the accepted mood stabilizers in treating PTSD. The exception is a double-blind, placebo-controlled trial of lamotrigine in 15 subjects with noncomorbid PTSD, which found a response rate of 50 percent compared with 25 percent for placebo (Hertzberg et al., 1999). With respect to lithium, it should be noted that bipolar disorder complicated by anxiety generally does not respond as well to the drug as does uncomplicated bipolar disorder; on the other hand, results of open trials and case reports suggest that lithium may be associated with a reduction in the arousal, anger, and irritability associated with noncomorbid PTSD (Forster et al., 1995). The results of open trials also suggest the efficacy of valproate in noncomorbid PTSD (Fesler, 1991). And open studies of carbamazepine have found reductions in intrusive memories, flashbacks, sleep disturbance, impulsivity, and violent behavior (Keck et al., 1992).

Various studies, both controlled and uncontrolled, have found adjunctive use of risperidone, olanzapine, and quetiapine to be effective in treating noncomorbid PTSD in patients not responding well to standard treatment (usually antidepressants) (Hutterfield et al., 2001; Hamner et al., 2003; Monnelly et al., 2003). Benzodiazepines, commonly used in bipolar disorder, have shown efficacy in treating some anxiety disorders, but they can increase the likelihood of developing PTSD when used during the acute post-trauma period and therefore should be avoided at those times.

As with other comorbid disorders seen in manic-depressive patients, psychotherapy has the advantage of providing an evidence-based intervention for PTSD apparently without the risks of potentially destabilizing drugs. Nevertheless, it is important to note that in some cases, psychotherapy carries risks of its own, and therapies shown to be effective in uncomplicated PTSD may not be effective in patients with comorbid bipolar disorder.

A recent consensus statement identified cognitive-behavioral therapy as an appropriate treatment for PTSD, although usually in combination with an SSRI antidepressant (Ballenger et al., 2004). There is also evidence for the efficacy of cognitive-behavioral therapy when used alone (Najavits et al., 1998).

Imaginal exposure therapy, which involves repeated recounting of the traumatic experience, has been shown to promote habituation of pathological anxiety and subsequent improvement in symptoms and functioning (Tarrier et al., 1999b). Some reports have suggested that imaginal exposure can be clinically problematic, however (Tarrier et al., 1999a). In particular, reexperiencing a traumatic event may be accompanied by shame, guilt, and anger. On the other hand, Foa and colleagues (2002) found that temporary exacerbation of symptoms during the course of treatment occurred in a minority of patients and tended to disappear during long-term follow-up. Moreover, patients who experienced temporary symptom exacerbation benefited from the treatment relative to other patients in this study. Despite generally reassuring data, however, this type of psychotherapy has not been tested in patients with comorbid PTSD and bipolar disorder. Because emotional upheaval can trigger mood episodes in bipolar patients and may result in destabilizing sleep loss, the risk associated with this treatment may be greater in comorbid patients. Yet given the substantial amount of data supporting its efficacy, imaginal exposure should not be avoided in patients with comorbid bipolar disorder; rather, it is prudent to use extra care and to remain vigilant for any signs of exacerbation of the clinical picture.

EATING AND PERSONALITY DISORDERS

The most common medications used in the management of eating disorders are the antidepressants, especially SSRIs; mood stabilizers have not been well studied in these disorders. Nevertheless, there are some limited data on the use of lithium to treat anorexia nervosa. A small double-blind, placebo-controlled trial of lithium in 16 young women with noncomorbid anorexia nervosa showed, not surprisingly, increased weight gain in the lithium group (Gross et al., 1981). The patients randomized to lithium showed significantly greater improvement on an item measuring "denial and minimization of illness." On the other hand, a larger study of depressed bulimic women showed a sizable placebo response and failed to demonstrate superiority for lithium in decreasing bulimic behavior (Hsu et al., 1991). In both studies, lithium was well tolerated, with no reports of serious adverse events.

Given its tendency to cause weight loss, topiramate has received some attention for the treatment of eating disorders associated with overconsumption of food. A controlled trial designed to evaluate topiramate in the treatment of noncomorbid binge eating disorder randomized 61 outpatients to receive placebo or flexible-dose topiramate (25 to 600 mg/day). Compared with placebo, topiramate was associated with a significantly greater reduction in binge frequency (McElroy et al., 2003). A separate placebo-controlled study also found a significant reduction in number of binge days per week among patients with noncomorbid bulimia nervosa who were treated with topiramate (Hoopes et al., 2003).

As noted earlier, zonisamide is another anticonvulsant that has been associated with weight loss, and it may have utility in the treatment of eating disorders. An open-label 12-week study of zonisamide in patients with noncomorbid binge eating disorder found significant decreases in binge eating, weight, and body mass index among patients who completed the study. There was a high dropout rate, however, with only 8 of 15 patients completing the study (McElroy et al., 2004).

Medication that causes weight gain may be useful in the treatment of anorexia nervosa. A short open trial of olanzapine in treating noncomorbid anorexia nervosa followed 17 patients for up to 6 weeks. Olanzapine was associated with a significant reduction in depression, anxiety, and core eating disorder symptoms and a significant increase in weight (Barbarich et al., 2004). A somewhat longer study (10 weeks) also found overall weight gain; 3 of 14 patients with anorexia nervosa who completed the study achieved their ideal body weight. Surprisingly, however, 4 of the 14 lost an average of 2.25 pounds (Powers et al., 2002).

Eating disorders are frequently comorbid with personality disorders (Braun et al., 1994; Zanarini et al., 2004). So, too, is bipolar disorder (see Chapter 10). Relatively little is known about the treatment of comorbid bipolar disorder and borderline personality disorder, although the treatment course is more problematic (Swartz et al., 2005). Anticonvulsant medications play a useful role in treating some patients with borderline personality disorder (Frankenburg and Zanarini, 2002; Bellino et al., 2005; MacKinnon and Pies, 2006), and there is evidence that some patients with both bipolar illness and borderline personality disorder show marked improvement with a combination of pharmacotherapy and psychotherapy (Bieling et al., 2003; Swartz et al., 2005).

GENERAL MEDICAL DISORDERS

Cardiovascular Disease

Patients with bipolar disorder and recurrent unipolar depression are at increased risk for cardiovascular disease; any evidence of such disease should be managed by a cardiac specialist. Beyond careful screening for conditions associated with heart disease, such as diabetes and dyslipidemia, treatment of these conditions is beyond the expertise of most mental health professionals.

Of significance, treatment with lithium may reduce excess cardiac mortality associated with bipolar disorder. An international multicenter trial found that cardiovascular mortality among patients who took lithium for 2 years or longer ($N = 641$) was the same as or only slightly higher than that found in the general population. Conversely, cardiovascular mortality remained high among those who took lithium for less than 2 years (Ahrens et al., 1995). Patients in this study who subsequently dropped out of lithium treatment lost the positive effects, however, and had a standardized mortality ratio (which included suicide mortality) 2.5 times higher than that in the general population (Muller-Oerlinghausen et al., 1996). SSRI use has also been associated with decreased morbidity and mortality in cardiovascular disease (Taylor et al., 2005; Tiihonen et al., 2006).

Obesity

The efficacy of most treatments for obesity is modest at best, and often temporary. Short-term caloric restriction, in particular, can lead to weight cycling. From the perspective of mood disorders, weight cycling is associated not only with physiological problems but also with psychological problems, such as diminished self-esteem and life satisfaction and a more negative body image (Friedman et al., 1998). From a dietary standpoint, the most effective approach to weight control among bipolar and recurrent unipolar patients is carbohydrate restriction.

Most agents used in the treatment of bipolar disorder are associated with weight gain, as well as with other components of the metabolic syndrome, such as insulin resistance and atherogenic dyslipidemia (see Chapter 20). Among the atypical antipsychotics used in the treatment of mania, ziprasidone and aripiprazole are relatively weight-neutral.[2] It is important to note that with this class of drugs, medical complications associated with obesity, such as insulin resistance, can occur even in the absence of obesity (Henderson et al., 2005). It remains to be seen whether the lack of weight gain associated with ziprasidone and aripiprazole is accompanied by a fully benign metabolic profile. Risperidone appears to cause fewer problems with glucose utilization compared with clozapine and olanzapine (Henderson et al., 2005). Among the established mood stabilizers, only lamotrigine does not cause weight gain, nor does it increase the risk of diabetes, atherogenic dyslipidemia, or other components of the metabolic syndrome.

As noted earlier, unlike many medications used in psychiatry, topiramate has been associated with weight loss rather than weight gain. Because so many mood stabilizers cause weight gain, topiramate may play a significant role as an antidote to iatrogenic weight gain in patients with bipolar disorder. A 6-month placebo-controlled, dose-ranging trial of topiramate for weight loss in obese patients found that all doses of the drug (64 to 384 mg/day) resulted in comparable weight loss, which was significantly greater than that observed with placebo. Mean weight loss from baseline to week 24 ranged from 4.8 to 6.3 percent of pretreatment body weight, compared with 2.6 percent with placebo (Bray et al., 2003). However, neurocognitive side effects, which are dose dependent, can interfere with patients' acceptance of topiramate; difficulty with memory, concentration, and attention were the most frequently observed of these effects.

Zonisamide has been associated with weight loss in patients with epilepsy; in a 16-week controlled trial involving 61 obese patients, zonisamide and a hypocaloric diet resulted in more weight loss than a hypocaloric diet alone (Gadde et al., 2003). The drug has also been reported to have therapeutic properties in a small number of open studies and case series of bipolar patients (see Chapter 18) (Kanba et al., 1994).

Bupropion was shown to be superior to placebo in facilitating weight loss in three controlled studies (Gadde et al., 2001; Anderson et al., 2002; Jain et al., 2002). In one of these, the weight loss was maintained for 48 weeks (Anderson et al., 2002). Moreover, in expert consensus guidelines, bupropion has been identified as a preferred antidepressant for patients with bipolar depression, although there is only limited supporting evidence from controlled trials.

Sibutramine, an antiobesity agent, is a serotonin–norepinephrine reuptake inhibitor that has been shown to improve depressed mood in patients with binge eating disorders (Appolinario et al., 2003). Although no studies have been done in patients with bipolar disorder, a dual reuptake inhibitor of this nature might be expected to lead to mood destabilization. Venlafaxine, an antidepressant dual reuptake inhibitor that has been associated with switches into mania, has not been associated with long-term weight loss. Duloxetine has not been formally evaluated for weight loss activity.

The most effective treatment for severe obesity is gastric bypass surgery, which leads to long-term loss of approximately 50 percent of excess body weight (Reinhold, 1994). This is a major abdominal surgery, however, associated with significant discomfort and medical complications. After the surgery, patients undergo extensive changes in their ability to tolerate food. They experience a drastic reduction in the amount of food they are able to consume, as well as a reduced ability to tolerate a wide variety of foods, including simple carbohydrates, foods with high fat content, and carbonated beverages. Patients who fail to follow a strict dietary regimen experience nausea, vomiting, and other aversive symptoms. The physical distress experienced by patients who do not adhere to the dietary rules may serve as a type of punishment, as characterized by the operant conditioning model, thereby facilitating long-term behavior change. It is interesting that despite the severity of the stress associated with this weight loss treatment, gastric bypass surgery has been found to lead to improvement in depressive symptoms (Dymek et al., 2001). This improvement is probably related directly to the treatment's success in bringing about long-term weight loss. Of course, with manic-depressive patients, especially the bipolar subgroup, the risks associated with major surgery (e.g., stress, disrupted sleep, temporary disruption of medications) need to be carefully weighed.

Thyroid Dysfunction

The thyroid gland produces two hormones—the prohormone thyroxine (T_4) and the more biologically active triiodothyronine (T_3). T_4 is partly converted into T_3 by deiodinases. Thyroid hormones enter the cell, bind to nuclear receptors, and alter the expression of specific genes that affect the synthesis of key enzymes required for neurotransmitter production, as well as glial cell proliferation and myelination.

As reviewed in Chapter 19, T_3 is used mainly in the adjunctive treatment of major depression and has been shown to accelerate the response to tricyclic antidepressants (Prange et al., 1969; Goodwin et al., 1982). Women in particular appear to benefit from the combination of T_3 and a tricyclic antidepressant. T_3 has also been used as an augmentation strategy in treatment-resistant depression (Aronson et al., 1996).

T_3, the most active thyroid hormone, carries the risk of inducing a hyperthyroid state. Because T_4 is the prohormone, the homeostatic mechanism of reduced conversion to T_3 allows the body to maintain a euthyroid state more easily. Unlike T_3, moreover, T_4 has not been associated with osteoporosis (Nuzzo et al., 1998).

Supraphysiological doses of T_4 were shown to be effective in the maintenance treatment of prophylaxis-resistant affective disorder in a prospective open-label study of 21 consecutively enrolled patients. The mean T$_4$ dose at the study's end was 378.6±90.2 μg/day. In this study, subjects with bipolar disorder benefited more from the T$_4$ treatment than did subjects with unipolar major depressive disorder (Bauer et al., 2002).

Despite some doubts that have been raised regarding the relationship between hypothyroidism and rapid cycling (Post et al., 1997), several open studies have demonstrated beneficial effects of high-dose T$_4$ augmentation in patients with rapid-cycling bipolar disorder resistant to conventional prophylactic drugs (Stancer and Persad, 1982; Leibow, 1983; Bauer and Whybrow, 1990). Double-blind studies are needed to confirm these results. (For more detail, see Chapter 20.)

There is a significant body of evidence supporting the connection between subclinical hypothyroidism and a less favorable course of illness in mood disorders (see Chapters 7 and 20). Unfortunately, controlled studies of thyroid supplementation for such patients have not been conducted.

CONCLUSIONS

Given the frequency of occurrence of comorbid conditions in manic-depressive illness, especially the bipolar subgroup, clinicians should screen specifically for comorbid substance abuse, anxiety disorders, obesity, eating disorders, and general medical disorders. All illnesses should be addressed individually when a treatment plan is developed. Depending on the relationship among the comorbid diagnoses, the successful treatment of one disorder may lead to improvement in the others. Nevertheless, this is not always the case, and the goal should always be full remission of each disorder individually. In the case of addiction, even if the substance abuse disorder was initially caused by symptoms of the mood disorder, the patient undergoes neurophysiological and psychological changes once the addiction is established that necessitate disease-specific interventions.

A mood stabilizer should always be initiated before other pharmacological options are considered. If the bipolar or recurrent unipolar disorder and the comorbid illness share some common pathophysiological processes, it is possible that the mood stabilizer will improve both conditions simultaneously.

For most of the comorbid disorders, the psychosocial component of treatment, ranging from 12-step programs for substance abuse to cognitive-behavioral therapy for comorbid anxiety, is a vital component of management. Further, psychotherapy alone can help some patients with comorbid anxiety disorders, enabling them to avoid the potentially destabilizing effects of antidepressants. Patients receive the most benefit from this kind of therapy once their bipolar disorder has been stabilized.

The pharmacological treatment of comorbid conditions requires careful weighing of risks and benefits. Treatment often involves using medications off label and venturing beyond the limited database of available evidence. Many patients are likely to require complex combinations of medications and psychotherapy for optimal response.

NOTES

1. Feltner et al., 2003; Pande et al., 2003; Pohl et al., 2005; Rickels et al., 2005.
2. Of these two atypical agents, ziprasidone is less likely to be associated with weight gain.

25 Clinical Management of Suicide Risk

Lithium . . . is the lightest of the solid elements and it is perhaps not surprising that it should in consequence possess certain modest magical qualities.

—*G. P. Hartigan (1959)*

Manic-depressive illness carries the risk of suicide throughout its course (see Chapter 8). The precise timing of suicide cannot be predicted, but there are almost always warning signs in the preceding days to weeks. The challenge for clinicians is to discern, from a complex and fluctuating clinical picture, suicidal intent in a patient, and to assess the presence of various risk factors for suicide, which may manifest as symptoms, stressful situations, and/or comorbidities. Specifically, treatment of manic-depressive patients to prevent suicide has three key elements: (1) clinical assessment of intent and overall suicide risk; (2) intensive treatment of those acute symptoms associated with an increased risk of suicide; and (3) careful clinical follow-up of patients with suicide risk factors, with renewed attention to treating the patient's underlying affective disorder and comorbidities. While no approach is foolproof, treatment in a maximally supportive clinical environment can reduce the risk of suicide and save lives (Rucci et al., 2002; Knox et al., 2003; Bruce et al., 2004).

In 1999, the U.S. Surgeon General declared that suicide is a *preventable* public health problem (U.S. Public Health Service, 1999). This embracing of a public health perspective on suicide was prompted by compelling evidence that (1) mental illness was undiagnosed in about 50 percent of suicides (see Chapter 8), (2) inadequate treatment characterized the majority of those individuals who had been diagnosed (Isometsa et al., 1994; Isacsson et al., 1997; Oquendo et al., 1999), and (3) the majority of those who killed themselves had had some type of contact with the health care system in the months leading up to their death. In the final month before the act alone, according to results of more than 40 studies, nearly 45 percent of suicide victims had had contact with a primary care physician and another 20 percent with a specialist (Luoma et al., 2002).

These findings strongly suggest that many lives might be saved by educating physicians and the public in how best to recognize, accurately diagnose, and correctly treat those at risk for suicide.

In this chapter, we begin by reviewing the various aspects of assessment of acute and chronic suicide risk. We then address the clinical management of those patients assessed as being at high risk for suicidal behaviors. This is followed by a review of the literature on medical and psychological treatments used for acute clinical management of suicidal patients and for long-term suicide prevention. The final section presents conclusions.

ASSESSMENT OF ACUTE AND CHRONIC SUICIDE RISK

Communication of Suicidal Intent

The clinician's ability to discern a patient's suicidal intent, which includes suicidal ideation, plans, and behaviors, is one important component of any effort to prevent suicide. All too often a breakdown in communication occurs between clinician and patient during the months preceding suicide. Final contacts with clinicians are often filled with miscues, miscommunications, and missed opportunities for intervention. Clinicians frequently fail to ask explicit questions, and patients often evade such questions and disguise or deny their intent (Institute of Medicine [IOM], 2002).

This failure of communication is one of the most enduring and disturbing findings of the literature on suicide. It should be pointed out that most of the evidence on this phenomenon comes from retrospective studies, which have methodological limitations and biases (see Busch et al.,

2003). Nevertheless, the available retrospective evidence on recent health care contacts is widely interpreted as suggesting that suicidal patients, while often motivated to seek help, are reluctant to disclose their full intent and plans. Likewise, it is clear that many clinicians are reluctant to ask explicit questions about suicide.

In a now classic retrospective study, Barraclough and colleagues (1974, p. 366) observed a trail of "unequivocal threats," not "enlightened hindsight" after studying warnings of suicide in 64 depressed patients. The authors found that 30 percent of those who killed themselves had left a direct threat; when indirect communications were taken into account, the total reached 51 percent.

In another landmark study, Robins and colleagues (1959, 1981) found, in a retrospective evaluation of 134 consecutive suicides, that 69 percent had communicated their intent to commit suicide within a year of their death; 41 percent had done so through a direct and specific statement. Suicidal ideation was expressed more frequently to spouses, relatives, and friends than to physicians. Nearly half (47 percent) of the study sample had been diagnosed with manic-depressive illness, which included severe recurrent depression as well as bipolar disorder. None of these patients were manic at the time of their suicide, a finding borne out by subsequent research showing that classic euphoric mania is not an acute risk factor for suicide (see Chapter 8).

More recent studies likewise have documented communication barriers. Isometsa and colleagues (1995) conducted a large psychological autopsy study of everyone in Finland who had committed suicide during a 12-month period and whose last medical or psychiatric appointment had been within 1 month of their suicide ($N=571$). The investigators found that only 30 percent of psychiatric inpatients and 39 percent of outpatients had communicated their intent to mental health providers during their final appointment. The problem is even worse in primary care settings; one large study found that only 19 percent of patients treated in such settings who committed suicide had communicated suicidal intent to their medical providers (Isometsa et al., 1994).

In light of patients' conflicting signals, it is no surprise that studies reveal the frequent failure of clinicians to identify those at greatest risk. Weeke (1979), studying clinicians' evaluations of suicide risk in patients who later killed themselves, reported that only 13 percent had been assessed as "seriously suicidal"; clinicians had rated 58 percent as "suicide possible, not likely," and 28 percent as "suicide quite unexpected." In a study of 76 inpatient suicides, Busch and colleagues (2003) found that approximately 30 percent had been on "no precautions" at the time of their suicide in the hospital (an additional 15 percent had been on pass or

---

BOX 25–1.   **Points at Which to Repeat Suicide Assessments**

- Prior to sustained therapeutic response—each visit
- First 6 months after hospital discharge—each visit
- In presence of a new, painful, or disabling medical condition
- In presence of a new or exacerbated comorbidity, especially anxiety, panic, or substance abuse
- At evidence of relapse or recurrence of symptoms
- At occurrence of major stresses, losses, threats, shame-inducing events
- With comorbid personality disorders: at times of vacations, reductions in treatment intensity (e.g., after hospital discharge), transfers of treatment or change of clinician
- On emergence of other acute risk factors not listed here (see Box 25–3)

---

recently discharged). This study also found that suicides occurred after suicidal intent had been expressly denied by patients. Fully 77 percent of hospital inpatients who committed suicide had, within 1 week of their suicide, denied suicidal ideation or intent in their last communication with physicians or staff. Similarly, a review of more than 30 cases of completed suicide revealed that in the majority of these cases, suicidal intent had been denied during the last communication to a clinician before the act was committed; the denial to the clinician had occurred despite earlier suicidal communications to a family member (J. Fawcett, personal communication, February 2004). Taken together, these studies suggest that many manic-depressive patients will not communicate, or will expressly deny, suicidal ideation or intent. This sobering reality means that the clinician must understand and be especially alert to other clinical risk factors, such as severe anxiety and panic, that are more predictive of suicide than expressed intent, at least in the short term, and that are amenable to direct pharmacological intervention (see the later discussion of acute versus chronic risk factors).

Goals and Timing of Suicide Assessment

The long-term management of affective illness requires that the clinician be constantly alert to the possibility of periods of increased suicide risk. We recommend that a complete suicide assessment be performed and documented during the initial evaluation of the patient and at certain points thereafter when suicide risk is likely to increase (Box 25–1). The initial suicide assessment should include family history of suicide, diagnosis, past history of suicide attempts, lethality, access to means, impulsiveness, substance abuse, and other areas of inquiry. The American Psychiatric

BOX 25–2. Questions That May be Helpful in Inquiring about Specific Aspects of Suicidal Thoughts, Plans, and Behaviors

Begin with questions that address the patient's feelings about living:

- Have you ever felt that life was not worth living?
- Did you ever wish you could go to sleep and not wake up?

Follow up with specific questions that ask about thoughts of death, self-harm, or suicide:

- Is death something you've thought about recently?
- Have things ever reached the point that you've thought of harming yourself?

For individuals who have thoughts of self-harm or suicide, ask:

- How often have those thoughts occurred (including frequency, persistence, obsessional quality, controllability)?
- How likely do you think it is that you will act on them in the future?
- What do you envision happening if you actually killed yourself (e.g., escape, reunion with significant other, rebirth, reactions of others)?
- Have you made a specific plan to harm or kill yourself? (If so, what does the plan include?)

For individuals who have attempted suicide or engaged in self-damaging actions, questions parallel to those in the previous section can address the prior attempts.

Additional questions can be asked in general terms or can refer to the specific method used and may include the following:

- Can you describe what happened (e.g., circumstances, precipitants, view of future, use of alcohol or other substances, method, intent, seriousness of injury)?

- What did you think would happen (e.g., going to sleep versus injury versus dying, getting a reaction out of a particular person)?
- How did you feel about surviving the attempt? Relieved? Disappointed? Indifferent?
- Did you receive treatment afterward (e.g., medical versus psychiatric, emergency department versus inpatient versus outpatient)?

For individuals with repeated suicidal thoughts or attempts, ask:

- About how often have you tried to harm (or kill) yourself?
- When was the most recent time?
- Can you describe your thoughts at the time you were thinking most seriously about suicide?

For individuals with psychosis, ask specifically about hallucinations and delusions:

- Have you ever done what the voices ask you to do? (What led you to obey the voices? If you tried to resist them, what made it difficult?)
- Have there been times when the voices told you to hurt or kill yourself? (How often? What happened?)
- Are there things that you've been feeling guilty about or blaming yourself for?

Consider assessing the patient's potential to harm others in addition to himself or herself:

- Are there others who you think may be responsible for what you're experiencing (e.g., persecutory ideas, passivity experiences)? Are you having any thought of harming them?
- Are there other people you would like to die with you?
- Are there others who you think would be unable to go on without you?

Source: Questions are selected from Table 3 of the American Psychiatric Association's *Practice Guideline for the Assessment and Treatment of Patients with Suicidal Behaviors.* See that table for additional questions. Reproduced with permission from the American Psychiatric Association.

Association's 2003 *Practice Guideline for the Assessment and Treatment of Patients with Suicidal Behaviors* gives examples of the kinds of questions that may be helpful to clinicians in inquiring about suicidal history and current intent (Box 25–2).

The goal of suicide assessment is to arrive at an overall qualitative estimate of the patient's risk of suicide in terms of both acute and chronic risk (Boxes 25–3 and 25–4, respectively). A risk estimate is a clinical judgment that integrates findings from the initial assessment with evaluation of risk factors and protective factors (Box 25–5). (Acute and chronic risk factors and protective factors are discussed in detail below.) Based in part on this assessment, the clinician should formulate a treatment plan for reducing the treatable risk factors, such as anxiety, insomnia, agitation, and psychosis.

Suicide assessment is not without its limitations. Research has failed to yield a set of criteria that predicts suicide risk in an individual patient.[1] Nor has any method of suicide assessment been adequately evaluated prospectively, in part because suicide is a statistically rare event (IOM, 2002). Assessment instruments are available, but no set of criteria can be sensitive enough to detect every patient at high risk while also avoiding a high false-positive identification rate. The current understanding of risk factors for suicide depends mainly on retrospective studies that lacked control groups and standardized measures of symptoms and behaviors; these studies may also suffer from bias introduced by the knowledge that a suicide occurred. Yet regardless of how imperfect clinical assessment may be, it can help prevent many suicides, and its imperfections cannot justify inattention or inaction on the part of the clinician.

BOX 25–3.   **Acute Risk Factors for Suicide in Manic-Depressive Illness**

- Recent onset of mania, depression, or mixed states
- Cycling within an episode (rapid mood fluctuations)
- Recent hospital discharge
- Recent suicide attempt
- Severe psychic anxiety—fearful ruminations occurring most of the time*
- Panic attacks*
- Episodes of agitation, depressive turmoil, mixed states, angry outbursts, tantrums*
- Global insomnia—trouble initiating sleep, middle waking, early awakening*
- Recent alcohol abuse
- Severe anhedonia
- Recent or anticipated loss of close personal relationship or job, financial loss, legal or criminal proceeding
- Acute psychosis with command hallucinations or paranoid fears of punishment, delusional guilt*

*Risk factors that are usually and rapidly modifiable with treatment.

BOX 25–4.   **Chronic Risk Factors for Suicide in Manic-Depressive Illness**

- History of frequent mood cycling
- History of mixed states
- Comorbidity—especially substance abuse and anxiety/panic; personality disorders (?)
- Family history of suicide
- Past suicide attempt
- Suicidal ideation—persistent, with specific plan and means
- Severe, sustained hopelessness
- Life dissatisfaction
- Few perceived reasons for living
- Absence of future orientation
- Loss of relationship, job
- Physical illness, chronic symptoms/pain*
- Firearms in the home*
- Help-rejection behavior
- Nonadherence to treatment
- History of impulsiveness and/or violence

*Risk factors that are usually and rapidly modifiable with intervention.

Evaluation of Patient History

A thorough history of the patient is an integral part of suicide assessment. In addition to the risk factors given in Boxes 25–3 and 25–4, the history should include the following points specific to the patient's illness:

BOX 25–5.   **Protective Factors against Suicide**

- Restricted access to highly lethal methods of suicide
- Children in the home; sense of responsibility to family
- Pregnancy
- Strong religious beliefs
- Life satisfaction; reality testing ability
- Positive coping and problem-solving skills
- Positive social support
- Access and adherence to care, with a positive therapeutic relationship

Note: Most factors come from clinical experience rather than a strong evidence base, because very little research has addressed the specific factors that might be protective in manic-depressive illlness.

Sources: Goodwin and Jamison, 1990; Malone et al., 2000; Jacobs et al., 2003.

- When in the *overall course of the illness* did past suicide attempts or severe suicidal ideation take place—in particular, how long after the onset of the illness, diagnosis, and preliminary treatment? The early stages of bipolar illness carry a significantly elevated risk of suicide (see Chapter 8).
- When in the *sequence of episodes* did attempts or ideation take place? For example, did the patient attempt suicide in a depressive episode that preceded or followed a manic episode?
- When in an *individual episode* did the patient appear to be most vulnerable to suicide?
  - In the transition from manic to depressive, depressive to manic, or manic to euthymic state? Were these states characterized by acute agitation?
  - Did increased suicidality occur relatively soon after the beginning of a depressive episode, well into it, or during the recovery period?
- How severe was the patient's suicidal ideation at the worst point in the illness?
- On the basis of past episodes (if any), when might the patient reasonably be expected to begin recovery? Has this period been associated with increased agitation and suicidality?
- If the patient is female, when in the menstrual cycle might the patient be in special jeopardy (e.g., in the premenstrual phase during a depressive or mixed episode)?
- When, in general, might the patient be at increased risk for suicide—for example, in the postpartum (puerperal) period, seasonally, or during transitions from one mood state into another?

The life-charting approach to recording data relevant to course (see Chapters 4, 11, and 20) is useful in tracking this information.

Acute versus Chronic Risk Factors

We recommend that assessment of suicide risk distinguish acute from chronic risk factors. By acute, we mean risk factors operating over days to months, whereas by chronic, we mean risk factors operating over months to years. The terms are somewhat overlapping and inexact, however; no precise lines can be drawn to demarcate when the acute period ends and the chronic one begins.

The importance of distinguishing acute from chronic risk factors was revealed in one of the few (and the largest) *prospective* suicide studies ever conducted, involving nearly 1,000 patients with major affective disorders followed for an average of 4 years, over which time 25 suicides occurred. Fawcett and colleagues (1987, 1990) observed that certain factors evaluated at study entry (e.g., severe psychic anxiety, panic attacks, global insomnia, alcohol abuse) were associated with a significantly higher suicide risk within 1 year of study entry (acute risk factors), while others (e.g., severe hopelessness, ideation) were correlated with higher risk within the second to tenth years (Table 25–1). Suicidal ideation and suicide attempts, contrary to the conventional wisdom based on retrospective studies, were not found to be acute predictors of suicide. Findings of other studies support mixed states, panic attacks, and agitation in the presence of depression and bipolar disorder as acute risk factors for suicide (Coryell, 1988; Busch et al., 2003). The main conclusion of the National Institute of Mental Health (NIMH)-sponsored prospective study of Fawcett and colleagues was that most standard suicide assessments, which focus on ideation, attempts, and hopelessness, are at best of limited value, and at worst are misleading because they overlook very real acute risk factors, most of which are treatable.

In bipolar disorder, mixed states, which are marked by intense irritability and agitation, heighten suicide risk (see Chapter 8). These states warrant particular attention because the criteria for the diagnosis of mixed states in the *Diagnostic and Statistical Manual* are far too narrow, while mixed states, broadly defined, are common (see Chapter 2), and their underdiagnosis leads to underestimation of acute suicide potential. Further, when agitation in patients manifesting a mixed–dysphoric mania is misdiagnosed as unipolar "agitated depression," inappropriate use of antidepressants

TABLE 25–1. Acute and Chronic Risk Factors for Suicide among Patients with Affective Disorder Who Committed Suicide ($N=25$) versus Patients Who Did Not Commit Suicide ($N=929$)

Symptom	Acute Risk Factor (p Value)[a]	Chronic Risk Factor (p Value)[a]
Hopelessness	.463	.007
Alcohol abuse	.029	.372
Loss of interest or pleasure (anhedonia)	.005	.223
Psychic anxiety/panic attacks	.012	.879
Suicidal ideation (persistent plan)	.613	.041
Suicide attempts	.815	.086
Obsessive-compulsive features	.063	.303
Indecisiveness	.085	.062
Diminished concentration	.028	.078
Global insomnia	.011	.765

Note: "Acute" refers to suicide occurring within 1 year of assessment; "chronic" refers to suicide occurring within 2–10 years of assessment.

[a]Probability values for Mann-Whitney U statistics.

Source: Fawcett et al., 1990. Reproduced with permission from the American Psychiatric Association.

may worsen the agitation and heighten the suicide risk (Koukopoulos et al., 1995; Akiskal et al., 2005; Baldessarini and Goodwin, 2005).

It is a matter of clinical judgment to arrive at a qualitative estimate of acute and chronic risk for suicide. Research suggests that some risk factors (e.g., pessimism, aggression/impulsivity) are additive (Oquendo et al., 2004), but they may also be synergistic. Clearly, however, certain risk factors, such as access to a firearm, pose a more immediate danger than others. Later we describe treatment of certain modifiable risk factors.

Protective Factors

> Minimum pathology in a suicidal person bereft of strengths may be lethal, while severe pathology in a person with unusual strengths may constitute only a moderate risk. (Motto, 1975, p. 239)

There can be little doubt that certain protective factors mitigate the risk factors for suicide, but it is unclear by how much or under what circumstances. Both sets of factors, which fluctuate over time, can constitute a delicate balance between the decision to live or die.

The focus on protective factors, a relatively recent phenomenon, is a direct outgrowth of the above-noted conceptualization of suicide as a preventable public health problem (IOM, 2002; Knox et al., 2004). For example, psychometric scales have been developed to measure resilience (e.g., Suicide Resilience Inventory; see Osman et al., 2004). One of the few formal studies of protective factors was conducted among psychiatric inpatients, who were administered the Reasons for Living scale, a self-report instrument measuring beliefs and attitudes thought to inhibit suicide, such as coping beliefs, a sense of responsibility to family, child-related concerns, and religious or moral objections to suicide (Malone et al., 2000). The investigators found that higher scores on this scale indicated protection from acting on suicidal thoughts, although it is unclear whether the severity of psychopathology affected the self-reporting of the study subjects.

Some of the same protective factors were observed in an earlier study by Motto (1975). Among the specific factors involved in the ability to survive suicidal inclinations, Motto cited the following: (1) the capacity to control behavior—that is, the ability to stand the pain or resist the impulse; (2) the capacity to relate readily and in a meaningful way to someone else, and the presence of family members and friends who are supportive; (3) a motivation to seek help and willingness to work actively on the problem; and (4) resources that facilitate the therapeutic process and the transition back to a stable life pattern, such as job skills, intelligence, physical health, communication skills, a capacity to trust, close ties to religion, and freedom from severe personality disturbance or addictive problems. To this list might be added financial resources (particularly important in gaining access to good medical treatment and psychotherapy, remedying financial excesses resulting from manic episodes, and meeting expenses during time lost from work); willingness and ability to follow a prescribed treatment regimen; and the kind of personality during normal times that accumulates a backlog of goodwill with friends, family, and colleagues. Manic-depressive illness strains and depletes relationships, and there is little restocking during periods of mania and depression. The support of family and friends—always crucial for depressed and suicidal individuals, particularly if they are to stay out of the hospital—depends largely on how well relationships were maintained before the depression began.

Some depressed people are better than others at garnering support. Hostile, paranoid, and irritable people are unlikely to do so, whereas those who are passive and sad when depressed will usually be offered help, especially if they normally are more outgoing when well. Unfortunately, the patient with the most dangerous depression—the most perturbed, volatile, irritable, and delusional—is often the most likely to drive away potential sources of support.

CLINICAL MANAGEMENT

The seriously suicidal person with manic-depressive illness, whether bipolar or recurrent unipolar, requires intensive clinical care. Suicide is prevented most effectively by a combination of immediate strategies to keep the patient safe by ameliorating acute risk factors, and long-term strategies to stabilize the patient's underlying illness and thereby prevent recurrences of potentially life-threatening affective episodes. The clinician may need to change or add medications, modify psychotherapeutic practices, and enlist support from the patient's family members and friends. A suicidal crisis while a patient is under psychiatric care often provides the opportunity and impetus to reappraise previous assumptions about diagnosis, psychiatric history, treatment response, and involvement in the treatment process of family members and other individuals of significance to the patient.

The immediate priorities with a suicidal patient are (1) to keep the patient safe by precluding or reducing access to common methods of suicide, such as firearms and medication overdose; (2) to establish a therapeutic alliance; and (3) to treat acute risk symptoms that can be clinically modified (e.g., recurrent severe anxiety/panic, mixed states, agitation, impulsivity, global insomnia, and substance abuse). The second priority is to develop and implement a systematic treatment plan for preventing future episodes of suicidal depression, mania, and mixed states. Chronic-risk patients usually do not warrant immediate care, but the clinician must be alert to the possibility that they may become acutely suicidal at any time if they experience a worsening of symptoms or situational setbacks or if they fail to respond to treatment. Once an acute risk of suicide is suspected, chronic-risk patients must be reassessed. The overall approach to acute- and chronic-risk patients is depicted in Figure 25–1.

In this section, we first address clinical management of acute and chronic suicide risk. We then examine a number of psychological and other aspects of treatment of patients deemed to be at risk of suicide.

Management of Acute Risk Factors

> . . . I have this almost terrible energy in mind and nothing seems to help. . . . I walk up and down the room—back and forth—and I feel like a caged tiger. (Anne Sexton[2])

The "terrible energy" described by the poet Anne Sexton, who ended her life by suicide, is typical of the physical and psychic agitation experienced by many patients in the midst of episodes of bipolar depression. Agitation—which, like several other acute risk factors, is usually modifiable with treatment—is marked by increased voluntary motor activity, such as pacing, handwriting, and pressured speech patterns, and a subjective sense of perturbation or feeling "wired" (see Chapter 2). The activity is typically repetitive, stereotyped, and purposeless. In suicidal states, agitation is often accompanied by, and difficult to distinguish from, severe anxiety. More severe, persistent, or recurrent anxiety, panic attacks, and agitation in the presence of unipolar or bipolar depression are all acute risk factors for suicide (Coryell, 1988; Fawcett et al., 1990; Busch et al., 2003). Prevalence data for the symptoms of agitation in bipolar disorder are sparse (Allen and Currier, 2004; Sachs, 2006), but their existence is common and potentially dangerous. These potentially dangerous symptoms can usually be reduced in a relatively brief period of time—a matter of hours to days—with appropriate pharmacological therapies. To the extent possible, patients who are agitated should

Figure 25–1. Overall approach to manic-depressive patients with acute and chronic risk factors for suicide.

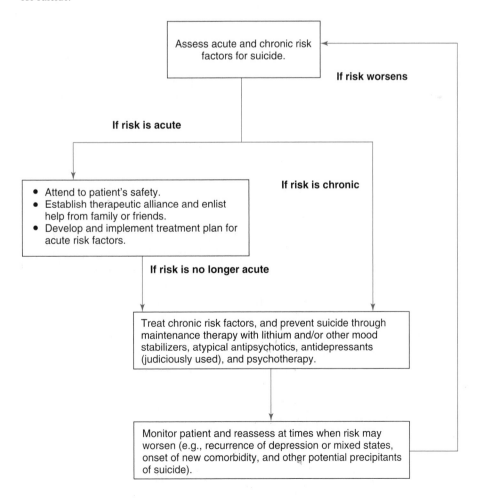

be isolated from external, exacerbating stimulation through the use of quiet or isolation rooms.

We recommend, at a minimum, regularly administered doses of benzodiazepines, such as clonazepam or lorazepam, for severe anxiety/panic, agitation, and global insomnia in a suicidal patient. For more severe anxiety/panic or insomnia, a typical or atypical antipsychotic or an anxiolytic anticonvulsant, such as valproate or gabapentin, is often appropriate (Battaglia, 2005; Marco and Vaughan, 2005; Marder, 2006). Benzodiazepines must be used cautiously because they may induce outbursts of anger and disinhibition. Atypical antipsychotics or some anticonvulsants may be helpful alternatives in these patients, especially when the risk of disinhibition is high.

The selective serotonin reuptake inhibitors (SSRIs) or serotonin/norepinephrine reuptake inhibitors (SNRIs) may be used for their anxiolytic effects, but with caution. First, SSRIs and other antidepressants have a gradual onset of efficacy (1 to several weeks), with most studies not showing significant decrements in severity of anxiety symptoms before 4 weeks. Second, bipolar patients prescribed antidepressants need to be carefully monitored, and they and their family members advised to be alert to the agitation and precipitous switches in mood that may be associated with use of these medications. Children and adolescents bear even closer monitoring, especially in the early stages of illness. Indeed, the U.S. Food and Drug Administration (FDA, 2004) has issued a black box warning on antidepressants for this age group because of the occasional occurrence of increased suicidal ideation or behavior as an antidepressant-related adverse event (see our later review of the literature on long-term suicide prevention). Some of these reports of suicidality no doubt represent treatment-induced activation of mixed states in young people with an unsuspected bipolar diathesis.[3]

Although there is danger of inducing mood cycling by administering antidepressants to a bipolar patient, the evidence appears to suggest that the risk is lower for the newer-generation SSRIs, SNRIs, and bupropion than for tricyclic antidepressants (see Chapter 19). In any case, to minimize the risk of inducing mood cycling or mixed states, mood stabilization should be established before antidepressant medications are introduced.

Acute suicidal depression in a manic-depressive patient, whether bipolar or recurrent unipolar, is one of the most compelling indications for the use of electroconvulsive therapy (ECT). This is particularly so given that antidepressants may worsen the course of illness in some bipolar patients, as well as induce mixed states (see Chapter 19), and that even the most up-to-date and effectively used pharmacological interventions will fail in 20 to 30 percent of suicidal patients (Prudic and Sackeim, 1999). Yet ECT continues to be under-used, particularly in the United States, because of the presence of obstructive legal and bureaucratic pressures that make the treatment difficult and cumbersome to employ; the risk of litigation by a small minority of patients; the availability of alternative antidepressant treatments; the influence of negative publicity from outside the medical field; and, within the psychiatric field, a relative lack of awareness of ECT's advantages in treating the acutely suicidal patient.

ECT has several advantages over pharmacotherapy: the antidepressant response is more rapid, thereby decreasing the immediate risk of suicide; there is less potential for worsening the course of the illness; and the interruption of the depressive episode allows time for the prophylactic effect of a mood stabilizer to take hold (Prudic and Sackeim, 1999). At the same time, however, some caveats are in order. First, ECT does not always relieve these symptoms quickly. Moreover, there may be delays in scheduling or accomplishing required medical tests and examinations, and during this period, the symptomatic patient remains at risk. Finally, ECT may be no more effective than other short-term treatments (see the later discussion).

Management of Chronic Risk Factors

The sophisticated use of medications and ECT in treating manic-depressive illness and preventing relapses is the single best prophylaxis against suicide, although it may not be sufficient; psychotherapy (discussed later) is often essential as well. In choosing pharmacological treatments, the most important considerations are efficacy, adverse events, and adherence. Accordingly, some of the recommendations made here summarize what has been covered in detail elsewhere (see Chapters 17 through 24).

Prevention of recurrent depressive or mixed episodes is the foremost deterrent to suicide; suicide rarely occurs during manic or euthymic states (see Chapter 8). When bipolar or recurrent unipolar patients at significant risk for suicide are maintained on lithium, alone or in combination with other mood stabilizers and/or atypical antipsychotics, the incidence of suicide can be significantly reduced. Carefully timed treatment with antidepressants may also reduce the risk of suicide; as noted previously, however, for bipolar patients antidepressants should generally be preceded by a mood stabilizer, preferably lithium because of its demonstrated antisuicidal effect.

Despite strong evidence of lithium's antisuicidal effect (discussed in detail in a later section), its prescription rate in the United States dropped beginning in the mid- to late 1990s in favor of anticonvulsants, for which there is no systematic evidence of antisuicidal efficacy. We recommend much greater awareness of lithium's value in suicide prevention, alone or in combination with other medication and, when appropriate, psychotherapy.

Psychological Aspects of Treatment

The psychological aspects of treating suicidal bipolar patients, although often emotionally draining and time-consuming for the clinician, are an essential component of preventing suicidal behavior. The suicidal bipolar patient, for example, has many problems that necessitate psychological support or therapy, reassurance, or general informational counseling. Moreover, ongoing professional assessment of suicide risk, as discussed earlier, is vital for those undergoing treatment, whether outpatient or inpatient. Because a suicidal depression often follows a manic episode, the depression is exacerbated by adverse circumstances generated while the patient was manic, such as financial or employment crises, marital problems, and legal difficulties. Other psychological problems arise from reactions to the illness itself (see Chapters 21 and 22) and the pervasive problem of treatment nonadherence (see Chapter 21). General psychotherapeutic issues are discussed more fully in Chapter 22. Here we discuss specific issues that arise during suicidal depressions, including therapeutic style, suicide-oriented therapies, the patient's need for reassurance and information, medication monitoring, clinician availability, and clinician attitudes engendered by the suicidal patient.

Therapeutic Style

Most clinicians agree that psychodynamic psychotherapy is contraindicated for suicidal patients, especially those who have bipolar disorder (Winokur et al., 1969; Hankoff, 1982). Clinical experience suggests that a direct and involved approach is the most effective and compassionate. The therapist should be willing to take more initiative with severely depressed patients than might be appropriate with others. Directness with a suicidal patient is imperative, because the gravity of the situation demands immediate action, and the patient's paralysis of will necessitates active intervention. Also, most suicidal bipolar patients are hyperalert and hypersensitive, as well as guarded and suspicious, and they often possess an uncanny ability to sense fear, irritation, and evasiveness in their therapists. Directness on the part of the clinician can help allay unnecessary anxiety and unwarranted speculation, decrease a pervasive sense of hopelessness, and establish a basis for trust that can extend into other aspects of clinical care. Along with directness, the therapist must demonstrate an ability to understand complex and painful feelings.

Because manic-depressive illness has biological roots, psychotherapeutically oriented clinicians often refer suicidal manic-depressive patients to psychopharmacologists, some of whom may not have the time, interest, or skill to provide psychotherapy and thus may tend to rely too heavily on medication. Conversely, clinicians who are primarily psychotherapists may tend to place too little emphasis on the importance of medication in alleviating short-term risk factors as well as treating the long-term course of the illness. This clinical problem is especially significant for suicidal patients, who have a particular need for integrated medical and psychotherapeutic care.

Suicide-Oriented Therapies

Contemporary randomized controlled trials of the long-term efficacy of psychotherapy in manic-depressive illness have focused on the bipolar subgroup (see Chapter 22). Disappointingly few of these studies have tested the efficacy of specific suicide-oriented therapies, and none have focused on decreasing suicide, or even "suicidality," per se. Indeed, most clinical trials that address suicidal behaviors have been directed at personality disorders or have grouped together patients with very different diagnoses (Brown et al., 2005). Further, the outcome measure has usually been deliberate self-harm, which encompasses both nonlethal and lethal intent and varying degrees of planning; it is an imperfect proxy for suicide. The primary problem is that most trials are underpowered to detect a decrease in suicide because of its relative rarity.

Systematic reviews of the efficacy and methodology of suicide-oriented clinical trials are available.[4] The types of therapies examined in such trials include particular cognitive-behavioral therapies (e.g., dialectical behavioral therapy for borderline personality disorder), psychodynamic interpersonal therapy, emergency cards (which allow emergency admission or contact with a physician), and problem-solving therapy. Recently, Miklowitz and Taylor (2006) proposed an adaptation of family-focused therapy for suicidal bipolar patients that holds promise for helping this at-risk group of patients. Given the limitations of the literature, clinical experience suggests that with suicidal bipolar patients, the quality of the relationship between therapist and patient is more important than any particular type of psychotherapy.

Providing Reassurance

The liberal and intelligent use of reassurance, an integral part of the treatment of manic-depressive illness, is particularly important when the patient is suicidal. Indeed, it is reasonable to offer hope when dealing with a generally treatable and spontaneously remitting illness. Winokur and colleagues (1969) suggested frequently reassuring patients and families first, that depression is an illness; second, that it is time-limited; and third, that the clinician is familiar with this kind of problem. While depressed, suicidal patients are unlikely to acknowledge that such reassurance is helpful, although after they have recovered, they often remark on how important the clinician's reassurance was to them (Coate, 1964; West, 1975; Jamison, 1995). Thus the clinician needs to have considerable skill and perseverance to maintain credibility while reassuring the patient. For example, it is helpful to acknowledge negativistic skepticism, with an understanding of the patient's current depression. By taking a stance of not overreacting and maintaining a positive outlook—knowing that if one treatment approach is not successful, the next may be—the therapist can sustain hope even in the face of failure of a therapeutic trial. The clinician's charge is to convince the patient that the treatment being administered may be able to help and to engage the patient's participation, if not belief, long enough to produce some symptom relief that will encourage continuation with the treatment. The patient needs to hear that the therapist is not going to give up even if initial efforts are unsuccessful. The protective factors discussed earlier, such as family and friends or strong religious beliefs, can be emphasized by the clinician. Certainly, whenever possible and clinically indicated, family members should be actively involved and educated in the patient's treatment.

Communicating Information

Explicit information about both the bipolar and recurrent unipolar forms of manic-depressive illness, their treatment, and their association with suicide is particularly important when dealing with suicidal patients, who may feel profound hopelessness and be severely cognitively impaired. Whenever feasible, information should be provided to such patients in both oral and written form. One of the first messages that must be clearly communicated concerns the limits on confidentiality between suicidal patients and their therapists. This message becomes highly significant for patients who are paranoid, irritable, and hostile or are experiencing mixed states and rapidly fluctuating moods. Other information for the patient and, where appropriate, for the family are listed in Box 25–6.

It is important to communicate consistently that although manic-depressive illness is serious, it can be treated successfully in the great majority of cases. Left untreated, however, particularly early in its course, it not infrequently results in suicide. The clinician must explain to both patient and family that denial of the possibility of recurrence is common, but it can also be dangerous. Such an explanation predicts thoughts and feelings and thereby lends credence to the clinician's recommendations.

The patient must be strongly and persuasively encouraged to take lithium or other medications as prescribed. In the case of lithium, the patient should be informed that the drug has been demonstrated to have a strong antisuicidal effect and that it can sometimes work as effectively against depression as it does against mania, but that it usually takes

---

> BOX **25–6.**   **Communicating Information to Suicidal Patients and Families**
>
> **General Issues**
>
> - Written information whenever possible
> - Ways of contacting clinician
> - Limits on confidentiality
> - Importance of postponing major life decisions
> - Treatable nature of affective illness
>
> **Medication Issues**
>
> - Availability of many effective medications
> - Imperative to take medications as prescribed
> - Importance of providing instructions in writing
> - Side effects usually transient and/or treatable
>
> **When to Contact Clinician**
>
> - Worsening of suicidal ideation
> - Worsening of symptoms, especially:
>   - Sleep loss
>   - Severe anxiety/panic
>   - Agitation, severe restlessness
>   - Delusions
>   - Feeling of violence, impulsivity
> - Problems with medication adherence
> - Increased impulsivity and aggressivity
>
> **Alcohol and Drugs**
>
> - Worsen sleep
> - Decrease impulse control and judgment
> - Potentiate or interfere with prescribed medications
> - Worsen course of illness
> - Increase the likelihood of mixed states
>
> **Recovery Issues**
>
> - High-risk nature of recovery period
> - Recovery likely to be frustrating and tumultuous
> - Uneven "sawtooth" pattern of recovery
> - Time course and recovery pattern with antidepressants (energy and the ability to execute a plan are likely to return more quickly than improved mood or cognition)

more time to have an effect on the former. The patient (and clinician) should not be discouraged by this delay. Patients should be advised as well that strict adherence to lithium therapy is very important because of the increased risk of suicide after stopping the medication (as discussed further below).

It is important to communicate explicitly that many side effects occurring with medications can be ameliorated, while others cannot. The clinician should be specific about possible side effects and how transitory or permanent they are likely to be. Patients who are started on a medication should be warned that the time course for a drug response may lead to a discrepancy between what their physician sees and what they themselves are experiencing. For example, the physician and family may see improvement because the patient has more energy and is sleeping better, and his face and body are more animated. These changes generally precede improvements in mood and thinking, changes that are likely to be more important to the patient. (Too, increased energy and capacity to act when combined with depressed mood can itself be dangerous.) Warning patients about this discrepancy in perception can lessen some of their discouragement, which is particularly important given that, as noted earlier, they may be at higher risk for suicide at this stage of the illness.

As the patient's condition begins to improve, the clinician should explain that recovery from a suicidal depression is exceptionally difficult, that a particularly frustrating and difficult period may lie ahead, and that temporary setbacks are common. The patient should be aware that alcohol generally worsens depression, interferes with sleep, impairs judgment and impulse control, and undermines the effects of medications (see Chapter 24). The patient should be advised as well to avoid significant occupational, social, or personal changes when depressed and to obtain a leave of absence from school or work rather than quit.

Medication Monitoring

The importance of prescribing only limited amounts of potentially lethal medications to suicidal patients cannot be overstated. Growing reliance on SSRI antidepressants has reduced the likelihood of lethal overdose because they are less toxic than monoamine oxidase inhibitors (MAOIs) and tricyclic antidepressants. In the pre-SSRI era, Murphy (1975) concluded that half of patients who killed themselves through an overdose had obtained their lethal antidepressant dose in a single prescription. Lithium is also potentially lethal and should be monitored accordingly (see Chapter 20).

Instructions regarding medications—dosages, timing, side effects, potentially dangerous adverse reactions, and potentiation/interference by alcohol and other drugs—should be explicit and in writing. If possible, another concerned individual (family member or friend) should become involved in monitoring the medications prescribed for a suicidal patient because confusion, hopelessness, and ambivalence about taking drugs can make depressed patients particularly susceptible to errors in taking medications. Plastic pill boxes with separate sections for each day of the week are helpful to many patients, particularly those who are confused as a result of their depression or are taking more than one medication.

Availability of Clinician

When patients are suicidal, they should be seen and contacted more frequently than usual. If financial or scheduling problems exist, the clinician should attempt to see the patient for shorter periods of time but more often. It may help to establish a time each day, or every few days, for a brief telephone conversation. Because the slowed anergic quality of bipolar depression often makes telephoning a difficult task for the patient, we find it helpful to initiate these contacts, asking the patient frequently and regularly to give his own assessment of suicidal ideation and obtaining as much information as possible from family members about the patient's behavior and suicidal intent.

The clinician's accessibility to the patient and the patient's understanding and acceptance of his alliance with the clinician are dimensions of care that are crucial to keeping the patient alive through the worst times. The patient must be told clearly how to reach the clinician in an emergency or during an acute exacerbation of suicidal thoughts and feelings. Directions for dealing with answering services, on-call systems, and coverage by other clinicians should be explicit and conveyed both orally and in writing. Depressive confusional states, as well as guilt or fear about overburdening and alienating clinicians, often prevent patients from indicating that they do not fully understand such practical details. Putting this information in writing, along with "Do not hesitate to call," can be both concrete and reassuring. The clinician needs to have a clear agreement with all suicidal patients stipulating that they will call if they are in danger of losing control of their feelings or actions, become acutely suicidal, or feel the need for immediate care. It generally is prudent as well to share this information with the closest family member or friend.

Clinician Attitudes

Therapists should always be sensitive to the feelings, thoughts, and actions engendered in them by a patient (see Chapter 22), but this is especially so when the patient is suicidal. The therapist's reactions often reflect the added stress, responsibility, and time commitments involved in treating a suicidal patient, who is frequently irritable and who conveys a sense of contagious hopelessness. The tendency for some therapists to overidentify with patients—professionally successful ones in particular—can increase the therapist's own psychological distress and lead to denial or overprotectiveness. The serious possibility of suicide reminds most therapists of their own limitations. As Cassem (1978, pp. 595–596) noted:

> The need to balance consideration for the patient's safety with the goal that he live his life independently . . . reminds

us how limited the therapist's powers are—that is, they are no stronger than the patient's desire to make use of help. The therapist who appreciates his ultimate inability to stop the person who really wants to kill himself is far more likely to be effective in restoring the person's sense of self-esteem and wholeness. . . . Clarifying these limitations with the patient helps convey respect for his autonomy and reminds the therapist that a completed suicide can occur despite complete fulfillment of his responsibility.

Suicidal manic-depressive patients can challenge and frustrate the clinician because of the need for complicated diagnostic judgments and sophisticated psychopharmacological decisions, as well as other problems in managing suicidal behavior, such as obstacles to hospitalization. Consultation with specialists in the pharmacological and psychotherapeutic treatment of affective illness can be helpful clinically, personally, and legally.

Other Aspects of Treatment

Involvement of Family Members and Friends

The involvement of family members and friends can lessen the need for hospitalization and increase the family's and patient's sense of control over a potentially devastating situation. By participating during a patient's acute-risk period, families can be actively involved in much of the decision making that takes place and learn ways to avert future crises. The clinician can alleviate family members' understandable sense of hopelessness and helplessness by providing information and reassurance, by giving them realistic expectations about likely difficulties in the acute and recovery phases, and by establishing clear contingency plans for serious problems that may arise. Families, like patients, should be given direct, preferably written, information about the patient's illness, medications, potentially dangerous adverse reactions, suicide risk, and ways of contacting the clinician.

The clinician can set up a suicide alert system by meeting with the patient, relevant family members, and a few close friends (if advisable) to coordinate an effective and direct method for noting particularly dangerous changes in the patient's mental condition and mood. At that meeting, the clinician should clarify the above-noted limits of confidentiality in situations of potential suicide and should stress that the ultimate responsibility for assessing lethality and making decisions about hospitalization rests with the clinician. Such clarification avoids confusion about responsibility and lessens family members' guilt should suicide or a severe attempt occur. The clinician must frequently assess the stress on all participants, as well as determine whether the patient needs to be hospitalized.

To facilitate communication, relatively new legal instruments, known as psychiatric advance directives, can be used by patients, when well, to document their instructions for care in times of suicidal crisis, including preferences for medication, hospitalization, and ECT and the designation of an individual authorized to make health care decisions on their behalf. More than 20 states have passed specific statutes for psychiatric advance directives. Forms can be downloaded through various gateway Web sites (e.g., Duke University, 2005) and through patient advocacy groups (see the suggested guidelines of the Depressive and Bipolar Support Alliance given in Box 22–1 in Chapter 22).

Hospitalization

The decision to admit a suicidal patient to a psychiatric hospital is often straightforward and reassuring. On the other hand, when a patient equates hospitalization with failure or symbolic defeat or when the stigma of hospitalization may have a severe and negative effect on work or personal relationships, the decision becomes more complicated. The psychological, social, financial, and clinical disadvantages to the patient must be weighed not only against the risk of suicide, but also against the pragmatic and emotional costs to the family and the clinician if the patient remains out of the hospital.

Hospitalization, although decreasing the risk of suicide, does not eliminate it. Robins and colleagues (1959) found that 7 percent of patients in their sample had committed suicide while in a psychiatric hospital. Weeke (1979) reported an even higher rate: 27 percent of manic-depressive patients killed themselves while under hospital care, although half of them were on a pass or had absconded. Weeke emphasized the need for special precautions to supplement hospitalization and the careful observation of such patients even when they appear substantially improved or recovered (see also Winokur et al., 1969; Roose et al., 1983). These measures are not always effective in preventing suicide, however. Busch and colleagues (2003) examined 76 cases of inpatient suicide and found that 42 percent had been on orders for suicide checks every 15 minutes or had been seen by staff within 15 minutes of their suicide. This finding underscores the potential inadequacy of one of the most commonly used precautions for those at acute risk of suicide.

Motto (1975) and Hawton and Catalan (1982) provided specific examples of ways to document evidence and improve communication among hospital staff members to prevent suicide:

- The degree of suicide risk should be carefully assessed and should be stated explicitly (for example, low, moderate, or high).

- The measures to be taken in dealing with the acutely suicidal patient should be stated in clear, specific terms. Most hospitals have devised suicide observation procedures that include detailed instructions to nurses and physicians.
- Nursing staff should be required to document on the patient's chart that the suicide prevention measures have been carried out.

It is especially important to specify whether the risk of suicide for a patient is acute or chronic. Once acute risk has been determined, efforts must be made to reduce that risk, such as by aggressively treating insomnia, agitation, and anxiety symptoms and providing the patient with one-on-one observation until the acute-risk state has ended.

Other factors important to preventing suicide in hospitalized patients are a high staff/patient ratio, a reduced number of exits on the ward or a locked ward, and an awareness that increased risk occurs during a change in nursing shifts and when a crisis on one part of the ward distracts staff attention from the suicidal patient (Hawton and Catalan, 1982). It is essential, when possible, to ask the patient's family members about expressed suicide intent since, as noted earlier, patients more often confide in family members than in their doctors.

Follow-Up Care

The chronic, recurrent, and serious nature of manic-depressive illness makes careful monitoring during the recovery period an essential part of treatment. Even in the early nineteenth century, Benjamin Rush (1812, p. 239) called attention to the danger of this period:

> We should be careful to distinguish between a return of reason and a certain cunning, which enables mad people to talk and behave correctly for a short time, and thereby to deceive their attendants, so as to obtain a premature discharge from their place of confinement. To prevent the evils that might arise from a mistake of this kind, they should be narrowly watched during their convalescence, nor should they be discharged until their recovery. . . .
> Three instances of suicide have occurred in patients soon after they left the Pennsylvania Hospital, and while they were receiving the congratulations of their friends upon their recovery.

Several studies (e.g., Roy, 1982; Fawcett et al., 1987) have found that the first 6 to 12 months after hospital discharge is a period of very high risk for suicide. Appleby and colleagues (1999) retrospectively studied 2,177 cases of suicide among patients who had had contact with mental health services within the year before their death. Of these suicides, 24 percent occurred within the first week of hospital discharge; 43 percent were in the highest-priority category for community care; and 26 percent had not adhered to treatment. The authors observed that earlier and more intensive follow-up in the community may be required for effective suicide prevention.

Many investigators (Fieve, 1975; Hankoff, 1982; Gitlin and Jamison, 1984) have noted the advantages of specialty affective disorder clinics in providing continuity of care. Because of their medical affiliations, these clinics are sometimes more free of stigma than other psychiatric programs. Such specialty clinics are also able to make rigorous diagnoses, provide highly specialized and up-to-date treatment, and treat a large number of patients with similar types of problems. Nonetheless, most patients with manic-depressive illness are not in fact treated in such facilities, and other settings, such as private practice, can provide some of these advantages as well. On the whole, continuity of care and expertise in diagnosis and treatment (through consultation when necessary) are most important in treating both the recurrent unipolar and bipolar subgroups of manic-depressive illness.

Impact of Suicide on Family Members

While the emphasis of this chapter is on treating and preventing suicidal behavior, suicide will still occur despite the dedicated efforts of clinicians, family members, and friends. The psychological impact of suicide on those left behind has received scant study, although there have been a few investigations. The existing research confirms clinical experience and the intuitive expectation that one of the highest priorities in the wake of a suicide is to attend to surviving relatives, who not only suffer terribly from the loss, but may themselves be at risk for developing psychiatric problems.

Relatives' nearly universal reactions to suicide—grief, guilt, devastation, and distress—are complicated by the stigma associated with the act and lingering questions of why, what if, and what else they could have done. Brent and colleagues (1996) found that most siblings of adolescents who commit suicide are themselves at heightened risk of developing depression within 6 months; within 3 years, however, they do not display excess psychopathology. On the other hand, mothers of children who have died by suicide continue to show long-lasting effects 3 years later, and nearly 30 percent develop depression. Another study, focused on children whose parents committed suicide, found that the anxiety, anger, and shame experienced during the first months after the event give way to behavioral and anxiety symptoms but, at least after 2 years, not to long-term psychopathology (Cerel et al., 1999). Children with preexisting psychopathology are, however, at long-term risk of exacerbation or the onset of new disorder. To avert long-term effects, children should be told the truth about the suicide, although the surviving parent's natural reaction is often otherwise. Shielding children leads to greater turmoil and potential long-term distress once they inevitably learn the truth from other children or adults. Clinicians, in addition to expressing their condolences and, if possible, attending the funeral or memorial services, should be available to families in the wake of suicide and should make appropriate referrals to other mental health professionals when necessary. Parents and family members can access help through several organizations listed in the appendix at the end of the volume.

Impact of Suicide on the Therapist

Therapists often portray losing a patient to suicide as the most anguishing time in their careers (Gitlin, 1999). Approximately one-half of psychiatrists and one-quarter of psychologists surveyed in the late 1980s reported experiencing a patient's suicide (Chemtob et al., 1988a,b). Therapists' immediate reactions to suicide include shock, grief, guilt, fear of blame, self-doubt, shame, anger, and a sense of betrayal, according to results of research sponsored by the American Foundation for Suicide Prevention (Hendin et al., 2000). About a third of those interviewed reported severe levels of distress, often lasting longer than a year. Severely affected therapists attributed their distress to their failure to hospitalize an acutely suicidal patient who later died, treatment decisions, negative reactions from institutions and peers, and fear of a lawsuit by the patient's family members (Hendin et al., 2004). These findings call for more collegial and institutional support for therapists after a patient's suicide, as well as for postmortem opportunities to learn more about suicide prevention.

REVIEW OF THE LITERATURE

In this section, we review in turn the literature on acute clinical management of suicidal patients and long-term suicide prevention, elaborating on the brief earlier discussion of various medical treatments.

Acute Clinical Management

Evidence concerning successful treatment of patients at acute risk of suicide is quite limited for several reasons. The first concerns ethical issues involved in conducting controlled studies in emergency clinical situations. The second is the limitation in statistical power that results from the relatively small numbers of actual suicides noted previously and the fact that the validity of using attempted suicide or suicidal ideation as a proxy measure is highly questionable (see Chapter 8). Third, the literature on suicide and its prevention generally does not distinguish acute from chronic risk; instead, it tends to address risk as a single category, perhaps as a result of the retrospective nature of most studies of suicide. Finally, most studies do not compare the incidence of risk factors in those who commit suicide with the incidence in a comparison group of those who do not, nor do they examine the time from the emergence of a putative risk factor to the occurrence of suicide.

Given this dearth of research evidence, it is difficult to assess the effectiveness of various clinical interventions in reducing the acute risk of suicide. The best evidence available is based on clinical trials that show a rapid reduction of high-risk symptoms, not of suicide or attempts per se. The value of this evidence is based on the reasonable, although as yet unproven, inference that reducing or reversing these symptoms will reduce the acute risk of suicide. Below we review this evidence for benzodiazepines, anticonvulsants and antipsychotics, antidepressants with rapid onset, and ECT.

Benzodiazepines

Results of several clinical trials suggest that adequate, regularly administered doses of benzodiazepines, such as clonazepam or lorazepam, can act fairly rapidly to reverse severe anxiety, panic attacks, and agitated states. Smith and colleagues (2002) presented data showing more rapid improvement in depression when clonazepam was added to fluvoxamine. Londborg and colleagues (2000) found over the first 3 weeks of treatment that fluoxetine plus clonazepam at night, versus fluoxetine plus placebo, worked better in reducing total Hamilton Rating Scale for Depression (HAM-D) scores, anxiety, and sleep disturbance. Treatment-emergent anxiety was reported for 25 percent of placebo but only 7 percent of cotherapy patients. An extension study assigned patients to the same dose (20 mg) of fluoxetine or an increased dose (40 mg) at 6 weeks (Smith et al., 2002). One week later, cotherapy (fluoxetine with clonazepam) was found to be superior to fluoxetine with placebo with respect to HAM-D and Clinical Global Impressions (CGI) ratings; response rates were 32 and 4 percent, respectively. Cotherapy with benzodiazepines was also found to be useful for rapid treatment of anxiety and insomnia.

There are caveats, however. The effects of benzodiazepines wear off rapidly, necessitating supervised use until basic antidepressant and/or mood-stabilizing treatment—with medications or ECT—has reduced the severity of depressive symptoms. Although giving one or two doses of anxiolytic medication can result in dramatic improvement in the acute state and thereby potentially lower acute suicidal risk, failure to repeat the dosage on a regular schedule until the underlying affective disorder has improved may result in a dangerous rebound of anxiety, which can in turn trigger suicide. Careful clinical supervision and follow-up are therefore necessary.

In general, because the treatment is time-limited, there is little risk of inducing dependency on benzodiazepines with proper supervision. At the same time, given that manic-depressive patients (especially the bipolar subgroup) frequently present with comorbid substance abuse (see Chapter 7), the increased risk of misuse of or dependency on benzodiazepines in these patients should be carefully weighed. In the case of recurring anxiety symptoms, especially panic attacks, more moderate doses may need to be continued. In the final analysis, death is a far greater danger than possible benzodiazepine dependency, which can usually be avoided through careful clinical management.

Anticonvulsants and Antipsychotics

The sleep disturbances that often accompany severe anxiety and panic and that represent an independent risk factor for suicide should be treated aggressively with sedative hypnotics, sedating atypical antipsychotics, or sedating and anxiolytic anticonvulsants, such as valproate or gabapentin.

Anticonvulsants and antipsychotics can be used to treat those patients who display disinhibition or outbursts of anger in response to fast-acting benzodiazepines. In these circumstances, anticonvulsants such as divalproex (Schatzberg, 1998), atypical antipsychotics, or sedating typical antipsychotics, such as thioridazine, may be useful, particularly in reducing agitation and anxiety. Indeed, these treatments can be life-saving in some high-risk patients. All of these medications are relatively safe if used skillfully and with the necessary amount of supervision and follow-up. It is important that they be given in sufficient doses, even if temporary sedation results, until the suicidal crisis has been brought under control. The atypical antipsychotics merit special mention because, as discussed later, the atypical clozapine is the only drug other than lithium for which there is replicated evidence of a reduction in suicide risk. (See Chapter 19 for discussion of the use of anticonvulsants and atypical antipsychotics in the treatment of bipolar depression.)

Antidepressants with Rapid Onset

There is suggestive evidence that antidepressants with a mechanism that blocks the type 2 serotonin (5-HT_2) receptor, such as mirtazapine (Nutt, 1999) and nefazodone (Fawcett and Barkin, 1998), may have a more rapid effect than other antidepressant medications in reducing agitation and anxiety. Most treatment algorithms for anxiety disorders, however, suggest SSRI antidepressants as a first-line treatment. The FDA has approved paroxetine for the treatment of panic disorder and social phobia and the SNRI venlafaxine for the treatment of anxiety disorders. The important point is that a rapid anxiolytic and antiagitation effect, within a time frame of hours, is called for in acutely suicidal patients, especially those who are particularly anxious and dysphoric. Identifying and managing a state of acute suicide risk can work to prevent a suicide only if both the immediate and follow-up treatments are successful. To this end, it is necessary to provide comprehensive treatment of the depressive episode or dysphoric–mixed state driving the suicidal state, as well as a maintenance medication regimen. In any patient who is believed to have been at acute risk for suicide, a long-term treatment strategy should be developed as the patient recovers from the episode.

Electroconvulsive Therapy

As noted earlier, the literature on the results of ECT in the prevention of suicide has generally shown that it can be highly effective in the short term; however, it may be no more effective than other short-term treatments (Prudic and Sackeim, 1999; Sharma, 1999, 2001). Despite the known effectiveness of ECT in depressed patients with severe agitation and anxiety, suicides have occurred while the treatment was under way or even soon after a completed course (Bradvik and Berglund, 2000). Prudic and Sackeim (1999) pointed out, however, that more acutely ill, more suicidal patients may tend to be given ECT (because treatment assignment is not randomized), leading to understatement of its broader effectiveness. Bradvik and Berglund (2000) conducted a study of treatment at last contact in 89 cases of suicide in individuals with severe depression matched to 89 individuals who did not commit suicide. No difference in ECT use and medication prescription could be found between the two groups. The authors did find that suicide after ECT was less common in those patients who received continued antidepressant therapy than in those who did not take maintenance antidepressants.

Long-Term Suicide Prevention

Lithium, antidepressants, and atypical antipsychotics are all used for the long-term prevention of suicide. In this section, we review the literature on each of these treatments, including the possible association between SSRIs and increased suicide risk.

Lithium

Several meta-analyses encompassing dozens of studies have shown that lithium is a powerful antisuicide agent. Tondo and Baldessarini (2000) analyzed 22 long-term investigations of lithium therapy published from 1974 to 1998. In the more than 5,600 patients studied (representing nearly

35,000 patient-years of risk), they found a suicide rate among those receiving long-term lithium treatment 9 times lower than that among patients who did not receive or who discontinued the drug. (Most patients in these studies had bipolar disorder, but some had recurrent depression only.) Baldessarini and colleagues (2001) updated this analysis by pooling findings from 33 studies published from 1970 to 2000. They found a 13-fold lower incidence of attempted and completed suicide among those undergoing long-term lithium treatment compared with those who did not receive or who discontinued the drug. Indeed, patients maintained on lithium had rates of attempted and completed suicide comparable to those found in the general population (Fig. 25–2).

In a subsequent analysis, Baldessarini and colleagues (2003) evaluated findings from 34 studies of patients receiving maintenance lithium (averaging 3.4 years of exposure) and 25 studies of patients not receiving such therapy (followed for 5.9 years). Risks for completed suicide were .17 versus .94 per 100 person-years, respectively—that is, the risk was 82 percent lower for patients receiving maintenance lithium. For suicide attempts, the corresponding rates were .31 and 4.65, a 93 percent difference. Risk reductions for recurrent unipolar depression, bipolar-II, and bipolar-I were 100, 82, and 67 percent, respectively. In

other words, patients with different affective diagnoses showed strong benefits, with those with recurrent unipolar depression appearing to benefit the most.

In the most recent update of the analysis, Baldessarini and colleagues (2006b) pooled 34 studies suitable for meta-analysis. These studies involved 85,636 person-years of exposure (60,094 with and 25,542 without lithium). Figure 25–3 shows risk ratios (RRs) and their 95 percent confidence intervals (CIs) based on random-effects meta-analysis of suicidal risk in these studies (rates of suicides and attempts per 100 person-years). Across all studies, the suicide risk was five-fold lower (RR=1.00; 95 percent CI=3.82–6.31; z=12.5, p<.0001) in those individuals treated versus those not treated with lithium. Of the 34 studies, 26 were open-label clinical studies, and 8 were randomized clinical trials of lithium versus placebo or another active agent. The pooled RRs are similar for the open trials (5.00; 95 percent CI=3.83–6.53; z=11.8; p<.0001) and for the randomized controlled trials (4.29; 95 percent CI=1.46–12.6 percent; z=2.64; p=.008). Table 25–2 shows that the degree of risk reduction was similar for suicide and attempted suicide as well as for bipolar and other affective disorders.

In a retrospective cohort study, Goodwin and colleagues (2003) compared the benefits of lithium and divalproex in a population-based sample of 20,638 bipolar-I

Figure 25–2. Rates of suicide and suicide attempts among patients with major affective disorders, without (Off) and with (On) long-term lithium maintenance treatment, and estimated rates in the general population. Rates are in terms of suicidal acts per 100 patient-years (% per year). Note that the suicide attempt rates for patients treated with lithium versus the general population do not differ significantly, but the rate for suicide among treated patients is 10 times higher than that among the general population. (*Source*: Baldessarini et al., 2006b. Reproduced with permission from the New York Academy of Sciences.)

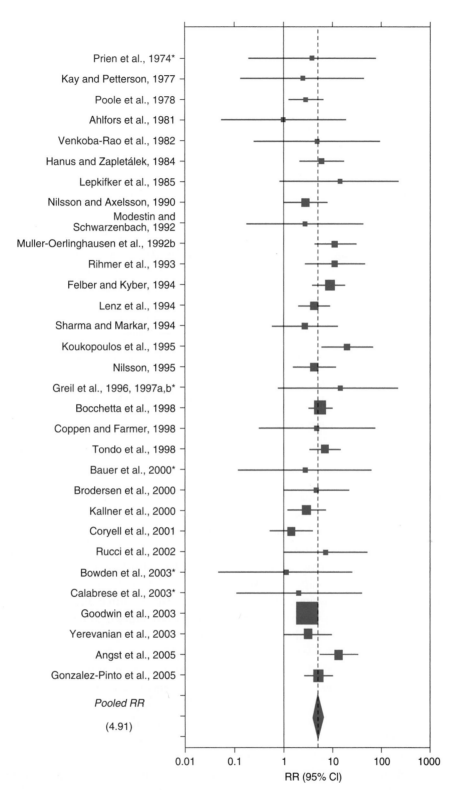

Figure 25–3. Overall random-effects meta-analysis of 31 studies of the risk of suicide and/or suicide attempts with and without lithium treatment. The risk ratio (RR) and 95 percent confidence interval (CI) for each study are shown (squares are proportional to study weight). The computed pooled RR (diamond) is 4.91 (95 percent CI = 3.82–6.31; z = 12.5, p < .0001). The vertical solid line represents the null hypothesis (RR = 100). Asterisks (*) denote randomized controlled trials. (*Source*: Baldessarini et al., 2006b. Reproduced with permission from the New York Academy of Sciences.)

TABLE 25–2. Summary of Meta-Analyses: Lithium Treatment vs. Risk for Suicide

Condition[a]	No. of Studies	Risk Ratio	(95% CI)	z	p Value
All two-armed studies[b]	31	4.91	(3.82–6.31)	12.5	<.0001
Omitting Goodwin et al., 2003[b]	30	5.34	(4.27–6.68)	14.7	<.0001
Suicides only	23	4.86	(3.36–7.02)	8.42	<.0001
Attempts only	17	4.98	(3.56–6.96)	9.42	<.0001
Bipolar disorder[c]	14	5.34	(3.59–7.93)	8.28	<.0001
Major affective disorders[c]	17	4.66	(3.43–6.33)	9.82	<.0001
Quality score ≥ 50%[d]	16	3.92	(2.94–5.23)	9.33	<.0001
Quality score < 50%[d]	15	5.56	(3.98–7.76)	10.1	<.0001

[a]Analyses are based on conservative, random-effects modeling.
[b]Results with Goodwin et al., 2003 omitted indicate that inclusion of this very large study did not alter the overall findings.
[c]For studies with bipolar disorder vs. major affective disorder patient samples: $\chi^2 = .91$, $df = 1$, $p = .34$; cases of bipolar-I and -II disorders and some schizoaffective disorders, in various combinations, are included.
[d]For studies with quality ratings at or above vs. below the median.
CI = confidence interval.
Source: Baldessarini et al., 2006b. Reproduced with permission from the New York Academy of Sciences.

patients treated in two large health maintenance organizations. A regression analysis, which controlled for age, gender, health plan, year of diagnosis, concomitant use of other psychotropic medications (e.g., antidepressants, antipsychotics), and comorbid diagnoses indicated that suicide was 2.7 times more likely among patients on divalproex versus lithium. Suicide attempts resulting in hospitalization or emergency department visits were 1.7 times more likely for those taking divalproex than among those on lithium. By far the primary determinant of which stabilizer was being used was the year of initial treatment: at the beginning of the period studied, 1994, more than 80 percent of the patients were prescribed lithium, but by 2001, about half were being given divalproex and half lithium, reflecting the trend in prescribing patterns in the United States during the 1990s (see Chapter 20). Taken together, the role of when patients entered treatment, along with the fact that comorbid diagnoses and coexisting medications were equivalent in the two groups, suggest that, any clinical differences in the patients chosen to receive the two drugs are unlikely to have contributed significantly to the differing suicide rates found.

Another recent meta-analysis that was restricted to randomized controlled trials found similar, albeit somewhat different, outcomes. Cipriani and colleagues (2005) analyzed 32 such trials comparing lithium with placebo ($n = 1,389$

patients) or with other pharmacological agents (the mood stabilizers carbamazepine, lamotrigine, and divalproex and the antidepressants imipramine and amitriptyline) ($n = 2,069$). The outcomes examined were suicide, deliberate self-harm (including attempted suicide), and death from all causes. The investigators found lithium to be more effective than the three other mood stabilizers as a group. Patients randomized to lithium experienced a 70 percent reduction in the risk of a composite of suicide and deliberate self-harm. The investigators concluded that "lithium remains the treatment with the most substantial evidence base for the prevention of relapse in bipolar disorder and should be a first-line therapy for patients with that disorder, including those at risk of suicidal behavior" (Cipriani et al., 2005, p. 1816).

A recent Danish observational cohort study compared the suicide risk in 13,186 patients who had purchased at least one prescription of lithium with that in 1.2 million subjects from the general population. Although the suicide rate was elevated in those who had purchased the drug, subjects from the general population who had purchased it at least twice had a 44 percent lower rate of suicide (95 percent CI = .28 to .70) than those who had purchased lithium only once (Kessing et al., 2005). The rate of suicide decreased with the number of prescriptions of lithium.

The authors, like Wolf and colleagues (1996) a decade earlier, emphasized the importance of taking into consideration the duration of lithium treatment given not only their own findings, but also those of earlier studies showing higher mortality rates when lithium treatment lasted only 2 to 5 years (Norton and Whalley, 1984; Vestergaard and Aagaard, 1991; Brodersen et al., 2000) versus 5 to 10 years (Coppen et al., 1990, 1991; Muller-Oerlinghausen et al., 1992a). The benefits of prolonged lithium treatment to some extent reflect a selection bias, of course: patients who respond better to lithium may be more likely to continue taking it, while those who respond less well or who otherwise are at increased risk for nonadherence (e.g., patients with substance abuse or personality disorder) may be more likely to stop taking their medication.

Adherence to lithium is key. In a recent 16-year follow-up study of lithium-treated patients with major affective disorders (who met the criterion of two to three affective episodes in a 5-year period), those who adhered to lithium had a standardized mortality ratio (SMR) of 8, while nonadherent patients had an SMR of 31, indicating that adherence reduced the risk of suicide about four-fold (Brodersen et al., 2000). Most of the suicides occurred among the "atypical" patients enrolled in the study (those with schizoaffective disorder, bipolar-II disorder, mixed episodes, and/or rapid cycling). The authors observed that the rate of nonadherence was about 40 percent in the first 2 years of treatment in this sample, but subsequently dropped to 5 to 10 percent. This finding calls for more clinical attention to adherence, especially during the early years of treatment (see Chapter 21). Adherence is particularly important for another reason, alluded to above. There is strong evidence that suicide and suicide attempts sharply increase after discontinuation of lithium, especially abrupt discontinuation (Baldessarini et al., 1999; Tondo and Baldessarini, 2000), as do episodes of affective illness (Faedda et al., 1993; Baldessarini et al., 1999; Baldessarini et al., 2003). Baldessarini and colleagues (1999, p. 81) concluded that "the first months after discontinuation of lithium may carry a particularly high risk of suicidal behavior and included multiple attempts and fatalities, sometimes in persons without previous suicidal acts. Moreover, the fatality rate due to suicide was 1.27 per 100 patient-years after discontinuation of lithium compared with 0.101 during lithium maintenance—an alarming 12.6-fold increase."

Lithium also has been studied in combination with other medications. Angst and colleagues (2002) provided evidence that a combination of lithium and antidepressant medications taken over a 6-month period can result in a significant reduction in the incidence of suicide in patients with recurrent affective disorders, especially those with bipolar disorder. This study is discussed in detail in the section on antidepressants.

Thus there is strong and consistent evidence of lithium's ability to prevent suicide in many bipolar patients, and almost certainly in those with recurrent unipolar depression as well. As alluded to earlier, however, psychological and medical autopsy studies suggest that patients at risk for suicide often are not prescribed and/or not taking the drug.[5] Other than its ability to stabilize mood, lithium's antisuicidal mechanism of action is not well understood, although the evidence points to its putative neurogenesis effects and capacity to reduce impulsivity or aggressiveness through its actions on serotonin and other neurotransmitters.[6]

Antidepressants

Antidepressants are efficacious for treating major depression and anxiety, but controversy exists as to whether they prevent suicide or can, under some circumstances, trigger it, and if the latter, in what age group and with what diagnosis or illness severity. We first consider the benefits of antidepressants for suicide prevention and then the possibility that suicide or suicidal behaviors may be precipitated by SSRI antidepressants in a small subgroup of particularly vulnerable individuals.

Most clinical trials of antidepressants have not meaningfully addressed potential efficacy in preventing suicide because they have expressly excluded suicidal patients or those with a history of suicide attempts, selected against severe forms of depression, and because they are of insufficient duration to detect a relatively rare event; they have relied instead on reports of suicidal ideation or attempts. Given the exclusion of high-risk patients, it is not surprising that adequately powered meta-analyses of clinical trials have found no significant difference in rates of suicide between antidepressant and placebo treatment (Khan et al., 2000a, 2003; Storosum et al., 2002). The absence of an observed antisuicide effect may also reflect the failure of antidepressants to reduce acute suicide risk over a relatively short period of treatment (1 to 8 weeks); the drugs may be more effective at reducing long-term risk. Results of epidemiological studies, on the other hand, reveal that suicide rates have been declining since the late 1980s, a time during which the prescribing of SSRIs for both adults and adolescents has risen dramatically.[7] Much of this increased prescribing has occurred in primary care settings (Pirraglia et al., 2003). A recent analysis of county-level U.S. vital statistics found that SSRIs were associated with lower rates of suicide, whereas tricyclic antidepressants were associated with higher rates (Gibbons et al., 2005). This finding reflects, at least in part, the toxicity of tricyclics when an overdose is taken. It may also reflect the fact that patients who were prescribed tricyclics almost certainly represented a more clinically ill population; the SSRIs have been prescribed over a broader range of severity. Moreover, there are, of course, limits to inferring causation from epidemiological studies. A recent study of 15,390 patients hospitalized because of a suicide attempt found that current use of antidepressants was associated with a 39 percent increase in suicide attempts but a 32 percent decrease in completed suicides (Tiihonen et al., 2006).

As noted earlier, there have been no clinical trials testing the antisuicide efficacy of antidepressants in patients with bipolar disorder. The only study to have expressly examined the effect of antidepressants in preventing suicide in bipolar patients was a large, nonrandomized, naturalistic one that included more than 30 years of follow-up (Angst et al., 2002). This study provided the best evidence to date that antidepressants, *in combination with lithium or other therapies,* may be effective in suicide prevention. Angst and colleagues in Switzerland studied the value of sustained treatment with antidepressants, particularly among bipolar patients, for prevention of suicide. Their sample included 186 unipolar and 220 bipolar patients, 61 percent of whom had manifested psychotic symptoms and all of whom had been hospitalized at least once. The severity of depression in these patients biased the group toward a higher risk of suicide. The patients were followed for 34 to 38 years; 99.3 percent of the sample could be tracked for the entire follow-up period. Of the original cohort, 76 percent had died by the time the study was completed. Treatment was assessed by obtaining records and calling the physicians responsible for clinical care. To be considered in treatment, a patient had to have been medicated for at least a 6-month period or for the entire period between two episodes. Treatment included lithium, antidepressants, and/or antipsychotics; the dose and duration of each treatment were not recorded. The authors noted that patients

with greater severity of illness tended to be in the treatment group.

The overall SMR for the sample was 1.61 (indicating a 61 percent increase over expected rates for the general population). The SMR for suicide in the patient group as a whole was 18.0 (13.5 for males and 21.9 for females). For bipolar patients specifically, the SMR for suicide was 12.3, and for unipolar patients it was 26.7. Treatment between episodes was much more frequent in bipolar than in unipolar patients—62 versus 38 percent. The suicide rates in treated and untreated unipolar patients were 7.1 and 18.1 percent, respectively; the corresponding rates for bipolar patients were 5.2 and 13.1 percent. Treated unipolar and bipolar patients showed a highly significant reduction in suicides, as well as a lower overall lower mortality rate (see Table 25–3).

With regard to specific treatments, 27.8 percent of the bipolar patients received lithium plus antipsychotics or antidepressants, 9.6 percent lithium alone, and 8.2 percent antipsychotics plus antidepressants (the remainder were untreated). The study design did not permit detail on the type of antipsychotic medication prescribed. Monotherapy with antidepressants was used in 9.1 percent of bipolar patients (compared with 15.6 percent of unipolar patients). Antipsychotic monotherapy was used in 10 percent of both groups. A logistic regression over all 305 unipolar and bipolar patients who had died showed significant effects of antidepressants in reducing suicide; similar effects were found for lithium, but only when it was used in combination with antidepressants or antipsychotics (perhaps because of the relatively small numbers of patients treated with lithium monotherapy—1.6 percent of unipolar and 10 percent of bipolar patients).

Although definitive conclusions cannot be drawn from nonrandomized data, the suggestion that patients receiving long-term antidepressant treatment had a significantly

TABLE 25–3. **Standardized Mortality Ratio (SMR) for Untreated vs. Treated[a] Unipolar ($n = 147$) and Bipolar ($n = 158$) Patients**

Condition	Untreated SMR	Treated SMR	Untreated vs. Treated p Value
Unipolar suicide	38.07	11.86	0.001[b]
Unipolar total mortality	1.67	1.56	0.001[c]
Bipolar suicide	29.19	6.43	0.001[c]
Bipolar total mortality	2.18	1.33	0.001[c]

[a]Treated with antidepressants, antipsychotics, and/or lithium over at least a 6-mo period or for the entire period between two episodes.
[b]Significant.
[c]With $p < .05$ (two-tailed) different from 1.0 (Poisson distribution).
Source: Angst et al., 2002.

lower overall mortality rate is important, especially given the difficulty of successfully following high-risk patients over 34 to 38 years. The apparent effect of treatment on suicide reduction was greater in the bipolar than in the unipolar group, but there was a significant effect in both conditions. As noted, this study was naturalistic; there was no control group or randomization, meaning that the patients who were kept on adjunctive antidepressants were likely to be those who were doing well on them. The authors pointed out that patients defined as being treated are likely to be more adherent to prescribed therapy, which in itself may mitigate against suicide. They also stressed that the treatment had to be received for longer than 6 months or over a full affective cycle until full remission had been attained.

These data do not prove a direct effect of antidepressant treatment on reducing suicide, but they do suggest that long-term adjunctive treatment with these medications may reduce suicide in some bipolar and to a lesser extent some unipolar patients.[8] Results of another naturalistic (non-randomized) follow-up study on the same sample, conducted in 2003, further support these conclusions, revealing that treatment significantly reduced suicides and that combined treatments were more effective than monotherapy (Angst et al., 2005).

Despite evidence for the effectiveness of antidepressants, they continue to be under prescribed in depressed patients at risk of suicide, according to a summary of seven American and European toxicological and autopsy studies (Jamison, 1999). Even fewer—typically less than half of medicated patients—were taking a therapeutic dose (see Fig. 25–4). The undertreatment of depression in general is consistent with research indicating that physicians fail to prescribe adequate doses of antidepressants (Isacsson et al., 1994; Isometsa et al., 1994). The reader is referred to Chapter 19 for a comprehensive discussion of the complex and controversial subject of the proper role of antidepressants in treating bipolar depression.

Antidepressants and Possible Increased Suicide Risk

The question of a possible increased risk of suicidal behavior associated with the use of SSRI antidepressants surfaced in the early 1990s in case reports of depressed adults[9] and children with obsessive-compulsive disorder (King et al., 1991). These case reports prompted regulatory agencies to reanalyze existing clinical trial data; however, no action was taken until more than a decade later after additional clinical trial data had become available, and one drug sponsor had submitted an analysis indicating that suicidal behavior was an adverse event with paroxetine use in young patients. After systematic evaluation of pooled data from clinical trials, drug regulators in both the United States and the United Kingdom issued strong warnings to physicians about the risk of suicidality and called for stronger monitoring of antidepressant use in young patients. The decade-long debate over the utility of these regulatory warnings has pitted those concerned about drug safety against others who are concerned that strong warnings may limit access to necessary and effective treatment. After regulatory warnings were issued in 2003 and 2004, according to reports from firms monitoring pharmaceutical

Figure 25–4. Antidepressant use at the time of suicide. An asterisk (*) indicates that no information is available about adequacy of dosage. (*Source*: Adapted from Jamison, 1999.)

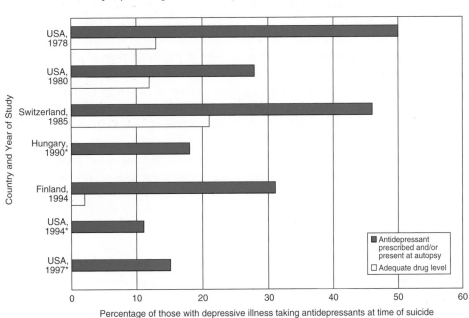

benefits, prescribing of SSRIs for young people decreased. The full impact on prescribing patterns is not yet known, nor is the impact on suicide rates.

Analysis of data from pediatric clinical trials by independent researchers has been hampered by the fact that the results of the majority of such trials are unpublished, and most of the trials had methodological limitations, particularly for extrapolation to bipolar illness. None specifically studied patients with bipolar or recurrent unipolar disorder. Rather, the trials involved patients with major depressive disorder with recurrence not specified (often with only moderate levels of depression given ethical constraints against exposing sick children to placebo, which makes it more difficult to evaluate treatment effects), obsessive-compulsive disorder, and attention-deficit hyperactivity disorder (ADHD). Exclusionary entry criteria, that is, excluding children and adolescents if they had previously attempted suicide or were actively suicidal, are a particularly problematic issue (Emslie et al., 2002; Wagner et al., 2004; Dubicka et al., 2006). The outcomes studied were suicidal ideation and suicide attempts; these are, as discussed earlier, quite limited predictors of completed suicide. Suicide itself was not studied, largely because the trials were conducted within a short time frame, and their entry criteria excluded suicidal patients.

The above methodological problems aside, one explanation for the emergence of suicidal behavior early in treatment with SSRIs stems from misdiagnosis of the depressive phase of bipolar disorder as unipolar depression. Use of antidepressant medications in patients who are in the depressive phase of bipolar disorder may trigger agitation and other behavior reflecting the induction of mixed states (see Chapter 19), which can be associated with an increased risk of suicide (see Chapter 8) (Shi et al., 2004; Fergusson et al., 2005; McElroy et al., 2006).

In 2004, the FDA evaluated pooled data from both unpublished and published clinical trials involving more than 4,000 children and adolescents. The FDA's conclusion was that although suicidal ideation or attempts were rare in these trials, the likelihood of such events occurring during antidepressant treatment was increased two-fold, from 2 percent with placebo to about 4 percent with the drugs (FDA, 2004). On the other hand, evidence for efficacy was not particularly strong, with only 3 of 15 randomized controlled trials (2 for fluoxetine) showing efficacy in treating depression (Advisory Committee to FDA, 2004). With less demonstrated efficacy (albeit from trials in which more severely depressed children were underrepresented) and a slight elevation in risk, the risk/benefit assessment in younger patients tilted in favor of risk (Leon, 2005).

This analysis led the FDA to require a black box warning for physicians and to extend that warning to *all* antide-

pressants sold in the United States—not just SSRIs. The warning states: "Antidepressants increased the risk of suicidal thinking and behavior (suicidality) in short-term studies in children and adolescents with Major Depressive Disorder (MDD) and other psychiatric disorders. Anyone considering the use of antidepressants in a child or adolescent must balance this risk with the clinical need. Patients who are started on therapy should be observed closely for clinical worsening, suicidality, or unusual changes in behavior." We strongly concur that patients and their families should be advised about potentially dangerous exacerbations of agitation and impulsivity early in the treatment of depression and that physicians must closely monitor patients in the early phases of treatment, but we are also very concerned that this black box warning may have a chilling effect on the legitimate and well-advised prescription of potentially life-saving medications.

Four recent studies bear mentioning. One, a large-scale investigation of computerized health plan records, identified 65,103 patients with 82,285 episodes of antidepressant treatment (Simon et al., 2006). The risk of suicide during the acute phase of treatment was approximately 1 in 3,000 treatment episodes; the risk of serious suicide attempts was 1 in 1,000. There was no indication of an increased risk of suicide or suicide attempts after starting antidepressant medications. Data on antidepressant medication prescription rates and U.S. county-level suicide rates for children ages 5 to 14 were examined for the years 1996–1998 (Gibbons et al., 2006). After adjustment for access to mental health care, as well as for gender, race, income level, and county-to-county variability in suicide rates, higher SSRI prescription rates (expressed as the number of pills prescribed per person) were associated with lower suicide rates in children and adolescents. Olfson and colleagues (2006) examined the risk of suicide and suicide attempts in Medicaid beneficiaries from all 50 states who received inpatient treatment for depression (the study specifically excluded bipolar patients). They concluded that antidepressant treatment in adults was not significantly associated with suicide or suicide attempts; in children and adolescents, however, treatment with antidepressants significantly increased the risk of both suicide and suicide attempts. Finally, Bauer and colleagues (2006a,b) prospectively studied 425 Systematic Treatment Enhancement Program for Bipolar Disorder (STEP-BD) participants who experienced a new-onset major depressive episode without initial suicidal ideation. They found no evidence that increased antidepressant exposure was associated with new-onset suicidality in this high-risk population. (New-onset suicidality was, on the other hand, associated with a history of a prior attempt and higher depressive or manic symptom ratings at index episode.) There was no association between antidepressant treatment and suicidality in the younger (age 21 or less) patients.

In summary, antidepressant medications are effective for treating major mood disorders, but their use should be monitored carefully by clinicians. This is particularly true for young patients, whose brain development is different from that of adults (see Chapter 23). Patients can worsen after the initiation of antidepressant treatment. Patients and their families should be warned of this possibility, and the prescribing physician should be contacted if symptoms, especially agitation and impulsivity, worsen after the initiation of treatment.

Atypical Antipsychotics

Several studies have found that clozapine reduces rates of suicide or attempted suicide in patients with schizophrenia or schizoaffective disorder. The first such study to be published was of 183 neuroleptic-resistant patients who had been consecutively hospitalized. After being prescribed clozapine, they were followed for periods of 6 months to 7 years. The number of suicide attempts with high lethality was reduced from five before the index hospitalization to zero afterward (Meltzer and Okayli, 1995). Walker and colleagues (1997) found a significant decrease in death rates from suicide in an epidemiologic sample of 67,072 users of clozapine. Likewise, Reid and colleagues (1998), comparing rates of suicide in a subset of patients treated with clozapine ($n = 1,310$) in a group of 30,000 schizophrenic patients treated in the Texas mental health system, found a marked reduction in the clozapine-treated group. More recently, Modestin and colleagues (2005) found that clozapine diminished the frequency of serious suicidal acts in a sample of 75 patients with schizophrenia, 14 with schizoaffective disorder, and 5 with affective illness. On the other hand, Sernyak and colleagues (2001), retrospectively studying a group of 1,415 schizophrenic patients treated with clozapine, found no reduction in suicide compared with a schizophrenic control group not treated with the drug.

There is some evidence that olanzapine, another atypical antipsychotic, also reduces suicide attempts. Olanzapine, as compared with haloperidol, was associated with a significant decrease in rates of attempted suicide in schizophrenic patients treated over 1 year (this study included schizoaffective patients) (Glazer, 1997). In a post hoc analysis of a randomized clinical trial, olanzapine given over a period of 28 weeks was found to be superior to risperidone in reducing suicide attempts (Tran et al., 1998). These findings suggest that olanzapine may have effects similar to those of clozapine in reducing suicide in schizophrenia. More recently, Houston and colleagues (2006) found that the addition of olanzapine (versus placebo) to lithium or divalproex monotherapy significantly reduced suicidal ideation (as measured by HAM-D-3 scores) in 58 bipolar-I mixed-state patients.

The comparative benefits of clozapine and olanzapine for suicide prevention were examined by Meltzer and colleagues (2003) in the International Suicide Prevention Trial. Over a 2-year period, that trial followed 980 patients with schizophrenia or schizoaffective disorder deemed to be at high risk for suicide. Suicide-related outcomes included suicide attempts, hospitalizations to prevent suicide, and a rating of "much worsening of suicidality." It was found that clozapine-treated patients had significantly fewer suicide attempts, hospitalizations, and rescue interventions. The study did not have sufficient power to compare suicide rates.

Although most studies of clozapine have been carried out in patients with schizophrenia, Ciapparelli and colleagues (2000) found in a naturalistic study that clozapine was also effective in patients with treatment-resistant schizoaffective disorder, as well as in psychotic bipolar patients, over a 24-month observation period. This finding suggests that the antisuicide effect seen with clozapine in schizophrenic patients may also be seen in those with bipolar disorder.

CONCLUSIONS

The seriously suicidal person with manic-depressive illness, whether bipolar or recurrent unipolar, requires intensive clinical care. Suicidal behavior is treated and prevented most effectively by a combination of immediate and long-term strategies. The immediate strategy is to keep the suicidal patient safe by ameliorating acute risk factors, such as global insomnia, agitation, and severe anxiety. The long-term strategy is to stabilize the patient's underlying illness, particularly recurrent depressive or mixed episodes. When bipolar or recurrent unipolar patients at chronic risk for suicide are maintained on lithium, alone or in combination with other mood stabilizers and/or atypical antipsychotics, the incidence of suicide can be significantly reduced. Lithium's antisuicidal effect has been demonstrated by meta-analyses of more than 30 studies that reveal an approximately five-fold reduction in suicide risk among patients treated with versus those not treated with lithium.

Careful treatment with antidepressants may also reduce the risk of suicide, but for bipolar patients antidepressants should generally be preceded by a mood stabilizer, preferably lithium because of its demonstrated antisuicidal effect. When administered alone, antidepressants may induce mood cycling or mixed states, which may in turn heighten the risk of suicide. Bipolar patients prescribed antidepressants, particularly children and adolescents, should be carefully monitored, and they and their family members advised to be alert to possible agitation and precipitous switches in mood.

Finally, the psychological aspects of treating suicidal manic-depressive patients are also an essential component of preventing suicidal behavior. Assessment of suicide risk should be performed during the initial patient evaluation and at certain points when the risk is likely to increase, such as in the presence of a new or exacerbated comorbidity or within 3 to 6 months after hospital discharge. The clinician's vigilance in suicide assessment and treatment with a combination of psychotherapeutic interventions can reduce the risk of suicide and save lives.

NOTES

1. MacKinnon and Farberow, 1976; Pokorny, 1983, 1991; Murphy et al., 1984; Goldstein et al., 1991; IOM, 2002.
2. Anne Sexton, probably 1977. Dr. Orne file, restricted collection. Cited in Middlebrook (1991, p. 36).
3. A very large percentage of adolescent-onset depression is bipolar (see Chapter 6), and psychiatrists initially misdiagnose 40 to 60 percent of bipolar patients as unipolar; primary care physicians and pediatricians miss an even larger percentage (see Chapter 3).
4. Hawton et al., 1998, 2000; IOM, 2002; Jacobs et al., 2003; Hepp et al., 2004; Soomro, 2004; Miklowitz and Taylor, 2006.
5. Isometsa and colleagues (1994), for example, identified 31 bipolar-I patients among all 1,397 suicides in Finland within a 12-month period. Of these patients, 74 percent were receiving psychiatric care at the time of their suicide, and 39 percent had explicitly communicated their intent to kill themselves to health personnel during the final 3 months of their lives, yet only 32 percent had received lithium (11 percent had received antidepressants, and none had received ECT). An international symposium evaluated current knowledge of the effects of medical treatment on suicidal behavior; one of its major conclusions was that there was a profound gap between the strong evidence base for lithium's effectiveness against suicidal behavior and what practicing clinicians knew (Baldessarini and Jamison, 1999). Likewise, Muller-Oerlinghausen (2003) found that lithium was infrequently prescribed in Germany.
6. Sheard, 1975, Treiser et al., 1981; Dixon and Hokin, 1998; Baldessarini et al., 2003; Brown et al., 2005.
7. Isacsson, 2000; Grunebaum et al., 2003; Olfson et al., 2003; Zito et al., 2003. Rihmer et al., 1995, 2004; Ludwig and Marcotte, 2005.
8. As reviewed in Chapter 19, only a minority of bipolar patients do well on long-term antidepressants; because Angst's patients were not randomized, we can assume that the patients who stayed on long-term antidepressants were those who had not been destabilized by them—which, according to the studies reviewed in Chapter 19, may represent about 20 percent of the bipolar group.
9. Teicher et al., 1990, 1993; Rothschild and Locke, 1992.

RESOURCES FOR INFORMATION ABOUT BIPOLAR DISORDER AND RELATED TOPICS

Organizations

American Academy of Child and Adolescent Psychiatry
3615 Wisconsin Avenue, N.W.
Washington, D.C. 20016-3007
Phone: 202-966-7300
Fax: 202-966-2891
http://www.aacap.org/

American Foundation for Suicide Prevention
(AFSP)
120 Wall Street, 22nd Floor
New York, NY 10005
Phone: 888-333-2377
Fax: 212-363-6237
www.afsp.org

Anxiety Disorders Association of America
8730 Georgia Avenue, Suite 600
Silver Spring, MD 20910-3604
Phone: 240-485-1001
Fax: 240-485-1035
www.adaa.org

American Psychiatric Association
1000 Wilson Blvd., Suite 1825
Arlington, VA 22209-3901
Phone: 888-357-7924
www.psych.org
www.healthyminds.org

American Psychological Association
750 First Street, N.E.
Washington, DC 20002-4242
Phone: 800-374-2721
www.apa.org
www.apahelpcenter.org

Bipolar Disorders Information Center
http://www.mhsource.com/bipolar/

Bipolar Kids
http://www.geocities.com/enchantedforest/1068/

Bipolar News
http://www.bipolarnews.org/

Bipolar Significant Others
http://www.bpso.org/

Centers for Disease Control and Prevention
National Center for Injury Control
and Prevention
Mailstop K65
4770 Buford Highway NE
Atlanta, GA 30341-3724
Phone: 800-232-4636
Fax: 770-488-1667
www.cdc.gov/ncipc

Center for Mental Health Services
P.O. Box 42557
Washington, DC 20015
Phone: 800-789-2647
Fax: 240-747-5470
http://www.mentalhealth.samhsa.gov/

Child and Adolescent Bipolar Foundation (CABF)
1000 Skokie Blvd., Suite 570
Wilmette, IL 60091
Phone: 847-256-8525
Fax: 847-920-9498
www.cabf.org

Depression and Bipolar Support Alliance (DBSA)
730 N. Franklin Street, Suite 501
Chicago, IL 60610-7224
Phone: 800-826-3632
Fax: 312-642-7243
http://www.dbsalliance.org

Depression and Related Affective Disorders
Association (DRADA)
8201 Greensboro Drive, Suite 300
McLean, VA 22102
Phone: 888-288-1104
http://www.drada.org/

Expert Consensus Guideline Series
http://www.psychguides.com/

International Foundation for Research
and Education on Depression (iFred)
7040 Bembe Beach Road, Suite 100
Annapolis, MD 21403
Phone: 800-789-2647
Fax: 443-782-0739
http://www.ifred.org/

Juvenile Bipolar Research Foundation (JBRF)
550 Ridgewood Road
Maplewood, NJ 07040
Phone: 866-333-5273
Fax: 973-275-0420
http://www.bpchildresearch.org/

Medscape Psychiatry & Mental Health
http://www.medscape.com/psychiatry

Mood Garden
www.moodgarden.org

National Alliance for Research on Schizophrenia
and Depression (NARSAD)
60 Cutter Mill Road, Suite 404
Great Neck, NY 11021
Phone: 800-829-8289
Fax: 516-487-6930
http://www.narsad.org/

National Alliance on Mental Illness (NAMI)
Colonial Place Three
2107 Wilson Blvd., Suite 300
Arlington, VA 22201-3042
Phone: 703-524-7600
Fax: 703-524-9094
www.nami.org

National Institute of Mental Health (NIMH)
Public Information and Communications Branch
6001 Executive Boulevard, Room 8184, MSC 9663
Bethesda, MD 20892-9663
Phone: 866-615-6464
Fax: 301-443-4279
www.nimh.nih.gov

National Institute on Alcohol Abuse
and Alcoholism (NIAAA)
5635 Fishers Lane, MSC 9304
Bethesda, MD 20892-9304
www.niaaa.nih.gov

National Institute on Drug Abuse
National Institutes of Health
6001 Executive Boulevard, Room 5213
Bethesda, MD 20892-9561
Phone: 301-443-1124
www.nida.nih.gov

National Mental Health Association (NMHA)
2000 N. Beauregard Street, 6th Floor
Alexandria, VA 22311
Phone: 703-684-7722
Fax: 703-684-5968
http://www.nmha.org/

Parents Med Guide
www.parentsmedguide.org.

Pendulum Resources
http://pendulum.org/

Screening for Mental Health, Inc.
One Washington Street, Suite 304
Wellesley Hills, MA 02481

Phone: 781-239-0071
Fax: 781-431-7447
www.nmisp.org

Stanley Medical Research Institute
8401 Connecticut Avenue, Suite 200
Chevy Chase, MD 20815
Phone: 301-571-0760
Fax: 301-571-0769
http://www.stanleyresearch.org/

Substance Abuse and Mental Health Services
Administration
1 Choke Cherry Road
Rockville, MD 20857
Phone: 800-273-8255
www.samhsa.gov

Suicide Awareness Voices of Education
9001 E. Bloomington Freeway, Suite 150
Bloomington, MN 55420
Phone: 952-946-7998
www.save.org

Suicide Prevention Action Network USA (SPAN USA)
1025 Vermont Avenue, N.W., Suite 1066
Washington, DC 20005
Phone: 202-449-3600
Fax: 202-449-3601
www.spanusa.org

Surgeon General of the United States
www.surgeongeneral.gov

Systemic Enhancement Program for Bipolar
Disorder (STEP-BD)
http://www.stepbd.org/

Recommended Reading for Patients and Families

Barondes, S.H. (1998). *Mood Genes: Hunting for Origins of Mania and Depression.* New York: Oxford University Press.

Basco, M.R., and Rush, A.J. (1996). *Cognitive-Behavioral Therapy for Bipolar Disorder.* New York: Guilford Press.

Bauer, M., and McBride, L. (1996). *Structured Group Psychotherapy for Bipolar Disorder: The Life Goals Program.* New York: Springer Publishing Company.

Beers, C. (1981). *A Mind that Found Itself.* Pittsburgh: University of Pittsburgh Press (first published, 1908).

Casey, N. (2001). *Unholy Ghost: Writers on Depression.* New York: Harper Collins.

Coate, M. (1964). *Beyond All Reason.* London: Constable.

Copeland, M.E. (1994). *Living without Depression and Manic-Depression: A Workbook for Maintaining Mood Stability.* Oakland, CA: New Harbinger Publications.

Cronkite, K. (1994). *On the Edge of Darkness: Conversations about Conquering Depression.* New York: Doubleday.

Custance, J. (1952). *Wisdom, Madness, and Folly: The Philosophy of a Lunatic.* New York: Farrar, Straus & Cudahy.

Danquah, M.N.-A. (1998). *Willow Weep for Me: A Black Woman's Journey through Depression.* New York: W. W. Norton.

Dees, M., Canfield, C., and Rowe, V. (1999). *Texas Medication Algorithm Project (TMAP) Consumer-to-Consumer Discussion Materials Peer Facilitator Guide.* Austin, TX: Texas Department of Mental Health and Mental Retardation (TDMHMR).

DePaulo, R., and Horvitz, L.A. (2002). *Understanding Depression: What We Know and What You Can Do About It.* New York: John Wiley & Sons.

Duke, P., and Hochman, G. (1992). *A Brilliant Madness: Living with Manic-Depressive Illness.* New York: Bantam Books.

Evans, D.L., and Andrews, L. W. (2005). *If Your Adolescent Has Depression or Bipolar Disorder: An Essential Resource for Parents.* New York: Oxford University Press.

Fieve, R.R. (1997). *Moodswing,* 2nd Edition. New York: Bantam Books.

Fitzgerald, F.S. (first published in 1936; reissued in 1965). *The Crack-Up. In: The Crack-Up with Other Pieces and Stories.* Middlesex, London: Penguin.

Goodwin, G. and Sachs, G. (2004). *Fast Facts: Bipolar Disorder.* Oxford: Health Press, UK.

Hamilton, I. (1982). *Robert Lowell: A Biography.* New York: Random House.

Head, J. (2004). *Standing in the Shadows: Black Men and Depression.* New York: Broadway.

Hinshaw, S.P. (2002). *The Years of Silence Are Past: My Father's Life with Bipolar Disorder.* Cambridge, MA: Cambridge University Press.

Irwin, C., with Evans, D.L., and Andrews, L.W. (2007). *Monochrome Days: A Firsthand Account of One Teenager's Experience with Depression.* New York: Oxford University Press.

Jamieson, P.E., with Rynn, M.A. (2006). *Mind Race: A Firsthand Account of One Teenager's Experience with Bipolar Disorder.* New York: Oxford University Press.

Jamison, K.R. (1993). *Touched with Fire: Manic-Depressive Illness and the Artistic Temperament.* New York: Free Press.

Jamison, K.R. (1995). *An Unquiet Mind: A Memoir of Moods and Madness.* New York: Alfred A. Knopf.

Jamison, K.R. (1999). *Night Falls Fast: Understanding Suicide.* New York: Alfred A. Knopf.

Logan, J. (1976). *Josh: My Up and Down, In and Out Life.* New York: Delacorte Press.

Manning, M. (1994). *Undercurrents: A Therapist's Reckoning with Her Own Depression.* New York: Harper Collins.

McDonnell, F. (2003). *Threads of Hope: Learning to Live with Depression.* London: Short Books.

McManamy, J. (2006). *Living Well with Depression and Bipolar Disorder: What Your Doctor Doesn't Tell You.* New York: Collins.

Miklowitz, D.J., and Goldstein, M.J. (2006). *Bipolar Disorder: A Family-Focused Treatment Approach.* New York: Guilford Press.

Milligan, S., and Clare, A. (1993). *Depression and How to Survive It.* London: Ebury Press.

Mondimore, F. (2006). *Depression: Mood Disease.* Baltimore: Johns Hopkins University Press.

Mondimore, F.M. (2006). *Bipolar Disorder: A Guide for Patients and Families.* Baltimore: Johns Hopkins Press Health Book.

O'Brien, S. (2004). *The Family Silver: A Memoir of Depression and Inheritance.* Chicago: University of Chicago Press.

Papolos, D., and Papolos, J. (2006). *The Bipolar Child: The Definitive and Reassuring Guide to Childhood's Most Misunderstood Disorder.* 3rd Edition. New York: Broadway Books (a division of Random House).

Phelps, J. (2006). *Why Am I Still Depressed? Recognizing and Managing the Ups and Downs of Bipolar II and Soft Bipolar Disorder.* New York: McGraw-Hill.

Raeburn, P. (2004). *Acquainted With the Night: A Parent's Quest to Understand Depression and Bipolar Disorder in his Children.* New York: Broadway.

Rosenthal, N. (2005). *Winter Blues: Seasonal Affective Disorder: What It Is and How to Overcome It.* New York: Guilford Press.

Sheffield, A. (1999). *How You Can Survive When They're Depressed: Living and Coping with Depression Fallout.* New York: HarperCollins.

Solomon, A. (2001). *The Noonday Demon: An Anatomy of Depression.* New York: Scribner.

Styron, W. (1990). *Darkness Visible: A Memoir of Madness.* New York: Random House.

Vonnegut, M. (1975). *The Eden Express.* New York: Laurel Books.

Waltz, M. (1999). *Bipolar Disorders: A Guide to Helping Children and Adolescents.* Sebastopol, CA: O'Reilly & Associates, Inc.

Whybrow, P.C. (1997). *A Mood Apart: The Thinker's Guide to Emotion and Its Disorders.* New York: HarperCollins.

Wolpert, L. (1999). *Malignant Sadness.* New York: Free Press.

Wyatt, R.J., and Chew, R.H. (2005). *Wyatt's Practical Psychiatric Practice.* Washington, DC: American Psychiatric Publishing.

REFERENCES

CHAPTER 1

Abrams, R., and Taylor, M.A. (1974). Unipolar mania: A preliminary report. *Arch Gen Psychiatry*, 30, 441–443.

Abrams, R., and Taylor, M.A. (1979). Differential EEG patterns in affective disorder and schizophrenia. *Arch Gen Psychiatry*, 36, 1355–1358.

Abrams, R., and Taylor, M.A. (1980). A comparison of unipolar and bipolar depressive illness. *Am J Psychiatry*, 137, 1084–1087.

Abrams, R., Taylor, M.A., Hayman, M.A., and Krishna, N.R. (1979). Unipolar mania revisited. *J Affect Disord*, 1, 59–68.

Ackerknecht, E.H. (1959). *A Short History of Psychiatry*. New York: Hafner Publishing Co.

Ackerknecht, E.H. (1982). *A Short History of Medicine*. Revised edition. Baltimore: Johns Hopkins University Press.

Agosti, V., and Stewart, J.W. (2001). Atypical and non-atypical subtypes of depression: Comparison of social functioning, symptoms, course of illness, co-morbidity and demographic features. *J Affect Disord*, 65(1), 75–79.

Akiskal, H.S. (1981). Subaffective disorders: Dysthymic, cyclothymic and bipolar II disorders in the "borderline" realm. *Psychiatr Clin North Am*, 4, 25–46.

Akiskal, H.S. (1983a). Dysthymic and cyclothymic disorders: A paradigm for high-risk research in psychiatry. In J.M. Davis and J.W. Mass (Eds.), *The Affective Disorders* (pp. 211–231). Washington, DC: The American Psychiatric Press.

Akiskal, H.S. (1983b). Diagnosis and classification of affective disorders: New insights from clinical and laboratory approaches. *Psychiatr Dev*, 2, 123–160.

Akiskal, H.S. (1983c). Dysthymic disorder: Psychopathology of proposed chronic depressive subtypes. *Am J Psychiatry*, 140, 11–20.

Akiskal, H.S. (1994). The temperamental borders of affective disorders. *Acta Psychiatr Scand Suppl*, 379), 32–37.

Akiskal, H.S. (1995). Toward a temperament-based approach to depression: Implications for neurobiologic research. *Adv Biochem Psychopharmacol*, 49, 99–112.

Akiskal, H.S. (1998). Toward a definition of generalized anxiety disorder as an anxious temperament type. *Acta Psychiatr Scand*, 98(Suppl. 393), 66–73.

Akiskal, H.S. (2000). *Mood Disorders: Clinical Features in Sadock & Sadock in Kaplan's Comprehensive Textbook of Psychiatry* (Edition VII). Baltimore: Williams & Wilkins, pp. 1338–1377.

Akiskal, H.S. (2001). Dysthymia and cyclothymia in psychiatric practice a century after Kraepelin. *J Affect Disord*, 62, 17–31.

Akiskal, H.S. (2003). Validating "hard" and "soft" phenotypes within the bipolar spectrum: Continuity or discontinuity? *J Affect Disord*, 73:1–5.

Akiskal, H.S., and Akiskal, K. (1988). Reassessing the prevalence of bipolar disorders: Clinical significance and artistic creativity. *Psychiatr Psychobiol*, 3, 29s–36s.

Akiskal, K.K., and Akiskal, H.S. (2005). The theoretical underpinnings of affective temperaments: Implications for evolutionary foundations of bipolar disorder and human nature. *J Affect Disord*, 85(1-2), 231–239.

Akiskal, H.S., and Benazzi, F. (2004). Validating Kraepelin's two types of depressive mixed states: "Depression with flight of ideas" and "excited depression." *World J Biol Psychiatry*, 5(2), 107–113.

Akiskal, H.S., and Benazzi F. (2005). Atypical depression: A variant of bipolar II or a bridge between unipolar and bipolar II? *J Affect Disord*, 84(2-3), 209–217.

Akiskal, H.S., and Benazzi, F. (2006). The DSM-IV and ICD-10 categories of recurrent (major) depressive and bipolar II disorders: Evidence that they lie on a dimensional spectrum. *J Affect Disord*, 92(1), 45–54.

Akiskal, H.S., and Mallya, G. (1987). Criteria for the "soft" bipolar spectrum: Treatment implications. *Psychopharmacol Bull*, 23, 68–73.

Akiskal, H.S., and Pinto, O. (1999). The evolving bipolar spectrum: Prototypes I, II, III, IV. *Psychiatr Clin North Am*, 22, 517–534.

Akiskal, H.S., Djenderedjian, A.H., Rosenthal, R.H., and Khani, M.K. (1977). Cyclothymic disorder: Validating criteria for inclusion in the bipolar affective group. *Am J Psychiatry*, 134, 1227–1233.

Akiskal, H.S., Bitar, A.H., Puzantian, V.R., Rosenthal, T.L., and Walker, P.W. (1978). The nosological status of neurotic depression: A prospective three-to-four-year follow-up examination in light of the primary–secondary and unipolar–bipolar dichotomies. *Arch Gen Psychiatry*, 35, 756–766.

Akiskal, H.S., Khani, M.K., and Scott-Strauss, A. (1979a). Cyclothymic temperamental disorders. *Psychiatr Clin North Am*, 2, 527–554.

Akiskal, H.S., Rosenthal, R.H., Rosenthal, T.L., Kashgarian, M., Khani, M.K., and Puzantian, V.R. (1979b). Differentiation of primary affective illness from situational, symptomatic, and secondary depressions. *Arch Gen Psychiatry*, 36, 635–643.

Akiskal, H.S., Walker, P., Puzantian, V.R., King, D., Rosenthal, T.L., and Dranon, M. (1983). Bipolar outcome in the course of depressive illness: Phenomenologic, familial, and pharmacologic predictors. *J Affect Disord*, 5, 115–128.

Akiskal, H.S., Downs, J., Jordan, P., Watson, S., Daugherty, D., and Pruitt, D.B. (1985). Affective disorders in referred children and younger siblings of manic-depressives: Mode of onset and prospective course. *Arch Gen Psychiatry*, 42, 996–1003.

Akiskal, H.S., Maser, J.D., Zeller, P.J., Endicott, J., Coryell, W., Keller, M., Warshaw, M., Clayton, P., and Goodwin, F.K. (1995). Switching from 'unipolar' to bipolar II. *Arch Gen Psychiatry*, 52, 114–123.

Akiskal, H.S., Hantouche, E., Bourgeois, M., Azorin, J.M., Sechter, D., Allilaire, J.F., Lancrenon, S., Fraud, J.P., and Chatenet-Duchene, L. (1998a). Gender, temperament and the clinical picture in dysphoric mixed mania: Findings from a French national study (EPIMAN). *J Affect Disord*, 50, 175–186.

Akiskal, H.S., Placidi, G.F., Signoretta, S., Liguori, A., Gervasi, R., Maremmani, I., Mallya, G., and Puzantian, V.R. (1998b). TEMPS-I: Delineating the most discriminant traits of cyclothymic, depressive, irritable and hyperthymic temperaments in a nonpatient population. *J Affect Disord*, 51, 7–19.

Akiskal, H.S., Bourgeois, M.L., Angst, J., Post, R., Moller, H.J., and Hirschfeld, R.M.A. (2000). Re-evaluating the prevalence of and diagnostic composition within the broad clinical spectrum of bipolar disorders. *J Affect Disord*, 59(Suppl. 1), 5s–30s.

Akiskal, H.S., Hantouche, E.G., Allilaire, J.F., Sechter, D., Bourgeois, M.L., Azorin, J.M., Chatenet-Duchene, L., and Lancrenon, S. (2003a). Validating antidepressant-associated hypomania (bipolar III): A systematic comparison with spontaneous hypomania (bipolar II). *J Affect Disord*, 73, 65–74.

Akiskal, H.S., Hantouche, E.G., and Lancrenon, S. (2003b). Bipolar II with and without cyclothymic temperament: "Dark" and "sunny" expressions of soft bipolarity. *J Affect Disord*, 73, 49–57.

Akiskal, H.S., Hantouche, E.G., and Allilaire J.F. (2003c). Bipolar II with and without cyclothymic temperament: "Dark" and "sunny" expressions of soft bipolarity. *J Affect Disord*, 73(1-2), 49–57.

Akiskal, H.S., Mendlowicz, M.V., Jean-Louis, G., Rapaport, M.H., Kelsoe, J.R., Gillin, J.C., and Smith, T.L. (2005). TEMPS-A: Validation of a short version of a self-rated instrument designed to measure variations in temperament. *J Affect Disord*, 85(1-2), 45–52.

Alda, M. (2004). The phenotypic spectra of bipolar disorder. *Eur Neuropsychopharmacol*, 14 (Suppl. 2), s94–s99.

Alexander, F.G., and Selesnick, S.T. (1966). *The History of Psychiatry: An Evaluation of Psychiatric Thought and Practice from Prehistoric Times to the Present*. New York: Harper & Row.

Altshuler, L.L., Gitlin, M.J., Mintz, J., Leight, K.L., and Frye, M.A. (2002). Subsyndromal depression is associated with functional impairment in patients with bipolar disorder. *J Clin Psychiatry*, 63, 807–811.

Andreasen, N.C., Grove, W.M., Shapiro, R.W., Keller, M.B., Hirschfeld, R.M.A., and McDonald-Scott, P. (1981). Reliability of lifetime diagnosis: A multicultural collaborative perspective. *Arch Gen Psychiatry*, 38, 400–405.

Andreasen, N.C., Grove, W.M., Coryell, W.H., Endicott, J., and Clayton, P.J. (1988). Bipolar versus unipolar and primary versus secondary affective disorder: Which diagnosis takes precedence? *J Affect Disord*, 15, 69–80.

Angst, J. (1966). *Zur Atiologie und Nosologie endogener depressiver Psychnose*. Berlin: Springer-Verlag.

Angst, J. (1978). The course of affective disorders: II. Typology of bipolar manic-depressive illness. *Arch Psychiatr Nervenkr*, 226, 65–73.

Angst, J. (1998). The emerging epidemiology of hypomania and bipolar II disorder. *J Affect Disord*, 50, 143–151.

Angst, J., and Marneros, A. (2001). Bipolarity from ancient to modern times: Conception, birth and rebirth. *J Affect Disord*, 67, 3–19.

Angst, J., Felder, W., Frey, R., and Stassen, H.H. (1978). The course of affective disorders: I. Change of diagnosis of monopolar, unipolar, and bipolar illness. *Arch Psychiatr Nervenkr*, 226, 57–64.

Angst, F., Stassen, H.H., Clayton, P.J., and Angst, J. (2002). Mortality of patients with mood disorders: Follow-up over 34–38 years. *J Affect Disord*, 68(2-3), 167–181.

Angst, J., Gamma, A., Benazzi, F., Ajdacic, V., Eich, D., and Rossler, W. (2003). Toward a re-definition of subthreshold bipolarity: Epidemiology and proposed criteria for bipolar-II, minor bipolar disorders and hypomania. *J Affect Disord*, 73, 133–146.

Angst, J., Gerber-Werder, R., Zuberbuhler, H.U., and Gamma, A. (2004). Is bipolar I disorder heterogeneous? *Eur Arch Psychiatry Clin Neurosci*, 254(2), 82–91.

Angst, J., Sellaro, R., Stassen, H., and Gamma, A. (2005). Diagnostic conversion from depression to bipolar disorders: Results of a long-term prospective study of hospital admissions. *J Affect Disord*, 84(2-3), 149–157.

Arato, M., Demeter, E., Rihmer, Z., and Somogyi, E. (1988). Retrospective psychiatric assessment of 200 suicides in Budapest. *Acta Psychiatr Scand*, 77(4), 454–456.

Baillarger, J. (1854). De la folie a double forme. *Annales Medico-Psychologiques*, 6, 369–391.

Baldessarini, R.J. (2000). A plea for integrity of the bipolar disorder concept. *Bipolar Disord*, 2(1), 3–7.

Baldessarini, R.J., Tondo, L., Floris, G., and Hennen, J. (2000). Effects of rapid cycling on response to lithium maintenance treatment in 360 bipolar I and II disorder patients. *J Affect Disord*, 61(1-2), 13–22.

Bauer, M.S., Simon, G.E., Ludman, E., and Unutzer, J. (2005). 'Bipolarity' in bipolar disorder: Distribution of manic and depressive symptoms in a treated population. *Br J Psychiatry*, 187, 87–88.

Beigel, A., and Murphy, D.L. (1971a). Assessing clinical characteristics of the manic state. *Am J Psychiatry*, 128, 688–694.

Beigel, A., and Murphy, D.L. (1971b). Unipolar and bipolar affective illness: Differences in clinical characteristics accompanying depression. *Arch Gen Psychiatry*, 24, 215–220.

Benazzi, F. (1997). Prevalence of bipolar II disorder in outpatient depression: A 203-case study in private practice. *J Affect Disord*, 46, 73–77.

Benazzi, F. (1999). A comparison of the age of onset of bipolar I and bipolar II outpatients. *J Affect Disord*, 54(3), 249–253.

Benazzi, F. (2001). Is 4 days the minimum duration of hypomania in bipolar II disorder? *Eur Arch Psychiatry Clin Neurosci*, 251, 32–34.

Benazzi, F. (2003a). Major depressive disorder with anger: A bipolar spectrum disorder? *Psychother Psychosom*, 72, 300–306.

Benazzi, F. (2003b). Unipolar depression with bipolar family history: Links with the bipolar spectrum. *Psychiatry Clin Neurosci*, 57(5), 497–503.

Benazzi, F., and Akiskal, H.S. (2001). Delineating bipolar II mixed states in the Ravenna–San Diego collaborative study: The relative prevalence and diagnostic significance of hypomanic features during major depressive episodes. *J Affect Disord*, 67, 115–122.

Benazzi, F., and Akiskal, H.S. (2003). Refining the evaluation of bipolar II: Beyond the strict SCID-CV guidelines for hypomania. *J Affect Disord*, 73, 33–38.

Benazzi, F., and Akiskal, H.S. (2005). A downscaled practical measure of mood lability as a screening tool for bipolar II. *J Affect Disord*, 84, 225–232.

Berrios, G.E., and Hauser, R. (1988). The early development of Kraepelin's ideas on classification: A conceptual history. *Psychol Med*, 18, 813–821.

Biondi, M., Picardi, A., Pasquini, M., Gaetano, P., and Pancheri, P. (2005). Dimensional psychopathology of depression: Detection of an 'activation' dimension in unipolar depressed outpatients. *J Affect Disord*, 84(2-3), 133–139.

Bleuler, E. (1924). *Textbook of Psychiatry* (4th German Edition). English edited by A.A. Brill. New York: Macmillan.

Brockington, I.F., Altman, E., Hillier, V., Meltzer, H.Y., and Nand, S. (1982). The clinical picture of bipolar affective disorder in its depressed phase: A report from London and Chicago. *Br J Psychiatry*, 141, 558–562.

Cantor, N., and Genero, N. (1986). Psychiatric diagnosis and natural categorization: A close analogy. In T. Millon and G.L. Klerman (Eds.), *Contemporary Directions in Psychopathology: Toward the DSM-IV* (pp. 233–256). New York: Guilford Press.

Cassano, G.B., Musetti, L., Perugi, G., Soriani, A., Mignani, V., McNair, D.M., and Akiskal, H.S. (1988). A proposed new approach to the clinical subclassification of depressive illness. *Pharmacopsychiatry*, 21, 19–23.

Cassano, G.B., Akiskal, H.S., Savino, M., Musetti, L., Perugi, G., and Soriani, A. (1992). Proposed subtypes of bipolar II and related disorders: With hypomanic episodes (or cyclothymia) and with hyperthymic temperament. *J Affect Disord*, 26, 127–140.

Cassano, G.B., Dell'Osso, L., Frank, E., Miniati, M., Fagiolini, A., Shear, K., Pini, S., and Maser, J. (1999). The bipolar spectrum: A clinical reality in search of diagnostic criteria and an assessment methodology. *J Affect Disord*, 54(3), 319–328.

Cassano, G.B., Frank, E., Miniati, M., Rucci, P., Fagiolini, A., Pini, S., Shear, M.K., and Maser, J.D. (2002). Conceptual underpinnings and empirical support for the mood spectrum. *Psychiatr Clin North Am*, 25(4), 699–712.

Cassano, G.B., Rucci, P., Frank, E., Fagiolini, A., Dell'Osso, L., Shear, M.K., and Kupfer, D.J. (2004). The mood spectrum in unipolar and bipolar disorder: Arguments for a unitary approach. *Am J Psychiatry*, 161(7), 1264–1269.

Coryell, W., Endicott, J., Reich, T., Andreasen, N., and Keller, M. (1984). A family study of bipolar II disorder. *Br J Psychiatry*, 145, 49–54.

Coryell, W., Endicott, J., Andreasen, N., and Keller, M. (1985). Bipolar I, bipolar II, and nonbipolar major depression among the relatives of affectively ill probands. *Am J Psychiatry*, 142, 817–821.

Coryell, W., Endicott, J., and Keller, M. (1992). Rapidly cycling affective disorder. Demographics, diagnosis, family history, and course. *Arch Gen Psychiatry*, 49(2), 126–131.

Coryell, W., Endicott, J., Maser, J.D., Keller, M.B., Leon, A.C., and Akiskal, H.S. (1995). Long-term stability of polarity distinctions in the affective disorders. *Am J Psychiatry*, 152, 385–390.

Coryell, W., Solomon, D., Turvey, C., Keller, M., Leon, A.C., Endicott, J., Schettler, P., Judd, L., and Mueller, T. (2003). The long-term course of rapid cycling bipolar disorder. *Arch Gen Psychiatry*, 60, 914–920.

Cutting, J. (1990). Relationship between cycloid psychosis and typical affective psychosis. *Psychopathology*, 23(4), 212–219.

Davenport, Y.B., Adland, M.L., Gold, P.W., and Goodwin, F.K. (1979). Manic-depressive illness: Psychodynamic features of multigenerational families. *Am J Orthopsychiatry*, 49, 24–35.

Davis, G.C., and Buchsbaum, B.S. (1981). Pain sensitivity and endorphins in functional psychoses. *Mod Probl Pharmacopsychiatry*, 17, 97–108.

Deckersbach, T., Perlis, R.H., Frankle, W.G., Gray, S.M., Grandin, L., Dougherty, D.D., Nierenberg, A.A., and Sachs, G.S. (2004). Presence of irritability during depressive episodes in bipolar disorder. *CNS Spectr*, 9, 227–231.

Deltito, J., Martin, L., Riefkohl, J., Austria, B., Kissilenko, A., Corless, C., and Morse, P. (2001). Do patients with borderline personality disorder belong to the bipolar spectrum? *J Affect Disord*, 67, 221–228.

Depue, R.A., and Klein, D.N. (1988). Identification of unipolar and bipolar affective conditions in nonclinical and clinical populations by the General Behavior Inventory. In D.L. Dunner, E.S. Gershon, and J.E. Barrett (Eds.), *Relatives at Risk for Mental Disorder* (pp. 179–204). New York: Raven Press.

Depue, R.A., Kleiman, R.M., Davis, P., Hutchinson, M., and Kraussm, S.O. (1981). The behavioral high risk paradigm and bipolar affective disorder: A conceptual framework with five validation studies. *J Abnorm Psychol Monograph*, 90, 381–437.

Depue, R.A., Krauss, S., Spoont, M.R., and Arbisi, P. (1989). General behavior inventory identification of unipolar and bipolar affective conditions in a nonclinical university population. *J Abnorm Psychol*, 98, 117–126.

Dilsaver, S.C., and Akiskal, H.S. (2005). High rate of unrecognized bipolar mixed states among destitute Hispanic adolescents referred for "major depressive disorder." *J Affect Disord*, 84(2-3), 179–186.

Duncan, W.C., Pettigrew, K.D., and Gillen, J.C. (1979). REM architecture changes in bipolar and unipolar depression. *Am J Psychiatry*, 136, 1424–1427.

Dunner, D.L. (1980). Unipolar and bipolar depression: Recent findings from clinical and biologic studies. In *The Psychobiology of Affective Disorders* (pp. 11–24). Pfizer Symposium Depression. Basel, Switzerland: Karger.

Dunner, D.L. (1987). Stability of bipolar II affective disorder as a diagnostic entity. *Psychiatr Ann*, 17, 18–20.

Dunner, D.L., and Tay, L.K. (1993). Diagnostic reliability of the history of hypomania in bipolar II patients and patients with major depression. *Compr Psychiatry*, 34(5), 303–307.

Dunner, D.L., Fleiss, J.L., and Fieve, R.R. (1976a). Depressive symptoms in patients with unipolar and bipolar affective disorder. *Compr Psychiatry*, 17, 447–451.

Dunner, D.L., Gershon, E.S., and Goodwin, F.K. (1976b). Heritable factors in the severity of affective illness. *Biol Psychiatry*, 11, 31–42.

Dunner, D.L., Hensel, B.M., and Fieve, R.R. (1979). Bipolar illness: Factors in drinking behavior. *Am J Psychiatry*, 136, 583–585.

Dunner, D.L., Murphy, D., Stallone, F., and Fieve, R.R. (1980). Affective episode frequency and lithium therapy. *Psychopharmacol Bull*, 16, 49–50.

Ebert, D., Barocka, A., Kalb, R., and Ott, G. (1993). Atypical depression as a bipolar spectrum disease: Evidence from a longitudinal study: The early course of atypical depression. *Psychiatria Danubina*, 5, 133–136.

Egeland, J.A., and Hotstetter, A.M. (1983). Amish study, I: Affective disorders among the Amish, 1976–1980. *Am J Psychiatry*, 140, 56–61.

Endicott, N.A. (1989). Psychophysiological correlates of 'bipolarity.' *J Affect Disord*, 17, 47–56.

Endicott, J., Nee, J., Andeason, N., Clayton P., Keller, M., and Coryell, W. (1985). Bipolar II: Combine or separate. *J Affect Disord*, 8, 17–28.

Fava, M., and Rosenbaum, J.F. (1999). Anger attacks in patients with depression. *J Clin Psychiatry*, 60(Suppl. 15), s21–S24.

Ferrier, I.N., MacMillan, I.C., and Young, A.H. (2001). The search for the wandering thymostat: A review of some developments in bipolar disorder research. *Br J Psychiatry*, 178(Suppl. 41), s103–s106.

Fieve, R.R., Go, R., Dunner, D.L., and Elston, R. (1984). Search for biological/genetic markers in a long-term epidemiological and morbid risk study of affective disorders. *J Psychiatr Res*, 18(4), 425–445.

Geller, B., Zimerman, B., Williams, M., Bolhofner, K., and Craney, J.L. (2001). Bipolar disorder at prospective follow-up of adults who had prepubertal major depressive disorder. *Am J Psychiatry*, 58(1), 125–127.

Gershon, E.S., Hamovit, J., Guroff, J.J., Dibble, E., Leckman, J.F., Sceery, W., Targum, S.D., Nurnberger, J.I., Goldin, L.R., and Bunney, W.E. (1982). A family study of schizoaffective, bipolar I, bipolar II, unipolar and normal control probands. *Arch Gen Psychiatry*, 39, 1157–1167.

Ghaemi, S.N., Sachs, G.S., Chiou, A.M., Pandurangi, A.K., and Goodwin, K. (1999). Is bipolar disorder still underdiagnosed? Are antidepressants overutilized? *J Affect Disord*, 52(1), 135–144.

Ghaemi, S.N., Ko, J.Y., and Goodwin, F.K. (2002). Cade's disease and beyond: Misdiagnosis, antidepressant use, and a proposed definition for bipolar spectrum disorder. *Can J Psychiatry*, 47, 125–134.

Ghaemi, S.N., Hsu, D.J., Ko, J.Y., Baldassano, C.F., Kontos, N.J., and Goodwin, F.K. (2004). Bipolar spectrum disorder: A pilot study. *Psychopathology*, 37(5), 222–226.

Goldberg, J.F., Harrow, M., and Whiteside, J.E. (2001). Risk for bipolar illness in patients initially hospitalized for unipolar depression. *Am J Psychiatry*, 158, 1265–1270.

Goodwin, F.K. (1977). Diagnosis of affective disorders. In M.E. Jarvik (Ed.), *Psychopharmacology in the Practice of Medicine* (pp. 219–228). New York: Appleton-Century-Crofts.

Goodwin, F.K., and Ghaemi, S.N. (2000). An introduction to and history of affective disorders. In M. Gelder, J. Lopez-Ibor, and N. Andreasen (Eds.), *New Oxford Textbook of Psychiatry*. New York: Oxford University Press, pp. 677–682.

Grayson, D.A. (1987). Can categorical and dimensional views of psychiatric illness be distinguished? *Br J Psychiatry*, 151, 355–361.

Greenhouse, S.W., and Geisser, S. (1959). On methods in the analysis of profile data. *Psychometrika*, 24, 95–112.

Griesinger, W. (1867). *Mental Pathology and Therapeutics*. Translated by C.L. Robertson and J. Rutherford. London: New Sydenhem Society.

Guze, S.B., Woodruff, R.A. Jr., and Clayton, P.J. (1975). The significance of psychotic affective disorders. *Arch Gen Psychiatry*, 32, 1147–1150.

Hantouche, E.G., and Akiskal, H.S. (2005). Bipolar II vs. unipolar depression: Psychopathologic differentiation by dimensional measures. *J Affect Disord*, 84(2-3), 127–132.

Hantouche, E.G., Akisakal, H.S., Lancrenon, S., Allilaire, J.F., Sechrer, D., Azorin, J.M., Bourgeois, M., Fraudm, J.P., and Chalenet-Duchene, L. (1998). Systemic clinical methodology for validating bipolar disorder data in mid stream from a French national multi-cite study (EPIDEP). *J Affect Disorder*, 50, 163–173.

Hantouche, E.G., Angst, J., and Akiskal, H.S. (2003a). Factor structure of hypomania: Interrelationships with cyclothymia and the soft bipolar spectrum. *J Affect Disord*, 73, 39–47.

Hantouche, E.G., Angst, J., Demonfaucon, C., Perugi, G., Lancrenon, S., and Akiskal, H.S. (2003b). Cyclothymic OCD: A distinct form? *J Affect Disord*, 75(1), 1–10.

Hartmann, E. (1968). Longitudinal studies of sleep and dream patterns in manic depressive patients. *Arch Gen Psychiatry*, 19, 312–329.

Heun, R., and Maier, W. (1993) The distinction of bipolar II disorder from bipolar I and recurrent unipolar depression: Results of a controlled family study. *Acta Psychiatr Scand*, 87(4), 279–284.

Himmelhoch, J.M., Detre, T., Kupfer, D.J., Swartzburg, M., and Byck, R. (1972). Treatment of previously intractable depressions with tranylcypromine and lithium. *J Nerv Mental Dis*, 155, 216–220.

Himmelhoch, J.M., Thase, M.E., Mallinger, A.G., and Houck, P. (1991). Tranylcypromine versus imipramine in anergic bipolar depression. *Am J Psychiatry*, 148(7), 910–916.

Horwath, E., Johnson, J., Weissman, M.M., and Hornig, C.D. (1992). The validity of major depression with atypical features based on a community study. *J Affect Disord*, 26(2), 117–125.

Jackson, S.W. (1986). *Melancholia and Depression: From Hippocratic Times to Modern Times*. New Haven, CT: Yale University Press.

Jamison, K.R. (2005). *Exuberance: The Passion for Life*. New York: Vintage Books.

Jelliffe, S.E. (1931). Some historical phases of the manic-depressive synthesis. *Research Publications Association for Research in Nervous and Mental Diseases*, 11, 3–47.

Joffe, R.T., Young, L.T., and MacQueen, G.M. (1999). A two-illness model of bipolar disorder. *Bipolar Disord*, 1(1), 25–30.

Judd, L.L., and Akiskal, H.S. (2000). Delineating the longitudinal structure of depressive illness: Beyond clinical subtypes and duration thresholds. *Pharmacopsychiatry*, 33, 3–7.

Judd, L.L., Akiskal, H.S., Schettler, P.J., Endicott, J., Maser, J., Solomon, D.A., Leon, A.C., Rice, J.A., and Keller, M.B. (2002). The long-term natural history of the weekly symptomatic status of bipolar I disorder. *Arch Gen Psychiatry*, 59, 530–537.

Judd, L.L., Akiskal, H.S., Coryell, W., Schettler, P., Maser, J., Rice, J., Solomon, D., and Keller, M. (2003a). The comparative clinical phenotype and long term longitudinal episode course of bipolar I and II: A clinical spectrum or distinct disorders? *J Affect Disord*, 73, 19–32.

Judd, L.L., Akiskal, H.S., Schettler, P., Endicott, J., Maser, J., Solomon, D., Leon, A., Coryell, W., and Keller, M. (2003b). A prospective naturalistic investigation of the long-term weekly symptomatic status of bipolar II disorder. *Arch Gen Psychiatry*, 60, 261–269.

Judd, L.L., Schettler, P.J., Akiskal, H.S., Maser, J., Coryell, W., Solomon, D., Endicott, J., and Keller, M. (2003c). Long-term symptomatic status of bipolar I vs. bipolar II disorders. *Int J Neuropsychopharmacol*, 6(2), 127–137.

Kadrmas, A., Winokur, G., and Crowe, R. (1979). Postpartum mania. *Br J Psychiatry*, 135, 551–554.

Kahlbaum, K.L. (1882). Uber cyclisches Irresein. *Der Irrenfreund*, 10, 145–157.

Katz, M.M., Robins, E., Croughan, J., Secunda, S., and Swann, A. (1982). Behavioral measurement and drug response characteristics of unipolar and bipolar depression. *Psychol Med*, 12, 25–36.

Kendell, R.E. (1968). *The Classification of Depressive Illness*. London: Oxford University Press.

Klein, D.N., Depue, R.A., and Slater, J.F. (1986). Inventory identification of cyclothymia: IX. Validation in offspring of bipolar I patients. *Arch General Psychiatry*, 43, 441–445.

Klerman, G.L. (1981). The spectrum of mania. *Compr Psychiatry*, 22, 11–20.

Kotin, J., and Goodwin, F.K. (1972). Depression during mania: Clinical observations and theoretical implications. *Am J Psychiatry*, 129, 679–686.

Koukopoulos, A. (2003). Ewald Hecker's description of cyclothymia as a cyclical mood disorder: Its relevance to the modern concept of bipolar II. *J Affect Disord*, 73, 199–205.

Koukopoulos, A. (2006). The primacy of mania. In H. Akiskal and M. Tohen (Eds.), *Bipolar Psychopharmacotherapy: Caring for the Patient*. New York: John Wiley and Sons.

Koukopoulos, A., and Koukopoulos, A. (1999). Agitated depression as a mixed state and the problem of melancholia. In H.S. Akiskal (Ed.), *Bipolarity: Beyond Classic Mania. Psychiatr Clin North Am*, 22, 547–564.

Koukopoulos, A., Caliari, B., Tundo, A., Minnai, G., Floris, G., Reginaldi, D., and Tondo, L. (1983). Rapid cyclers, temperament, and antidepressants. *Compr Psychiatry*, 24, 249–258.

Kovacs, M., Akiskal, H.S., Gatsonis, C., and Parrone, P.L. (1994). Childhood-onset dysthymic disorder: Clinical features and prospective naturalistic outcome. *Arch Gen Psychiatry*, 51, 365–374.

Kraemer, H., Noda, A., and O'Hara, R. (2004). Categorical versus dimensional approaches to diagnosis: Methodological challenges. *J Psychiatr Res*, 38, 17–25.

Kraepelin, E. (1899). *Manic Depressive Insanity and Paranoia*. Edinburgh: E. & S. Livingstone.

Kraepelin, E. (1921). *Manic-Depressive Insanity and Paranoia*. Edinburgh: E. & S. Livingstone. Originally published as *Psychiatrie. Ein Lehrbuch fur Studierende und Arzte. ed. 2. Klinische Psychiatrie. II*. Leipzig: Johann Ambrosius Barth, 1899.

Kupfer, D.J., Himmelhoch, J.M., Swartzburg, M., Anderson, C., Byck, R., and Detre, T.P. (1972). Hyperinsomnia in manic-depressive disease (a preliminary report). *Dis Nerv Syst*, 33, 720–724.

Kupfer, D.J., Weiss, B.L., Foster, F.G., Detre, T.P., Delgado, J., and McPartland, R. (1974). Psychomotor activity in affective states. *Arch Gen Psychiatry*, 30, 765–768.

Kupfer, D.J., Pakcar, D., Himmelhoch, J.M., and Detre, T.P. (1975). Are there two types of unipolar depression? *Arch Gen Psychiatry*, 32, 866–871.

Leff, J. (1977). International variations in the diagnosis of psychiatric illness. *Br J Psychiatry*, 131, 329–338.

Leonhard, K. (1957). Pathogenesis of manic-depressive disease. *Nervenarzt*, 28(6), 271–272.

Leonhard, K. (1979). *The Classification of Endogenous Psychoses*, 5th edition. E. Robins (Ed.), R. Berman (Trans.). New York: Irvington Publishers, Inc., (pp. 3–4). Originally published as *Aufteilung der Endogenen Psychosen*, 1st edition. Berlin: Akademie-Verlag, 1957.

Levitan, R.D., Lesage, A., Parikh, S.V., Goering, P., and Kennedy, S.H. (1997). Reversed neurovegetative symptoms of depression: A community study of Ontario. *Am J Psychiatry*, 154(7), 934–940.

Lewis, A.J. (1936). Prognosis in the manic depressive psychosis. *Lancet*, 2, 997–999.

Mainia, G., Albert, U., Ceregato, A., and Bogetto, F. (2002). *Re-evaluating the prevalence of bipolar spectrum disorders in a clinical sample referred to a mood disorder unit: From DSM-IV criteria to a broad clinical spectrum of bipolar disorder* (Abstract). Philadelphia: American Psychiatric Association, p. 123.

Maj, M., Pirozzi, R, Formicola, A.M., and Tortorella, A. (1999). Reliability and validity of four alternative definitions of rapid cycling bipolar disorder. *Am J Psychiatry*, 156, 1421–1424.

Maj, M., Pirozzi, R., Magliano, L., and Bartoli, L. (2003). Agitated depression in bipolar I disorder: Prevalence, phenomenology, and outcome. *Am J Psychiatry*, 160(12), 2134–2140.

Manning, J.S., Haykal, R.F., Connor, P.D., and Akiskal, H.S. (1997). On the nature of depressive and anxious states in a family practice setting: The high prevalence of bipolar II and related disorders in a cohort followed longitudinally. *Compr Psychiatry*, 38, 102–108.

Marneros, A. (2001). Origin and development of concepts of bipolar mixed states. *J Affect Disord*, 67(1–3), 229–240.

Maser, J.D., and Akiskal, H.S. (2002). Spectrum concepts in major mental disorders. *Psychiatr Clin North Am*, 25(4), 685–885.

Mayer-Gross, W., Slater, E., and Roth, M. (1955). *Clinical Psychiatry*. Baltimore: Williams and Wilkens.

Mendel, E. (1881). *Die Manie*. Vienna: Urban and Schwazenberg.

Mendels, J. (1976). Lithium in the treatment of depression. *Am J Psychiatry*, 133, 373–378.

Mendelson, W.B., Sack, D.A., James, S.P., Martin, J.V., Wagner, R., Garnett, D., Milton, J., and Wehr, T.A. (1987). Frequency analysis of the sleep EEG in depression. *Psychiatry Res*, 21, 89–94.

Meyer, A. (1866–1950). *Collected Papers of Adolf Myer*. E.E. Winters (Ed.). Baltimore: Johns Hopkins University Press.

Mitchell, P.B., Parker, G., Jamieson, K., Wilhelm, K., Hickie, I., Brodaty, H., Boyce, P., Hadzi-Pavlovic, D., and Roy, K. (1992). Are there any differences between bipolar and unipolar melancholia? *J Affect Disord*, 25, 97–105.

Mitchell, P.B., Wilhelm, K., Parker, G., Austin, M.P., Ritgers, P., and Malhi, G.S. (2001). The clinical features of bipolar depression: A comparison with matched major depressive disorder patients. *J Clin Psychiatry*, 62, 212–216.

Moorhead, S.R., and Young, A.H. (2003). Evidence for a late onset bipolar-I disorder sub-group from 50 years. *J Affect Disord*, 73, 271–277.

Nurnberger, J. Jr., Roose, S.P., Dunner, D.L., and Fieve, R.R. (1979). Unipolar mania: A distinct clinical entity? *Am J Psychiatry*, 136(11), 1420–1423.

Papadimitriou, G.N., Dikeos, D.G., Daskalopoulou, E.G., and Soldatos, C.R. (2002). Co-occurrence of disturbed sleep and appetite loss differentiates between unipolar and bipolar depressive episodes. *Prog Neuropsychopharmacol Biol Psychiatry*, 26, 1041–1045.

Parker, G., Roy, K., Wilhelm, K., Mitchell, P., and Hadzi-Pavlovic, D. (2000). The nature of bipolar depression: Implications for the definition of melancholia. *J Affect Disord*, 59, 217–224.

Perlis, R.H., Smoller, J.W., Fava, M., Rosenbaum, J.F., Nierenberg, A.A., and Sachs, G.S. (2004). The prevalence and clinical correlates of anger attacks during depressive episodes in bipolar disorder. *J Affect Disord*, 79, 291–295.

Perlis, R.H., Brown, E., Baker, R.W., and Nierenberg, A.A. (2006). Clinical features of bipolar depression versus major depressive disorder in large multicenter trials. *Am J Psychiatry*, 163(2), 175–176.

Perris, C. (Ed.). (1966). A study of bipolar (manic-depressive) and unipolar recurrent depressive psychoses. *Acta Psychiatr Scand*, 42(Suppl. 194).

Perris, C. (1968). The course of depressive psychoses. *Acta Psychiatr Scand*, 44, 238–248.

Perris, C. (1971). The course of depressive psychoses. *Acta Psychiatr Scand*, (Suppl. 221), 43–51.

Perugi, G., Akiskal, H.S., Lattanzi, L., Cecconi, D., Mastrocinque, C., Patronelli, A., and Vignoli, S. (1998a). The high prevalence of soft bipolar (II) features in atypical depression. *Compr Psychiatry*, 39, 63–71.

Perugi, G., Akiskal, H.S., Rossi, L., Paiano, A., Quilici, C., Madaro, D., Musetti, L., and Cassano, G.B. (1998b). Chronic mania: Family history, prior course, clinical picture and social consequences. *Br J Psychiatry*, 173, 514–518.

Perugi, G., Akiskal, H.S., Ramacciotti, S., Nassini, S., Toni, C., Milanfranchi, A., and Musetti, L. (1999). Depressive comorbidity of panic, social phobic and obsessive-compulsive disorders: Is there a bipolar II connection? *J Psychiatr Res*, 33, 53–61.

Perugi, G., Akiskal, H.S., Toni, C., Simonini, E., and Gemignani A. (2001). The temporal relationship between anxiety disorders and (hypo)mania: A retrospective examination of 63 panic, social phobic and obsessive-compulsive patients with comorbid bipolar disorder. *J Affect Disord*, 67, 199–206.

Perugi, G., Toni, C., Travierso, M.C., and Akiskal, H.S. (2003). The role of cyclothymia in atypical depression: Toward a data-based reconceptualization of the borderline-bipolar II connection. *J Affect Disord*, 73, 87–98.

Pichot, P. (1988). European perspectives on the classification of depression. *Br J Psyciatry*, 153(Suppl. 3), 11–15.

Pichot, P. (1995). The birth of the bipolar disorder. *Eur Psychiatry*, 10, 1–10.

Pirozzi, M.M., Magliano, L., Fiorillo, A., and Bartoli, L. (2006). Agitated "unipolar" major depression: Prevalence, phenomenology, and outcome. *J Clin Psychiatry*, 67(5), 712–719.

Placidi, G.F., Signoretta, S., Liguori, A., Gervasi, R., Maremmani, I., and Akiskal, H.S. (1998). The semi-structured affective temperament interview (TEMPS-I): Reliability and psychometric properties in 1010 14–26 year students. *J Affect Disord*, 47, 1–10.

Popescu, C., Ionescu, R., Jipescu, I., and Popa, S. (1991). Psychomotor functioning in unipolar and bipolar affective disorders. *Rom J Neurol Psychiatry*, 29(1-2), 17–33.

Posternak, M.A., and Zimmerman, M. (2002). Lack of association between seasonality and psychopathology in psychiatric outpatients. *Psychiatry Res*, 112(3), 187–194.

Rao, U., Ryan, N.D., Birmaher, B., Dahl, R., Williamson, D., Kaufman, J., Rao, R., and Nelson, B. (1995). Unipolar depression in adolescents: Clinical outcome in adulthood. *J Am Acad Child Adolesc Psychiatry*, 34(5), 566–578.

Rao, U., Dahl, R.E., Ryan, N.D., Birmaher, B., Williamson, D.E., Rao, R., and Kaufman, J. (2002). Heterogeneity in EEG sleep findings in adolescent depression: Unipolar versus bipolar clinical course. *J Affect Disord*, 70(3), 273–280.

Raskin, A., and Crook, T.H. (1976). The endogenous-neurotic distribution as a predictor of response to antidepressant drug. *Psychol Med*, 6, 59–70.

Regier, D.A., Farmer, M.E., Rae, D.S., Locke, B.Z., Keith, S.J., Judd, L.L., and Goodwin, F.K. (1990). Comorbidity of mental disorders with alcohol and other drug abuse. Results from the Epidemiologic Catchment Area (ECA) Study. *JAMA*, 264(19), 2511–2518.

Reich, T., and Winokur, G. (1970). Postpartum psychoses in patients with manic depressive disease. *J Nerv Ment Dis*, 151, 60–68.

Rice, J.P., McDonald-Scott, P., Endocott, J., Coryell, W., Grove, W.M., Keller, M.B., and Altis, D. (1986). The stability of diagnosis with an application to bipolar II disorder. *Psychiatry Res*, 19, 285–296.

Rihmer, Z., and Pestality, P. (1999). Bipolar II disorder and suicidal behavior. *Psychiatr Clin North Am*, 22(3), 667–673.

Ritti, A. (1892). Circular insanity. In D. Hack Tuke (Ed.), *A Dictionary of Psychological Medicine Giving the Definition, Etymology and Synonyms of Terms Used in Medical Psychology, with the Symptoms, Treatment and Pathology of Insanity and the Law of Lunacy in Great Britain and Ireland* (p. 214), 2 volumes. Philadelphia: P. Blakiston.

Robertson, H.A., Lam, R.W., Stewart, J.N., Yatham, L.N., Tam, E.M., and Zis, A.P. (1996). Atypical depressive symptoms and clusters in unipolar and bipolar depression. *Acta Psychiatr Scand*, 94, 421–427.

Roccatagliata, G. (1986). *A History of Ancient Psychiatry*. New York: Greenwood Press.

Roth, M. (1983). Depression and affective disorder in later life. In J. Angst (Ed.), *The Origins of Depression: Current Concepts and Approaches* (pp. 39–75). Berlin: Springer-Verlag.

Rybakowski, J.K., Suwalska, A., Lojko, D., Rymaszewska, J., and Kiejna, A. (2005). Bipolar mood disorders among Polish psychiatric outpatients treated for major depression. *J Affect Disord*, 84(2-3), 141–147.

Sass, H., Herpertz, S., and Steinmeyer, E.M. (1993). Subaffective personality disorders. *Int Clin Psychopharmacol*, 8(Suppl. 1), 39–46.

Sato, T., Bottlender, R., Schroter, A., and Moller, H.J. (2003). Frequency of manic symptoms during a depressive episode and unipolar 'depressive mixed state' as bipolar spectrum. *Acta Psychiatr Scand*, 107, 268–274.

Sato, T., Bottlender, R., Kleindienst, N., and Moller, H.J. (2005). Irritable psychomotor elation in depressed inpatients: A factor validation of mixed depression. *J Affect Disord*, 84(2-3), 187–196.

Serretti, A., and Olgiati, P. (2005). Profiles of "manic" symptoms in bipolar I, bipolar II and major depressive disorders. *J Affect Disord*, 84(2-3), 159–166.

Sharma, V., Khan, M., and Smith, A. (2005). A closer look at treatment resistant depression: Is it due to a bipolar diathesis? *J Affect Disord*, 84(2-3), 251–257.

Serretti, A., Lattuada, E., Cusin, C., Macciardi, F., and Smeraldi, E. (1998). Analysis of depressive symptomatology in mood disorders. *Depress Anxiety*, 8(2), 80–85.

Shulman, K., and Post, F. (1980). Bipolar affective disorder in old age. *Br J Psychiatry*, 136, 26–32.

Shulman, K.I., and Tohen, M. (1994). Unipolar mania reconsidered: Evidence from an elderly cohort. *Br J Psychiatry*, 164(4), 547–549.

Signoretta, S., Maremmani, I., Liguori, A., Perugi, G., and Akiskal, H.S. (2005). Affective temperament traits measured by TEMPS-I and emotional-behavioral problems in clinically-well children, adolescents, and young adults. *J Affect Disord*, 85, 169–180.

Simpson, S.G., Folstein, S.E., Meyers, D.A., McMahon, F.J., Brusco, D.M., and DePaulo, J.R. (1993). Bipolar II: The most common bipolar phenotype? *Am J Psychiatry*, 150, 901–903.

Simpson, S.G., McMahon, F.J., McInnis, M.G., MacKinnon, D.F., Edwin, D., Folstein, S.E., and DePaulo, J.R. (2002). Diagnostic reliability of bipolar II disorder. *Arch Gen Psychiatry*, 59, 736–740.

Smith, D.J., Harrison, N., Muir, W., and Blackwood, D.H. (2005). The high prevalence of bipolar spectrum disorders in young adults with recurrent depression: Toward an innovative diagnostic framework. *J Affect Disord*, 84(2-3), 167–178.

Solomon, D.A., Leon, A.C., Endicott, J., Coryell, W.H., Mueller, T.I., Posternak, M.A., and Keller, M. (2003). Unipolar mania over the course of a 20-year follow-up study. *Am J Psychiatry*, 60(11), 2049–2051.

Sullivan, P.F., Prescott, C.A., and Candler, K.S. (2002). Subtypes of major depression in a twin registry. *J Affect Disorder*, 68, 273–284.

Toni, C., Perugi, G., Mata, B., Madaro, D., Maremmani, I., and Akiskal, H.S. (2001). Is mood-incongruent manic psychosis a distinct subtype? *Eur Arch Psychiatry Clin Neurosci*, 251, 12–17.

Tsuang, M.T., Faraone, S.V., and Fleming, J.A. (1985). Familial transmission of major affective disorders: Is there evidence supporting the distinction between unipolar and bipolar disorders? *Br J Psychiatry*, 146, 268–271.

Vahip, S., Kesebir, S., Alkan, M., Yazici, O., Akiskal, K.K., and Akiskal, H.S. (2005). Affective temperaments in clinically-well subjects in Turkey: Initial psychometric data on the TEMPS-A. *J Affect Disord*, 85, 113–125.

VanEerdewegh, M.M., Van Eerdewegh, P., Coryell, W., Clayton, P.J., Endicott, J., Koepke, J., and Rochberg, N. (1987). Schizoaffective disorders: Bipolar-unipolar subtyping. Natural history variables: A discriminant analysis approach. *J Affect Disord*, 12, 223–232.

van Praag, H.M. (1993). What is self-evident but does not occur as a matter-of-course; observations on the report about biological psychiatry. *Ned Tijdschr Geneeskd*, 13, 137(7), 366–368.

Vieta, E., and Barcia, D. (2000). *El trastorno bipolar en el siglo XVIII*. Burdeos, Spain: Mra ediciones.

Vieta, E., Gasto, C., Otero, A., Nieto, E., and Vallejo, J. (1997). Differential features between bipolar I and bipolar II disorder. *Compr Psychiatry*, 38(2), 98–101.

Waters, B.G.H. (1979). Early symptoms of bipolar affective psychosis: Research and clinical implications. *Can Psychiatr Assoc J*, 2, 55–60.

Weissman, M.M., Bland, R.C., Canino, G.J., Faravelli, C., Greenwald, S., Hwu, H.G., Joyce, P.R., Karam, E.G., Lee, C.K., Lellouch, J., Lepine, J.P., Newman, S.C., Rubio-Stipec, M., Wells, J.E., Wickramaratne, P.J., Wittchen, H., and Yeh, E.K. (1996). Cross-national epidemiology of major depression and bipolar disorder. *JAMA*, 276(4), 293–299.

Whitwell, J.R. (1936). *Historical Notes on Psychiatry (Early Times–End of the 16th Century)*. London: HK Lewis & Co.

Wicki, W., and Angst, J. (1991). The Zurich study. X. Hypomania in a 28- to 30-year-old cohort. *EurArch Psychiatr Clin Neurosci*, 40, 339–348.

Wightman, W.P.D. (1971). *The Emergence of Scientific Medicine*. Edinburgh: Oliver and Boyd.

Winokur. G. (1979). Unipolar depression: Is it divisible into autonomous subtypes? *Arch Gen Psychiatry*, 36, 47–52.

Winokur, G. (1980). Is there a common genetic factor in bipolar and unipolar affective disorder? *Compr Psychiatry*, 21, 460–468.

Winokur, G., and Clayton, P. (1967). Family history studies: I. Two types of affective disorders separated according to genetic and clinical factors. In J. Worris (Ed.), *Recent Advances in Biological Psychiatry* (Vol. 10) (pp. 35–50). New York: Plenum Press.

Winokur, G., Clayton, P.J., and Reich, T. (1969). *Manic Depressive Illness*. St. Louis: C.V. Mosby.

Winokur, G., Coryell, W., Endicott, J., and Akiskal, H. (1993). Further distinctions between manic-depressive illness (bipolar disorder) and primary depressive disorder (unipolar depression). *Am J Psychiatry*, 150, 1176–1181.

Winokur, G., Coryell, W., Akiskal, H.S., Endicott, J., Keller, M., and Mueller, T. (1994). Manic-depressive illness: The course in light of a prospective ten-year follow-up. *Acta Psychiatr Scand*, 89, 102–110.

Winokur, G., Coryell, W., Keller, M., Endicott, J., and Leon, A. (1995). A family study of manic-depressive (bipolar I) disease. Is it a distinct illness separable from primary unipolar depression? *Arch Gen Psychiatry*, 52, 367–373.

Winokur, G., Turvey, C., Akiskal, H., Coryell, W., Solomon, D., Leon, A., Mueller, T., Endicott, J., Maser, J., and Keller, M. (1998). Alcoholism and drug abuse in three groups—bipolar I, unipolars and their acquaintances. *J Affect Disord*, 50(2-3), 81–89.

Yazici, O., Kora, K., Ucok, A., Saylan, M., Ozdemir, O., Kiziltan, E., and Ozpulat, T. (2002). Unipolar mania: A distinct disorder? *J Affect Disord*, 71(1-3), 97–103.

Zilboorg, G. (1941). *A History of Medical Psychology*. New York: W.W. Norton.

CHAPTER 2

Abrams, R., and Taylor, M.A. (1976). Mania and schizoaffective disorder, manic type: A comparison. *Am J Psychiatry*, 133, 1445–1447.

Abrams, R., and Taylor, M.A. (1981). Importance of schizophrenic symptoms in the diagnosis of mania. *Am J Psychiatry*, 138, 658–661.

Abrams, R., and Taylor, M.A. (1983) The importance of mood-incongruent psychotic symptoms in melancholia. *J Affect Disord*, 5, 179–181.

Adler, D., and Harrow, M. (1974). Idiosyncratic thinking and personally overinvolved thinking in schizophrenic patients during partial recovery. *Compr Psychiatry*, 15, 57–67.

Akiskal, H.S. (1992a). Delineating irritable-choleric and hyperthymic temperaments as variants of cyclothymia. *J Person Disord*, 6, 326–342.

Akiskal, H.S. (1992b). The distinctive mixed states of bipolar I, II and III. *Clin Neuropharmacol*, 15(Suppl 1A), 632–633.

Akiskal, H.S. (Ed). (1999). Bipolarity: Beyond classic mania. *Psychiatr Clin North Am*, 22(3), 517–703.

Akiskal, H.S., and Mallya, G. (1987). Criteria for the "soft" bipolar spectrum: Treatment implications. *Psychopharmacol Bull*, 23, 68–73.

Akiskal, H.S., and Puzantian, V.R. (1979). Psychotic forms of depression and mania. *Psychiatr Clin North Am*, 2, 419–439.

Akiskal, H.S., Djenderedjian, A.H., Rosenthal, R.H., and Khani, M.K. (1977). Cyclothymic disorder: Validating criteria for inclusion in the bipolar affective group. *Am J Psychiatry*, 134, 1227–1233.

Akiskal, H.S., Khani, M.K., and Scott-Strauss, A. (1979a). Cyclothymic temperament disorders. *Psychiatr Clin North Am*, 2, 527–554.

Akiskal, H.S., Rosenthal, R.H., Rosenthal, T.L., Kashgarian, M., Khani, M.K., and Puzantian, V.R. (1979b). Differentiation of primary affective illness from situational, symptonmatic, and secondary depressions. *Arch Gen Psychiatry*, 36, 635–643.

Akiskal, H.S., Waker, P., Puzantian, V.R., King, D., Rosenthal, T.L., and Dranon, M. (1983). Bipolar outcome in the course of depressive illness: Phenomenologic, familial, and pharmacologic predictors. *J Affect Disord*, 5, 115–128.

Akiskal, H.S., Hantouche, E., Bourgeois, M., Azorin, J.M., Sechter, D., Allilaire, J.F., Lancrenon, S., Fraud, J.P., and Chatenet-Duchene, L. (1998a). Gender, temperament and the clinical picture in dysphoric mixed mania: Findings from a French national study (EPIMAN). *J Affect Disord*, 50, 175–186.

Akiskal, H.S., Placidi, G.F., Maremmani, I., Signoretta, S., Liguori, A., Gervasi, R., Mallya, G., and Puzantian, V.R. (1998b). TEMPS-I: Delineating the most discriminant traits of the cyclothymic, depressive, hyperthymic and irritable temperaments in a nonpatient population. *J Affect Disord*, 51, 7–19.

Akiskal, H.S., Bourgeois, M.L., Angst, J., Post, R., Moller, H.J., and Hirschfeld, R.M.A. (2000). Re-evaluating the prevalence of and diagnostic composition within the broad clinical spectrum of bipolar disorders. *J Affect Disord*, 59(Suppl 1), 5s–30s.

Akiskal, H.S., Hantouche, E.G., Bourgeois, M.L., Azorin, J.M., Sechter, D., Allilair, J.F., Chatenet-Duchene, L., and Lancrenon, S. (2001). Toward a refined phenomenology of DSM-IV mania: Combining clinician-assessment and self-report in the French EPIMAN study. *J Affect Disord*, 67, 89–96.

Akiskal, H.S., Azorin, J.F., and Hantouche, E.G. (2003a). A proposed multidimensional structure of mania: Beyond the euphoric–dysphoric dichotomy. *J Affect Disord*, 73, 7–18.

Akiskal, H.S., Hantouche, E.G., Alliliaire, J.F., Sechter, D., Bourgeois, M.L., Azorin, J.M., Chatenet-Duchene, L., and Lancrenon, S. (2003b). Validating antidepressant-associated hypomania (bipolar III): A systematic comparison with spontaneous hypomania (bipolar II). *J Affect Disord*, 73, 65–74.

Allison, J.B., and Wilson, W.P. (1960). Sexual behaviors of manic patients: A preliminary report. *South Med J*, 53, 870–874.

Andreasen, N.C. (1979a). Thought, language, and communication disorders: I. Clinical assessment, definition of terms, and evaluation of their reliability. *Arch Gen Psychiatry*, 36, 1315–1321.

Andreasen, N.C. (1979b). Thought, language, and communication disorders: II. Diagnostic significance. *Arch Gen Psychiatry*, 36, 1325–1330.

Andreasen, N.C. (1984). *The clinical significance of "thought disorder."* Hibbs Award Lecture, 137th Annual Meeting of the American Psychiatric Association, May.

Andreasen, N.C., and Pfohl, B. (1976). Linguistic analysis of speech in affective disorders. *Arch Gen Psychiatry*, 33, 1361–1367.

Andreasen, N.C., and Powers, P.S. (1975). Creativity and psychosis: An examination of conceptual style. *Arch Gen Psychiatry*, 32, 70–73.

Aretaeus. (1856). *The Extant Works of Aretaeus, the Cappadocian.* London: Sydenham Society.

Aronson, T.A., Shukla, S., Hoff, A., and Cook, B. (1988). Proposed delusional depression subtypes: Preliminary evidence from a retrospective study of phenomenology and treatment course. *J Affect Disord*, 14, 69–74.

Astrup, C., Fossum, A., and Holmboe, R. (1959). A follow–up study of 270 patients with acute affective psychoses. *Acta Psychiatr Neurol Scand*, 34(Suppl 135), 11–65.

Azorin, J.M. (2000) Acute phase of schizophrenia: Impact of atypical antipsychotics. *Int Clin Psychopharmacol*, 15, S5–S9.

Baethge, C., Baldessarini, R.J., Freudenthal, K., Streetuwitz, A., Bauer, M., and Bschor, T. (2005). Hallucinations in bipolar disorder: Characteristics and comparison to unipolar depression and schizophrenia. *Bipolar Disord*, 7, 136–145.

Bauer, M.S., Whybrow, P.C., Gyulai, L., Gonnel, J., and Yeh, H.S. (1994). Testing definitions of dysphoric mania and hypomania: Prevalence, clinical characteristics and inter-episode stability. *J Affect Disord*, 32, 201–211.

Bauer, M.S., Simon, G.E., Ludman, E., and Unützer, J. (2005). 'Bipolarity' in bipolar disorder: Distribution of manic and depressive symptoms in a treated population. *Br J Psychiatry*, 187, 87–88.

Beck, A.T. (1967). *Depression: Causes and Treatment.* Philadelphia: University of Pennsylvania Press.

Beigel, A., and Murphy, D.L. (1971a). Assessing clinical characteristics of the manic state. *Am J Psychiatry*, 128, 688–694.

Beigel, A., and Murphy, D.L. (1971b). Unipolar and bipolar affective illness: Differences in clinical characteristics accompanying depression. *Arch Gen Psychiatry*, 24, 215–220.

Beigel, A., Murphy, D.L., and Bunney, W.E. (1971). The manic–state rating scale: Scale construction, reliability, and validity. *Arch Gen Psychiatry*, 25, 256–262.

Bell, L. (1849). On a form of disease resembling some advanced stages of mania and fever, but so contradistinguished from any ordinarily observed or described combination of symptoms as to render it probable that it may be an overlooked and hitherto unrecorded malady. *Am J Insanity*, 6, 97–127.

Benazzi, F. (2000a). Depression with DSM-IV atypical features: A marker for bipolar II disorder. *Eur Arch Psychiatry Clin Neurosci*, 250, 53–55.

Benazzi, F. (2000b). Depressive mixed states: Unipolar and bipolar II. *Eur Arch Psychiatry Clin Neurosci*, 250, 249–253.

Benazzi, F. (2001). Is 4 days the minimum duration of hypomania in bipolar II disorder? *Eur Arch Psychiatry Clin Neurosci*, 251, 32–34.

Benazzi F. (2003). Depression with racing thoughts. *Psychiatry Res*, 15, 273–282.

Benazzi F. (2004). Is depressive mixed state a transition between depression and hypomania? *Eur Arch Psychiatry Clin Neurosci*, 254, 69–75.

Benazzi, F. (2005). A. Marneros, and F. Goodwin (Eds.), *Bipolar Disorders: Mixed States, Rapid Cycling and Atypical Forms*. New York: Cambridge University Press.

Benazzi, F. (2006). Symptoms of depression as possible markers for bipolar II disorder. *Prog Neuropsychopharmacol Biol Psychiatry*, 30, 471–477.

Benazzi, F. (2007). Is overactivity the core feature of hypomania in bipolar II disorder? *Psychopathology*, 40, 54–60.

Benazzi, F., and Akiskal, H.S. (2001). Delineating bipolar II mixed states in the Ravenna–San Diego collaborative study: The relative prevalence and diagnostic significance of hypomanic features during major depressive episodes. *J Affect Disord*, 67, 115–122.

Benazzi, F., and Akiskal, H.S. (2003). Refining the evaluation of bipolar II: Beyond the strict SCID-CV guidelines for hypomania. *J Affect Disord*, 73, 33–38.

Benazzi, F., and Akiskal, H.S. (2005). Irritable-hostile depression: Further validation as a bipolar depressive mixed state. *J Affect Dis*, 84, 197–207.

Berlioz, H.L. (1966). *Memoirs of Hector Berlioz from 1803 to 1865*. Paris: Michel Lévy Bros, Annotated and translated by E. Newman. New York: Dover.

Berlioz, H.L. (1969). *Memoirs*. Translated by D. Cairns. London: Granada.

Berner, P., Gabriel, E., Katsching, H., Kieffer, W., Koehler, K., Lenz, G., Nutzinger, D., Schanda, H., and Simhandl, C. (1992). *Diagnostic Criteria for Functional Psychoses* (2nd Edition). Cambridge, England: Cambridge University Press.

Biondi, M., Picardi, A., Pasquini, M., Gaetano, P., and Pancheri, P. (2005). Dimensional psychopathology of depression: Detection of an 'activation' dimension in unipolar depressed outpatients. *J Affect Disord*, 84, 133–139.

Black, D.W., and Nasrallah, A. (1989). Hallucinations and delusions in 1,715 patients with unipolar and bipolar affective disorders. *Psychopathology*, 22, 28–34.

Bleuler, E. (1924). *Textbook of Psychiatry* (4th German Edition). A.A. Brill (Ed.). New York: The Macmillan Co.

Bond, T.C. (1980). Recognition of acute delirious mania. *Arch Gen Psychiatry*, 37, 553–554.

Bowman, K.M., and Raymond, A.F. (1931–1932a). A statistical study of delusions in the manic–depressive psychoses. *Am J Psychiatry*, 88, 111–121.

Bowman, K.M., and Raymond, A.F. (1931–1932b). A statistical study of hallucinations in the manic–depressive psychoses. *Am J Psychiatry*, 88, 299–309.

Braden, W., and Ho, C.K. (1981). Racing thoughts in psychiatric inpatients. *Arch Gen Psychiatry*, 38, 71–75.

Braden, W., and Qualls, C.B. (1979). Racing thoughts in depressed patients. *J Clin Psychiatry*, 40, 336–339.

Braunig, P., Kruger, S., and Shugar, G. (1998). Prevalence and clinical significance of catatonic symptoms in mania. *Compr Psychiatry*, 39(1), 35–46.

Breakey, W.R., and Goodell, H. (1972). Thought disorder in mania and schizophrenia evaluated by Bannister's Grid Test for schizophrenic thought disorder. *Br J Psychiatry*, 120, 391–395.

Brieger, P. (2000). Comorbidity in bipolar disorder. In A. Marneros and J. Angst (Eds.), *Bipolar Disorders: 100 Years after Manic-Depressive Insanity*. Dordrecht: Kluwer Academic Publishers, pp. 215–229.

Brieger, P., Roettig, S., Ehrt, U., Wenzel, A., Bloink, R., and Marneros, A. (2003). TEMPS-A scale in 'mixed' and 'pure' manic episodes: New data and methodological considerations on the relevance of joint anxious–depressive temperament traits. *J Affect Disord*, 73(1-2), 99–104.

Brockington, I.F., Wainwright, S., and Kendell, R.E. (1980). Manic patients with schizophrenic or paranoid symptoms. *Psychol Med*, 10, 73–83.

Brockington, I.F., Hillier, V.F., Francis, A.F., Helzer, J.E., and Wainwright, S. (1983). Definitions of mania: Concordance and prediction of outcome. *Am J Psychiatry*, 140, 435–439.

Bunney, W.E. Jr., Murphy, D., Goodwin, F.K., and Borge, G.F. (1972a). The "switch process" in manic depressive illness: I. A systematic study of sequential behavior change. *Arch Gen Psychiatry*, 27, 295–302.

Bunney, W.E. Jr., Goodwin, F.K., Murphy, D.L., House, K.M., and Gordon, E.K. (1972b). The "switch process" in manic–depressive illness: II. Relationship to catecholamines, REM sleep, and drugs. *Arch Gen Psychiatry*, 27, 304–309.

Bunney, W.E. Jr., Goodwin, F.K., and Murphy, D.L. (1972c). The "switch process" in manic–depressive illness: III. Theoretical implications. *Arch Gen Psychiatry*, 27, 312–317.

Burns, R. (1985). *The Letters of Robert Burns* (Volume 2, 1790–1796). G.R. Roy (Ed.). Letter to Mrs. W. Riddell, December, 1793. Oxford, England: Oxford University Press.

Byron, G.G. (1819, August 23). Letter to John Cam Hobhouse. In *Byron's Letters and Journals* (p. 214), Vol. 6. L. Marchand (Ed.). London: John Murray.

Calev, A., Nigal, D., and Chazan, S. (1989). Retrieval from semantic memory using meaningful and meaningless constructs by depressed, stable bipolar and manic patients. *Br J Clin Psychol*, 28, 67–73.

Campbell, J.D. (1953). *Manic–Depressive Disease: Clinical and Psychiatric Significance*. Philadelphia: Lippincott.

Carlson, G.A., and Goodwin, F.K. (1973). The stages of mania: A longitudinal analysis of the manic episode. *Arch Gen Psychiatry*, 28, 221–228.

Carlson, G., and Strober, M. (1979). Affective disorders in adolescence. *Psychiatr Clin North Am*, 2, 511–526.

Carpenter, W.T., Strauss, J.S., and Mulch, S. (1973). Are there pathognomonic symptoms in schizophrenia? An empiric investigation of Schneider's first rank symptoms. *Arch Gen Psychiatry*, 28, 847–852.

Casper, R.C., Redmond, E. Jr., Katz, M.M., Schaffer, C.B., Davis, J.M., and Koslow, S.H. (1985). Somatic symptoms in primary affective disorder: Presence and relationship to the classification of depression. *Arch Gen Psychiatry*, 42, 1098–1104.

Cassidy, F., and Carroll, B.J. (2002). Hypocholesterolemia during mixed manic episodes. *Eur Arch Psychiatry Clin Neurosci*, 252, 110–114.

Cassidy, F., Murry, E., Forest, K., and Carroll, B.J. (1998). Signs and symptoms of mania in pure and mixed episodes. *J Affect Disord*, 50, 187–201.

Cassidy, F., McEvoy, J.P., Yang, Y.K., and Wilson, W.H. (2001a). Insight is greater in mixed than in pure manic episodes of bipolar I disorder. *J Nerv Ment Dis*, 180, 398–399.

Cassidy, F., Ahearn, E., and Carroll, B.J. (2001b). A prospective study of inter-episode consistency of manic and mixed subtypes of bipolar disorder. *J Affect Disord*, 67, 181–185.

Cassidy, F., Ahearn, E.P., and Carrol, B.J. (2001c). Substance abuse in bipolar disorder. *Bipolar Disord*, 3, 181–188.

Cassidy, F., Ahearn, E.P., and Carroll, B.J. (2002). Symptom profile consistency in recurrent manic episodes. *Compr Psychiatr*, 43(3), 179–181.

Charney, D.S., and Nelson, J.C. (1981). Delusional and nondelusional unipolar depression: Further evidence for distinct subtypes. *Am J Psychiatry*, 138, 328–333.

Chiaroni, P., Hantouche, E.G., Gouvernet, J., Azorin, J.M., and Akiskal, H.S. (2005). The cyclothymic temperament in healthy controls and familially at risk individuals for mood disorder: Endophenotype for genetic studies? *J Affect Dis*, 85, 135–145.

Clayton, P., Pitts, F.N. Jr., and Winokur, G. (1965). Affective disorder: IV. Mania. *Compr Psychiatry*, 6, 313–322.

Cloninger, C.R. (1987). *The tridimensional personality questionnaire* (Version IV). St. Louis: Washington University School of Medicine.

Coate, M. (1964). *Beyond All Reason*. London: Constable & Co.

Coryell, W., and Tsuang, M.T. (1982). Primary unipolar depression and the prognostic importance of delusions. *Arch Gen Psychiatry*, 39, 1181–1184.

Coryell, W., Keller, M., Lavori, P., Endicott, J. (1990). Affective syndromes, psychotic features, and prognosis. II. Mania. *Arch Gen Psychiatry*, 47, 658–662.

Coryell, W., Leon, A.C., Turvey, C., Akiskal, H.S., Mueller, T., and Endicott, J. (2001). The significance of psychotic features in manic episodes: A report from the NIMH collaborative study. *J Affect Disord*, 67, 79–88.

Custance, J. (1952). *Wisdom, Madness, and Folly: The Philosophy of a Lunatic*. New York: Farrar, Straus & Cudahy.

Deckersbach, T., Perlis, R.H., Frankle, W.G., Gray, S.M., Grandin, L., Dougherty, D.D., Nierenberg, A.A., and Sachs, G.S. (2004). Presence of irritability during depressive episodes in bipolar disorder. *CNS Spectr*, 9, 227–231.

Dell'Osso, L., Nassi, R., Freer, P., Placidi, G.F., Cassano, G.B., and Akiskal, H.S. (1991). The manic-depressive mixed state: Familial, temperamental and psychopathologic characteristics in 108 female inpatients. *Eur Arch Psychiatry Clin Neurosci*, 240, 234–239.

Dell'Osso, L., Pini, S., Tundo, A., Sarno, N., Musetti, L., and Cassano, G.B. (2000). Clinical characteristics of mania, mixed mania, and bipolar depression with psychotic features. Compr Psychiatry, 41, 242–247.

Depue, R.A., Slater, J.F., Wolfstetter–Kausch, H., Klein, D., Goplerud, E., and Farr, D. (1981). A behavioral paradigm for identifying persons at risk for bipolar depressive disorder: A conceptual framework and five validation studies. *J Abnorm Psychol Monograph*, 90, 381–437.

Dewhurst, K. (1962). A seventeenth–century symposium on manic–depressive psychosis. *Br J Med Psychol*, 35, 113–125.

Dilsaver, S.C., Chen, R., Shoaib, A.M., and Swann, A.C. (1999). Phenomenology of mania: Evidence for distinct depressed, dysphoric, and euphoric presentations. *Am J Psychiatry*, 156, 426–430.

Dilsaver, S.C., Benazzi, F., Rihmer, Z., Akiskal, K.K., and Akiskal, H.S. (2005). Gender, suicidality and bipolar mixed states in adolescents. *J Affect Disord*, 87, 11–16.

Docherty, N.M., DeRosa, M., and Andreasen, N.C. (1996). Communication disturbances in schizophrenia and mania. *Arch Gen Psychiatry*, 53, 358–364.

Double. D. B. (1990). The factor structure of manic rating scales. *J Affect Disord*, 18, 113–119.

Double, D.B. (1991). A cluster analysis of manic states. *Compr Psychiatry*, 32, 187–194.

Endicott, J., Nee, J., Coryell, W., Keller, M., Andreasen, N., and Croughan, J. (1986). Schizoaffective, psychotic, and non–psychotic depression: Differential familial association. *Compr Psychiatry*, 27, 1–13.

Esquirol, J.E.D. (1838). *Des maladies mentales*. Paris: Balliére. Translated by E.K. Hunt as *Mental Maladies: A Treatise on Insanity*. Philadelphia: Lea and Blachard, 1845 (facsimile edition London, England: Hafner, 1966).

Falret, J.P. (1854). Mémoire sur la folie circulaire, forme de maladie mentale caractérisée par la reproduction successive et régulière de l' état maniaque, de l' état mélancolique, e d'un intervalle lucide plus ou moins prolongé. *Bulletin de l'Académie de Médecine*, 19, 382–415.

Fava, M., and Rosenbaum, J.F. (1999). Anger attacks in patients with depression. *J Clin Psychiatry*, 60(Suppl 15), 21–24.

Fennig, S., Bromet, E.J., Karant, M.T., Ram, R., and Jandorf, L. (1996). Mood-congruent versus mood-incongruent psychotic symptoms in first-admission patients with affective disorder. *J Affect Disord*, 37, 23–29.

Fink, M. (1999). Delirious mania. *Bipolar Disord*, 1, 54–60.

Fitzgerald, F.S. (1956). *The Crack–Up*. New York: New Directions (essays first published in 1936).

Fox, N.A., Henderson, H.A., Rubin, K.H., Calkins, S.D., and Schmidt, L.A. (2001). Continuity and discontinuity of behavioral inhibition and exuberance: Psychophysiological and behavioral influences across the first four years of life. *Child Dev*, 72, 1–21.

Frances, A., Brown, R.P., Kocsis, J.H., and Mann, J.J. (1981). Psychotic depression: A separate entity? *Am J Psychiatry*, 138, 831–833.

Francis, A., Divadeenam, K.M., Bush, G., and Petrides, G. (1997). Consistency of symptoms in recurrent catatonia. *Compr Psychiatry*, 38, 56–60.

Frangos, E., Athanassenas, G., Tsitourides, S., Psilolignos, P., and Katsanou, N. (1983). Psychotic depressive disorder: A separate entity? *J Affect Disord*, 5, 259–265.

Fraser, W.I., King, K.M., Thomas, P., and Kendell, R.E. (1986). The diagnosis of schizophrenia by language analysis. *Br J Psychiatry*, 148, 275–278.

Garety, P. (1985). Delusions: Problems in definition and measurement. *Br J Med Psychol*, 58, 25–34.

Garner, A. (1997). *The Voice that Thunders: Essays and Lectures*. London: Harvill Press.

Ghaemi, S.N., Stoll, A.L., and Pope, H.G. (1995). Lack of insight in bipolar disorder: The acute manic episode. *J Nerv Ment Dis*, 183, 464–467.

Glassman, A.H., and Roose, S.P. (1981). Delusional depression: A distinct clinical entity? *Arch Gen Psychiatry*, 38, 424–427.

Goes, F.S., Sadler, B., Toolan, J., Zamoiski, R.D., Mondimore, F.M., MacKinnon, D.F., Schweizer, B., Bipolar Disorder Phenome Group, DePaulo, J.R., and Potash, J.B. (in press). Psychotic features in bipolar and unipolar depression. *J Bipolar Disord*.

Goldberg, J.F., Harrow, M., and Grossman, L.S. (1995). Recurrent affective syndromes in bipolar and unipolar mood disorders at follow-up. *Br J Psychiatry*, 166, 382–385.

Goldberg, J.F., Garno, J.L., Leon, A.C., Kocsis, J.H., and Portera, L. (1999). A history of substance abuse complicates remission from acute mania in bipolar disorder. *J Clin Psychiatry, 60,* 733–740.

González-Pinto, A., Ballesteros, J., Aldama, A., Pérez de Heredia, J.L., Gutierrez, M., Mosquera, F., and González-Pinto, A. (2003). Principal components of mania. *J Affect Disord, 76,* 95–102.

Goodwin, F.K., Murphy, D.L., and Bunney, W.F. Jr. (1969). Lithium carbonate treatment in depression and mania: A longitudinal double-blind study. *Arch Gen Psychiatry, 21,* 486–496.

Goodwin, D.W., Alderson, P., and Rosenthal, R. (1971) Clinical significance of hallucinations in psychiatric disorders: A study of 116 hallucinatory patients. *Arch. Gen. Psychiatry, 24,* 76–80.

Griesinger, W. (1845). *Pathologie und Therapie der psychischen Krankheiten.* Stuttgart: Adolf Krabbe Verlag.

Griesinger, W. (1867). *Mental Pathology and Therapeutics.* Translated by C.L. Robertson and J. Rutherford. London: New Sydenham Society.

Grossman, L.S., Harrow, M., Lazar, B., Kettering, R., Meltzer, H.Y., and Lechert, J. (1981). *Do thought disorders persist in manic patients?* Abstract of paper presented at the 134th Annual Meeting of the American Psychiatric Association, May.

Grossman, L.S., Harrow, M., and Sands, J.R. (1986). Features associated with thought disorder in manic patients at 2–4 year follow–up. *Am J Psychiatry, 143,* 306–311.

Grunebaum, M.F., Oquendo, M.A., Harkavy-Friedman, J.M., Ellis, S.P., Li, S., and Haas, G.L. (2001). Delusions and suicidality. *Am J Psychiatry, 158,* 743–747.

Guze, S.B., Woodruff, R.A. Jr., and Clayton, P.J. (1975). The significance of psychotic affective disorders. *Arch Gen Psychiatry, 32,* 1147–1150.

Hantouche, E.G., Akiskal, H.S., Lancrenon, S., Allilaire, J.F., Sechter, D., Azorin, J.M., Bourgeois, M., Fraud, J.P., and Châtenet-Duchêne, L. (1998). Systematic clinical methodology for validating bipolar-II disorder: Data in mid-stream from a French national multisite study (EPIDEP). *J Affect Disord, 50,* 63–173.

Hantouche, E.G., Angst, J., and Akiskal, H.S. (2003). Factor structure of hypomania: Interrelationships with cyclothymia and the soft bipolar spectrum. *J Affect Disord, 73,* 39–47.

Hare, E. (1981). The two manias: A study of the evolution of the modern concept of mania. *Br J Psychiatry, 138,* 89–99.

Harrow, M., and Prosen, M. (1978). Intermingling and disordered logic as influences on schizophrenic thought disorders. *Arch Gen Psychiatry, 35,* 1213–1218.

Harrow, M., and Quinlan, D. (1977). Is disordered thinking unique to schizophrenia? *Arch Gen Psychiatry, 34,* 15–21.

Harrow, M., Himmelhoch, J., Tucker, G., Hersh, J., and Quinlan, D. (1972a). Overinclusive thinking in acute schizophrenic patients. *J Abnorm Psychol, 79,* 161–168.

Harrow, M., Tucker, G.J., and Adler, D. (1972b). Concrete and idiosyncratic thinking in acute schizophrenic patients. *Arch Gen Psychiatry, 26,* 433–439.

Harrow, M., Grossman, L.S., Silverstein, M.L., and Meltzer, H.Y. (1982). Thought pathology in manic and schizophrenic patients: Its occurrence at hospital admission and seven weeks later. *Arch Gen Psychiatry, 39,* 665–671.

Harrow, M., Lanin-Kettering, I., Prosen, M., and Miller, J.G. (1983). Disordered thinking in schizophrenia: Intermingling and loss of set. *Schizophr Bull, 9,* 354–367.

Harrow, M., Grossman, L.S., Silverstein, M.L., Meltzer, H.Y., and Kettering, R.L. (1986). A longitudinal study of thought disorder in manic patients. *Arch Gen Psychiatry, 43,* 781–785.

Harrow, M., Goldberg, J.F., Grossman, L.S., and Meltzer, H.Y. (1990). Outcome in manic disorders: A naturalistic follow–up study. *Arch Gen Psychiatry, 47,* 665–671.

Harvey, P.D. (1983). Speech competence in manic and schizophrenic psychoses: The association between clinically rated thought disorder and cohesion and reference performance. *J Abnorm Psychol, 92,* 368–377.

Hawton, K., Sutton, L., Haw, C., Sinclair, J., and Harris, L. (2005). Suicide and attempted suicide in bipolar disorder: A systematic review of risk factors. *J Clin Psychiatry, 66,* 693–704.

Heckers, S. (2002). How many bipolar mixed states are there? *Harvard Rev Psychiatry, 10,* 276–279.

Heinroth, J.C.A. (1818). *Lehrbuch der Stoerungen des Seelenlebens.* Leipzig: Vogel.

Helms, P.M., and Smith, R.E. (1983). Recurrent psychotic depression: Evidence of diagnostic stability. *J Affect Disord, 5,* 51–54.

Henderson, D., and Gillespie, R.D. (1956). *A Text–book of Psychiatry for Students and Practitioners* (8th Edition). London: Oxford University Press.

Himmelhoch, J.M. (1979). Mixed states, manic-depressive illness, and the nature of mood. *Psychiatr Clin North Am, 2,* 449–459.

Himmelhoch, J.M., Harrow, M., Hersh, J., and Tucker, G.J. (1973). *Manual for Assessment of Selected Aspects of Thinking: Object Sorting Test.* ASIS/NAPS #02206, New York: Microfiche Publications.

Himmelhoch, J.M., Mulla, D., Neil, J.F., Detre, T.P., and Kupfer, D.J. (1976a). Incidence and significance of mixed affective states in a bipolar population. *Arch Gen Psychiatry, 33,* 1062–1066.

Himmelhoch, J.M., Coble, P., Kupfer, D.J., and Ingenito, J. (1976b). Agitated psychotic depression associated with severe hypomanic episodes: A rare syndrome. *Am J Psychiatry, 133,* 765–771.

Hoffman, R.E., Stopek, S., and Andreasen, N.C. (1986). A comparative study of manic vs schizophrenic speech disorganization. *Arch Gen Psychiatry, 43,* 831–835.

Holzman, P.S., Solovay, M.R., and Shenton, M.E. (1985). Thought disorder specificity in functional psychoses. In M. Alpert (Ed.), *Controversies in Schizophrenia: Changes and Constancies* (pp. 228–252). New York: Guilford Press.

Ianzito, B.M., Cadoret, R.J., and Pugh, D.D. (1974). Thought disorder in depression. *Am J Psychiatry, 131,* 703–707.

James, W. (1902). *The Varieties of Religious Experience: A Study in Human Nature.* Middlesex, England: Penguin.

Jamison, K.R. (1993). *Touched with Fire: Manic-Depressive Illness and the Artistic Temperament.* New York: Free Press.

Jamison, K.R. (1995). *An Unquiet Mind: A Memoir of Moods and Madness.* New York: Alfred A. Knopf.

Jamison, K.R. (2004). *Exuberance: The Passion for Life.* New York: Alfred A. Knopf.

Jamison, K.R., Gerner, R.H., Hammen, C., and Padesky, C. (1980). Clouds and silver linings: Positive experiences associated with primary affective disorders. *Am J Psychiatry, 137,* 198–202.

Jampala, V.C., Taylor, M.A., and Abrams, R. (1989). The diagnostic implications of formal thought disorder in mania and schizophrenia: A reassessment. *Am J Psychiatry, 146,* 459–463.

Jaspers, K. (1913). *General Psychopathology.* Translated by J. Hoenig and M.W. Hamilton. Chicago: University of Chicago Press.

Jaspers, K. (1997). *General Psychopathology*. Translated by J. Hoenig and M.W. Hamilton. Chicago: University of Chicago Press, 1968. Republished by Johns Hopkins University Press, 1997.

Jelliffe, S.E. (1931). Some historical phases of the manic–depressive synthesis. *Research Publications Association for Research in Nervous and Mental Diseases*, 11, 3–47.

Johnston, M.H., and Holzman, P.S. (1979). *Assessing Schizophrenic Thinking*. San Francisco: Josey–Bass.

Juruena, M.F., Weingarthner, N., Marquardt, A.R., Fleig, S.S., Machado Viera, R., Busnello, E.A., and Broilo, L. (submitted). Bipolar II vs. bipolar I: More differences than previously thought.

Kagan, J. (1989). Temperamental contributions to social behavior. *Am Psychologist*, 44, 688–674.

Kagan, D.L., and Oltmanns, T.F. (1981). Matched tasks for measuring single–word, referent communication: The performance of patients with schizophrenic and affective disorders. *J Abnorm Psychol*, 90, 204–212.

Kagan, J., and Snidman, N. (1991). Infant predictors of inhibited and uninhibited profiles. *Psychol Sci*, 2, 40–44.

Kagan, J., Resnick, J.S., and Snidman, N. (1988). Biological basis of childhood shyness. *Science*, 240, 167–171.

Kagan, J., Snidman, N., and Arcus, D.M. (1992). Initial reactions to unfamiliarity. *Current Directions in Psychological Science*, 1, 171–174.

Kawa, I., Carter, J.D., Joyce, P.R., Doughty, C.J., Frampton, C.M., Wells, J.E., Walsh, A.E.S., and Olds, R.J. (2005). Gender differences in bipolar disorder: Age of onset, course, comorbidity, and symptom presentation. *Bipolar Disord*, 7, 119–125.

Keck, P.E., McElroy, S.L., Havens, J.R., Altshuler, L., Nolen, W.A., Frye, M.A., Suppes, T., Denicoff, K.D., Kupka, R., Leverich, G.S., Rush, J.A., and Post, R.M. (2003). Psychosis in bipolar disorder: Phenomenology and impact on morbidity and course of illness. *Compr Psychiatry*, 44, 263–269.

Kochman, F.J., Hantouche, E.G., Ferrari, P., Lancrenon, S., Bayart, D., and Akiskal, H.S. (2005). Cyclothymic temperament as a prospective predictor of bipolarity and suicidality in children and adolescents with major depressive disorder. *J Affect Disord*, 85, 181–189.

Kotin, J., and Goodwin, F.K. (1972). Depression during mania: Clinical observations and theoretical implications. *Am J Psychiatry*, 129, 679–686.

Koukopoulos, A. (2003). Ewald Hecker's description of cyclothymia as a cyclical mood disorder: Its relevance to the modern concept of bipolar II. *J Affect Disord*, 73, 199–205.

Koukopoulos, A. (2005). The primacy of mania. In H. Akiskal and M. Tohen (Eds.), *Bipolar Psychopharmacotherapy: Caring for the Patient*. New York: John Wiley.

Koukopoulos, A., and Koukopoulos, A. (1999). Agitated depression as a mixed state and the problem of melancholia. In: H.S. Akiskal (Ed.), *Bipolarity: Beyond Classic Mania. Psychiatr Clin North Am*, 22, 547–564.

Koukopoulos, A., Faedda, G., Proietti, R., D'Amico, S., De Pisa, E., and Simonetto, C. (1992). A mixed depressive syndrome. *Encéphale*, 18, 19–21.

Kraepelin, E. (1921). *Manic-Depressive Insanity and Paranoia*. Edinburgh: E & S Livingstone.

Kretschmer, E. (1936). *Physique and Character*. New York: Macmillan.

Krüger, S., Cooke, R.G., Spegg, C.C., and Bräunig, P. (2003). Relevance of the catatonic syndrome to the mixed manic episode. *J Affect Disord*, 74, 279–285.

Lange, J. (1922). *Katatonische Erscheinungen im Rahmen manischer Erkrankungen* Berlin: Julius Springer.

Leff, J.P., Fischer, M., and Bertelsen, A.C. (1976). A cross–national epidemiological study of mania. *Br J Psychiatry*, 129, 428–442.

Lerner, Y. (1980). The subjective experience of mania. In R.H. Belmaker and H.M. Van Praag (Eds.), *Mania: An Evolving Concept* (pp. 77–88). New York: Spectrum Publications.

Lewis, A.J. (1934). Melancholia: A clinical survey of depressive states. *J Ment Sci*, 80, 277–378.

Lott, P.R., Guggenbühl, S., Schneeberer, A., Pulver, A.E., and Stassen, H.H. (2002). Linguistic analysis of the speech output of schizophrenic, bipolar, and depressive patients. *Psychopathology*, 35, 220–227.

Loudon, J.B., Blackburn, I.M., and Ashworth, C.M. (1977). A study of the symptomatology and course of manic illness using a new scale. *Psychol Med*, 7, 723–729.

Lowe, G.R. (1973). The phenomenology of hallucinations as an aid to differential diagnosis. *Br J Psychiatry*, 123, 621–633.

Lundquist, G. (1945). Prognosis and course in manic–depressive psychoses: A follow–up study of 319 first admissions. *Acta Psychiatr Neurol*, (Suppl 35), 1–96.

Lykouras, E., Christodoulou, G.N., and Malliaras D. (1985). Type and content of delusions in unipolar psychotic depression. *J Affect Disord*, 9, 249–252.

Mammen, O.K., Pilkonis, P.A., Chengappa, K.N.R., and Kupfer, D.J. (2004). Anger attacks in bipolar depression: Predictors and response to citalopram added to mood stabilizers. *J Clin Psychiatry*, 65, 627–633.

Mann, S.C., Caroff, S.N., Bleier, H.R., Welz, W.K., Kling, M.A., and Hayashida, M. (1986). Lethal catatonia. *Am J Psychiatry*, 143, 1374–1381.

Mantere, O., Suominen, K., Leppämäki, S., Valtonen, H., Arvilommi, P., and Isometsä, E. (2004). The clinical characteristics of DSM-IV bipolar I and II disorders: Baseline findings from the Jorvi Bipolar Study (JoBS). *Bipolar Disord*, 6(5), 395–405.

Mantere, O., Suominen, K., Avrilommi, P., Valtonen, H., Leppämäki, S., and Isometsä, E. (2006). Clinical predictors of unrecognized bipolar I and II disorders. *J Affect Disord*, 91S, S42, S72, S73.

Maremmani, I., Akiskal, H.S., Signoretta, S., Liguori, A., Perugi, G., and Cloninger, R. (2005). The relationship of Kraepelinian affective temperaments (as measured by TEMPS-I) to the tridimensional personality questionnaire (TPQ). *J Affect Disord*, 85, 17–27.

Markov, V. (1975). *The Longer Poems of Velimir Khlebnikov*. Westport, CT: Greenwood Press.

Marneros, A. (2001). Expanding the group of bipolar disorders. *J Affect Disord*, 62, 39–44.

Marneros, A., and Angst, J. (Eds.). (2000). *Bipolar Disorders: 100 Years after Manic-Depressive Insanity*. London: Kluwer Academic Publishers.

Marneros, A., and Goodwin, F. (Eds). (2003). *Mixed States, Rapid Cycling and Atypical Bipolar Disorders*. London: Cambridge University Press.

Marneros, A., Deister, A., and Rohde, A. (1991a). *Affektive, schizoaffective und schizofrene Psychosen. Eine vergleichende Langzeitstudie*. Berlin: Springer-Verlag.

Marneros, A., Röttig, S., Wenzel, A., Blöink, R., and Brieger, P. (2004). Affective and schizoaffective mixed states. *Eur Arch Psychiatry Clin Neurosci*, 254, 76–81.

Mayer-Gross, W., Slater, E., and Roth, M. (1960). *Clinical Psychiatry* (2nd Edition). London: Cassell & Co.

McElroy, S.L., Keck, P.E., Pope, H.G., Hudson, J.I., Faedda, G.L., and Swann, A.C. (1992). Clinical and research implications of the diagnosis of dysphoric or mixed mania or hypomania. *Am J Psychiatry*, 149, 1633–1644.

McElroy, S.L., Strakowski, S.M., Keck, P.E., Tugrul, K.L., West, S.A., and Lonczak, H.S. (1995). Differences and similarities in mixed and pure mania. *Compr Psychiatry*, 36, 184–194.

McElroy, S.L., Strakowski, S.M., West, S.A., Keck, P.E., and McConville, B.S. (1997). Phenomenology of adolescent and adult mania in hospitalized patients with bipolar disorder. *Am J Psychiatry*,154, 44–49.

Miklowitz, D. (1992). Longitudinal outcome and medication noncompliance among manic patients with and without mood-incongruent features. *J Nerv Ment Dis*, 180, 703–711.

Mitchell, P.B., Wilhelm, K., Parker, G., Austin, M.P., Rutgers, P., and Malhi, G.S. (2001). The clinical features of bipolar depression: a comparison with matched major depressive disorder patients. *J Clin Psychiatry*, 62(3), 212–216.

Morice, R.D., and Ingram, J.C. (1983). Language complexity and age of onset of schizophrenia. *Psychol Res*, 9, 233–242.

Morice, R.D., and McNicol, D. (1986). Language changes in schizophrenia: A limited replication. *Schizophr Bull*, 12, 239–251.

Murphy, D.L., and Beigel, A. (1974). Depression, elation, and lithium carbonate responses in manic patient subgroups. *Arch Gen Psychiatry*, 31, 643–648.

Nelson, W.H., Khan, A., and Orr, W.W. (1984). Delusional depression: Phenomenology, neuroendocrine function, and tricyclic antidepressant response. *J Affect Disord*, 6, 297–306.

Niecks, F. (1925). *Robert Schumann: A Supplementary and Corrective Biography*. London: JM Dent & Sons.

Nunn, C.M.H. (1979). Mixed affective states and the natural history of manic-depressive psychosis. *Br J Psychiatry*, 134, 153–160.

Orvaschel, H., Thompson, W.D., Belanger, A., Prusoff, B.A., and Kidd, K.K. (1982). Comparison of the family history method to direct interview: Factors affecting the diagnosis of depression. *J Affect Disord*, 4, 45–59.

Othmer, E., DeSouza, C.M., Penick, E.C., Nickel, E.J., Hunter, E.E., Othmer, S.C., Gabrielli, W.F., Read, M.F., Krambeer, L.L., and Powell, B.J. (in press). Psychotic features in major depressive disorder are associated with mania.

Pease, E. (1912). A note on the prognostic value of hallucinations in the manic-depressive psychosis. *Am J Insanity*, 69, 1–36.

Perlis, R.H., Smoller, J.W., Fava, M., Rosenbaum, J.F., Nierenberg, A.A., and Sachs, G.S. (2004). The prevalence and clinical correlates of anger attacks during depressive episodes in bipolar disorder. *J Affect Disord*, 79, 291–295.

Perugi, G., and Akiskal, H.S. (2002). The soft bipolar spectrum redefined: Focus on the anxious-senstitive, impulse-dyscontrol and binge-eating connection in bipolar II and related conditions. *Psychiatr Clin North Am*, 25, 713–737.

Perugi, G., Akiskal, H.S., Micheli, C., Musetti, L., Paiano, A., Quilici, C., Rossi, L., and Cassano, G.B. (1997). Clinical subtypes of bipolar mixed states: Validating a broader European definition in 143 cases. *J Affect Disord*, 43, 169–180.

Perugi, G., Akiskal, H.S., Lattanzi, L., Cecconi, D., Mastrocinque, C., Patronelli, A., and Vignoli, S. (1998a). The high prevalence of soft bipolar (II) features in atypical depression. *Compr Psychiatry*, 39, 63–71.

Perugi, G., Akiskal, H.S., Rossi, L., Paiano, A., Quilici, C., Madaro, D., Musetti, L., and Cassano, G.B. (1998b). Chronic mania: Family history, prior course, clinical picture and social consequences. *Br J Psychiatry*, 173, 514–518.

Perugi, G., Akiskal, H.S., Ramacciotti, S., Nassini, S., Toni, C., Milanfranchi, A., and Musetti, L. (1999). Depressive comorbidity of panic, social phobic and obsessive-compulsive disorders: Is there a bipolar II connection? *J Psychiatr Res*, 33, 53–61.

Perugi, G., Micheli, C., Akiskal, H.S., Modaro, D., Socci, C., Quilci, C., and Musetti, L. (2000). Polarity and course of manic-depressive illness: A retrospective analysis of 320 bipolar I patients. *Compr Psychiatry*, 41, 13–18.

Perugi, G., Akiskal, H.S., Micheli, C., Toni, C., and Madaro, D. (2001a). Clinical characterization of depressive mixed state in bipolar-I patients: Pisa–San Diego collaboration. *J Affect Disord*, 67, 105–114.

Perugi, G., Maremmani, I., Toni, C., Madaro, D., Mata, B., and Akiskal, H.S. (2001b). The contrasting influence of depressive and hyperthymic temperaments on psychometrically derived manic subtypes. *Psychiatry Res*, 101, 249–258.

Pinel, P. (1801). *Traité médico–philosophique sur l'aliénation mentale, ou La manie*. Paris: Brosson. Translated by D.D. Davis as *A Treatise on Insanity*. Sheffield, United Kingdom: Cadell and Davis (facsimile edition, New York: Hafner, 1962).

Placidi, G.F., Maremmani, I., Signoretta, S., Liguori, A., and Akiskal, H.S. (1998). The semi-structured affective temperament interview (TEMPS-I). Reliability and psychometric properties in 1010 14–26-year old students. *J Affect Disord*, 51, 199–208.

Plath, S. (1971). *The Bell Jar*. New York: Harper & Row, 1971.

Plath, S. (1982). *The Journals of Sylvia Plath*. T. Hughes and F. McCullough (Eds.). New York: Dial Press.

Pope, H.G. Jr., and Lipinski, J.S. Jr. (1978). Diagnosis in schizophrenia and manic–depressive illness: A reassessment of the specificity of "schizophrenic" symptoms in light of current research. *Arch Gen Psychiatry*, 35, 811–828.

Post, R.M., Rubinow, D.R., Uhde, T.W., Roy–Byrne, P.P., Linnoila, M., Rosoff, A., and Cowdry, R. (1989). Dysphoric mania: Clinical and biological correlates. *Arch Gen Psychiatry*, 46, 353–358.

Price, L.H., Nelson, J.C., Charney, D.S., and Quinlan, D.M. (1984). Family history in delusional depression. *J Affect Disord*, 6, 109–114.

Prien, R.F., Himmelhoch, J.M., and Kupfer, D.J. (1988). Treatment of mixed mania. *J Affect Disord*, 15, 9–15.

Ragin, A.B., and Oltmanns, T.F. (1983). Predictability as an index of impaired verbal communication in schizophrenic and affective disorders. *Br J Psychiatry*, 143, 578–583.

Ragin, A.B., and Oltmanns, T.F. (1987). Communicability and thought disorder in schizophrenics and other diagnostic groups. A follow–up study. *Br J Psychiatry*, 150, 494–500.

Rapaport, D., Gill, M.M., and Schafer, R. (1968). *Diagnostic Psychological Testing*. New York: International Universities Press.

Reiss, E. (1910). *Konstitutionelle Verstimmung und manisch–depressives Irresein: Klinische Untersuchungen über den Zusammenhang von Veranlagung und Psychose*. Berlin: J. Springer.

Rennie, T.A.C. (1942). Prognosis in manic-depressive psychoses. *Am J Psychiatry*, 98, 801–814.

Resnick, H.S., and Oltmanns, T.F. (1984). Hesitation patterns in the speech of thought-disordered schizophrenic and manic patients. *J Abnorm Psychol*, 93, 80–86.

Robertson, H.A., Lam, R.W., Stewart, J.N., Yatham, L.N., Tam, E.M., and Zis, A.P. (1996). Atypical depressive symptoms and clusters in unipolar and bipolar depression. *Acta Psychiatr Scand*, 94, 421–427.

Roccatagliata, G. (1986). *A History of Ancient Psychiatry*. New York: Greenwood Press.

Roose, S.P., and Glassman, A.H. (1988). Delusional depression. In A. Georgotas and R. Cancro (Eds.), *Depression and Mania* (pp. 76–85). New York: Elsevier.

Rosen, L.N., Rosenthal, N.E., Dunner, D.L., and Fieve, R.R. (1983a). Social outcome compared in psychotic and nonpsychotic bipolar I patients. *J Nerv Ment Dis*, 171, 272–275.

Rosen, L.N., Rosenthal, N.E., VanDusen, P.H., Dunner, D.L., and Fieve, R.R. (1983b). Age at onset and number of psychotic symptoms in bipolar I and schizoaffective disorder. *Am J Psychiatry*, 140, 1523–1524.

Rosenberg, J.D. (1986). *The Darkening Glass: A Portrait of Ruskin's Genius*. New York: Columbia University Press.

Rosenthal, N.E., Rosenthal, L.N., Stallone, F., Fleiss, J., Dunner, D.L., and Fieve, R.R. (1979). Psychosis as a predictor of response to lithium maintenance treatment in bipolar affective disorder. *J Affect Disord*, 1, 237–245.

Rosenthal, N.E., Rosenthal, L.N., Stallone, F., Dunner, D.L., and Fieve, R.R. (1980). Toward the validation of RDC schizoaffective disorder. *Arch Gen Psychiatry*, 37, 804–810.

Rush, B. (1812). *Medical Inquiries and Observations upon the Diseases of the Mind*. Philadelphia: Kimber and Richardson.

Sato, T., Bottlender, R., Kleindienst, N., and Möller, H.J. (2002). Syndromes and phenomenological subtypes underlying acute mania: A factor analytic study of 576 manic patients. *Am J Psychiatry*, 159, 968–974.

Sato, T., Bottlender, R., Schroter, A., and Möller, H.J. (2003). Frequency of manic symptoms during a depressive episode and unipolar 'depressive mixed state' as bipolar spectrum. *Acta Psychiatr Scand*, 107, 268–274.

Sato, T., Bottlender, R., Sievers, M., Schröter, A., and Möller, H.J. (2004). Evaluating the inter-episode stability of depressive mixed states. *J Affect Disord*, 81, 103–113.

Sato, T., Bottlender, R., Sievers, M., and Möller, H.-J. (2006). Distinct seasonality of depressive episodes differentiates unipolar depressive patients with and without depressive mixed states. *J Affect Disord*, 90, 1–5.

Schneider, K. (1959). *Clinical Psychopathology*. Translated by M.W. Hamilton. New York: Grune and Stratton.

Schott, A. (1904). Klinischer Beitrag zur Lehre von der chronischen Manie. *Monatschrift für Psychiatrie und Neurologie*, 15, 1–19.

Schwartz, R.C., Reynolds, C.A., Austin, J.F., and Petersen, S. (2003). Homicidality in schizophrenia: A replication study. *Am J Orthopsychiatry*, 73, 74–77.

Seager, A. (1991). *The Glass House: The Life of Theodore Roethke*. Ann Arbor, MI: University of Michigan Press.

Sedler, M.J. (1983). Falret's discovery: The origin of the concept of bipolar affective illness. *Am J Psychiatry*, 140, 1127–1133.

Serretti, A., and Olgiati, P. (2005). Profiles of "manic" symptoms in bipolar I, bipolar II and major depressive disorders. *J Affect Disord*, 84, 159–166.

Serretti, A., Mandelli, L., Lattuada, E., Cusin, C., and Smeraldi, E. (2002). Clinical and demographic features of mood disorder subtypes. *Psychiatry Res*, 15, 195–210.

Sharma, V., Khan, M., and Smith, A. (2005). A closer look at treatment resistant depression: Is it due to a bipolar diathesis? *J Affect Disord*, 84, 251–257.

Shenton, M.E., Solovay, M.R., and Holzman, P. (1987). Comparative studies of thought disorders: II. Schizoaffective disorder. *Arch Gen Psychiatry*, 44, 21–30.

Signoretta, S., Maremmani, I., Liguori, A., Perugi, G., and Akiskal, H.S. (2005). Affective temperament traits measured by TEMPS-I and emotional-behavioral problems in clinically-well children, adolescents, and young adults. *J Affect Disord* 85, 169–180.

Silberman, E.K., Post, R.M., Nurnberger, J., Theodore, W., and Boulenger, J.P. (1985). Transient sensory, cognitive and affective phenomena in affective illness: A comparison with complex partial epilepsy. *Br J Psychiatry*, 146, 81–89.

Simpson, D.M., and Davis, G.C. (1985). Measuring thought disorder with clinical rating scales in schizophrenic and nonschizophrenic patients. *Psychiatry Res*, 15, 313–318.

Slater, E., and Roth, M. (1969). *Clinical Psychiatry* (3rd Edition). Baltimore: Williams and Wilkins.

Solovay, M.R., Shenton, M.E., and Holzman, P.S. (1987). Comparative studies of thought disorders: I. Mania and schizophrenia. *Arch Gen Psychiatry*, 44, 13–20.

Sonne, S.C., Brady, K.T., and Morton, W.A. (1994). Substance abuse and bipolar affective disorder. *J Nerv Ment Dis*, 182, 349–352.

Spiker, D.G., Weiss, J.C., Dealy, R.S., Griffin, S.J., Hanin, I., Neil, J.F., Perel, J.M., Rossi, A.J., and Soloff, P.H. (1985). The pharmacological treatment of delusional depression. *Am J Psychiatry*, 142, 430–436.

Strakowski, S.M., McElroy, S.L., Keck, P.E., and West, S.A. (1996). Suicidality among patients with mixed and manic bipolar disorder. *Am J Psychiatry*, 153, 674–676.

Strakowski, S.M., Williams, J.R., Sax, K.W., Fleck, D.E., DelBello, M.P., and Bourne, M.L. (2000). Is impaired outcome following a first manic episode due to mood-incongruent psychosis? *J Affect Disord*, 61, 87–94.

Suppes, T., Leverich, G.S., Keck, P.E., Nolen, W.A., Denicoff, K.D., Altshuler, L.L., McElroy, S.L., Rush, A.J., Kupka, R., Frye, M.A., Bickel, M., and Post, R.M. (2001). The Stanley Foundation Bipolar Treatment Outcome Network II. Demographics and illness characteristics of the first 261 patients. *J Affect Disord*, 67, 45–49.

Suppes, T., Mintz, J., McElroy, S.L., Altshulet, L.L., Kupka, R.W., Frye, M.A., Keck, P.E., Nolen, W.A., Leverich, G.S., Grunze, H., Rush, A.J., and Post, R.M. (2005). Mixed hypomania in 908 patients with bipolar disorder evaluated prospectively in the Stanley Foundation Bipolar Treatment Network. *Arch Gen Psychiatry*, 62, 1089–1096.

Swann, A., Janicak, P., Calabrese, J., Bowden, C., Dilsaver, S., Morris, D., Petty, F., and Davis, J. (2001). Structure of mania: Depressive, irritable and psychotic clusters with different retrospectively assessed course patterns of illness in randomized clinical trial participants. *J Affect Disord*, 67, 123–132.

Taylor, M.A., and Abrams, R. (1973). The phenomenology of mania: A new look at some old patients. *Arch Gen Psychiatry*, 29, 520–522.

Taylor, M.A., and Abrams, R. (1975). Acute mania: Clinical and genetic study of responders and nonresponders to treatment. *Arch Gen Psychiatry*, 32, 863–865.

Taylor, M.A., and Abrams, R. (1977). Catatonia: Prevalence and importance in the manic phase of manic-depressive illness. *Arch Gen Psychiatry*, 34, 1223–1225.

Taylor, M.A., and Abrams, R. (1983). Schizo-affective disorder, manic type. A clinical, laboratory, and genetic study. *Psychiatr Clin (Basel)*, 16, 234–244.

Tetsuya, S., Bottlender, R., Sievers, M., and Möller, H.-J. (2006). Distinct seasonality of depressive episodes differentiates unipolar depressive patients with and without depressive mixed states. *J Affect Disord,* 90, 1–5.

Thomas, P., Kearney, G., Napier, E., Ellis, E., Leuder, I., and Johnson, M. (1996). Speech and language in first onset psychosis differences between people with schizophrenia, mania, and controls. *Br J Psychiatry*, 168, 337–343.

Tohen, M., Waternaux, C.M., and Tsuang, M.T. (1990). Outcome in mania. A 4-year prospective follow-up of 75 patients utilizing survival analysis. *Arch Gen Psychiatry*, 47, 1106–1111.

Tohen, M., Tsuang, M.T., and Goodwin, D.C. (1992). Prediction of outcome in mania by mood-congruent or mood-incongruent psychotic features. *Am J Psychiatry*, 149, 1580–1581.

Toni, C., Perugi, G., Mata, B., Madaro, D., Maremmani, I., and Akiskal, H.S. (2001). Is mood-incongruent manic psychosis a distinct subtype? *Eur Arch Psychiatry Clin Neurosci*, 251, 12–17.

Tuke, D.H. (1892). *A Dictionary of Psychological Medicine.* Philadelphia: P. Blakiston, Son & Co.

Vieta, E., Gasto, C., Otero, A., Nieto, E., and Vallejo, J. (1997). Differential features between bipolar I and bipolar II disorder. *Compr Psychiatry*, 38, 98–101.

Walker, F. (1968). *Hugo Wolf: A Biography.* London: JM Dent & Sons.

Waters, B.G.H. (1979). Early symptoms of bipolar affective psychosis: Research and clinical implications. *Can Psychiatr Assoc J*, 2, 55–60.

Watkins, J.G., and Stauffacher, J.C. (1952). An index of pathological thinking in the Rorschach. *J Projective Techniques*, 16, 276–286.

Wellner, J., and Marstal, H.B. (1964). Symptoms in mania, an analysis of 279 attacks of manic depressive elation. In B. Jansson (Ed.), Report on the Fourteenth Congress of Scandinavian Psychiatrist. *Acta Psychiatr Scand*, 40(Suppl 180), 175–176.

Wertham, F.I. (1929). A group of benign psychoses: Prolonged manic excitements: With a statistical study of age, duration and frequency in 2000 manic attacks. *Am J Psychiatry*, 9, 17–78.

Weygandt, W. (1899). *Uber die Mischzustande des manisch-depressiven Irreseins.* Munich: J.F. Lehmann.

Winokur, G. (1984). Psychosis in bipolar and unipolar affective illness with special reference to schizo-affective disorder. *Br J Psychiatry*, 145, 236–242.

Winokur, G., and Kadrmas, A. (1989). A polyepisodic course in bipolar illness: Possible clinical relationships. *Compr Psychiatry*, 30, 121–127.

Winokur, G., and Tsuang, M.T. (1975). Elation versus irritability in mania. *Compr Psychiatry*, 16, 435–436.

Winokur, G., Clayton, P.J., and Reich T. (1969). *Manic Depressive Illness.* St. Louis: CV Mosby.

Winokur, G., Scharfetter, C., and Angst, J. (1985). Stability of psychotic symptomatology (delusions, hallucinations), affective syndromes, and schizophrenic symptoms (thought disorder, incongruent affect) over episodes in remitting psychoses. *Eur Arch Psychiatry Neurol Sci*, 234, 303–307.

Winokur, G., Crowe, R., and Kadrmas, A. (1986). Genetic approach to heterogeneity in psychoses: Relationship of a family history of mania or depression to course in bipolar illness. *Psychopathology*, 19, 80–84.

Woods, S.W., Money, R., and Baker, C.B. (2001). Does the manic/mixed episode distinction in bipolar disorder patients run true over time? *Am J Psychiatry*, 158, 1324–1326.

Young, R.C., and Klerman, G.L. (1992) Mania in late life: focus on age at onset. *Am J Psychiatry*, 149, 867–876.

Young, R.C., Schreiber, M.T., and Nysewander, R.W. (1983). Psychotic mania. *Biol Psychiatry*, 18, 1167–1173.

CHAPTER 3

Akiskal, H.S. (1996). The prevalent clinical spectrum of bipolar disorders: Beyond DSM-IV. *J Clin Psychopharmacol*, 16(2 Suppl. 1), 4S–14S.

Akiskal, H.S. (2002). The bipolar spectrum: The shaping of a new paradigm in psychiatry. *Curr Psychiatry Rep*, 4(1), 1–3.

Akiskal, H.S. (2005). Searching for behavioral indicators of bipolar II in patients presenting with major depressive episodes: The "red sign," the "rule of three" and other biographic signs of temperamental extravagance, activism, and hypomania. *J Affect Disord,* 84, 279–290.

Akiskal, H.S., and Benazzi, F. (2003). Family history validation of the bipolar nature of depressive mixed states. *J Affect Disord*, 73(1-2), 113–122.

Akiskal, H.S., and Benazzi, F. (2005). Atypical depression: A variant of bipolar II or a bridge between unipolar and bipolar II? *J Affect Disord*, 84(2-3), 209–217.

Akiskal, H.S., Maser, J.D., Zeller, P.J., Endicott, J., Coryell, W., Keller, M., Warshaw, M., Clayton, P., and Goodwin, F. (1995). Switching from 'unipolar' to bipolar II. An 11-year prospective study of clinical and temperamental predictors in 559 patients. *Arch Gen Psychiatry*, 52(2), 114–123.

Akiskal, H.S., Hantouche, E.G., Allilaire, J.F., Sechter, D., Bourgeois, M.L., Azorin, J.M., Chatenet-Duchene, L., and Lancrenon, S. (2003). Validating antidepressant-associated hypomania (bipolar III): A systematic comparison with spontaneous hypomania (bipolar II). *J Affect Disord*, 73(1-2), 65–74.

Amador, X.F., Flaum, M., Andreasen, N.C., Strauss, D.H., Yale, S.A., Clark, S.C., and Gorman, J.M. (1994). Awareness of illness in schizophrenia and schizoaffective and mood disorders. *Arch Gen Psychiatry*, 51(10), 826–836.

American Psychiatric Association. (2005). *DSM-V prelude project: Research and outreach.* Available: http://www.dsm5.org/ [July 1, 2005].

Amin, S., Singh, S.P., Brewin, J., Jones, P.B., Medley, I., and Harrison, G. (1999). Diagnostic stability of first-episode psychosis. Comparison of ICD-10 and DSM-III-R systems. *Br J Psychiatry*, 175, 537–543.

Andreasen, N.C. (1982). Negative symptoms in schizophrenia: Definition and reliability. *Arch Gen Psychiatry*, 39, 784–788.

Andreasen, N.C., and Grove, W.M. (1982). The classification of depression: Traditional versus mathematical approaches. *Am J Psychiatry*, 139, 45–52.

Andreasen, N.C., Grove, W.M., Shapiro, R.W., Keller, M.B., Hirschfeld, R.M.A., and McDonald-Scott, P. (1981). Reliability of lifetime diagnosis: A multicenter collaborative perspective. *Arch Gen Psychiatry*, 38, 400–405.

Angst, J. (1980). Verlauf unipolar depressiver, bipolar manisch-depressiver und schizo-affektiver Erkrankungen und Psychosen: Ergebnisse einer prospektiven Studie. *Fortschr Neurol Psychiatr*, 48, 3–30.

Angst, J. (1998). The emerging epidemiology of hypomania and bipolar II disorder. *J Affect Disord*, 50(2-3), 143–151.

Angst, J., and Cassano, G. (2005). The mood spectrum: Improving the diasnosis of bipilor disorder. *Bipolar Disord*, 7 (Suppl 4), 4–12.

Angst, J., Gamma, A., Benazzi, F., Ajacic, V., Eich, D., and Rossler, W. (2003). Toward a re-definition of subthreshold bipolarity: Epidemiology and proposed criteria for bipolar-II, minor bipolar disorders and hypomania. *J Affect Disord*, 73(1-2), 133–146.

Angst, J., Sellaro, R., Stassen, H.H., and Gamma, A. (2005). Diagnostic conversion from depression to bipolar disorders: Results of a long-term prospective study of hospital admissions. *J Affect Disord*, 84, 149–157.

Atre-Vaidya, N., and Hussain, S.M. (1999). Borderline personality disorder and bipolar mood disorder: Two distinct disorders or a continuum? *J Nerv Ment Dis*, 187, 313–315.

Benazzi, F. (1999). Bipolar II disorder is common among depressed outpatients. *Psychiatry Clin Neurosci*, 53, 607–609.

Benazzi, F. (2000a). Borderline personality disorder and bipolar II disorder in private practice depressed outpatients. *Compr Psychiatry*, 41(2), 106–110.

Benazzi, F. (2000b). Depression with DSM-IV atypical features: A marker for bipolar II disorder. *Eur Arch Psychiatry Clin Neurosci*, 250(1), 53–55.

Benazzi, F. (2001). Is the minimum duration of hypomania in bipolar II disorder 4 days? *Can J Psychiatry*, 46, 86.

Benazzi, F., and Akiskal, H.S. (2005). A downscaled practical measure of mood lability as a screening tool for bipolar II. *J Affect Disord*, 84, 225–232.

Benazzi, F., and Rihmer, Z. (2000). Sensitivity and specificity of DSM-IV atypical features for bipolar II disorder diagnosis. *Psychiatry Res*, 93(3), 257–262.

Berns, S., Jaeger, J., Iannuzzo, R., et al. (2003). *A comparison of medical chart diagnosis with SCID consensus diagnosis among bipolar disorder patients* (abstract). Presented at the 5th International Conference on Bipolar Disorder, Pittsburgh, PA.

Blacker, D., and Tsuang, M.T. (1992). Contested boundaries of bipolar disorder and the limits of categorical diagnosis in psychiatry. *Am J Psychiatry*, 149, 1473–1483.

Bleuler, E. (1911). *Dementia Praecox or the Group of Schizophrenias*. Translated by J. Zinkin. New York: International Universities Press, 1950. (Originally published in German as a volume of *Aschaffenburg's Handbuch, Dementia Praecox oder die Gruppe der Schizophrenien*.)

Bleuler, M. (1968). Significance of the current theory of depression in general practice. *Ther Umsch*, 25(1), 3–4.

Bridge, T.P., Mirsky, A.F., and Goodwin, F.K. (Eds.). (1988). *Psychological, Neuropsychiatric and Substance Abuse Aspects in AIDS: Advances in Biochemical Psychopharmacology*. Vol. 44. New York: Raven Press.

Brockington, I.F., and Jeff, J.P. (1979). Schizo-affective psychoses: Definitions and incidence. *Psychol Med*, 9, 91–99.

Brockington, I.F., Kendell, R.E., and Wainwright, S. (1980). Depressed patients with schizophrenic or paranoid symptoms. *Psychol Med*, 10(4), 665–675.

Cantor, N., Smith, E.E., French, R.S., and Mezzich, J. (1980). Psychiatric diagnosis as prototype categorization. *J Abnorm Psychol*, 89(2), 181–193.

Carlson, G.A., and Goodwin, F.K. (1973). The stages of mania. A longitudinal analysis of the manic episode. *Arch Gen Psychiatry*, 28(2), 221–228.

Cassidy, F., Murry, E., Forest, K., and Carroll, B.J. (1998). Signs and symptoms of mania in pure and mixed episodes. *J Affect Disord*, 50(2-3), 187–201.

Cassidy, F., Ahearn, E., and Carroll, B.J. (2001a). A prospective study of inter-episode consistency of manic and mixed subtypes of bipolar disorder. *J Affect Disord*, 67, 181–185.

Cassidy, F., Pieper, C.F., and Carroll, B.J. (2001b). Subtypes of mania determined by grade of membership analysis. *Neuropsychopharmacology*, 25(3), 373–383.

Cassidy, F., Ahearn, E.P., and Carroll, B.J. (2002). Symptom profile consistency in recurrent manic episodes. *Compr Psychiatry*, 43(3), 179–181.

Citrome, L., and Goldberg, J.F. (2005). The many faces of bipolar disorder. How to tell them part. *Postgrad Med*, 117(2), 15–16, 19–23.

Cluss, P.A., Marcus, S.C., Kelleher, K.J., Thase, M.E., Arvay, L.A., and Kupfer, D.J. (1999). Diagnostic certainty of a voluntary bipolar disorder case registry. *J Affect Disord*, 52, 93–99.

Copper, J.E., Kendell, R.E., Gurland, B.J., Sharpe, L., Copeland, J.R.M., and Simon, R. (1972). Psychiatric diagnosis in New York and London: A comparative study of mental hospital admissions. Maudsley Monograph No. 20. London: Oxford University Press.

Coryell, W., Keller, M., Endicott, J., Andreasen, N., Clayton, P., and Hirschfeld, R. (1989). Bipolar II illness: Course and outcome over a five-year period. *Psychol Med*, 19(1), 129–141.

Coryell, W., Keller, M., Lavori, P., and Endicott, J. (1990). Affective syndromes, psychotic features, and prognosis. II. Mania. *Arch Gen Psychiatry*, 47(7), 658–662.

Craddock, N., and Owen, M.J. (2005). The beginning of the end for the Kraepelinian dichotomy. *Br J Psychiatry*, 186, 364–366.

Crow, T.J. (1990). The continuum of psychosis and its genetic origins. The sixty-fifth Maudsley lecture. *Br J Psychiatry*, 156, 788–797.

Crow, T.J. (1998). From Kraepelin to Kretschmer leavened by Schneider: The transition from categories of psychosis to dimensions of variation intrinsic to Homo sapiens. *Arch Gen Psychiatry*, 55(6), 502–504.

Cutting, J. (1990). Relationship between cycloid psychosis and typical affective psychosis. *Psychopathology*, 23(4-6), 212–219.

Danielson, C.K., Youngstrom, E.A., Findling, R.L., and Calabrese, J.R. (2003). Discriminative validity of the general behavior inventory using youth report. *J Abnorm Child Psychol*, 31(1), 29–39.

DeBattista, C., Sofuoglu, M., and Schatzberg, A.F. (1998). Serotonergic synergism: The risks and benefits of combining the selective serotonin reuptake inhibitors with other serotonergic drugs. *Biol Psychiatry*, 44(5), 341–347.

Dikeos, D.G., Wickham, H., McDonald, C., Walshe, M., Sigmundsson, T., Bramon, E., Grech, A., Toulopoulou, T., Murray, R., and Sham, P.C. (2006). Distribution of symptom dimensions across Kraepelinian divisions. *Br J Psychiatry*, 189, 346–353.

Dunner, D.L. (1992). Differential diagnosis of bipolar disorder. *J Clin Psychopharmacol*, 12(Suppl. 1), 7S–12S.

Dunner, D.L. (1998). Diagnostic revisions for DSM-IV. In P.J. Goodnick (Ed.), *Mania. Clinical and Research Perspectives* (pp. 3–10). Washington, DC: American Psychiatric Press.

Dunner, D.L., and Tay, L.K. (1993). Diagnostic reliability of the history of hypomania in bipolar II patients and patients with major depression. *Compr Psychiatry*, 34(5), 303–307.

Evans, J.D., Heaton, R.K., Paulsen, J.S., McAdams, L.A., Heaton, S.C., and Jeste, D.V. (1999). Schizoaffective disorder: A form of schizophrenia or affective disorder? *J Clin Psychiatry*, 60(12), 874–882.

Feighner, J.P., Robins, E., Guze, S.B., Woodruff, R.A., Jr., Winokur, G., and Munoz, R. (1972). Diagnostic criteria for use in psychiatric research. *Arch Gen Psychiatry*, 26(1), 57–63.

Fennig, S., Kovasznay, C., Rich, R., Ram, C., Pato, A., Miller, J., Rubinstein, G., Carlson, J.E., Schwartz, and Phelan, J. (1994). Six-month stability of psychiatric diagnoses in first-admission patients with psychosis. *Am J Psychiatry*, 151, 1200–1208.

Fergus, E.L., Miller, R.B., Luckenbaugh, D.A., Leverich, G.S., Findling, R.L., Speer, A.M., and Post, R.M. (2003). Is there progression from irritability/dyscontrol to major depressive and manic symptoms? A retrospective community survey of parents of bipolar children. *J Affect Disord*, 77(1), 71–78.

Fink, M. (1999). Delirious mania. *Bipolar Disord*, 1(1), 54–60.

Flor-Henry, P. (1969). Schizophrenic-like reactions and affective psychoses associated with temporal lobe epilepsy: Etiological factors. *Am J Psychiatry*, 126(3), 400–404.

Gabel, R.H., Barnard, N., Norko, M., and O'Connell, R.A. (1986). AIDS presenting as mania. *Compr Psychiatry*, 27(3), 251–254.

Gershon, E.S., Hamovit, J., Guroff, J.J., Dibble, E., Leckman, J.F., Sceery, W., Targum, S.D., Nurnberger, J.I., Jr., Goldin, L.R., and Bunney, W.E., Jr. (1982). A family study of schizoaffective, bipolar I, bipolar II, unipolar, and normal control probands. *Arch Gen Psychiatry*, 39(10), 1157–1167.

Ghaemi, S.N., Stoll, A.L., and Pope, H.G., Jr. (1995). Lack of insight in bipolar disorder. The acute manic episode. *J Nerv Ment Dis*, 183(7), 464–467.

Ghaemi, S.N., Sachs, G.S., Chiou, A.M., Pandurangi, A.K., and Goodwin, K. (1999). Is bipolar disorder still underdiagnosed? Are antidepressants overutilized? *J Affect Disord*, 52(1-3), 135–144.

Ghaemi, S.N., Boiman, E.E., and Goodwin, F.K. (2000). Diagnosing bipolar disorder and the effect of antidepressants: A naturalistic study. *J Clin Psychiatry*, 61(10), 804–808; quiz 809.

Ghaemi, S.N., Ko, J.Y., and Goodwin, F.K. (2002). Cade's disease and beyond: Misdiagnosis, antidepressant use, and a proposed definition for bipolar spectrum disorder. *Can J Psychiatry*, 47(2), 125–134.

Ghaemi, S.N., Hsu, D.J., Ko, J.Y., Baldassano, C.F., Kontos, N.J., and Goodwin, F.K. (2004). Bipolar spectrum disorder: A pilot study. *Psychopathology*, 37(5), 222–226.

Gibbs, F.A., and Gibbs, E.L. (1952). *Atlas of Electroencephalography*. Vol. 2, Epilepsy. Cambridge, MA: Addison-Wesley Press.

Goldberg, J.F., Harrow, M., and Grossman, L. (1995). Course and outcome in bipolar affective disorder: A longitudinal follow-up study. *Am J Psychiatry*, 152(3), 379–384.

Goldberg, J.F., Harrow, M., and Whiteside, J.E. (2001). Risk for bipolar illness in patients initially hospitalized for unipolar depression. *Am J Psychiatry*, 158, 1265–1270.

Goodwin, F.K., and Bunney, W.E., Jr. (1971). Depressions following reserpine: A reevaluation. *Semin Psychiatry*, 3, 435–448.

Goodwin, F.K., and Ghaemi, S.N. (1998). Understanding manic-depressive illness. *Arch Gen Psychiatry*, 55, 23–25.

Guy, W., and Ban, T.A. (Eds.). (1982). *The AMDP System: Manual for the Assessment and Documentation of Psychopathology*. Berlin: Springer-Verlag.

Hantouche, E.G., Allilaire, J.P., Bourgeois, M.L., Azorin, J.M., Sechter, D., Chatenet-Duchene, L., Lancrenon, S., and Akiskal, H.S. (2001). The feasibility of self-assessment of dysphoric mania in the French national EPIMAN study. *J Affect Disord*, 67(1-3), 97–103.

Hirschfeld, R.M., Williams, J.B., Spitzer, R.L., Calabrese, J.R., Flynn, L., Keck, P.E., Jr., Lewis, L., McElroy, S.L., Post, R.M., Rapport, D.J., Russell, J.M., Sachs, G.S., and Zajecka, J. (2000). Development and validation of a screening instrument for bipolar spectrum disorder: The Mood Disorder Questionnaire. *Am J Psychiatry*, 157(11), 1873–1875.

Hirschfeld, R.M., Lewis, L., and Vornik, L.A. (2003). Perceptions and impact of bipolar disorder: How far have we really come? Results of the national depressive and manic-depressive association 2000 survey of individuals with bipolar disorder. *J Clin Psychiatry*, 64(2), 161–174.

Jampala, V.C., Abrams, R., and Taylor, M.A. (1985). Mania with emotional blunting: Affective disorder or schizophrenia? *Am J Psychiatry*, 142(5), 608–612.

Jampala, V.C., Taylor, M.A., and Abrams, R. (1989). The diagnostic implications of formal thought disorder in mania and schizophrenia: A reassessment. *Am J Psychiatry*, 146, 459–463.

Jaspers, K. (1913). *General Psychology*. Translated by J. Hoenig and M.W. Hamilton. Baltimore: Johns Hopkins University Press, 1997.

Jorm, A.F. (2000). Is depression a risk factor for dementia or cognitive decline? A review. *Gerontology*, 46(4), 219–227.

Kanner, A.M. (2004). Recognition of the various expressions of anxiety, psychosis, and aggression in epilepsy. *Epilepsia*, 45(Suppl. 2), 22–27.

Kasanin, J. (1933). The acute schizoaffective psychoses. *Am J Psychiatry*, 17, 877–883.

Keitner, G.I., Solomon, D.A., Ryan, C.E., Miller, I.W., Mallinger, A., Kupfer, D.J., and Frank, E. (1996). Prodromal and residual symptoms in bipolar I disorder. *Compr Psychiatry*, 37(5), 362–367.

Keller, M.B., and Baker, L.A. (1991). Bipolar disorder: Epidemiology, course, diagnosis, and treatment. *Bull Menninger Clin*, 55(2), 172–181.

Keller, M.B., Lavori, P.W., McDonald-Scott, P., Scheftner, W.A., Andreasen, N.C., Shapiro, R.W., and Croughan, J. (1981). Reliability of lifetime diagnosis and symptoms in patients with a current psychiatric disorder. *J Psychiatr Res*, 4, 229–240.

Kendler, K.S. (1986). Kraepelin and the differential diagnosis of dementia praecox and manic-depressive insanity. *Compr Psychiatry*, 27, 549–558.

Kendler, K.S., Gruenberg, A.M., and Tsuang, M.T. (1986). A DSM-III family study of nonschizophrenic psychotic disorders. *Am J Psychiatry*, 143, 1098–1105.

Kendler, K.S., McGuire, M., Gruenberg, A.M., O'Hare, A., Spellman, M., and Walsh, D. (1993). The Roscommon family study. I. Methods, diagnosis of probands, and risk of schizophrenia in relatives. *Arch Gen Psychiatry*, 50(7), 527–540.

Kendler, K.S., Gallagher, T.J., Abelson, J.M., and Kessler, R.C. (1996). Lifetime prevalence, demographic risk factors, and diagnostic validity of nonaffective psychosis as assessed in a U.S. community sample. The National Comorbidity Survey. *Arch Gen Psychiatry, 53*(11), 1022–1031.

Kendler, K.S., Karkowski, L.M., and Walsh, D. (1998). The structure of psychosis: Latent class analysis of probands from the Roscommon Family Study. *Arch Gen Psychiatry, 55*(6), 492–499.

Keri, S., Kelemen, O., Benedek, G., and Janka, Z. (2001). Different trait markers for schizophrenia and bipolar disorder: A neurocognitive approach. *Psychol Med, 31*(5), 915–922.

Kessing, L. (2005). Diagnostic stability in bipolar disorder in clinical practice as according to ICD-10. *J Affect Disord, 85*(3), 293–299.

Kessler, R.C., Adler, L., Barkley, R., Biederman, J., Conners, C.K., Demler, O., Faraone, S.V., Greenhill, L.L., Howes, M.J., Secnik, K., Spencer, T., Ustun, T.B., Walters, E.E., and Zaslavsky, A.M. (2006). The prevalence and correlates of adult ADHD in the United States: Results from the National Comorbidity Survey Replication. *Am J Psychiatry, 163*(4), 716–723.

Ketter, T.A., Wang, P.W., Becker, O.V., Nowakowska, C., and Yang, Y.S. (2003). The diverse roles of anticonvulsants in bipolar disorders. *Ann Clin Psychiatry, 15*(2), 95–108.

Ketter, T.A., Wang, P.W., Becker, O.V., Nowakowska, C., and Yang, Y. (2004). Psychotic bipolar disorders: Dimensionally similar to or categorically different from schizophrenia? *J Psychiatr Res, 38*(1), 47–61.

Koukopoulos, A. (2001). *Treating the complex patient* (abstract). Presented at 4th Annual International Conference on Bipolar Disorder, Pittsburgh, PA.

Koukopoulos, A., Faedda, G., Proietti, R., D'Amico, S., de Pisa, E., and Simonetto, C. (1992). Mixed depressive syndrome. *Encephale, 18* Spec(1), 19–21.

Koukopoulos, A., Albert, M.J., Sani, G., Koukopoulos, A.E., and Girardi, P. (2005). Mixed depressive states: Nosologic and therapeutic issues. *Int Rev Psychiatry, 17*(1), 12–37.

Kraepelin, E. (1896). *Ein Lehrbuch fur Studirende and Aerzte. Psychiatrie.* Leipzig: J.A. Barth, 8th ed. published in 1913. Reprinted in 1976, New York: Arno Press.

Kraepelin, E. (1913). *Psychiatrie. Ein Lehrbuch fur Studirende und Aerzte,* 8th edition. (Leipzig: JA Barth, 1896). Reprinted New York: Arno Press, 1976.

Kraepelin, E. (1921). *Manic-Depressive Insanity and Paranoia.* Edinburgh: E & S Livingstone.

Krauthammer, C., and Klerman, G.L. (1978). Secondary mania: Manic syndromes associated with antecedent physical illness or drugs. *Arch Gen Psychiatry, 35*(11), 1333–1339.

Kudo, T., Ishida, S., Kubota, H., and Yagi, K. (2001). Manic episode in epilepsy and bipolar I disorder: A comparative analysis of 13 patients. *Epilepsia, 42*(8), 1036–1042.

Leonhard, K. (1957). *Aufteilung der Endogenen Psychosen,* 1st edition. Berlin: Akademie-Verlag. Translated by R. Berman as *The Classification of Endogenous Psychoses,* 5th edition. Edited by E. Robins. New York: Irvington Publishers, 1979.

Lewis, L. (2001). *The use of surveys as an advocacy tool* (abstract). Presented at 4th International Conference for Bipolar Disorder, Pittsburgh, PA.

Lish, J.D., Dime-Meenan, S., Whybrow, P.C., Price, R.A., and Hirschfeld, R.M. (1994). The National Depressive and Manic-Depressive Association (DMDA) survey of bipolar members. *J Affect Disord, 31*(4), 281–294.

Lyketsos, C.G., Schwartz, J., Fishman, M., and Treisman, G. (1997). AIDS mania. *J Neuropsychiatry Clin Neurosci, 9*(2), 277–279.

Maj, M., Pirozzi, R., and Starace, F. (1989). Previous pattern of course of the illness as a predictor of response to lithium prophylaxis in bipolar patients. *J Affect Disord, 17,* 237–241.

Manning, J.S., Haykal, R.F., Connor, P.D., and Akiskal, H.S. (1997). On the nature of depressive and anxious states in a family practice setting: The high prevalence of bipolar II and related disorders in a cohort followed longitudinally. *Compr Psychiatry, 38*(2), 102–108.

Marneros, A. (2001). Origin and development of concepts of bipolar mixed states. *J Affect Disord, 67*(1-3), 229–240.

Marneros, A., Deister, A., Rohde, A., Junemann, H., and Fimmers, R. (1988). Long-term course of schizoaffective disorders. Part I: Definitions, methods, frequency of episodes and cycles. *Eur Arch Psychiatry Neurol Sci, 237*(5), 264–275.

Marneros, A., Rohde, A., Deister, A., and Steinmeyer, E.M. (1989). Premorbid and social markers of patients with schizoaffective psychoses. *Fortschr Neurol Psychiatr, 57*(5), 205–212.

Marneros, A., Deister, A., and Rohde, A. (1991). Stability of diagnoses in affective, schizoaffective and schizophrenic disorders. Cross-sectional versus longitudinal diagnosis. *Eur Arch Psychiatry Clin Neurosci, 241*(3), 187–192.

Marneros, A., Pillmann, F., Haring, A., and Balzuweit, S. (2000). Acute and transient psychotic disorders. *Fortschr Neurol Psychiatr, 68*(Suppl. 1), S22–S25.

McElroy, S.L., Keck, P.E., Jr., Pope, H.G., Jr., Hudson, J.I., Faedda, G.L., and Swann, A.C. (1992). Clinical and research implications of the diagnosis of dysphoric or mixed mania or hypomania. *Am J Psychiatry, 149*(12), 1633–1644.

McKenna, P.J., Kane, J.M., and Parrish, K. (1985). Psychotic syndromes in epilepsy. *Am J Psychiatry, 142*(8), 895–904.

Melton, S.T., Kirkwood, C.K., and Ghaemi, S.N. (1997). Pharmacotherapy of HIV dementia. *Ann Pharmacother, 31*(4), 457–473.

Miller, A., Fox, N.A., Cohn, J.F., Forbes, E.E., Sherrill, J.T., and Kovacs, M. (2002). Regional patterns of brain activity in adults with a history of childhood-onset depression: Gender differences and clinical variability. *Am J Psychiatry, 159*(6), 934–940.

Miller, C.J., Klugman, J., Berv, D.A., Rosenquist, K.J., and Ghaemi, S.N. (2004). Sensitivity and specificity of mood disorder questionnaire for detecting bipolar disorder. *J Affect Disord, 81*(2), 167–171.

Mitchell, P., Parker, G., Jamieson, K., Wilhelm, K., Hickie, I., Brodaty, H., Boyce, P., Hadzi-Pavlovic, D., and Roy, K. (1992). Are there any differences between bipolar and unipolar melancholia? *J Affect Disord, 25*(2), 97–105.

Mitsuda, H. (1965). The concept of "atypical psychoses" from the aspect of clinical genetics. *Acta Psychiatr Scand, 41,* 372–377.

Nierenberg, A.A., Miyahara, S., Spencer, T., Wisniewski, S.R., Otto, M.W., Simon, N., Pollack, M.H., Ostacher, M.J., Yan, L., Siegel, R., Sachs, G.S., and STEP-BD Investigators (2005). Clinical and diagnostic implications of lifetime attention-deficit/hyperactivity disorder comorbidity in adults with bipolar disorder. *Biol Psychiatry, 57*(11), 146–1473.

Parker, G., Parker, K., Malhi, G., Wilhelm, K., and Mitchell, P. (2004). Studying personality characteristics in bipolar depressed subjects: How comparator group selection can dictate results. *Acta Psychiatr Scand, 109*(5), 376–382.

Perris, C. (1988). The concept of cycloid psychotic disorder. *Psychiatr Dev, 6*(1), 37–56.

Perris, C. (1990). The importance of Karl Leonhard's classification of endogenous psychoses. *Psychopathology, 23*(4-6), 282–290.

Perugi, G., Akiskal, H.S., Micheli, C., Musetti, L., Paiano, A., Quilici, C., Rossi, L., and Cassano, G.B. (1997). Clinical subtypes of bipolar mixed states: Validating a broader European definition in 143 cases. *J Affect Disord*, 43(3), 169–180.

Perugi, G., Akiskal, H.S., Micheli, C., Toni, C., and Madaro, D. (2001). Clinical characterization of depressive mixed state in bipolar-I patients: Pisa–San Diego collaboration. *J Affect Disord*, 67(1-3), 105–114.

Pfuhlmann, B., Jabs, B., Althaus, G., Schmidtke, A., Bartsch, A., Stober, G., Beckmann, H., and Franzek, E. (2004). Cycloid psychoses are not part of a bipolar affective spectrum: Results of a controlled family study. *J Affect Disord*, 83(1), 11–19.

Phelps, J.R., and Ghaemi, S.N. (2006). Improving the diagnosis of bipolar disorder: Predictive value of screening tests. *J Affect Disord*, 92(2-3), 141–148.

Pope, H.G. (1983). Distinguishing bipolar disorder from schizophrenia in clinical practice: Guidelines and case reports. *Hosp Community Psychiatry*, 34, 322–328.

Pope, H.G., Jr., and Lipinski, J.F., Jr. (1978). Diagnosis in schizophrenia and manic-depressive illness: A reassessment of the specificity of 'schizophrenic' symptoms in the light of current research. *Arch Gen Psychiatry*, 35(7), 811–828.

Post, R.M., and Weiss, S.R. (2004). Convergences in course of illness and treatments of the epilepsies and recurrent affective disorders. *Clin EEG Neurosci*, 35(1), 14–24.

Price, L.H., Charney, D.S., Rubin, A.L., and Heninger, G.R. (1986). Alpha 2-adrenergic receptor function in depression: The cortisol response to yohimbine. *Arch Gen Psychiatry*, 43, 849–858.

Prien, R.F., Himmelhoch, J.M., and Kupfer, D.J. (1988). Treatment of mixed mania. *J Affect Disord*, 15(1), 9–15.

Rice, J.P., Rochberg, N., Endicott, J., Lavori, P.W., and Miller, C. (1992). Stability of psychiatric diagnoses. An application to the affective disorders. *Arch Gen Psychiatry*, 49, 824–830.

Sachs, G.S., Baldassano, C.F., Truman, C.J., and Guille, C. (2000). Comorbidity of attention deficit hyperactivity disorder with early- and late-onset bipolar disorder. *Am J Psychiatry*, 157(3), 466–468.

Salvatore, P., Baldessarini, R.J., Centorrino, F., Egli, S., Albert, M., Gerhard, A., and Maggini, C. (2002). Weygandt's on the mixed states of manic-depressive insanity: A translation and commentary on its significance in the evolution of the concept of bipolar disorder. *Harv Rev Psychiatry*, 10(5), 255–275.

Sato, T., Bottlender, R., Kleindienst, N., Tanabe, A., and Moller, H.J. (2002). The boundary between mixed and manic episodes in the ICD-10 classification. *Acta Psychiatr Scand*, 106(2), 109–116.

Schatzberg, A.F., and Rothschild, A.J. (1992). Psychotic (delusional) major depression: Should it be included as a distinct syndrome in DSM-IV? *Am J Psychiatry*, 149(6), 733–745.

Scheffer, R.E., and Niskala Apps, J.A. (2004). The diagnosis of preschool bipolar disorder presenting with mania: Open pharmacological treatment. *J Affect Disord*, 82(Suppl. 1), S25–S34.

Schneider, K. (1959). *Clinical Psychopathology*. Translated by M.W. Hamilton. New York: Grune and Stratton.

Serretti, A., Rietschel, M., Lattuada, E., Krauss, H., Schulze, T.G., Muller, D.J., Maier, W., and Smeraldi, E. (2001). Major psychoses symptomatology: Factor analysis of 2241 psychotic subjects. *Eur Arch Psychiatry Clin Neurosci*, 251(4), 193–198.

Smith, D., Harrison, N., Muir, W., and Blackwood D. (2005). The high prevalence of bipolar spectrum in young adults with recurrent depression: Toward an innovative diagnostic framework. *J Affect Disord*, 84, 167–178.

Spitzer, R.L., Endicott, J., Robins, E. (1978). Research diagnostic criteria: Rationale and reliability. *Arch Gen Psychiatry*, 35(6), 773–782.

Sprock, J. (1988). Classification of schizoaffective disorder. *Compr Psychiatry*, 29(1), 55–71.

Stoll, A.L., Banov, M., Kolbrener, M., Mayer, P.V., Tohen, M., Strakowski, S.M., Castillo, J., Suppes, T., and Cohen, B.M. (1994). Neurologic factors predict a favorable valproate response in bipolar and schizoaffective disorders. *J Clin Psychopharmacol*, 14(5), 311–313.

Surtees, P.G., and Kendell, R.E. (1979). The hierarchy model of psychiatric symptomatology: An investigation based on present state examination ratings. *Br J Psychiatry*, 135, 43–443.

Swann, A.C. (2000). Depression, mania, and feeling bad: The role of dysphoria in mixed states. *Bipolar Disord*, 2(4), 325–327.

Swann, A.C., Secunda, S.K., Katz, M.M., Croughan, J., Bowden, C.L., Koslow, S.H., Berman, N., and Stokes, P.E. (1993). Specificity of mixed affective states: Clinical comparison of dysphoric mania and agitated depression. *J Affect Disord*, 28(2), 81–89.

Swann, A.C., Bowden, C.L., Morris, D., Calabrese, J.R., Petty, F., Small, J., Dilsaver, S.C., and Davis, J.M. (1997). Depression during mania. Treatment response to lithium or divalproex. *Arch Gen Psychiatry*, 54(1), 37–42.

Swann, A.C., Janicak, P.L., Calabrese, J.R., Bowden, C.L., Dilsaver, S.C., Morris, D.D., Petty, F., and Davis, J.M. (2001). Structure of mania: Depressive, irritable, and psychotic clusters with different retrospectively-assessed course patterns of illness in randomized clinical trial participants. *J Affect Disord*, 67(1-3), 123–132.

Swann, A.C., Pazzaglia, P., Nicholls, A., Dougherty, D.M., and Moeller, F.G. (2003). Impulsivity and phase of illness in bipolar disorder. *J Affect Disord*, 73(1-2), 105–111.

Toomey, R., Faraone, S.V., Simpson, J.C., and Tsuang, M.T. (1998). Negative, positive, and disorganized symptom dimensions in schizophrenia, major depression, and bipolar disorder. *J Nerv Ment Dis*, 186(6), 470–476.

Tsuang, D., and Coryell, W. (1993). An 8-year follow-up of patients with DSM-III-R psychotic depression, schizoaffective disorder, and schizophrenia. *Am J Psychiatry*, 150(8), 1182–1188.

Tsuang, M.T., and Simpson, J.C. (1984). Schizoaffective disorder: Concept and reality. *Schizophr Bull*, 10(1), 14–25.

Tsuang, M.T., Winokur, G., and Crowe, R.R. (1980). Morbidity risks of schizophrenia and affective disorders among first-degree relatives of patients with schizophrenia, mania, depression and surgical conditions. *Br J Psychiatry*, 137, 497–504.

Tsuang, M.T., Woolson, R.F., and Simpson, J.C. (1981). An evaluation of the Feighner criteria for schizophrenia and affective disorders using long-term outcome data. *Psychol Med*, 11, 281–287.

Van Os, J., Castle, D.J., Takei, N., Der, G., and Murray, R.M. (1996). Psychotic illness in ethnic minorities: Clarification from the 1991 census. *Psychol Med*, 26(1), 203–208.

Van Os, J., Jones, P., Sham, P., Bebbington, P., and Murray, R.M. (1998). Risk factors for inset and persistence of psychosis. *Soc Psychiatry Psychiatr Epidemiol*, 33(12), 596–605.

van Praag, H.M. (1993). *Make-Believes in Psychiatry: Or the Perils of Progress*. New York: Brunner/Mazel.

Ventura, J., Nuechterlein, K.H., Subotnik, K.L., Gutkind, D., and Gilbert, E.A. (2000). Symptom dimensions in recent-onset schizophrenia and mania: A principal components analysis of the 24-item Brief Psychiatric Rating Scale. *Psychiatry Res,* 97(2-3), 129–135.

Vieta, E., and Salva, J. (1997). Diagnostico diferencial de los trastornos bipolares. In E. Vieta, and C. Gasto (Eds.), *Trastornos Bipolares* (pp. 175–193). Barcelona: Springer.

Vieta, E., Gasto, C., Otero, A., Nieto, E., and Vallejo, J. (1997). Differential features between bipolar I and bipolar II disorder. *Compr Psychiatry,* 38(2), 98–101.

Viguera, A.C., and Cohen, L.S. (1998). The course and management of bipolar disorder during pregnancy. *Psychopharmacol Bull,* 34(3), 339–346.

Whyte, E.M., and Mulsant, B.H. (2002). Post-stroke depression: Epidemiology, pathophysiology, and biological treatment. *Biol Psychiatry,* 52(3), 253–264.

Wilens, T.E., Biederman, J., Wozniak, J., Gunawardene, S., Wong, J., and Monuteaux, M. (2003). Can adults with attention-deficit/hyperactivity disorder be distinguished from those with comorbid bipolar disorder? Findings from a sample of clinically referred adults. *Biol Psychiatry,* 54(1), 1–8.

Wing, J., and Nixon, J. (1975). Discriminating symptoms in schizophrenia. A report from the international pilot study of schizophrenia. *Arch Gen Psychiatry,* 32(7), 853–859.

Yang, C.Y., Su, T.P., Wong, W.W., Guo, W.Y., and Su, Y.L. (2005). Association of AIDS and bipolar mania with rapid progression to dementia and death. *J Chin Med Assoc,* 68(2), 92–95.

Zimmerman, M., Posternak, M.A., Chelminski, I., and Solomon, D.A. (2004). Using questionnaires to screen for psychiatric disorders: A comment on a study of screening for bipolar disorder in the community. *J Clin Psychiatry,* 65(5), 605–610.

CHAPTER 4

Ahrens, B., Berghofer, A., Wolf, T., and Muller-Oerlinghausen, B. (1995). Suicide attempts, age and duration of illness in recurrent affective disorders. *J Affect Disord,* 36(1-2), 43–49.

Akdeniz, F., Vahip, S., Pirildar, S., Vahip, I., Doganer, I., and Bulut, I. (2003). Risk factors associated with childbearing-related episodes in women with bipolar disorder. *Psychopathology,* 36(5), 234–238.

Akiskal, H.S., Maser, J.D., Zeller, P.J., Endicott, J., Coryell, W., Keller, M., Warshaw, M., Clayton, P., and Goodwin, F. (1995). Switching from "unipolar" to bipolar II: An 11-year prospective study of clinical and temperamental predictors in 559 patients. *Arch Gen Psychiatry,* 52(2), 114–123.

Akiskal, H.S., Hantouche, E.G., Bourgeois, M.L., Azorin, J.M., Sechter, D., Allilaire, J.F., Lancrenon, S., Fraud, J.P., and Chatenet-Duchene, L. (1998). Gender, temperament, and the clinical picture in dysphoric mixed mania: Findings from a French national study (EPIMAN). *J Affect Disord,* 50(2-3), 175–186.

Almeida, O.P., and Fenner, S. (2002). Bipolar disorder: Similarities and differences between patients with illness onset before and after 65 year of age. *Int Psychogeriatr,* 14(3), 311–322.

Altshuler, L.L., Conrad, A., Hauser, P., Li, X.M., Guze, B.H., Denikoff, K., Tourtellotte, W., and Post, R. (1991). Reduction of temporal lobe volume in bipolar disorder: A preliminary report of magnetic resonance imaging. *Arch Gen Psychiatry,* 48(5), 482–483.

Altshuler, L.L., Post, R.M., Leverich, G.S., Mikalauskas, K., Rosoff, A., and Ackerman, L. (1995). Antidepressant-induced mania and cycle acceleration: A controversy revisited. *Am J Psychiatry,* 152, 1130–1138.

Altshuler, L.L., Kiriakos, L., Calcagno, J., Goodman, R., Gitlin, M., Frye, M., and Mintz, J. (2001). The impact of antidepressant discontinuation versus antidepressant continuation on 1-year risk for relapse of bipolar depression: A retrospective chart review. *J Clin Psychiatry,* 62, 612–616.

Altshuler, L.L., Gitlin, M.J., Mintz, J., Leight, K.L., and Frye, M.A. (2002). Subsyndromal depression is associated with functional impairment in patients with bipolar disorder. *J Clin Psychiatry,* 63(9), 807–811.

Ambelas, A. (1979). Psychologically stressful events in the precipitation of manic episodes. *Br J Psychiatry,* 135, 15–21.

Angst, F., Stassen, H.H., Clayton, P.J., Angst J. (2002). Mortality of patients with mood disorders: Follow-up over 34–38 years. *Affect Disord,* 68, 167–181.

Angst, J. (1978). The course of affective disorders: II. Typology of bipolar manic-depressive illness. *Arch Psychiatr Nervenkr,* 226, 65–73.

Angst, J. (1980). Verlauf unipolar depressiver, bipolar manisch-depressiver und schizo-affektiver Erkrankungen and Psychosen: Ergebnisse einer prospektiven Studie. *Fortschr Neurol Psychiatr,* 48, 3–30.

Angst, J. (1981a). Clinical indications for a prophylactic treatment of depression. *Adv Biol Psychiatry,* 7, 218–229.

Angst, J. (1981b). Course of affective disorders. In H.M. Van Praag, M.H. Lader, O.J. Rafaelsen, E.J. Sachar (Eds.), *Handbook of Biological Psychiatry* (pp. 225–242). New York: Marcel Dekker.

Angst, J. (1985). Switch from depression to mania: A record study over decades between 1920 and 1982. *Psychopathology,* 18, 140–154.

Angst, J. (1986c). The course of schizoaffective disorders. In M.T. Tsuang, A. Maneros (Eds.), *Schizoaffective Psychoses.* Berlin-Heidelberg: Springer-Verlag.

Angst, J. (1986d). The course of affective disorders. *Psychopath,* 19(Suppl. 2), 47–52.

Angst, J. (1988). *Suicides among depressive and bipolar patients.* Abstract of paper presented at the 141st annual meeting of the American Psychiatric Association, May 7–12, Montreal, Canada.

Angst, J., and Preisig, M. (1995). Course of a clinical cohort of unipolar, bipolar and schizoaffective patients: Results of a prospective study from 1959 to 1985. *Schweiz Arch Neurol Psychiatr,* 146, 5–16.

Angst, J., and Sellaro, R. (2000). Historical perspectives and natural history of bipolar disorder. *Biological Psychiatry,* 48, 445–457.

Angst, J., and Weis, P. (1967). Periodicity of depressive psychoses. In H. Brill, J.O. Cole, P. Deniker (Eds.), *Neuropsychopharmacology: Proceedings of the Fifth Internal Congress of the Collegium Internationale Neuro-pscyho-pharmalogicum* (pp. 703–710). Amsterdam: Excerpta Medica.

Angst, J., Weis, P., Grof, P., Baastrup, P.C., and Schou, M. (1970). Lithium prophylaxis in recurrent affective disorders. *Br J Psychiatry,* 116, 604–614.

Angst, J., Baastrup, P., Grof, P., Hippius, H., Poldinger, W., and Weis, P. (1973). The course of monopolar depression and bipolar psychoses. *Psychiatr Neurol Neurochir,* 76, 489–500.

Angst, J., Felder, W., Frey, R., and Stassen, H.H. (1978). The course of affective disorders: I. Change of diagnosis of monopolar, unipolar, and bipolar illness. *Arch Psychiatr Nervenkr,* 226(1), 57–64.

Angst, J., Felder, W., and Frey, R. (1979). The course of unipolar and bipolar affective disorders. In: M. Schou and E. Strömgren (Eds.), *Origin, Prevention and Treatment of Affective Disorders*. New York: Academic Press, pp. 215–226.

Angst, J., Angst, F., and Stassen, H.H. (1999). Suicide risk in patients with major depressive disorder. *J Clin Psychiatry*, 60(Suppl 2), 57–62; discussion 75–76, 113–116.

Angst, J., Gamma, A., Neuenschwander, M., Ajdacic-Gross, V., Eich, D., Rossler, W., and Merikangas, K.R. (2005). Prevalence of mental disorders in the Zurich Cohort Study: A twenty year prospective study. *Epidemiol Psichiatr Soc*, 14(2), 68–76.

Aronson, T.A., and Shukla, S. (1987). Life events and relapse in bipolar disorder: The impact of a catastrophic event. *Acta Psychiatr Scand*, 75, 571–576.

Baethge, C., Baldessarini, R.J., Freudenthal, K., Streeruwitz, A., Bauer, M., and Bschor, T. (2005). Hallucinations in bipolar disorder: Characteristics and comparison to unipolar depression and schizophrenia. *Bipolar Disord*, 7(2), 136–145.

Baldassano et al. (2002). *Gender differences in bipolar disorder*. Systematic Treatment Enhancement Program First 500 (STEP-BD), 155th annual meeting of the American Psychiatric Association, May 18–23, Philadelphia, PA.

Baldessarini, R.J., Tondo, L., Hennen, J., and Floris, G. (1999). Latency and episodes before treatment: Response to lithium maintenance in bipolar I and II disorders. *Bipolar Disorders*, 2, 91–97.

Baldessarini, R.J., Tondo, L., Floris, G., and Hennen, J. (2000). Effects of rapid cycling on response to lithium maintenance treatment in 360 bipolar I and II disorder patients. *J Affect Disord*, 61, 13–22.

Baron, M., Mendlewicz, J., and Klotz, J. (1981). Age-of-onset and genetic transmission in affective disorders. *Acta Psychiatr Scand*, 64(5), 373–380.

Bauer, M., and Whybrow, P. (1988). Thyroid hormones and the central nervous system in affective illness: Interactions that may have clinical significance. *Integrative Psychiatry*, 6, 75–100.

Bauer, M.S., Calabrese, J., Dunner, D.L., Post, R., Whybrow, P.C., Gyulai, L., Tay, L.K., Younkin, S.R., Bynum, D., and Lavori, P. (1994). Multisite data reanalysis of the validity of rapid cycling as a course modifier for bipolar disorder in DSM-IV. *Am J Psychiatry*, 151(4), 506–515.

Bellivier, F., Golmard, J.L., Henry, C., Leboyer, M., and Schurhoff, F. (2001). Admixture analysis of age at onset in bipolar I affective disorder. *Arch Gen Psychiatry*, 58(5), 510–512.

Bellivier, F., Leroux, M., Henry, C., Rayah, F., Rouillon, F., Laplanche, J.L., and Leboyer, M. (2002). Serotonin transporter gene polymorphism influences age at onset in patients with bipolar affective disorder. *Neurosci Lett*, 334(1), 17–20.

Bellivier, F., Golmard, J.L., Rietschel, M., Schulze, T.G., Malafosse, A., Preisig, M., McKeon, P., Mynett-Johnson, L., Henry, C., and Leboyer, M. (2003). Age at onset in bipolar I affective disorder: Further evidence for three subgroups. *Am J Psychiatry*, 160(5), 999–1001.

Benazzi, F. (1999). A comparison of the age of onset of bipolar I and bipolar II outpatients. *J Affect Disord*, 54, 249–253.

Benedetti, F., Lucca, A., Brambilla, F., Colombo, C., and Smeraldi, E. (2002). Interleukin-6 serum levels correlate with response to antidepressant sleep deprivation and sleep phase advance. *Prog Neuropsychopharmacol Biol Psychiatry*, 26(6), 1167–1170.

Berghofer, A., Wolf, T., and Muller-Oerlinghausen, B. (1995). Suicide attempts, age and duration of illness in recurrent affective disorders. *J Affect Disord*, 36(1–2), 43–49.

Bidzinska, E.J. (1984). Stress factors in affective diseases. *Br J Psychiatry*, 144, 161–166.

Black, D.W., Winokur, G., and Nasrallah, A. (1987a). Is death from natural causes still excessive in psychiatric patients? A follow-up of 1593 patients with major affective disorder. *J Nerv Ment Dis*, 175, 674–680.

Black, K.J., and Perlmutter, J.S. (1997). Septuagenarian Sydenham's with secondary hypomania. *Neuropsychiatry Neuropsychol Behav Neurol*, 10(2), 147–150.

Blumenthal, R.L., Egeland, J.A., Sharpe, L., Nee, J., and Endicott, J. (1987). Age of onset in bipolar and unipolar illness with and without delusions or hallucinations. *Compr Psychiatry*, 28(6), 547–554.

Bourgeois, M., and Campagne, A. (1967). Maniaco-depressive et syndrome de Garcin. *Ann Med Psychol*, 125(Suppl. 2), 451–460.

Bratfos, O., and Haug, J.O. (1968). The course of manic-depressive psychosis: A follow up investigation of 215 patients. *Acta Psychiatr Scand*, 44, 89–112.

Bratfos, O., Eitinger, L., and Tau, T. (1968). Mental illness and crime in adopted children and adoptive parents. *Acta Psychiatr Scand*, 44, 376–384.

Brieger, P., Roettig, S., Ehrt, U., Wenzel, A., Bloink, R., and Marneros, A. (2003). TEMPS-A scale in "mixed" and "pure" manic episodes: New data and methodological considerations on the relevance of joint anxious-depressive temperament traits. *J Affect Disord*, 73(1–2), 99–104.

Brody, E.B. (1973). *The lost ones*. New York: International Universities Press.

Bromet, E.J., Jandorf, L., Fennig, S., Lavelle, J., Kovasznay, B., Ram, R., Tanenberg-Karant, M., and Craig, T. (1996). The Suffolk County Mental Health Project: Demographic, premorbid and clinical correlates of 6-month outcome. *Psychol Med*, 26(5), 953–962.

Burke, K.C., Burke, J.D., Regier, D.A., and Rae, D.S. (1990). Age at onset of selected mental disorders in five community populations. *Arch Gen Psychiatry*, 47(6), 511–518.

Cannon, M., Jones, P., Gilvarry, C., Rifkin, L., McKenzie, K., Foerster, A., and Murray, R.M. (1997). Premorbid social functioning in schizophrenia and bipolar disorder: Similarities and differences. *Am J Psychiatry*, 154(11), 1544–1550.

Carlson, G.A., Kotin, J., Davenport, Y.B., and Adland, M. (1974). Follow-up of 53 bipolar manic-depressive patients. *Br J Psychiatry*, 124(579), 134–139.

Carlson, G.A., Davenport, Y.B., and Jamison, K. (1977). A comparison of outcome in adolescent- and late-onset bipolar manic-depressive illness. *Am J Psychiatry*, 134, 919–922.

Carlson, G.A., Bromet, E.J., and Sievers, S. (2000). Phenomenology and outcome of subjects with early- and adult-onset psychotic mania. *Am J Psychiatry*, 157, 213–219.

Carlson, G.A., Bromet, E.J., Driessons, C., Mojtabai, R., and Schwartz, J.E. (2002). Age at onset, childhood psychopathology, and 2-year outcome in psychotic bipolar disorder. *Am J Psychiatry*, 159(2), 307–309.

Carter, T.D., Mundo, E., Parikh, S.V., and Kennedy, J.L. (2003). Early age at onset as a risk factor for poor outcome of bipolar disorder. *J Psychiatr Res*, 37(4), 297–303.

Casanova, M.F., Kruesi, M., and Mannheim, G. (1996). Multiple sclerosis and bipolar disorder: A case report with autopsy findings. *J Neuropsychiatry Clin Neurosci*, 8(2), 206–208.

Chase, T.N., Holden, E.M., and Brody, J.A. (1973). Levodopa-induced dyskinesias. Comparison in Parkinsonism-dementia and amyotrophic lateral sclerosis. *Arch Neurol*, 29(5), 328–333.

Chaturvedi, S.K., and Upadhyaya, M. (1988). Secondary mania in a patient receiving isonicotinic acid hydrazide and pyridoxine: Case report. *Can J Psychiatry*, 33, 675–676.

Chengappa, R., Kupfer, D.J., Frank, E., Houck, P.R., Grochocinski, V.J., Cluss, P.A., and Stapf, D.A. (2003). Relationship of birth cohort and early age at onset of illness in a bipolar disorder case registry. *Am J Psychiatry*, 160, 1636–1642.

Cicero, D., El-Mallakh, R.S., Holman, J., and Robertson, J. (2003). Antidepressant exposure in bipolar children. *Psychiatry*, 66, 317–322.

Cooper, A.J. (1967). Hypomanic psychosis precipitated by hemodialysis. *Compr Psychiatry*, 8, 168–172.

Corn, T.H., and Checkley, S.A. (1983). A case of recurrent mania with recurrent hyperthyroidism. *Br J Psychiatry*, 143, 74–76.

Coryell, W., and Norten, S.G. (1980). Mania during adolescence: The pathoplastic significance of age. *J Nerv Ment Dis*, 168(10), 611–613.

Coryell, W., Keller, M., Endicott, J., Andreasen, N., Clayton, P., and Hirschfeld, R. (1989). Bipolar II illness: Course and outcome over a five-year period. *Psychol Med*, 19, 129–141.

Coryell, W., Endicott, J., and Keller, M. (1990). Outcome of patients with chronic affective disorder: A five-year follow-up. *Am J Psychiatry*, 147(12), 1627–1633.

Coryell, W., Endicott, J., and Keller, M. (1992). Rapid cycling affective disorder: Demographics, diagnosis, family history, and course. *Arch Gen Psychiatry*, 49, 126–131.

Coryell, W., Scheftner, W., Keller, M., Endicott, J., Maser, J., and Klerman, G.L. (1993). The enduring psychosocial consequences of mania and depression. *Am J Psychiatry*, 150, 720–727.

Coryell, W., Winokur, G., Maser, J.D., Akiskal, H.S., Keller, M.B., and Endicott, J. (1994). Recurrently situational (reactive) depression: A study of course, phenomenology and familial psychopathology. *J Affect Disord*, 31(3), 203–210.

Coryell, W., Endicott, J., Maser, J.D., Keller, M.B., Leon, A.C., and Akiskal, H.S. (1995). Long-term stability of polarity distinctions in the affective disorders. *Am J Psychiatry*, 152(3), 385–390.

Coryell, W., Leon, A.C., Turvey, C., Akiskal, H.S., Mueller, T., and Endicott, J. (2001). The significance of psychotic features in manic episodes: A report from the NIMH collaborative study. *J Affect Disord*, 67(1–3), 79–88.

Crane, G.E. (1956). The psychiatric side effects of iproniazid. *Am J Psychiatry*, 112, 494–501.

Cummings, J.L., and Mendez, M.F. (1984). Secondary mania with focal cerebrovascular lesions. *Am J Psychiatry*, 141, 1084–1087.

Cusin, C., Serretti, A., Lattuada, E., Mandelli, L., and Smeraldi, E. (2000). Impact of clinical variables on illness time course in mood disorders. *Psychiatry Res*, 97, 217–227.

Cutler, N.R., and Post, R.M. (1982a). Life course of illness in untreated manic-depressive patients. *Comp Psychiatry*, 23, 101–115.

Dauncey, K. (1988). Mania in the early stages of AIDS. *Br J Psychiatry*, 152, 716–717.

Deister, A., and Marneros, A. (1993). Predicting the long-term outcome of affective disorders. *Acta Psychiatr Scand*, 88(3), 174–177.

Dell'Osso, L., Akiskal, H.S., Freer, P., Barberi, M., Placidi, G.F., and Cassano, G.B. (1993). Psychotic and nonpsychotic bipolar mixed states: Comparisons with manic and schizoaffective disorders. *Eur Arch Psychiatry Clin Neurosci*, 243(2), 75–81.

Depue, R.A., Slater, J.F., Wolfstetter-Kausch, H., Klein, D., Goplerud, E., and Farr, D. (1981). A behavioral paradigm for identifying persons at risk for bipolar depressive disorder: A conceptual framework and five validation studies. *J Abnorm Psychol Monograph*, 90, 381–437.

Derby, I.M. (1933). Manic-depressive "exhaustion" deaths: An analysis of "exhaustion" case histories. *Psychiatr Q*, 7, 435–449.

Dittmann, S., Biedermann, N.C., Grunze, H., Hummel, B., Scharer, L.O., Kleindienst, N., Forsthoff, A., Matzner, N., Walser, S., and Walden, J. (2002). The Stanley Foundation Bipolar Network: Results of the naturalistic follow-up study after 2.5 years of follow-up in the German centres. *Neuropsychobiology*, 46(Suppl. 1), 2–9.

Donaldson, S., Goldstein, L.H., Landau, S., Raymont, V., and Frangou, S. (2003). The Maudsley Bipolar Disorder Project: The effect of medication, family history, and duration of illness on IQ and memory in bipolar I disorder. *J Clin Psychiatry*, 64(1), 86–93.

Dunner, D.L., Fleiss, J.L., and Fieve, R.R. (1976b). The course of development of mania in patients with recurrent depression. *Am J Psychiatry*, 133, 905–908.

Dunner, D.L., Murphy, D., Stallone, F., and Fieve, R.R. (1979b). Episode frequency prior to lithium treatment in bipolar manic-depressive patients. *Compr Psychiatry*, 20, 511–515.

Dunner, D.L., Murphy, D., Stallone, F., and Fieve, R.R. (1980). Affective episode frequency and lithium therapy. *Psychopharmacol Bull*, 16, 49–50.

Eaton, W.W., Anthony, J.C., Gallo, J., Cai, G., Tien, A., Romanoski, A., Lyketsos, C., and Chen L.S. (1997). Natural history of Diagnostic Interview Schedule/DSM-IV major depression. The Baltimore Epidemiologic Catchment Area follow-up. *Arch Gen Psychiatry*, 54, 993–999.

Egeland, J.A., Blumenthal, R.L., Nee, J., Sharpe, L., and Endicott, J. (1987a). Reliability and relationship of various ages of onset criteria for major affective disorder. *J Affect Disord*, 12(2), 159–165.

Ellicott, A.G. (1988). *A prospective study of stressful life events and bipolar illness.* Unpublished doctoral dissertation, University of California, Los Angeles.

Engstrom, C., Brandstrom, S., Sigvardsson, S., Cloninger, R., and Nylander, P.O. (2003). Bipolar disorder: II. Personality and age of onset. *Bipolar Disord*, 5(5), 340–348.

Ernst, C.L., and Goldberg, J.F. (2004). Clinical features related to age at onset in bipolar disorder. *J Affect Disord*, 82(1), 21–27.

Faedda, G.L., Tondo, L., Baldessarini, R.J., Suppes, T., and Tohen, M. (1993). Outcome after rapid vs. gradual discontinuation of lithium treatment in bipolar disorders. *Arch Gen Psychiatry*, 50(6), 448–455.

Faraone, S.V., Glatt, S.J., Su, J., and Tsuang, M.T. (2004). Three potential susceptibility loci shown by a genomic-wide scan for regions influencing the age at onset of mania. *Am J Psychiatry*, 161, 625–630.

Fisfalen, M.E., Schulze, T.G., DePaulo, J.R., DeGroot, L.J., Badner, J.A., and McMahon, F.J. (2005). Familial variation in episode frequency in bipolar affective disorder. *Am J Psychiatry*, 162(7), 1266–1272.

Fogarty, F., Russell, J.M., Newman, S.C., and Bland, R.C. (1994). Epidemiology of psychiatric disorders in Edmonton mania. *Acta Psychiatr Scand Suppl*, 376, 16–23.

France, R.D., and Krishnan, K.R. (1984). Alprazolam-induced manic reaction. *Am J Psychiatry*, 1127–1128.

Freinhar, J.P., and Alvarez, W.H. (1985b). Androgen-induced hypomania. Letter. *J Clin Psychiatry*, 46, 354–355.

Fujikawa, T., Yamawaki, S., and Touhouda, Y. (1995). Silent cerebral infarctions in patients with late-onset mania. *Stroke*, 26(6), 946–949.

Fukuda, K., Etoh, T., Iwadate, T., and Ishii, A. (1983). The course and prognosis of manic-depressive psychosis: A quantitative analysis of episodes and intervals. *Tohoku J Exp Med*, 139, 299–307.

Gabel, R.H., Barnard, N., Norko, M., and O'Connell, R.A. (1986). AIDS presenting as mania. *Compr Psychiatry*, 27, 251–254.

Geller, B., and Cook, E.H. Jr. (2000). Ultradian rapid cycling in prepubertal and early adolescent bipolarity is not in transmission disequilibrium with val/met COMT alleles. *Biol Psychiatry*, 47, 605–609.

Geller, B., Zimerman, B., Williams, M., Bolhofner, K., and Craney, J.L. (2001). Bipolar disorder at prospective follow-up of adults who had prepubertal major depressive disorder. *Am J Psychiatry*, 158, 125–127.

Geller, B., Tillman, R., Craney, J.L., and Bolhofner, K. (2004). Four-year prospective outcome and natural history of mania in children with a prepubertal and early adolescent bipolar disorder phenotype. *Arch Gen Psychiatry*, 61, 459–467.

Gershon, E.S., Hamovit, J., Guroff, J.J., Dibble, E., Leckman, J.F., Sceery, W., Targum, S.D., Nurnberger, J.I., Goldin, L.R., and Bunney, W.E. (1982). A family study of schizoaffective, bipolar I, bipolar II, unipolar, and normal control probands. *Arch Gen Psychiatry*, 39(10), 1157–1167.

Ghaemi, S.N., Sachs, G.S., Chiou, A.M., Pandurangi, A.K., and Goodwin, F.K. (1999). Is bipolar disorder still underdiagnosed? Are antidepressants overutilized? *J Affect Dis*, 52, 135–144.

Ghaemi, S.N., Boiman, E.E., and Goodwin, F.K. (2000). Diagnosing bipolar disorder and the effect of antidepressants: A naturalistic study. *J Clin Psychiatry*, 61, 804–808.

Gitlin, M.J., Swendsen, J., Heller, T.L., and Hammen, C. (1995). Relapse and impairment in bipolar disorder. *Am J Psychiatry*, 152(11), 1635–1640.

Gitlin, M., Boerlin, H., Fairbanks, L., and Hammen, C. (2003). The effect of previous mood states on switch rates: A naturalistic study. *Bipolar Disord*, 5(2), 150–152.

Glaser, G.H. (1953). Psychotic reactions induced by corticotropin (ACTH) and cortisone. *Psychosom Med*, 15, 280–291.

Glassner, B., and Haldipur, C.V. (1983). Life events and early and late onset of bipolar disorder. *Am J Psychiatry*, 140, 215–217.

Goggans, F.C. (1984). A case of mania secondary to vitamin B12 deficiency. *Am J Psychiatry*, 141, 300–301.

Goldberg, J.F. (2001). Spontaneous depression versus biphasic cycling. Letter to the editor. *Am J Psychiatry*, 158(2), 325–326.

Goldberg, J.F., and Harrow, M. (1994). Kindling in bipolar disorders: A longitudinal follow-up study. *Biol Psychiatry*, 35, 70–72.

Goldberg, J.F., and Harrow, M. (1999). *Bipolar disorders: Clinical course and outcome*. Washington, DC: American Psychiatric Press.

Goldberg, J.F., Harrow, M., and Grossman, L.S. (1995). Course and outcome in bipolar affective disorder: A longitudinal follow-up study. *American Journal of Psychiatry*, 152, 379–384.

Goldberg, J.F., Harrow, M., and Whiteside, J.E. (2001). Risk for bipolar illness in patients initially hospitalized for unipolar depression. *Am J Psychiatry*, 158, 1265–1270.

Goldberg, T.E., Gold, J.M., Greenberg, R., Griffin, S., Schulz, S.C., Pickar, D., Kleinman, J.E., and Weinberger, D.R. (1993).

Contrasts between patients with affective disorders and patients with schizophrenia on a neuropsychological test battery. *Am J Psychiatry*, 150, 1355–1362.

Goldstein, B.I., and Levitt, A.J. (2006). Further evidence for a developmental subtype of bipolar disorder defined by age at onset: Results from the national epidemiologic survey on alcohol and related conditions. *Am J Psychiatry*, 163(9), 1633–1636.

Goldstein, E.T., and Preskorn, S.H. (1989). Mania triggered by a steroid nasal spray in a patient with stable bipolar disorder. *Am J Psychiatry*, 146, 1076–1077.

Goodwin, F.K., and Ghaemi, S.N. (1998). Understanding manic-depressive illness. *Arch Gen Psychiatry*, 55(1), 23–25.

Goodwin, F.K., and Jamison, K.R. (1984). The natural course of manic-depressive illness. In R.M. Post, J.C. Ballenger (Eds.), *Neurobiology of mood disorders* (pp. 20–37). Baltimore: Williams & Wilkins.

Goolker, P., and Schein, J. (1953). Psychic effects of ACTH and cortisone. *Psychosom Med*, 15, 589–597.

Greenberg, D.B., and Brown, G.L. (1985). Mania resulting from brainstem tumor. *J Nerv Ment Dis*, 173, 434–436.

Grigoroiu-Serbanescu, M., Martinez, M., Nothen, M.M., Grinberg, M., Sima, D., Propping, P., Marinescu, E., and Hrestic, M. (2001). Different familial transmission patterns in bipolar I disorder with onset before and after age 25. *Am J Med. Genet*, 105, 765–773.

Grof, P., Alda, M., and Ahrens, B. (1995). Clinical course of affective disorders: Were Emil Kraepelin and Jules Angst wrong? *Psychopathology*, 28, 73–80.

Guttman, E., and Hermann, K. (1932). Ueber psychische Storungen bei Hirnstammerkrankungen und das Automatosesyndrom. *Z Ges Neurol Pscyhiatr*, 140, 439–472.

Guze, S.B., and Robins, E. (1970). Suicide and primary affective disorders. *Br J Psychiatry*, 117, 437–438.

Haghighat, R. (1996). Lifelong development of risk of recurrence in depressive disorders. *J Affect Disord*, 41(2), 141–147.

Harrow, M., Goldberg, J.F., Grossman, L.S., and Meltzer, H.Y. (1990). Outcome in manic disorders: A naturalistic follow-up study. *Arch Gen Psychiatry*, 47, 665–671.

Heila, H., Turpeinen, P., and Erkinjuntti, T. (1995). Case study: Mania associated with multiple sclerosis. *J Am Acad Child Adolesc Psychiatry*, 34(12), 1591–1595.

Hendrick, V., Altshuler, L.L., Gitlin, M.J., Delrahim, S., and Hammen, C. (2000). Gender and bipolar illness. *J Clin Psychiatry*, 61(5), 93–96; quiz 397.

Henry, C., Lacoste, J., Bellivier, F., Verdoux, H., Bourgeois, M.L., and Leboyer, M. (1999). Temperament in bipolar illness: Impact on prognosis. *J Affect Disord*, 56, 103–108.

Hlastala, S.A., Frank, E., Kowalski, J., Sherrill, J.T., Tu, X.M., Anderson, B., and Kupfer, D.J. (2000). Stressful life events, bipolar disorder, and the "kindling model." *J Abnorm Psychol*, 109, 777–786.

Honig, A., Hendriks, C.H., Akkerhuis, G.W., and Nolen, W.A. (2001). Usefulness of the retrospective Life-Chart method manual in outpatients with a mood disorder: A feasibility study. *Patient Educ Couns*, 43(1), 43–48.

Horrigan, J.P., and Barnhill, L.J. (1999). Guanfacine and secondary mania in children. *J Affect Disord*, 54(3), 309–314.

Hoyer, E.H., Mortensen, P.B., and Olesen, A.V. (2000). Mortality and causes of death in a total national sample of patients with affective disorders admitted for the first time between 1973 and 1993. *Br J Psychiatry*, 176, 76–82.

Hubain, P.P., Sobolski, J., and Mendlewicz, J. (1982). Cimetidine-induced mania. *Neuropsychobiology*, 8, 223–224.

Huber, M.T., Braun, H.A., and Krieg, J.C. (2001). On the impact of episode sensitization on the course of recurrent affective disorders. *J Psychiatr Res*, 35, 49–57.

Hunt, N., Bruce-Jones, W., and Silverstone, T. (1992). Life events and relapse in bipolar affective disorder. *J Affect Disord*, 25(1), 13–20.

Hyun, M., Friedman, S.D., and Dunner, D.L. (2000). Relationship of childhood physical and sexual abuse to adult bipolar disorder. *Bipolar Disord*, 2, 131–135.

Jackson, A., Cavanagh, J., and Scott, J. (2003). A systematic review of manic and depressive prodromes. *J Affect Disord*, 74(3), 209–217.

Jackson, S.L. (1957). Psychosis due to isoniazid. *Br Med J*, 2, 743–746.

Jacobson, J.E. (1965). The hypomanic alert: A program designed for greater therapeutic control. *Am J Psychiatry*, 122, 295–299.

Jampala, V.C., and Abrams, R. (1983). Mania secondary to left and right hemisphere damage. *Am J Psychiatry*, 140, 1197–1199.

Johnson, F.Y., and Naraqi, S. (1993). Manic episode secondary to cryptococcal meningitis in a previously healthy adult. *P N G Med J*, 36(1), 59–62.

Johnson, L., Andersson-Lundman, G., Aberg-Wistedt, A., and Mathe, A.A. (2000). Age of onset in affective disorder: Its correlation with hereditary and psychosocial factors. *J Affect Disord*, 59, 139–148.

Johnson, S.L., and Miller, I. (1997). Negative life events and time to recovery from episodes of bipolar disorder. *J Abnorm Psychol*, 106, 449–457.

Jorge, R.E., Robinson, R.G., Starkstein, S.E., Arndt, S.V., Forrester, A.W., and Geisler, F.H. (1993). Secondary mania following traumatic brain injury. *Am J Psychiatry*, 150(6), 916–921.

Judd, L.L., Akiskal, H.S., Maser, J.D., Zeller, P.J., Endicott, J., Coryell, W., Paulus, M.P., Kunovac, J.L., Leon, A.C., Mueller, T.I., Rice, J.A., and Keller, M.B. (1998). A prospective 12-year study of subsyndromal and syndromal depressive symptoms in unipolar major depressive disorders. *Arch Gen Psychiatry*, 55(8), 694–700.

Judd, L.L., Akiskal, H.S., Schettler, P.J., Endicott, J., Maser, J., Solomon, D.A., Leon, A.C., Rice, J.A., and Keller, M.B. (2002). The long-term natural history of the weekly symptomatic status of bipolar I disorder. *Arch Gen Psychiatry*, 59(6), 530–537.

Judd, L.L., Akiskal, H.S., Schettler, P.J., Coryell, W., Maser, J., Rice, J.A., Solomon, D.A., and Keller, M.B. (2003). The comparative clinical phenotype and long term longitudinal episode course of bipolar I and II: A clinical spectrum or distinct disorders? *J Affect Disord*, 73(1–2), 19–32.

Kadrmas, A., Winokur, G., and Crowe, R. (1979). Postpartum mania. *Br J Psychiatry*, 135, 551–554.

Kallner, G., Lindelius, R., Petterson, U., Stockman, O., and Tham, A. (2000). Mortality in 497 patients with affective disorders attending a lithium clinic or after having left it. *Pharmacopsychiatry*, 33, 8–13.

Kanai, T., Takeuchi, H., Furukawa, T.A., Yoshimura, R., Imaizumi, T., Kitamura, T., and Takahashi, K. (2003). Time to recurrence after recovery from major depressive episodes and its predictors. *Psychol Med*, 33(5), 839–845.

Kane, F.J., and Taylor, T.W. (1963). Mania associated with the use of INH and cocaine. *Am J Psychiatry*, 119, 1098–1099.

Kay, J.H., Altshuler, L.L., Ventura, J., and Mintz, J. (2002). Impact of axis II comorbidity on the course of bipolar illness in men: A retrospective chart review. *Bipolar Disord*, 4(4), 237–242.

Keck, P.E. Jr., McElroy, S.L., Strakowski, S.M., West, S.A., Hawkins, J.M., Huber, T.J., Newman, R.M., and DePriest, M. (1995). Outcome and comorbidity in first- compared with multiple-episode mania. *J Nerv Ment Dis*, 183, 320–324.

Keck, P.E. Jr., McElroy, S.L., Strakowski, S.M., West, S.A., Sax, K.W., Hawkins, J.M., Bourne, M.L., and Haggard, P. (1998). 12-Month outcome of patients with bipolar disorder following hospitalization for a manic or mixed episode. *Am J Psychiatry*, 155, 646–652.

Keck, P.E. Jr., McElroy, S.L., Havens, J.R., Altshuler, L.L., Nolen, W.A., Frye, M.A., Suppes, T., Denicoff, K.D., Kupka, R., Leverich, G.S., Rush, A.J., and Post, R.M. (2003). Psychosis in bipolar disorder: Phenomenology and impact on morbidity and course of illness. *Compr Psychiatry*, 44, 263–269.

Keitner, G.I., Solomon, D.A., Ryan, C.E., Miller, I.W., Mallinger, A., Kupfer, D.J., and Frank, E. (1996). Prodromal and residual symptoms in bipolar I disorder. *Comprehensive Psychiatry*, 37, 362–367.

Keller, M.B., and Boland, R.J. (1998). Implications of failing to achieve successful long-term maintenance treatment of recurrent unipolar major depression. *Biol Psychiatry*, 44(5), 348–360.

Keller, M.B., Shapiro, R.W., Lavori, P.W., and Wolfe, N. (1982). Relapse in major depressive disorder: Analysis with the life table. *Arch Gen Psychiatry*, 39, 911–915.

Keller, M.B., Lavori, P.W., Endicott, J., Coryell, W., and Klerman, G.L. (1983). "Double-depression": Two-year follow-up. *Am J Psychiatry*, 140, 689–694.

Keller, M.B., Lavori, P.W., Friedman, B., Nielsen, E., Endicott, J., McDonald-Scott, P., and Andreasen, N.C. (1987). The longitudinal interval follow-up evaluation: A comprehensive method for assessing outcome in prospective longitudinal studies. *Arch Gen Psychiatry*, 44(6), 540–548.

Keller, M.B., Lavori, P.W., Coryell, W., Endicott, J., and Mueller, T.I. (1993). Bipolar I: A five-year prospective follow-up. *J Nerv Ment Dis*, 181(4), 238–245.

Kendell, R.E., Wainwright, S., Hailey, A., and Shannon, B. (1976). Influence of childbirth on psychiatric morbidity. *Psychol Med*, 6, 297–302.

Kendell, R.E., Chalmers, J.C., and Platz, C. (1987). Epidemiology of puerperal psychoses. *Br J Psychiatry*, 150, 662–673.

Kendler, K.S., and Karkowski-Shuman, L. (1997). Stressful life events and genetic liability to major depression: Genetic control of exposure to the environment? *Psychol Med*, 27, 539–547.

Kendler, K.S., Thornton, L.M., and Gardner, C.O. (2000). Stressful life events and previous episodes in the etiology of major depression in women: An evaluation of the "kindling" hypothesis. *Am J Psychiatry*, 157(8), 1243–1251.

Kennedy, S., Thompson, R., Stancer, H.C., Roy, A., and Persad, E. (1983). Life events precipitating mania. *Br J Psychiatry*, 142, 398–403.

Kermani, E.J., Borod, J.C., Brown, P.H., and Tunnell, G. (1985). New psychopathologic findings in AIDS: Case report. *J Clin Psychiatry*, 46, 240–241.

Kessing, L.V. (1999). The effect of the first manic episode in affective disorder: A case register study of hospitalised episodes. *J Affect Disord*, 53, 233–239.

Kessing, L.V. (2006). Gender differences in subtypes of late-onset depression and mania. *Int Psychogeriatr*, 18, 727–738.

Kessing, L.V., and Andersen, P.K. (1999). The effect of episodes on recurrence in affective disorder: A case register study. *J Affect Disord*, 53, 225–231.

Kessing, L.V., Andersen, P.K., Mortensen, P.B., and Bolwig, T.G. (1998a). Recurrence in affective disorder: I. Case register study. *Br J Psychiatry*, 172, 23–28.

Kessing, L.V., Mortensen, P.B., and Bolwig, T.G. (1998b). Clinical consequences of sensitisation in affective disorder: A case register study. *J Affect Disord*, 47, 41–47.

Kessing, L.V., Andersen, P.K., and Mortensen, P.B. (1998c). Predictors of recurrence in affective disorder. A case register study. *J Affect Disord*, 49(2), 101–108.

Kessing, L.V., Hansen, M.G., Andersen, P.K., and Angst, J. (2004). The predictive effect of episodes on the risk of recurrence in depressive and bipolar disorders: A life-long perspective. *Acta Psychiatr Scand*, 109(5), 339–344.

Kessler, R.C., McGonagle, K.A., Swartz, M., Blazer, D.G., and Nelson, C.B. (1993). Sex and depression in the National Comorbidity Survey. I: Lifetime prevalence, chronicity and recurrence. *J Affect Disord*, 29(2-3), 85–96.

Khanna, R., Gupta, N., and Shanker, S. (1992). Course of bipolar disorder in eastern India. *J Affect Disord*, 24(1), 35–41.

Kirov, G., Murphy, K.C., Arranz, M.J., Jones, I., McCandless, F., Kunugi, H., Murray, R.M., McGuffin, P., Collier, D.A., Owen, M.J., and Craddock, N. (1998). Low activity allele of catechol-O-methyltransferase gene associated with rapid cycling bipolar disorder. *Mol Psychiatry*, 3(4), 342–345.

Klein, D.N., Taylor, E.B., Harding, K., and Dickstein, S. (1988). Double depression and episodic major depression: Demographic, clinical, familial, personality, and socioenvironmental characteristics and short-term outcome. *Am J Psychiatry*, 145(10), 1226–1231.

Koehler-Troy, C., Strober, M., and Malenbaum, R. (1986). Methylphenidate-induced mania in a prepubertal child. *J Clin Psychiatry*, 47, 566–567.

Kogan, J.N., Otto, M.W., Bauer, M.S., Dennehy, E.B., Miklowitz, D.J., Zhang, H.W., Ketter, T., Rudorfer, M.V., Wisniewski, S.R., Thase, M.E., Calabrese, J., Sachs, G.S., and STEP-BD Investigators (2004). Demographic and diagnostic characteristics of the first 1000 patients enrolled in the Systematic Treatment Enhancement Program for Bipolar Disorder (STEP-BD). *Bipolar Disord*, 6(6), 460–469.

Koukopoulos, A., and Reginaldi, D. (1973). Does lithium prevent depressions by suppressing manias? *Int Pharmacopsychiatry*, 8, 152–158.

Koukopoulos, A., Reginaldi, D., Laddomada, P., Floris, G., Serra, G., and Tondo, L. (1980). Course of the manic-depressive cycle and changes caused by treatments. *Pharmakopsychiatr Neuropsychopharmakol*, 13, 156–167.

Koukopoulos, A., Caliari, B., Tundo, A., Minnai, G., Floris, G., Reginaldi, D., and Tondo, L. (1983). Rapid cyclers, temperament, and antidepressants. *Compr Psychiatry*, 24, 249–258.

Koukopoulos, A., Sni, G., Koukopoulos, A., and Girardi, P. (2000). Cyclicity and manic-depressive illness. In A. Marneros, J. Angst (Eds.), *Bipolar Disorders: 100 Years after Manic-depressive Insanity* (pp. 315–334). London, England: Kluwer Academic Publishers.

Kraepelin, E. (1921). *Manic-depressive Insanity and Paranoia*. Translated by R. M. Barclay. Edinburgh, Scotland: E & S Livingstone.

Krauthammer, C., and Klerman, G.L. (1978). Secondary mania: Manic syndromes associated with antecedent physical illness or drugs. *Arch Gen Psychiatry*, 35, 1333–1339.

Krishnan, K.R.R., Swartz, M.S., Larson, M.J., and Santoliquido, G. (1984). Funeral mania in recurrent bipolar affective disorders: Reports on three cases. *J Clin Psychiatry*, 45, 310–311.

Kulisevsky, J., Berthier, M.L., and Pujol, J. (1993). Hemiballismus and secondary mania following a right thalamic infarction. *Neurology*, 43(7), 1422–1424.

Kupfer, D.J., Frank, E., Grochocinski, V.J., Cluss, P.A., Houck, P.R., and Stapf, D.A. (2002). Demographic and clinical characteristics of individuals in a bipolar disorder case registry. *J Clin Psychiatry*, 63(2), 120–125.

Kupka, R.W., Luckenbaugh, D.A., Post, R.M., Suppes, T., Altshuler, L.L., Keck, P.E., Frye, M.A., Denicoff, K.D., Grunze, H., Leverich, G.S., McElroy, S.L., Walden, J., and Nolen, W.A. (2005). Comparison of rapid-cycling and non-rapid-cycling bipolar disorder based on prospective mood ratings in 539 outpatients. *Am J Psychiatry*, 162(7), 1273–1280.

Kwentus, J.A., Silverman, J.J., and Sprague, M. (1984). Manic syndrome after metrizamide myelography. *Am J Psychiatry*, 141, 700–702.

Labbate, L.A., and Holzgang, A.J. (1989). Manic syndrome after discontinuation of methyldopa. *Am J Psychiatry*, 146, 1075–1076.

Lat, J. (1973). The analysis of habituation. *Acta Neurobiol Exp (Warsz)*, 33(4), 771–789.

Lazare, A. (1979). Manic behavior. In A. Lazare (Ed.), *Outpatient Psychiatry: Diagnosis and Treatment* (pp. 261–264). Baltimore: Williams & Wilkins.

Leboyer, M., Henry, C., Paillere-Martinot, M.L., and Bellivier, F. (2005). Age at onset in bipolar affective disorders: A review. *Bipolar Disord*, 7(2), 111–118.

Lee, H.J., Kim, L., Joe, S.H., and Suh, K.Y. (2002). Effects of season and climate on the first manic episode of bipolar affective disorder in Korea. *Psychiatry Res*, 113(1–2), 151–159.

Lendvai, I., Saravay, S.M., and Steinberg, M.D. (1999). Creutzfeldt-Jakob disease presenting as secondary mania. *Psychosomatics*, 40(6), 524–525.

Leverich, G.S., Nolen, W.A., Rush, A.J., McElroy, S.L., Keck, P.E., Denicoff, K.D., Suppes, T., Altshuler, L.L., Kupka, R., Kramlinger, K.G., and Post, R.M. (2001). The Stanley Foundation Bipolar Treatment Outcome Network: I. Longitudinal methodology, *J Affect Disord*, 67(1–3), 33–44.

Liegghio, N.E., and Yeragani, Y.K. (1988). Buspirone-induced hypomania. *J Clin Psychopharmacol*, 8, 226–227.

Lin, P.I., McInnis, M.G., Potash, J.B., Willour, V., MacKinnon, D.F., DePaulo, J.R., and Zandi, P.P. (2006). Clinical correlates and familial aggregation of age at onset in bipolar disorder. *Am J Psychiatry*, 163(2), 240–246.

Lish, J.D., Gyulai, L., Resnick, S.M., Kirtland, A., Amsterdam, J.D., Whybrow, P.C., and Price, R.A. (1993). A family history study of rapid-cycling bipolar disorder. *Psychiatry Res*, 48(1), 37–46.

Lish, J.D., Dime-Meenan, S., Whybrow, P.C., Price, R.A., and Hirschfeld, R.M. (1994). The National Depressive and Manic-depressive Association (DMDA) survey of bipolar members. *J Affect Disord*, 31, 281–294.

Loranger, A.W., and Levine, P.M. (1978). Age at onset of bipolar affective illness. *Arch Gen Psychiatry*, 35(11), 1345–1348.

Lundquist, G. (1945). Prognosis and course in manic-depressive psychoses: A follow-up study of 319 first admissions. *Acta Psychiatr Neurol* (Suppl. 35), 1–96.

MacDonald, J.B. (1918). Prognosis in manic-depressive insanity. *J Nerv Ment Dis*, 17, 20–30.

Maj, M., Pirozzi, R., and Starace, F. (1989). Previous pattern of course of the illness as a predictor of response to lithium prophylaxis in bipolar patients. *J Affective Disord*, 17, 237–241.

Maj, M., Magliano, L., Pirozzi, R., Marasco, C., and Guarneri, M. (1994). Validity of rapid cycling as a course specifier for bipolar disorder. *Am J Psychiatry*, 151(7), 1015–1019.

Maj, M., Pirozzi, R., and Magliano, L. (1995). Nonresponse to re-instituted lithium prophylaxis in previously responsive bipolar patients: Prevalence and predictors. *Am J Psychiatry*, 152(12), 1810–1811.

Maj, M., Pirozzi, R., Magliano, L., and Bartoli, L. (2002). The prognostic significance of "switching" in patients with bipolar disorder: A 10-year prospective follow-up study. *Am J Psychiatry*, 159(10), 1711–1717.

Maj, M., Pirozzi, R., Magliano, L., and Bartoli, L. (2003). Agitated depression in bipolar I disorder: Prevalence, phenomenology, and outcome. *Am J Psychiatry*, 160(12), 2134–2140.

Mann, A.M., and Hutchinson, J.L. (1967). Manic reaction associated with procarbazine hydrochloride therapy of Hodgkin's disease. *Can Med Assoc J*, 97, 1350–1353.

Mantere, O., Suominen, K., Leppamaki, S., Valtonen, H., Arvilommi, P., and Isometa, E. (2004). The clinical characteristics of DSM-IV bipolar I and II disorders: Baseline findings from the Jorvi Bipolar Study (JoBS). *Bipolar Disorders*, 6, 395–405.

Marneros, A., Deister, A., and Rohde, A. (1990). The concept of distinct but voluminous groups of bipolar and unipolar diseases: III. Bipolar and unipolar comparison. *Eur Arch Psychiatry Clin Neurosci*, 240(2), 90–95.

Maurizi, C.P. (1985). Influenza and mania: A possible connection with the locus ceruleus. *South Med J*, 78, 207–209.

Maxwell, S., Scheftner, W.A., Kessler, H.A., and Busch, K. (1988). Manic syndrome associated with zidovudine. *JAMA*, 259, 3406–3407.

McClellan, J., Breiger, D., McCurry, C., and Hlastala, S.A. (2003). Premorbid functioning in early-onset psychotic disorders. *J Am Acad Child Adolesc Psychiatry*, 42, 666–672.

McElroy, S.L., Strakowski, S.M., Keck, P.E. Jr., Tugrul, K.L., West, S.A., and Lonczak, H.S. (1995). Differences and similarities in mixed and pure mania. *Compr Psychiatry*, 36(3), 187–194.

McElroy, S.L., Strakowski, S.M., West, S.A., Keck, P.E., and McConville, B.J. (1997). Phenomenology of adolescent and adult mania in hospitalized patients with bipolar disorder. *Am J Psychiatry*, 154(1), 44–49.

McElroy, S.L., Altshuler, L.L., Suppes, T., Keck, P.E. Jr., Frye, M.A., Denicoff, K.D., Nolen, W.A., Kupka, R.W., Leverich, G.S., Rochussen, J.R., Rush, A.J., and Post, R.M. (2001). Axis I psychiatric comorbidity and its relationship to historical illness variables in 288 patients with bipolar disorder. *Am J Psychiatry*, 158(3), 420–426.

McGlashan, T.H. (1988). Adolescent versus adult onset of mania. *Am J Psychiatry*, 145(2), 221–223.

McKeown, S.P., and Jani, C.J. (1987). Mania following head injury. *Br J Pscyhiatry*, 151, 867–868.

McMahon, F.J., Stine, O.C., Chase, G.A., Meyers, D.A., Simpson, S.G., and DePaulo, J.R. (1994). Influence of clinical subtype, sex, and lineality on age at onset of major affective disorder in a family sample. *Am J Psychiatry*, 151(2), 210–215.

Mebane, A.H. (1984). L-Glutamine and mania. *Am J Psychiatry*, 141, 1302–1303.

Meeks, S. (1999). Bipolar disorder in the latter half of life: Symptom presentation, global functioning and age of onset. *J Affect Disord*, 52(1–3), 161–167.

Mendlewicz, J., Fieve, R.R., Rainer, J., and Fleiss, J.L. (1972a). Manic-depressive illness: A comparative study of patients with and without a family history. *Br J Psychiatry*, 120, 523–530.

Meyer, S.E., Carlson, G.A., Wiggs, E.A., Ronsaville, D.S., Martinez, P.E., Klimes-Dougan, B., Gold, P.W., and Radke-Yarrow, M. (2006). A prospective high-risk study of the association among maternal negativity, apparent frontal lobe dysfunction, and the development of bipolar disorder. *Dev Psychopathol*, 18(2), 573–589.

Mick, E., Biederman, J., Faraone, S.V., Murray, K., and Wozniak, J. (2003). Defining a developmental subtype of bipolar disorder in a sample of nonreferred adults by age at onset. *J Child Adolesc Psychopharmacol*, 13, 453–462.

Mijch, A.M., Judd, F.K., Lyketsos, C.G., Ellen, S., and Cockram, A. (1999). Secondary mania in patients with HIV infection: Are antiretrovirals protective? *J Neuropsychiatry Clin Neurosci*, 11(4), 475–480.

Molnar, G.J., Feeney, M.G., and Fava, G.A. (1988). Duration and symptoms of bipolar prodromes. *Am J Psychiatry*, 145, 1576–1578.

Moore, G.J., Bebchuk, J.M., Wilds, I.B., Chen, G., and Manji, H.K. (2000). Lithium-induced increase in human brain grey matter. Letter. *Lancet*, 356(9237), 1241–1242.

Morris, R. (2002). Clinical importance of inter-episode symptoms in patients with bipolar affective disorder. *J Affect Disord*, 72(Suppl. 1), S3–S13.

Morselli, P.L., Elgie, R., and Cesana, B.M. (2004). GAMIAN-Europe/BEAM survey II: Cross-national analysis of unemployment, family history, treatment satisfaction and impact of the bipolar disorder on life style. *Bipolar Disord*, 6(6), 487–497.

Mueller, T.I., Leon, A.C., Keller, M.B., Solomon, D.A., Endicott, J., Coryell, W., Warshaw, M., and Maser, J.D. (1999). Recurrence after recovery from major depressive disorder during 15 years of observational follow-up. *Am J Psychiatry*, 156, 1000–1006.

Muller-Oerlinghausen, B., Wolf, T., Ahrens, B., Glaenz, T., Schou, M., Grof, E., Grof, P., Lenz, G., Simhandl, C., Thau, K., Vestergaard, P., and Wolf R. (1996). Mortality of patients who dropped out from regular lithium prophylaxis: A collaborative study by the International Group for the Study of Lithium-treated patients (IGSLI). *Acta Psychiatr Scand*, 94, 344–347.

Muncie, W. (1934). Postoperative states of excitement. *Arch Neurol Psychiatry*, 34, 681–703.

Nierenberg, A.A., Miyahara, S., Spencer, T., Wisniewski, S.R., Otto, M.W., Simon, N., Pollack, M.H., Ostacher, M.J., Yan, L., Siegel, R., and Sachs, G.S. (2005). Clinical and diagnostic implications of lifetime attention-deficit/hyperactivity disorder comorbidity in adults with bipolar disorder: Data from the first 1000 STEP-BD participants. *Biol Psychiatry*, 57(11), 1467–1473.

Nolen, W.A., Luckenbaugh, D.A., Altshuler, L.L., Suppes, T., McElroy, S.L., Frye, M.A., Kupka, R.W., Keck, P.E. Jr., Leverich, G.S., and Post, R.M. (2004). Correlates of 1-year prospective outcome in bipolar disorder: Results from the Stanley Foundation Bipolar Network. *Am J Psychiatry*, 161(8), 1447–1454.

Nurnberger, J.I. Jr., Guroff, J.J., Hamovit, J., Berrettini, W., and Gershon, E.S. (1988b). A family study of rapid-cycling bipolar illness. *J Affective Disord*, 15, 87–91.

O'Brien, C.P., DiGiacomo, J.N., and Fahn, S. (1971). Mental effects of high-dosage levodopa. *Arch Gen Psychiatry*, 24, 61–64.

O'Connell, R.A., Mayo, J.A., Flatow, L., Cuthbertson, B., and O'Brien, B.E. (1991). Outcome of bipolar disorder on long-term treatment with lithium. *Br J Psychiatry*, 159, 123–129.

O'Dowd, M.A., and McKegney, F.P. (1988). Manic syndrome associated with zidovudine. *JAMA*, 260, 3587.

Oepen, G., Baldessarini, R.J., Salvatore, P., and Slater, E. (2004). On the periodicity of manic-depressive insanity, by Eliot Slater (1938): Translated excerpts and commentary. *J Affect Disord*, 78(1), 1–9.

Okuma, T., and Shimoyama, N. (1972). Course of endogenous manic-depressive psychosis, precipitating factors and pre-morbid personality: A statistical study. *Folia Psychiatr Neurol Japonica*, 26, 19–33.

Oppler, W. (1950). Manic psychosis in a case of parasagittal meningioma. *Arch Neurol Psychiatry*, 64, 417–430.

Osby, U., Brandt, L., Correia, N., Ekbom, A., Sparen, P. (2001). Excess mortality in bipolar and unipolar disorder in Sweden. *Arch Gen Psychiatry*, 8, 44–50.

Papolos, D.F., Veit, S., Faedda, G.L., Saito, T., and Lachman, H.M. (1998). Ultra-ultra rapid cycling bipolar disorder is associated with the low activity catecholamine-O-methyltransferase allele. *Mol Psychiatry*, 3(4), 346–349.

Patel, N.C., Delbello, M.P., and Strakowski, S.M. (2006). Ethnic differences in symptom presentation of youths with bipolar disorder. *Bipolar Disord*, 8(1), 95–99.

Perlis, R.H., Miyahara, S., Marangell, L.B., Wisniewski, S.R., Ostacher, M., DelBello, M.P., Bowden, C.L., Sachs, G.S., Nierenberg, A.A., and STEP-BD Investigators. (2004). Long-term implications of early onset in bipolar disorder: Data from the first 1000 participants in the Systematic Treatment Enhancement Program for Bipolar Disorder (STEP-BD). *Biol Psychiatry*, 55, 875–881.

Perris, C. (1968). The course of depressive psychoses. *Acta Psychiatr Scand*, 44, 238–248.

Perris, C., and d'Elia, G. (1966). A study of bipolar (manic-depressive) and unipolar recurrent depressive psychoses: X. Mortality, suicide, and life cycles. *Acta Psychiatr Scand*, 42(Suppl. 194), 172–183.

Perris, C., Eisemann, M., von Knorring, L., and Perris, H. (1984). Presentation of a subscale for the rating of depression and some additional items to the Comprehensive Psychopathological Rating Scale. *Acta Psychiatr Scand*, 70(3), 261–274.

Perugi, G., Micheli, C., Akiskal, H.S., Madaro, D., Socci, C., Quilici, C., and Musetti, L. (2000). Polarity of the first episode, clinical characteristics, and course of manic depressive illness: A systematic retrospective investigation of 320 bipolar I patients. *Compr Psychiatry*, 41, 13–18.

Pollock, H.M. (1931). Recurrence of attacks in manic-depressive psychoses. *Am J Psychiatry*, 11, 568–573.

Pope, H.G., and Katz, D.L. (1988). Affective and psychotic symptoms associated with anabolic steroid use. *Am J Psychiatry*, 145, 487–490.

Post, R.M. (1990). Sensitization and kindling perspectives for the course of affective illness: Toward a new treatment with the anticonvulsant carbamazepine. *Pharmacopsychiatry*, 23, 3–17.

Post, R.M., and Weiss, S.R. (1989). Sensitization, kindling, and anticonvulsants in mania. *J Clin Psychiatry*, 50(Suppl.), 23–30; discussion 45–47.

Post, R.M., Rubinow, D.R., Ballenger, J.C. (1986a). Conditioning and sensitisation in the longitudinal course of affective illness. *Br J Psychiatry*, 149, 191–201.

Post, R.M., Roy-Byrne, P.P., and Uhde, T.W. (1988). Graphic representation of the life course of illness in patients with affective disorder. *Am J Psychiatry*, 145(7), 844–848.

Post, R.M., Weiss, S.R., Smith, M., Rosen, J., and Frye, M. (1995). Stress, conditioning, and the temporal aspects of affective disorders. *Ann N Y Acad Sci*, 771, 677–696.

Post, R.M., Leverich, G.S., Xing, G., and Weiss, R.B. (2001). Developmental vulnerabilities to the onset and course of bipolar disorder. *Dev Psychopathol*, 13(3), 581–598.

Post, R.M., Leverich, G.S., Altshuler, L.L., Frye, M.A., Suppes, T.M., Keck, P.E. Jr., McElroy, S.L., Kupka, R., Nolen, W.A., Grunze, H., and Walden, J. (2003). An overview of recent findings of the Stanley Foundation Bipolar Network (Part I). *Bipolar Disord*, 5(5), 310–319.

Price, W.A., and Bielefeld, M. (1989). Buspirone-induced mania. *J Clin Psychopharmacol*, 9, 150–151.

Rego, M.D., and Giller, E.L. (1989). Mania secondary to amantadine treatment of neuroleptic-induced hyperprolactinemia. *J Clin Psychiatry*, 50, 143–144.

Reich, T., and Winokur, G. (1970). Postpartum psychoses in patients with manic depressive disease. *J Nerv Ment Dis*, 151, 60–68.

Reichart, C.G., van der Ende, J., Wals, M., Hillegers, M.H., Ormel, J., Nolen, W.A., and Verhulst, F.C. (2004). The use of the GBI in a population of adolescent offspring of parents with a bipolar disorder. *J Affect Disord*, 80(2–3), 263–267.

Reichenberg, A., Weiser, M., Rabinowitz, J., Caspi, A., Schmeidler, J., Mark, M., Kaplan, Z., and Davidson, M. (2002). A population-based cohort study of premorbid intellectual, language, and behavioral functioning in patients with schizophrenia, schizoaffective disorder, and nonpsychotic bipolar disorder. *Am J Psychiatry*, 159(12), 2027–2035.

Rennie, T.A.C. (1942). Prognosis in manic-depressive psychoses. *Am J Psychiatry*, 98, 801–814.

Revicki, D.A., Matza, L.S., Flood, E., and Lloyd, A. (2005). Bipolar disorder and health-related quality of life: Review of burden of disease and clinical trials. *Pharmacoeconomics*, 23(6), 583–594.

Rigby, J., Harvey, M., and Davies, D.R. (1989). Mania precipitated by benzodiazepine withdrawal. *Acta Psychiatr Scan*, 79, 406–407.

Rosenbaum, A.H., and Barry, M.J. (1975). Positive therapeutic response to lithium in hypomania secondary to organic brain syndrome. *Am J Psychiatry*, 132, 1072–1073.

Rousseva, A., Henry, C., van den Bulke, D., Fournier, G., Laplanche, J.L., Leboyer, M., Bellivier, F., Aubry, J.M., Baud, P., Boucherie, M., Buresi, C., Ferrero, F., and Malafosse, A. (2003). Antidepressant-induced mania, rapid cycling and the serotonin transporter gene polymorphism. *Pharmacogenomics J*, 3(2), 101–104.

Roy-Byrne, P., Post, R., Uhde, T., Porcu, T., and Davis, D. (1985a). The longitudinal course of recurrent affective illness: Life chart data from research patients at the NIMH. *Acta Psychiatr Scand*, 71, 1–34.

Ryback, R.S., and Schwab, R.S. (1971). Manic response to levodopa therapy: Report of a case. *N Engl J Med*, 285, 788–789.

Salazar-Calderon Perriggo, V.H., Oommen, K.J., and Sobonya, R.E. (1993). Silent solitary right parietal chondroma resulting in secondary mania. *Clin Neuropathol*, 12(6), 325–329.

Saran, B.M. (1970). The course of recurrent depressive illness in selected patients from a defined population. *Int Pharmacopsychiatry*, 5, 119–131.

Sax, K.W., Strakowski, S.M., Keck, P.E., McElroy, S.L., West, S.A., Bourne, M.L., and Larson, E.R. (1997). Comparison of patients with early-, typical-, and late-onset affective psychosis. *Am J Psychiatry*, 154(9), 1299–1301.

Sayed, A.J. (1976). Mania and bromism: A case report and a look to the future. *Am J Psychiatry*, 133, 228–229.

Schaerf, F.W., Miller, R., Pearlson, G.D., Kaminsky, M.J., and Weaver, D. (1988). Manic syndrome associated with zidovudine. *JAMA*, 260, 3587–3588.

Schulze, T.G., Muller, D.J., Krauss, H., Gross, M., Fangerau-Lefevre, H., Illes, F., Ohlraun, S., Cichon, S., Held, T., Propping, P., Nothen, M.M., Maier, W., and Rietschel, M. (2002). Further evidence for age of onset being an indicator for severity in bipolar disorder. *J Affect Disord*, 68(2–3), 343–345.

Schurhoff, F., Bellivier, F., Jouvent, R., Mouren-Simeoni, M.C., Bouvard, M., Allilaire, J.F., and Leboyer, M. (2000). Early and late onset bipolar disorders: Two different forms of manic-depressive illness? *J Affect Disord*, 58(3), 215–221.

Schwartz, R.B. (1974). Manic psychosis in connection with Q-fever. *Br J Psychiatry*, 124, 140–143.

Sharma, R., and Markar, H.R. (1994). Mortality in affective disorder. *J Affect Disord*, 31(2), 91–96.

Shulman, K., and Post, F. (1980). Bipolar affective disorder in old age. *Br J Psychiatry*, 136, 26–32.

Sierra, P., Livianos, L., and Rojo, L. (2005). Quality of life for patients with bipolar disorder: Relationship with clinical and demographic variables. *Bipolar Disord*, 7(2), 159–165.

Skop, B.P., and Masterson, B.J. (1995). Mania secondary to lisinopril therapy. *Psychosomatics*, 36(5), 508–509.

Slater, E. (1938a). Zur periodik des manische-depressiven irreseins. *Ztschr Neurol Psychiatr*, 162, 794–801.

Smeraldi, E., Gasperini, M., Macciardi, F., Bussoleni, C., and Morabito, A. (1982–1983). Factors affecting the distribution of age at onset in patients with affective disorders. *J Psychiatr Res*, 17(3), 309–317.

Sotsky, S.M., and Tossell, J.W. (1984). Tolmetin induction of mania. *Psychosomatics*, 25, 626–628.

Spencer, T.J., Biederman, J., Wozniak, J., Faraone, S.V., Wilens, T.E., and Mick, E. (2001). Parsing pediatric bipolar disorder from its associated comorbidity with the disruptive behavior disorder. *Biol Psychiatry*, 49(12), 1062–1070.

Spicer, C.C., Hare, E.H., and Slater, E. (1973). Neurotic and psychotic forms of depressive illness: Evidence from age-incidence in a national sample. *Br J Psychiatry*, 123, 535–541.

Staner, L., Tracy, A., Dramaix, M., Genevrois, C., Vanderelst, M., Vilane, A., Bauwens, F., Pardoen, D., and Mendlewicz, J. (1997). Clinical and psychosocial predictors of recurrence in recovered bipolar and unipolar depressives: A one-year controlled prospective study. *Psychiatry Res*, 69, 39–51.

Steinberg, D., Hirsch, S.R., Marston, S.D., Reynolds, K., and Sutton, R.N. (1972). Influenza infection causing manic psychosis. *Br J Psychiatry*, 120, 531–535.

Stenstedt, Å. (1952). A study in manic-depressive psychosis: Clinical, social, and genetic investigations. *Acta Psychiatr et Neurol* (Suppl. 79), 1–111.

Stephens, J.H., and McHugh, P.R. (1991). Characteristics and long-term follow-up of patients hospitalized for mood disorders in the Phipps Clinic, 1913–1940. *J Nerv Ment Dis*, 179, 64–73.

Stern, K., and Dancey, T. (1942). Giloma of the diencephalon in a manic patient. *Am J Psychiatry*, 98, 716.

Stone, K. (1989). Mania in the elderly. *Br J Psychiatry*, 155, 220–224.

Strakowski, S.M., Sax, K.W., McElroy, S.L., Keck, P.E. Jr., Hawkins, J.M., and West, S.A. (1998). Course of psychiatric and substance abuse syndromes co-occurring with bipolar disorder after a first psychiatric hospitalization. *J Clin Psychiatry*, 59(9), 465–471.

Strakowski, S.M., DelBello, M.P., Adler, C., Cecil, D.M., and Sax, K.W. (2000). Neuroimaging in bipolar disorder. *Bipolar Disord*, 2(3 Pt. 1), 148–164.

Strakowski, S.M., DelBello, M.P., Zimmerman, M.E., Getz, G.E., Mills, N.P., Ret, J., Shear, P., and Adler, C.M. (2002). Ventricular and periventricular structural volumes in first- versus multiple-episode bipolar disorder. *Am J Psychiatry*, 159(11), 1841–1847.

Sultzer, D.L., and Cummings, J.L. (1989). Drug-induced mania—Causative agents, clinical characteristics and management: A retrospective analysis of the literature. *Med Toxicol Adverse Drug Exper*, 4, 127–143.

Suppes, T., Leverich, G.S., Keck, P.E., Nolen, W.A., Denicoff, K.D., Altshuler, L.L., McElroy, S.L., Rush, A.J., Kupka, R., Frye, M.A., Bickel, M., and Post R.M. (2001). The Stanley Foundation Bipolar Treatment Outcome Network: II. Demographics and illness characteristics of the first 261 patients. *J Affect Disord*, 67(1–3), 45–59.

Swann, A.C., Secunda, S.K., Stokes, P.E., Croughan, J., Davis, J.M., Koslow, S.H., Maas, J.W. (1990). Stress, depression, and mania: Relationship between perceived role of stressful events and clinical and biochemical characteristics. *Acta Psychiatr Scand*, 81(4), 389–397.

Swann, A.C., Janicak, P.L., Calabrese, J.R., Bowden, C.L., Dilsaver, S.C., Morris, D.D., Petty, F., and Davis, J.M. (2001). Structure of mania: Depressive, irritable, and psychotic clusters with different retrospectively-assessed course patterns of illness in randomized clinical trial participants. *J Affect Disord*, 67(1–3), 123–132.

Swift, H.M. (1907). The prognosis of recurrent insanity of manic-depressive type. *Am J Insanity*, 64, 311–326.

Taschev, T. (1974). The course and prognosis of depression on the basis of 652 patients deceased. In J. Angst (Ed.), *Classification and Prediction of Outcome of Depression* (pp. 157–172). Symposium Schloss Reinhartshausen/Rhein. Symposia Medica Hoeschst 8. Stuttgart: FK Schattauer.

Taylor, M.A., and Abrams, R. (1973a). Manic states: A genetic study of early and late onset affective disorders. *Arch Gen Psychiatry*, 28, 656–658.

Tham, A., Engelbrektson, K., Mathe, A.A., Johnson, L., Olsson, E., and Aberg-Wistedt, A. (1997). Impaired neuropsychological performance in euthymic patients with recurring mood disorders. *J Clin Psychiatry*, 58, 26–29.

Tohen, M., Waternaux, C.M., and Tsuang, M. (1990). Outcome in mania: A 4-year prospective follow-up of 75 patients utilizing survival analysis. *Arch Gen Psychiatry*, 47, 1106–1111.

Tohen, M., Stoll, A.L., Strakowski, S.M., Faedda, G.L., Mayer, P.V., Goodwin, D.C., Kolbrener, M.L., and Madigan, A.M. (1992). The McLean First-Episode Psychosis Project: Six-month recovery and recurrence outcome. *Schizophr Bull*, 18(2), 273–282.

Tohen, M., Shulman, K.I., and Satlin, A. (1994). First-episode mania in late life. *Am J Psychiatry*, 151(1), 130–132.

Tohen, M., Hennen, J., Zarate, C.J., Baldessarini, R., Strakowski, S., Stoll, A., Faedda, G., Suppes, T., Gebre-Medhin, A., and Cohen, B. (2000). The McLean first episode project: Two-year syndromal and functional recovery in 219 cases of major affective disorders with psychotic features. *Am J Psychiatry*, 157(2), 220–228.

Tohen, M., Zarate, C., Hennen, J., Khalsa, H.M., Strakowski, S.M., Gebre-Medhin, P., Salvatore, P., and Baldessarini, R.J. (2003). The McLean-Harvard First-Episode Mania Study: Prediction of recovery and first recurrence. *Am J Psychiatry*, 160(12), 2099–2107.

Tondo, L., Ghiani, C., and Albert, M. (2001). Pharmacologic interventions in suicide prevention. *J Clin Psychiatry*, 62(Suppl. 25), 51–55.

Tsai, S.J., Wang, Y.C., and Hong, C.J. (2001). Association study between cannabinoid receptor gene (CNR1) and pathogenesis and psychotic symptoms of mood disorders. *Am J Med Genet*, 105, 219–221.

Tsuang, M.T. (1978). Suicide in schizophrenics, manics, depressives and surgical controls: A comparison with general suicide mortality. *Arch Gen Psychiatry*, 35, 153–155.

Tsuang, M.T., Woolson, R., and Fleming, J.A. (1979). Long-term outcome of major psychoses: I. Schizophrenia and affective disorders compared with psychiatrically symptom-free surgical conditions. *Arch Gen Psychiatry*, 36, 1295–1301.

Tsuang, M.T., Woolson, R.F., and Fleming, J.A. (1980). Causes of death in schizophrenia and manic-depression. *Br J Psychiatry*, 136, 239–242.

Turvey, C.L., Coryell, W.H., Solomon, D.A., Leon, A.C., Endicott, J., Mueller, T., Keller, M., and Akiskal, H. (1999). Long-term prognosis of bipolar I disorder. *Acta Psychiatr Scand*, 99, 110–119.

van Gorp, W.G., Altshuler, L., Theberge, D.C., Wilkins, J., and Dixon, W. (1998). Cognitive impairment in euthymic bipolar patients with and without prior alcohol dependence: A preliminary study. *Arch Gen Psychiatry*, 55(1), 41–46.

van Os, J., Takei, N., Castle, D.J., Wessely, S., Der, G., and Murray, R.M. (1995). Premorbid abnormalities in mania, schizomania, acute schizophrenia and chronic schizophrenia. *Soc Psychiatry Psychiatr Epidemiol*, 30(6), 274–278.

Van Woert, M.H., Ambani, L.M., and Weintraub, M.I. (1971). Manic behavior and levodopa. *N Engl J Med*, 285, 1326.

Venkatarangam, S.H.M., Kutcher, S.P., and Notkin, R.M. (1988). Secondary mania with steroid withdrawal. *Can J Psychiatry*, 33, 631–632.

Verdoux, H., and Bourgeois, M. (1993). A comparison of manic patient subgroups. *J Affect Disord*, 27(4), 267–272.

Vieta, E., Gasto, C., Otero, A., Nieto, E., and Vallejo, J. (1997). Differential features between bipolar I and bipolar II disorder. *Compr Psychiatry*, 38(2), 98–101.

Viguera, A.C., and Cohen, L.S. (1998). The course and management of bipolar disorder during pregnancy. *Psychopharmacol Bull*, 34, 339–346.

Viguera, A.C., Cohen, L.S., Baldessarini, R.J., and Nonacs, R. (2002). Managing bipolar disorder during pregnancy: Weighing the risks and benefits. *Can J Psychiatry*, 47, 426–436.

Viswanathan, R., and Glickman, L. (1989). Clonazepam in the treatment of steroid-induced mania in a patient after renal transplantation. *N Engl J Med*, 320, 319–320.

Vocisano, C., Klein, D.N., Keefe, R., Dienst, E.R., and Kincaid, M.M. (1996). Demographics, family history, premorbid functioning, developmental characteristics, and course of patients with deteriorated affective disorder. *Am J Psychiatry*, 153(2), 248–255.

Vuilleumier, P., Ghika-Schmid, F., Bogousslavsky, J., Assal, G., and Regli, F. (1998). Persistent recurrence of hypomania and prosopoaffective agnosia in a patient with right thalamic infarct. *Neuropsychiatry Neuropsychol Behav Neurol*, 11(1), 40–44.

Walton, R.G. (1986). Seizure and mania after high intake of aspartame. *Psychosomatics*, 27, 218–220.

Waters, B.G.H., and Lapierre, Y.D. (1981). Secondary mania associated with sympathomimetic drug use. *Am J Psychiatry*, 138, 837–838.

Wehr, T.A., and Goodwin, F.K. (1979). Rapid cycling in manic-depressives induced by tricyclic antidepressants. *Arch Gen Psychiatry*, 36, 555–559.

Wehr, T.A., and Goodwin, F.K. (1987). Can antidepressants cause mania and worsen the course of affective illness? *Am J Psychiatry*, 144, 1403–1411.

Wehr, T.A., Sack, D.A., and Rosenthal, N.E. (1987a). Sleep reduction as a final common pathway in the genesis of mania. *Am J Psychiatry*, 144, 201–204.

Wehr, T.A., Sack, D.A., Rosenthal, N.E., and Cowdry, R.W. (1988). Rapid cycling affective disorder: Contributing factors and treatment responses in 51 patients. *Am J Psychiatry*, 145, 179–184.

Weilburg, J.B., Sachs, G., and Falk, W.E. (1987). Triazolam-induced brief episodes of secondary mania in a depressed patient. *J Clin Psychiatry*, 48, 492–493.

Weisert, K.N., and Hendrie, H.C. (1977). Secondary mania? A case report. *Am J Psychiatry*, 134, 929–930.

Weiss, R.D., Ostacher, M.J., Otto, M.W., Calabrese, J.R., Fossey, M., Wisniewski, S.R., Bowden, C.L., Nierenberg, A.A., Pollack, M.H., Salloum, I.M., Simon, N.M., Thase, M.E., and Sachs, G.S. (2005). Does recovery from substance use disorder matter in patients with bipolar disorder? *J Clin Psychiatry*, 66(6), 730–735.

Weiss, S.R., Post, R.M., Costello, M., Nutt, D.J., and Tandeciarz, S. (1990). Carbamazepine retards the development of cocaine-kindled seizures but not sensitization to cocaine-induced hyperactivity. *Neuropsychopharmacology*, 3, 273–281.

Weissman, M.M., Bland, R.C., Canino, G.J., Faravelli, C., Greenwald, S., Hwu, H.G., Joyce, P.R., Karam, E.G., Lee, C.K., Lellouch, J., Lepine, J.P., Newman, S.C., Rubio-Stipec, M., Wells, J.E., Wickramaratne, P.J., Wittchen, H., and Yeh, E.K. (1996). Cross-national epidemiology of major depression and bipolar disorder. *JAMA*, 276(4), 293–299.

Winokur, G. (1974). Genetic and clinical factors associated with course in depression. Contributions to genetic aspects. *Pharmakopsychiatr Neuropsychopharmakol*, 7(2), 122–126.

Winokur, G. (1975). The Iowa 500: Heterogeneity and course of manic-depressive illness (bipolar). *Compr Psychiatry*, 16, 125–131.

Winokur, G. (1976). Duration of illness prior to hospitalization (onset) in the affective disorders. *Neuropsychobiology*, 2, 87–93.

Winokur, G., and Kadrmas, A. (1989). A polyepisodic course in bipolar illness: Possible clinical relationships. *Compr Psychiatry*, 30, 121–127.

Winokur, G., and Tsuang, M. (1975b). The Iowa 500: Suicide in mania, depression, and schizophrenia. *Am J Psychiatry*, 132, 650–651.

Winokur, G., Clayton, P.J., and Reich, T. (1969). *Manic depressive illness.* St. Louis: CV Mosby.

Winokur, G., Coryell, W., Keller, M., Endicott, J., and Akiskal, H. (1993). A prospective follow-up of patients with bipolar and primary unipolar affective disorder. *Arch Gen Psychiatry,* 50(6), 457–465.

Wright, J.M., Sachdev, P.S., Perkins, R.J., and Rodriguez, P. (1989). Zidovudine-related mania. *Med J Aust,* 150, 339–341.

Wylie, M.E., Mulsant, B.H., Pollock, B.G., Sweet, R.A., Zubenko, G.S., Begley, A.E., Gregor, M., Frank, E., Reynolds, C.F., and Kupfer, D.J. (1999). Age at onset in geriatric bipolar disorder. Effects on clinical presentation and treatment outcomes in an inpatient sample. *Am J Psychiatry,* 7(1), 77–83.

Yassa, R., Nair, V., Nastase, C., Camille, Y., and Belzile, L. (1988a). Prevalence of bipolar disorder in a psychogeriatric population. *J Affect Disord,* 14(3), 197–201.

Yatham, L.N., Lecrubier, Y., Fieve, R.R., Davis, K.H., Harris, S.D., and Krishnan, A.A. (2004). Quality of life in patients with bipolar I depression: Data from 920 patients. *Bipolar Disord,* 6(5), 379–385.

Zis, A.P., and Goodwin, F.K. (1979). Major affective disorder as a recurrent illness: A critical review. *Arch Gen Psychiatry,* 36, 835–839.

Zis, A.P., Grof, P., and Goodwin, F.K. (1979). The natural course of affective disorders: Implications for lithium prophylaxis. In T.B. Cooper, S. Gershon, N.S. Kline, and M. Schou (Eds.), *Lithium: Controversies and Unresolved Issues* (pp. 381–398). Amsterdam: Exerpta Medica.

Zis, A.P., Grof, P., Webster, M., and Goodwin, F.K. (1980). Prediction of relapse in recurrent affective disorder. *Psychopharmacol Bull,* 16, 47–49.

CHAPTER 5

Aalto-Setälä, T., Marttunen, M., Tuulio-Henriksson, A., Poikolainen, K., and Lönnqvist, J. (2001). One-month prevalence of depression and other DSM-IV disorders among young adults. *Psychol Med,* 31, 791–801.

Abood, Z., Sharkey, A., Webb, M., Kelly, A., and Gill, M. (2002). Are patients with bipolar affective disorder socially disadvantaged? A comparison with a control group. *Bipolar Disorders,* 4, 243–248.

Achenbach, T.M. (1991a). *Manual for the Child Behavior Checklist/4-18 and 1991 Profile.* Burlington, MA: University of Vermont Department of Psychiatry.

Achenbach, T.M. (1991b). *Integrative Guide for the 1991 CBCL/8-14, YSR and TRF profile.* Burlington, MA: University of Vermont Department of Psychiatry.

Ahrens, B., Berghofer, A., Wolf, T., and Muller-Oerlinghausen, B. (1995). Suicide attempts, age and duration of illness in recurrent affective disorders. *J Affect Disord,* 36(1–2), 43–49.

Akiskal, H.S. (1995). Developmental pathways to bipolarity: Are juvenile onset depressions pre-bipolar? *J Am Acad Child Adolesc Psychiatry,* 34, 754–763.

Akiskal, H.S. (1996). The prevalent clinical spectrum of bipolar disorders: Beyond DSM-IV. *J Clin Psychopharmacol,* 16, 4S–14S.

Akiskal, H.S., Bourgeois, M.L., Angst, J., Post, R., Möller, H-J., and Hirschfeld, R. (2000). Re-evaluating the prevalence of and diagnostic composition within the broad clinical spectrum of bipolar disorders. *J Affect Disord,* 59, S5–S30.

American Psychiatric Association. (1980). *Diagnostic and Statistical Manual of Mental Disorders.* 3rd ed. Washington, DC: American Psychiatric Association.

American Psychiatric Association. (1986). *Diagnostic and Statistical Manual of Mental Disorders.* 3rd ed., revised. Washington, DC: American Psychiatric Association.

American Psychiatric Association. (1994). *Diagnostic and Statistical Manual of Mental Disorders.* 4th ed. Washington, DC: American Psychiatric Association.

Andrade, L., Walters, E.E., Gentil, V., and Laurenti, R. (2002). Prevalence of ICD-10 mental disorders in a catchment area in the city of São Paulo, Brazil. *Soc Psychiat Psychiatric Epidemiol,* 37, 316–325.

Andreason, N.C. (1982). Negative symptoms in schizophrenia. *Arch Gen Psychiatry,* 39, 784–788.

Andrews, G., Sanderson, K., and Beard, J. (1998). Burden of disease: Methods of calculating disability from mental disorder. *Brit J Psychiatry,* 173, 123–131.

Angold, A. (1988). Childhood and adolescent depression: II. Research in clinical populations. *Br J Psychiatry,* 153, 476–492.

Angold, A., Costello, E.J., Worthman, C.M. (1998). Puberty and depression: The roles of age, pubertal status and pubertal timing. *Psychol Med,* 28, 51–61.

Angold, A., Costello, E.J., Erkanli, A., and Worthman, C.M. (1999). Pubertal changes in hormone levels and depression in girls. *Psychol Med,* 29, 1043–1053.

Angst, J. (1978). The course of affective disorders: II. Typology of bipolar manic-depressive illness. *Arch Psychiatr Nervenkr,* 226, 65–73.

Angst, J. (1995). Epidemiologie du spectre bipolarie. *L'Encephale,* 6, 37–42.

Angst, J. (1998). The emerging epidemiology of hypomania and bipolar II disorder. *J Affect Disord,* 50, 143–151.

Angst, J., and Gamma, A. (2002). Prevalence of bipolar disorders: Traditional and novel approaches. *Clinical Approaches in Bipolar Disorders,* 1, 10–14.

Angst, J., and Merikangas, K.R. (1992). Headache and personality. *Clin Neuropharmacol,* 15 (Suppl. 1, Pt. A), 273A–274A.

Angst, J., Dobler-Mikola, A., and Binder, A. (1984). The Zurich study: A prospective epidemiologic study of depressive, neurotic and psychomatic symptoms. I: Problem, methodology. *Eur Arch Psychiatry Neurol Sci,* 234, 13–20.

Angst, J., Degonda, M., and Ernst, C. (1992). The Zurich study: XV. Suicide attempts in a cohort from age 20–30. *Eur Arch Psychiatr Clin Neurosci,* 242, 135–141.

Angst, J., Gamma, A., and Lewinsohn, P. (2002). The evolving epidemiology of bipolar disorder. *World Psychiatry,* 1(3), 146–148.

Anthony, J.C., Folstein, M., Romanoski, A.J., Von Korff, M.R., Nestadt, G.R., Chahal, R., Merchant, A., Brown, C.H., Shapiro, S., Kramer, M., and Gruenberg, E.M. (1985). Comparison of the lay Diagnostic Interview Schedule and a standardized psychiatric diagnosis. *Arch Gen Psychiatry,* 42, 667–675.

Arce, A.A., and Vergare, M.J. (1984). Identifying and characterizing the mentally ill among the homeless. In H.R. Lamb (Ed.), *The Homeless Mentally ill: A Task Force Report of the American Psychiatric Association* (pp. 75–89). Washington, DC: American Psychiatric Association.

Babidge, N.C., Buhrich, N., and Butler, T. (2002). Mortality among homeless people with schizophrenia in Sydney, Australia: A 10-year follow-up. *Acta Psychiatr Scand,* 103, 105–110.

Badawi, M.A., Eaton, W.W., Myllyluoma, J., Weimer, L.G., and Gallo, J. (1999). Psychopathology and attrition in the Baltimore ECA 15-year follow-up 1981–1996. *Soc Psychiat Psychiatric Epidemiol*, 34, 91–98.

Bagley, C. (1973). Occupational status and symptoms of depression. *Soc Sci Med*, 7, 327–339.

Baldwin, P.A., Scully, P.J., Quinn, J.F., Morgan, M.G., Kinsella, A., O'Callaghan, E., Owens, J.M., and Waddington, J.L. (2002). First episode bipolar disorder: Systematic comparison of incidence with other affective and non-affective psychoses among an epidemiologically complete, rural population. *Bipolar Disorders*, 4(Suppl. 1), 39–40.

Benazzi, F. (1997). Prevalence of bipolar II disorder in outpatient depression: A 203 case study in private practice. *J Affect Dis*, 43, 163–166.

Biederman, J. (1995). Developmental subtypes of juvenile bipolar disorder. *Harvard Rev Psychiatry*, 327–330.

Biederman, J., Wozniak, J., Kiely, K., Ablon, S., Faraone, S., Mick, E., Mundy, E., and Kraus, I. (1995). CBCL clinical scales discriminate prepubertal children with structured-interview derived diagnosis of mania from those with ADHD. *J Am Acad Child Adolesc Psychiatry*, 34, 464–471.

Biederman, J., Farone, S.V., Wozniak, J., Mick, E., Kwon, A., and Aleardi, M. (2004). Further evidence of unique developmental phenotypic correlates of pediatric bipolar disorder: Findings from a large sample of clinically referred preadolescent children assessed over the last 7 years. *J Affect Dis*, 82(Suppl. 1), 517–523.

Bijl, R.V., de Graaf, R., Ravelli, A., Smit, F., and Vollebergh, W.A.M. (2002). Gender and age-specific first incidence of DSM-III-R psychiatric disorders in the general population. *Soc Psychiatry Psychiatr Epidemiol*, 37, 372–379.

Blazer, D. (1985). The epidemiology of psychiatric disorders in the elderly. Editorial. *J Am Geriatr Soc*, 33, 226–227.

Blehar, M.C., DePaulo, J., Gershon, E.S., Reich, T., Simpson, S.G., and Nurnberger, J.J. (1998). Women with bipolar disorder: Findings from the NIMH Genetics Initiative sample. *Psychopharmacol Bulletin*, 34, 239–243.

Breslow, N.E., and Day, N.E. (1987). *Statistical Methods in Cancer Research. Volume II: The Design and Analysis of Cohort Studies.* Lyon, France: International Agency for Research on Cancer.

Brewin, J., Cantwell, R., Dalkin, T., Fox, R., Medley, I., Glazebrook, C., Kwiecinski, R., and Harrison, G. (1997). Incidence of schizophrenia in Nottingham: A comparison of two cohorts, 1978–80 and 1992–94. *Br J Psychiatry*, 71, 140–144.

Buhrich, N., Hodder, T., and Teesson, M. (2000). Prevalence of cognitive impairment among homeless people in inner Sydney. *Psychiatry Services*, 51, 520–521.

Calabrese, J.R., Hirschfeld, R.M.A., Reed, M., Davies, M.A., Frye, M.A., Keck, P.E., Lewis, L., McElroy, S.L., McNulty, J.P., and Wagner, K.D. (2002). Impact of bipolar disorders on a U.S. community sample. *J Clin Psychiatry*.

Canino, G.J., Bird, H.R., Shrout, P.E., Rubio-Stipec, M., Bravo, M., Martinez, R., Sesman, M., and Guevara, L.M. (1987). The prevalence of specific psychiatric disorders in Puerto Rico. *Arch Gen Psychiatry*, 44, 727–735.

Carlson, G.A. (1996). Clinical features and pathogenesis of child and adolescent mania. In K.I. Schulman, M. Tohen (Eds.), *Mood Disorders across the Lifespan*. New York: Wiley-Liss.

Carney, P.A., Fitzgerald, C.T., and Monaghan, C.E. (1988). Influence of climate on the prevalence of mania. *Br J Psychiatry*, 152, 820–823.

Cassano, G.B., McElroy, S.L., Brady, K., Nolen, W.A., and Placidi, G.F. (2000). Current issues in the identification and management of bipolar spectrum disorders in "special populations." *J Affect Disord*, 59, S69–S79.

Chambers, W.J., Puig-Antich, J., Hirsch, M., Paez, P., Ambrosini, P., Tabrizi, M., and Davies, M. (1985). The assessment of affective disorders in children and adolescents by semi-structured interviews. *Arch Gen Psychiatry*, 42, 696–702.

Chen, C.N., Wong, J., Lee, N., Chan-Ho, M.W., Lau, T.F., and Fung, M. (1993). The Shatin community mental health survey in Hong Kong. *Arch Gen Psychiatry*, 50, 125–133.

Coryell, W., Endicott, J., Keller, M., Andreason, N., Grove, W., Hirschfeld, R.M.A., and Scheftner, W. (1989). Bipolar affective disorder and high achievement: A familial association. *Am J Psychiatry*, 146, 983–988.

Coryell, W., Endicott, J., Maser, J.D., Keller, M.B., Leon, A.C., and Akiskal, H.S. (1995). Long-term stability of polarity distinctions in the affective disorders. *Am J Psychiatry*, 152, 385–390.

Cowley, P., and Wyatt, J.R. (1993). Schizophrenia and manic-depressive illness. In D.T. Jamison, W.H. Mosley, A.R. Measham, J.L. Bobadilla (Eds.), *Disease Control Priorities in Developing Countries* (pp. 661–670). Oxford: Oxford University Press.

Cross-National Collaborative Group. (1992). The changing rate of major depression: Cross-national comparisons. *J Am Med Assoc*, 268, 3098–3106.

de Graaf, R., Bijl, R.V., Smit, F., Vollebergh, W.A.M., and Spijker, J. (2002). Risk factors for 12-month comorbidity of mood, anxiety and substance use disorders: Findings from the Netherlands Mental Health Survey and Incidence study. *Am J Psychiatry*, 159(4), 620–629.

Dilling, H., and Weyerer, S. (1984). Prevalence of mental disorders in the smalltown-rural region of Traunstein (Upper Bavaria). *Acta Psychiatr Scand*, 69, 60–79.

Dilsaver, S.C., and Akiskal, H.S. (2005). High rate of unrecognized bipolar mixed states among destitute Hispanic adolescents referred for "major depressive disorder." *J Affect Disord*, 84, 179–186.

Dunner, D.L., and Tay, L.K. (1993). Diagnostic reliability of the history of hypomania in bipolar II patients and patients with major depression. *Compr Psychiatry*, 34, 303–307.

Dunner, D.L., Russek, F.D., Russek, B., and Fieve, R.R. (1982). Classification of bipolar affective disorder subtypes. *Compr Psychiatry*, 23, 186–189.

Eaton, W.W., Kramer, M., Anthony, A., Dryman, S., Shapiro, S., and Locke, B.Z. (1989). The incidence of specific DIS/DSM-III mental health disorders: Data from the NIMH Epidemiologic Catchment Area Program. *Acta Psychiatr Scand*, 79, 163–178.

Egeland, J.A., and Hostetter, A.M. (1983). Amish study: I. Affective disorder among the Amish, 1976–1980. *Am J Psychiatry*, 140, 56–61.

Egeland, J.A., Hostetter, A.M., and Eshleman, S.K. III. (1983). Amish Study: III. The impact of cultural factors on diagnosis of bipolar illness. *Am J Psychiatry*, 140, 67–71.

Endicott, J., and Spitzer, R.L. (1978). A diagnostic interview: The Schedule for Affective Disorders and Schizophrenia. *Arch Gen Psychiatry*, 35, 837–844.

Faraone, S.V., Biederman, J., Mennin, D., Wozniak, J., and Spencer, T. (1997). Attention-deficit hyperactivity disorder with bipolar disorder: A familial subtype. *J Am Acad Child Adolesc Psychiatry*, 36, 1378–1387.

Faravelli, C., and Incerpi, G. (1985). Epidemiology of affective disorders in Florence. *Acta Psychiatr Scand*, 72, 331–333.

Faravelli, C., Degl'Innocenti, B.G., Aiazzi, L., Incerpi, G., and Pallanti, S. (1990). Epidemiology of mood disorders: A community survey in Florence. *J Affect Disord*, 20, 135–141.

Faravelli, C., Rosi, S., Scarpato, M.A., Lampronti, L., Amedei, S.G., and Rana, N. (2006). Threshold and subthreshold bipolar disorders in the Sesto Fiorentino Study. *J Affect Disord*, 94, 111–119.

Faris, R.E.L., and Dunham, H.W. (1939). *Mental Disorders in Urban Areas: An Ecological Study of Schizophrenia and Other Psychoses*. Chicago: University of Chicago Press.

Feinman, J.A., and Dunner, D.L. (1996). The effect of alcohol and substance abuse on the course of bipolar affective disorder. *J Affect Disord*, 12, 37(1), 43–49.

Fichter, M.M., and Quadflieg, N. (2001). Prevalence of mental illness in homeless men in Munich, Germany: Results from a representative sample. *Acta Psychiatr Scand*, 103, 94–104.

Gagrat, D.D., and Spiro, H.R. (1980). Social, cultural, and epidemiological aspects of mania. In R.H. Belmaker, H.M. van Praag (Eds.), *Mania: An Evolving Concept* (pp. 291–307). Jamaica, NY: Spectrum Publications.

Geller, B., Warner, K., Williams, M., and Zimmerman, B. (1998). Prepubertal and young adolescent bipolarity versus ADHD: Assessment and validity using the WASH-U-KSADS, CBCL, and TRF. *J Affect Disord*, 51, 93–100.

Geller, B., Zimmerman, B., Williams, M., Del Bello, M.P., Frazier, J., and Beringer, L. (2002). Phenomenology of prepubertal and early adolescent bipolar disorder: Examples of elated mood, grandiose behaviors, decreased need for sleep, racing thoughts, and hypersexuality. *J Child Adolesc Psychopharm*, 12, 3–9.

Gershon, E.S. (2000). Bipolar illness and schizophrenia as oliogenic diseases: Implications for the future. *Biol Psychiatry*, 47, 240–244.

Gershon, E.S., and Liebowitz, J.H. (1975). Sociocultural and demographic correlates of affective disorder in Jerusalem. *J Psychiatr Res*, 12, 37–50.

Gershon, E.S., Hamovit, J.H., Guroff, J.J., and Nurnberger, J.I. (1987). Birth-cohort changes in manic and depressive disorders in relatives of bipolar and schizoaffective patients. *Arch Gen Psychiatry*, 44, 314–319.

Gershon, E.S., Badner, J.A., Goldin, L.R., Sanders, A.R., Cravchik, A., and Detera-Wadleigh, S.D. (1998). Closing in on genes for manic-depressive illness and schizophrenia. *Neuropsychopharmacology*, 18, 233–242.

Glassman, A.H. (1993). Cigarette smoking: Implications for psychiatric illness. *Am J Psychiatry*, 150(4), 546–553.

Gonzalez-Pinto, A., Gutierrex, M., Ezcurra, J., Aizpuru, F., Nosquera, F., Lopez, P., and deLeon, J. (1998). Tobacco smoking and bipolar disorder. *J Clin Psychiatr*, 59, 225–228.

Gould, M.S., King, R., Greenwald, S., Fisher, P., Schwab-Stone, M., Kramer, R., Flisher, A.J., Goodman, S., Canino, G., and Shaffer, D. (1998). Psychopathology associated with suicidal ideation and attempts among children and adolescents. *J Am Acad Child Adolesc Psychiatry*, 37, 915–923.

Hare, E.H. (1968). *Bethlem Royal Hospital and the Maudsley Hospital Triennial Statistical Report: 1964–1966*. Triennial Statistical Reports. Stat Soc Ser A.

Helzer, J.E. (1975). Bipolar affective disorder in black and white men: A comparison of symptoms and familial illness. *Arch Gen Psychiatry*, 32, 1140–1143.

Helzer, J.E., and Pryzbeck, T.R. (1988). The co-occurrence of alcoholism with other psychiatric disorders in the general population and its impact on treatment. *J Stud Alcohol*, 49, 219–224.

Helzer, J.E., Robins, L.N., McEvoy, L.T., Spitznagel, E.L., Stoltzman, R.K., Farmer, A., and Brockington, I.F. (1985). A comparison of clinical and Diagnostic Interview Schedule diagnoses. *Arch Gen Psychiatry*, 42, 657–666.

Henderson, S., Andrews, G.H., and Hall, W. (2000). Australia's mental health: An overview of the general population survey. *Aust N Z J Psychiatry*, 34, 197–205.

Heun, R., and Maier, W. (1993). The distinction of bipolar II disorder from bipolar I and recurrent unipolar depression: Results of a controlled family study. *Acta Psychiatr Scand*, 87(4), 279–284.

Hibbeln, J.R. (1998). Fish consumption and major depression. *The Lancet*, 351, 1213.

Hirschfeld, R.M.A., Calabrese, J.R., Weissman, M.M., Reed, M., Davies, M.A., Frye, M.A., Keck, P.E., Lewis, L., McElroy, S.L., McNulty, J.P., and Wagner, K.D. (2001). Lifetime prevalence of bipolar spectrum disorder in the United States. Submitted. Hirschfeld, R.M.A., Calabrese, J.R., Weissman, M.M., Frye, M.A., Keck, P.E., Jr., and Wagner, K.D. *Lifetime prevalence of bipolar I & II disorders in United States*. American Psychiatric Association Annual Meeting, New Research Abstract 247, Philadelphia, PA, May 18–23, 2002.

Hirschfeld, R.M.A., Calabrese, J.R., Weissman, M.M., Reed, M., Davies, M.A., Frye, M.A., Keck, P.E., Lewis, L., McElroy, S.L., McNulty, J.P., and Wagner, K.D. (2003a). Screening for bipolar disorder in the community. *J Clin Psychiatry*, 64, 53–59.

Hirschfeld, R.M.A., Holzer, C., Calabrese, J.R., Weissman, M.M., Reed, M., Davies, M.A., Frye, M.A., Keck, P.E., McElroy, S., Lewis, L., Tierce, J., Wagner, K.D., and Hazard, E. (2003b). Validity of the Mood Disorder Questionnaire: A general population study. *Am J Psychiatry*, 160, 178–180.

Hollingshead, A.B., and Redlich, F.C. (1958). *Social Class and Mental Illness: A Community Study*. New York: J. Wiley & Sons.

Hostetter, A.M., Egeland, J.A., and Endicott, J. (1983). Amish study: II. Consensus diagnosis and reliability results. *Am J Psychiatry*, 140, 62–66.

Hwu, H.G., Yeh, E.K., and Chang, L.Y. (1989). Prevalence of psychiatric disorders in Taiwan defined by the Chinese Diagnostic Interview Schedule. *Acta Psychiatr Scand*, 79, 136–147.

Isometsa, E., Henriksson, M., Aro, H., Heikkinen, M., Kuoppasalmi, K., and Lonnqvist, J. (1994). Suicide in psychotic major depression. *J Affect Disord*, 31, 187–191.

Jenkins, R., Lewis, G., Bebbington, P., Brugha, T., Farrell, M., Gill, B., and Meltzer, H. (2003). The National Psychiatry Morbidity Surveys of Great Britian: Initial findings from the household survey. *Int Rev Psychiatry*, 15, 29–42.

Judd, L.L., and Akiskal, H.S. (2003). The prevalence and disability of bipolar spectrum disorders in the US population: Reanalysis of the ECA database taking into account subthreshhold cases. *J Affect Disord*, 73(1-2), 123–131.

Karam, E.G. (1992). Depression et Guerres du Liban: Methodologies d'une Recherche. *Annales de Psychologie et des Sciences de l'Education*. Beyrouth, Lebanon: Université St. Joseph.

Keller, M.B., Lavori, P.W., Friedman, B., Nielsen, E., Endicott, J., and McDonald-Scott, P.A. (1987). The Longitudinal Enterval Follow-up Evaluation: A comprehensive method for assessing outcome in prospective longitudinal studies. *Arch Gen Psychiatry*, 44, 540–548.

Kelsoe, J.R. (2000). Mood disorders: Genetic. In B.J. Sadock, V.A. Sadock (Eds.), *Comprehensive Textbook of Psychiatry*. 7th ed. New York: Lippincott Williams & Wilkins.

Kennedy, N., Boydell, J., van Os, J., and Murray, R.M. (2004). Ethnic differences in first clinical presentation of bipolar disorder: Results from an epidemiological study. *J Affec Dis*, 83, 161–168.

Kessler, R. (1995). Development of modifications for the Composite International Diagnostic Interview (UM-CIDI) and prevalence estimates from its use in the National Comorbidity Survey (NCS). Presented at the World Psychiatric Association on May 17, New York, NY.

Kessler, R.C., McGonagle, K.A., Zhao, S., Nelson, C.B., Hughes, M., Eshleman, S., Wittchen, H.U., and Kendler, K.S. (1994). Lifetime and 12-month prevalence of DSM-III-R psychiatric disorders in the United States: Results from the National Comorbidity Study. *Arch Gen Psychiatry*, 51, 8–19.

Kessler, R.C., Rubinow, D.R., Holmes, C., Abelson, J.M., and Zhao, S. (1997). The epidemiology of DSM-III-R bipolar I disorder in a general population survey. *Psychol Med*, 27, 1079–1089.

Kessler, R.C., Berglund, P., Demler, O., Jin, R., and Walters, E.E. (2005a). Lifetime prevalence and age-of-onset distributions of DSM-IV disorders in the National Comorbidity Survey Replication. *Arch Gen Psychiatry*, 62, 593–602.

Kessler, R.C., Chiu, W.T., Demler, O., and Walters, E.E. (2005b). Prevalence, severity, and comorbidity of 12-month DSM-IV disorders in the National Comorbidity Survey Replication. *Arch Gen Psychiatry*, 62, 617–627.

Klerman, G.L. (1981). The spectrum of mania. *Compr Psychiatry*, 22, 11–20.

Klerman, G.L., and Weissman, M.M. (1989). Increasing rates of depression. *JAMA*, 261, 2229–2235.

Koegel, P., Burnam, M.A., and Farr, R.K. (1988). The prevalence of specific psychiatric disorders among homeless individuals in the inner city of Los Angeles. *Arch Gen Psychiatry*, 45, 1085–1092.

Koukopoulos, A., and Koukopoulos, A. (1999). Agitated depression as a mixed state and the problem of melancholia. *Psychiatr Clin North Am*, 22(3), 547–564.

Kovess, V., and Lazarus, C.M. (1999). The prevalence of psychiatric disorders and use of care by homeless people in Paris. *Soc Psychiatry Psychiatr Epidemiol*, 34, 580–587.

Kramer, M., von Korff, M., and Kessler, L. (1980). The lifetime prevalence of mental disorders: Estimation, uses, and limitations. *Psychol Med*, 10, 429.

Krauthammer, C., and Klerman, G.L. (1979). The epidemiology of mania. In B. Shopsin (Ed.), *Manic Illness* (pp. 11–28). New York: Raven Press.

Kringlen, E., Torgersen, S., and Cramer, V. (2001). A norwegian psychiatric epidemiological study. *Am J Psychiatry*, 158, 1091–1098.

Lahey, B.B., Flagg, E.W., Bird, H.R., Schwab-Stone, M.E., Canino, G., Dulcan, M.K., Leaf, P.J., Davies, M., Brogan, D., Bourdon, K., Horwitz, S.M., Rubio-Stipec, M., Freeman, D.H., Lichtman, J.H., Shaffer, D., Goodman, S.H., Narrow, W.E., Weissman, M.M., Kandel, D.B., Jensen, P.S., Richters, J.E., and Regier, D.A. (1996). The NIMH Methods for the Epidemiology of Child and Adolescent Mental Disorders (MECA) study: Background and methodology. *J Am Acad Child Adolesc Psychiatry*, 35, 855–864.

Lasch, K., Weissman, M., Wickramaratne, P., and Bruce, M.L. (1990). Birth-cohort changes in the rates of mania. *Psychiatry Res*, 33, 31–37.

Lasser, K., Boyd, J.W., Woolhandler, S., Himmelstein, D.U., McCormick, D., and Bor, D.H. (2000). Smoking and mental illness: A population-based prevalence study. *JAMA*, 284(20), 2606–2610.

Lee, C.K., Kwak Y.S., Yamamoto, J., Rhee, H., Kim, Y.S., Han, J.H., Choi, J.O., and Lee, Y.H. (1990a). Psychiatric epidemiology in Korea: Part I. Gender and age differences in Seoul. *J Nerv Ment Disord*, 178, 242–246.

Lee, C.K., Kwak, Y.S., Yamamoto, J., Rhee, H., Kim, Y.S., Han, J.H., Choi, J.O., and Lee, Y.H. (1990b). Psychiatric epidemiology in Korea: Part II. Urban and rural differences in Seoul. *J Nerv Ment Disord*, 178, 247–252.

Leibenluft, E. (1996). Women with bipolar illness: Clinical and research issues. *Am J Psychiatry*, 153, 163–173.

Lépine, J.P., Lellouch, J., Lovell, A., Teherani, M., Ha, C., Verdier-Taillefer, M.H., Rambourg, N., and Lemperiere, T. (1989). Anxiety and depressive disorders in a French population: Methodology and preliminary results. *Psychiatr Psychobiol*, 4, 267–274.

Lester, D. (1993). Suicidal behavior in bipolar and unipolar affective disorders: A meta-analysis. *J Affect Disord*, 27, 117–121.

Levav, J., Kohn, R., Dohrenwend, B.P., Shrout, P.E., Skodol, A.E., Schwartz, S., Link, B.G., and Naveh, G. (1993). An epidemiological study of mental disorders in a 10-year cohort of young adults in Israel. *Psychol Med*, 23, 691–707.

Lewinsohn, P.M., Klein, D.N., and Seeley, M.S. (1995). Bipolar disorders in a community sample of older adolescents: Prevalence, phenomenology, comorbidity and course. *J Am Acad Child Adolesc Psychiatry*, 34, 454–463.

Lewinsohn, P.M., Klein, D.N., and Seeley, M.S. (2000). Bipolar disorder during adolescence and young adulthood in a community sample. *Bipolar Disorders*, 2, 281–293.

Lewinsohn, P.M., Seeley, J.R., and Klein, D.N. (2003). Bipolar disorder during adolescence. *Acta Psychiatr Scand*, 108(Suppl. 418), 47–50.

Lewis, N.D., and Hubbard, L.D. (1931). Manic-depressive reactions in Negroes. *Res Pub Assoc Res Nerv Ment Dis*, 11, 779–817.

Link, B.G., Susser, E., Stueve, A., Phelan, J., Moore, R.E., and Struening, E. (1994). Lifetime and five-year prevalence of homelessness in the United States. *Am J Publ Health*, 84, 1907–1912.

MacKinnon, D.F., Jianfeng, X., McMahon, F.J., Simpson, S.G., Stine, O.C., McInnis, M.G., and DePaulo, J.R. (1998). Bipolar disorder and panic disorder in families: An analysis of chromosome 18 data. *Am J Psychiatry*, 155, 829–831.

Mathers, C.D., Lopez, A.D., and Murray, C.J.L. (2006). The burden of disease and mortality by condition: Data, methods, and results for 2001. In A.D. Lopez, C.D. Mathers, M. Ezzati, D.T. Jamison, and C.J.L. Murray (Eds.), *Global Burden of Disease and Risk Factors*. New York: Oxford University Press.

Melse, J.M., Essink-Bot, M.L., Kramers, P.G., and Hoeymans, N. on behalf of the Dutch Burden of Disease Group. (2000). A national burden of disease calculation: Dutch disability-adjusted life-years. *Am J Public Health*, 90, 1241–1247.

Merikangas, K.R., and Angst, J. (1992). Migraine and psychopathology: Epidemiologic and genetic aspects. *Clin Neuropharmacol*, 15(Suppl. 1, Pt. A), 275A–276A.

Mino, Y., Oshima, I., and Okagami, K. (2000). Seasonality of birth in patients with mood disorders in Japan. *J Affect Disord*, 59, 41–46.

Mitchell, P.B., Slade, T., and Andrews, G. (2004). Twelve-month prevalence and disability of DSM-IV bipolar disorder in an Australian population survey. *Psychol Med*, 34, 777–785.

Morens, D.H., and Andrade, L.H. (2005). The lifetime prevalence, health services utilization and risk of suicide of bipolar spectrum subjects, including subthreshold categories in the São Paulo ECA study. *J Affect Dis*, 87, 231–241.

Muñoz, M., Vázquez, C., Koegel, P., Sanz, J., and Burnam, M.A. (1998). Differential patterns of mental disorders among the homeless in Madrid (Spain) and Los Angeles (USA). *Soc Psychiatry Psychiatr Epidemiol*, 33, 514–520.

Murphy, J.M., Laird, N.M., Monson, R.R., Sobol, A.M., and Leighton, A.H. (2000). A 40-year perspective on the prevalence of depression: The Stirling County Study. *Arch Gen Psychiatry*, 57, 209–215.

Murray, C.J.L., and Lopez, A.D. (1996). *The Global Burden of Disease: Summary*. Geneva: World Health Organization.

Murray, C.J., and Lopez, A.D. (2000). Progress and directions in refining the global burden of disease approach: A response to Williams. *Health Econ*, 9(1), 69–82.

Murray, C.J.L., Lopez, A.D., and Jamison, D.T. (1994). The global burden of disease in 1990: Summary, results, sensitivity analyses, and future directions. *Bull World Health Organ*, 72, 495–508.

Nair, S.R.N., O'Reardon, J.P., Sethi, S.S., and Amsterdam, J.D. (2000). Bipolar disorder: For women a mixed picture. *Psychiatr Ann*, 30, 463–471.

Narrow, W.E., Regier, D.A., Rae, D.S., Manderscheid, M., and Locke, B.Z. (1993). Use of services by persons with mental and addictive disorders. Findings from the National Institute of Mental Health Epidemiologic Catchment Area Program. *Arch Gen Psychiatry*, 50, 95–107.

Narrow, W.E., Rae, D.S., Robins, L.N., and Regier, D.A. (2002). Revised prevalence estimates of mental disorders in the United States. *Arch Gen Psychiatry*, 59, 115–123.

Negash, A., Alem, A., Kebede, D., Deyessa, N., Shibre, T., and Kullgren, G. (2005). Prevalence and clinical characteristics of bipolar I disorder in Butajira, Ethiopia: A community-based study. *J Affect Dis*, 87, 193–201.

Nurnberger, J.I., Blehar, M.C., Kaufmann, C.A., York-Cooler, C., Simpson, S.G., Harkavy-Friedman, J., Severe, J.B., Malaspina, D., and Reich, T. (1994). Diagnostic Interview for Genetic Studies: Rationale, unique features and training. *Arch Gen Psychiatry*, 51, 849–859.

Oliver, J.M., and Simmons, M.E. (1985). Affective disorders and depression as measured by the Diagnostic Interview Schedule and the Beck Depression Inventory in an unselected adult population. *J Clin Psychol*, 41(4), 469–477.

Orn, H., Newman, S.C., and Bland, R.C. (1988). Design and field methods of the Edmonton survey of psychiatric disorders. *Acta Psychiatr Scand Suppl*, 338, 17–23.

Parker, J.B., Spielberger, C.D., Wallace, D.K., and Becker, J. (1959). Factors in manic-depressive reactions. *Dis Nerv Syst*, 20, 505–511.

Petterson, U. (1977). Manic-depressive illness: A clinical, social and genetic study. *Acta Psychiatr Scand*, 9(Suppl. 269), 1–93.

Phelan, J.C., and Link, B.G. (1999). Who are "the homeless"? Reconsidering the stability and composition of the homeless population. *Am J Public Health*, 89(9), 1334–1338.

Rao, M.S.S. (1966). Socio-economic groups and mental disorders. *Psychiatr Q*, 40, 677–691.

Rao, U., Ryan, N.D., Birmaher, B., Dahl, R.E., Williamson, D.E., Kaufman, J., Rao, R., and Nelson, B. (1995). Unipolar depression in adolescents: Clinical outcome in adulthood. *J Am Acad Child Adolesc Psychiatry*, 34, 566–578.

Regeer, E.J., Rosso, M.L., Have, M., Vollebergh, W., and Nolen, W.A. (2002). Prevalence of bipolar disorder: A further study in the Netherlands. *Bipolar Disorders*, 4(Suppl. 1), 37–38.

Regier, D.A., and Burke, J.D. (2000). Epidemiology. In B.J. Sadock, V.A. Sadock (Eds.), *Kaplan and Sadock's Comprehensive Textbook of Psychiatry*. 7th ed. New York: Lippincott Williams & Wilkins.

Regier, D.A., Meyers, J.M., Kramer, M., Robins, L.N., Blazer, D.G., Hough, R.L., Eaton, W.W., and Locke, B.Z. (1984). The NIMH Epidemiologic Catchment Area Program. *Arch Gen Psychiatry*, 41, 934–941.

Regier, D.A., Narrow, W.E., Rae, D.S., Manderscheid, R.W., Locke, B.Z., and Goodwin, F.K. (1993). The de facto U.S. mental and addictive disorders service system: Epidemiologic Catchment Area prospective 1-year prevalence rates of disorders and services. *Arch Gen Psychiatry*, 50, 85–94.

Regier, D.A., Kaelber, C.T., Rae, D.S., Farmer, M.E., Knauper, B., Kessler, R.C., Norquist, G.S. (1998). Limitations of diagnostic criteria and assessment instruments for mental disorders. *Arch Gen Psychiatry*, 55, 109–115.

Robbins, D.R., Alessi, N.E., Cook, S.C., Poznanski, E.O., and Yanchyshyn, G.W. (1982). The use of the Research Diagnostic Criteria (RDC) for depression in adolescent psychiatric inpatients. *J Am Acad Child Psychiatry*, 21(3), 251–255.

Robins, L.N., and Regier, D.A. (1991). *Psychiatric Disorders in America: The Epidemiologic Catchment Area Study*. New York: Free Press.

Robins, L.N., Helzer, J.E., Croughan, J., and Ratcliff, K. (1981). National Institute of Mental Health Diagnostic Interview Schedule: Its history, characteristics, and validity. *Arch Gen Psychiatry*, 38, 381–389.

Rothman, K.J., and Greenland, S. (1998). *Modern Epidemiology*. 2nd ed. Philadelphia: Lippincott-Raven.

Rowitz, L., and Levy, L. (1968). Ecological analysis of treated mental disorders in Chicago. *Arch Gen Psychiatry*, 19(5), 571–579.

Rybakowski, J.K., Suwalska, A., Lojko, D., Rymaszewska, J., and Kiejna, A. (2005). Bipolar mood disorders among Polish psychiatric outpatients treated for major depression. *J Affect Dis*, 84, 141–147.

Sanchez, L., Hagino, O., Weller, E., and Weller, R. (1999). Bipolarity in children. *Psychiatr Clin North Am*, 22, 629–648.

Scully, P.J., Owens, J.M., Kinsella, A., and Waddington, J.L. (2000). Small area variation in the rate of schizophrenia vs. bipolar disorder by place of birth vs. place at onset within an Irish rural catchment area population. *Schizophr Res*, 41, 64.

Scully, P.J., Owens, J.M., Kinsella, A., and Waddington, J.L. (2002a). Dimensions of psychopathology in bipolar disorder versus other affective and non-affective psychoses among an epidemiologically complete population. *Bipolar Disorders*, 4(Suppl. 1), 43–44.

Scully, P.J., Quinn, J.F., Morgan, M.G., Kinsella, A., O'Callaghan, E., Owen, J.M., and Waddington, J.L. (2002b). First-episode schizophrenia, bipolar disorder and other psychoses in a rural Irish catchment area: Incidence and gender in the Cavan-Monaghan study at 5 years. *Br J Psychiatry*, 181(Suppl. 43), S3–S9.

Sharma, V., Khan, M., and Smith, A. (2005). A closer look at treatment resistant depression: Is it due to a bipolar diathesis? *J Affect Disord*, 84, 251–257.

Shulman, K.I., and Hermann, N. (1999). The nature and management of mania in old age. *Psychiatr Clin North Am*, 22, 649–665.

Simpson, S.G., Folstein, S.E., Meyers, D.A., McMahon, F.J., Brusco, D.M., and DePaulo, J.R. Jr. (1993). Bipolar II: The most common bipolar phenotype? *Am J Psychiatry*, 150, 901–903.

Snowdon, J. (1991). A retrospective case-note study of bipolar disorder in old age. *Br J Psychiatry*, 158, 485–490.

Soldani, F., Sullivan, P.F., and Pedersen, N.L. (2005). Mania in the Swedish Twin Registry: Criterion validity and prevalence. *Aust N Z J Psychiatry*, 39, 235–243.

Spitzer, R.L., Endicott, J., and Robins, E. (1978). Research Diagnostic Criteria: Rationale and reliability. *Arch Gen Psychiatry*, 35, 773–782.

Stefansson, E., Lindal, E., Bjornsson, J.K., and Gudmundsdottir, A. (1991). Lifetime prevalence of specific mental disorders among people born in Iceland in 1931. *Acta Psychiatr Scand*, 84, 142–149.

Stoll, A.L., Severus, W.E., Freeman, M.P., Rueter, S., Zboyan, H.A., Diamond, E., Cress, K.K., and Marangell, L.B. (1999). Omega 3 fatty acids in bipolar disorder: A preliminary double-blind, placebo-controlled trial. *Arch Gen Psychiatry*, 56(5), 407–412.

Strober, M., Lampert, C., Schmidt, S., and Morrell, W. (1993). The course of major depressive disorder in adolescents: I. Recovery and risk of manic switching in a follow-up of psychotic and nonspsychotic subtypes. *J Am Acad Child Adolesc Psychiatry*, 32, 34–42.

Szadoczky, E., Papp, Z.S., Vitrai, J., Rihmer, Z., and Furedi, J. (1998). The prevalence of major depressive and bipolar disorders in Hungary: Results from a national epidemiologic survey. *J Affect Disord*, 50, 153–162.

Tanskanen, A., Hibbeln, J.R., Tuomilehto, J., Uutela, A., Viinamäki, H., Lehtonen, J., and Vartianen, E. (2001). Fish consumption and depressive symptoms in the general population in Finland. *Psychiatr Serv*, 52(4), 529–531.

Thayer, W.S. (1920). Osler, the teacher. In H.M. Thomas (Ed.), *Sir William Osler, Bart*. Baltimore: Johns Hopkins University Press.

Torrey, E.F., Miller, J., Rawlings, R., and Yolken, R.H. (1997). Seasonality of births in schizophrenia and bipolar disorder: A review of the literature. *Schizophr Res*, 28, 1–38.

Tsai, S.Y., Chen, C.C., and Yeh, E.K. (1997). Alcohol problems and long-term psychosocial outcome in Chinese patients with bipolar disorder. *J Affect Disord*, 46, 143–150.

Tsuang, M.T., Tohen, M., and Zahner, G.E.P. (1995). *Textbook in Psychiatric Epidemiology*. New York: Wiley-Liss.

Tsuchiya, K.J., Agerbo, E., Byrne, M., and Mortensen, P.B. (2004). Higher socio-economic status of parents may increase risk for bipolar disorder in the offspring. *Psychol Med*, 34, 787–793.

U.S. Department of Health and Human Services. (1992). *National Health Interview Survey, 1992*. Hyattsville, MD: Centers for Disease Control and Prevention.

U.S. Department of Health and Human Services. (1996). *National Health Interview Survey, 1996*. Data File (CD-ROM Series 10, No. 11A). Hyattsville, MD: Centers for Disease Control and Prevention.

U.S. Department of Health and Human Services. (1998). *Third National Health and Nutrition Examination Survey, 1988–1994*. NHANES III Second Laboratory Data File (CD-ROM Series II, No. 2A). Hyattsville, MD: Centers for Disease Control and Prevention.

U.S. Department of Health and Human Services. (1999). *National Household Survey on Drug Abuse, 1997*. [Computer file]. ICPSR version. Research Triangle Park, NC, and Ann Arbor, MI: Research Triangle Institute [producer] and Inter-university Consortium for Political and Social Research [distributor].

Varanka, T.M., Weller, E.B., Weller, R.A., and Fristad, M.A. (1988). Lithium treatment of psychotic features in prepubertal children. *Am J Psychiatry*, 145, 1557–1559.

Vázquez, C., Muñoz, M., and Sanz, J. (1997). Lifetime and 12-month prevalence of DSM-III-R mental disorders among the homeless in Madrid: A European study using the CIDI. *Acta Psychiatr Scand*, 95, 523–530.

Verdoux, H., and Bourgeois, M. (1995). Social class in unipolar and bipolar probands and relatives. *J Affect Disord*, 33, 181–187.

Vicente, B., Kohn, R., Rioseco, P., Saldivia, S., Levav, I., and Torres, S. (2006). Lifetime and 12-month prevalence of DSM-III-R disorders in the Chile Psychiatric Prevalence Study. *Am J Psychiatry*, 163, 1362–1370.

Vos, T., and Mathers, C.D. (2000). The burden of mental disorders: A comparison of methods between the Australian Burden of Disease study and the Global Burden of Disease study. *Bul World Health Organ*, 78, 427–438.

Wakefield, J.C., and Spitzer, R.L. (2002). Lowered estimates—but of what? *Arch Gen Psychiatry*, 59, 129–130.

Weissman, M.M., and Klerman, G.L. (1978). Epidemiology of mental disorders: Emerging trends in the United States. *Arch Gen Psychiatry*, 35, 705–712.

Weissman, M.M., and Myers, J.K. (1978). Affective disorders in a U.S. urban community: The use of Research Diagnostic Criteria in an epidemiological survey. *Arch Gen Psychiatry*, 35, 1304–1311.

Weissman, M.M., Bland, R., Canino, G., Faravelli, C., Greenwald, S., Hwu, H.G., Joyce, P.R., Karam, E.G., Lee, C.K., Lellouch, J., Lepine, J.P., Newman, S., Rubio-Stipec, M., Wells, J.E., Wickramaratne, P., Wittchen, H.U., and Yeh, E.K. (1996). Cross national epidemiology of major depression and bipolar disorder. *JAMA*, 276, 293–299.

Weissman, M.M., Wolk, S., Goldstein, B., Moreau, D., Adams, P., Greenwald, S., Klier, C.M., Ryan, N.D., Dahl, R.E., and Wickramaratne, P. (1999a). Depressed adolescents grown up. *JAMA*, 281, 1707–1713.

Weissman, M.M., Wolk, S., Wickramaratne, P., Goldstein, B., Adams, P., Greenwald, S., Ryan, N., Dahl, R.E., and Steinberg, D. (1999b). Children with prepubertal-onset major depressive disorder and anxiety grown up. *Arch Gen Psychiatry*, 56, 794–801.

Wells, J.E., Bushnell, J.A., Hornblow, A.R., Joyce, P.R., and Oakley-Brown, M.A. (1989). Christchurch Psychiatric Epidemiology Study, part I: Methodology and lifetime prevalence for specific psychiatric disorders. *Aust N Z J Psychiatry*, 23, 315–326.

Winokur, G., Coryell, W., Akiskal, H.S., Endicott, J., Keller M., and Mueller T. (1994). Manic-depressive (bipolar) disorder: The course in light of a prospective ten-year follow-up of 131 patients. *Acta Psychiatr Scand*, 89, 102–110.

Wittchen, H.U., Essau, C.A., von Zeressen, D., Krieg, J.D., and Zaudig, M. (1992). Lifetime and six-month prevalence of mental disorders in the Munich Follow-Up Study. *Eur Arch Psychiatry Clin Neurosci*, 241, 247–258.

Wittchen, H.U., Lachner, G., Wunderlich, U., and Pfister, H. (1998a). Test-retest reliability of the computerized DSM-IV version of the Munich-Composite International Diagnostic Interview (M-CIDI). *Soc Psychiatry Psychiatr Epidemiol*, 33, 568–578.

Wittchen, H.U., Nelson, C.B., and Lachner, G. (1998b). Prevalence of mental disorders and psychosocial impairments in adolescents and young adults. *Psychol Med*, 28, 109–126.

Wittkower, E.D., and Rin, H. (1965). Transcultural psychiatry. *Arch Gen Psychiatry*, 13, 387–398.

World Bank, and Reich, M.R. (1993a). *World Development Report 1993: Investing in Health*. New York: Oxford University Press.

World Bank, Jamison, D.T., Mosley, W.H., Measham, A.R., Bobadilla, J.L. (Eds.). (1993b). *Disease Control Priorities in Developing Countries*. New York: Oxford University Press.

World Health Organization. (1990). *Composite International Diagnostic Interview (CIDI)*. Version 1.0. Geneva: World Health Organization.

World Health Organization. (1991). Mental health and behavioural disorders (including disorders of psychological development). In *International Classification of Diseases*. 10th revision. Geneva: World Health Organization.

World Health Organization. (1994). *Schedule for Clinical Assessment in Neuropsychiatry* (Version 2). Geneva: World Health Organization.

World Health Organization International Consortium of Psychiatric Epidemiology. (2000). Cross-national comparisons of mental disorders. *Bull World Health Organ*, 78, 414–426.

Wozniak, J., Biederman, J., Kiely, S., Ablon, J.S., Faraone, S.V., Mundy, W., and Mennin, D. (1995). Mania-like symptoms suggestive of childhood-onset bipolar disorder in clinically referred children. *J Am Acad Child Adolesc Psychiatry*, 34, 867–876.

Yassa, R., Nair, V., Nastase, C., Camille, Y., and Belzile, L. (1988). Prevalence of bipolar disorder in a psychogeriatric population. *J Affect Disord*, 14, 197–201.

Chapter 6

Achenbach, T.M. (1991). *Manual for the Child Behavior Checklist/4–18 and 1991 Profile*. Burlington, VT: University of Vermont Department of Psychiatry.

Akiskal, H.S., Downs, J., Jordan, P., Watson, S., Daugherty, D., and Pruitt, D.B. (1985). Affective disorders in referred children and younger siblings of manic-depressives. *Arch Gen Psychiatry*, 42, 996–1003.

Anderson, C.A., and Hammen, C.L. (1993). Psychosocial outcomes of children of unipolar depressed, bipolar, medically ill, and normal women: A longitudinal study. *J Consult Clin Psychol*, 61, 448–454.

Anthony, E.J., and Scott, P. (1960). Manic-depressive psychosis in childhood. *J Child Psychol Psychiatry*, 1, 53–72.

Angst, J., Gamma, A., Sellaro, A., Zhang, H., and Merikangas, K. (2003). Toward validation of atypical depression in the community: Results of the Zurich cohort study. *J Affect Disord*, 73, 133–146.

Axelson, D., Birmaher, B., Strober, M., Gill, M.K., Valeri, S., Chiappetta, L., Ryan, N., Leonard, H., Hunt, J., Iyengar, S., Bridge, J., and Keller, M. (2006). Phenomenology of children and adolescents with bipolar spectrum disorders. *Arch Gen Psychiatry*, 63, 1139–1148.

Benes, F. (1999). Neurodevelopmental approach to the study of mental illness. *Dev Neuropsychol*, 16, 359–360.

Biederman, J. (1998). Resolved: Mania is mistaken for ADHD in prepubertal children. *J Am Acad Child Adolesc Psychiatry*, 37, 1091–1093.

Biederman, J., Faraone, S., Mick, E., Wozniak, J., Chen, L., Ouellette, C., Marrs, A., Moore, P., Garcia, J., Mennin, D., and Lelon, E. (1996). Attention-deficit hyperactivity disorder and juvenile mania: An overlooked comorbidity? *J Am Acad Child Adolesc Psychiatry*, 35, 997–1008.

Biederman, J., Russell, R., Soriano, J., Wozniak, J., and Faraone, S.V. (1998). Clinical features of children with both ADHD and mania: Does ascertainment source make a difference? *J Affect Disord*, 51, 101–112.

Biederman, J., Faraone, S.V., Wozniak, J., and Monuteaux, M.C. (2000a). Parsing the association between bipolar, conduct, and substance use disorders: A familial risk analysis. *Biol Psychiatry*, 48, 1037–1044.

Biederman, J., Mick, E., Faraone, S., Spencer, T., Wilens, T., and Wozniak, J. (2000b). Pediatric mania: A developmental subtype of bipolar disorder? *Biol Psychiatry*, 48, 458–466.

Biederman, J., Spencer, T.J., Wozniak, J., Faraone, S.V., and Mick, E. (2001). Attention-deficit/hyperactivity disorder and pediatric-onset bipolar disorder. *TEN: Economics of Neuroscience*, 3, 45–48.

Biederman, J., Faraone, S.V., Woniak, J., Mick, E., Kwon, A., and Aleardi, M. (2004a). Further evidence of unique developmental phenotypic correlates of pediatric bipolar disorder: Findings from a large sample of clinically referred preadolescent children assessed over the last 7 years. *J Affect Disord*, 82(Suppl. 1), S45–S58.

Biederman, J., Kwon, A., Wozniak, J., Mick, E., Markowitz, S., Fazio, V., and Faraone, S.V. (2004b). Absence of gender differences in pediatric bipolar disorder: Findings from a large sample of referred youth. *J Affect Disord*, 83, 207–214.

Biederman, J., Mick, E., Faraone, S.V., and Wozniak, J. (2004c). Pediatric bipolar disorder or disruptive behavior disorder? *Primary Psychiatry*, 11, 36–41.

Biederman, J., Mick, E., Faraone, S.V., Van Patten, S., Burback, M., and Wozniak, J. (2004d). A prospective follow-up study of pediatric bipolar disorder in boys with attention-deficit/hyperactivity disorder. *J Affect Disord*, 82(Suppl. 1), S17–S23.

Birmaher, B., Kennah, A., Brent, D., Ehmann, M., Bridge, J., and Axelson, D. (2002). Is bipolar disorder specifically associated with panic disorder in youths? *J Clin Psychiatry*, 63, 414–419.

Birmaher, B., Axelson, D., Monk, K., Kalas, C., Ehmann, M., Pan, R., Bridge, J., Iyengar, S., Kupfer, D., and Brent, D. (2003). Psychiatric disorders in children of bipolar parents. Child and Adolescent Program of the 43rd Annual National Institutes of Health Boca Raton, FL, Mayo

Birmaher, B., Axelson, D., Strober, M., Gill, M.K., Valeri, S., Chiappetta, L., Ryan, N., Leonard, H., Hunt, J., Iyengar, S., and Keller, M. (2006). Clinical course of children and adolescents with bipolar spectrum disorders. *Arch Gen Psychiatry*, 63, 175–183.

Blumberg, H.P., Kaufman, J., Martin, A., Whiteman, R., Zhang, J.H., Gore, J.C., Charney, D.S., Krystal, J.H., and Peterson, B.S. (2003a). Amygdala and hippocampal volumes in adolescents and adults with bipolar disorder. *Arch Gen Psychiatry*, 60, 1201–1208.

Blumberg, H.P., Martin, A., Kaufman, J., Leung, H-C., Skudlarski, P., Lacadie, C., Fulbright, R.K., Gore, J.C., Charney, D.S., Krystal, J.H., and Peterson, B.S. (2003b). Frontostriatal abnormalities in adolescents with bipolar disorder: Preliminary observations from functional MRI. *Am J Psychiatry*, 160, 1345–1347.

Botteron, K., Vannier, M., Geller, B., Todd, R., and Lee, B. (1995). Preliminary study of magnetic resonance imaging characteristics in 8- to 16-year-olds with mania. *J Am Acad Child Adolesc Psychiatry*, 34, 742–749.

Breslau, N. (1987). Inquiring about the bizarre: False positives in Diagnostic Interview Schedule for Children (DISC) ascertainment of obsessions, compulsions, and psychotic symptoms. *J Am Acad Child Adolesc Psychiatry*, 26, 639–644.

Carlson, G.A. (1998). Mania and ADHD: Comorbidity or confusion. *J Affect Disord*, 51, 177–187.

Carlson, G.A. (1999). Juvenile mania vs. ADHD [Letter to the editor]. *J Am Acad Child Adolesc Psychiatry*, 38, 353.

Carlson, G.A. (2005). Early onset bipolar disorder: Clinical and research considerations. *J Clinical Child Adolescent Psychology*, 34, 333–343.

Carlson, G.A., and Goodwin, F.K. (1973). The stages of mania: A longitudinal analysis of the manic episode. *Arch Gen Psychiatry*, 28, 221–228.

Carlson, G.A., and Kelley, K.L. (1998). Manic symptoms in psychiatrically hospitalized children: What do they mean? *J Affect Disord*, 51, 123–135.

Carlson, G.A., and Mick, E. (2003). Drug-induced disinhibition in psychiatrically hospitalized children. *J Child Adolesc Psychopharmacol*, 13, 153–163.

Carlson, G., and Strober, M. (1979). Affective disorders in adolescence. *Psychiatr Clin North Am*, 2, 511–526.

Carlson, G.A., and Weintraub, S. (1993). Childhood behavior problems and bipolar disorder: Relationship or coincidence? *J Affect Disord*, 28, 143–153.

Carlson, G.A., and Youngstrom, E.A. (2003). Clinical implications of pervasive manic symptoms in children. *Bio Psychiatry*, 53, 1050–1058.

Carlson, G.A., Loney, J., Salisbury, H., and Volpe, R.J. (1998). Young referred boys with DICA-P manic symptoms vs. two comparison groups. *J Affect Disord*, 121, 113–121.

Carlson, G.A., Bromet, E.J., and Sievers, S. (2000). Phenomenology and outcome of subjects with early- and adult-onset psychotic mania. *Am J Psychiatry*, 157, 213–219.

Carlson, G.A., Bromet, E.J., Driessens, C., Mojtabai, R., and Schwartz, J.E. (2002). Age at onset, childhood psychopathology, and 2-year outcome in psychotic bipolar disorder. *Am J Psychiatry*, 159, 307–309.

Cecil, K.M., DelBello, M.P., Sellars, M.C., and Strakowski, S.M. (2003). Proton magnetic resonance spectroscopy of the frontal lobe and cerebellar vermis in children with a mood disorder and a familial risk for bipolar disorders. *J Child Adolesc Psychopharmacol*, 13, 545–555.

Chambers, C.A., Smith, A.H., and Naylor, G.J. (1982). The effect of digoxin on the response to lithium therapy in mania. *Psychol Med*, 12, 57–60.

Chang, K.D., Steiner, H., and Ketter, T. (2000). Psychiatric phenomenology of child and adolescent bipolar offspring. *J Am Acad Child Adolesc Psychiatry*, 39, 453–460.

Chang, K.D., Blasey, C.M., Ketter, T.A., and Steiner, H. (2003). Temperament characteristics of child and adolescent. *J Affect Disord*, 77, 11–19.

Chengappa, K.N.R., Kupfer, D.J., Frank, E., Houck, P.R., Grochocinski, V.J., Cluss, P.A., and Stapf, D.A. (2003). Relationship of birth cohort and early age of onset of illness in a bipolar disorder case registry. *Am J Psychiatry*, 160, 1636–1642.

Conners, C.K., Himmelhoch, J., Goyette, C.H., Ulrich, R., and Neil, J.F. (1979). Children of parents with affective illness. *J Am Acad Child Psychiatry*, 18, 503–504.

Correll, C.U., Penzer, J., Kafantaris, V., Nakayama, E., Auther, A., Lencz, T., and Cornblatt, B. (2005). Searching for prodromal symptoms in early-onset bipolar disorder. Poster presented at the American Psychiatric Association. Annual Meeting, Atlanta, GA, May.

Coyle, J., Pine, D., Charney, D., Lewis, L., Nemeroff, C., Carlson, G., and The Depression and Bipolar Support Alliance Consensus Development Panel. (2003). Depression and Bipolar Support Alliance consensus statement on the unmet needs in diagnosis and treatment of mood disorders in children and adolescents. *J Am Acad Child Adolesc Psychiatry*, 42, 1494–1503.

Craney, J.L., and Geller, B. (2003). A prepubertal and early adolescent bipolar disorder-I phenotype: Review of phenomenology and longitudinal course. *Bipolar Disord*, 5, 243–256. *J Affect Disord*, 77, 11–19.

Cytryn, L., McKnew, D.H., Bartko, J.J., Lamour, M., and Hamovit, J. (1982). Offspring of patients with affective disorders: Part 2. *J Am Acad Child Psychiatry*, 21, 389–391.

Davanzo, P., Yue, K., Thomas, M.A., Belin, T., Mintz, J., Venkatraman, T.N., Santoro, E., Barnett, S., and McCracken, J. (2003). Proton magnetic resonance spectroscopy of bipolar disorder versus intermittent explosive disorder in children and adolescents. *Am J Psychiatry*, 160, 1442–1452.

Decina, P., Kestenbaum, C.J., Farber, S., Kron, L., Gargan, M., Sackeim, H.A., and Fieve, R.R. (1983). Clinical and psychological assessment of children of bipolar probands. *Am J Psychiatry*, 140, 548–553.

DelBello, M.P., Soutullo, C.A., Hendricks, W., Niemeier, R.T., McElroy, S.L., and Strakowski, S.M. (2001). Prior stimulant treatment in adolescents with bipolar disorder: Association with age at onset. *Bipolar Disord*, 3, 53–57.

DelBello, M.P., Carlson, G., Tohen, M., Bromet, E., Schwiers, M., and Strakowski, S. (2003). Rates and predictors of developing a manic or hypomanic episode 1 to 2 years following a first hospitalization for major depression with psychotic features. *J Child Adolesc Psychopharmacol*, 13, 173–185.

DelBello, M.P., Zimmerman, M.E., Mills, N.P., Getz, G.E., and Strakowski, S.M. (2004). Magnetic resonance imaging analysis of amygdala and other subcortical brain regions in adolescents with bipolar disorder. *Bipolar Disord*, 6, 43–52.

Dickstein, D.P., Treland, J.E., Snow, J., McClure, E.B., Mehta, M.S., Towbin, K.E., *Pine, D.S.*, and *Leibenluft, E.* (2004). Neuropsychological performance in pediatric bipolar disorder. *Biol Psychiatry*, 55, 32–39.

Doyle, A., Wilens, T., Kwon, A., Seidman, L., Faraone, S.V., Fried, R., Swezey, A., Snyder L., and Biederman, J. (2005). Neuropsychological functioning in youth with bipolar disorder. *Biol Psychiatry*, 58, 540–548.

Duffy, A., Alda, M., Kutcher, S., Fusee, C., and Grof, P. (1998). Psychiatric symptoms and syndromes among adolescent children of parents with lithium-responsive or lithium-nonresponsive bipolar disorder. *Am J Psychiatry*, 155, 431–433.

Duffy, A., Alda, M., Kutcher, S., Cavazzoni, P., Robertson, C., Grof, E., and Grof, P. (2002). A prospective study of the offspring of bipolar parents responsive and nonresponsive to lithium treatment. *J Clin Psychiatry*, 63(12), 1171–1178.

Dupont, R.M., Jernigan, T.L., Butters, N., Delis, D.C., Hesselink, J.R., Heindel, W., and Gillin, J.C. (1990). Subcortical abnormalities detected in bipolar affective disorder using magnetic resonance imaging: Clinical and neuropsychological significance. *Arch Gen Psychiatry*, 47, 55–59.

Eaton, W.E., Mortensen, P.B., Thomsen, P.H., and Frydenberg, M. (2001). Obstetric complications and risk for severe psychopathology in childhood. *J Autism Dev Disord*, 31, 279–285.

Egeland, J.A., Shaw, J.A., Endicott, J., Pauls, D.L., Allen, C.R., Hostetter, A.M., and Sussex, J.N. (2003). Prospective study of prodromal features for bipolarity in well Amish children. *J Am Acad Child Adolesc Psychiatry*, 42, 786–796.

Faedda, G.L., Baldessarini, R., Suppes, T., Tondo, L., Becker, I., and Lipschitz, D. (1995). Pediatric-onset bipolar disorder: A neglected clinical and public health problem. *Harvard Rev Psychiatry*, 3, 171–195.

Faedda, G.L., Baldessarini, R.J., Glovinsky, I.P., and Austin, N.B. (2004). Pediatric bipolar disorder: Phenomenology and course of illness. *Bipolar Disorders*, 6, 305–313.

Faraone, S.V., Biederman, J., Mennin, D., Wozniak, J., and Spencer, T. (1997a). Attention-deficit hyperactivity disorder with bipolar disorder: A familial subtype? *J Am Acad Child Adolesc Psychiatry*, 36, 1378–1387.

Faraone, S.V., Biederman, J., Wozniak, J., Mundy, E., Mennin, D., and O'Donnell, D. (1997b). Is comorbidity with ADHD a marker for juvenile-onset mania? *J Am Acad Child Adolesc Psychiatry*, 36, 1046–1055.

Fergus, E.L., Miller, R.B., Luckenbaugh, D.A., Leverich, G.S., Findling, R.L., Speer, A.M., and Post, R.M. (2003). Is there progression from irritability/dyscontrol to major depressive and manic symptoms? A retrospective community survey of parents of bipolar children. *J Affect Disord*, 77, 71–78.

Findling, R.L., Gracious, B.L., McNamara, N.K., Youngstrom, E.A., Demeter, C.A., Branicky, L.A., and Calabrese, J.R. (2001). Rapid, continuous cycling and psychiatric co-morbidity in pediatric bipolar-I disorder. *Bipolar Disord*, 3, 202–210.

Findling, R.L., Youngstrom, E.A., Danielson, C.K., DelPorto-Bedoya, D., Papish-David, R., Townsend, L., and Calabrese, J.R. (2002). Clinical decision-making using the General Behavior Inventory in juvenile bipolarity. *Bipolar Disord*, 4, 34–42.

Frazier, J.A., Biederman, J., Tohen, M., Feldman, P.D., Jacobs, T.G., Toma, V., Rater, M.A., Tarazi, R.A., Kim, G.S., Garfield, S.B., Sohma, M., Gonzalez-Heydrich, J., Risser, R.C., and Nowlin, Z.M. (2001). A prospective open-label treatment trial of olanzapine monotherapy in children and adolescents with bipolar disorder. *J Child Psychopharmacol*, 11(3), 239–250.

Friedman, R.C., Hurt, S.W., Clarken, J.F., and Corn, R. (1983). Primary and secondary affective disorders in adolescents and young adults. *Acta Psychiatr Scand*, 67(4), 226–235.

Friedman, L., Findling, R.L., Kenny, J.T., Swales, T.P., Stuve, T.A., Jesberger, J.A., Lewin, J.S., and Schulz, S.C. (1999). An MRI study of adolescent patients with either schizophrenia or bipolar disorder as compared to healthy control subjects. *Biol Psychiatry*, 46, 77–88.

Geller, B., and Luby, J. (1997). Child and adolescent bipolar disorder: Review of the past 10 years. *J Am Acad Child Adolesc Psychiatry*, 36, 1168–1176.

Geller, B., Fox, L.W., and Clark, K.A. (1994). Rate and predictors of prepubertal bipolarity during follow-up of 6- to 12-year-old depressed children. *J Am Acad Child Adolesc Psychiatry*, 33, 461–468.

Geller, B., Warner, K., Williams, M., and Zimerman, B. (1998a). Prepubertal and young adolescent bipolarity versus ADHD: Assessment and validity using the WASH-U-KSADs, CBCL and TRF. *J Affect Disord*, 51, 93–100.

Geller, B., Williams, M., Zimerman, B., Frazier, J., Beringer, L., and Warner, K. (1998b). Prepubertal and early adolescent bipolarity differentiate from ADHD by manic symptoms, grandiose delusions, ultra-rapid or ultradian cycling. *J Affect Disord*, 51, 81–91.

Geller, B., Bolhofner, K., Craney, J.L., Williams, M., DelBello, M.P., and Gundersen, K. (2000a). Psychosocial functioning in a prepubertal and early adolescent bipolar disorder phenotype. *J Am Acad Child Adolesc Psychiatry*, 39, 1543–1548.

Geller, B., Zimerman, B., Williams, M., Bolhofner, K., Craney, J.L., DelBello, M.P., and Soutullo, C. (2000b). Diagnostic characteristics of 93 cases of a prepubertal and early adolescent bipolar disorder phenotype by gender, puberty and co-morbid attention deficit hyperactivity disorder. *J Child Adolesc Psychopharmacol*, 10, 157–164.

Geller, B., Craney, J.L., Bolhofner, K., DelBello, M.P., Williams, M., and Zimerman, B. (2001a). One-year recovery and relapse rates of children with a prepubertal and early adolescent bipolar disorder phenotype. *Am J Psychiatry*, 158, 303–305.

Geller, B., Zimerman, B., Williams, M., Bolhofner, K., and Craney, J. (2001b). Bipolar disorder at prospective follow-up of adults who had prepubertal major depressive disorder. *Am J Psychiatry*, 158, 125–127.

Geller, B., Zimerman, B., Williams, M., Bolhofner, K., Craney, J.L., DelBello, M.P., and Soutullo, C. (2001c). Reliability of the Washington University in St. Louis Kiddie Schedule for Affective Disorders and Schizophrenia (WASH-U-KSADS) mania and rapid cycling sections. *J Am Acad Child Adolesc Psychiatry*, 40, 450–455.

Geller, B., Craney, J.L., Bolhofner, K., Nickelsburg, M.J., Williams, M., and Zimerman, B. (2002a). Two-year prospective follow-up of children with a prepubertal and early adolescent bipolar disorder phenotype. *Am J Psychiatry*, 159, 927–933.

Geller, B., Zimerman, B., Williams, M., DelBello, M., Bolhofner, K., Craney, J.L., Frazier, J., Beringer, L., and Nickelsburg, M.J. (2002b). DSM-IV mania symptoms in a prepubertal and early adolescent bipolar disorder phenotype compared to attention-deficit hyperactive and normal controls. *J Child Adolesc Psychopharmacol*, 12, 11–25.

Geller, B., Zimerman, B., Williams, M., DelBello, M.P., Frazier, J., and Beringer, L. (2002c). Phenomenology of prepubertal and early adolescent bipolar disorder: Examples of elated mood, grandiose behaviors, decreased need for sleep, racing thoughts and hypersexuality. *J Child Adolesc Psychopharmacol*, 12, 3–9.

Geller, B., Tillman, R., Craney, J.L., and Bolhofner, K. (2004). Four-year prospective and natural history of mania in children with a prepubertal and early adolescent bipolar disorder phenotype. *Arch Gen Psychiatry*, 61, 459–467.

Geller, B., Tillman, R., Bolhofner, K., Zimerman, B., Strauss, N.A., and Kaufmann, P. (2006). Controlled, blindly rated, direct-interview family study of a prepubertal and early-adolescent bipolar I disorder phenotype. *Arch Gen Psychiatry*, 63, 1139–1138.

Gershon, E.S., McKnew, D., Cytryn, L., Hamovit, J., Schreiber, J., Hibbs, E., and Pellegrini, D. (1985). Diagnoses in school-age children of bipolar affective disorder patients and normal controls. *J Affect Disord*, 8, 283–291.

Goldberg, J.F., Harrow, M., and Whiteside, J.E. (2001). Risk for bipolar illness in patients initially hospitalized for unipolar depression. *Am J Psychiatry*, 158, 1265–1270.

Goldstein, T.R., Miklowitz, D.J., and Mullen, K.L. (2006). Social skills knowledge and performance among adolescents with bipolar disorder. *Bipolar Disord*, 8, 350–361.

Greenhill, L.L., Shopsin, B., and Temple, H. (1980). Children of affectively ill parents: Psychiatric status determined by structured interview. *Psychopharmacol Bull*, 16, 23–24.

Grigoroiu-Serbanescu, M., Christodorescu, D., Jipescu, I., Totoescu, A., Marinescu, E., and Ardelean, V. (1989). Psychopathology in children aged 10–17 of bipolar parents: Psychopathology rate and correlates of the severity of the psychopathology. *J Affect Disord*, 16, 167–179.

Grigoroiu-Serbanescu, M., Christodorescu, D., Totoescu, A., and Jipescu, I. (1991). Depressive disorders and depressive personality traits in offspring aged 10–17 of bipolar and of normal parents. *J Youth Adolescence*, 20, 135–148.

Hammen, C. (1991). *Depression Runs in Families: The Social Context of Risk and Resilience in Children of Depressed Mothers*. New York: Springer-Verlag.

Hammen, C., Gordon, D., Burge, D., Adrian, C., Jaenicke, C., and Hiroto, D. (1987). Maternal affective disorders, illness, and stress: Risk for children's psychopathology. *Am J Psychiatry*, 144(6), 736–741.

Hammen, C., Burge, D., Burney, E., and Adrian, C. (1990). Longitudinal study of diagnoses in children of women with unipolar and bipolar affective disorder. *Arch Gen Psychiatry*, 47, 1112–1117.

Hammersley, P., Dias, A., Todd, G., Bowen-Jones, K., Reilly, B., and Bentall, R.P. (2003). Childhood trauma and hallucinations in bipolar affective disorder: Preliminary investigation. *Br J Psychiatry*, 182, 543–547.

Harpold, T.L., Wozniak, J., Kwon, A., Gilbert, J., Wood, J., Smith, L., and Biederman, J. (2005). Examining the association between pediatric bipolar disorder and anxiety disorders in psychiatrically referred children and adolescents. *J Affect Disord*, 88, 19–26.

Harrington, R., and Myatt, T. (2003). Is preadolescent mania the same condition as adolescent mania? A British perspective. *Biol Psychiatry*, 53, 961–969.

Hazell, P.L., Carr, V., Lewin, T.J., and Sly, K. (2003). Manic symptoms in young males with ADHD predict functioning but not diagnosis after 6 years. *J Am Acad Child Adolesc Psychiatry*, 42, 552–560.

Hellender, M. (2003). Pediatric bipolar disorder: The parent advocacy perspective. *Biol Psychiatry*, 53(11), 935–937.

Hellander, M.E., and Burke, T. (1999). Children with bipolar disorder [Letter to the editor]. *J Am Acad Child Adolesc Psychiatry*, 38, 495–496.

Hillegers, M.H.J., Reichart, G.G., Wals, M., Verhulst, F.C., Ormel, J., and Nolen, W.A. (2005). Five year prospective outcome of psychopathology in the adolescent offspring of bipolar patients. *Bipolar Disord*, 7, 344–350.

Hirshfeld-Becker, D.R., Biederman, J., Henin, A., Faraone, S.V., Cayton, G.A., and Rosenbaum, J.F. (2006). Laboratory-observed behavioral disinhibition in the young offspring of parents with bipolar disorder: A high-risk pilot study. *Am J Psychiatry*, 163, 265–271.

Hodgins, S., Faucher, B., Zarac, A., and Ellenbogen, M. (2002). Children of parents with bipolar disorder: A population at high risk for major affective disorders. *Child Adolesc Psychiatr Clin North Am*, 11, 533–553.

Hyun, M., Friedman, S.D., and Dunner, D.L. (2000). Relationship of childhood physical and sexual abuse to adult bipolar disorder. *Bipolar Disord*, 2, 131–135.

Jaideep, T., Reddy, Y.C.J., and Srinath, S. (2006). Comorbidity of attention deficit hyperactivity disorder in juvenile bipolar disorder. *Bipolar Disord*, 8, 182–187.

Jamison, K.R. (1995). *An Unquiet Mind: A Memoir of Moods and Madness*. New York: Alfred A. Knopf.

Jones, S.H., Tai, S., Evershed, K., Knowles, R., and Bentall, R. (2006). Early detection of bipolar disorder: A pilot familial high-risk study of parents with bipolar disorder and their adolescent children. *Bipolar Disord*, 8, 362–372.

Judd, L.J., and Akiskal, H.S. (2003). The prevalence and disability of bipolar spectrum disorders in the U.S. population: Reanalysis of the ECA database taking into account subthreshold cases. *J Affect Disord*, 73, 123–131.

Kafantaris, V., Coletti, D.J., Dicker, R., Padula, G., and Pollack S. (1998). Are childhood psychiatric histories of bipolar adolescents associated with family history, psychosis, and response to lithium treatment? *J Affect Disord*, 51, 153–164.

Kent, L., and Craddock, N. (2003). Is there a relationship between attention deficit hyperactivity disorder and bipolar disorder? *J Affect Disord*, 73, 211–221.

Kessler, R.C., Berglund, P., Demler, O., Jin, R., Merikangas, K.R., and Walters, E.E. (2005). Lifetime prevalence and age-of-onset distributions of DSM-IV disorders in the National Comorbidity Survey Replication. *Arch Gen Psychiatry*, 62, 593–602.

Kestenbaum, C.J. (1997). Children at risk for manic-depressive illness: Possible predictors. *Am J Psychiatry*, 136, 1206–1208.

Kim, E.Y., and Miklowitz, D.J. (2002). Childhood mania, attention deficit hyperactivity disorder and conduct disorder: A critical review of diagnostic dilemmas. *Bipolar Disord*, 4, 215–225.

Kirov, G., and Murray, R.M. (1999). Ethnic differences in the presentation of bipolar disorder. *Eur Psychiatry*, 14, 199–204.

Klein, D.N., Depue, R.A., and Slater, J.F. (1985). Cyclothymia in the adolescent offspring of parents with bipolar affective disorder. *J Abnorm Psychol*, 94, 115–127.

Klein, D.N., Lewinsohn, P.M., and Seeley, J.R. (1996). Hypomanic personality traits in a community sample of adolescents. *J Affect Disord*, 38, 135–143.

Klimes-Dougan, B., Ronsaville, D., Wiggs, E.A., and Martinez, P.E., (2006). Neuropsychological functioning in adolescent children of mothers with a history of bipolar or major depressive disorders. *Biol Psychiatry*, 60, 957–965.

Kovacs, M. (1996). Presentation and course of major depressive disorder during childhood and later years of the life span. *J Am Acad Child Adolesc Psychiatry*, 35, 705–715.

Kowatch, R.A., Suppes, T., Carmody, T.J., Bucci, J.P., Hume, J.H., Kromelis, M., Emslie, G.J., Weinberg, W.A., and Rush, A.J. (2000). Effect size of lithium, divalproex sodium, and carbamazepine in children and adolescents with bipolar disorder. *J Am Acad Child Adolesc Psychiatry*, 39(6), 713–720.

Kowatch, R.A., Fristad, M., Birmaher, B., Wagner, K.D., Findling, R.L., Hellander, M., and the Child Psychiatric Workgroup on Bipolar Disorder. (2005). Treatment guidelines for children and adolescents with bipolar disorder. *J Am Acad Child Adolesc Psychiatry*, 44, 213–235.

Kraepelin, E. (1921). *Manic-Depressive Insanity and Paranoia*. Translated by R.M. Barclay. Edinburgh: E. & S. Livingstone. Originally published as *Psychiatrie. Ein Lehrbuch fur Studierende und Ärzte*. ed. 2. *Klinische Psychiatrie*. II. Leipzig: Johann Ambrosius Barth, 1899.

Kron, L., Decina, P., Kestenbaum, C.J., Farber, S., Gargan, M., and Fieve, R. (1982). The offspring of bipolar manic-depressives: Clinical features. *Adolesc Psychiatry*, 10, 273–291.

Kutcher, S.P. (2000). Adolescent-onset bipolar illness. In A. Marneros and J. Angst (Eds.), *Bipolar Disorders: 100 Years after Manic-Depressive Insanity* (pp. 139–152). London: Kluwer Academic Publishers.

Kutcher, S.P., Marton, P., and Korenblum, M. (1990). Adolescent bipolar illness and personality disorder. *J Am Acad Child Adolesc Psychiatry*, 29, 355–358.

Kutcher, S.P., Robertson, H.A., and Bird, D. (1998). Premorbid functioning in adolescent onset bipolar I disorder: A preliminary report from an ongoing study. *J Affect Disord*, 51, 137–144.

Kuyler, P.L., Rosenthal, L., Igel, G., Dunner, D.L., and Fieve, R.R. (1980). Psychopathology among children of manic-depressive patients. *Biol Psychiatry*, 15, 589–597.

Lapalme, M., Hodgins, S., and LaRoche, C. (1997). Children of parents with bipolar disorder: A meta-analysis of risk for mental disorders. *Can J Psychiatry*, 42, 623–631.

Laroche, C., Sheiner, R., Lester, E., Benierakis, C., Marrache, M., Engelsmann, F., and Cheifetz, P. (1987). Children of parents with manic-depressive illness: A follow-up study. *Can J Psychiatry*, 32, 563–569.

Leibenluft, E., Charney, D.S., and Pine, D.S. (2003a). Researching the pathophysiology of pediatric bipolar disorder. *Biol Psychiatry*, 53, 1009–1020.

Leibenluft, E., Charney, D.S., Towbin, K.E., Bhangoo, R.K., and Pine, D.S. (2003b). Defining clinical phenotypes of juvenile mania. *Am J Psychiatry*, 160, 430–437.

Lenzenweger, M.F., and Dworkin, R.H. (Eds.). (1998). *Origins and Development of Schizophrenia*. Washington, DC: American Psychological Association Press.

Leverich, G.S., McElroy, S.L., Suppes, T., Keck, P.E., Denicoff, K.D., Nolen, W.A., Altshuler, L.A., Rush, A.J., Kupka, R., Frye, M.A., Autio, K.A., and Post, R.M. (2002). Early physical and sexual abuse associated with an adverse course of bipolar illness. *Biol Psychiatry*, 51, 288–297.

Lewinsohn, P.M., Klein, D.N., and Seeley, J.R. (1995). Bipolar disorders in a community sample of older adolescents: Prevalence, phenomenology, comorbidity, and course. *J Am Acad Child Adolesc Psychiatry*, 34, 454–463.

Lewinsohn, P.M., Klein, D.N., and Seeley, J.R. (2000). Bipolar disorder during adolescence and young adulthood in a community sample. *Bipolar Disord*, 2, 281–293.

Lewinsohn P.M., Seeley, J.R., and Klein, D.N. (2003). Bipolar disorders during adolescence. *Acta Psychiatr Scand*, 108(Suppl. 418), 47–50.

Lish, J.D., Dime-Meenan, S., Whybrow, P.C., Price, R.A., and Hirschfeld, R.M.A. (1994). The National Depressive and Manic-Depressive Association (DMDA) survey of bipolar members. *J Affect Disord*, 31, 281–294.

Luby, J., and Mrakotsky, C. (2003). Depressed preschoolers with bipolar family history: A group at high risk for later switching to mania? *J Child Adolesc Psychopharmacol*, 13, 187–197.

Masi, G., Toni, C., Perugi, G., Mucci, M., Millepiedi, S., and Akiskal, H.S. (2001). Anxiety disorders in children and adolescents with bipolar disorder: A neglected comorbidity. *Can J Psychiatry*, 46, 797–802.

Masi, G., Toni, C., Perugi, G., Travierso, M.C., Millepiedi, S., Mucci, M., Akiskal, H.S. (2003). Externalizing disorders in consecutively referred children and adolescents with bipolar disorder. *Compr Psychiatry*, 44, 184–189.

Masi, G., Perugi, G., Toni, C., Millepiedi, S., Mucci, M., Bertini, N., and Pfanner, C. (2006). Attention-deficit hyperactivity disorder—Bipolar cormobidity in children and adolescents. *Bipolar Disord*, 8, 373–381.

McClellan, J., and Werry, J.S. (1997). Practice parameters for the assessment and treatment of children and adolescents with bipolar disorder. *J Am Acad Child Adolesc Psychiatry*, 36(Suppl. 10), 157s–176s.

McClellan, J., McCurry, C., Snell, J., and DuBose, A. (1999). Early-onset psychotic disorders: Course and outcome over a 2-year period. *J Am Acad Child Adolesc Psychiatry*, 38, 1380–1388.

McClure, E.B., Treland, J.E., Snow, J., Dickstein, D.P., Towbin, K.E., Charney, D.S., Pine, D.S., and Leibenluft, E. (2005). Memory and learning in pediatric bipolar disorder. *J Am Acad Child Adolesc Psychiatry*, 44, 461–469.

McElroy, S.L., Strakowski, S.M., West, S.A., Keck, P.E., and McConville, B.J. (1997). Phenomenology of adolescent and adult mania in hospitalized patients with bipolar disorder. *Am J Psychiatry*, 154, 44–49.

McKnew, D.H., Cytryn, L., Efron, A.M., Gershon, E.S., and Bunney, W.E. (1979). Offspring of patients with affective disorders. *Br J Psychiatry*, 134, 148–152.

Miklowitz, D.J., Goldstein, M.J., Nuechterlein, K.H., Snyder, K.S., and Mintz, J. (1988). Family factors and the course of bipolar affective disorder. *Arch Gen Psychiatry*, 45(3), 225–231.

Meyer, S., Ronsaville, D.S., Gold, P.W., Radke-Yarrow, M., and Martinez, P.E. (2001). A prospective study of children at risk for mood disorder. In G.A. Carlson (Chair), *Juvenile Bipolar Disorder*. Symposium conducted at the meeting of the International Society for Research on Child and Adolescent Psychopathology, Vancouver, B.C.

Meyer, S., Carlson, G., Wiggs, E., Martinez, P., Ronsaville, D., Klimes-Dougan, B., Gold, P., and Radke-Yarrow, M. (2004a). Predictors of apparent frontal lobe dysfunction among adolescents at risk for bipolar disorders. Manuscript under review.

Meyer, S., Carlson, G., Wiggs, E., Martinez, P., Ronsaville, D., Klimes-Dougan, B., Gold, P., and Radke-Yarrow, M. (2004). A prospective study of the association among impaired executive functioning, childhood attentional problems, and the development of bipolar disorder. *Dev Psychopathol*, 16, 416–476.

Milberger, S., Biederman, J., Faraone, S.V., Murphy, J., and Tsuang, M.T. (1995). Attention deficit hyperactivity disorder and comorbid disorders: Issues of overlapping symptoms. *Am J Psychiatry*, 152, 1793–1799.

National Institute of Mental Health Research Roundtable on Prepubertal Bipolar Disorder. (2001). *J Am Acad Child Adolesc Psychiatry*, 40, 871–878.

Nurnberger, J.I., Hamovit, J., Hibbs, E.D., Pellegrini, D., Guroff, J.J., Maxwell, M.E., Smith, A., and Gershon, E.S. (1988). A high-risk study of primary affective disorder: Selection of subjects, initial assessment, and 1- to 2-year follow-up. In D.L. Dunner, E.S. Gershon, and J.E. Barrett (Eds.), *Relatives at Risk for Mental Disorder* (pp. 161–177). New York: Raven Press.

Osher, Y., Mandel, B., Shapiro, E., and Belmaker, R. (2000). Rorschach markers in offspring of manic-depressive patients. *J Affect Disord*, 59, 231–236.

Papolos, D.F. (2003). Bipolar disorder and comorbid disorders: The case for a dimensional nosology. In B. Geller and M. DelBello (Eds.), *Child and Early Adolescent Bipolar Disorder: Theory, Assessment, and Treatment*. New York: Guilford Publications.

Papolos, D., and Papolos, J. (2002). *The Bipolar Child: The Definitive and Reassuring Guide to Childhood's Most Misunderstood Disorder*. New York: Broadway Books.

Patel, N.C., DelBello, M.P., and Strakowski, S.M. (2006). Ethnic differences in symptom presentation of youths with bipolar disorder. *Bipolar Disord*, 8, 95–99.

Pavuluri, M.N., Herbener, E.S., and Sweeney, J.A. (2004). Psychotic symptoms in pediatric bipolar disorder. *J Affect Disord*, 80(1), 19–28.

Pavuluri, M.N., O'Connor, M.M., Harral, E.M., Moss, M., and Sweeney, J.A. (2006). Impact of neurocognitive function on academic difficulties in pediatric bipolar disorder: A clinical translation. *Biol Psychiatry*, 60, 951–956.

Pellegrini, D., Kosisky, S., Nackman, D., Cytryn, L., McKnew, D.H., Gershon, E., Hamovit, J., and Cammuso, K. (1986). Personal and social resources in children of patients with bipolar affective disorder and children of normal control subjects. *Am J Psychiatry*, 143, 856–861.

Post, R.M., Leverich, G.S., Fergus, E., Miller, R., and Luckenbaugh, D. (2002). Parental attitudes towards early intervention in children at high risk for affective disorders. *J Affect Disord*, 70(2), 117–124.

Quackenbush, D., Kutcher, S., Roberson, H.A., Boulos, C., and Chaban, P. (1996). Premorbid and postmorbid school functioning in bipolar adolescent description and suggested academic interventions. *Can J Psychiatry*, 41, 16–22.

Radke-Yarrow, M. (1998). *Children of Depressed Mothers: From Early Childhood to Maturity*. Cambridge, England: Cambridge University Press.

Radke-Yarrow, M., Nottelmann, E., Martinez, P., Fox, M.B., and Belmont, B. (1992). Young children of affectively ill parents: A longitudinal study of psychosocial development. *J Am Acad Child Adolesc Psychiatry*, 31, 68–77.

Rajeev, J., Srinath, S., Reddy, Y.C.J., Shashikiran, M.G., Girimaji, S.C., Seshadri, S.P., and Subbakrishna, D.K. (2003). The index manic episode in juvenile-onset bipolar disorder: The pattern of recovery. *Can J Psychiatry*, 48, 52–55.

Reichart, C.G., van der Ende, J., Wals, M., Hillegers, M.H.J., Nolen, W.A., Ormel, J., and Verhulst, F.C. (2005). The use of GBI as predictor of bipolar disorder in a population of adolescent offspring of parents with a bipolar disorder. *J Affect Disord*, 89(1-3), 147–155.

Rucklidge, J.J. (2006). Impact of ADHD on the neurocognitive functioning of adolescents with bipolar disorder. *Biol Psychiatry*, 60, 921–928.

Sachs, G.S., Baldassano, C.F., Truman, C.J., and Guille, C. (2000). Comorbidity of attention deficit hyperactivity disorder with early- and late-onset bipolar disorder. *Am J Psychiatry*, 157, 466–468.

Schneck, C.D., Miklowitz, D.J., Calabrese, J.R., Allen, M.H., Thomas, M.R., Wisniewski, S.R., Miyahara, S., Shelton, M.D., Ketter, T.A., Goldberg, J.F., Bowden, C.L., and Sachs, G.S. (2004). Phenomenology of rapid-cycling bipolar disorder: Data from the first 500 participants in the systematic treatment enhancement program. *Am J Psychiatry*, 161, 1902–1908.

Schurhoff, F., Bellivier, F., Jouvent, R., Mouren-Simeoni, M.-C., Bouvard, M., Allilaire, J.-F., and Leboyer, M. (2000). Early and late onset bipolar disorders: Two different forms of manic-depressive illness? *J Affect Disord*, 58, 215–221.

Shaffer, D. (2002). *Juvenile Mania: Newly Observed? Newly Invited? The Challenge of Adapting Adult Mood Disorder Criteria for Children*. Yokohama, Japan: World Congress of Psychiatry.

Sigurdsson, E., Fombonne, E., Sayal, K., and Checkley, S. (1999). Neurodevelopmental antecedents of early-onset bipolar affective disorder. *Br J Psychiatry*, 174, 121–127.

Smith, D.J., Harrison, N., Muir, W., and Blackwood, D.H.R. (2005). The high prevalence of bipolar spectrum disorders in young adults with recurrent depression: Toward an innovative diagnostic framework. *J Affect Disord*, 84, 167–178.

Soutullo, C.A., DelBello, M.P., Ochsner, J.E., McElroy, S.L., Taylor, S.A., Strakowski, S.M., and Keck, P.E. Jr. (2002). Severity of bipolarity in hospitalized manic adolescents with history of stimulant or antidepressant treatment. *J Affect Disord*, 70(3), 323–327.

State, R.C., Altshuler, L.L., and Frye, M.A. (2002). Mania and attention deficit hyperactivity disorder in a prepubertal child: Diagnostic and treatment challenges. *Am J Psychiatry*, 159, 918–925.

Staton, D., and Lysne, D. (1999, May). Children with bipolar disorder [Letter to the editor]. *J Am Acad Child Adolesc Psychiatry*, 38, 496.

Strakowski, S.M., McElroy, S.L., Keck, P.E., and West, S.A. (1996). Racial influence on diagnosis in psychotic manis. *J Affect Disord*, 39, 157–162.

Strober, M., and Carlson, G. (1982). Bipolar illness in adolescents with major depression: Clinical, genetic, and psychopharmacologic predictors in a three- to four-year prospective follow-up investigation. *Arch Gen Psychiatry*, 39, 549–555.

Strober, M., Schmidt-Lackner, S., Freeman, R., Bower, S., Lampert, C., and DeAntonio, M. (1995). Recovery and relapse in adolescents with bipolar affective illness: A five-year naturalistic, prospective follow-up. *J Am Acad Child Adolesc Psychiatry*, 34, 724–731.

Strober, M., DeAntonio, M., Schmidt-Lackner, S., Freeman, R., Lampert, C., and Diamond, J. (1998). Early childhood attention deficit hyperactivity disorder predicts poorer response to acute lithium therapy in adolescent mania. *J Affect Disord*, 51, 145–151.

Tillman, R., and Geller, B. (2003). Definitions of rapid, ultrarapid, and ultradian cycling and of episode duration in pediatric and adult bipolar disorders: A proposal to distinguish episodes from cycles. *J Child Adolesc Psychopharmacol*, 13, 267–271.

Tillman, R., Geller, B., Bolhofner, K., Craney, J.L., Williams, M., and Zimerman, B. (2003). Ages of onset and rates of syndromal and subsyndromal comorbid DSM-IV diagnoses in a prepubertal and early adolescent bipolar disorder phenotype. *J Am Acad Child Psychiatry*, 42(12), 1486–1493.

Tillman, R., Geller, B., Craney, J.L., Bolhofner, K., Williams, M., and Zimerman, B. (2004). Relationship of parent and child informants to prevalence of mania symptoms in children with a prepubertal and early adolescent bipolar disorder phenotype. *Am J Psychiatry*, 161, 1278–1284.

Todd, R.D., and Botteron, K.N. (2002). Etiology and genetics of early-onset mood disorders. *Child Adolesc Psychiatr Clin North Am*, 11, 499–518.

Todd, R.D., Reich, W., Petti, T.A., Joshi, P., DePaulo, J.R., Nurnberger, J., and Reich, T. (1996). Psychiatric diagnoses in the child and adolescent members of extended families identified through adult bipolar affective disorder probands. *J Am Acad Child Adolesc Psychiatry*, 35, 664–671.

Tohen, M., Greenfield, S.F., Weiss, R.D., Zarate, C.A., and Vagge, L.M. (1998). The effect of comorbid substance use disorders on the course of bipolar disorder: A review. *Harvard Rev Psychiatry*, 6, 133–141.

Walker, E.F. (2002). Adolescent neurodevelopment and psychopathology. *Curr Dir Psychol Sci*, 11, 24–28.

Wals, M., Hillegers, M.H.J., Reichart, C.G., Ormel, J., Nolen, W.A., and Verhulst, F.C. (2001). Prevalence of psychopathology in children of a bipolar parent. *J Am Acad Child Adolesc Psychiatry*, 40, 1094–1102.

Wals, M., Reichart, C.G., Hillegers, M.H.J., Van Os, J., Verhulst, F.C., Nolen, W.A., and Ormel, J. (2003). Impact of birth weight and genetic liability on psychopathology in children of bipolar parents. *J Am Acad Child Adolesc Psychiatry*, 42, 1116–1121.

Wals, M., Hillegers, M.H.J., Reichart, C.G., Verhulst, F.C., Nolen, W.A., and Ormel, J. (2005). Stressful life events and onset of mood disorders in children of bipolar parents during 14-month follow-up. *J Affect Disord*, 87, 253–263.

Waters, B.G.H., Marchenko, I., and Smiley, D. (1983). Affective disorder, paranatal, and educational factors in the offspring of bipolar manic-depressives. *Can J Psychiatry*, 28, 527–531.

Weintraub, S. (1987). Risk factors in schizophrenia: The Stony Brook High-Risk Project. *Schizophrenia Bull*, 13, 439–450.

Weintraub, S., and Neale, J.M. (1984). The Stony Brook High-Risk Project. In N.F. Watt, and J. Anthony (Eds.), *Children at Risk for Schizophrenia* (pp. 243–263). Cambridge, England: Cambridge University Press.

Weissman, M.M., Wolk, S., Goldstein, R.B., Moreau, D., Adams, P., Greenwald, S., Klier, C.M., Ryan, N.D., Dahl, R.E., and Wickramaratne, P. (1999a). Depressed adolescents grown up. *JAMA*, 281, 1707–1713.

Weissman, M.M., Wolk, S., Wickramaratne, P., Goldstein, R., Adams, P., Greenwald, S., Ryan, N., Dahl, R., and Steinberg, D. (1999b). Children with prepubertal-onset major depressive disorder and anxiety grown up. *Arch Gen Psychiatry*, 56, 794–801.

Worland, J., Lander, H., and Hesselbrock, V. (1979). Psychological evaluation of clinical disturbance in children at risk for psychopathology. *J Abnorm Psychol*, 88, 13–26.

Wozniak, J., Biederman, J., Kiely, K., Ablon, J. S., Faraone, S.V., Mundy, E., and Mennin, D. (1995). Mania-like symptoms suggestive of childhood-onset bipolar disorder in clinically referred children. *J Am Acad Child Adolesc Psychiatry*, 34, 867–876.

Wozniak, J., Biederman, J., Faraone, S.V., Blier, H., and Monuteaux, M.C. (2001). Heterogeneity of childhood conduct disorder: Further evidence of a subtype of conduct disorder linked to bipolar disorder. *J Affect Disord*, 64, 121–131.

Wozniak, J., Biederman, J., Monuteaux, M.C., Richards, J., and Faraone, S.V. (2002). Parsing the comorbidity between bipolar disorder and anxiety disorders: A familial risk analysis. *J Child Adolesc Psychopharmacol*, 12, 101–111.

Wozniak, J., Spencer, T., Biederman, J., Kwon, A., Monuteaux, M., Rettew, J., and Lail, K. (2004). The clinical characteristics of unipolar vs. bipolar major depression in ADHD youth. *J Affect Disord*, 82(Suppl. 1), S59–S69.

Youngstrom, E.A., Findling, R.L., Danielson, C.K., and Calabrese, J.R. (2001). Discriminative validity of parent report of hypomanic and depressive symptoms on the General Behavioral Inventory. *Psychol Assess*, 13, 267–276.

Youngstrom, E.A., Gracious, B.L., Danielson, C.K., Findling, R.L., and Calabrese, J.R. (2003). Toward an integration of parent and clinician report on the Young Mania Rating Scale. *J Affect Disord*, 77, 179–190.

Youngstrom, E., Findling, R.L., and Calabrese, J.R. (2004). Effects of adolescent manic symptoms on agreement between youth, parent, and teacher ratings of behavior problems. *J Affect Disord*, 825, S5–S16.

Zahn-Waxler, C., Cummings, E.M., McKnew, D.H., and Radke-Yarrow, M. (1984a). Altruism, aggression, and social interactions in young children with a manic-depressive parent. *Child Dev*, 55, 112–122.

Zahn-Waxler, C., McKnew, D.H., Cummings, E.M., Davenport, Y.B., and Radke-Yarrow, M. (1984b). Problem behaviors and peer interactions of young children with a manic-depressive parent. *Am J Psychiatry*, 141, 236–240.

Zahn-Waxler, C., Chapman, M., and Cummings, E.M. (1984c). Cognitive and social development in infants and toddlers with a bipolar parent. *Child Psychiatry Hum Dev*, 15, 75–85.

Zahn-Waxler, C., Mayfield, A., Radke-Yarrow, M., McKnew, D.H., Cytryn, L., and Davenport, Y.B. (1988). A follow-up investigation of offspring of parents with bipolar disorder. *Am J Psychiatry*, 145, 506–509.

Zito, J.M., Safer, D.J., dosReis, S., Gardner, J.F., Soeken, K., Boles, M., and Lynch, F. (2002). Rising prevalence of antidepressants among U.S. youths. *Pediatrics*, 109, 721–727.

CHAPTER 7

Ackerknecht, E.A. (1959). *A Short History of Psychiatry*. New York: Hafner.

American Diabetes Association, American Psychiatric Association, American Association of Clinical Endocrinologists, and North American Association for the Study of Obesity. (2004). Consensus development conference on antipsychotic drugs and obesity and diabetes. *Diabetes Care*, 27, 596–601.

Angst, F., Stassen, H.H., Clayton, P.J., and Angst, J. (2002). Mortality of patients with mood disorders: Follow-up over 34–38 years. *J Affect Disord*, 68, 167–181.

Angst, J. (1998). The emerging epidemiology of hypomania and bipolar II disorder. *J Affect Disord*, 50, 143–151.

Baldassano, C.F., Marangell, L.B., Gyulai, L., Ghaemi, S.N., Joffe, H., Kim, D.R., Sagduyu, K., Truman, C.J., Wisniewski, S.R., Sachs, G.S., and Cohen, L.S. (2005). Gender differences in bipolar disorder: Retrospective data from the first 500 STEP-BD participants. *Bipolar Disord*, 7, 465–470.

Bandelow, B., Sengos, G., Wedekind, D., Huether, G., Pilz, J., Broocks, A., Hajak, G., and Ruther, E. (1997). Urinary excretion of cortisol, norepinephrine, testosterone, and melatonin in panic disorder. *Pharmacopsychiatry*, 30, 113–117.

Bauer, M.S., Whybrow, P.C., and Winokur, A. (1990). Rapid cycling bipolar affective disorder: I. Association with grade I hypothyroidism. *Arch Gen Psychiatry*, 47, 427–432.

Bauer, M.S., Altshuler, L., Evans, D.R., Beresford, T., Williford, W.O., and Hauger, R. (2005). Prevalence and distinct correlates of anxiety, substance, and combined comorbidity in a multi-site public sector sample with bipolar disorder. *J Affect Disord*, 85, 301–315.

Bernadt, M.W., and Murray, R.M. (1986). Psychiatric disorder, drinking and alcoholism: What are the links? *Br J Psychiatry*, 148, 393–400.

Berrettini, W.H., Nurnberger, J.I., Jr., Scheinin, M., Seppala, T., Linnoila, M., Narrow, W., Simmons-Alling, S., and Gershon, E.S. (1985). Cerebrospinal fluid and plasma monoamines and their metabolites in euthymic bipolar patients. *Biol Psychiatry*, 20, 257–269.

Blehar, M.C., DePaulo, J.R., Gershon, E.S., Reich, T., Simpson, S.G., and Nurnberger, J.I. (1998). Women with bipolar disorder: Findings from the NIMH Genetics Initiative sample. *Psychopharmacol Bull*, 34(3), 239–243.

Bovasso, G.B. (2001). Cannabis abuse as a risk factor for depressive symptoms. *Am J Psychiatry*, 158, 2033–2037.

Bowen, R., South, M., and Hawkes, J. (1994). Mood swings in patients with panic disorder. *Can J Psychiatry*, 39, 91–94.

Bowers, M.B. Jr. (1977). Psychoses precipitated by psychotomimetic drugs: A follow-up study. *Arch Gen Psychiatry*, 34, 832–835.

Brieger, P. (2005). Comorbidity in mixed states and rapid-cycling forms of bipolar disorders. In A. Marneros and F.K. Goodwin (Eds.), *Bipolar Disorders: Mixed States, Rapid Cycling, and Atypical Forms*. Cambridge, UK: Cambridge University Press, pp. 263–276.

Brown, E.S., Beard, L., Dobbs, L., and Rush, A.J. (2006). Naltrexone in patients with bipolar disorder and alcohol dependence. *Depress Anxiety*, 23, 492–495.

Brownlie, B.E., Rae, A.M., Walshe, J.W., and Wells, J.E. (2000). Psychoses associated with thyrotoxicosis—"thyrotoxic psychosis": A report of 18 cases, with statistical analysis of incidence. *Eur J Endocrinol*, 142, 438–444.

Cade, J.F. (1979). *Mending the Mind: A Short History of Twentieth Century Psychiatry*. Melbourne, FL: Sun.

Calabrese, J.R., and Delucchi, G.A. (1990). Spectrum of efficacy of valproate in 55 patients with rapid-cycling bipolar disorder. *Am J Psychiatry*, 147, 431–434.

Calabrese, J.R., Hirschfeld, R.M., Reed, M., Davies, M.A., Frye, M.A., Keck, P.E., Lewis, L., McElroy, S.L., McNulty, J.P., and Wagner, K.D. (2003). Impact of bipolar disorder on a U.S. community sample. *J Clin Psychiatry*, 64(4), 425–432.

Carpenter, K.M., Hasin, D.S., Allison, D.B., and Faith, M.S. (2000). Relationships between obesity and DSM-IV major depressive disorder, suicide ideation, and suicide attempts: Results from a general population study. *Am J Public Health*, 90, 251–257.

Cassano, G.B., Pini, S., Saettoni, M., Rucci, P., and Dell'Osso, L. (1998). Occurrence and clinical correlates of psychiatric comorbidity in patients with psychotic disorders. *J Clin Psychiatry*, 59(2), 60–68.

Cassidy, F., Murry, E., Forest, K., and Carroll, B.J. (1998). Signs and symptoms of mania in pure and mixed episodes. *J Affect Disord*, 50, 187–201.

Cassidy, F., Ahearn, E., and Carroll, B.J. (1999). Elevated frequency of diabetes mellitus in hospitalized manic-depressive patients. *Am J Psychiatry*, 156, 1417–1420.

Cassidy, F., Ahearn, E.P., and Carroll, B.J. (2001). Substance abuse in bipolar disorder. *Bipolar Disord*, 3, 181–188.

Cassidy, F., Ahearn, E.P., and Carroll, B.J. (2002). Thyroid function in mixed and pure manic episodes. *Bipolar Disord*, 4(6), 393–397.

Castaneda, R., Galanter, M., and Franco, H. (1989). Self-medication among addicts with primary psychiatric disorders. *Compr Psychiatry*, 30, 80–83.

Chen, Y.W., and Dilsaver, S.C. (1995a). Comorbidity for obsessive-compulsive disorder in bipolar and unipolar disorders. *Psychiatry Res*, 59, 57–64.

Chen, Y.W., and Dilsaver, S.C. (1995b). Comorbidity of panic disorder in bipolar illness: Evidence from the Epidemiologic Catchment Area Survey. *Am J Psychiatry*, 152, 280–282.

Chengappa, K.N., Levine, J., Gershon, S., and Kupfer, D.J. (2000). Lifetime prevalence of substance or alcohol abuse and dependence among subjects with bipolar I and II disorders in a voluntary registry. *Bipolar Disord*, 2, 191–195.

Cole, D.P., Thase, M.E., Mallinger, A.G., Soares, J.C., Luther, J.F., Kupfer, D.J., and Frank, E. (2002). Slower treatment response in bipolar depression predicted by lower pretreatment thyroid function. *Am J Psychiatry*, 159, 116–121.

Davidson, J.R., Rothbaum, B.O., van der Kolk, B.A., Sikes, C.R., and Farfel, G.M. (2001). Multicenter, double-blind comparison of sertraline and placebo in the treatment of posttraumatic stress disorder. *Arch Gen Psychiatry*, 58, 485–492.

de Graaf, R., Bijl, R.V., Smit, F., Vollebergh, W.A., and Spijker, J. (2002). Risk factors for 12-month comorbidity of mood, anxiety, and substance use disorders: Findings from the Netherlands Mental Health Survey and Incidence Study. *Am J Psychiatry*, 159, 620–629.

Derby, I.M. (1933). Manic-depressive "exhaustion" deaths: An analysis of "exhaustion" case histories. *Psychiatr Q*, 7, 435–449.

Dilsaver, S.C., Chen, Y.W., Swann, A.C., Shoaib, A.M., Tsai-Dilsaver, Y., and Krajewski, K.J. (1997). Suicidality, panic disorder and psychosis in bipolar depression, depressive-mania and pure-mania. *Psychiatry Res*, 73, 47–56.

Donahue, R.P., Abbott, R.D., Bloom, E., Reed, D.M., and Yano, K. (1987). Central obesity and coronary heart disease in men. *Lancet*, 1, 821–824.

Doughty, C.J., Elisabeth Wells, J., Joyce, P.R., Olds, R.J., and Walsh, A.E. (2004). Bipolar-panic disorder comorbidity within bipolar disorder families: A study of siblings. *Bipolar Disord*, 6, 245–252.

Edmonds, L.K., Mosley, B.J., Admiraal, A.J., Olds, R.J., Romans, S.E., Silverstone, T., and Walsh, A.E. (1998). Familial bipolar disorder: Preliminary results from the Otago Familial Bipolar Genetic Study. *Aust N Z J Psychiatry*, 32(6), 823–829.

El-Guebaly, N. (1975). Manic-depressive psychosis and drug abuse. *Can Psychiatr Assoc J*, 20, 595–598.

Ellinwood, E.H., and Petrie, W.M. (1979). Drug-induced psychoses. In R.W. Pickens, L.L. Heston (Eds.), *Psychiatric Factors in Drug Abuse* (pp. 301–336). New York: Grune and Stratton.

Elmslie, J.L., Silverstone, J.T., and Mann, J.I. (2000). Prevalence of overweight and obesity in bipolar patients. *J Clin Psychiatry*, 61, 179–184.

Elmslie, J.L., Mann, J.I., and Silverstone, J.T. (2001). Determinants of overweight and obesity in patients with bipolar disorders. *J Clin Psychiatry*, 62, 486–491.

Engum, A., Bjoro, T., Mykletun, A., and Dahl, A.A. (2002). An association between depression, anxiety and thyroid function: A clinical fact or an artifact? *Acta Psychiatr Scand*, 106, 27–34.

Erard, R., Luisada, P.V., and Peele, R. (1980). The PCP psychosis: Prolonged intoxication or drug-precipitated functional illness? *J Psychedelic Drugs*, 12, 235–251.

Estroff, T.W., Dackis, C.A., Gold, M.S., and Pottash, A.L. (1985). Drug abuse and bipolar disorders. *Int J Psychiatry Med*, 15, 37–40.

Fagiolini, A., Frank, E., Houck, P.R., Mallinger, A.G., Swartz, H.A., Buysse, D.J., Ombao, H., and Kupfer, D.J. (2002). Prevalence of obesity and weight change during treatment in patients with bipolar I disorder. *J Clin Psychiatry*, 63, 528–533.

Fasmer, O.B. (2001). The prevalence of migraine in patients with bipolar and unipolar affective disorders. *Cephalalgia*, 21(9), 894–899.

Fava, M., Labbate, L.A., Abraham, M.E., and Rosenbaum, J.F. (1995). Hypothyroidism and hyperthyroidism in major depression revisited. *J Clin Psychiatry*, 56(5), 186–192.

Feinman, J.A., and Dunner, D.L. (1996). The effect of alcohol and substance abuse on the course of bipolar affective disorder. *J Affect Disord*, 37, 43–49.

Findling, R.L., Gracious, B.L., McNamara, N.K., Youngstrom, E.A., Demeter, C.A., Branicky, L.A., and Calabrese, J.R. (2001). Rapid, continuous cycling and psychiatric co-morbidity in pediatric bipolar I disorder. *Bipolar Disord*, 3, 202–210.

Flegal, K.M., Carroll, M.D., Ogden, C.L., and Johnson, C.L. (2002). Prevalence and trends in obesity among US adults, 1999–2000. *JAMA*, 288, 1723–1727.

Flynn, R.W., MacDonald, T.M., Morris, A.D., Jung, R.T., and Leese, G.P. (2004). The thyroid epidemiology, audit, and research study: Thyroid dysfunction in the general population. *J Clin Endocrinol Metab*, 89, 3879–3884.

Fogarty, F., Russell, J.M., Newman, S.C., and Bland, R.C. (1994). Epidemiology of psychiatric disorders in Edmonton: Mania. *Acta Psychiatr Scand Suppl*, 376, 16–23.

Frank, E., Cyranowski, J.M., Rucci, P., Shear, M.K., Fagiolini, A., Thase, M.E., Cassano, G.B., Grochocinski, V.J., Kostelnik, B., and Kupfer, D.J. (2002). Clinical significance of lifetime panic spectrum symptoms in the treatment of patients with bipolar I disorder. *Arch Gen Psychiatry*, 59, 905–911.

Freed, E.X. (1969). Alcohol abuse by manic patients. *Psychol Rep*, 25, 280.

Freeman, M.P., Freeman, S.A., and McElroy, S.L. (2002). The comorbidity of bipolar and anxiety disorders: Prevalence, psychobiology, and treatment issues. *J Affect Disord*, 68, 1–23.

Frye, M.A., Denicoff, K.D., Bryan, A.L., Smith-Jackson, E.E., Ali, S.O., Luckenbaugh, D., Leverich, G.S., and Post, R.M. (1999). Association between lower serum free T4 and greater mood instability and depression in lithium-maintained bipolar patients. *Am J Psychiatry*, 156, 1909–1914.

Frye, M.A., Altshuler, L.L., McElroy, S.L., Suppes, T., Keck, P.E., Denicoff, K., Nolen, W.A., Kupka, R., Leverich, G.S., Pollio, C., Grunze, H., Walden, J., Post, R.M. (2003). Gender differences in prevalence, risk, and clinical correlates of alcoholism comorbidity in bipolar disorder. *Am J Psychiatry*, 160, 883–889.

Gawin, F.H., and Kleber, H.D. (1986). Abstinence symptomatology and psychiatric diagnosis in cocaine abusers: Clinical observations. *Arch Gen Psychiatry*, 43, 107–113.

Gaziano, J.M., Gaziano, T.A., Glynn, R.J., Sesso, H.D., Ajani, U.A., Stampfer, M.J., Manson, J.E., Hennekens, C.H., and Buring, J.E. (2000). Light-to-moderate alcohol consumption and mortality in the Physicians' Health Study enrollment cohort. *J Am Coll Cardiol*, 35, 96–105.

Gibb, B., Coles, M., and Heimberg, R. (2005). Differentiating symptoms of social anxiety and depression in adults with social anxiety disorder. *J Behav Ther Exp Psychol*, 36, 99–109.

Gijsman, H.J., Geddes, J.R., Rendell, J.M., Nolen, W.A., and Goodwin, G.M. (2004). Antidepressants for bipolar depression: A systematic review of randomized, controlled trials. *Am J Psychiatry*, 161, 1537–1547.

Gold, P.W., Goodwin, F.K., Wehr, T., and Rebar, R. (1977). Pituitary thyrotropin response to thyrotropin-releasing hormone in affective illness: Relationship to spinal fluid amine metabolites. *Am J Psychiatry*, 134, 1028–1031.

Goldberg, J.F., and Whiteside, J.E. (2002). The association between substance abuse and antidepressant-induced mania in bipolar disorder: A preliminary study. *J Clin Psychiatry*, 63, 791–795.

Goldberg, J.F., Garno, J.L., Leon, A.C., Kocsis, J.H., and Portera, L. (1999). A history of substance abuse complicates remission from acute mania in bipolar disorder. *J Clin Psychiatry*, 60, 733–740.

Goldstein, B.I., and Levitt, A.J. (2006). Factors associated with temporal priority in comorbid bipolar I disorder and alcohol use disorders: Results from the National Epidemiologic Survey on Alcohol and Related Conditions. *J Clin Psychiatry*, 67, 643–649.

Goldstein, B.I., Velyvis, V.P., and Parikh, S.V. (2005). *Does Moderate Alcohol Use in Bipolar Disorder Impact Course and Symptom Burden?* Presented at the annual meeting of the American Psychiatric Association, Atlanta.

Goldstein, B.I., Herrmann, N., and Shulman, K.I. (2006). Comorbidity in bipolar disorder among the elderly: Results from an epidemiological community sample. *Am J Psychiatry*, 163, 319–321.

Goodwin, R.D., and Hoven, C.W. (2002). Bipolar-panic comorbidity in the general population: Prevalence and associated morbidity. *J Affect Disord*, 70, 27–33.

Gortmaker, S.L., Must, A., Perrin, J.M., Sobol, A.M., and Dietz, W.H. (1993). Social and economic consequences of overweight in adolescence and young adulthood. *N Engl J Med*, 329, 1008–1012.

Gould, T.D., Chen, G., and Manji, H.K. (2004). In vivo evidence in the brain for lithium inhibition of glycogen synthase kinase-3. *Neuropsychopharmacology*, 29, 32–38.

Guo, J.J., Keck, P.E., Jang, R., Li, H., Corey Lisle, P., and Jiang, D. (2005). *Prevalence and Key Comorbidities among Patients with Bipolar Disorders in a Large Managed Care Population.* Presented at the annual meeting of the American Psychiatric Association, Atlanta.

Haggerty, J.J. Jr., Stern, R.A., Mason, G.A., Beckwith, J., Morey, C.E., and Prange, A.J. Jr. (1993). Subclinical hypothyroidism: A modifiable risk factor for depression? *Am J Psychiatry*, 150, 508–510.

Harris, E.C., and Barraclough, B. (1997). Suicide as an outcome for mental disorders: A meta analysis. *Br J Psychiatry*, 170, 205–228.

Haywood, T.W., Kravitz, H.M., Grossman, L.S., Cavanaugh, J.L. Jr., Davis, J.M., and Lewis, D.A. (1995). Predicting the "revolving door" phenomenon among patients with schizophrenic, schizoaffective, and affective disorders. *Am J Psychiatry*, 152, 856–861.

Helzer, J.E., and Pryzbeck, T.R. (1988). The co-occurrence of alcoholism with other psychiatric disorders in the general population and its impact on treatment. *J Stud Alcohol*, 49, 219–224.

Henderson, D.C., Cagliero, E., Copeland, P.M., Borba, C.P., Evins, E., Hayden, D., Weber, M.T., Anderson, E.J., Allison, D.B., Daley, T.B., Schoenfeld, D., and Goff, D.C. (2005). Glucose metabolism in patients with schizophrenia treated with atypical antipsychotic agents: A frequently sampled intravenous glucose tolerance test and minimal model analysis. *Arch Gen Psychiatry*, 62, 19–28.

Henquet, C., Krabbendam, L., de Graaf, R., ten Have, M., and van Os, J. (2006). Cannabis use and expression of mania in the general population. *J Affect Disord*, 95, 103–110.

Henry, C., Van den Bulke, D., Bellivier, F., Etain, B., Rouillon, F., and Leboyer, M. (2003). Anxiety disorders in 318 bipolar patients: Prevalence and impact on illness severity and response to mood stabilizer. *J Clin Psychiatry*, 64, 331–335.

Hensel, B., Dunner, D.L., and Fieve, R.R. (1979). The relationship of family history of alcoholism to primary affective disorder. *J Affect Disord*, 1, 105–113.

Hesselbrock, M.N., Meyer, R.E., and Keener, J.J. (1985). Psychopathology in hospitalized alcoholics. *Arch Gen Psychiatry*, 42, 1050–1055.

Hetman, M., Cavanaugh, J.E., Kimelman, D., and Xia, Z. (2000). Role of glycogen synthase kinase-3β in neuronal apoptosis induced by trophic withdrawal. *J Neurosci*, 20, 2567–2574.

Hides, L., Dawe, S., Kavanagh, D.J., and Young, R. (2006). Psychotic symptom and cannabis relapse in recent-onset psychosis. *Br J Psychiatry*, 189, 137–143.

Himmelhoch, J.M. (1998). Social anxiety, hypomania and the bipolar spectrum: Data, theory and clinical issues. *J Affect Disord*, 50, 203–213.

Himmelhoch, J.M., and Garfinkel, M.E. (1986). Sources of lithium resistance in mixed mania. *Psychopharmacol Bull*, 22, 613–620.

Himmelhoch, J.M., Mulla, D., Neil, J.F., Detre, T.P., and Kupfer, D.J. (1976). Incidence and significance of mixed affective states in a bipolar population. *Arch Gen Psychiatry*, 33, 1062–1066.

Himmelhoch, J.M., Hill, S., Steinberg, B., and May, S. (1983). Lithium, alcoholism, and psychiatric diagnosis. *J Psychiatr Treat Eval*, 5, 83–88.

Howland, R.H. (1993). Thyroid dysfunction in refractory depression: Implications for pathophysiology and treatment. *J Clin Psychiatry*, 54, 47–54.

Hu, M., Wu, H., and Chao, C. (1997). Assisting effects of lithium on hypoglycemic treatment in patients with diabetes. *Biol Trace Elem Res*, 60, 131–137.

Hudson, J.I., Pope, H.G. Jr., Wurtman, J., Yurgelun-Todd, D., Mark, S., and Rosenthal, N.E. (1988). Bulimia in obese individuals: Relationship to normal-weight bulimia. *J Nerv Ment Dis*, 176, 144–152.

Institute of Medicine (IOM). (2002). *Reducing Suicide: A National Imperative*. Washington, DC: National Academy Press.

Isojarvi, J.I., Pakarinen, A.J., and Myllyla, V.V. (1989). Thyroid function in epileptic patients treated with carbamazepine. *Arch Neurol*, 46, 1175–1178.

Jamison, K.R. (2004). *Exuberance: The Passion for Life*. New York: Alfred A. Knopf.

Johannessen, L., Strudsholm, U., Foldager, L., and Munk-Jorgensen, P. (2006). Increased risk of hypertension in patients with bipolar disorder and patients with anxiety compared to background population and patients with schizophrenia. *J Affect Disord*, 95(1–3), 13–17.

Johnson, S.L., Winett, C.A., Meyer, B., Greenhouse, W.J., and Miller, I. (1999). Social support and the course of bipolar disorder. *J Abnorm Psychol*, 108, 558–566.

Judd, L.L., Akiskal, H.S., Schettler, P.J., Coryell, W., Maser, J., Rice, J.A., Solomon, D.A., and Keller, M.B. (2003a). The comparative clinical phenotype and long term longitudinal episode course of bipolar I and II: A clinical spectrum or distinct disorders? *J Affect Disord*, 73, 19–32.

Judd, L.L., Schettler, P.J., Akiskal, H.S., Maser, J., Coryell, W., Solomon, D., Endicott, J., and Keller, M. (2003b). Long-term symptomatic status of bipolar I vs. bipolar II disorders. *Int J Neuropsychopharmacol*, 6, 127–137.

Kathol, R.G., Turner, R., and Delahunt, J. (1986). Depression and anxiety associated with hyperthyroidism: Response to antithyroid therapy. *Psychosomatics*, 27, 501–505.

Kawa, I., Carterm, J., Joyce, P., Doughty, C., Frampton, C., Well, E.J., Walsh, A., and Olds, R. (2005). Gender differences in bipolar disorder: Age of onset, course, comorbidity, and symptom presentation. *Bipolar Disord*, 7, 119–125.

Keck, P.E. Jr., McElroy, S.L., Strakowski, S.M., West, S.A., Hawkins, J.M., Huber, T.J., Newman, R.M., and DePriest, M. (1995). Outcome and comorbidity in first- compared with multiple-episode mania. *J Nerv Ment Dis*, 183, 320–324.

Keck, P.E. Jr., McElroy, S.L., Strakowski, S.M., Bourne, M.L., and West, S.A. (1997). Compliance with maintenance treatment in bipolar disorder. *Psychopharmacol Bull*, 33, 87–91.

Keeler, M.H., Taylor, C.I., and Miller, W.C. (1979). Are all recently detoxified alcoholics depressed? *Am J Psychiatry*, 136, 586–588.

Kessler, R. (2004). *Prevalence of adult ADHD in the United States: Results from the National Comorbidity Survey Replication (NCS)*. Presented at the annual meeting of the American Psychiatric Association, New York.

Kessler, R.C., McGonagle, K.A., Zhao, S., Nelson, C.B., Hughes, M., Eshleman, S., Wittchen, H.U., and Kendler, K.S. (1994). Lifetime and 12-month prevalence of DSM-III-R psychiatric disorders in the United States: Results from the National Comorbidity Survey. *Arch Gen Psychiatry*, 51, 8–19.

Kessler, R.C., Sonnega, A., Bromet, E., Hughes, M., and Nelson, C.B. (1995). Posttraumatic stress disorder in the National Comorbidity Survey. *Arch Gen Psychiatry*, 52, 1048–1060.

Kessler, R.C., Nelson, C.B., McGonagle, K.A., Edlund, M.J., Frank, R.G., and Leaf, P.J. (1996). The epidemiology of co-occurring addictive and mental disorders: Implications for prevention and service utilization. *Am J Orthopsychiatry*, 66, 17–31.

Kessler, R.C., Rubinow, D.R., Holmes, C., Abelson, J.M., and Zhao, S. (1997). The epidemiology of DSM-III-R bipolar I disorder in a general population survey. *Psychol Med*, 27, 1079–1089.

Khantzian, E.J. (1974). Opiate addiction: A critique of theory and some implications for treatment. *Am J Psychother*, 28, 59–70.

Khantzian, E.J. (1985). The self-medication hypothesis of addictive disorders: Focus on heroin and cocaine dependence. *Am J Psychiatry*, 142, 1259–1264.

Kogan, J.N., Otto, M.W., Bauer, M.S., Dennehy, E.B., Miklowitz, D.J., Zhang, H.W., Ketter, T., Rudorfer, M.V., Wisniewski, S.R., Thase, M.E., Calabrese, J., Sachs, G.S., and STEP-BD Investigators. (2004). Demographic and diagnostic characteristics of the first 1000 patients enrolled in the Systematic Treatment Enhancement Program for Bipolar Disorder (STEP-BD). *Bipolar Disord*, 6, 460–469.

Kosten, T.R., and Rounsaville, B.J. (1986). Psychopathology in opioid addicts. *Psychiatr Clin North Am*, 9, 515–532.

Kosten, T.R., Mason, J.W., Giller, E.L., Ostroff, R.B., and Harkness, L. (1987). Sustained urinary norepinephrine and epinephrine elevation in post-traumatic stress disorder. *Psychoneuroendocrinology*, 12, 13–20.

Kraepelin, E. (1921). *Manic-depressive insanity and paranoia*. Edinburgh, Scotland: E & S Livingstone.

Krüger, S., Cooke, R.G., Hasey, G.M., Jorna, T., and Persad, E. (1995). Comorbidity of obsessive compulsive disorder in bipolar disorder. *J Affect Disord*, 34, 117–120.

Krüger, S., Shugar, G., and Cooke, R.G. (1996). Comorbidity of binge eating disorder and the partial binge eating syndrome with bipolar disorder. *Int J Eat Disord*, 19, 45–52.

Krüger, S., Braunig, P., and Cooke, R.G. (2000). Comorbidity of obsessive-compulsive disorder in recovered inpatients with bipolar disorder. *Bipolar Disord*, 2, 71–74.

Kusalic, M. (1992). Grade II and grade III hypothyroidism in rapid-cycling bipolar patients. *Neuropsychobiology*, 25, 177–181.

Lazarus, J.H. (1998). The effects of lithium therapy on thyroid and thyrotropin-releasing hormone. *Thyroid*, 8, 909–913.

Leino-Arjas, P., Liira, J., Mutanen, P., Malmivaara, A., and Matikainen, E. (1999). Predictors and consequences of unemployment among construction workers: Prospective cohort study. *BMJ*, 319, 600–605.

Lensi, P., Cassano, G.B., Correddu, G., Ravagli, S., Kunovac, J.L., and Akiskal, H.S. (1996). Obsessive-compulsive disorder: Familial-developmental history, symptomatology, comorbidity and course with special reference to gender-related differences. *Br J Psychiatry*, 169, 101–107.

Lewinsohn, P.M., Striegel-Moore, R.H., Seeley, J.R. (2000). Epidemiology and natural course of eating disorders in young women from adolescence to young adulthood. *J Am Acad Child Adolesc Psychiatry*, 39, 1284–1292.

Lewis, A. (1936). Prognosis in the manic-depressive psychosis. *Lancet*, 997–999.

Liskow, B., Mayfield, D., and Thiele, J. (1982). Alcohol and affective disorder: Assessment and treatment. *J Clin Psychiatry*, 43, 144–147.

MacKinnon, D.F., McMahon, F.J., Simpson, S.G., McInnis, M.G., and DePaulo, J.R. (1997). Panic disorder with familial bipolar disorder. *Biol Psychiatry*, 42, 90–95.

MacKinnon, D.F., Zandi, P.P., Cooper, J., Potash, J.B., Simpson, S.G., Gershon, E., Nurnberger, J., Reich, T., and DePaulo, J.R. (2002). Comorbid bipolar disorder and panic disorder in families with a high prevalence of bipolar disorder. *Am J Psychiatry*, 159, 30–35.

MacKinnon, D.F., Zandi, P.P., Gershon, E., Nurnberger, J.I. Jr., Reich, T., and DePaulo, J.R. (2003). Rapid switching of mood in families with multiple cases of bipolar disorder. *Arch Gen Psychiatry*, 60, 921–928.

MacQueen, G.M., Marriott, M., Begin, H., Robb, J., Joffe, R.T., and Young, L.T. (2003). Subsyndromal symptoms assessed in longitudinal, prospective follow-up of a cohort of patients with bipolar disorder. *Bipolar Disord*, 5(5), 349–355.

Maes, M., Lin, A.H., Verkerk, R., Delmeire, L., Van Gastel, A., Van der Planken, M., and Scharpe, S. (1999). Serotonergic and noradrenergic markers of post-traumatic stress disorder with and without major depression. *Neuropsychopharmacology*, 20, 188–197.

Mahmood, T., Romans, S., and Silverstone, T. (1999). Prevalence of migraine in bipolar disorder. *J Affect Disord*, 52(1–3), 239–241.

Mantere, O., Melartin, T.R., Suominen, K., Rytsala, H.J., Valtonen, H.M., Arvilommi, P., Leppamaki, S., and Isometsa, E.T. (2006). Differences in axis-I and -II comorbidity between bipolar I and II disorders and major depressive disorder. *J Clin Psychiatry*, 67, 584–593.

Maremmani, I., Perugi, G., Pacini, M., and Akiskal, H.S. (2006). Toward a unitary perspective on the bipolar spectrum and substance abuse: Opiate addiction as a paradigm. *J Affect Disord*, 93(1-3), 1–12.

Marneros, A., and Goodwin, F.K. (Eds.). (2005). *Mixed States, Rapid Cycling and Atypical Forms*. Cambridge, MA: Cambridge University Press.

Mayfield, D.G., and Coleman, L.L. (1968). Alcohol use and affective disorder. *Dis Nerv Syst* 29, 467–474.

McElroy, S.L., Strakowski, S.M., Keck, J., Paul, E., Tugrul, K.L., West, S.A., and Lonczak, H.S. (1995). Differences and similarities in mixed and pure mania. *Compr Psychiatry*, 36, 187–194.

McElroy, S.L., Altshuler, L.L., Suppes, T., Keck, P.E. Jr., Frye, M.A., Denicoff, K.D., Nolen, W.A., Kupka, R.W., Leverich, G.S., Rochussen, J.R., Rush, A.J., and Post, R.M. (2001). Axis I psychiatric comorbidity and its relationship to historical illness variables in 288 patients with bipolar disorder. *Am J Psychiatry*, 158, 420–426.

McElroy, S.L., Frye, M.A., Suppes, T., Dhavale, D., Keck, P.E. Jr., Leverich, G.S., Altshuler, L., Denicoff, K.D., Nolen, W.A., Kupka, R., Grunze, H., Walden, J., and Post, R.M. (2002). Correlates of overweight and obesity in 644 patients with bipolar disorder. *J Clin Psychiatry*, 63, 207–213.

McElroy, S.L., Kotwal, R., Keck, P.E., and Akiskal, H.S. (2005). Comorbidity of bipolar and eating disorders: Distinct or related disorders with shared dysregulations? *J Affect Dis*, 86, 107–127.

McIntyre, R., Konarski, J., Wilkins, K., Bouffard, B., Soczynska, J.D., and Kennedy, S. (2006). The prevalence and impact of migraine headache in bipolar disorder: Results from the Canadian Community Health Survey. *Headache*, 6, 973–982.

Milkman, H., and Frosch, W.A. (1973). On the preferential abuse of heroin and amphetamine. *J Nerv Ment Dis*. 156, 242–248.

Miller, F.T., Busch, F, and Tanenbaum, J.H. (1989). Drug abuse in schizophrenia and bipolar disorder. *Am J Drug Alcohol Abuse*, 15, 291–295.

Minski, L. (1938). Psychopathology and psychoses associated with alcohol. *J Mental Sci*, 84, 985–990.

Mirin, S.M., Weiss, R.D., Sollogub, A., and Michael, J. (1984). Affective illness in substance abusers. In S.M. Mirin (Ed.), *Substance Abuse and Psychopathology* (pp. 57–78). Washington, DC: American Psychiatric Press.

Morrison, J.R. (1974). Bipolar affective disorder and alcoholism. *Am J Psychiatry*, 131, 1130–1133.

Mueser, K.T., Goodman, L.B., Trumbetta, S.L., Rosenberg, S.D., Osher, C., Vidaver, R., Auciello, P., and Foy, D.W. (1998). Trauma and posttraumatic stress disorder in severe mental illness. *J Consult Clin Psychol*, 66, 493–499.

Musselman, D.L., Tomer, A., Manatunga, A.K., Knight, B.T., Porter, M.R., Kasey, S., Marzec, U., Harker, L.A., and Nemeroff, C.B. (1996). Exaggerated platelet reactivity in major depression. *Am J Psychiatry*, 153, 1313–1317.

Narrow, W.E., Rae, D.S., Robins, L.N., and Regier, D.A. (2002). Revised prevalence estimates of mental disorders in the United States: Using a clinical significance criterion to reconcile 2 surveys' estimates. *Arch Gen Psychiatry*, 59, 115–123.

Neria, Y., Bromet, E.J., Sievers, S., Lavelle, J., and Fochtmann, L.J. (2002). Trauma exposure and posttraumatic stress disorder in psychosis: Findings from a first-admission cohort. *J Consult Clin Psychol*, 70, 246–251.

Norton, B., and Whalley, L.J. (1984). Mortality of a lithium-treated population. *Br J Psychiatry*, 145, 277–282.

Oedegaard, K.J., and Fasmer, O.B. (2005). Is migraine in unipolar depressed patients a bipolar spectrum trait? *J Affect Disord*, 84(2-3), 233–242.

Oedegaard, K.J., Neckelmann, D., and Fasmer, O.B. (2005). Type A behavior differentiates bipolar II from unipolar depressed patients. *J Affect Disord*, 90, 7–13.

Office of Applied Studies. (2001). *Summary of Findings from the 2000 National Household Survey on Drug Abuse*. Rockville, MD: Substance Abuse and Mental Health Services Administration.

Olfson, M., Guardino, M., Struening, E., Schneier, F.R., Hellman, F., and Klein, D.F. (2000). Barriers to the treatment of social anxiety. *Am J Psychiatry*, 157, 521–527.

Orena, S.J., Torchia, A.J., and Garofalo, R.S. (2000). Inhibition of glycogen-synthase kinase 3 stimulates glycogen synthase and glucose transport by distinct mechanisms in 3T3-L1 adipocytes. *J Biol Chem*, 275, 15765–15772.

Osby, U., Brandt, L., Correia, N., Ekbom, A., and Sparen, P. (2001). Excess mortality in bipolar and unipolar disorder in Sweden. *Arch Gen Psychiatry* 58(9), 844–850.

Otto, M.W., Perlman, C.A., Wernicke, R., Reese, H.E., Bauer, M.S., and Pollack, M.H. (2004). Posttraumatic stress disorder in patients with bipolar disorder: A review of prevalence, correlates, and treatment strategies. *Bipolar Disord*, 6, 470–479.

Otto, M.W., Simon, N.M., Wisniewski, S.R., Miklowitz, D.J., Kogan, J.N.., Reilly-Harrington, N.A., Frank, E., Nierenberg, A.A., Marangell, L.B., Sagduyu, K., Weiss, R.D., Miyahara, S., Thase, M.E., Sachs, G.S., and Pollack, M.H. (2006). Prospective 12-month course of bipolar disorder in outpatients with and without comorbid anxiety disorders. *Br J Psychiatry*, 189, 20–25.

Perlick, D.A., Rosenheck, R.A., Kaczynski, R., and Kozma, L. (2004). Medication non-adherence in bipolar disorder: A patient-centered review of research findings. *Clinical Approaches in Bipolar Disorders*, 3, 56–64.

Perlis, R.H., Miyahara, S., Marangell, L.B., Wisniewski, S.R., Ostacher, M., DelBello, M.P., Bowden, C.L., Sachs, G.S., Nierenberg, A.A., and STEP-BD Investigators. (2004). Long-term implications of early onset in bipolar disorder: Data from the first 1000 participants in the Systematic Treatment Enhancement Program for Bipolar Disorder (STEP-BD). *Biol Psychiatry*, 55, 875–881.

Perry, C.G., Spiers, A., Cleland, S.J., Lowe, G.D., Petrie, J.R., and Connell, J.M. (2003). Glucocorticoids and insulin sensitivity: Dissociation of insulin's metabolic and vascular actions. *J Clin Endocrinol Metab*, 88, 6008–6014.

Perugi, G., Akiskal, H.S., Pfanner, C., Presta, S., Gemignani, A., Milanfranchi, A., Lensi, P., Ravagli, S., and Cassano, G.B. (1997). The clinical impact of bipolar and unipolar affective comorbidity on obsessive-compulsive disorder. *J Affect Disord*, 46, 15–23.

Perugi, G., Akiskal, H.S., Ramacciotti, S., Nassini, S., Toni, C., Milanfranchi, A., and Musetti, L. (1999). Depressive comorbidity of panic, social phobic, and obsessive-compulsive disorders re-examined: Is there a bipolar II connection? *J Psychiatr Res*, 33, 53–61.

Perugi, G., Akiskal, H.S., Toni, C., Simonini, E., and Gemignani, A. (2001). The temporal relationship between anxiety disorders and (hypo)mania: A retrospective examination of 63 panic, social phobic and obsessive-compulsive patients with comorbid bipolar disorder. *J Affect Disord*, 67, 199–206.

Perugi, G., Toni, C., Frare, F., Travierso, M.C., Hantouche, E., and Akiskal, H.S. (2002). Obsessive-compulsive–bipolar comorbidity: A systematic exploration of clinical features and treatment outcome. *J Clin Psychiatry*, 63(12), 1129–1134.

Pine, D.S., Goldstein, R.B., Wolk, S., and Weissman, M.M. (2001). The association between childhood depression and adulthood body mass index. *Pediatrics*, 107, 1049–1056.

Pini, S., Cassano, G.B., Simonini, E., Savino, M., Russo, A., and Montgomery, S.A. (1997). Prevalence of anxiety disorders comorbidity in bipolar depression, unipolar depression and dysthymia. *J Affect Disord*, 42, 145–153.

Pini, S., Dell'Osso, L., Mastrocinque, C., Marcacci, G., Papasogli, A., Vignoli, S., Pallanti, S., and Cassano, G. (1999). Axis I comorbidity in bipolar disorder with psychotic features. *Br J Psychiatry*, 175, 467–471.

Placidi, G.P., Boldrini, M., Patronelli, A., Fiore, E., Chiovato, L., Perugi, G., and Marazziti, D. (1998). Prevalence of psychiatric disorders in thyroid diseased patients. *Neuropsychobiology*, 38, 222–225.

Poe, E.A. (1848). *The Letters of Edgar Allan Poe* (Vol. 2, p. 356). J. Wand Ostrom (Ed.). Cambridge, MA: Harvard University Press.

Post, R.M., Kotin, J., and Goodwin, F.K. (1974). The effects of cocaine on depressed patients. *Am J Psychiatry*, 131, 511–517.

Post, R.M., Rubinow, D.R., and Ballenger, J.C. (1984). Conditioning, sensitization and kindling: Implications for the course of affective illness. In R.M. Post, J.C. Ballenger (Eds.), *The Neurobiology of Mood Disorders* (pp. 432–466). New York: Williams & Wilkins.

Post, R.M., Kramlinger, K.G., Joffe, R.T., Roy-Byrne, P.P., Rosoff, A., Frye, M.A., and Huggins, T. (1997). Rapid cycling bipolar affective disorder: Lack of relation to hypothyroidism. *Psychiatry Res*, 72, 1–7.

Potash, J.B., Willour, V.L., Chiu, Y.F., Simpson, S.G., MacKinnon, D.F., Pearlson, G.D., DePaulo, J.R. Jr., and McInnis, M.G. (2001). The familial aggregation of psychotic symptoms in bipolar disorder pedigrees. *Am J Psychiatry*, 158, 1258–1264.

Prien, R.F., Klett, C.J., and Caffey, E.M. Jr. (1973). Lithium carbonate and imipramine in prevention of affective episodes: A comparison in recurrent affective illness. *Arch Gen Psychiatry*, 29, 420–425.

Reed, C., Goetz, I., van Os, J., and Tohen, M. (2005). Comorbid Cannabis Use in Patients with Acute Mania: Functional Status. Presented at the annual meeting of the American Psychiatric Association, Atlanta.

Regier, D.A., Boyd, J.H., Burke, J.D., Jr., Rae, D.S., Myers, J.K., Kramer, M., Robins, L.N., George, L.K., Karno, M., and Locke, B.Z. (1988). One-month prevalence of mental disorders in the United States: Based on five Epidemiologic Catchment Area sites. *Arch Gen Psychiatry*, 45, 977–986.

Regier, D.A., Farmer, M.E., Rae, D.S., Locke, B.Z., Keith, S.J., Judd, L.L., and Goodwin, F.K. (1990). Comorbidity of mental disorders with alcohol and other drug abuse: Results from the Epidemiologic Catchment Area (ECA) Study. *JAMA*, 264, 2511–2518.

Reich, L.H., Davies, R.K., and Himmelhoch, J.M. (1974). Excessive alcohol use in manic-depressive illness. *Am J Psychiatry*, 131, 83–86.

Robins, L.N., and Regier, D.A. (1991). *Psychiatric Disorders in America: The Epidemiologic Catchment Area Study*. New York: Free Press.

Rounsaville, B.J., Weissman, M.M., Kleber, H., and Wilber, C. (1982). Heterogeneity of psychiatric diagnosis in treated opiate addicts. *Arch Gen Psychiatry*, 39, 161–166.

Ruzickova, M., Slaney, C., Garnham, J., and Alda, M. (2003). Clinical features of bipolar disorder with and without comorbid diabetes mellitus. *Can J Psychiatry*, 48, 458–461.

Salloum, I.M., Cornelius, J.R., Douaihy, A., Kirisci, L., Daley, D., Kelly, T. (2005). Patient characteristic and treatment implications of marijuana abuse among bipolar alcoholics: Results from a double blind, placebo-controlled study. *Addict Behav* 30(9), 1702–1708.

Sasson, Y., Chopra, M., Harrari, E., Amitai, K., and Zohar, J. (2003). Bipolar comorbidity: From diagnostic dilemmas to therapeutic challenge. *Int J Neuropsychopharmacol*, 6, 139–144.

Savino, M., Perugi, G., Simonini, E., Soriani, A., Cassano, G.B., and Akiskal, H.S. (1993). Affective comorbidity in panic disorder: Is there a bipolar connection? *J Affect Disord*, 28, 155–163.

Schneck, C.D., Miklowitz, D.J., Calabrese, J.R., Allen, M.H., Thomas, M.R., Wisniewski, S.R., Miyahara, S., Shelton, M.D., Ketter, T.A., Goldberg, J.F., Bowden, C.L., and Sachs, G.S. (2004). Phenomenology of rapid-cycling bipolar disorder: Data from the first 500 participants in the Systematic Treatment Enhancement Program. *Am J Psychiatry*, 161, 1902–1908.

Schnurr, P.P., Friedman, M.J., and Rosenberg, S.D. (1993). Premilitary MMPI scores as predictors of combat-related PTSD symptoms. *Am J Psychiatry*, 150, 479–483.

Schuckit, M.A. (1986). Genetic and clinical implications of alcoholism and affective disorder. *Am J Psychiatry*, 143, 140–147.

Schuckit, M.A., Tipp, J.E., Anthenelli, R.M., Bucholz, K.K., Hesselbrock, V.M., and Nurnberger, J.I. Jr. (1996). Anorexia nervosa and bulimia nervosa in alcohol-dependent men and women and their relatives. *Am J Psychiatry*, 153(1), 74–82.

Secnik, K., Swensen, A., and Lage, M.J. (2005). Comorbidities and costs of adult patients diagnosed with attention-deficit hyperactivity disorder. *Pharmacoeconomics*, 23, 93–102.

Sharma, R., and Markar, H.R. (1994). Mortality in affective disorder. *J Affect Disord*, 31, 91–96.

Silberman, E.K., Reus, V.I., Jimerson, D.C., Lynott, A.M., and Post, R.M. (1981). Heterogeneity of amphetamine response in depressed patients. *Am J Psychiatry*, 138, 1302–1307.

Simon, N.M., Smoller, J.W., Fava, M., Sachs, G., Racette, S.R., Perlis, R., Sonawalla, S., and Rosenbaum, J.F. (2003). Comparing anxiety disorders and anxiety-related traits in bipolar disorder and unipolar depression. *J Psychiatr Res*, 37, 187–192.

Simon, N.M., Otto, M.W., Weiss, R.D., Bauer, M.S., Miyahara, S., Wisniewski, S.R., Thase, M.E., Kogan, J., Frank, E., Nierenberg, A.A., Calabrese, J.R., Sachs, G.S., Pollack, M.H., and STEP-BD Investigators. (2004a). Pharmacotherapy for bipolar disorder and comorbid conditions: Baseline data from STEP-BD. *J Clin Psychopharmacol*, 24, 512–520.

Simon, N.M., Otto, M.W., Wisniewski, S.R., Fossey, M., Sagduyu, K., Frank, E., Sachs, G.S., Nierenberg, A.A., Thase, M.E., and Pollack, M.H. (2004b). Anxiety disorder comorbidity in bipolar disorder patients: Data from the first 500 participants in the Systematic Treatment Enhancement Program for Bipolar Disorder (STEP-BD). *Am J Psychiatry*, 161, 2222–2229.

Simpson, S.G., al-Mufti, R., Andersen, A.E., and DePaulo, J.R. Jr. (1992). Bipolar II affective disorder in eating disorder inpatients. *J Nerv Ment Dis*, 180, 719–722.

Spitzer, R.L., Yanovski, S., Wadden, T., Wing, R., Marcus, M.D., Stunkard, A., Devlin, M., Mitchell, J., Hasin, D., and Horne, R.L. (1993). Binge eating disorder: Its further validation in a multisite study. *Int J Eat Disord*, 13, 137–153.

Strakowski, S.M., Tohen, M., Stoll, A.L., Faedda, G.L., and Goodwin, D.C. (1992). Comorbidity in mania at first hospitalization. *Am J Psychiatry*, 149(4), 554–556.

Strakowski, S.M., Stoll, A.L., Tohen, M., Faedda, G.L., and Goodwin, D.C. (1993). The Tridimensional Personality Questionnaire as a predictor of six-month outcome in first episode mania. *Psychiatry Res*, 48(1), 1–8.

Strakowski, S.M., Sax, K.W., McElroy, S.L., Keck, P.E. Jr., Hawkins, J.M., and West, S.A. (1998). Course of psychiatric and substance abuse syndromes co-occurring with bipolar disorder after a first psychiatric hospitalization. *J Clin Psychiatry*, 59, 465–471.

Strakowski, S.M., DelBello, M.P., Fleck, D.E., and Arndt, S. (2000). The impact of substance abuse on the course of bipolar disorder. *Biol Psychiatry*, 48, 477–485.

Strakowski, S.M., DelBello, M.P., and Fleck, D.E. (2005). Effects of co-occurring alcohol abuse on the course of bipolar disorder following a first hospitalization for mania. *Arch Gen Psychiatry*, 62, 851–858.

Swann, A.C., Secunda, S., Davis, J.M., Robins, E., Hanin, I., Koslow, S.H., and Maas, J.W. (1983). CSF monoamine metabolites in mania. *Am J Psychiatry*, 140, 396–400.

Swartz, K.L., Pratt, L.A., Armenian, H.K., Lee, L.C., and Eaton, W.W. (2000). Mental disorders and the incidence of migraine headaches in a community sample: Results from the Baltimore Epidemiologic Catchment Area Follow-Up Study. *Arch Gen Psychiatry*, 57(10), 945–950.

Swartz, M.S., Swanson, J.W., Hiday, V.A., Borum, R., Wagner, R., and Burns, B.J. (1998). Taking the wrong drugs: The role of substance abuse and medication noncompliance in violence among severely mentally ill individuals. *Soc Psychiatry Psychiatr Epidemiol*, 33(Suppl 1), S75–S80.

Szadoczky, E., Papp, Z., Vitrai, J., Rihmer, Z., and Furedi, J. (1998). The prevalence of major depressive and bipolar disorders in Hungary: Results from a national epidemiologic survey. *J Affect Disord*, 50, 153–162.

Tabata, I., Schluter, J., Gulve, E.A., and Holloszy, J.O. (1994). Lithium increases susceptibility of muscle glucose transport to stimulation by various agents. *Diabetes*, 43, 903–907.

Thomsen, A.F., and Kessing, L.V. (2005). Increased risk of hyperthyroidism among patients hospitalized with bipolar disorder. *Bipolar Disord*, 7, 351–357.

Toalson, P., Ahmed, S., Hardy, T., and Kabinoff, G. (2004). The metabolic syndrome in patients with severe mental illnesses. *J Clin Psychiatry*, 6, 152–158.

Trzepacz, P.T., McCue, M., Klein, I., Levey, G.S., and Greenhouse, J. (1988). A psychiatric and neuropsychological study of patients with untreated Graves' disease. *Gen Hosp Psychiatry*, 10, 49–55.

Tucker, P., Zaninelli, R., Yehuda, R., Ruggiero, L., Dillingham, K., and Pitts, C.D. (2001). Paroxetine in the treatment of chronic posttraumatic stress disorder: Results of a placebo-controlled, flexible-dosage trial. *J Clin Psychiatry*, 62, 860–868.

Valle, J., Ayuso-Gutierrez, J.L., Abril, A., and Ayuso-Mateos, J.L. (1999). Evaluation of thyroid function in lithium-naive bipolar patients. *Eur Psychiatry*, 14, 341–345.

Vieta, E., Colom, F., Corbella, B., Martinez-Aran, A., Reinares, M., Benabarre, A., and Gasto, C. (2001). Clinical correlates of psychiatric comorbidity in bipolar I patients. *Bipolar Disord*, 3(5), 253–258.

Weber-Hamann, B., Hentschel, F., Kniest, A., Deuschle, M., Colla, M., Lederbogen, F., Heuser, I. (2002). Hypercortisolemic depression is associated with increased intra-abdominal fat. *Psychosom Med*, 64, 274–277.

Weeke, A. (1979). Causes of death in manic-depressives. In M. Schou, E. Strömgren (Eds.), *Origin, Prevention and Treatment of Affective Disorders*. London: Academic Press.

Weiller, E., Bisserbe, J.C., Boyer, P., Lepine, J.P., and Lecrubier, Y. (1996). Social phobia in general health care: An unrecognised undertreated disabling disorder. *Br J Psychiatry*, 168, 169–174.

Weiss, R.D., and Mirin, S.M. (1984). Drug, host, and environmental factors in the development of chronic cocaine abuse. In S.M. Mirin (Ed.), *Substance Abuse and Psychopathology* (pp. 41–56). Washington, DC: American Psychiatric Press.

Weiss, R.D., and Mirin, S.M. (1986). Subtypes of cocaine abusers. *Psychiatr Clin North Am*, 9, 491–501.

Weiss, R.D., and Mirin, S.M. (1987). Substance abuse as an attempt at self-medication. *Psychiatr Med*, 3, 357–367.

Weiss, R.D., Mirin, S.M., Michael, J.L., and Sollogub, A.C. (1986). Psychopathology in chronic cocaine abusers. *Am J Drug Alcohol Abuse*, 12, 17–29.

Weiss, R.D., Mirin, S.M., Griffin, M.L., and Michael, J.L. (1988). Psychopathology in cocaine abusers: Changing trends. *J Nerv Ment Dis*, 176, 719–725.

Weiss, R.D., Kolodziej, M., Griffin, M.L., Najavits, L.M., Jacobson, L.M., and Greenfield, S.F. (2004). Substance use and perceived symptom improvement among patients with bipolar disorder and substance dependence. *J Affect Disord*, 79, 279–283.

Wenzel, K.W., Meinhold, H., Raffenberg, M., Adlkofer, F., and Schleusener, H. (1974). Classification of hypothyroidism in evaluating patients after radioiodine therapy by serum cholesterol, T3-uptake, total T4, FT4-index, total T3, basal TSH and TRH-test. *Eur J Clin Invest*, 4, 141–148.

Whitwell, J.R. (1936). *Historical Notes on Psychiatry (Early times–End of 16th Century)*. London: H.K. Lewis.

Wilens, T.E., Biederman, J., Wozniak, J., Gunawardene, S., Wong, J., and Monuteaux, M. (2003). Can adults with attention-deficit/hyperactivity disorder be distinguished from those with comorbid bipolar disorder? Findings from a sample of clinically referred adults. *Biol Psychiatry*, 54, 1–8.

Winokur, G., Clayton, P.J., and Reich, T. (1969). *Manic Depressive Illness*. St. Louis: C.V. Mosby.

Winokur, G., Coryell, W., Akiskal, H.S., Maser, J.D., Keller, M.B., Endicott, J., and Mueller, T. (1995). Alcoholism in manic-depressive (bipolar) illness: Familial illness, course of illness, and the primary-secondary distinction. *Am J Psychiatry*, 152, 365–372.

Winokur, G., Turvey, C., Akiskal, H., Coryell, W., Solomon, D., and Leon, A. (1998). Alcoholism and drug abuse in three groups: Bipolar I, unipolars, and their acquaintances. *J Affect Dis*, 50, 81–89.

Wise, T., and Fernandez, F. (1979). Psychological profiles of candidates seeking surgical correction for obesity. *Obesity/Bariatric Med*, 8, 83–86.

Wurmser, L. (1974). Pscyhoanalytic considerations of the etiology of compulsive drug use. *J Am Psychoanal Assoc*, 22, 820–843.

Yates, W.R., and Wallace, R. (1987). Cardiovascular risk factors in affective disorder. *J Affect Disord*, 12, 129–134.

Young, L.T., Cooke, R.G., Robb, J.C., Levitt, A.J., and Joffe, R.T. (1993). Anxious and non-anxious bipolar disorder. *J Affect Disord*, 29, 49–52.

Young, L.T., Warsh, J.J., Kish, S.J., Shannak, K., and Hornykeiwicz, O. (1994). Reduced brain 5-HT and elevated NE turnover and metabolites in bipolar affective disorder. *Biol Psychiatry*, 35, 121–127.

Zilboorg, G. (1941). *A History of Medical Psychology*. New York: W.W. Norton.

Zisook, S., and Schuckit, M.A. (1987). Male primary alcoholics with and without family histories of affective disorder. *J Stud Alcohol*, 48, 337–344.

CHAPTER 8

Alvarez, J.C., Cremniter, D., Bluck, N., Quintin, P., Leboyer, M., Berlin, I., Therond, P., and Spreux-Varoquaux, O. (2000). Low serum cholesterol in violent but not in non-violent suicide attempters. *Psychiatry Res*, 21, 95(2), 103–108.

Angst, F., Strassen, H.H., Clayton, P.J., and Angst, J. (2002). Mortality of patients with mood disorders: Follow-up over 34–38 years. *J Affect Disord*, 68(2–3), 167–181.

Angst, J., Sellaro, R., and Angst, F. (1998). Long-term outcome and mortality of treated versus untreated bipolar and depressed patients: A preliminary report. *Int J Psychiatry Clin*, Practice 2, 115–119.

Angst, J., Angst, F., and Strassen, H.H. (1999). Suicide risk in patients with major depressive disorder. *J Clin Psychiatry*, 60(Suppl 2), 57–62; discussion 75–76, 113–116.

Appleby, L., Shaw, J., Amos, T., McDonnell, R., Harris, C., McCann, K., Kiernan, K., Davies, S., Bickley, H., and Parsons, R. (1999). Suicide within 12 months of contact with mental health services: National clinical survey. *BMJ*, 318(7193), 1235–1239.

Arango, V., Underwood, M.D., Gubbi, A.V., and Mann, J.J. (1995). Localized alterations in pre- and postsynaptic serotonin binding sites in the ventrolateral prefrontal cortex of suicide victims. *Brain Res*, 688(1–2), 121–133.

Arango, V., Underwood, M.D., and Mann, J.J. (1997). Postmortem findings in suicide victims: Implications for in vivo imaging studies. *Ann N Y Acad Sci*, 836, 269–287.

Arato, M., Banki, C.M., Bissette, G., and Nemeroff, C.B. (1989). Elevated CSF-CRF in suicide victims. *Biol Psychiatry*, 25(3), 355–359.

Asberg, M., Bertilsson, L., Cronholm, B., Harfast, A., Sjoqvist, F., and Tuck, D. (1972). Studies of indolamine metabolites in cerebrospinal fluid in depression. *Nord Psykiatr Tidsskr*, 26(6), 351–357.

Aschoff, J. (1981). Annual rhythms in man. In J. Aschoff (Ed.), *Handbook of Behavioral Neurobiology*. Vol. 4: *Biological Rhythms* (pp. 475–487). New York: Plenum Press.

Baca-Garcia, E., Vaquero, C., Diaz-Sastre, C., Ceverino, A., Saiz-Ruiz, J., Fernandez-Piquera, J., and de Leon, J. (2003). A pilot study on a gene-hormone interaction in female suicide attempts. *Eur Arch Psychiatry Clin Neurosci*, 253(6), 281.

Baca-Garcia, E., Vaquero, C., Diaz-Sastre, C., Garcia-Resa, E., Saiz-Ruiz, J., Fernandez-Piqueras, J., and De Leon, J. (2004). Lack of association between the serotonin transporter promoter gene polymorphism and impulsivity or aggressive behavior among suicide attempters and healthy volunteers. *Psychiatry Res*, 126(2), 99–106.

Balazs, J., Lecrubier, Y., Csiszer, N., Kosztak, J., and Bitter, I. (2003). Prevalence and comorbidity of affective disorders in persons making suicide attempts in Hungary: Importance of the first depressive episodes and of bipolar II diagnoses. *J Affect Disord*, 76(1–3), 113–119.

Baldessarini, R.J., and Hennen, J. (2004). Genetics of suicide: An overview. *Harv Rev Psychiatry*, 12(1), 1–13.

Ballenger, J.C., Goodwin, F.K., Major, L.F., and Brown, G.L. (1979). Alcohol and central serotonin metabolism in man. *Arch Gen Psychiatry*, 36, 224–227.

Barner-Rasmussen, P. (1986). Suicide in psychiatric patients in Denmark, 1971–1981. II: Hospital utilization and risk groups. *Acta Psychiatr Scand*, 73(4), 449–455.

Barraclough, B. (1970). The diagnostic classification and psychiatric treatment of 100 suicides. In R. Fox (Ed.), *Proceedings of the Fifth International Conference for Suicide Prevention* (pp. 129–132). Vienna, Austria: IASP.

Barraclough, B., Bunch, J., Nelson, B., and Sainsbury, P. (1974). A hundred cases of suicide: Clinical aspects. *Br J Psychiatry*, 125, 355–373.

Bauer, M.S., Calabrese, J., Dunner, D.L., Post, R., Whybrow, P.C., Gyulai, L., Tay, L.K., Younkin, S.R., Bynum, D., and Lavori, P. (1994). Multisite data reanalysis of the validity of rapid cycling as a course modifier for bipolar disorder in DSM-IV. *Am J Psychiatry*, 151(4), 506–515.

Beck, A.T., Brown, G.K., Steer, R.A., Dahlsgaard, K.K., and Grisham, J.R. (1999). Suicide ideation at its worst point: A predictor of eventual suicide in psychiatric outpatients. *Suicide Life Threat Behav*, 29(1), 1–9.

Behall, K.M., Scholfield, D.J., Hallfrisch, J.G., Kelsay, J.L., and Reiser, S. (1984). Seasonal variation in plasma glucose and hormone levels in adult men and women. *Am J Clin Nutr*, 40, 1352–1356.

Bertolote, J.M., and Fleischmann, A. (2002). Suicide rates in China. *Lancet*, 359(9325), 2274.

Black, D.W., Winokur, G., and Nassrallah, A. (1988). Effects of psychosis on suicide risk in 1593 patients with unipolar and bipolar affective disorders. *Am J Psychiatry*, 145, 849–852.

Bocchetta, A., Chillotti, C., Carboni, G., Oi, A., Ponti, M., and Del Zompo, M. (2001). Association of personal and familial suicide risk with low serum cholesterol concentration in male lithium patients. *Acta Psychiatr Scand*, 104(1), 37–41.

Bondy, B., Erfurth, A., de Jonge, S., Kruger, M., and Meyer, H. (2000). Possible association of the short allele of the serotonin transporter promoter gene polymorphism (5-HTTLPR) with violent suicide. *Mol Psychiatry*, 5(2), 193–195.

Bonnier, B., Garwood, P., Harmon, M., Surfeit, Y., Bony, C., and Hardy-Bale, M.C. (2002). Association of 5-HT(2A) receptor gene polymorphism with major affective disorders: The case of a subgroup of bipolar disorder with low suicide risk. *Biol Psychiatry*, 51(9), 762–765.

Boston, P.F., Durson, S.M., and Reveley, M.A. (1996). Cholesterol and mental disorder. *Br J Psychiatry*, 169, 682–689.

Bostwick, J.M., and Pankratz, V.S. (2000). Affective disorders and suicide risk: A reexamination. *Am J Psychiatry*, 157(12), 1925–1932.

Bottlender, R., Jager, M., Strauss, A., and Moller, H.J. (2000). Suicidality in bipolar compared to unipolar depressed inpatients. *Eur Arch Psychiatry Clin Neurosci*, 250(5), 257–261.

Brent, D.A., Bridge, J., Johnson, B.A., and Connolly, J. (1996). Suicidal behavior runs in families: A controlled family study of adolescent suicide victims. *Arch Gen Psychiatry*, 53(2), 1145–1152.

Brent, D.A., Oquendo, M., Birmaher, B., Greenhill, L., Kolko, D., Stanley, B., Zelazny, J., Brodsky, B., Firinciogullari, S., Ellis, S.P., and Mann, J.J. (2003). Peripubertal suicide attempts in offspring of suicide attempters siblings concordant for suicidal behavior. *Am J Psychiatry*, 160(8), 1486–1493.

Brodersen, A., Licht, R.W., Vestergaard, P., Olesen, A.V., and Mortensen, P.B. (2000). *Br J Psychiatry*, 176, 429–433.

Brown, G.K., Beck, A.T., Steer, R.A., and Grisham, J.R. (2000). Risk factors for suicide in psychiatric outpatients: A 20-year prospective study. *J Consult Clin Psychol*, 68(3), 371–377.

Brown, R.P., Mason, B., Stoll, P., Brizer, D., Kocsis, J., Stokes, P.E., and Mann, J.J. (1986). Consistency of pituitary-adrenocortical function across multiple psychiatric hospitalizations. *Psychiatry Research*. 17, 317–323.

Brunner, J., and Bronisch, T. (1999). Neurobiological correlates of suicidal behavior. *Fortschr Neurol Psychiatr*, 67(9), 391–412.

Bulik, C.M., Carpenter, L.L., Kupfer, D.J., and Frank, E. (1990). Features associated with suicide attempts in recurrent major depression. *J Affect Disord*, 18(1), 29–37.

Bunney, W.E., and Fawcett, J.A. (1965). Possibility of a biochemical test for suicidal potential: An analysis of endocrine findings prior to three studies. *Arch Gen Psychiatry* 13, 232–239.

Bunney, W.E. Jr., Fawcett, J.A., Davis, J.M., and Gifford, S. (1969). Further evaluation of urinary 17-hydroxycorticosteroids in suicidal patients. *Arch Gen Psychiatry*, 21(2), 138–150.

Busch, K.A., Fawcett, J., and Jacobs, D.G. (2003). Clinical correlates of inpatient suicide. *J Clin Psychiatry*, 64(1), 14–19.

Caetano, S.C., Olvera, R.L., Hunter, K., Hatch, J.P., Najt, P., Bowden, C., Pliszka, S., and Soares, J.C. (2006). Association of psychosis with suicidality in pediatric bipolar I, II and bipolar NOS patients. *J Affect Disord*, 91, 33–37.

Carlsson, A., Svennerholm, L., and Winblad, B. (1979). Seasonal and circadian monoamine variations in human brains examined postmorten. *Acta Psychiatr Scand*, 280, 75–83.

Caspi, A., Sugden, K., Moffitt, T.E., Taylor, A., Craig, I.W., Harrington, H., McClay, J., Mill, J., Martin, J., Braithwaite, A., and Poulton, R. (2003). Influence of life stress on depression: Moderation by a polymorphism in the 5-HTT gene. *Science*, 301(5631), 386–389.

Cassano, G.B., Akiskal, H.S., Savino, M., Musetti, S.M., and Perugi, G. (1992). Proposed subtypes of bipolar II and related disorders: With hypomanic episodes (or cyclothymia) and with hyperthymic temperament. *J Affect Disord*, 26(2), 127–140.

Cassidy, F., and Carroll, B.J. (2002a). Hypocholesterolemia during mixed manic episodes. *Eur Arch Psychiatry Clin Neurosci*, 252(3), 110–114.

Cassidy, F., and Carroll, B.J. (2002b). Seasonal variation of mixed and pure episodes of bipolar disorder. *J Affect Disord*, 68(1), 25–31.

Cheng, A.T., Chen, T.H., Chen, C.C., and Jenkins, R. (2000). Psychosocial and psychiatric risk factors for suicide: Case-control psychological autopsy study. *Br J Psychiatry*, 177, 360–365.

Chew, K.S., and McCleary, R. (1995). The spring peak in suicides: A cross-national analysis. *Soc Sci Med*, 40(2), 223–230.

Clark, D.A. (1991). *Crisis Intervention and Suicide Prevention from a Rural Perspective*. New York: NLN. NLN Publication 21-2408, pp. 165–172.

Cloninger, C.R. (2000). A practical way to diagnose personality disorder: A proposal. *J Personal Disord*, 14(2), 99–108.

Cloninger, C.R., Svrakic, D.M., and Przybeck, T.R. (1993). A psychobiological model of temperament and character. *Arch Gen Psychiatry*, 50(12), 975–990.

Cloninger, C.R., Van Eerdewegh, P., Goate, A., Edenberg, H.J., Blangero, J., Hesselbrock, V., Reich, T., Nurnberger, J. Jr., Schuckit, M., Porjesz, B., Crowe, R., Rice, J.P., Foroud, T., Przybeck, T.R., Almasy, L., Bucholz, K., Wu, W., Shears, S., Carr, K., Crose, C., Willig, C., Zhao, J., Tischfield, J.A., Li, T.K., and Conneally, P.M. (1998). Anxiety proneness linked to epistatic loci in genome scan of human personality traits. *Am J Med Genet*, 81(4), 313–317.

Cornelius, J.R., Salloum, I.M., Mezzich, J., Cornelius, M.D., Fabrega, H. Jr., Ehler, J.G., Ulrich, R.F., Thast, M.E., and Mann, J.J. (1995). Disproportionate suicidality in patients with co-morbid major depression and alcoholism. *Am J Psychiatry*, 152(3), 358–364.

Coryell, W. (1990). DST abnormality as a predictor of course in major depression. *J Affect Disord*, 19(3), 163–169.

Coryell, W., and Schlesser, M. (2001). The dexamethasone suppression test and suicide prediction. *Am J Psychiatry*, 158(5), 748–753.

Coryell, W., and Tsuang, M.T. (1982). Primary unipolar depression and the prognostic importance of delusions. *Arch Gen Psychiatry*, 39, 1181–1184.

Coryell, W., Andreasen, N.C., Endicott, J., and Keller, M. (1987). The significance of past mania or hypomania in the course and outcome of major depression. *Am J Psychiatry*, 144(3), 309–315.

Coryell, W., Solomon, D., Turvey, C., Keller, M., Leon, A.C., Endicott, J., Schettler, P., Judd, L., and Mueller, T. (2003). The long-term course of rapid-cycling bipolar disorder. *Arch Gen Psychiatry*, 60(9), 914–920.

Courtet, P., Picot, M.C., Bellivier, F., Torres, S., Jollant, F., Michelon, C., Castelnau, D., Astruc, B., Buresi, C., and Malafosse, A. (2004). Serotonin transporter gene may be involved in short-term risk of subsequent suicide attempts. *Biol Psychiatry*, 55(1), 46–51.

D'Hondt, P., Maes, M., Leysen, J.E., Gommeren, W., Scharpe, S., and Cosyns, P. (1994). Binding of [3H]paroxetine to platelets of depressed patients: Seasonal differences and effects of diagnostic classification. *J Affect Disord*, 32(1), 27–35.

D'Mello, D.A., McNeil, J.A., and Msibi, B. (1995). Seasons and bipolar disorder. *Ann Clin Psychiatry*, 7(1), 11–18.

De Vriese, S.R., Christophe, A.B., and Maes, M. (2004). In humans, the seasonal variation in poly-unsaturated fatty acids is related to the seasonal variation in violent suicide and serotonergic markers of violent suicide. *Prostaglandins Leukot Essent Fatty Acids*, 71(1), 13–18.

Desai, R.A., Dausey, D.J., and Rosenheck, R.A. (2005). Mental health service delivery and suicide risk: The role of individual patient and facility factors. *Am J Psychiatry*, 162(2), 311–318.

Dilsaver, S.C., and Chen, Y.W. (2003). Social phobia, panic disorder and suicidality in subjects with pure and depressive mania. *J Affect Disord*, 77(2), 173–177.

Dilsaver, S.C., Chen, Y.W., Swann, A.C., Shoaib, A.M., and Krajewski, K.J. (1994). Suicidality in patients with pure and depressive mania. *Am J Psychiatry*, 151(9), 1312–1315.

Dilsaver, S.C., Chen, Y.W., Swann, A.C., Shoaib, A.M., Tsai-Dilsaver, Y., and Krajewski, K.J. (1997). Suicidality, panic disorder and psychosis in bipolar depression, depressive-mania and pure-mania. *Psychiatry Res*, 73(1-2), 47–56.

Dilsaver, S.C., Benazzi, F., Rihmer, Z., Akiskal, K.K., and Akiskal, H.S. (2005). Gender, suicidality and bipolar mixed states in adolescents. *J Affect Disord*, 87, 11–16.

Dorovini-Zis, K., and Zis, A.P. (1987). Increased adrenal weight in victims of violent suicide. *Am J Psychiatry*, 144(9), 1214–1215.

Dorpat, T.L., and Ripley, H.S. (1960). A study of suicide in the Seattle area. *Compr Psychiatry*, 1, 349–359.

Dunner, D.L., Gershon, E.S., and Goodwin, F.K. (1976). Heritable factors in the severity of affective illness. *Biol Psychiatry*, 11(1), 31–42.

Egeland, J.A., and Sussex, J.N. (1985). Suicide and family loading for affective disorders. *JAMA*, 254(7), 915–918.

Ellison, L.F., and Morrison, H.I. (2001). Low serum cholesterol concentration and risk of suicide. *Epidemiology*, 12(2), 168–172.

Endicott, J., Nee, J., Andreasen, N., Clayton, P., Keller, M., and Coryell, W. (1985). Bipolar II: Combine or keep separate? *J Affect Disord*, 8(1), 17–28.

Engstrom, C., Brandstrom, S., Sigvardsson, S., Cloninger, R., and Nylander, P.O. (2003). Bipolar disorder II: Personality and age of onset. *Bipolar Disord*, 5(5), 340–348.

Fawcett, J., and Bunney, W.E. (1967). Pituitary adrenal function and depression: An outline for research. *Arch Gen Psychiatry*, 16, 517–535.

Fawcett, J., Edwards, J.H., Kravitz, H.M., and Jeffriess, H. (1987). Alprazolam: An antidepressant? Alprazolam, desipramine, and an alprazolam-desipramine combination in the treatment of adult depressed outpatients. *J Clin Psychopharmacol*, 7(5), 295–310.

Fawcett, J., Scheftner, W.A., Fogg, L., Clark, D.C., Young, M.A., Hedeker, D. (1990). Gibbons, R. Time-related predictors of suicide in major affective disorder. *Am J Psychiatry*, 147(9), 1189–1194.

Fawcett, J., Busch, K.A., Jacobs, D., Kravitz, H.M., and Fogg, L. (1997). Suicide: A four-pathway clinical-biochemical model. *Ann N Y Acad Sci*, 836, 288–301.

Fisher, A.J., Parry, C.D., Bradshaw, D., and Juritz, J.M. (1997). Seasonal variation of suicide in South Africa. *Psychiatry Res*, 66(1), 13–22.

Fitch, D., Lesage, A., Seguin, M., Trousignant, M., Bankelfat, C., Rouleau, G.A., and Turecki, G. (2001). Suicide and the serotonin transporter gene. *Mol Psychiatry*, 6(2), 127–128.

Foster, T., Gillespie, K., McClelland, R., and Patterson, C. (1999). Risk factors for suicide independent of DSM-III-R Axis I disorder: Case-control psychological autopsy study in Northern Ireland. *Br J Psychiatry*, 175, 175–179.

Frangos, E., Athanassenas, G., Tsitourides, S., Psilolignos, P., and Katsanou, N. (1983). Psychotic depressive disorder: A separate entity? *J Affective Disord*, 5, 259–265.

Frank, J.D., and Frank, J.B. (1991). *Persuasion and Healing: A Comparative Study of Psychotherapy*, 3rd ed. Baltimore: Johns Hopkins University Press.

Fruehwald, S., Frottler, P., Matschnig, T., Loenig, F., Lehr, S., and Eher, R. (2004). Do monthly or seasonal variations exist in suicides in a high-risk setting? *Psychiatry Res*, 121(3), 301–302.

Fu, Q., Heath, A., Bucholz, K.K., Nelson, E.C., Glowinski, A., Goldberg, J., Lyons, M.J., Tsuang, M.T., Jacob, T., True, M.R., and Eisen, S.A. (2002). A twin study of genetic and environmental influences on suicidality in men. *Psychol Med*, 32, 11–24.

Galfalvy, H., Oquendo, M.A., Carballo, J.J., Sher, L., Grunebaum, M.F., Burke, A., and Mann, J.J. (2006). Clinical predictors of suicidal acts after major depression in bipolar disorder: A prospective study. *Bipolar Disord*, 8, 586–595.

Geddes, J.R., and Juszczak, E. (1995). Period trends in rate of suicide in first 28 days after discharge from psychiatric hospital in Scotland, 1968–1992. *BMJ*, 311(7001), 357–360.

Geddes, J.R., Juszczak, E., O'Brien, F., and Kendrick, S. (1997). Suicide in the 12 months after discharge from psychiatric inpatient care, Scotland 1968–1992. *J Epidemiol Community Health*, 51(4), 430–434.

Geijer, T., Frisch, A., Persson, M.L., Wasserman, D., Rockah, R., Michaelovsky, E., Apter, A., Jonsson, E.G., Nothen, M.M., and Weizman, A. (2000). Search for association between suicide attempt and serotonergic polymorphisms. *Psychiatr Genet*, 10(1), 19–26.

Glowinski, A.L., Bucholtz, K.K., Nelson, E.C., Fu, Q., Madden, P.A., Reich, W., Heath, A.C. (2001). Suicide attempts in an adolescent female twin sample. *J Am Acad Child Adolesc Psychiatry*, 40(11), 1300–1307.

Goldberg, J.F., and Ernst, C.L. (2004). Clinical correlates of childhood and adolescent adjustment in adult patients with bipolar disorder. *J Nerv Ment Dis*, 192(3), 187–192.

Goldberg, J.F., Garno, J.L., Leon, A.C., Kocsis, J.H., and Portera, L. (1998). Association of recurrent suicidal ideation with nonremission from acute mixed mania. *Am J Psychiatry*, 155(12), 1753–1755.

Goldberg, J.F., Garno, J.L., Portera, L., Leon, A.C., Kocsis, J.H., Whiteside, J.E. (1999). Correlates of suicidal ideation in dysphoric mania. *J Affect Disord*, 56(1), 75–81.

Goldstein, R.B., Black, D.W., Nasrallah, A., and Winokur, G. (1991). The prediction of suicide: Sensitivity, specificity, and predictive value of a multivariate model applied to suicide among 1906 patients with affective disorders. *Arch Gen Psychiatry*, 48(5), 418–422.

Golomb, B.A., Tenkanen, L., Alikoski, T., Niskanen, T., Manninen, V., Huttunen, M., and Mednick, S.A. (2002). Insulin sensitivity markers: Predictors of accidents and suicides in Helsinki Heart Study screenees. *J Clin Epidemiol*, 55(8), 767–773.

Gonzalez-Maeso, J., Rodriguez-Puertas, R., Meana, J.J., Garcia-Sevilla, J.A., and Guimon, J. (2002). Neurotransmitter receptor-mediated activation of G-proteins in brains of suicide victims with mood disorders: Selective supersensitivity of alpha (2A)-adrenoceptors. *Mol Psychiatry*, 7(7), 755–767.

Gonzalez-Pinto, A., Mosquera, F., Alonso, M., Lopez, P., Ramirez, F., Vieta, E., and Baldessarini, R.J. (2006). Suicidal risk in bipolar I disorder patients and adherence to long-term lithium treatment. *Bipolar Disord*, 8, 618–624.

Gordon, D.J., Trost, D.C., Hyde, J., Whaley, F.S., Hannan, P.J., Jacobs, D.R., and Ekelund, L.-G. (1987). Seasonal cholesterol cycles: The lipid research clinics coronary primary prevention trial placebo group. *Circulation*, 76, 1224–1231.

Granberg, D., and Westerberg, C. (1999). On abandoning life when it is least difficult. *Soc Biol*, 46(1–2), 154–162.

Greening, L., and Stoppelbein, L. (2002). Religiosity, attributional style, and social support as psychosocial buffers for African American and white adolescents' perceived risk for suicide. *Suicide Life Threat Behav*, 32(4), 404–417.

Grunebaum, M.F., Galfalvy, H.C., Oquendo, M.A., Burke, A.K., and Mann, J.J. (2004). Melancholia and the probability and lethality of suicide attempt. *Br J Psychiatry*, 184, 534–535.

Grunebaum, M.F., Ramsay, S.R., Galfalvy, H.C., Ellis, S.P., Burke, A.K., Sher, L., Printz, D.J., Kahn, D.A., Mann, J.J., and

Oquendo, M.A. (2006). Correlates of suicide attempt history in bipolar disorder: A stress-diathesis perspective. *Bipolar Disord*, 8, 551–557.

Guze, S.B., and Robins, E. (1970). Suicide and primary affective disorders. *Br J Psychiatry*, 117(539), 437–439.

Haberlandt, W.F. (1967). Contribution to the genetics of suicide. Data in twins and familial findings. *Folia Clin Int (Barc)*, 17(6), 319–322.

Hagnell, O., Lanke, J., and Rorsman, B. (1981). Suicide rates in the Lundby Study: Mental illness as a risk factor for suicide. *Neuropsychobiology*, 7, 248–253.

Hakko, H., Rasanen, P., and Tiihonen, J. (1998). Seasonal variation in suicide occurrence in Finland. *Acta Psychiatr Scand*, 98(2), 92–97.

Hall, R.C., Platt, D.E., and Hall, R.C. (1999). Suicide risk assessment: A review of risk factors for suicide in 100 patients who made severe suicide attempts. Evaluation of suicide risk in a time of managed care. *Psychosomatics*, 40(1), 18–27.

Harris, E.C., and Barraclough, B. (1997). Suicide as an outcome for mental disorders. A meta-analysis. *Br J Psychiatry*, 170, 205–228.

Hawton, K., Sutton, L., Haw, C., Sinclair, J., and Harriss, L. (2005). Suicide and attempted suicide in bipolar disorder: A system review of risk factors. *J Clin Psychiatry*, 66, 693–704.

Heikkinen, M.E., Henriksson, M.M., Isometsa, E.T., Marttunen, M.H., Aro, H.M., and Lonnqvist, J.K. (1997). Recent life events and suicide in personality disorders. *J Nerv Ment Dis*, 185(6), 373–381.

Heim, C., and Nemeroff, C.B. (1999). The impact of early adverse experiences on brain systems involved in the pathophysiology of anxiety and affective disorders. *Biol Psychiatry*, 46(11), 1509–1522.

Heim, C., and Nemeroff, C.B. (2002). Neurobiology of early life stress: Clinical studies. *Semin Clin Neuropsychiatry*, 7(2), 147–159.

Henriksson, M.M., Aro, H.M., Marttunen, M.J., Heikkinen, M.E., Isometsa, E.T., Kuoppasalmi, K.I., and Lonnqvist, J.K. (1993). Mental disorders and comorbidity in suicide. *Am J Psychiatry*, 150(6), 935–940.

Hibbeln, J.R. (1998). Fish consumption and major depression. *Lancet*, 351, 1213.

Hillbrand, M., and Spitz, R.T. (Eds.) (1992). *Lipids, Health, and Behavior*. Washington, DC: American Psychiatric Association.

Hiroi, N., Wong, M.L., Licino, J., Park, C., Young, M., Gold, P.W., Chrousos, G.P., and Bornstein, S.R. (2001). Expression of corticotropin releasing hormone receptors type I and type II mRNA in suicide victims and controls. *Mol Psychiatry*, 6(5), 540–546.

Hucks, D., Lowther, S., Cromptom, M.R., Katona, C.L., and Horton, R.W. (1997). Corticotropin-releasing factor binding sites in cortex of depressed suicides. *Psychopharmacology (Berl)*, 134(2), 174–178.

Inskip, H.M., Harris, E.C., and Barraclough, B. (1998). Lifetime risk of suicide for affective disorder, alcoholism and schizophrenia. *Br J Psychiatry*, 172, 35–37.

Institute of Medicine (IOM). (2002). *Reducing Suicide: A National Imperative*. Washington, DC: National Academy Press.

Isometsa, E.T., Henriksson, M.M., Aro, H.M., and Lonnqvist, J.K. (1994a). Suicide in bipolar disorder in Finland. *Am J Psychiatry*, 151(7), 1020–1024.

Isometsa, E.T., Henriksson, M.M., Aro, H.M., Heikkinen, M.E., Kuoppasalmi, K.I., and Lönnqvist, J.K. (1994b). Suicide in major depression. *Am J Psychiatry*, 151, 530–536.

Jacobs, D.G., Baldessarini, R.J., Conwell, Y., Fawcett, J., Horton, L., Meltzer, H., Pfeffer, C.R., and Simon, R.L. (2003). Practice guideline for the assessment and treatment of patients with suicide behaviors. American Psychiatric Association. Available: http://www.psych.org/psych_pract/treatg/pg/suicidalbehaviors_05-15-06.pdf (accessed 12/1/06).

Jameison, G.R. (1936). Suicide and mental disease: A clinical analysis of one hundred cases. *Arch Neurol Psychiatry*, 36, 1–12.

Jameison, G.R., and Wall, J.H. (1933). Some psychiatric aspects of suicide. *Psychiatr Q*, 7, 211–229.

Jamison, K.R. (1999). *Night Falls Fast: Understanding Suicide.* New York: Alfred A. Knopf.

Johnson, B.A., Brent, D.A., Bridge, J., and Connolly, J. (1998). The familial aggregation of adolescent suicide attempts. *Acta Psychiatr Scan*, 97(1), 18–24.

Johnson, G.F., and Hunt, G. (1979). Suicidal behavior in bipolar manic-depressive patients and their families. *Compr Psychiatry*, 20, 159–164.

Johnson, J.L., and Cameron, M.C. (2001). Barriers to providing effective mental health services to American Indians. *Ment Health Serv Res*, 3(4), 215–223.

Joiner, T.E., Jr., Conwell, Y., Fitzpatrick, K.K., Witte, T.K., Schmidt, N.B., Berlim, M.T., Fleck, M.P.A., and Rudd, M.D. (2005). Four studies on how past and current suicidology relate even when "everything but the kitchen sink" is covaried. *J Abnorm Psychol*, 114, 291–303.

Juurlink, D.N., Herrmann, N., Szalai, J.P., Kopp, A., and Redelmeier, D.A. (2004). Medical illness and the risk of suicide in the elderly. *Arch Intern Med*, 164(11), 1179–1184.

Kaslow, N.J., Thompson, M.P., Meadows, L., Chance, S., Puett, R., Hollins, L., Jessee, S., and Kellermann A. (2000). Risk factors for suicide attempts among African American women. *Depress Anxiety*, 12(1), 13–20.

Kaslow, N.J., Price, A.W., Wyckoff, S., Bender Grall, M., Sherry, A., Young, S., Scholl, L., Millington Upshaw, V., Rashid, A., Jackson, E.B., and Bethea, K. (2004). Person factors associated with suicidal behavior among African American women and men. *Cultur Divers Ethnic Minor Psychol*, 10(1), 5–22.

Keilp, J.G., Sackeim, H.A., Brodsky, B.S., Oquendo, M.A., Malone, K.M., and Mann, J.J. (2001). Neuropsychological dysfunction in depressed suicide attempters. *Am J Psychiatry*, 158(5), 735–741.

Keith-Spiegel, P., and Spiegel, D.E. (1967). Affective states of patients immediately preceding suicide. *J Psychiatr Res*, 5(2), 89–93.

Keith-Spiegel, P., and Spiegel, D.E. (1979). Affective states of patients immediately preceding suicide. *J Psychiatr Res*, 5, 89–93.

Kety, S.S. (1987). The significance of genetic factors in the etiology of schizophrenia: Results from the national study of adoptees in Denmark. *J Psychiart Res*, 21(4), 423–429.

Kety, S.S., Rosenthal, D., Wender, P.H., and Schulsinger, F. (1968). The types and prevalence of mental illness in the biological and adoptive families of adopted schizophrenics. *J Psychiatr Res*, 6, 345–362.

Kim, C., Lesage, A., Seguin, M., Chawky, N., Vanier, C., Lipp, O., and Turecki, G. (2003). Patterns of co-morbidity in male suicide completers. *Psychol Med*, 33(7), 1299–1309.

Kotin, J., and Goodwin, F.K. (1972). Depression during mania: Clinical observations and theoretical implications. *Am J Psychiatry*, 129, 679–686.

Koukopoulos, A., and Koukopoulos, A. (1999). Agitated depression as a mixed state and the problem of melancholia. *Psychiatr Clin North Am*, 22(3), 547–564.

Kraepelin, E. (1921). *Manic-Depressive Insanity and Paranoia.* Translated by R.M. Barclay. Edinburgh, Scotland: E & S Livingstone.

Krieger, G. (1970). Biochemical predictors of suicide. *Dis Nerv Syst*, 31(7), 478–482.

Kunugi, H., Ishida, S., Kato, T., Sakai, T., Tatsumi, M., Hirose, T., and Nanko, S. (1999). No evidence for an association of polymorphisms of the tryptophan hydroxylase gene with affective disorders or attempted suicide among Japanese patients. *Am J Psychiatry*, 156(5), 774–776.

Lacoste, V., and Wirz-Justice, A. (1989). Seasonal variation in normal subjects: An update of variables current in depression research. In N. Rosenthal, M. Blehar (Eds.), *Seasonal Affective Disorders and Phototherapy* (pp. 167–229). New York: Guilford Press.

Lalovic, A., Sequeira, A., DeGuzman, R., Chawky, N., Lesage, A., Seguin, M., and Turecki, G. (2004). Investigation of completed suicide and genes involved in cholesterol metabolism. *J Affect Disord*, 79(1–3), 25–32.

Lee, H.-C., Lin, H.-C., Tsai, S.-Y., Li, C.-Y., Chen, C.-C., and Huang, C.-C. (2006). Suicide rates and the association with climate: A population-based study. *J Affect Disord*, 92, 221–226.

Lesch, K.P., Bengel, D., Heils, A., Sabol, S.Z., Greenberg, B.D., Petri, S., Benjamin, J., Muller, C.R., Hamer, D.H., Murphy, D.L. (1996). Association of anxiety-related traits with a polymorphism in the serotonin transporter gene regulatory region. *Science*, 274(5292), 1527–1531.

Lester, D. (1992). The dexamethasone suppression test as an indicator of suicide: A meta-analysis. *Pharmacopsychiatry*, 25(6), 265–270.

Lester, D. (1995). The concentration of neurotransmitter metabolites in the cerebrospinal fluid of suicidal individuals: A meta-analysis. *Pharmacopsychiatry*, 28(2), 45–50.

Lester, D. (2002). Serum cholesterol levels and suicide: A meta-analysis. *Suicide Life Threat Behav*, 32(3), 333–346.

Leverich, G.S., McElroy, S.L., Suppes, T., Keck, P.E. Jr., Denicoff, K.D., Nolen, W.A., Altshuler, L.L., Rush, A.J., Kupka, R., Frye, M.A., Autio, K.A., and Post, R.M. (2002). Early physical and sexual abuse associated with an adverse course of bipolar illness. *Biol Psychiatry*, 51(4), 288–297.

Leverich, G.S., Altshuler, L.L., Frye, M.A., Suppes, T., Keck, P.E. Jr., McElroy, S.L., Denicoff, K.D., Obrocea, G., Nolen, W.A., Kupka, R., Walden, J., Grunze, H., Perez, S., Luckenbaugh, D.A., and Post, R.M. (2003). Factors associated with suicide attempts in 648 patients with bipolar disorder in the Stanley Foundation Bipolar Network. *J Clin Psychiatry*, 64(5), 506–515.

Levy, B., and Hansen, E. (1969). Failure of the urinary test for suicide potential: Analysis of urinary 17-OHCS steroid findings prior to suicide in two patients. *Arch Gen Psychiatry*, 20(4), 415–418.

Lin, P.Y., and Tsai, G. (2004). Association between serotonin transporter gene promoter polymorphism and suicide: Results of a meta-analysis. *Biol Psychiatry*, 55(10), 1023–1030.

Linkowski, P., Martin, F., and De Maertelaer, V. (1992). Effect of some climatic factors on violent and non-violent suicides in Belgium. *J Affect Disord*, 25(3), 161–166.

Linnoila, V.M., and Virkkunen, M. (1992). Aggression, suicidality, and serotonin. *J Clin Psychiatry*, 53(Suppl), 46–51.

Losonczy, M.F., Mohs, R.C., and Davis, K.L. (1984). Seasonal variations of human lumbar CSF neurotransmitter metabolite concentrations. *Psychiatry Res*, 12, 79–87.

Luoma, J.B., Martin, C.E., and Pearson, J.L. (2002). Contact with mental health and primary care providers before suicide: A review of the evidence. *Am J Psychiatry*, 159(6), 909–916.

MacKinnon, D.F., Potash, J.B., McMahon, F.J., Simpson, S.G., and DePaulo, R. (2005). Rapid moon switching and suicidality in familial bipolar disorder. *Bipolar Disord*, 7, 441–448.

MacQueen, G.M., and Young, L.T. (2001). Bipolar II disorder: Symptoms, course, and response to treatment. *Psychiatr Serv*, 52(3), 358–361.

Maes, M., Cosyns, P., Meltzer, H.Y., De Meyer, F., and Peeters, D. (1993a). Seasonality in violent suicide but not in nonviolent suicide or homicide. *Am J Psychiatry*, 150(9), 1380–1385.

Maes, M., Meltzer, H.Y., Suy, E., De Meyer, F. (1993b). Seasonality in severity of depression: Relationships to suicide and homicide occurrence. *Acta Psychiatr Scand*, 88(3), 156–161.

Maes, M., De Meyer, F., Thompson, P., Peeters, D., and Cosyns, P. (1994). Synchronized annual rhythms in violent suicide rate, ambient temperature and the light-dark span. *Acta Psychiatr Scand*, 90(5), 391–396.

Maes, M., Scharpe, S., Verkerk, R., D'Hondt, P., Peeters, D., Cosyns, P., Thompson, P., De Meyer, F., Wauters, A., and Neels, H. (1995). Seasonal variation in plasma L-tryptophan availability in healthy volunteers: Relationships to violent suicide occurrence. *Arch Gen Psychiatry*, 52(11), 937–946.

Maj, M., Magliano, L., Pirozzi, R., Marasco, C., and Guarneri, M. (1994). Validity of rapid cycling as a course specifier for bipolar disorder. *Am J Psychiatry*, 151(7), 1015–1019.

Maldonado, G., and Kraus, J.F. (1991). Variation in suicide occurrence by time of day, day of the week, month, and lunar phase. *Suicide Life Threat Behav*, 21(2), 174–187.

Manfredini, R., Caracciolo, S., Salmi, R., Boari, B., Tomelli, A., and Gallerani, M. (2000). The association of low serum cholesterol with depression and suicidal behaviors: New hypotheses for the missing link. *J Int Med Res*, 28(6), 247–257.

Mann, J.J. (1998). The neurobiology of suicide. *Nat Med*, 4(1), 25–30.

Mann, J.J. (2002). A current perspective of suicide and attempted suicide. *Ann Intern Med* 136(4), 302–311.

Mann, J.J., McBride, P.A., Brown, R.P., Linnoila, M., Leon, A.C., DeMeo, M., Mieczkowski, T., Myers, J.E., and Stanley, M. (1992). Relationship between central and peripheral serotonin indexes in depressed and suicidal psychiatric inpatients. *Arch Gen Psychiatry*, 49(6), 442–446.

Mann, J.J., Waternaux, C., Haas, G.L., and Malone, K.M. (1999). Toward a clinical model of suicidal behavior in psychiatric patients. *Am J Psychiatry*, 156(2), 181–189.

Mann, J.J., Huang, Y.Y., Underwood, M.D., Kassir, S.A., Oppenheim, S., Kelly, T.M., Dwork, A.J., and Arango, V. (2000). A serotonin transporter gene promoter polymorphism (5-HTTLPR) and prefrontal cortical binding in major depression and suicide. *Arch Gen Psychiatry*, 57(8), 729–738.

Marangell, L.B., Bauer, M.S., Dennehy, E.B., Wisniewski, S.R., Allen, M.H., Miklowitz, D.J., Oquendo, M.A., Frank, E., Perlis, R.H., Martinez, J.M., Fagiolini, A., Otto, M.W., Chessick, C.A., Zboyan, H.A., Miyahara, S., Sachs, G., and Thase, M.E. (2006). Prospective predictors of suicide and suicide attempts in 1,556

patients with bipolar disorders followed for up to 2 years. *Bipolar Disord*, 8, 566–575.

Marion, S.A., Agbayewa, M.O., and Wiggins, S. (1999). The effect of season and weather on suicide rates in the elderly in British Columbia. *Can J Public Health*, 90(6), 418–422.

Martin, S.J., Kelly, I.W., and Saklofske, D.H. (1992). Suicide and lunar cycles: A critical review over 28 years. *Psychol Rep*, 71(3, Pt 1), 787–795.

Mathers, C.D., Lopez, A.D., and Murray, C.J.L. (2006). The burden of disease and mortality by condition: Data, methods, and results for 2001. In A.D. Lopez, C.D. Mathers, M. Ezzate, D.T. Jamison, and C.J.L. Murral (Eds.), *Global Burden of Disease and Risk Factors*. New York: Oxford University Press.

McElroy, S.L., Keck, P.E. Jr., Pope, H.G. Jr., Hudson, J.I., Faedda, G.L., and Swann, A. (1992). Clinical and research implications of the diagnosis of dysphoric mixed mania or hypomania. *Am J Psychiatry*, 149(12), 1633–1644.

McElroy, S.L., Strakowski, S.M., Keck, P.E. Jr., Tugrul, K.L., West, S.A., and Loneza, H.S. (1995). Differences and similarities in mixed and pure mania. *Compr Psychiatry*, 36(3), 187–194.

McElroy, S.L., Altshuler, L.L., Suppes, T., Keck, P.E. Jr., Frye, M.A., Denicoff, K.D., Nolen, W.A., Kupka, R.W., Leverich, G.S., Rochussen, J.R., Rush, A.J., and Post, R.M. (2001). Axis I psychiatric comorbidity and its relationship to historical illness variables in 288 patients with bipolar disorder. *Am J Psychiatry*, 158(3), 420–426.

Micciolo, R., Zimmermann-Tansella, C., Williams, P., and Tansella, M. (1989). Seasonal variation in suicide: Is there a sex difference? *Psychol Med*, 19(1), 199–203.

Micciolo, R., Williams, P., Zimmermann-Tansella, C., and Tansella, M. (1991). Geographical and urban-rural variation in the seasonality of suicide: Some further evidence. *J Affect Disord*, 21(1), 39–43.

Michaelis, B.H., Goldberg, J.F., Davis, G.P., Singer, T.M., Garno, J.L., and Wenze, S.J. (2004). Dimensions of impulsivity and aggression associated with suicide attempts among bipolar patients: A preliminary study. *Suicide Life Threat Behav*, 34, 172–176.

Modai, I., Malmgren, R., Wetterberg, L., Eneroth, P., Valevski, A., and Asberg, M. (1992). Blood levels of melatonin, serotonin, cortisol, and prolactin in relation to the circadian rhythm of platelet serotonin uptake. *Psychiatry Res*, 43, 161–166.

Morken, G., Lilleeng, S., and Linaker, O.M. (2002). Seasonal variation in suicides and in admissions to hospital for mania and depression. *J Affect Disord*, 69(1-3), 39–45.

Morrison, J.R. (1975). The family histories of manic-depressive patients with and without alcoholism. *J Nerv Ment Dis*, 160, 227–229.

Motto, J.A. (1985). The recognition and management of the suicidal patient. In F.F. Flach, S.C. Draghi (Eds.), *The Nature and Treatment of Depression* (pp. 229–254). New York: John Wiley & Sons.

Mulder, R.T., Cosgriff, J.P., Smith, A.M., and Joyce, P.R. (1990). Seasonality of mania in New Zealand. *Aust N Z J Psychiatry*, 24(2), 187–190.

Muldoon, M.F., Manuck, S.B., Mendelsohn, A.B., Kaplan, J.R., and Belle, S.H. (2001). Cholesterol reduction and non-illness mortality: Meta-analysis of randomised clinical trials. *BMJ*, 322(7277), 11–15.

Murphy, G.E. (1988). Suicide and substance abuse. *Arch Gen Psychiatry*, 45(6), 593–594.

National Center for Injury Prevention and Control (NCIPC). (2005). Web-based injury statistics query and reporting system. Available: http://www.cdc.gov/ncipc/wisqars/ (accessed August 31, 2006).

Neeleman, J., Wessely, S., and Lewis, G. (1998). Suicide acceptability in African- and white Americans: The role of religion. *J Nerv Ment Dis*, 186(1), 12–16.

Nemeroff, C.B., Owens, M.J., Bissette, G., Andorn, A.C., and Stanley, M. (1988). Reduced corticotropin releasing factor binding sites in the frontal cortex of suicide victims. *Arc Gen Psychiatry*, 45(6), 577–579.

Nordstrom, P., Asberg, M., Aberg-Wistedt, A., and Nordin, C. (1995a). Attempted suicide predicts suicide risk in mood disorders. *Acta Psychiatr Scand*, 92, 345–350.

Nordstrom, P., Samuelsson, M., and Asberg, M. (1995b). Survival analyses of suicide risk after attempted suicide. *Acta Psychiatr Scand*, 91, 336–340.

Norman, W.H., Brown, W.A., Miller, I.W., Keitner, G.I., and Overholser, J.C. (1990). The dexamethasone suppression test and completed suicide. *Acta Psychiatr Scand*, 81(2), 120–125.

Oddie, T.H., Klein, A.H., Foley, T.P., and Fisher, D.A. (1979). Variation in values for iodothyronine hormones, thyrotropin, and thyroxine-binding globulin in normal umbilical cord serum with season and duration of storage. *Clinical Chemistry*, 25(7), 1251–1253.

Ono, H., Shirakawa, O., Nishiguchi, N., Nishimura, A., Nushida, H., Ueno, Y., Maeda, K. (2000). Tryptophan hydroxylase gene polymorphisms are not associated with suicide. *Am J Med Genet*, 96(6), 861–863.

Ono, H., Shirakawa, O., Nushida, H., Ueno, Y., and Maeda, K. (2004). Association between catechol-O-methyltransferase functional polymorphism and male suicide completers. *Neuropsychopharmacology*, 29(7), 1374–1377.

Oquendo, M.A., and Mann, J.J. (2000). The biology of impulsivity and suicidality. *Psychiatr Clin North Am*, 23(1), 11–25.

Oquendo, M.A., and Mann, J.J. (2001). Identifying and managing suicide risk in bipolar patients. *J Clin Psychiatry*, 62(Suppl 25), 31–34.

Oquendo, M.A., Placidi, G.P., Malone, K.M., Campbell, C., Keilp, J., Brodsky, B., Kegeles, L.S., Cooper, T.B., Parsey, R.V., van Heertum, R.L., and Mann, J.J. (2003). Positron emission tomography of regional brain metabolic responses to a serotonergic challenge and lethality of suicide attempts in major depression. *Arch Gen Psychiatry*, 60(1), 14–22.

Oquendo, M.A., Galfalvy, H., Russo, S., Ellis, S.P., Grunebaum, M.F., Burke, A., and Mann, J.J. (2004). Prospective study of clinical predictors of suicidal acts after a major depressive episode in patients with major depressive disorder or bipolar disorder. *Am J Psychiatry*, 161(8), 1433–1441.

Oravecz, R., Rocchi, M.B., Sisti, D., Zorko, M., Marusic, A., and Preti, A. (2006). Changes in the seasonality of suicides over time in Slovenia, 1971 to 2002. *J Affect Disord*, 95(1–3), 135–140.

Ordway, G.A. (1997). Pathophysiology of the locus coeruleus in suicide. *Ann N Y Acad Sci*, 836, 233–252.

Osby, U., Brandt, L., Correia, N., Ekbom, A., and Sparen, P. (2001). Excess mortality in bipolar and unipolar disorder in Sweden. *Arch Gen Psychiatry*, 58(9), 844–850.

Osby, U., Brandt, L., Correia, N., Ekbom, A., and Sparen, P. (2005). *Excess Mortality in Bipolar and Unipolar Disorder*. Paper presented to the annual meeting of the American Psychiatric Association, Atlanta.

Pandey, G.N., Dwivedi, Y., Rizavl, H.S., Ren, X., Pandey, S.C., Pesold, C., Robert, R.C., Conley, R.R., and Tamminga, C.A. (2002). Higher expression of serotonin 5-HT(2A) receptors in the postmortem brains of teenage suicide victims. *Am J Psychiatry*, 159(3), 419–429.

Papadopoulos, F.C., Frangakis, C.E., Skalkidou, A., Petridou, E., Stevens, R.G., and Trichopoulos, D. (2005). Exploring lag and duration effect of sunshine in triggering suicide. *J Affect Disord*, 88, 287–297.

Papolos, D., Hennen, J., and Cockerham, M.S. (2005). Factors associated with patient-reported suicide threats by children and adolescents with community-diagnosed bipolar disorder. *J Affect Dis*, 86, 267–275.

Parker, G., and Walter, S. (1982). Seasonal variation in depressive disorders and suicidal deaths in New South Wales. *Br J Psychiatry*, 140, 626–632.

Parker, G., Gao, F., and Machin, D. (2001). Seasonality of suicide in Singapore: Data from the equator. *Psychol Med*, 31(7), 1323–1325.

Partonen, T., Haukka, J., Virtamo, J., Taylor, P.R., and Lonnqvist, J. (1999). Association of low serum total cholesterol with major depression and suicide. *Br J Psychiatry*, 175, 259–262.

Perez, P.R., Lopez, J.G., Makeos, I.P., Escribano, A.D., and Sanchez, M.L.S. (1980). Seasonal variations in thyroid hormones in plasma. *Revista Clínica Española*, 156, 245–247.

Perlis, R.H., Miyahara, S., Marangell, L.B., Wisniewski, S.R., Ostacher, M., DelBello, M.P., Bowden, C.L., Sachs, G.S., and Nierenberg, A.A. (2004). STEP-BD investigators: Long-term implications of early onset in bipolar disorder. Data from the first 1000 participants in the Systematic Treatment Enhancement Program for Bipolar Disorder (STEP-BD). *Biol Psychiatry*, 55(9), 875–881.

Petridou, E., Papadopoulos, F.C., Frangakis, C.E., Skalkidou, A., and Trichopoulos, D. (2002). A role of sunshine in the triggering of suicide. *Epidemiology*, 13(1), 106–109.

Pfeffer, C.R., Normandin, L., and Kakuma, T. (1994). Suicidal children grow up: suicidal behavior and psychiatric disorders among relatives. *J Am Acad Child Adolesc Psychiatry*, 33(8), 1087–1097.

Pfeffer, C.R., Normandin, L., and Kakuma, T. (1998). Suicidal children grow up: Relations between family psychopathology and adolescents' lifetime suicidal behavior. *J Nerv Ment Dis*, 186(5), 269–275.

Pine, D.S., Trautman, P.D., Shaffer, D., Cohen, L., Davies, M., Stanley, M., and Parsons, B. (1995). Seasonal rhythm of platelet [^{3}H]imipramine binding in adolescents who attempted suicide. *Am J Psychiatry*, 152(6), 923–925.

Pini, S., Dell'Osso, L., Mastrocinque, C., Marcacci, G., Papasogli, A., Vignoli, S., Pallanti, S., and Cassano, G. (1999). Axis I comorbidity in bipolar disorder with psychotic features. *Br J Psychiatry*, 175, 467–471.

Pokorny, A.D. (1983). Prediction of suicide in psychiatric patients: Report of a prospective study. *Arch Gen Psychiatry*, 40(3), 249–257.

Pokorny, L.J. (1991). A summary measure of client level of functioning: Progress and challenges for use within mental health agencies. *J Ment Health Admin*, 18(2), 80–87.

Pooley, E.C., Houston, K., Hawton, K., and Harrison, P.J. (2003). Deliberate self-harm is associated with allelic variation in the tryptophan hydroxylase gene (TPH A779C), but not with polymorphisms in five other serotonergic genes. *Psychol Med*, 33(5), 775–783.

Potash, J.B., Kane, H.S., Chiu, Y.F., Simpson, S.G., MacKinnon, D.F., McInnis, M.G., McMahon, F.J., and DePaulo, J.R. Jr. (2000). Attempted suicide and alcoholism in bipolar disorder: Clinical and familial relationships. *Am J Psychiatry*, 157(12), 2048–2050.

Preti, A., and Miotto, P. (1998). Seasonality in suicides: The influence of suicide method, gender and age on suicide distribution in Italy. *Psychiatry Res*, 81(2), 219–231.

Preti, A., Miotto, P., and De Coppi, M. (2000). Season and suicide: Recent findings from Italy. *Crisis*, 21(2), 59–70.

Qin, P., and Nordentoft, M. (2005). Suicide risk in relation to psychiatric hospitalization: Evidence based on longitudinal registers. *Arch Gen Psychiatry*, 667, 427–432.

Qin, P., Agerbo, E., and Mortensen, P.B. (2002). Suicide risk in relation to family history of completed suicide and psychiatric disorders: A nested case-control study based on longitudinal registers. *Lancet*, 360(9340), 1126–1130.

Rasanen, P., Hakko, H., Jokelainen, J., Tihonen, J. (2002). Seasonal variation in specific methods of suicide: A national register study of 20,234 Finnish people. *J Affect Disord*, 71, 51–59.

Reich, J. (1998). The relationship of suicide attempts, borderline personality traits and major depressive disorder in a veteran outpatient population. *J Affect Disord*, 49(2), 151–156.

Retamal, P., and Humphreys, D. (1998). Occurrence of suicide and seasonal variation. *Rev Saude Publica*, 32(5), 408–412.

Rich, C.L., Ricketts, J.E., Fowler, R.C., and Young, D. (1988). Some differences between men and women who commit suicide. *Am J Psychiatry*, 145, 718–722.

Rihmer, Z., and Kiss, K. (2002). Bipolar disorders and suicidal behaviour. *Bipolar Disord*, 4(Suppl. 1), 21–25.

Rihmer, Z., and Pestality, P. (1999). Bipolar II disorder and suicidal behavior. *Psychiatr Clin North Am*, 22(3), 667–673, ix–x.

Rihmer, Z., Barsi, J., Arato, M., and Demeter, E. (1990). Suicide in subtypes of primary depression. *J Affect Disord*, 18(3), 221–225.

Rihmer, Z., Rutz, W., and Pihlgren, H. (1995). Depression and suicide on Gotland: An intensive study of all suicides before and after a depression-training programme for general practitioners. *J Affect Disord*, 35(4), 147–152.

Rihmer, Z., Rutz, W., Pihlgren, H., and Pestality, P. (1998). Decreasing tendency of seasonality in suicide may indicate lowering rate of depressive suicides in the population. *Psychiatry Res*, 81(2), 233–240.

Robins, E. (1981). *The Final Months: A Study of the Lives of 134 Persons Who Committed Suicide.* New York: Oxford University Press.

Robins, E., Murphy, G.E., Wilkinson, R.H. Jr., Gassner, S., and Kayes, J. (1959). Some clinical considerations in the prevention of suicide based on a study of 134 successful suicides. *Am J Public Health*, 49(7), 888–899.

Rock, D., Greenberg, D.M., and Hallmayer, J.F. (2003). Increasing seasonality of suicide in Australia 1970–1999. *Psychiatry Res*, 120(1), 43–51.

Roose, S.P., Glassman, A.H., Walsh, B.T., Woodring, S., Vital-Herne, J. (1983). Depression, delusions, and suicide. *Am J Psychiatry*, 140(9), 1159–1162.

Rosenthal, N.E., Davenport, Y., Cowdry, R.W., Webster, M.H., and Goodwin, F.K. (1980). Monamine metabolite in cerebrospinal fluid of depressive subgroups. *Psychiatry Research*, 2, 113–119.

Roy, A. (1994). Recent biologic studies on suicide. *Suicide Life Threat Behav*, 24(1), 10–14.

Roy, A., Segal, N.L., Centerwall, B.S., and Robinette, C.D. (1991). Suicide in twins. *Arch Gen Psychiatry*, 48(1), 29–32.

Roy, A., Nielsen, D., Rylander, G., Sarchiapone, M., and Segal, N. (1999). Genetics of suicide in depression. *J Clin Psychiatry*, 60(Suppl 2), 12–17; discussion 18–20, 113–116.

Rudd, M.D., Dahm, P.F., and Rajab, M.H. (1993). Diagnostic comorbidity in persons with suicidal ideation and behavior. *Am J Psychiatry*, 150(6), 928–934.

Runeson, B. (1989). Mental disorder in youth suicide. DSM-III-R Axes I and II. *Acta Psychiatr Scand*, 79(5), 490–497.

Rush, B. (1812). *Medical Inquiries and Observations upon the Diseases of the Mind.* Philadelphia: Kimber and Richardson.

Russ, M.J., Lachman, H.M., Kashdan, T., Saito, T., and Bajmakovic-Kacila, S. (2000). Analysis of catechol-O-methyltransferase and 5-hydroxytryptamine transporter polymorphisms in patients at risk for suicide. *Psychiatry Res*, 93(1), 73–78.

Rutter, P.A., and Behrendt, A.E. (2004). Adolescent suicide risk: Four psychosocial factors. *Adolescence*, 39, 295–302.

Salib, E. (1997). Elderly suicide and weather conditions: Is there a link? *Int J Geriatr Psychiatry*, 12(9), 937–941.

Sarrias, M.J., Artigas, F., Martinez, E., and Gelpi, E. (1989). Seasonal changes of plasma serotonin and related parameters: Correlation with environmental measures. *Biol Psychiatry*, 26, 695–706.

Sato, T., Bottlender, R., Tanabe, A., and Moller, H.J. (2004). Cincinnati criteria for mixed mania and suicidality in patients with acute mania. *Compr Psychiatry*, 45(1), 62–69.

Schmauss, C. (2003). Serotonin 2C receptors: Suicide, serotonin, and runaway RNA editing. *Neuroscientist*, 9(4), 237–242.

Schnyder, U., Valach, L., Bichsel, K., and Michel, K. (1999). Attempted suicide: Do we understand the patients' reasons? *Gen Hosp Psychiatry*, 21(1), 62–69.

Schulsinger, F., Kety, S.S., Rosenthal, D., and Wender, P.H. (1979). A family study of suicide. In M. Schou, E. Strömgren (Eds.), *Origin, Prevention, and Treatment of Affective Disorders* (pp. 277–287). London: Academic Press.

Schweizer, E., Dever, A., and Clary, C. (1988). Suicide upon recovery from depression: A clinical note. *J Nerv Ment Dis*, 176, 633–636.

Sharma, R., and Markar, H.R. (1994). Mortality in affective disorder. *J Affect Disord*, 31(2), 91–96.

Sher, L., Carballo, J.J., Grunebaum, M.F., Burke, A.K., Zalsman, G., Huang, Y.-Y., Mann, J.J., and Oquendo, M.A. (2006). A prospective study of the association of cerebrospinal fluid monoamine metabolite levels with lethality of suicide attempts in patients with bipolar disorder. *Bipolar Disord*, 8, 543–550.

Simkin, S., Hawton, K., Yip, P.S., Yam, C.H. (2003). Seasonality in suicide: A study of farming suicides in England and Wales. *Crisis*, 24(3), 93–97.

Simon, N.M., Otto, M.W., Wisniewski, S.R., Fossey, M., Sagduyu, K., Frank, E., Sachs, G.S., Nierenberg, A.A., Thase, M.E., and Pollack, M.H. (2004). Anxiety disorder comorbidity in bipolar disorder patients: Data from the first 500 participants in the Systematic Treatment Enhancement Program for Bipolar Disorder (STEP-BD). *Am J Psychiatry*, 161(12), 2222–2229.

Simpson, S.G., and Jamison, K.R. (1999). The risk of suicide in patients with bipolar disorders. *J Clin Psychiatry*, 60(Suppl 2), 53–56; discussion 75–76, 113–116.

Slater, E., and Roth, M. (1969). *Clinical Psychiatry* (3rd edition). Baltimore: Williams & Wilkins.

Sokero, T.P., Melartin, T.K., Rytsälä, H.J., Leskelä, U.S., Lestelä–Mielonen, L.A., and Isometsä, E.T. (2005). Prospective study of risk factors for attempted suicide among patients with DSM-IV major depressive disorder. *Br J Psychiat*, 186, 314–318.

Souêtre, E., Salvati, E., Belugou, J.L., Douillet, P., Braccini, T., and Darcourt, G. (1989). Seasonal variation of serotonin function in humans: Research and clinical implications. *Ann Clin Psychiatry*, 1, 153–164.

Strakowski, S.M., McElroy, S.L., Keck, P.E. Jr., West, S.A. (1996). Suicidality among patients with mixed and manic bipolar disorder. *Am J Psychiatry*, 153(5), 674–676.

Statham, D.J., Heath, A.C., Madden, P.A., Bucholz, K.K., Bierut, L., Dinwiddie, S.H., Slutske, W.S., Dunne, M.P., and Martin, N.G. (1998). Suicidal behavior: An epidemiological and genetic study. *Psychol Med*, 28(4), 839–855.

Swann, A.C., Dougherty, D.M., Pazzaglia, P.J., Pham, M., and Moeller, F.G. (2004). Impulsivity: A link between bipolar disorder and substance abuse. *Bipolar Disord*, 6(3), 204–212.

Swann, A.C., Doughery, D.M., Pazzaglia, P.J., Pham, M., Steinberg, J.L. and Moeller, F.G. (2005). Increased impulsivity associated with severity of suicide attempt history in patients with bipolar disorder. *Am J Psychiatry*, 162, 1680–1687.

Szigethy, E., Conwell, Y., Forbes, N.T., Cox, C., and Caine, E.D. (1994). Adrenal weight and morphology in victims of completed suicide. *Biol Psychiatry*, 36(6), 374–380.

Takahashi, E. (1964). Seasonal variation of conception and suicide. *Tohoku J Exp Med*, 84, 215–227.

Takei, N., O'Callaghan, E., Sham, P., Glover, G., Tamura, A., Murray, R. (1992). Seasonality of admissions in the psychoses: Effect of diagnosis, sex, and age at onset. *Br J Psychiatry*, 161, 506–511.

Tanskanen, A., Tuomilehto, J., and Vinamaki, H. (2000). Cholesterol, depression and suicide. *Br J Psychiatry*, 176, 398–399.

Tietjen, G.H., Kripke, D.F. (1994). Suicides in California (1968–1977): Absence of seasonality in Los Angeles and Sacramento counties. *Psychiatry Res*, 53(2), 161–172.

Timonen, M., Viilo, K., Hakko, H., Sarkioja, T., Meyer-Rochow, V.B., Vaisanen, E., Rasanen, P. (2004). Is seasonality of suicides stronger in victims with hospital-treated atopic disorders? *Psychiatry Res*, 126(2), 167–175.

Tondo, L., Baldessarini, R.J., Hennen, J., Minnai, G.P., Salis, P., Scamonatti, L., Masia, M., Ghiani, C., and Mannu, P. (1999). Suicide attempts in major affective disorder patients with comorbid substance use disorders. *J Clin Psychiatry*, 60(Suppl 2), 63–69, discussion 75–76, 113–116.

Tondo, L., Isacsson, G., and Baldessarini, R. (2003). Suicidal behaviour in bipolar disorder: Risk and prevention. *CNS Drugs*, 17(7), 491–511.

Tsai, S.Y., Kuo, C.J., Chen, C.C., and Lee, H.C. (2002). Risk factors for completed suicide in bipolar disorder. *J Clin Psychiatry*, 63(6), 469–476.

Tsuang, M.T. (1977). Genetic factors in suicide. *Dis Nerv Syst*, 38(7), 498–501.

Tsuang, M.T. (1983). Risk of suicide in the relatives of schizophrenics, manics, depressives, and controls. *J Clin Psychiatry*, 44(11), 396–400.

Tsuang, M.T., and Woolson, R.F. (1977). Mortality in patients with schizophrenia, mania, depression and surgical conditions. *Br J Pscyhiatry*, 130, 162–166.

Turecki, G., Zhu, Z., Tzenova, J., Lesage, A., Seguin, M., Tousignant, M., Chawky, N., Vanier, C., Lipp, O., Alda, M., Joober, R., Benkelfat, C., Rouleau, G.A. (2001). TPH and suicidal behavior: A study in suicide completers. *Mol Psychiatry*, 6(1), 98–102.

Turecki, G., Dequeira, A., Gingras, Y., Seguin, M., Lesage, A., Tousignant, M., Chawky, N., Vanier, C., Lipp, O., Benkelfat, C., Rouleau, G.A. (2003). Suicide and serotonin: Study of variation at seven serotonin receptor genes in suicide completers. *Am J Med Genet*, 118B(1), 36–40.

U.S. Department of Health and Human Services. (2000). *In Harm's Way: Suicide in America*. Washington, DC: U.S. Public Health Service.

U.S. Public Health Service. (1999). *Office of the Surgeon General: The Surgeon General's Call to Action to Prevent Suicide*. Washington, DC: U.S. Public Health Service.

Valtonen, H.M., Suominen, K., Mantere, O., Leppämäki, S., Arvilommi, P., and Isometsä, E.T. (2006). Prospective study of risk factors for attempted suicide among patients with bipolar disorder. *Bipolar Disord*, 8, 576–585.

Verkes, R.J., Kerkhof, G.A., Beld, E., Hengeveld, M.W., and van Kempen, G.M.J. (1996). Suicidality, circadian activity rhythms and platelet serotonergic measures in patients with recurrent suicidal behaviour. *Acta Psychiatr Scand*, 93, 27–34.

Vieta, E., Benabarre, A., Colom, F., Gasto, C., Nieto, E., Otero, A., Vallejo, J. (1997). Suicidal behavior in bipolar I and bipolar II disorder. *J Nerv Ment Dis*, 185(6), 407–409.

Vieta, E., Colom, F., Martinez-Aran, A., Benabarre, A., Reinares, M., and Gastro, C. (2000). Bipolar II disorder and comorbidity. *Compr Psychiatry*, 41(5), 339–343.

Vieta, E., Colom, F., Corbella, B., Martinez-Aran, A., Reinares, M., Benabarre, A., and Gasto, C. (2001). Clinical correlates of psychiatric comorbidity in bipolar I patients. *Bipolar Disord*, 3(5), 253–258.

Virkkunen, M., and Linnoila, M. (1993). Brain serotonin, type II alcoholism and impulsive violence. *J Stud Alcohol Suppl*, 11, 163–169.

Waller, S.J., Lyons, J.S., and Costantini-Ferrando, M.F. (1999). Impact of comorbid affective and alcohol use disorders on suicidal ideation and attempts. *J Clin Psychol*, 55(5), 585–595.

Weeke, A. (1979). Causes of death in manic-depressives. In M. Schou, E. Strömgren (Eds.), *Origin, Prevention and Treatment of Affective Disorders* (pp. 289–299). London: Academic Press.

Wehr, T.A. (1992). In short photoperiods, human sleep is biphasic. *J Sleep Res*, 1(2), 103–107.

Wender, P.H., Kety, S.S., Rosenthal, D., Schulsinger, F., Ortmann, J., and Lunde, I. (1986). Psychiatric disorders in the biological and adoptive families of adopted individuals with affective disorders. *Arch Gen Psychiatry*, 43(10), 923–929.

Wetterberg, L., Eriksson, D., Friberg, Y., and Vango, B. (1978). Melatonin in humans: Physiological and clinical studies. *Clin Chim Acta*, 86, 169–177.

Whitney, D.K., Sharma, V., and Kueneman, K. (1999). Seasonality of manic depressive illness in Canada. *J Affect Disord*, 55(2–3), 99–105.

Winokur, G., Clayton, P.J., and Reich, T. (1969). Manic depressive illness. St. Louis: C.V. Mosby.

World Health Organization. (2001a). *The World Report on Violence and Health*. Geneva: World Health Organization.

World Health Organization [WHO] (2001b). *Mental Health and Brain Disorders, Suicide Rates (Per 100,000)*. Geneva: World Health Organization. [Online]. Available: http://www.who.int/mental_health/Topic_Suicide/ Suicide_rates.html [accessed January 7, 2002].

Wu, L.H., and Dunner, D.L. (1993). Suicide attempts in rapid cycling bipolar disorder patients. *J Affect Disord*, 29(1), 57–61.

Yip, P.S., Chao, A., and Ho, T.P. (1998). Are-examination of seasonal variation in suicides in Australia and New Zealand. *J Affect Disord*, 47(1–3), 141–150.

Young, M.A., Fogg, L.F., Scheftner, W., Fawcett, J., Akiskal, H., and Maser, J. (1996). Stable trait components of hopelessness: Baseline and sensitivity to depression. *J Abnorm Psychol*, 105(2), 155–165.

Zajicek, K.B., Price, C.S., Shoaf, S.E., Mehlman, P.T., Suomi, S.J., Linnoila, M., and Dee Higgley, J. (2000). Seasonal variation in CSF 5-HIAA concentrations in male rhesus macaques. *Neuropsychopharmacology*, 22(3), 240–250.

CHAPTER 9

Addington, J., and Addington, D. (1998). Facial affect recognition and information processing in schizophrenia and bipolar disorder. *Schizophr Res,* 32, 171–181.

Agarwal, A.K., Kalra, R., Natu, M.V., Dadhich, A.P., and Deswal, R.S. (2002). Psychomotor performance of psychiatric inpatients under therapy: Assessment by paper and pencil tests. *Hum Psychopharmacol*, 17(2), 91–93.

Ahearn, E.P., Steffens, D.C., Cassidy, F., Van Meter, S.A., Provenzale, J.M., Seldin, M.F., Weisler, R.H., and Krishnan, K.R. (1998). Familial leukoencephalopathy in bipolar disorder. *Am J Psychiatry*, 155, 1605–1607.

Ahn, K.H., Lyoo, I.K., Lee, H.K., Song, I.C., Oh, J.S., Hwang, J., Kwon, J., Kim, M.J., Kim, M., and Renshaw, P.F. (2004). White matter hyperintensities in subjects with bipolar disorder. *Psychiatry Clin Neurosci*, 58, 516–521.

Albus, M., Hubmann, W., Wahlheim, C., Sobizack, N., Franz, U., and Mohr, F. (1996). Contrasts in neuropsychological test profile between patients with first-episode schizophrenia and first-episode affective disorders. *Acta Psychiatr Scand*, 94, 87–93.

Alema, G., and Donini, G. (1960). On the clinical and electroencephalographic changes caused by the intracarotid administration of sodium 5-isoamyl-5-ethylbarbiturate in man. *Bollettino–Societa Italiana Biologia Sperimentale*, 36, 900–904.

Ali, S.O., Denicoff, K.D., Altshuler, L.L., Hauser, P., Li, X., Conrad, A.J., Mirsky, A.F., Smith-Jackson, E.E., and Post, R.M. (2000). A preliminary study of the relation of neuropsychological performance to neuroanatomic structures in bipolar disorder. *Neuropsychiatry Neuropsychol Behav Neurol*, 13(1), 20–28.

Alpert, M., Pouget, E.R., and Silva, R.R. (2001). Reflections of depression in acoustic measures of the patient's speech. *J Affect Disord*, 66, 59–69.

Altshuler, L.L. (1993). Bipolar disorder: Are repeated episodes associated with neuroanatomic and cognitive changes? *Biol Psychiatry*, 33, 563–565.

Altshuler, L.L., Ventura, J., van Gorp, W.G., Green, M.F., Theberge, D.C., and Mintz, J. (2004). Neurocognitive function in clinically stable men with bipolar I disorder or schizophrenia and normal control subjects. *Biol Psychiatry*, 56, 560–569.

Amminger, G.P., Edwards, J., Brewer, W.J., Harrigan, S., and McGorry, P.D. (2002). Duration of untreated psychosis and cognitive deterioration in first-episode schizophrenia. *Schizophr Res*, 54, 223–230.

Andersen, G., Vestergaard, K., and Riis, J.O. (1993). Citalopram for post-stroke pathological crying. *Lancet*, 342, 837–839.

Andreasen, N.C. (1987). Creativity and mental illness: Prevalence rates in writers and their first-degree relatives. *Am J Psychiatry*, 144, 1288–1292.

Andreasen, N.C., and Glick, I.D. (1988). Bipolar affective disorder and creativity: Implications and clinical management. *Compr Psychiatry*, 29, 207–217.

Arroyo, S., Lesser, R.P., Gordon, B., Uematsu, S., Hart, J., Schwerdt, P., Andreasson, K., and Fisher, R.S. (1993). Mirth, laughter and gelastic seizures. *Brain*, 116(Pt. 4), 757–780.

Asarnow, R.F., and MacCrimmon, D.J. (1981). Span of apprehension deficits during the postpsychotic stages of schizophrenia: A replication and extension. *Arch Gen Psychiatry*, 38, 1006–1011.

Ashton, E.A., Berg, M.J., Parker, K.J., Weisberg, J., Chen, C.W., and Ketonen, L. (1995). Segmentation and feature extraction techniques, with applications to MRI head studies. *Magn Reson Med*, 33, 670–677.

Atre-Vaidya, N., Taylor, M.A., Seidenberg, M., Reed, R., Perrine, A., and Glick-Oberwise, F. (1998). Cognitive deficits, psychopathology, and psychosocial functioning in bipolar mood disorder. *Neuropsychiatry Neuropsychol Behav Neurol*, 11, 120–126.

Austin, M.P., Mitchell, P., Hadzi-Pavlovic, D., Hickie, I., Parker, G., Chan, J., and Eyers, K. (2000). Effect of apomorphine on motor and cognitive function in melancholic patients: A preliminary report. *Psychiatry Res*, 97, 207–215.

Aylward, E.H., Roberts-Twillie, J.V., Barta, P.E., Kumar, A.J., Harris, G.J., Geer, M., Peyser, C.E., and Pearlson, G.D. (1994). Basal ganglia volumes and white matter hyperintensities in patients with bipolar disorder. *Am J Psychiatry*, 151, 687–693.

Baddeley, A. (1986). *Working Memory*. Oxford, England: Clarendon.

Baldwin, R.C., Walker, S., Simpson, S.W., Jackson, A., and Burns, A. (2000). The prognostic significance of abnormalities seen on magnetic resonance imaging in late life depression: Clinical outcome, mortality and progression to dementia at three years. *Int J Geriatr Psychiatry*, 15, 1097–1104.

Baloh, R.W., Yue, Q., Socotch, T.M., and Jacobson, K.M. (1995). White matter lesions and disequilibrium in older people: I. Case-control comparison. *Arch Neurol*, 52, 970–974.

Barona, A., Reynolds, C., and Chastain, R. (1984). A demographically based index of premorbid intelligence for the WAIS-R. *J Consult Clin Psychol*, 52, 885–887.

Bayles, K.A., Trosset, M.W., Tomoeda, C.K., Montgomery, E.B. Jr., and Wilson, J. (1993). Generative naming in Parkinson disease patients. *J Clin Exper Neuropsychol*, 15, 547–562.

Bayley, P.J., Salmon, D.P., Bondi, M.W., Bui, B.K., Olichney, J., Delis, D.C., Thomas, R.G., and Thal, L.J. (2000). Comparison of the serial position effect in very mild Alzheimer's disease, mild Alzheimer's disease, and amnesia associated with electroconvulsive therapy. *J Int Neuropsychol Soc*, 6, 290–298.

Bearden, C.E., Hoffman, K.M., and Cannon, T.D. (2001). The neuropsychology and neuroanatomy of bipolar affective disorder: A critical review. *Bipolar Disord*, 3, 106–150; discussion 151–103.

Becerra, R., Amos, A., and Jongenelis, S. (2002). Organic alexithymia: A study of acquired emotional blindness. *Brain Injury*, 16, 633–645.

Beck, A.T., Steer, R.A., and Brown, G.K. (1996). *Beck Depression Inventory Manual* (2nd edition). San Antonio, TX: Psychological Corporation.

Beck, L.H., Bransome, E.D. Jr., Mirsky, A.F., Rosvold, H.E., and Sarason, I. (1956). A continuous performance test of brain damage. *J Consult Psychol*, 20, 343–350.

Bejjani, B.P., Damier, P., Arnulf, I., Thivard, L., Bonnet, A.M., Dormont, D., Cornu, P., Pidoux, B., Samson, Y., and Agid, Y.

(1999). Transient acute depression induced by high-frequency deep-brain stimulation. *N Engl J Med,* 340, 1476–1480.

Bench, C.J., Friston, K.J., Brown, R.G., Scott, L.C., Frackowiak, R.S., and Dolan, R.J. (1992). The anatomy of melancholia: Focal abnormalities of cerebral blood flow in major depression. *Psychol Med,* 22, 607–615.

Benedek, D.M., and Peterson, K.A. (1995). Sertraline for treatment of pathological crying. *Am J Psychiatry,* 152, 953–954.

Berney, A., Vingerhoets, F., Perrin, A., Guex, P., Villemure, J.G., Burkhard, P.R., Benkelfat, C., and Ghika, J. (2002). Effect on mood of subthalamic DBS for Parkinson's disease: A consecutive series of 24 patients. *Neurology,* 59, 1427–1429.

Black, D.W. (1982). Pathological laughter: A review of the literature. *J Nerv Ment Dis,* 170, 67–71.

Blackburn, I.M. (1975). Mental and psychomotor speed in depression and mania. *Br J Psychiatry,* 132, 329–335.

Blaney, P.H. (1986). Affect and memory: A review. *Psychol Bull,* 99, 229–246.

Boone, K.B., Miller, B.L., Lesser, I.M., Mehringer, C.M., Hill-Gutierrez, E., Goldberg, M.A., and Berman, N.G. (1992). Neuropsychological correlates of white-matter lesions in healthy elderly subjects: A threshold effect. *Arch Neurol,* 49, 549–554.

Borod, J.C., Koff, E., Lorch, M.P., Nicholas, M., and Welkowitz, J. (1988). Emotional and non-emotional facial behaviour in patients with unilateral brain damage. *J Neurol Neurosurg Psychiatry,* 51, 826–832.

Botteron, K.N., Vannier, M.W., Geller, B., Todd, R.D., and Lee, B.C. (1995). Preliminary study of magnetic resonance imaging characteristics in 8- to 16-year-olds with mania. *J Am Acad Child Adolesc Psychiatry,* 34, 742–749.

Bouhuys, A.L., and Mulder-Hajonides van der Meulen, W.R. (1984). Speech timing measures of severity, psychomotor retardation, and agitation in endogenously depressed patients. *J Commun Disord,* 17, 277–288.

Bouhuys, A.L., Bloem, G.M., and Groothuis, T.G. (1995). Induction of depressed and elated mood by music influences the perception of facial emotional expressions in healthy subjects. *J Affect Disord,* 33, 215–226.

Bozikas, V.P., Tonia, T., Fokas, K., Karavatos, A., and Kosmidis, M.H. (2006). Impaired emotion processing in remitted patients with bipolar disorder. *J Affect Disord,* 91, 53–56.

Branch, C., Milner, B., and Rasmussen, T. (1964). Intracarotid sodium amytal for the lateralization of cerebral speech dominance: Observations in 123 patients. *J Neurosurg,* 21, 399–405.

Breeze, J.L., Hesdorffer, D.C., Hong, X., Frazier, J.A., and Renshaw, P.F. (2003). Clinical significance of brain white matter hyperintensities in young adults with psychiatric illness. *Harv Rev Psychiatry,* 11, 269–283.

Breslow, R., Kocsis, J., and Belkin, B. (1980). Memory deficits in depression: Evidence utilizing the Wechsler Memory Scale. *Percept Motor Skills,* 51, 541–542.

Breslow, R., Kocsis, J., and Belkin, B. (1981). Contribution of the depressive perspective to memory function in depression. *Am J Psychiatry,* 138, 227–230.

Breteler, M.M., van Swieten, J.C., Bots, M.L., Grobbee, D.E., Claus, J.J., van den Hout, J.H., van Harskamp, F., Tanghe, H.L., de Jong, P.T., and van Gijn, J. (1994). Cerebral white matter lesions, vascular risk factors, and cognitive function in a population-based study: The Rotterdam Study. *Neurology,* 44, 1246–1252.

Brown, E.S., Rush, A.J., and McEwen, B.S. (1999). Hippocampal remodeling and damage by corticosteroids: Implications for mood disorders. *Neuropsychopharmacology,* 21, 474–484.

Brown, F.W., Lewine, R.J., Hudgins, P.A., and Risch, S.C. (1992). White matter hyperintensity signals in psychiatric and nonpsychiatric subjects. *Am J Psychiatry,* 149, 620–625.

Burt, D.B., Zembar, M.J., and Niederehe, G. (1995). Depression and memory impairment: A meta-analysis of the association, its pattern, and specificity. *Psychol Bull,* 117, 285–305.

Burt, T., Prudic, J., Peyser, S., Clark, J., and Sackeim, H.A. (2000). Learning and memory in bipolar and unipolar major depression: Effects of aging. *Neuropsychiatry Neuropsychol Behav Neurol,* 13, 246–253.

Burt, T., Lisanby, S.H., and Sackeim, H.A. (2002). Neuropsychiatric applications of transcranial magnetic stimulation: A meta analysis. *Int J Neuropsychopharmacol,* 5, 73–103.

Buschke, H. (1973). Selective reminding for analysis of memory and learning. *J Verbal Learning Verbal Behav,* 12, 543–550.

Cadelo, M., Inzitari, D., Pracucci, G., and Mascalchi, M. (1991). Predictors of leukoaraiosis in elderly neurological patients. *Cerebrovasc Dis,* 1, 345–351.

Calev, A., and Erwin, P. (1985). Recall and recognition in depressives: Use of matched tasks. *Br J Clin Psychol,* 24, 127–128.

Caligiuri, M.P., and Ellwanger, J. (2000). Motor and cognitive aspects of motor retardation in depression. *J Affect Disord,* 57, 83–93.

Caligiuri, M.P., Brown, G.G., Meloy, M.J., Eberson, S.C., Kindermann, S.S., Frank, L.R., Zorrilla, L.E., and Lohr, J.B. (2003). An fMRI study of affective state and medication on cortical and subcortical brain regions during motor performance in bipolar disorder. *Psychiatry Res,* 123, 171–182.

Caligiuri, M.P., Brown, G.G., Meloy, M.J., Eyler, L.T., Kindermann, S.S., Eberson, S., Frank, L.R., and Lohr, J.B. (2004). A functional magnetic resonance imaging study of cortical asymmetry in bipolar disorder. *Bipolar Disord,* 6, 183–196.

Cannizzaro, M., Harel, B., Reilly, N., Chappell, P., and Snyder, P.J. (2004). Voice acoustical measurement of the severity of major depression. *Brain Cognition,* 56, 30–35.

Carson, A.J., MacHale, S., Allen, K., Lawrie, S.M., Dennis, M., House, A., and Sharpe, M. (2000). Depression after stroke and lesion location: A systematic review. *Lancet,* 356, 122–126.

Cavanagh, J.T., Van Beck, M., Muir, W., and Blackwood, D.H. (2002). Case-control study of neurocognitive function in euthymic patients with bipolar disorder: An association with mania. *Br J Psychiatry,* 180, 320–326.

Chamberlain, S.R., and Sahakian, B.J. (2004). Cognition in mania and depression: Psychological models and clinical implications. *Curr Psychiatry Rep,* 6, 451–458.

Chapman, L.J., and Chapman, J.P. (1973). *Disordered Thought in Schizophrenia.* Englewood Cliffs, NJ: Prentice Hall.

Christensen, H., Griffiths, K., Mackinnon, A., and Jacomb, P. (1997). A quantitative review of cognitive deficits in depression and Alzheimer-type dementia. *J Int Neuropsychol Soc,* 3, 631–651.

Christodoulou, G.N., Kokkevi, A., Lykouras, E.P., Stefanis, C.N., and Papadimitriou, G.N. (1981). Effects of lithium on memory. *Am J Psychiatry,* 138, 847–848.

Clark, D.M., and Teasdale, J.D. (1982). Diurnal variation in clinical depression and accessibility of memories of positive and negative experiences. *J Abnorm Psychology,* 91, 87–95.

Clark, L., Iversen, S.D., and Goodwin, G.M. (2001). A neuropsychological investigation of prefrontal cortex involvement in acute mania. *Am J Psychiatry*, 158, 1605–1611.

Clark, L., Iversen, S.D., Goodwin, G.M. (2002). Sustained attention deficit in bipolar disorder. *Br J Psychiatry*, 180, 313–319.

Clark, L., Kempton, M.J., Scarna, A., Grasby, P.M., and Goodwin, G.M. (2005). Sustained attention-deficit confirmed in euthymic bipolar disorder but not in first-degree relatives of bipolar patients or euthymic unipolar depression. *Biol Psychiatry*, 57, 183–187.

Coffey, C.E., Figiel, G.S., Djang, W.T., and Weiner, R.D. (1990). Subcortical hyperintensity on magnetic resonance imaging: A comparison of normal and depressed elderly subjects. *Am J Psychiatry*, 147, 187–189.

Coffey, C.E., Wilkinson, W.E., Weiner, R.D., Parashos, I.A., Djang, W.T., Webb, M.C., Figiel, G.S., and Spritzer, C.E. (1993). Quantitative cerebral anatomy in depression: A controlled magnetic resonance imaging study. *Arch Gen Psychiatry*, 50, 7–16.

Coffman, J.A., Bornstein, R.A., Olson, S.C., Schwarzkopf, S.B., and Nasrallah, H.A. (1990). Cognitive impairment and cerebral structure by MRI in bipolar disorder. *Biol Psychiatry*, 27, 1188–1196.

Cohen, N., and Squire, L. (1980). Preserved learning and retention of pattern-analyzing skill in amnesia: Dissociation of knowing how and knowing that. *Science*, 210, 207–210.

Cohen, R., Weingartner, H., Smallberg, S., Pickar, D., and Murphy, D. (1982). Effort and cognition in depression. *Arch Gen Psychiatry*, 39, 593–597.

Cohen-Gadol, A.A., Westerveld, M., Alvarez-Carilles, J., and Spencer, D.D. (2004). Intracarotid Amytal memory test and hippocampal magnetic resonance imaging volumetry: Validity of the Wada test as an indicator of hippocampal integrity among candidates for epilepsy surgery. *J Neurosurgery*, 101, 926–931.

Colvin, C.R., and Block, J. (1994). Do positive illusions foster mental health? An examination of the Taylor and Brown formulation. *Psychol Bull*, 116, 3–20.

Cools, R., and Robbins, T.W. (2004). Chemistry of the adaptive mind. *Philos Transact A Math Phys Eng Sci*, 362, 2871–2888.

Corwin, J., Peselow, E., Feenan, K., Rotrosen, J., and Fieve, R. (1990). Disorders of decision in affective disease: An effect of beta-adrenergic dysfunction? *Biol Psychiatry*, 27, 813–833.

Coryell, W., Endicott, J., Reich, T., Andreasen, N., and Keller, M. (1984). A family study of bipolar II disorder. *Br J Psychiatry*, 145, 49–54.

Coryell, W., Endicott, J., Keller, M., Andreasen, N., Grove, W., Hirschfeld, R.M., and Scheftner, W. (1989). Bipolar affective disorder and high achievement: A familial association. *Am J Psychiatry*, 146(8), 983–988.

Coyne, J.C., and Gotlib, I.H. (1983). The role of cognition in depression: A critical appraisal. *Psychol Bull*, 94, 472–505.

Craik, F.I., and Jennings, J.M. (1992). Human memory. In F.I.M. Crisk, T.A. Salthouse (Eds.), *The Handbook of Aging and Cognition* (pp. 51–110). Hillsdale, NJ: Erlbaum.

Craik, F.I., and Tulving, E. (1975). Depth of processing and the retention of words in episodic memory. *J Exp Psychol (Gen)*, 1, 268–294.

Cronholm, B., and Ottosson, J.-O. (1961). Memory functions in endogenous depression: Before and after electroconvulsive therapy. *Arch Gen Psychiatry*, 5, 193–199.

Cronholm, B., and Ottosson, J.-O. (1963). The experience of memory function after electroconvulsive therapy. *Br J Psychiatry*, 109, 251–258.

Cummings, J.L., and Mendez, M.F. (1984). Secondary mania with focal cerebrovascular lesions. *Am J Psychiatry*, 141, 1084–1087.

Custance, J. (1952). *Wisdom, Madness and Folly: The Philosophy of a Lunatic.* London: Pellegrini & Cudahy.

Dahabra, S., Ashton, C.H., Bahrainian, M., Britton, P.G., Ferrier, I.N., McAllister, V.A., Marsh, V.R., and Moore, P.B. (1998). Structural and functional abnormalities in elderly patients clinically recovered from early- and late-onset depression. *Biol Psychiatry*, 44, 34–46.

Dalby J.T., and Williams, R. (1986). Preserved reading and spelling ability in psychotic disorders. *Psychol Med*, 16, 171–175.

Daly, D.D., and Mulder, D.W. (1957). Gelastic epilepsy. *Neurology*, 7, 189–192.

Daly, J.J., Prudic, J., Devanand, D.P., Nobler, M.S., Lisanby, S.H., Peyser, S., Roose, S.P., and Sackeim, H.A. (2001). ECT in bipolar and unipolar depression: Differences in speed of response. *Bipolar Disord*, 3, 95–104.

David, A.S., and Cutting, J.C. (1990). Affect, affective disorder and schizophrenia: A neuropsychological investigation of right hemisphere function. *Br J Psychiatry*, 156, 491–495.

Davidson, M. (1939). Studies in the application of mental tests to psychotic patients. *Br J Med Psychol*, 18, 44–52.

Davidson, R.J. (1995). Cerebral asymmetry, emotion, and affective style. In R.J. Davidson, K. Hugdahl (Eds.), *Brain Asymmetry* (pp. 361–387). Cambridge, MA: MIT Press.

Davison, C., and Kelman, H. (1939). Pathological laughing and crying. *Arch Neurol Psychiatry*, 42, 595–643.

Decina, P., Kestenbaum, C.J., Farber, S., Kron, L., Gargan, M., Sackeim, H.A., and Fieve, R.R. (1983). Clinical and psychological assessment of children of bipolar probands. *Am J Psychiatry*, 140, 548–553.

DelBello, M.P., Adler, C.M., Amicone, J., Mills, N.P., Shear, P.K., Warner, J., and Strakowski, S.M. (2004). Parametric neurocognitive task design: A pilot study of sustained attention in adolescents with bipolar disorder. *J Affect Disord*, 82(Suppl. 1), S79–S88.

Demers, R.G., and Heninger, G.R. (1971). Visual-motor performance during lithium treatment: A preliminary report. *J Clin Pharmacol New Drugs*, 11, 274–279.

Den Hartog, H.M., Derix, M.M., Van Bemmel, A.L., Kremer, B., and Jolles, J. (2003). Cognitive functioning in young and middle-aged unmedicated out-patients with major depression: Testing the effort and cognitive speed hypotheses. *Psychol Med*, 33, 1443–1451.

Denicoff, K.D., Ali, S.O., Mirsky, A.F., Smith-Jackson, E.E., Leverich, G.S., Duncan, C.C., Connell, E.G., and Post, R.M. (1999). Relationship between prior course of illness and neuropsychological functioning in patients with bipolar disorder. *J Affect Disord*, 56, 67–73.

Deptula, D., Manevitz, A., and Yozawitz, A. (1991). Asymmetry of recall in depression. *J Clin Exper Neuropsychol*, 13, 854–870.

Dhingra, U., and Robins, P.V. (1991). Mania in the elderly: A 5–7 year follow-up. *J Am Geriatr Soc*, 39, 581–583.

Dickstein, D.P., Treland, J.E., Snow, J., McClure, E.B., Mehta, M.S., Towbin, K.E., Pine, D.S., and Leibenluft, E. (2004). Neuropsychological performance in pediatric bipolar disorder. *Biol Psychiatry*, 55, 32–39.

Dixon, T., Kravariti, E., Frith, C., Murray, R.M., and McGuire, P.K. (2004). Effect of symptoms on executive function in bipolar illness. *Psychol Med*, 34, 811–821.

Docherty, N.M., Hawkins, K.A., Hoffman, R.E., Quinlan, D.M., Rakfeldt, J., and Sledge, W.H. (1996). Working memory, attention, and communication disturbances in schizophrenia. *J Abnorm Psychol*, 105(2), 212–219.

Dolan, R.J., Bench, C.J., Liddle, P.F., Friston, K.J., Frith, C.D., Grasby, P.M., and Frackowiak, R.S. (1993). Dorsolateral prefrontal cortex dysfunction in the major psychoses; Symptom or disease specificity? *J Neurol Neurosurg Psychiatry*, 56(12), 1290–1294.

Dolan, R.J., Bench, C.J., Brown, R.G., Scott, L.C., and Frackowiak, R.S. (1994). Neuropsychological dysfunction in depression: The relationship to regional cerebral blood flow. *Psychol Med*, 24, 849–857.

Donnelly, E.F., Murphy, D.L., Goodwin, F.K., and Waldman, I.N. (1982). Intellectual function in primary affective disorder. *Br J Psychiatry*, 140, 633–636.

Drevets, W.C., Bogers, W., and Raichle, M.E. (2002). Functional anatomical correlates of antidepressant drug treatment assessed using PET measures of regional glucose metabolism. *Eur Neuropsychopharmacol*, 12, 527–544.

Dunner, D.L., Dwyer, T., and Fieve, R.R. (1976). Depressive symptoms in patients with unipolar and bipolar affective disorder. *Compr Psychiatry*, 17, 447–451.

Dupont, R.M., Jernigan, T.L., Gillin, J.C., Butters, N., Delis, D.C., and Hesselink, J.R. (1987). Subcortical signal hyperintensities in bipolar patients detected by MRI. *Psychiatry Res*, 21, 357–358.

Dupont, R.M., Jernigan, T.L., Butters, N., Delis, D., Hesselink, J.R., Heindel, W., and Gillin, J.C. (1990). Subcortical abnormalities detected in bipolar affective disorder using magnetic resonance imaging: Clinical and neuropsychological significance [see comments]. *Arch Gen Psychiatry*, 47, 55–59.

Dupont, R.M., Butters, N., Schafer, K., Wilson, T., Hesselink, J., and Gillin, J.C. (1995). Diagnostic specificity of focal white matter abnormalities in bipolar and unipolar mood disorder. *Biol Psychiatry*, 38, 482–486.

Ebmeier, K.P., Prentice, N., Ryman, A., Halloran, E., Rimmington, J.E., Best, J.K., and Goodwin, G.M. (1997). Temporal lobe abnormalities in dementia and depression: A study using high resolution single photon emission tomography and magnetic resonance imaging. *J Neurol Neurosurg Psychiatry*, 63, 597–604.

Eisemann, M. (1986). Social class and social mobility in depressed patients. *Acta Psychiatr Scand*, 73(4), 399–402.

el Massioui, F., and Lesevre, N. (1988). Attention impairment and psychomotor retardation in depressed patients: An event-related potential study. *Electroencephalogr Clin Neurophysiol*, 70, 46–55.

El-Badri, S.M., Ashton, C.H., Moore, P.B., Marsh, V.R., and Ferrier, I.N. (2001). Electrophysiological and cognitive function in young euthymic patients with bipolar affective disorder. *Bipolar Disord*, 3, 79–87.

Ellenbogen, M.A., Young, S.N., Dean, P., Palmour, R.M., and Benkelfat, C. (1996). Mood response to acute tryptophan depletion in healthy volunteers: Sex differences and temporal stability. *Neuropsychopharmacology*, 15, 465–474.

Engel, J., Kuhl, D.E., and Phelps, M.E. (1982). Patterns of human local cerebral glucose metabolism during epileptic seizures. *Science*, 218, 64–66.

Engelsmann, F., Katz, J., Ghadirian, A.M., and Schachter, D. (1988). Lithium and memory: A long-term follow-up study. *J Clin Psychopharmacol*, 8, 207–212.

Erkinjuntti, T., Gao, F., Lee, D.H., Eliasziw, M., Merskey, H., and Hachinski, V.C. (1994). Lack of difference in brain hyperintensities between patients with early Alzheimer's disease and control subjects. *Arch Neurol*, 51, 260–268.

Ferrier, I.N., Stanton, B.R., Kelly, T.P., and Scott, J. (1999). Neuropsychological function in euthymic patients with bipolar disorder. *Br J Psychiatry*, 175, 246–251.

Ferrier, I.N., Chowdhury, R., Thompson, J.M., Watson, S., and Young, A.H. (2004). Neurocognitive function in unaffected first-degree relatives of patients with bipolar disorder: A preliminary report. *Bipolar Disord*, 6, 319–322.

Fleck, D.E., Shear, P.K., Zimmerman, M.E., Getz, G.E., Corey, K.B., Jak, A., Lebowitz, B.K., and Strakowski, S.M. (2003). Verbal memory in mania: Effects of clinical state and task requirements. *Bipolar Disord*, 5(5), 375–380.

Fleminger, J.J., Dalton, R., and Standage, K.F. (1977). Handedness in psychiatric patients. *Br J Psychiatry*, 131, 448–452.

Flor-Henry, P. (1976). Lateralized temporal-limbic dysfunction and psychopathology. *Ann N Y Acad Sci*, 280, 777–797.

Flor-Henry, P. (1979). On certain aspects of the localization of the cerebral systems regulating and determining emotion. *Biol Psychiatry*, 14, 677–698.

Flor-Henry, P. (1983). *The Cerebral Basis of Psychopathology*. Boston: John Wright.

Flor-Henry, P., and Gruzalier, J. (1983). *Laterality and Psychopathology*, Amsterdam: Elsevier.

Flor-Henry, P., and Yeudall, L.T. (1979). Neuropsychological investigation of schizophrenia and manic-depressive psychoses. In J. Gruzelier, P. Flor-Henry (Eds.), *Hemispheric Asymmetries of Function in Psychopathology* (pp. 341–362). Amsterdam: Elsevier.

Foster, F.G., and Kupfer, D.J. (1975). Psychomotor activity as a correlate of depression and sleep in acutely disturbed psychiatric inpatients. *Am J Psychiatry*, 132, 928–931.

Frangou, S., Donaldson, S., Hadjulis, M., Landau, S., and Goldstein, L.H. (2006). The Maudsley Bipolar Disorder Project: Executive dysfunction in bipolar disorder I and its clinical correlates. *Biol Psychiatry*, 58, 859–864.

Frith, C., Stevens, M., Johnstone, E., Deakin, J., Lawler, P., and Crow, T.J. (1983). Effects of ECT and depression on various aspects of memory. *Br J Psychiatry*, 142, 610–617.

Fujikawa, T., Yamawaki, S., and Touhouda, Y. (1995). Silent cerebral infarctions in patients with late-onset mania. *Stroke*, 26, 946–949.

Gainotti, G. (1970). Emotional behavior of patients with right and left brain damage in neuropsychological test conditions. *Archivio di Psicologia, Neurologia e Psichiatria*, 31, 457–480.

Gainotti, G. (1972). Emotional behavior and hemispheric side of the lesion. *Cortex*, 8, 41–55.

Gascon, G.G., and Lombroso, C.T. (1971). Epileptic (gelastic) laughter. *Epilepsia*, 12, 63–76.

Gass, C.S., and Russell, E.W. (1986). Differential impact of brain damage and depression on memory test performance. *J Consult Clin Psychol*, 54, 261–263.

Geschwind, N. (1965). Disconnexion syndromes in animals and man. *Brain*, 88, 273–294, 584–644.

Getz, G.E., Shear, P.K., and Strakowski, S.M. (2003). Facial affect recognition deficits in bipolar disorder. *J Int Neuropsychol Soc*, 9, 623–632.

Ghacibeh, G.A., and Heilman, K.M. (2003). Progressive affective aprosodia and prosoplegia. *Neurology, 60*, 1192–1194.

Ghadirian, A.M., Engelsmann, F., and Ananth, J. (1983). Memory functions during lithium therapy. *J Clin Psychopharmacol, 3*, 313–315.

Gildengers, A.G., Butters, M.A., Seligman, K., McShea, M., Miller, M.D., Mulsant, B.H., Kupfer, D.J., and Reynolds, C.F. III. (2004). Cognitive functioning in late-life bipolar disorder. *Am J Psychiatry, 161*(4), 736–738.

Godfrey, H.P., and Knight, R.G. (1984). The validity of actometer and speech activity measures in the assessment of depressed patients. *Br J Psychiatry, 145*, 159–163.

Goldman-Rakic, P.S. (1987). Circuitry of primate prefrontal cortex and regulation of behavior by representational memory. In F. Plum, V. Mountcastle (Eds.), *The Handbook of Physiology: Section 1. The Nervous System: Vol. 5. Higher Functions of the Brain: Part 1* (pp. 373–417). Bethesda, MD: American Physiological Society.

Goode, D.J., Meltzer, H.Y., Moretti, R., Kupfer, D.J., and McPartland, R.J. (1979). The relationship between wrist-monitored motor activity and serum CPK activity in psychiatric inpatients. *Br J Psychiatry, 135*, 62–66.

Goswami, U., Sharma, A., Khastigir, U., Ferrier, I.N., Young, A.H., Gallagher, P., Thompson, J.M., and Moore, P.B. (2006). Neuropsychological dysfunction, soft neurological signs and social disability in euthymic patients with bipolar disorder. *Br J Psychiatry, 188*, 366–373.

Gotlib, I.H. (1981). Self-reinforcement and recall: Differential deficits in depressed and nondepressed psychiatric inpatients. *J Abnorm Psychol, 90*, 521–530.

Gotlib, I.H., and Olson, J.M. (1983). Depression, psychopathology, and self-serving attributions. *Br J Clin Psychol, 22*(Pt. 4), 309–310.

Gourovitch, M.L., Torrey, E.F., Gold, J.M., Randolph, C., Weinberger, D.R., and Goldberg, T.E. (1999). Neuropsychological performance of monozygotic twins discordant for bipolar disorder. *Biol Psychiatry, 45*, 639–646.

Greden, J.F. (1982). Biological markers of melancholia and reclassification of depressive disorders. *Encephale, 8*, 193–202.

Greden, J.F., and Carroll, B.J. (1980). Decrease in speech pause times with treatment of endogenous depression. *Biol Psychiatry, 15*, 575–587.

Greden, J.F., Albala, A.A., Smokler, I.A., Gardner, R., and Carroll, B.J. (1981). Speech pause time: A marker of psychomotor retardation among endogenous depressives. *Biol Psychiatry, 16*, 851–859.

Green, A., Nutt, D., and Cowen, P. (1982). Increased seizure threshold following convulsion. In M. Sandler (Ed.), *Psychopharmacology of Anticonvulsants* (pp. 16–26). Oxford, England: Oxford University Press.

Green, M., and Walker, E. (1986). Attentional performance in positive- and negative-symptom schizophrenia. *J Nerv Ment Dis, 174*(4), 208–213.

Greenwald, B.S., Kramer-Ginsberg, E., Krishnan, K.R., Ashtari, M., Auerbach, C., and Patel, M. (1998). Neuroanatomic localization of magnetic resonance imaging signal hyperintensities in geriatric depression. *Stroke, 29*, 613–617.

Gruzelier, J., Seymour, K., Wilson, L., Jolley, A., and Hirsch, S. (1988). Impairments on neuropsychologic tests of temporo-hippocampal and frontohippocampal functions and word fluency in remitting schizophrenia and affective disorders. *Arch Gen Psychiatry, 45*(7), 623–629.

Haldane, M., and Frangou, S. (2004). New insights help define the pathophysiology of bipolar affective disorder: Neuroimaging and neuropathology findings. *Prog Neuropsychopharmacology Biol Psychiatry, 28*, 943–960.

Hammar, A. (2003). Automatic and effortful information processing in unipolar major depression. *Scand J Psychol, 44*, 409–413.

Hammar, A., Lund, A., and Hugdahl, K. (2003a). Long-lasting cognitive impairment in unipolar major depression: A 6-month follow-up study. *Psychiatry Res, 118*, 189–196.

Hammar, A., Lund, A., and Hugdahl, K. (2003b). Selective impairment in effortful information processing in major depression. *J Int Neuropsychol Soc, 9*, 954–959.

Hardy, P., Jouvent, R., and Widlocher, D. (1984). Speech pause time and the retardation rating scale for depression (ERD): Towards a reciprocal validation. *J Affect Disord, 6*, 123–127.

Harmer, C.J., Clark, L., Grayson, L., and Goodwin, G.M. (2002). Sustained attention deficit in bipolar disorder is not a working memory impairment in disguise. *Neuropsychologia, 40*, 1586–1590.

Hartlage, S., Alloy, L.B., Vazquez, C., and Dykman, B. (1993). Automatic and effortful processing in depression. *Psycho Bul, 113*, 247–278.

Harvey, P.D., and Brault, J. (1986). Speech performance in mania and schizophrenia: The association of positive and negative thought disorders and reference failures. *J Commun Disord, 19*(3), 161–173.

Harvey, P.D., and Serper, M.R. (1990). Linguistic and cognitive failures in schizophrenia. A multivariate analysis. *J Nerv Ment Dis, 178*(8), 487–493.

Harvey, P.D., Earle-Boyer, E.A., Weilgus, M.S., and Levinson, J.C. (1986). Encoding, memory, and thought disorder in schizophrenia and mania. *Schizaphr Bull, 12*(2), 252–261.

Hasher, L., and Zacks, R. (1979). Automatic and effortful processes in memory. *J Exp Psychol (Gen), 108*, 356–388.

Hawkins, K.A., Hoffman, R.E., Quinlan, D.M., Rakfeldt, J., Docherty, N.M., and Sledge, W.H. (1997). Cognition, negative symptoms, and diagnosis: A comparison of schizophrenic, bipolar, and control samples. *J Neuropsychiatry Clin Neurosci, 9*(1), 81–89.

Head, H. (1921). Release of function in the nervous system. *Proc R Soc Lond Biol, 92*, 184–209.

Heilman, K.M., Scholes, R., and Watson, R.T. (1975). Auditory affective agnosia: Disturbed comprehension of affective speech. *J Neurol Neurosurg Psychiatry, 38*, 69–72.

Henry, M.E., Schmidt, M.E., Matochik, J.A., Stoddard, E.P., and Potter, W.Z. (2001). The effects of ECT on brain glucose: A pilot FDG PET study. *J ECT, 17*, 33–40.

Hickie, I., Parsonage, B., and Parker, G. (1990a). Prediction of response to electroconvulsive therapy: Preliminary validation of a sign-based typology of depression. *Br J Psychiatry, 157*, 65–71.

Hickie, I., Parsonage, B., and Parker, G. (1990b). Prediction of response to electroconvulsive therapy: Preliminary validation of a sign-based typology of depression. *Br J Psychiatry, 157*, 65–71.

Hickie, I., Scott, E., Mitchell, P., Wilhelm, K., Austin, M.P., and Bennett, B. (1995). Subcortical hyperintensities on magnetic resonance imaging: Clinical correlates and prognostic significance in patients with severe depression. *Biol Psychiatry, 37*, 151–160.

Hickie, I., Mason, C., Parker, G., and Brodaty, H. (1996). Prediction of ECT response: Validation of a refined sign-based

(CORE) system for defining melancholia. *Br J Psychiatry*, 169, 68–74.

Hickie, I., Scott, E., Wilhelm, K., and Brodaty, H. (1997). Subcortical hyperintensities on magnetic resonance imaging in patients with severe depression: A longitudinal evaluation. *Biol Psychiatry*, 42, 367–374.

Hoffmann, G.M., Gonze, J.C., and Mendlewicz, J. (1985). Speech pause time as a method for the evaluation of psychomotor retardation in depressive illness. *Br J Psychiatry*, 146, 535–538.

Hoffman, R.E., Quinlan, D.M., Mazure, C.M., and McGlashan, T.M. (2001). Cortical instability and the mechanism of mania: A neural network simulation and perceptual text. *Biol Psychiatry*, 49(6), 500–509.

Holtzheimer, P.E., III, Russo, J., and Avery, D.H. (2001). A meta-analysis of repetitive transcranial magnetic stimulation in the treatment of depression. *Psychopharmacol Bull*, 35, 149–169.

Hommes, O.R. (1965). Semming sanomalien als neurologisch symptoom. *Nederlands Tijdschrift Voor Geneeskunde*, 109, 588–589.

House, A.O., Hackett, M.L., Anderson, C.S., and Horrocks, J.A. (2004). Pharmaceutical interventions for emotionalism after stroke. *Cochrane Database Syst Rev* CD003690.

Hughlings Jackson, J. (1958). *Selected Writings of John Hughling Jackson*. New York: Classics of Neurology and Neurosurgery. Richmond, VA: Staples Publishing.

Iverson, G.L. (2004). Objective assessment of psychomotor retardation in primary care patients with depression. *J Behav Med*, 27, 31–37.

James, W. (1890). *The Principles of Psychology* [microform]. New York: H. Holt.

Jamison, K.R. (1993). Manic-depressive illness and creativity. *Scientific American*. Available: http://www.sciamdigital.com/index.cfm?fa=Products.ViewIssuePreview&ARTICLEID_CHAR=3C9F2798-2B35-221B-6FA853B375CBA8C4.

Jenkins, M., Malloy, P., Salloway, S., Cohen, R., Rogg, J., Tung, G., Kohn, R., Westlake, R., Johnson, E.G., and Richardson, E. (1998). Memory processes in depressed geriatric patients with and without subcortical hyperintensities on MRI. *J Neuroimaging*, 8, 20–26.

Jeret, J.S. (1997). Treatment of poststroke pathological crying. *Stroke*, 28, 2321–2322.

Joanette, I., and Goulet, P. (1986). Criterion-specific reduction of verbal fluency in right brain-damaged right handers. *Neuropsychologia*, 24, 857–879.

Joffe, R.T., MacDonald, C., and Kutcher, S.P. (1988). Lack of differential cognitive effects of lithium and carbamazapine in bipolar affective disorder. *J Clin Psychopharmacol*, 8(6), 425–428.

Jorge, R.E., Robinson, R.G., Starkstein, S.E., Arndt, S.V., Forrester, A.W., and Geisler, F.H. (1993). Secondary mania following traumatic brain injury. *Am J Psychiatry*, 150, 916–921.

Judd, L.L. (1979). Effect of lithium on mood, cognition, and personality function in normal subjects. *Arch Gen Psychiatry*, 36, 860–866.

Junqué, C., Pujol, J., Vendrell, P., Bruna, O., Jódar, M., Ribas, J.C., Viñas, J., Capdevila, A., and Marti-Vilalta, J.L. (1990). Leuko-araiosis on magnetic resonance imaging and speed of mental processing. *Arch Neurol*, 47, 151–156.

Kano, M., Fukudo, S., Gyoba, J., Kamachi, M., Tagawa, M., Mochizuki, H., Itoh, M., Hongo, M., and Yanai, K. (2003). Specific brain processing of facial expressions in people with alexithymia: An H2 15O-PET study. *Brain*, 126, 1474–1484.

Kaprinis, G., Nimatoudis, J., Karavatos, A., Kandylis, D., and Kaprinis, S. (1995). Functional brain organization in bipolar affective patients during manic phase and after recovery: A digit dichotic listening study. *Percept Motor Skills*, 80(3 Pt. 2), 1275–1282.

Karniol, I.G., Dalton, J., and Lader, M.H. (1978). Acute and chronic effects of lithium chloride on physiological and psychological measures in normals. *Psychopharmacology*, 57, 289–294.

Kaschka, W.P., Meyer, A., Schier, K.R., and Froscher, W. (2001). Treatment of pathological crying with citalopram. *Pharmacopsychiatry*, 34, 254–258.

Keilp, J.G., Sackeim, H.A., Brodsky, B.S., Oquendo, M.A., Malone, K.M., and Mann, J.J. (2001). Neuropsychological dysfunction in depressed suicide attempters. *Am J Psychiatry*, 158, 735–741.

Keri, S., Kelemen, O., Benedek, G., and Janka, Z. (2001). Different trait markers for schizophrenia and bipolar disorder: A neurocognitive approach. *Psychol Med*, 31, 915–922.

Kessing, L.V. (1998). Cognitive impairment in the euthymic phase of affective disorder. *Psychol Med*, 28, 1027–1038.

Kestenbaum, C.J. (1979). Children at risk for manic-depressive illness: Possible predictors. *Am J Psychiatry*, 136(9), 1206–1208.

Kety, S.S., Woodford, R.B., Harmel, M.H., Freyhan, F.A., Appel, K.E., and Schmidt, C.F. (1948). Cerebral blood flow and metabolism in schizophrenia. *Am J Psychiatry*, 104, 765–770.

Kimbrell, T.A., Little, J.T., Dunn, R.T., Frye, M.A., Greenberg, B.D., Wassermann, E.M., Repella, J.D., Danielson, A.L., Willis, M.W., Benson, B.E., Speer, A.M., Osuch, E., George, M.S., and Post, R.M. (1999). Frequency dependence of antidepressant response to left prefrontal repetitive transcranial magnetic stimulation (rTMS) as a function of baseline cerebral glucose metabolism. *Biol Psychiatry*, 46, 1603–1613.

Kjellman, B.F., Karlberg, B.E., and Thorell, L.H. (1980). Cognitive and affective functions in patients with affective disorders treated with lithium: An assessment by questionnaire. *Acta Psychiatr Scand*, 62, 32–46.

Klein, D., Gittelman, R., Quitkin, F., and Rifkin, A. (1980). *Diagnosis and Drug Treatment of Psychiatric Disorders: Adults and Children*. Baltimore: Williams and Wilkins.

Kluger, A., and Goldberg, E. (1990). IQ patterns in affective disorder, lateralized and diffuse brain damage. *J Clin Exper Neuropsychol*, 12, 182–194.

Kocsis, J.H., Shaw, E.D., Stokes, P.E., Wilner, P., Elliot, A.S., Sikes, C., Myers, B., Manevitz, A., and Parides, M. (1993). Neuropsychologic effects of lithium discontinuation. *J Clin Psychopharmacol*, 13, 268–275.

Kolb, B., and Milner, B. (1981). Observations on spontaneous facial expression after focal cerebral excisions and after intracarotid injection of sodium amytal. *Neuropsychologia*, 19, 505–514.

Kolur, U.S., Reddy, Y.C.J., John, J.P., Kandavel, T., and Jain, S. (2006). Sustained attention and executive functions in euthymic young people with bipolar disorder. *Br J Psychiatry*, 189, 453–458.

Kopelman, M.D. (2002). Disorders of memory. *Brain*, 125, 2152–2190.

Kotin, J., and Goodwin, F.K. (1972). Depression during mania: Clinical observations and theoretical implications. *Am J Psychiatry*, 129, 679–686.

Krabbendam, L., Honig, A., Wiersma, J., Vuurman, E.F., Hofman, P.A., Derix, M.M., Nolen, W.A., and Jolles, J. (2000).

Cognitive dysfunctions and white matter lesions in patients with bipolar disorder in remission. *Acta Psychiatr Scand*, 101, 274–280.

Kraemer, G.W., and McKinney, W.T. (1979). Interactions of pharmacological agents which alter biogenic amine metabolism and depression: An analysis of contributing factors within a primate model of depression. *J Affect Disord*, 1, 33–54.

Kraepelin, E. (1896). *Dementia Praecox and Paraphrenia*. Reprinted (1971) (Trans. R.M. Barclay). Melbourne, FL: Krieger.

Kremen, W.S., Seidman, L.J., Faraone, S.V., and Tsuang, M.T. (2003). Is there disproportionate impairment in semantic or phonemic fluency in schizophrenia? *J Int Neuropsychol Soc*, 9(1), 79–88.

Krishnan, K.R., Taylor, W.D., McQuoid, D.R., MacFall, J.R., Payne, M.E., Provenzale, J.M., and Steffens, D.C. (2004). Clinical characteristics of magnetic resonance imaging-defined subcortical ischemic depression. *Biol Psychiatry*, 55, 390–397.

Kriss, A., Blumhardt, L., Halliday, A., and Pratt, R. (1978). Neurological asymmetries immediately after unilateral ECT. *J Neurol Neurosurg Psychiatry*, 41, 1135–1144.

Kropf, D., and Muller-Oerlinghausen, B. (1979). Changes in learning, memory, and mood during lithium treatment: Approach to a research strategy. *Acta Psychiatr Scand*, 59, 97–124.

Kumar, A., Jin, Z., Bilker, W., Udupa, J., and Gottlieb, G. (1998). Late-onset minor and major depression: Early evidence for common neuroanatomical substrates detected by using MRI. *Proc Natl Acad Sci U S A*, 95, 7654–7658.

Kupfer, D.J., and Foster, F.G. (1973). Sleep and activity in a psychotic depression. *J Nerv Ment Dis*, 156, 341–348.

Kupfer, D.J., Weiss, B.L., Foster, G., Detre, T.P., and McPartland, R. (1974). Psychomotor activity in affective states. *Arch Gen Psychiatry*, 30, 765–768.

Kupfer, D.J., Foster, F.G., Detre, T.P., and Himmelhoch, J. (1975). Sleep EEG and motor activity as indicators in affective states. *Neuropsychobiology*, 1, 296–303.

Kurthen, M., Linke, D.B., Reuter, B.M., Hufnagel, A., and Elger, C.E. (1991). Severe negative emotional reactions in intracarotid sodium amytal procedures: Further evidence for hemispheric asymmetries? *Cortex*, 27, 333–337.

Kyte, Z.A., Carlson, G.A., and Goodyer, I.M. (2006). Clinical and neuropsychological characteristics of child and adolescent bipolar disorder. *Psychol Med*, 36(9), 1197–1211.

Larsen, J.K., Brand, N., Bermond, B., and Hijman, R. (2003). Cognitive and emotional characteristics of alexithymia: A review of neurobiological studies. *J Psychosom Res*, 54, 533–541.

Lesser, I.M., Hill-Gutierrez, E., Miller, B.L., and Boone, K.B. (1993). Late-onset depression with white matter lesions. *Psychosomatics*, 34, 364–367.

Lesser, I.M., Boone, K.B., Mehringer, C.M., Wohl, M.A., Miller, B.L., and Berman, N.G. (1996). Cognition and white matter hyperintensities in older depressed patients. *Am J Psychiatry*, 153, 1280–1287.

Lewis, D.A. (1983). Unrecognized chronic lithium neurotoxic reactions. *JAMA*, 250, 2029–2030.

Lezak, M.D. (1995). *Neuropsychological Assessment* (3rd edition). New York: Oxford University Press.

Lisanby, S.H., Bazil, C.W., Resor, S.R., Nobler, M.S., Finck, D.A., and Sackeim, H.A. (2001). ECT in the treatment of status epilepticus. *J ECT*, 17, 210–215.

Lishman, W.A. (1968). Brain damage in relation to psychiatric disability after head injury. *Br J Psychiatry*, 114, 373–410.

Liu, S.K., Chiu, C.H., Chang, C.J., Hwang, T.J., Hwu, H.G., and Chen, W.J. (2002). Deficits in sustained attention in schizophrenia and affective disorders: Stable versus state-dependent markers. *Am J Psychiatry*, 159, 975–982.

Lohr, J.B., and Caligiuri, M.P. (1995). Motor asymmetry, a neurobiologic abnormality in the major psychoses. *Psychiatry Res*, 57, 279–282.

Lohr, J.B., and Caligiuri, M.P. (1997). Lateralized hemispheric dysfunction in the major psychotic disorders: Historical perspectives and findings from a study of motor asymmetry in older patients. *Schizophr Res*, 27, 191–198.

Lund, Y., Nissen, M., and Rafaelsen, O.J. (1982). Long-term lithium treatment and psychological functions. *Acta Psychiatr Scand*, 65, 233–244.

Lupien, S.J., Nair, N.P., Briere, S., Maheu, F., Tu, M.T., Lemay, M., McEwen, B.S., and Meaney, M.J. (1999). Increased cortisol levels and impaired cognition in human aging: Implication for depression and dementia in later life. *Rev Neurosci*, 10, 117–139.

Lyoo, I.K., Lee, H.K., Jung, J.H., Noam, G.G., and Renshaw, P.F. (2002). White matter hyperintensities on magnetic resonance imaging of the brain in children with psychiatric disorders. *Compr Psychiatry*, 43, 361–368.

MacQueen, G.M., Campbell, S., McEwen, B.S., Macdonald, K., Amano, S., Joffe, R.T., Nahmias, C., and Young, L.T. (2003). Course of illness, hippocampal function, and hippocampal volume in major depression. *Proc Natl Acad Sci U S A*, 100, 1387–1392.

Madsen, T.M., Greisen, M.H., Nielsen, S.M., Bolwig, T.G., and Mikkelsen, J.D. (2000). Electroconvulsive stimuli enhance both neuropeptide Y receptor Y1 and Y2 messenger RNA expression and levels of binding in the rat hippocampus. *Neuroscience*, 98, 33–39.

Mandzia, J.L., Black, S.E., McAndrews, M.P., Grady, C., and Graham, S. (2004). fMRI differences in encoding and retrieval of pictures due to encoding strategy in the elderly. *Hum Brain Mapp*, 21, 1–14.

Manji, H.K., Moore, G.J., and Chen, G. (2000a). Clinical and preclinical evidence for the neurotrophic effects of mood stabilizers: Implications for the pathophysiology and treatment of manic-depressive illness. *Biol Psychiatry*, 48, 740–754.

Manji, H.K., Moore, G.J., Rajkowska, G., and Chen, G. (2000b). Neuroplasticity and cellular resilience in mood disorders. *Mol Psychiatry*, 5, 578–593.

Mann, J.J., Waternaux, C., Haas, G.L., and Malone, K.M. (1999). Toward a clinical model of suicidal behavior in psychiatric patients. *Am J Psychiatry*, 156, 181–189.

Martinez-Arán, A., Vieta, E., Colom, F., Reinares, M., Benabarre, A., Gasto, C., and Salamero, M. (2000). Cognitive dysfunctions in bipolar disorder: Evidence of neuropsychological disturbances. *Psychother Psychosom*, 69, 2–18.

Martinez-Arán, A., Penades, R., Vieta, E., Colom, F., Reinares, M., Benabarre, A., Salamero, M., and Gasto, C. (2002a). Executive function in patients with remitted bipolar disorder and schizophrenia and its relationship with functional outcome. *Psychother Psychosom*, 71, 39–46.

Martinez-Arán, A., Vieta, E., Colom, F., Reinares, M., Benabarre, A., Torrent, C., Goikolea, J.M., Corbella, B., Sanchez-Moreno, J., and Salamero, M. (2002b). Neuropsychological performance in depressed and euthymic bipolar patients. *Neuropsychobiology*, 46(Suppl. 1), 16–21.

Martinez-Arán, A., Vieta, E., Colom, F., Torrent, C., Sanchez-Moreno, J., Reinares, M., Benabarre, A., Goikolea, J.M., Brugue, E., Daban, C., and Salamero, M. (2004a). Cognitive impairment in euthymic bipolar patients: Implications for clinical and functional outcome. *Bipolar Disord*, 6, 224–232.

Martinez-Arán, A., Vieta, E., Reinares, M., Colom, F., Torrent, C., Sanchez-Moreno, J., Benabarre, A., Goikolea, J.M., Comes, M., and Salamero, M. (2004b). Cognitive function across manic or hypomanic, depressed, and euthymic states in bipolar disorder. *Am J Psychiatry*, 161, 262–270.

Marvel, C.L., and Paradiso, S. (2004). Cognitive and neurological impairment in mood disorders. *Psychiatr Clin North Am*, 27, 19–36, vii–viii.

Mason, C.F. (1956). Pre-illness intelligence of mental hospital patients. *J Consult Psychol*, 20, 297–300.

Matarazzo, J.D. (1980). Behavioral health and behavioral medicine: Frontiers for a new health psychology. *Am Psychol*, 35(9), 807–817.

Mayberg, H.S., Liotti, M., Brannan, S.K., McGinnis, S., Mahurin, R.K., Jerabek, P.A., Silva, J.A., Tekell, J.L., Martin, C.C., Lancaster, J.L., and Fox, P.T. (1999). Reciprocal limbic-cortical function and negative mood: Converging PET findings in depression and normal sadness. *Am J Psychiatry*, 156, 675–682.

McCarthy, J., Arrese, D., McGlashan, A., Rappaport, B., Kraseski, K., Conway, F., Mule, C., and Tucker, J. (2004). Sustained attention and visual processing speed in children and adolescents with bipolar disorder and other psychiatric disorders. *Psychol Rep*, 95, 39–47.

McCullagh, S., and Feinstein, A. (2000). Treatment of pathological affect: Variability of response for laughter and crying. *J Neuropsychiatry Clin Neurosci*, 12, 100–102.

McElhiney, M.C., Moody, B.J., Steif, B.L., Prudic, J., Devanand, D.P., Nobler, M.S., and Sackeim, H.A. (1995). Autobiographical memory and mood: Effects of electroconvulsive therapy. *Neuropsychology*, 9, 501–517.

McKay, A.P., Tarbuck, A.F., Shapleske, J., and McKenna, P.J. (1995). Neuropsychological function in manic-depressive psychosis: Evidence for persistent deficits in patients with chronic, severe illness. *Br J Psychiatry*, 167, 51–57.

McNamara, B., Ray, J.L., Arthurs, O.J., and Boniface, S. (2001). Transcranial magnetic stimulation for depression and other psychiatric disorders. *Psychol Med*, 31, 1141–1146.

McPartland, R.J., Kupfer, D.J., Foster, F.G., Reisler, K.L., and Matthews, G. (1975). Objective measurement of human motor activity: A preliminary normative study. *Biotelemetry*, 2, 317–323.

Merrin, E.L. (1984). Motor and sighting dominance in chronic schizophrenics: Relationship to social competence, age at first admission, and clinical course. *Br J Psychiatry*, 145, 401–406.

Mesulam, M.M. (2000). *Principles of Behavioral and Cognitive Neurology* (2nd edition). Oxford, New York: Oxford University Press.

Meyer, S., Carlson, G., Wiggs, E., Martinez, P., Ronsaville, D., Klimes-Dougan, B., Gold, P., and Radke-Yarrow, M. (2004). Predictors of apparent frontal lobe dysfunction among adolescents at risk for bipolar disorders. *Dev Psychopathol*, 16(2), 461–476.

Miller, W.R. (1975). Psychological deficit in depression. *Psychol Bull*, 82, 238–260.

Mills, C.K. (1912). The cerebral mechanisms of emoitonal expression. *Trans Coll Physicians Philadelphia*, 34, 147–185.

Mitchell, P., Parker, G., Jamieson, K., Wilhelm, K., Hickie, I., Brodaty, H., Boyce, P., Hadzi-Pavlovic, D., and Roy, K. (1992). Are there any differences between bipolar and unipolar melancholia? *J Affect Disord*, 25, 97–105.

Mitchell, P., Hadzi-Pavlovic, D., Parker, G., Hickie, I., Wilhelm, K., Brodaty, H., and Boyce, P. (1996). Depressive psychomotor disturbance, cortisol, and dexamethasone. *Biol Psychiatry*, 40, 941–950.

Mitchell, P.B., Wilhelm, K., Parker, G., Austin, M.P., Rutgers, P., and Malhi, G.S. (2001). The clinical features of bipolar depression: A comparison with matched major depressive disorder patients. *J Clin Psychiatry*, 62, 212–216; quiz 217.

Moore, G.J., Bebchuk, J.M., Wilds, I.B., Chen, G., Manji, H.K., and Menji, H.K. (2000). Lithium-induced increase in human brain grey matter. *Lancet*, 356, 1241–1242.

Morice, R. (1990). Cognitive inflexibility and pre-frontal dysfunction in schizophrenia and mania. *Br J Psychiatry*, 157, 50–54.

Moscovitch, M. (1994). Memory and working with memory: Evaluation of a component process model and comparisons with other models. In D.L. Schacter, E. Tulving (Eds.), *Memory Systems 1994* (pp. 269–310). Cambridge, MA: MIT Press.

Mukherjee, S., Sackeim, H.A., and Schnur, D.B. (1994). Electroconvulsive therapy of acute manic episodes: A review of 50 years' experience. *Am J Psychiatry*, 151, 169–176.

Murphy, F.C., and Sahakian, B.J. (2001). Neuropsychology of bipolar disorder. *Br J Psychiatry Suppl*, 41, s120–s127.

Murphy, F.C., Sahakian, B.J., Rubinsztein, J.S., Michael, A., Rogers, R.D., Robbins, T.W., and Paykel, E.S. (1999). Emotional bias and inhibitory control processes in mania and depression. *Psychol Med*, 29, 1307–1321.

Murray, L.A., Whitehouse, W.G., and Alloy, L.B. (1999). Mood congruence and depressive deficits in memory: A forced-recall analysis. *Memory*, 7, 175–196.

Narushima, K., Kosier, J.T., and Robinson, R.G. (2003). A reappraisal of poststroke depression, intra- and inter-hemispheric lesion location using meta-analysis. *J Neuropsychiatry Clin Neurosci*, 15, 422–430.

Nehra, R., Chakrabarti, S., Pradham, B.D., and Khehra, N. (2005). Comparison of cognitive functions between first- and multi-episode bipolar affective disorders. *J Affect Disord*, 93, 185–192.

Nelson, L.D., Cicchetti, D., Satz, P., Sowa, M., and Mitrushina, M. (1994). Emotional sequelae of stroke: A longitudinal perspective. *J Clin Exper Neuropsychol*, 16, 796–806.

Nelson, R.E., and Craighead, W.E. (1977). Selective recall of positive and negative feedback, self-control behaviors, and depression. *J Abnorm Psychol*, 86, 379–388.

Newell, B.R., and Andrews, S. (2004). Levels of processing effects on implicit and explicit memory tasks: Using question position to investigate the lexical-processing hypothesis. *Exp Psychol*, 51, 132–144.

Nilsonne, A. (1987). Acoustic analysis of speech variables during depression and after improvement. *Acta Psychiatr Scand*, 76, 235–245.

Nilsonne, A. (1988). Speech characteristics as indicators of depressive illness. *Acta Psychiatr Scand*, 77, 253–263.

Nobler, M.S., Sackeim, H.A., Solomou, M., Luber, B., Devanand, D.P., and Prudic, J. (1993). EEG manifestations during ECT: Effects of electrode placement and stimulus intensity. *Biol Psychiatry*, 34, 321–330.

Nobler, M.S., Sackeim, H.A., Prohovnik, I., Moeller, J.R., Mukherjee, S., Schnur, D.B., Prudic, J., and Devanand, D.P.

(1994). Regional cerebral blood flow in mood disorders: III. Treatment and clinical response. *Arch Gen Psychiatry, 51,* 884–897.

Nobler, M.S., Teneback, C.C., Nahas, Z., Bohning, D.E., Shastri, A., Kozel, F.A., and George, M.S. (2000). Structural and functional neuroimaging of electroconvulsive therapy and transcranial magnetic stimulation. *Depression Anxiety, 12,* 144–156.

Nobler, M.S., Oquendo, M.A., Kegeles, L.S., Malone, K.M., Campbell, C.C., Sackeim, H.A., and Mann, J.J. (2001). Decreased regional brain metabolism after ECT. *Am J Psychiatry, 158,* 305–308.

Norman, R.M., and Malla, A.K. (2001). Duration of untreated psychosis: A critical examination of the concept and its importance. *Psychol Med, 31,* 381–400.

Okun, M.S., Raju, D.V., Walter, B.L., Juncos, J.L., DeLong, M.R., Heilman, K., McDonald, W.M., and Vitek, J.L. (2004). Pseudobulbar crying induced by stimulation in the region of the subthalamic nucleus. *J Neurol Neurosurg Psychiatry, 75,* 921–923.

Oltmanns, T.F. (1978). Selective attention in schizophrenic and manic psychoses: The effect of distraction on information processing. *J Abnorm Psychol, 87*(2), 212–225.

Oquendo, M.A., and Mann, J.J. (2001). Identifying and managing suicide risk in bipolar patients. *J Clin Psychiatry, 62*(Suppl. 25), 31–34.

Oquendo, M.A., Galfalvy, H., Russo, S., Ellis, S.P., Grunebaum, M.F., Burke, A., and Mann, J.J. (2004). Prospective study of clinical predictors of suicidal acts after a major depressive episode in patients with major depressive disorder or bipolar disorder. *Am J Psychiatry, 161,* 1433–1441.

Paradiso, S., Lamberty, G.J., Garvey, M.J., and Robinson, R.G. (1997). Cognitive impairment in the euthymic phase of chronic unipolar depression. *J Nerv Ment Dis, 185*(12), 748–754.

Park, S. (1997). Association of an oculomotor delayed response task and the Wisconsin card sort test in schizophrenic patients. *Int J Psychophysiol, 27*(2), 147–151.

Park, S., and Holzman, P.S. (1992). Schizophrenics show spatial working memory deficits. *Arch Gen Psychiatry, 49*(12), 975–982.

Parker, G., and Hadzi-Pavlovic, D. (1993). Prediction of response to antidepressant medication by a sign-based index of melancholia. *Aust N Z J Psychiatry, 27,* 56–61.

Parker, G., Hadzi-Pavlovic, D., Brodaty, H., Boyce, P., Mitchell, P., Wilhelm, K., Hickie, I., and Eyers, K. (1993). Psychomotor disturbance in depression: Defining the constructs. *J Affect Disord, 27*(4), 255–265.

Parker, G., Hadzi-Pavlovic, D., Austin, M.P., Mitchell, P., Wilhelm, K., Hickie, I., Boyce, P., and Eyers, K. (1995a). Sub-typing depression: I. Is psychomotor disturbance necessary and sufficient to the definition of melancholia? *Psychol Med, 25,* 815–823.

Parker, G., Hadzi-Pavlovic, D., Hickie, I., Brodaty, H., Boyce, P., Mitchell, P., and Wilhelm, K. (1995b). Sub-typing depression: III. Development of a clinical algorithm for melancholia and comparison with other diagnostic measures. *Psychol Med, 25,* 833–840.

Parker, G., Roy, K., Wilhelm, K., Mitchell, P., and Hadzi-Pavlovic, D. (2000). The nature of bipolar depression: Implications for the definition of melancholia. *J Affect Disord, 59,* 217–224.

Pavuluri, M.N., Schenkel, L.S., Aryal, S., Harral, E.M., Hill, S.K., Herbener, E.S., and Sweeney, J.A. (2006). Neurocognitive function in unmedicated manic and medicated euthymic pediatric bipolar patients. *Am J Psychiatry, 163,* 286–293.

Penfield, W., and Jasper, H. (1954). *Epilepsy and the Functional Anatomy of the Human Brain.* Boston: Little, Brown.

Perera, T.D., Luber, B., Nobler, M.S., Prudic, J., Anderson, C., and Sackeim, H.A. (2004). Seizure expression during electroconvulsive therapy: Relationships with clinical outcome and cognitive side effects. *Neuropsychopharmacology, 29*(4), 813–825.

Petterson, U. (1977). Manic-depressive illness: A clinical, social and genetic study. *Acta Psychiatr Scand Suppl* (269), 1–93.

Phillips, M.L., Drevets, W.C., Rauch, S.L., and Lane, R. (2003a). Neurobiology of emotion perception: I. The neural basis of normal emotion perception. *Biol Psychiatry, 54,* 504–514.

Phillips, M.L., Drevets, W.C., Rauch, S.L., and Lane, R. (2003b). Neurobiology of emotion perception: II. Implications for major psychiatric disorders. *Biol Psychiatry, 54,* 515–528.

Pier, M.P., Hulstijn, W., and Sabbe, B.G. (2004). Psychomotor retardation in elderly depressed patients. *J Affect Disord, 81,* 73–77.

Pillai, J.J., Friedman, L., Stuve, T.A., Trinidad, S., Jesberger, J.A., Lewin, J.S., Findling, R.L., Swales, T.P., and Schulz, S.C. (2002). Increased presence of white matter hyperintensities in adolescent patients with bipolar disorder. *Psychiatr Res, 114,* 51–56.

Politis, A., Lykouras, L., Mourtzouchou, P., and Christodoulou, G.N. (2004). Attentional disturbances in patients with unipolar psychotic depression: A selective and sustained attention study. *Compr Psychiatry, 45,* 452–459.

Post, F. (1996). Verbal creativity, depression and alcoholism: An investigation of one hundred American and British writers. *Br J Psychiatry, 168,* 545–555.

Post, R.M. (1990). Sensitization and kindling perspectives for the course of affective illness: Toward a new treatment with the anticonvulsant carbamazepine. *Pharmacopsychiatry, 23,* 3–17.

Post, R.M. (2002). Do the epilepsies, pain syndromes, and affective disorders share common kindling-like mechanisms? *Epilepsy Res, 50,* 203–219.

Pratt, R., and Warrington, E. (1972). The assessment of cerebral dominance with unilateral ECT. *Br J Psychiatry, 121,* 327–328.

Pratt, R., Warrington, E., and Halliday, A. (1971). Unilateral ECT as a test for cerebral dominance, with a strategy for treating left-handers. *Br J Psychiatry, 119,* 79–83.

Quraishi, S., and Frangou, S. (2002). Neuropsychology of bipolar disorder: A review. *J Affect Disord, 72,* 209–226.

Reus, V.I., Targum, S.D., Weingarter, H., and Post, R.M. (1979). Effect of lithium carbonate on memory processes of bipolar affectively ill patients. *Psychopharmacology, 63,* 39–42.

Rey, A. (1941). L'examen psychologique dans les cas d'encephalopathie traumatique. *Archives de Psychologie, 28,* 286–340.

Richell, R.A., and Anderson, M. (2004). Reproducibility of negative mood induction: A self-referent plus musical mood induction procedure and a controllable/uncontrollable stress paradigm. *J Psychopharmacol, 18,* 94–101.

Robertson, G., and Taylor, P.J. (1985). Some cognitive correlates of affective disorders. *Psychol Med, 15*(2), 297–309.

Robinson, L.J., Thompson, J.M., Gallagher, P., Goswami, U., Young, A.H., Ferrier, I.N., and Moore, P.B. (2006). A meta-analysis of cognitive deficits in euthymic patients with bipilor disorder. *J Affect Disord, 93,* 105–115.

Robinson, R.G. (1997). Neuropsychiatric consequences of stroke. *Ann Rev Med, 48,* 217–229.

Robinson, R.G., and Szetela, B. (1981). Mood change following left hemispheric brain injury. *Ann Neurol, 9,* 447–453.

Robinson, R.G., Kubos, K.L., Starr, L.B., Rao, K., and Price, T.R. (1984). Mood disorders in stroke patients: Importance of location of lesion. *Brain*, 107(Pt. 1), 81–93.

Rogers, M.A., Bradshaw, J.L., Phillips, J.G., Chiu, E., Vaddadi, K., Presnel, I., and Mileshkin, C. (2000). Parkinsonian motor characteristics in unipolar major depression. *J Clin Exper Neuropsychol*, 22, 232–244.

Rogers, M.A., Kasai, K., Koji, M., Fukuda, R., Iwanami, A., Nakagome, K., Fukuda, M., and Kato, N. (2004). Executive and prefrontal dysfunction in unipolar depression: A review of neuropsychological and imaging evidence. *Neurosci Res*, 50, 1–11.

Rosadini, G., and Rossi, G.F. (1967). On the suggested cerebral dominance for consciousness. *Brain*, 90, 101–112.

Rosenberg, R., Vorstrup, S., Anderson, A., and Bolwig, T.G. (1988). Effect of ECT on cerebral blood flow in melancholia assessed with SPECT. *Convulsive Ther*, 4, 62–73.

Rossi, G.F., and Rosadini, G. (1967). Experimental analysis of cerebral dominance. In C.H. Millikan (Ed.), *Brain Mechanisms Underlying Speech and Language* (pp. 167–184). New York: Grune and Stratton.

Rossi, A., Arduini, L., Daneluzzo, E., Bustini, M., Prosperini, P., and Stratta, P. (2000). Cognitive function in euthymic bipolar patients, stabilized schizophrenic patients, and healthy controls. *J Psychiatr Res*, 34(4–5), 333–339.

Rothenberg, A. (2001). Bipolar illness, creativity, and treatment. *Psychiatr Q*, 72, 131–147.

Roy-Byrne, P.P., Weingartner, H., Bierer, L.M., Thompson, K., and Post, R.M. (1986). Effortful and automatic cognitive processes in depression. *Arch Gen Psychiatry*, 43, 265–267.

Royant-Parola, S., Borbely, A.A., Tobler, I., Benoit, O., and Widlocher, D. (1986). Monitoring of long-term motor activity in depressed patients. *Br J Psychiatry*, 149, 288–293.

Rubinsztein, J.S., Michael, A., Paykel, E.S., and Sahakian, B.J. (2000). Cognitive impairment in remission in bipolar affective disorder. *Psychol Med*, 30, 1025–1036.

Rush, A.J., Schlesser, M.A., Roffwarg, H.P., Giles, D.E., Orsulak, P.J., and Fairchild, C. (1983). Relationships among the TRH, REM latency, and dexamethasone suppression tests: Preliminary findings. *J Clin Psychiatry*, 44(8 Pt. 2), 23–29.

Sackeim, H.A. (1986). A neuropsychodynamic perspective on the self: Brain, thought, emotion. In L.M. Hartman and K.R. Blankstein (Eds.), *Perception of Self in Emotional Disorder and Psychotherapy* (pp. 51–83). New York: Plenum.

Sackeim, H.A. (1999). The anticonvulsant hypothesis of the mechanisms of action of ECT: Current status. *J ECT*, 15, 5–26.

Sackeim, H.A. (2000a). Memory and ECT: From polarization to reconciliation. *J ECT*, 16, 87–96.

Sackeim, H.A. (2000b). Repetitive transcranial magnetic stimulation: What are the next steps? *Biol Psychiatry*, 48, 959–961.

Sackeim, H.A. (2004). The convulsant and anticonvulsant properties of electroconvulsive therapy: Towards a focal form of brain stimulation. *Clin Neurosci Rev*, 4, 39–57.

Sackeim, H.A., and Decina, P. (1983). Lateralized neuropsychological abnormalities in bipolar adults and in children of bipolar probands. In P. Flor-Henry, J. Gruzelier (Eds.), *Laterality and Psychopathology* (pp. 103–128). New York: Elsevier.

Sackeim, H.A., and Prohovnik, I. (1993). Brain imaging studies in depressive disorders. In J.J. Mann, D. Kupfer (Eds.), *Biology of Depressive Disorders* (pp. 205–258). New York: Plenum.

Sackeim, H.A., and Wegner, A.Z. (1986). Attributional patterns in depression and euthymia. *Arch Gen Psychiatry*, 43, 553–560.

Sackeim, H.A., Gur, R.C., and Saucy, M.C. (1978). Emotions are expressed more intensely on the left side of the face. *Science*, 202, 434–436.

Sackeim, H.A., Greenberg, M.S., Weiman, A.L., Gur, R.C., Hungerbuhler, J.P., and Geschwind, N. (1982). Hemispheric asymmetry in the expression of positive and negative emotions: Neurologic evidence. *Arch Neurol*, 39, 210–218.

Sackeim, H.A., Decina, P., Prohovnik, I., Malitz, S., and Resor, S.R. (1983a). Anticonvulsant and antidepressant properties of electroconvulsive therapy: A proposed mechanism of action. *Biol Psychiatry*, 18, 1301–1310.

Sackeim, H.A., Prohovnik, I., Decina, P., Malitz, S., and Resor, S. (1983b). Anticonvulsant properties of electroconvulsive therapy: Theory and case report. In M. Baldy-Moulinier, D.H. Ingvar, B.S. Meldrum (Eds.), *Current Problems in Epilepsy: Cerebral Blood Flow, Metabolism, and Epilepsy* (pp. 370–377). London: Libbey.

Sackeim, H.A., Decina, P., Portnoy, S., Neeley, P., and Malitz, S. (1987). Studies of dosage, seizure threshold, and seizure duration in ECT. *Biol Psychiatry*, 22, 249–268.

Sackeim, H.A., Freeman, J., McElhiney, M., Coleman, E., Prudic, J., and Devanand, D.P. (1992). Effects of major depression on estimates of intelligence. *J Clin Exp Neuropsychol*, 14, 268–288.

Sackeim, H.A., Prudic, J., Devanand, D.P., Kiersky, J.E., Fitzsimons, L., Moody, B.J., McElhiney, M.C., Coleman, E.A., and Settembrino, J.M. (1993). Effects of stimulus intensity and electrode placement on the efficacy and cognitive effects of electroconvulsive therapy. *N Engl J Med*, 328, 839–846.

Sackeim, H.A., Luber, B., Katzman, G.P., Moeller, J.R., Prudic, J., Devanand, D.P., and Nobler, M.S. (1996). The effects of electroconvulsive therapy on quantitative electroencephalograms: Relationship to clinical outcome. *Arch Gen Psychiatry*, 53, 814–824.

Sackeim, H.A., Prudic, J., Devanand, D.P., Nobler, M.S., Lisanby, S.H., Peyser, S., Fitzsimons, L., Moody, B.J., and Clark, J. (2000b). A prospective, randomized, double-blind comparison of bilateral and right unilateral electroconvulsive therapy at different stimulus intensities. *Arch Gen Psychiatry*, 57, 425–434.

Salloway, S., Malloy, P., Kohn, R., Gillard, E., Duffy, J., Rogg, J., Tung, G., Richardson, E., Thomas, C., and Westlake, R. (1996). MRI and neuropsychological differences in early- and late-life-onset geriatric depression. *Neurology*, 46, 1567–1574.

Sanacora, G., Mason, G.F., Rothman, D.L., Hyder, F., Ciarcia, J.J., Ostroff, R.B., Berman, R.M., and Krystal, J.H. (2003). Increased cortical GABA concentrations in depressed patients receiving ECT. *Am J Psychiatry*, 160, 577–579.

Sapin, L.R., Berrettini, W.H., Nurnberger, J.I., and Rothblat, L.A. (1987). Mediational factors underlying cognitive changes and laterality in affective illness. *Biol Psychiatry*, 22, 979–986.

Savard, R.J., Rey, A.C., and Post, R.M. (1980). Halstead-Reitan Category Test in bipolar and unipolar affective disorders: Relationship to age and phase of illness. *J Nerv Ment Dis*, 168, 297–304.

Sax, K.W., Strakowski, S.M., Zimmerman, M.E., DelBello, M.P., Keck, P.E. Jr., and Hawkins, J.M. (1999). Frontosubcortical neuroanatomy and the continuous performance test in mania. *Am J Psychiatry*, 156(1), 139–141.

Schachter, S., and Singer, J. (1962). Cognitive, social and physiological determinants of emotional state. *Psych Review, 69,* 379–407.

Schaefer, A., Collette, F., Philippot, P., van der Linden, M., Laureys, S., Delfiore, G., Degueldre, C., Maquet, P., Luxen, A., and Salmon, E. (2003). Neural correlates of "hot" and "cold" emotional processing: A multilevel approach to the functional anatomy of emotion. *Neuroimage, 18,* 938–949.

Schlosser, R., Hutchinson, M., Joseffer, S., Rusinek, H., Saarimaki, A., Stevenson, J., Dewey, S.L., and Brodie, J.D. (1998). Functional magnetic resonance imaging of human brain activity in a verbal fluency task. *J Neurol Neurosurg Psychiatry, 64,* 492–498.

Seidman, L.J., Kremen, W.S., Koren, D., Faraone, S.V., Goldstein, J.M., and Tsuang, M.T. (2002). A comparative profile analysis of neuropsychological functioning in patients with schizophrenia and bipolar psychoses. *Schizophr Res, 53*(1–2), 31–44.

Seidman, L.J., Lanca, M., Kremen, W.S., Faraone, S.V., and Tsuang, M.T. (2003). Organizational and visual memory deficits in schizophrenia and bipolar psychoses using the Rey-Osterrieth complex figure: Effects of duration of illness. *J Clin Exp Neuropsychol, 25*(7), 949–964.

Seminowicz, D.A., Mayberg, H.S., McIntosh, A.R., Goldapple, K., Kennedy, S., Segal, Z., and Rafi-Tari, S. (2004). Limbic-frontal circuitry in major depression: A path modeling metanalysis. *Neuroimage, 22,* 409–418.

Shallice, T. (1982). Specific impairments of planning. *Philos Trans R Soc Lond B Biol Sci, 298,* 199–209.

Shansis, F.M., Busnello, J.V., Quevedo, J., Forster, L., Young, S., Izquierdo, I., and Kapczinski, F. (2000). Behavioural effects of acute tryptophan depletion in healthy male volunteers. *J Psychopharmacol, 14,* 157–163.

Shaw, E.D., Mann, J.J., Stokes, P.E., and Manevitz, A.Z. (1986). Effects of lithium carbonate on associative productivity and idiosyncrasy in bipolar outpatients. *Am J Psychiatry, 143,* 1166–1169.

Shaw, E.D., Stokes, P.E., Mann, J.J., and Manevitz, A.Z. (1987). Effects of lithium carbonate on the memory and motor speed of bipolar outpatients. *J Abnorm Psychology, 96,* 64–69.

Sheline, Y.I., Wang, P.W., Gado, M.H., Csernansky, J.G., and Vannier, M. (1996). Hippocampal atrophy in recurrent major depression. *Proc Natl Acad Sci U S A, 93*(9), 3908–3913.

Sheline, Y.I., Sanghavi, M., Mintun, M.A., and Gado, M.H. (1999). Depression duration but not age predicts hippocampal volume loss in medically healthy women with recurrent major depression. *J Neurosci, 19,* 5034–5043.

Silfverskiöld, P., and Risberg, J. (1989). Regional cerebral blood flow in depression and mania. *Arch Gen Psychiatry, 46,* 253–259.

Silverstone, T., McPherson, H., Li, Q., and Doyle, T. (2003). Deep white matter hyperintensities in patients with bipolar depression, unipolar depression and age-matched control subjects. *Bipolar Disord, 5,* 53–57.

Simpson, S., Talbot, P.R., Snowden, J.S., and Neary, D. (1997a). Subcortical vascular disease in elderly patients with treatment resistant depression [Letter]. *J Neurol Neurosurg Psychiatry, 62,* 196–197.

Simpson, S.W., Jackson, A., Baldwin, R.C., and Burns, A. (1997b). 1997 IPA/Bayer Research Awards in Psychogeriatrics. Subcortical hyperintensities in late-life depression: Acute response to treatment and neuropsychological impairment. *Int Psychogeriatr, 9,* 257–275.

Simpson, S., Baldwin, R.C., Jackson, A., and Burns, A.S. (1998). Is subcortical disease associated with a poor response to antidepressants? Neurological, neuropsychological and neuroradiological findings in late-life depression. *Psychol Med, 28,* 1015–1026.

Small, J.G., Milstein, V., Kellams, J.J., Miller, M.J., Woodham, G.C., and Small, I.F. (1993). Hemispheric components of ECT response in mood disorders and shizophrenia. In C.E. Coeffey (Ed.), *The Clinical Science of Electroconvulsive Therapy* (pp. 111–123). Washington, DC: American Psychiatric Press.

Smith, A.G., Montealegre-Orjuela, M., Douglas, J.E., and Jenkins, E.A. (2003). Venlafaxine for pathological crying after stroke. *J Clin Psychiatry, 64,* 731–732.

Snyder, P.J., and Harris, L.J. (1997). The intracarotid amobarbital procedure: An historical perspective. *Brain Cognition, 33,* 18–32.

Soares, J.C., and Mann, J.J. (1997). The functional neuroanatomy of mood disorders. *J Psychiatr Res, 31,* 393–432.

Sobczak, S., Riedel, W.J., Booij, I., Aan Het Rot, M., Deutz, N.E., and Honig, A. (2002). Cognition following acute tryptophan depletion: Difference between first-degree relatives of bipolar disorder patients and matched healthy control volunteers. *Psychol Med, 32,* 503–515.

Sobin, C., and Sackeim, H.A. (1997). Psychomotor symptoms of depression. *Am J Psychiatry, 154,* 4–17.

Souza, V.B., Muir, W.J., Walker, M.T., Glabus, M.F., Roxborough, H.M., Sharp, C.W., Dunan, J.R., and Blackwood, D.H. (1995). Auditory p300 event-related potentials and neuropsychological performance in schizophrenia and bipolar affective disorder. *Biol Psychiatry, 37*(5), 300–310.

Speer, A.M., Kimbrell, T.A., Wassermann, E.M., J, D.R., Willis, M.W., Herscovitch, P., and Post, R.M. (2000). Opposite effects of high and low frequency rTMS on regional brain activity in depressed patients. *Biol Psychiatry, 48,* 1133–1141.

Spence, S.A., Liddle, P.F., Stefan, M.D., Hellewell, J.S., Sharma, T., Friston, K.J., Hirsch, S.R., Frith, C.D., Murray, R.M., Deakin, J.F., and Grasby, P.M. (2000). Functional anatomy of verbal fluency in people with schizophrenia and those at genetic risk: Focal dysfunction and distributed disconnectivity reappraised. *Br J Psychiatry, 176,* 52–60.

Spitzer, R.L., Endicott, J., and Robins, E. (1978). Research diagnostic criteria: Rationale and reliability. *Arch Gen Psychiatry, 35,* 773–782.

Spreen, O., and Strauss, E. (1998). *A Compendium of Neuropsychological Tests: Administration, Norms, and Commentary* (2nd edition). New York: Oxford University Press.

Squire, L.R., Judd, L.L., Janowsky, D.S., and Huey, L.Y. (1980). Effects of lithium carbonate on memory and other cognitive functions. *Am J Psychiatry, 137,* 1042–1046.

Squire, L.R., Stark, C.E., and Clark, R.E. (2004). The medial temporal lobe. *Ann Rev Neurosci, 27,* 279–306.

Starkstein, S.E., Boston, J.D., and Robinson, R.G. (1988). Mechanisms of mania after brain injury: 12 case reports and review of the literature. *J Nerv Ment Dis, 176,* 87–100.

Stefurak, T., Mikulis, D., Mayberg, H., Lang, A.E., Hevenor, S., Pahapill, P., Saint-Cyr, J., and Lozano, A. (2003). Deep brain stimulation for Parkinson's disease dissociates mood and motor circuits: A functional MRI case study. *Movement Disord, 18,* 1508–1516.

Steif, B., Sackeim, H., Portnoy, S., Decina, P., and Malitz, S. (1986). Effects of depression and ECT on anterograde memory. *Biol Psychiatry, 21,* 921–930.

Steingart, A., Hachinski, V., Lau, C., Fox, A.J., Diaz, F., Cape, R., Lee, D., Inzitari, D., and Merskey, H. (1987). Cognitive and neurologic findings in subjects with diffuse white matter lucencies on computed tomographic scans (leuko-araiosis). *Arch Neurol*, 44, 32–35.

Stern, Y., and Sackeim, H.A. (2002). The neuropsychology of memory and amnesia. In S.C. Yudofsky, R.E. Hales (Eds.), *The American Psychiatric Press Textbook of Neuropsychiatry and Clinical Neurosciences* (4th edition, pp. 597–622). Washington, DC: American Psychiatric Press.

Stern, Y., Sano, M., Pauson, J., and Mayeux, R. (1987). Modified mini-mental status examination: Validity and reliability. *Neurology*, 37(Suppl. 1), 179.

Sternberg, D.E., and Jarvik, M.E. (1976). Memory function in depression: Improvement with antidepressant medication. *Arch Gen Psychiatry*, 33, 219–224.

Stoll, A.L., Locke, C.A., Vuckovic, A., and Mayer, P.V. (1996). Lithium-associated cognitive and functional deficits reduced by a switch to divalproex sodium: A case series. *J Clin Psychiatry*, 57, 356–359.

Strakowksi, S.M., Adler, C.M., Holland, S.K., Mills, N.P., DelBello, M.P., and Eliassen, J.C. (2005). Abnormal fMRI brain activation in euthymic bipolar disorder patients during a counting stroop interference task. *Am J Psychiatry*, 162, 1697–1705.

Strömgren, L. (1977). The influence of depression on memory. *Acta Psychiatr Scand*, 56, 109–128.

Suppes, T., Webb, A., Carmody, T., Gordon, E., Gutierrez-Esteinou, R., Hudson, J.I., and Pope, H.G.J. (1996). Is postictal electrical silence a predictor of response to electroconvulsive therapy? *J Affect Disord*, 41, 55–58.

Swann, A.C., Katz, M.M., Bowden, C.L., Berman, N.G., and Stokes, P.E. (1999). Psychomotor performance and monoamine function in bipolar and unipolar affective disorders. *Biol Psychiatry*, 45, 979–988.

Swann, A.C., Pazzaglia, P., Nicholls, A., Dougherty, D.M., and Moeller, F.G. (2003). Impulsivity and phase of illness in bipolar disorder. *J Affect Disord*, 73(1–2), 105–111.

Swanson, J., Castellanos, F.X., Murias, M., LaHoste, G., and Kennedy, J. (1998). Cognitive neuroscience of attention deficit hyperactivity disorder and hyperkinetic disorder. *Curr Opin Neurobiol*, 8, 263–271.

Swayze, V.W.D., Andreasen, N.C., Alliger, R.J., Ehrhardt, J.C., and Yuh, W.T. (1990). Structural brain abnormalities in bipolar affective disorder: Ventricular enlargement and focal signal hyperintensities. *Arch Gen Psychiatry*, 47, 1054–1059.

Sweeney, J.A., Kmiec, J.A., and Kupfer, D.J. (2000). Neuropsychologic impairments in bipolar and unipolar mood disorders on the CANTAB neurocognitive battery. *Biol Psychiatry*, 48, 674–684.

Szabadi, E., Bradshaw, C.M., and Besson, J.A. (1976). Elongation of pause-time in speech: A simple, objective measure of motor retardation in depression. *Br J Psychiatry*, 129, 592–597.

Takayama, M., Miyamoto, S., Ikeda, A., Mikuni, N., Takahashi, J.B., Usui, K., Satow, T., Yamamoto, J., Matsuhashi, M., Matsumoto, R., Nagamine, T., Shibasaki, H., and Hashimoto, N. (2004). Intracarotid propofol test for speech and memory dominance in man. *Neurology*, 63, 510–515.

Tanaka, M., and Sumitsuji, N. (1991). Electromyographic study of facial expressions during pathological laughing and crying. *Electromyogr Clin Neurophysiol*, 31, 399–406.

Tateno, A., Jorge, R.E., and Robinson, R.G. (2004). Pathological laughing and crying following traumatic brain injury. *J Neuropsychiatry Clin Neurosci*, 16, 426–434.

Tavares, J.V., Drevets, W.C., and Sahakian, B.J. (2003). Cognition in mania and depression. *Psychol Med*, 33, 959–967.

Taylor, M.A., and Abrams, R. (1983). Schizo-affective disorder, manic type. A clinical, laboratory, and genetic study. *Psychiatr Clin (Basel)*, 16(2–4), 234–244.

Taylor, S.E., and Brown, J.D. (1988). Illusion and well-being: A social psychological perspective on mental health. *Psychol Bull*, 103, 193–210.

Taylor, S.E., and Brown, J.D. (1994). Positive illusions and well-being revisited: Separating fact from fiction. *Psychol Bull*, 116, 21–27; discussion 28.

Teicher, M.H., Lawrence, J.M., Barber, N.I., Finklestein, S.P., Lieberman, H.R., and Baldessarini, R.J. (1988). Increased activity and phase delay in circadian motility rhythms in geriatric depression: Preliminary observations. *Arch Gen Psychiatry*, 45, 913–917.

Telford, R., and Worrall, E.P. (1978). Cognitive functions in manic-depressives: Effects of lithium and physostigmine. *Br J Psychiatry*, 133, 424–428.

Teneback, C.C., Nahas, Z., Speer, A.M., Molloy, M., Stallings, L.E., Spicer, K.M., Risch, S.C., and George, M.S. (1999). Changes in prefrontal cortex and paralimbic activity in depression following two weeks of daily left prefrontal TMS. *J Neuropsychiatry Clin Neurosci*, 11, 426–435.

Terao, Y., and Ugawa, Y. (2002). Basic mechanisms of TMS. *J Clin Neurophysiol*, 19, 322–343.

Terzian, H. (1964). Behavioural and EEG effects of intracarotid sodium amytal injection. *Acta Neurochirurgica*, 12, 230–239.

Terzian, H., and Cecotto, C. (1959). Determination and study of hemispheric dominance by means of intracarotid injection of sodium amytal in man: I. Clinical modifications. *Bollettino–Societa Italiana Biologia Sperimentale*, 35, 1623–1626.

Tham, A., Engelbrektson, K., Mathe, A.A., Johnson, L., Olsson, E., and Aberg-Wistedt, A. (1997). Impaired neuropsychological performance in euthymic patients with recurring mood disorders. *J Clin Psychiatry*, 58, 26–29.

Thomas, P., Kearney, G., Napier, E., Ellis, E., Leuder, I., and Johnson, M. (1996). Speech and language in first onset psychosis differences between people with schizophrenia, mania, and controls. *Br J Psychiatry*, 168(3), 337–343.

Thomas, P., Goudemand, M., and Rousseaux, M. (1999). Attentional resources in major depression. *Eur Arch Psychiatry Clin Neurosci*, 249, 79–85.

Tohen, M., Waternaux, C.M., and Tsuang, M.T. (1990a). Outcome in Mania: A 4-year prospective follow-up of 75 patients utilizing survival analysis. *Arch Gen Psychiatry*, 47, 1106–1111.

Tohen, M., Waternaux, C.M., Tsuang, M.T., and Hunt, A.T. (1990b). Four-year follow-up of twenty-four first-episode manic patients. *J Affect Disord*, 19, 79–86.

Tohen, M., Hennen, J., Zarate, C.M. Jr., Baldessarini, R.J., Strakowski, S.M., Stoll, A.L., Faedda, G.L., Suppes, T., Gebre-Medhin, P., and Cohen, B.M. (2000). Two-year syndromal and functional recovery in 219 cases of first-episode major affective disorder with psychotic features. *Am J Psychiatry*, 157, 220–228.

Torrent, C., Martinez-Aran, A., Daban, C., Sanchez-Moreno, J., Comes, M., Goikolea, J.M., Salamero, M., and Vieta, E. (2006). Cognitive impairment in bipolar II disorder. *Br J Psychiatry*, 189, 254–259.

Tortella, F.C., and Long, J.B. (1985). Endogenous anticonvulsant substance in rat cerebrospinal fluid after a generalized seizure. *Science*, 228, 1106–1108.

Umbricht, D., Koller, R., Schmid, L., Skrabo, A., Grubel, C., Huber, T., and Stassen, H. (2003). How specific are deficits in mismatch negativity generation to schizophrenia? *Biol Psychiatry*, 53(12), 1120–1131.

van Gorp, W.G., Altshuler, L., Theberge, D.C., Wilkins, J., and Dixon, W. (1998). Cognitive impairment in euthymic bipolar patients with and without prior alcohol dependence: A preliminary study. *Arch Gen Psychiatry*, 55, 41–46.

van Gorp, W.G., Altshuler, L., Theberge, D.C., and Mintz, J. (1999). Declarative and procedural memory in bipolar disorder. *Biol Psychiatry*, 46, 525–531.

van Vugt, J.P., Siesling, S., Piet, K.K., Zwinderman, A.H., Middelkoop, H.A., van Hilten, J.J., and Roos, R.A. (2001). Quantitative assessment of daytime motor activity provides a responsive measure of functional decline in patients with Huntington's disease. *Movement Disord*, 16, 481–488.

Velten, E. Jr. (1968). A laboratory task for induction of mood states. *Behav Res Ther*, 6, 473–482.

Videbech, P. (1997). MRI findings in patients with affective disorder: A meta-analysis. *Acta Psychiatr Scand*, 96, 157–168.

Volkers, A.C., Tulen, J.H., van den Broek, W.W., Bruijn, J.A., Passchier, J., and Pepplinkhuizen, L. (2003). Motor activity and autonomic cardiac functioning in major depressive disorder. *J Affect Disord*, 76, 23–30.

Volkow, N.D., Bellar, S., Mullani, N., Jould, L., and Dewey, S. (1988). Effects of electroconvulsive therapy on brain glucose metabolism: A preliminary study. *Convulsive Ther*, 4, 199–205.

Vuilleumier, P., Ghika-Schmid, F., Bogousslavsky, J., Assal, G., and Regli, F. (1998). Persistent recurrence of hypomania and prosopoaffective agnosia in a patient with right thalamic infarct. *Neuropsychiatry Neuropsychol Behav Neurol*, 11, 40–44.

Wada, J.A. (1997). Clinical experimental observations of carotid artery injections of sodium amytal. *Brain Cognition*, 33, 11–13.

Wassermann, E.M., Pascual-Leone, A., Valls-Sole, J., Toro, C., Cohen, L.G., and Hallett, M. (1993). Topography of the inhibitory and excitatory responses to transcranial magnetic stimulation in a hand muscle. *Electroencephalogr Clin Neurophysiol*, 89, 424–433.

Wechsler, D. (1981). *Wechsler Adult Intelligence Scale—Revised*. New York: Psychological Corporation.

Weingartner, H., Miller, H., and Murphy, D.L. (1977). Mood-state-dependent retrieval of verbal associations. *J Abnorm Psychol*, 86, 276–284.

Weingartner, H., Cohen, R.M., Murphy, D.L., Martello, J., and Gerdt, C. (1981). Cognitive processes in depression. *Arch Gen Psychiatry*, 38, 42–47.

Weiss, B.L., Foster, F.G., Reynolds, C.F. III, and Kupfer, D.J. (1974a). Psychomotor activity in mania. *Arch Gen Psychiatry*, 31, 379–383.

Weiss, B.L., Kupfer, D.J., Foster, F.G., and Delgado, J. (1974b). Psychomotor activity, sleep, and biogenic amine metabolites in depression. *Biol Psychiatry*, 9, 45–54.

Whitehead, A. (1973a). The pattern of WAIS performance in elderly psychiatric patients. *Br J Social Clin Psychol*, 12, 435–436.

Whitehead, A. (1973b). Verbal learning and memory in elderly depressives. *Br J Psychiatry*, 123, 203–208.

Wickelgren, W. (1973). The long and short of of memory. *Psychol Bull*, 80, 425–438.

Widlocher, D.J. (1983). Psychomotor retardation: Clinical, theoretical, and psychometric aspects. *Psychiatr Clin North Am*, 6, 27–40.

Wielgus, M.S., and Harvey, P.D. (1988). Dichotic listening and recall in schizophrenia and mania. *Schizophr Bull*, 14(4), 689–700.

Winter, L., Lawton, M.P., Casten, R.J., and Sando, R.L. (2000). The relationship between external events and affect states in older people. *Int J Aging Hum Dev*, 50, 85–96.

Wolfe, J., Granholm, E., Butters, N., Saunders, E., and Janowsky, D. (1987). Verbal memory deficits associated with major affective disorders: A comparison of unipolar and bipolar patients. *J Affect Disord*, 13, 83–92.

Wolff, E.A. III, Putnam, F.W., and Post, R.M. (1985). Motor activity and affective illness: The relationship of amplitude and temporal distribution to changes in affective state. *Arch Gen Psychiatry*, 42, 288–294.

Woodruff, R., Robins, L., and Winokur, G. (1968). Educational and occupational achievement in primary affective disorder. *Am J Psychiatry*, 124, 57–64.

Woodruff, R.J., Robins, L.N., Winokur, G., and Reich, T. (1971). Manic depressive illness and social achievement. *Acta Psychiatr Scand*, 47, 237–249.

Woods, D.L., Knight, R.T., and Scabini, D. (1993). Anatomical substrates of auditory selective attention: Behavioral and electrophysiological effects of posterior association cortex lesions. *Brain Res Cognitive Brain Res*, 1, 227–240.

Wu, J.C., Gillin, J.C., Buchsbaum, M.S., Hershey, T., Johnson, J.C., and Bunney, W.E.J. (1992). Effect of sleep deprivation on brain metabolism of depressed patients. *Am J Psychiatry*, 149, 538–543.

Wu, J., Buchsbaum, M.S., Gillin, J.C., Tang, C., Cadwell, S., Wiegand, M., Najafi, A., Klein, E., Hazen, K., Bunney, W.E.J., Fallon, J.H., and Keator, D. (1999). Prediction of antidepressant effects of sleep deprivation by metabolic rates in the ventral anterior cingulate and medial prefrontal cortex. *Am J Psychiatry*, 156, 1149–1158.

Wu, L., Goto, Y., Taniwaki, T., Kinukawa, N., and Tobimatsu, S. (2002). Different patterns of excitation and inhibition of the small hand and forearm muscles from magnetic brain stimulation in humans. *Clin Neurophysiol*, 113, 1286–1294.

Wyatt, R.J. (1991). Neuroleptics and the natural course of schizophrenia. *Schizophrenia Bull*, 17, 325–351.

Wyatt, R.J. (1995). Early intervention for schizophrenia: Can the course of the illness be altered? *Biol Psychiatry*, 38, 1–3.

Yan, S.M., Flor-Henry, P., Chen, D.Y., Li, T.G., Qi, S.G., and Ma, Z.X. (1985). Imbalance of hemispheric functions in the major psychoses: A study of handedness in the People's Republic of China. *Biol Psychiatry*, 20, 906–917.

Yang, J.A., and Rehm, L.P. (1993). A study of autobiographical memories in depressed and nondepressed elderly individuals. *Int J Aging Hum Devel*, 36, 39–55.

Yen, C.F., Chung, L.C., and Chen, C.S. (2002). Insight and neuropsychological functions in bipolar outpatients in remission. *J Nerv Ment Dis*, 190, 713–715.

Yovell, Y., Sackeim, H.A., Epstein, D.G., Prudic, J., Devanand, D.P., McElhiney, M.C., Settembrino, J.M., and Bruder, G.E. (1995). Hearing loss and asymmetry in major depression. *J Neuropsychiatry Clin Neurosci*, 7, 82–89.

Yu, L., Liu, C.K., Chen, J.W., Wang, S.Y., Wu, Y.H., and Yu, S.H. (2004). Relationship between post-stroke depression and lesion location: A meta-analysis. *Kaohsiung J Med Sci*, 20, 372–380.

Zakzanis, K.K., Leach, L., and Kaplan, E. (1998). On the nature and pattern of neurocognitive function in major depressive disorder. *Neuropsychiatry Neuropsychol Behav Neurol*, 11, 111–119.

Zalla, T., Joyce, C., Szoke, A., Schurhoff, F., Pillon, B., Komano, O., Perez-Diaz, F., Bellivier, F., Alter, C., Dubois, B., Rouillon, F., Houde, O., and Leboyer, M. (2004). Executive dysfunctions as potential markers of familial vulnerability to bipolar disorder and schizophrenia. *Psychiatry Res*, 121, 207–217.

Zarate, C.A. Jr., Tohen, M., Land, M., and Cavanagh, S. (2000). Functional impairment and cognition in bipolar disorder. *Psychiatr Q*, 71, 309–329.

Zubenko, G.S., Sullivan, P., Nelson, J.P., Belle, S.H., Huff, F.J., and Wolf, G.L. (1990). Brain imaging abnormalities in mental disorders of late life. *Arch Neurol*, 47, 1107–1111.

Zubieta, J.K., Huguelet, P., O'Neil, R.L., and Giordani, B.J. (2001). Cognitive function in euthymic bipolar I disorder. *Psychiatry Res*, 102, 9–20.

CHAPTER 10

Abou-Saleh, M.T., and Coppen, A. (1984). Classification of depressive illness: Clinico-psychological correlates. *J Affect Disord*, 6(1), 53–66.

Abraham, K. (1911). Notes on the psycho-analytical investigation and treatment of manic-depressive insanity and allied conditions. In D. Bryan, A. Strachey (Translators), *Selected Papers of Karl Abraham, M.D.* (pp. 137–156). London, England: Hogarth Press, 1927.

Abraham, K. (1924). A short study of the development of the libido, viewed in the light of mental disorders. In D. Bryan, A. Strachey (Translators), *Selected Papers of Karl Abraham, M.D.* (pp. 418–480). London, England: Hogarth Press, 1927.

Akiskal, H.S., Djenderedjian, A.M., Rosenthal, R.H., and Khani, M.K. (1977). Cyclothymic disorder: Validating criteria for inclusion in the bipolar affective group. *Am J Psychiatry*, 134(11), 1227–1233.

Akiskal, H.S., Hirschfeld, R.M., and Yerevanian, B.I. (1983). The relationship of personality to affective disorders. *Arch Gen Psychiatry*, 40(7), 801–810.

Akiskal, H.S., Chen, S.E., Davis, G.C., Puzantian, V.R., Kashgarian, M., and Bolinger, J.M. (1985). Borderline: An adjective in search of a noun. *J Clin Psychiatry*, 46(2), 41–48.

Akiskal, H.S., Bourgeois, M.L., Angst, J., Post, R., Moller, H., and Hirschfeld, R. (2000). Re-evaluating the prevalence of and diagnostic composition within the broad clinical spectrum of bipolar disorders. *J Affect Disord*, 59(Suppl. 1), S5–S30.

Akiskal, H.S., Kilzieh, N., Maser, J.D., Clayton, P.J., Schettler, P.J., Shea, M.T., Endicott, J., Scheftner, W., Hirschfeld, R.M.A., and Keller, M.B. (2006). The distinct temperament profiles of bipolar I, bipolar II and unipolar patients. *J Affect Disord*, 92, 19–33.

Alexander, F. (1948). *Fundamentals of Psychoanalysis*. New York: WW Norton.

Allison, J.B., and Wilson, W.P. (1960). Sexual behaviors of manic patients: A preliminary report. *South Med J*, 53, 870–874.

Allport, G.W. (1961). *Pattern and Growth in Personality*. New York: Holt, Rinehart and Winston.

Anderson, C.A., and Hammen, C.L. (1993). Psychosocial outcomes of children of unipolar depressed, bipolar, medically ill, and normal women: A longitudinal study. *J Consult Clin Psychol*, 61(3), 448–454.

Anderson, P., Beach, S.R.H., and Kaslow, N.J. (1999). Marital discord and depression: The potential of attachment theory to guide integrative clinical intervention. In T. Joiner, C.C. Coyne (Eds.), *The Interactional Nature of Depression* (pp. 271–297). Washington, DC: American Psychological Association.

Arieti, S. (1959). Manic-depressive psychoses. In S. Arieti (Ed.), *American Handbook of Psychiatry*. New York: Basic Books.

Barbato, N., and Hafner, R.J. (1998). Comorbidity of bipolar and personality disorder. *Aust N Z J Psychiatry*, 32(2), 276–280.

Bauer, M.S., Kirk, G.F., Gavin, C., and Williford, W.O. (2001). Determinants of functional outcome and healthcare costs in bipolar disorder: A high-intensity follow-up study. *J Affect Disord*, 65(3), 231–241.

Bauwens, F., Tracy, A., Pardoen, D., Vander Elst, M., and Mendlewicz, J. (1991). Social adjustment of remitted bipolar and unipolar out-patients: A comparison with age- and sex-matched controls. *Br J Psychiatry*, 159, 239–244.

Beach, S.R.H., and Jones, D. (2002). Marital and family therapy for depression in adults. In I. Gotlib, C. Hammen (Eds.), *Handbook of Depression* (pp. 422–440). New York: Guilford Press.

Beardslee, W.R., Versage, E.M., and Gladstone, T.R. (1998). Children of affectively ill parents: A review of the past 10 years. *J Am Acad Child Adolesc Psychiatry*, 37(11), 1134–1141.

Bech, P., Shapiro, R.W., Sihm, F., Nielsen, B.M., Sorensen, B., and Rafaelsen, O.J. (1980). Personality in unipolar and bipolar manic-malancholic patients. *Acta Psychiatr Scand*, 62(3), 245–257.

Beigel, A., Murphy, D.L., and Bunney, W.E. (1971). The Manic-State Rating Scale: Scale construction, reliability, and validity. *Arch Gen Psychiatry*, 25, 256–262.

Belmaker, R.H., Lehrer, R., Ebstein, R.P., Lettik, H., and Kugelmass, S. (1979). A possible cardiovascular effect of lithium. *Am J Psychiatry*, 136, 577–579.

Benazzi, F. (2000). Exploring aspects of DSM-IV interpersonal sensitivity in bipolar II. *J Affect Disord* 60(1), 43–46.

Benazzi, F., and Akiskal, H.S. (2005). A downscaled practical measure of mood lability as a screening tool for bipolar II. *J Affect Disord*, 84, 225–232.

Bieling, P.J., MacQueen, G.M., Marriot, M.J., Robb, J.C., Begin, H., Joffe, R.T., and Young, L.T. (2003). Longitudinal outcome in patients with bipolar disorder assessed by life-charting is influenced by DSM-IV personality disorder symptoms. *Bipolar Disord*, 5(1), 14–21.

Billings, A.G., and Moos, R.H. (1985). Psychosocial processes of remission in unipolar depression: Comparing depressed patients with matched community controls. *J Consult Clin Psychol*, 53(3), 314–325.

Blairy, S., Linotte, S., Souery, D., Papadimitriou, G.N., Dikeos, D., Lerer, B., Kaneva, R., Milanova, V., Serretti, A., Macciardi, F., and Mendlewicz, J. (2004). Social adjustment and self-esteem of bipolar patients: A multicenter study. *J Affect Disord*, 79, 97–103.

Blalock, J.R. (1936). Psychology of the manic phase of the manic-depressive psychoses. *Psychiatr Q*, 10, 263–344.

Bleuler, E. (1924). *Textbook of Psychiatry* (4th German Edition). A.A. Brill (Ed.). New York: Macmillan.

Bonetti, U., Johansson, F., Von Knorring, L., Perris, C., and Strandman, E. (1977). Prophylactic lithium and personality variables: An international collaborative study. *Int Pharmacopsychiatry*, 12, 14–19.

Brieger, P., Ehrt, U., and Marneros, A. (2003). Frequency of co-morbid personality disorders in bipolar and unipolar affective disorders. *Compr Psychiatry*, 44(1), 28–34.

Brodie, H.K., and Leff, M.J. (1971). Bipolar depression: A comparative study of patient characteristics. *Am J Psychiatry*, 127(8), 1086–1090.

Brown, G.W., and Harris, T. (1986). Establishing causal links: The Bedford College studies of depression. In H. Katschnig (Ed.), *Life Events and Psychiatric Disorders: Controversial Issues* (pp. 107–187). Cambridge, England: Cambridge University Press.

Campbell, J.D. (1953). *Manic-Depressive Disease: Clinical and Psychiatric Significance*. Philadelphia: JB Lippincott.

Cannon, M., Jones, P., Gilvarry, C., Rifkin, L., McKenzie, K., Foerster, A., and Murray, R.M. (1997). Premorbid social functioning in schizophrenia and bipolar disorder: Similarities and differences, *Am J Psychiatry*, 154(11), 1544–1550.

Carpenter, D., Clarkin, J.F., Glick, I.D., and Wilner, P.J. (1995). Personality pathology among married adults with bipolar disorder. *J Affect Disord*, 34(4), 269–274.

Carpenter, D., Clarkin, J.F., Isman, L., and Patten, M. (1999). The impact of neuroticism upon married bipolar patients. *J Personal Disord*, 13(1), 60–66.

Carpenter, K.M., and Hittner, J.B. (1995). Dimensional characteristics of the SCL-90-R: Evaluation of gender differences in dually diagnosed inpatients. *J Clin Psychol*, 51(3), 383–390.

Casper, R.C., Redmond, E. Jr., Katz, M.M., Schaffer, C.B., Davis, J.M., and Koslow, S.H. (1985). Somatic symptoms in primary affective disorder: Presence and relationship to the classification of depression. *Arch Gen Psychiatry*, 42, 1098–1104.

Cassano, G.B., Akiskal, H.S., Savino, M., Musetti, L., and Perugi, G. (1992). Proposed subtypes of bipolar II and related disorders; with hypomanic episodes (or cyclothymia) and with hyperthymic temperament. *J Affect Disord*, 26, 127–140.

Chakrabarti, S., and Gill, S. (2002). Coping and its correlates among caregivers of patients with bipolar disorder: A preliminary study. *Bipolar Disord*, 4(1), 50–60.

Chang, K.D., Blasey, C., Ketter, T.A., and Steiner, H. (2001). Family environment of children and adolescents with bipolar parents. *Bipolar Disord*, 3(2), 73–78.

Chang, K.D., Blascy, C.M., Ketter, T.A., and Steiner, H. (2003). Temperament characteristics of child and adolescent bipolar offspring. *J Affect Disord*, 77, 11–19.

Chodoff, P. (1972). The depressive personality: A critical review. *Arch Gen Psychiatry*, 27(5), 666–673.

Clark, L.A., Watson, D., and Mineka, S. (1994). Temperament, personality, and the mood and anxiety disorders. *J Abnorm Psychol*, 103(1), 103–116.

Clarkin, J.F., Carpenter, D., Hull, J., Wilner, P., and Glick, I. (1998). Effects of psychoeducational intervention for married patients with bipolar disorder and their spouses. *Psychiatr Serv*, 49(4), 531–533.

Clayton, P.J., Ernst, C., and Angst, J. (1994). Premorbid personality traits of men who develop unipolar or bipolar disorders. *Eur Arch Psychiatry Clin Neurosci*, 243(6), 340–346.

Cloninger, C.R. (1987). A systematic method for clinical description and classification of personality variants. A proposal. *Arch Gen Psychiatry*, 44(6), 573–588.

Cohen, A.N., Hammen, C., Henry, R.M., and Daley, S.E. (2004). Effects of stress and social support on recurrence in bipolar disorder. *J Affect Disord*, 82(1), 143–147.

Cohen, M.B., Baker, G., Cohen, R.A., Fromm-Reichmann, F., and Weigert, E.V. (1954). An intensive study of twelve cases of manic-depressive psychosis. *Psychiatry*, 17, 103–137.

Colombo, M., Cox, G., and Dunner, D.L. (1990). Assortative mating in affective and anxiety disorders: Preliminary findings. *Psychiatr Genet*, 1, 35–44.

Cooke, R.G., Robb, J.C., Young, L.T., and Joffe, R.T. (1996). Well-being and functioning in patients with bipolar disorder assessed using the MOS 20-ITEM short form (SF-20). *J Affect Disord*, 39(2), 93–97.

Coryell, W., Endicott, J., and Keller, M. (1992). Major depression in a nonclinical sample. Demographic and clinical risk factors for first onset. *Arch Gen Psychiatry*, 49(2), 117–125.

Coryell, W., Scheftner, W., Keller, M., Endicott, J., Maser, J., and Klerman, G.L. (1993). The enduring psychosocial consequences of mania and depression. *Am J Psychiatry*, 150(5), 720–727.

Coryell, W., Turvey, C., Endicott, J., Leon, A.C., Mueller, T., Solomon, D., and Keller, M. (1998). Bipolar I affective disorder: Predictors of outcome after 15 years. *J Affect Disord*, 50(2–3), 109–116.

Costa, P.T., and McCrae, R.R. (1985). *The NEO-Personality Inventory Manual*. Odessa, FL: Psychological Assessment Resources.

Costa, P.T., and McCrae, R.R. (1992). *NEO PI-R Professional Manual: Revised NEO Personality Inventory (NEO PI-R) and NEO Five-Factor Inventory (NEO-FFI)*. Odessa, FL: Psychological Assessment Resources.

Coyne, J.C. (1976). Depression and the response of others. *J Abnorm Psychol*, 85(2), 186–193.

Coyne, J.C., Kessler, R.C., Tal, M., Turnbull, J., Wortman, C.B., and Greden, J.F. (1987). Living with a depressed person. *J Consult Clin Psychol*, 55(3), 347–352.

Cronin, C., and Zuckerman, M. (1992). Sensation seeking and bipolar affective disorder. *Pers Individ Dif*, 13, 385–387.

Custance, J. (1952). *Wisdom, Madness, and Folly: The Philosophy of a Lunatic*. New York: Farrar, Straus, & Cudahy.

Dax, E.C. (1953). *Experimental Studies in Psychiatric Art*. London: Faber & Faber.

Deltito, J., Martin, L., Riefkohl, J., Austria, B., Kissilenko, A., Corless, C., and Morse, P. (2001). Do patients with borderline personality disorder belong to the bipolar spectrum? *J Affect Disord*, 67(1–3), 221–228.

Demers, R.G., and Davis, L.S. (1971). The influence of prophylactic lithium treatment on the marital adjustment of manic-depressives and their spouses. *Compr Psychiatry*, 12(4), 348–353.

DePaulo, J.R., Correa, E.I., and Folstein, M.F. (1983). Does lithium stabilize mood? *Biol Psychiatry*, 18, 1093–1097.

Depue, R.A., and Iacono, W.G. (1988). Neurobehavioral aspects of affective disorders. *Ann Rev Psychol*, 40, 457–492.

Depue, R.A., Slater, J.F., Wolfstetter-Kausch, H., Klein, D., Goplerud, E., and Farr, D. (1981). A behavioral paradigm for identifying persons at risk for bipolar depressive disorder: A conceptual framework and five validation studies. *J Abnorm Psychol*, 90(5), 381–437.

Depue, R.A., Luciana, M., Arbisi, P., Collins, P., and Leon, A. (1994). Dopamine and the structure of personality: Relation of agonist-induced dopamine activity to positive emotionality. *J Pers Soc Psychol*, 67(3), 485–498.

Dickerson, F.B., Sommerville, J., Origoni, A.E., Ringel, N.B., and Parente, F. (2001). Outpatients with schizophrenia and bipolar I disorder: Do they differ in their cognitive and social functioning? *Psychiatry Res*, 102(1), 21–27.

Donnelly, E.F., and Murphy, D.L. (1973). Primary affective disorder: MMPI differences between unipolar and bipolar depressed subjects. *J Clin Psychol*, 29(3), 303–306.

Donnelly, E.F., and Murphy, D.L. (1974). Primary affective disorder: Bender-Gestalt sequence of placement as an indicator of impulse control. *Percept Motor Skills*, 38(3), 1079–1082.

Donnelly, E.F., Murphy, D.L., and Goodwin, F.K. (1976). Cross-sectional and longitudinal comparisons of bipolar and unipolar depressed groups on the MMPI. *J Consult Clin Psychol*, 44(2), 233–237.

Dooley, L. (1921). A psychoanalytic study of manic depressive psychoses. *Psychoanal Rev*, 8, 144–167.

Dore, G., and Romans, S.E. (2001). Impact of bipolar affective disorder on family and partners. *J Affect Disord*, 67(1–3), 147–158.

Dorz, S., Borgherini, G., Cognolato, S., Conforti, D., Fiorellini, A.L., Scarso, C., and Magni, G. (2002). Social adjustment in in-patients with affective disorders: Predictive factors. *J Affect Disord*, 70(1), 49–56.

Downey, G., and Coyne, J.C. (1990). Children of depressed parents: An integrative review. *Psychol Bull*, 108(1), 50–76.

Dunayevich, E., Strakowski, S.M., Sax, K.W., Sorter, M.T., Keck, P.E. Jr., McElroy, S.L., and McConville, B.J. (1996). Personality disorders in first- and multiple-episode mania. *Psychiatry Res*, 64(1), 69–75.

Dunayevich, E., Sax, K.W., Keck, P.E. Jr., McElroy, S.L., Sorter, M.T., McConville, B.J., and Strakowski, S.M. (2000). Twelve-month outcome in bipolar patients with and without personality disorders. *J Clin Psychiatry*, 61(2), 134–139.

English, O.S. (1949). Observation of trends in manic-depressive psychosis. *Psychiatry*, 12, 125–133.

Engström, C., Brändström, S., Sigvardsson, S., Cloninger, R., Nylander, P.-O. (2003). Bipolar disorder: II. Personality and age of onset. *Bipolar Disord*, 5, 340–348.

Evans, L., Akiskal, H.S., Keck, P.E., McElroy, S.L., Sadovnick, A.D., Remick, R.A., and Kelsoe, J.R. (2005). Familialry of temperament in bipolar disorder: Support for a genetic spectrum. *J Affect Disord*, 85, 153–168.

Eysenck, H.J. (1956). The questionnaire measurement of neuroticism and extraversion. *Revista di Psicologia*, 50, 113–140.

Eysenck, H.J. (1959). *The Manual of the Maudsley Personality Inventory*. London: University of London Press.

Eysenck, H.J., and Eysenck, S.B.G. (1963a). *Eysenck Personality Inventory*. San Diego: Educational and Industrial Testing Service.

Eysenck, H.J., and Eysenck, S.B.G. (1963b). *Manual of the Eysenck Personality Inventory*. San Diego: Educational and Industrial Testing Service.

Fadden, G., Bebbington, P., and Kuipers, L. (1987). Caring and its burdens. A study of the spouses of depressed patients. *Br J Psychiatry*, 151, 660–667.

Fenichel, O. (1945). *The Psychoanalytic Theory of Neuroses*. New York: WW Norton.

Flick, S.N., Roy-Byrne, P.P., Cowley, D.S., Shores, M.M., and Dunner, D.L. (1993). DSM-III-R personality disorders in a mood and anxiety disorders clinic: Prevalence, comorbidity, and clinical correlates. *J Affect Disord*, 27(2), 71–79.

Folstein, M.F., DePaulo, J.R. Jr., and Trepp, K. (1982). Unusual mood stability in patients taking lithium. *Br J Psychiatry*, 140, 188–191.

Frank, E., Targum, S.D., Gershon, E.S., Anderson, C., Stewart, B.D., Davenport, Y., Ketchum, K.L., and Kupfer, D.J. (1981). A comparison of nonpatient and bipolar patient–well spouse couples. *Am J Psychiatry*, 138(6), 764–768.

Freud, S. (1917). Mourning and melancholia. In W. Gaylin (Ed.), *The Meaning of Despair: Psychoanalytic Contributions to the Understanding of Depression*. New York: Science House, 1968.

Frey, R. (1977). Die prämorbide Persönlichkeit von monopolar und bipolar Depressiven: Ein Vergleich aufgrund von Persönlichkeitstests. *Archiv Psychiatr Nervenkr*, 224, 161–173.

Fromm-Reichmann, F. (1949). Intensive psychotherapy of manic-depressives: A preliminary report. *Confina Neurologica*, 9, 158–165.

Garma, A. (1968). The deceiving superego and the masochistic ego in mania. *Psychoanal Q*, 37(1), 63–79.

Gelfand, D.M., and Teti, D.M. (1990). The effects of maternal depression on children. *Clin Psychol Rev*, 10, 320–354.

George, E.L., Miklowitz, D.J., Richards, J.A., Simoneau, T.L., and Taylor, D.O. (2003). The comorbidity of bipolar disorders and axis II personality disorders: Prevalence and clinical correlates. *Bipolar Disord*, 5(2), 115–122.

Gerö, G. (1936). Construction of depression. *Int J Psychoanal*, 17, 423–461.

Gershon, E.S., McKnew, D., Cytryn, L., Hamovit, J., Schreiber, J., Hibbs, E., and Pellegrini, D. (1985). Diagnoses in school-age children of bipolar affective disorder patients and normal controls. *J Affect Disord*, 8(3), 283–291.

Gibson, R.W., Cohen, M.B., and Cohen, R.A. (1959). On the dynamics of the manic-depressive personality. *Am J Psychiatry*, 115, 1101–1107.

Gitlin, M.J., Swendsen, J., Heller, T.L., and Hammen, C. (1995). Relapse and impairment in bipolar disorder. *Am J Psychiatry*, 152(11), 1635–1640.

Goodman, S.H., and Gotlib, I.H. (1999). Risk for psychopathology in the children of depressed mothers: A developmental model for understanding mechanisms of transmission. *Psychol Rev*, 106(3), 458–490.

Gordon, D., Burge, D., Hammen, C., Adrian, C., Jaenicke, C., and Hiroto, D. (1989). Observations of interactions of depressed women with their children. *Am J Psychiatry*, 146(1), 50–55.

Gotlib, I.H., and Whiffen, V.E. (1989). Depression and marital functioning: An examination of specificity and gender differences. *J Abnorm Psychol*, 98(1), 23–30.

Grant, B.F., Stinson, F.S., Hasin, D.S., Dawson, D.A., Chou, P., Ruan, W.J., and Huang, B. (2005). Prevalence, correlates, and comorbidity of bipolar I disorder and axis I and II disorders: Results from the National Epidemiologic Survey on Alcohol and Related Conditions. *J Clin Psychiatry*, 66, 1205–1215.

Gray, J.A. (1982). *The Neuropsychology of Anxiety: An Enquiry into the Functions of the Septa-Hippocampal System*. Oxford, England: Clarendon Press.

Grigoroiu-Serbanescu, M., Christodorescu, D., Jipescu, I., Totoescu, A., Marinescu, E., and Ardelean, V. (1989). Psychopathology in children aged 10–17 of bipolar parents: Psychopathology rate and correlates of the severity of the psychopathology. *J Affect Disord*, 16(2–3), 167–179.

Grigoroiu-Serbanescu, M., Christodorescu, D., Totoescu, A., and Jipescu, I. (1991). Depressive disorders and depressive personality traits in offspring aged 10–17 of bipolar and of normal parents. *Journal of Youth and Adolescence*, 20, 135–148.

Grotstein, J.S. (1986). The psychology of powerlessness: Disorders of self-regulation and interactional regulation as a newer paradigm for psychopathology. *Psychoanal Inq*, 6, 93–118.

Gunderson, J.G., Weinberg, I., Daversa, M.T., Kueppenbender, K.D., Zanarini, M.C., Shea, M.T., Skodol, A.E., Sanislow, C.A., Yen, S., Morey, L.C., Grilo, C.M., McGlashan, T.H., Stout, R.L., and Dyck, I.D. (2006). Descriptive and longitudinal observations on the relationship of borderline personality disorder and bipolar disorder. *Am J Psychiatry*, 163, 1173–1178.

Gurtman, M.B. (1986). Depression and the response of others: Reevaluating the reevaluation. *J Abnorm Psychol*, 95(1), 99–101.

Hall, C.S., and Lindzey, G. (1970). *Theories of Personality*. New York: John Wiley & Sons.

Hamilton, M. (1982). Symptoms and assessment of depression. In E.S. Paykel (Ed.), *Handbook of Affective Disorders* (pp. 3–11). Edinburgh, Scotland: Churchill Livingstone.

Hammen, C.L. (1991). *Depression Runs in Families: The Social Context of Risk and Resilience in Children of Depressed Mothers*. New York: Springer-Verlag.

Hammen, C. (1997). *Depression*. London: Psychology Press.

Hammen, C., and Brennan, P.A. (2002). Interpersonal dysfunction in depressed women: Impairments independent of depressive symptoms. *J Affect Disord*, 72(2), 145–156.

Hantouche, E.G., Akiskal, H.S., Lancrenon, S, Allilaire, J.F., Sechter, D., Azorin, J.M., Bourgeois, M., Fraud, J.P., and Chatenet-Duchene, L. (1998). Systematic clinical methodology for validating bipolar-II disorder: Data in mid-stream from a French national multi-site study. *J Affect Disord*, 50, 163–173.

Harrow, M., Goldberg, J.F., Grossman, L.S., and Meltzer, H.Y. (1990). Outcome in manic disorders: A naturalistic follow-up study. *Arch Gen Psychiatry*, 47(7), 665–671.

Hipwell, A.E., and Kumar, R. (1996). Maternal psychopathology and prediction of outcome based on mother–infant interaction ratings (BMIS). *Br J Psychiatry*, 169(5), 655–661.

Hirschfeld, R.M.A. (1985). Personality and bipolar disorder. Paper presented at the Symposium on New Results in Depression Research. Munich.

Hirschfeld, R.M.A., and Klerman, G.L. (1979). Personality attributes and affective disorders. *Am J Psychiatry*, 136, 67–70.

Hirschfeld, R.M.A., Klerman, G.L., Clayton, P.J., Keller, M.B., McDonald-Scott, P., and Larkin, B.H. (1983). Assessing personality: Effects of the depressive state on trait measurement. *Am J Psychiatry*, 140(6), 695–699.

Hirschfeld, R.M.A., Klerman, G.L., Keller, M.B., Andreasen, N.C., and Clayton, P.J. (1986). Personality of recovered patients with bipolar affective disorder. *J Affect Disord*, 11(1), 81–89.

Holinger, P.C., and Wolpert, E.A. (1979). A ten year follow-up of lithium use. *IMJ Ill Med J*, 156, 99–104.

Hooley, J.M., Richters, J.E., Weintraub, S., and Neale, J.M. (1987). Psychopathology and marital distress: The positive side of positive symptoms. *J Abnorm Psychol*, 96(1), 27–33.

Hoover, C.F., and Fitzgerald, R.G. (1981). Marital conflict of manic-depressive patients. *Arch Gen Psychiatry*, 38(1), 65–67.

Jacobson, E. (1953). Contribution of the metapsychology of cyclothymic depression. In P. Greenacre (Ed.), *Affective Disorders: Psychoanalytic Contribution to Their Study* (pp. 49–83). New York: International Universities Press.

Jamison, K.R. (2004). *Exuberance: The Passion for Life*. New York: Alfred A. Knopf.

Jamison, K.R., Gerner, R.H., Hammen, C., and Padesky, C. (1980). Clouds and silver linings: Positive experiences associated with primary affective disorders. *Am J Psychiatry*, 137, 198–202.

Jamison, K.R., Litman-Adizes, T., Gitlin, M.J., and Fieve, R.R. (Unpublished data). Personality and attitudinal patterns in affective illness.

Janowsky, D.S., Leff, M., and Epstein, R.S. (1970). Playing the manic game: Interpersonal maneuvers of the acutely manic patient. *Arch Gen Psychiatry*, 22(3), 252–261.

Janowsky, D.S., El-Yousef, M.K., and Davis, J.M. (1974). Interpersonal maneuvers of manic patients. *Am J Psychiatry*, 131, 250–255.

Janowsky, D.S., Morter, S., Hong, L., and Howe, L. (1999). Myers Briggs Type Indicator and Tridimensional Personality Questionnaire differences between bipolar patients and unipolar depressed patients. *Bipolar Disord*, 1(2), 98.

Janowsky, D.S., El-Yousef, M.K., and Davis, J.M. (2003). Interpersonal maneuvers of manic patients. *Focus*, 1, 58–63.

Jelliffe, S.E. (1931). Some historical phases of the manic-depressive synthesis. *Res Publ Assoc Res Nerv Ment Dis*, 11, 3–47.

Johnson, L., Lundstroem, O., Aberg-Wistedt, A., and Mathe, A.A. (2003). Social support in bipolar disorder: Its revelance to remission and relapse. *Bipolar Disord*, 5(2), 129–137.

Johnson, S.L., and Jacob, T. (1997). Marital interactions of depressed men and women. *J Consult Clin Psychol*, 65(1), 15–23.

Johnson, S.L., Meyer, B., Winett, C., and Small, J. (2000). Social support and self-esteem predict changes in bipolar depression but not mania. *J Affect Disord*, 58(1), 79–86.

Johnson, S.L., Winters, R., and Meyer, B. (in press). A polarity-specific model of bipolar disorder. In T. Joiner (Ed.), *A Festschrift for Jack Hokanson*. Washington, DC: American Psychological Association Press.

Joiner, T., and Coyne J.C. (1999). *The Interactional Nature of Depression: Advances in Interpersonal Approaches*. Washington, DC: American Psychological Association.

Judd, L.L., Hubbard, B., Janowsky, D.S., Huey, L.Y., and Attewell, P.A. (1977). The effect of lithium carbonate on affect, mood, and personality of normal subjects. *Arch Gen Psychiatry*, 34, 346–351.

Kay, J.H., Altshuler, L.L., Ventura, J., and Mintz, J. (1999). Prevalence of axis II comorbidity in bipolar patients with and without alcohol use disorders. *Ann Clin Psychiatry*, 11(4), 187–195.

Kay, J.H., Altshuler, L.L., Ventura, J., and Mintz, J. (2002). Impact of axis II comorbidity on the course of bipolar illness in men: A retrospective chart review. *Bipolar Disord*, 4(4), 237–242.

Keller, M.B., Lavori, P.W., Coryell, W., Endicott, J., and Mueller, T.I. (1993). Bipolar I: A five-year prospective follow-up. *J Nerv Ment Dis*, 181(4), 238–245.

Kim, E.Y., and Miklowitz, D.J. (2004). Expressed emotion as a predictor of outcome among bipolar patients undergoing family therapy. *J Affect Disord*, 82, 343–352.

Klein, D.N., and Depue, R.A. (1985). Obsessional personality traits and risk for bipolar affective disorder: An offspring study. *J Abnorm Psychol*, 94(3), 291–297.

Klein, D.N., Depue, R.A., and Krauss, S.P. (1986). Social adjustment in the offspring of parents with bipolar affective disorder. *J Psychopathol Behav Assess*, 8, 355–366.

Klerman, G.L. (1973). The relationships between personality and clinical depressions: Overcoming the obstacles to verifying psychodynamic theories. *Int J Psychiatry*, 11(2), 227–233.

Klerman, G.L., Weissman, M.M., Rounsaville, B.J., and Chevron, E.S. (1984). *Interpersonal Psychotherapy of Depression*. New York: Basic Books.

Kotin, J., and Goodwin, F.K. (1972). Depression during mania: Clinical observations and theoretical implications. *Am J Psychiatry*, 129(6), 679–686.

Kraepelin, E. (1921). *Manic-Depressive Insanity and Paranoia*. R.M. Barclay (Translator), G.M. Robertson (Ed.). Edinburgh, Scotland: E & S Livingstone.

Kretschmer, E. (1936). *Physique and Character*. New York: Macmillan.

Kron, L., Decina, P., Kestenbaum, C.J., Farber, S., Gargan, M., and Fieve, R. (1982). The offspring of bipolar manic-depressives: Clinical features. *Adolesc Psychiatry*, 10, 273–291.

Kropf, D., and Müller-Oerlinghausen, B. (1975). The influence of lithium long-term medication on personality and mood. *Pharmacopsychiatry*, 18, 104–105.

Kropf, D., and Müller-Oerlinghausen, B. (1979). Changes in learning, memory, and mood during lithium treatment: Approach to a research strategy. *Acta Psychiatr Scand*, 59, 97–124.

Kulhara, P., Basu, D., Mattoo, S.K., Sharan, P., and Chopra, R. (1999). Lithium prophylaxis of recurrent bipolar affective disorder: Long-term outcome and its psychosocial correlates. *J Affect Disord*, 54(1–2), 87–96.

Kutcher, S.P., Marton, P., and Korenblum, M. (1990). Adolescent bipolar illness and personality disorder. *J Am Acad Child Adolesc Psychiatry*, 29(3), 355–358.

Lam, D., and Wong, G. (1997). Prodromes, coping strategies, insight and social functioning in bipolar affective disorders. *Psychol Med*, 27(5), 1091–1100.

Lam, D., Donaldson, C., Brown, Y., and Malliaris, Y. (2005). Burden and marital and sexual satisfaction in the partners of bipolar patients. *Bipolar Disord*, 7, 431–440.

Leonhard, K. (1957). *Aufteilung der Endogenen Psychosen* (1st edition). Berlin: Akademie-Verlag.

Lepkifker, E., Horesh, N., and Floru, S. (1988). Life satisfaction and adjustment in lithium-treated affective patients in remission. *Acta Psychiatr Scand*, 78(3), 391–395.

Levkovitz, V., Fennig, S., Horesh, N., Barak, V., and Treves, I. (2000). Perception of ill spouse and dyadic relationship in couples with affective disorder and those without. *J Affect Disord*, 58(3), 237–240.

Lewis, N.D.C. (1931). Mental dynamisms and psychotherapeutic modifications in manic-depressive psychoses. *Res Publ Assoc Res Nerv Ment Dis*, 11, 754–776.

Liebowitz, M.R., Stallone, F., Dunner, D.L., and Fieve, R.F. (1979). Personality features of patients with primary affective disorder. *Acta Psychiatr Scand*, 60(2), 214–224.

Lion, J.R. (1975). Conceptual issues in the use of drugs for the treatment of aggression in man. *J Nerv Ment Dis*, 160, 76–82.

Lorimy, F., Lôo, H., and Deniker, P. (1977). Effets cliniques des traitements prolongés par les sels de lithium sur le sommeil, l'appétit et la sexualité. *L'Encéphale*, 3, 227–239.

Lozano, B.E., and Johnson, S.L. (2001). Can personality traits predict increases in manic and depressive symptoms? *J Affect Disord*, 63(1–3), 103–111.

Lumry, A.E., Gottesman, I.I., and Tuason, V.B. (1982). MMPI state dependency during the course of bipolar psychosis. *Psychiatry Res*, 7(1), 59–67.

MacKinnon, D.F., and Pies, R. (2006). Affective instability as rapid cycling: Theoretical and clinical implications for borderline personality and bipolar spectrum disorders. *Bipolar Disord*, 8, 1–14.

Mathews, C.A., and Reus, V.I. (2001). Assortative mating in the affective disorders: A systematic review and meta-analysis. *Compr Psychiatry*, 42(4), 257–262.

Matsumoto, S., Akiyama, T., Tsuda, H., Miyake, Y., Kawamura, Y., Noda, T., Akiskal, K.K., and Akiskal, H.S. (2005). Reliability and validity of TEMPS-A in a Japanese non-clinical population: Application to unipolar and bipolar depressives. *J Affect Disord*, 85, 83–92.

Matussek, P., and Feil, W.B. (1983). Personality attributes of depressive patients: Results of group comparisons. *Arch Gen Psychiatry*, 40, 783–790.

Mayer-Gross, W., Slater, E., and Roth, M. (1955). *Clinical Psychiatry*. Baltimore: Williams & Wilkins.

McKnight, D.L., Nelson-Grey, R.O., and Gullick, E. (1989). Interactional patterns of bipolar patients and their spouses. *J Psychopathol Behav Assess* 11, 269–289.

Mendlewicz, M.V., Jean-Louis, G., Kelsoe, J.R., and Akiskal, H.S. (2005). A comparison of recovered bipolar patients, healthy relatives of bipolar probands, and normal controls using the short TEMPS-A. *J Affect Disord*, 85(1-2), 147–151.

Merikangas, K.R., and Spiker, D.G. (1982). Assortative mating among in-patients with primary affective disorder. *Psychol Med*, 12(4), 753–764.

Miklowitz, D.J., and Goldstein, M.J. (1997). *Bipolar Disorder: A Family-Focused Treatment Approach*. New York: Guilford Press.

Miklowitz, D.J., Goldstein, M.J., Nuechterlein, K.H., Snyder, K.S., and Mintz, J. (1988). Family factors and the course of bipolar affective disorder. *Arch Gen Psychiatry*, 45(3), 225–231.

Miklowitz, D.J., George, E.L., Richards, J.A., Simoneau, T.L., and Suddath, R.L. (2003). A randomized study of family-focused psychoeducation and pharmacotherapy in the outpatient management of bipolar disorder. *Arch Gen Psychiatry*, 60, 904–912.

Millingen, J. (1831). *Memoirs of the Affairs of Greece: Containing an Account of the Military and Political Events which Occurred in 1823 and Following Years. With Various Anecdotes Relating to Lord Byron, and an Account of His Last Illness and Death*. London: John Rodwell, p. 16.

Millon, T. (1987). *Millon Clinical Multiaxial Inventory-II Manual*. Minneapolis: National Computer Systems.

Mundt, C., Kronmuller, K., and Backenstrass, M. (2000). Interactional styles in bipolar disorder. In A. Marneros, J. Angst (Eds.), *Bipolar Disorders: 100 Years after Manic-Depressive Insanity* (pp. 201–213). London: Kluwer Academic Publishers.

Murphy, D.L., Beigel, A., Weingartner, H., and Bunney, W.E. Jr. (1974). The quantitation of manic behavior. *Mod Probl Pharmacopsychiatry*, 7, 203–220.

Murray, L.G., and Blackburn, I.M. (1974). Personality differences in patients with depressive illness and anxiety neurosis. *Acta Psychiatr Scand*, 50(2), 183–191.

NICHD Early Child Care Research Network. (1999). Chronicity of maternal depressive symptoms, maternal sensitivity, and child functioning at 36 months. *Dev Psychol*, 35(5), 1297–1310.

Nowakowska, C., Strong, C.M., Santosa, C.M., Wang, P.W., and Ketter, T.A., (2005). Temperamental commonalities and differences in euthymic mood disorder patients, creative controls, and healthy controls. *J Affect Disord*, 85, 207–215.

Nurnberger, J. Jr., Guroff, J.J., Hamovit, J., Berrettini, W., and Gershon, E. (1988). A family study of rapid-cycling bipolar illness. *J Affect Disord*, 15(1), 87–91.

O'Connell, R.A., and Mayo, J.A. (1981). A biopsychosocial perspective. *Compr Psychiatry*, 22, 87–93.

O'Connell, R.A., Mayo, J.A., Eng, L.K., Jones, J.S., and Gabel, R.H. (1985). Social support and long-term lithium outcome. *Br J Psychiatry*, 147, 272–275.

O'Connell, R.A., Mayo, J.A., Flatow, L., Cuthbertson, B., and O'Brien, B.E. (1991). Outcome of bipolar disorder on long-term treatment with lithium. *Br J Psychiatry*, 159, 123–129.

Oedegaard, K.J., Neckelmann, D., and Fasmer, O.B. (2006). Type A behaviour differentiates bipolar II from unipolar depressed patients. *J Affect Dis*, 90, 7–13.

Osher, Y., Cloninger, C.R., and Belmaker, R.H. (1996). TPQ in euthymic manic-depressive patients. *J Psychiatr Res*, 30(5), 353–357.

Parker, G., Parker, K., Malhi, G., Wilhelm, K., and Mitchell, P. (2004). Studying personality characteristics in bipolar depressed subjects: How comparator group selection can dictate results. *Acta Psychiatr Scand*, 109, 376–382.

Perlick, D., Clarkin, J.F., Sirey, J., Raue, P., Greenfield, S., Struening, E., and Rosenheck, R. (1999). Burden experienced by care-givers of persons with bipolar affective disorder. *Br J Psychiatry*, 175, 56–62.

Perlick, D.A., Rosenheck, R.R., Clarkin, J.F., Raue, P., and Sirey, J. (2001). Impact of family burden and patient symptom status on clinical outcome in bipolar affective disorder. *J Nerv Ment Dis*, 189(1), 31–37.

Perris, C. (1971). Personality patterns in patients with affective disorders. *Acta Psychiatr Scand Suppl*, 221, 43–45.

Perugi, G., Akiskal, H.S., Lattanzi, L., Cecconi, D., Mastrocinque, C., Patronelli, A., Vignoli, S., and Bemi, E. (1998). The high prevalence of "soft" bipolar (II) features in atypical depression. *Compr Psychiatry*, 39, 63–71.

Peselow, E.D., Sanfilipo, M.P., and Fieve, R.R. (1995). Relationship between hypomania and personality disorders before and after successful treatment. *Am J Psychiatry*, 152(2), 232–238.

Platman, S.R., Plutchik, R., Fieve, R.R., and Lawlor, W.G. (1969). Emotion profiles associated with mania and depression. *Arch Gen Psychiatry*, 20(2), 210–214.

Popescu, C., Totoescu, A., Christodorescu, D., and Ionescu, R. (1985). Personality attributes in unipolar and bipolar affective disorders. *Neurol Psychiatr (Bucur)*, 23(4), 231–242.

Radke-Yarrow, M. (1998). *Children of Depressed Mothers: From Early Childhood to Maturity*. Cambridge, England: Cambridge University Press.

Rado, S. (1928). The problem of melancholia. *Int J Psychoanal*, 9, 420–438.

Romans, S.E., and McPherson, H.M. (1992). The social networks of bipolar affective disorder patients. *J Affect Disord*, 25(4), 221–228.

Rossi, A., Daneluzzo, E., Arduini, L., Di Domenico, M., Pollice, R., and Petruzzi, C. (2001). A factor analysis of signs and symptoms of the manic episode with Bech-Rafaelsen Mania and Melancholia Scales. *J Affect Disord*, 64(2–3), 267–270.

Rowe, C.J., and Daggett, D.R. (1954). Prepsychotic personality traits in manic depressive disease. *J Nerv Ment Dis*, 119, 412–420.

Ruestow, P., Dunner, D.L., Bleecker, B., and Fieve, R.R. (1978). Marital adjustment in primary affective disorder. *Compr Psychiatry*, 19(6), 565–571.

Sauer, H., Richter, P., Czernik, A., Ludwig-Mayerhofer, W., Schöchlin, C., Greil, W., and von Zerssen, D. (1997). Personality differences between patients with major depression and

bipolar disorder—The impact of minor symptoms on self-ratings of personality. *J Affect Disord*, 42, 169–177.

Savitz, J.B., and Ramesar, R.S. (2006). Personality: Is it a viable endophenotype for genetic studies of bipolar affective disorder? *Bipolar Disord*, 8, 322–337.

Schou, M. (1968). Lithium in psychiatric therapy and prophylaxis. *J Psychiatr Res*, 6, 67–95.

Schwartz, D.A. (1961). Some suggestions for a unitary formulation of the manic-depressive reactions. *Psychiatry*, 24, 238–245.

Sheard, M.H. (1971). Effect of lithium on human aggression. *Nature*, 230, 113–114.

Sheard, M.H. (1975). Lithium in the treatment of aggression. *J Nerv Ment Dis*, 160, 108–118.

Simoneau, T.L., Miklowitz, D.J., Richards, J.A., Saleem, R., and George, E.L. (1999). Bipolar disorder and family communication: Effects of a psychoeducational treatment program. *J Abnorm Psychol*, 108(4), 588–597.

Smith, D.J., Muir, W.J., and Blackwood, D.H.R. (2005). Borderline personality disorder characteristics in young adults with recurrent mood disorders: A comparison of bipolar and unipolar depression. *J Affect Dis*, 87, 17–23.

Smith, J.H. (1960). The metaphor of the manic-depressive. *Psychiatry*, 123, 375–383.

Solomon, D.A., Shea, M.T., Leon, A.C., Mueller, T.I., Coryell, W., Maser, J.D., Endicott, J., and Keller, M.B. (1996). Personality traits in subjects with bipolar I disorder in remission. *J Affect Disord*, 40(1–2), 41–48.

Spalt, L. (1975). Sexual behavior and affective disorders. *Dis Nerv Syst*, 36, 974–977.

Stefos, G., Bauwens, F., Staner, L., Pardoen, D., and Mendlewicz, J. (1996). Psychosocial predictors of major affective recurrences in bipolar disorder: A 4-year longitudinal study of patients on prophylactic treatment. *Acta Psychiatr Scand*, 93(6), 420–426.

Stoddard, F.J., Post, R.M., and Bunney, W.E. (1977). Slow and rapid psychobiological alterations in a manic-depressive patient: Clinical phenomenology. *Br J Psychiatry*, 130, 72–78.

Stone, M.H. (1978). Toward early detection of manic-depressive illness in psychoanalytic patients: I. Patients who later develop a manic illness. *Am J Psychother*, 32(3), 427–439.

Strakowski, S.M., Faedda, G.L., Tohen, M., Goodwin, D.C., and Stoll, A.L. (1992). Possible affective-state dependence of the Tridimensional Personality Questionnaire in first-episode psychosis. *Psychiatry Res*, 41(3), 215–226.

Strakowski, S.M., Stoll, A.L., Tohen, M., Faedda, G.L., and Goodwin, D.C. (1993). The Tridimensional Personality Questionnaire as a predictor of six-month outcome in first episode mania. *Psychiatry Res*, 48(1), 1–8.

Strandman, E. (1978). Psychogenic needs in patients with affective disorders. *Acta Psychiatr Scand*, 58(1), 16–29.

Suppes, T., Leverich, G.S., Keck, P.E., Nolen, W.A., Denicoff, K.D., Altshuler, L.L., McElroy, S.L., Rush, A.J., Kupka, R., Frye, M.A., Bickel, M., and Post, R.M. (2001). The Stanley Foundation Bipolar Treatment Outcome Network: II. Demographics and illness characteristics of the first 261 patients. *J Affect Disord*, 67(1–3), 45–59.

Targum, S.D., Dibble, E.D., Davenport, Y.B., and Gershon, E.S. (1981). The Family Attitudes Questionnaire: Patients' and spouses' views of bipolar illness. *Arch Gen Psychiatry*, 38(5), 562–568.

Tohen, M., Waternaux, C.M. and Tsuang, M.T. (1990). Outcome in mania: A 4-year prospective follow-up of 75 patients utilizing survival analysis. *Arch Gen Psychiatry*, 47(12), 1106–1111.

Tuke, D.H. (1892). *A Dictionary of Psychological Medicine.* Philadelphia: P. Blakiston, Son & Co.

Ucok, A., Karaveli, D., Kundakci, T., and Yazici, O. (1998). Comorbidity of personality disorders with bipolar mood disorders. *Compr Psychiatry*, 39(2), 72–74.

Vieta, E., Colom, F., Martinez-Aran, A., Benabarre, A., and Gasto, C. (1999). Personality disorders in bipolar II patients. *J Nerv Ment Dis*, 187(4), 245–248.

von Zerssen, D. (1977). Premorbid personality and affective psychoses. In G.D. Burrows (Ed.), *Handbook of Studies on Depression*. Amsterdam: Excerpta Medica.

Watson, D., Clark, L.A., and Harkness, A.R. (1994). Structures of personality and their relevance to psychopathology. *J Abnorm Psychol*, 103(1), 18–31.

Weissman, M.M. (1987). Advances in psychiatric epidemiology: Rates and risks for major depression. *Am J Public Health*, 77(4), 445–451.

Weissman, M.M. (1993). The epidemiology of personality disorders: A 1990 update. *J Pers Disord* 7(Suppl. 1), 44–62.

Weissman, M.M., and Paykel, E.S. (1974). *The Depressed Woman: A Study of Social Relationships*. Chicago: University of Chicago Press.

Weissman, M.M, Warner, V., Wickramaratne, P., Moreau, D., and Olfson, M. (1997). Offspring of depressed parents: 10 years later. *Arch Gen Psychiatry*, 54, 932–940.

Weissman, M.M., Markowitz, J.C., and Klerman, G.L. (2000). *Comprehensive Guide to Interpersonal Psychotherapy*. New York: Basic Books.

Wetzler, S., Khadivi, A., and Oppenheim, S. (1995). The psychological assessment of depression: Unipolars versus bipolars. *J Pers Assess*, 65(3), 557–566.

Whisman, M.A. (2001). The association between depression and marital dissatisfaction. In S.R.H. Beach (Ed.), *Marital and Family Processes in Depression: A Scientific Foundation for Clinical Practice* (pp. 3–24). Washington, DC: American Psychological Association.

White, K., Bohart, R., Whipple, K., and Boyd, J. (1979). Lithium effects on normal subjects: Relationships to plasma and RBC lithium levels. *Int Pharamacopsychiatry*, 14, 176–183.

Widiger, T., and Rogers, J.H. (1989). Prevalence and comorbidity of personality disorders. *Psychiatric Ann*, 19, 132–136.

Wilson, D.C. (1951). Families of manic depressives. *Dis Nerv Sys*, 12, 362–369.

Winokur, G., Clayton, P.J., and Reich, T. (1969). *Manic Depressive Illness*. St. Louis: CV Mosby.

Winters, K.C., and Neale, J.M. (1985). Mania and low self-esteem. *J Aborm Psychol*, 94, 282–290.

Worland, J., Lander, H., and Hesselbrock, V. (1979). Psychological evaluation of clinical disturbance in children at risk for psychopathology. *J Abnorm Psychol*, 88(1), 13–26.

Yan, L.J., Hammen, C., Cohen, A.N., Daley, S.E., and Henry, R.M. (2004). Expressed emotion versus relationship quality variables in the prediction of recurrence in bipolar patients. *J Affect Disord*, 83, 199–206.

Yazici, O., Kora, K., Ucok, A., Tunali, D., and Turan, N. (1999). Predictors of lithium prophylaxis in bipolar patients. *J Affect Disord*, 55(2–3), 133–142.

Young, L.T., Bagby, R.M., Cooke, R.G., Parker, J.D., Levitt, A.J., and Joffe, R.T. (1995). A comparison of Tridimensional Personality Questionnaire dimensions in bipolar disorder and unipolar depression. *Psychiatry Res*, 58(2), 139–143.

CHAPTER 11

Ahearn, E.P., and Carroll, B.J. (1996). Short-term variability of mood ratings in unipolar and bipolar depressed patients. *J Affect Disord*, 36(3–4), 107–115.

Akiskal, H.S., Hantouche, E.G., Bourgeois, M.L., Azorin, J.M., Sechter, D., Allilaire, J.F., Chatenet-Duchene, L., and Lancrenon, S. (2001). Toward a refined phenomenology of mania: Combining clinician-assessment and self-report in the French EPIMAN study. *J Affect Disord*, 67(1–3), 89–96.

Akiskal, H.S., Mendlowicz, M.V., Jean-Louis, G., Rapaport, M.H., Kelsoe, J.R., Gillin, J.C., and Smith, T.L. (2005a). TEMPS-A: Validation of a short version of a self-rated instrument designed to measure variations in temperament. *J Affect Disord*, 85, 45–52.

Akiskal, H.S., Akiskal, K.K., Haykal, R.F., Manning J.S., and Connor, P.D. (2005b). TEMPS-A: Progress towards validation of a self-rated clinical version of the Temperament Evaluation of the Memphis, Pisa, Paris, and San Diego Autoquestionnaire. *J Affect Disord*, 85, 3–16.

Akiskal, H.S., Akiskal, K., Allilaire, J.-F., Azorin, J.-M., Bourgeois, M.L., Sechter, D., Fraud, J.-P., Chatenêt-Duchêne, L., Lancrenon, S., Perugi, G., and Hantouche, E.G. (2005c). Validating affective temperaments in their subaffective and socially positive attributes: Psychometric, clinical and familial data from a French national study. *J Affect Disord*, 85, 29–36.

Akiyama, T., Tsuda, H., Matsumoto, S., Miyake, Y., Kawamura, Y., Noda, T., Akiskal, K.K., and Akiskal, H.S. (2005). The proposed factor structure of temperament and personality in Japan: Combining traits from TEMPS-A and MPT. *J Affect Disord*, 85, 93–100.

Altman, E.G., Hedeker, D.R., Janicak, P.G., Peterson, J.L., and Davis, J.M. (1994). The Clinician-Administered Rating Scale for Mania (CARS-M): Development, reliability, and validity. *Biol Psychiatry*, 36(2), 124–134.

Altman, E.G., Hedeker, D., Peterson, J.L., and Davis, J.M. (1997). The Altman Self-Rating Mania Scale. *Biol Psychiatry*, 42(10), 948–955.

Altman, E., Hedeker, D., Peterson, J.L., and Davis, J.M. (2001). A comparative evaluation of three self-rating scales for acute mania. *Biol Psychiatry*, 50(6), 468–471.

Ambrosini, P.J. (2000). A review of pharmacotherapy of major depression in children and adolescents. *Psychiatr Serv*, 51(5), 627–633.

Asberg, M., Montgomery, S.A., Perris, C., Schalling, D., and Sedvall, G. (1978). A comprehensive psychopathological rating scale. *Acta Psychiatr Scand Suppl* (271), 5–27.

Baldessarini, R.J. (2003). Assessment of treatment response in mania: Commentary and new findings. *Bipolar Disord*, 5(2), 79–84.

Bauer, M.S., Crits-Christoph, P., Ball, W.A., Dewees, E., McAllister, T., Alahi, P., Cacciola, J., and Whybrow, P.C. (1991). Independent assessment of manic and depressive symptoms by self-rating: Scale characteristics and implications for the study of mania. *Arch Gen Psychiatry*, 48(9), 807–812.

Bauer, M.S., Vojta, C., Kinosian, B., Altshuler, L., and Glick, H. (2000). The Internal State Scale: Replication of its discriminating abilities in a multisite, public sector sample. *Bipolar Disord*, 2(4), 340–346.

Bech, P. (1981). Rating scales for affective disorders: Their validity and consistency. *Acta Psychiatr Scand Suppl*, 295, 1–101.

Bech, P. (2002). The Bech-Rafaelsen Mania Scale in clinical trials of therapies for bipolar disorder: A 20-year review of its use as an outcome measure. *CNS Drugs*, 16(1), 47–63.

Bech, P., and Rafaelsen, O.J. (1980). The use of rating scales exemplified by a comparison of the Hamilton and the Bech-Rafaelsen Melancholia Scale. *Acta Psychiatr Scand Suppl*, 285, 128–132.

Bech, P., Bolwig, T.G., Kramp, P., and Rafaelsen, O.J. (1979). The Bech-Rafaelsen Mania Scale and the Hamilton Depression Scale. *Acta Psychiatr Scand*, 59(4), 420–430.

Bech, P., Kastrup, M., and Rafaelsen, O.J. (1986). Mini-compendium of rating scales for states of anxiety depression mania schizophrenia with corresponding DSM-III syndromes. *Acta Psychiatr Scand Suppl*, 326, 1–37.

Bech, P., Rasmussen, N.A., Olsen, L.R., Noerholm, V., and Abildgaard, W. (2001). The sensitivity and specificity of the Major Depression Inventory, using the Present State Examination as the index of diagnostic validity. *J Affect Disord*, 66(2–3), 159–164.

Beck, A.T., Ward, C.H., Mendelsohn, M., Mock, J., and Erbaugh, J. (1961). An inventory for measuring depression. *Arch Gen Psychiatry*, 4, 561–571.

Beck, A.T., Steer, R.A., and Garbin, M.G. (1988). Psychometric properties of the Beck Depression Inventory: Twenty-five years of evaluation. *Clin Psychol Rev*, 8, 77–100.

Beck, A.T., Steer, R.A., and Brown, G.K. (1996). *Manual for the BDI-II*. San Antonio, TX: The Psychological Corporation.

Beigel, A., and Murphy, D.L. (1971). Assessing clinical characteristics of the manic state. *Am J Psychiatry*, 128(6), 688–694.

Beigel, A., Murphy, D.L., and Bunney, W.E. (1971). The Manic-State Rating Scale: Scale construction, reliability, and validity. *Arch Gen Psychiatry*, 25, 256–262.

Berk, M., Malhi, G.S., Mitchell, P.B., Cahill, C.M., Carman, A.C., Hadzi-Pavlovic, D., Hawkins, M.T., and Tohen, M. (2004). Scale matters: The need for a Bipolar Depression Rating Scale (BDRS). *Acta Psychiatr Scand*, 100(Suppl. 422), 39–45.

Blackburn, I.M., Loudon, J.B., and Ashworth, C.M. (1977). A new scale for measuring mania. *Psychol Med*, 7(3), 453–458.

Bosc, M., Dubini, A., and Polin, V. (1997). Development and validation of a social functioning scale, the Social Adaptation Self-evaluation Scale. *Eur Neuropsychopharmacol*, 7(Suppl. 1), S57–S70, discussion S71–S73.

Boyle, M.H., and Pickles, A.R. (1997). Influence of maternal depressive symptoms on ratings of childhood behavior. *J Abnorm Child Psychol*, 25(5), 399–412.

Braunig, P., Shugar, G., and Kruger, S. (1996). An investigation of the Self-Report Manic Inventory as a diagnostic and severity scale for mania. *Compr Psychiatry*, 37, 52–55.

Bunney, W.E., and Hamburg, D.A. (1963). Methods for reliable longitudinal observation of behavior. *Arch Gen Psychiatry*, 9, 280–294.

Burnam, M.A., Wells, K.B., Leake, B., and Landsverk, J. (1988). Development of a brief screening instrument for detecting depressive disorders. *Med Care*, 26, 775–789.

Carney, M.W.P., Roth, M., and Garside, R.F. (1965). The diagnosis of depressive syndromes and the prediction of E.C.T. response. *Br J Psychiatry*, 111, 659–674.

Carroll, B.J. (1991). Psychopathology and neurobiology of manic-depressive disorders. In B.J. Carroll, J.E. Barrett (Eds.), *Psychopathology and the Brain* (pp. 265–285). New York: Raven Press.

Carroll, B. (1998). *Carroll Depression Scales-Revised (CDS-R): Technical Manual*. Toronto: Multi-Health Systems.

Carroll, B.J., Feinberg, M., Smouse, P.E., Rawson, S.G., and Greden, J.F. (1981). The Carroll rating scale for depression: I. Development, reliability and validation. *Br J Psychiatry*, 138, 194–200.

Chapman, L.J., Chapman, J.P., Numbers, J.S., Edell, W.S., Carpenter, B.N., and Beckfield, D. (1984). Impulsive nonconformity as a trait contributing to the prediction of psychotic-like and schizotypal symptoms. *J Nerv Ment Dis*, 172(11), 681–691.

Cooke, R.G., Kruger, S., and Shugar, G. (1996). Comparative evaluation of two self-report Mania Rating Scales. *Biol Psychiatry*, 40(4), 279–283.

Corruble, E., Legrand, J.M., Duret, C., Charles, G., and Guelfi, J.D. (1999). IDS-C and IDS-SR: Psychometric properties in depressed in-patients. *J Affect Disord*, 56(2–3), 95–101.

Craddock, N., Jones, I., Kirov, G., and Jones, L. (2004). The Bipolar Affective Disorder Dimension Scale (BADDS): A dimensional scale for rating lifetime psychopathology in bipolar spectrum disorders. *BMC Psychiatry*, 4, 19.

Cronholm, B., and Ottosson, J.O. (1996). Experimental studies of the therapeutic action of electroconvulsive therapy in endogenous depression: The role of the electrical stimulation and of the seizure studied by variation of stimulus intensity and modification by lidocaine of seizure discharge. *Acta Psychiatr Neurol Scand Suppl*, 12 (3), 172–194.

Das, A.K., Olfson, M., Gameroff, M.J., Pilowsky, D.J., Blanco, C., Feder, A., Gross, R., Neria, Y., Lantigua, R., Shea, S., and Weissman, M.M. (2005). Screening for bipolar disorder in a primary care practice. *JAMA*, 23(293), 8.

Davidson, J., Turnbull, C.D., Strickland, R., Miller, R., and Graves, K. (1986). The Montgomery-Asberg Depression Scale: Reliability and validity. *Acta Psychiatr Scand*, 73(5), 544–548.

Denicoff, K.D., Smith-Jackson, E.E., Disney, E.R., Suddath, R.L., Leverich, G.S., and Post, R.M. (1997). Preliminary evidence of the reliability and validity of the prospective life-chart methodology (LCM-p). *J Psychiatr Res*, 31(5), 593–603.

Depue, R.A., Slater, J.F., Wolfstetter-Kausch, H., Klein, D., Goplerud, E., and Farr, D. (1981). A behavioral paradigm for identifying persons at risk for bipolar depressive disorder: A conceptual framework and five validation studies. *J Abnorm Psychol*, 90(5), 381–437.

Depue, R.A., Krauss, S., Spoont, M.R., and Arbisi, P. (1989). General behavior inventory identification of unipolar and bipolar affective conditions in a nonclinical university population. *J Abnorm Psychol*, 98(2), 117–126.

Eckblad, M., and Chapman, L.J. (1986). Development and validation of a scale for hypomanic personality. *J Abnorm Psychol*, 95(3), 214–222.

Ellicott, A., Hammen, C., Gitlin, M., Brown, G., and Jamison, K. (1990). Life events and the course of bipolar disorder. *Am J Psychiatry*, 147(9), 1194–1198.

Endicott, J., Spitzer, R.L., Fleiss, J.L., and Cohen, J. (1976). The global assessment scale: A procedure for measuring overall severity of psychiatric disturbance. *Arch Gen Psychiatry*, 33(6), 766–771.

Erfurth, A., Gerlach, A.L., Michael, N., Boenigk, I., Hellweg, I., Signoretta, S., Akiskal, K., and Akiskal, H.S. (2005a). Distribution and gender effects of the subscales of a German version of the temperament autoquestionnaire brief TEMPS-M in a university student population. *J Affect Disord*, 85, 71–76.

Erfurth, A., Gerlach, A.L., Hellweg, I., Boenigk, I., Michael, N., and Akiskal, H.S. (2005b). Studies on a German (Münster) version of the temperament auto-questionnaire TEMPS-A: Construction and validation of the brief TEMPS-M. *J Affect Disord*, 85, 53–69.

Feighner, J.P., Meredith, C.H., Stern, W.C., Hendrickson, G., and Miller, L.L. (1984). A double-blind study of bupropion and placebo in depression. *Am J Psychiatry*, 141(4), 525–529.

Feinberg, M., Carroll, B.J., Smouse, P.E., and Rawson, S.G. (1981). The Carroll rating scale for depression: III. Comparison with other rating instruments. *Br J Psychiatry*, 138, 205–209.

Fergusson, D.M., Lynskey, M.T., and Horwood, L.J. (1993). The effect of maternal depression on maternal ratings of child behavior. *J Abnorm Child Psychol*, 21(3), 245–269.

Findling, R.L., Youngstrom, E.A., Danielson, C.K., DelPorto-Bedoya, D., Papish-David, R., Townsend, L., and Calabrese, J.R. (2002). Clinical decision-making using the General Behavior Inventory in juvenile bipolarity. *Bipolar Disord*, 4(1), 34–42.

Folstein, M.F., and Luria, R. (1973). Reliability, validity, and clinical application of the Visual Analogue Mood Scale. *Psychol Med*, 3(4), 479–486.

Frank, E., Swartz, H.A., Mallinger, A.G., Thase, M.E., Weaver, E.V., and Kupfer, D.J. (1999). Adjunctive psychotherapy for bipolar disorder: Effects of changing treatment modality. *J Abnorm Psychol*, 108(4), 579–587.

Furukawa, T., Anraku, K., Hiroe, T., Takahashi, K., Kitamura, T., Hirai, T., and Iida, M. (1997). Screening for depression among first-visit psychiatric patients: Comparison of different scoring methods for the Center for Epidemiologic Studies Depression Scale using receiver operating characteristic analyses. *Psychiatry Clin Neurosci*, 51(2), 71–78.

Geller, B., Zimerman, B., Williams, M., Bolhofner, K., Craney, J.L., DelBello, M.P., and Soutullo, C. (2001). Reliability of the Washington University in St. Louis Kiddie Schedule for Affective Disorders and Schizophrenia (WASH-U-KSADS) mania and rapid cycling sections. *J Am Acad Child Adolesc Psychiatry*, 40(4), 450–455.

Ghaemi, S.N., Miller, C.J., Berv, D.A., Klugman, J., Rosenquist, K.J., and Pies, R.W. (2005). Sensitivity and specificity of a new bipolar spectrum diagnostic scale. *J Affect Disord*, 84, 273–277.

Gitlin, M.J., Swendsen, J., Heller, T.L., and Hammen, C. (1995). Relapse and impairment in bipolar disorder. *Am J Psychiatry*, 152(11), 1635–1640.

Glick, H.A., McBride, L., and Bauer, M.S. (2003). A manic-depressive symptom self-report in optical scanable format. *Bipolar Disorders*, 5(5), 366–369.

Gracious, B., Youngstrom, E., Findling, R., and Calabrese, J. (2002). Discriminative validity of a parent version of the Young Mania Rating Scale. *J Am Acad Child Adolesc Psychiatry*, 41, 1350–1359.

Hamilton, M. (1960). A rating scale for depression. *J Neurol Neurosurg Psychiatry*, 12, 56–62.

Hamilton, M. (1976). Clinical evaluation of depressions: Clinical criteria and rating scales, including a Guttman Scale. In D.M. Gallant, G.M. Simpson (Eds.), *Depression: Behavioral, Biochemical, Diagnostic and Treatment Concepts* (pp. 155–179). New York: Spectrum Publications.

Hamilton, M. (1988). Assessment of depression and mania. In A. Georgotas, R. Cancro (Eds.), *Depression and Mania* (pp. 625–637). New York: Elsevier.

Hammen, C., Ellicott, A., Gitlin, M., and Jamison, K.R. (1989). Sociotropy/autonomy and vulnerability to specific life events in patients with unipolar depression and bipolar disorders. *J Abnorm Psychol*, 98(2), 154–160.

Hammen, C., Davila, J., Brown, G., Gitlin, M., and Ellicott, A. (1992). Stress as a mediator of the effects of psychiatric history on severity of unipolar depression. *J Abnorm Psychol*, 101, 45–52.

Hammen, C., Gitlin, M., and Altshuler, L. (2000). Predictors of work adjustment in bipolar I patients: A naturalistic longitudinal follow-up. *J Consult Clin Psychol*, 68(2), 220–225.

Hantouche, E.G., Allilaire, J.P., Bourgeois, M.L., Azorin, J.M., Sechter, D., Chatenet-Duchene, L., Lancrenon, S., and Akiskal, H.S. (2001). The feasibility of self-assessment of dysphoric mania in the French national EPIMAN study. *J Affect Disord*, 67(1–3), 97–103.

Harrow, M., Goldberg, J.F., Grossman, L.S., and Meltzer, H.Y. (1990). Outcome in manic disorders: A naturalistic follow-up study. *Arch Gen Psychiatry*, 47(7), 665–671.

Hayes, M.H.S., and Patterson, D.G. (1921). Experimental development of the graphic rating method. *Psychol Bull*, 18, 98–99.

Hays, R.D., Wells, K.B., Sherbourne, C.D., Rogers, W., and Spritzer, K. (1995). Functioning and well-being outcomes of patients with depression compared with chronic general medical illnesses. *Arch Gen Psychiatry*, 52(1), 11–19.

Hedlund, J.L., and Vieweg, B.W. (1979). The Hamilton Rating Scale for Depression: A comprehensive review. *J Operational Psychiatry*, 10, 149–165.

Hett, W.S. (Transl.) (1936). *Aristotle, Problems II: Books XXII-XXXVIII.* Cambridge, MA: Harvard University Press, pp. 155–157.

Hirschfeld, R.M. (2002). The mood disorder questionnaire: A simple, patient-rated screening instrument for bipolar disorder. *Prim Care Companion J Clin Psychiatry*, 4(1), 9–11.

Hirschfeld, R.M., Williams, J.B., Spitzer, R.L., Calabrese, J.R., Flynn, L., Keck, P.E. Jr., Lewis, L., McElroy, S.L., Post, R.M., Rapport, D.J., Russell, J.M., Sachs, G.S., and Zajecka, J. (2000). Development and validation of a screening instrument for bipolar spectrum disorder: The Mood Disorder Questionnaire. *Am J Psychiatry*, 157(11), 1873–1875.

Hirschfeld, R.M., Calabrese, J.R., Weissman, M.M., Reed, M., Davies, M.A., Frye, M.A., Keck, P.E. Jr., Lewis, L., McElroy, S.L., McNulty, J.P., and Wagner, K.D. (2003a). Screening for bipolar disorder in the community. *J Clin Psychiatry*, 64(1), 53–59.

Hirschfeld, R.M., Holzer, C., Calabrese, J.R., Weissman, M., Reed, M., Davies, M., Frye, M.A., Keck, P., McElroy, S., Lewis, L., Tierce, J., Wagner, K.D., and Hazard, E. (2003b). Validity of the mood disorder questionnaire: A general population study. *Am J Psychiatry*, 160(1), 178–180.

Hofmann, B.U., and Meyer, T.D. (2006). Mood fluctuations in people putatively at risk for bipolar disorders. *Br J Clin Psychol*, 45, 105–110.

Jones, S., Mansell, W., and Waller, L. (2006). Appraisal of hypomania-relevant experiences: Development of a questionnaire to assess positive self-dispositional appraisals in bipolar and behavioural high risk samples. *J Affect Disord*, 93, 19–28.

Judd, L.L., Akiskal, H.S., Zeller, P.J., Paulus, M., Leon, A.C., Maser, J.D., Endicott, J., Coryell, W., Kunovac, J.L., Mueller, T.I., Rice, J.P., and Keller, M.B. (2000). Psychosocial disability during the long-term course of unipolar major depressive disorder. *Arch Gen Psychiatry*, 57(4), 375–380.

Katz, M.M., and Itil, T.M. (1974). Video methodology for research in psychopathology and psychopharmacology: Rationale and application. *Arch Gen Psychiatry*, 31(2), 204–210.

Keller, M.B., Lavori, P.W., Friedman, B., Nielsen, E., Endicott, J., McDonald-Scott, P., and Andreasen, N.C. (1987). The Longitudinal Interval Follow-up Evaluation: A comprehensive method for assessing outcome in prospective longitudinal studies. *Arch Gen Psychiatry*, 44(6), 540–548.

Khan, A., Brodhead, A.E., and Kolts, R.L. (2004). Relative sensitivity of the Montgomery-Asberg Depression Rating Scale, the Hamilton Depression Rating Scale and the Clinical Global Impressions Rating Scale in antidepressant clinical trials: A replication analysis. *Int Clin Psychopharmacol*, 19(3), 157–160.

Klein, D.N., and Depue, R.A. (1984). Continued impairment in persons at risk for bipolar affective disorder: Results of a 19-month follow-up study. *J Abnorm Psychol*, 93(3), 345–347.

Klein, D.N., Depue, R.A., and Slater, J.F. (1986). Inventory identification of cyclothymia: IX. Validation in offspring of bipolar I patients. *Arch Gen Psychiatry*, 43(5), 441–445.

Klein, D.N., Lewinsohn, P.M., and Seeley, J.R. (1996). Hypomanic personality traits in a community sample of adolescents. *J Affect Disord*, 38(2–3), 135–143.

Kovacs, M. (1981). Rating scales to assess depression in school-aged children. *Acta Paedopsychiatrica*, 46, 305–315.

Kraepelin, E. (1921). *Manic-Depressive Insanity and Paranoia.* R.M. Barclay (Translator), G.M. Robertson (Ed.). Edinburgh, Scotland: E & S Livingstone.

Kramlinger, K.G., and Post, R.M. (1996). Ultra-rapid and ultradian cycling in bipolar affective illness. *Br J Psychiatry*, 168(3), 314–323.

Kwapil, T.R., Miller, M.B., Zinser, M.C., Chapman, L.J., Chapman, J., and Eckblad, M. (2000). A longitudinal study of high scorers on the hypomanic personality scale. *J Abnorm Psychol*, 109(2), 222–226.

Leverich, G.S., Nolen, W.A., Rush, A.J., McElroy, S.L., Keck, P.E., Denicoff, K.D., Suppes, T., Altshuler, L.L., Kupka, R., Kramlinger, K.G., and Post, R.M. (2001). The Stanley Foundation Bipolar Treatment Outcome Network: I. Longitudinal methodology. *J Affect Disord*, 67(1–3), 33–44.

Licht, R.W., and Jensen, J. (1997). Validation of the Bech-Rafaelsen Mania Scale using latent structure analysis. *Acta Psychiatr Scand*, 96, 67–72.

Livianos-Aldana, L., and Rojo-Moreno, L. (2001). Rating and quantification of manic syndromes. *Acta Psychiatr Scand Suppl*, (409), 2–33.

Lorr, M. (1974). Assessing psychotic behavior by the IMPS. *Mod Probl Pharmacopsychiatry*, 7(0), 50–63.

Loudon, J.B., Blackburn, I.M., and Ashworth, C.M. (1977). A study of the symptomatology and course of manic illness using a new scale. *Psychol Med*, 7(4), 723–729.

Lubin, B. (1994). *State Trait-Dependent Adjective Check Lists: Professional Manual.* Odessa, FL: Psychological Assessment Resources.

Luria, R.E. (1975). The validity and reliability of the visual analogue mood scale. *J Psychiatr Res*, 12(1), 51–57.

Mansell, W., and Jones, S.H. (2006). The Brief-HAPPI: A questionnaire to assess cognitions that distinguish between individuals with a diagnosis of bipolar disorder and non-clinical controls. *J Affect Disord*, 93, 29–34.

Matsumoto, S., Akiyama, T., Tsuda, H., Miyake, Y., Kawamura, Y., Noda, T., Akiskal, K.K., and Akiskal, H.S. (2005). Reliability and validity of TEMPS-A in a Japanese non-clinical population: Application to unipolar and bipolar depressives. *J Affect Disord*, 85, 85–92.

Mendels, J., Weinstein, N., and Cochrane, C. (1972). The relationship between depression and anxiety. *Arch Gen Psychiatry*, 27(5), 649–653.

Mendlowicz, M.V., Akiskal, H.S., Kelsoe, J.R., Rapaport, M.H., Jean-Louis, G., and Gillin, J.C. (2005). Temperament in the clinical differentiation of depressed bipolar and unipolar major depressive patients. *J Affect Disord*, 84, 219–223.

Meyer, T.D., and Hautzinger, M. (2003). Screening for bipolar disorders using the Hypomanic Personality Scale. *J Affect Disord*, 75, 149–154.

Mintz, J., Mintz, L.I., Arruda, M.J., and Hwang, S.S. (1992). Treatments of depression and the functional capacity to work. *Arch Gen Psychiatry*, 49(10), 761–768.

Montgomery, S.A., and Asberg, M. (1979). A new depression scale designed to be sensitive to change. *Br J Psychiatry*, 134, 382–389.

Montgomery, S., Asberg, M., Jornestedt, L., Thoren, P., Traskman, L., McAuley, R., Montgomery, D., and Shaw, P. (1978a). Reliability of the CPRS between the disciplines of psychiatry, general practice, nursing and psychology in depressed patients. *Acta Psychiatr Scand Suppl*, 271, 29–32.

Montgomery, S., Asberg, M., Traskman, L., and Montgomery, D. (1978b). Cross cultural studies on the use of CPRS in English and Swedish depressed patients. *Acta Psychiatr Scand Suppl*, (271), 33–37.

Murphy, D.L., Beigel, A., Weingartner, H., Bunney, W.E. Jr. (1974). The quantitation of manic behavior. *Mod Probl Pharmacopsychiatry*, 7(0), 203–220.

Murphy D.L., Pickar D., and Alterman, I.S. (1982). Methods for the quantitative assessment of depressive and manic behavior. In E.I. Burdock, A. Sudilovsky, S. Gershon (Eds.), *The Behavior of Psychiatric Patients: Quantitative Techniques for Evaluation* (pp. 355–392). New York: Marcel Dekker.

Nezu, A.M., Ronan, G.F., Meadows, E.A., and McClure, K.S. (2000). *Practitioner's Guide to Empirically Based Measures of Depression.* New York: Kluwer Academic/Plenum Publishers.

Paykel, E.S., and Prusoff, B.A. (1973). Response set and observer set in the assessment of depressed patients. *Psychol Med*, 3(2), 209–216.

Paykel, E.S., and Weissman, M.M. (1973). Social adjustment and depression: A longitudinal study. *Arch Gen Psychiatry*, 28(5), 659–663.

Paykel, E.S., Prusoff, B.A., Klerman, G.L., and DiMascio, A. (1973). Self-report and clinical interview ratings in depression. *J Nerv Ment Dis*, 156(3), 166–182.

Perris, C. (1979). Reliability and validity studies of the comprehensive Psychopathological Rating Scale (CPRS). *Prog Neuropsychopharmacol*, 3(4), 413–421.

Petterson, U., Fyro, B., and Sedvall, G. (1973). A new scale for the longitudinal rating of manic states. *Acta Psychiatr Scand*, 49(3), 248–256.

Phelps, J.R., and Ghaemi, S.N. (2006). Improving the diagnosis of bipolar disorder: Predictive value of screening tests. *J Affect Disord*, 92, 141–148.

Pinard, G., and Tetreault, L. (1974). Concerning semantic problems in psychological evaluation. *Mod Probl Pharmacopsychiatry*, 7(0), 8–22.

Platman, S.R., Plutchik, R., Fieve, R.R., and Lawlor, W.G. (1969). Emotion profiles associated with mania and depression. *Arch Gen Psychiatry*, 20(2), 210–214.

Plutchik, R., Platman, S.R., Tilles, R., and Fieve, R.R. (1970). Construction and evaluation of a test for measuring mania and depression. *J Clin Psychol*, 26(4), 499–503.

Prusoff, B.A., Klerman, G.L., and Paykel, E.S. (1972a). Pitfalls in the self-report assessment of depression. *Can Psychiatr Assoc J*, 17(2), SS101.

Prusoff, B.A., Klerman, G.L., and Paykel, E.S. (1972b). Concordance between clinical assessments and patients' self-report in depression. *Arch Gen Psychiatry*, 26(6), 546–552.

Radloff, L.S. (1977). The CED-D Scale: A self-report depression scale for research in the general population. *Appl Psychol Measure*, 1, 385–401.

Rafaelsen, O.J., Bech, P., Bolwig, T.G., Kramp P., and Gjerris, A. (1980). The Bech-Rafaelsen combined rating scale for mania and melancholia. In K. Achte, V. Aalberg, J. Lonnqvist (Eds.), *Psychopathology of Depression: Proceedings of the Symposium by the Section of Clinical Psychopathology of the World Psychiatric Association* (pp. 327–331). Helsinki: Psychiatric Fennica.

Raskin, A., Schulterbrandt, J.G., Reatig, N., and McKeon, J.J. (1970). Differential response to chlorpromazine, imipramine, and placebo: A study of subgroups of hospitalized depressed patients. *Arch Gen Psychiatry*, 23(2), 164–173.

Reichart, C.G., van der Ende, J., Wals, M., Hillegers, M.H.J., Nolen, W.A., Ormel, J., and Verhulst, F.C. (2005). The use of the GBI as predictor of bipolar disorder in a population of adolescent offspring of parents with a bipolar disorder. *J Affect Disord*, 89, 147–155.

Renouf, A.G., and Kovacs, M. (1994). Concordance between mothers' reports and children's self-reports of depressive symptoms: A longitudinal study. *J Am Acad Child Adolesc Psychiatry*, 33(2), 208–216.

Reynolds, W.M., and Kobak, K.A. (1995). *Hamilton Depression Inventory (HDI): Professional Manual*. Odessa, FL: Psychological Assessment Resources.

Reynolds, W.M., and Kobak, K.A. (1998). *Reynolds Depression Screening Inventory: Professional Manual*. Odessa, FL: Psychological Assessment Resources.

Richters, J.E. (1992). Depressed mothers as informants about their children: A critical review of the evidence for distortion. *Psychol Bull*, 112(3), 485–499.

Rickels, K., Gordon, P.E., Mecklenburg, R., Sablosky, L., Whalen, E.M., and Dion, H. (1968). Iprindole in neurotic depressed general practice patients: A controlled study. *Psychosomatics*, 9(4), 208–214.

Ronan, G.F., Dreer, L.E., and Dollard, K.M. (2000). Measuring patient symptom change on rural psychiatry units: Utility of the symptom checklist-90 revised. *J Clin Psychiatry*, 61(7), 493–497.

Rossi, A., Daneluzzo, E., Arduini, L., Di Domenico, M., Pollice, R., and Petruzzi, C. (2001). A factor analysis of signs and symptoms of the manic episode with Bech-Rafaelsen Mania and Melancholia Scales, *J Affect Disord* 64(2–3): 267–270.

Roth, M., Gurney, C., and Mountjoy, C.Q. (1983). The newcastle rating scales. *Acta Psychiatr Scand Suppl*, 310, 42–54.

Rouget, W.B., Gervasoni, N., Dubuis, V., Gex-Fabry, M., Bondolfi, G., and Aubry, J.M. (2005). Screening for bipolar disorders using a French version of the Mood Disorder Questionnaire (MDQ). *J Affect Disord*, 88, 103–108.

Roy-Byrne, P., Post, R.M., Uhde, T.W., Porcu, T., and Davis, D. (1985). The longitudinal course of recurrent affective illness: Life chart data from research patients at the NIMH. *Acta Psychiatr Scand Suppl*, 317, 1–34.

Rush, A.J., Giles, D.E., Schlesser, M.A., Fulton, C.L., Weissenburger, J., and Burns, C. (1986). The Inventory for Depressive Symptomatology (IDS): Preliminary findings. *Psychiatry Res*, 18(1), 65–87.

Rush, A.J., Giles, D.E., Schlesser, M.A., Orsulak, P.J., Parker, C.R. Jr., Weissenburger, J.E., Crowley, G.T., Khatami, M., and Vasavada, N. (1996a). The dexamethasone suppression test in patients with mood disorders. *J Clin Psychiatry*, 57(10), 470–484.

Rush, A.J., Gullion, C.M., Basco, M.R., Jarrett, R.B., and Trivedi, M.H. (1996b). The Inventory of Depressive Symptomatology (IDS): Psychometric properties. *Psychol Med*, 26(3), 477–486.

Rush, A.J., Trivedi, M.H., Ibrahim, H.M., Carmody, T.J., Arnow, B., Klein, D.N., Markowitz, J.C., Ninan, P.T., Kornstein, S., Manber, R., Thase, M.E., Kocsis, J.H., and Keller, M.B. (2003). The 16-item Quick Inventory of Depressive Symptomatology (QIDS), clinician rating (QIDS-C), and self-report (QIDS-SR): A psychometric evaluation in patients with chronic major depression. *Biol Psychiatry*, 54(5), 573–583.

Scharer, L.O., Hartweg, V., Valerius, G., Graf, M., Hoern, M., Biedermann, C., Walser, S., Boensch, A., Dittmann, S., Forsthoff, A., Hummel, B., Grunze, H., and Walden, J. (2002). Life charts on a palmtop computer: First results of a feasibility study with an electronic diary for bipolar patients. *Bipolar Disord*, 4(Suppl. 1), 107–108.

Schou, M. (1979). Artistic productivity and lithium prophylaxis in manic-depressive illness. *Br J Psychiatry*, 135, 97–103.

Secunda, S.K., Katz, M.M., Swann, A., Koslow, S.H., Maas, J.W., Chuang, S., and Croughan, J. (1985). Mania: Diagnosis, state measurement and prediction of treatment response. *J Affect Disord*, 8(2), 113–121.

Shaffer, D., Fisher, P., Lucas, C.P., Dulcan, M.K., and Schwab-Stone, M.E. (2000). NIMH Diagnostic Interview Schedule for Children Version IV (NIMH DISC-IV): Description, differences from previous versions, and reliability of some common diagnoses. *J Am Acad Child Adolesc Psychiatry*, 39(1), 28–38.

Shugar, G., Schertzer, S., Toner, B., and DiGasbarro, I. (1992). Development, use, and factor analysis of a self-report inventory for mania. *Comprehensive Psychiatry*, 33(5), 325–331.

Smouse, P.E., Feinberg, M., Carroll, B.J., Park, M.H., and Rawson, S.G. (1981). The Carroll rating scale for depression: II. Factor analyses of the feature profiles. *Br J Psychiatry*, 138, 201–204.

Snaith, P. (1993). What do depression rating scales measure? *Br J Psychiatry*, 163, 293–298.

Snaith, R.P. (1981). Rating scales. *Br J Psychiatry*, 138, 512–514.

Solomon, D.A., Keller, M.B., Leon, A.C., Mueller, T.I., Lavori, P.W., Shea, M.T., Coryell, W., Warshaw, M., Turvey, C., Maser, J.D., and Endicott, J. (2000). Multiple recurrences of major depressive disorder. *Am J Psychiatry*, 157(2), 229–233.

Solomon, D.A., Leon, A.C., Maser, J.D., Truman, C.J., Coryell, W., Endicott, J., Teres, J.J., and Keller, M.B. (2006). Distinguishing bipolar major depression from unipolar major depression with the Screening Assessment of Depression-Polarity (SAD-P). *J Clin Psychiatry*, 67, 434–442.

Spearing, M.K., Post, R.M., Leverich, G.S., Brandt, D., and Nolen, W. (1997). Modification of the Clinical Global Impressions (CGI) Scale for use in bipolar illness (BP): The CGI-BP. *Psychiatry Res*, 73(3), 159–171.

Spitzer, R.L., and Endicott, J. (1978). *Schedule for Affective Disorders and Schizophrenia.* New York, NY: Biometrics Research, Evaluation Section, New York State Psychiatric Institute.

Squillace, K., Post, R.M., Savard, R., and Erwin-Gorman, M. (1984). Life charting of the longitudinal course of recurrent affective illness. In R.M. Post, J.C. Ballenger (Eds.), *Neurobiology of Mood Disorders* (pp. 38–59). Baltimore: Williams & Wilkins.

Svanborg, P., and Asberg, M. (2001). A comparison between the Beck Depression Inventory (BDI) and the self-rating version of the Montgomery Asberg Depression Rating Scale (MADRS). *J Affect Disord*, 64(2–3), 203–216.

Tandon, R., Flegel, P., and Greden, J.F. (1986). *Carroll and Hamilton Rating Scales for Depression* (Abstract). Washington, DC: American Psychiatric Association.

Thalbourne, M.A., and Bassett, D.L. (1998). The Manic Depressiveness Scale: A preliminary effort at replication and extension. *Psychol Rep*, 83(1), 75–80.

Thalbourne, M.A., Delin, P.S., and Bassett, D.L. (1994). An attempt to construct short scales measuring manic-depressive-like experience and behaviour. *Br J Clin Psychol*, 33(Pt. 2), 205–207.

Thase, M.E., Hersen, M., Bellack, A.S., Himmelhoch, J.M., and Kupfer, D.J. (1983). Validation of a Hamilton subscale for endogenomorphic depression. *J Affect Disord*, 5(3), 267–278.

Tillman, R., and Geller, B. (2005). A brief screening tool for a prepubertal and early adolescent bipolar disorder phenotype. *Am J Psychiatry*, 162, 1214–1216.

Tillman, R., Geller, B., Craney, J.L., Bolhofner, K., Williams, M., and Zimerman, B. (2004). Relationship of parent and child informants to prevalence of mania symptoms in children with a prepubertal and early adolescent bipolar disorder phenotype. *Am J Psychiatry*, 151, 1278–1284.

Tohen, M., Jacobs, T.G., Grundy, S.L., McElroy, S.L., Banov, M.C., Janicak, P.G., Sanger, T., Risser, R., Zhang, F., Toma, V., Francis, J., Tollefson, G.D., and Breier, A. (2000). Efficacy of olanzapine in acute bipolar mania: A double-blind, placebo-controlled study. The Olanzipine HGGW Study Group. *Arch Gen Psychiatry*, 57(9), 841–849.

Trivedi, M.H., Rush, A.J., Ibrahim, H.M., Carmody, T.J., Biggs, M.M., Suppes, T., Crismon, M.L., Shores-Wilson, K., Toprac, M.G., Dennehy, E.B., Witte, B., and Kashner, T.M. (2004). The Inventory of Depressive Symptomatology, Clinician Rating (IDS-C) and Self-Report (IDS-SR), and the Quick Inventory of Depressive Symptomatology, Clinician Rating (QIDS-C) and Self-Report (QIDS-SR) in public sector patients with mood disorders: A psychometric evaluation. *Psychol Med*, 34(1), 73–82.

Tyrer, S.P., and Shopsin, B. (1982). Symptoms and assessment of mania. In E.S. Paykel (Ed.), *Handbook of Affective Disorders* (pp. 12–23). Edinburgh, Scotland: Churchill Livingstone.

Vojta, C., *Kinosian, B., Glick, H., Altshuler, L., and Bauer, M.S.* (2001). Self-reported quality of life across mood states in bipolar disorder. *Compr Psychiatry*, 42(3), 190–195.

von Zerssen, D., and Cording, C. (1978). The measurement of change in endogenous affective disorders. *Arch Psychiatr Nervenkr*, 226(2), 95–112.

Ware, J.E. Jr., and Sherbourne, C.D. (1992). The MOS 36-item short-form health survey (SF-36): I. Conceptual framework and item selection. *Med Care*, 30(6), 473–483.

Warren, W.L. (1994). *Revised Hamilton Rating Scale for Depression (RHRSD): Manual.* Los Angeles: Western Psychological Services.

Warshaw, M.G., Keller, M.B., and Stout, R.L. (1994). Reliability and validity of the longitudinal interval follow-up evaluation for assessing outcome of anxiety disorders. *J Psychiatr Res*, 28(6), 531–545.

Weissman, M.M. (1997). Beyond symptoms: Social functioning and the new antidepressants. *J Psychopharmacol*, 11(Suppl. 4), S5–S8.

Weissman, M.M., and Bothwell, S. (1976). Assessment of social adjustment by patient self-report. *Arch Gen Psychiatry*, 33(9), 1111–1115.

Weissman, M.M., Sholomskas, D., Pottenger, M., Prusoff, B.A., and Locke, B.Z. (1977). Assessing depressive symptoms in five psychiatric populations: A validation study. *Am J Epidemiol*, 106(3), 203–214.

Weissman, M.M., Prusoff, B.A., Thompson, W.D., Harding, P.S., and Myers, J.K. (1978). Social adjustment by self-report in a community sample and in psychiatric outpatients. *J Nerv Ment Dis*, 166(5), 317–326.

Weissman, M.M., Sholomskas, D., and John, K. (1981). The assessment of social adjustment: An update. *Arch Gen Psychiatry*, 38(11), 1250–1258.

Wells, K.B., Stewart, A., Hays, R.D., Burnam, M.A., Rogers, W., Daniels, M., Berry, S., Greenfield, S., and Ware, J. (1989). The functioning and well-being of depressed patients: Results from the Medical Outcomes Study. *JAMA*, 262(7), 914–919.

Whybrow, P.C., Grof, P., Gyalai, L., Rasgon, N., Glenn, T., and Bauer, M. (2003). The electronic assessment of the longitudinal course of bipolar disorder: The ChronoRecord software. *Pharmaco*, 36(Suppl. 3), S244–S249.

Williams, J.B.W. (2000). Mental health status, functioning, and disabilities measures. In *Handbook of Psychiatric Measures* (pp. 93–115). Washington, DC: American Psychiatric Association.

Williamson, D., Brown, E., Perlis, R.H., Ahl, J., Baker, R.W., and Tohen, M. (2006). Clinical relevance of depressive symptom improvement in bipolar I depressed patients. *J Affect Disord*, 92, 261–266.

Young, R.C., Biggs, J.T., Ziegler, V.E., and Meyer, D.A. (1978). A rating scale for mania: Reliability, validity and sensitivity. *Br J Psychiatry*, 133, 429–435.

Youngstrom, E.A., Findling, R.L., Danielson, C.K., and Calabrese, J.R. (2001). Discriminative validity of parent report of hypomanic and depressive symptoms on the General Behavior Inventory. *Psychol Assess*, 13(2), 267–276.

Youngstrom, E., Danielson, C., Findling, R., Gracious, B., and Calabrese, J. (2002). Factor structure of the Young Mania Rating Scale for use with youths aged 5 to 17 years. *J Clin Child Adolesc Psychol*, 31, 567–572.

Youngstrom, E., Gracious, B., Danielson, C., Findling, R., and Calabrese, J. (2003). Toward an integration of parent and clinician report on the Young Mania Rating Scale. *J Affect Disord*, 77, 179–190.

Youngstrom, E.A., Findling, R.L., and Calabrese, J.R. (2004). Effects of adolescent manic symptoms on agreement between youth, parent, and teacher ratings of behavior problems. *J Affect Disord*, 828, S5–S16.

Zealley, A.K., and Aitken, R.C. (1969). Measurement of mood. *Proc R Soc Med*, 62(10), 993–996.

Zimmerman, M., Coryell, W., Corenthal, C., and Wilson, S. (1986). A self-report scale to diagnose major depressive disorder. *Arch Gen Psychiatry*, 43(11), 1076–1081.

Zimmerman, M., Sheeran, T., and Young, D. (2004a). The diagnostic inventory for depression: A self-report scale to diagnose

DSM-IV major depressive disorder. *J Clin Psychol*, 60(1), 87–110.

Zimmerman, M., Posternak, M.A., Chelminski, I., and Solomon, D.A. (2004b). *Using Questionnaires to Screen for Psychiatric Disorders: A Comment on a Study of Screening for Bipolar Disorder in the Community*. Providence, RI: Physicians Postgraduate Press.

Zung, W.W. (1974). The measurement of affects: Depression and anxiety. *Mod Probl Pharmacopsychiatry*, 7(0), 170–188.

Zung, W.W., Richards, C.B., and Short, M.J. (1965). Self-rating depression scale in an outpatient clinic: Further validation of the SDS. *Arch Gen Psychiatry*, 13(6), 508–515.

CHAPTER 12

Akiskal, K.K., Savino, M., and Akiskal, H.S. (2005). Temperament profiles in physicians, lawyers, managers, industrialists, architects, journalists, and artists: A study in psychiatric outpatients. *J Affect Disord*, 85, 201–206.

Andreasen, N.C. (1980). Mania and creativity. In R.H. Belmaker and H.M. Praag (Eds.), *Mania: An Evolving Concept*. New York: Spectrum, pp. 377–386.

Andreasen, N.C. (1987). Creativity and mental illness: Prevalence rates in writers and their first-degree relatives. *Am J Psychiatry*, 144, 1288–1292.

Andreasen, N.C., and Canter, A. (1974). The creative writer: Psychiatric symptoms and family history. *Compr Psychiatry*, 15, 123–131.

Andreasen, N.C., and Glick, I.D. (1988). Bipolar affective disorder and creativity: Implications and clinical management. *Compr Psychiatry*, 29(3), 207–217.

Andreasen, N.C., and Powers, P.S. (1975). Creativity and psychosis: An examination of conceptual style. *Arch Gen Psychiatry*, 32, 70–73.

Aristotle. (1936). *Problems II: Books XXII–XXXVIII*. Translated by W.S. Hett. Cambridge, MA: Harvard University Press.

Babcock, W.L. (1895). On the morbid heredity and predisposition to insanity of the Man of Genius. *J Ment Nerv Disorders*, 20, 749–769.

Berryman, J. (1976). *Writers at Work: The Paris Review Interviews*. G. Plimpton (Ed.). New York: Viking Press, p. 322.

Bett, W.R. (1952). *The Infirmities of Genius*. London: Johnson.

Bleuler, E. (1924). *Textbook of Psychiatry*. A.A. Brill (Transl.). New York: Macmillan.

Bold, A. (1983). *Byron: Wrath and Rhyme*. London: Vision Press.

Brody, J.F. (2001). Evolutionary recasting: ADHD, mania and its variants. *J Affect Disord*, 65, 197–215.

Carson, S.H., Peterson, J.B., and Higgins, D.M. (2003). Decreased latent inhibition is associated with increased creative achievement in high-functioning individuals. *J Pers Soc Psychol*, 85, 499–506.

Collins, F. (1990, September 17). Tracking down killer genes. *Time*. p. 12.

Coryell, W., Endicott, J., Keller, M., Andreasen, N., Grove, W., Hirschfeld, R.M.A., and Scheftner, W. (1989). Bipolar affective disorder and high achievement: A familial association. *Am J Psychiatry*, 146, 983–988.

Czeizel, E. (2001). Aki költo akar lenni, pokolra kell annak menni? Magyar költo-géniuszok testi és lelki betegségei. GMR Reklámügynökség, Budapest.

Dax, E.C. (1953). *Experimental Studies in Psychiatric Art*. London: Faber & Faber.

Donnelly, E.F., Murphy, D.L., Goodwin, F.K., and Waldman, I.N. (1982). Intellectual function in primary affective disorder. *Br J Psychiatry*, 140, 633–636.

Enâchescu, C. (1971). Aspects of pictorial creation in manic-depressive psychosis. *Confin Psychiatr*, 14, 133–142.

Fodor, E.M. (1999). Subclinical inclination toward manic-depression and creative performance on the Remote Associates Test. *Person Individual Differences*, 27, 1273–1283.

Fodor, E.M., and Laird, B.A. (2004). Therapeutic intervention, bipolar inclination, and literary creativity. *Creativity Res J*, 16, 149–161.

Folley, B.S., Doop, M.L., and Park. S. (2003). Psychoses and creativity: Is the missing link a biological mechanism related to phospholipids turnover? *Prostoglandins Leukot Essent Fatty Acids*, 69, 467–476.

Galton, F. (1892). *Hereditary Genius*. London: Walter Scott.

Gardner, H. (1993). *Creating Minds*. New York: Basic Books.

Gardner, R. Jr. (1982). Mechanisms in manic-depressive disorder: An evolutionary model. *Arch Gen Psychiatry*, 39(12), 1436–1441.

George, M.S., Melvin, J.A., and Mossman, D. (1988). Mental illness and creativity. *Am J Psychiatry*, 145, 908.

Getzels, J.W., and Jackson, P.W. (1963). The highly intelligent and the highly creative adolescent: A summary of some research findings. In C.W. Taylor and F. Barron (Eds.), *Scientific Creativity: Its Recognition and Development*. New York: John Wiley & Sons, pp. 161–172.

Ghacibeh, G.A., Shenker, J.I., Shenal, B., Uthman, B.M., and Heilman, K.M. (2006). Effect of vagus nerve stimulation on creativity and cognitive flexibility. *Epilepsy Behav*, 8, 720–725.

Gilbert, P. (2004). Depression: A biopsychosocial, integrative and evolutionary approach. In M. Power (Ed.), *Mood Disorders: A Handbook of Science and Practice*. Chichester: John Wiley, pp. 99–142.

Gilbert, P. (2006). Evolution and depression: Issues and implications. *Psychol Med*, 36, 287–297.

Giroux, R. (Ed.). (1987). *Robert Lowell: Collected Prose*. New York: Farrar, Straus, Giroux.

Greene, T.R., and Noice, H. (1988). Influence of positive affect upon creative thinking and problem solving in children. *Psychol Rep*, 63, 895–898.

Guilford, J.P. (1957). A revised structure of intellect. *Report of the Psychological Laboratory, University of Southern California* (No. 19).

Guilford, J.P. (1959). Traits of creativity. In H.H. Anderson (Ed.), *Creativity and Its Cultivation*. New York: Harper, pp. 142–161.

Henry, G.M., Weingartner, H., and Murphy, D.L. (1971). Idiosyncratic patterns of learning and word association during mania. *Am J Psychiatry*, 128, 564–574.

Hoffman, R.E., Quinlan, D.M., Mazure, C.M., and McGlashan, T.M. (2001). Cortical instability and the mechanism of mania: A neural network simulation and perceptual test. *Soc Biol Psychiatry*, 49, 500–509.

Hudson, L. (1966). *Contrary Imaginations: A Psychological Study of the English Schoolboy*. Middlesex, England: Penguin Books.

Isen, A.M. (1999). On creative problem solving. In S. Russ (Ed.), *Affect, Creative Experience, and Psychological Adjustment*. Philadelphia: Taylor and Francis, pp. 3–17.

Isen, A.M., and Daubman, K.A. (1984). The influence of affect on categorization. *J Pers Soc Psychol*, 47, 1206–1217.

Isen, A.M., Johnson, M.S., Mertz, E., and Robinson, G.F. (1985). The influence of positive affect on the unusualness of word associations. *J Pers Soc Psychol*, 48, 1413–1426.

Isen, A.M., Daubman, K.A., and Nowicki, G.P. (1987). Positive affect facilitates creative problem solving. *J Pers Soc Psychol*, 52, 1122–1131.

Jacobson, A.C. (1912). Literary genius and manic depressive insanity. *Med Rec*, 82, 937–939.

James, W. (1902). *The Varieties of Religious Experience: A Study in Human Nature*.

Jamison, K.R. (1989). Mood disorders and seasonal patterns in British writers and artists. *Psychiatry*, 52, 125–134.

Jamison, K.R. (1993). *Touched with Fire: Manic-Depressive Illness and the Artistic Temperament*. New York: Free Press.

Jamison, K.R. (2004). *Exuberance: The Passion for Life*. New York: Alfred A. Knopf.

Juda, A. (1949). The relationship between highest mental capacity and psychic abnormalities. *Am J Psychiatry*, 106, 296–307.

Judd, L.L., Hubbard, B., Janowsky, D.S., Huey, L.Y., and Takahashi, K.I. (1977). The effect of lithium carbonate on the cognitive functions of normal subjects. *Arch Gen Psychiatry*, 34, 355–357.

Karlsson, J.L. (1970). Genetic association of giftedness and creativity with schizophrenia. *Hereditas*, 66, 177–182.

Keller, M.C., and Miller G. (2006). Resolving the paradox of common harmful, heritable mental disorders: Which evolution genetic models work best? *Behavioral and Brain Sciences*, 29, 385–452.

Keller, M.C., and Nesse, R.M. (2005). Is low mood an adaptation? Evidence for subtypes with symptoms that match precipitants. *J Affect Disord*, 86, 27–35.

Kocsis, J.H., Shaw, E.D., Stokes, P.E., Wilner, P., Elliot, A.S., Sikes, C., Myers, B., Manevitz, A., and Parides, M. (1993). Neuropsycholic effects of lithium discontinuation. *J Clin Psychopharmacol*, 13, 268–276.

Koukopoulos, A., and Koukopoulos, A. (1999). Agitated depression as a mixed state and the problem of melancholia. *Psychiatr Clin North Am*, 22(3), 547–564.

Kraepelin E. (1921). *Manic-Depressive Insanity and Paranoia*. R.M. Barclay (Ed.), G.M. Robertson (Transl.). Edinburgh: E & S Livingstone. Reprinted New York: Arno Press, 1976.

Lamb, C. (1987). *Elia and the Last Essays of Elia*. New York: Oxford University Press, pp. 212–213.

Lange-Eichbaum, W. (1932). *The Problem of Genius*. Translated by E. Paul and C. Paul. New York: Macmillan.

Larsen, R.J., Diener E., and Cropanzano, R.S. (1987). Cognitive operations associated with the characteristic of Intense Emotional Responsiveness. *J Pers Soc Psychol*, 53, 767–774.

Levine, J., Schild, K., Kimhi, R., and Schreiber, G. (1996). Word associative production in affective versus schizophrenic psychoses. *Psychopathology*, 29, 7–13.

Lombroso, C. (1891). *The Man of Genius*, 2nd Edition. London: Walter Scott. New York: Charles Scribners Sons (1905).

Ludwig, A.M. (1992). Creative achievement and psychopathology: Comparison among professions. *Am J Psychother*, 46(3), 330–356.

Ludwig, A.M. (1994). Mental illness and creative activity in female writers. *Am J Psychiatry*, 151, 1650–1656.

Ludwig, A.M. (1995). *The Price of Greatness: Resolving the Creativity and Madness Controversy*. New York: Guilford Press.

Luxenburger, H. (1933). Berufsgliederun und soziale Schichtung in den Familien erblich Geisteskranker. *Eugenik*, 3, 34–40.

MacKinnon, D.W. (1962). The personality correlates of creativity: A study of American architects. *Proceedings of the Fourteenth Congress on Applied Psychology*, 2, 11–39.

Marshall, M.H., Neumann, C.P., and Robinson, M. (1970). Lithium, creativity, and manic-depressive illness: Review and prospectus. *Psychosomatics*, 11, 406–488.

Martindale, C. (1972). Father's absence, psychopathology, and poetic eminence. *Psychol Rep*, 31(3), 843–847.

McNeil, T.F. (1971). Prebirth and postbirth influence on the relationship between creative ability and recorded mental illness. *J Pers*, 39, 391–406.

Moore, T. (1832). *The Works of Lord Byron: With His Letters and Journals and His Life*. R.H. Stoddard (Ed.). (Reprint, London: Francis A. Nicholls, 1900), Vol. 16, p. 237.

Murphy, G. (1923). Types of word-association in dementia praecox, manic-depressives, and normal persons. *Am J Psychiatry*, 79, 539–571.

Myerson, A., and Boyle, R. (1941). The incidence of manic-depressive psychosis in certain socially important families. *Am J Psychiatry*, 98, 11–21.

Nowakowska, C., Strong, C.M., Santosa, C.M., Wang, P.W., and Ketter, T.A. (2005). Temperamental commonalities and differences in euthymic mood disorder patients, creative controls, and healthy controls. *J Affect Disord*, 85, 207–215.

Ochse, R. (1990). *Before the Gates of Excellence: The Determinants of Creative Genius*. Cambridge, UK: Cambridge University Press.

Piirto, J. (1994). *Talented Children and Adults: Their Development and Education*. New York: Macmillan.

Plato. (1974). *Phaedrus and the Seventh and Eighth Letters*. Translated by W. Hamilton. Middlesex, England: Penguin.

Plokker, J.J. (1965). *Art from the Mentally Disturbed, the Scattered Vision of Schizophrenics*. Boston: Little Brown.

Polatin, P., and Fieve, R.R. (1971). Patient rejection of lithium carbonate prophylaxis. *JAMA*, 218, 864–866.

Pons, L., Nurberger, J.I. Jr., and Murphy, D.L. (1985). Mood-independent aberrancies in associative processes in bipolar affective disorder: An apparent stabilizing effect of lithium. *Psychiatry Res*, 14, 315–322.

Post, F. (1994). Creativity and psychopathology: A study of 291 world-famous men. *Br J Psychiatry*, 165, 22–34.

Post, F. (1996). Verbal creativity, depression and alcoholism: An investigation of one hundred American and British writers. *Br J Psychiatry*, 168, 545–555.

Price, J.S. (1967). Hypothesis: The dominance hierarchy and the evolution of mental illness. *Lancet*, ii, 243–246.

Price, J.S. (1972). Genetic and phylogenetic aspects of mood variation. *Int J Ment Health*, 1, 124–144.

Price, J., Sloman, L., Gardner, R., Gilbert, P., and Rohde, P. (1994). The social competition hypothesis of depression. *Br J Psychiatry*, 164, 309–315.

Reid, E.C. (1912). Manifestations of manic-depressive insanity in literary genius. *Am J Insanity*, 68, 595–632.

Reitman, F. (1950). *Psychotic Art*. London: Rutledge and Kegan Paul.

Richards, R.L. (1981). Relationships between creativity and psychopathology: An evaluation and interpretation of the evidence. *Genet Psychol Monogr*, 103, 261–324.

Richards, R., and Kinney, D.K. (1990). Mood swings and creativity. *Creativity Res J*, 3, 202–217.

Richards, R.L., Kinney, D.K., Lunde, I., Benet, M., and Merzel, A.P. (1988). Creativity in manic-depressives, cyclothymes, their normal relatives, and control subjects. *J Abnorm Psychol*, 97, 281–288.

Robins, L.N., Helzer, J.E., Weissman, M.M., Orvaschel, H., Gruenberg, E., Burk, J.D. Jr., and Regier, D.A. (1984). Lifetime prevalence of specific psychiatric disorders in three sites. *Arch Gen Psychiatry*, 41, 949–958.

Roe, A. (1946). The personality of artists. *Educat Psychol Measurement*, 6, 401–408.

Roe, A. (1951). A psychological study of eminent biologists. *Psychol Monogr*, 65, 1–68.

Roe, A. (1952). A psychologist examines sixty-four eminent scientists. *Sci Am*, 187, 21–25.

Rush, B. (1812). *Medical Inquiries and Observations upon the Diseases of the Mind*. Philadelphia: Kimber and Richardson, pp. 153–154.

Schildkraut, J.J., and Hirshfeld, A.J. (1995). Mind and mood in modern art I: Miro and "Melancolie." *Creativity Res J*, 8, 139–156.

Schildkraut, J.J., Hirshfeld, A.J., and Murphy, J.M. (1994). Mind and mood in modern art, II: Depressive disorders, spirituality, and early deaths in the Abstract Expressionist Artists of the New York School. *Am J Psychiatry*, 151, 482–488.

Schou, M. (1968). Lithium in psychiatric therapy and prophylaxis. *J Psychiatr Res*, 6, 67–95.

Schou, M. (1979). Artistic productivity and lithium prophylaxis in manic-depressive illness. *Br J Psychiatry*, 135, 97–103.

Schuldberg, D. (1990). Schizotypal and hypomanic traits, creativity, and psychological health. *Creativity Res J*, 3, 218–230.

Sexton, L.G., and Ames, L. (Eds). (1977). *Anne Sexton: A Self-Portrait in Letters*. Boston: Houghton Mifflin.

Shaw, E.D., Mann, J.J., Stokes, P.E., and Manevitz, A.Z. (1986). Effects of lithium carbonate on associative productivity and idiosyncrasy in bipolar outpatients. *Am J Psychiatry*, 143, 1166–1169.

Shenton, M.E., Solovay, M.R., and Holzman, P. (1987). Comparative studies of thought disorders: II. Schizoaffective disorder. *Arch Gen Psychiatry*, 44, 21–30.

Simeonova, D.I., Chang, K.D., Strong, C., and Ketter, T.A. (2005). Creativity in familial bipolar disorder. *J Psychiatr Res*, 39, 623–631.

Simonton, D.K. (1994). *Greatness: Who Makes History and Why*. New York: Guilford Press.

Solovay, M.R., Shenton, M.E., and Holzman, P.S. (1987). Comparative studies of thought disorders: I. Mania and schizophrenia. *Arch Gen Psychiatry*, 44, 13–20.

Steffan, T.G. (1971). *Byron's Don Juan: The Making of a Masterpiece*. Austin, TX: University of Texas Press, p. 345.

Stoll, A.L., Locke, C.A., Vuckovic, A., and Mayer, P.V. (1996). Lithium-associated cognitive and functional deficits reduced by a switch to divalproex sodium: A case series. *J Clin Psychiatry*, 57, 356–359.

Trethowan, W.H. (1977). Music and mental disorder. In M. Critchley and R.E. Henson (Eds.), *Music and the Brain*. London: Heinemann, pp. 398–442.

Wadeson, H.S., and Carpenter, W.T. Jr. (1976). A comparative study of art expression of schizophrenic, unipolar depressive, and bipolar manic-depressive patients. *J Nerv Ment Dis*, 162, 334–344.

Watson, P.J., and Andrews, P.W. (2002). Toward a revised evolutionary adaptationist analysis of depression: The social navigation hypothesis. *J Affect Disord*, 72, 1–14.

Welch, L., Diethelm, O., and Long, L. (1946). Measurement of hyper-associative activity during elation. *J Psychol*, 21, 113–126.

Welsh, G.S. (1977). Personality correlates of intelligence and creativity in gifted adolescents. In J.C. Stanley, W.C. George, and C.H. Solano (Eds.), *The Gifted and the Creative: A Fifty-Year Perspective*. Baltimore: Johns Hopkins University Press, pp. 197–221.

White, R.K. (1930). Note on the psychopathology of genius. *J Soc Psychol*, I, 311–315.

Wills, G.I. (2003). Forty lives in the bebop business: Mental health in a group of eminent jazz musicians. *Br J Psychiatry*, 183, 255–259.

Wilson, D.R. (1993). Evolutionary epidemiology: Darwinian theory in the service of medicine and psychiatry. *Acta Biotheoretica*, 41, 205–218.

Winner, E. (1996). *Gifted Children: Myths and Realities*. New York: Basic Books.

Woodruff, R.A. Jr., Robins, L.N., Winokur, G., and Reich, T. (1971). Manic depressive illness and social achievement. *Acta Psychiatry*, 119, 33–38.

Zimmerman, J., and Garfinkle, L. (1942). Preliminary study of the art productions of the adult psychotic. *Psychiatr Q*, 16, 313–318.

CHAPTER 13

Abkevich, V., Camp, N.J., Hensel, C.H., Neff, C.D., Russell, D.L., Hughes, D.C., Plenk, A.M., Lowry, M.R., Richards, R.L., Carter, C., Frech, G.C., Stone, S., Rowe, K., Chau, C.A., Cortado, K., Hunt, A., Luce, K., O'Neil, G., Poarch, J., Potter, J., Poulsen, G.H., Saxton, H., Bernat-Sestak, M., Thompson, V., Gutin, A., Skolnick, M.H., Shattuck, D., and Cannon-Albright, L. (2003). Predisposition locus for major depression at chromosome 12q22-12q23.2. *Am J Hum Genet*, 73(6), 1271–1281.

Abrams, R., and Taylor, M.A. (1980). A comparison of unipolar and bipolar depressive illness. *Am J Psychiatry*, 137, 658–661.

Adams, L.J., Mitchell, P.B., Fielder, S.L., Rosso, A., Donald, J.A., and Schofield, P.R. (1998). A susceptibility locus for bipolar affective disorder on chromosome 4q35. *Am J Hum Genet*, 62(5), 1084–1091.

Ahearn, E.P., Speer, M.C., Chen, Y.T., Steffens, D.C., Cassidy, F., Van Meter, S., Provenzale, J.M., Weisler, R.H., and Krishnan, K.R. (2002). Investigation of Notch3 as a candidate gene for bipolar disorder using brain hyperintensities as an endophenotype. *Am J Med Genet*, 114(6), 652–658.

Albrecht, U., Sutcliffe, J.S., Cattanach, B.M., Beechey, C.V., Armstrong, D., Eichele, G., and Beaudet, A.L. (1997). Imprinted expression of the murine Angelman syndrome gene, *Ube3a*, in hippocampal and Purkinje neurons. *Nat Genet*, 17(1), 75–78.

Alda, M., Turecki, G., Grof, P., Cavazzoni, P., Duffy, A., Grof, E., Ahrens, B., Berghofer, A., Muller-Oerlinghausen, B., Dvorakova, M., Libigerova, E., Vojtechovsky, M., Zvolsky, P., Joober, R., Nilsson, A., Prochazka, H., Licht, R.W., Rasmussen, N.A., Schou, M., Vestergaard, P., Holzinger, A., Schumann, C., Thau, K., and Rouleau, G.A. (2000). Association and linkage studies of CRH and PENK genes in bipolar disorder: A collaborative IGSLI study. *Am J Med Genet*, 96(2), 178–181.

Andreasen, N.C., Grove, W.M., Shapiro, R.W., Keller, M.B., Hirschfeld, R.M., and McDonald-Scott, P. (1981). Reliability of lifetime diagnosis: A multicenter collaborative perspective. *Arch Gen Psychiatry*, 38(4), 400–405.

Andreasen, N.C., Hoffman, R.E., and Grove, W.M. (1985). Mapping abnormalities in language and cognition. In M. Alpert (Ed.), *Controversies in Schizophrenia: Changes and Constancies* (pp. 199–227). New York: Guilford Press.

Andreasen, N.C., Rice, J., Endicott, J., Reich, T., and Coryell, W. (1986). The family history approach to diagnosis. How useful is it? *Arch Gen Psychiatry*, 43(5), 421–429.

Andreasen, N.C., Rice, J., Endicott, J., Coryell, W., Grove, W.M., and Reich, T. (1987). Familial rates of affective disorder. A report from the national institute of mental health collaborative study. *Arch Gen Psychiatry*, 44(5), 461–469.

Andrews, G., Stewart, G., Allen, R., and Henderson, A.S. (1990) The genetics of six neurotic disorders: A twin study. *J Affect Disord*, 19(1), 23–29.

Angst, J. (1961). A clinical analysis of the effects of tranfranil in depression. Longitudinal and follow-up studies. Treatment of blood relations. *Psychopharmacologia*, 2, 381–407.

Angst, J. (1964). Antidepressive Effekt und genetische Faktoren. *Arzneimittelforschung*, 14(Suppl.), 496–500.

Arai, M., Itokawa, M., Yamada, K., Toyota, T., Arai, M., Haga, S., Ujike, H., Sora, I., Ikeda, K., and Yoshikawa, T. (2004). Association of neural cell adhesion molecule 1 gene polymorphisms with bipolar affective disorder in Japanese individuals. *Biol Psychiatry*, 55(8), 804–810.

Arinami, T., Itokawa, M., Aoki, J., Shibuya, H., Ookubo, Y., Iwawaki, A., Ota, K., Shimizu, H., Hamaguchi, H., and Toru, M. (1996). Further association study on dopamine D2 receptor variant S311C in schizophrenia and affective disorders. *Am J Med Genet*, 67(2), 133–138.

Arranz, M.J., Erdmann, J., Kirov, G., Rietschel, M., Sodhi, M., Albus, M., Ball, D., Maier, W., Davies, N., Franzek, E., Abusaad, I., Weigelt, B., Murray, R., Shimron-Abarbanell, D., Kerwin, R., Propping, P., Sham, P., Nothen, M.M., and Collier, D.A. (1997). 5-HT2A receptor and bipolar affective disorder: Association studies in affected patients. *Neurosci Lett*, 224(2), 95–98.

Asghari, V., Sanyal, S., Buchwaldt, S., Paterson, A., Jovanovic, V., and Van Tol, H.H. (1995). Modulation of intracellular cyclic AMP levels by different human dopamine D4 receptor variants. *J Neurochem*, 65(3), 1157–1165.

Asherson, P., Mant, R., Williams, N., Cardno, A., Jones, L., Murphy, K., Collier, D.A., Nanko, S., Craddock, N., Morris, S., Muir, W., Blackwood, B., McGuffin, P., and Owen, M.J. (1998). A study of chromosome 4p markers and dopamine D5 receptor gene in schizophrenia and bipolar disorder. *Mol Psychiatry*, 3(4), 310–320.

Avramopoulos, D., Willour, V.L., Zandi, P.P., Huo, Y., MacKinnon, D.F., Potash, J.B., DePaulo, J.R. Jr., and McInnis, M.G. (2004). Linkage of bipolar affective disorder on chromosome 8q24: Follow-up and parametric analysis. *Mol Psychiatry*, 9(2), 191–196.

Badenhop, R.F., Moses, M.J., Scimone, A., Mitchell, P.B., Ewen-White, K.R., Rosso, A., Donald, J.A., Adams, L.J., and Schofield, P.R. (2002). A genome screen of 13 bipolar affective disorder pedigrees provides evidence for susceptibility loci on chromosome 3 as well as chromosomes 9, 13 and 19. *Mol Psychiatry*, 7(8), 851–859.

Badner, J.A., and Gershon, E.S. (2002). Meta-analysis of whole-genome linkage scans of bipolar disorder and schizophrenia. *Mol Psychiatry*, 7(4):405–411.

Banse, D. (1929). Zum Problem der Erbprognosebestimmung. Die Erkrankungsaussuchten der Vettern und Basen von Manisch-Depressiven. [The problem of empirical hereditary risk. The morbidity risk of cousins of manic depressive patients]. *Z Ges Neurol Psychiatrie*, 119, 576–612.

Baron, M., Mendlewicz, J., and Klotz, J. (1981). Age-of-onset and genetic transmission in affective disorders. *Acta Psychiatr Scand*, 64(5), 373–380.

Baron, M., Barkai, A., Asnis, L., and Kane, J. (1982). Schizoaffective illness, schizophrenia and affective disorders: Morbidity risk and genetic transmission. *Acta Psychiatr Scand*, 65, 253–262.

Baron, M., Risch, N., Hamburger, R., Mandel, B., Kushner, S., Newman, M., Drumer, D., and Belmaker, R.H. (1987). Genetic linkage between X-chromosome markers and bipolar affective illness. *Nature*, 326(6110), 289–292.

Baron, M., Freimer, N.F., Risch, N., Lerer, B., Alexander, J.R., Straub, R.E., Asokan, S., Das, K., Peterson, A., and Amos, J. (1993). Diminished support for linkage between manic depressive illness and X-chromosome markers in three Israeli pedigrees [see comments]. *Nat Genet*, 3(1), 49–55.

Battersby, S., Ogilvie, A.D., Smith, C.A., Blackwood, D.H., Muir, W.J., Quinn, J.P., Fink, G., Goodwin, G.M., and Harmar, A.J. (1996). Structure of a variable number tandem repeat of the serotonin transporter gene and association with affective disorder. *Psychiatr Genet*, 6(4), 177–181.

Bellivier, F., Henry, C., Szoke, A., Schurhoff, F., Nosten-Bertrand, M., Feingold, J., Launay, J.M., Leboyer, M., and Laplanche, J.L. (1998a). Serotonin transporter gene polymorphisms in patients with unipolar or bipolar depression. *Neurosci Lett*, 255(3), 143–146.

Bellivier, F., Leboyer, M., Courtet, P., Buresi, C., Beaufils, B., Samolyk, D., Allilaire, J.F., Feingold, J., Mallet, J., and Malafosse, A. (1998b). Association between the tryptophan hydroxylase gene and manic-depressive illness. *Arch Gen Psychiatry*, 55(1), 33–37.

Bellivier, F., Szoke, A., Henry, C., Lacoste, J., Bottos, C., Nosten-Bertrand, M., Hardy, P., Rouillon, F., Launay, J.M., Laplanche, J.L., and Leboyer, M. (2000). Possible association between serotonin transporter gene polymorphism and violent suicidal behavior in mood disorders. *Biol Psychiatry*, 48(4), 319–322.

Belmaker, R.H., Henry, C., Szoke, A., Schurhoff, F., Nosten-Bertrand, M., Feingold, J., Launay, J.M., Leboyer, M., and Laplanche, J.L. (2002). Reduced inositol content in lymphocyte-derived cell lines from bipolar patients. *Bipolar Disord*, 4(1), 67–69.

Bennett, P., Segurado, R., Jones, I., Bort, S., McCandless, F., Lambert, D., Heron, J., Comerford, C., Middle, F., Corvin, A., Pelios, G., Kirov, G., Larsen, B., Mulcahy, T., Williams, N., O'-Connell, R., O'Mahony, E., Payne, A., Owen, M., Holmans, P., Craddock, N., and Gill, M. (2002). The Wellcome trust UK-Irish bipolar affective disorder sibling-pair genome screen: First stage report. *Mol Psychiatry*, 7(2), 189–200.

Berrettini, W.H. (2000). Are schizophrenic and bipolar disorders related? A review of family and molecular studies. *Biol Psychiatry*, 48(6), 531–538.

Berrettini, W.H., Goldin, L.R., Gelernter, J., Gejman, P.V., Gershon, E.S., and Detera-Wadleigh, S. (1990). X-chromosome markers and manic-depressive illness. Rejection of linkage to Xq28 in nine bipolar pedigrees [see comments]. *Arch Gen Psychiatry*, 47(4), 366–373.

Berrettini, W.H., Ferraro, T.N., Goldin, L.R., Weeks, D.E., Detera-Wadleigh, S., Nurnberger, J.I. Jr., and Gershon, E.S. (1994). Chromosome 18 DNA markers and manic-depressive illness: evidence for a susceptibility gene. *Proc Natl Acad Sci USA*, 91(13), 5918–5921.

Bertelsen, A., Harvald, B., and Hauge, M. (1977). A Danish twin study of manic-depressive disorders. *Br J Psychiatry*, 130, 330–351.

Bezchlibnyk, Y.B., Wang, J.F., McQueen, G.M., and Young, L.T. (2001). Gene expression differences in bipolar disorder revealed by cDNA array analysis of post-mortem frontal cortex. *J Neurochem*, 79(4), 826–834.

Bierut, L.J., Heath, A.C., Bucholz, K.K., Dinwiddie, S.H., Madden, P.A., Statham, D.J., Dunne, M.P., and Martin, N.G. (1999). Major depressive disorder in a community-based twin sample: Are there different genetic and environmental contributions for men and women? *Arch Gen Psychiatry*, 56(6), 557–563.

Billings, P.R., Hubbard, R., and Newman, S.A. (1999). Human germline gene modification: A dissent. *Lancet*, 353(9167), 1873–1875.

Biomed European Bipolar Collaborative Group. (1997). No association between bipolar disorder and alleles at a functional polymorphism in the COMT gene. *Br J Psychiatry*, 170, 526–528.

Blackwood, D.H., He, L., Morris, S.W., McLean, A., Whitton, C., Thomson, M., Walker, M.T., Woodburn, K., Sharp, C.M., Wright, A.F., Shibasaki, Y., St. Clair, D.M., Porteous, D.J., and Muir, W.J. (1996). A locus for bipolar affective disorder on chromosome 4p. *Nat Genet*, 12(4), 427–430.

Blackwood, D.H., Fordyce, A., Walker, M.T., St. Clair, D.M., Porteous, D.J., and Muir, W.J. (2001). Schizophrenia and affective disorders—cosegregation with a translocation at chromosome 1q42 that directly disrupts brain-expressed genes: Clinical and P300 findings in a family. *Am J Hum Genet*, 69(2), 428–433.

Bland, R.C., Newman, S.C., and Orn, H. (1986). Recurrent and nonrecurrent depression. A family study. *Arch Gen Psychiatry*, 43(11), 1085–1089.

Blouin, J.L., Dombroski, B.A., Nath, S.K., Lasseter, V.K., Wolyniec, P.S., Nestadt, G., Thornquist, M., Ullrich, G., McGrath, J., Kasch, L., Lamacz, M., Thomas, M.G., Gehrig, C., Radhakrishna, U., Snyder, S.E., Balk, K.G., Neufeld, K., Swartz, K.L., DeMarchi, N., Papadimitriou, G.N., Dikeos, D.G., Stefanis, C.N., Chakravarti, A., Childs, B., Housman, D.E., Kazazian, H.H., Antonarakis, S., and Pulver, A.E. (1998). Schizophrenia susceptibility loci on chromosomes 13q32 and 8p21. *Nat Genet*, 20(1), 70–73.

Bocchetta, A., Piccardi, M.P., Palmas, M.A., Chillotti, C., Oi, A., Del Zompo, M. (1999). Family-based association study between bipolar disorder and DRD2, DRD4, DAT, and SERT in Sardinia. *Am J Med Genet*, 88(5), 522–526.

Bondy, B., Erfurth, A., de Jonge, S., Kruger, M., and Meyer, H. (2000). Possible association of the short allele of the serotonin transporter promoter gene polymorphism (5-HTTLPR) with violent suicide. *Mol Psychiatry*, 5(2), 193–195.

Borglum, A.D., Bruun, T.G., Kjeldsen, T.E., Ewald, H., Mors, O., Kirov, G., Russ, C., Freeman, B., Collier, D.A., and Kruse, T.A. (1999). Two novel variants in the DOPA decarboxylase gene: Association with bipolar affective disorder. *Mol Psychiatry*, 4(6), 545–551.

Borglum, A.D., Kirov, G., Craddock, N., Mors, O., Muir, W., Murray, V., McKee, I., Collier, D.A., Ewald, H., Owen, M.J., Blackwood, D., and Kruse, T.A. (2003). Possible parent-of-origin effect of Dopa decarboxylase in susceptibility to bipolar affective disorder. *Am J Med Genet*, 117B(1), 18–22.

Botstein, D., and Risch, N. (2003). Discovering genotypes underlying human phenotypes: Past successes for mendelian disease, future approaches for complex disease. *Nat Genet*, 33(Suppl.), 228–237.

Botstein, D., White, R.L., Skolnick, M., and Davis, R.W. (1980). Construction of a genetic linkage map in man using restriction fragment length polymorphisms. *Am J Hum Genet*, 32(3), 314–331.

Bowen, T., Ashworth, L., Kirov, G., Guy, C.A., Jones, I.R., McCandless, F., Craddock, N., O'Donovan, M.C., and Owen, M.J. (2000). No evidence of association from transmission disequilibrium analysis of the hKCa3 gene in bipolar disorder. *Bipolar Disord*, 2(4), 328–331.

Brunner, H.G., Nelen, M., Breakefield, X.O., Ropers, H.H., and van Oost, B.A. (1993). Abnormal behavior associated with a point mutation in the structural gene for monoamine oxidase A. *Science*, 262(5133), 578–580.

Brzustowicz, L.M., Honer, W.G., Chow, E.W., Little, D., Hogan, J., Hodgkinson, K., and Bassett, A.S. (1999). Linkage of familial schizophrenia to chromosome 13q32. *Am J Hum Genet*, 65(4), 1096–1103.

Bucher, K.D., Elston, R.C., Green, R., Whybrow, P., Helzer, J., Reich, T., Clayton, P., and Winokur, G. (1981). The transmission of manic depressive illness: II. Segregation analysis of three sets of family data. *J Psychiatr Res*, 16(1), 65–78.

Bunzel, R., Blumcke, I., Cichon, S., Normann, S., Schramm, J., Propping, P., and Nothen, M.M. (1998). Polymorphic imprinting of the serotonin-2A (5-HT2A) receptor gene in human adult brain. *Brain Res Mol Brain Res*, 59(1), 90–92.

Burgert, E., Crocq, M.A., Bausch, E., Macher, J.P., and Morris-Rosendahl, D.J. (1998). No association between the tyrosine hydroxylase microsatellite marker HUMTH01 and schizophrenia or bipolar I disorder. *Psychiatr Genet*, 8(2), 45–48.

Burton, R. (1621). *The Anatomy of Melancholy*. Republished 2001, New York: New York Review of Books.

Caberlotto, L., Jimenez, P., Overstreet, D.H., Hurd, Y.L., Mathe, A.A., and Fuxe, K. (1999). Alterations in neuropeptide Y levels and Y1 binding sites in the Flinders Sensitive Line rats, a genetic animal model of depression. *Neurosci Lett*, 265(3), 191–194.

Cadoret, R.J., O'Gorman, T.W., Heywood, E., and Troughton, E. (1985). Genetic and environmental factors in major depression. *J Affect Disord*, 9(2), 155–164.

Cardno, A.G., Marshall, E.J., Coid, B., Macdonald, A.M., Ribchester, T.R., Davies, N.J., Venturi, P., Jones, L.A., Lewis, S.W., Sham, P.C., Gottesman, I.I., Farmer, A.E., McGuffin, P., Reveley, A.M., and Murray, R.M. (1999). Heritability estimates for psychotic disorders: The Maudsley twin psychosis series. *Arch Gen Psychiatry*, 56(2), 162–168.

Cardno, A.G., Rijsdijk, F.V., Sham, P.C., Murray, R.M., and McGuffin, P. (2002). A twin study of genetic relationships between psychotic symptoms. *Am J Psychiatry*, 159(4), 539–545.

Carmelli, D., DeCarli, C., Swan, G.E., Jack, L.M., Reed, T., Wolf, P.A., and Miller, B.L. (1998). Evidence for genetic variance in white matter hyperintensity volume in normal elderly male twins. *Stroke*, 29(6), 1177–1181.

Carrasquillo, M.M., McCallion, A.S., Puffenberger, E.G., Kashuk, C.S., Nouri, N., and Chakravarti, A. (2002). Genome-wide association study and mouse model identify interaction between RET and EDNRB pathways in Hirschsprung disease. *Nat Genet*, 32(2), 237–244.

Caspi, A., Sugden, K., Moffitt, T.E., Taylor, A., Craig, I.W., Harrington, H., McClay, J., Mill, J., Martin, J., Braithwaite, A., and Poulton, R. (2003). Influence of life stress on depression: Moderation by a polymorphism in the 5-HTT gene. *Science*, 301(5631), 386–389.

Cavazzoni, P., Alda, M., Turecki, G., Rouleau, G., Grof, E., Martin, R., Duffy, A., and Grof, P. (1996). Lithium-responsive affective disorders: no association with the tyrosine hydroxylase gene. *Psychiatry Res*, 64(2), 91–96.

Chakravarti, A. (1999). Population genetics: Making sense out of sequence. *Nat Genet*, 21(Suppl. 1), 56–60.

Chandy, K.G., Fantino, E., Wittekindt, O., Kalman, K., Tong, L.L., Ho, T.H., Gutman, G.A., Crocq, M.A., Ganguli, R., Nimgaonkar, V., Morris-Rosendahl, D.J., and Gargus, J.J. (1998). Isolation of a novel potassium channel gene hSKCa3 containing a polymorphic CAG repeat: A candidate for schizophrenia and bipolar disorder? *Mol Psychiatry*, 3(1), 32–37.

Chang, K.D., Steiner, H., and Ketter, T.A. (2000). Psychiatric phenomenology of child and adolescent bipolar offspring. *J Am Acad Child Adolesc Psychiatry*, 39(4), 453–460.

Chee, I.S., Lee, S.W., Kim, J.L., Wang, S.K., Shin, Y.O., Shin, S.C., Lee, Y.H., Hwang, H.M., and Lim, M.R. (2001). 5-HT2A receptor gene promoter polymorphism-1438A/G and bipolar disorder. *Psychiatr Genet*, 11(3), 111–114.

Chen, Y.S., Akula, N., Detera-Wadleigh, S.D., Schulze, T.G., Thomas, J., Potash, J.B., DePaulo, J.R., McInnis, M.G., Cox, N.J., and McMahon, F.J. (2004). Findings in an independent sample support an association between bipolar affective disorder and the G72/G30 locus on chromosome 13q33. *Mol Psychiatry*, 9(1), 87–92; image 5.

Cheung, V.G., Conlin, L.K., Weber, T.M., Arcaro, M., Jen, K.Y., Morley, M., and Spielman, R.S. (2003). Natural variation in human gene expression assessed in lymphoblastoid cells. *Nat Genet*, 33(3), 422–425.

Chumakov, I., Blumenfeld, M., Guerassimenko, O., Cavarec, L., Palicio, M., Abderrahim, H., Bougueleret, L., Barry, C., Tanaka, H., La Rosa, P., Puech, A., Tahri, N., Cohen-Akenine, A., Delabrosse, S., Lissarrague, S., Picard, F.P., Maurice, K., Essioux, L., Millasseau, P., Grel, P., Debailleul, V., Simon, A.M., Caterina, D., Dufaure, I., Malekzadeh, K., Belova, M., Luan, J.J., Bouillot, M., Sambucy, J.L., Primas, G., Saumier, M., Boubkiri, N., Martin-Saumier, S., Nasroune, M., Peixoto, H., Delaye, A., Pinchot, V., Bastucci, M., Guillou, S., Chevillon, M., Sainz-Fuertes, R., Meguenni, S., Aurich-Costa, J., Cherif, D., Gimalac, A., Van Duijn, C., Gauvreau, D., Ouellette, G., Fortier, I., Raelson, J., Sherbatich, T., Riazanskaia, N., Rogaev, E., Raeymaekers, P., Aerssens, J., Konings, F., Luyten, W., Macciardi, F., Sham, P.C., Straub, R.E., Weinberger, D.R., Cohen, N., and Cohen, D. (2002). Genetic and physiological data implicating the new human gene G72 and the gene for D-amino acid oxidase in schizophrenia. *Proc Natl Acad Sci USA*, 99(21), 13675–13680.

Cichon, S., Nothen, M.M., Rietschel, M., Korner, J., and Propping, P. (1994). Single-strand conformation analysis (SSCA) of the dopamine D1 receptor gene (DRD1) reveals no significant mutation in patients with schizophrenia and manic depression. *Biol Psychiatry*, 36(12), 850–853.

Cichon, S., Nothen, M.M., Stober, G., Schroers, R., Albus, M., Maier, W., Rietschel, M., Korner, J., Weigelt, B., Franzek, E., Wildenauer, D., Fimmers, R., and Propping, P. (1996). Systematic screening for mutations in the 5'-regulatory region of the human dopamine D1 receptor (DRD1) gene in patients with schizophrenia and bipolar affective disorder. *Am J Med Genet*, 67(4), 424–428.

Cichon, S., Schumacher, J., Muller, D.J., Hurter, M., Windemuth, C., Strauch, K., Hemmer, S., Schulze, T.G., Schmidt-Wolf, G., Albus, M., Borrmann-Hassenbach, M., Franzek, E., Lanczik, M., Fritze, J., Kreiner, R., Reuner, U., Weigelt, B., Minges, J., Lichtermann, D., Lerer, B., Kanyas, K., Baur, M.P., Wienker, T.F., Maier, W., Rietschel, M., Propping, P., and Nothen, M.M. (2001). A genome screen for genes predisposing to bipolar affective disorder detects a new susceptibility locus on 8q. *Hum Mol Genet*, 10(25), 2933–2944.

Cichon, S., Buervenich, S., Kirov, G., Akula, N., Dimitrova, A., Green, E., Schumacher, J., Klopp, N., Becker, T., Ohlraun, S., Schulze, T.G., Tullius, M., Gross, M.M., Jones, L., Krastev, S., Nikolov, I., Hamshere, M., Jones, I., Czerski, P.M., Leszczynska-Rodziewicz, A., Kapelski, P., Bogaert, A.V., Illig, T., Hauser, J., Maier, W., Berrettini, W., Byerley, W., Coryell, W., Gershon, E.S., Kelsoe, J.R., McInnis, M.G., Murphy, D.L., Nurnberger, J.I., Reich, T., Scheftner, W., O'Donovan, M.C., Propping, P., Owen, M.J., Rietschel, M., Nothen, M.M., McMahon, F.J., and Craddock, N. (2004). Lack of support for a genetic association of the XBP1 promoter polymorphism with bipolar disorder in probands of European origin. *Nat Genet*, 36(8), 783–784.

Collier, D.A., Arranz, M.J., Sham, P., Battersby, S., Vallada, H., Gill, P., Aitchison, K.J., Sodhi, M., Li, T., Roberts, G.W., Smith, B., Morton, J., Murray, R.M., Smith, D., and Kirov, G. (1996a). The serotonin transporter is a potential susceptibility factor for bipolar affective disorder. *Neuroreport*, 7(10), 1675–1679.

Collier, D.A., Stober, G., Li, T., Heils, A., Catalano, M., Di Bella, D., Arranz, M.J., Murray, R.M., Vallada, H.P., Bengel, D., Muller, C.R., Roberts, G.W., Smeraldi, E., Kirov, G., Sham, P., and Lesch, K.P. (1996b). A novel functional polymorphism within the promoter of the serotonin transporter gene: Possible role in susceptibility to affective disorders. *Mol Psychiatry*, 1(6), 453–460.

Coon, H., Jensen, S., Hoff, M., Holik, J., Plaetke, R., Reimherr, F., Wender, P., Leppert, M., and Byerley, W. (1993). A genome-wide search for genes predisposing to manic-depression, assuming autosomal dominant inheritance. *Am J Hum Genet*, 52(6), 1234–1249.

Coon, H., Hoff, M., Holik, J., Hadley, D., Fang, N., Reimherr, F., Wender, P., and Byerley, W. (1996). Analysis of chromosome 18 DNA markers in multiplex pedigrees with manic depression. *Biol Psychiatry*, 39(8), 689–696.

Coryell, W., Endicott, J., and Keller, M. (1992). Rapidly cycling affective disorder. Demographics, diagnosis, family history, and course. *Arch Gen Psychiatry*, 49(2), 126–131.

Coryell, W., Akiskal, H., Leon, A.C., Turvey, C., Solomon, D., and Endicott, J. (2000). Family history and symptom levels during treatment for bipolar I affective disorder. *Biol Psychiatry*, 47(12), 1034–1042.

Coryell, W., Leon, A.C., Turvey, C., Akiskal, H.S., Mueller, T., and Endicott, J. (2001). The significance of psychotic features in manic episodes. *J Affect Disord*, 67, 79–88.

Courtet, P., Baud, P., Abbar, M., Boulenger, J.P., Castelnau, D., Mouthon, D., Malafosse, A., and Buresi, C. (2001). Association between violent suicidal behavior and the low activity allele of the serotonin transporter gene. *Mol Psychiatry*, 6(3), 338–341.

Craddock, N., Owen, M., Burge, S., Kurian, B., Thomas, P., and McGuffin, P. (1994). Familial cosegregation of major affective disorder and Darier's disease (keratosis follicularis) [see comments]. *Br J Psychiatry*, 164(3), 355–358.

Craddock, N., Daniels, J., Roberts, E., Rees, M., McGuffin, P., and Owen, M.J. (1995a). No evidence for allelic association between bipolar disorder and monoamine oxidase A gene polymorphisms. *Am J Med Genet, 60*(4), 322–324.

Craddock, N., Khodel, V., Van Eerdewegh, P., and Reich, T. (1995b). Mathematical limits of multilocus models: The genetic transmission of bipolar disorder. *Am J Hum Genet, 57*(3), 690–702.

Craddock, N., Roberts, Q., Williams, N., McGuffin, P., and Owen, M.J. (1995c). Association study of bipolar disorder using a functional polymorphism (Ser311→Cys) in the dopamine D2 receptor gene. *Psychiatr Genet, 5*(2), 63–65.

Craddock, N., Dave, S., and Greening, J. (2001). Association studies of bipolar disorder. *Bipolar Disord, 3*(6), 284–298.

Curtis, D., Kalsi, G., Brynjolfsson, J., McInnis, M., O'Neill, J., Smyth, C., Moloney, E., Murphy, P., McQuillin, A., Petursson, H., and Gurling, H. (2003). Genome scan of pedigrees multiply affected with bipolar disorder provides further support for the presence of a susceptibility locus on chromosome 12q23-q24, and suggests the presence of additional loci on 1p and 1q. *Psychiatr Genet, 13*(2), 77–84.

da Fonseca A. (1959). Analise Heredo-Clinca Das Perturbacoes Afectivas (Estudio De 60 Pares De Gemeos, e Sues Conganguin Neos). Proto: Impresna Protuguesa.

Dawson, E., Gill, M., Curtis, D., Castle, D., Hunt, N., Murray, R., and Powell, J. (1995). Genetic association between alleles of pancreatic phospholipase A2 gene and bipolar affective disorder. *Psychiatr Genet, 5*(4), 177–180.

DeBaun, M.R., Niemitz, E.L., and Feinberg, A.P. (2003). Association of in vitro fertilization with Beckwith-Wiedemann syndrome and epigenetic alterations of LIT1 and H19. *Am J Hum Genet, 72*(1), 156–160.

de Bruyn, A., Mendelbaum, K., Sandkuijl, L.A., Delvenne, V., Hirsch, D., Staner, L., Mendlewicz, J., and Van Broeckhoven, C. (1994). Nonlinkage of bipolar illness to tyrosine hydroxylase, tyrosinase, and D2 and D4 dopamine receptor genes on chromosome 11. *Am J Psychiatry, 151*(1), 102–106.

de Bruyn, A., Souery, D., Mendelbaum, K., Mendlewicz, J., and Van Broeckhoven, C. (1996). Linkage analysis of families with bipolar illness and chromosome 18 markers. *Biol Psychiatry, 39*(8), 679–688.

Decina, P., Kestenbaum, C.J., Farber, S., Kron, L., Gargan, M., Sackeim, H.A., and Fieve, R.R. (1983). Clinical and psychological assessment of children of bipolar probands. *Am J Psychiatry, 140*(5), 548–553.

Deckert, J., Nothen, M.M., Albus, M., Franzek, E., Rietschel, M., Ren, H., Stiles, G.L., Knapp, M., Weigelt, B., Maier, W., Beckmann, H., and Propping, P. (1998). Adenosine A1 receptor and bipolar affective disorder: Systematic screening of the gene and association studies. *Am J Med Genet, 81*(1), 18–23.

Del Favero, J., Gestel, S.V., Borglum, A.D., Muir, W., Ewald, H., Mors, O., Ivezic, S., Oruc, L., Adolfsson, R., Blackwood, D., Kruse, T., Mendlewicz, J., Schalling, M., and Van Broeckhoven, C. (2002). European combined analysis of the CTG18.1 and the ERDA1 CAG/CTG repeats in bipolar disorder. *Eur J Hum Genet, 10*(4), 276–280.

DeLisi, L.E., Goldin, L.R., Maxwell, M.E., Kazuba, D.M., and Gershon, E.S. (1987). Clinical features of illness in siblings with schizophrenia or schizoaffective disorder. *Arch Gen Psychiatry, 44*(10), 891–896.

Detera-Wadleigh, S.D., Berrettini, W.H., Goldin, L.R., Boorman, D., Anderson, S., and Gershon, E.S. (1987). Close linkage of c-Harvey-ras-1 and the insulin gene to affective disorder is ruled out in three North American pedigrees. *Nature, 325*(6107), 806–808.

Detera-Wadleigh, S.D., Badner, J.A., Goldin, L.R., Berrettini, W.H., Sanders, A.R., Rollins, D.Y., Turner, G., Moses, T., Haerian, H., Muniec, D., Nurnberger, J.I. Jr., and Gershon, E.S. (1996). Affected-sib-pair analyses reveal support of prior evidence for a susceptibility locus for bipolar disorder, on 21q. *Am J Hum Genet, 58*(6), 1279–1285.

Detera-Wadleigh, S.D., Badner, J.A., Yoshikawa, T., Sanders, A.R., Goldin, L.R., Turner, G., Rollins, D.Y., Moses, T., Guroff, J.J., Kazuba, D., Maxwell, M.E., Edenberg, H.J., Foroud, T., Lahiri, D., Nurnberger, J.I. Jr., Stine, O.C., McMahon, F., Meyers, D.A., MacKinnon, D., Simpson, S., McInnis, M., DePaulo, J.R., Rice, J., Goate, A., and Gershon, E.S. (1997). Initial genome scan of the NIMH genetics initiative bipolar pedigrees: chromosomes 4, 7, 9, 18, 19, 20, and 21q. *Am J Med Genet, 74*(3), 254–262.

Detera-Wadleigh, S.D., Badner, J.A., Berrettini, W.H., Yoshikawa, T., Goldin, L.R., Turner, G., Rollins, D.Y., Moses, T., Sanders, A.R., Karkera, J.D., Esterling, L.E., Zeng, J., Ferraro, T.N., Guroff, J.J., Kazuba, D., Maxwell, M.E., Nurnberger, J.I. Jr., and Gershon, E.S. (1999). A high-density genome scan detects evidence for a bipolar-disorder susceptibility locus on 13q32 and other potential loci on 1q32 and 18p11.2. *Proc Natl Acad Sci USA, 96*(10), 5604–5609.

Di Bella, D., Catalano, M., Cichon, S., and Nothen, M.M. (1996). Association study of a null mutation in the dopamine D4 receptor gene in Italian patients with obsessive-compulsive disorder, bipolar mood disorder and schizophrenia. *Psychiatr Genet, 6*(3), 119–121.

Dick, D.M., Foroud, T., Edenberg, H.J., Miller, M., Bowman, E., Rau, N.L., DePaulo, J.R., McInnis, M., Gershon, E., McMahon, F., Rice, J.P., Bierut, L.J., Reich, T., and Nurnberger, J. Jr. (2002). Apparent replication of suggestive linkage on chromosome 16 in the NIMH genetics initiative bipolar pedigrees. *Am J Med Genet, 114*(4), 407–412.

Dick, D.M., Foroud, T., Flury, L., Bowman, E.S., Miller, M.J., Rau, N.L., Moe, P.R., Samavedy, N., El-Mallakh, R., Manji, H., Glitz, D.A., Meyer, E.T., Smiley, C., Hahn, R., Widmark, C., McKinney, R., Sutton, L., Ballas, C., Grice, D., Berrettini, W., Byerley, W., Coryell, W., DePaulo, R., MacKinnon, D.F., Gershon, E.S., Kelsoe, J.R., McMahon, F.J., McInnis, M., Murphy, D.L., Reich, T., Scheftner, W., and Nurnberger, J.I. Jr. (2003). Genomewide linkage analyses of bipolar disorder: A new sample of 250 pedigrees from the National Institute of Mental Health Genetics Initiative. *Am J Hum Genet, 73*(1), 107–114. Erratum in: *Am J Hum Genet, 73*(4), 979.

Dimitrova, A., Georgieva, L., Nikolov, I., Poriazova, N., Krastev, S., Toncheva, D., Owen, M.J., and Kirov, G. (2002). Major psychiatric disorders and the serotonin transporter gene (SLC6A4): Family-based association studies. *Psychiatr Genet, 12*(3), 137–141.

Duffy, A., Turecki, G., Grof, P., Cavazzoni, P., Grof, E., Joober, R., Ahrens, B., Berghofer, A., Muller-Oerlinghausen, B., Dvorakova, M., Libigerova, E., Vojtechovsky, M., Zvolsky, P., Nilsson, A., Licht, R.W., Rasmussen, N.A., Schou, M., Vestergaard, P., Holzinger, A., Schumann, C., Thau, K., Robertson, C., Rouleau, G.A., and Alda, M. (2000). Association and linkage studies of candidate genes involved in GABAergic neurotransmission in lithium-responsive bipolar disorder. *J Psychiatry Neurosci, 25*(4), 353–358.

Eastwood, S.L., Burnet, P.W., and Harrison, P.J. (2000). Expression of complexin I and II mRNAs and their regulation by antipsychotic drugs in the rat forebrain. *Synapse,* 36(3), 167–177.

Edenberg, H.J., Foroud, T., Conneally, P.M., Sorbel, J.J., Carr, K., Crose, C., Willig, C., Zhao, J., Miller, M., Bowman, E., Mayeda, A., Rau, N.L., Smiley, C., Rice, J.P., Goate, A., Reich, T., Stine, O.C., McMahon, F., DePaulo, J.R., Meyers, D., Detera-Wadleigh, S.D., Goldin, L.R., Gershon, E.S., Blehar, M.C., and Nurnberger, J.I. Jr. (1997). Initial genomic scan of the NIMH genetics initiative bipolar pedigrees: Chromosomes 3, 5, 15, 16, 17, and 22. *Am J Med Genet,* 74(3), 238–246.

Egeland, J.A., Gerhard, D.S., Pauls, D.L., Sussex, J.N., Kidd, K.K., Allen, C.R., Hostetter, A.M., and Housman, D.E. (1987). Bipolar affective disorders linked to DNA markers on chromosome 11. *Nature,* 325(6107), 783–787.

Ekholm, J.M., Kieseppa, T., Hiekkalinna, T., Partonen, T., Paunio, T., Perola, M., Ekelund, J., Lonnqvist, J., Pekkarinen-Ijas, P., and Peltonen, L. (2003). Evidence of susceptibility loci on 4q32 and 16p12 for bipolar disorder. *Hum Mol Genet,* 12(15), 1907–1915.

Endicott, J., and Spitzer, R.L. (1978). A diagnostic interview: the schedule for affective disorders and schizophrenia. *Arch Gen Psychiatry,* 35(7), 837–844.

Erdmann, J., Shimron-Abarbanell, D., Cichon, S., Albus, M., Maier, W., Lichtermann, D., Minges, J., Reuner, U., Franzek, E., and Ertl, M.A. (1995). Systematic screening for mutations in the promoter and the coding region of the 5-HT1A gene. *Am J Med Genet,* 60(5), 393–399.

Erdmann, J., Nothen, M.M., Shimron-Abarbanell, D., Rietschel, M., Albus, M., Borrmann, M., Maier, W., Franzek, E., Korner, J., Weigelt, B., Fimmers, R., and Propping, P. (1996). The human serotonin 7 (5-HT7) receptor gene: Genomic organization and systematic mutation screening in schizophrenia and bipolar affective disorder. *Mol Psychiatry,* 1(5), 392–397.

Erlenmeyer-Kimling, L., and Cornblatt, B.A. (1992). A summary of attentional findings in the New York High-Risk Project. *J Psychiatr Res,* 26(4), 405–426.

Erlenmeyer-Kimling, L., Adamo, U.H., Rock, D., Roberts, S.A., Bassett, A.S., Squires-Wheeler, E., Cornblatt, B.A., Endicott, J., Pape, S., and Gottesman, I.I. (1997). The New York High-Risk Project. Prevalence and comorbidity of axis I disorders in offspring of schizophrenic parents at 25-year follow-up. *Arch Gen Psychiatry,* 54(12), 1096–1102.

Esterling, L.E., Yoshikawa, T., Turner, G., Badner, J.A., Bengel, D., Gershon, E.S., Berrettini, W.H., and Detera-Wadleigh, S.D. (1998). Serotonin transporter (5-HTT) gene and bipolar affective disorder. *Am J Med Genet,* 81(1), 37–40.

Etain, B., Rousseva, A., Roy, I., Henry, C., Malafosse, A., Buresi, C., Preisig, M., Rayah, F., Leboyer, M., and Bellivier, F. (2004). Lack of association between 5HT2A receptor gene haplotype, bipolar disorder and its clinical subtypes in a West European sample. *Am J Med Genet B Neuropsychiatr Genet,* 129(1), 29–33.

Evans, K.L., Le Hellard, S., Morris, S.W., Lawson, D., Whitton, C., Semple, C.A., Fantes, J.A., Torrance, H.S., Malloy, M.P., Maule, J.C., Humphray, S.J., Ross, M.T., Bentley, D.R., Muir, W.J., Blackwood, D.H., and Porteous, D.J. (2001). A 6.9-Mb high-resolution BAC/PAC contig of human 4p15.3-p16.1, a candidate region for bipolar affective disorder. *Genomics,* 71(3), 315–323.

Ewald, H., Mors, O., Flint, T., Koed, K., Eiberg, H., and Kruse, T.A. (1995a). A possible locus for manic depressive illness on chromosome 16p13. *Psychiatr Genet,* 5(2), 71–81.

Ewald, H., Mors, O., Flint, T., Friedrich, U., Eiberg, H., and Kruse, T.A. (1995b). Linkage analysis between manic-depressive illness and markers on the long arm of chromosome 11. *Am J Med Genet,* 60(5), 386–392.

Ewald, H., Mors, O., Koed, K., Eiberg, H., and Kruse, T.A. (1997). Susceptibility loci for bipolar affective disorder on chromosome 18? A review and a study of Danish families. *Psychiatr Genet,* 7(1), 1–12.

Ewald, H., Degn, B., Mors, O., and Kruse, T.A. (1998). Significant linkage between bipolar affective disorder and chromosome 12q24. *Psychiatr Genet,* 8(3), 131–140.

Falconer, D.S. (1965). The inheritance of liability to certain diseases, estimated from the incidence among relatives. *Ann Hum Genet,* 29, 51–76.

Fallin, M.D., Lasseter, V.K., Wolyniec, P.S., McGrath, J.A., Nestadt, G., Valle, D., Liang, K.Y., and Pulver, A.E. (2004). Genomewide linkage scan for bipolar-disorder susceptibility loci among Ashkenazi Jewish families. *Am J Hum Genet,* 75(2), 204–219.

Faraone, S.V., Tsuang, M.T., and Gutierrez, J.M. (1987). Long-term outcome and family psychiatric illness in unipolar and bipolar disorders. *Psychopharmacol Bull,* 23(3), 465–467.

Faraone, S.V., Biederman, J., Mennin, D., Wozniak, J., and Spencer, T. (1997). Attention-deficit hyperactivity disorder with bipolar disorder: a familial subtype? *J Am Acad Child Adolesc Psychiatry,* 36(10), 1378–1387.

Faraone, S.V., Matise, T., Svrakic, D., Pepple, J., Malaspina, D., Suarez, B., Hampe, C., Zambuto, C.T., Schmitt, K., Meyer, J., Markel, P., Lee, H., Harkavy Friedman, J., Kaufmann, C., Cloninger, C.R., and Tsuang, M.T. (1998). Genome scan of European-American schizophrenia pedigrees: Results of the NIMH Genetics Initiative and Millennium Consortium. *Am J Med Genet,* 81(4), 290–295.

Faraone, S.V., Doyle, A.E., Mick, E., and Biederman, J. (2001a). Meta-analysis of the association between the 7-repeat allele of the dopamine D(4) receptor gene and attention deficit hyperactivity disorder. *Am J Psychiatry,* 158(7), 1052–1057.

Faraone, S.V., Biederman, J., and Monuteaux, M.C. (2001b). Attention deficit hyperactivity disorder with bipolar disorder in girls: Further evidence for a familial subtype? *J Affect Disord,* 64(1), 19–26.

Faraone, S.V., Glatt, S.J., Su, J., and Tsuang, M.T. (2004). Three potential susceptibility loci shown by a genome-wide scan for regions influencing the age at onset of mania. *Am J Psychiatry,* 161(4), 625–630.

Farmer, A.E., McGuffin, P., and Gottesman, I.I. (1987). Twin concordance for DSM-III schizophrenia. Scrutinizing the validity of the definition. *Arch Gen Psychiatry,* 44(7), 634–641.

Farmer, A., Breen, G., Brewster, S., Craddock, N., Gill, M., Korszun, A., Maier, W., Middleton, L., Mors, O., Owen, M., Perry, J., Preisig, M., Rietschel, M., Reich, T., Jones, L., Jones, I., and McGuffin, P. (2004). The Depression Network (DeNT) Study: Methodology and sociodemographic characteristics of the first 470 affected sibling pairs from a large multi-site linkage genetic study. *BMC Psychiatry,* 4(1), 42.

Ferrier, I.N., and Thompson, J.M. (2002). Cognitive impairment in bipolar affective disorder: Implications for the bipolar diathesis. *Br J Psychiatry,* 180, 293–295.

Foroud, T., Castelluccio, P.F., Koller, D.L., Edenberg, H.J., Miller, M., Bowman, E., Rau, N.L., Smiley, C., Rice, J.P., Goate, A., Armstrong, C., Bierut, L.J., Reich, T., Detera-Wadleigh, S.D., Goldin, L.R., Badner, J.A., Guroff, J.J., Gershon, E.S., McMahon, F.J.,

Simpson, S., MacKinnon, D., McInnis, M., Stine, O.C., De-Paulo, J.R., Blehar, M.C., and Nurnberger, J.I. Jr. (2000). Suggestive evidence of a locus on chromosome 10p using the NIMH genetics initiative bipolar affective disorder pedigrees. *Am J Med Genet*, 96(1), 18–23.

Franks, E., Guy, C., Jacobsen, N., Bowen, T., Owen, M.J., O'Donovan, M.C., and Craddock, N. (1999). Eleven trinucleotide repeat loci that map to chromosome 12 excluded from involvement in the pathogenesis of bipolar disorder. *Am J Med Genet*, 88(1), 67–70.

Freimer, N.B., Reus, V.I., Escamilla, M.A., McInnes, L.A., Spesny, M., Leon, P., Service, S.K., Smith, L.B., Silva, S., Rojas, E., Gallegos, A., Meza, L., Fournier, E., Baharloo, S., Blankenship, K., Tyler, D.J., Batki, S., Vinogradov, S., Weissenbach, J., Barondes, S.H., and Sandkuijl, L.A. (1996). Genetic mapping using haplotype, association and linkage methods suggests a locus for severe bipolar disorder (BPI) at 18q22–q23. *Nat Genet*, 12(4), 436–441.

Friddle, C., Koskela, R., Ranade, K., Hebert, J., Cargill, M., Clark, C.D., McInnis, M., Simpson, S., McMahon, F., Stine, O.C., Meyers, D., Xu, J., MacKinnon, D., Swift-Scanlan, T., Jamison, K., Folstein, S., Daly, M., Kruglyak, L., Marr, T., DePaulo, J.R., and Botstein, D. (2000). Full-genome scan for linkage in 50 families segregating the bipolar affective disease phenotype. *Am J Hum Genet*, 66(1), 205–215.

Furlong, R.A., Coleman, T.A., Ho, L., Rubinsztein, J.S., Walsh, C., Paykel, E.S., and Rubinsztein, D.C. (1998a). No association of a functional polymorphism in the dopamine D2 receptor promoter region with bipolar or unipolar affective disorders. *Am J Med Genet*, 81(5), 385–387.

Furlong, R.A., Ho, L., Rubinsztein, J.S., Walsh, C., Paykel, E.S., and Rubinsztein, D.C. (1998b). No association of the tryptophan hydroxylase gene with bipolar affective disorder, unipolar affective disorder, or suicidal behaviour in major affective disorder. *Am J Med Genet*, 81(3), 245–247.

Furlong, R.A., Ho, L., Walsh, C., Rubinsztein, J.S., Jain, S., Paykel, E.S., Easton, D.F., and Rubinsztein, D.C. (1998c). Analysis and meta-analysis of two serotonin transporter gene polymorphisms in bipolar and unipolar affective disorders. *Am J Med Genet*, 81(1), 58–63.

Furlong, R.A., Ho, L., Rubinsztein, J.S., Walsh, C., Paykel, E.S., and Rubinsztein, D.C. (1999a). Analysis of the monoamine oxidase A (MAOA) gene in bipolar affective disorder by association studies, meta-analyses, and sequencing of the promoter. *Am J Med Genet*, 88(4), 398–406.

Furlong, R.A., Rubinsztein, J.S., Ho, L., Walsh, C., Coleman, T.A., Muir, W.J., Paykel, E.S., Blackwood, D.H., and Rubinsztein, D.C. (1999b). Analysis and metaanalysis of two polymorphisms within the tyrosine hydroxylase gene in bipolar and unipolar affective disorders. *Am J Med Genet*, 88(1), 88–94.

Gabriel, S.B., Schaffner, S.F., Nguyen, H., Moore, J.M., Roy, J., Blumenstiel, B., Higgins, J., DeFelice, M., Lochner, A., Faggart, M., Liu-Cordero, S.N., Rotimi, C., Adeyemo, A., Cooper, R., Ward, R., Lander, E.S., Daly, M.J., and Altshuler, D. (2002). The structure of haplotype blocks in the human genome. *Science*, 296(5576), 2225–2229.

Gass, P., Reichardt, H.M., Strekalova, T., Henn, F., and Tronche, F. (2001). Mice with targeted mutations of glucocorticoid and mineralocorticoid receptors: Models for depression and anxiety? *Physiol Behav*, 73(5), 811–825.

Geller, B., and Cook, E.H. Jr. (2000). Ultradian rapid cycling in prepubertal and early adolescent bipolarity is not in transmission disequilibrium with val/met COMT alleles. *Biol Psychiatry*, 47(7), 605–609.

Geller, B., Badner, J.A., Tillman, R., Christian, S.L., Bolhofner, K., and Cook, E.H. Jr. (2004). Linkage disequilibrium of the brain-derived neurotrophic factor Val66Met polymorphism in children with a prepubertal and early adolescent bipolar disorder phenotype. *Am J Psychiatry*, 161(9), 1698–1700.

Georgieva, L., Dimitrova, A., Nikolov, I., Koleva, S., Tsvetkova, R., Owen, M.J., Toncheva, D., and Kirov, G. (2002). Dopamine transporter gene (DAT1) VNTR polymorphism in major psychiatric disorders: Family-based association study in the Bulgarian population. *Acta Psychiatr Scand*, 105(5), 396–399.

Gershon, E.S., and Goldin, L.R. (1989). Linkage data on affective disorders in an epidemiologic context. *Genet Epidemiol*, 6(1), 201–209.

Gershon, E.S., Hamovit, J., Guroff, J.J., Dibble, E., Leckman, J.F., Sceery, W., Targum, S.D., Nurnberger, J.I. Jr., Goldin, L.R., and Bunney, W.E. Jr. (1982). A family study of schizoaffective, bipolar I, bipolar II, unipolar, and normal control probands. *Arch Gen Psychiatry*, 39(10), 1157–1167.

Gershon, E.S., McKnew, D., Cytryn, L., Hamovit, J., Schreiber, J., Hibbs, E., and Pellegrini, D. (1985). Diagnoses in school-age children of bipolar affective disorder patients and normal controls. *J Affect Disord*, 8(3), 283–291.

Gershon, E.S., Weissman, M.M., Guroff, J.J., Prusoff, B.A., and Leckman, J.F. (1986). Validation of criteria for major depression through controlled family study. *J Affect Disord*, 11(2), 125–131.

Gershon, E.S., DeLisi, L.E., Hamovit, J., Nurnberger, J.I. Jr., Maxwell, M.E., Schreiber, J., Dauphinais, D., Dingman, C.W. II, and Guroff, J.J. (1988). A controlled family study of chronic psychoses. Schizophrenia and schizoaffective disorder. *Arch Gen Psychiatry*, 45(4), 328–336.

Gershon, E.S., Goldin, L.R., Guroff, J.J., and Hamovit, J.R. (1989). Description of the National Institute of Mental Health family study of affective disorders. *Genet Epidemiol*, 6(1), 183–185.

Gill, M., Castle, D., Hunt, N., Clements, A., Sham, P., and Murray, R.M. (1991). Tyrosine hydroxylase polymorphisms and bipolar affective disorder. *J Psychiatr Res*, 25(4), 179–184.

Gill, M., Vallada, H., Collier, D., Sham, P., Holmans, P., Murray, R., McGuffin, P., Nanko, S., Owen, M., Antonarakis, S., Housman, D., Kazazian, H., Nestadt, G., Pulver, A.E., Straub, R.E., MacLean, C.J., Walsh, D., Kendler, K.S., DeLisi, L., Polymeropoulos, M., Coon, H., Byerley, W., Lofthouse, R., Gershon, E., and Read, C.M. (1996). A combined analysis of D22S278 marker alleles in affected sib-pairs: Support for a susceptibility locus for schizophrenia at chromosome 22q12. Schizophrenia Collaborative Linkage Group (Chromosome 22). *Am J Med Genet*, 67(1), 40–45.

Ginns, E.I., St. Jean, P., Philibert, R.A., Galdzicka, M., Damschroder-Williams, P., Thiel, B., Long, R.T., Ingraham, L.J., Dalwaldi, H., Murray, M.A., Ehlert, M., Paul, S., Remortel, B.G., Patel, A.P., Anderson, M.C., Shaio, C., Lau, E., Dymarskaia, I., Martin, B.M., Stubblefield, B., Falls, K.M., Carulli, J.P., Keith, T.P., Fann, C.S., Lacy, L.G., Allen, C.R., Hostetter, A.M., Elston, R.C., Schork, N.J., Egeland, J.A., and Paul, S.M. (1998). A genome-wide search for chromosomal loci linked to mental health wellness in relatives at high risk for bipolar affective disorder among the Old Order Amish. *Proc Natl Acad Sci USA*, 95(26), 15531–15536.

Goldin, L.R., Gershon, E.S., Targum, S.D., Sparkes, R.S., and McGinniss, M. (1983). Segregation and linkage analyses in families of patients with bipolar, unipolar, and schizoaffective mood disorders. *Am J Hum Genet*, 35(2), 274–287.

Goldstein, J.M., Faraone, S.V., Chen, W.J., and Tsuang, M.T. (1993). The role of gender in understanding the familial transmission of schizoaffective disorder. *Br J Psychiatry*, 163, 763–768.

Gomez-Casero, E., Perez de Castro, I., Saiz-Ruiz, J., Llinares, C., and Fernandez-Piqueras, J. (1996). No association between particular DRD3 and DAT gene polymorphisms and manic-depressive illness in a Spanish sample. *Psychiatr Genet*, 6(4), 209–212.

Goossens, D., Del Favero, J., and Van Broeckhoven, C. (2001). Trinucleotide repeat expansions: Do they contribute to bipolar disorder? *Brain Res Bull*, 56(3–4), 243–257.

Gourovitch, M.L., Torrey, E.F., Gold, J.M., Randolph, C., Weinberger, D.R., and Goldberg, T.E. (1999). Neuropsychological performance of monozygotic twins discordant for bipolar disorder. *Biol Psychiatry*, 45(5), 639–646.

Griffith, A.J., and Friedman, T.B. (1999). Making sense out of sound [news]. *Nat Genet*, 21(4), 347–349.

Grigoroiu-Serbanescu, M., Wickramaratne, P.J., Hodge, S.E., Milea, S., and Mihailescu, R. (1997). Genetic anticipation and imprinting in bipolar I illness. *Br J Psychiatry*, 170, 162–166.

Grigoroiu-Serbanescu, M., Martinez, M., Nothen, M.M., Grinberg, M., Sima, D., Propping, P., Marinescu, E., and Hrestic, M. (2001). Different familial transmission patterns in bipolar I disorder with onset before and after age 25. *Am J Med Genet*, 105(8), 765–773.

Grof, P., Duffy, A., Cavazzoni, P., Grof, E., Garnham, J., MacDougall, M., O'Donovan, C., and Alda, M. (2002). Is response to prophylactic lithium a familial trait? *J Clin Psychiatry*, 63(10), 942–947.

Guidotti, A., Auta, J., Davis, J.M., Di-Giorgi-Gerevini, V., Dwivedi, Y., Grayson, D.R., Impagnatiello, F., Pandey, G., Pesold, C., Sharma, R., Uzunov, D., and Costa, E. (2000). Decrease in reelin and glutamic acid decarboxylase67 (GAD67) expression in schizophrenia and bipolar disorder: A postmortem brain study. *Arch Gen Psychiatry*, 57(11), 1061–1069. Erratum in: Arch Gen Psychiatry, 2002, 59(1), 12.

Gutierrez, B., Arranz, M., Fananas, L., Valles, V., Guillamat, R., van Os, J., and Collier, D. (1995). 5HT2A receptor gene and bipolar affective disorder [letter]. *Lancet*, 346(8980), 969.

Gutierrez, B., Fananas, L., Arranz, M.J., Valles, V., Guillamat, R., van Os, J., and Collier, D. (1996). Allelic association analysis of the 5-HT2C receptor gene in bipolar affective disorder. *Neurosci Lett*, 212(1), 65–67.

Gutierrez, B., Bertranpetit, J., Guillamat, R., Valles, V., Arranz, M.J., Kerwin, R., and Fananas, L. (1997). Association analysis of the catechol-O-methyltransferase gene and bipolar affective disorder. *Am J Psychiatry*, 154(1), 113–115.

Gutierrez, B., Arranz, M.J., Collier, D.A., Valles, V., Guillamat, R., Bertranpetit, J., Murray, R.M., and Fanas, L. (1998). Serotonin transporter gene and risk for bipolar affective disorder: An association study in Spanish population. *Biol Psychiatry*, 43(11), 843–847.

Gutierrez, B., Arias, B., Papiol, S., Rosa, A., and Fananas, L. (2001). Association study between novel promoter variants at the 5-HT2C receptor gene and human patients with bipolar affective disorder. *Neurosci Lett*, 309(2), 135–137.

Guy, C.A., Bowen, T., Williams, N., Jones, I.R., McCandless, F., McGuffin, P., Owen, M.J., Craddock, N., and O'Donovan, M.C. (1999). No association between a polymorphic CAG repeat in the human potassium channel gene hKCa3 and bipolar disorder. *Am J Med Genet*, 88(1), 57–60.

Haines, J.L., and Pericak-Vance, M.A. (1998). Overview of mapping common and genetically complex human disease traits. In J.L. Haines and M.A. Pericak-Vance (Eds.), *Approaches to Gene Mapping in Complex Human Diseases*. New York: John Wiley and Sons.

Hariri, A.R., Mattay, V.S., Tessitore, A., Kolachana, B., Fera, F., Goldman, D., Egan, M.F., and Weinberger, D.R. (2002). Serotonin transporter genetic variation and the response of the human amygdala. *Science*, 297(5580), 400–403.

Hashimoto, K., Maruyama, H., Nishiyama, M., Asaba, K., Ikeda, Y., Takao, T., Iwasaki, Y., Kumon, Y., Suehiro, T., Tanimoto, N., Mizobuchi, M., and Nakamura, T. (2005). Susceptibility alleles and haplotypes of human leukocyte antigen DRB1, DQA1, and DQB1 in autoimmune polyglandular syndrome type III in Japanese population. *Horm Res*, 64(5), 253–260.

Hattori, E., Yamada, K., Ebihara, M., Toyota, T., Nankai, M., Shibuya, H., and Yoshikawa, T. (2002). Association study of the short tandem repeat in the 5' upstream region of the cholecystokinin gene with mood disorders in the Japanese population. *Am J Med Genet*, 114(5), 523–526.

Hattori, E., Liu, C., Badner, J.A., Bonner, T.I., Christian, S.L., Maheshwari, M., Detera-Wadleigh, S.D., Gibbs, R.A., and Gershon, E.S. (2003). Polymorphisms at the G72/G30 gene locus, on 13q33, are associated with bipolar disorder in two independent pedigree series. *Am J Hum Genet*, 72(5), 1131–1140.

Hauser, E.R., Boehnke, M., Guo, S.W., and Risch, N. (1996). Affected-sib-pair interval mapping and exclusion for complex genetic traits: sampling considerations. *Genet Epidemiol*, 13(2), 117–137.

Hawi, Z., Mynett-Johnson, L., Murphy, V., Straub, R.E., Kendler, K.S., Walsh, D., McKeon, P., and Gill, M. (1999). No evidence to support the association of the potassium channel gene hSKCa3 CAG repeat with schizophrenia or bipolar disorder in the Irish population. *Mol Psychiatry*, 4(5), 488–491.

Hayward, B.E., Moran, V., Strain, L., and Bonthron, D.T. (1998). Bidirectional imprinting of a single gene: GNAS1 encodes maternally, paternally, and biallelically derived proteins. *Proc Natl Acad Sci USA*, 95(26), 15475–15480.

Heath, A.C., Berg, K., Eaves, L.J., Solaas, M.H., Corey, L.A., Sundet, J., Magnus, P., and Nance, W.E. (1985). Education policy and the heritability of educational attainment. *Nature*, 314(6013), 734–736.

Heckers, S., Stone, D., Walsh, J., Shick, J., Koul, P., and Benes, F.M. (2002). Differential hippocampal expression of glutamic acid decarboxylase 65 and 67 messenger RNA in bipolar disorder and schizophrenia. *Arch Gen Psychiatry*, 59(6), 521–529.

Heiden, A., Schussler, P., Itzlinger, U., Leisch, F., Scharfetter, J., Gebhardt, C., Fuchs, K., Willeit, M., Nilsson, L., Miller-Reiter, E., Stompe, T., Meszaros, K., Sieghart, W., Hornik, K., Kasper, S., and Aschauer, H.N. (2000). Association studies of candidate genes in bipolar disorders. *Neuropsychobiology*, 42(Suppl. 1), 18–21.

Hettema, J.M., Neale, M.C., and Kendler, K.S. (1995). Physical similarity and the equal-environment assumption in twin studies of psychiatric disorders. *Behav Genet*, 25(4), 327–335.

Heun, R., and Maier, W. (1993). The distinction of bipolar II disorder from bipolar I and recurrent unipolar depression: Results of a controlled family study. *Acta Psychiatr Scand*, 87(4), 279–284.

Hodgkinson, S., Gurling, H.M., Marchbanks, R.H., McInnis, M., and Petursson, H. (1987a). Minisatellite mapping in manic depression. *J Psychiatr Res*, 21(4), 589–596.

Hodgkinson, S., Sherrington, R., Gurling, H., Marchbanks, R., Reeders, S., Mallet, J., McInnis, M., Petursson, H., and Brynjolfsson, J. (1987b). Molecular genetic evidence for heterogeneity in manic depression. *Nature*, 325(6107), 805–806.

Hodgkinson, C.A., Goldman, D., Jaeger, J., Persaud S., Kane, J.M., Lipsky, R.H., and Malhotra, A.K. (2004). Disrupted in schizophrenia 1 (DISC1): Association with schizophrenia, schizoaffective disorder, and bipolar disorder. *Am J Hum Genet*, 75(5), 862–872.

Hoehe, M.R., Wendel, B., Grunewald, I., Chiaroni, P., Levy, N., Morris-Rosendahl, D., Macher, J.P., Sander, T., and Crocq, M.A. (1998). Serotonin transporter (5-HTT) gene polymorphisms are not associated with susceptibility to mood disorders. *Am J Med Genet*, 81(1), 1–3

Hoffmann, H. (1921). *Die Nachkommenschaft bei endogenen Psychosen*. Berlin: Springer-Verlag.

Holmans, P., Zubenko, G.S., Crowe, R.R., DePaulo, J.R. Jr., Scheftner, W.A., Weissman, M.M., Zubenko, W.N., Boutelle, S., Murphy-Eberenz, K., MacKinnon, D., McInnis, M.G., Marta, D.H., Adams, P., Knowles, J.A., Gladis, M., Thomas, J., Chellis, J., Miller, E., and Levinson, D.F. (2004). Genomewide significant linkage to recurrent, early-onset major depressive disorder on chromosome 15q. *Am J Hum Genet*, 74(6), 1154–1167.

Holmes, A., Yang, R.J., Murphy, D.L., and Crawley, J.N. (2002). Evaluation of antidepressant-related behavioral responses in mice lacking the serotonin transporter. *Neuropsychopharmacology*, 27(6), 914–923.

Hong, C.J., Tsai, S.J., Cheng, C.Y., Liao, W.Y., Song, H.L., and Lai, H.C. (1999). Association analysis of the 5-HT(6) receptor polymorphism (C267T) in mood disorders. *Am J Med Genet*, 88(6), 601–602.

Hong, C.J., Liu, H.C., Liu, T.Y., Lin, C.H., Cheng, C.Y., and Tsai, S.J. (2003). Brain-derived neurotrophic factor (BDNF) Val66Met polymorphisms in Parkinson's disease and age of onset. *Neurosci Lett*, 353(1), 75–77.

Horikawa, Y., Oda, N., Cox, N.J., Li, X., Orho-Melander, M., Hara, M., Hinokio, Y., Lindner, T.H., Mashima, H., Schwarz, P.E., del Bosque-Plata, L., Horikawa, Y., Oda, Y., Yoshiuchi, I., Colilla, S., Polonsky, K.S., Wei, S., Concannon, P., Iwasaki, N., Schulze, J., Baier, L.J., Bogardus, C., Groop, L., Boerwinkle, E., Hanis, C.L., and Bell, G.I. (2000). Genetic variation in the gene encoding calpain-10 is associated with type 2 diabetes mellitus. *Nat Genet*, 26(2), 163–175.

Horikawa, Y., Oda, N., Yu, L., Imamura, S., Fujiwara, K., Makino, M., Seino, Y., Itoh, M., and Takeda, J. (2003). Genetic variations in calpain-10 gene are not a major factor in the occurrence of type 2 diabetes in Japanese. *J Clin Endocrinol Metab*, 88(1), 244–247.

Horiuchi, Y., Nakayama, J., Ishiguro, H., Ohtsuki, T., Detera-Wadleigh, S.D., Toyota, T., Yamada, K., Nankai, M., Shibuya, H., Yoshikawa, T., and Arinami, T. (2004). Possible association between a haplotype of the GABA-A receptor alpha 1 subunit gene (GABRA1) and mood disorders. *Biol Psychiatry*, 55(1), 40–45.

Hou, S.J., Yen, F.C., Cheng, C.Y., Tsai, S.J., and Hong, C.J. (2004). X-box binding protein 1 (XBP1) C—116G polymorphisms in bipolar disorders and age of onset. *Neurosci Lett*, 367(2), 232–234.

Huang, Y.Y., Oquendo, M.A., Friedman, J.M., Greenhill, L.L., Brodsky, B., Malone, K.M., Khait, V., and Mann, J.J. (2003). Substance abuse disorder and major depression are associated with the human 5-HT1B receptor gene (HTR1B) G861C polymorphism. *Neuropsychopharmacology*, 28(1), 163–169.

Humm, D.G. (1932). Mental disorders in siblings. *Am J Psychiatry*, 89, 239–284.

Hurd, Y.L. (2002). Subjects with major depression or bipolar disorder show reduction of prodynorphin mRNA expression in discrete nuclei of the amygdaloid complex. *Mol Psychiatry*, 7(1), 75–81.

Inayama, Y., Yoneda, H., Sakai, T., Ishida, T., Kobayashi, S., Nonomura, Y., Kono, Y., Koh, J., and Asaba, H. (1993). Lack of association between bipolar affective disorder and tyrosine hydroxylase DNA marker. *Am J Med Genet*, 48(2), 87–89.

Ishiguro, H., Ohtsuki, T., Okubo, Y., Kurumaji, A., and Arinami, T. (2001). Association analysis of the pituitary adenyl cyclase activating peptide gene (PACAP) on chromosome 18p11 with schizophrenia and bipolar disorders. *J Neural Transm*, 108(7), 849–854.

Itokawa, M., Yamada, K., Iwayama-Shigeno, Y., Ishitsuka, Y., Detera-Wadleigh, S., and Yoshikawa, T. (2003). Genetic analysis of a functional GRIN2A promoter (GT)n repeat in bipolar disorder pedigrees in humans. *Neurosci Lett*, 345(1), 53–56.

Iwamoto, K., Kakiuchi, C., Bundo, M., Ikeda, K., and Kato T. (2004). Molecular characterization of bipolar disorder by comparing gene expression profiles of postmortem brains of major mental disorders. *Mol Psychiatry*, 9(4), 406–416.

Iwamoto, K., Bundo, M., and Kato, T. (2005). Altered expression of mitochondria-related genes in postmortem brains of patients with bipolar disorder or schizophrenia, as revealed by large-scale DNA microarray analysis. *Hum Mol Genet*, 14(2), 241–253.

Jacobsen, N., Daniels, J., Moorhead, S., Harrison, D., Feldman, E., McGuffin, P., Owen, M.J., and Craddock, N. (1996). Association study of bipolar disorder at the phospholipase A2 gene (PLA2A) in the Darier's disease (DAR) region of chromosome 12q23-q24.1. *Psychiatr Genet*, 6(4), 195–199.

Jahnes, E., Muller, D.J., Schulze, T.G., Windemuth, C., Cichon, S., Ohlraun, S., Fangerau, H., Held, T., Maier, W., Propping, P., Nothen, M.M., and Rietschel, M. (2002). Association study between two variants in the DOPA decarboxylase gene in bipolar and unipolar affective disorder. *Am J Med Genet*, 114(5), 519–522.

Jakimow-Venulet, B. (1981). Hereditary factors in the pathogenesis of affective illnesses. *Br J Psychiatry*, 139, 450–456.

James, N.M., and Chapman, C.J. (1975). A genetic study of bipolar affective disorder. *Br J Psychiatry*, 126, 449–456.

Jamison, K.R. (1993). *Touched with Fire: Manic-Depressive Illness and the Artistic Temperament*. New York: The Free Press.

Jin, D.K., Hwang, H.Z., Oh, M.R., Kim, J.S., Lee, M., Kim, S., Lim, S.W., Seo, M.Y., Kim, J.H., and Kim, D.K. (2001). CAG repeats of CTG18.1 and KCNN3 in Korean patients with bipolar affective disorder. *J Affect Disord*, 66(1), 19–24.

Johnson, G.F., and Leeman, M.M. (1977). Analysis of familial factors in bipolar affective illness. *Arch Gen Psychiatry*, 34(9), 1074–1083.

Johnston, N.L., Cervenak, J., Shore, A.D., Torrey, E.F., and Yolken, R.H. (1997). Multivariate analysis of RNA levels from postmortem human brains as measured by three different methods of RT-PCR. Stanley Neuropathology Consortium. *J Neurosci Methods*, 77(1), 83–92.

Jones, I., Middle, F., McCandless, F., Coyle, N., Robertson, E., Brockington, I., Lendon, C., and Craddock, N. (2000). Molecular genetic studies of bipolar disorder and puerperal psychosis at two polymorphisms in the estrogen receptor alpha gene (ESR 1). *Am J Med Genet*, 96(6), 850–853.

Jones, I., Scourfield, J., McCandless, F., and Craddock, N. (2002). Attitudes towards future testing for bipolar disorder susceptibility genes: A preliminary investigation. *J Affect Disord*, 71(1–3), 189–193.

Jun, T.Y., Lee, K.U., Pae, C.U., Kweon, Y.S., Chae, J.H., Bahk, W.M., Kim, K.S., Lew, T.Y., and Han, H. (2004). No evidence for an association of the CTLA4 gene with bipolar I disorder. *Psychiatry Clin Neurosci*, 58(1), 21–24.

Jung, S.K., Hong, M.S., Suh, G.J., Jin, S.Y., Lee, H.J., Kim, B.S., Lim, Y.J., Kim, M.K., Park, H.K., Chung, J.H., and Yim, S.V. (2004). Association between polymorphism in intron 1 of cocaine- and amphetamine-regulated transcript gene with alcoholism, but not with bipolar disorder and schizophrenia in Korean population. *Neurosci Lett*, 365(1), 54–57.

Kakiuchi, C., Iwamoto, K., Ishiwata, M., Bundo, M., Kasahara, T., Kusumi, I., Tsujita, T., Okazaki, Y., Nanko, S., Kunugi, H., Sasaki, T., and Kato, T. (2003). Impaired feedback regulation of XBP1 as a genetic risk factor for bipolar disorder. *Nat Genet*, 35(2), 171–175.

Kallmann, F.J. (1953). *Heredity in Health and Mental Disorder*. New York: W.W. Norton and Company.

Kallmann, F.J. (1954). Genetic principles in manic-depressive psychosis. In P.H. Hoch and J. Zubin (Eds.), *Depression*. New York: Grune and Stratton.

Kato, M.V., Shimizu, T., Nagayoshi, M., Kaneko, A., Sasaki, M.S., and Ikawa, Y. (1996a). Genomic imprinting of the human serotonin-receptor (HTR2) gene involved in development of retinoblastoma. *Am J Hum Genet*, 59(5), 1084–1090.

Kato, T., Winokur, G., Coryell, W., Keller, M.B., Endicott, J., and Rice, J. (1996b). Parent-of-origin effect in transmission of bipolar disorder. *Am J Med Genet*, 67(6), 546–550.

Kato, T., Kunugi, H., Nanko, S., and Kato, N. (2000). Association of bipolar disorder with the 5178 polymorphism in mitochondrial DNA. *Am J Med Genet*, 96(2), 182–186.

Kato, T., Kunugi, H., Nanko, S., and Kato, N. (2001). Mitochondrial DNA polymorphisms in bipolar disorder. *J Affect Disord*, 62(3), 151–164.

Kato, T., Iwamoto, K., Washizuka, S., Mori, K., Tajima, O., Akiyama, T., Nanko, S., Kunugi, H., and Kato, N. (2003). No association of mutations and mRNA expression of WFS1/wolframin with bipolar disorder in humans. *Neurosci Lett*, 338(1), 21–24.

Kawada, Y., Hattori, M., Dai, X.Y., and Nanko, S. (1995a). Possible association between monoamine oxidase A gene and bipolar affective disorder [letter; comment] [see comments]. *Am J Hum Genet*, 56(1), 335–336.

Kawada, Y., Hattori, M., Fukuda, R., Arai, H., Inoue, R., and Nanko, S. (1995b). No evidence of linkage or association between tyrosine hydroxylase gene and affective disorder. *J Affect Disord*, 34(2), 89–94.

Kealey, C., Reynolds, A., Mynett-Johnson, L., Claffey, E., and McKeon, P. (2001). No evidence to support an association between the oestrogen receptor beta gene and bipolar disorder. *Psychiatr Genet*, 11(4), 223–226.

Kelsoe, J.R., Spence, M.A., Loetscher, E., Foguet, M., Sadovnick, A.D., Remick, R.A., Flodman, P., Khristich, J., Mroczkowski-Parker, Z., Brown, J.L., Masser, D., Ungerleider, S., Rapaport, M.H., Wishart, W.L., and Luebbert, H. (1989). Re-evaluation of the linkage relationship between chromosome 11p loci and the gene for bipolar affective disorder in the Old Order Amish [see comments]. *Nature*, 342(6247), 238–243.

Kelsoe, J.R., Spence, M.A., Loetscher, E., Foguet, M., Sadovnick, A.D., Remick, R.A., Flodman, P., Khristich, J., Mroczkowski-Parker, Z., Brown, J.L., Masser, D., Ungerleider, S., Rapaport, M.H., Wishart, W.L., and Luebbert, H. (2001). A genome survey indicates a possible susceptibility locus for bipolar disorder on chromosome 22. *Proc Natl Acad Sci USA*, 98(2), 585–590.

Kendler, K.S. (1986). Kraepelin and the differential diagnosis of dementia praecox and manic-depressive insanity. *Compr Psychiatry*, 27, 549–558.

Kendler, K.S. (2001). Twin studies of psychiatric illness: An update. *Arch Gen Psychiatry*, 58(11), 1005–1014.

Kendler, K.S., and Prescott, C.A. (1999). A population-based twin study of lifetime major depression in men and women. *Arch Gen Psychiatry*, 56(1), 39–44. Erratum in: *Arch Gen Psychiatry*, 57(1), 94–95.

Kendler, K.S., and Walsh, D. (1995). Gender and schizophrenia. Results of an epidemiologically based family study. *Br J Psychiatry*, 167(2), 184–192.

Kendler, K.S., Gruenberg, A.M., and Tsuang, M.T. (1985). Psychiatric illness in first-degree relatives of schizophrenic and surgical control patients. A family study using DSM-III criteria. *Arch Gen Psychiatry*, 42(8), 770–779.

Kendler, K.S., Gruenberg, A.M., and Tsuang, M.T. (1986). A DSM-III family study of the nonschizophrenic psychotic disorders. *Am J Psychiatry*, 143(9), 1098–1105.

Kendler, K.S., McGuire, M., Gruenberg, A.M., O'Hare, A., Spellman, M., and Walsh, D. (1993a). The Roscommon Family Study. I. Methods, diagnosis of probands, and risk of schizophrenia in relatives. *Arch Gen Psychiatry*, 50(7), 527–540.

Kendler, K.S., McGuire, M., Gruenberg, A.M., O'Hare, A., Spellman, M., and Walsh, D. (1993b). The Roscommon Family Study. IV. Affective illness, anxiety disorders, and alcoholism in relatives. *Arch Gen Psychiatry*, 50(12), 952–960.

Kendler, K.S., Neale, M.C., Kessler, R.C., Heath, A.C., and Eaves, L.J. (1993c). A test of the equal-environment assumption in twin studies of psychiatric illness. *Behav Genet*, 23(1), 21–27.

Kendler, K.S., Karkowski-Shuman, L., O'Neill, F.A., Straub, R.E., MacLean, C.J., and Walsh, D. (1997). Resemblance of psychotic symptoms and syndromes in affected sibling pairs from the Irish Study of High-Density Schizophrenia Families: Evidence for possible etiologic heterogeneity. *Am J Psychiatry*, 154(2), 191–198.

Kendler, K.S., Myers, J., and Prescott, C.A. (2000). Parenting and adult mood, anxiety and substance use disorders in female twins: An epidemiological, multi-informant, retrospective study. *Psychol Med*, 30(2), 281–294.

Kent, L., and Craddock, N. (2003). Is there a relationship between attention deficit hyperactivity disorder and bipolar disorder? *J Affect Disord*, 73(3), 211–221.

Keverne, E.B., Fundele, R., Narasimha, M., Barton, S.C., and Surani, M.A. (1996). Genomic imprinting and the differential roles of parental genomes in brain development. *Brain Res Dev Brain Res*, 92(1), 91–100.

Kevles, D.J. (1995). *In the Name of Eugenics: Genetics and the Uses of Human Heredity*. Cambridge, MA: Harvard University Press.

Kim, D.K., Lim, S.W., Lee, S., Sohn, S.E., Kim, S., Hahn, C.G., and, Carroll, B.J. (2000). Serotonin transporter gene polymorphism and antidepressant response. *Neuroreport*, 11(1), 215–219.

Kirk, R., Furlong, R.A., Amos, W., Cooper, G., Rubinsztein, J.S., Walsh, C., Paykel, E.S., and Rubinsztein, D.C. (1999). Mitochondrial genetic analyses suggest selection against maternal lineages in bipolar affective disorder. *Am J Hum Genet*, 65(2), 508–518.

Kirov, G., Murphy, K.C., Arranz, M.J., Jones, I., McCandles, F., Kunugi, H., Murray, R.M., McGuffin, P., Collier, D.A., Owen, M.J., and Craddock, N. (1998). Low activity allele of catechol-O-methyltransferase gene associated with rapid cycling bipolar disorder. *Mol Psychiatry*, 3(4), 342–345.

Kirov, G., Jones, I., McCandless, F., Craddock, N., and Owen, M.J. (1999a). Family-based association studies of bipolar disorder with candidate genes involved in dopamine neurotransmission: DBH, DAT1, COMT, DRD2, DRD3 and DRD5. *Mol Psychiatry*, 4(6), 558–565.

Kirov, G., Norton, N., Jones, I., McCandless, F., Craddock, N., and Owen, M.J. (1999b). A functional polymorphism in the promoter of monoamine oxidase A gene and bipolar affective disorder. *Int J Neuropsychopharmcol*, 2(4), 293–298.

Kirov, G., Rees, M., Jones, I., MacCandless, F., Owen, M.J., and Craddock, N. (1999c). Bipolar disorder and the serotonin transporter gene: A family-based association study. *Psychol Med*, 29(5), 1249–1254.

Kirov, G., Lowry, C.A., Stephens, M., Oldfield, S., O'Donovan, M.C., Lightman, S.L., and Owen, M.J. (2001). Screening ABCG1, the human homologue of the *Drosophila* white gene, for polymorphisms and association with bipolar affective disorder. *Mol Psychiatry*, 6(6), 671–677.

Koh, P.O., Undie, A.S., Kabbani, N., Levenson, R., Goldman-Rakic, P.S., and Lidow, M.S. (2003). Up-regulation of neuronal calcium sensor-1 (NCS-1) in the prefrontal cortex of schizophrenic and bipolar patients. *Proc Natl Acad Sci USA*, 100(1), 313–317.

Koido, K., Koks, S., Nikopensius, T., Maron, E., Altmae, S., Heinaste, E., Vabrit, K., Tammekivi, V., Hallast, P., Kurg, A., Shlik, J., Vasar, V., Metspalu, A., and Vasar, E. (2005). Polymorphisms in wolframin (WFS1) gene are possibly related to increased risk for mood disorders. *Int J Neuropsychopharmacol*, 8(2), 235–244.

Konradi, C., Eaton, M., MacDonald, M.L., Walsh, J., Benes, F.M., and Heckers, S. (2004). Molecular evidence for mitochondrial dysfunction in bipolar disorder. *Arch Gen Psychiatry*, 61(3), 300–308. Erratum in: *Arch Gen Psychiatry*, 2004, 61(6), 538.

Kornberg, J.R., Brown, J.L., Sadovnick, A.D., Remick, R.A., Keck, P.E. Jr., McElroy, S.L., Rapaport, M.H., Thompson, P.M., Kaul, J.B., Vrabel, C.M., Schommer, S.C., Wilson, T., Pizzuco, D., Jameson, S., Schibuk, L., and Kelsoe, J.R. (2000). Evaluating the parent-of-origin effect in bipolar affective disorder. Is a more penetrant subtype transmitted paternally? *J Affect Disord*, 59(3), 183–192.

Korner, J., Fritze, J., and Propping, P. (1990). RFLP alleles at the tyrosine hydroxylase locus: No association found to affective disorders. *Psychiatry Res*, 32(3), 275–280.

Korner, J., Rietschel, M., Hunt, N., Castle, D., Gill, M., Nothen, M.M., Craddock, N., Daniels, J., Owen, M., Fimmers, R. (1994). Association and haplotype analysis at the tyrosine hydroxylase locus in a combined German-British sample of manic depressive patients and controls. *Psychiatr Genet*, 4(3), 167–175.

Kraepelin, E. (1899). *Manic-Depressive Insanity and Paranoia*. Edinburgh: E. & S. Livingstone.

Kraepelin, E (1921). *Manic-Depressive Insanity and Paranoia*. Translated by R.M. Barclay, edited by G.M. Robertson. Edinburgh: E. & S. Livingstone. Originally published as *Psychiatrie. Ein Lehrbuch fur Studierende und Ärzte. ed. 2. Klinische Psychiatrie*. II. Leipzig: Johann Ambrosius Barth, 1899.

Kringlen, E. (1967). *Heredity and Environment in the Functional Psychoses* (Vol. 1, pp. 27–47). Oslo: Universitetsforlaget.

Kunugi, H., Hattori, M., Kato, T., Tatsumi, M., Sakai, T., Sasaki, T., Hirose, T., and Nanko, S. (1997a). Serotonin transporter gene polymorphisms: Ethnic difference and possible association with bipolar affective disorder. *Mol Psychiatry*, 2(6), 457–462.

Kunugi, H., Vallada, H.P., Hoda, F., Kirov, G., Gill, M., Aitchison, K.J., Ball, D., Arranz, M.J., Murray, R.M., and Collier, D.A. (1997b). No evidence for an association of affective disorders with high- or low- activity allele of catechol-O-methyltransferase gene. *Biol Psychiatry*, 42(4), 282–285.

Kunugi, H., Ishida, S., Kato, T., Tatsumi, M., Sakai, T., Hattori, M., Hirose, T., and Nanko, S. (1999). A functional polymorphism in the promoter region of monoamine oxidase-A gene and mood disorders. *Mol Psychiatry*, 4(4), 393–395.

Kunugi, H., Kato, T., Fukuda, R., Tatsumi, M., Sakai, T., and Nanko, S. (2002). Association study of C825T polymorphism of the G-protein b3 subunit gene with schizophrenia and mood disorders. *J Neural Transm*, 109(2), 213–218.

Kunugi, H., Iijima, Y., Tatsumi, M., Yoshida, M., Hashimoto, R., Kato, T., Sakamoto, K., Fukunaga, T., Inada, T., Suzuki, T., Iwata, N., Ozaki, N., Yamada, K., and Yoshikawa, T. (2004). No association between the Val66Met polymorphism of the brain-derived neurotrophic factor gene and bipolar disorder in a Japanese population: A multicenter study. *Biol Psychiatry*, 56(5), 376–378.

Kurumaji, A., Nomoto, H., Yamada, K., Yoshikawa, T., and Toru, M. (2001). No association of two missense variations of the benzodiazepine receptor (peripheral) gene and mood disorders in a Japanese sample. *Am J Med Genet*, 105(2), 172–175.

Lachman, H.M., Kelsoe, J., Moreno, L., Katz, S., and Papolos, D.F. (1997). Lack of association of catechol-O-methyltransferase (COMT) functional polymorphism in bipolar affective disorder. *Psychiatr Genet*, 7(1), 13–17.

Lander, E., and Kruglyak, L. (1995). Genetic dissection of complex traits: Guidelines for interpreting and reporting linkage results. *Nat Genet*, 11(3), 241–247.

Lasky-Su, J.A., Faraone, S.V., Glatt, S.J., and Tsuang, M.T. (2005). Meta-analysis of the association between two polymorphisms in the serotonin transporter gene and affective disorders. *Am J Med Genet B Neuropsychiatr Genet*, 133(1), 110–115.

Leboyer, M., Malafosse, A., Boularand, S., Campion, D., Gheysen, F., Samolyk, D., Henriksson, B., Denise, E., des Lauriers, A., and Lepine, J.P. (1990). Tyrosine hydroxylase polymorphisms associated with manic-depressive illness. *Lancet*, 335(8699), 1219.

Leboyer, M., Bellivier, F., McKeon, P., Albus, M., Borrman, M., Perez-Diaz, F., Mynett-Johnson, L., Feingold, J., and Maier, W. (1998). Age at onset and gender resemblance in bipolar siblings. *Psychiatry Res*, 81(2), 125–131.

Lerer, B., Macciardi, F., Segman, R.H., Adolfsson, R., Blackwood, D., Blairy, S., Del Favero, J., Dikeos, D.G., Kaneva, R., Lilli, R., Massat, I., Milanova, V., Muir, W., Noethen, M., Oruc, L., Petrova, T.,

Papadimitriou, G.N., Rietschel, M., Serretti, A., Souery, D., Van Gestel, S., Van Broeckhoven, C., and Mendlewicz, J. (2001). Variability of 5-HT2C receptor cys23ser polymorphism among European populations and vulnerability to affective disorder. *Mol Psychiatry*, 6(5), 579–585.

Lesch, K.P., Bengel, D., Heils, A., Sabol, S.Z., Greenberg, B.D., Petri, S., Benjamin, J., Muller, C.R., Hamer, D.H., and Murphy, D.L. (1996). Association of anxiety-related traits with a polymorphism in the serotonin transporter gene regulatory region. *Science*, 274(5292), 1527–1531.

Leszczynska-Rodziewicz, A., Czerski, P.M., Kapelski, P., Godlewski, S., Dmitrzak-Weglarz, M., Rybakowski, J., and Hauser, J. (2002). A polymorphism of the norepinephrine transporter gene in bipolar disorder and schizophrenia: Lack of association. *Neuropsychobiology*, 45(4), 182–185.

Levinson, D.F. (2006). The genetics of depression: A review. *Biol Psychiatry*, 60, 84–92.

Li, T., Vallada, H., Curtis, D., Arranz, M., Xu, K., Cai, G., Deng, H., Liu, J., Murray, R., Liu, X., and Collier, D.A. (1997). Catechol-O-methyltransferase Val158Met polymorphism: Frequency analysis in Han Chinese subjects and allelic association of the low activity allele with bipolar affective disorder. *Pharmacogenetics*, 7(5), 349–353.

Li, L., Keverne, E.B., Aparicio, S.A., Ishino, F., Barton, S.C., and Surani, M.A. (1999a). Regulation of maternal behavior and offspring growth by paternally expressed Peg3. *Science*, 284(5412), 330–333.

Li, T., Liu, X., Sham, P.C., Aitchison, K.J., Cai, G., Arranz, M.J., Deng, H., Liu, J., Kirov, G., Murray, R.M., and Collier, D.A. (1999b). Association analysis between dopamine receptor genes and bipolar affective disorder. *Psychiatry Res*, 86(3), 193–201.

Licinio, J., and Wong, M.L. (2002). Brain-derived neurotrophic factor (BDNF) in stress and affective disorders. *Mol Psychiatry*, 7(6), 519.

Liddell, M.B., Lovestone, S., and Owen, M.J. (2001). Genetic risk of Alzheimer's disease: Advising relatives. *Br J Psychiatry*, 178(1), 7–11.

Lim, L.C., Nothen, M.M., Korner, J., Rietschel, M., Castle, D., Hunt, N., Propping, P., Murray, R., and Gill, M. (1994). No evidence of association between dopamine D4 receptor variants and bipolar affective disorder. *Am J Med Genet*, 54(3), 259–263.

Lim, L.C., Powell, J., Sham, P., Castle, D., Hunt, N., Murray, R., and Gill, M. (1995). Evidence for a genetic association between alleles of monoamine oxidase A gene and bipolar affective disorder. *Am J Med Genet*, 60(4), 325–331.

Lin, J.P., and Bale, S.J. (1997). Parental transmission and D18S37 allele sharing in bipolar affective disorder. *Genet Epidemiol*, 14(6), 665–668.

Lin, M.W., Sham, P., Hwu, H.G., Collier, D., Murray, R., and Powell, J.F. (1997). Suggestive evidence for linkage of schizophrenia to markers on chromosome 13 in Caucasian but not Oriental populations. *Hum Genet*, 99(3), 417–420.

Lin, C.N., Tsai, S.J., and Hong, C.J. (2001). Association analysis of a functional G protein beta3 subunit gene polymorphism (C825T) in mood disorders. *Neuropsychobiology*, 44(3), 118–121.

Lin, P.-I., McInnis, M.G., Potash, J.B., Willour, V.L., MacKinnon, D.F., Miao, K., DePaulo, J.R., and Zandi, P.P. (2005). Assessment of the age at onset on linkage to bipolar disorder: Evidence on chromosomes 18p and 21q. *Am J Hum Genet*, 77, 545–555.

Lin, P.-I., McInnis, M.G., Potash, J.B., Willour, V., MacKinnon, D.F., DePaulo, J.R., and Zandi, P.P. (2006). Clinical correlates and familial aggregation of age at onset in bipolar disorder. *Am J Psychiatry*, 163(2), 240–246.

Lish, J.D., Gyulai, L., Resnick, S.M., Kirtland, A., Amsterdam, J.D., Whybrow, P.C., and Price, R.A. (1993). A family history study of rapid-cycling bipolar disorder. *Psychiatry Res*, 48(1), 37–46.

Liu, W., Gu, N., Feng, G., Li, S., Bai, S., Zhang, J., Shen, T., Xue, H., Breen, G., St., Clair, D., and He, L. (1999). Tentative association of the serotonin transporter with schizophrenia and unipolar depression but not with bipolar disorder in Han Chinese. *Pharmacogenetics*, 9(4), 491–495.

Liu, C., Badner, J.A., Christian, S.L., Guroff, J.J., Detera-Wadleigh, S.D., and Gershon, E.S. (2001a). Fine mapping supports previous linkage evidence for a bipolar disorder susceptibility locus on 13q32. *Am J Med Genet*, 105(4), 375–380.

Liu, J., Juo, S.H., Terwilliger, J.D., Grunn, A., Tong, X., Brito, M., Loth, J.E., Kanyas, K., Lerer, B., Endicott, J., Penchaszadeh, G., Gilliam, T.C., and Baron, M. (2001b). A follow-up linkage study supports evidence for a bipolar affective disorder locus on chromosome 21q22. *Am J Med Genet*, 105(2), 189–194.

Liu, J., Juo, S.H., Dewan, A., Grunn, A., Tong, X., Brito, M., Park, N., Loth, J.E., Kanyas, K., Lerer, B., Endicott, J., Penchaszadeh, G., Knowles, J.A., Ott, J., Gilliam, T.C., and Baron, M. (2003). Evidence for a putative bipolar disorder locus on 2p13-16 and other potential loci on 4q31, 7q34, 8q13, 9q31, 10q21-24, 13q32, 14q21 and 17q11-12. *Mol Psychiatry*, 8(3), 333–342.

Lucotte, G., Landoulsi, A., Berriche, S., David, F., and Babron, M.C. (1992). Manic depressive illness is linked to factor IX in a French pedigree [see comments]. *Ann Genet*, 35(2), 93–95.

Luxenburger, H. (1928). Vorlaufiger Bericht uber psychiatrische Serinumtersuchungen an Zwillinger. *Z Ges Neurol Psychiatrie*, 116, 297–326.

Luxenburger, H. (1930). Psychiatrisch-neurologisch Zwillingspathologie. *Z Ges Neurol Psychiatrie*, 56, 145–180.

Luxenburger, H. (1942). *Handbuch der Erbkrankheiten*. Leipzig: Georg Thieme Verlag.

Lyons, M.J., Eisen, S.A., Goldberg, J., True, W., Lin, N., Meyer, J.M., Toomey, R., Faraone, S.V., Merla-Ramos, M., and Tsuang, M.T. (1998). A registry-based twin study of depression in men. *Arch Gen Psychiatry*, 55(5), 468–472.

Lytton, H., Martin, N.G., and Eaves, L. (1977). Environmental and genetical causes of variation in ethological aspects of behavior in two-year-old boys. *Soc Biol*, 24(3), 200–211.

Macgregor, S., Visscher, P.M., Knott, S.A., Thomson, P., Porteous, D.J., Millar, J.K., Devon, R.S., Blackwood, D., and Muir, W.J. (2004). A genome scan and follow-up study identify a bipolar disorder susceptibility locus on chromosome 1q42. *Mol Psychiatry*, 9(12), 1083–1090.

MacKenzie, A., and Quinn, J. (1999). A serotonin transporter gene intron 2 polymorphic region, correlated with affective disorders, has allele-dependent differential enhancer-like properties in the mouse embryo. *Proc Natl Acad Sci USA*, 96(26), 15251–15255.

MacKinnon, D.F., McMahon, F.J., Simpson, S.G., McInnis, M.G., and DePaulo, J.R. (1997). Panic disorder with familial bipolar disorder. *Biol Psychiatry*, 42(2), 90–95.

MacKinnon, D.F., Zandi, P.P., Cooper, J., Potash, J.B., Simpson, S.G., Gershon, E., Nurnberger, J., Reich, T., and DePaulo, J.R.

(2002). Comorbid bipolar disorder and panic disorder in families with a high prevalence of bipolar disorder. *Am J Psychiatry*, 159(1), 30–35.

MacKinnon, D.F., Zandi, P.P., Gershon, E., Nurnberger, J.I. Jr., Reich, T., and DePaulo, J.R. (2003a). Rapid switching of mood in families with multiple cases of bipolar disorder. *Arch Gen Psychiatry*, 60(9), 921–928.

MacKinnon, D.F., Zandi, P.P., Gershon, E.S., Nurnberger, J.I. Jr., and DePaulo, J.R. Jr. (2003b). Association of rapid mood switching with panic disorder and familial panic risk in familial bipolar disorder. *Am J Psychiatry*, 160(9), 1696–1698.

MacQueen, G.M., Ramakrishnan, K., Croll, S.D., Siuciak, J.A., Yu, G., Young, L.T., and Fahnestock, M. (2001). Performance of heterozygous brain-derived neurotrophic factor knockout mice on behavioral analogues of anxiety, nociception, and depression. *Behav Neurosci*, 115(5), 1145–1153.

Mahieu, B., Souery, D., Lipp, O., Mendelbaum, K., Verheyen, G., De Maertelaer, V., Van Broeckhoven, C., and Mendlewicz, J. (1997). No association between bipolar affective disorder and a serotonin receptor (5-HT2A) polymorphism. *Psychiatry Res*, 70(2), 65–69.

Maier, W., Lichtermann, D., Minges, J., Hallmayer, J., Heun, R., Benkert, O., and Levinson, D.F. (1993). Continuity and discontinuity of affective disorders and schizophrenia. Results of a controlled family study. *Arch Gen Psychiatry*, 50(11), 871–883.

Malafosse, A., Leboyer, M., d'Amato, T., Amadeo, S., Abbar, M., Campion, D., Canseil, O., Castelnau, D., Gheysen, F., Granger, B., Henrikson, B., Poirier, M.F., Sabate, O., Samolyk, D., Feingold, J., and Mallet, J. (1997). Manic-depressive illness and tyrosine hydroxylase gene: linkage heterogeneity and association. *Neurobiol Dis*, 4(5), 337–349.

Manki, H., Kanba, S., Muramatsu, T., Higuchi, S., Suzuki, E., Matsushita, S., Ono, Y., Chiba, H., Shintani, F., Nakamura, M., Yagi, G., and Asai, M. (1996). Dopamine D2, D3 and D4 receptor and transporter gene polymorphisms and mood disorders. *J Affect Disord*, 40(1–2), 7–13.

Massat, I., Souery, D., Lipp, O., Blairy, S., Papadimitriou, G., Dikeos, D., Ackenheil, M., Fuchshuber, S., Hilger, C., Kaneva, R., Milanova, V., Verheyen, G., Raeymaekers, P., Staner, L., Oruc, L., Jakovljevic, M., Serretti, A., Macciardi, F., Van Broeckhoven, C., and Mendlewicz, J. (2000). A European multicenter association study of HTR2A receptor polymorphism in bipolar affective disorder. *Am J Med Genet*, 96(2), 136–140.

Massat, I., Souery, D., Del-Favero, J., Oruc, L., Noethen, M.M., Blackwood, D., Thomson, M., Muir, W., Papadimitriou, G.N., Dikeos, D.G., Kaneva, R., Serretti, A., Lilli, R., Smeraldi, E., Jakovljevic, M., Folnegovic, V., Rietschel, M., Milanova, V., Valente, F., Van Broeckhoven, C., and Mendlewicz, J. (2002a). Excess of allele1 for alpha3 subunit GABA receptor gene (GABRA3) in bipolar patients: A multicentric association study. *Mol Psychiatry*, 7(2), 201–207.

Massat, I., Souery, D., Del-Favero, J., Van Gestel, S., Serretti, A., Macciardi, F., Smeraldi, E., Kaneva, R., Adolfsson, R., Nylander, P.O., Blackwood, D., Muir, W., Papadimitriou, G.N., Dikeos, D., Oruc, L., Segman, R.H., Ivezic, S., Aschauer, H., Ackenheil, M., Fuchshuber, S., Dam, H., Jakovljevic, M., Peltonen, L., Hilger, C., Hentges, F., Staner, L., Milanova, V., Jazin, E., Lerer, B., Van Broeckhoven, C., and Mendlewicz, J. (2002b). Positive association of dopamine D2 receptor polymorphism with bipolar affective disorder in a European Multicenter Association Study of affective disorders. *Am J Med Genet*, 114(2), 177–185.

Maziade, M., Roy, M.A., Rouillard, E., Bissonnette, L., Fournier, J.P., Roy, A., Garneau, Y., Montgrain, N., Potvin, A., Cliché, D., Dion, C., Wallot, H., Fournier, A., Nicole, L., Lavallee, J.C., and Merette, C. (2001). A search for specific and common susceptibility loci for schizophrenia and bipolar disorder: A linkage study in 13 target chromosomes. *Mol Psychiatry*, 6(6), 684–693.

Maziade, M., Roy, M.A., Chagnon, Y.C., Cliché, D., Fournier, J.P., Montgrain, N., Dion, C., Lavallee, J.C., Garneau, Y., Gingras, N., Nicole, L., Pires, A., Ponton, A.M., Potvin, A., Wallot, H., and Merette, C. (2005). Shared and specific susceptibility loci for schizophrenia and bipolar disorder: A dense genome scan in Eastern Quebec families. *Mol Psychiatry*, 10(5), 486–499.

McGuffin, P., Katz, R., and Bebbington, P. (1987). Hazard, heredity and depression. A family study. *J Psychiatr Res*, 21(4), 365–375.

McGuffin, P., Katz, R., Watkins, S., and Rutherford, J. (1996). A hospital-based twin register of the heritability of DSM-IV unipolar depression. *Arch Gen Psychiatry*, 53(2), 129–136.

McHugh, P.R., and Slavney, P.R. (1998). *The Perspectives of Psychiatry*, Second Edition. Baltimore: Johns Hopkins University Press.

McInnes, L.A., Escamilla, M.A., Service, S.K., Reus, V.I., Leon, P., Silva, S., Rojas, E., Spesny, M., Baharloo, S., Blankenship, K., Peterson, A., Tyler, D., Shimayoshi, N., Tobey, C., Batki, S., Vinogradov, S., Meza, L., Gallegos, A., Fournier, E., Smith, L.B., Barondes, S.H., Sandkuijl, L.A., and Freimer, N.B. (1996). A complete genome screen for genes predisposing to severe bipolar disorder in two Costa Rican pedigrees. *Proc Natl Acad Sci USA*, 93(23), 13060–13065.

McInnes, L.A., Service, S.K., Reus, V.I., Barnes, G., Charlat, O., Jawahar, S., Lewitzky, S., Yang, Q., Duong, Q., Spesny, M., Araya, C., Araya, X., Gallegos, A., Meza, L., Molina, J., Ramirez, R., Mendez, R., Silva, S., Fournier, E., Batki, S.L., Mathews, C.A., Neylan, T., Glatt, C.E., Escamilla, M.A., Luo, D., Gajiwala, P., Song, T., Crook, S., Nguyen, J.B., Roche, E., Meyer, J.M., Leon, P., Sandkuijl, L.A., Freimer, N.B., and Chen, H. (2001). Fine-scale mapping of a locus for severe bipolar mood disorder on chromosome 18p11.3 in the Costa Rican population. *Proc Natl Acad Sci USA*, 98(20), 11485–11490.

McInnis, M.G., McMahon, F.J., Chase, G.A., Simpson, S.G., Ross, C.A., and DePaulo, J.R. Jr. (1993). Anticipation in bipolar affective disorder. *Am J Hum Genet*, 53(2), 385–390.

McInnis, M.G., Breschel, T.S., Margolis, R.L., Chellis, J., MacKinnon, D.F., McMahon, F.J., Simpson, S.G., Lan, T.H., Chen, H., Ross, C.A., and DePaulo, J.R. (1999). Family-based association analysis of the hSKCa3 potassium channel gene in bipolar disorder. *Mol Psychiatry*, 4(3), 217–219.

McInnis, M.G., Swift-Scanlanl, T., Mahoney, A.T., Vincent, J., Verheyen, G., Lan, T.H., Oruc, L., Riess, O., Van Broeckhoven, C., Chen, H., Kennedy, J.L., MacKinnon, D.F., Margolis, R.L., Simpson, S.G., McMahon, F.J., Gershon, E., Nurnberger, J., Reich, T., DePaulo, J.R., and Ross, C.A. (2000). Allelic distribution of CTG18.1 in Caucasian populations: Association studies in bipolar disorder, schizophrenia, and ataxia. *Mol Psychiatry*, 5(4), 439–442.

McInnis, M.G., Lan, T.H., Willour, V.L., McMahon, F.J., Simpson, S.G., Addington, A.M., MacKinnon, D.F., Potash, J.B., Mahoney, A.T., Chellis, J., Huo, Y., Swift-Scanlan, T., Chen, H., Koskela, R., Stine, O.C., Jamison, K.R., Holmans, P., Folstein, S.E., Ranade, K., Friddle, C., Botstein, D., Marr, T., Beaty, T.H.,

Zandi, P., and DePaulo, J.R. (2003). Genome-wide scan of bipolar disorder in 65 pedigrees: Supportive evidence for linkage at 8q24, 18q22, 4q32, 2p12, and 13q12. *Mol Psychiatry*, 8(3), 288–298.

McKnew, D.H., Cytryn, L., Buchsbaum, M.S., Hamovit, J., Lamour, M., Rapoport, J.L., and Gershon, E.S. (1981). Lithium in children of lithium-responding parents. *Psychiatry Res*, 4(2), 171–180.

McMahon, F.J., Stine, O.C., Meyers, D.A., Simpson, S.G., and DePaulo, J.R. (1995). Patterns of maternal transmission in bipolar affective disorder [see comments]. *Am J Hum Genet*, 56(6), 1277–1286.

McMahon, F.J., Hopkins, P.J., Xu, J., McInnis, M.G., Shaw, S., Cardon, L., Simpson, S.G., MacKinnon, D.F., Stine, O.C., Sherrington, R., Meyers, D.A., and DePaulo, J.R. (1997). Linkage of bipolar affective disorder to chromosome 18 markers in a new pedigree series. *Am J Hum Genet*, 61(6), 1397–1404.

McMahon, F.J., Chen, Y.S., Patel, S., Kokoszka, J., Brown, M.D., Torroni, A., DePaulo, J.R., and Wallace, D.C. (2000). Mitochondrial DNA sequence diversity in bipolar affective disorder. *Am J Psychiatry*, 157(7), 1058–1064.

McMahon, F.J., Simpson, S.G., McInnis, M.G., Badner, J.A., MacKinnon, D.F., and DePaulo, J.R. (2001). Linkage of bipolar disorder to chromosome 18q and the validity of bipolar II disorder. *Arch Gen Psychiatry*, 58(11), 1025–1031.

McQueen, M.B., Devlin, B., Faraone, S.V., Nimgaonkar, V.L., Sklar, P., Smoller, J.W., Abou, J.R., Albus, M., Bacanu, S.A., Baron, M., Barrett, T.B., Berrettini, W., Blacker, D., Byerley, W., Cichon, S., Coryell, W., Craddock, N., Daly, M.J., DePaulo, J.R., Edenberg, H.J., Foroud, T., Gill, M., Gilliam, T.C., Hamshere, M., Jones, I., Jones, L., Juo, S.H., Kelsoe, J.R., Lambert, D., Lange, C., Lerer, B., Liu, J., Maier, W., Mackinnon, J.D., McInnis, M.G., McMahon, F.J., Murphy, D.L., Nothen, M.M., Nurnberger, J.I., Pato, C.N., Pato, M.T., Potash, J.B., Propping, P., Pulver, A.E., Rice, J.P., Rietschel, M., Scheftner, W., Schumacher, J., Segurado, R., Van Steen, K., Xie, W., Zandi, P.P., and Laird, N.M. (2005). Combined analysis from eleven linkage studies of bipolar disorder provides strong evidence of susceptibility loci on chromosomes 6q and 8q. *Am J Hum Genet*, 77(4), 582–595.

McQuillin, A., Lawrence, J., Curtis, D., Kalsi, G., Smyth, C., Hannesdottir, S., and Gurling, H. (1999). Adjacent genetic markers on chromosome 11p15.5 at or near the tyrosine hydroxylase locus that show population linkage disequilibrium with each other do not show allelic association with bipolar affective disorder. *Psychol Med*, 29(6), 1449–1454.

Meira-Lima, I.V., and Vallada, H. (2003). Genes related to phospholipid metabolism as risk factors related to bipolar affective disorder. *Rev Bras Psiquiatr*, 25(1), 51–55.

Meira-Lima, I.V., Pereira, A.C., Mota, G.F., Krieger, J.E., and Vallada, H. (2000). Angiotensinogen and angiotensin converting enzyme gene polymorphisms and the risk of bipolar affective disorder in humans. *Neurosci Lett*, 293(2), 103–106.

Meira-Lima, I.V., Zhao, J., Sham, P., Pereira, A.C., Krieger, J.E., and Vallada, H. (2001). Association and linkage studies between bipolar affective disorder and the polymorphic CAG/CTG repeat loci ERDA1, SEF2-1B, MAB21L and KCNN3. *Mol Psychiatry*, 6(5), 565–569.

Meira-Lima, I.V., Pereira, A.C., Mota, G.F., Floriano, M., Araujo, F., Mansur, A.J., Krieger, J.E., and Vallada, H. (2003a). Analysis of a polymorphism in the promoter region of the tumor necrosis factor alpha gene in schizophrenia and bipolar disorder: Further support for an association with schizophrenia. *Mol Psychiatry*, 8(8), 718–720.

Meira-Lima, I., Jardim, D., Junqueira, R., Ikenaga, E., Vallada, H. (2003b). Allelic association study between phospholipase A2 genes and bipolar affective disorder. *Bipolar Disord*, 5(4), 295–299.

Mellon, C.D. (1996). Hereditary Madness: The Evolution of Psychiatric Genetic Thought. Placitas, NM: Genetics Heritage Press.

Meloni, R., Leboyer, M., Bellivier, F., Barbe, B., Samolyk, D., Allilaire, J.F., and Mallet, J. (1995). Association of manic-depressive illness with tyrosine hydroxylase microsatellite marker. *Lancet*, 345(8954), 932.

Mendes de Oliveira J.R., Otto, P.A., Vallada, H., Lauriano, V., Elkis, H., Lafer, B., Vasquez, L., Gentil, V., Passos-Bueno, M.R., and Zatz, M. (1998). Analysis of a novel functional polymorphism within the promoter region of the serotonin transporter gene (5-HTT) in Brazilian patients affected by bipolar disorder and schizophrenia. *Am J Med Genet*, 81(3), 225–227.

Mendlewicz, J., and Rainer, J.D. (1974). Morbidity risk and genetic transmission in manic-depressive illness. *Am J Hum Genet*, 26(6), 692–701.

Mendlewicz, J., and Rainer, J.D. (1977). Adoption study supporting genetic transmission in manic–depressive illness. *Nature*, 268(5618), 327–329.

Mendlewicz, J., Fleiss, J.L., and Fieve, R.R. (1972). Evidence for X-linkage in the transmission of manic-depressive illness. *JAMA*, 222(13), 1624–1627.

Mendlewicz, J., Linkowski, P., Guroff, J.J., and Van Praag, H.M. (1979). Color blindness linkage to bipolar manic-depressive illness. New evidence. *Arch Gen Psychiatry*, 36(13), 1442–1447.

Mendlewicz, J., Linkowski, P., and Wilmotte, J. (1980). Linkage between glucose-6-phosphate dehydrogenase deficiency and manic-depressive psychosis. *Br J Psychiatry*, 137, 337–342.

Mendlewicz, J., Simon, P., Sevy, S., Charon, F., Brocas, H., Legros, S., and Vassart, G. (1987). Polymorphic DNA marker on X chromosome and manic depression. *Lancet*, 1(8544), 1230–1232.

Mendlewicz, J., Massat, I., Souery, D., Del-Favero, J., Oruc, L., Nothen, M.M., Blackwood, D., Muir, W., Battersby, S., Lerer, B., Segman, R.H., Kaneva, R., Serretti, A., Lilli, R., Lorenzi, C., Jakovljevic, M., Ivezic, S., Rietschel, M., Milanova, V., Van Broeckhoven, C. (2004). Serotonin transporter 5HTTLPR polymorphism and affective disorders: No evidence of association in a large european multicenter study. *Eur J Hum Genet*, 12(5), 377–382.

Merette, C., Roy-Gagnon, M.H., Ghazzali, N., Savard, F., Boutin, P., Roy, M.A., and Maziade, M. (2000). Anticipation in schizophrenia and bipolar disorder controlling for an information bias. *Am J Med Genet*, 96(1), 61–68.

Merikangas, K.R., Leckman, J.F., Prusoff, B.A., Pauls, D.L., and Weissman, M.M. (1985). Familial transmission of depression and alcoholism. *Arch Gen Psychiatry*, 42(4), 367–372.

Middle, F., Jones, I., McCandless, F., Barrett, T., Khanim, F., Owen, M.J., Lendon, C., and Craddock, N. (2000). Bipolar disorder and variation at a common polymorphism (A1832G) within exon 8 of the Wolfram gene. *Am J Med Genet*, 96(2), 154–157.

Middleton, F.A., Pato, M.T., Gentile, K.L., Morley, C.P., Zhao, X., Eisener, A.F., Brown, A., Petryshen, T.L., Kirby, A.N., Medeiros, H., Carvalho, C., Macedo, A., Dourado, A., Coelho, I., Valente, J., Soares, M.J., Ferreira, C.P., Lei, M., Azevedo, M.H., Kennedy, J.L., Daly, M.J., Sklar, P., and Pato, C.N.

(2004). Genomewide linkage analysis of bipolar disorder by use of a high-density single-nucleotide-polymorphism (SNP) genotyping assay: A comparison with microsatellite marker assays and finding of significant linkage to chromosome 6q22. *Am J Hum Genet*, 74(5), 886–897.

Miki, Y., Swensen, J., Shattuck-Eidens, D., Futreal, P.A., Harshman, K., Tavtigian, S., Liu, Q., Cochran, C., Bennett, L.M., and Ding, W. (1994). A strong candidate for the breast and ovarian cancer susceptibility gene BRCA1. *Science*, 266(5182), 66–71.

Mimmack, M.L., Ryan, M., Baba, H., Navarro-Ruiz, J., Iritani, S., Faull, R.L., McKenna, P.J., Jones, P.B., Arai, H., Starkey, M., Emson, P.C., and Bahn, S. (2002). Gene expression analysis in schizophrenia: Reproducible up-regulation of several members of the apolipoprotein L family located in a high-susceptibility locus for schizophrenia on chromosome 22. *Proc Natl Acad Sci USA*, 99(7), 4680–4685.

Montkowski, A., Barden, N., Wotjak, C., Stec, I., Ganster, J., Meaney, M., Engelmann, M., Reul, J.M., Landgraf, R., and Holsboer, F. (1995). Long-term antidepressant treatment reduces behavioural deficits in transgenic mice with impaired glucocorticoid receptor function. *J Neuroendocrinol*, 7(11), 841–845.

Morison, I.M., and Reeve, A.E. (1998). A catalogue of imprinted genes and parent-of-origin effects in humans and animals. *Hum Mol Genet*, 7(10), 1599–1609.

Morissette, J., Villeneuve, A., Bordeleau, L., Rochette, D., Laberge, C., Gagne, B., Laprise, C., Bouchard, G., Plante, M., Gobeil, L., Shink, E., Weissenbach, J., and Barden, N. (1999). Genome-wide search for linkage of bipolar affective disorders in a very large pedigree derived from a homogeneous population in Quebec points to a locus of major effect on chromosome 12q23-q24. Am J Med Genet, 88(5), 567–587.

Muglia, P., Petronis, A., Mundo, E., Lander, S., Cate, T., and Kennedy, J.L. (2002). Dopamine D4 receptor and tyrosine hydroxylase genes in bipolar disorder: Evidence for a role of DRD4. *Mol Psychiatry*, 7(8), 860–866.

Muir, W.J., Thomson, M.L., McKeon, P., Mynett-Johnson, L., Whitton, C., Evans, K.L., Porteous, D.J., and Blackwood, D.H. (2001). Markers close to the dopamine D5 receptor gene (DRD5) show significant association with schizophrenia but not bipolar disorder. *Am J Med Genet*, 105(2), 152–158.

Mundo, E., Walker, M., Tims, H., Macciardi, F., and Kennedy, J.L. (2000). Lack of linkage disequilibrium between serotonin transporter protein gene (SLC6A4) and bipolar disorder. *Am J Med Genet*, 96(3), 379–383.

Mundo, E., Walker, M., Cate, T., Macciardi, F., and Kennedy, J.L. (2001a). The role of serotonin transporter protein gene in antidepressant-induced mania in bipolar disorder: Preliminary findings. *Arch Gen Psychiatry*, 58(6), 539–544.

Mundo, E., Zai, G., Lee, L., Parikh, S.V., and Kennedy, J.L. (2001b). The 5HT1Dbeta receptor gene in bipolar disorder: A family-based association study. *Neuropsychopharmacology*, 25(4), 608–613.

Muramatsu, T., Matsushita, S., Kanba, S., Higuchi, S., Manki, H., Suzuki, E., and Asai, M. (1997). Monoamine oxidase genes polymorphisms and mood disorder. *Am J Med Genet*, 74(5), 494–496.

Murphy, V.E., Mynett-Johnson, L.A., Claffey, E., Shields, D.C., and McKeon, P. (2001). No association between 5HT-2A and bipolar disorder irrespective of genomic imprinting. *Am J Med Genet*, 105(5), 422–425.

Murphy, G.M. Jr., Hollander, S.B., Rodrigues, H.E., Kremer, C., and Schatzberg, A.F. (2004). Effects of the serotonin transporter gene promoter polymorphism on mirtazapine and paroxetine efficacy and adverse events in geriatric major depression. *Arch Gen Psychiatry*, 61(11), 1163–1169.

Mynett-Johnson, L.A., Murphy, V.E., Claffey, E., Shields, D.C., and McKeon, P. (1998). Preliminary evidence of an association between bipolar disorder in females and the catechol-O-methyltransferase gene. *Psychiatr Genet*, 8(4), 221–225.

Mynett-Johnson, L., Kealey, C., Claffey, E., Curtis, D., Bouchier-Hayes, L., Powell, C., and McKeon, P. (2000). Multimarker haplotypes within the serotonin transporter gene suggest evidence of an association with bipolar disorder. *Am J Med Genet*, 96(6), 845–849.

Nakamura, M., Ueno, S., Sano, A., and Tanabe, H. (2000). The human serotonin transporter gene linked polymorphism (5-HTTLPR) shows ten novel allelic variants. *Mol Psychiatry*, 5(1), 32–38.

Nakata, K., Ujike, H., Sakai, A., Uchida, N., Nomura, A., Imamura, T., Katsu, T., Tanaka, Y., Hamamura, T., and Kuroda, S. (2003). Association study of the brain-derived neurotrophic factor (BDNF) gene with bipolar disorder. *Neurosci Lett*, 337(1), 17–20.

Nemanov, L., Ebstein, R.P., Belmaker, R.H., Osher, Y., and Agam, G. (1999). Effect of bipolar disorder on lymphocyte inositol monophosphatase mRNA levels. *Int J Neuropsychopharmcol*, 2(1), 25–29.

Neves-Pereira, M., Mundo, E., Muglia, P., King, N., Macciardi, F., and Kennedy, J.L. (2002). The brain-derived neurotrophic factor gene confers susceptibility to bipolar disorder: Evidence from a family-based association study. *Am J Hum Genet*, 71(3), 651–655.

Ni, X., Trakalo, J.M., Mundo, E., Lee, L., Parikh, S., and Kennedy, J.L. (2002a). Family-based association study of the serotonin-2A receptor gene (5-HT2A) and bipolar disorder. *Neuromol Med*, 2(3), 251–259.

Ni, X., Trakalo, J.M., Mundo, E., Macciardi, F.M., Parikh, S., Lee, L., and Kennedy, J.L. (2002b). Linkage disequilibrium between dopamine D1 receptor gene (DRD1) and bipolar disorder. *Biol Psychiatry*, 52(12), 1144–1150.

Niculescu, A.B., III, Segal, D.S., Kuczenski, R., Barrett, T., Hauger, R.L., and Kelsoe, J.R. (2000). Identifying a series of candidate genes for mania and psychosis: A convergent functional genomics approach. *Physiol Genomics*, 4(1), 83–91.

Noga, J.T., Vladar, K., and Torrey, E.F. (2001). A volumetric magnetic resonance imaging study of monozygotic twins discordant for bipolar disorder. *Psychiatry Res*, 106(1), 25–34.

Nothen, M., Korner, J., Lanczik, M., Fritze, J., and Propping, P. (1990). Tyrosine hydroxylase polymorphisms and manic-depressive illness. *Lancet*, 336(8714), 575.

Nothen, M.M., Erdmann, J., Korner, J., Lanczik, M., Fritze, J., Fimmers, R., Grandy, D.K., O'Dowd, B., and Propping, P. (1992). Lack of association between dopamine D1 and D2 receptor genes and bipolar affective disorder. *Am J Psychiatry*, 149(2), 199–201.

Nothen, M.M., Eggermann, K., Albus, M., Borrmann, M., Rietschel, M., Korner, J., Maier, W., Minges, J., Lichtermann, D., and Franzek, E. (1995). Association analysis of the monoamine oxidase A gene in bipolar affective disorder by using family-based internal controls. *Am J Hum Genet*, 57(4), 975–978.

Nothen, M.M., Cichon, S., Rohleder, H., Hemmer, S., Franzek, E., Fritze, J., Albus, M., Borrmann-Hassenbach, M., Kreiner,

R., Weigelt, B., Minges, J., Lichtermann, D., Maier, W., Craddock, N., Fimmers, R., Holler, T., Baur, M.P., Rietschel, M., and Propping, P. (1999). Evaluation of linkage of bipolar affective disorder to chromosome 18 in a sample of 57 German families. *Mol Psychiatry*, 4(1), 76–84.

Nurnberger, J. Jr., Guroff, J.J., Hamovit, J., Berrettini, W., and Gershon, E. (1988). A family study of rapid-cycling bipolar illness. *J Affect Disord*, 15(1), 87–91.

Nyegaard, M., Borglum, A.D., Bruun, T.G., Collier, D.A., Russ, C., Mors, O., Ewald, H., and Kruse, T.A. (2002). Novel polymorphisms in the somatostatin receptor 5 (SSTR5) gene associated with bipolar affective disorder. *Mol Psychiatry*, 7(7), 745–754.

Nylander, P.O., Engstrom, C., Chotai, J., Wahlstrom, J., and Adolfsson, R. (1994). Anticipation in Swedish families with bipolar affective disorder. *J Med Genet*, 31(9), 686–689.

Ogura, Y., Bonen, D.K., Inohara, N., Nicolae, D.L., Chen, F.F., Ramos, R., Britton, H., Moran, T., Karaliuskas, R., Duerr, R.H., Achkar, J.P., Brant, S.R., Bayless, T.M., Kirschner, B.S., Hanauer, S.B., Nunez, G., and Cho, J.H. (2001). A frameshift mutation in NOD2 associated with susceptibility to Crohn's disease. *Nature*, 411(6837), 603–606.

Ohara, K., Suzuki, Y., Ushimi, Y., Yoshida, K., and Ohara, K. (1998a). Anticipation and imprinting in Japanese familial mood disorders. *Psychiatry Res*, 79(3), 191–198.

Ohara, K., Nagai, M., and Suzuki, Y. (1998b). Low activity allele of catechol-O-methyltransferase gene and Japanese unipolar depression. *Neuroreport*, 9(7), 1305–1308.

Ohtsuki, T., Ishiguro, H., Detera-Wadleigh, S.D., Toyota, T., Shimizu, H., Yamada, K., Yoshitsugu, K., Hattori, E., Yoshikawa, T., and Arinami, T. (2002). Association between serotonin 4 receptor gene polymorphisms and bipolar disorder in Japanese case-control samples and the NIMH Genetics Initiative Bipolar Pedigrees. *Mol Psychiatry*, 7(9), 954–961.

Omahony, E., Corvin, A., O'Connell, R., Comerford, C., Larsen, B., Jones, R., McCandless, F., Kirov, G., Cardno, A.G., Craddock, N., and Gill, M. (2002). Sibling pairs with affective disorders: Resemblance of demographic and clinical features. *Psychol Med*, 32(1), 55–61.

Ophoff, R.A., Escamilla, M.A., Service, S.K., Spesny, M., Meshi, D.B., Poon, W., Molina, J., Fournier, E., Gallegos, A., Mathews, C., Neylan, T., Batki, S.L., Roche, E., Ramirez, M., Silva, S., De Mille, M.C., Dong, P., Leon, P.E., Reus, V.I., Sandkuijl, L.A., and Freimer, N.B. (2002). Genomewide linkage disequilibrium mapping of severe bipolar disorder in a population isolate. *Am J Hum Genet*, 71(3), 565–574.

Oruc, L., Furac, I., Croux, C., Jakovljevic, M., Kracun, I., Folnegovic, V., and Van Broeckhoven, C. (1996). Association study between bipolar disorder and candidate genes involved in dopamine–serotonin metabolism and GABAergic neurotransmission: A preliminary report. *Psychiatr Genet*, 6(4), 213–217.

Oruc, L., Verheyen, G.R., Furac, I., Jakovljevic, M., Ivezic, S., Raeymaekers, P., and Van Broeckhoven, C. (1997a). Analysis of the tyrosine hydroxylase and dopamine D4 receptor genes in a Croatian sample of bipolar I and unipolar patients. *Am J Med Genet*, 74(2), 176–178.

Oruc, L., Verheyen, G.R., Furac, I., Jakovljevic, M., Ivezic, S., Raeymaekers, P., and Van Broeckhoven, C. (1997b). Association analysis of the 5-HT2C receptor and 5-HT transporter genes in bipolar disorder. *Am J Med Genet*, 74(5), 504–506.

Ospina-Duque, J., Duque, C., Carvajal-Carmona, L., Ortiz-Barrientos, D., Soto, I., Pineda, N., Cuartas, M., Calle, J., Lopez, C., Ochoa, L., Garcia, J., Gomez, J., Agudelo, A., Lozano, M., Montoya, G., Ospina, A., Lopez, M., Gallo, A., Miranda, A., Serna, L., Montoya, P., Palacio, C., Bedoya, G., McCarthy, M., Reus, V., Freimer, N., and Ruiz-Linares, A. (2000). An association study of bipolar mood disorder (type I) with the 5-HTTLPR serotonin transporter polymorphism in a human population isolate from Colombia. *Neurosci Lett*, 292(3), 199–202.

Oswald, P., Del-Favero, J., Massat, I., Souery, D., Claes, S., Van Broeckhoven, C., and Mendlewicz, J. (2004). Non-replication of the brain-derived neurotrophic factor (BDNF) association in bipolar affective disorder: A Belgian patient–control study. *Am J Med Genet B Neuropsychiatr Genet*, 129(1), 34–35.

Ozeki, Y., Tomoda, T., Kleiderlein, J., Kamiya, A., Bord, L., Fujii, K., Okawa, M., Yamada, N., Hatten, M.E., Snyder, S.H., Ross, C.A., and Sawa, A. (2003). Disrupted-in-Schizophrenia-1 (DISC-1): Mutant truncation prevents binding to NudE-like (NUDEL) and inhibits neurite outgrowth. *Proc Natl Acad Sci USA*, 100(1), 289–294.

Pae, C.U., Yu, H.S., Kim, T.S., Lee, C.U., Lee, S.J., Jun, T.Y., Lee, C., Serretti, A., and Paik, I.H. (2004). Monocyte chemoattractant protein-1 (MCP1) promoter-2518 polymorphism may confer a susceptibility to major depressive disorder in the Korean population. *Psychiatry Res*, 127(3), 279–281.

Papadimitriou, G.N., Dikeos, D.G., Karadima, G., Avramopoulos, D., Daskalopoulou, E.G., Vassilopoulos, D., and Stefanis, C.N. (1998). Association between the GABA(A) receptor alpha5 subunit gene locus (GABRA5) and bipolar affective disorder. *Am J Med Genet*, 81(1), 73–80.

Papadimitriou, G.N., Dikeos, D.G., Karadima, G., Avramopoulos, D., Daskalopoulou, E.G., and Stefanis, C.N. (2001). GABA-A receptor beta3 and alpha5 subunit gene cluster on chromosome 15q11-q13 and bipolar disorder: A genetic association study. *Am J Med Genet*, 105(4), 317–320.

Papolos, D.F., Veit, S., Faedda, G.L., Saito, T., and Lachman, H.M. (1998). Ultra-ultra rapid cycling bipolar disorder is associated with the low activity catecholamine-O-methyltransferase allele. *Mol Psychiatry*, 3(4), 346–349.

Pare, C.M., and Mack, J.W. (1971). Differentiation of two genetically specific types of depression by the response to antidepressant drugs. *J Med Genet*, 8(3), 306–309.

Pare, C.M., Rees, B.L., and Sainsbury, M.J. (1962). Differentiation of two genetically specific types of depression by the response to anti-depressants. Lancet, 2, 1340–1343.

Park, N., Juo, S.H., Cheng, R., Liu, J., Loth, J.E., Lilliston, B., Nee, J., Grunn, A., Kanyas, K., Lerer, B., Endicott, J., Gilliam, T.C., and Baron, M. (2004). Linkage analysis of psychosis in bipolar pedigrees suggests novel putative loci for bipolar disorder and shared susceptibility with schizophrenia. *Mol Psychiatry*, 9(12), 1091–1099.

Parsian, A., and Todd, R.D. (1997). Genetic association between monoamine oxidase and manic-depressive illness: Comparison of relative risk and haplotype relative risk data. *Am J Med Genet*, 74(5), 475–479.

Parsian, A., Chakraverty, S., and Todd, R.D. (1995). Possible association between the dopamine D3 receptor gene and bipolar affective disorder. *Am J Med Genet*, 60(3), 234–237.

Pauls, D.L., Morton, L.A., and Egeland, J.A. (1992). Risks of affective illness among first-degree relatives of bipolar I old-order Amish probands. *Arch Gen Psychiatry*, 49(9), 703–708.

Pauls, D.L., Bailey, J.N., Carter, A.S., Allen, C.R., and Egeland, J.A. (1995). Complex segregation analyses of old order Amish families ascertained through bipolar I individuals. *Am J Med Genet,* 60(4), 290–297.

Pauls, J., Bandelow, B., Ruther, E., and Kornhuber, J. (2000). Polymorphism of the gene of angiotensin converting enzyme: Lack of association with mood disorder. *J Neural Transm,* 107(11), 1361–1366.

Pekkarinen, P., Terwilliger, J., Bredbacka, P.E., Lonnqvist, J., and Peltonen, L. (1995). Evidence of a predisposing locus to bipolar disorder on Xq24-q27.1 in an extended Finnish pedigree. *Genome Res,* 5(2), 105–115.

Perez de Castro, I., Torres, P., Fernandez-Piqueras, J., Saiz-Ruiz, J., and Llinares, C. (1994). No association between dopamine D4 receptor polymorphism and manic depressive illness. *J Med Genet,* 31(11), 897–898.

Perez de Castro, I., Santos, J., Torres, P., Visedo, G., Saiz-Ruiz, J., Llinares, C., and Fernandez-Piqueras, J. (1995). A weak association between TH and DRD2 genes and bipolar affective disorder in a Spanish sample. *J Med Genet,* 32(2), 131–134.

Peters, E.J., Slager, S.L., McGrath, P.J., Knowles, J.A., and Hamilton, S.P. (2004). Investigation of serotonin-related genes in antidepressant response. *Mol Psychiatry,* 9(9), 879–889.

Petronis, A. (2001). Human morbid genetics revisited: Relevance of epigenetics. *Trends Genet,* 17(3), 142–146.

Piccardi, M.P., Severino, G., Bocchetta, A., Palmas, M.A., Ruiu, S., and Del Zompo, M. (1997). No evidence of association between dopamine D3 receptor gene and bipolar affective disorder. *Am J Med Genet,* 74(2), 137–139.

Piccardi, M.P., Ardau, R., Chillotti, C., Deleuze, J.F., Mallet, J., Meloni, R., Oi, A., Severino, G., Congiu, D., Bayorek, M., and Del Zompo, M. (2002). Manic-depressive illness: An association study with the inositol polyphosphate 1-phosphatase and serotonin transporter genes. *Psychiatr Genet,* 12(1), 23–27.

Pollock, B.G., Ferrell, R.E., Mulsant, B.H., Mazumdar, S., Miller, M., Sweet, R.A., Davis, S., Kirshner, M.A., Houck, P.R., Stack, J.A., Reynolds, C.F., and Kupfer, D.J. (2000). Allelic variation in the serotonin transporter promoter affects onset of paroxetine treatment response in late-life depression. *Neuropsychopharmacology,* 23(5), 587–590.

Pollock, H.M., Malzberg, B., and Fuller, R.G. (1939). *Hereditary and Environmental Factors in the Causation of Manic-Depressive Psychoses and Dementia Praecox.* Utica, NY: State Hospital Press.

Potash, J.B., Willour, V.L., Chiu, Y.F., Simpson, S.G., MacKinnon, D.F., Pearlson, G.D., DePaulo, J.R. Jr., and McInnis, M.G. (2001). The familial aggregation of psychotic symptoms in bipolar disorder pedigrees. *Am J Psychiatry,* 158(8), 1258–1264.

Potash, J.B., Chiu, Y.F., MacKinnon, D.F., Miller, E.B., Simpson, S.G., McMahon, F.J., McInnis, M.G., and DePaulo, J.R. Jr. (2003a). Familial aggregation of psychotic symptoms in a replication set of 69 bipolar disorder pedigrees. *Am J Med Genet,* 160, 680–686.

Potash, J.B., Zandi, P.P., Willour, V.L., Lan, T.H., Huo, Y., Avramopoulos, D., Shugart, Y.Y., MacKinnon, D.F., Simpson, S.G., McMahon, F.J., DePaulo, J.R. Jr., and McInnis, M.G. (2003b). Suggestive linkage to chromosomal regions 13q31 and 22q12 in families with psychotic bipolar disorder. *Am J Psychiatry,* 160(4), 680–686.

Prathikanti, S., Schulze, T.G., Chen, Y.S., Harr, B., Akula, N., Hennessy, K., Potluri, S., Lyons, J., Nguyen, T., and McMahon, F.J. (2004). Neither single-marker nor haplotype analyses support an association between genetic variation near NOTCH4 and bipolar disorder. *Am J Med Genet B Neuropsychiatr Genet,* 131(1), 10–15.

Preisig, M., Bellivier, F., Fenton, B.T., Baud, P., Berney, A., Courtet, P., Hardy, P., Golaz, J., Leboyer, M., Mallet, J., Matthey, M.L., Mouthon, D., Neidhart, E., Nosten-Bertrand, M., Stadelmann-Dubuis, E., Guimon, J., Ferrero, F., Buresi, C., and Malafosse, A. (2000). Association between bipolar disorder and monoamine oxidase A gene polymorphisms: Results of a multicenter study. *Am J Psychiatry,* 157(6), 948–955.

Puertollano, R., Visedo, G., Saiz-Ruiz, J., Llinares, C., and Fernandez-Piqueras, J. (1995). Lack of association between manic-depressive illness and a highly polymorphic marker from GABRA3 gene. *Am J Med Genet,* 60(5), 434–435.

Puertollano, R., Visedo, G., Zapata, C., and Fernandez-Piqueras, J. (1997). A study of genetic association between manic-depressive illness and a highly polymorphic marker from the GABRbeta-1 gene. *Am J Med Genet,* 74(3), 342–344.

Pulver, A.E., Mulle, J., Nestadt, G., Swartz, K.L., Blouin, J.L., Dombroski, B., Liang, K.Y., Housman, D.E., Kazazian, H.H., Antonarakis, S.E., Lasseter, V.K., Wolyniec, P.S., Thornquist, M.H., and McGrath, J.A. (2000). Genetic heterogeneity in schizophrenia: Stratification of genome scan data using co-segregating related phenotypes. *Mol Psychiatry,* 5(6), 650–653.

Ranade, S.S., Mansour, H., Wood, J., Chowdari, K.V., Brar, L.K., Kupfer, D.J., and Nimgaonkar, V.L. (2003). Linkage and association between serotonin 2A receptor gene polymorphisms and bipolar I disorder. *Am J Med Genet B Neuropsychiatr Genet,* 121(1), 28–34.

Rasmussen, S.K., Urhammer, S.A., Berglund, L., Jensen, J.N., Hansen, L., Echwald, S.M., Borch-Johnsen, K., Horikawa, Y., Mashima, H., Lithell, H., Cox, N.J., Hansen, T., Bell, G.I., and Pedersen, O. (2002). Variants within the calpain-10 gene on chromosome 2q37 (NIDDM1) and relationships to type 2 diabetes, insulin resistance, and impaired acute insulin secretion among Scandinavian Caucasians. *Diabetes,* 51(12), 3561–3567.

Rausch, J.L., Johnson, M.E., Fei, Y.J., Li, J.Q., Shendarkar, N., Hobby, H.M., Ganapathy, V., and Leibach, F.H. (2002). Initial conditions of serotonin transporter kinetics and genotype: Influence on SSRI treatment trial outcome. *Biol Psychiatry,* 51(9), 723–732.

Rees, M., Norton, N., Jones, I., McCandless, F., Scourfield, J., Holmans, P., Moorhead, S., Feldman, E., Sadler, S., Cole, T., Redman, K., Farmer, A., McGuffin, P., Owen, M.J., and Craddock, N. (1997). Association studies of bipolar disorder at the human serotonin transporter gene (hSERT; 5HTT). *Mol Psychiatry,* 2(5), 398–402.

Reich, D.E., and Lander, E.S. (2001). On the allelic spectrum of human disease. *Trends Genet,* 17(9), 502–510.

Reich, T., Clayton, P.J., and Winokur, G. (1969). Family history studies: V. The genetics of mania. *Am J Psychiatry,* 125(10), 1358–1369.

Reich, T., Van Eerdewegh, P., Rice, J., Mullaney, J., Endicott, J., and Klerman, G.L. (1987). The familial transmission of primary major depressive disorder. *J Psychiatr Res,* 21(4), 613–624.

Rice, J., Reich, T., Andreasen, N.C., Endicott, J., Van Eerdewegh, M., Fishman, R., Hirschfeld, R.M., and Klerman, G.L. (1987). The familial transmission of bipolar illness. *Arch Gen Psychiatry,* 44(5), 441–447.

Rice, J.P., Goate, A., Williams, J.T., Bierut, L., Dorr, D., Wu, W., Shears, S., Gopalakrishnan, G., Edenberg, H.J., Foroud, T.,

Nurnberger, J. Jr., Gershon, E.S., Detera-Wadleigh, S.D., Goldin, L.R., Guroff, J.J., McMahon, F.J., Simpson, S., Mac-Kinnon, D., McInnis, M., Stine, O.C., DePaulo, J.R., Blehar, M.C., and Reich, T. (1997). Initial genome scan of the NIMH genetics initiative bipolar pedigrees: Chromosomes 1, 6, 8, 10, and 12. *Am J Med Genet,* 74(3), 247–253.

Rietschel, M., Nothen, M.M., Lannfelt, L., Sokoloff, P., Schwartz, J.C., Lanczik, M., Fritze, J., Cichon, S., Fimmers, R., and Korner, J. (1993). A serine to glycine substitution at position 9 in the extracellular N-terminal part of the dopamine D3 receptor protein: No role in the genetic predisposition to bipolar affective disorder. *Psychiatry Res,* 46(3), 253–259.

Rietschel, M., Schorr, A., Albus, M., Franzek, E., Kreiner, R., Held, T., Knapp, M., Muller, D.J., Schulze, T.G., Propping, P., Maier, W., and Nothen, M.M. (2000). Association study of the tryptophan hydroxylase gene and bipolar affective disorder using family-based internal controls. *Am J Med Genet,* 96(3), 310–311.

Risch, N. (1990). Linkage strategies for genetically complex traits. I. Multilocus models. *Am J Hum Genet,* 46(2), 222–228.

Risch, N.J. (2000). Searching for genetic determinants in the new millennium. *Nature,* 405(6788), 847–856.

Roberts, S.B., MacLean, C.J., Neale, M.C., Eaves, L.J., and Kendler, K.S. (1999). Replication of linkage studies of complex traits: An examination of variation in location estimates. *Am J Hum Genet,* 65(3), 876–884.

Rohrmeier, T., Putzhammer, A., Schoeler, A., Sartor, H., Dallinger, P., Nothen, M.M., Propping, P., Knapp, M., Albus, M., Borrmann, M., Knothe, K., Kreiner, R., Franzek, E., Lichtermann, D., Rietschel, M., Maier, W., Klein, H.E., and Eichhammer, P. (1999). hSKCa3: No association of the polymorphic CAG repeat with bipolar affective disorder and schizophrenia. *Psychiatr Genet,* 9(4), 169–175.

Roll, A., and Entres, J.L. (1936). Zum Problem der Erbprognosebestimmung. *Z Ges Neurol Psychiatrie,* 156, 169–202.

Rosanoff, A.J., Handy, L., and Plesset, I.R. (1935). The etiology of manic-depressive syndromes with special reference to their occurrence in twins. *Am J Psychiatry,* 91, 725–762.

Rosenthal, D. (1970). *Genetic Theory and Abnormal Behavior.* New York: McGraw-Hill.

Rotondo, A., Mazzanti, C., Dell'Osso, L., Rucci, P., Sullivan, P., Bouanani, S., Gonnelli, C., Goldman, D., and Cassano, G.B. (2002). Catechol-O-methyltransferase, serotonin transporter, and tryptophan hydroxylase gene polymorphisms in bipolar disorder patients with and without comorbid panic disorder. *Am J Psychiatry,* 159(1), 23–29.

Rubinsztein, D.C., Leggo, J., Goodburn, S., Walsh, C., Jain, S., and Paykel, E.S. (1996). Genetic association between monoamine oxidase A microsatellite and RFLP alleles and bipolar affective disorder: Analysis and meta-analysis. *Hum Mol Genet,* 5(6), 779–782.

Rujescu, D., Giegling, I., Sato, T., and Moeller, H.J. (2001). A polymorphism in the promoter of the serotonin transporter gene is not associated with suicidal behavior. *Psychiatr Genet,* 11(3), 169–172.

Saleem, Q., Ganesh, S., Vijaykumar, M., Reddy, Y.C., Brahmachari, S.K., and Jain, S. (2000a). Association analysis of 5HT transporter gene in bipolar disorder in the Indian population. *Am J Med Genet,* 96(2), 170–172.

Saleem, Q., Sreevidya, V.S., Sudhir, J., Savithri, J.V., Gowda, Y., B-Rao, C., Benegal, V., Majumder, P.P., Anand, A., Brahmachari, S.K., and Jain, S. (2000b). Association analysis of

CAG repeats at the KCNN3 locus in Indian patients with bipolar disorder and schizophrenia. *Am J Med Genet,* 96(6), 744–748.

Savoye, C., Laurent, C., Amadeo, S., Gheysen, F., Leboyer, M., Lejeune, J., Zarifian, E., and Mallet, J. (1998). No association between dopamine D1, D2, and D3 receptor genes and manic-depressive illness. *Biol Psychiatry,* 44(7), 644–647.

Scharfetter, C. (1981). Subdividing the functional psychoses: A family hereditary approach. *Psychol Med,* 11(3), 637–640.

Schizophrenia Collaborative Linkage Group for Chromosome 22. (1998). A transmission disequilibrium and linkage analysis of D22S278 marker alleles in 574 families: Further support for a susceptibility locus for schizophrenia at 22q12. *Schizophr Res,* 32(2), 115–121.

Schulze, T.G., Chen, Y.S., Badner, J.A., McInnis, M.G., DePaulo, J.R. Jr., and McMahon, F.J. (2003). Additional, physically ordered markers increase linkage signal for bipolar disorder on chromosome 18q22. *Biol Psychiatry,* 53(3), 239–243.

Schulze, T.G., Buervenich, S., Badner, J.A., Steele, C.J., Detera-Wadleigh, S.D., Dick, D., Foroud, T., Cox, N.J., MacKinnon, D.F., Potash, J.B., Berrettini, W.H., Byerley, W., Coryell, W., DePaulo, J.R. Jr., Gershon, E.S., Kelsoe, J.R., McInnis, M.G., Murphy, D.L., Reich, T., Scheftner, W., Nurnberger, J.I. Jr., and McMahon, F.J. (2004). Loci on chromosomes 6q and 6p interact to increase susceptibility to bipolar affective disorder in the National Institute of Mental Health genetics initiative pedigrees. *Biol Psychiatry,* 56(1), 18–23.

Schulze, T.G., Ohlraun, S., Czerski, P.M., Schumacher, J., Kassem, L., Deschner, M., Gross, M., Tullius, M., Heidmann, V., Kovalenko, S., Jamra, R.A., Becker, T., Leszczynska-Rodziewicz, A., Hauser, J., Illig, T., Klopp, N., Wellek, S., Cichon, S., Henn, F.A., McMahon, F.J., Maier, W., Propping, P., Nothen, M.M., and Rietschel, M. (2005). Genotype–phenotype studies in bipolar disorder showing association between the DAOA/G30 locus and persecutory delusions: A first step toward a molecular genetic classification of psychiatric phenotypes. *Am J Psychiatry,* 162, 2101–2108.

Schumacher, J., Jamra, R.A., Freudenberg, J., Becker, T., Ohlraun S., Otte, A.C., Tullius, M., Kovalenko, S., Bogaert, A.V., Maier, W., Rietschel, M., Propping, P., Nothen, M.M., and Cichon, S. (2004). Examination of G72 and D-amino-acid oxidase as genetic risk factors for schizophrenia and bipolar affective disorder. *Mol Psychiatry,* 9(2), 203–207.

Schurhoff, F., Szoke, A., Meary, A., Bellivier, F., Rouillon, F., Pauls, D., and Leboyer, M. (2003). Familial aggregation of delusional proneness in schizophrenia and bipolar pedigrees. *Am J Psychiatry,* 160(7), 1313–1319.

Schwab, S.G., Hallmayer, J., Lerer, B., Albus, M., Borrmann, M., Honig, S., Strauss, M., Segman, R., Lichtermann, D., Knapp, M., Trixler, M., Maier, W., and Wildenauer, D.B. (1998). Support for a chromosome 18p locus conferring susceptibility to functional psychoses in families with schizophrenia, by association and linkage analysis. *Am J Hum Genet,* 63(4), 1139–1152.

Schwab, S.G., Hallmayer, J., Albus, M., Lerer, B., Eckstein, G.N., Borrmann, M., Segman, R.H., Hanses, C., Freymann, J., Yakir, A., Trixler, M., Falkai, P., Rietschel, M., Maier, W., and Wildenauer, D.B. (2000). A genome-wide autosomal screen for schizophrenia susceptibility loci in 71 families with affected siblings: Support for loci on chromosome 10p and 6. *Mol Psychiatry,* 5(6), 638–649.

Segman, R.H., Shapira, Y., Modai, I., Hamdan, A., Zislin, J., Heresco-Levy, U., Kanyas, K., Hirschmann, S., Karni, O., Finkel, B., Schlafman, M., Lerner, A., Shapira, B., Macciardi, F., and Lerer, B. (2002). Angiotensin converting enzyme gene insertion/deletion polymorphism: Case–control association studies in schizophrenia, major affective disorder, and tardive dyskinesia and a family-based association study in schizophrenia. *Am J Med Genet*, 114(3), 310–314.

Segurado, R., Detera-Wadleigh, S.D., Levinson, D.F., Lewis, C.M., Gill, M., Nurnberger, J.I. Jr., Craddock, N., DePaulo, J.R., Baron, M., Gershon, E.S., Ekholm, J., Cichon, S., Turecki, G., Claes, S., Kelsoe, J.R., Schofield, P.R., Badenhop, R.F., Morissette, J., Coon, H., Blackwood, D., McInnes, L.A., Foroud, T., Edenberg, H.J., Reich, T., Rice, J.P., Goate, A., McInnis, M.G., McMahon, F.J., Badner, J.A., Goldin, L.R., Bennett, P., Willour, V.L., Zandi, P.P., Liu, J., Gilliam, C., Juo, S.H., Berrettini, W.H., Yoshikawa, T., Peltonen, L., Lonnqvist, J., Nothen, M.M., Schumacher, J., Windemuth, C., Rietschel, M., Propping, P., Maier, W., Alda, M., Grof, P., Rouleau, G.A., Del-Favero, J., Van Broeckhoven, C., Mendlewicz, J., Adolfsson, R., Spence, M.A., Luebbert, H., Adams, L.J., Donald, J.A., Mitchell, P.B., Barden, N., Shink, E., Byerley, W., Muir, W., Visscher, P.M., Macgregor, S., Gurling, H., Kalsi, G., McQuillin, A., Escamilla, M.A., Reus, V.I., Leon, P., Freimer, N.B., Ewald, H., Kruse, T.A., Mors, O., Radhakrishna, U., Blouin, J.L., Antonarakis, S.E., and Akarsu, N. (2003). Genome scan meta-analysis of schizophrenia and bipolar disorder, part III: Bipolar disorder. *Am J Hum Genet*, 73(1), 49–62.

Sen, S., Nesse, R.M., Stoltenberg, S.F., Li, S., Gleiberman, L., Chakravarti, A., Weder, A.B., and Burmeister, M. (2003). A BDNF coding variant is associated with the NEO personality inventory domain neuroticism, a risk factor for depression. *Neuropsychopharmacology*, 28(2), 397–401.

Serretti, A., Macciardi, F., Cusin, C., Verga, M., Pedrini, S., and Smeraldi, E. (1998). Tyrosine hydroxylase gene in linkage disequilibrium with mood disorders. *Mol Psychiatry*, 3(2), 169–174.

Serretti, A., Lilli, R., Di Bella, D., Bertelli, S., Nobile, M., Novelli, E., Catalano, M., and Smeraldi, E. (1999a). Dopamine receptor D4 gene is not associated with major psychoses. *Am J Med Genet*, 88(5), 486–491.

Serretti, A., Lilli, R., Lorenzi, C., Gasperini, M., and Smeraldi, E. (1999b). Tryptophan hydroxylase gene and response to lithium prophylaxis in mood disorders. *J Psychiatr Res*, 33(5), 371–377.

Serretti, A., Lilli, R., Mandelli, L., Lorenzi, C., and Smeraldi, E. (2001). Serotonin transporter gene associated with lithium prophylaxis in mood disorders. *Pharmacogenomics*, J1(1), 71–77.

Serretti, A., Cristina, S., Lilli, R., Cusin, C., Lattuada, E., Lorenzi, C., Corradi, B., Grieco, G., Costa, A., Santorelli, F., Barale, F., Nappi, G., and Smeraldi, E. (2002). Family-based association study of 5-HTTLPR, TPH, MAO-A, and DRD4 polymorphisms in mood disorders. *Am J Med Genet*, 114(4), 361–369.

Serretti, A., Lilli, R., and Smeraldi, E. (2002c). Pharmacogenetics in affective disorders. *Eur J Pharmacol*, 438(3), 117–128.

Serretti, A., Cusin, C., Cristina, S., Lorenzi, C., Lilli, R., Lattuada, E., Grieco, G., Costa, A., Santorelli, F., Barale, F., Smeraldi, E., and Nappi, G. (2003). Multicentre Italian family-based association study on tyrosine hydroxylase, catechol-O-methyl transferase and Wolfram syndrome 1 polymorphisms in mood disorders. *Psychiatr Genet*, 13(2), 121–126.

Serretti, A., Cusin, C., Rossini, D., Artioli, P., Dotoli, D., and Zanardi, R. (2004). Further evidence of a combined effect of SERTPR and TPH on SSRIs response in mood disorders. *Am J Med Genet B Neuropsychiatr Genet*, 129(1), 36–40.

Shaikh, S., Ball, D., Craddock, N., Castle, D., Hunt, N., Mant, R., Owen, M., Collier, D., and Gill, M. (1993). The dopamine D3 receptor gene: no association with bipolar affective disorder. *J Med Genet*, 30(4), 308–309.

Sham, P.C., MacLean, C.J., and Kendler, K.S. (1994). A typological model of schizophrenia based on age at onset, sex and familial morbidity. *Acta Psychiatr Scand*, 89(2), 135–141.

Sham, P.C., Castle, D.J., Wessely, S., Farmer, A.E., and Murray, R.M. (1996). Further exploration of a latent class typology of schizophrenia. *Schizophr Res*, 20(1-2), 105–115.

Shimon, H., Agam, G., Belmaker, R.H., Hyde, T.M., and Kleinman, J.E. (1997). Reduced frontal cortex inositol levels in postmortem brain of suicide victims and patients with bipolar disorder. *Am J Psychiatry*, 154(8), 1148–1150.

Shorter, E. (1996). A History of Psychiatry: From the Era of the Asylum to the Age of Prozac. New York: John Wiley and Sons.

Simpson, S.G., Folstein, S.E., Meyers, D.A., McMahon, F.J., Brusco, D.M., and DePaulo, J.R. Jr. (1993). Bipolar II: The most common bipolar phenotype? *Am J Psychiatry*, 150(6), 901–903.

Simpson, S.G., McMahon, F.J., McInnis, M.G., MacKinnon, D.F., Edwin, D., Folstein, S.E., and DePaulo, J.R. (2002). Diagnostic reliability of bipolar II disorder. *Arch Gen Psychiatry*, 59(8), 736–740.

Sjögren, T. (1948). Genetic-statistical and psychiatric investigations of a West Swedish population. *Acta Psychiatr Neurol*, 24 (Suppl.), 269–271.

Sjoholt, G., Ebstein, R.P., Lie, R.T., Berle, J.O., Mallet, J., Deleuze, J.F., Levinson, D.F., Laurent, C., Mujahed, M., Bannoura, I., Murad, I., Molven, A., and Steen, V.M. (2004). Examination of IMPA1 and IMPA2 genes in manic-depressive patients: Association between IMPA2 promoter polymorphisms and bipolar disorder. *Mol Psychiatry*, 9(6), 621–629.

Sklar, P., Gabriel, S.B., McInnis, M.G., Bennett, P., Lim, Y.M., Tsan, G., Schaffner, S., Kirov, G., Jones, I., Owen, M., Craddock, N., DePaulo, J.R., and Lander, E.S. (2002). Family-based association study of 76 candidate genes in bipolar disorder: BDNF is a potential risk locus. Brain-derived neutrophic factor. *Mol Psychiatry*, 7(6), 579–593.

Skuse, D.H., James, R.S., Bishop, D.V., Coppin, B., Dalton, P., Aamodt-Leeper, G., Bacarese-Hamilton, M., Creswell, C., McGurk, R., and Jacobs, P.A. (1997). Evidence from Turner's syndrome of an imprinted X-linked locus affecting cognitive function [see comments]. *Nature*, 387(6634), 705–708.

Slater, E. (1936a). The inheritance of manic-depressive insanity. *Proc R Soc Med*, 29, 981–990.

Slater, E. (1936b). The inheritance of manic-depressive insanity and its relation to mental defect. *J Ment Sci*, 82:626–634.

Slater, E. (1938). Erbpathologie des manisch-depressiven Irreseins. Die Eltern und Kinder von Manisch-Depressiven. [Hereditary pathology of manic-depressive illness. Parents and offspring of manic-depressives]. *Z Ges Neurol Psychiatrie*, 163, 1–47.

Slater, E., and Shields, J. (1953). Psychotic and neurotic illnesses in twins. In: *Medical Research Current Special Report*, Series #ZN8. London: HMSO.

Smeraldi, E., Negri, F., and Melica, A.M. (1977). A genetic study of affective disorders. *Acta Psychiatr Scand*, 56(5), 382–398.

Smeraldi, E., Zanardi, R., Benedetti, F., Di Bella, D., Perez, J., and Catalano, M. (1998). Polymorphism within the promoter of the serotonin transporter gene and antidepressant efficacy of fluvoxamine. *Mol Psychiatry*, 3(6), 508–511.

Smith, D.J., Stevens, M.E., Sudanagunta, S.P., Bronson, R.T., Makhinson, M., Watabe, A.M., O'Dell, T.J., Fung, J., Weier, H.U., Cheng, J.F., and Rubin, E.M. (1997). Functional screening of 2 Mb of human chromosome 21q22.2 in transgenic mice implicates minibrain in learning defects associated with Down syndrome. *Nat Genet*, 16(1), 28–36.

Smith, L.B., Sapers, B., Reus, V.I., and Freimer, N.B. (1996). Attitudes towards bipolar disorder and predictive genetic testing among patients and providers. *J Med Genet*, 33(7), 544–549.

Souery, D., Lipp, O., Mahieu, B., Mendelbaum, K., De Bruyn, A., De Maertelaer, V., Van Broeckhoven, C., and Mendlewicz, J. (1996a). Excess tyrosine hydroxylase restriction fragment length polymorphism homozygosity in unipolar but not bipolar patients: A preliminary report. *Biol Psychiatry*, 40(4), 305–308.

Souery, D., Lipp, O., Mahieu, B., Mendelbaum, K., De Martelaer, V., Van Broeckhoven, C., and Mendlewicz, J. (1996b). Association study of bipolar disorder with candidate genes involved in catecholamine neurotransmission: DRD2, DRD3, DAT1, and TH genes. *Am J Med Genet*, 67(6), 551–555.

Souery, D., Lipp, O., Rivelli, S.K., Massat, I., Serretti, A., Cavallini, C., Ackenheil, M., Adolfsson, R., Aschauer, H., Blackwood, D., Dam, H., Dikeos, D., Fuchshuber, S., Heiden, M., Jakovljevic, M., Kaneva, R., Kessing, L., Lerer, B., Lonnqvist, J., Mellerup, T., Milanova, V., Muir, W., Nylander, P.O., Oruc, L., and Mendlewicz, J. (1999). Tyrosine hydroxylase polymorphism and phenotypic heterogeneity in bipolar affective disorder: A multicenter association study. *Am J Med Genet*, 88(5), 527–532.

Souery, D., Van Gestel, S., Massat, I., Blairy, S., Adolfsson, R., Blackwood, D., Del-Favero, J., Dikeos, D., Jakovljevic, M., Kaneva, R., Lattuada, E., Lerer, B., Lilli, R., Milanova, V., Muir, W., Nothen, M., Oruc, L., Papadimitriou, G., Propping, P., Schulze, T., Serretti, A., Shapira, B., Smeraldi, E., Stefanis, C., Thomson, M., Van Broeckhoven, C., and Mendlewicz, J. (2001). Tryptophan hydroxylase polymorphism and suicidality in unipolar and bipolar affective disorders: A multicenter association study. *Biol Psychiatry*, 49(5), 405–409.

Speight, G., Turic, D., Austin, J., Hoogendoorn, B., Cardno, A.G., Jones, L., Murphy, K.C., Sanders, R., McCarthy, G., Jones, I., McCandless, F., McGuffin, P., Craddock, N., Owen, M.J., Buckland, P., and O'Donovan, M.C. (2000). Comparative sequencing and association studies of aromatic L-amino acid decarboxylase in schizophrenia and bipolar disorder. *Mol Psychiatry*, 5(3), 327–331.

Spence, M.A., Flodman, P.L., Sadovnick, A.D., Bailey-Wilson, J.E., Ameli, H., and Remick, R.A. (1995). Bipolar disorder: Evidence for a major locus [see comments]. *Am J Med Genet*, 60(5), 370–376.

Spielman, R.S., McGinnis, R.E., and Ewens, W.J. (1993). Transmission test for linkage disequilibrium: The insulin gene region and insulin-dependent diabetes mellitus (IDDM). *Am J Hum Genet*, 52(3), 506–516.

Spitzer, R.L., and Endicott, J. (1975). *Research Diagnostic Criteria (RDC) for a Selected Group of Functional Disorders*. New York: New York State Psychiatric Institute, Biometrics Research.

Stenstedt, Å. (1952). A study in manic-depressive psychosis: Clinical, social, and genetic investigations. *Acta Psychiatr Neurol*, (Suppl. 79), 1–111.

St. George-Hyslop, P.H. (2000). Molecular genetics of Alzheimer's disease. *Biol Psychiatry*, 47(3), 183–199.

Stine, O.C., Xu, J., Koskela, R., McMahon, F.J., Gschwend, M., Friddle, C., Clark, C.D., McInnis, M.G., Simpson, S.G., and Breschel, T.S. (1995). Evidence for linkage of bipolar disorder to chromosome 18 with a parent-of-origin effect. *Am J Hum Genet*, 57(6), 1384–1394.

Stine, O.C., McMahon, F.J., Chen, L., Xu, J., Meyers, D.A., MacKinnon, D.F., Simpson, S., McInnis, M.G., Rice, J.P., Goate, A., Reich, T., Edenberg, H.J., Foroud, T., Nurnberger, J.I. Jr., Detera-Wadleigh, S.D., Goldin, L.R., Guroff, J., Gershon, E.S., Blehar, M.C., and DePaulo, J.R. (1997). Initial genome screen for bipolar disorder in the NIMH genetics initiative pedigrees: Chromosomes 2, 11, 13, 14, and X. *Am J Med Genet*, 74(3), 263–269.

Stober, G., Nothen, M.M., Porzgen, P., Bruss, M., Bonisch, H., Knapp, M., Beckmann, H., and Propping, P. (1996). Systematic search for variation in the human norepinephrine transporter gene: Identification of five naturally occurring missense mutations and study of association with major psychiatric disorders. *Am J Med Genet*, 67(6), 523–532.

Stober, G., Jatzke, S., Heils, A., Jungkunz, G., Knapp, M., Mossner, R., Riederer, P., and Lesch, K.P. (1998). Insertion/deletion variant (−141C Ins/Del) in the 5' regulatory region of the dopamine D2 receptor gene: Lack of association with schizophrenia and bipolar affective disorder. Short communication. *J Neural Transm*, 105(1), 101–109.

Straub, R.E., Lehner, T., Luo, Y., Loth, J.E., Shao, W., Sharpe, L., Alexander, J.R., Das, K., Simon, R., and Fieve, R.R. (1994). A possible vulnerability locus for bipolar affective disorder on chromosome 21q22.3. *Nat Genet*, 8(3), 291–296.

Straub, R.E., MacLean, C.J., Martin, R.B., Ma, Y., Myakishev, M.V., Harris-Kerr, C., Webb, B.T., O'Neill, F.A., Walsh, D., and Kendler, K.S. (1998). A schizophrenia locus may be located in region 10p15-p11. *Am J Med Genet*, 81(4), 296–301.

Strober, M., Morrell, W., Burroughs, J., Lampert, C., Danforth, H., and Freeman, R. (1988). A family study of bipolar I disorder in adolescence. Early onset of symptoms linked to increased familial loading and lithium resistance. *J Affect Disord*, 15(3), 255–268.

Strömgren, E. (1938) Beitrage zur psychiatrischen Erblehre. Copenhagen: Munksgaard.

Sullivan, P.F., Neale, M.C., and Kendler, K.S. (2000). Genetic epidemiology of major depression: Review and meta-analysis. *Am J Psychiatry*, 157(10), 1552–1562.

Sun, Y., Zhang, L., Johnston, N.L., Torrey, E.F., and Yolken, R.H. (2001). Serial analysis of gene expression in the frontal cortex of patients with bipolar disorder. *Br J Psychiatry*, (Suppl. 41), s137–s141.

Swift-Scanlan, T., Lan, T.H., Fallin, M.D., Coughlin, J.M., Potash, J.B., DePaulo, J.R., and McInnis, M.G. (2002). Genetic analysis of the (CTG)n NOTCH4 polymorphism in 65 multiplex bipolar pedigrees. *Psychiatr Genet*, 12(1), 43–47.

Syagailo, Y.V., Stober, G., Grassle, M., Reimer, E., Knapp, M., Jungkunz, G., Okladnova, O., Meyer, J., and Lesch, K.P. (2001). Association analysis of the functional monoamine oxidase A gene promoter polymorphism in psychiatric disorders. *Am J Med Genet*, 105(2), 168–171.

Tadokoro, K., Hashimoto, R., Tatsumi, M., Kamijima, K., and Kunugi, H. (2004). Analysis of enhancer activity of a dinucleotide repeat polymorphism in the neurotrophin-3 gene and its association with bipolar disorder. *Neuropsychobiology*, 50(3), 206–210.

Tanna, V.L., and Winokur, G. (1968). A study of association and linkage of ABO blood types and primary affective disorder. *Br J Psychiatry*, 114(514), 1175–1181.

Tkachev, D., Mimmack, M.L., Ryan, M.M., Wayland, M., Freeman, T., Jones, P.B., Starkey, M., Webster, M.J., Yolken, R.H., and Bahn, S. (2003). Oligodendrocyte dysfunction in schizophrenia and bipolar disorder. *Lancet*, 362(9386), 798–805.

Todd, R.D., and O'Malley, K.L. (1989). Population frequencies of tyrosine hydroxylase restriction fragment length polymorphisms in bipolar affective disorder. *Biol Psychiatry*, 25(5), 626–630.

Todd, R.D., Lobos, E.A., Parsian, A., Simpson, S., and DePaulo, J.R. (1996). Manic-depressive illness and tyrosine hydroxylase markers. Bipolar Disorder Working Group. *Lancet*, 347(9015), 1634.

Torgersen, S. (1986). Genetic factors in moderately severe and mild affective disorders. *Arch Gen Psychiatry*, 43(3), 222–226.

Toyota, T., Watanabe, A., Shibuya, H., Nankai, M., Hattori, E., Yamada, K., Kurumaji, A., Karkera, J.D., Detera-Wadleigh, S.D., and Yoshikawa, T. (2000). Association study on the DUSP6 gene, an affective disorder candidate gene on 12q23, performed by using fluorescence resonance energy transfer-based melting curve analysis on the LightCycler. *Mol Psychiatry*, 5(5), 489–494.

Toyota, T., Hattori, E., Meerabux, J., Yamada, K., Saito, K., Shibuya, H., Nankai, M., and Yoshikawa, T. (2002). Molecular analysis, mutation screening, and association study of adenylate cyclase type 9 gene (ADCY9) in mood disorders. *Am J Med Genet*, 114(1), 84–92.

Tremolizzo, L., Carboni, G., Ruzicka, W.B., Mitchell, C.P., Sugaya, I., Tueting, P., Sharma, R., Grayson, D.R., Costa, E., and Guidotti, A. (2002). An epigenetic mouse model for molecular and behavioral neuropathologies related to schizophrenia vulnerability. *Proc Natl Acad Sci USA*, 99(26), 17095–17100.

Trippitelli, C.L., Jamison, K.R., Folstein, M.F., Bartko, J.J., and DePaulo, J.R. (1998). Pilot study on patients' and spouses' attitudes toward potential genetic testing for bipolar disorder. *Am J Psychiatry*, 155(7), 899–904.

Tsai, S.J., Hong, C.J., Hsu, C.C., Cheng, C.Y., Liao, W.Y., Song, H.L., and Lai, H.C. (1999). Serotonin-2A receptor polymorphism (102T/C) in mood disorders. *Psychiatry Res*, 87(2–3), 233–237.

Tsai, S.J., Wang, Y.C., and Hong, C.J. (2001). Association study between cannabinoid receptor gene (CNR1) and pathogenesis and psychotic symptoms of mood disorders. *Am J Med Genet*, 105(3), 219–221.

Tsai, S.J., Cheng, C.Y., Yu, Y.W., Chen, T.J., and Hong, C.J. (2003). Association study of a brain-derived neurotrophic-factor genetic polymorphism and major depressive disorders, symptomatology, and antidepressant response. *Am J Med Genet B Neuropsychiatr Genet*, 123(1), 19–22.

Tsuang, M.T., and Faraone, S.V. (1990). *The Genetics of Mood Disorders*. Baltimore: Johns Hopkins University Press.

Tsuang, M.T., Woolson, R., and Fleming, J.A. (1980). Causes of death in schizophrenia and manic-depression. *Br J Psychiatry*, 136, 239–242.

Turecki, G., Alda, M., Grof, P., Martin, R., Cavazzoni, P.A., Duffy, A., Maciel, P., and Rouleau, G.A. (1996). No association between chromosome-18 markers and lithium-responsive affective disorders. *Psychiatry Res*, 63(1), 17–23.

Turecki, G., Grof, P., Cavazzoni, P., Duffy, A., Grof, E., Ahrens, B., Berghofer, A., Muller-Oerlinghausen, B., Dvorakova, M., Libigerova, E., Vojtechovsky, M., Zvolsky, P., Joober, R., Nilsson, A., Prochazka, H., Licht, R.W., Rasmussen, N.A., Schou, M., Vestergaard, P., Holzinger, A., Schumann, C., Thau, K., Rouleau, GA., and Alda, M. (1998). Evidence for a role of phospholipase C-gamma1 in the pathogenesis of bipolar disorder. *Mol Psychiatry*, 3(6), 534–538.

Turecki, G., Grof, P., Cavazzoni, P., Duffy, A., Grof, E., Ahrens, B., Berghofer, A., Muller-Oerlinghausen, B., Dvorakova, M., Libigerova, E., Vojtechovsky, M., Zvolsky, P., Joober, R., Nilsson, A., Prochazka, H., Licht, R.W., Rasmussen, N.A., Schou, M., Vestergaard, P., Holzinger, A., Schumann, C., Thau, K., Rouleau, G.A., and Alda, M. (1999). MAOA: Association and linkage studies with lithium responsive bipolar disorder. *Psychiatr Genet*, 9(1), 13–16.

Turecki, G., Grof, P., Grof, E., D'Souza, V., Lebuis, L., Marineau, C., Cavazzoni, P., Duffy, A., Betard, C., Zvolsky, P., Robertson, C., Brewer, C., Hudson, T.J., Rouleau, G.A., and Alda, M. (2001). Mapping susceptibility genes for bipolar disorder: A pharmacogenetic approach based on excellent response to lithium. *Mol Psychiatry*, 6(5), 570–578.

Tut, T.G., Wang, J.L., and Lim, C.C. (2000). Negative association between T102C polymorphism at the 5-HT2A receptor gene and bipolar affective disorders in Singaporean Chinese. *J Affect Disord*, 58(3), 211–214.

Ujike, H., Yamamoto, A., Tanaka, Y., Takehisa, Y., Takaki, M., Taked, T., Kodama, M., and Kuroda, S. (2001). Association study of CAG repeats in the KCNN3 gene in Japanese patients with schizophrenia, schizoaffective disorder and bipolar disorder. *Psychiatry Res*, 101(3), 203–207.

Van Tol, H.H., Bunzow, J.R., Guan, H.C., Sunahara, R.K., Seeman, P., Niznik, H.B., and Civelli, O. (1991). Cloning of the gene for a human dopamine D4 receptor with high affinity for the antipsychotic clozapine. *Nature*, 350(6319), 610–614.

Van Tol, H.H., Wu, C.M., Guan, H.C., Ohara, K., Bunzow, J.R., Civelli, O., Kennedy, J., Seeman, P., Niznik, H.B., and Jovanovic, V. (1992). Multiple dopamine D4 receptor variants in the human population. *Nature*, 358(6382), 149–152.

Vawter, M.P., Thatcher, L., Usen, N., Hyde, T.M., Kleinman, J.E., and Freed, W.J. (2002). Reduction of synapsin in the hippocampus of patients with bipolar disorder and schizophrenia. *Mol Psychiatry*, 7(6), 571–578.

Venken, T., Claes, S., Sluijs, S., Paterson, A.D., van Duijn, C., Adolfsson, R., Del-Favero, J., and Van Broeckhoven, C. (2005). Genomewide scan for affective disorder susceptibility Loci in families of a northern Swedish isolated population. *Am J Hum Genet*, 76(2), 237–248.

Vincent, J.B., Masellis, M., Lawrence, J., Choi, V., Gurling, H.M., Parikh, S.V., and Kennedy, J.L. (1999). Genetic association analysis of serotonin system genes in bipolar affective disorder. *Am J Psychiatry*, 156(1), 136–138.

Vogt, I.R., Shimron-Abarbanell, D., Neidt, H., Erdmann, J., Cichon, S., Schulze, T.G., Muller, D.J., Maier, W., Albus, M., Borrmann-Hassenbach, M., Knapp, M., Rietschel, M., Propping, P., and Nothen, M.M. (2000). Investigation of the human serotonin 6 [5-HT6] receptor gene in bipolar affective disorder and schizophrenia. *Am J Med Genet*, 96(2), 217–221.

von Knorring, A.L., Cloninger, C.R., Bohman, M., and Sigvardsson, S. (1983). An adoption study of depressive disorders and substance abuse. *Arch Gen Psychiatry*, 40(9), 943–950.

Waldman, I.D., Robinson, B.F., and Feigon, S.A. (1997). Linkage disequilibrium between the dopamine transporter gene (DAT1) and bipolar disorder: Extending the transmission disequilibrium test (TDT) to examine genetic heterogeneity. *Genet Epidemiol*, 14(6), 699–704.

Washizuka, S., Ikeda, A., Kato, N., and Kato, T. (2003). Possible relationship between mitochondrial DNA polymorphisms and lithium response in bipolar disorder. *Int J Neuropsychopharmacol*, 6(4), 421–424.

Weber, M.M. (1996). Ernst Rudin, 1874–1952: A German psychiatrist and geneticist. *Am J Med Genet*, 67(4), 323–331.

Weinberg, I., and Lobstein, J. (1936). Beitrag zur Vererbung des manisch-depressiven Irreseins. *Psychiatr Neurol*, 1, 337.

Weiss, J., Magert, H.J., Cieslak, A., and Forssmann, W.G. (1996). Association between different psychotic disorders and the DRD4 polymorphism, but no differences in the main ligand binding region of the DRD4 receptor protein compared to controls. *Eur J Med Res*, 1(9), 439–445.

Weissman, M.M., Gershon, E.S., Kidd, K.K., Prusoff, B.A., Leckman, J.F., Dibble, E., Hamovit, J., Thompson, W.D., Pauls, D.L., and Guroff, J.J. (1984). Psychiatric disorders in the relatives of probands with affective disorders. The Yale University–National Institute of Mental Health collaborative study. *Arch Gen Psychiatry*, 41(1), 13–21.

Weissman, M.M., Wickramaratne, P., Adams, P.B., Lish, J.D., Horwath, E., Charney, D., Woods, S.W., Leeman, E., and Frosch, E. (1993). The relationship between panic disorder and major depression. A new family study. *Arch Gen Psychiatry*, 50(10), 767–780.

Weksberg, R., Shuman, C., Caluseriu, O., Smith, A.C., Fei, Y.L., Nishikawa, J., Stockley, T.L., Best, L., Chitayat, D., Olney, A., Ives, E., Schneider, A., Bestor, T.H., Li, M., Sadowski, P., and Squire, J. (2002). Discordant KCNQ1OT1 imprinting in sets of monozygotic twins discordant for Beckwith-Wiedemann syndrome. *Hum Mol Genet*, 11(11), 1317–1325.

Wender, P.H., Kety, S.S., Rosenthal, D., Schulsinger, F., Ortmann, J., and Lunde, I. (1986). Psychiatric disorders in the biological and adoptive families of adopted individuals with affective disorders. *Arch Gen Psychiatry*, 43(10), 923–929.

Williams, R.S., Cheng, L., Mudge, A.W., and Harwood, A.J. (2002). A common mechanism of action for three mood-stabilizing drugs. *Nature*, 417(6886), 292–295.

Willour, V.L., Zandi, P.P., Huo, Y., Diggs, T.L., Chellis, J.L., MacKinnon, D.F., Simpson, S.G., McMahon, F.J., Potash, J.B., Gershon, E.S., Reich, T., Foroud, T., Nurnberger, J.I. Jr., DePaulo, J.R. Jr., and McInnis, M.G. (2003). Genome scan of the fifty-six bipolar pedigrees from the NIMH genetics initiative replication sample: Chromosomes 4, 7, 9, 18, 19, 20, and 21. *Am J Med Genet B Neuropsychiatr Genet*, 121(1), 21–27.

Winokur, G., and Clayton, P. (1967). Family history studies: I. Two types of affective disorders separated according to genetic and clinical factors. In J. Wortis (Ed.), Recent Advances in Biological Psychiatry (Vol. 10). New York: Plenum Press, pp. 35–50

Woo, T.U., Walsh, J.P., and Benes, F.M. (2004). Density of glutamic acid decarboxylase 67 messenger RNA-containing neurons that express the *N*-methyl-D-aspartate receptor subunit NR2A in the anterior cingulate cortex in schizophrenia and bipolar disorder. *Arch Gen Psychiatry*, 61(7), 649–657.

Wooster, R., Neuhausen, S.L., Mangion, J., Quirk, Y., Ford, D., Collins, N., Nguyen, K., Seal, S., Tran, T., Averill, D. (1994). Localization of a breast cancer susceptibility gene, BRCA2, to chromosome 13q12-13. *Science*, 265(5181), 2088–2090.

Wozniak, J., Biederman, J., Mundy, E., Mennin, D., and Faraone, S.V. (1995). A pilot family study of childhood-onset mania. *J Am Acad Child Adolesc Psychiatry*, 34 (12), 1577–1583.

Wozniak, J., Biederman, J., Monuteaux, M.C., Richards, J., and Faraone, S.V. (2002). Parsing the comorbidity between bipolar disorder and anxiety disorders: A familial risk analysis. *J Child Adolesc Psychopharmacol*, 12(2), 101–111.

Wright, A.F., Carothers, A.D., and Pirastu, M. (1999). Population choice in mapping genes for complex diseases. *Nat Genet*, 23(4), 397–404.

Xian, H., Scherrer, J.F., Eisen, S.A., True, W.R., Heath, A.C., Goldberg, J., Lyons, M.J., and Tsuang, M.T. (2000). Self-Reported zygosity and the equal-environments assumption for psychiatric disorders in the Vietnam Era Twin Registry. *Behav Genet*, 30(4), 303–310.

Xing, G., Russell, S., Hough, C., O'Grady, J., Zhang, L., Yang, S., Zhang, L.X., and Post, R. (2002). Decreased prefrontal CaMKII alpha mRNA in bipolar illness. *Neuroreport*, 13(4), 501–505.

Yamamoto, A., Lucas, J.J., and Hen, R. (2000). Reversal of neuropathology and motor dysfunction in a conditional model of Huntington's disease. *Cell*, 101(1), 57–66.

Yang, Q., Khoury, M.J., Botto, L., Friedman, J.M., and Flanders, W.D. (2003). Improving the prediction of complex diseases by testing for multiple disease-susceptibility genes. *Am J Hum Genet*, 72(3), 636–649.

Yen, F.C., Hong, C.J., Hou, S.J., Wang, J.K., and Tsai, S.J. (2003). Association study of serotonin transporter gene VNTR polymorphism and mood disorders, onset age and suicide attempts in a Chinese sample. *Neuropsychobiology*, 48(1), 5–9.

Yoon, I.S., Li, P.P., Siu, K.P., Kennedy, J.L., Macciardi, F., Cooke, R.G., Parikh, S.V., and Warsh, J.J. (2001). Altered TRPC7 gene expression in bipolar-I disorder. *Biol Psychiatry*, 50(8), 620–626.

Yoshida, K., Ito, K., Sato, K., Takahashi, H., Kamata, M., Higuchi, H., Shimizu, T., Itoh, K., Inoue, K., Tezuka, T., Suzuki, T., Ohkubo, T., Sugawara, K., and Otani, K. (2002). Influence of the serotonin transporter gene–linked polymorphic region on the antidepressant response to fluvoxamine in Japanese depressed patients. *Prog Neuropsychopharmacol Biol Psychiatry*, 26(2), 383–386.

Yoshida, K., Takahashi, H., Higuchi, H., Kamata, M., Ito, K., Sato, K., Naito, S., Shimizu, T., Itoh, K., Inoue, K., Suzuki, T., and Nemeroff, C.B. (2004). Prediction of antidepressant response to milnacipran by norepinephrine transporter gene polymorphisms. *Am J Psychiatry*, 161(9), 1575–1580.

Young, L.T., Asghari, V., Li, P.P., Kish, S.J., Fahnestock, M., and Warsh, J.J. (1996). Stimulatory G-protein alpha-subunit mRNA levels are not increased in autopsied cerebral cortex from patients with bipolar disorder. *Brain Res Mol Brain Res*, 42(1), 45–50.

Young, L.E., Sinclair, K.D., and Wilmut, I. (1998). Large offspring syndrome in cattle and sheep. *Rev Reprod*, 3(3), 155–163.

Yu, Y.W., Tsai, S.J., Chen, T.J., Lin, C.H., and Hong, C.J. (2002). Association study of the serotonin transporter promoter polymorphism and symptomatology and antidepressant response in major depressive disorders. *Mol Psychiatry*, 7(10), 1115–1119.

Zanardi, R., Benedetti, F., Di Bella, D., Catalano, M., Smeraldi, E. (2000). Efficacy of paroxetine in depression is influenced by a functional polymorphism within the promoter of the serotonin transporter gene. *J Clin Psychopharmacol*, 20(1), 105–107.

Zanardi, R., Artigas, F., Moresco, R., Colombo, C., Messa, C., Gobbo, C., Smeraldi, E., and Fazio, F. (2001). Increased 5-hydroxytryptamine-2 receptor binding in the frontal cortex of depressed patients responding to paroxetine treatment: A position emission tomography scan study. *J Clin Psychopharmacol*, 21(1), 53–58.

Zandi, P.P., Willour, V.L., Huo, Y., Chellis, J., Potash, J.B., MacKinnon, D.F., Simpson, S.G., McMahon, F.J., Gershon, E., Reich, T., Foroud, T., Nurnberger, J., Jr., DePaulo, J.R. Jr., McInnis, M.G., and National Institute of Mental Health Genetics Initiative Bipolar Group. (2003). Genome scan of a second wave of NIMH genetics initiative bipolar pedigrees: chromosomes 2, 11, 13, 14, and X. *Am J Med Genet B Neuropsychiatr Genet*, 119(1), 69–76.

Zhang, H.Y., Ishigaki, T., Tani, K., Chen, K., Shih, J.C., Miyasato, K., Ohara, K., and Ohara, K. (1997). Serotonin2A receptor gene polymorphism in mood disorders. *Biol Psychiatry*, 41(7), 768–773.

Zubenko, G.S., Hughes, H.B. III, Maher, B.S., Stiffler, J.S., Zubenko, W.N., and Marazita, M.L. (2002). Genetic linkage of region containing the CREB1 gene to depressive disorders in women from families with recurrent, early-onset, major depression. *Am J Med Genet*, 114(8), 980–987.

Zubenko, G.S., Maher, B., Hughes, H.B. III, Zubenko, W.N., Stiffler, J.S., Kaplan, B.B., and Marazita, M.L. (2003). Genome-wide linkage survey for genetic loci that influence the development of depressive disorders in families with recurrent, early-onset, major depression. *Am J Med Genet B Neuropsychiatr Genet*, 123(1), 1–18.

Chapter 14

Abarca, C., Albrecht, U., and Spanagel, R. (2002). Cocaine sensitization and reward are under the influence of circadian genes and rhythm. *Proc Natl Acad Sci USA*, 99, 9026–9030.

Aberg-Wistedt, A., Hasselmark, L., Stain-Malmgren, R., Aperia, B., Kjellman, B.F., and Mathe, A.A. (1998). Serotonergic "vulnerability" in affective disorder: a study of the tryptophan depletion test and relationships between peripheral and central serotonin indexes in citalopram-responders. *Acta Psychiatr Scand*, 97, 374–380.

Abou-Saleh, M.T., and Coppen, A. (1989). The efficacy of low-dose lithium: Clinical, psychological and biological correlates. *J Psychiatr Res*, 23, 157–162.

Adams, J.M., and Cory, S. (1998). The Bcl-2 protein family: Arbiters of cell survival. *Science*, 281, 1322–1326.

Aguiar, M.S., and Brandao, M.L. (1996). Effects of microinjections of the neuropeptide substance P in the dorsal periqueductal grey on the behaviour of rats in the plus mazetest. *Physiol Behav*, 60, 1183–1186.

Ahluwalia, P., and Singhal, R.L. (1980). Effect of low-dose lithium administration and subsequent withdrawal on biogenic amines in rat brain. *Br J Pharmacol*, 71, 601–607.

Ahluwalia, P., Grewaal, D.S., and Singhal, R.L. (1981). Brain GABAergic and dopaminergic systems following lithium treatment and withdrawal. *Prog Neuropsychopharmacol*, 5, 527–530.

Aigner, T., Weiss, S.R.B., and Post, R.M. (1990). Carbamazepine attenuates i.v. cocaine self-administration in rhesus monkeys. *Am Coll Neuropsychopharmacol San Juan*, 181.

Akagawa, K., Watanabe, M., and Tsukada, Y. (1980). Activity of erythrocyte Na,K-ATPase in manic patients. *J Neurochem*, 35, 258–260.

Albert, I., Cicala, G.A., and Siegel, J. (1970). The behavioral effects of REM sleep deprivation in rats. *Psychophysiology*, 6, 550–560.

Albright, P.S., and Burnham, W.M. (1980). Development of a new pharmacological seizure model: Effects of anticonvulsants on cortical- and amygdala-kindled seizures in the rat. *Epilepsia*, 21, 681–689.

Alda, M., Turecki, G., Grof, P., Cavazzoni, P., Duffy, A., Grof, E., Ahrens, B., Berghofer, A., Muller-Oerlinghausen, B., Dvorakova, M., Libigerova, E., Vojtechovsky, M., Zvolsky, P., Joober, R., Nilsson, A., Prochazka, H., Licht, R.W., Rasmussen, N.A., Schou, M., Vestergaard, P., Holzinger, A., Schumann, C., Thau, K., and Rouleau, G.A. (2000). Association and linkage studies of CRH and PENK genes in bipolar disorder: A collaborative IGSLI study. *Am J Med Genet*, 96, 178–181.

Alda, M., Keller, D., Grof, E., Turecki, G., Cavazzoni, P., Duffy, A., Rouleau, G.A., Grof, P., and Young, L.T. (2001). Is lithium response related to G(s)alpha levels in transformed lymphoblasts from subjects with bipolar disorder? *J Affect Disord*, 65(2), 117–122.

Alexander, D.R., Deeb, M., Bitar, F., and Antun, F. (1986). Sodium-potassium, magnesium, and calcium ATPase activities in erythrocyte membranes from manic-depressive patients responding to lithium. *Biol Psychiatry*, 21, 997–1007.

Allada, R., Emery, P., Takahashi, J.S., and Rosbash, M. (2001). Stopping time: The genetics of fly and mouse circadian clocks. *Annu Rev Neurosci*, 24, 1091–1119.

Allard, P., and Norlén, M. (1997). Unchanged density of caudate nucleus dopamine uptake sites in depressed suicide victims. *J Neural Transm*, 104, 1353–1360.

Allison, J.H., and Stewart, M.A. (1971). Reduced brain inositol in lithium-treated rats. *Nat New Biol*, 233, 267–268.

Alrecht, J., and Muller-Oerlinghausen, B. (1976). Clinical relevance of lithium determination in RBC: Results of a catamnestic study [in German]. *Arzneimittelforschung*, 26(6), 1145–1147.

Altamura, C.A., Mauri, M.C., Ferrara, A., Moro, A.R., D'Andrea, G., and Zamberlan, F. (1993). Plasma and platelet excitatory amino acids in psychiatric disorders. *Am J Psychiatry*, 150, 1731–1733.

Altshuler, L.L., Casanova, M.F., Goldberg, T.E., and Kleinman, J.E. (1990). The hippocampus and parahippocampus in schizophrenic, suicide, and control brains. *Arch Gen Psychiatry*, 47, 1029–1034.

Alvarez, G., Munoz-Montano, J.R., Satrustegui, J., Avila, J., Bogonez, E., and Diaz-Nido, J. (1999). Lithium protects cultured neurons against beta-amyloid-induced neurodegeneration. *FEBS Lett*, 453, 260–264.

Amsterdam, J.D. (1991). Use of high dose tranylcypromine in resistant depression. In J.D. Amsterdam (Ed.), *Advances in Neuropsychiatry and Psychopharmacology: Refractory Depression* (Vol. 2) (pp. 123–130). New York: Raven Press.

Amsterdam, J.D., Winokur, A., Caroff, S., and Mendels, J. (1981). Thyrotropin-releasing hormone's mood-elevating effects in depressed patients, anorectic patients, and normal volunteers. *Am J Psychiatry*, 138, 115–116.

Anand, A., Darnell, A., Miller, H.L., Berman, R.M., Cappiello, A., Oren, D.A., Woods, S.W., and Charney, D.S. (1999). Effect of catecholamine depletion on lithium-induced long-term remission of bipolar disorder. *Biol Psychiatry*, 45, 972–978.

Anand, A., Charney, D.S., Oren, D.A., Berman, R.M., Hu, X.S., Cappiello, A., and Krystal, J.H. (2000a). Attenuation of the neuropsychiatric effects of ketamine with lamotrigine: Support for hyperglutamatergic effects of N-methyl-D-aspartate receptor antagonists. *Arch Gen Psychiatry*, 57, 270–276.

Anand, A., Verhoeff, P., Seneca, N., Zoghbi, S.S., Seibyl, J.P., Charney, D.S., and Innis, R.B. (2000b). Brain SPECT imaging of amphetamine-induced dopamine release in euthymic bipolar disorder patients. *Am J Psychiatry*, 157, 1108–1114.

Andersen, P.H., and Geisler, A. (1984). Lithium inhibition of forskolin-stimulated adenylate cyclase. *Neuropsychobiology*, 12, 1–3.

Anderson, G.M., and Horne, W.C. (1992). Activators of protein kinase C decrease serotonin transport in human platelets. *Biochim Biophys Acta*, 1137, 331–337.

Andersson, A., Eriksson, A., and Marcusson, J. (1992). Unaltered number of brain serotonin uptake sites in suicide victims. *J Psychopharmacol*, 6, 509–513.

Angers, A., Fioravante, D., Chin, J., Cleary, L.J., Bean, A.J., and Byrne, J.H. (2002). Serotonin stimulates phosphorylation of aplysia synapsin and alters its subcellular distribution in sensory neurons. *J Neurosci*, 22, 5412–5422.

Angst, J., Autenreith, V., Brem, F., Koukkou, M., Meyer, H., Stassen, H.H., and Storck, U. (1979). Preliminary results of treatment with β-endorphin in depression. In E. Usdin, W.E., Bunney, and N.S. Kline (Eds.), *Endorphins in Mental Health Research* (pp. 518–528). New York: Oxford University Press.

Anlezark, G.M., Horton, R.W., Meldrum, B.S., Sawaya, M.C., and Stephenson, J.D. (1976). Proceedings: Gamma-aminobutyric acid metabolism and the anticonvulsant action of ethanolamine-O-sulphate and di-N-propylacetate. *Br J Pharmacol*, 56, 383P–384P.

Ansseau, M., von Frenckell, R., Cerfontaine, J.L., Papart, P., Franck, G., Timsit-Berthier, M., Geenen, V., and Legros, J.J. (1987). Neuroendocrine evaluation of catecholaminergic neurotransmission in mania. *Psychiatry Res*, 22, 193–206.

Ansseau, M., Von Frenckell, R., Cerfontaine, J.L., Papart, P., Franck, G., Timsit-Berthier, M., Geenen, V., and Legros, J.J. (1988). Blunted response of growth hormone to clonidine and apomorphine in endogenous depression. *Br J Psychiatry*, 153, 65–71.

Antelman, S.M., and Caggiula, A.R. (1996). Oscillation follows drug sensitization: Implications. *Crit Rev Neurobiol*, 10, 101–117.

Antelman, S.M., Caggiula, A.R., Kiss, S., Edwards, D.J., Kocan, D., and Stiller, R. (1995). Neurochemical and physiological effects of cocaine oscillate with sequential drug treatment: Possibly a major factor in drug variability. *Neuropsychopharmacology*, 12(4), 297–306.

Antelman, S.M., Caggiula, A.R., Kucinski, B.J., Fowler, H., Gershon, S., Edwards, D.J., Austin, M.C., Stiller, R., Kiss, S., and Kocan, D. (1998). The effects of lithium on a potential cycling model of bipolar disorder. *Prog Neuropsychopharmacol Biol Psychiatry*, 22, 495–510.

Antoniou, K., Kafetzopoulos, E., Papadopoulou-Daifoti, Z., Hyphantis, T., and Marselos, M. (1998). D-amphetamine, cocaine and caffeine: A comparative study of acute effects on locomotor activity and behavioural patterns in rats. *Neurosci Biobehav Rev*, 23, 189–196.

Apparsundaram, S., Galli, A., DeFelice, L.J., Hartzell, H.C., and Blakely, R.D. (1998). Acute regulation of norepinephrine transport: I. Protein kinase C–linked muscarinic receptors influence transport capacity and transporter density in SK-N-SH cells. *J Pharmacol Exp Ther*, 287, 733–743.

Arana, G.W., Barreira, P.J., Cohen, B.M., Lipinski, J.F., and Fogelson, D. (1983). The dexamethasone suppression test in psychotic disorders. *Am J Psychiatry*, 140, 1521–1523.

Arango, V., Ernsberger, P., Marzuk, P.M., Chen, J.S., Tierney, H., Stanley, M., Reis, D.J., and Mann, J.J. (1990). Autoradiographic demonstration of increased serotonin 5-HT$_2$ and beta-adrenergic receptor binding sites in the brain of suicide victims. *Arch Gen Psychiatry*, 47, 1038–1047.

Arango, V., Ernsberger, P., Sved, A.F., and Mann, J.J. (1993). Quantitative autoradiography of alpha 1- and alpha 2-adrenergic receptors in the cerebral cortex of controls and suicide victims. *Brain Res*, 630(1-2), 271–282.

Arango, V., Underwood, M.D., Gubbi, A.V., and Mann, J.J. (1995). Localized alterations in pre- and postsynaptic serotonin binding sites in the ventrolateral prefrontal cortex of suicide victims. *Brain Res*, 688, 121–133.

Arango, V., Underwood, M.D., and Mann, J.J. (1996a). Fewer pigmented locus coeruleus neurons in suicide victims: Preliminary results. *Biol Psychiatry*, 39(2), 112–120.

Arango, V., Underwood, M.D., Pauler, D.K., Kass, R.E., and Mann, J.J. (1996b). Differential age-related loss of pigmented locus coeruleus neurons in suicides, alcoholics, and alcoholic suicides. *Alcohol Clin Exp Res*, 20(7), 1141–1147.

Arato, M., Tekes, K., Tothfalusi, L., Magyar, K., Palkovits, M., Demeter, E., and Falus, A. (1987). Serotonergic split brain and suicide. *Psychiatry Res*, 21, 355–356.

Arato, M., Banki, C.M., Bissette, G., and Nemeroff, C.B. (1989). Elevated CSF CRF in suicide victims. *Biol Psychiatry*, 25, 355–359.

Arendt, T., Lehmann, K., Seeger, G., and Gartner, U. (1999). Synergistic effects of tetrahydroaminoacridine and lithium on cholinergic function after excitotoxic basal forebrain lesions in rat. *Pharmacopsychiatry*, 32, 242–247.

Arnsten, A.F., Mathew, R., Ubriani, R., Taylor, J.R., and Li, B.M. (1999). Alpha-1 noradrenergic receptor stimulation impairs prefrontal cortical cognitive function. *Biol Psychiatry*, 45, 26–31.

Arora, R.C., and Meltzer, H.Y. (1989a). 3H-imipramine binding in the frontal cortex of suicides. *Psychiatry Res*, 30, 125–135.

Arora, R.C., and Meltzer, H.Y. (1989b). Increased serotonin2 (5-HT$_2$) receptor binding as measured by 3H-lysergic acid diethylamide (3H-LSD) in the blood platelets of depressed patients. *Life Sci*, 44, 725–734.

Arora, R.C., and Meltzer, H.Y. (1991). Laterality and 3H-imipramine binding: Studies in the frontal cortex of normal controls and suicide victims. *Biol Psychiatry*, 29, 1016–1022.

Arora, R.C., and Meltzer, H.Y. (1993). Serotonin2 receptor binding in blood platelets of schizophrenic patients. *Psychiatry Res*, 47, 111–119.

Arranz, B., Blennow, K., Eriksson, A., Mansson, J.E., and Marcusson, J. (1997). Serotonergic, noradrenergic, and dopaminergic measures in suicide brains. *Biol Psychiatry*, 41, 1000–1009.

Artigas, F., Sarrias, M.J., Martinez, E., Gelpi, E., Alvarez, E., and Udina, C. (1989). Increased plasma free serotonin but unchanged platelet serotonin in bipolar patients treated chronically with lithium. *Psychopharmacology (Berl)*, 99, 328–332.

Arystarkhova, E., and Sweadner, K.J. (1996). Isoform-specific monoclonal antibodies to Na,K-ATPase alpha subunits. Evidence for a tissue-specific post-translational modification of the alpha subunit. *J Biol Chem*, 271, 23407–23417.

Asberg, M., Bertilsson, L., Tuck, D., Cronholm, B., and Sjoqvist, F. (1973). Indoleamine metabolites in the cerebrospinal fluid of depressed patients before and during treatment with nortriptyline. *Clin Pharmacol Ther*, 14, 277–286.

Asberg, M., Bertilsson, L., and Martensson, B. (1984). CSF monoamine metabolites, depression, and suicide. *Adv Biochem Psychopharmacol*, 39, 87–97.

Asghar, S.J., Tanay, V.A., Baker, G.B., Greenshaw, A., and Silverstone, P.H. (2003). Relationship of plasma amphetamine levels to physiological, subjective, cognitive and biochemical measures in healthy volunteers. *Hum Psychopharmacol*, 18(4), 291–299.

Ashcroft, G.W., Blackburn, I.M., Eccleston, D., Glen, A.I., Hartley, W., Kinloch, N.E., Lonergan, M., Murray, L.G., and Pullar, I.A. (1973). Changes on recovery in the concentrations of tryptophan and the biogenic amine metabolites in the cerebrospinal fluid of patients with affective illness. *Psychol Med*, 3, 319–325.

Asnis, G.M., Sachar, E.J., Halbreich, U., Nathan, R.S., Ostrow, L., and Halpern, F.S. (1981). Cortisol secretion and dexamethasone response in depression. *Am J Psychiatry*, 138, 1218–1221.

Aston, C., Jiang, L., and Sokolov, B.P. (2004). Microarray analysis of postmortem temporal cortex from patients with schizophrenia. *J Neurosci Res*, 77(6), 858–866.

Aston, C., Jiang, L., and Sokolov, B.P. (2005). Transcriptional profiling reveals evidence for signaling and oligodendroglial abnormalities in the temporal cortex from patients with major depressive disorder. *Mol Psychiatry*, 10(3), 309–322.

Atack, J.R. (1996). Inositol monophosphatase, the putative therapeutic target for lithium. *Brain Res Brain Res Rev*, 22(2), 183–190.

Atkinson, J.H., Jr., Kremer, E.F., Risch, S.C., and Janowsky, D.S. (1986). Basal and post-dexamethasone cortisol and prolactin concentrations in depressed and non-depressed patients with chronic pain syndromes. *Pain*, 25, 23–34.

Attar-Levy, D., Martinot, J.L., Blin, J., Dao-Castellana, M.H., Crouzel, C., Mazoyer, B., Poirier, M.F., Bourdel, M.C., Aymard, N., Syrota, A., and Feline, A. (1999). The cortical serotonin2 receptors studied with positron-emission tomography and [18F]-setoperone during depressive illness and antidepressant treatment with clomipramine. *Biol Psychiatry*, 45, 180–186.

Auer, D.P., Putz, B., Kraft, E., Lipinski, B., Schill, J., and Holsboer, F. (2000). Reduced glutamate in the anterior cingulate cortex in depression: An in vivo proton magnetic resonance spectroscopy study. *Biol Psychiatry*, 47, 305–313.

Aujla, H., and Beninger, R.J. (2003). Intra-accumbens protein kinase C inhibitor NPC 15437 blocks amphetamine-produced conditioned place preference in rats. *Behav Brain Res*, 147(1-2), 41–48.

Austin, J., Hoogendoorn, B., Buckland, P., Jones, I., McCandless, F., Williams, N., Middle, F., Owen, M.J., Craddock, N., and O'Donovan, M.C. (2000). Association analysis of the proneurotensin gene and bipolar disorder. *Psychiatr Genet*, 10(1), 51–54.

Avissar, S., Barki-Harrington, L., Nechamkin, Y., Roitman, G., and Schreiber, G. (1996). Reduced beta-adrenergic receptor-coupled Gs protein function and Gs alpha immunoreactivity in mononuclear leukocytes of patients with depression. *Biol Psychiatry*, 39, 755–760.

Avissar, S., Nechamkin, Y., Barki-Harrington, L., Roitman, G., and Schreiber, G. (1997). Differential G protein measures in mononuclear leukocytes of patients with bipolar mood disorder are state dependent. *J Affect Disord*, 43, 85–93.

Axelrod, J., and Reisine, T.D. (1984). Stress hormones: Their interaction and regulation. *Science*, 224, 452–459.

Azorin, J.M., Tramoni, V. (1987). Kindling models and antikindling effects of mood normalizers. *Pharmacopsychiatry*, 20, 189–191.

Bach, R.O., and Gallicchio, V.S. (1990). *Lithium and Cell Physiology* (June Edition). New York: Springer Verlag.

Bachmann, C.G., Linthorst, A.C., Holsboer, F., and Reul, J.M. (2003). Effect of chronic administration of selective glucocorticoid receptor antagonists on the rat hypothalamic–pituitary–adrenocortical axis. *Neuropsychopharmacology*, 28(6), 1056–1067.

Bachmann, R.F., Schloesser, R.J., Gould, T.D., and Manji, H.K. (2005). Mood stabilizers target cellular plasticity and resilience cascades: Implications for the development of novel therapeutics. *Mol Neurobiol*, 32(2), 173–202.

Bachus, S.E., Hyde, T.M., Akil, M., Weickert, C.S., Vawter, M.P., and Kleinman, J.E. (1997). Neuropathology of suicide. A review and an approach. *Ann NY Acad Sci*, 836, 201–219.

Backstrom, P., and Hyytia, P. (2003). Attenuation of cocaine-seeking behaviour by the AMPA/kainate receptor antagonist CNQX in rats. *Psychopharmacology (Berl)*, 166(1), 69–76.

Baghai, T.C., Schule, C., Zwanzger, P., Minov, C., Zill, P., Ella, R., Eser, D., Oezer, S., Bondy, B., and Rupprecht, R. (2002). Hypothalamic–pituitary–adrenocortical axis dysregulation in patients with major depression is influenced by the insertion/deletion polymorphism in the angiotensin I-converting enzyme gene. *Neurosci Lett*, 328, 299–303.

Bahr, B.A., Bendiske, J., Brown, Q.B., Munirathinam, S., Caba, E., Rudin M., Urwyler, S., Sauter, A., and Rogers, G. (2002). Survival signaling and selective neuroprotection through glutamatergic transmission. *Exp Neurol*, 174, 37–47.

Bakchine, S., Lacomblez, L., Benoit, N., Parisot, D., Chain, F., and Lhermitte, F. (1989). Manic-like state after bilateral orbitofrontal and right temporoparietal injury: Efficacy of clonidine. *Neurology*, 39, 777–781.

Baker, E.F. (1971). Sodium transfer to cerebrospinal fluid in functional psychiatric illness. *Can Psychiatr Assoc J*, 16, 167–170.

Baker, K.A., Hong, M., Sadi, D., and Mendez, I. (2000). Intrastriatal and intranigral grafting of hNT neurons in the 6-OHDA rat model of Parkinson's disease. *Exp Neurol*, 162, 350–360.

Ballenger, J.C., Post, R.M., Gold, P.W., Goodwin, F.K., Bunney, W.E., and Robertson, G. (1980). *Endocrine correlates of personality and cognition in normals* (pp. 144–145). 133rd Annual Meeting of the American Psychiatric Association.

Baltuch, G.H., Couldwell, W.T., Villemure, J.G., and Yong, V.W. (1993). Protein kinase C inhibitors suppress cell growth in established and low-passage glioma cell lines. A comparison between staurosporine and tamoxifen. *Neurosurgery*, 33:495–501; discussion 501.

Banay-Schwartz, M., DeGuzman, T., Faludi, G., Lajtha, A., and Palkovits, M. (1998). Alteration of protease levels in different brain areas of suicide victims. *Neurochem Res*, 23, 953–959.

Banerjee, S.P., Kung, L.S., Riggi, S.J., and Chanda, S.K. (1977). Development of beta-adrenergic receptor subsensitivity by antidepressants. *Nature*, 268, 455–456.

Banki, C.M., Bissette, G., Arato, M., O'Connor, L., and Nemeroff, C.B. (1987). CSF corticotropin-releasing factor-like immunoreactivity in depression and schizophrenia. *Am J Psychiatry*, 144, 873–877.

Banki, C.M., Bissette, G., Arato, M., and Nemeroff, C.B. (1988). Elevation of immunoreactive CSF TRH in depressed patients. *Am J Psychiatry*, 145, 1526–1531.

Banki, C.M., Karmacsi, L., Bissette, G., and Nemeroff, C.B. (1992). CSF corticotropin-releasing hormone and somatostatin in major depression: Response to antidepressant treatment and relapse. *Eur Neuropsychopharmacol*, 2, 107–113.

Baptista, T., Weiss, S.R., Post, R.M. (1993). Carbamazepine attenuates cocaine-induced increases in dopamine in the nucleus accumbens: An in vivo dialysis study. *Eur J Pharmacol*, 236, 39–42.

Barbini, B., Colombo, C., Benedetti, F., Campori, E., Bellodi, L., and Smeraldi, E. (1998). The unipolar–bipolar dichotomy and the response to sleep deprivation. *Psychiatry Res*, 79, 43–50.

Barnes, R.F., Veith, R.C., Borson, S., Verhey, J., Raskind, M.A., and Halter, J.B. (1983). High levels of plasma catecholamines in dexamethasone-resistant depressed patients. *Am J Psychiatry*, 140, 1623–1625.

Bartalena, L., Pellegrini, L., Meschi, M., Antonangeli, L., Bogazzi, F., Dell'Osso, L., Pinchera, A., and Placidi, G.F. (1990). Evaluation of thyroid function in patients with rapid-cycling and non-rapid-cycling bipolar disorder. *Psychiatry Res*, 34, 13–17.

Basturk, M., Karaaslan, F., Esel, E., Sofuoglu, S., Tutus, A., and Yabanoglu, I. (2001). Effects of short- and long-term lithium treatment on serum prolactin levels in patients with bipolar affective disorder. *Prog Neuropsychopharmacol Biol Psychiatry*, 25, 315–322.

Bauer, M.S., and Whybrow, P.C. (1988). *Rapid cycling bipolar affective disorder: Thyroid function and response to adjuvant treatment with high-dose thyroxine.* 43rd Annual meeting of the Society of Biological Psychiatry.

Bauer, M.S., and Whybrow, P.C. (1990). Rapid cycling bipolar affective disorder. II. Treatment of refractory rapid cycling with high-dose levothyroxine: A preliminary study. *Arch Gen Psychiatry*, 47, 435–440.

Bauer, M.S., Whybrow, P.C., and Winokur, A. (1990). Rapid cycling bipolar affective disorder. I. Association with grade I hypothyroidism. *Arch Gen Psychiatry*, 47(5), 427–432.

Bauer, M.S., Hellweg, R., Graf, K.J., and Baumgartner, A. (1998a). Treatment of refractory depression with high-dose thyroxine. *Neuropsychopharmacology*, 18, 444–455.

Bauer, M.S., Hellweg, R., and Baumgartner, A. (1998b). High dosage thyroxine treatment in therapy and prevention refractory patients with affective psychoses. *Nervenarzt*, 69(11), 1019–1022.

Bauman, A.L., Apparsundaram, S., Ramamoorthy, S., Wadzinski, B.E., Vaughan, R.A., and Blakely, R.D. (2000). Cocaine and antidepressant-sensitive biogenic amine transporters exist in regulated complexes with protein phosphatase 2A. *J Neurosci*, 20, 7571–7578.

Baumann, B., Danos, P., Krell, D., Diekmann, S., Wurthmann, C., Bielau, H., Bernstein, H.G., and Bogerts, B. (1999a). Unipolar–bipolar dichotomy of mood disorders is supported by noradrenergic brainstem system morphology. *J Affect Disord*, 54, 217–224.

Baumann, B., Danos, P., Krell, D., Diekmann, S., Leschinger, A., Stauch, R., Wurthmann, C., Bernstein, H.G., and Bogerts, B. (1999b). Reduced volume of limbic system–affiliated basal ganglia in mood disorders: Preliminary data from a postmortem study. *J Neuropsychiatry Clin Neurosci*, 11, 71–78.

Baumgartner, A., Graf, K. J., Kurten, I., Meinhold, H., and Scholz, P. (1990a). Neuroendocrinological investigations during sleep deprivation in depression. I. Early morning levels of thyrotropin, TH, cortisol, prolactin, LH, FSH, estradiol, and testosterone. *Biol Psychiatry*, 28(7), 556–568.

Baumgartner, A., Riemann, D., and Berger, M. (1990b). Neuroendocrinological investigations during sleep deprivation in depression. II. Longitudinal measurement of thyrotropin, TH, cortisol, prolactin, GH, and LH during sleep and sleep deprivation. *Biol Psychiatry*, 28(7), 569–587.

Baumgartner, A., Bauer, M., and Hellweg, R. (1994). Treatment of intractable non-rapid cycling bipolar affective disorder with high-dose thyroxine: An open clinical trial. *Neuropsychopharmacology*, 10, 183–189.

Bebchuk, J.M., Arfken, C.L., Dolan-Manji, S., Murphy, J., Hasanat, K., and Manji, H.K. (2000). A preliminary investigation of a protein kinase C inhibitor in the treatment of acute mania. *Arch Gen Psychiatry*, 57, 95–97.

Bech, P., Kirkegaard, C., Bock, E., Johannesen, M., and Rafaelsen, O.J. (1978). Hormones, electrolytes, and cerebrospinal fluid proteins in manic-melancholic patients. *Neuropsychobiology*, 4, 99–112.

Beckmann, H., and Jakob, H. (1991). Prenatal disturbances of nerve cell migration in the entorhinal region: A common vulnerability factor in functional psychoses? *J Neural Transm*, 84, 155–164.

Beckmann, H., St.-Laurent, J., and Goodwin, F.K. (1975). The effect of lithium on urinary MHPG in unipolar and bipolar depressed patients. *Psychopharmacologia*, 42, 277–282.

Belanoff, J.K., Kalehzan, M., Sund, B., Fleming Ficek, S.K., and Schatzberg, A.F. (2001). Cortisol activity and cognitive changes in psychotic major depression. *Am J Psychiatry*, 158(10), 1612–1616.

Belanoff, J.K., Rothschild, A.J., Cassidy, F., DeBattista, C., Baulieu, E.E., Schold, C., and Schatzberg, A.F. (2002). An open label trial of c-1073 (mifepristone) for psychotic major depression. *Biol Psychiatry*, 52(5), 386–392.

Bellivier, F., Henry, C., Szoke, A., Schurhoff, F., Nosten-Bertrand, M., Feingold, J., Launay, J.M., Leboyer, M., and Laplanche, J.L. (1998a). Serotonin transporter gene polymorphisms in patients with unipolar or bipolar depression. *Neurosci Lett*, 255, 143–146.

Bellivier, F., Leboyer, M., Courtet, P., Buresi, C., Beaufils, B., Samolyk, D., Allilaire, J.F., Feingold, J., Mallet, J., and Malafosse, A. (1998b). Association between the tryptophan hydroxylase gene and manic-depressive illness. *Arch Gen Psychiatry*, 55, 33–37.

Benazzi, F. (1998). Mania associated with donepezil. *Int J Geriatr Psychiatry*, 13, 814–815.

Benazzi, F. (1999). Mania associated with donepezil. *J Psychiatry Neurosci*, 24, 468–469.

Benedetti, F., Colombo, C., Barbini, B., Campori, E., and Smeraldi, E. (1999). Ongoing lithium treatment prevents relapse after total sleep deprivation. *J Clin Psychopharmacol*, 19, 240–245.

Benes, F.M., Kwok, E.W., Vincent, S.L., and Todtenkopf, M.S. (1998). A reduction of nonpyramidal cells in sector CA2 of schizophrenics and manic depressives. *Biol Psychiatry*, 44, 88–97.

Benes, F.M., Todtenkopf, M.S., Logiotatos, P., and Williams, M. (2000). Glutamate decarboxylase(65)-immunoreactive terminals in cingulate and prefrontal cortices of schizophrenic and bipolar brain. *J Chem Neuroanat*, 20, 259–269.

Benes, F.M., Vincent, S.L., and Todtenkopf, M. (2001). The density of pyramidal and nonpyramidal neurons in anterior cingulate cortex of schizophrenic and bipolar subjects. *Biol Psychiatry*, 50(6), 395–406.

Benes, F.M., Matzilevich, D., Burke, R.E., and Walsh, J. (2006). The expression of proapoptosis genes is increased in bipolar disorder, but not in schizophrenia. *Mol Psychiatry*, 11(3), 241–251.

Benkelfat, C., Seletti, B., Palmour, R.M., Hillel, J., Ellenbogen, M., and Young, S.N. (1995). Tryptophan depletion in stable lithium-treated patients with bipolar disorder in remission. *Arch Gen Psychiatry*, 52, 154–156.

Berger, M., Riemann, D., Hochli, D., and Spiegel, R. (1989). The cholinergic rapid eye movement sleep induction test with RS-86. State or trait marker of depression? *Arch Gen Psychiatry*, 46, 421–428.

Berger, M., Riemann, D., and Krieg, C. (1991). Cholinergic drugs as diagnostic and therapeutic tools in affective disorders. *Acta Psychiatr Scand Suppl*, 366, 52–60.

Berggren, U. (1985). Effects of chronic lithium treatment on brain monoamine metabolism and amphetamine-induced locomotor stimulation in rats. *J Neural Transm*, 64, 239–250.

Bergquist, J., Bergquist, S., Axelsson, R., and Ekman, R. (1993). Demonstration of immunoglobulin G with affinity for dopamine in cerebrospinal fluid from psychotic patients. *Clin Chim Acta*, 217, 129–142.

Bergstrom, D.A., and Kellar, K.J. (1979). Effect of electroconvulsive shock on monoaminergic receptor binding sites in rat brain. *Nature*, 278, 464–466.

Berk, M. (1999). Lamotrigine and the treatment of mania in bipolar disorder. *Eur Neuropsychopharmacol*, 9(Suppl. 4), S119–S123.

Berk, M., Bodemer, W., van Oudenhove, T., and Butkow, N. (1994). Dopamine increases platelet intracellular calcium in bipolar affective disorder and controls. *Int Clin Psychopharmacol*, 9(4), 291–293.

Berk, M., Kirchmann, N.H., and Butkow, N. (1996). Lithium blocks 45Ca^{2+} uptake into platelets in bipolar affective disorder and controls. *Clin Neuropharmacol*, 19(1), 48–51.

Berk, M., Plein, H., and Ferreira, D. (2001). Platelet glutamate receptor supersensitivity in major depressive disorder. *Clin Neuropharmacol*, 24, 129–132.

Berman, R.M., Cappiello, A., Anand, A., Oren, D.A., Heninger, G.R., Charney, D.S., and Krystal, J.H. (2000). Antidepressant effects of ketamine in depressed patients. *Biol Psychiatry*, 47, 351–354.

Bernasconi, R. (1982). The GABA hypothesis of affective illness: Influence of clinically effective antimanic drugs on GABA turnover. In H.M. Emrich, J.B. Aldenhoff, H.D., and Lux (Eds.), *Basic Mechanisms in the Action of Lithium* (pp. 183–192). Amsterdam: Excerpta Medica.

Bernstein, H.G., Stanarius, A., Baumann, B., Henning, H., Krell, D., Danos, P., Falkai, P., and Bogerts, B. (1998). Nitric oxide synthase–containing neurons in the human hypothalamus: Reduced number of immunoreactive cells in the paraventricular nucleus of depressive patients and schizophrenics. *Neuroscience*, 83, 867–875.

Berrettini, W.H., and Post, R.M. (1984). GABA in affective illness. In *Neurobiology of Mood Disorders* (pp. 673–685). Baltimore: Williams & Wilkins.

Berrettini, W.H., Umberkoman-Wiita, B., Nurnberger, J.I., Jr., Vogel, W.H., Gershon, E.S., and Post, R.M. (1982). Platelet GABA-transaminase in affective illness. *Psychiatry Res*, 7, 255–260.

Berrettini, W.H., Nurnberger, J.I. Jr., Hare, T.A., Simmons-Alling, S., Gershon, E.S., and Post, R.M. (1983). Reduced plasma and CSF gamma-aminobutyric acid in affective illness: Effect of lithium carbonate. *Biol Psychiatry*, 18, 185–194.

Berrettini, W.H., Nurnberger, J.I. Jr., Gold, P.W., Chretien, M., Chrousos, G.P., Chan, J.S., Goldin, L.R., and Gershon, E.S. (1985a). Neuropeptides in human cerebrospinal fluid. *Life Sci*, 37, 1265–1270.

Berrettini, W.H., Nurnberger, J.I. Jr., Scheinin, M., Seppala, T., Linnoila, M., Narrow, W., Simmons-Alling, S., and Gershon, E.S. (1985b). Cerebrospinal fluid and plasma monoamines and their metabolites in euthymic bipolar patients. *Biol Psychiatry*, 20, 257–269.

Berrettini, W.H., Runinow, D.R., Nurnberger, J.I., Simmons-Alling, S., Post, R.M., and Gershon, E.S. (1985c). CSF substance P immunoreactivity in affective disorders. *Biol Psychiatry*, 20(9), 965–970.

Berrettini, W.H., Nurnberger, J.I. Jr., Hare, T.A., Simmons-Alling, S., and Gershon, E.S. (1986). CSF GABA in euthymic manic-depressive patients and controls. *Biol Psychiatry*, 21, 844–846.

Berrettini, W.H., Nurnberger, J.I. Jr., Zerbe, R.L., Gold, P.W., Chrousos, G.P., and Tomai, T. (1987). CSF neuropeptides in euthymic bipolar patients and controls. *Br J Psychiatry*, 150, 208–212.

Berridge, M.J., and Irvine, R.F. (1989). Inositol phosphates and cell signalling. *Nature*, 341, 197–205.

Berridge, M.J., Downes, C.P., and Hanley, M.R. (1982). Lithium amplifies agonist-dependent phosphatidylinositol responses in brain and salivary glands. *Biochem J*, 206, 587–595.

Berridge, M.J., Downes, C.P., and Hanley, M.R. (1989). Neural and developmental actions of lithium: A unifying hypothesis. *Cell*, 59, 411–419.

Berton, O., and Nestler, E.J. (2006). New approaches to antidepressant drug discovery: Beyond monoamines. *Nat Rev Neurosci*, 7(2), 137–151.

Beskow, J., Gottfries, C.G., Roos, B.E., and Winblad, B. (1976). Determination of monoamine and monoamine metabolites in the human brain: Post mortem studies in a group of suicides and in a control group. *Acta Psychiatr Scand*, 53, 7–20.

Beyer, J.L., and Krishnan, K.R. (2002). Volumetric brain imaging findings in mood disorders. *Bipolar Disord*, 4, 89–104.

Bezchlibnyk, Y., and Young, L.T. (2002). The neurobiology of bipolar disorder: Focus on signal transduction pathways and the regulation of gene expression. *Can J Psychiatry*, 47, 135–148.

Bhalla, U.S., and Iyengar, R. (1999). Emergent properties of networks of biological signaling pathways. *Science*, 283, 381–387.

Biegon, A., and Fieldust, S. (1992). Reduced tyrosine hydroxylase immunoreactivity in locus coeruleus of suicide victims. *Synapse*, 10, 79–82.

Biegon, A., and Israeli, M. (1988). Regionally selective increases in beta-adrenergic receptor density in the brains of suicide victims. *Brain Res*, 442, 199–203.

Biegon, A., Weizman, A., Karp, L., Ram, A., Tiano, S., and Wolff, M. (1987). Serotonin 5-HT$_2$ receptor binding on blood platelets—a peripheral marker for depression? *Life Sci*, 41, 2485–2492.

Biegon, A., Essar, N., Israeli, M., Elizur, A., Bruch, S., and Bar-Nathan, A.A. (1990a). Serotonin 5-HT$_2$ receptor binding on blood platelets as a state dependent marker in major affective disorder. *Psychopharmacology (Berl)*, 102, 73–75.

Biegon, A., Grinspoon, A., Blumenfeld, B., Bleich, A., Apter, A., and Mester, R. (1990b). Increased serotonin 5-HT$_2$ receptor binding on blood platelets of suicidal men. *Psychopharmacology (Berl)*, 100, 165–167.

Biggs, C.S., Pearce, B.R., Fowler, L.J., and Whitton, P.S. (1992). Regional effects of sodium valproate on extracellular concentrations of 5-hydroxytryptamine, dopamine, and their metabolites in the rat brain: An in vivo microdialysis study. *J Neurochem*, 59, 1702–1708.

Bijur, G.N., De Sarno, P., and Jope, R.S. (2000). Glycogen synthase kinase-3β facilitates staurosporine- and heat shock-induced apoptosis. Protection by lithium. *J Biol Chem*, 275, 7583–7590.

Binder, E.B., Kinkead, B., Owens, M.J., and Nemeroff, C.B. (2001). The role of neurotensin in the pathophysiology of schizophrenia and the mechanism of action of antipsychotic drugs. *Biol Psychiatry*, 50, 856–872.

Birkett, J.T., Arranz, M.J., Munro, J., Osbourn, S., Kerwin, R.W., and Collier, D.A. (2000). Association analysis of the 5-HT5A gene in depression, psychosis and antipsychotic response. *Neuroreport*, 11, 2017–2020.

Birnbaum, S., Yuan, P.X., Wang, M., Vijayraghaven, S., Bloom, A.K., Davis, D.J., Gobeske, K.T., Sweatt, J.D., Manji, H.K., and Arnsten, A. (2004). Protein kinase C overactivity impairs prefrontal cortical regulation of working memory. *Science*, 306, 882–884.

Biver, F., Lotstra, F., Monclus, M., Dethy, S., Damhaut, P., Wikler, D., Luxen, A., and Goldman, S. (1997). In vivo binding of [18F]altanserin to rat brain 5HT2 receptors: A film and electronic autoradiographic study. *Nucl Med Biol*, 24, 357–360.

Blakely, R.D., Ramamoorthy, S., Schroeter, S., Qian, Y., Apparsundaram, S., Galli, A., and DeFelice, L.J. (1998). Regulated phosphorylation and trafficking of antidepressant-sensitive serotonin transporter proteins. *Biol Psychiatry*, 44, 169–178.

Blancquaert, J.P., Lefebvre, R.A., and Willems, J.L. (1987). Anti-aversive properties of opioids in the conditioned taste aversion test in the rat. *Pharmacol Biochem Behav*, 27, 437–441.

Blehar, M.C., DePaulo, J.R. Jr., Gershon, E.S., Reich, T., Simpson, S.G., and Nurnberger, J.I. Jr. (1998). Women with bipolar disorder: Findings from the NIMH genetics initiative sample. *Psychopharmacol Bull*, 34, 239–243.

Blier, P., and De Montigny, C. (1985). Short-term lithium administration enhances serotonergic neurotransmission: Electrophysiological evidence in the rat CNS. *Eur J Pharmacol*, 113, 69–77.

Blier, P., de Montigny, C., and Tardif, D. (1987). Short-term lithium treatment enhances responsiveness of postsynaptic 5-HT$_{1A}$ receptors without altering 5-HT autoreceptor sensitivity: An electrophysiological study in the rat brain. *Synapse*, 1, 225–232.

Bligh-Glover, W., Kolli, T.N., Shapiro-Kulnane, L., Dilley, G.E., Friedman, L., Balraj, E., Rajkowska, G., and Stockmeier, C.A. (2000). The serotonin transporter in the midbrain of suicide victims with major depression. *Biol Psychiatry*, 47, 1015–1024.

Bloch, M., Schmidt, P.J., Danaceau, M.A., Adams, L.F., and Rubinow, D.R. (1999). Dehydroepiandrosterone treatment of midlife dysthymia. *Biol Psychiatry*, 45(12), 1533–1541.

Bloom, F.E., Baetge, G., Deyo, S., Ettenberg, A., Koda, L., Magistretti, P.J., Shoemaker, W.J., and Staunton, D.A. (1983). Chemical and physiological aspects of the actions of lithium and antidepressant drugs. *Neuropharmacology*, 22(Spec No. 3), 359–365.

Board, F., Wadeson, R., and Persky, H. (1957). Depressive affect and endocrine functions; blood levels of adrenal cortex and thyroid hormones in patients suffering from depressive reactions. *AMA Arch Neurol Psychiatry*, 78, 612–620.

Bodick, N.C., Offen, W.W., Levey, A.I., Cutler, N.R., Gauthier, S.G., Satlin, A., Shannon, H.E., Tollefson, G.D., Rasmussen, K., Bymaster, F.P., Hurley, D.J., Potter, W.Z., and Paul, S.M. (1997). Effects of xanomeline, a selective muscarinic receptor agonist, on cognitive function and behavioral symptoms in Alzheimer disease. *Arch Neurol*, 54, 465–473.

Boerlin, H.L., Gitlin, M.J., Zoellner, L.A., and Hammen, C.L. (1998). Bipolar depression and antidepressant-induced mania: A naturalistic study. *J Clin Psychiatry*, 59, 374–379.

Bohus, B., Kovacs, G.L., and de Wied, D. (1978). Oxytocin, vasopressin and memory: Opposite effects on consolidation and retrieval processes. *Brain Res*, 157, 414–417.

Bond, P.A., Jenner, F.A., and Sampson, G.A. (1972). Daily variations of the urine content of 3-methoxy-4-hydroxyphenylglycol in two manic-depressive patients. *Psychol Med*, 2, 81–85.

Bonnier, B., Gorwood, P., Hamon, M., Sarfati, Y., Boni, C., and Hardy-Bayle, M.C. (2002). Association of 5-HT(2A) receptor gene polymorphism with major affective disorders: The case of a subgroup of bipolar disorder with low suicide risk. *Biol Psychiatry*, 51, 762–765.

Borglum, A.D., Bruun, T.G., Kjeldsen, T.E., Ewald, H., Mors, O., Kirov, G., Russ, C., Freeman, B., Collier, D.A., and Kruse, T.A. (1999). Two novel variants in the DOPA decarboxylase gene: Association with bipolar affective disorder. *Mol Psychiatry*, 4, 545–551.

Born, G.V., Grignani, G., and Martin, K. (1980). Long-term effect of lithium on the uptake of 5-hydroxytryptamine by human platelets. *Br J Clin Pharmacol*, 9, 321–325.

Borsini, F., and Meli, A. (1988). Is the forced swimming test a suitable model for revealing antidepressant activity? *Psychopharmacology (Berl)*, 94, 147–160.

Bothwell, R.A., Eccleston, D., and Marshall, E. (1994). Platelet intracellular calcium in patients with recurrent affective disorders. *Psychopharmacology (Berl)*, 114(2), 375–381.

Bottlender, R., Rudolf, D., Strauss, A., and Moller, H.J. (2000). Are low basal serum levels of the thyroid stimulating hormone (b-TSH) a risk factor for switches into states of expansive syndromes (known in Germany as "maniform syndromes") in bipolar I depression? *Pharmacopsychiatry*, 33, 75–77.

Bouras, C., Kovari, E., Hof, P.R., Riederer, B.M., and Giannakopoulos, P. (2001). Anterior cingulate cortex pathology schizophrenia and bipolar disorder. *Acta Neuopathol*, 102, 373–379.

Bourne, H.R., and Nicoll, R. (1993). Molecular machines integrate coincident synaptic signals. *Cell*, 72(Suppl.), 65–75.

Bourne, H.R., Bunney, W.E. Jr., Colburn, R.W., Davis, J.M., Davis, J.N., Shaw, D.M., and Coppen, A.J. (1968). Noradrenaline, 5-hydroxytryptamine, and 5-hydroxyindoleacetic acid in hindbrains of suicidal patients. *Lancet*, 2, 805–808.

Bousquet, P., and Feldman, J. (1987). The blood pressure effects of alpha-adrenoceptor antagonists injected in the medullary site of action of clonidine: The nucleus reticularis lateralis. *Life Sci*, 40, 1045–1052.

Bowden, C.L., Huang, L.G., Javors, M.A., Johnson, J.M., Seleshi, E., McIntyre, K., Contreras, S., and Maas, J.W. (1988). Calcium function in affective disorders and healthy controls. *Biol Psychiatry*, 23, 367–376.

Bowden, C.L., Brugger, A.M., Swann, A.C., Calabrese, J.R., Janicak, P.G., Petty, F., Dilsaver, S.C., Davis, J.M., Rush, A.J., and Small, J.G. (1994). Efficacy of divalproex vs. lithium and placebo in the treatment of mania. The Depakote Mania Study Group. *JAMA*, 271, 918–924.

Bowden, C., Cheetham, S.C., Lowther, S., Katona, C.L., Crompton, M.R., and Horton, R.W. (1997a). Dopamine uptake sites, labelled with [3H]GBR12935, in brain samples from depressed suicides and controls. *Eur Neuropsychopharmacol*, 7, 247–252.

Bowden, C., Theodorou, A.E., Cheetham, S.C., Lowther, S., Katona, C.L., Crompton, M.R., and Horton, R.W. (1997b). Dopamine D1 and D2 receptor binding sites in brain samples from depressed suicides and controls. *Brain Res*, 752, 227–233.

Bowden, C., Cheetham, S.C., Lowther, S., Katona, C.L., Crompton, M.R., and Horton, R.W. (1997c). Reduced dopamine turnover in the basal ganglia of depressed suicides. *Brain Res*, 769, 135–140.

Bowden, C.L., Davis, J., Morris, D., Swann, A., Calabrese, J., Lambert, M., and Goodnick, P. (1997d). Effect size of efficacy measures comparing divalproex, lithium and placebo in acute mania. *Depress Anxiety*, 6, 26–30.

Bowen, D.M., Najlerahim, A., Procter, A.W., Francis, P.T., and Murphy, E. (1989). Circumscribed changes of the cerebral cortex in neuropsychiatric disorders of later life. *Proc Natl Acad Sci USA*, 86, 9504–9508.

Bowers, M.B. Jr., and Heninger, G.R. (1977). Lithium: Clinical effects and cerebrospinal fluid acid monoamine metabolites. *Commun Psychopharmacol*, 1, 135–145.

Bowers, M.B. Jr., Mazure, C.M., Nelson, J.C., and Jatlow, P.I. (1992). Lithium in combination with perphenazine: Effect on plasma monoamine metabolites. *Biol Psychiatry*, 32, 1102–1107.

Boyer, P., Davila, M., Schaub, C., Kanowski, S., and Nasset, J. (1986). Growth hormone response to clonidine stimulation in depressive states. Part I. *Psychiatr Psychobiol*, 1, 189–195.

Brake, W.G., Alves, S.E., Dunlop, J.C., Lee, S.J., Bulloch, K., Allen, P.B., Greengard, P., and McEwen, B.S. (2001). Novel target sites for estrogen action in the dorsal hippocampus: An examination of synaptic proteins. *Endocrinology*, 142, 1284–1289.

Browman, K.E., Kantor, L., Richardson, S., Badiani, A., Robinson, T.E., and Gnegy, M.E. (1998). Injection of the protein kinase C inhibitor ro31-8220 into the nucleus accumbens attenuates the acute response to amphetamine: Tissue and behavioral studies. *Brain Res*, 814(1-2), 112–119.

Brown, D.W. (1993). Abnormal fluctuations of acetylcholine and serotonin. *Med Hypotheses*, 40, 309–310.

Brown, W.A., Johnston, R., and Mayfield, D. (1979). The 24-hour dexamethasone suppression test in a clinical setting: Relationship to diagnosis, symptoms, and response to treatment. *Am J Psychiatry*, 136, 543–547.

Brown, A.S., Mallinger, A.G., and Renbaum, L.C. (1993). Elevated platelet membrane phosphatidylinositol-4,5-bisphosphate in bipolar mania. *Am J Psychiatry*, 150, 1252–1254.

Brown, E.S., Rush, A.J., and McEwen, B.S. (1999). Hippocampal remodeling and damage by corticosteroids: Implications for mood disorders. *Neuropsychopharmacology*, 21(4), 474–484.

Brown, E.S., Suppes, T., Khan, D.A., and Carmody, T.J. III. (2002). Mood changes during prednisone bursts in outpatients with asthma. *J Clin Psychopharmacol*, 22(1), 55–61.

Bruckheimer, E.M., Cho, S.H., Sarkiss, M., Herrmann, J., and McDonnell, T.J. (1998). The Bcl-2 gene family and apoptosis. *Adv Biochem Eng Biotechnol*, 62, 75–105.

Bruno, V., Sortino, M.A., Scapagnini, U., Nicoletti, F., and Canonico, P.L. (1995). Antidegenerative effects of Mg(2+)-valproate in cultured cerebellar neurons. *Funct Neurol*, 10, 121–130.

Brunson, K.L., Eghbal-Ahmadi, M., Bender, R., Chen, Y., and Baram, T.Z. (2001). Long-term, progressive hippocampal cell loss and dysfunction induced by early-life administration of corticotropin-releasing hormone reproduce the effects of early-life stress. *Proc Natl Acad Sci USA*, 98, 8856–8861.

Brusov, O.S., Beliaev, B.S., Katasonov, A.B., Zlobina, G.P., Factor, M.I., and Lideman, R.R. (1989). Does platelet serotonin receptor supersensitivity accompany endogenous depression? *Biol Psychiatry*, 25, 375–381.

Bschor, T., Berghofer, A., Strohle, A., Kunz, D., Adli, M., Muller-Oerlinghausen, B., and Bauer, M. (2002). How long should the lithium augmentation strategy be maintained? A 1-year follow-up of a placebo-controlled study in unipolar refractory major depression. *J Clin Psychopharmacol*, 22(4), 427–430.

Bschor, T., Baethge, C., Adli, M., Eichmann, U., Ising, M., Uhr, M., Modell, S., Kunzel, H., Muller-Oerlinghausen, B., and Bauer, M. (2003). Association between response to lithium augmentation and the combined DEX/CRH test in major depressive disorder. *J Psychiatr Res*, 37(2), 135–143.

Buervenich, S., Carmine, A., Arvidsson, M., Xiang, F., Zhang, Z., Sydow, O., Jonsson, E.G., Sedvall, G.C., Leonard, S., Ross, R.G., Freedman, R., Chowdari, K.V., Nimgaonkar, V.L., Perlmann, T., Anvret, M., and Olson, L. (2000). *NURR1* mutations in cases of schizophrenia and manic-depressive disorder. *Am J Med Genet*, 96, 808–813.

Buervenich, S., Xiang, F., Sydow, O., Jonsson, E.G., Sedvall, G.C., Anvret, M., and Olson, L. (2001). Identification of four novel polymorphisms in the calcitonin/alpha-CGRP (CALCA) gene and an investigation of their possible associations with Parkinson disease, schizophrenia, and manic depression. *Hum Mutat*, 17(5), 435–436.

Bunney, W.E. Jr., and Davis, J.M. (1965). Norepinephrine in depressive reactions. A review. *Arch Gen Psychiatry*, 13, 483–494.

Bunney, W.E. Jr., and Garland, B. (1982). A second generation catecholamine hypothesis. *Pharmacopsychiatry*, 15(4), 111–115.

Bunney, W.E. Jr., and Garland, B.L. (1983). Possible receptor effects of chronic lithium administration. *Neuropharmacology*, 22, 367–372.

Bunney, W.E. Jr., and Garland-Bunney, B.L. (1987). Mechanisms of action of lithium in affective illness: Basic and clinical implications. In H.Y. Meltzer (Ed.), *Psychopharmacology: The Third Generation of Progress* (pp. 553–565). New York: Raven Press.

Bunney, W.E. Jr., Mason, J.W., and Hamburg, D.A. (1965). Correlations between behavioral variables and urinary 17-hydroxycorticosteroids in depressed patients. *Psychosom Med*, 27, 299–308.

Bunney, W.E. Jr., Brodie, H.K.H., Murphy, D.L., and Goodwin, F.K. (1970). *Psychopharmacological differentiation between two subgroups of depressed patients*. Abstract of a paper presented at the 125th Annual Meeting of the American Psychiatric Association, May.

Bunney, W.E. Jr., Murphy, D., Goodwin, F.K., and Borge, G.F. (1972a). The "switch process" in manic-depressive illness: I. A systematic study of sequential behavior change. *Arch Gen Psychiatry*, 27, 295–302.

Bunney, W.E. Jr., Goodwin, F.K., Murphy, D.L., House, K.M., and Gordon, E.K. (1972b). The "switch process" in manic-depressive illness: II. Relationship to catecholamines, REM sleep, and drugs. *Arch Gen Psychiatry*, 27, 304–309.

Bunney, W.E. Jr., Goodwin, F.K., and Murphy, D.L. (1972c). The "switch process" in manic-depressive illness: III. Theoretical implications. *Arch Gen Psychiatry*, 27, 312–317.

Burnet, P.W., and Harrison, P.J. (2000). Substance P (NK1) receptors in the cingulate cortex in unipolar and bipolar mood disorder and schizophrenia. *Biol Psychiatry*, 47, 80–83.

Burns, G., Herz, A., and Nikolarakis, K.E. (1990). Stimulation of hypothalamic opioid peptide release by lithium is mediated by opioid autoreceptors: Evidence from a combined in vitro, ex vivo study. *Neuroscience*, 36(3), 691–697.

Burt, T., Sachs, G.S., and Demopulos, C. (1999). Donepezil in treatment-resistant bipolar disorder. *Biol Psychiatry*, 45, 959–964.

Busa, W.B., and Gimlich, R.L. (1989). Lithium-induced teratogenesis in frog embryos prevented by a polyphosphoinositide cycle intermediate or a diacylglycerol analog. *Dev Biol*, 132, 315–324.

Bylund, D.B., Ray-Prenger, C., and Murphy, T.J. (1988). Alpha-2A and alpha-2B adrenergic receptor subtypes: Antagonist binding in tissues and cell lines containing only one subtype. *J Pharmacol Exp Ther*, 245, 600–607.

Caberlotto, L., and Hurd, Y.L. (1999). Reduced neuropeptide Y mRNA expression in the prefrontal cortex of subjects with bipolar disorder. *Neuroreport*, 10, 1747–1750.

Caberlotto, L., and Hurd, Y.L. (2001). Neuropeptide Y Y(1) and Y(2) receptor mRNA expression in the prefrontal cortex of psychiatric subjects. Relationship of Y(2) subtype to suicidal behavior. *Neuropsychopharmacology*, 25, 91–97.

Caggiula, A.R., Antelman, S.M., Palmer, A.M., Kiss, S., Edwards, D.J., and Docan, D. (1996). The effects of ethanol on striatal dopamine and frontal cortical D-[3H]aspartate efflux oscillate with repeated treatment. Relevance to individual differences in drug responsiveness. *Neuropsychopharmacology*, 15, 125–132.

Caggiula, A.R., Antelman, S.M., Kucinski, B.J., Fowler, H., Edwards, D.J., Austin, M.C., Gershon, S., and Stiller, R. (1998). Oscillatory-sensitization model of repeated drug exposure: Cocaine's effects on shock-induced hypoalgesia. *Prog Neuropsychopharmacol Biol Psychiatry*, 22(3), 511–521.

Calabrese, J.R., Bowden, C.L., Sachs, G.S., Ascher, J.A., Monaghan, E., and Rudd, G.D. (1999). A double-blind placebo-controlled study of lamotrigine monotherapy in outpatients with bipolar I depression. Lamictal 602 Study Group. *J Clin Psychiatry*, 60, 79–88.

Calabresi, P., Siniscalchi, A., Pisani, A., Stefani, A., Mercuri, N.B., and Bernardi, G. (1996). A field potential analysis on the effects of lamotrigine, GP 47779, and felbamate in neocortical slices. *Neurology*, 47, 557–562.

Caldji, C., Francis, D., Sharma, S., Plotsky, P.M., and Meaney, M.J. (2000). The effects of early rearing environment on the development of GABAA and central benzodiazepine receptor levels and novelty-induced fearfulness in the rat. *Neuropsychopharmacology*, 22, 219–229.

Callado, L.F., Meana, J.J., Grijalba, B., Pazos, A., Sastre, M., and Garcia-Sevilla, J.A. (1998). Selective increase of a2A-adrenoceptor agonist binding sites in brains of depressed suicide victims. *J Neurochem*, 70, 1114–1123.

Callahan, A.M., Frye, M.A., Marangell, L.B., George, M.S., Ketter, T.A., L'Herrou, T., and Post, R.M. (1997). Comparative antidepressant effects of intravenous and intrathecal thyrotropin-releasing hormone: Confounding effects of tolerance and implications for therapeutics. *Biol Psychiatry*, 41, 264–272.

Calogero, A.E., Gallucci, W.T., Chrousos, G.P., and Gold, P.W. (1988). Interaction between GABAergic neurotransmission and rat hypothalamic corticotropin-releasing hormone secretion in vitro. *Brain Res*, 463, 28–36.

Calogero, A.E., Gallucci, W.T., Kling, M.A., Chrousos, G.P., and Gold, P.W. (1989). Cocaine stimulates rat hypothalamic corticotropin-releasing hormone secretion in vitro. *Brain Res*, 505, 7–11.

Cameron, H.A., and McKay, R.D. (1999). Restoring production of hippocampal neurons in old age. *Nat Neurosci*, 2, 894–897.

Canessa, M., Adragna, N., Solomon, H.S., Connolly, T.M., and Tosteson, D.C. (1980). Increased sodium-lithium countertransport in red cells of patients with essential hypertension. *N Engl J Med*, 302, 772–776.

Canessa, M., Brugnara, C., and Escobales, N. (1987). The Li+-Na+ exchange and Na+-K+-Cl- cotransport systems in essential hypertension. *Hypertension*, 10, I4–10.

Cappeliez, P., and Moore, E. (1990). Effects of lithium on an amphetamine animal model of bipolar disorder. *Prog Neuropsychopharmacol Biol Psychiatry*, 14, 347–358.

Cappiello, A., Malison, R.T., McDougle, C.J., Vegso, S.J., Charney, D.S., Heninger, G.R., and Price, L.H. (1996). Seasonal variation in neuroendocrine and mood responses to i.v. L-tryptophan in depressed patients and healthy subjects. *Neuropsychopharmacology*, 15, 475–483.

Cappiello, A., Sernyak, M.J., Malison, R.T., McDougle, C.J., Heninger, G.R., and Price, L.H. (1997). Effects of acute tryptophan depletion in lithium-remitted manic patients: A pilot study. *Biol Psychiatry*, 42(11), 1076–1078.

Carletti, R., Corsi, M., Melotto, S., and Caberlotto, L. (2005). Down-regulation of amygdala preprotachykinin A mRNA but not 3H-SP receptor binding sites in subjects affected by mood disorders and schizophrenia. *Eur J Neurosci*, 21(6), 1712–1718.

Carli, M., Morissette, M., Hebert, C., Di Paolo, T., and Reader, T.A. (1997). Effects of a chronic lithium treatment on central dopamine neurotransporters. *Biochem Pharmacol*, 54, 391–397.

Carlson, P.J., Singh, J.B., Zarazte, C.A., Drevets, W.C., and Manji, H.K. (2006). Neural circuitry and neuroplasticity in mood disorders: Insights for novel therapeutic targets. *Neurotherapeutics*, 3, 22–41.

Carman, J.S., Wyatt, E.S., Smith, W., Post, R.M., and Ballenger, J.C. (1984). Calcium and calcitonin in bipolar affective disorder. In R.M. Post and J.C. Ballinger (Eds.), *Neurobiology of Mood Disorders* (pp. 340–355). Baltimore: Williams & Wilkins.

Carmeliet, E.E. (1964). Influence of lithium ions on the transmembrane potential and cation content of cardiac cells. *J Gen Physiol*, 47, 501–530.

Carroll, B.J. (1972). Sodium and potassium transfer to cerebrospinal fluid in severe depression. In B. Davies, B.J. Caroll, and R.M. Mowbray (Eds.), *Depressive Illness: Some Research Studies* (pp. 247–257). Springfield, IL: Charles C. Thomas.

Carroll, B.J. (1976). Limbic system–adrenal cortex regulation in depression and schizophrenia. *Psychosom Med*, 38, 106–121.

Carroll, B.J. (1980). Dexamethasone suppression test in depression. *Lancet*, 2, 1249.

Carroll, B.J. (1982). Clinical applications of the dexamethasone suppression test for endogenous depression. *Pharmacopsychiatria*, 15, 19–25.

Carroll, B.J., Martin, F.I., and Davies, B. (1968). Resistance to suppression by dexamethasone of plasma 11-O.H.C.S. levels in severe depressive illness. *BMJ*, 3, 285–287.

Carstens, M.E., Engelbrecht, A.H., Russell, V.A., van Zyl, A.M., and Taljaard, J.J. (1988). Biological markers in juvenile depression. *Psychiatry Res*, 23, 77–88.

Casebolt, T.L., and Jope, R.S. (1989). Long-term lithium treatment selectively reduces receptor-coupled inositol phospholipid hydrolysis in rat brain. *Biol Psychiatry*, 25, 329–340.

Cassidy, F., Murry, E., and Carroll, B.J. (1998a). Tryptophan depletion in recently manic patients treated with lithium. *Biol Psychiatry*, 43, 230–232.

Cassidy, F., Ritchie, J.C., and Carroll, B.J. (1998b). Plasma dexamethasone concentration and cortisol response during manic episodes. *Biol Psychiatry*, 43, 747–754.

Castillo, M., Kwock, L., Courvoisie, H., and Hooper, S.R. (2000). Proton MR spectroscopy in children with bipolar affective disorder: Preliminary observations. *AJNR Am J Neuroradiol*, 21, 832–838.

Catherino, W.H., Jeng, M.H., and Jordan, V.C. (1993). Norgestrel and gestodene stimulate breast cancer cell growth through an oestrogen receptor mediated mechanism. *Br J Cancer*, 67(5), 945–952.

Cazzullo, C.L., Smeraldi, E., Scchetti, E., and Bottinelli, S. (1975). Letter: Intracellular lithium concentration and clinical response. *Br J Psychiatry*, 126, 298–300.

Cervantes, P., Gelber, S., Kin, F.N., Nair, V.N., and Schwartz, G. (2001). Circadian secretion of cortisol in bipolar disorder. *J Psychiatry Neurosci*, 26(5), 411–416.

Chalecka-Franaszek, E., and Chuang, D.M. (1999). Lithium activates the serine/threonine kinase Akt-1 and suppresses glutamate-induced inhibition of Akt-1 activity in neurons. *Proc Natl Acad Sci USA*, 96, 8745–8750.

Chana, G., Landau, S., Beasley, C., Everall, I.P., and Cotter, D. (2003). Two-dimensional assessment of cytoarchitecture in the anterior cingulate cortex in major depressive disorder, bipolar disorder, and schizophrenia: Evidence for decreased neuronal somal size and increased neuronal density. *Biol Psychiatry*, 53, 1086–1098.

Chang, D.C., and Reppert, S.M. (2001). The circadian clocks of mice and men. *Neuron*, 29(3), 555–558.

Chang, M.C., Grange, E., Rabin, O., Bell, J.M., Allen, D.D., and Rapoport, S.I. (1996). Lithium decreases turnover of arachidonate in several brain phospholipids. *Neurosci Lett*, 220, 171–174.

Chang, M.C., Contreras, M.A., Rosenberger, T.A., Rintala, J.J., Bell, J.M., and Rapoport, S.I. (2001). Chronic valproate treatment decreases the in vivo turnover of arachidonic acid in brain phospholipids: A possible common effect of mood stabilizers. *J Neurochem*, 77, 796–803.

Charles, H.C., Lazeyras, F., Krishnan, K.R., Boyko, O.B., Payne, M., and Moore, D. (1994). Brain choline in depression: In vivo detection of potential pharmacodynamic effects of antidepressant therapy using hydrogen localized spectroscopy. *Prog Neuropsychopharmacol Biol Psychiatry*, 18, 1121–1127.

Charlton, B.G., Leake, A., Wright, C., Gairbairn, A.F., McKeith, U.G., Candy, J.M., and Ferrier, I.N. (1988). Somatostatin content and receptors in the cerebral cortex of depressed and control subjects. *J Neurol Neurosurg Psychiatry*, 51, 719–721.

Charney, D.S., and Heninger, G.R. (1986). Abnormal regulation of noradrenergic function in panic disorders. Effects of clonidine in healthy subjects and patients with agoraphobia and panic disorder. *Arch Gen Psychiatry*, 43, 1042–1054.

Charney, D.S., and Manji, H.K. (2004). Life stress, genes, and depression: Multiple pathways lead to increased risk and new opportunities for intervention. *Sci STKE*, 2004(225), re5.

Charney, D.S., Heninger, G.R., Sternberg, D.E., Hafstad, K.M., Giddings, S., and Landis, D.H. (1982). Adrenergic receptor sensitivity in depression. Effects of clonidine in depressed patients and healthy subjects. *Arch Gen Psychiatry*, 39, 290–294.

Charney, D.S., Heninger, G.R., and Redmond, D.E. Jr. (1983). Yohimbine induced anxiety and increased noradrenergic function in humans: Effects of diazepam and clonidine. *Life Sci*, 33(1), 19–29.

Chazot, G., Claustrat, B., Brun, J., and Olivier, M. (1985). Rapid antidepressant activity of destyr gamma endorphin: Correlation with urinary melatonin. *Biol Psychiatry*, 20, 1026–1030.

Checkley, S.A., Slade, A.P., and Shur, E. (1981). Growth hormone and other responses to clonidine in patients with endogenous depression. *Br J Psychiatry*, 138, 51–55.

Checkley, S.A., Glass, I.B., Thompson, C., Corn, T., and Robinson, P. (1984). The GH response to clonidine in endogenous as compared with reactive depression. *Psychol Med*, 14, 773–777.

Checkley, S.A., Thompson, C., Burton, S., Franey, C., and Arendt, J. (1985). Clinical studies of the effect of (+) and (−) oxaprotiline upon noradrenaline uptake. *Psychopharmacology (Berl)*, 87(1), 116–118.

Chee, I.S., Lee, S.W., Kim, J.L., Wang, S.K., Shin, Y.O., Shin, S.C., Lee, Y.H., Hwang, H.M., and Lim, M.R. (2001). 5-HT2A receptor gene promoter polymorphism −1438A/G and bipolar disorder. *Psychiatr Genet*, 11, 111–114.

Cheetham, S.C., Crompton, M.R., Katona, C.L., and Horton, R.W. (1988). Brain 5-HT2 receptor binding sites in depressed suicide victims. *Brain Res*, 443, 272–280.

Cheetham, S.C., Crompton, M.R., Czudek, C., Horton, R.W., Katona, C.L., and Reynolds, G.P. (1989). Serotonin concentrations and turnover in brains of depressed suicides. *Brain Res*, 502, 332–340.

Cheetham, S.C., Crompton, M.R., Katona, C.L., and Horton, R.W. (1990). Brain 5-HT1 binding sites in depressed suicides. *Psychopharmacology*, 102, 544–548.

Chen, A.C., Shirayama, Y., Shin, K.H., Neve, R.L., and Duman, R.S. (2001). Expression of the cAMP response element binding protein (CREB) in hippocampus produces an antidepressant effect. *Biol Psychiatry*, 49, 753–762.

Chen, B., Dowlatshahi, D., MacQueen, G.M., Wang, J.F., and Young, L.T. (2001). Increased hippocampal BDNF immunoreactivity in subjects treated with antidepressant medication. *Biol Psychiatry*, 50, 260–265.

Chen, D.F., Schneider, G.E., Martinou, J.C., and Tonegawa, S. (1997). Bcl-2 promotes regeneration of severed axons in mammalian CNS. *Nature*, 385, 434–439.

Chen, G., and Manji, H.K. (2006). The extracellular signal-regulated kinase pathway: An emerging promising target for mood stabilizers. *Curr Opin Psychiatry*, 19(3), 313–323.

Chen, G., Manji, H.K., Hawver, D.B., Wright, C.B., and Potter, W.Z. (1994). Chronic sodium valproate selectively decreases protein kinase C alpha and epsilon in vitro. *J Neurochem*, 63, 2361–2364.

Chen, G., Manji, H.K., Wright, C.B., Hawver, D.B., and Potter, W.Z. (1996a). Effects of valproic acid on beta-adrenergic receptors, G-proteins, and adenylyl cyclase in rat C6 glioma cells. *Neuropsychopharmacology*, 15, 271–280.

Chen, G., Pan, B., Hawver, D.B., Wright, C.B., Potter, W.Z., and Manji, H.K. (1996b). Attenuation of cyclic AMP production by carbamazepine. *J Neurochem*, 67, 2079–2086.

Chen, G., Yuan, P.X., Jiang, Y.M., Huang, L.D., and Manji, H.K. (1998). Lithium increases tyrosine hydroxylase levels both in vivo and in vitro. *J Neurochem*, 70, 1768–1771.

Chen, G., Hasanat, K.A., Bebchuk, J.M., Moore, G.J., Glitz, D., and Manji, H.K. (1999). Regulation of signal transduction pathways and gene expression by mood stabilizers and antidepressants. *Psychosom Med*, 61, 599–617.

Chen, G., Masana, M.I., and Manji, H.K. (2000). Lithium regulates PKC-mediated intracellular cross-talk and gene expression in the CNS in vivo. *Bipolar Disord*, 2, 217–236.

Chen, G., Einat, H., Yuan, P., and Manji, H. (2002). Evidence for the involvement of the MAP/ERK signaling pathway in mood modulation. *Biol Psychiatry*, 51, 126S.

Chen, R.W., and Chuang, D.M. (1999). Long-term lithium treatment suppresses p53 and bax expression but increases bcl-2 expression. A prominent role in neuroprotection against excitotoxicity. *J Biol Chem*, 274(10), 6039–6042.

Chen, T.J., Zitter, R.N., Tao, R., Hunter, W.R., and Rife, J.C. (1995). Optical constants of lithium triborate crystals in the 55–71 ev region. *Phys Rev B Condensed Matter*, 52(19), 13703–13706.

Chi, P., Greengard, P., and Ryan, T.A. (2001). Synapsin dispersion and reclustering during synaptic activity. *Nat Neurosci*, 4, 1187–1193.

Chiaroni, P., Azorin, J.M., Dassa, D., Henry, J.M., Giudicelli, S., Malthiery, Y., and Planells, R. (2000). Possible involvement of the dopamine D3 receptor locus in subtypes of bipolar affective disorder. *Psychiatr Genet*, 10, 43–49.

Cho, J.T., Bone, S., Dunner, D.L., Colt, E., and Fieve, R.R. (1979). The effect of lithium treatment on thyroid function in patients with primary affective disorder. *Am J Psychiatry*, 136, 115–116.

Choi, S.J., Taylor, M.A., and Abrams, R. (1977). Depression, ECT, and erythrocyte adenosinetriphosphatase activity. *Biol Psychiatry*, 12, 75–81.

Choi, Y.R., and Akera, T. (1977). Kinetics studies on the interaction between ouabain and (Na+,K+)-ATPase. *Biochim Biophys Acta*, 481, 648–659.

Chouinard, G., Steinberg, S., and Steiner, W. (1987). Estrogen–progesterone combination: Another mood stabilizer? *Am J Psychiatry*, 144(6), 826.

Chronwall, B.M., and Zukowska, Z. (2004). Neuropeptide Y, ubiquitous and elusive. *Peptides*, 25(3), 359–363.

Chuang, D.M. (1989). Inositol lipids and transmembrane signalling. In M.J. Berridge and R.H. Michell (Eds.), *Inositol Lipids and Transmembrane Signalling* (pp. 40–53). London: Scholium Intl.

Cirelli, C. (2002). How sleep deprivation affects gene expression in the brain: A review of recent findings. *J Appl Physiol*, 92, 394–400.

Cirelli, C., and Tononi, G. (2000a). Differential expression of plasticity-related genes in waking and sleep and their regulation by the noradrenergic system. *J Neurosci*, 20, 9187–9194.

Cirelli, C., and Tononi, G. (2000b). On the functional significance of c-fos induction during the sleep-waking cycle. *Sleep*, 23(4), 453–469.

Cirelli, C., and Tononi, G. (2000c). Gene expression in the brain across the sleep-waking cycle. *Brain Res*, 885(2), 303–321.

Clark, L.D., Quarton, G.C., Cobb, S., and Bauer, W. (1953). Further observations on mental disturbances associated with cortisone and acth therapy. *N Engl J Med*, 249(5), 178–183.

Cochran, E., Robins, E., and Grote, S. (1976). Regional serotonin levels in brain: A comparison of depressive suicides and alcoholic suicides with controls. *Biol Psychiatry*, 11, 283–294.

Coffman, J.F., and Petty, F. (1986). Plasma GABA: A potential indicator of altered GABAergic function in psychiatric illness.

In G.L. Bartholinim, P.L. Morselli, (Eds.), *GABA and Mood Disorders: Experimental and Clinical Research* (pp. 179–185). New York: Raven Press.

Cohen, P., and Frame, S. (2001). The renaissance of GSK3. *Nat Rev Mol Cell Biol*, 2, 769–776.

Cohn, C.K., Dunner, D.L., and Axelrod, J. (1970). Reduced catechol-O-methyltransferase activity in red blood cells of women with primary affective disorder. *Science*, 170, 1323–1324.

Colin, S.F., Chang, H.C., Mollner, S., Pfeuffer, T., Reed, R.R., Duman, R.S., and Nestler, E.J. (1991). Chronic lithium regulates the expression of adenylate cyclase and Gi-protein alpha subunit in rat cerebral cortex. *Proc Natl Acad Sci USA*, 88, 10634–10637.

Collard, K.J. (1978). The effect of lithium on the increase in forebrain 5-hydroxyindoleacetic acid produced by raphe stimulation. *Br J Pharmacol*, 62, 137–142.

Collard, K.J., and Roberts, M.H. (1977). Effects of lithium on the elevation of forebrain 5-hydroxyindoles by tryptophan. *Neuropharmacology*, 16, 671–673.

Collier, D.A., Arranz, M.J., Sham, P., Battersby, S., Vallada, H., Gill, P., Aitchison, K.J., Sodhi, M., Li, T., Roberts, G.W., Smith, B., Morton, J., Murray, R.M., Smith, D., and Kirov, G. (1996a). The serotonin transporter is a potential susceptibility factor for bipolar affective disorder. *Neuroreport*, 7, 1675–1679.

Collier, D.A., Stober, G., Li, T., Heils, A., Catalano, M., Di Bella, D., Arranz, M.J., Murray, R.M., Vallada, H.P., Bengel, D., Muller, C.R., Roberts, G.W., Smeraldi, E., Kirov, G., Sham, P., and Lesch, K.P. (1996b). A novel functional polymorphism within the promoter of the serotonin transporter gene: Possible role in susceptibility to affective disorders. *Mol Psychiatry*, 1, 453–460.

Conn, P., and Sweatt, J. (1994). Protein kinase C in the nervous system. In J. Kuo (Ed.), *Protein Kinase C* (pp. 199–235). New York: Oxford University Press.

Consogno, E., Racagni, G., and Popoli, M. (2001a). Modifications in brain CaM kinase II after long-term treatment with desmethylimipramine. *Neuropsychopharmacology*, 24, 21–30.

Consogno, E., Tiraboschi, E., Iuliano, E., Gennarelli, M., Racagni, G., and Popoli, M. (2001b). Long-term treatment with S-adenosylmethionine induces changes in presynaptic CaM kinase II and synapsin I. *Biol Psychiatry*, 50, 337–344.

Cooney, J.M., Lucey, J.V., and Dinan, T.G. (1997). Enhanced growth hormone responses to pyridostigmine challenge in patients with panic disorder. *Br J Psychiatry*, 170, 159–161.

Cooper, S.J., Kelly, J.G., and King, D.J. (1985). Adrenergic receptors in depression. Effects of electroconvulsive therapy. *Br J Psychiatry*, 147, 23–29.

Coppen, A. (1960). Abnormality in the blood: Cerebrospinal fluid barrier of patients suffering from a depressive illness. *J Neurol Neuroserg Psychiatry*, 23, 156–161.

Coppen, A., and Shaw, D.M. (1963). Mineral metabolism in melancholia. *BMJ*, 2, 1439–1444.

Coppen, A., Shaw, D.M., Malleson, A., and Costain, R. (1966). Mineral metabolism in mania. *BMJ*, 5479, 71–75.

Coppen, A., Prange, A.J. Jr., Hill, C., Whybrow, P.C., and Noguera, R. (1972). Abnormalities of indoleamines in affective disorders. *Arch Gen Psychiatry*, 26, 474–478.

Coppen, A., Swade, C., and Wood, K. (1980). Lithium restores abnormal platelet 5-HT transport in patients with affective disorders. *Br J Psychiatry*, 136, 235–238.

Cordeiro, M.L., Umbach, J.A., and Gundersen, C.B. (2000). Lithium ions up-regulate mRNAs encoding dense-core vesicle proteins in nerve growth factor-differentiated PC12 cells. *J Neurochem*, 75, 2622–2625.

Corona, G.L., Cucchi, M.L., Santagostino, G., Frattini, P., Zerbi, F., Fenoglio, L., and Savoldi, F. (1982). Blood noradrenaline and 5-HT levels in depressed women during amitriptyline or lithium treatment. *Psychopharmacology (Berl)*, 77, 236–241.

Corrigan, M.H., Denahan, A.Q., Wright, C.E., Ragual, R.J., and Evans, D.L. (2000). Comparison of pramipexole, fluoxetine, and placebo in patients with major depression. *Depress Anxiety*, 11, 58–65.

Corvol, J.C., Studler, J.M., Schonn, J.S., Girault, J.A., and Herve, D. (2001). Gα(olf) is necessary for coupling D1 and A2a receptors to adenylyl cyclase in the striatum. *J Neurochem*, 76, 1585–1588.

Costa, E., Davis, J., Grayson, D.R., Guidotti, A., Pappas, G.D., and Pesold, C. (2001). Dendritic spine hypoplasticity and downregulation of reelin and GABAergic tone in schizophrenia vulnerability. *Neurobiol Dis*, 8, 723–742.

Costa, E., Chen, Y., Davis, J., Dong, E., Noh, J.S., Tremolizzo, L., Veldic, M., Grayson, D.R., and Guidotti, A. (2002). REELIN and schizophrenia: A disease at the interface of the genome and the epigenome. *Mol Intervent*, 2, 47–57.

Cotter, D., Mackay, D., Landau, S., Kerwin, R., and Everall, I. (2001). Reduced glial cell density and neuronal size in the anterior cingulate cortex in major depressive disorder. *Arch Gen Psychiatry*, 58, 545–553.

Cotter, D., Landau, S., Beasley, C., Stevenson, R., Chana, G., MacMillan, L., and Everall, I. (2002a). The density and spatial distribution of GABAergic neurons, labelled using calcium binding proteins, in the anterior cingulate cortex in major depressive disorder, bipolar disorder, and schizophrenia. *Biol Psychiatry*, 51, 377–386.

Cotter, D., Mackay, D., Chana, G., Beasley, C., Landau, S., and Everall, I.P. (2002b). Reduced neuronal size and glial cell density in area 9 of the dorsolateral prefrontal cortex in subjects with major depressive disorder. *Cereb Cortex*, 12, 386–394.

Couldwell, W.T., Weiss, M.H., DeGiorgio, C.M., Weiner, L.P., Hinton, D.R., Ehresmann, G.R., Conti, P.S., and Apuzzo, M.L. (1993). Clinical and radiographic response in a minority of patients with recurrent malignant gliomas treated with high-dose tamoxifen. *Neurosurgery*, 32(3), 485–489; discussion 489–490.

Couldwell, W.T., Hinton, D.R., Surnock, A.A., DeGiorgio, C.M., Weiner, L.P., Apuzzo, M.L., Masri, L., Law, R.E., and Weiss, M.H. (1996). Treatment of recurrent malignant gliomas with chronic oral high-dose tamoxifen. *Clin Cancer Res*, 2(4), 619–622.

Coull, M.A., Lowther, S., Katona, C.L., and Horton, R.W. (2000). Altered brain protein kinase C in depression: A post-mortem study. *Eur Neuropsychopharmacol*, 10, 283–288.

Cowan, W.M., Kopnisky, K.L., and Hyman, S.E. (2002). The human genome project and its impact on psychiatry. *Annu Rev Neurosci*, 25, 1–50.

Cowdry, R.W., Wehr, T.A., Zis, A.P., and Goodwin, F.K. (1983). Thyroid abnormalities associated with rapid-cycling bipolar illness. *Arch Gen Psychiatry*, 40, 414–420.

Cowell, H.E., and Garrod, D.R. (1999). Activation of protein kinase C modulates cell–cell and cell–substratum adhesion of a human colorectal carcinoma cell line and restores 'normal' epithelial morphology. *Int J Cancer*, 80(3), 455–464.

Cowen, P.J. (2000). Psychopharmacology of 5-HT(1A) receptors. *Nucl Med Biol*, 27, 437–439.

Cowen, P.J., Charig, E.M., Fraser, S., and Elliott, J.M. (1987). Platelet 5-HT receptor binding during depressive illness and tricyclic antidepressant treatment. *J Affect Disord*, 13, 45–50.

Cowen, P.J., Parry-Billings, M., and Newsholme, E.A. (1989). Decreased plasma tryptophan levels in major depression. *J Affect Disord*, 16, 27–31.

Coyle, J.T., and Manji, H.K. (2002). Getting balance: Drugs for bipolar disorder share target. *Nat Med*, 8, 557–558.

Coyle, J.T., and Schwarcz, R. (2000). Mind glue: Implications of glial cell biology for psychiatry. *Arch Gen Psychiatry*, 57, 90–93.

Coyle, N., Jones, I., Robertson, E., Lendon, C., and Craddock, N. (2000). Variation at the serotonin transporter gene influences susceptibility to bipolar affective puerperal psychosis. *Lancet*, 356, 1490–1491.

Craddock, N., O'Donovan, M.C., and Owen, M.J. (2005). The genetics of schizophrenia and bipolar disorder: Dissecting psychosis. *J Med Genet*, 42(3), 193–204.

Cremona, O., Di Paolo, G., Wenk, M.R., Luthi, A., Kim, W.T., Takei, K., Daniell, L., Nemoto, Y., Shears, S.B., Flavell, R.A., McCormick, D.A., and De Camilli, P. (1999). Essential role of phosphoinositide metabolism in synaptic vesicle recycling. *Cell*, 99, 179–188.

Cross, D.A., Culbert, A.A., Chalmers, K.A., Facci, L., Skaper, S.D., and Reith, A.D. (2001). Selective small-molecule inhibitors of glycogen synthase kinase-3 activity protect primary neurones from death. *J Neurochem*, 77, 94–102.

Crow, T.J., Cross, A.J., Cooper, S.J., Deakin, J.F., Ferrier, I.N., Johnson, J.A., Joseph, M.H., Owen, F., Poulter, M., and Lofthouse, R. (1984). Neurotransmitter receptors and monoamine metabolites in the brains of patients with Alzheimer-type dementia and depression, and suicides. *Neuropharmacology*, 23, 1561–1569.

Crowder, R.J., and Freeman, R.S. (2000). Glycogen synthase kinase-3 beta activity is critical for neuronal death caused by inhibiting phosphatidylinositol 3-kinase or Akt but not for death caused by nerve growth factor withdrawal. *J Biol Chem*, 275, 34266–34271.

Crunelli, V., Bernasconi, S., and Samanin, R. (1979). Evidence against serotonin involvement in the tonic component of electrically induced convulsions and in carbamazepine anticonvulsant activity. *Psychopharmacology (Berl)*, 66(1), 79.

Cusin, C., Serretti, A., Lattuada, E., Lilli, R., Lorenzi, C., Mandelli, L., Pisati, E., and Smeraldi, E. (2001). Influence of 5-HTTLPR and TPH variants on illness time course in mood disorders. *J Psychiatr Res*, 35, 217–223.

Cutler, N.R., and Post, R.M. (1982). State-related cyclical dyskinesias in manic-depressive illness. *J Clin Psychopharmacol*, 2, 350–354.

Czeh, B., Michaelis, T., Watanabe, T., Frahm, J., de Biurrun, G., van Kampen, M., Bartolomucci, A., and Fuchs, E. (2001). Stress-induced changes in cerebral metabolites, hippocampal volume, and cell proliferation are prevented by antidepressant treatment with tianeptine. *Proc Natl Acad Sci USA*, 98, 12796–12801.

Dafflon, M., Decosterd, L.A., Biollaz, J., Preisig, M., Dufour, H., and Buclin, T. (1999). Trace lithium in mood disorders. *J Affect Disord*, 54(1-2), 199–203.

Dagher, G., Gay, C., Brossard, M., Feray, J.C., Olie, J.P., Garay, R.P., Loo, H., and Meyer, P. (1984). Lithium, sodium and potassium transport in erythrocytes of manic-depressive patients. *Acta Psychiatr Scand*, 69(1), 24–36.

Daigen, A., Akiyama, K., Itoh, T., Kohira, I., Sora, I., Morimoto, K., and Otsuki, S. (1991). Long-lasting enhancement of the membrane-associated protein kinase C activity in the hippocampal kindled rat. *Jpn J Psychiatry Neurol*, 45, 297–301.

Dailey, J.W., Cheong, J.H., Ko, K.H., Adams-Curtis, L.E., and Jobe, P.C. (1995). Anticonvulsant properties of D-20443 in genetically epilepsy-prone rats: prediction of clinical response. *Neurosci Lett*, 195, 77–80.

D'Aquila, P.S., Collu, M., Devoto, P., and Serra, G. (2000). Chronic lithium chloride fails to prevent imipramine-induced sensitization to the dopamine D(2)-like receptor agonist quinpirole. *Eur J Pharmacol*, 395, 157–160.

D'Aquila, P.S., Peana, A.T., Tanda, O., and Serra, G. (2001). Carbamazepine prevents imipramine-induced behavioural sensitization to the dopamine D(2)-like receptor agonist quinpirole. *Eur J Pharmacol*, 416, 107–111.

Davanzo, P., Thomas, M.A., Yue, K., Oshiro, T., Belin, T., Strober, M., and McCracken, J. (2001). Decreased anterior cingulate myo-inositol/creatine spectroscopy resonance with lithium treatment in children with bipolar disorder. *Neuropsychopharmacology*, 24, 359–369.

David, M.M., Owen, J.A., Abraham, G., Delva, N.J., Southmayd, S.E., Wooltorton, E., and Lawson, J.S. (2000). Thyroid function and response to 48-hour sleep deprivation in treatment-resistant depressed patients. *Biol Psychiatry*, 48(4), 323–326.

Davies, J.A. (1995). Mechanisms of action of antiepileptic drugs. *Seizure*, 4, 267–271.

Davis, G.C., Bunney, W.E., Buchsbaum, M., DeFraties, E.G., Duncan, W., Gillin, J.C., Van Kammen, D.P., Kleinman, J., Murphy, D.L., Post, R.M., Reus, V., and Wyatt, R.J. (1979). Use of narcotic antagonists to study the role of endorphins in normal and psychiatric patients. In E. Usdin, W.E. Bunney, and N.S. Kline (Eds.), *Endorphins in Mental Health Research* (pp. 393–406). New York: Oxford University Press.

Davis, G.C., Extein, I., Reus, V.I., Hamilton, W., Post, R.M., Goodwin, F.K., and Bunney, W.E. Jr. (1980). Failure of naloxone to reduce manic symptoms. *Am J Psychiatry*, 137, 1583–1585.

Davis, J.M., and Bresnahan, D.B. (1987). Psychopharmacology in clinical psychiatry. In R.E. Hales and A.J. Frances (Eds), *American Psychiatric Association Annual Review* (Vol. 6) (pp. 159–187). Washington, DC: American Psychiatric Press.

Davis, J.M., Koslow, S.H., Gibbons, R.D., Maas, J.W., Bowden, C.L., Casper, R., Hanin, I., Javaid, J.I., Chang, S.S., and Stokes, P.E. (1988). Cerebrospinal fluid and urinary biogenic amines in depressed patients and healthy controls. *Arch Gen Psychiatry*, 45, 705–717.

Davis, K.L., Berger, P.A., Hollister, L.E., and Defraites, E. (1978). Physostigmine in mania. *Arch Gen Psychiatry*, 35, 119–122.

Deakin, J.F., Pennell, I., Upadhyaya, A.J., and Lofthouse, R. (1990). A neuroendocrine study of 5-HT function in depression: Evidence for biological mechanisms of endogenous and psychosocial causation. *Psychopharmacology (Berl)*, 101, 85–92.

Dean, B., Pavey, G., McLeod, M., Opeskin, K., Keks, N., and Copolov, D. (2001). A change in the density of [(3)H]flumazenil, but not [(3)H]muscimol binding, in Brodmann's area 9 from subjects with bipolar disorder. *J Affect Disord*, 66, 147–158.

Dean, B., Scarr, E., and McLeod, M. (2005). Changes in hippocampal GABAA receptor subunit composition in bipolar 1 disorder. *Brain Res Mol Brain Res*, 138(2), 145–155.

Dean, C., Williams, R.J., and Brockington, I.F. (1989). Is puerperal psychosis the same as bipolar manic-depressive disorder? A family study. *Psychol Med*, 19(3), 637–647.

Deans, Z.C., Dawson, S.J., Kilimann, M.W., Wallace, D., Wilson, M.C., and Latchman, D.S. (1997). Differential regulation of genes encoding synaptic proteins by the Oct-2 transcription factor. *Brain Res Mol Brain Res*, 51, 1–7.

DeBattista, C., Posener, J.A., Kalehzan, B.M., and Schatzberg, A.F. (2000). Acute antidepressant effects of intravenous hydrocortisone and CRH in depressed patients: A double-blind, placebo-controlled study. *Am J Psychiatry*, 157, 1334–1337.

DeBattista, C., Solvason, H.B., Poirier, J., Kendrick, E., and Schatzberg, A.F. (2003). A prospective trial of bupropion sr augmentation of partial and non-responders to serotonergic antidepressants. *J Clin Psychopharmacol*, 23(1), 27–30.

Degkwitz, R., Koufen, H., Consbruch, U., Becker, W., and Knauf, H. (1979). Lithium balance in mania. *Int Pharmacopsychiatry*, 14, 199–212.

Delgado, P.L., Charney, D.S., Price, L.H., Aghajanian, G.K., Landis, H., and Heninger, G.R. (1990). Serotonin function and the mechanism of antidepressant action. Reversal of antidepressant-induced remission by rapid depletion of plasma tryptophan. *Arch Gen Psychiatry*, 47, 411–418.

Delgado, P.L., Price, L.H., Miller, H.L., Salomon, R.M., Licinio, J., Krystal, J.H., Heninger, G.R., and Charney, D.S. (1991). Rapid serotonin depletion as a provocative challenge test for patients with major depression: Relevance to antidepressant action and the neurobiology of depression. *Psychopharmacol Bull*, 27, 321–330.

Delgado, P.L., Miller, H.L., Salomon, R.M., Licinio, J., Krystal, J.H., Moreno, F.A., Heninger, G.R., and Charney, D.S. (1999). Tryptophan-depletion challenge in depressed patients treated with desipramine or fluoxetine: Implications for the role of serotonin in the mechanism of antidepressant action. *Biol Psychiatry*, 46, 212–220.

Del Vecchio, M., Farzati, B., Maj, M., Minucci, P., Guida, L., and Kemali, D. (1981). Cell membrane predictors of response to lithium prophylaxis of affective disorders. *Neuropsychobiology*, 7(5), 243–247.

Demeester-Mirkine, N., and Dumont, J.E. (1980). The hypothalamo-pituitary thyroid axis. In M. deVisscher (Ed.), *The Thyroid Gland* (pp. 145–152). New York: Raven Press.

DeMet, E.M., and Sokolski, K.N. (1999). Sodium valproate increases pupillary responsiveness to a cholinergic agonist in responders with mania. *Biol Psychiatry*, 46, 432–436.

Demitrack, M.A., and Gold, P.W. (1988). Oxytocin: Neurobiologic considerations and their implications for affective illness. *Prog Neuropsychopharmacol Biol Psychiatry*, 12(Suppl.), S23–S51.

de Montigny, C. (1981). Enhancement of the 5-HT neurotransmission by antidepressant treatments. *J Physiol (Paris)*, 77(2-3), 455–461.

de Montigny, C., Grunberg, F., Mayer, A., and Deschenes, J.P. (1981). Lithium induces rapid relief of depression in tricyclic antidepressant drug non-responders. *Br J Psychiatry*, 138, 252–256.

de Montigny, C., Cournoyer, G., Morissette, R., Langlois, R., and Caille, G. (1983). Lithium carbonate addition in tricyclic antidepressant-resistant unipolar depression. Correlations with the neurobiologic actions of tricyclic antidepressant drugs and lithium ion on the serotonin system. *Arch Gen Psychiatry*, 40(12), 1327–1334.

DeMontis, M.G., Fadda, P., Devoto, P., Martellotta, M.C., and Fratta, W. (1990). Sleep deprivation increases dopamine D1 receptor antagonist [3H]SCH 23390 binding and dopamine-stimulated adenylate cyclase in the rat limbic system. *Neurosci Lett*, 117, 224–227.

De Paermentier, F., Cheetham, S.C., Crompton, M.R., Katona, C.L., and Horton, R.W. (1990). Brain beta-adrenoreceptor binding sites in antidepressant-free depressed suicide victims. *Brain Res*, 525, 71–77.

De Paermentier, F., Cheetham, S.C., Crompton, M.R., Katona, C.L., and Horton, R.W. (1991). Brain beta-adrenoreceptor binding sites in depressed suicide victims: Effects of antidepressant treatment. *Psychopharmacology*, 105, 283–288.

De Paermentier, F., Lowther, S., Crompton, M.R., Katona, C.L., and Horton, R.W. (1997a). Beta-adrenoceptors in human pineal glands are unaltered in depressed suicides. *J Psychopharmacol*, 11, 295–299.

De Paermentier, F., Mauger, J.M., Lowther, S., Crompton, M.R., Katona, C.L., and Horton, R.W. (1997b). Brain alpha-adrenoceptors in depressed suicides. *Brain Res*, 757, 60–68.

Depue, R.A., Kleiman, R.M., Davis, P., Hutchinson, M., and Krauss, S.P. (1985). The behavioral high-risk paradigm and bipolar affective disorder: VIII. Serum free cortisol in nonpatient cyclothymic subjects selected by the General Behavior Inventory. *Am J Psychiatry*, 142, 175–181.

Deshauer, D., Grof, E., Alda, M., and Grof, P. (1999). Patterns of DST positivity in remitted affective disorders. *Biol Psychiatry*, 45, 1023–1029.

Deuschle, M., Schweiger, U., Gotthardt, U., Weber, B., Korner, A., Schmider, J., Standhardt, H., Lammers, C.H., Krumm, B., and Heuser, I. (1998). The combined dexamethasone/corticotropin-releasing hormone stimulation test is more closely associated with features of diurnal activity of the hypothalamo-pituitary-adrenocortical system than the dexamethasone suppression test. *Biol Psychiatry*, 43, 762–766.

Devanand, D.P., Lo, I., Sackeim, H.A., Halbreich, U., Ross, F., and Cooper, T. (1987). *Acute and subacute effects of electroconvulsive therapy on plasma oxytocin and vasopressin in depressed patients.* 42nd Annual meeting of the Society of Biological Psychiatry.

de Villiers, A.S., Russell, V.A., Carstens, M.E., Searson, J.A., van Zyl, A.M., Lombard, C.J., and Taljaard, J.J. (1989). Noradrenergic function and hypothalamic–pituitary–adrenal axis activity in adolescents with major depressive disorder. *Psychiatry Res*, 27(2), 101–109.

De Wied, D., Bohus, B., and Van Wimersma, Tj.B. (1975). Memory deficit in rats with hereditary diabetes insipidus. *Brain Research*, 85(1), 152–156.

D'Haenen, H.A., and Bossuyt, A. (1994). Dopamine D2 receptors in depression measured with single photon emission computed tomography. *Biol Psychiatry*, 35(2), 128–132.

D'Haenen, H., Bossuyt, A., Mertens, J., Bossuyt-Piron, C., Gijsemans, M., and Kaufman, L. (1992). SPECT imaging of serotonin2 receptors in depression. *Psychiatry Res*, 45, 227–237.

Diacicov, S., and Tudorache, B. (1990). Clonidine treatment in manic episodes. *Rev Med Int Neurol Psihiatr Neurochir Dermatovenerol Neurol Psihiatr Neurochir*, 35, 29–32.

Dick, D.A.T., Naylor, G.J., and Dick, E.G. (1978). Effects of Lithium on sodium transport across membranes. In F.N. Johnson, S. Johnson (Eds.), *Lithium in Medical Practice* (pp. 173–182). Baltimore: University Park Press.

Dillon, K.A., Gross-Isseroff, R., Israeli, M., and Biegon, A. (1991). Autoradiographic analysis of serotonin 5-HT1A receptor binding in the human brain postmortem: Effects of age and alcohol. *Brain Res*, 554, 56–64.

Dilsaver, S.C., and Coffman, J.A. (1989). Cholinergic hypothesis of depression: A reappraisal. *J Clin Psychopharmacol*, 9, 173–179.

Dilsaver, S.C., and Hariharan, M. (1988). Amitriptyline-induced supersensitivity of a central muscarinic mechanism: Lithium blocks amitriptyline-induced supersensitivity. *Psychiatry Res*, 25, 181–186.

Dilsaver, S.C., and Hariharan, M. (1989). Chronic treatment with lithium produces supersensitivity to nicotine. *Biol Psychiatry*, 25, 795–799.

Dilsaver, S.C., Peck, J.A., Traumata, D., and Swan, A.C. (1993). Treatment with carbamazepine may enhance alpha 2-noradrenergic autoreceptor sensitivity. *Biol Psychiatry*, 34, 551–557.

Dinan, T.G., Yatham, L.N., O'Keane, V., and Barry, S. (1991). Blunting of noradrenergic-stimulated growth hormone release in mania. *Am J Psychiatry*, 148, 936–938.

Dinan, T.G., O'Keane, V., and Thakore, J. (1994). Pyridostigmine induced growth hormone release in mania: focus on the cholinergic/somatostatin system. *Clin Endocrinol (Oxf)*, 40, 93–96.

Divish, M.M., Sheftel, G., Boyle, A., Kalasapudi, V.D., Papolos, D.F., and Lachman, H.M. (1991). Differential effect of lithium on fos protooncogene expression mediated by receptor and postreceptor activators of protein kinase C and cyclic adenosine monophosphate: Model for its antimanic action. *J Neurosci Res*, 28, 40–48.

Dixon, J.F., and Hokin, L.E. (1997). The antibipolar drug valproate mimics lithium in stimulating glutamate release and inositol 1,4,5-trisphosphate accumulation in brain cortex slices but not accumulation of inositol monophosphates and bisphosphates. *Proc Natl Acad Sci USA*, 94, 4757–4760.

Dixon, J.F., and Hokin, L.E. (1998). Lithium acutely inhibits and chronically up-regulates and stabilizes glutamate uptake by presynaptic nerve endings in mouse cerebral cortex. *Proc Natl Acad Sci USA*, 95(14), 8363–8368.

D'Mello, S.R., Anelli, R., and Calissano, P. (1994). Lithium induces apoptosis in immature cerebellar granule cells but promotes survival of mature neurons. *Exp Cell Res*, 211, 332–338.

Dobner, P.R., Tischler, A.S., Lee, Y.C., Bloom, S.R., and Donahue, S.R. (1988). Lithium dramatically potentiates neurotensin/neuromedin N gene expression. *J Biol Chem*, 263, 13983–13986.

Doraiswamy, P.M., MacFall, J., Krishnan, K.R., O'Connor, C., Wan, X., Benaur, M., Lewandowski, M., and Fortner, M. (1999). Magnetic resonance assessment of cerebral perfusion in depressed cardiac patients: Preliminary findings. *Am J Psychiatry*, 156, 1641–1643.

Doran, A.R., Rubinow, D.R., Roy, A., and Pickar, D. (1986). CSF somatostatin and abnormal response to dexamethasone administration in schizophrenic and depressed patients. *Arch Gen Psychiatry*, 43, 365–369.

Dowlatshahi, D., MacQueen, G.M., Wang, J.F., and Young, L.T. (1998). Increased temporal cortex CREB concentrations and antidepressant treatment in major depression. *Lancet*, 352, 1754–1755.

Drevets, W.C. (2000). Neuroimaging studies of mood disorders. *Biol Psychiatry*, 48, 813–829.

Drevets, W.C. (2001). Neuroimaging and neuropathological studies of depression: Implications for the cognitive-emotional features of mood disorders. *Curr Opin Neurobiol*, 11, 240–249.

Drevets, W.C., Frank, E., Price, J.C., Kupfer, D.J., Holt, D., Greer, P.J., Huang, Y., Gautier, C., and Mathis, C. (1999). PET imaging of serotonin 1A receptor binding in depression. *Biol Psychiatry*, 46, 1375–1387.

Drevets, W.C., Frank, E., Price, J.C., Kupfer, D.J., Greer, P.J., and Mathis, C. (2000). Serotonin type-1A receptor imaging in depression. *Nucl Med Biol*, 27, 499–507.

Drevets, W.C., Price, J.L., Bardgett, M.E., Reich, T., Todd, R.D., and Raichle, M.E. (2002). Glucose metabolism in the amygdala in depression: Relationship to diagnostic subtype and plasma cortisol levels. *Pharmacol Biochem Behav*, 71, 431–447.

D'Sa, C., and Duman, R.S. (2002). Antidepressants and neuroplasticity. *Bipolar Disord*, 4, 183–194.

Du, J., Gray, N., Falke, C., Yuan, P., Szabo, S., and Manji, H. (2003). Structurally dissimilar antimanic agents modulate synaptic plasticity by regulating AMPA glutamate receptor subunit GluR1 synaptic expression. *Ann NY Acad Sci*, 1003, 378–380.

Dubovsky, S.L., Christiano, J., Daniell, L.C., Franks, R.D., Murphy, J., Adler, L., Baker, N., and Harris, R.A. (1989). Increased platelet intracellular calcium concentration in patients with bipolar affective disorders. *Arch Gen Psychiatry*, 46, 632–638.

Dubovsky, S.L., Lee, C., Christiano, J., and Murphy, J. (1991). Elevated platelet intracellular calcium concentration in bipolar depression. *Biol Psychiatry*, 29, 441–450.

Dubovsky, S.L., Murphy, J., Christiano, J., and Lee, C. (1992a). The calcium second messenger system in bipolar disorders: Data supporting new research directions. *J Neuropsychiatry Clin Neurosci*, 4, 3–14.

Dubovsky, S.L., Murphy, J., Thomas, M., and Rademacher, J. (1992b). Abnormal intracellular calcium ion concentration in platelets and lymphocytes of bipolar patients. *Am J Psychiatry*, 149, 118–120.

Dubovsky, S.L., Thomas, J., Hijazi, A., and Murphy, J. (1994). Intracellular calcium signaling in peripheral cells of patients with bipolar affective disorder. *Eur Arch Psychiatry Clin Neurosci*, 243, 229–234.

Ducottet, C., Griebel, G., and Belzung, C. (2003). Effects of the selective nonpeptide corticotropin-releasing factor receptor 1 antagonist antalarmin in the chronic mild stress model of depression in mice. *Prog Neuropsychopharmacol Biol Psychiatry*, 27(4), 625–631.

Duman, RS. (2004). Role of neurotrophic factors in the etiology and treatment of mood disorders. *Neuromol Med*, 5(1), 11–25.

Duman, R.S., Heninger, G.R., and Nestler, E.J. (1997). A molecular and cellular theory of depression. *Arch Gen Psychiatry*, 54, 597–606.

Duman, R.S., Malberg, J., and Thome, J. (1999). Neural plasticity to stress and antidepressant treatment. *Biol Psychiatry*, 46, 1181–1191.

Duman, R.S., Malberg, J., Nakagawa, S., and D'Sa, C. (2000). Neuronal plasticity and survival in mood disorders. *Biol Psychiatry*, 48, 732–739.

Dunner, D.L., Levitt, M., Kumbaraci, T., and Fieve, R.R. (1977). Erythrocyte catechol-O-methyltransferase activity in primary affective disorder. *Biol Psychiatry*, 12, 237–244.

Duval, F., Macher, J.P., and Mokrani, M.C. (1990). Difference between evening and morning thyrotropin responses to protirelin in major depressive episode. *Arch Gen Psychiatry*, 47, 443–448.

Dwivedi, Y., and Pandey, G.N. (1999). Administration of dexamethasone up-regulates protein kinase C activity and the expression of gamma and epsilon protein kinase C isozymes in the rat brain. *J Neurochem*, 72, 380–387.

Eastwood, S.L., and Harrison, P.J. (2001). Synaptic pathology in the anterior cingulate cortex in schizophrenia and mood disorders. A review and a Western blot study of synaptophysin, GAP-43 and the complexins. *Brain Res Bull*, 55, 569–78.

Ebert, D., and Ebmeier, K.P. (1996). The role of the cingulate gyrus in depression: From functional anatomy to neurochemistry. *Biol Psychiatry*, 39, 1044–1050.

Ebstein, R.P., Lerer, B., Shlaufman, M., and Belmaker, R.H. (1983). The effect of repeated electroconvulsive shock treatment and chronic lithium feeding on the release of norepinephrine from rat cortical vesicular preparations. *Cell Mol Neurobiol*, 3, 191–201.

Ebstein, R.P., Moscovich, D., Zeevi, S., Amiri, Z., and Lerer, B. (1987). Effect of lithium in vitro and after chronic treatment on human platelet adenylate cyclase activity: Postreceptor modification of second-messenger signal amplification. *Psychiatry Res*, 21, 221–228.

Ebstein, R.P., Lerer, B., Bennett, E.R., Shapira, B., Kindler, S., Shemesh, Z., and Gerstenhaber, N. (1988). Lithium modulation of second messenger signal amplification in man: Inhibition of phosphatidylinositol-specific phospholipase C and adenylate cyclase activity. *Psychiatry Res*, 24, 45–52.

Eckermann, K., Beasley, A., Yang, P., Gaytan, O., Swann, A., and Dafny, N. (2001). Methylphenidate sensitization is modulated by valproate. *Life Sci*, 69, 47–57.

Eden Evins, A., Demopulos, C., Nierenberg, A., Culhane, M.A., Eisner, L., and Sachs, G. (2006). A double-blind, placebo-controlled trial of adjunctive donepezil in treatment-resistant mania. *Bipolar Disord*, 8, 75–80.

Egan, M.F., Goldberg, T.E., Kolachana, B.S., Callicott, J.H., Mazzanti, C.M., Straub, R.E., Goldman, D., and Weinberger, D.R. (2001). Effect of COMT Val108/158 Met genotype on frontal lobe function and risk for schizophrenia. *Proc Natl Acad Sci USA*, 98, 6917–6922.

Egan, M.F., Kojima, M., Callicott, J.H., Goldberg, T.E., Kolachana, B.S., Bertolino, A., Zaitsev, E., Gold, B., Goldman, D., Dean, M., Lu, B., and Weinberger, D.R. (2003). The BDNF val66met polymorphism affects activity-dependent secretion of BDNF and human memory and hippocampal function. *Cell*, 112(2), 257–269.

Egeland, J.A., Kidd, J.R., Frazer, A., Kidd, K.K., and Neuhauser, V.I. (1984). Amish study: V. Lithium-sodium countertransport and catechol O-methyltransferase in pedigrees of bipolar probands. *Am J Psychiatry*, 141, 1049–1054.

Ehrlich, B.E., and Diamond, J.M. (1979). Lithium fluxes in human erythrocytes. *Am J Physiol*, 237, C102–C110.

Ehrlich, B.E., and Diamond, J.M. (1980). Lithium, membranes, and manic-depressive illness. *J Membr Biol*, 52, 187–200.

Ehrlich, B.E., Diamond, J.M., and Gosenfeld, L. (1981). Lithium-induced changes in sodium-lithium countertransport. *Biochem Pharmacol*, 30, 2539–2543.

Ehrlich, B.E., Diamond, J.M., Fry, V., and Meier, K. (1983). Lithium's inhibition of erythrocyte cation countertransport involves a slow process in the erythrocyte. *J Membr Biol*, 75, 233–240.

Eilam, D., and Szechtman, H. (1989). Biphasic effect of D2 agonist quinpirole on locomotion and movements. *Eur J Pharmacol*, 161, 151–157.

Eilam, D., and Szechtman, H. (1990). Dosing regimen differentiates sensitization of locomotion and mouthing to D2 agonist quinpirole. *Pharmacol Biochem Behav*, 36, 989–991.

Einat, H., Einat, D., Allan, M., Talangbayan, H., Tsafnat, T., and Szechtman, H. (1996). Associational and nonassociational mechanisms in locomotor sensitization to the dopamine agonist quinpirole. *Psychopharmacology (Berl)*, 127, 95–101.

Einat, H., Kofman, O., and Belmaker, R.H. (2000). Animal models of bipolar disorder: From a single episode to progressive cycling models. In I. Weiner (Ed.), *Contemporary Issues in Modeling Psychopharmacology* (pp. 165–180). Boston: Kluwer Academic Publishers.

Einat, H., Belmaker, R.H., Zangen, A., Overstreet, D.H., and Yadid, G. (2002a). Chronic inositol treatment reduces depression-like immobility of Flinders Sensitive Line rats in the forced swim test. *Depress Anxiety*, 15, 148–151.

Einat, H., Chen, G., and Manji, H.K. (2002b). Does the ERK map kinase signaling cascade play a role in the pathophysiology and treatment of bipolar disorder? *Biol Psychiatry*, 51, 376s.

Einat, H., Belmaker, R.H., and Manji, H.K. (2003a). New aproaches to modeling bipolar disorder. *Psychopharmacol Bull*, 37, 47–63.

Einat, H., Yuan, P., Gould, T.D., Li, J., Du, J., Zhang, L., Manji, H.K., and Chen, G. (2003b). The role of the extracellular signal-regulated kinase signaling pathway in mood modulation. *J Neurosci*, 23, 7311–7316.

Elizur, A., Shopsin, B., Gershon, S., and Ehlenberger, A. (1972). Intra-extracellular lithium ratios and clinical course in affective states. *Clin Pharmacol Ther*, 13, 947–953.

Ellinwood, E.H. Jr., Sudilovsky, A., and Nelson, L. (1972). Behavioral analysis of chronic amphetamine intoxication. *Biol Psychiatry*, 4, 215–230.

Ellis, J., and Lenox, R.H. (1990). Chronic lithium treatment prevents atropine-induced supersensitivity of the muscarinic phosphoinositide response in rat hippocampus. *Biol Psychiatry*, 28, 609–619.

Ellis, P.M., and Salmond, C. (1994). Is platelet imipramine binding reduced in depression? A meta-analysis. *Biol Psychiatry*, 36:292–299.

El-Mallakh, R.S. (1983). The Na,K-ATPase hypothesis for manic-depression. II. The mechanism of action of lithium. *Med Hypotheses*, 12, 269–282.

El-Mallakh, R.S., and Jaziri, W.A. (1990). Calcium channel blockers in affective illness: Role of sodium-calcium exchange. *J Clin Psychopharmacol*, 10, 203–206.

Elphick, M., Yang, J.D., and Cowen, P.J. (1990). Effects of carbamazepine on dopamine- and serotonin-mediated neuroendocrine responses. *Arch Gen Psychiatry*, 47, 135–140.

Emamghoreishi, M., Schlichter, L., Li, P.P., Parikh, S., Sen, J., Kamble, A., and Warsh, J.J. (1997). High intracellular calcium concentrations in transformed lymphoblasts from subjects with bipolar I disorder. *Am J Psychiatry*, 154, 976–982.

Emamghoreishi, M., Li, P.P., Schlichter, L., Parikh, S.V., Cooke, R., and Warsh, J.J. (2000). Associated disturbances in calcium homeostasis and G protein–mediated cAMP signaling in bipolar I disorder. *Biol Psychiatry*, 48(7), 665–673.

Emrich, H.M., Cording, C., Piree, S., Kölling, A., Möller, H.J., VonZerssen, D., and Herz, A. (1979). Actions of naloxone in different types of psychosis. In E. Usdin, W.E. Bunney, and N.S. Kline (Eds.), *Endorphins in Mental Health Research* (pp. 452–460). New York: Oxford University Press.

Emrich, H.M., Aldenhoff, J.B., and Lux, H.D. (1982). *Basic Mechanisms in the Action of Lithium*. Amsterdam: Excerpta Medica.

Engel, J., and Berggren, U. (1980). Effects of lithium on behaviour and central monoamines. *Acta Psychiatr Scand Suppl*, 280, 133–143.

Erfurth, A., Michael, N., Stadtland, C., and Arolt, V. (2002). Bupropion as add-on strategy in difficult-to-treat bipolar depressive patients. *Neuropsychobiology*, 45(Suppl. 1), 33–36.

Eriksson, P.S., Perfilieva, E., Bjork-Eriksson, T., Alborn, A.M., Nordborg, C., Peterson, D.A., and Gage, F.H. (1998). Neurogenesis in the adult human hippocampus. *Nat Med*, 4(11), 1313–1317.

Eroglu, L., Hizal, A., and Koyuncuoglu, H. (1981). The effect of long-term concurrent administration of chlorpromazine and lithium on the striatal and frontal cortical dopamine metabolism in rats. *Psychopharmacology (Berl)*, 73, 84–86.

Esler, M. (1982). Assessment of sympathetic nervous function in humans from noradrenaline plasma kinetics. *Clin Sci (Lond)*, 62, 247–254.

Esler, M., Turbott, J., Schwarz, R., Leonard, P., Bobik, A., Skews, H., and Jackman, G. (1982). The peripheral kinetics of norepinephrine in depressive illness. *Arch Gen Psychiatry*, 39(3), 295–300.

Evans, D.L., and Nemeroff, C.B. (1983). The dexamethasone suppression test in mixed bipolar disorder. *Am J Psychiatry*, 140, 615–617.

Evans, M.S., Zorumski, C.F., and Clifford, D.B. (1990). Lithium enhances neuronal muscarinic excitation by presynaptic facilitation. *Neuroscience*, 38, 457–468.

Everitt, B.J., Hokfelt, T., Terenius, L., Tatemoto, K., Mutt, V., and Goldstein, M. (1984). Differential co-existence of neuropeptide Y (NPY)-like immunoreactivity with catecholamines in the central nervous system of the rat. *Neuroscience*, 11(2), 443–462.

Extein, I.L. (2000). High doses of levothyroxine for refractory rapid cycling. *Am J Psychiatry*, 157, 1704–1705.

Extein, I., Goodwin, F.K., Lewy, A.J., Schoenfeld, R.I., and Fakhur, L.R. (1979a). Behavioral and biochemical effects of FK 33-824, a parenterally and orally active enkephalin analog. In E. Usdin, W.E. Bunney, and N.S. Kline (Eds.), *Endorphins in Mental Health Research* (pp. 279–292). New York: Oxford University Press.

Extein, I., Lo, C., Goodwin, F.K., and Schoenfeld, R.I. (1979b). Dopamine-mediated behavior produced by the enkephalin analogue FK 33-824. *Psychiatry Res*, 1, 333–339.

Fadda, P., Tortorella, A., and Fratta, W. (1991). Sleep deprivation decreases mu and delta opioid receptor binding in the rat limbic system. *Neurosci Lett*, 129, 315–317.

Fadda, P., Martellotta, M.C., De Montis, M.G., Gessa, G.L., and Fratta, W. (1992). Dopamine D1 and opioid receptor binding changes in the limbic system of sleep deprived rats. *Neurochem Int*, 20, 153S–156S.

Fadic, R., and Johns, D.R. (1996). Clinical spectrum of mitochondrial diseases. *Semin Neurol*, 16(1), 11–20.

Fahn, S. (1978). Post-anoxic action myoclonus: Improvement with valproic acid. *N Engl J Med*, 299, 313–314.

Fahndrich, E., Coper, H., Christ, W., Helmchen, H., Muller-Oerlinghausen, B., and Pietzcker, A. (1980). Erythrocyte COMT-activity in patients with affective disorders. *Acta Psychiatr Scand*, 61, 427–437.

Farley, I.J., Price, K.S., McCullough, E., Deck, J.H., Hordynski, W., and Hornykiewicz, O. (1978). Norepinephrine in chronic paranoid schizophrenia: Above-normal levels in limbic fore-brain. *Science*, 200, 456–458.

Fatemi, S.H. (2002). The role of Reelin in pathology of autism. *Mol Psychiatry*, 7, 919–920.

Fatemi, S.H., Earle, J.A., and McMenomy, T. (2000a). Hippocampal CA4 Reelin-positive neurons. *Mol Psychiatry*, 5, 571.

Fatemi, S.H., Earle, J.A., and McMenomy, T. (2000b). Reduction in Reelin immunoreactivity in hippocampus of subjects with schizophrenia, bipolar disorder and major depression. *Mol Psychiatry*, 5, 571, 654–663.

Fatemi, S.H., Earle, J.A., Stary, J.M., Lee, S., and Sedgewick, J. (2001a). Altered levels of the synaptosomal associated protein SNAP-25 in hippocampus of subjects with mood disorders and schizophrenia. *Neuroreport*, 12, 3257–3262.

Fatemi, S.H., Kroll, J.L., and Stary, J.M. (2001b). Altered levels of Reelin and its isoforms in schizophrenia and mood disorders. *Neuroreport*, 12, 3209–3215.

Fatemi, S.H., Stary, J.M., and Egan, E.A. (2002). Reduced blood levels of reelin as a vulnerability factor in pathophysiology of autistic disorder. *Cell Mol Neurobiol*, 22, 139–152.

Feinberg, M., and Carroll, B.J. (1984). Biological 'markers' for endogenous depression. Effect of age, severity of illness, weight loss, and polarity. *Arch Gen Psychiatry*, 41, 1080–1085.

Fernstrom, J.D. (1983). Role of precursor availability in control of monoamine biosynthesis in brain. *Physiol Rev*, 63, 484–546.

Fernstrom, J.D., and Wurtman, R.J. (1997). Brain serotonin content: Physiological regulation by plasma neutral amino acids. *Obes Res*, 5(4), 377–380.

Ferrari, E., Bossolo, P.A., Vailati, A., Martinelli, I., Rea, A., and Nosari, I. (1977). Effects of a vagolytic substance on the circadian rhythm of the ACTH-secreting system in man. *Ann Endocrinol (Paris)*, 38, 203–213.

Ferrendelli, J.A., and Kinscherf, D.A. (1979). Inhibitory effects of anticonvulsant drugs on cyclic nucleotide accumulation in brain. *Ann Neurol*, 5, 533–538.

Ferris, C.F., Lu, S.F., Messenger, T., Guillon, C.D., Heindel, N., Miller, M., Koppel, G., Robert Bruns, F., and Simon, N.G. (2006). Orally active vasopressin V1a receptor antagonist, SRX251, selectively blocks aggressive behavior. *Pharmacol Biochem Behav*, 83(2), 169–174.

Fields, A., Li, P.P., Kish, S.J., and Warsh, J.J. (1999). Increased cyclic AMP-dependent protein kinase activity in postmortem brain from patients with bipolar affective disorder. *J Neurochem*, 73, 1704–1710.

File, S.E. (1997). Anxiolytic action of a neurokinin1 receptor antagonist in the social interaction test. *Pharmacol Biochem Behav*, 58(3), 747–752.

Filser, J.G., Spira, J., Fischer, M., Gattaz, W.F., and Muller, W.E. (1988). The evaluation of 4-hydroxy-3-methoxyphenylglycol sulfate as a possible marker of central norepinephrine turnover. Studies in healthy volunteers and depressed patients. *J Psychiatr Res*, 22, 171–181.

Fink, M., Papakostas, Y., Lee, J., Meehan, T., and Johnson, L. (1981). Clinical trials with des-tyr-gamma-endorphin (GK-78). In C. Perris, G. Struwe, and B. Jansson (Eds.), *Biological Psychiatry 1981* (pp. 398–401). Amsterdam: Elsevier.

Fischer, W., and Muller, M. (1988). Pharmacological modulation of central monoaminergic systems and influence on the anticonvulsant effectiveness of standard antiepileptics in maximal electroshock seizure. *Biomed Biochim Acta*, 47, 631–645.

Fisher, S.K., Heacock, A.M., and Agranoff, B.W. (1992). Inositol lipids and signal transduction in the nervous system: An update. *J Neurochem*, 58, 18–38.

Fishman, S.M., Catarau, E.M., Sachs, G., Stojanovic, M., and Borsook, D. (1996). Corticosteroid-induced mania after single regional application at the celiac plexus. *Anesthesiology*, 85(5), 1194–1196.

Foley, K.M., Kourides, I.A., Inturrisi, C.E., Kaiko, R.F., Zaroulis, C.G., Posner, J.B., Houde, R.W., and Li, C.H. (1979). Beta-endorphin: Analgesic and hormonal effects in humans. *Proc Natl Acad Sci USA*, 76, 5377–5381.

Forstner, U., Bohus, M., Gebicke-Harter, P.J., Baumer, B., Berger, M., and van Calker, D. (1994). Decreased agonist-stimulated Ca2+ response in neutrophils from patients under chronic lithium therapy. *Eur Arch Psychiatry Clin Neurosci*, 243(5), 240–243.

France, R.D., Urban, B., Krishnan, K.R., Bissett, G., Banki, C.M., Nemeroff, C., and Speilman, F.J. (1988). CSF corticotropin-releasing factor-like immunoactivity in chronic pain patients with and without major depression. *Biol Psychiatry*, 23, 86–88.

Frances, H., Maurin, Y., Lecrubier, Y., Puech, A.J., and Simon, P. (1981). Effect of chronic lithium treatment on isolation-induced behavioral and biochemical effects in mice. *Eur J Pharmacol*, 72, 337–341.

Francis, D., Diorio, J., Liu, D., and Meaney, M.J. (1999). Nongenomic transmission across generations of maternal behavior and stress responses in the rat. *Science*, 286, 1155–1158.

Fratta, W., Collu, M., Martellotta, M.C., Pichiri, M., Muntoni, F., and Gessa, G.L. (1987). Stress-induced insomnia: Opioid-dopamine interactions. *Eur J Pharmacol*, 142, 437–440.

Frazer, A., Mendels, J., Brunswick, D., London, J., Pring, M., Ramsey, T.A., and Rybakowski, J. (1978). Erythrocyte concentrations of the lithium ion: Clinical correlates and mechanisms of action. *Am J Psychiatry*, 135, 1065–1069.

Frazer, A., Ramsey, T.A., Swann, A., Bowden, C., Brunswick, D., Garver, D., and Secunda, S. (1983). Plasma and erythrocyte electrolytes in affective disorders. *J Affect Disord*, 5, 103–113.

Freedman, R.R., Embury, J., Migaly, P., Keegan, D., Pandey, G.N., Javaid, J.I., and Davis, J.M. (1990). Stress-induced desensitization of alpha 2-adrenergic receptors in human platelets. *Psychosom Med*, 52, 624–630.

Friedman, E., and Gershon, S. (1973). Effect of lithium on brain dopamine. *Nature*, 243, 520–521.

Friedman, E., and Wang, H.Y. (1988). Effect of chronic lithium treatment on 5-hydroxytryptamine autoreceptors and release of 5-[3H]hydroxytryptamine from rat brain cortical, hippocampal, and hypothalamic slices. *J Neurochem*, 50, 195–201.

Friedman, E., and Wang, H.Y. (1996). Receptor-mediated activation of G proteins is increased in postmortem brains of bipolar affective disorder subjects. *J Neurochem*, 67, 1145–1152.

Friedman, E., Dallob, A., and Levine, G. (1979). The effect of long-term lithium treatment on reserpine-induced supersensitivity in dopaminergic and serotonergic transmission. *Life Sci*, 25, 1263–1266.

Friedman, E., Hoau Yan, W., Levinson, D., Connell, T.A., and Singh, H. (1993). Altered platelet protein kinase C activity in bipolar affective disorder, manic episode. *Biol Psychiatry*, 33, 520–525.

Frye, M.A., Denicoff, K.D., Bryan, A.L., Smith-Jackson, E.E., Ali, S.O., Luckenbaugh, D., Leverich, G.S., and Post, R.M. (1999a). Association between lower serum free T4 and greater mood instability and depression in lithium-maintained bipolar patients. *Am J Psychiatry*, 156, 1909–1914.

Frye, M.A., Dunn, R.T., Gary, K.A., Kimbrell, T.A., Callahan, A.M., Luckenbaugh, D.A., Cora-Locatelli, G., Vanderham, E., Winokur, A., and Post, R.M. (1999b). Lack of correlation between cerebrospinal fluid thyrotropin-releasing hormone (TRH) and TRH-stimulated thyroid-stimulating hormone in patients with depression. *Biol Psychiatry*, 45, 1049–1052.

Furlong, R.A., Ho, L., Walsh, C., Rubinsztein, J.S., Jain, S., Paykel, E.S., Easton, D.F., and Rubinsztein, D.C. (1998). Analysis and meta-analysis of two serotonin transporter gene polymorphisms in bipolar and unipolar affective disorders. *Am J Med Genet*, 81, 58–63.

Fyro, B., Petterson, U., and Sedvall, G. (1975). The effect of lithium treatment on manic symptoms and levels of monoamine metabolites in cerebrospinal fluid of manic depressive patients. *Psychopharmacologia*, 44, 99–103.

Gabriel, S.M., Knott, P.J., and Haroutunian, V. (1995). Alterations in cerebral cortical galanin concentrations following neurotransmitter-specific subcortical lesions in the rat. *J Neurosci*, 15(8), 5526–5534.

Gaillard, W.D., Zeffiro, T., Fazilat, S., DeCarli, C., and Theodore, W.H. (1996). Effect of valproate on cerebral metabolism and blood flow: An 18F-2-deoxyglucose and 15O water positron emission tomography study. *Epilepsia*, 37, 515–521.

Gallager, D.W., Pert, A., and Bunney, W.E. Jr. (1978). Haloperidol-induced presynaptic dopamine supersensitivity is blocked by chronic lithium. *Nature*, 273, 309–312.

Galva, M.D., Bondiolotti, G.P., Olasmaa, M., and Picotti, G.B. (1995). Effect of aging on lazabemide binding, monoamine oxidase activity and monoamine metabolites in human frontal cortex. *J Neural Transm Gen Sect*, 101, 83–94.

Gann, H., Riemann, D., Hohagen, F., Strauss, L.G., Dressing, H., Muller, W.E., and Berger, M. (1993). 48-hour rapid cycling: Results of psychopathometric, polysomnographic, PET imaging and neuroendocrine longitudinal investigations in a single case. *J Affect Disord*, 28, 133–140.

Garcia-Sevilla, J.A., and Fuster, M.J. (1986). Labelling of human platelet alpha 2-adrenoceptors with the full agonist [3H](-)adrenaline. *Eur J Pharmacol*, 124, 31–41.

Garcia-Sevilla, J.A., Ugedo, L., Ulibarri, I., and Gutierrez, M. (1986a). Heroin increases the density and sensitivity of platelet alpha 2-adrenoceptors in human addicts. *Psychopharmacology (Berl)*, 88(4), 489–492.

Garcia-Sevilla, J.A., Guimon, J., Garcia-Vallejo, P., and Fuster, M.J. (1986b). Biochemical and functional evidence of supersensitive platelet alpha 2-adrenoceptors in major affective disorder. Effect of long-term lithium carbonate treatment. *Arch Gen Psychiatry*, 43(1), 51–57.

Garcia-Sevilla, J.A., Padro, D., Giralt, M.T., Guimon, J., and Areso, P. (1990). Alpha 2-adrenoceptor-mediated inhibition of platelet adenylate cyclase and induction of aggregation in major depression. Effect of long-term cyclic antidepressant drug treatment. *Arch Gen Psychiatry*, 47, 125–132.

Garcia-Sevilla, J.A., Escriba, P.V., Busquets, X., Walzer, C., and Guimon, J. (1996). Platelet imidazoline receptors and regulatory G proteins in patients with major depression. *Neuroreport*, 8, 169–172.

Garcia-Sevilla, J.A., Escriba, P.V., Ozaita, A., La Harpe, R., Walzer, C., Eytan, A., and Guimon, J. (1999). Up-regulation of immunolabeled alpha2A-adrenoceptors, Gi coupling proteins, and regulatory receptor kinases in the prefrontal cortex of depressed suicides. *J Neurochem*, 72, 282–291.

Garlow, S., Mussellman, D., and Nemeroff, C. (1999). The neurochemistry of mood disorders. In B.S. Bunney (Ed.), *Neurobiology of Mental Illness* (pp. 348–364). New York: Oxford University Press.

Gass, P., Kretz, O., Wolfer, D.P., Berger, S., Tronche, F., Reichardt, H.M., Kellendonk, C., Lipp, H.P., Schmid, W., and Schutz, G. (2000). Genetic disruption of mineralocorticoid receptor leads to impaired neurogenesis and granule cell degeneration in the hippocampus of adult mice. *EMBO Rep*, 1, 447–451.

Geracioti, T.D. Jr., Loosen, P.T., Ekhator, N.N., Schmidt, D., Chambliss, B., Baker, D.G., Kasckow, J.W., Richtand, N.M., Keck, P.E. Jr., and Ebert, M.H. (1997). Uncoupling of serotonergic and noradrenergic systems in depression: Preliminary evidence from continuous cerebrospinal fluid sampling. *Depress Anxiety*, 6, 89–94.

Gerner, R.H., and Hare, T.A. (1981). CSF GABA in normal subjects and patients with depression, schizophrenia, mania, and anorexia nervosa. *Am J Psychiatry*, 138, 1098–1101.

Gerner, R.H., and Wilkins, J.N. (1983). CSF cortisol in patients with depression, mania, or anorexia nervosa and in normal subjects. *Am J Psychiatry*, 140, 92–94.

Gerner, R.H., and Yamada, T. (1982). Altered neuropeptide concentrations in cerebrospinal fluid of psychiatric patients. *Brain Res*, 238(1), 298–302.

Gerner, R.H., Post, R.M., and Bunney, W.E. Jr. (1976). A dopaminergic mechanism in mania. *Am J Psychiatry*, 133, 1177–1180.

Gerner, R.H., Post, R.M., Gillin, J.C., and Bunney, W.E. Jr. (1979). Biological and behavioral effects of one night's sleep deprivation in depressed patients and normals. *J Psychiatr Res*, 15, 21–40.

Gerner, R.H., Catlin, D.H., Gorelick, D.A., Hui, K.K., and Li, C.H. (1980). Beta-endorphin: Intravenous infusion causes behavioral change in psychiatric inpatients. *Arch Gen Psychiatry*, 37, 642–647.

Gerner, R.H., Fairbanks, L., Anderson, G.M., Young, J.G., Scheinin, M., Linnoila, M., Hare, T.A., Shaywitz, B.A., and Cohen, D.J. (1984). CSF neurochemistry in depressed, manic, and schizophrenic patients compared with that of normal controls. *Am J Psychiatry*, 141, 1533–1540.

Gershon, E.S., and Jonas, W.Z. (1975). Erythrocyte soluble catechol-O-methyl transferase activity in primary affective disorder. A clinical and genetic study. *Arch Gen Psychiatry*, 32, 1351–1356.

Gesing, A., Bilang-Bleuel, A., Droste, S.K., Linthorst, A.C., Holsboer, F., and Reul, J.M. (2001). Psychological stress increases hippocampal mineralocorticoid receptor levels: Involvement of corticotropin-releasing hormone. *J Neurosci*, 21, 4822–4829.

Gessa, G.L., Pani, L., Serra, G., and Fratta, W. (1995). Animal models of mania. *Adv Biochem Psychopharmacol*, 49, 43–66.

Giambalvo, C.T. (1992a). Protein kinase C and dopamine transport: 1. Effects of amphetamine in vivo. *Neuropharmacology*, 31, 1201–1210.

Giambalvo, C.T. (1992b). Protein kinase C and dopamine transport: 2. Effects of amphetamine in vitro. *Neuropharmacology*, 31, 1211–1222.

Gibbons, J.L. (1964). Cortisol secretion rate in depressive illness. *Arch Gen Psychiatry*, 10, 572–575.

Gillin, J.C., Wyatt, R.J., Fram, D., and Snyder, F. (1978). The relationship between changes in REM sleep and clinical improvement in depressed patients treated with amitriptyline. *Psychopharmacology (Berl)*, 59, 267–272.

Gjerris, A., Fahrenkrug, J., Bojhold, S., and Rafaelsen, O.J. (1981). Vasoactive intestinal polypeptide in cerebrospinal fluid in psychiatric disorders. In C. Perris, G. Struwe, and B. Jansson (Eds.), *Biological Psychiatry 1981* (pp. 359–362). Amsterdam: Elsevier.

Gjerris, A., Rafaelsen, O.J., Vendsborg, P., Fahrenkrug, J., and Rehfeld, J.F. (1984). Vasoactive intestinal polypeptide decreased in cerebrospinal fluid (CSF) in atypical depression. Vasoactive intestinal polypeptide, cholecystokinin and gastrin in CSF in psychiatric disorders. *J Affect Disord*, 7, 325–337.

Gjerris, A., Hammer, M., Vendsborg, P., Christensen, N.J., and Rafaelsen, O.J. (1985). Cerebrospinal fluid vasopressin—changes in depression. *Br J Psychiatry*, 147, 696–701.

Gjessing, R. (1938). Disturbance of somatic functions in catatonia with periodic course, and their compensation. *J Ment Sci*, 84, 608–621.

Glen, A.I., and Reading, H.W. (1973). Regulatory action of lithium in manic-depressive illness. *Lancet*, 2, 1239–1241.

Glen, A.I., Ongley, G.C., and Robinson, K. (1968). Diminished membrane transport in manic-depressive psychosis and recurrent depression. *Lancet*, 2, 241–243.

Glitz, D.A., Manji, H.K., and Moore, G.J. (2002). Mood disorders: Treatment-induced changes in brain neurochemistry and structure. *Semin Clin Neuropsychiatry*, 7, 269–280.

Glue, P.W., Cowen, P.J., Nutt, D.J., Kolakowska, T., and Grahame-Smith, D.G. (1986). The effect of lithium on 5-HT-mediated neuroendocrine responses and platelet 5-HT receptors. *Psychopharmacology (Berl)*, 90, 398–402.

Gnegy, M.E., Hong, P., and Ferrell, S.T. (1993). Phosphorylation of neuromodulin in rat striatum after acute and repeated, intermittent amphetamine. *Brain Res Mol Brain Res*, 20, 289–298.

Godfrey, P.P., McClue, S.J., White, A.M., Wood, A.J., and Grahame-Smith, D.G. (1989). Subacute and chronic in vivo lithium treatment inhibits agonist- and sodium fluoride-stimulated inositol phosphate production in rat cortex. *J Neurochem*, 52, 498–506.

Godwin, C.D., Greenberg, L.B., and Shukla, S. (1984). Consistent dexamethasone suppression test results with mania and depression in bipolar illness. *Am J Psychiatry*, 141, 1263–1265.

Gold, M.S., Pottash, A.L., and Extein, I. (1981). Hypothyroidism and depression. Evidence from complete thyroid function evaluation. *JAMA*, 245, 1919–1922.

Gold, M.S., Pottash, A.L., and Extein, I. (1982). "Symptomless" autoimmune thyroiditis in depression. *Psychiatry Res*, 6, 261–269.

Gold, P.W., and Chrousos, G.P. (1985). Clinical studies with corticotropin releasing factor: Implications for the diagnosis and pathophysiology of depression, Cushing's disease, and adrenal insufficiency. *Psychoneuroendocrinology*, 10, 401–419.

Gold, P.W., and Chrousos, G.P. (2002). Organization of the stress system and its dysregulation in melancholic and atypical depression: High vs. low CRH/NE states. *Mol Psychiatry*, 7, 254–275.

Gold, P.W., Goodwin, F.K., and Reus, V.I. (1978). Vasopressin in affective illness. *Lancet*, 1, 1233–1236.

Gold, P.W., Weingartner, H., Ballenger, J.C., Goodwin, F.K., and Post, R.M. (1979). Effects of 1-desamo-8-D-arginine vasopressin on behaviour and cognition in primary affective disorder. *Lancet*, 2, 992–994.

Gold, P.W., Goodwin, F.K., Post, R.M., and Robertson, G.L. (1981). Vasopressin function in depression and mania [proceedings]. *Psychopharmacol Bull*, 17, 7–9.

Gold, P.W., Ballenger, J.C., Robertson, G.L., Wingartner, H., Rubinow, D.R., Hoban, M.C., Goodwin, F.K., and Post, R.M. (1984a). Vasopressin in affective illness: Direct measurement, clinical trials, and response to hypertonic saline. In R.M. Post and J.C. Ballenger (Eds.), *Neurobiology of Mood Disorders* (pp. 323–339). Baltimore: Williams and Wilkins.

Gold, P.W., Chrousos, G., Kellner, C., Post, R., Roy, A., Augerinos, P., Schulte, H., Oldfield, E., and Loriaux, D.L. (1984b). Psychiatric implications of basic and clinical studies with corticotropin-releasing factor. *Am J Psychiatry*, 141, 619–627.

Gold, P.W., Calabrese, J.R., Kling, M.A., Avgerinos, P., Khan, I., Gallucci, W.T., Tomai, T.P., and Chrousos, G.P. (1986). Abnormal ACTH and cortisol responses to ovine corticotropin releasing factor in patients with primary affective disorder. *Prog Neuropsychopharmacol Biol Psychiatry*, 10, 57–65.

Gold, P.W., Goodwin, F.K., and Chrousos, G.P. (1988). Clinical and biochemical manifestations of depression. Relation to the neurobiology of stress (2). *N Engl J Med*, 319, 413–420.

Goldberg, J.F., Burdick, K.E., and Endick, C.J. (2004). Preliminary randomized, double-blind, placebo-controlled trial of pramipexole added to mood stabilizers for treatment-resistant bipolar depression. *Am J Psychiatry*, 161(3), 564–566.

Goldstein, D.S., Brush, J.E. Jr., Eisenhofer, G., Stull, R., and Esler, M. (1988). In vivo measurement of neuronal uptake of norepinephrine in the human heart. *Circulation*, 78, 41–48.

Goldstein, E.T., and Preskorn, S.H. (1989). Mania triggered by a steroid nasal spray in a patient with stable bipolar disorder. *Am J Psychiatry*, 146, 1076–1077.

Goldstein, J., Van Cauter, E., Linkowski, P., Vanhaelst, L., and Mendlewicz, J. (1980). Thyrotropin nyctohemeral pattern in primary depression: Differences between unipolar and bipolar women. *Life Sci*, 27, 1695–1703.

Goldstein, M., Fuxe, K., Meller, E., Seyfried, C.A., Agnati, L., and Mascagni, F.M. (1987). The characterization of the dopaminergic profile of EMD 23,448, and indolyl-3-butylamine: Selective actions on presynaptic and supersensitive postsynaptic DA receptor populations. *J Neural Transm*, 70, 193–215.

Gomez-Pinilla, F., So, V., and Kesslak, J.P. (2001). Spatial learning induces neurotrophin receptor and synapsin I in the hippocampus. *Brain Res*, 904, 13–19.

Gonzalez-Pinto, A., Imaz, H., De Heredia, J.L., Gutierrez, M., and Mico, J.A. (2001). Mania and tramadol-fluoxetine combination. *Am J Psychiatry*, 158(6), 964–965.

Goodnick, P.J. (1990). Bupropion in chronic fatigue syndrome. *Am J Psychiatry*, 147(8), 1091.

Goodnick, P., and Gershon, S. (1984). Chemotherapy of cognitive disorders in geriatric subjects. *J Clin Psychiatry*, 45, 196–209.

Goodnick, P.J., and Meltzer, H.Y. (1984). Neurochemical changes during discontinuation of lithium prophylaxis. I. Increases in clonidine-induced hypotension. *Biol Psychiatry*, 19, 883–889.

Goodwin, F.K., and Ghaemi, S.N. (1998). Understanding manic-depressive illness. *Arch Gen Psychiatry*, 55(1), 23–25.

Goodwin, F.K., and Jamison, K.R. (1990). *Manic-Depressive Illness*. New York: Oxford University Press.

Goodwin, F., and Sack, R.L. (1973). Affective disorders: The catecholamine hypothesis revisited. In E. Usdin and S. Snyder (Eds.), *Frontiers in Catecholamine Research* (pp. 1157–1164). New York: Pergamon Press.

Goodwin, F.K., and Sack, R.L. (1974). Central dopamine function in affective illness: Evidence from precursors, enzyme inhibitors, and studies of central dopamine turnover. *Adv Biochem Psychopharmacol*, 12(0), 261–279.

Goodwin, F.K., Murphy, D.L., Brodie, H.K., and Bunney, W.E. Jr. (1970). L-DOPA, catecholamines, and behavior: A clinical and biochemical study in depressed patients. *Biol Psychiatry*, 2, 341–366.

Goodwin, F.K., Post, R.M., Dunner, D.L., and Gordon, E.K. (1973). Cerebrospinal fluid amine metabolites in affective illness: The probenecid technique. *Am J Psychiatry*, 130, 73–79.

Goodwin, F.K., Muscettola, G., Gold, P.W., and Wehr, T.A. (1978). Biochemical and pharmacological differentiation of affective disorders: An overview. In H.S. Akiskal and W.L. Webb (Eds.), *Psychiatric Diagnoses: Exploration of Biological Predictors* (pp. 313–336). New York: SP Medical and Scientific Books.

Goodwin, F.K., Prange, A.J. Jr., Post, R.M., Muscettola, G., and Lipton, M.A. (1982). Potentiation of antidepressant effects by L-triiodothyronine in tricyclic nonresponders. *Am J Psychiatry*, 139, 34–38.

Goodwin, G.M., De Souza, R.J., Wood, A.J., and Green, A.R. (1986a). The enhancement by lithium of the 5-HT$_{1A}$ mediated serotonin syndrome produced by 8-OH-DPAT in the rat: Evidence for a post-synaptic mechanism. *Psychopharmacology (Berl)*, 90, 488–493.

Goodwin, G.M., DeSouza, R.J., Wood, A.J., and Green, A.R. (1986b). Lithium decreases 5-HT$_{1A}$ and 5-HT$_2$ receptor and alpha 2-adrenoceptor mediated function in mice. *Psychopharmacology (Berl)*, 90, 482–487.

Gorkin, R.A., and Richelson, E. (1981). Lithium transport by mouse neuroblastoma cells. *Neuropharmacology*, 20, 791–801.

Gottesfeld, Z., Ebstein, B.S., and Samuel, D. (1971). Effect of lithium on concentrations of glutamate and GABA levels in amygdala and hypothalamus of rat. *Nat New Biol*, 234, 124–125.

Gottesman, I.I., and Gould, T.D. (2003). The endophenotype concept in psychiatry: Etymology and strategic intentions. *Am J Psychiatry*, 160(4), 636–645.

Gottesman, I.I., and Shields, J. (1973). Genetic theorizing and schizophrenia. *Br J Psychiatry*, 122(566), 15–30.

Gould, E., Tanapat, P., Rydel, T., and Hastings, N. (2000). Regulation of hippocampal neurogenesis in adulthood. *Biol Psychiatry*, 48, 715–720.

Gould, G.G., Mehta, A.K., Frazer, A., and Ticku, M.K. (2003). Quantitative autoradiographic analysis of the new radioligand [^{3}H](2E)-(5-hydroxy-5,7,8,9-tetrahydro-6H-benzo[a][7]annulen-6-ylidene) ethanoic acid ([^{3}H]NCS-382) at gamma-hydroxybutyric acid (GHB) binding sites in rat brain. *Brain Res*, 979, 51–56.

Gould, T.D., and Manji, H.K. (2002a). Signaling networks in the pathophysiology and treatment of mood disorders. *J Psychosom Res*, 53, 687–697.

Gould, T.D., and Manji, H.K. (2002b). The Wnt signaling pathway in bipolar disorder. *Neuroscientist*, 8(5), 497–511.

Gould, T.D., and Manji, H.K. (2004). The molecular medicine revolution and psychiatry: Bridging the gap between basic neuroscience research and clinical psychiatry. *J Clin Psychiatry*, 65, 598–604.

Gould, T.D., and Manji, H.K. (2005). Glycogen synthase kinase-3: A putative molecular target for lithium mimetic drugs. *Neuropsychopharmacology*, 30(7), 1223–1237.

Gould, T.D., Gray, N.A., and Manji, H.K. (2003). The cellular neurobiology of severe mood and anxiety disorders: Implications for the development of novel therapeutics. In D.S. Charney (Ed.), *Molecular Neurobiology for the Clinician* (pp. 123–227). Washington, DC: American Psychiatric Press.

Gould, T.D., Chen, G., and Manji, H.K. (2004a). In vivo evidence in the brain for lithium inhibition of glycogen synthase kinase-3. *Neuropsychopharmacology*, 29, 32–38.

Gould, T.D., Einat, E., Bhat, R., and Manji, H.K. (2004b). AR-A014418, a selective GSK-3 inhibitor, produces antidepressant-like effects in the forced swim test. *Int J Neuropsychopharmacol*, 7, 1–4.

Gould, T.D., Quiroz, J., Singh, J., Zarate, C., and Manji, H.K. (2004c). Emerging experimental therapeutics for bipolar disorder: Novel insights from the molecular and cellular mechanisms of action of mood stabilizers. *Mol Psychiatry*, 9, 734–755.

Graham, P.M., Booth, J., Boranga, G., Galhenage, S., Myers, C.M., Teoh, C.L., and Cox, L.S. (1982). The dexamethasone suppression test in mania. *J Affect Disord*, 4, 201–211.

Graham, Y.P., Heim, C., Goodman, S.H., Miller, A.H., and Nemeroff, C.B. (1999). The effects of neonatal stress on brain development: Implications for psychopathology. *Dev Psychopathol*, 11, 545–565.

Grahame-Smith, D.G., and Green, A.R. (1974). The role of brain 5-hydroxytryptamine in the hyperactivity produced in rats by lithium and monoamine oxidase inhibition. *Br J Pharmacol*, 52, 19–26.

Gram, L., Larsson, O.M., Johnsen, A.H., and Schousboe, A. (1988). Effects of valproate, vigabatrin and aminooxyacetic acid on release of endogenous and exogenous GABA from cultured neurons. *Epilepsy Res*, 2, 87–95.

Gray, N.A., Zhou, R., Du, J., Moore, G.J., and Manji, H.K. (2003). The use of mood stabilizers as plasticity enhancers in the treatment of neuropsychiatric disorders. *J Clin Psychiatry*, 64(Suppl. 5), 3–17.

Gray, T.S., and Morley, J.E. (1986). Neuropeptide Y: Anatomical distribution and possible function in mammalian nervous system. *Life Sci*, 38(5), 389–401.

Greden, J.F. (1982). Biological markers of melancholia and reclassification of depressive disorders. *Encephale*, 8, 193–202.

Greden, J.F., Price, H.L., Genero, N., Feinberg, M., and Levine, S. (1984). Facial emg activity levels predict treatment outcome in depression. *Psychiatry Res*, 13(4), 345–352.

Greengard, P., Valtorta, F., Czernik, A.J., and Benfenati, F. (1993). Synaptic vesicle phosphoproteins and regulation of synaptic function. *Science*, 259, 780–785.

Greenspan, K., Schildkraut, J.J., Gordon, E.K., Baer, L., Aronoff, M.S., and Durell, J. (1970). Catecholamine metabolism in affective disorders. 3. MHPG and other catecholamine metabolites in patients treated with lithium carbonate. *J Psychiatr Res*, 7, 171–183.

Greenwood, T.A., Alexander, M., Keck, P.E., McElroy, S., Sadovnick, A.D., Remick, R.A., and Kelsoe, J.R. (2001). Evidence for linkage disequilibrium between the dopamine transporter and bipolar disorder. *Am J Med Genet*, 105, 145–151.

Greil, W., Eisenried, F., Becker, B.F., and Duhm, J. (1977). Interindividual differences in the Na+-dependent Li+ countertransport system and in the Li+ distribution ratio across the red cell membrane among Li+-treated patients. *Psychopharmacology (Berl)*, 53, 19–26.

Griebel, G., Simiand, J., Steinberg, R., Jung, M., Gully, D., Roger, P., Geslin, M., Scatton, B., Maffrand, J.P., and Soubrie, P. (2002). 4-(2-chloro-4-methoxy-5-methylphenyl)-n-[(1s)-2-cyclopropyl-1-(3-fluoro-4-methylphenyl)ethyl]5-methyl-n-(2-propynyl)-1, 3-thiazol-2-amine hydrochloride (ssr125543a), a potent and selective corticotrophin-releasing factor(1) receptor antagonist. II. Characterization in rodent models of stress-related disorders. *J Pharmacol Exp Ther*, 301(1), 333–345.

Griffiths, E.C. (1985). Thyrotrophin releasing hormone: Endocrine and central effects. *Psychoneuroendocrinology*, 10, 225–235.

Grignon, S., Levy, N., Couraud, F., and Bruguerolle, B. (1996). Tyrosine kinase inhibitors and cycloheximide inhibit Li+ protection of cerebellar granule neurons switched to non-depolarizing medium. *Eur J Pharmacol*, 315, 111–114.

Grillo, C., Piroli, G., Gonzalez, S.L., Angulo, J., McEwen, B.S., and De Nicola, A.F. (1994). Glucocorticoid regulation of mRNA encoding (Na+K) ATPase alpha 3 and beta 1 subunits in rat brain measured by in situ hybridization. *Brain Res*, 657, 83–91.

Grimes, C.A., and Jope, R.S. (1999). Cholinergic stimulation of early growth response-1 DNA binding activity requires protein kinase C and mitogen-activated protein kinase kinase activation and is inhibited by sodium valproate in SH-SY5Y cells. *J Neurochem*, 73, 1384–1392.

Grof, E., Brown, G.M., Grof, P., and Van Loon, G.R. (1986). Effects of lithium administration on plasma catecholamines. *Psychiatry Res*, 19, 87–92.

Gross-Isseroff, R., Israeli, M., and Biegon, A. (1989). Autoradiographic analysis of tritiated imipramine binding in the human brain post mortem: Effects of suicide. *Arch Gen Psychiatry*, 46, 237–241.

Gross-Isseroff, G., Salama, D., Israeli, M., and Biegon, A. (1990a). Autoradiographic analysis of [3H]ketanserin binding in the human brain postmortem: Effect of suicide. *Brain Res*, 507, 208–215.

Gross-Isseroff, R., Dillon, K.A., Fieldust, S.J., and Biegon, A. (1990b). Autoradiographic analysis of α1-noradrenergic receptors in the human brain postmortem. Effect of suicide. *Arch Gen Psychiatry*, 47: 1049–1053.

Gross-Isseroff, R., Dillon, K.A., Israeli, M., and Biegon, A. (1990c). Regionally selective increases in mu opioid receptor density in the brains of suicide victims. *Brain Res*, 530, 312–316.

Grossman, F., and Potter, W.Z. (1999). Catecholamines in depression: A cumulative study of urinary norepinephrine and its major metabolites in unipolar and bipolar depressed patients versus healthy volunteers at the NIMH. *Psychiatry Res*, 87, 21–27.

Grote, S.S., Moses, S.G., Robins, E., Hudgens, R.W., and Croninger, A.B. (1974). A study of selected catecholamine metabolizing enzymes: A comparison of depressive suicides and alcoholic suicides with controls. *J Neurochem*, 23, 791–802.

Grunhage, F., Schulze, T.G., Muller, D.J., Lanczik, M., Franzek, E., Albus, M., Borrmann-Hassenbach, M., Knapp, M., Cichon, S., Maier, W., Rietschel, M., Propping, P., and Nothen, M.M. (2000). Systematic screening for DNA sequence variation in the coding region of the human dopamine transporter gene (DAT1). *Mol Psychiatry*, 5, 275–282.

Guerri, C., Ribelles, M., and Grisolia, S. (1981). Effects of lithium, and lithium and alcohol administration on (Na + K)-ATPase. *Biochem Pharmacol*, 30, 25–30.

Guidotti, A., Auta, J., Davis, J.M., Di-Giorgi-Gerevini, V., Dwivedi, Y., Grayson, D.R., Impagnatiello, F., Pandey, G.,

Pesold, C., Sharma, R., Uzunov, D., and Costa, E. (2000). Decrease in reelin and glutamic acid decarboxylase67 (GAD67) expression in schizophrenia and bipolar disorder. A post-mortem brain study. *Arch Gen Psychiatry*, 57, 1061–1069.

Gurevich, E.V., and Joyce, J.N. (1996). Comparison of [3H]paroxetine and [3H]cyanoimipramine for quantitative measurement of serotonin transporter sites in human brain. *Neuropsychopharmacology*, 14, 309–323.

Gutierrez, B., Fananas, L., Arranz, M.J., Valles, V., Guillamat, R., van Os, J., and Collier, D. (1996). Allelic association analysis of the 5-HT2C receptor gene in bipolar affective disorder. *Neurosci Lett*, 212, 65–67.

Habib, K.E., Weld, K.P., Rice, K.C., Pushkas, J., Champoux, M., Listwak, S., Webster, E.L., Atkinson, A.J., Schulkin, J., Contoreggi, C., Chrousos, G.P., McCann, S.M., Suomi, S.J., Higley, J.D., and Gold, P.W. (2000). Oral administration of a corticotropin-releasing hormone receptor antagonist significantly attenuates behavioral, neuroendocrine, and autonomic responses to stress in primates. *Proc Natl Acad Sci USA*, 97(11), 6079–6084.

Haggerty, J.J. Jr., Silva, S.G., Marquardt, M., Mason, G.A., Chang, H.Y., Evans, D.L., Golden, R.N., and Pedersen, C. (1997). Prevalence of antithyroid antibodies in mood disorders. *Depress Anxiety*, 5, 91–96.

Hahn, C.G., and Friedman, E. (1999). Abnormalities in protein kinase C signaling and the pathophysiology of bipolar disorder. *Bipolar Disord*, 1, 81–86.

Halaris, A.E. (1978). Plasma 3-methoxy-4-hydroxyphenylglycol in manic psychosis. *Am J Psychiatry*, 135, 493–494.

Hall, A.C., Brennan, A., Goold, R.G., Cleverley, K., Lucas, F.R., Gordon-Weeks, P.R., and Salinas, P.C. (2002). Valproate regulates GSK-3-mediated axonal remodeling and synapsin I clustering in developing neurons. *Mol Cell Neurosci*, 20, 257–270.

Hallcher, L.M., and Sherman, W.R. (1980). The effects of lithium ion and other agents on the activity of myo-inositol-1-phosphatase from bovine brain. *J Biol Chem*, 255, 10896–10901.

Halper, J.P., Brown, R.P., Sweeney, J.A., Kocsis, J.H., Peters, A., and Mann, J.J. (1988). Blunted beta-adrenergic responsivity of peripheral blood mononuclear cells in endogenous depression. Isoproterenol dose-response studies. *Arch Gen Psychiatry*, 45, 241–244.

Hamilton, S.R., Liu, B., Parsons, R.E., Papadopoulos, N., Jen, J., Powell, S.M., Krush, A.J., Berk, T., Cohen, Z., and Tetu B. (1995). The molecular basis of Turcot's syndrome. *N Engl J Med*, 332, 839–847.

Hao, Y.L., Creson, T., Zhang, L., Li, P., Yuan, P.X., Gould, T.D., Manji, H.K., and Chen, G. (2004). Mood-stabilizer valproate promotes ERK pathway dependent cortical neuronal growth and neurogenesis. *J Neurosci*, 24, 6590–6599.

Harder, R., and Bonisch, H. (1985). Effects of monovalent ions on the transport of noradrenaline across the plasma membrane of neuronal cells (PC-12 cells). *J Neurochem*, 45, 1154–1162.

Harrison-Read, P.E. (1979). Evidence from behavioural reactions to fenfluramine, 5-hydroxytryptophan, and 5-methoxy-N,N-dimethyltryptamine for differential effects of short-term and long-term lithium on indoleaminergic mechanisms in rats [proceedings]. *Br J Pharmacol*, 66, 144P–145P.

Harro, J., Tonissaar, M., and Eller, M. (2001). The effects of CRA 1000, a non-peptide antagonist of corticotropin-releasing factor receptor type 1, on adaptive behaviour in the rat. *Neuropeptides*, 35(2), 100–109.

Hashimoto, H., Onishi, H., Koide, S., Kai, T., and Yamagami, S. (1996). Plasma neuropeptide Y in patients with major depressive disorder. *Neurosci Lett*, 216(1), 57–60.

Hashimoto, R., Hough, C., Nakazawa, T., Yamamoto, T., and Chuang, D.M. (2002). Lithium protection against glutamate excitotoxicity in rat cerebral cortical neurons: Involvement of NMDA receptor inhibition possibly by decreasing NR2B tyrosine phosphorylation. *J Neurochem*, 80(4), 589–597.

Haskett, R.F. (1985). Diagnostic categorization of psychiatric disturbance in Cushing's syndrome. *Am J Psychiatry*, 142, 911–916.

Hasler, G., Drevets, W.C., Gould, T.D., Gottesman, I.I., and Manji, H.K. (2006). Toward constructing an endophenotype strategy for bipolar disorders. *Biol Psychiatry*, 60(2), 93–105.

Hassel, B., Iversen, E.G., Gjerstad, L., and Tauboll, E. (2001). Up-regulation of hippocampal glutamate transport during chronic treatment with sodium valproate. *J Neurochem*, 77, 1285–1292.

Hatterer, J.A., Kocsis, J.H, and Stokes, P.E. (1988). Thyroid function in patients maintained on lithium. *Psychiatry Res*, 26, 249–257.

Hayashi, T., Umemori, H., Mishina, M., and Yamamoto, T. (1999). The AMPA receptor interacts with and signals through the protein tyrosine kinase Lyn. *Nature*, 397, 72–76.

Haydon, P.G. (2001). GLIA: Listening and talking to the synapse. *Nat Rev Neurosci*, 2, 185–193.

Healy, D., Carney, P.A., and Leonard, B.E. (1983). Monoamine-related markers of depression: Changes following treatment. *J Psychiatr Res*, 17, 251–260.

Healy, D., Carney, P.A., O'Halloran, A., and Leonard, B.E. (1985). Peripheral adrenoceptors and serotonin receptors in depression. Changes associated with response to treatment with trazodone or amitriptyline. *J Affect Disord*, 9, 285–296.

Heckers, S., Stone, D., Walsh, J., Shick, J., Koul, P., and Benes, F.M. (2002). Differential hippocampal expression of glutamic acid decarboxylase 65 and 67 messenger RNA in bipolar disorder and schizophrenia. *Arch Gen Psychiatry*, 59, 521–529.

Hedge, G.A., and de Wied, D. (1971). Corticotropin and vasopressin secretion after hypothalamic implantation of atropine. *Endocrinology*, 88, 1257–1259.

Hedge, G.A., and Smelik, P.G. (1968). Corticotropin release: Inhibition by intrahypothalamic implantation of atropine. *Science*, 159, 891–892.

Hedlund, B., Abens, J., and Bartfai, T. (1983). Vasoactive intestinal polypeptide and muscarinic receptors: Supersensitivity induced by long-term atropine treatment. *Science*, 220, 519–521.

Heilig, M., and Widerlöv, E. (1990). Neuropeptide Y: An overview of central distribution, functional aspects, and possible involvement in neuropsychiatric illnesses. *Acta Psychiatr Scand*, 82(2), 95–114.

Heilig, M., Wahlestedt, C., Ekman, R., and Widerlöv, E. (1988a). Antidepressant drugs increase the concentration of neuropeptide Y (NPY)-like immunoreactivity in the rat brain. *Eur J Pharmacol*, 147, 465–467.

Heilig, M., Wahlestedt, C., and Widerlöv, E. (1988b). Neuropeptide Y (NPY)-induced suppression of activity in the rat: Evidence for NPY receptor heterogeneity and for interaction with alpha-adrenoceptors. *Eur J Pharmacol*, 157, 205–213.

Hein, M.D., and Jackson, I.M. (1990). Review: Thyroid function in psychiatric illness. *Gen Hosp Psychiatry*, 12, 232–244.

Hendrick, V., Altshuler, L., and Whybrow, P. (1998). Psycho-neuroendocrinology of mood disorders. The hypothalamic–pituitary–thyroid axis. *Psychiatr Clin North Am*, 21, 277–292.

Heninger, G.R., Charney, D.S., and Sternberg, D.E. (1983). Lithium carbonate augmentation of antidepressant treatment. An effective prescription for treatment-refractory depression. *Arch Gen Psychiatry*, 40, 1335–1342.

Heninger, G.R., Charney, D.S., and Price, L.H. (1988). Alpha 2-Adrenergic receptor sensitivity in depression. The plasma MHPG, behavioral, and cardiovascular responses to yohimbine. *Arch Gen Psychiatry*, 45, 718–726.

Henn, F.A., and McKinney, W.T. (1987). Animal models in psychiatry. In H.Y. Meltzer (Ed.), *Psychopharmacology: The Third Generation of Progress* (pp. 687–695). New York: Raven Press.

Hermoni, M., Lerer, B., Ebstein, R.P., and Belmaker, R.H. (1980). Chronic lithium prevents reserpine-induced supersensitivity of adeylate cyclase. *J Pharm Pharmacol*, 32, 510–511.

Hermoni, M., Barzilai, A., and Rahamimoff, H. (1987). Modulation of the Na+-Ca2+ antiport by its ionic environment: The effect of lithium. *Isr J Med Sci*, 23, 44–48.

Hertz, M. (1964). On rhythmic phenomenon in thyroidectomized patients. *Acta Psychiatr Scand*, 40, 449–456.

Herve, D., Levi-Strauss, M., Marey-Semper, I., Verney, C., Tassin, J.P., Glowinski, J., and Girault, J.A. (1993). G(olf) and Gs in rat basal ganglia: possible involvement of G(olf) in the coupling of dopamine D1 receptor with adenylyl cyclase. *J Neurosci*, 13, 2237–2248.

Herzog, E.D., Aton, S.J., Numano, R., Sakaki, Y., and Tei, H. (2004). Temporal precision in the mammalian circadian system: A reliable clock from less reliable neurons. *J Biol Rhythms*, 19(1), 35–46.

Hesketh, J., and Glen, I. (1978). Lithium transport from cerebrospinal fluid. *Biochem Pharmacol*, 27(5), 813–814.

Hesketh, J.C., Glen, A.I.M., and Reading, H.W. (1977). Membrane ATPase activities in depressive illness. *J Neurochem*, 28, 1401–1402.

Hetman, M., Cavanaugh, J.E., Kimelman, D., and Xia, Z. (2000). Role of glycogen synthase kinase-3beta in neuronal apoptosis induced by trophic withdrawal. *J Neurosci*, 20, 2567–2574.

Heuser, I., Yassouridis, A., and Holsboer, F. (1994). The combined dexamethasone/CRH test: A refined laboratory test for psychiatric disorders. *J Psychiatr Res*, 28, 341–356.

Hicks, R.A., Moore, J.D., Hayes, C., Phillips, N., and Hawkins, J. (1979). REM sleep deprivation increases aggressiveness in male rats. *Physiol Behav*, 22, 1097–1100.

Hilfiker, S., Pieribone, V.A., Czernik, A.J., Kao, H.T., Augustine, G.J., and Greengard, P. (1999a). Synapsins as regulators of neurotransmitter release. *Philos Trans R Soc Lond B Biol Sci*, 354, 269–279.

Hilfiker, S., Pieribone, V.A., Nordstedt, C., Greengard, P., and Czernik, A.J. (1999b). Regulation of synaptotagmin I phosphorylation by multiple protein kinases. *J Neurochem*, 73, 921–932.

Himmelhoch, J.M., Thase, M.E., Mallinger, A.G., and Houck, P. (1991). Tranylcypromine versus imipramine in anergic bipolar depression. *Am J Psychiatry*, 148, 910–916.

Hirvonen, M.R., Paljarvi, L., Naukkarinen, A., Komulainen, H., and Savolainen, K.M. (1990). Potentiation of malaoxon-induced convulsions by lithium: early neuronal injury, phosphoinositide signaling, and calcium. *Toxicol Appl Pharmacol*, 104, 276–289.

Hitzemann, R. (2000). Animal models of psychiatric disorders and their relevance to alcoholism. *Alcohol Res Health*, 24, 149–158.

Hitzemann, R., Mark, C., Hirschowitz, J., and Garver, D. (1989). RBC lithium transport in the psychoses. *Biol Psychiatry*, 25, 296–304.

Ho, A.K., and Tsai, C.S. (1975). Lithium and ethanol preference. *J Pharm Pharmacol*, 27, 58–59.

Ho, A.K., Loh, H.H., Craves, F., Hitzemann, R.J., and Gershon, S. (1970). The effect of prolonged lithium treatment on the synthesis rate and turnover of monoamines in brain regions of rats. *Eur J Pharmacol*, 10, 72–78.

Hoehe, M., Valido, G., and Matussek, N. (1988). Growth hormone, noradrenaline, blood pressure and cortisol responses to clonidine in healthy male volunteers: Dose–response relations and reproducibility. *Psychoneuroendocrinology*, 13, 409–418.

Hoesche, C., Bartsch, P., and Kilimann, M.W. (1995). The CRE consensus sequence in the synapsin I gene promoter region confers constitutive activation but no regulation by cAMP in neuroblastoma cells. *Biochim Biophys Acta*, 1261, 249–256.

Hofmann, P., Gangadhar, B.N., Probst, C., Koinig, G., and Hatzinger, R. (1994). TSH response to TRH and ECT. *J Affect Disord*, 32, 127–131.

Hokfelt, T., Lundberg, J.M., Tatemoto, K., Mutt, V., Terenius, L., Polak, J., Bloom, S., Sasek, C., Elde, R., and Goldstein, M. (1983). Neuropeptide y (NPY)- and FMRFamide neuropeptide-like immunoreactivities in catecholamine neurons of the rat medulla oblongata. *Acta Physiol Scand*, 117(2), 315–318.

Hokin-Neaverson, M., and Jefferson, J.W. (1989a). Erythrocyte sodium pump activity in bipolar affective disorder and other psychiatric disorders. *Neuropsychobiology*, 22, 1–7.

Hokin-Neaverson, M., and Jefferson, J.W. (1989b). Deficient erythrocyte Na,K-ATPase activity in different affective states in bipolar affective disorder and normalization by lithium therapy. *Neuropsychobiology*, 22, 18–22.

Hokin-Neaverson, M., Spiegel, D.A., and Lewis, W.C. (1974). Deficiency of erythrocyte sodium pump activity in bipolar manic-depressive psychosis. *Life Sci*, 15, 1739–1748.

Hokin-Neaverson, M., Burckhardt, W.A., and Jefferson, J.W. (1976). Increased erythrocyte Na+ pump and NaK-ATPase activity during lithium therapy. *Res Commun Chem Pathol Pharmacol*, 14, 117–126.

Holemans, S., De Paermentier, F., Horton, R.W., Crompton, M.R., Katona, C.L., and Maloteaux, J.M. (1993). NMDA glutamatergic receptors, labelled with [3H]MK-801, in brain samples from drug-free depressed suicides. *Brain Res*, 616, 138–143.

Holian, O., and Nelson, R. (1992). Action of long-chain fatty acids on protein kinase C activity: Comparison of omega-6 and omega-3 fatty acids. *Anticancer Res*, 12, 975–980.

Holmes, A., Kinney, J.W., Wrenn, C.C., Li, Q., Yang, R.J., Ma, L., Vishwanath, J., Saavedra, M.C., Innerfield, C.E., Jacoby, A.S., Shine, J., Iismaa, T.P., and Crawley, J.N. (2003). Galanin GAL-R1 receptor null mutant mice display increased anxiety-like behavior specific to the elevated plus-maze. *Neuropsychopharmacology*, 28(6), 1031–1044.

Holsboer, F. (2000). The stress hormone system is back on the map. *Curr Psychiatry Rep*, 2(6), 454–456.

Holsboer, F. (2001). Stress, hypercortisolism and corticosteroid receptors in depression: Implications for therapy. *J Affect Disord*, 62(1-2), 77–91.

Holsboer, F., Gerken, A., Stalla, G.K., and Muller, O.A. (1985). ACTH, cortisol, and corticosterone output after ovine corticotrophin-releasing factor challenge during depression and after recovery. *Biol Psychiatry*, 20(3), 276–286.

Holsboer, F., Lauer, C.J., Schreiber, W., and Krieg, J.C. (1995). Altered hypothalamic–pituitary–adrenocortical regulation in healthy subjects at high familial risk for affective disorders. *Neuroendocrinology*, 62(4), 340–347.

Holzbauer, M., and Youdim, M.B. (1973). The oestrous cycle and monoamine oxidase activity. *Br J Pharmacol*, 48(4), 600–608.

Honchar, M.P., Olney, J.W., and Sherman, W.R. (1983). Systemic cholinergic agents induce seizures and brain damage in lithium-treated rats. *Science*, 220, 323–325.

Honer, C., Nam, K., Fink, C., Marshall, P., Ksander, G., Chatelain, R.E., Cornell, W., Steele, R., Schweitzer, R., and Schumacher, C. (2003). Glucocorticoid receptor antagonism by cyproterone acetate and ru486. *Mol Pharmacol*, 63(5), 1012–1020.

Honer, W.G., Falkai, P., Bayer, T.A., Xie, J., Hu, L., Li, H.Y., Arango, V., Mann, J.J., Dwork, A.J., and Trimble, W.S. (2002). Abnormalities of SNARE mechanism proteins in anterior frontal cortex in severe mental illness. *Cereb Cortex*, 12, 349–356.

Hong, J.S., Tilson, H.A., and Yoshikawa, K. (1983). Effects of lithium and haloperidol administration on the rat brain levels of substance P. *J Pharmacol Exp Ther*, 224, 590–593.

Hong, S.E., Shugart, Y.Y., Huang, D.T., Shahwan, S.A., Grant, P.E., Hourihane, J.O., Martin, N.D., and Walsh, C.A. (2000). Autosomal recessive lissencephaly with cerebellar hypoplasia is associated with human *RELN* mutations. *Nat Genet*, 26, 93–96.

Horgan, K., Cooke, E., Hallett, M.B., and Mansel, R.E. (1986). Inhibition of protein kinase C mediated signal transduction by tamoxifen. Importance for antitumour activity. *Biochem Pharmacol*, 35(24), 4463–4465.

Hotsenpiller, G., Giorgetti, M., and Wolf, M.E. (2001). Alterations in behaviour and glutamate transmission following presentation of stimuli previously associated with cocaine exposure. *Eur J Neurosci*, 14(11), 1843–1855.

Hotta, I., and Yamawaki, S. (1988). Possible involvement of presynaptic 5-HT autoreceptors in effect of lithium on 5-HT release in hippocampus of rat. *Neuropharmacology*, 27, 987–992.

Hough, C.J., Irwin, R.P., Gao, X.M., Rogawski, M.A., and Chuang, D.M. (1996). Carbamazepine inhibition of *N*-methyl-D-aspartate-evoked calcium influx in rat cerebellar granule cells. *J Pharmacol Exp Ther*, 276, 143–149.

Hough, C., Lu, S.J., Davis, C.L., Chuang, D.M., and Post, R.M. (1999). Elevated basal and thapsigargin-stimulated intracellular calcium of platelets and lymphocytes from bipolar affective disorder patients measured by a fluorometric microassay. *Biol Psychiatry*, 46, 247–255.

Hovatta, I., Tennant, R.S., Helton, R., Marr, R.A., Singer, O., Redwine, J.M., Ellison, J.A., Schadt, E.E., Verma, I.M., Lockhart, D.J., and Barlow, C. (2005). Glyoxalase 1 and glutathione reductase 1 regulate anxiety in mice. *Nature*, 438(7068), 662–666.

Hrdina, P.D., Demeter, E., Vu, T.B., Sotonyi, P., and Palkovits, M. (1993). 5-HT uptake sites and 5-HT2 receptors in brain of antidepressant-free suicide victims/depressives: Increase in 5-HT2 sites in cortex and amygdala. *Brain Res*, 614, 37–44.

Hrdina, P.D., Bakish, D., Chudzik, J., Ravindran, A., and Lapierre, Y.D. (1995). Serotonergic markers in platelets of patients with major depression: Upregulation of 5-HT$_2$ receptors. *J Psychiatry Neurosci*, 20, 11–19.

Hrdina, P.D., Faludi, G., Li, Q., Bendotti, C., Tekes, K., Sotonyi, P., and Palkovits, M. (1998). Growth-associated protein (GAP-43), its mRNA, and protein kinase C (PKC) isoenzymes in brain regions of depressed suicides. *Mol Psychiatry*, 3, 411–418.

Huang, L.T., Liou, C.W., Yang, S.N., Lai, M.C., Hung, P.L., Wang, T.J., Cheng, S.C., and Wu, C.L. (2002). Aminophylline aggravates long-term morphological and cognitive damages in status epilepticus in immature rats. *Neurosci Lett*, 321(3), 137–140.

Huang, X., Wu, D.Y., Chen, G., Manji, H., and Chen, D.F. (2003). Support of retinal ganglion cell survival and axon regeneration by lithium through a Bcl-2-dependent mechanism. *Invest Ophthalmol Vis Sci*, 44, 347–354.

Hucks, D., Lowther, S., Crompton, M.R., Katona, C.L., and Horton, R.W. (1997). Corticotropin-releasing factor binding sites in cortex of depressed suicides. *Psychopharmacology (Berl)*, 134, 174–178.

Huey, L.Y., Janowsky, D.S., Judd, L.L., Abrams, A., Parker, D., and Clopton, P. (1981). Effects of lithium carbonate on methylphenidate-induced mood, behavior, and cognitive processes. *Psychopharmacology (Berl)*, 73, 161–164.

Hughes, J.H., Dunne, F., and Young, A.H. (2000). Effects of acute tryptophan depletion on mood and suicidal ideation in bipolar patients symptomatically stable on lithium. *Br J Psychiatry*, 177, 447–451.

Hunter, R., Christie, J.E., Whalley, L.J., Bennie, J., Carroll, S., Dick, H., Goodwin, G.M., Wilson, H., and Fink, G. (1989). Luteinizing hormone responses to luteinizing hormone releasing hormone (LHRH) in acute mania and the effects of lithium on LHRH and thyrotrophin releasing hormone tests in volunteers. *Psychol Med*, 19(1), 69–77.

Hurd, Y.L. (2002). Subjects with major depression or bipolar disorder show reduction of prodynorphin mRNA expression in discrete nuclei of the amygdaloid complex. *Mol Psychiatry*, 7, 75–81.

Hurd, Y.L., Herman, M.M., Hyde, T.M., Bigelow, L.B., Weinberger, D.R., and Kleinman, J.E. (1997). Prodynorphin mRNA expression is increased in the patch versus matrix compartment of the caudate nucleus in suicide subjects. *Mol Psychiatry*, 2, 495–500.

Hurley, S.C. (2002). Lamotrigine update and its use in mood disorders. *Ann Pharmacother*, 36, 860–873.

Husum, H., Vasquez, P.A., and Mathe, A.A. (2001). Changed concentrations of tachykinins and neuropeptide Y in brain of a rat model of depression: Lithium treatment normalizes tachykinins. *Neuropsychopharmacology*, 24, 183–191.

Ichikawa, J., and Meltzer, H.Y. (1999). Valproate and carbamazepine increase prefrontal dopamine release by 5-HT$_{1A}$ receptor activation. *Eur J Pharmacol*, 380, R1–R3.

Ichikawa, J., Dai, J., and Meltzer, H.Y. (2001). DOI, a 5-HT2A/2C receptor agonist, attenuates clozapine-induced cortical dopamine release. *Brain Res*, 907(1-2), 151–155.

Ichimiya, T., Suhara, T., Sudo, Y., Okubo, Y., Nakayama, K., Nankai, M., Inoue, M., Yasuno, F., Takano, A., Maeda, J., and Shibuya, H. (2002). Serotonin transporter binding in patients with mood disorders: A PET study with [11C](+)McN5652. *Biol Psychiatry*, 51(9), 715–722.

Ikeda, Y., Ijima, M., and Nomura, S. (1982). Serum dopamine-beta-hydroxylase in manic-depressive psychosis. *Br J Psychiatry*, 140, 209–210.

Ikonomov, O.C., and Manji, H.K. (1999). Molecular mechanisms underlying mood stabilization in manic-depressive illness: The phenotype challenge. *Am J Psychiatry*, 156(10), 1506–1514.

Impagnatiello, F., Guidotti, A.R., Pesold, C., Dwivedi, Y., Caruncho, H., Pisu, M.G., Uzunov, D.P., Smalheiser, N.R., Davis, J.M., Pandey, G.N., Pappas, G.D., Tueting, P., Sharma, R.P., and Costa, E. (1998). A decrease of reelin expression as a putative vulnerability factor in schizophrenia. *Proc Natl Acad Sci USA*, 95, 15718–15723.

Ingbar, S.H., and Braverman, L.E. (Eds.). (1986). *Werner's, the Thyroid: A Fundamental and Clinical Text* (5th Edition). New York: Lippincott.

Inoue, T., Tsuchiya, K., and Koyama, T. (1996). Serotonergic activation reduces defensive freezing in the conditioned fear paradigm. *Pharmacol Biochem Behav*, 53, 825–831.

Inouye, M., Yamamura, H., and Nakano, A. (1995). Lithium delays the radiation-induced apoptotic process in external granule cells of mouse cerebellum. *J Radiat Res (Tokyo)*, 36, 203–208.

Insel, T.R., Kalin, N.H., Guttmacher, L.B., Cohen, R.M., and Murphy, D.L. (1982). The dexamethasone suppression test in patients with primary obsessive-compulsive disorder. *Psychiatry Res*, 6, 153–160.

Insel, T.R., Hamilton, J.A., Guttmacher, L.B., and Murphy, D.L. (1983). D-amphetamine in obsessive-compulsive disorder. *Psychopharmacology (Berl)*, 80(3), 231–235.

Irwin, M., Brown, M., Patterson, T., Hauger, R., Mascovich, A., and Grant, I. (1991). Neuropeptide Y and natural killer cell activity: Findings in depression and Alzheimer caregiver stress. *FAESB J*, 5, 3100–3107.

Iwata, S., Hewlett, G.H., and Gnegy, M.E. (1997a). Amphetamine increases the phosphorylation of neuromodulin and synapsin I in rat striatal synaptosomes. *Synapse*, 26, 281–291.

Iwata, S.I., Hewlett, G.H., Ferrell, S.T., Kantor, L., and Gnegy, M.E. (1997b). Enhanced dopamine release and phosphorylation of synapsin I and neuromodulin in striatal synaptosomes after repeated amphetamine. *J Pharmacol Exp Ther*, 283, 1445–1452.

Jacobs, B.L., Praag, H., and Gage, F.H. (2000). Adult brain neurogenesis and psychiatry: A novel theory of depression. *Mol Psychiatry*, 5, 262–269.

Jacobs, D., and Silverstone, T. (1986). Dextroamphetamine-induced arousal in human subjects as a model for mania. *Psychol Med*, 16, 323–329.

Jahn, H., Schick, M., Kiefer, F., Kellner, M., Yassouridis, A., and Wiedemann, K. (2004). Metyrapone as additive treatment in major depression: A double-blind and placebo-controlled trial. *Arch Gen Psychiatry*, 61(12), 1235–1244.

Janowsky, D.S., and Overstreet, D.H. (1995). The role of acetylcholine mechanisms in mood disorders. In D.J. Kupfer (Ed.), *Psychopharmacology: The Fourth Generation of Progress* (pp. 945–956). New York: Raven Press.

Janowsky, D.S., and Risch, S.C. (1984). Choinomimetic and anticholinergic drugs used to investigate an acetylcholine hypothesis of affective disorders and stress. *Drug Dev Res*, 125–142.

Janowsky, D.S., el-Yousef, K., Davis, J.M., and Sekerke, H.J. (1973). Parasympathetic suppression of manic symptoms by physostigmine. *Arch Gen Psychiatry*, 28(4), 542–547.

Janowsky, D., Judd, L., Huey, L., Roitman, N., Parker, D., and Segal, D. (1978). Naloxone effects on manic symptoms and growth-hormone levels. *Lancet*, 2, 320.

Janowsky, D., Judd, L., Huey, L., Roitman, N., and Parker, D. (1979). Naloxone effects on serum growth hormone and prolactin in man. *Psychopharmacology (Berl)*, 65, 95–97.

Janowsky, D.S., Overstreet, D.H., and Nurnberger, J.I. Jr. (1994). Is cholinergic sensitivity a genetic marker for the affective disorders? *Am J Med Genet*, 54, 335–344.

Jensen, J.B., and Mork, A. (1997). Altered protein phosphorylation in the rat brain following chronic lithium and carbamazepine treatments. *Eur Neuropsychopharmacol*, 7, 173–179.

Jensen, J.B., Mikkelsen, J.D., and Mork, A. (2000). Increased adenylyl cyclase type 1 mRNA, but not adenylyl cyclase type 2 in the rat hippocampus following antidepressant treatment. *Eur Neuropsychopharmacol*, 10, 105–111.

Jimenez-Vasquez, P.A., Overstreet, D.H., and Mathe, A.A. (2000). Neuropeptide Y in male and female brains of Flinders Sensitive Line, a rat model of depression. Effects of electroconvulsive stimuli. *J Psychiatr Res*, 34, 405–412.

Jimerson, D.C., Post, R.M., Carman, J.S., van Kammen, D.P., Wood, J.H., Goodwin, F.K., and Bunney, W.E. Jr. (1979). CSF calcium: Clinical correlates in affective illness and schizophrenia. *Biol Psychiatry*, 14, 37–51.

Jimerson, D.C., Nurnberger, J.I. Jr., Post, R.M., Gershon, E.S., and Kopin, I.J. (1981). Plasma MHPG in rapid cyclers and healthy twins. *Arch Gen Psychiatry*, 38, 1287–1290.

Jimerson, D.C., van Kammen, D.P., Post, R.M., Docherty, J.P., and Bunney, W.E. Jr. (1982). Diazepam in schizophrenia: A preliminary double-blind trial. *Am J Psychiatry*, 139(4), 489–491.

Jimerson, D.C., Insel, T.R., Reus, V.I., and Kopin, I.J. (1983). Increased plasma MHPG in dexamethasone-resistant depressed patients. *Arch Gen Psychiatry*, 40(2), 173–176.

Joffe, H., and Cohen, L.S. (1998). Estrogen, serotonin, and mood disturbance: Where is the therapeutic bridge? *Biol Psychiatry*, 44, 798–811.

Joffe, R.T., Roy-Byrne, P.P., Udhe, T.W., and Post, R.M. (1984). Thyroid function and affective illness: A reappraisal. *Biol Psychiatry*, 19(12), 1685–1691.

Joffe, R.T., Post, R.M., and Uhde, T.W. (1986). Effects of carbamazepine on serum electrolytes in affectively ill patients. *Psychol Med*, 16, 331–335.

Joffe, R.T., Kutcher, S., and MacDonald, C. (1988). Thyroid function and bipolar affective disorder. *Psychiatry Res*, 25, 117–121.

Joffe, R.T., Young, L.T., Cooke, R.G., and Robb, J. (1994). The thyroid and mixed affective states. *Acta Psychiatr Scand*, 90, 131–132.

Johannessen, C.U. (2000). Mechanisms of action of valproate: A commentatory. *Neurochem Int*, 37, 103–110.

Johannessen, C.U., Petersen, D., Fonnum, F., and Hassel, B. (2001). The acute effect of valproate on cerebral energy metabolism in mice. *Epilepsy Res*, 47, 247–256.

Johnson, F.N. (1980). *Handbook of Lithium Therapy*. Baltimore: University Park Press.

Johnson, L., El-Khoury, A., Aberg-Wistedt, A., Stain-Malmgren, R., and Mathe, A.A. (2001). Tryptophan depletion in lithium-stabilized patients with affective disorder. *Int J Neuropsychopharmacol*, 4, 329–336.

Johnston-Wilson, N.L., Sims, C.D., Hofmann, J.P., Anderson, L., Shore, A.D., Torrey, E.F., and Yolken, R.H. (2000). Disease-specific alterations in frontal cortex brain proteins in schizophrenia, bipolar disorder, and major depressive disorder. The Stanley Neuropathology Consortium. *Mol Psychiatry*, 5, 142–149.

Jones, F.D., Maas, J.W., Dekirmenjian, H., and Fawcett, J.A. (1973). Urinary catecholamine metabolites during behavioral changes in a patient with manic-depressive cycles. *Science*, 179, 300–302.

Jope, R.S. (1979). High affinity choline transport and acetylCoA production in brain and their roles in the regulation of acetylcholine synthesis. *Brain Res*, 180, 313–344.

Jope, R.S. (1993). Lithium selectively potentiates cholinergic activity in rat brain. *Prog Brain Res*, 98, 317–322.

Jope, R.S. (1999). A bimodal model of the mechanism of action of lithium. *Mol Psychiatry*, 4, 21–25.

Jope, R.S., and Song, L. (1997). AP-1 and NF-kappaB stimulated by carbachol in human neuroblastoma SH-SY5Y cells are differentially sensitive to inhibition by lithium. *Brain Res Mol Brain Res*, 50, 171–180.

Jope, R.S., and Williams, M.B. (1994). Lithium and brain signal transduction systems. *Biochem Pharmacol*, 47, 429–441.

Jope, R.S., Jenden, D.J., Ehrlich, B.E., and Diamond, J.M. (1978). Choline accumulates in erythrocytes during lithium therapy. *N Engl J Med*, 299, 833–834.

Jope, R.S., Jenden, D.J., Ehrlich, B.E., Diamond, J.M., and Gosenfeld, L.F. (1980). Erythrocyte choline concentrations are elevated in manic patients. *Proc Natl Acad Sci USA*, 77, 6144–6146.

Jope, R.S., Morrisett, R.A., and Snead, O.C. (1986). Characterization of lithium potentiation of pilocarpine-induced status epilepticus in rats. *Exp Neurol*, 91, 471–480.

Jope, R.S., Song, L., Li, P.P., Young, L.T., Kish, S.J., Pacheco, M.A., and Warsh, J.J. (1996). The phosphoinositide signal transduction system is impaired in bipolar affective disorder brain. *J Neurochem*, 66, 2402–2409.

Jordan, V.C. (1994). Molecular mechanisms of antiestrogen action in breast cancer. *Breast Cancer Res Treat*, 31(1), 41–52.

Jordan, V.C. (2003). Targeting antihormone resistance in breast cancer: A simple solution. *Ann Oncol*, 14(7), 969–970.

Josephson, A.M., and Mackenzie, T.B. (1979). Appearance of manic psychosis following rapid normalization of thyroid status. *Am J Psychiatry*, 136, 846–847.

Josephson, A.M., and Mackenzie, T.B. (1980). Thyroid-induced mania in hypothyroid patients. *Br J Psychiatry*, 137, 222–228.

Joyce, J.N., Lexow, N., Kim, S.J., Artymyshyn, R., Senzon, S., Lawrence, D., Cassanova, M.F., Kleinman, J.E., Bird, E.D., and Winokur, A. (1992). Distribution of beta-adrenergic receptor subtypes in human post-mortem brain: Alterations in limbic regions of schizophrenics. *Synapse*, 10, 228–246.

Joyce, J.N., Shane, A., Lexow, N., Winokur, A., Casanova, M.F., and Kleinman, J.E. (1993). Serotonin uptake sites and serotonin receptors are altered in the limbic system of schizophrenics. *Neuropsychopharmacology*, 8, 315–336.

Joyce, P.R. (1991). The prognostic significance of thyroid function in mania. *J Psychiatr Res*, 25(1-2), 1–6.

Joyce, P.R., and Paykel, E.S. (1989). Predictors of drug response in depression. *Arch Gen Psychiatry*, 46, 89–99.

Joyce, P.R., Fergusson, D.M., Woollard, G., Abbott, R.M., Horwood, L.J., and Upton, J. (1995). Urinary catecholamines and plasma hormones predict mood state in rapid cycling bipolar affective disorder. *J Affect Disord*, 33, 233–243.

Juckel, G., Hegerl, U., Mavrogiorgou, P., Gallinat, J., Mager, T., Tigges, P., Dresel, S., Schroter, A., Stotz, G., Meller, I., Greil, W., and Moller, H.J. (2000). Clinical and biological findings in a case with 48-hour bipolar ultrarapid cycling before and during valproate treatment. *J Clin Psychiatry*, 61, 585–593.

Judd, L.L., Janowsky, D.S., Segal, D.S., and Huey, L.Y. (1980). Naloxone-induced behavioral and physiological effects in normal and manic subjects. *Arch Gen Psychiatry*, 37, 583–586.

Kafka, M.S., and Paul, S.M. (1986). Platelet alpha 2-adrenergic receptors in depression. *Arch Gen Psychiatry*, 43, 91–95.

Kafka, M.S., Wirz-Justice, A., Naber, D., Marangos, P.J., O'Donohue, T.L., and Wehr, T.A. (1982). Effect of lithium on circadian neurotransmitter receptor rhythms. *Neuropsychobiology*, 8, 41–50.

Kakiuchi, C., Iwamoto, K., Ishiwata, M., Bundo, M., Kasahara, T., Kusumi, I., Tsujita, T., Okazaki, Y., Nanko, S., Kunugi, H., Sasaki, T., and Kato, T. (2003). Impaired feedback regulation of XBP1 as a genetic risk factor for bipolar disorder. *Nat Genet*, 35, 171–175.

Kakiuchi, C., Ishiwata, M., Kametani, M., Nelson, C., Iwamoto, K., and Kato, T. (2005). Quantitative analysis of mitochondrial DNA deletions in the brains of patients with bipolar disorder and schizophrenia. *Int J Neuropsychopharmacol*, 8(4), 515–522.

Kalin, N.H., Gibbs, D.M., Barksdale, C.M., Shelton, S.E., and Carnes, M. (1985). Behavioral stress decreases plasma oxytocin concentrations in primates. *Life Sci*, 36, 1275–1280.

Kao, H.T., Song, H.J., Porton, B., Ming, G.L., Hoh, J., Abraham, M., Czernik, A.J., Pieribone, V.A., Poo, M.M., and Greengard, P. (2002). A protein kinase A–dependent molecular switch in synapsins regulates neurite outgrowth. *Nat Neurosci*, 5, 431–437.

Karege, F., Bovier, P., Gaillard, J.M., and Tissot, R. (1987). The decrease of erythrocyte catechol-O-methyltransferase activity in depressed patients and its diagnostic significance. *Acta Psychiatr Scand*, 76, 303–308.

Karege, F., Bovier, P., Widmer, J., Gaillard, J.M., and Tissot, R. (1992). Platelet membrane alpha 2-adrenergic receptors in depression. *Psychiatry Res*, 43(3), 243–252.

Karege, F., Golaz, J., Schwald, M., and Malafosse, A. (1999). Lithium and haloperidol treatments differently affect the mononuclear leukocyte Gαs protein levels in bipolar affective disorder. *Neuropsychobiology*, 39(4), 181–186.

Karson, C.N., Mrak, R.E., Schluterman, K.O., Sturner, W.Q., Sheng, J.G., and Griffin, W.S. (1999). Alterations in synaptic proteins and their encoding mRNAs in prefrontal cortex in schizophrenia: A possible neurochemical basis for 'hypofrontality.' *Mol Psychiatry*, 4, 39–45.

Kasper, S., Sack, D.A., Wehr, T.A., Kick, H., Voll, G., and Vieira, A. (1988). Nocturnal TSH and prolactin secretion during sleep deprivation and prediction of antidepressant response in patients with major depression. *Biol Psychiatry*, 24, 631–641.

Kastin, A.J., Ehrensing, R.H., Schalch, D.S., and Anderson, M.S. (1972). Improvement in mental depression with decreased thyrotropin response after administration of thyrotropin-releasing hormone. *Lancet*, 2, 740–742.

Kato, T. (2001). The other, forgotten genome: Mitochondrial DNA and mental disorders. *Mol Psychiatry*, 6(6), 625–633.

Kato, T., and Kato, N. (2000). Mitochondrial dysfunction in bipolar disorder. *Bipolar Disord*, 2(3 Pt. 1), 180–190.

Kato, T., Hamakawa, H., Shioiri, T., Murashita, J., Takahashi, Y., Takahashi, S., and Inubushi, T. (1996). Choline-containing compounds detected by proton magnetic resonance spectroscopy in the basal ganglia in bipolar disorder. *J Psychiatry Neurosci*, 21, 248–254.

Kato, T., Ishiwata, M., Mori, K., Washizuka, S., Tajima, O., Akiyama, T., and Kato, N. (2003). Mechanisms of altered CA2+ signalling in transformed lymphoblastoid cells from patients with bipolar disorder. *Int J Neuropsychopharmacol*, 6(4), 379–389.

Katona, C.L., Theodorou, A.E., and Horton, R.W. (1987). Alpha 2-adrenoceptors in depression. *Psychiatr Dev*, 5, 129–49.

Katz, M.M., Maas, J.W., Frazer, A., Koslow, S.H., Bowden, C.L., Berman, N., Swann, A.C., and Stokes, P.E. (1994). Drug-induced actions on brain neurotransmitter systems and changes in the behaviors and emotions of depressed patients. *Neuropsychopharmacology*, 11(2), 89–100.

Katzenellenbogen, J.A., O'Malley, B.W., and Katzenellenbogen, B.S. (1996). Tripartite steroid hormone receptor pharmacology: Interaction with multiple effector sites as a basis for the cell- and promoter-specific action of these hormones. *Mol Endocrinol*, 10, 119–131.

Katzman, R., and Pappius, H.M. (1973). *Brain Electrolytes and Fluid Metabolism*. Baltimore: Williams & Wilkins.

Kaufmann, C.A., Gillin, J.C., Hill, B., O'Laughlin, T., Phillips, I., Kleinman, J.E., and Wyatt, R.J. (1984). Muscarinic binding in suicides. *Psychiatry Res*, 12, 47–55.

Kay, G., Sargeant, M., McGuffin, P., Whatley, S., Marchbanks, R., Baldwin, D., Montgomery, S., and Elliott, J.M. (1993). The lymphoblast beta-adrenergic receptor in bipolar depressed patients: Characterization and down-regulation. *J Affect Disord*, 27, 163–172.

Kay, G., Sargeant, M., McGuffin, P., Whatley, S., Marchbanks, R., Bullock, T., Montgomery, S., and Elliott, J.M. (1994). The lymphoblast beta-adrenergic receptor in bipolar depressed patients: Effect of chronic incubation with lithium chloride. *J Affect Disord*, 30, 185–192.

Keck, M.E., Welt, T., Muller, M.B., Uhr, M., Ohl, F., Wigger, A., Toschi, N., Holsboer, F., and Landgraf, R. (2003). Reduction of hypothalamic vasopressinergic hyperdrive contributes to clinically relevant behavioral and neuroendocrine effects of chronic paroxetine treatment in a psychopathological rat model. *Neuropsychopharmacology*, 28(2), 235–243.

Kelly, W.F., Kelly, M.J., and Faragher, B. (1996). A prospective study of psychiatric and psychological aspects of cushing's syndrome. *Clin Endocrinol (Oxf)*, 45(6), 715–720.

Kempermann, G. (2002). Why new neurons? Possible functions for adult hippocampal neurogenesis. *J Neurosci*, 22, 635–638.

Kempermann, G., and Gage, F.H. (1999). Experience-dependent regulation of adult hippocampal neurogenesis: Effects of long-term stimulation and stimulus withdrawal. *Hippocampus*, 9, 321–332.

Kempermann, G., Kuhn, H.G., and Gage, F.H. (1997). More hippocampal neurons in adult mice living in an enriched environment. *Nature*, 386, 493–495.

Kendall, D.A., and Nahorski, S.R. (1987). Acute and chronic lithium treatments influence agonist and depolarization-stimulated inositol phospholipid hydrolysis in rat cerebral cortex. *J Pharmacol Exp Ther*, 241, 1023–1027.

Kendall, D.A., Stancel, G.M., and Enna, S.J. (1982). The influence of sex hormones on antidepressant-induced alterations in neurotransmitter receptor binding. *J Neurosci*, 2, 354–360.

Kennedy, S.H., Tighe, S., McVey, G., and Brown, G.M. (1989). Melatonin and cortisol "switches" during mania, depression, and euthymia in a drug-free bipolar patient. *J Nerv Ment Dis*, 177, 300–303.

Kessler, R.C., McGonagle, K.A., Swartz, M., Blazer, D.G., and Nelson, C.B. (1993). Sex and depression in the National Comorbidity Survey. I: Lifetime prevalence, chronicity and recurrence. *J Affect Disord*, 29, 85–96.

Keynes, R.D., and Swan, R.C. (1959). The permeability of frog muscle fibres to lithium ions. *J Physiol*, 147, 626–638.

Khaitan, L., Calabrese, J.R., and Stockmeier, C.A. (1994). Effects of chronic treatment with valproate on serotonin-1A receptor binding and function. *Psychopharmacology (Berl)*, 113, 539–542.

Kilbey, M.M., and Ellinwood, E.H. Jr. (1977). Reverse tolerance to stimulant-induced abnormal behavior. *Life Sci*, 20, 1063–1075.

Kilts, C.D. (2001). Imaging the roles of the amygdala in drug addiction. *Psychopharmacol Bull*, 35(1), 84–94.

Kim, C.H., Chung, H.J., Lee, H.K., and Huganir, R.L. (2001). Interaction of the AMPA receptor subunit GluR2/3 with PDZ domains regulates hippocampal long-term depression. *Proc Natl Acad Sci USA*, 98, 11725–11730.

Kim, J.S., Chang, M.Y., Yu, I.T., Kim, J.H., Lee, S.H., Lee, Y.S., and Son, H. (2004). Lithium selectively increases neuronal differentiation of hippocampal neural progenitor cells both in vitro and in vivo. *J Neurochem*, 89(2), 324–336.

Kim, M.H., and Neubig, R.R. (1987). Membrane reconstitution of high-affinity alpha 2 adrenergic agonist binding with guanine nucleotide regulatory proteins. *Biochemistry*, 26, 3664–3672.

Kim, Y.B., Dunner, D.L., Meltzer, H.L., and Fieve, R.R. (1978). Lithium erythrocyte: Plasma ratio in primary affective disorder. *Compr Psychiatry*, 19(2), 129–134.

Kiriike, N., Izumiya, Y., Nishiwaki, S., Maeda, Y., Nagata, T., and Kawakita, Y. (1988). TRH test and DST in schizoaffective mania, mania, and schizophrenia. *Biol Psychiatry*, 24, 415–422.

Kirkegaard, C., Faber, J., Hummer, L., and Rogowski, P. (1979). Increased levels of TRH in cerebrospinal fluid from patients with endogenous depression. *Psychoneuroendocrinology*, 4, 227–235.

Kirov, G., Murphy, K.C., Arranz, M.J., Jones, I., McCandles, F., Kunugi, H., Murray, R.M., McGuffin, P., Collier, D.A., Owen, M.J., and Craddock, N. (1998). Low activity allele of catechol-O-methyltransferase gene associated with rapid cycling bipolar disorder. *Mol Psychiatry*, 3(4), 342–345.

Kirov, G., Rees, M., Jones, I., MacCandless, F., Owen, M.J., and Craddock, N. (1999). Bipolar disorder and the serotonin transporter gene: A family-based association study. *Psychol Med*, 29, 1249–1254.

Kjellman, B.F., Beck-Friis, J., Ljunggren, J.G., and Wetterberg, L. (1984). Twenty-four-hour serum levels of TSH in affective disorders. *Acta Psychiatr Scand*, 69(6), 491–502.

Kjellman, B.F., Beck-Friis, J., Ljunggren, J.G., Ross, S.B., Unden, F., and Wetterberg, L. (1986). Serum dopamine-beta-hydroxylase activity in patients with major depressive disorders. *Acta Psychiatr Scand*, 73, 266–270.

Klaiber, E.L., Kobayashi, Y., Broverman, D.M., and Hall, F. (1971). Plasma monoamine oxidase activity in regularly menstruating women and in amenorrheic women receiving cyclic treatment with estrogens and a progestin. *J Clin Endocrinol Metab*, 33, 630–638.

Klawans, H.L., Weiner, W.J., and Nausieda, P.A. (1977). The effect of lithium on an animal model of tardive dyskinesia. *Prog Neuropsychopharmacol*, 1, 53–60.

Klein, P.S., and Melton, D.A. (1996). A molecular mechanism for the effect of lithium on development. *Proc Natl Acad Sci USA*, 93, 8455–8459.

Klein, E., Lerer, B., Newman, M., Belmaker, R.H., and Bhargava, H.N. (1984). Effect of cyclo(Leu-Gly) on reserpine-induced hypomotility and increases in cortical beta-adrenergic receptors. *Psychopharmacology (Berl)*, 83, 76–78.

Klemfuss, H. (1992). Diminishing toxic effects of lithium administration. *Am J Psychiatry*, 149(6), 846.

Kline, N.S., and Lehmann, H.E. (1979). β-Endorphin therapy in psychiatric patients. In E. Usdin, W.E. Bunney, and N.S. Kline (Eds.), *Endorphins in Mental Health Research* (pp. 500–517). New York: Oxford University Press.

Kling, M.A., Rubinow, D.R., Doran, A.R., Roy, A., Davis, C.L., Calabrese, J.R., Nieman, L.K., Post, R.M., Chrousos, G.P., and Gold, P.W. (1993). Cerebrospinal fluid immunoreactive somatostatin concentrations in patients with Cushing's disease and major depression: Relationship to indices of corticotrophin-releasing hormone and cortisol secretion. *Neuroendocrinology*, 57(1), 79–88.

Klysner, R., Geisler, A., and Rosenberg, R. (1987). Enhanced histamine- and beta-adrenoceptor-mediated cyclic AMP formation in leukocytes from patients with endogenous depression. *J Affect Disord*, 13, 227–232.

Knapp, S., and Mandell, A.J. (1973). Short- and long-term lithium administration: Effects on the brain's serotonergic biosynthetic systems. *Science*, 180, 645–670.

Koenig, R.J., Leonard, J.L., Senator, D., Rappaport, N., Watson, A.Y., and Larsen, P.R. (1984). Regulation of thyroxine 5'-deiodinase activity by 3,5,3'-triiodothyronine in cultured rat anterior pituitary cells. *Endocrinology*, 115, 324–329.

Kofman, O., and Belmaker, R.H. (1990). Intracerebroventricular myo-inositol antagonizes lithium-induced suppression of rearing behaviour in rats. *Brain Res*, 534, 345–347.

Kofman, O., and Belmaker, R.H. (1991). Animal models of mania and bipolar affective disorders. In P. Soubrie. (Ed.), *Anxiety, Depression and Mania*. New York: Karger.

Kofman, O., and Belmaker, R.H. (1993). Ziskind-Somerfeld Research Award 1993. Biochemical, behavioral, and clinical studies of the role of inositol in lithium treatment and depression. *Biol Psychiatry*, 34, 839–852.

Kofman, O., Belmaker, R.H., Grisaru, N., Alpert, C., Fuchs, I., Katz, V., and Rigler, O. (1991). Myo-inositol attenuates two specific behavioral effects of acute lithium in rats. *Psychopharmacol Bull*, 27, 185–190.

Kofman, O., Bersudsky, Y., Vinnitsky, I., Alpert, C., and Belmaker, R.H. (1993). The effect of peripheral inositol injection on rat motor activity models of depression. *Isr J Med Sci*, 29, 580–586.

Kofman, O., Li, P.P., and Warsh, J.J. (1998). Lithium, but not carbamazepine, potentiates hyperactivity induced by intra-accumbens cholera toxin. *Pharmacol Biochem Behav*, 59, 191–200.

Konradi, C., Eaton, M., MacDonald, M.L., Walsh, J., Benes, F.M., and Heckers, S. (2004). Molecular evidence for mitochondrial dysfunction in bipolar disorder. *Arch Gen Psychiatry*, 61(3), 300–308.

Kontaxakis, V., Markianos, M., Markidis, M., and Stefanis, C. (1989). Clonidine in the treatment of mixed bipolar disorder. *Acta Psychiatr Scand*, 79, 108.

Kopin, I.J. (1985). Catecholamine metabolism: Basic aspects and clinical significance. *Pharmacol Rev*, 37, 333–364.

Korpi, E.R., Kleinman, J.E., Goodman, S.I., Phillips, I., DeLisi, L.E., Linnoila, M., and Wyatt, R.J. (1986). Serotonin and 5-hydroxyindoleacetic acid in brains of suicide victims: Comparison in chronic schizophrenic patients with suicide as cause of death. *Arch Gen Psychiatry*, 43, 594–600.

Korpi, E.R., Kleinman, J.E., and Wyatt, R.J. (1988). GABA concentrations in forebrain areas of suicide victims. *Biol Psychiatry*, 23, 109–114.

Korte, M., Griesbeck, O., Gravel, C., Carroll, P., Staiger, V., Thoenen, H., and Bonhoeffer, T. (1996). Virus-mediated gene transfer into hippocampal CA1 region restores long-term potentiation in brain-derived neurotrophic factor mutant mice. *Proc Natl Acad Sci USA*, 93, 12547–12552.

Koslow, S.H., Maas, J.W., Bowden, C.L., Davis, J.M., Hanin, I., and Javaid, J. (1983). CSF and urinary biogenic amines and metabolites in depression and mania. A controlled, univariate analysis. *Arch Gen Psychiatry*, 40, 999–1010.

Kostic, V., Jackson-Lewis, V., de Bilbao, F., Dubois-Dauphin, M., and Przedborski, S. (1997). Bcl-2: Prolonging life in a transgenic mouse model of familial amyotrophic lateral sclerosis. *Science*, 277(5325), 559–562.

Kraemer, G.W., Ebert, M.H., Lake, C.R., and McKinney, W.T. (1984). Cerebrospinal fluid measures of neurotransmitter changes associated with pharmacological alteration of the despair response to social separation in rhesus monkeys. *Psychiatry Res*, 11, 303–315.

Kramer, M.S., Cutler, N., Feighner, J., Shrivastava, R., Carman, J., Sramek, J.J., Reines, S.A., Liu, G., Snavely, D., Wyatt-Knowles, E., Hale, J.J., Mills, S.G., MacCoss, M., Swain, C.J., Harrison, T., Hill, R.G., Hefti, F., Scolnick, E.M., Cascieri, M.A., Chicchi, G.G., Sadowski, S., Williams, A.R., Hewson, L., Smith, D., Carlson, E.J., Hargreaves, R.J., and Rupniak, N.M. (1998). Distinct mechanism for antidepressant activity by blockade of central substance P receptors. *Science*, 281, 1640–1645.

Krell, R.D., and Goldberg, A.M. (1973). Effect of acute and chronic administration of lithium on steady-state levels of mouse brain choline and acetylcholine. *Biochem Pharmacol*, 22, 3289–3291.

Krieger, D.T., Silverberg, A.I., Rizzo, F., and Krieger, H.P. (1968). Abolition of circadian periodicity of plasma 17-OHCS levels in the cat. *Am J Physiol*, 215, 959–967.

Krishnan, R.R., Maltbie, A.A., and Davidson, J.R. (1983). Abnormal cortisol suppression in bipolar patients with simultaneous manic and depressive symptoms. *Am J Psychiatry*, 140, 203–205.

Krystal, A., Krishnan, K.R., Raitiere, M., Poland, R., Ritchie, J.C., Dunnick, N.R., Hanada, K., and Nemeroff, C.B. (1990). Differential diagnosis and pathophysiology of Cushing's syndrome and primary affective disorder. *J Neuropsychiatry Clin Neurosci*, 2(1), 34–43.

Krystal, J.H., Sanacora, G., Blumberg, H., Anand, A., Charney, D.S., Marek, G., Epperson, C.N., Goddard, A., and Mason, G.F. (2002). Glutamate and GABA systems as targets for novel antidepressant and mood-stabilizing treatments. *Mol Psychiatry*, 7(Suppl. 1), S71–S80.

Kucinski, B.J., Antelman, S.M., Caggiula, A.R., Fowler, H., Gershon, S., and Edwards, D.J. (1999). Cocaine-induced oscillation is conditionable. *Pharmacol Biochem Behav*, 63, 449–455.

Kuhn, H.G., Biebl, M., Wilhelm, D., Li, M., Friedlander, R.M., and Winkler, J. (2005). Increased generation of granule cells in adult Bcl-2-overexpressing mice: A role for cell death during continued hippocampal neurogenesis. *Eur J Neurosci*, 22(8), 1907–1915.

Kuhs, H., Farber, D., and Tolle, R. (1996). Serum prolactin, growth hormone, total corticoids, thyroid hormones and thyrotropine during serial therapeutic sleep deprivation. *Biol Psychiatry*, 39(10), 857–864.

Künig, G., Niedermeyer, B., Deckert, J., Gsell, W., Ransmayr, G., and Riederer, P. (1998). Inhibition of [3H]alpha-amino-3-hydroxy-5-methyl-4-isoxazole-propionic acid [AMPA] binding by the anticonvulsant valproate in clinically relevant concentrations: An autoradiographic investigation in human hippocampus. *Epilepsy Res*, 31, 153–157.

Kunugi, H., Hattori, M., Kato, T., Tatsumi, M., Sakai, T., Sasaki, T., Hirose, T., and Nanko, S. (1997). Serotonin transporter gene polymorphisms: Ethnic difference and possible association with bipolar affective disorder. *Mol Psychiatry*, 2, 457–462.

Kunzel, H.E., Zobel, A.W., Nickel, T., Ackl, N., Uhr, M., Sonntag, A., Ising, M., and Holsboer, F. (2003). Treatment of depression with the CRH-1-receptor antagonist R121919: Endocrine changes and side effects. *J Psychiatr Res*, 37(6), 525–533.

Kuriyama, K., and Kakita, K. (1980). Cholera toxin induced epileptogenic focus: An animal model for studying roles of cyclic AMP in the establishment of epilepsy. *Prog Clin Biol Res*, 39, 141–155.

Kuruvilla, A., and Uretsky, N.J. (1981). Effect of sodium valproate on motor function regulated by the activation of GABA receptors. *Psychopharmacology (Berl)*, 72(2), 167–172.

Kusalic, M. (1992). Grade II and grade III hypothyroidism in rapid-cycling bipolar patients. *Neuropsychobiology*, 25, 177–181.

Kusalic, M., and Engelsmann, F. (1996). Effect of lithium maintenance treatment on hypothalamic pituitary gonadal axis in bipolar men. *J Psychiatry Neurosci*, 21, 181–186.

Kusumi, I., Koyama, T., and Yamashita, I. (1991). Effects of various factors on serotonin-induced Ca2+ response in human platelets. *Life Sci*, 48, 999–1010.

Kusumi, I., Koyama, T., and Yamashita, I. (1994a). Serotonin-induced platelet intracellular calcium mobilization in depressed patients. *Psychopharmacology (Berl)*, 113, 322–327.

Kusumi, I., Koyama, T., and Yamashita, I. (1994b). Effect of mood stabilizing agents on agonist-induced calcium mobilization in human platelets. *J Psychiatr Neurosci*, 19, 222–225.

Kusumi, I., Suzuki, K., Sasaki, Y., Kameda, K., and Koyama, T. (2000). Treatment response in depressed patients with enhanced Ca mobilization stimulated by serotonin. *Neuropsychopharmacology*, 23, 690–696.

Laakso, M.L., and Oja, S.S. (1979). Transport of tryptophan and tyrosine in rat brain slices in the presence of lithium. *Neurochem Res*, 4, 411–423.

Lachman, H.M., Morrow, B., Shprintzen, R., Veit, S., Parsia, S.S., Faedda, G., Goldberg, R., Kucherlapati, R., and Papolos, D.F. (1996). Association of codon 108/158 catechol-O-methyltransferase gene polymorphism with the psychiatric manifestations of velo-cardio-facial syndrome. *Am J Med Genet*, 67, 468.

Ladd, C.O., Huot, R.L., Thrivikraman, K.V., Nemeroff, C.B., Meaney, M.J., and Plotsky, P.M. (2000). Long-term behavioral and neuroendocrine adaptations to adverse early experience. *Prog Brain Res*, 122, 81–103.

Laeng, P., Pitts, R.L., Lemire, A.L., Drabik, C.E., Weiner, A., Tang, H., Thyagarajan, R., Mallon, B.S., and Altar, C.A. (2004). The mood stabilizer valproic acid stimulates GABA neurogenesis from rat forebrain stem cells. *J Neurochem*, 91(1), 238–251.

Laruelle, M., Abi-Dargham, A., Casanova, M.F., Toti, R., Weinberger, D.R., and Kleinman, J.E. (1993). Selective abnormalities of prefrontal serotonergic receptors in schizophrenia. A postmortem study. *Arch Gen Psychiatry*, 50, 810–818.

Lattanzi, L., Dell'Osso, L., Cassano, P., Pini, S., Rucci, P., Houck, P.R., Gemignani, A., Battistini, G., Bassi, A., Abelli, M., and Cassano, G.B. (2002). Pramipexole in treatment-resistant depression: A 16-week naturalistic study. *Bipolar Disord*, 4, 307–314.

Lauterborn, J.C., Lynch, G., Vanderklish, P., Arai, A., and Gall, C.M. (2000). Positive modulation of AMPA receptors increases neurotrophin expression by hippocampal and cortical neurons. *J Neurosci*, 20, 8–21.

Lawrence, K.M., De Paermentier, F., Cheetham, S.C., Crompton, M.R., Katona, C.L., and Horton, R.W. (1990). Brain 5-HT uptake sites, labelled with [3H]paroxetine, in antidepressant-free depressed suicides. *Brain Res*, 526, 17–22.

Lawrence, K.M., De Paermentier, F., Lowther, S., Crompton, M.R., Katona, C.L., and Horton, R.W. (1997). Brain 5-hydroxytryptamine uptake sites labeled with [3H]paroxetine in antidepressant drug-treated depressed suicide victims and controls. *J Psychiatry Neurosci*, 22, 185–191.

Lawrence, K.M., Kanagasundaram, M., Lowther, S., Katona, C.L., Crompton, M.R., and Horton, R.W. (1998). [3H]imipramine binding in brain samples from depressed suicides and controls: 5-HT uptake sites compared with sites defined by desmethylimipramine. *J Affect Disord*, 47, 105–112.

Lawrence, M.S., Ho, D.Y., Sun, G.H., Steinberg, G.K., and Sapolsky, R.M. (1996). Overexpression of bcl-2 with herpes simplex virus vectors protects cns neurons against neurological insults in vitro and in vivo. *J Neurosci*, 16(2), 486–496.

Lazarus, J.H., and Muston, H.L. (1978). The effect of lithium on the iodide concentrating mechanism in mouse salivary gland. *Acta Pharmacol Toxicol (Copenh)*, 43, 55–58.

Leach, M.J., Marden, C.M., and Miller, A.A. (1986). Pharmacological studies on lamotrigine, a novel potential antiepileptic drug: II. Neurochemical studies on the mechanism of action. *Epilepsia*, 27, 490–497.

Leake, A., Fairbairn, A.F., McKeith, I.G., and Ferrier, I.N. (1991). Studies on the serotonin uptake binding site in major depressive disorder and control post-mortem brain: Neurochemical and clinical correlates. *Psychiatry Res*, 39, 155–165.

Leboyer, M., Quintin, P., Manivet, P., Varoquaux, O., Allilaire, J.F., and Launay, J.M. (1999). Decreased serotonin transporter binding in unaffected relatives of manic depressive patients. *Biol Psychiatry*, 46, 1703–1706.

Lechin, F., van der Dijs, B., Jakubowicz, D., Camero, R.E., Villa, S., Arocha, L., and Lechin, A.E. (1985). Effects of clonidine on blood pressure, noradrenaline, cortisol, growth hormone, and prolactin plasma levels in high and low intestinal tone depressed patients. *Neuroendocrinology*, 41, 156–162.

Lecuona, E., Luquin, S., Avila, J., Garcia-Segura, L.M., and Martin-Vasallo, P. (1996). Expression of the beta 1 and beta 2(AMOG) subunits of the Na,K-ATPase in neural tissues: Cellular and developmental distribution patterns. *Brain Res Bull*, 40, 167–174.

Lee, P.L. (1974). Single-column system for accelerated amino acid analysis of physiological fluids using five lithium buffers. *Biochem Med*, 10, 107–121.

Legutko, B., Li, X., and Skolnick, P. (2001). Regulation of BDNF expression in primary neuron culture by LY392098, a novel AMPA receptor potentiator. *Neuropharmacology*, 40, 1019–1027.

Leibenluft, E. (1996). Women with bipolar illness: Clinical and research issues. *Am J Psychiatry*, 153, 163–173.

Leibenluft, E., Ashman, S.B., Feldman-Naim, S., and Yonkers, K.A. (1999). Lack of relationship between menstrual cycle phase and mood in a sample of women with rapid cycling bipolar disorder. *Biol Psychiatry*, 46, 577–580.

Leiderman, D.B., Balish, M., Bromfield, E.B., and Theodore, W.H. (1991). Effect of valproate on human cerebral glucose metabolism. *Epilepsia*, 32, 417–422.

Lenox, R.H., and Hahn, C.G. (2000). Overview of the mechanism of action of lithium in the brain: Fifty-year update. *J Clin Psychiatry*, 61, 5–15.

Lenox, R.H., and Manji, H.K. (1995). Lithium. In A.F. Schatzberg, C.B. Nemeroff (Eds.), *The American Psychiatric Press Textbook of Psychopharmacology* (pp. 303–349). Washington, DC: American Psychiatric Press.

Lenox, R.H., and Manji, H. (1998). Drugs for treatment of bipolar disorder: Lithium. In C.B. Nemeroff (Ed.), *Textbook of psychopharmacology* (2nd Edition) (pp. 379–429). Washington, DC: American Psychiatry Press.

Lenox, R.H., Watson, D.G., Patel, J., and Ellis, J. (1992). Chronic lithium administration alters a prominent PKC substrate in rat hippocampus. *Brain Res*, 570, 333–340.

Lenox, R.H., Gould, T.D., and Manji, H.K. (2002). Endophenotypes in bipolar disorder. *Am J Med Genet*, 114, 391–406.

Lerer, B., and Stanley, M. (1985). Does lithium stabilize muscarinic receptors? *Biol Psychiatry*, 20, 1247–1250.

Lerer, B., Globus, M., Brik, E., Hamburger, R., and Belmaker, R.H. (1984). Effect of treatment and withdrawal from chronic lithium in rats on stimulant-induced responses. *Neuropsychobiology*, 11, 28–32.

Lerer, B., Macciardi, F., Segman, R.H., Adolfsson, R., Blackwood, D., Blairy, S., Del Favero, J., Dikeos, D.G., Kaneva, R., Lilli, R., Massat, I., Milanova, V., Muir, W., Noethen, M., Oruc, L., Petrova, T., Papadimitriou, G.N., Rietschel, M., Serretti, A., Souery, D., Van Gestel, S., Van Broeckhoven, C., and Mendlewicz, J. (2001). Variability of 5-HT2C receptor cys23ser polymorphism among European populations and vulnerability to affective disorder. *Mol Psychiatry*, 6, 579–585.

Leverich, G.S., Altshuler, L.L., Frye, M.A., Suppes, T., Keck, P.E. Jr., McElroy, S.L., Denicoff, K.D., Obrocea, G., Nolen, W.A., Kupka, R., Walden, J., Grunze, H., Perez, S., Luckenbaugh, D.A., and Post, R.M. (2003). Factors associated with suicide attempts in 648 patients with bipolar disorder in the Stanley Foundation Bipolar Network. *J Clin Psychiatry*, 64(5), 506–515.

Leviel, V., and Naquet, R. (1977). A study of the action of valproic acid on the kindling effect. *Epilepsia*, 18, 229–234.

Levine, J., Panchalingam, K., Rapoport, A., Gershon, S., McClure, R.J., and Pettegrew, J.W. (2000). Increased cerebrospinal fluid glutamine levels in depressed patients. *Biol Psychiatry*, 47, 586.

Levitt, M., Dunner, D.L., Mendlewicz, J., Frewin, D.B., Lawlor, W., Fleiss, J.L., Stallone, F., and Fieve, R.R. (1976). Plasma dopamine beta hydroxylase activity in affective disorders. *Psychopharmacologia*, 46, 205–210.

Levy, A., Zohar, J., and Belmaker, R.H. (1982). The effect of chronic lithium pretreatment on rat brain muscarinic receptor regulation. *Neuropharmacology*, 21(11), 1199–1201.

Lewin, E., and Bleck, V. (1977). Cyclic AMP accumulation in cerebral cortical slices: Effect of carbamazepine, phenobarbital, and phenytoin. *Epilepsia*, 18, 237–242.

Lewis, D.A., and Smith, R.E. (1983). Steroid-induced psychiatric syndromes. A report of 14 cases and a review of the literature. *J Affect Disord*, 5(4), 319–332.

Lewis, L.D., and Cochrane, G.M. (1983). Psychosis in a child inhaling budesonide. *Lancet*, 2(8350), 634.

Leyton, M., Young, S.N., and Benkelfat, C. (1997). Relapse of depression after rapid depletion of tryptophan. *Lancet*, 349, 1840–1841.

Li, R., and El-Mallakh, R.S. (2000). A novel evidence of different mechanisms of lithium and valproate neuroprotective action on human sy5y neuroblastoma cells: Caspase-3 dependency. *Neurosci Lett*, 294(3), 147–150.

Li, R., Shen, Y., and El-Mallahk, R.S. (1994). Lithium protects against ouabain-induced cell death. *Lithium*, 5, 211–216.

Li, T., Vallada, H., Curtis, D., Arranz, M., Xu, K., Cai, G., Deng, H., Liu, J., Murray, R., Liu, X., and Collier, D.A. (1997). Catechol-O-methyltransferase Val158Met polymorphism: Frequency analysis in Han Chinese subjects and allelic association of the low activity allele with bipolar affective disorder. *Pharmacogenetics*, 7, 349–353.

Li, T., Liu, X., Sham, P.C., Aitchison, K.J., Cai, G., Arranz, M.J., Deng, H., Liu, J., Kirov, G., Murray, R.M., and Collier, D.A. (1999). Association analysis between dopamine receptor genes and bipolar affective disorder. *Psychiatry Res*, 86(3), 193–201.

Li, X., Tizzano, J.P., Griffey, K., Clay, M., Lindstrom, T., and Skolnick, P. (2001). Antidepressant-like actions of an AMPA receptor potentiator (LY392098). *Neuropharmacology*, 40, 1028–1033.

Li, X., Bijur, G.N., and Jope, R.S. (2002). Glycogen synthase kinase-3beta, mood stabilizers, and neuroprotection. *Bipolar Disord*, 4(2), 137–144.

Li, Y.W., Hill, G., Wong, H., Kelly, N., Ward, K., Pierdomenico, M., Ren, S., Gilligan, P., Grossman, S., Trainor, G., Taub, R., McElroy, J., and Zazcek, R. (2003). Receptor occupancy of nonpeptide corticotropin-releasing factor 1 antagonist DMP696: Correlation with drug exposure and anxiolytic efficacy. *J Pharmacol Exp Ther*, 305(1), 86–96.

Lieberman, K.W., and Stokes, P. (1980). Lithium distribution ratios in psychiatrically normal subjects. *Pharmacol Biochem Behav*, 13(2), 205–208.

Lieblich, I., and Yirmiya, R. (1987). Naltrexone reverses a longterm depressive effect of a toxic lithium injection on saccharin preference. *Physiol Behav*, 39, 547–550.

Lingsch, C., and Martin, K. (1976). An irreversible effect of lithium administration to patients. *Br J Pharmacol*, 57, 323–327.

Linkowski, P., Kerkhofs, M., Van Onderbergen, A., Hubain, P., Copinschi, G., L'Hermite-Baleriaux, M., Leclercq, R., Brasseur, M., Mendlewicz, J., and Van Cauter, E. (1994). The 24-hour profiles of cortisol, prolactin, and growth hormone secretion in mania. *Arch Gen Psychiatry*, 51(8), 616–624.

Linnoila, M., Karoum, F., and Potter, W.Z. (1983a). Effects of antidepressant treatments on dopamine turnover in depressed patients. *Arch Gen Psychiatry*, 40, 1015–1017.

Linnoila, M., Karoum, F., Rosenthal, N., and Potter, W.Z. (1983b). Electroconvulsive treatment and lithium carbonate. Their effects on norepinephrine metabolism in patients with primary, major depressions. *Arch Gen Psychiatry*, 40, 677–680.

Linnoila, M., Miller, T.L., Bartko, J., and Potter, W.Z. (1984). Five antidepressant treatments in depressed patients. Effects on urinary serotonin and 5-hydroxyindoleacetic acid output. *Arch Gen Psychiatry*, 41, 688–692.

Linnoila, M., Guthrie, S., Lane, E.A., Karoum, F., Rudorfer, M., and Potter, W.Z. (1986). Clinical studies on norepinephrine metabolism: how to interpret the numbers. *Psychiatry Res*, 17, 229–239.

Little, K., Clark, T.B., Ranc, J., and Duncan, G.E. (1993). Beta-adrenergic receptor binding in frontal cortex from suicide victims. *Biol Psychiatry*, 34, 596–605.

Little, K.Y., McLauglin, D.P., Ranc, J., Gilmore, J., Lopez, J.F., Watson, S.J., Carroll, F.I., and Butts, J.D. (1997). Serotonin transporter binding sites and mRNA levels in depressed persons committing suicide. *Biol Psychiatry*, 41, 1156–1164.

Lloyd, K.G., Farley, I.J., Deck, J.H., and Hornykiewicz, O. (1974). Serotonin and 5-hydroxyindoleacetic acid in discrete areas of the brainstem of suicide victims and control patients. *Adv Biochem Psychopharmacol*, 11, 387–397.

Lloyd, K.G., Morselli, P.L., and Bartholini, G. (1987). GABA and affective disorders. *Med Biol*, 65, 159–165.

Lloyd, R.L., Pekary, A.E., Sattin, A., and Amundson, T. (2001). Antidepressant effects of thyrotropin-releasing hormone analogues using a rodent model of depression. *Pharmacol Biochem Behav*, 70, 15–22.

Looney, S.W., and el-Mallakh, R.S. (1997). Meta-analysis of erythrocyte Na,K-ATPase activity in bipolar illness. *Depress Anxiety*, 5(2), 53–65.

Loosen, P.T., Marciniak, R., and Thadani, K. (1987). TRH-induced TSH response in healthy volunteers: Relationship to psychiatric history. *Am J Psychiatry*, 144(4), 455–459.

López, J.F., Palkovits, M., Arato, M., Mansour, A., Akil, H., and Watson, S.J. (1992). Localization and quantification of pro-opiomelanocortin mRNA and glucocorticoid receptor mRNA in pituitaries of suicide victims. *Neuroendocrinology*, 56, 491–501.

López, J.F., Chalmers, D.T., Little, K.Y., and Watson, S.J. (1998). A.E. Bennett Research Award. Regulation of serotonin1A, glucocorticoid, and mineralocorticoid receptor in rat and human hippocampus: Implications for the neurobiology of depression. *Biol Psychiatry*, 43, 547–573.

Loscher, W. (1993). Effects of the antiepileptic drug valproate on metabolism and function of inhibitory and excitatory amino acids in the brain. *Neurochem Res*, 18, 485–502.

Loscher, W. (1999). Valproate: A reappraisal of its pharmacodynamic properties and mechanisms of action. *Prog Neurobiol*, 58, 31–59.

Loscher, W., and Honack, D. (1996). Valproate and its major metabolite E-2-en-valproate induce different effects on behaviour and brain monoamine metabolism in rats. *Eur J Pharmacol*, 299, 61–67.

Loscher, W., and Schmidt, D. (1980). Increase of human plasma GABA by sodium valproate. *Epilepsia*, 21, 611–615.

Loscher, W., and Siemes, H. (1984). Valproic acid increases gamma-aminobutyric acid in CSF of epileptic children. *Lancet*, 2, 225.

LoTurco, J.J. (2000). Neural circuits in the 21st century: Synaptic networks of neurons and glia. *Proc Natl Acad Sci USA*, 97, 8196–8197.

Louis, W.J., Doyle, A.E., and Anavekar, S.N. (1975). Plasma noradrenaline concentration and blood pressure in essential hypertension, phaeochromocytoma and depression. *Clin Sci Mol Med Suppl*, 2, 239s–242s.

Lowther, S., Crompton, M.R., Katona, C.L., and Horton, R.W. (1996). GTP gamma S and forskolin-stimulated adenylyl cyclase activity in post-mortem brain from depressed suicides and controls. *Mol Psychiatry*, 1, 470–477.

Lowther, S., De Paermentier, F., Cheetham, S.C., Crompton, M.R., Katona, C.L., and Horton, R.W. (1997a). 5-HT1A receptor binding sites in post-mortem brain samples from depressed suicides and controls. *J Affect Disord*, 42, 199–207.

Lowther, S., Katona, C.L., Crompton, M.R., and Horton, R.W. (1997b). 5-HT1D and 5-HT1E/1F binding sites in depressed suicides: Increased 5-HT1D binding in globus pallidus but not cortex. *Molec Psychiatry*, 2, 314–321.

Lowther, S., Katona, C.L., Crompton, M.R., and Horton, R.W. (1997c). Brain [3H]cAMP binding sites are unaltered in depressed suicides, but decreased by antidepressants. *Brain Res*, 758, 223–228.

Lu, R., Song, L., and Jope, R.S. (1999). Lithium attenuates p53 levels in human neuroblastoma SH-SY5Y cells. *Neuroreport*, 10, 1123–1125.

Lucas, F.R., and Salinas, P.C. (1997). WNT-7a induces axonal remodeling and increases synapsin I levels in cerebellar neurons. *Dev Biol*, 192, 31–44.

Lucca, A., Lucini, V., Piatti, E., Ronchi, P., and Smeraldi, E. (1992). Plasma tryptophan levels and plasma tryptophan/neutral amino acids ratio in patients with mood disorder, patients with obsessive-compulsive disorder, and normal subjects. *Psychiatry Res*, 44, 85–91.

Lucki, I. (1997). The forced swimming test as a model for core and component behavioral effects of antidepressant drugs. *Behav Pharmacol*, 8(6-7), 523–532.

Ludvig, N., and Moshe, S.L. (1989). Different behavioral and electrographic effects of acoustic stimulation and dibutyryl cyclic AMP injection into the inferior colliculus in normal and in genetically epilepsy-prone rats. *Epilepsy Res*, 3185–3190.

Lyon, M. (1991). Animal models of mania and schizophrenia. In P. Willner (Ed.), *Behavioral Models in Psychopharmacology: Theoretical, Industrial and Clinical Perspectives* (pp. 253–310). Cambridge, MA: Cambridge University Press.

Lyons, D.M. (2002). Stress, depression, and inherited variation in primate hippocampal and prefrontal brain development. *Psychopharmacol Bull*, 36, 27–43.

Lyons, D.M., Yang, C., Sawyer-Glover, A.M., Moseley, M.E., and Schatzberg, A.F. (2001). Early life stress and inherited variation in monkey hippocampal volumes. *Arch Gen Psychiatry*, 58, 1145–1151.

Lyttkens, L., Soderberg, U., and Wetterberg, L. (1976). Relation between erythrocyte and plasma lithium concentrations as an index in psychiatric disease. *Ups J Med Sci*, 81(2), 123.

Maas, J.W. (1972). Adrenocortical steroid-hormones, electrolytes, and disposition of catecholamines with particular reference to depressive states. *J Psychiatr Res*, 9, 227–241.

Maas, J.W., Koslow, S.H., Katz, M.M., Bowden, C.L., Gibbons, R.L., Stokes, P.E., Robins, E., and Davis, J.M. (1984). Pretreatment neurotransmitter metabolite levels and response to tricyclic antidepressant drugs. *Am J Psychiatry*, 141, 1159–1171.

Maas, J.W., Koslow, S.H., Davis, J., Katz, M., Frazer, A., Bowden, C.L., Berman, N., Gibbons, R., Stokes, P., and Landis, D.H. (1987). Catecholamine metabolism and disposition in healthy and depressed subjects. *Arch Gen Psychiatry*, 44(4), 337–344.

Machado-Vieira, R., Kapczinski, F., and Soares, J.C. (2004). Perspectives for the development of animal models of bipolar disorder. *Prog Neuropsychopharmacol Biol Psychiatry*, 28(2), 209–224.

MacMillan, V., Leake, J., Chung, T., and Bovell, M. (1987). The effect of valproic acid on the 5-hydroxyindoleacetic, homovanillic and lactic acid levels of cerebrospinal fluid. *Brain Res*, 420, 268–276.

MacQueen, G.M., Campbell, S., McEwen, B.S., Macdonald, K., Amano, S., Joffe, R.T., Nahmias, C., and Young, L.T. (2003). Course of illness, hippocampal function, and hippocampal volume in major depression. *Proc Natl Acad Sci USA*, 100(3), 1387–1392.

Maes, M.H., De Ruyter, M., and Suy, E. (1987). Prediction of subtype and severity of depression by means of dexamethasone suppression test, l-tryptophan: Competing amino acid ratio, and mhpg flow. *Biol Psychiatry*, 22(2), 177–188.

Maes, M., Vandewoude, M., Schotte, C., Martin, M., D'Hondt, P., Scharpe, S., and Blockx, P. (1990). The decreased availability of L-tryptophan in depressed females: Clinical and biological correlates. *Prog Neuropsychopharmacol Biol Psychiatry*, 14, 903–919.

Maes, M., Meltzer, H., D'Hondt, P., Cosyns, P., and Blockx, P. (1995). Effects on serotonin precursors on the negative feedback effects of glucocorticoids on hypothalamic–pituitary–adrenal axis function in depression. *Psychoneuroendocrinology*, 20, 149–167.

Maes, M., Calabrese, J., Jayathilake, K., and Meltzer, H.Y. (1997). Effects of subchronic treatment with valproate on l-5-HTP-induced cortisol responses in mania: Evidence for increased central serotonergic neurotransmission. *Psychiatry Res*, 71(2), 67–76.

Maes, M., Verkerk, R., Vandoolaeghe, E., Lin, A., and Scharpe, S. (1998). Serum levels of excitatory amino acids, serine, glycine, histidine, threonine, taurine, alanine and arginine in treatment-resistant depression: Modulation by treatment with antidepressants and prediction of clinical responsivity. *Acta Psychiatr Scand*, 97, 302–308.

Maggi, A., and Enna, S.J. (1980). Regional alterations in rat brain neurotransmitter systems following chronic lithium treatment. *J Neurochem*, 34, 888–892.

Maggirwar, S.B., Sarmiere, P.D., Dewhurst, S., and Freeman, R.S. (1998). Nerve growth factor–dependent activation of NF-kappaB contributes to survival of sympathetic neurons. *J Neurosci*, 18, 10356–10365.

Magistretti, P.J., and Pellerin, L. (1996). Cellular mechanisms of brain energy metabolism. Relevance to functional brain imaging and to neurodegenerative disorders. *Ann NY Acad Sci*, 777, 380–387.

Magliozzi, J.R., Gietzen, D., Maddock, R.J., Haack, D., Doran, A.R., Goodman, T., and Weiler, P.G. (1989). Lymphocyte beta-adrenoreceptor density in patients with unipolar depression and normal controls. *Biol Psychiatry*, 26(1), 15–25.

Mahan, L.C., Burch, R.M., Monsma, F.J. Jr., and Sibley, D.R. (1990). Expression of striatal D1 dopamine receptors coupled to inositol phosphate production and Ca2+ mobilization in *Xenopus* oocytes. *Proc Natl Acad Sci USA*, 87, 2196–2200.

Mahmood, T., and Silverstone, T. (2001). Serotonin and bipolar disorder. *J Affect Disord*, 66, 1–11.

Mahmood, T., Silverstone, T., Connor, R., and Herbison, P. (2002). Sumatriptan challenge in bipolar patients with and without migraine: A neuroendocrine study of 5-HT1D receptor function. *Int Clin Psychopharmacol*, 17, 33–36.

Maisel, A.S., Harris, T., Rearden, C.A., and Michel, M.C. (1990). Beta-adrenergic receptors in lymphocyte subsets after exercise. Alterations in normal individuals and patients with congestive heart failure. *Circulation*, 82, 2003–2010.

Maitre, L., Baltzer, V., Mondadori, C., Olpe, H.R., Baumann, P.A., and Waldmeier, P.C. (1984). Psychopharmacological and behavioral effects of anti-epileptic drugs in animals. In A.A. Muller (Ed.), *Anticonvulsants in Affective Disorders* (pp. 3–13). Amsterdam: Elsevier.

Maizels, E.T., Miller, J.B., Cutler, R.E. Jr., Jackiw, V., Carney, E.M., Mizuno, K., Ohno, S., and Hunzicker-Dunn, M. (1992). Estrogen modulates Ca(2+)-independent lipid-stimulated kinase in the rabbit corpus luteum of pseudopregnancy. Identification of luteal estrogen-modulated lipid-stimulated kinase as protein kinase C delta. *J Biol Chem*, 267, 17061–17068.

Maj, J., and Wedzony, K. (1985). Repeated treatment with imipramine or amitriptyline increases the locomotor response of rats to (+)-amphetamine given into the nucleus accumbens. *J Pharm Pharmacol*, 37, 362–364.

Maj, M., Ariano, M.G., Arena, F., and Kemali, D. (1984). Plasma cortisol, catecholamine and cyclic AMP levels, response to dexamethasone suppression test and platelet MAO activity in manic-depressive patients. A longitudinal study. *Neuropsychobiology*, 11, 168–173.

Maj, J., Chojnacka-Wojcik, E., Lewandowska, A., Tatarczynska, E., and Wiczynska, B. (1985). The central action of carbamazepine as a potential antidepressant drug. *Pol J Pharmacol Pharm*, 37(1), 47–56.

Malik, N., Canfield, V.A., Beckers, M.C., Gros, P., and Levenson, R. (1996). Identification of the mammalian Na,K-ATPase 3 subunit. *J Biol Chem*, 271, 22754–22758.

Malison, R.T., Anand, A., Pelton, G.H., Kirwin, P., Carpenter, L., McDougle, C.J., Heninger, G.R., and Price, L.H. (1999). Limited efficacy of ketoconazole in treatment-refractory major depression. *J Clin Psychopharmacol*, 19(5), 466–470.

Mallinger, A.G., Mallinger, J., Himmelhoch, J.M., Neil, J.F., and Hanin, I. (1980). Transmembrane distribution of lithium and sodium in erythrocytes of depressed patients. *Psychopharmacology (Berl)*, 68(3), 249.

Mallinger, A.G., Mallinger, J., Himmelhoch, J.M., Rossi, A., and Hanin, I. (1983). Essential hypertension and membrane lithium transport in depressed patients. *Psychiatry Res*, 10, 11–16.

Mallinger, A.G., Hanin, I., Himmelhoch, J.M., Thase, M.E., and Knopf, S. (1987). Stimulation of cell membrane sodium transport activity by lithium: Possible relationship to therapeutic action. *Psychiatry Res*, 22, 49–59.

Mallinger, A.G., Frank, E., Thase, M.E., Dippold, C.S., and Kupfer, D.J. (1997). Low rate of membrane lithium transport during treatment correlates with outcome of maintenance pharmacotherapy in bipolar disorder. *Neuropsychopharmacology*, 16(5), 325–332.

Malone, K.M., Thase, M.E., Mieczkowski, T., Myers, J.E., Stull, S.D., Cooper, T.B., and Mann, J.J. (1993). Fenfluramine challenge test as a predictor of outcome in major depression. *Psychopharmacol Bull*, 29, 155–161.

Manev, H., Uz, T., Smalheiser, N.R., and Manev, R. (2001). Antidepressants alter cell proliferation in the adult brain in vivo and in neural cultures in vitro. *Eur J Pharmacol*, 411, 67–70.

Manji, H.K. (1992). G proteins: Implications for psychiatry. *Am J Psychiatry*, 149, 746–760.

Manji, H.K., and Chen, G. (2000). Post-receptor signaling pathways in the pathophysiology and treatment of mood disorders. *Curr Psychiatry Rep*, 2, 479–489.

Manji, H., and Duman, R. (2001). Impairments of neuroplasticity and cellular resilience in severe mood disorder: Implications for the development of novel therapeutics. *Psychopharmacol Bull*, 35, 5–49.

Manji, H.K., and Lenox, R.H. (1994). Long-term action of lithium: A role for transcriptional and posttranscriptional factors regulated by protein kinase C. *Synapse*, 16, 11–28.

Manji, H.K., and Lenox, R.H. (1998). Lithium: A molecular transducer of mood-stabilization in the treatment of bipolar disorder. *Neuropsychopharmacology*, 19, 161–166.

Manji, H.K., and Lenox, R.H. (1999). Ziskind-Somerfeld Research Award. Protein kinase C signaling in the brain: Molecular transduction of mood stabilization in the treatment of manic-depressive illness. *Biol Psychiatry*, 46, 1328–1351.

Manji, H.K., and Lenox, R.H. (2000a). The nature of bipolar disorder. *J Clin Psychiatry*, 61(Suppl. 13), 42–57.

Manji, H.K., and Lenox, R.H. (2000b). Signaling: Cellular insights into the pathophysiology of bipolar disorder. *Biol Psychiatry*, 48, 518–530.

Manji, H.K., and Potter, W. (1997). Monoaminergic mechanisms in bipolar disorder. In R.T. Joffe (Ed.), *Bipolar Disorder: Biological Models and Their Clinical Application* (pp. 235–254). New York: Marcel Dekker.

Manji, H.K., Chen, G.A., Bitran, J.A., and Potter, W.Z. (1991a). Down-regulation of beta receptors by desipramine in vitro involves PKC/phospholipase A2. *Psychopharmacol Bull*, 27, 247–253.

Manji, H.K., Hsiao, J.K., Risby, E.D., Oliver, J., Rudorfer, M.V., and Potter, W.Z. (1991b). The mechanisms of action of lithium. I. Effects on serotoninergic and noradrenergic systems in normal subjects. *Arch Gen Psychiatry*, 48, 505–512.

Manji, H.K., Etcheberrigaray, R., Chen, G., and Olds, J.L. (1993). Lithium decreases membrane-associated protein kinase C in hippocampus: selectivity for the alpha isozyme. *J Neurochem*, 61, 2303–2310.

Manji, H.K., Chen, G., Shimon, H., Hsiao, J.K., Potter, W.Z., and Belmaker, R.H. (1995a). Guanine nucleotide-binding proteins in bipolar affective disorder. Effects of long-term lithium treatment. *Arch Gen Psychiatry*, 52, 135–144.

Manji, H.K., Potter, W.Z., and Lenox, R.H. (1995b). Signal transduction pathways. Molecular targets for lithium's actions. *Arch Gen Psychiatry*, 52, 531–543.

Manji, H.K., Bersudsky, Y., Chen, G., Belmaker, R.H., and Potter, W.Z. (1996). Modulation of protein kinase C isozymes and substrates by lithium: The role of myo-inositol. *Neuropsychopharmacology*, 15, 370–381.

Manji, H.K., Chen, G., Potter, W., and Kosten, T.R. (1997a). Guanine nucleotide binding proteins in opioid-dependent patients. *Biol Psychiatry*, 41(2), 130–134.

Manji, H.K., Moore, G.J., and Bebchuk, J.M. (1997b). Modulation of brain phosphoinositide signaling by lithium: Relationship to therapeutic response. *Biol Psychiatry*, 42, 290S.

Manji, H.K., McNamara, R., Chen, G., and Lenox, R.H. (1999a). Signalling pathways in the brain: Cellular transduction of mood stabilisation in the treatment of manic-depressive illness. *Aust N Z J Psychiatry*, 33(Suppl.), S65–S83.

Manji, H.K., Moore, G.J., and Chen, G. (1999b). Lithium at 50: Have the neuroprotective effects of this unique cation been overlooked? *Biol Psychiatry*, 46, 929–940.

Manji, H.K., Moore, G.J., and Chen, G. (2000a). Clinical and preclinical evidence for the neurotrophic effects of mood stabilizers: Implications for the pathophysiology and treatment of manic-depressive illness. *Biol Psychiatry*, 48(8), 740–754.

Manji, H.K., Moore, G.J., and Chen, G. (2000b). Lithium upregulates the cytoprotective protein Bcl-2 in the CNS in vivo: A role for neurotrophic and neuroprotective effects in manic-depressive illness. *J Clin Psychiatry*, 61(Suppl. 9), 82–96.

Manji, H.K., Drevets, W.C., and Charney, D.S. (2001a). The cellular neurobiology of depression. *Nat Med*, 7, 541–547.

Manji, H.K., Moore, G.J., and Chen, G. (2001b). Bipolar disorder: Leads from the molecular and cellular mechanisms of action of mood stabilizers. *Br J Psychiatry Suppl*, 41, s107–s119.

Manji, H.K., Gottesman, I.I., and Gould, T.D. (2003a). Signal transduction and genes-to-behaviors pathways in psychiatric diseases. *Sci STKE*, 207, pe49.

Manji, H.K., Quiroz, J.A., Sporn, J., Payne, J.L., Denicoff, K.A., Gray, N., Zarate, C.A. Jr., and Charney, D.S. (2003b). Enhancing neuronal plasticity and cellular resilience to develop novel, improved therapeutics for difficult-to-treat depression. *Biol Psychiatry*, 53, 707–742.

Mann, J.J., and Stanley, M. (1984). Postmortem monoamine oxidase enzyme kinetics in the frontal cortex of suicide victims and controls. *Acta Psychiatr Scand*, 69, 135–139.

Mann, J.J., Brown, R.P., Halper, J.P., Sweeney, J.A., Kocsis, J.H., Stokes, P.E., and Bilezikian, J.P. (1985). Reduced sensitivity of lymphocyte beta-adrenergic receptors in patients with endogenous depression and psychomotor agitation. *N Engl J Med*, 313, 715–720.

Mann, J.J., Stanley, M., McBride, P.A., and McEwen, B.S. (1986). Increased serotonin2 and beta-adrenergic receptor binding in the frontal cortices of suicide victims. *Arch Gen Psychiatry*, 43(10), 954–959.

Mann, J.J., McBride, P.A., Brown, R.P., Linnoila, M., Leon, A.C., DeMeo, M., Mieczkowski, T., Myers, J.E., and Stanley, M. (1992). Relationship between central and peripheral serotonin indexes in depressed and suicidal psychiatric inpatients. *Arch Gen Psychiatry*, 49, 442–446.

Mann, J.J., Henteleff, R.A., Lagattuta, T.F., Perper, J.A., Li, S., and Arango, V. (1996a). Lower 3H-paroxetine binding in cerebral cortex of suicide victims is partly due to fewer high affinity, non-transporter sites. *J Neural Transm*, 103, 1337–1350.

Mann, J.J., Arango, V., Henteleff, R.A., Lagattuta, T.F., and Wong, D.T. (1996b). Serotonin 5-HT3 receptor binding kinetics in the cortex of suicide victims are normal. *J Neural Transm*, 103, 165–171.

Mannel, M., Muller-Oerlinghausen, B., Czernik, A., and Sauer, H. (1997). 5-HT brain function in affective disorder: d,l-fenfluramine-induced hormone release and clinical outcome in long-term lithium/carbamazepine prophylaxis. *J Affect Disord*, 46, 101–113.

Mansbach, R.S., Brooks, E.N., and Chen, Y.L. (1997). Antidepressant-like effects of CP-154,526, a selective CRF1 receptor antagonist. *Eur J Pharmacol*, 323, 21–26.

Marangell, L.B., George, M.S., Callahan, A.M., Ketter, T.A., Pazzaglia, P.J., L'Herrou, T.A., Leverich, G.S., and Post, R.M. (1997). Effects of intrathecal thyrotropin-releasing hormone (protirelin) in refractory depressed patients. *Arch Gen Psychiatry*, 54, 214–222.

Marazziti, D., Lenzi, A., Galli, L., San Martino, S., and Cassano, G.B. (1991). Decreased platelet serotonin uptake in bipolar I patients. *Int Clin Psychopharmacol*, 6, 25–30.

Mark, R.J., Ashford, J.W., Goodman, Y., and Mattson, M.P. (1995). Anticonvulsants attenuate amyloid beta-peptide neurotoxicity, Ca2+ deregulation, and cytoskeletal pathology. *Neurobiol Aging*, 16, 187–198.

Martinek, S., Inonog, S., Manoukian, A.S., and Young, M.W. (2001). A role for the segment polarity gene *shaggy/GSK-3* in the *Drosophila* circadian clock. *Cell*, 105, 769–779.

Masana, M.I., Bitran, J.A., Hsiao, J.K., and Potter, W.Z. (1992). In vivo evidence that lithium inactivates Gi modulation of adenylate cyclase in brain. *J Neurochem*, 59, 200–205.

Masand, P.S., Pickett, P., and Murray, G.B. (1995). Hypomania precipitated by psychostimulant use in depressed medically ill patients. *Psychosomatics*, 36(2), 145–147.

Mason, J.W., Giller, E.L., and Kosten, T.R. (1988). Serum testosterone differences between patients with schizophrenia and those with affective disorder. *Biol Psychiatry*, 23, 357–366.

Massat, I., Souery, D., Del-Favero, J., Oruc, L., Noethen, M.M., Blackwood, D., Thomson, M., Muir, W., Papadimitriou, G.N., Dikeos, D.G., Kaneva, R., Serretti, A., Lilli, R., Smeraldi, E., Jakovljevic, M., Folnegovic, V., Rietschel, M., Milanova, V., Valente, F., Van Broeckhoven, C., and Mendlewicz, J. (2002). Excess of allele1 for alpha3 subunit GABA receptor gene (GABRA3) in bipolar patients: A multicentric association study. *Mol Psychiatry*, 7, 201.

Mastronardi, L., Puzzilli, F., and Ruggeri, A. (1998). Tamoxifen as a potential treatment of glioma. *Anticancer Drugs*, 9(7), 581–586.

Mathe, A.A., Jousisto-Hanson, J., Stenfors, C., and Theodorsson, E. (1990). Effect of lithium on tachykinins, calcitonin gene-related peptide, and neuropeptide Y in rat brain. *J Neurosci Res*, 26, 233–237.

Mathe, A.A., Agren, H., Lindstrom, L., and Theodorsson, E. (1994). Increased concentration of calcitonin gene-related peptide in cerebrospinal fluid of depressed patients. A possible trait marker of major depressive disorder. *Neurosci Lett*, 182(2), 138–142.

Mathews, R., Li, P.P., Young, L.T., Kish, S.J., and Warsh, J.J. (1997). Increased G alpha q/11 immunoreactivity in postmortem occipital cortex from patients with bipolar affective disorder. *Biol Psychiatry*, 41, 649–656.

Mathis, P., Schmitt, L., Benatia, M., Granier, F., Ghisolfi, J., and Moron, P. (1988). Plasma amino acid disturbances and depression. *Encephale*, 14, 77–82.

Matsubara, S., Arora, R.C., and Meltzer, H.Y. (1991). Serotonergic measures in suicide brain: 5-HT$_{1A}$ binding sites in frontal cortex of suicide victims. *J Neural Transm Gen Sect*, 85, 181–194.

Mattson, M.P., LaFerla, F.M., Chan, S.L., Leissring, M.A., Shepel, P.N., and Geiger, J.D. (2000). Calcium signaling in the ER: Its role in neuronal plasticity and neurodegenerative disorders. *Trends Neurosci*, 23(5), 222–229.

Matussek, N., Ackenheil, M., Hippius, H., Muller, F., Schroder, H.T., Schultes, H., and Wasilewski, B. (1980). Effect of clonidine on growth hormone release in psychiatric patients and controls. *Psychiatry Res*, 2, 25–36.

Mauri, M.C., Ferrara, A., Boscati, L., Bravin, S., Zamberlan, F., Alecci, M., and Invernizzi, G. (1998). Plasma and platelet amino acid concentrations in patients affected by major depression and under fluvoxamine treatment. *Neuropsychobiology*, 37, 124–129.

McBride, P.A., Brown, R.P., DeMeo, M., Keilp, J., Mieczkowski, T., and Mann, J.J. (1994). The relationship of platelet 5-HT$_2$ receptor indices to major depressive disorder, personality traits, and suicidal behavior. *Biol Psychiatry*, 35, 295–308.

McCance, S.L., Cohen, P.R., and Cowen, P.J. (1989). Lithium increases 5-HT-mediated prolactin release. *Psychopharmacology (Berl)*, 99, 276–281.

McCullumsmith, R.E., and Meador-Woodruff, J.H. (2002). Striatal excitatory amino acid transporter transcript expression in schizophrenia, bipolar disorder, and major depressive disorder. *Neuropsychopharmacology*, 26, 368–375.

McDonald, W.M., Tupler, L.A., Marsteller, F.A., Figiel, G.S., DiSouza, S., Nemeroff, C.B., and Krishnan, K.R. (1999). Hyperintense lesions on magnetic resonance images in bipolar disorder. *Biol Psychiatry*, 45, 965–971.

McEwen, B.S. (1999a). Stress and the aging hippocampus. *Front Neuroendocrinol*, 20(1), 49–70.

McEwen, B.S. (1999b). Stress and hippocampal plasticity. *Annu Rev Neurosci*, 22, 105–122.

McEwen, B.S. (2000). The neurobiology of stress: From serendipity to clinical relevance. *Brain Res*, 886, 172–189.

McEwen, B.S. (2003). Interacting mediators of allostasis and allostatic load: Towards an understanding of resilience in aging. *Metabolism*, 52(10 Suppl. 2), 10–16.

McEwen, B.S., and Magarinos, A.M. (2001). Stress and hippocampal plasticity: Implications for the pathophysiology of affective disorders. *Hum Psychopharmacol*, 16, S7–S19.

McGrath, P.J., Stewart, J.W., Harrison, W., and Quitkin, F.M. (1987). Treatment of tricyclic refractory depression with a monoamine oxidase inhibitor antidepressant. *Psychopharmacol Bull*, 23, 169–172.

McGrath, P.J., Stewart, J.W., Nunes, E.V., Ocepek-Welikson, K., Rabkin, J.G., Quitkin, F.M., and Klein, D.F. (1993). A double-blind crossover trial of imipramine and phenelzine for outpatients with treatment-refractory depression. *Am J Psychiatry*, 150, 118–123.

McGrath, P.J., Quitkin, F.M., and Klein, D.F. (1995). Bromocriptine treatment of relapses seen during selective serotonin reuptake inhibitor treatment of depression. *J Clin Psychopharmacol*, 15, 289–291.

McKinney, W.T. (1986). Electroconvulsive therapy and animal models of depression. *Ann NY Acad Sci*, 462, 65–69.

McKinney, W.T. (1988). *Models of Mental Disorders: A New Comparative Psychiatry*. New York: Plenum Medical Book Co.

McKinney, W.T. (2001). Overview of the past contributions of animal models and their changing place in psychiatry. *Semin Clin Neuropsychiatry*, 6, 68–78.

McKinney, W.T., Jr., Young, L.D., Suomi, S.J., and Davis, J.M. (1973). Chlorpromazine treatment of disturbed monkeys. *Arch Gen Psychiatry*, 29, 490–494.

McMahon, F.J., Buervenich, S., Charney, D., Lipsky, R., Rush, A.J., Wilson, A.F., Sorant, A.J., Papanicolaou, G.J., Laje, G., Fava, M., Trivedi, M.H., Wisniewski, S.R., and Manji, H. (2006). Variation in the gene encoding the serotonin 2a receptor is associated with outcome of antidepressant treatment. *Am J Hum Genet*, 78(5), 804–814.

McManamy, J. (2006). *Living Well with Depression and Bipolar Disorder: What Your Doctor Doesn't Tell You*. New York: Collins.

McNamara, R.K., Hyde, T.M., Kleinman, J.E., and Lenox, R.H. (1999). Expression of the myristoylated alanine-rich C kinase substrate (MARCKS) and MARCKS-related protein (MRP) in the prefrontal cortex and hippocampus of suicide victims. *J Clin Psychiatry*, 60(Suppl. 2), 21–26.

McTavish, S.F., McPherson, M.H., Harmer, C.J., Clark, L., Sharp, T., Goodwin, G.M., and Cowen, P.J. (2001). Antidopaminergic effects of dietary tyrosine depletion in healthy subjects and patients with manic illness. *Br J Psychiatry*, 179, 356–360.

Meador-Woodruff, J.H., Hogg, A.J. Jr., and Smith, R.E. (2001). Striatal ionotropic glutamate receptor expression in schizophrenia,

bipolar disorder, and major depressive disorder. *Brain Res Bull*, 55, 631–640.

Meagher, J.B., O'Halloran, A., Carney, P.A., and Leonard, B.E. (1990). Changes in platelet 5-hydroxytryptamine uptake in mania. *J Affect Disord*, 19, 191–196.

Meana, J.J., and Garcia-Sevilla, J.A. (1987). Increased alpha 2-adrenoceptor density in the frontal cortex of depressed suicide victims. *J Neural Transm*, 70, 377–381.

Meana, J.J., Barturen, F., and García-Sevilla, J.A. (1992). α2-Adrenoceptors in the brain of suicide victims: Increased receptor density associated with major depression. *Biol Psychiatry*, 31, 471–490.

Meaney, M.J., Diorio, J., Francis, D., LaRocque, S., O'Donnell, D., Smythe, J.W., Sharma, S., and Tannenbaum, B. (1994). Environmental regulation of the development of glucocorticoid receptor systems in the rat forebrain. The role of serotonin. *Ann NY Acad Sci*, 746, 260–273; discussion 274, 289–293.

Medini, L., Colli, S., Mosconi, C., Tremoli, E., and Galli, C. (1990). Diets rich in n-9, n-6 and n-3 fatty acids differentially affect the generation of inositol phosphates and of thromboxane by stimulated platelets, in the rabbit. *Biochem Pharmacol*, 39, 129–133.

Mellerup, E.T., and Rafaelsen, O.J. (1981). Depression and cerebrospinal fluid citrate. *Acta Psychiatr Scand*, 63, 57–60.

Meltzer, H.Y., and Lowy, M.T. (1987). The serotonin hypothesis of depression. In H.Y. Meltzer (Ed.), *Psychopharmacology: The Third Generation of Progress* (pp. 513–526). New York: Raven Press.

Meltzer, H.Y., Arora, R.C., Baber, R., and Tricou, B.J. (1981). Serotonin uptake in blood platelets of psychiatric patients. *Arch Gen Psychiatry*, 38, 1322–1326.

Meltzer, H.Y., Tueting, P., and Jackman, H. (1982). The effect of lithium on platelet monoamine oxidase activity in bipolar and schizoaffective disorders. *Br J Psychiatry*, 140, 192–198.

Meltzer, H.Y., Arora, R.C., and Goodnick, P. (1983). Effect of lithium carbonate on serotonin uptake in blood platelets of patients with affective disorders. *J Affect Disord*, 5, 215–21.

Meltzer, H.Y., Umberkoman-Wiita, B., Robertson, A., Tricou, B.J., Lowy, M., and Perline, R. (1984). Effect of 5-hydroxytryptophan on serum cortisol levels in major affective disorders. I. Enhanced response in depression and mania. *Arch Gen Psychiatry*, 41, 366–374.

Mendels, J., and Frazer, A. (1973). Intracellular lithium concentration and clinical response: Towards a membrane theory of depression. *J Psychiatr Res*, 10, 9–18.

Mendlewicz, J., Verbanck, P., Linkowski, P., and Wilmotte, J. (1978). Lithium accumulation in erythrocytes of manic-depressive patients: An in vivo twin study. *Br J Psychiatry*, 133, 436–444.

Merry, D.E., and Korsmeyer, S.J. (1997). Bcl-2 gene family in the nervous system. *Annu Rev Neurosci*, 20, 245–267.

Meurs, E., Rougeot, C., Svab, J., Laurent, A.G., Hovanessian, A.G., Robert, N., Gruest, J., Montagnier, L., and Dray, F. (1982). Use of an anti-human leukocyte interferon monoclonal antibody for the purification and radioimmunoassay of human alpha interferon. *Infect Immun*, 37(3), 919–926.

Meyer, J.H., Kapur, S., Houle, S., DaSilva, J., Owczarek, B., Brown, G.M., Wilson, A.A., and Kennedy, S.H. (1999). Prefrontal cortex 5-HT$_2$ receptors in depression: An [18F]setoperone PET imaging study. *Am J Psychiatry*, 156, 1029–1034.

Meyerson, L.R., Wennogle, L.P., Abel, M.S., Coupet, J., Lippa, A.S., Rauh, C.E., and Beer, B. (1982). Human brain receptor alterations in suicide victims. *Pharmacol Biochem Behav*, 17, 159–163.

Michael-Titus, A.T., Bains, S., Jeetle, J., and Whelpton, R. (2000). Imipramine and phenelzine decrease glutamate overflow in the prefrontal cortex: A possible mechanism of neuroprotection in major depression? *Neuroscience*, 100(4), 681.

Michel, A.D., Loury, D.N., and Whiting, R.L. (1990). Assessment of imiloxan as a selective alpha 2B-adrenoceptor antagonist. *Br J Pharmacol*, 99, 560–564.

Miguel-Hidalgo, J., and Rajkowska, G. (2002). Reduction of glia in the prefrontal cortex: A hypothesis of its role in the pathophysiology of major depressive disorder. *Biol Psychiatry*, 51, 98S.

Miguel-Hidalgo, J.J., Baucom, C., Dilley, G., Overholser, J.C., Meltzer, H.Y., Stockmeier, C.A., and Rajkowska, G. (2000). Glial fibrillary acidic protein immunoreactivity in the prefrontal cortex distinguishes younger from older adults in major depressive disorder. *Biol Psychiatry*, 48(8), 861–873.

Miki, M., Hamamura, T., Ujike, H., Lee, Y., Habara, T., Kodama, M., Ohashi, K., Tanabe, Y., and Kuroda, S. (2001). Effects of subchronic lithium chloride treatment on G-protein subunits (G_{olf}, $G\gamma7$) and adenylyl cyclase expressed specifically in the rat striatum. *Eur J Pharmacol*, 428, 303–309.

Miller, H.L., Delgado, P.L., Salomon, R.M., Berman, R., Krystal, J.H., Heninger, G.R., and Charney, D.S. (1996). Clinical and biochemical effects of catecholamine depletion on antidepressant-induced remission of depression. *Arch Gen Psychiatry*, 53(2), 117–128.

Milligan, G., and Wakelam, M. (1992). *G Proteins: Signal Transduction and Disease*. San Diego: Academic Press.

Minabe, Y., Tanii, Y., Tsunoda, M., and Kurachi, M. (1987). Acute effect of TRH, flunarizine, lithium and zotepine on amygdaloid kindled seizures induced with low-frequency stimulation. *Jpn J Psychiatry Neurol*, 41, 685–691.

Minabe, Y., Emori, K., and Kurachi, M. (1988). Effects of chronic lithium treatment on limbic seizure generation in the cat. *Psychopharmacology (Berl)*, 96, 391–394.

Minden, S.L., Orav, J., and Schildkraut, J.J. (1988). Hypomanic reactions to ACTH and prednisone treatment for multiple sclerosis. *Neurology*, 38(10), 1631–1634.

Mineka, S., and Suomi, S.J. (1978). Social separation in monkeys. *Psychol Bull*, 85, 1376–1400.

Miner, J.N., Tyree, C., Hu, J., Berger, E., Marschke, K., Nakane, M., Coghlan, M.J., Clemm, D., Lane, B., and Rosen, J. (2003). A nonsteroidal glucocorticoid receptor antagonist. *Mol Endocrinol*, 17(1), 117–127.

Minneman, K.P., Dibner, M.D., Wolfe, B.B., and Molinoff, P.B. (1979). Beta1- and beta2-adrenergic receptors in rat cerebral cortex are independently regulated. *Science*, 204, 866–868.

Mirnikjoo, B., Brown, S.E., Kim, H.F., Marangell, L.B., Sweatt, J.D., and Weeber, E.J. (2001). Protein kinase inhibition by omega-3 fatty acids. *J Biol Chem*, 276, 10888–10896.

Mitchell, P.B., and Smythe, G. (1990). Hormonal responses to fenfluramine in depressed and control subjects. *J Affect Disord*, 19, 43–51.

Mitchell, P.B., Manji, H.K., Chen, G., Jolkovsky, L., Smith-Jackson, E., Denicoff, K., Schmidt, M., and Potter, W.Z. (1997). High levels of Gs alpha in platelets of euthymic patients with bipolar affective disorder. *Am J Psychiatry*, 154, 218–223.

Mizuno, K., Okada, M., Murakami, T., Kamata, A., Zhu, G., Kawata, Y., Wada, K., and Kaneko, S. (2000). Effects of carbamazepine on acetylcholine release and metabolism. *Epilepsy Res*, 40, 187–195.

Mizuta, T., and Segawa, T. (1989). Chronic effects of imipramine and lithium on 5-HT receptor subtypes in rat frontal cortex, hippocampus and choroid plexus: Quantitative receptor autoradiographic analysis. *Jpn J Pharmacol*, 50, 315–326.

Modell, S., Lauer, C.J., Schreiber, W., Huber, J., Krieg, J.C., and Holsboer, F. (1998). Hormonal response pattern in the combined DEX-CRH test is stable over time in subjects at high familial risk for affective disorders. *Neuropsychopharmacology*, 18, 253–262.

Modestin, J., Hunger, J., and Schwartz, R.B. (1973a). Depressive effects of physostigmine. *Arch Psychiatr Nervenkr*, 218, 67–77.

Modestin, J., Schwartz, R.B., and Hunger, J. (1973b). Investigation about an influence of physostigmine on schizophrenic symptoms. *Pharmakopsychiatr Neuropsychopharmakol*, 6, 300–304.

Moises, H.C., Smith, C.B., Spengler, R.N., and Hollingsworth, P.J. (1986). Presynaptic alpha 2 adrenoreceptor function in dependent rats before and after morphine withdrawal. *NIDA Res Monogr*, 75, 579–582.

Molchan, S.E., Lawlor, B.A., Hill, J.L., Mellow, A.M., Davis, C.L., Martinez, R., and Sunderland, T. (1991). The TRH stimulation test in Alzheimer's disease and major depression: Relationship to clinical and CSF measures. *Biol Psychiatry*, 30, 567–576.

Moller, S.E., de Beurs, P., Timmerman, L., Tan, B.K., Leijnse-Ybema, H.J., Stuart, M.H., and Petersen, H.E. (1986). Plasma tryptophan and tyrosine ratios to competing amino acids in relation to antidepressant response to citalopram and maprotiline. A preliminary study. *Psychopharmacology (Berl)*, 88, 96–100.

Mooney, J.J., Samson, J.A., McHale, N.L., Colodzin, R., Alpert, J., Koutsos, M., and Schildkraut, J.J. (1998). Signal transduction by platelet adenylate cyclase: Alterations in depressed patients may reflect impairment in the coordinated integration of cellular signals (coincidence detection). *Biol Psychiatry*, 43, 574–583.

Moore, C.M., Breeze, J.L., Kukes, T.J., Rose, S.L., Dager, S.R., Cohen, B.M., and Renshaw, P.F. (1999a). Effects of myo-inositol ingestion on human brain myo-inositol levels: A proton magnetic resonance spectroscopic imaging study. *Biol Psychiatry*, 45, 1197–1202.

Moore, C.M., Frederick, B.B., and Renshaw, P.F. (1999b). Brain biochemistry using magnetic resonance spectroscopy: Relevance to psychiatric illness in the elderly. *J Geriatr Psychiatry Neurol*, 12, 107–117.

Moore, C.M., Biederman, J., Wozniak, J., Mick, E., Aleardi, M., Wardrop, M., Dougherty, M., Harpold, T., Hammerness, P., Randall, E., and Renshaw, P.F. (2006). Differences in brain chemistry in children and adolescents with attention deficit hyperactivity disorder with and without comorbid bipolar disorder: A proton magnetic resonance spectroscopy study. *Am J Psychiatry*, 163(2), 316–318.

Moore, G.J., and Galloway, M.P. (2002). Magnetic resonance spectroscopy: Neurochemistry and treatment effects in affective disorders. *Psychopharmacol Bull*, 36, 5–23.

Moore, G.J., Bebchuk, J.M., Parrish, J.K., Faulk, M.W., Arfken, C.L., Strahl-Bevacqua, J., and Manji, H.K. (1999). Temporal dissociation between lithium-induced changes in frontal lobe myo-inositol and clinical response in manic-depressive illness. *Am J Psychiatry*, 156, 1902–1908.

Moore, G.J., Bebchuk, J.M., Hasanat, K., Chen, G., Seraji-Bozorgzad, N., Wilds, I.B., Faulk, M.W., Koch, S., Glitz, D.A.,

Jolkovsky, L., and Manji, H.K. (2000). Lithium increases N-acetyl-aspartate in the human brain: In vivo evidence in support of Bcl-2's neurotrophic effects? *Biol Psychiatry*, 48, 1–8.

Moore, P., Gillin, C., Bhatti, T., DeModena, A., Seifritz, E., Clark, C., Stahl, S., Rapaport, M., and Kelsoe, J. (1998). Rapid tryptophan depletion, sleep electroencephalogram, and mood in men with remitted depression on serotonin reuptake inhibitors. *Arch Gen Psychiatry*, 55, 534–539.

Moore, P.B., Shepherd, D.J., Eccleston, D., Macmillan, I.C., Goswami, U., McAllister, V.L., and Ferrier, I.N. (2001). Cerebral white matter lesions in bipolar affective disorder: Relationship to outcome. *Br J Psychiatry*, 178, 172–176.

Mora, A., Gonzalez-Polo, R.A., Fuentes, J.M., Soler, G., and Centeno, F. (1999). Different mechanisms of protection against apoptosis by valproate and Li+. *Eur J Biochem*, 266, 886–891.

Mora, A., Sabio, G., Gonzalez-Polo, R.A., Cuenda, A., Alessi, D.R., Alonso, J.C., Fuentes, J.M., Soler, G., and Centeno, F. (2001). Lithium inhibits caspase 3 activation and dephosphorylation of PKB and GSK3 induced by K+ deprivation in cerebellar granule cells. *J Neurochem*, 78, 199–206.

Morden, B., Mullins, R., Levine, S., Cohen, H., and Dement, W. (1968). Effect of REM deprivation on the mating behavior of male rats. *Psychophysiology*, 5, 241.

Mori, S., Tardito, D., Dorigo, A., Zanardi, R., Smeraldi, E., Racagni, G., and Perez, J. (1998). Effects of lithium on cAMP-dependent protein kinase in rat brain. *Neuropsychopharmacology*, 19, 233–240.

Mork, A., and Geisler, A. (1989). The effects of lithium in vitro and ex vivo on adenylate cyclase in brain are exerted by distinct mechanisms. *Neuropharmacology*, 28, 307–311.

Mork, A., Klysner, R., and Geisler, A. (1990). Effects of treatment with a lithium-imipramine combination on components of adenylate cyclase in the cerebral cortex of the rat. *Neuropharmacology*, 29, 261–267.

Mork, A., Geisler, A., and Hollund, P. (1992). Effects of lithium on second messenger systems in the brain. *Pharmacol Toxicol*, 71(Suppl. 1), 4–17.

Morris, P.J., Lakin, N.D., Dawson, S.J., Ryabinin, A.E., Kilimann, M.W., Wilson, M.C., and Latchman, D.S. (1996). Differential regulation of genes encoding synaptic proteins by members of the Brn-3 subfamily of POU transcription factors. *Brain Res Mol Brain Res*, 43, 279–285.

Moscovich, D.G., Belmaker, R.H., Agam, G., and Livne, A. (1990). Inositol-1-phosphatase in red blood cells of manic-depressive patients before and during treatment with lithium. *Biol Psychiatry*, 27(5), 552–555.

Moses, S.G., and Robins, E. (1975). Regional distribution of norepinephrine and dopamine in brains of depressive suicides and alcoholic suicides. *Psychopharmacol Commun*, 1, 327–337.

Mota de Freitas, D., Silberberg, J., Espanol, M.T., Dorus, E., Abraha, A., Dorus, W., Elenz, E., and Whang, W. (1990). Measurement of lithium transport in RBC from psychiatric patients receiving lithium carbonate and normal individuals by 7Li NMR spectroscopy. *Biol Psychiatry*, 28, 415–424.

Motohashi, N., Ikawa, K., and Kariya, T. (1989). GABAB receptors are up-regulated by chronic treatment with lithium or carbamazepine. GABA hypothesis of affective disorders? *Eur J Pharmacol*, 166, 95–99.

Moudy, A.M., Handran, S.D., Goldberg, M.P., Ruffin, N., Karl, I., Kranz-Eble, P., DeVivo, D.C., and Rothman, S.M. (1995). Abnormal calcium homeostasis and mitochondrial polarization in a human encephalomyopathy. *Proc Natl Acad Sci USA*, 92(3), 729–733.

Mucha, R.F., Millan, M.J., and Herz, A. (1985). Aversive properties of naloxone in non-dependent (naive) rats may involve blockade of central beta-endorphin. *Psychopharmacology (Berl)*, 86, 281–285.

Muhlbauer, H.D. (1984). The influence of fenfluramine stimulation on prolactin plasma levels in lithium long-term-treated manic-depressive patients and healthy subjects. *Pharmacopsychiatry*, 17(6), 191–193.

Muhlbauer, H.D., and Muller-Oerlinghausen, B. (1985). Fenfluramine stimulation of serum cortisol in patients with major affective disorders and healthy controls: Further evidence for a central serotonergic action of lithium in man. *J Neural Transm*, 61, 81–94.

Muller, W., Brunner, H., and Misgeld, U. (1989). Lithium discriminates between muscarinic receptor subtypes on guinea pig hippocampal neurons in vitro. *Neurosci Lett*, 100, 135.

Mullins, L.J., and Brinley, F.J. Jr. (1967). Some factors influencing sodium extrusion by internally dialyzed squid axons. *J Gen Physiol*, 50, 2333–2355.

Mundo, E., Walker, M., Cate, T., Macciardi, F., and Kennedy, J.L. (2001). The role of serotonin transporter protein gene in antidepressant-induced mania in bipolar disorder: Preliminary findings. *Arch Gen Psychiatry*, 58, 539–544.

Munzer, J.S., Daly, S.E., Jewell-Motz, E.A., Lingrel, J.B., and Blostein, R. (1994). Tissue- and isoform-specific kinetic behavior of the Na,K-ATPase. *J Biol Chem*, 269, 16668–16676.

Murakami, T., Okada, M., Kawata, Y., Zhu, G., Kamata, A., and Kaneko, S. (2001). Determination of effects of antiepileptic drugs on SNAREs-mediated hippocampal monoamine release using in vivo microdialysis. *Br J Pharmacol*, 134, 507–520.

Murashita, J., Kato, T., Shioiri, T., Inubushi, T., and Kato, N. (2000). Altered brain energy metabolism in lithium-resistant bipolar disorder detected by photic stimulated 31P-MR spectroscopy. *Psychol Med*, 30(1), 107–115.

Murphy, B.E., Filipini, D., and Ghadirian, A.M. (1993). Possible use of glucocorticoid receptor antagonists in the treatment of major depression: Preliminary results using RU486. *J Psychiatry Neurosci*, 18(5), 209–213.

Murphy, D.L., Brodie, H.K., Goodwin, F.K., and Bunney, W.E. Jr. (1971). Regular induction of hypomania by L-dopa in "bipolar" manic-depressive patients. *Nature*, 229, 135–136.

Murphy, D.L., Donnelly, C., and Moskowitz, J. (1974). Catecholamine receptor function in depressed patients. *Am J Psychiatry*, 131, 1389–1391.

Murphy, D.L., Lipper, S., Campbell, I.C., Major, M.F., Slater, S., and Buchsbaum, M.S. (1979). Comparative studies of MAO-A and MAO-B inhibitors in man. In T.P. Singer, R.W. Von Korff, and D.L. Murphy (Eds.), *Monamine Oxidase: Structure Function and Altered Functions* (pp. 457–475). New York: Academic Press.

Murphy, D.L., Coursey, R.D., Haenel, T., Aloi, J., and Buchsbaum, M.S. (1982a). Platelet monoamine oxidase as a biological marker in the affective disorders and alcoholism. In E.H. Usdin (Ed.), *Biological Markers in Psychiatry and Neurology* (pp. 123–134). Oxford: Pergamon Press.

Murphy, D.L., Pickar, D., and Alterman, I.S. (1982b). Methods for the quantitative assessment of depressive and manic behavior. In E.I. Burdock, A. Sudilovsky, and S. Gershon (Eds.), *The Behavior of Psychiatric Patients: Quantitative Techniques for Evaluation* (pp. 355–392). New York: Marcel Dekker.

Murray, M., and Greenberg, M.L. (2000). Expression of yeast INM1 encoding inositol monophosphatase is regulated by inositol, carbon source and growth stage and is decreased by lithium and valproate. *Mol Microbiol*, 36, 651–661.

Muscettola, G., Potter, W.Z., Pickar, D., and Goodwin, F.K. (1984). Urinary 3-methoxy-4-hydroxyphenylglycol and major affective disorders. A replication and new findings. *Arch Gen Psychiatry*, 41, 337–342.

Musselman, D.L., and Nemeroff, C.B. (1996). Depression and endocrine disorders: Focus on the thyroid and adrenal system. *Br J Psychiatry Suppl*, 123–128.

Musselman, D.L., Evans, D.L., and Nemeroff, C.B. (1998). The relationship of depression to cardiovascular disease: epidemiology, biology, and treatment. *Arch Gen Psychiatry*, 55, 580–592.

Mynett-Johnson, L.A., Murphy, V.E., Claffey, E., Shields, D.C., and McKeon, P. (1998). Preliminary evidence of an association between bipolar disorder in females and the catechol-O-methyltransferase gene. *Psychiatr Genet*, 8, 221–225.

Mynett-Johnson, L., Kealey, C., Claffey, E., Curtis, D., Bouchier-Hayes, L., Powell, C., and McKeon, P. (2000). Multimarker haplotypes within the serotonin transporter gene suggest evidence of an association with bipolar disorder. *Am J Med Genet*, 96(6), 845–849.

Naber, D., Sand, P., and Heigl, B. (1996). Psychopathological and neuropsychological effects of 8-days' corticosteroid treatment. A prospective study. *Psychoneuroendocrinology*, 21(1), 25–31.

Nahorski, S.R., Ragan, C.I., and Challiss, R.A. (1991). Lithium and the phosphoinositide cycle: An example of uncompetitive inhibition and its pharmacological consequences. *Trends Pharmacol Sci*, 12, 297–303.

Nahorski, S.R., Jenkinson, S., and Challiss, R.A. (1992). Disruption of phosphoinositide signalling by lithium. *Biochem Soc Trans*, 20, 430–434.

Nakamura, S. (1990). Antidepressants induce regeneration of catecholaminergic axon terminals in the rat cerebral cortex. *Neurosci Lett*, 111, 64–68.

Nalepa . (1993). The effects of chlorpromazine and haloperidol on second messenger systems related to adrenergic receptors. *Pol J Pharmacol*, 45, 399–412.

Nalep I. (1994). The effect of psychotropic drugs on the interaction of protein kinase C with second messenger systems in the rat cerebral cortex. *Pol J Pharmacol*, 46, 1–14.

Narita, M., Aoki, T., Ozaki, S., Yajima, Y., and Suzuki, T. (2001). Involvement of protein kinase Cγ isoform in morphine-induced reinforcing effects. *Neuroscience*, 103(2), 309–314.

Nau, H., and Loscher, W. (1982). Valproate: Brain and plasma levels of the drug and its metabolites, anticonvulsant effects and gamma-aminobutyric acid (GABA) metabolism in the mouse. *J Pharmacol Exp Ther*, 220, 654–659.

Naylor, G.J., and Smith, A.H. (1981). Vanadium: A possible aetiological factor in manic depressive illness. *Psychol Med*, 11, 249–256.

Naylor, G.J., McNamee, H.B., and Moody, J.P. (1970). The plasma control of erythrocyte sodium and potassium metabolism in depressive illness. *J Psychosom Res*, 14, 179–186.

Naylor, G.J., McNamee, H.B., and Moody, J.P. (1971). Changes in erythrocyte sodium and potassium on recovery from a depressive illness. *Br J Psychiatry*, 118, 219–223.

Naylor, G.J., Dick, D.A., Dick, E.G., and Moody, J.P. (1974a). Lithium therapy and erythrocyte membrane cation carrier. *Psychopharmacologia*, 37, 81–86.

Naylor, G.J., Donald, J.M., Le Poidevin, D., and Reid, A.H. (1974b). A double-blind trial of long-term lithium therapy in mental defectives. *Br J Psychiatry*, 124, 52–57.

Naylor, G.J., Reid, A.H., Dick, D.A.T., and Dick, E.G. (1976). A biochemical study of short-cycle manic-depressive psychosis in mental defectives. *Br J Psychiatry*, 128, 1690–1180.

Naylor, G.J., Smith, A.H., Dick, E.G., Dick, D.A., McHarg, A.M., and Chambers, C.A. (1980). Erythrocyte membrane cation carrier in manic-depressive psychosis. *Psychol Med*, 10, 521–525.

Nemanov, L., Ebstein, R.P., Belmaker, R.H., Osher, Y., and Agam, G. (1999). Effect of bipolar disorder on lymphocyte inositol monophosphatase mRNA levels. *Int J Neuropsychopharmcol*, 2, 25–29.

Nemeroff, C.B., Kalivas, P.W., Golden, R.N., and Prange, A.J. Jr. (1984a). Behavioral effects of hypothalamic hypophysiotropic hormones, neurotensin, substance P and other neuropeptides. *Pharmacol Ther*, 24, 1–56.

Nemeroff, C.B., Widerlöv, E., Bissette, G., Walleus, H., Karlsson, I., Eklund, K., Kilts, C.D., Loosen, P.T., and Vale, W. (1984b). Elevated concentrations of CSF corticotropin-releasing factor-like immunoreactivity in depressed patients. *Science*, 226, 1342–1344.

Nemeroff, C.B., Simon, J.S., Haggerty, J.J. Jr., and Evans, D.L. (1985). Antithyroid antibodies in depressed patients. *Am J Psychiatry*, 142, 840–843.

Nemeroff, C.B., Owens, M.J., Bissette, G., Andorn, A.C., and Stanley, M. (1988). Reduced corticotropin releasing factor binding sites in the frontal cortex of suicide victims. *Arch Gen Psychiatry*, 45, 577–579.

Nemeroff, C.B., Bissette, G., Akil, H., and Fink, M. (1991). Neuropeptide concentrations in the cerebrospinal fluid of depressed patients treated with electroconvulsive therapy. Corticotrophin-releasing factor, beta-endorphin and somatostatin. *Br J Psychiatry*, 158, 59–63.

Nemeroff, C.B., Evans, D.L., Gyulai, L., Sachs, G.S., Bowden, C.L., Gergel, I.P., Oakes, R., and Pitts, C.D. (2001). Double-blind, placebo-controlled comparison of imipramine and paroxetine in the treatment of bipolar depression. *Am J Psychiatry*, 158, 906–912.

Nestler, E.J., Terwilliger, R.Z., and Duman, R.S. (1989). Chronic antidepressant administration alters the subcellular distribution of cyclic AMP–dependent protein kinase in rat frontal cortex. *J Neurochem*, 53, 1644–1647.

Nestler, E.J., Terwilliger, R.Z., and Duman, R.S. (1995). Regulation of endogenous ADP-ribosylation by acute and chronic lithium in rat brain. *J Neurochem*, 64, 2319–2324.

Nestler, E.J., Barrot, M., DiLeone, R.J., Eisch, A.J., Gold, S.J., and Monteggia, L.M. (2002a). Neurobiology of depression. *Neuron*, 34, 13–25.

Nestler, E.J., Gould, E., Manji, H., Buncan, M., Duman, R.S., Greshenfeld, H.K., Hen, R., Koester, S., Lederhendler, I., Meaney, M., Robbins, T., Winsky, L., and Zalcman, S. (2002b). Preclinical models: status of basic research in depression. *Biol Psychiatry*, 52, 503–528.

Neubig, R.R., Gantzos, R.D., and Thomsen, W.J. (1988). Mechanism of agonist and antagonist binding to alpha 2 adrenergic receptors: Evidence for a precoupled receptor-guanine nucleotide protein complex. *Biochemistry*, 27, 2374–2384.

Neumeister, A. (2003). Tryptophan depletion, serotonin, and depression: Where do we stand? *Psychopharmacol Bull*, 37, 99–115.

Neumeister, A., Praschak-Rieder, N., Hesselmann, B., Vitouch, O., Rauh, M., Barocka, A., and Kasper, S. (1997). Rapid tryptophan depletion in drug-free depressed patients with seasonal affective disorder. *Am J Psychiatry*, 154(8), 1153–1155.

Neumeister, A., Praschak-Rieder, N., Hesselmann, B., Vitouch, O., Rauh, M., Barocka, A., Tauscher, J., and Kasper, S. (1998). Effects of tryptophan depletion in drug-free depressed patients who responded to total sleep deprivation. *Arch Gen Psychiatry*, 55, 167–172.

Neumeister, A., Young, T., and Stastny, J. (2004). Implications of genetic research on the role of the serotonin in depression: Emphasis on the serotonin type 1a receptor and the serotonin transporter. *Psychopharmacology (Berl)*, 174(4), 512–524.

Newman, M.E., and Belmaker, R.H. (1987). Effects of lithium in vitro and ex vivo on components of the adenylate cyclase system in membranes from the cerebral cortex of the rat. *Neuropharmacology*, 26, 211–217.

Newman, M.E., Drummer, D., and Lerer, B. (1990). Single and combined effects of desimipramine and lithium on serotonergic receptor number and second messenger function in rat brain. *J Pharmacol Exp Ther*, 252, 826–831.

Newman, M.E., Shapira, B., and Lerer, B. (1998). Evaluation of central serotonergic function in affective and related disorders by the fenfluramine challenge test: A critical review. *Int J Neuropsychopharmcol*, 1, 49–69.

Nibuya, M., Morinobu, S., and Duman, R.S. (1995). Regulation of BDNF and TrkB mRNA in rat brain by chronic electroconvulsive seizure and antidepressant drug treatments. *J Neurosci*, 15, 7539–7547.

Nibuya, M., Nestler, E.J., and Duman, R.S. (1996). Chronic antidepressant administration increases the expression of cAMP response element binding protein (CREB) in rat hippocampus. *J Neurosci*, 16, 2365–2372.

Nibuya, M., Takahashi, M., Russell, D.S., and Duman, R.S. (1999). Repeated stress increases catalytic TrkB mRNA in rat hippocampus. *Neurosci Lett*, 267, 81–84.

Nicholas, L., Dawkins, K., and Golden, R.N. (1998). Psychoneuroendocrinology of depression. Prolactin. *Psychiatr Clin North Am*, 21, 341–358.

Niesler, B., Flohr, T., Nothen, M.M., Fischer, C., Rietschel, M., Franzek, E., Albus, M., Propping, P., and Rappold, G.A. (2001). Association between the 5' UTR variant C178T of the serotonin receptor gene HTR3A and bipolar affective disorder. *Pharmacogenetics*, 11, 471–475.

Nikaido, T., Akiyama, M., Moriya, T., and Shibata, S. (2001). Sensitized increase of period gene expression in the mouse caudate/putamen caused by repeated injection of methamphetamine. *Mol Pharmacol*, 59(4), 894–900.

Nilsson, C., Karlsson, G., Blennow, K., Heilig, M., and Ekman, R. (1996). Differences in the neuropeptide Y–like immunoreactivity of the plasma and platelets of human volunteers and depressed patients. *Peptides*, 17(3), 359–362.

Nilsson, M., Hansson, E., and Ronnback, L. (1990). Transport of valproate and its effects on GABA uptake in astroglial primary culture. *Neurochem Res*, 15, 763–767.

Nishizuka, Y. (1992). Intracellular signaling by hydrolysis of phospholipids and activation of protein kinase C. *Science*, 258, 607–614.

Noble, A.B., McKinney, W.T. Jr., Mohr, C., and Moran, E. (1976). Diazepam treatment of socially isolated monkeys. *Am J Psychiatry*, 133, 1165–1170.

Noga, J.T., Hyde, T.M., Herman, M.M., Spurney, C.F., Bigelow, L.B., Weinberger, D.R., and Kleinman, J.E. (1997). Glutamate receptors in the postmortem striatum of schizophrenic, suicide, and control brains. *Synapse*, 27, 168–176.

Nolen, W.A., van de Putte, J.J., Dijken, W.A., Kamp, J.S., Blansjaar, B.A., Kramer, H.J., and Haffmans, J. (1988). Treatment strategy in depression. II. MAO inhibitors in depression resistant to cyclic antidepressants: Two controlled crossover studies with tranylcypromine versus L-5-hydroxytryptophan and nomifensine. *Acta Psychiatr Scand*, 78, 676–683.

Nolen-Hoeksema, S. (1987). Sex differences in unipolar depression: Evidence and theory. *Psychol Bull*, 101, 259–282.

Nonaka, S., and Chuang, D.M. (1998). Neuroprotective effects of chronic lithium on focal cerebral ischemia in rats. *Neuroreport*, 9, 2081–2084.

Nonaka, S., Hough, C.J., and Chuang, D.M. (1998). Chronic lithium treatment robustly protects neurons in the central nervous system against excitotoxicity by inhibiting N-methyl-D-aspartate receptor-mediated calcium influx. *Proc Natl Acad Sci USA*, 95, 2642–2647.

Nowak, G., Trullas, R., Layer, R.T., Skolnick, P., and Paul, I.A. (1993). Adaptive changes in the N-methyl-D-aspartate receptor complex after chronic treatment with imipramine and 1-aminocyclopropanecarboxylic acid. *J Pharmacol Exp Ther*, 265, 1380–1386.

Nowak, G., Ordway, G.A., and Paul, I.A. (1995a). Alterations in the N-methyl-D-aspartate (NMDA) receptor complex in the frontal cortex of suicide victims. *Brain Res*, 675, 157–164.

Nowak, G., Redmond, A., McNamara, M., and Paul, I.A. (1995b). Swim stress increases the potency of glycine at the N-methyl-D-aspartate receptor complex. *J Neurochem*, 64, 925–927.

Nurnberger, J.I. Jr., Jimerson, D.C., Allen, J.R., Simmons, S., and Gershon, E. (1982). Red cell ouabain-sensitive Na⁺-K⁺-adenosine triphosphatase: Astate marker in affective disorder inversely related to plasma cortisol. *Biol Psychiatry*, 17, 981–992.

Nurnberger, J.I. Jr., Jimerson, D.C., Simmons-Alling, S., Tamminga, C., Nadi, N.S., Lawrence, D., Sitaram, N., Gillin, J.C., and Gershon, E.S. (1983). Behavioral, physiological, and neuroendocrine responses to arecoline in normal twins and "well state" bipolar patients. *Psychiatry Res*, 9, 191–200.

Nurnberger, J.I. Jr., Berrettini, W., Mendelson, W., Sack, D., and Gershon, E.S. (1989). Measuring cholinergic sensitivity: I. Arecoline effects in bipolar patients. *Biol Psychiatry*, 25, 610–617.

Nurnberger, J.I. Jr., Berrettini, W., Simmons-Alling, S., Lawrence, D., and Brittain, H. (1990). Blunted ACTH and cortisol response to afternoon tryptophan infusion in euthymic bipolar patients. *Psychiatry Res*, 31, 57–67.

Nurnberger, J.I., Adkins, S., Lahiri, D.K., Mayeda, A., Hu, K., Lewy, A., Miller, A., Bowman, E.S., Miller, M.J., Rau, L., Smiley, C., and Davis-Singh, D. (2000). Melatonin suppression by light in euthymic bipolar and unipolar patients. *Arch Gen Psychiatry*, 57(6), 572–579.

Nutt, D.J. (1989). Altered central alpha 2-adrenoceptor sensitivity in panic disorder. *Arch Gen Psychiatry*, 46, 165–169.

O'Brian, C.A., Ward, N.E., and Anderson, B.W. (1988). Role of specific interactions between protein kinase C and triphenylethylenes in inhibition of the enzyme. *J Natl Cancer Inst*, 80(20), 1628–1633.

Odagaki, Y., Koyama, T., Matsubara, S., Matsubara, R., and Yamashita, I. (1990). Effects of chronic lithium treatment on serotonin binding sites in rat brain. *J Psychiatr Res*, 24, 271–277.

Ohmori, T., Arora, R.C., and Meltzer, H.Y. (1992). Serotonergic measures in suicide brain: The concentration of 5-HIAA, HVA, and tryptophan in frontal cortex of suicide victims. *Biol Psychiatry*, 32, 57–71.

Okamoto, Y., Kagaya, A., Shinno, H., Motohashi, N., and Yamawaki, S. (1995). Serotonin-induced platelet calcium mobilization is enhanced in mania. *Life Sci*, 56, 327–332.

Okuyama, S., Chaki, S., Kawashima, N., Suzuki, Y., Ogawa, S., Nakazato, A., Kumagai, T., Okubo, T., and Tomisawa, K. (1999). Receptor binding, behavioral, and electrophysiological profiles of nonpeptide corticotropin-releasing factor subtype 1 receptor antagonists CRA1000 and CRA1001. *J Pharmacol Exp Ther*, 289(2), 926–935.

Olive, M.F., Mehmert, K.K., Messing, R.O., and Hodge, C.W. (2000). Reduced operant ethanol self-administration and in vivo mesolimbic dopamine responses to ethanol in PKCepsilon-deficient mice. *Eur J Neurosci*, 12, 4131–4140.

Ongur, D., Drevets, W.C., and Price, J.L. (1998). Glial reduction in the subgenual prefrontal cortex in mood disorders. *Proc Natl Acad Sci USA*, 95, 13290–13295.

Oomen, H.A., Schipperijn, A.J., and Drexhage, H.A. (1996). The prevalence of affective disorder and in particular of a rapid cycling of bipolar disorder in patients with abnormal thyroid function tests. *Clin Endocrinol (Oxf)*, 45, 215–223.

Oppenheim, G., Ebstein, R.P., and Belmaker, R.H. (1979). Effect of lithium on the physostigmine-induced behavioral syndrome and plasma cyclic GMP. *J Psychiatr Res*, 15, 133–138.

Ordway, G.A., Smith, K.S., and Haycock, J.W. (1994a). Elevated tyrosine hydroxylase in the locus coeruleus of suicide victims. *J Neurochem*, 62, 680–685.

Ordway, G.A., Widdowson, P.S., Smith, K.S., and Halaris, A. (1994b). Agonist binding to α2-adrenoceptors is elevated in the locus coeruleus from victims of suicide. *J Neurochem*, 63, 617–624.

Ordway, G.A., Farley, J.T., Dilley, G.E., Overholser, J.C., Meltzer, H.Y., Balraj, E.K., Stockmeier, C.A., and Klimek, V. (1999). Quantitative distribution of monoamine oxidase A in brainstem monoamine nuclei is normal in major depression. *Brain Res*, 847, 71–79.

Orlovskaya, D.D., Vostrikov, V.M., Rachmanova, V.I., and Uranova, N.A. (2000). Decreased numerical density of oligodendroglial cells in postmortem prefrontal cortex in schizophrenia, bipolar affective disorder and major depression. *Schizophr Res*, 41, 105.

Ormandy, G.C., and Jope, R.S. (1991). Pertussis toxin potentiates seizures induced by pilocarpine, kainic acid and N-methyl-D-aspartate. *Brain Res*, 553, 51–57.

Orr, K.G., Mostert, J., and Castle, D.J. (1998). Mania associated with codeine and paracetamol. *Aust N Z J Psychiatry*, 32, 586–588.

Orth, D.N., Shelton, R.C., Nicholson, W.E., Beck-Peccoz, P., Tomarken, A.J., Persani, L., and Loosen, P.T. (2001). Serum thyrotropin concentrations and bioactivity during sleep deprivation in depression. *Arch Gen Psychiatry*, 58, 77–83.

Oruc, L., Verheyen, G.R., Furac, I., Jakovljevic, M., Ivezic, S., Raeymaekers, P., and Van Broeckhoven C. (1997). Association analysis of the 5-HT2C receptor and 5-HT transporter genes in bipolar disorder. *Am J Med Genet*, 74(5), 504–506.

Oshima, A., Yamashita, S., Owashi, T., Murata, T., Tadokoro, C., Miyaoka, H., Kamijima, K., and Higuchi, T. (2000). The differential ACTH responses to combined dexamethasone/CRH administration in major depressive and dysthymic disorders. *J Psychiatr Res*, 34(4-5), 325–328.

Ostrow, D.G., Pandey, G.N., Davis, J.M., Hurt, S.W., and Tosteson, D.C. (1978). A heritable disorder of lithium transport in erythrocytes of a subpopulation of manic-depressive patients. *Am J Psychiatry*, 135, 1070–1078.

Ostrow, D.G., and Davis, J.M. (1982). Laboratory measurements in the clinical use of lithium. *Clin Neuropharmacol*, 5(3), 317–336.

Owen, F., Cross, A.J., Crow, T.J., Deakin, J.F., Ferrier, I.N., Lofthouse, R., and Poulter, M. (1983). Brain 5-HT2 receptors and suicide. *Lancet*, ii, 1256.

Owen F., Chambers, D.R., Cooper, S.J., Crow, T.J., Johnson, J.A., Lofthouse, R., and Poulter, M. (1986). Serotonergic mechanisms in brains of suicide victims. *Brain Res*, 362, 185–188.

Owens, D.F., and Kriegstein, A.R. (2002). Is there more to GABA than synaptic inhibition? *Nat Rev Neurosci*, 3(9), 715–727.

Owens, M.J., and Nemeroff, C.B. (1998). The serotonin transporter and depression. *Depress Anxiety*, 8(Suppl. 1), 5–12.

Oyama, T., Yamaya, R., Jin, T., and Kudo, T. (1982). Effect of exogenous beta-endorphin on anterior pituitary hormone secretion in man. *Acta Endocrinol (Copenh)*, 99, 9–13.

Ozaki, N., and Chuang, D.M. (1997). Lithium increases transcription factor binding to AP-1 and cyclic AMP-responsive element in cultured neurons and rat brain. *J Neurochem*, 69, 2336–2344.

Pacheco, M.A., Stockmeier, C., Meltzer, H.Y., Overholser, J.C., Dilley, G.E., and Jope, R.S. (1996). Alterations in phosphoinositide signaling and G-protein levels in depressed suicide brain. *Brain Res*, 723, 37–45.

Palmer, G.C. (1979). Interactions of antiepileptic drugs on adenylate cyclase and phosphodiesterases in rat and mouse cerebrum. *Exp Neurol*, 63, 322–335.

Palmer, A.M., Burns, M.A., Arango, V., and Mann, J.J. (1994). Similar effects of glycine, zinc and an oxidizing agent on [3H]dizocilpine binding to the N-methyl-D-aspartate receptor in neocortical tissue from suicide victims and controls. *J Neural Transm Gen Sect*, 96, 1–8.

Pandey, G.N., and Davis, J.M. (1986). Leukocyte β-adrenergic receptors: A marker for central β-adrenergic receptor function in depression. *Clin Neuropharmacol*, 14(Suppl. 9), 353–355.

Pandey, G.N., Ostrow, D.G., Haas, M., Dorus, E., Casper, R.C., Davis, J.M., and Tosteson, D.C. (1977). Abnormal lithium and sodium transport in erythrocytes of a manic patient and some members of his family. *Proc Natl Acad Sci USA*, 74(8), 3607–3611.

Pandey, G.N., Dysken, M.W., Garver, D.L., and Davis, J.M. (1979). Beta-adrenergic receptor function in affective illness. *Am J Psychiatry*, 136, 675–678.

Pandey, G.N., Sudershan, P., and Davis, J.M. (1985). Beta-adrenergic receptor function in depression and the effect of antidepressant drugs. *Acta Pharmacol Toxicol (Copenh)*, 56 (Suppl. 1), 66–79.

Pandey, G.N., Janicak, P.G., and Davis, J.M. (1987). Decreased beta-adrenergic receptors in the leukocytes of depressed patients. *Psychiatry Res*, 22, 265–273.

Pandey, G.N., Janicak, P.G., Javaid, J.I., and Davis, J.M. (1989). Increased 3H-clonidine binding in the platelets of patients with depressive and schizophrenic disorders. *Psychiatry Res*, 28, 73–88.

Pandey, G.N., Pandey, S.C., Janicak, P.G., Marks, R.C., and Davis, J.M. (1990). Platelet serotonin-2 receptor binding sites in depression and suicide. *Biol Psychiatry*, 28, 215–222.

Pandey, G.N., Pandey, S.C., Dwivedi, Y., Sharma, R.P., Janicak, P.G., and Davis, J.M. (1995). Platelet serotonin-2A receptors: A potential biological marker for suicidal behavior. *Am J Psychiatry*, 152, 850–855.

Pandey, G.N., Dwivedi, Y., Pandey, S.C., Conley, R.R., Roberts, R.C., and Tamminga, C.A. (1997a). Protein kinase C in the postmortem brain of teenage suicide victims. *Neurosci Lett*, 228, 111–114.

Pandey, G.N., Conley, R.R., Pandey, S.C., Goel, S., Roberts, R.C., Tamminga, C.A., Chute, D., and Smialek, J. (1997b). Benzodiazepine receptors in the post-mortem brain of suicide victims and schizophrenic subjects. *Psychiatry Res*, 71, 137–149.

Pap, M., and Cooper, G.M. (1998). Role of glycogen synthase kinase-3 in the phosphatidylinositol 3-kinase/Akt cell survival pathway. *J Biol Chem*, 273, 19929–19932.

Papadimitriou, G.N., Dikeos, D.G., Karadima, G., Avramopoulos, D., Daskalopoulou, E.G., Vassilopoulos, D., and Stefanis, C.N. (1998). Association between the GABA(A) receptor alpha5 subunit gene locus (GABRA5) and bipolar affective disorder. *Am J Med Genet*, 81, 73–80.

Papolos, D.F., Veit, S., Faedda, G.L., Saito, T., and Lachman, H.M. (1998). Ultra-ultra rapid cycling bipolar disorder is associated with the low activity catecholamine-O-methyltransferase allele. *Mol Psychiatry*, 3, 346–349.

Papp, M., Willner, P., and Muscat, R. (1991). An animal model of anhedonia: Attenuation of sucrose consumption and place preference conditioning by chronic unpredictable mild stress. *Psychopharmacology (Berl)*, 104, 255–259.

Pare, C.M.B., Yeung, D.P., Price, K., and Stacey, R.S. (1969). 5-Hydroxytryptamine, noradrenaline, and dopamine in brainstem, hypothalamus, and caudate nucleus of controls and of patients committing suicide by coal-gas poisoning. *Lancet*, ii, 133–135.

Parekh, P.I., Ketter, T.A., Altshuler, L., Frye, M.A., Callahan, A., Marangell, L., and Post, R.M. (1998). Relationships between thyroid hormone and antidepressant responses to total sleep deprivation in mood disorder patients. *Biol Psychiatry*, 43, 392–394.

Parry, B.L., Hauger, R., LeVeau, B., Mostofi, N., Cover, H., Clopton, P., and Gillin, J.C. (1996). Circadian rhythms of prolactin and thyroid-stimulating hormone during the menstrual cycle and early versus late sleep deprivation in premenstrual dysphoric disorder. *Psychiatry Res*, 62(2), 147–160.

Parsian, A., Chakraverty, S., and Todd, R.D. (1995). Possible association between the dopamine D3 receptor gene and bipolar affective disorder. *Am J Med Genet*, 60, 234–237.

Pascual, T., and Gonzalez, J.L. (1995). A protective effect of lithium on rat behaviour altered by ibotenic acid lesions of the basal forebrain cholinergic system. *Brain Res*, 695, 289–292.

Patel, P.D., Lopez, J.F., Lyons, D.M., Burke, S., Wallace, M., and Schatzberg, A.F. (2000). Glucocorticoid and mineralocorticoid receptor mRNA expression in squirrel monkey brain. *J Psychiatr Res*, 34, 383–392.

Patsalos, P.N., and Lascelles, P.T. (1981). Changes in regional brain levels of amino acid putative neurotransmitters after prolonged treatment with the anticonvulsant drugs diphenylhydantoin, phenobarbitone, sodium valproate, ethosuximide, and sulthiame in the rat. *J Neurochem*, 36, 688–695.

Paul, I.A., Trullas, R., Skolnick, P., and Nowak, G. (1992). Downregulation of cortical beta-adrenoceptors by chronic treatment with functional NMDA antagonists. *Psychopharmacology (Berl)*, 106, 285–287.

Paul, S.M., Rehavi, M., Skolnick, P., and Goodwin, F.K. (1984). High affinity binding of antidepressants to biogenic amine transport sites in human brain and platelet: Studies in depression. In M. Post and J.C. Ballenger (Eds.), *Neurobiology of Mood Disorders* (pp. 846–853). Baltimore: Williams & Wilkins.

Payne, J.L., Quiroz, J.A., Carlos, A., Zarate, J., and Manji, H.K. (2002). Timing is everything: Does the robust upregulation of noradrenergically regulated plasticity genes underlie the rapid antidepressant effects of sleep deprivation? *Biol Psychiatry*, 52, 921–926.

Pearlson, G.D., Wong, D.F., Tune, L.E., Ross, C.A., Chase, G.A., Links, J.M., Dannals, R.F., Wilson, A.A., Ravert, H.T., and Wagner, H.N. Jr. (1995). In vivo D2 dopamine receptor density in psychotic and nonpsychotic patients with bipolar disorder. *Arch Gen Psychiatry*, 52, 471–477.

Peckys, D., and Hurd, Y.L. (2001). Prodynorphin and kappa opioid receptor mRNA expression in the cingulate and prefrontal cortices of subjects diagnosed with schizophrenia or affective disorders. *Brain Res Bull*, 55, 619–624.

Pepe, S., Bogdanov, K., Hallaq, H., Spurgeon, H., Leaf, A., and Lakatta, E. (1994). Omega 3 polyunsaturated fatty acid modulates dihydropyridine effects on L-type Ca2+ channels, cytosolic Ca2+, and contraction in adult rat cardiac myocytes. *Proc Natl Acad Sci USA*, 91, 8832–8836.

Pepper, G.M., and Krieger, D.T. (1984). Hypothalamic–pituitary–adrenal abnormalities in affective illness. In R.M. Post and J.C. Ballenger (Eds.), *Neurobiology of the Mood Disorders*, Vol. I (pp. 245–270). Baltimore: Williams and Wilkins.

Perera, T.F., Coplan, J.D., Lisanby, S.H., et al. (2006, submitted). ECS induced neurogenesis in the adult monkey dentate gyrus. Submitted to *Proc Natl Acad Sci USA*.

Perez, J., Zanardi, R., Mori, S., Gasperini, M., Smeraldi, E., and Racagni, G. (1995). Abnormalities of cAMP dependent endogenous phosphorylation in platelets from patients with bipolar disorder. *Am J Psychiatry*, 152(8), 1204–1206.

Perez, J., Tardito, D., Mori, S., Racagni, G., Smeraldi, E., and Zanardi, R. (2000). Altered Rap1 endogenous phosphorylation and levels in platelets from patients with bipolar disorder. *J Psychiatr Res*, 34, 99–104.

Perez de Castro, I., Santos, J., Torres, P., Visedo, G., Saiz-Ruiz, J., Llinares, C., and Fernandez-Piqueras, J. (1995). A weak association between TH and DRD2 genes and bipolar affective disorder in a Spanish sample. *J Med Genet*, 32, 131–134.

Perlman, W.R., Webster, M.J., Kleinman, J.E., and Weickert, C.S. (2004). Reduced glucocorticoid and estrogen receptor alpha messenger ribonucleic acid levels in the amygdala of patients with major mental illness. *Biol Psychiatry*, 56(11), 844–852.

Perlow, M.J., Reppert, S.M., Artman, H.A., Fisher, D.A., Self, S.M., and Robinson, A.G. (1982). Oxytocin, vasopressin, and estrogen-stimulated neurophysin: Daily patterns of concentration in cerebrospinal fluid. *Science*, 216, 1416–1418.

Pernow, J., Lundberg, J.M., and Kaijser, L. (1988). Alpha-adrenoceptor influence on plasma levels of neuropeptide Y–like immunoreactivity and catecholamines during rest and sympathoadrenal activation in humans. *J Cardiovasc Pharmacol*, 12(5), 593–599.

Persico, A.M., D'Agruma, L., Maiorano, N., Totaro, A., Militerni, R., Bravaccio, C., Wassink, T.H., Schneider, C., Melmed, R., Trillo, S., Montecchi, F., Palermo, M., Pascucci, T., Puglisi-Allegra, S., Reichelt, K.L., Conciatori, M., Marino, R., Quattrocchi, C.C., Baldi, A., Zelante, L., Gasparini, P., Keller, F., and Collaborative Linkage Study of Autism. (2001). *Reelin* gene alleles and haplotypes as a factor predisposing to autistic disorder. *Mol Psychiatry*, 6, 150–159.

Persinger, M.A., Makarec, K., and Bradley, J.C. (1988). Characteristics of limbic seizures evoked by peripheral injections of lithium and pilocarpine. *Physiol Behav*, 44, 27–37.

Pert, A., Rosenblatt, J.E., Sivit, C., Pert, C.B., and Bunney, W.E. Jr. (1978). Long-term treatment with lithium prevents the development of dopamine receptor supersensitivity. *Science*, 201(4351), 171–173.

Pert, C.B., and Snyder, S.H. (1973). Properties of opiate-receptor binding in rat brain. *Proc Natl Acad Sci USA*, 70(8), 2243–2247.

Perugi, G., Toni, C., Ruffolo, G., Frare, F., and Akiskal, H. (2001). Adjunctive dopamine agonists in treatment-resistant bipolar II depression: An open case series. *Pharmacopsychiatry*, 34, 137–141.

Pesold, C., Impagnatiello, F., Pisu, M.G., Uzunov, D.P., Costa, E., Guidotti, A., and Caruncho, H.J. (1998a). Reelin is preferentially expressed in neurons synthesizing gamma-aminobutyric acid in cortex and hippocampus of adult rats. *Proc Natl Acad Sci USA*, 95, 3221–3226.

Pesold, C., Pisu, M.G., Impagnatiello, F., Uzunov, D.P., and Caruncho, H.J. (1998b). Simultaneous detection of glutamic acid decarboxylase and reelin mRNA in adult rat neurons using in situ hybridization and immunofluorescence. *Brain Res Brain Res Protoc*, 3, 155–160.

Petronis, A. (2003). Epigenetics and bipolar disorder: New opportunities and challenges. *Am J Med Genet C Semin Med Genet*, 123(1), 65–75.

Petronis, A. (2004). The origin of schizophrenia: Genetic thesis, epigenetic antithesis, and resolving synthesis. *Biol Psychiatry*, 55(10), 965–970.

Petty, F., and Schlesser, M.A. (1981). Plasma GABA in affective illness. A preliminary investigation. *J Affect Disord*, 3, 339–343.

Petty, F., and Sherman, A.D. (1981). A pharmacologically pertinent animal model of mania. *J Affect Disord*, 3, 381–387.

Petty, F., and Sherman, A.D. (1984). Plasma GABA levels in psychiatric illness. *J Affect Disord*, 6, 131–138.

Petty, F., Kramer, G.L., Dunnam, D., and Rush, A.J. (1990). Plasma GABA in mood disorders. *Psychopharmacol Bull*, 26, 157–161.

Petty, F., Kramer, G.L., Fulton, M., Moeller, F.G., and Rush, A.J. (1993). Low plasma GABA is a trait-like marker for bipolar illness. *Neuropsychopharmacology*, 9, 125–132.

Petty, F., Rush, A.J., Davis, J.M., Calabrese, J.R., Kimmel, S.E., Kramer, G.L., Small, J.G., Miller, M.J., Swann, A.E., Orsulak, P.J., Blake, M.E., and Bowden, C.L. (1996). Plasma GABA predicts acute response to divalproex in mania. *Biol Psychiatry*, 39, 278–284.

Phelan, M.C. (1989). Beclomethasone mania. *Br J Psychiatry*, 155, 871–872.

Phelps, J. (2006). *Why Am I Still Depressed? Recognizing and Managing the Ups and Downs of Bipolar II and Soft Bipolar Disorder*. New York: McGraw-Hill.

Phiel, C.J., and Klein, P.S. (2001). Molecular targets of lithium action. *Annu Rev Pharmacol Toxicol*, 41, 789–813.

Pickar, D., Sweeney, D.R., Maas, J.W., and Heninger, G.R. (1978). Primary affective disorder, clinical state change, and MHPG excretion: A longitudinal study. *Arch Gen Psychiatry*, 35, 1378–1383.

Pickar, D., Davis, G.C., Schulz, S.C., Extein, I., Wagner, R., Naber, D., Gold, P.W., van Kammen, D.P., Goodwin, F.K., Wyatt, R.J.,

Li, C.H., and Bunney, W.E. Jr. (1981). Behavioral and biological effects of acute beta-endorphin injection in schizophrenic and depressed patients. *Am J Psychiatry*, 138, 160–166.

Pickar, D., Naber, D., Post, R.M., van Kammen, D.P., Kaye, W., Rubinow, D.R., Ballenger, J.C., and Bunney, W.E. Jr. (1982a). Endorphins in the cerebrospinal fluid of psychiatric patients. *Ann NY Acad Sci*, 398, 399–412.

Pickar, D., Vartanian, F., Bunney, W.E. Jr., Maier, H.P., Gastpar, M.T., Prakash, R., Sethi, B.B., Lideman, R., Belyaev, B.S., Tsutsulkovskaja, M.V., Jungkunz, G., Nedopil, N., Verhoeven, W., and van Praag, H. (1982b). Short-term naloxone administration in schizophrenic and manic patients. A World Health Organization collaborative study. *Arch Gen Psychiatry*, 39, 313–319.

Pickar, D., Dubois, M., and Cohen, M.R. (1984). Behavioral change in a cancer patient following intrathecal beta-endorphin administration. *Am J Psychiatry*, 141, 103–104.

Pilc, A., Branski, P., Palucha, A., and Aronowski, J. (1999). The effect of prolonged imipramine and electroconvulsive shock treatment on calcium/calmodulin-dependent protein kinase II in the hippocampus of rat brain. *Neuropharmacology*, 38, 597–603.

Piletz, J.E., Schubert, D.S., and Halaris, A. (1986). Evaluation of studies on platelet alpha 2 adrenoreceptors in depressive illness. *Life Sci*, 39, 1589–1616.

Piletz, J.E., Halaris, A., Saran, A., and Marler, M. (1990). Elevated 3H-para-aminoclonidine binding to platelet purified plasma membranes from depressed patients. *Neuropsychopharmacology*, 3, 201–210.

Pilgrim, C., and Hutchison, J.B. (1994). Developmental regulation of sex differences in the brain: Can the role of gonadal steroids be redefined? *Neuroscience*, 60, 843–855.

Plotsky, P.M., Owens, M.J., and Nemeroff, C.B. (1995). Neuropeptide alterations in mood disorder. In R.E. Bloom, D.J. Kupfer (Eds.), *Psychopharmacology: The Fourth Generation of Progress* (pp. 971–981). New York: Raven Press.

Plyte, S.E., Hughes, K., Nikolakaki, E., Pulverer, B.J., and Woodgett, J.R. (1992). Glycogen synthase kinase-3: Functions in oncogenesis and development. *Biochim Biophys Acta*, 1114, 147–162.

Poirier, M.F., Galzin, A.M., Pimoule, C., Schoemaker, H., Le Quan Bui, K.H., Meyer, P., Gay, C., Loo, H., and Langer, S.Z. (1988). Short-term lithium administration to healthy volunteers produces long-lasting pronounced changes in platelet serotonin uptake but not imipramine binding. *Psychopharmacology (Berl)*, 94, 521–526.

Poirier-Littre, M.F., Loo, H., Dennis, T., and Scatton, B. (1993). Lithium treatment increases norepinephrine turnover in the plasma of healthy subjects. *Arch Gen Psychiatry*, 50, 72–73.

Poitou, P., and Bohuon, C. (1975). Catecholamine metabolism in the rat brain after short- and long-term lithium administration. *J Neurochem*, 25, 535–537.

Pollack, I.F., DaRosso, R.C., Robertson, P.L., Jakacki, R.L., Mirro, J.R. Jr., Blatt, J., Nicholson, S., Packer, R.J., Allen, J.C., Cisneros, A., and Jordan, V.C. (1997). A phase I study of high-dose tamoxifen for the treatment of refractory malignant gliomas of childhood. *Clin Cancer Res*, 3(7), 1109–1115.

Poncelet, M., Dangoumau, L., Soubrie, P., and Simon, P. (1987). Effects of neuroleptic drugs, clonidine and lithium on the expression of conditioned behavioral excitation in rats. *Psychopharmacology (Berl)*, 92, 393–397.

Pontzer, N.J., and Crews, F.T. (1990). Desensitization of muscarinic stimulated hippocampal cell firing is related to phosphoinositide hydrolysis and inhibited by lithium. *J Pharmacol Exp Ther*, 253, 921–929.

Pope, H.G. Jr., and Katz, D.L. (1988). Affective and psychotic symptoms associated with anabolic steroid use. *Am J Psychiatry*, 145, 487–490.

Pope, H.G., Kourie, E.M., and Hudson, J.I. (2000). Effects of supraphysiologic doses of testosterone on mood and aggression in normal men. *Arch Gen Psychiatry*, 57, 133–140.

Popoli, M., Vocaturo, C., Perez, J., Smeraldi, E., and Racagni, G. (1995). Presynaptic Ca2+/calmodulin-dependent protein kinase II: Autophosphorylation and activity increase in the hippocampus after long-term blockade of serotonin reuptake. *Mol Pharmacol*, 48, 623–629.

Popoli, M., Brunello, N., Perez, J., and Racagni, G. (2000). Second messenger–regulated protein kinases in the brain: Their functional role and the action of antidepressant drugs. *J Neurochem*, 74, 21–33.

Porsolt, R.D. (2000). Animal models of depression: Utility for transgenic research. *Rev Neurosci*, 11, 53–58.

Post, R.M., and Ballenger, J.C. (1981). *Kindling Models for the Progressive Development of Psychopathology. Handbook of Biological Psychiatry*. New York: Dekker.

Post, R., and Kopanda, R.T. (1976). Cocaine, kindling, and psychosis. *Am J Psychiatry*, 133, 627–634.

Post, R.M., and Weiss, S.R. (1989). Sensitization, kindling, and anticonvulsants in mania. *J Clin Psychiatry*, 50, 23–30; discussion 45–47.

Post, R.M., and Weiss, S.R. (1992). Ziskind-Somerfeld Research Award 1992. Endogenous biochemical abnormalities in affective illness: Therapeutic versus pathogenic. *Biol Psychiatry*, 32, 469–484.

Post, R.M., and Weiss, S.R. (1996). A speculative model of affective illness cyclicity based on patterns of drug tolerance observed in amygdala-kindled seizures. *Mol Neurobiol*, 13, 33–60.

Post, R.M., and Weiss, S.R. (1997). Emergent properties of neural systems: How focal molecular neurobiological alterations can affect behavior. *Dev Psychopathol*, 9, 907–929.

Post, R.M., Kotin, J., and Goodwin, F.K. (1976). Effect of sleep deprivation on mood and central amine metabolism in depressed patients. *Arch Gen Psychiatry*, 33, 627–632.

Post, R.M., Cramer, H., and Goodwin, F.K. (1977). Cyclic AMP in cerebrospinal fluid of manic and depressive patients. *Psychol Med*, 7, 599–605.

Post, R.M., Gerner, R.H., Carman, J.S., Gillin, J.C., Jimerson, D.C., Goodwin, F.K., and Bunney, W.E. Jr. (1978). Effects of a dopamine agonist piribedil in depressed patients: Relationship of pretreatment homovanillic acid to antidepressant response. *Arch Gen Psychiatry*, 35, 609–615.

Post, R.M., Ballenger, J.C., Hare, T.A., and Bunney, W.E. Jr. (1980a). Lack of effect of carbamazepine on gamma-aminobutyric acid in cerebrospinal fluid. *Neurology* 30, 1008–1011.

Post, R.M., Jimerson, D.C., Bunney, W.E., Jr., and Goodwin, F.K. (1980b). Dopamine and mania: Behavioral and biochemical effects of the dopamine receptor blocker pimozide. *Psychopharmacology (Berl)*, 67, 297–305.

Post, R.M., Lockfeld, A., Squillace, K.M., and Contel, N.R. (1981). Drug–environment interaction: Context dependency of cocaine-induced behavioral sensitization. *Life Sci*, 28(7), 755–760.

Post, R.M., Contel, N.R., and Gold, P. (1982a). Impaired behavioral sensitization to cocaine in vasopressin-deficient rats. *Life Sci*, 31(24), 2745–2750.

Post, R.M., Ballenger, J.C., Uhde, T.W., Smith, C., Rubinow, D.R., and Bunney, W.E. (1982b). Effect of carbamazepine on cyclic nucleotides in CSF of patients with affective illness. *Biol Psychiatry*, 17, 1037–1045.

Post, R.M., Jimerson, D.C., Ballenger, J.C., Lake, C.R., Uhde, T.W., and Goodwin, F.K. (1984a). Cerebrospinal fluid norepinephrine and its metabolites in manic-depressive illness. In R.M. Post and J.C. Ballenger (Eds.), *Neurobiology of Mood Disorders* (pp. 539–553). Baltimore: Williams & Wilkins.

Post, R.M., Putnam, F., Contel, N.R., and Goldman, B. (1984b). Electroconvulsive seizures inhibit amygdala kindling: Implications for mechanisms of action in affective illness. *Epilepsia*, 25, 234–239.

Post, R.M., Rubinow, D.R., and Ballenger, J.C. (1984c). Conditioning, sensitization, and kindling: Implications for the course of affective illness. In R.M. Post and J.C. Ballenger (Eds.), *The Neurobiology of Mood Disorders* (pp. 432–466). Baltimore: Williams & Wilkins.

Post, R.M., Uhde, T.W., and Ballenger, J.C. (1984d). The efficacy of carbamazepine in affective illness. *Adv Biochem Psychopharmacol*, 39, 421–437.

Post, R.M., Weiss, S.R., and Pert, A. (1984e). Differential effects of carbamazepine and lithium on sensitization and kindling. *Prog Neuropsychopharmacol Biol Psychiatry*, 8, 425–434.

Post, R.M., Rubinow, D.R., Uhde, T.W., Ballenger, J.C., Lake, C.R., Linnoila, M., Jimerson, D.C., and Reus, V. (1985). Effects of carbamazepine on noradrenergic mechanisms in affectively ill patients. *Psychopharmacology (Berl)*, 87, 59–63.

Post, R.M., Uhde, T.W., Rubinow, D.R., and Huggins, T. (1987). Differential time course of antidepressant effects after sleep deprivation, ECT, and carbamazepine: Clinical and theoretical implications. *Psychiatry Res*, 22, 11–19.

Post, R.M., Rubinow, D.R., Uhde, T.W., Roy-Byrne, P.P., Linnoila, M., Rosoff, A., and Cowdry, R. (1989). Dysphoric mania. Clinical and biological correlates. *Arch Gen Psychiatry*, 46(4), 353–358.

Post, R.M., Ketter, T.A., Joffe, R.T., and Kramlinger, K.L. (1991). Lack of beneficial effects of l-baclofen in affective disorder. *Int Clin Psychopharmacol*, 6(4), 197–207.

Post, R.M., Weiss, S.R., Smith, M., Rosen, J., and Frye, M. (1995). Stress, conditioning, and the temporal aspects of affective disorders. *Ann N Y Acad Sci*, 771, 677–696.

Post, R.M., Kramlinger, K.G., Joffe, R.T., Roy-Byrne, P.P., Rosoff, A., Frye, M.A., and Huggins, T. (1997). Rapid cycling bipolar affective disorder: Lack of relation to hypothyroidism. *Psychiatry Res*, 72(1), 1–7.

Post, R.M., Weiss, S.R., Li, H., Smith, M.A., Zhang, L.X., Xing, G., Osuch, E.A., and McCann, U.D. (1998). Neural plasticity and emotional memory. *Dev Psychopathol*, 10, 829–855.

Potter, W.Z., and Linnoila, M. (1989). Biochemical classifications of diagnostic subgroups and D-type scores. *Arch Gen Psychiatry*, 46(3), 269–271.

Potter, W.Z., and Manji, H.K. (1994). Catecholamines in depression: An update. *Clin Chem*, 40(2), 279–287.

Potter, W.Z., Rudorfer, M.V., and Goodwin, F.K. (1987). Biological findings in bipolar disorders. In D. Francis (Ed.), *American Psychiatric Association Annual Review* (Vol. 6) (pp. 32–60). Washington, DC: American Psychiatric Press.

Prange, A.J., Jr., Lara, P.P., Wilson, I.C., Alltop, L.B., and Breese, G.R. (1972). Effects of thyrotropin-releasing hormone in depression. *Lancet*, 2, 999–1002.

Prange, A.J.W., Lara, P.P., and Alltop, P.P. (1974). Effects of thyrotropin-releasing hormones in depression. In A.J. Prange (Ed.), *The Thyroid Axis, Drugs and Behavior* (pp. 135–145). New York: Raven Press.

Preisig, M., Bellivier, F., Fenton, B.T., Baud, P., Berney, A., Courtet, P., Hardy, P., Golaz, J., Leboyer, M., Mallet, J., Matthey, M.L., Mouthon, D., Neidhart, E., Nosten-Bertrand, M., Stadelmann-Dubuis, E., Guimon, J., Ferrero, F., Buresi, C., and Malafosse, A. (2000). Association between bipolar disorder and monoamine oxidase A gene polymorphisms: Results of a multicenter study. *Am J Psychiatry*, 157, 948–955.

Price, L.H., Charney, D.S., Rubin, A.L., and Heninger, G.R. (1986). Alpha 2-adrenergic receptor function in depression. The cortisol response to yohimbine. *Arch Gen Psychiatry*, 43, 849–858.

Price, L.H., Charney, D.S., Delgado, P.L., and Heninger, G.R. (1989). Lithium treatment and serotoninergic function. Neuroendocrine and behavioral responses to intravenous tryptophan in affective disorder. *Arch Gen Psychiatry*, 46, 13–19.

Price, L.H., Charney, D.S., Delgado, P.L., and Heninger, G.R. (1990). Lithium and serotonin function: Implications for the serotonin hypothesis of depression. *Psychopharmacology (Berl)*, 100, 3–12.

Price, L.H., Charney, D.S., Delgado, P.L., and Heninger, G.R. (1991). Serotonin function and depression: Neuroendocrine and mood responses to intravenous L-tryptophan in depressed patients and healthy comparison subjects. *Am J Psychiatry*, 148, 1518–1525.

Price, W.A., and DeMarzio, L. (1986). Premenstrual tension syndrome in rapid-cycling bipolar affective disorder. *J Clin Psychiatry*, 47, 415–417.

Purba, J.S., Hoogendijk, W.J., Hofman, M.A., and Swaab, D.F. (1996). Increased number of vasopressin- and oxytocin-expressing neurons in the paraventricular nucleus of the hypothalamus in depression. *Arch Gen Psychiatry*, 53, 137–143.

Purdy, R.E., Julien, R.M., Fairhurst, A.S., and Terry, M.D. (1977). Effect of carbamazepine on the in vitro uptake and release of norepinephrine in adrenergic nerves of rabbit aorta and in whole brain synaptosomes. *Epilepsia*, 18, 251–257.

Puzynski, S., Rode, A., and Zaluska, M. (1983). Studies on biogenic amine metabolizing enzymes (DBH, COMT, MAO) and pathogenesis of affective illness. I. Plasma dopamine-β-hydroxylase activity in endogenous depression. *Acta Psychiatr Scand*, 67, 89–95.

Quattrone, A., and Samanin, R. (1977). Decreased anticonvulsant activity of carbamazepine in 6-hydroxydopamine-treated rats. *Eur J Pharmacol*, 41, 336.

Quattrone, A., Crunelli, V., and Samanin, R. (1978). Seizure susceptibility and anticonvulsant activity of carbamazepine, diphenylhydantoin and phenobarbital in rats with selective depletions of brain monoamines. *Neuropharmacology*, 17, 643–647.

Quattrone, A., Annunziato, L., Aguglia, U., and Preziosi, P. (1981). Carbamazepine, phenytoin and phenobarbital do not influence brain catecholamine uptake, in vivo, in male rats. *Arch Int Pharmacodyn Ther*, 252, 180–185.

Quigley, H.A., Nickells, R.W., Kerrigan, L.A., Pease, M.E., Thibault, D.J., and Zack, D.J. (1995). Retinal ganglion cell death in experimental glaucoma and after axotomy occurs by apoptosis. *Invest Ophthalmol Vis Sci*, 36, 774–786.

Quintin, P., Benkelfat, C., Launay, J.M., Arnulf, I., Pointereau-Bellenger, A., Barbault, S., Alvarez, J.C., Varoquaux, O., Perez-Diaz, F., Jouvent, R., and Leboyer, M. (2001). Clinical and neurochemical effect of acute tryptophan depletion in unaffected relatives of patients with bipolar affective disorder. *Biol Psychiatry*, 50, 184–190.

Quiroz, J., Singh, J., Gould, T.D., Denicoff, K., Zarate, C., and Manji, H.K. (2004). Emerging experimental therapeutics for bipolar disorder: Clues from the molecular neurobiology of the disorder. *Mol Psychiatry*, 9, 756–776.

Raadsheer, F.C., Hoogendijk, W.J., Stam, F.C., Tilders, F.J., and Swaab, D.F. (1994). Increased numbers of corticotropin-releasing hormone expressing neurons in the hypothalamic paraventricular nucleus of depressed patients. *Neuroendocrinology*, 60(4), 436–444.

Racine, R. (1978). Kindling: The first decade. *Neurosurgery*, 3, 234–252.

Raeburn, P. (2004). *Acquainted with the Right: A Parent's Quest to Understand Depression and Bipolar Disorder in His Children.* New York: Broadway.

Rahman, S., Li, P.P., Young, L.T., Kofman, O., Kish, S.J., and Warsh, J.J. (1997). Reduced [3H]cyclic AMP binding in postmortem brain from subjects with bipolar affective disorder. *J Neurochem*, 68, 297–304.

Rajkowska, G. (1997). Morphometric methods for studying the prefrontal cortex in suicide victims and psychiatric patients. *Ann NY Acad Sci*, 836, 253–268.

Rajkowska, G. (2000). Postmortem studies in mood disorders indicate altered numbers of neurons and glial cells. *Biol Psychiatry*, 48, 766–777.

Rajkowska, G. (2002a). Cell pathology in bipolar disorder. *Bipolar Disord*, 4, 105–116.

Rajkowska, G. (2002b). Cell pathology in mood disorders. *Semin Clin Neuropsychiatry*, 7, 281–292.

Rajkowska, G., Miguel-Hidalgo, J.J., Wei, J., Dilley, G., Pittman, S.D., Meltzer, H.Y., Overholser, J.C., Roth, B.L., and Stockmeier, C.A. (1999). Morphometric evidence for neuronal and glial prefrontal cell pathology in major depression. *Biol Psychiatry*, 45, 1085–1098.

Rajkowska, G., Halaris, A., and Selemon, L.D. (2001). Reductions in neuronal and glial density characterize the dorsolateral prefrontal cortex in bipolar disorder. *Biol Psychiatry*, 49(9), 741–752.

Rajkowska, G., Stockmeier, C.A., Mahajan, G.J., and Konick, L.C. (2004). Cellular changes in the postmortem hippocampus in major depression. *Biol Psychiatry*, 56(9), 640–650.

Ram, A., Guedj, F., Cravchik, A., Weinstein, L., Cao, Q., Badner, J.A., Goldin, L.R., Grisaru, N., Manji, H.K., Belmaker, R.H., Gershon, E.S., and Gejman, P.V. (1997). No abnormality in the gene for the G protein stimulatory alpha subunit in patients with bipolar disorder. *Arch Gen Psychiatry*, 54, 44–48.

Ramsey, T.A., Frazer, A., Mendels, J., and Dyson, W.L. (1979). The erythrocyte lithium-plasma lithium ratio in patients with primary affective disorder. *Arch Gen Psychiatry*, 36, 457–461.

Rana, R.S., and Hokin, L.E. (1990). Role of phosphoinositides in transmembrane signaling. *Physiol Rev*, 70, 115–164.

Rasenick, M.M., Chen, J., and Ozawa, H. (2000). Effects of antidepressant treatments on the G protein–adenylyl cyclase axis as the possible basis of therapeutic action. In R.H. Belmaker

(Ed.), *Bipolar Medications: Mechanisms of Action* (1st Edition) (pp. 87–108). Washington, DC: American Psychiatric Press.

Rasmusson, A.M., Southwick, S.M., Hauger, R.L., and Charney, D.S. (1998). Plasma neuropeptide Y (NPY) increases in humans in response to the alpha 2 antagonist yohimbine. *Neuropsychopharmacology*, 19(1), 95–98.

Rausch, J.L., Janowsky, D.S., Risch, S.C., and Huey, L.Y. (1986). A kinetic analysis and replication of decreased platelet serotonin uptake in depressed patients. *Psychiatry Res*, 19, 105–112.

Rebas, E., Lachowicz, A., and Lachowicz, L. (1995). Estradiol and pregnenolone sulfate could modulate PMA-stimulated and Ca2+/calmodulin-dependent synaptosomal membrane protein phosphorylation from rat brain in vivo. *Biochem Biophys Res Commun*, 207, 606–612.

Reddy, P.L., Khanna, S., Subhash, M.N., Channabasavanna, S.M., and Rao, B.S. (1989). Erythrocyte membrane Na-K ATPase activity in affective disorder. *Biol Psychiatry*, 26, 533–537.

Reddy, P.L., Khanna, S., Subhash, M.N., Channabasavanna, S.M., and Rao, B.S. (1992). Erythrocyte membrane sodium-potassium adenosine triphosphatase activity in affective disorders. *J Neural Transm [Gen Sect]*, 89, 209–218.

Redei, E., Organ, M., and Hart, S. (1999). Antidepressant-like properties of prepro-TRH 178–199: Acute effects in the forced swim test. *Neuroreport*, 10, 3273–3276.

Redmond, D.E. Jr., Katz, M.M., Maas, J.W., Swann, A., Casper, R., and Davis, J.M. (1986). Cerebrospinal fluid amine metabolites. Relationships with behavioral measurements in depressed, manic, and healthy control subjects. *Arch Gen Psychiatry*, 43, 938–947.

Rees, M., Norton, N., Jones, I., McCandless, F., Scourfield, J., Holmans, P., Moorhead, S., Feldman, E., Sadler, S., Cole, T., Redman, K., Farmer, A., McGuffin, P., Owen, M.J., and Craddock, N. (1997). Association studies of bipolar disorder at the human serotonin transporter gene (hSERT; 5HTT). *Mol Psychiatry*, 2, 398–402.

Reiach, J.S., Li, P.P., Warsh, J.J., Kish, S.J., and Young, L.T. (1999). Reduced adenylyl cyclase immunolabeling and activity in postmortem temporal cortex of depressed suicide victims. *J Affect Disord*, 56(23), 141–151.

Reich, T., and Winokur, G. (1970). Postpartum psychoses in patients with manic depressive disease. *J Nerv Ment Dis*, 151, 60–68.

Reisine, T.D. (1984). Cellular mechanisms regulating adrenocorticotropin release. *J Recept Res*, 4, 291–300.

Ren, M., Senatorov, V.V., Chen, R.W., and Chuang, D.M. (2003). Postinsult treatment with lithium reduces brain damage and facilitates neurological recovery in a rat ischemia/reperfusion model. *Proc Natl Acad Sci USA*, 100(10), 6210–6215.

Ren, M., Leng, Y., Jeong, M., Leeds, P.R., and Chuang, D.M. (2004). Valproic acid reduces brain damage induced by transient focal cerebral ischemia in rats: Potential roles of histone deacetylase inhibition and heat shock protein induction. *J Neurochem*, 89(6), 1358–1367.

Renshaw, P.F., and Cohen, B.M. (1993). Functional brain imaging in the elderly. *J Nucl Med*, 34, 1101–1102.

Reppert, S.M., and Weaver, D.R. (2001). Molecular analysis of mammalian circadian rhythms. *Annu Rev Physiol*, 63, 647–676.

Reul, J.M., and Holsboer, F. (2002). Corticotropin-releasing factor receptors 1 and 2 in anxiety and depression. *Curr Opin Pharmacol*, 2, 23–33.

Reus, V.I., Joseph, M., and Dallman, M. (1983). Regulation of ACTH and cortisol in depression. *Peptides*, 4, 785–788.

Reynolds, G.P., Beasley, C.L., and Zhang, Z.J. (2002). Understanding the neurotransmitter pathology of schizophrenia: Selective deficits of subtypes of cortical GABAergic neurons. *J Neural Transm*, 109, 881–889.

Reynolds, J.N., and Wickens, J.R. (2000). Substantia nigra dopamine regulates synaptic plasticity and membrane potential fluctuations in the rat neostriatum, in vivo. *Neuroscience*, 99(2), 199–203.

Richelson, E. (1977). Lithium ion entry through the sodium channel of cultured mouse neuroblastoma cells: A biochemical study. *Science*, 196, 1001–1002.

Richelson, E., Snyder, K., Carlson, J., Johnson, M., Turner, S., Lumry, A., Boerwinkle, E., and Sing, C.F. (1986). Lithium ion transport by erythrocytes of randomly selected blood donors and manic-depressive patients: Lack of association with affective illness. *Am J Psychiatry*, 143, 457–462.

Riddell, F.G., Patel, A., and Hughes, M.S. (1990). Lithium uptake rate and lithium: Lithium exchange rate in human erythrocytes at a nearly pharmacologically normal level monitored by 7Li NMR. *J Inorg Biochem*, 39(3), 187–192.

Rihmer, Z., Bagdy, G., and Arato, M. (1983). Serum dopamine-beta-hydroxylase activity and family history of patients with bipolar manic-depressive illness. *Acta Psychiatr Scand*, 68, 140–141.

Rimon, R., Terenius, L., Averbuch, I., and Belmaker, R.H. (1983). High-dose haloperidol increases CSF opioid activity in patients with chronic schizophrenia. *Pharmacopsychiatria*, 16, 9–12.

Rimon, R., Le Greves, P., Nyberg, F., Heikkila, L., Salmela, L., and Terenius, L. (1984). Elevation of substance P–like peptides in the CSF of psychiatric patients. *Biol Psychiatry*, 19(4), 509–516.

Risby, E.D., Hsiao, J.K., Manji, H.K., Bitran, J., Moses, F., Zhou, D.F., and Potter, W.Z. (1991). The mechanisms of action of lithium. II. Effects on adenylate cyclase activity and beta-adrenergic receptor binding in normal subjects. *Arch Gen Psychiatry*, 48, 513–524.

Risch, S.C., Cohen, R.M., Janowsky, D.S., Kalin, N.H., and Murphy, D.L. (1980). Mood and behavioral effects of physostigmine on humans are accompanied by elevations in plasma beta-endorphin and cortisol. *Science*, 209, 1545–1546.

Risch, S.C., Cohen, R.M., Janowsky, D.S., Kalin, N.H., Sitaram, N., Gillin, J.C., and Murphy, D.L. (1981). Physostigmine induction of depressive symptomatology in normal human subjects. *Psychiatry Res*, 4, 89–94.

Risch, S.C., Janowsky, D.S., and Gillin, J.C. (1983). Muscarinic supersensitivity of anterior pituitary ACTH and β-endorphin release in major depressive illness. *Peptides*, 4, 789–792.

Ritchie, E.A. (1956). Toxic psychosis under cortisone and corticotrophin. *J Ment Sci*, 102(429), 830–837.

Ritchie, J.M., and Straub, R.W. (1980). Observations on the mechanism for the active extrusion of lithium in mammalian non-myelinated nerve fibres. *J Physiol*, 304, 123–134.

Rizzo, N.D., Fox, H.M., Laidlaw, J.C., and Thorn, G.W. (1954). Concurrent observations of behavior changes and of adrenocortical variations in a cyclothymic patient during a period of 12 months. *Ann Intern Med*, 41, 798–815.

Robbins, T.W., and Sahakian, B.J. (1980). Animal models of mania. In R.H. Belmaker (Ed.), *Mania, an Evolving Concept* (pp. 143–216). Jamaica: MTP Press/Spectrum Publications.

Robinson, P.J. (1991). The role of protein kinase C and its neuronal substrates dephosphin, B-50, and MARCKS in neurotransmitter release. *Mol Neurobiol*, 5(2-4), 87–130.

Robinson, T.E., and Becker, J.B. (1986). Enduring changes in brain and behavior produced by chronic amphetamine administration: A review and evaluation of animal models of amphetamine psychosis. *Brain Res*, 396, 157–198.

Rochet, T., Tonon, M.C., Kopp, N., Vaudry, H., and Miachon, S. (1998). Evaluation of endozepine-like immuoreactivity in the frontal cortex of suicide victims. *Neuroreport*, 9, 53–56.

Ronai, A.Z., and Vizi, S.E. (1975). The effect of lithium treatment on the acetylcholine content of rat brain. *Biochem Pharmacol*, 24, 1819–1820.

Rose, A.M., Mellett, B.J., Valdes, R. Jr., Kleinman, J.E., Herman, M.M., Li, R., and el-Mallakh, R.S. (1998). Alpha 2 isoform of the Na,K-adenosine triphosphatase is reduced in temporal cortex of bipolar individuals. *Biol Psychiatry*, 44, 892–897.

Rosel, P., Arranz, B., Vallejo, J., Oros, M., Menchon, J.M., Alvarez, P., and Navarro, M.A. (1997). High affinity [3H]imipramine and [3H]paroxetine binding sites in suicide brains. *J Neural Transm*, 104, 921–929.

Rosel, P., Arranz, B., Vallejo, J., Oros, M., Crespo, J.M., Menchon, J.M., and Navarro, M.A. (1998). Variations in [3H]imipramine and 5-HT2A but not [3H]paroxetine binding sites in suicide brains. *Psychiatry Res Neuroimaging Sect*, 82, 161–170.

Rosenblatt, J.E., Pert, C.B., Tallman, J.F., Pert, A., and Bunney, W.E. Jr. (1979). The effect of imipramine and lithium on alpha- and beta-receptor binding in rat brain. *Brain Res*, 160, 186–191.

Rosenblatt, J.E., Pert, A., Layton, B., and Bunney, W.E. Jr. (1980). Chronic lithium reduces [3H]spiroperidol binding in rat striatum. *Eur J Pharmacol*, 67, 321–322.

Rothman, S.M. (1999). Mutations of the mitochondrial genome: Clinical overview and possible pathophysiology of cell damage. *Biochem Soc Symp*, 66, 111–122.

Rothschild, A.J., Schatzberg, A.F., Rosenbaum, A.H., Stahl, J.B., and Cole, J.O. (1982). The dexamethasone suppression test as a discriminator among subtypes of psychotic patients. *Br J Psychiatry*, 141, 471–474.

Rotondo, A., Mazzanti, C., Dell'Osso, L., Rucci, P., Sullivan, P., Bouanani, S., Gonnelli, C., Goldman, D., and Cassano, G.B. (2002). Catechol O-methyltransferase, serotonin transporter, and tryptophan hydroxylase gene polymorphisms in bipolar disorder patients with and without comorbid panic disorder. *Am J Psychiatry*, 159(1), 23–29.

Rousseva, A., Henry, C., van den Bulke, D., Fournier, G., Laplanche, J.L., Leboyer, M., Bellivier, F., Aubry, J.M., Baud, P., Boucherie, M., Buresi, C., Ferrero, F., and Malafosse, A. (2003). Antidepressant-induced mania, rapid cycling and the serotonin transporter gene polymorphism. *Pharmacogenomics J*, 3(2), 101–104.

Rowntree, D.W., Neven, S., and Wilson, A. (1950). The effect of diisopropylfluorophosphonate in schizophrenia and manic depressive psychosis. *J Neurol Neuroserg Psychiatry*, 47–62.

Roy, A., Pickar, D., Linnoila, M., and Potter, W.Z. (1985). Plasma norepinephrine level in affective disorders. Relationship to melancholia. *Arch Gen Psychiatry*, 42, 1181–1185.

Roy, A., Jimerson, D.C., and Pickar, D. (1986). Plasma MHPG in depressive disorders and relationship to the dexamethasone suppression test. *Am J Psychiatry*, 143, 846–851.

Roy, A., Everett, D., Pickar, D., Paul, S.M. (1987a). Platelet tritiated imipramine binding and serotonin uptake in depressed patients and controls. *Arch Gen Psychiatry*, 44, 320–327.

Roy, A., Guthrie, S., Pickar, D., and Linnoila, M. (1987b). Plasma norepinephrine responses to cold challenge in depressed patients and normal controls. *Psychiatry Res*, 21, 161–168.

Roy, A., Pickar, D., Paul, S., Doran, A., Chrousos, G.P., and Gold, P.W. (1987c). CSF corticotrophin-releasing hormone in depressed patients and normal control subjects. *Am J Psychiatry*, 144, 641–645.

Roy, A., Guthrie, S., Karoum, F., Pickar, D., and Linnoila, M. (1988). High intercorrelations among urinary outputs of norepinephrine and its major metabolites. A replication in depressed patients and controls. *Arch Gen Psychiatry*, 45(2), 158–161.

Roy, A., Wolkowitz, O.M., Bissette, G., and Nemeroff, C.B. (1994). Differences in CSF concentrations of thyrotropin-releasing hormone in depressed patients and normal subjects: Negative findings. *Am J Psychiatry*, 151, 600–602.

Rubin, A.L., Price, L.H., Charney, D.S., and Heninger, G.R. (1985). Noradrenergic function and the cortisol response to dexamethasone in depression. *Psychiatry Res*, 15, 5–15.

Rubin, R.T., O'Toole, S.M., Rhodes, M.E., Sekula, L.K., and Czambel, R.K. (1999). Hypothalamo–pituitary–adrenal cortical responses to low-dose physostigmine and arginine vasopressin administration: Sex differences between major depressives and matched control subjects. *Psychiatry Res*, 89, 1–20.

Rubinow, D.R. (1986). Cerebrospinal fluid somatostatin and psychiatric illness. *Biol Psychiatry*, 21, 341–365.

Rubinow, D.R., Gold, P.W., Post, R.M., Ballenger, J.C., Cowdry, R., Bollinger, J., and Reichlin, S. (1983). CSF somatostatin in affective illness. *Arch Gen Psychiatry*, 40, 409–412.

Rubinow, D.R., Post, R.M., Savard, R., and Gold, P.W. (1984). Cortisol hypersecretion and cognitive impairment in depression. *Arch Gen Psychiatry*, 41, 279–283.

Rudorfer, M.V., Golden, R.N., and Potter, W.Z. (1984). Second-generation antidepressants. *Psychiatr Clin North Am*, 7, 519–534.

Rudorfer, M.V., Ross, R.J., Linnoila, M., Sherer, M.A., and Potter, W.Z. (1985). Exaggerated orthostatic responsivity of plasma norepinephrine in depression. *Arch Gen Psychiatry*, 42, 1186–1192.

Rudorfer, M.V., Sherer, M.A., Lane, E.A., Golden, R.N., Linnoila, M., and Potter, W.Z. (1991). Acute noradrenergic effects of desipramine in depression. *J Clin Psychopharmacol*, 11, 22–27.

Rush, A.J., Giles, D.E., Schlesser, M.A., Orsulak, P.J., Parker, C.R. Jr., Weissenburger, J.E., Crowley, G.T., Khatami, M., and Vasavada, N. (1996). The dexamethasone suppression test in patients with mood disorders. *J Clin Psychiatry*, 57(10), 470–484.

Rush, A.J., Giles, D.E., Schlesser, M.A., Orsulak, P.J., Weissenburger, J.E., Fulton, C.L., Fairchild, C.J., and Roffwarg, H.P. (1997). Dexamethasone response, thyrotropin-releasing hormone stimulation, rapid eye movement latency, and subtypes of depression. *Biol Psychiatry*, 41, 915–928.

Russell, R.W., Pechnick, R., and Jope, R.S. (1981). Effects of lithium on behavioral reactivity: Relation to increases in brain cholinergic activity. *Psychopharmacology (Berl)*, 73, 120–125.

Ryabinin, A.E., Sato, T.N., Morris, P.J., Latchman, D.S., and Wilson, M.C. (1995). Immediate upstream promoter regions required for neurospecific expression of SNAP-25. *J Mol Neurosci*, 6, 201–210.

Ryan, W.G., Richards, J.M., and Lee, J.Y. (1989). Characteristics of the in vivo RBC: Plasma lithium ratio in a clinical setting. *Biol Psychiatry*, 26(5), 537–540.

Rybakowski, J.K., and Twardowska, K. (1999). The dexamethasone/corticotropin-releasing hormone test in depression in bipolar and unipolar affective illness. *J Psychiatr Res*, 33, 363–370.

Rybakowski, J., Chlopocka, M., Kapelski, Z., Hernacka, B., Szajnerman, Z., and Kasprzak, K. (1974). Red blood cell lithium index in patients with affective disorders in the course of lithium prophylaxis. *Int Pharmacopsychiatry*, 9(3), 166–171.

Rybakowski, J., Frazer, A., Mendels, J., and Ramsey, T.A. (1978). Erythrocyte accumulation of the lithium ion in control subjects and patients with primary affective disorder. *Commun Psychopharmacol*, 2(2), 99–104.

Rybakowski, J., Potok, E., and Strzyzewski, W. (1981). Erythrocyte membrane adenosine triphosphatase activities in patients with endogenous depression and healthy subject. *Eur J Clin Invest*, 11, 61–64.

Rybakowski, J.K., Borkowska, A., Czerski, P.M., Skibinska, M., and Hauser, J. (2003). Polymorphism of the brain-derived neurotrophic factor gene and performance on a cognitive prefrontal test in bipolar patients. *Bipolar Disord*, 5(6), 468–472.

Ryves, W.J., and Harwood, A.J. (2001). Lithium inhibits glycogen synthase kinase-3 by competition for magnesium. *Biochem Biophys Res Commun*, 80, 720–725.

Sachar, E.J., Hellman, L., Roffwarg, H.P., Halpern, F.S., Fukushima, D.K., and Gallagher, T.F. (1973). Disrupted 24-hour patterns of cortisol secretion in psychotic depression. *Arch Gen Psychiatry*, 28, 19–24.

Sack, D.A., Duncan, W., Rosenthal, N.E., Mendelson, W.E., and Wehr, T.A. (1988). The timing and duration of sleep in partial sleep deprivation therapy of depression. *Acta Psychiatr Scand*, 77, 219–224.

Sahin-Erdemli, I., Medford, R.M., and Songu-Mize, E. (1995). Regulation of Na+,K(+)-ATPase alpha-subunit isoforms in rat tissues during hypertension. *Eur J Pharmacol*, 292, 163–171.

Saito, T., Parsia, S., Papolos, D.F., and Lachman, H.M. (2000). Analysis of the pseudoautosomal X-linked gene *SYBL1* in bipolar affective disorder: Description of a new candidate allele for psychiatric disorders. *Am J Med Genet*, 96, 317–323.

Saito, T., Guan, F., Papolos, D.F., Lau, S., Klein, M., Fann, C.S., and Lachman, H.M. (2001a). Mutation analysis of *SYNJ1*: A possible candidate gene for chromosome 21q22-linked bipolar disorder. *Mol Psychiatry*, 6, 387–395.

Saito, T., Guan, F., Papolos, D.F., Rajouria, N., Fann, C.S., and Lachman, H.M. (2001b). Polymorphism in SNAP29 gene promoter region associated with schizophrenia. *Mol Psychiatry*, 6, 193–201.

Sanacora, G., Mason, G.F., Rothman, D.L., Behar, K.L., Hyder, F., Petroff, O.A., Berman, R.M., Charney, D.S., and Krystal, J.H. (1999). Reduced cortical gamma-aminobutyric acid levels in depressed patients determined by proton magnetic resonance spectroscopy. *Arch Gen Psychiatry*, 56, 1043–1047.

Sanacora, G., Gueorguieva, R., Epperson, C.N., Wu, Y.T., Appel, M., Rothman, D.L., Krystal, J.H., and Mason, G.F. (2004). Subtype-specific alterations of gamma-aminobutyric acid and glutamate in patients with major depression. *Arch Gen Psychiatry*, 61(7), 705–713.

Sanchez, M.M., Young, L.J., Plotsky, P.M., and Insel, T.R. (2000). Distribution of corticosteroid receptors in the rhesus brain: Relative absence of glucocorticoid receptors in the hippocampal formation. *J Neurosci*, 20, 4657–4668.

Sanchez, R.S., Murthy, G.G., Mehta, J., Shreeve, W.W., and Singh, F.R. (1976). Pituitary–testicular axis in patients on lithium therapy. *Fertil Steril*, 27, 667–669.

Sands, S.A., Guerra, V., and Morilak, D.A. (2000). Changes in tyrosine hydroxylase mRNA expression in the rat locus coeruleus following acute or chronic treatment with valproic acid. *Neuropsychopharmacology*, 22(1), 27–35.

Santarelli, L., Saxe, M., and Gross, C. (2003). Requirement of hippocampal neurogenesis for the behavioral effects of antidepressants. *Science*, 301(5634), 805–809.

Sapolsky, R.M. (1996). Stress, glucocorticoids, and damage to the nervous system: The current state of confusion. *Stress*, 1, 1–19.

Sapolsky, R.M. (2000a). The possibility of neurotoxicity in the hippocampus in major depression: A primer on neuron death. *Biol Psychiatry*, 48, 755–765.

Sapolsky, R.M. (2000b). Glucocorticoids and hippocampal atrophy in neuropsychiatric disorders. *Arch Gen Psychiatry*, 57, 925–935.

Sapolsky, R.M., Romero, L.M., and Munck, A.U. (2000). How do glucocorticoids influence stress responses? Integrating permissive, suppressive, stimulatory, and preparative actions. *Endocr Rev*, 21, 55–89.

Sarai, M., Taniguchi, N., Kagomoto, T., Kameda, H., Uema, T., and Hishikawa, Y. (1982). Major depressive episode and low dose dexamethasone suppression test. *Folia Psychiatr Neurol Jpn*, 36(2), 109–114.

Sargent, P.A., Kjaer, K.H., Bench, C.J., Rabiner, E.A., Messa, C., Meyer, J., Gunn, R.N., Grasby, P.M., and Cowen, P.J. (2000). Brain serotonin1A receptor binding measured by positron emission tomography with [11C]WAY-100635: Effects of depression and antidepressant treatment. *Arch Gen Psychiatry*, 57, 174–180.

Sarkadi, B., Alifimoff, J.K., Gunn, R.B., and Tosteson, D.C. (1978). Kinetics and stoichiometry of Na-dependent Li transport in human red blood cells. *J Gen Physiol*, 72, 249–265.

Sastre, M., and García-Sevilla, J.A. (1997). Densities of I2-imidazoline receptors, α2-adrenoceptors and monoamine oxidase B in brains of suicide victims. *Neurochem Int*, 30, 63–72.

Sastre, M., Escriba, P.V., Reis, D.J., and Garcia-Sevilla, J.A. (1995). Decreased number and immunoreactivity of I2-imidazoline receptors in the frontal cortex of suicide victims. *Ann NY Acad Sci*, 763, 520–522.

Sattin, A. (1999). The role of TRH and related peptides in the mechanism of action of ECT. *J ECT*, 15, 76–92.

Saunders, J., and Williams, J. (2003). Antagonists of the corticotropin releasing factor receptor. *Prog Med Chem*, 41, 195–247.

Sawaya, M.C., Horton, R.W., and Meldrum, B.S. (1975). Effects of anticonvulsant drugs on the cerebral enzymes metabolizing GABA. *Epilepsia*, 16, 649–655.

Scappa, S., Teverbaugh, P., and Ananth, J. (1993). Episodic tardive dyskinesia and parkinsonism in bipolar disorder patients. *Can J Psychiatry*, 38, 633–634.

Schaefer, E., Leimer, I., Haeselbarth, V., and Meier, D. (1996). Tolerability of pramipexole in patients hospitalized for major depressive disorder: An open-label study to assess the maximum tolerated dose of pramipexole with repeated dosing. Clinical Report No. U96-0084, February 5, 1996.

Schatzberg, A.F., and Schildkraut, J.J. (1995). Recent studies on norepinephrine systems in mood disorders. In D.J. Kupfer (Ed.), *Psychopharmacology: The Fourth Generation of Progress* (pp. 957–969). New York: Raven Press.

Schatzberg, A.F., Orsulak, P.J., Rosenbaum, A.H., Maruta, T., Kruger, E.R., Cole, J.O., and Schildkraut, J.J. (1982). Toward a biochemical classification of depressive disorders: V. Heterogeneity of unipolar depressions. *Am J Psychiatry*, 139, 471–475.

Schatzberg, A.F., Samson, J.A., Bloomingdale, K.L., Orsulak, P.J., Gerson, B., Kizuka, P.P., Cole, J.O., and Schildkraut, J.J. (1989). Toward a biochemical classification of depressive disorders. X. Urinary catecholamines, their metabolites, and D-type scores in subgroups of depressive disorders. *Arch Gen Psychiatry*, 46, 260–268.

Schildkraut, J.J. (1965). The catecholamine hypothesis of affective disorders: A review of supporting evidence. *Am J Psychiatry*, 122, 509–522.

Schildkraut, J.J. (1973). Norepinephrine metabolites as biochemical criteria for classifying depressive disorders and predicting responses to treatment: Preliminary findings. *Am J Psychiatry*, 130, 695–699.

Schildkraut, J.J. (1974). The effects of lithium on norepinephrine turnover and metabolism: Basic and clinical studies. *J Nerv Ment Dis*, 158, 348–360.

Schildkraut, J.J., Schanberg, S.M., and Kopin, I.J. (1966). The effects of lithium ion on H3-norepinephrine metabolism in brain. *Life Sci*, 5, 1479–1483.

Schildkraut, J.J., Logue, M.A., and Dodge, G.A. (1969). The effects of lithium salts on the turnover and metabolism of norepinephrine in rat brain. *Psychopharmacologia*, 14, 135–141.

Schildkraut, J.J., Keeler, B.A., Grab, E.L., Kantrowich, J., and Hartmann, E. (1973). M.H.P.G. excretion and clinical classification in depressive disorders. *Lancet*, 1, 1251–1252.

Schmider, J., Lammers, C.H., Gotthardt, U., Dettling, M., Holsboer, F., and Heuser, I.J. (1995). Combined dexamethasone/corticotropin-releasing hormone test in acute and remitted manic patients, in acute depression, and in normal controls: I. *Biol Psychiatry*, 38, 797–802.

Schmidt, P.J., Daly, R.C., Bloch, M., Smith, M.J., Danaceau, M.A., St Clair, L.S., Murphy, J.H., Haq, N., and Rubinow, D.R. (2005). Dehydroepiandrosterone monotherapy in midlife-onset major and minor depression. *Arch Gen Psychiatry*, 62(2), 154–162.

Schoch, S., Deak, F., Konigstorfer, A., Mozhayeva, M., Sara, Y., Sudhof, T.C., and Kavalali, E.T. (2001). SNARE function analyzed in synaptobrevin/VAMP knockout mice. *Science*, 294(5544), 1117–1122.

Schreiber, G., Avissar, S., Danon, A., and Belmaker, R.H. (1991). Hyperfunctional G proteins in mononuclear leukocytes of patients with mania. *Biol Psychiatry*, 29(3), 273–280.

Schreiber, S., and Lerer, B. (1997). "Failure to thrive" in elderly depressed patients: A new concept or a different name for an old problem? *Isr J Psychiatry Relat Sci*, 34(2), 108–114.

Schultz, J.E., Siggins, G.R., Schocker, F.W., Turck, M., and Bloom, F.E. (1981). Effects of prolonged treatment with lithium and tricyclic antidepressants on discharge frequency, norepinephrine responses and beta receptor binding in rat cerebellum: Electrophysiological and biochemical comparison. *J Pharmacol Exp Ther*, 216, 28–38.

Scott, M., and Reading, H.W. (1978). A comparison of platelet membrane and erythrocyte membrane adenosine triphosphatase-specific activities in affective disorders. *Biochem Soc Trans*, 6, 642–644.

Scott, M., Reading, H.W., and Loudon, J.B. (1979). Studies on human blood platelets in affective disorder. *Psychopharmacology (Berl)*, 60, 131–135.

Segal, D.S., Callaghan, M., and Mandell, A.J. (1975). Alterations in behaviour and catecholamine biosynthesis induced by lithium. *Nature*, 254, 58–59.

Seligman, M.E., and Maier, S.F. (1967). Failure to escape traumatic shock. *J Exp Psychol*, 74, 1–9.

Senatorov, V.V., Ren, M., Kanai, H., Wei, H., and Chunag, D.M. (2004). Short-term lithium treatment promotes neuronal survival and proliferation in rat striatum infused with quinolinic acid, and excitotoxic model of Huntington's disease. *Mol Psychiatry*, 9, 371–385.

Sengupta, N., Datta, S.C., Sengupta, D., and Bal, S. (1980). Platelet and erythrocyte-membrane adenosine triphosphatase activity in depressive and manic-depressive illness. *Psychiatry Res*, 3, 337–344.

Serretti, A., Macciardi, F., Verga, M., Cusin, C., Pedrini, S., and Smeraldi, E. (1998). Tyrosine hydroxylase gene associated with depressive symptomatology in mood disorder. *Am J Med Genet*, 81, 127–130.

Serretti, A., Lattuada, E., Lorenzi, C., Lilli, R., and Smeraldi, E. (2000). Dopamine receptor D2 Ser/Cys 311 variant is associated with delusion and disorganization symptomatology in major psychoses. *Mol Psychiatry*, 5, 270–274.

Serretti, A., Lilli, R., Lorenzi, C., Lattuada, E., Cusin, C., and Smeraldi, E. (2001). Tryptophan hydroxylase gene and major psychoses. *Psychiatry Res*, 103, 79–86.

Seymour, P.A., Schmidt, A.W., and Schulz, D.W. (2003). The pharmacology of CP-154,526, a non-peptide antagonist of the CRH1 receptor: A review. *CNS Drug Rev*, 9(1), 57–96.

Shah, P.J., Ogilvie, A.D., Goodwin, G.M., and Ebmeier, K.P. (1997). Clinical and psychometric correlates of dopamine D2 binding in depression. *Psychol Med*, 27, 1247–1256.

Shaldubina, A., Einat, H., Szechtman, H., Shimon, H., and Belmaker, R.H. (2002). Preliminary evaluation of oral anticonvulsant treatment in the quinpirole model of bipolar disorder. *J Neural Transm*, 109, 433–440.

Shapira, B., Cohen, J., Newman, M.E., and Lerer, B. (1993). Prolactin response to fenfluramine and placebo challenge following maintenance pharmacotherapy withdrawal in remitted depressed patients. *Biol Psychiatry*, 33, 531–535.

Sharfstein, S.S., Sack, D.S., and Fauci, A.S. (1982). Relationship between alternate-day corticosteroid therapy and behavioral abnormalities. *JAMA*, 248(22), 2987–2989.

Sharma, R., Venkatasubramanian, P.N., Barany, M., and Davis, J.M. (1992). Proton magnetic resonance spectroscopy of the brain in schizophrenic and affective patients. *Schizophr Res*, 8, 43–49.

Shaughnessy, R., Greene, S.C., Pandey, G.N., and Dorus, E. (1985). Red-cell lithium transport and affective disorders in a multigeneration pedigree: Evidence for genetic transmission of affective disorders. *Biol Psychiatry*, 20, 451–454.

Shaw, D.M., Camps, F.E., and Eccleston, E.G. (1967). 5-Hydroxytryptamine in the hind-brain of depressive suicides. *Br J Psychiatry*, 113, 1407–1411.

Sheffield, A. (1999). *How You Can Survive When They're Depressed: Living and Coping with Depression Fallout*. New York: HarperCollins.

Sheline, Y.I., Black, K.J., Bardgett, M.E., and Csernansky, J.G. (1995). Platelet binding characteristics distinguish placebo responders from nonresponders in depression. *Neuropsychopharmacology*, 12, 315–322.

Sheline, Y.I., Wang, P.W., Gado, M.H., Csernansky, J.G., and Vannier, M.W. (1996). Hippocampal atrophy in recurrent major depression. *Proc Natl Acad Sci USA*, 93(9), 3908–3913.

Sheline, Y.I., Gado, M.H., and Kraemer, H.C. (2003). Untreated depression and hippocampal volume loss. *Am J Psychiatry*, 160(8), 1516–1518.

Sherif, F., Marcusson, J., and Oreland, L. (1991). Brain gamma-aminobutyrate transaminase and monoamine oxidase activities in suicide victims. *Eur Arch Psychiatry Clin Neurosci*, 241, 139–144.

Sherman, W.R., Munsell, L.Y., Gish, B.G., and Honchar, M.P. (1985). Effects of systemically administered lithium on phosphoinositide metabolism in rat brain, kidney, and testis. *J Neurochem*, 44(3), 798–807.

Sherman, W.R., Gish, B.G., Honchar, M.P., and Munsell, L.Y. (1986). Effects of lithium on phosphoinositide metabolism in vivo. *Fed Proc*, 45(11), 2639–2646.

Shiah, I.S., and Yatham, L.N. (2000). Serotonin in mania and in the mechanism of action of mood stabilizers: A review of clinical studies. *Bipolar Disord*, 2, 77–92.

Shiah, I.S., Yatham, L.N., Lam, R.W., and Zis, A.P. (1997). Effects of divalproex sodium on 5-HT$_{1A}$ receptor function in healthy human males: Hypothermic, hormonal, and behavioral responses to ipsapirone. *Neuropsychopharmacology*, 17, 382–390.

Shibata, K., Morita, K., Kitayama, S., Okamoto, H., and Dohi, T. (1996). Ca2+ entry induced by calcium influx factor and its regulation by protein kinase C in rabbit neutrophils. *Biochem Pharmacol*, 52, 167–171.

Shimon, H., Agam, G., Belmaker, R.H., Hyde, T.M., and Kleinman, J.E. (1997). Reduced frontal cortex inositol levels in postmortem brain of suicide victims and patients with bipolar disorder. *Am J Psychiatry*, 154, 1148–1150.

Shippenberg, T.S., and Herz, A. (1991). Influence of chronic lithium treatment upon the motivational effects of opioids: Alteration in the effects of mu- but not kappa-opioid receptor ligands. *J Pharmacol Exp Ther*, 256, 1101–1106.

Shippenberg, T.S., Millan, M.J., Mucha, R.F., and Herz, A. (1988). Involvement of beta-endorphin and mu-opioid receptors in mediating the aversive effect of lithium in the rat. *Eur J Pharmacol*, 154, 135–144.

Shukla, G.S. (1985). Combined lithium and valproate treatment and subsequent withdrawal: Serotonergic mechanism of their interaction in discrete brain regions. *Prog Neuropsychopharmacol Biol Psychiatry*, 9, 153–156.

Siegel, J.M., and Rogawski, M.A. (1988). A function for REM sleep: Regulation of noradrenergic receptor sensitivity. *Brain Res*, 472(3), 213–233.

Siever, L.J. (1987). Role of noradrenergic mechanisms in the etiology of the affective disorders. In H.Y. Meltzer (Ed.), *Psychopharmacology: The Third Generation of Progress* (pp. 493–504). New York: Raven Press.

Siever, L.J., and Uhde, T.W (1984). New studies and perspectives on the noradrenergic receptor system in depression: Effects of the alpha 2-adrenergic agonist clonidine. *Biol Psychiatry*, 19, 131–156.

Siever, L.J., Uhde, T.W., Silberman, E.K., Jimerson, D.C., Aloi, J.A., Post, R.M., and Murphy, D.L. (1982). Growth hormone response to clonidine as a probe of noradrenergic receptor responsiveness in affective disorder patients and controls. *Psychiatry Res*, 6, 171–183.

Siever, L.J., Insel, T.R., Jimerson, D.C., Lake, C.R., Uhde, T.W., Aloi, J., and Murphy, D.L. (1983). Growth hormone response to clonidine in obsessive-compulsive patients. *Br J Psychiatry*, 142, 184–187.

Siever, L.J., Uhde, T.W., Jimerson, D.C., Lake, C.R., Silberman, E.R., Post, R.M., and Murphy, D.L. (1984). Differential inhibitory noradrenergic responses to clonidine in 25 depressed patients and 25 normal control subjects. *Am J Psychiatry*, 141, 733–741.

Silverstone, T. (1978). Dopamine, mood and manic-depressive psychosis. In S. Garattini (Ed.), *Depressive Disorders* (pp. 419–430). Stuttgart: FK Schattauer Verlag.

Silverstone, T. (1984). Response to bromocriptine distinguishes bipolar from unipolar depression. *Lancet*, 1, 903–904.

Simmons, N.E., Alden, T.D., Thorner, M.O., and Laws, E.R. Jr. (2001). Serum cortisol response to transsphenoidal surgery for cushing disease. *J Neurosurg*, 95(1), 1–8.

Simon, J.R., and Kuhar, M.J. (1976). High-affinity choline uptake: Ionic and energy requirements. *J Neurochem*, 27, 93–99.

Simpkins, J.W., Green, P.S., Gridley, K.E., Singh, M., de Fiebre, N.C., and Rajakumar, G. (1997). Role of estrogen replacement therapy in memory enhancement and the prevention of neuronal loss associated with Alzheimer's disease. *Am J Med*, 103, 19S–25S.

Simpson, H.B., Nee, J.C., and Endicott, J. (1997). First-episode major depression. Few sex differences in course. *Arch Gen Psychiatry*, 54, 633–639.

Singh, M., Meyer, E.M., and Simpkins, J.W. (1995). The effect of ovariectomy and estradiol replacement on brain-derived neurotrophic factor messenger ribonucleic acid expression in cortical and hippocampal brain regions of female Sprague-Dawley rats. *Endocrinology*, 136, 2320–2324.

Sirois, F. (2003). Steroid psychosis: A review. *Gen Hosp Psychiatry*, 25(1), 27–33.

Si-Tahar, M., Renesto, P., Falet, H., Rendu, F., and Chignard, M. (1996). The phospholipase C/protein kinase C pathway is involved in cathepsin G-induced human platelet activation: Comparison with thrombin. *Biochem J*, 313(Pt. 2), 401–408.

Sitaram, N., Wyatt, R.J., Dawson, S., and Gillin, J.C. (1976). REM sleep induction by physostigmine infusion during sleep. *Science*, 191, 1281–1283.

Sitaram, N., Moore, A.M., and Gillin, J.C. (1978a). Experimental acceleration and slowing of REM sleep ultradian rhythm by cholinergic agonist and antagonist. *Nature*, 274, 490–492.

Sitaram, N., Moore, A.M., and Gillin, J.C. (1978b). Induction and resetting of REM sleep rhythm in normal man by arecoline: Blockade by scopolamine. *Sleep*, 1, 83–90.

Sitaram, N., Weingartner, H., and Gillin, J.C. (1978c). Human serial learning: Enhancement with arecholine and choline impairment with scopolamine. *Science*, 201, 274–276.

Sitaram, N., Moore, A.M., and Gillin, J.C. (1979). Scopolamine-induced muscarinic supersensitivity in normal man: Changes in sleep. *Psychiatry Res*, 1, 9–16.

Sitaram, N., Nurnberger, J.I. Jr., Gershon, E.S., and Gillin, J.C. (1980). Faster cholinergic REM sleep induction in euthymic patients with primary affective illness. *Science*, 208, 200–202.

Sitaram, N., Nurnberger, J.I. Jr., Gershon, E.S., and Gillin, J.C. (1982). Cholinergic regulation of mood and REM sleep: Potential model and marker of vulnerability to affective disorder. *Am J Psychiatry*, 139, 571–576.

Sitaram, N., Dube, S., Keshavan, M., Davies, A., and Reynal, P. (1987). The association of supersensitive cholinergic REM-induction and affective illness within pedigrees. *J Psychiatr Res*, 21, 487–497.

Sivam, S.P., Breese, G.R., Napier, T.C., Mueller, R.A., and Hong, J.S. (1986). Dopaminergic regulation of proenkephalin-A gene expression in the basal ganglia. *NIDA Res Monogr*, 75, 389–392.

Sivam, S.P., Takeuchi, K., Li, S., Douglass, J., Civelli, O., Calvetta, L., Herbert, E., McGinty, J.F., and Hong, J.S. (1988). Lithium increases dynorphin A(1-8) and prodynorphin mRNA levels in the basal ganglia of rats. *Brain Res*, 427, 155–163.

Sivam, S.P., Krause, J.E., Takeuchi, K., Li, S., McGinty, J.F., and Hong, J.S. (1989). Lithium increases rat striatal beta- and gamma-preprotachykinin messenger RNAs. *J Pharmacol Exp Ther*, 248(3), 1297–1301.

Skolnick, P. (1999). Antidepressants for the new millennium. *Eur J Pharmacol*, 375, 31–40.

Skolnick, P., Legutko, B., Li, X., and Bymaster, F.P. (2001). Current perspectives on the development of non-biogenic amine-based antidepressants. *Pharmacol Res*, 43, 411–423.

Slater, S.J., Kelly, M.B., Taddeo, F.J., Ho, C., Rubin, E., and Stubbs, C.D. (1994). The modulation of protein kinase C activity by membrane lipid bilayer structure. *J Biol Chem*, 269, 4866–4871.

Smeraldi, E., Benedetti, F., Barbini, B., Campori, E., and Colombo, C. (1999). Sustained antidepressant effect of sleep deprivation combined with pindolol in bipolar depression. A placebo-controlled trial. *Neuropsychopharmacology*, 20, 380–385.

Smith, A.D., and Winkler, H. (1972). Fundamental mechanisms in the release of Catecholamines. In H. Blaschko and E. Muscholl (Eds.), *Handbook of Experimental Pharmacology, Vol. 33 Catecholamines* (pp. 538–617). Berlin: Springer-Verlag.

Smith, D.F. (1988). Lithium attenuates clonidine-induced hypoactivity: Further studies in inbred mouse strains. *Psychopharmacology (Berl)*, 94, 428–430.

Smith, M.A., Makino, S., Kvetnansky, R., and Post, R.M. (1995). Stress and glucocorticoids affect the expression of brain-derived neurotrophic factor and neurotrophin-3 mRNAs in the hippocampus. *J Neurosci*, 15, 1768–1777.

Smith, R.C., Chua, J.W., Lipetsker, B., and Bhattacharyya, A. (1996). Efficacy of risperidone in reducing positive and negative symptoms in medication-refractory schizophrenia: An open prospective study. *J Clin Psychiatry*, 57, 460–466.

Smith, R.E., and Helms, P.M. (1982). Adverse effects of lithium therapy in the acutely ill elderly patient. *J Clin Psychiatry*, 43(3), 94–99.

Soares, J.C., and Mallinger, A.G. (1997). Intracellular phosphatidylinositol pathway abnormalities in bipolar disorder patients. *Psychopharmacol Bull*, 33(4), 685–691.

Soares, J.C., Dippold, C.S., and Mallinger, A.G. (1997). Platelet membrane phosphatidylinositol-4,5-bisphosphate alterations in bipolar disorder—evidence from a single case study. *Psychiatry Res*, 69(2-3), 197–202.

Soares, J.C., Mallinger, A.G., Dippold, C.S., Frank, E., and Kupfer, D.J. (1999). Platelet membrane phospholipids in euthymic bipolar disorder patients: Are they affected by lithium treatment? *Biol Psychiatry*, 45(4), 453–457.

Soares, J.C., Mallinger, A.G., Dippold, C.S., Forster Wells, K., Frank, E., and Kupfer, D.J. (2000a). Effects of lithium on platelet membrane phosphoinositides in bipolar disorder patients: A pilot study. *Psychopharmacology (Berl)*, 149(1), 12–16.

Soares, J.C., Chen, G., Dippold, C.S., Wells, K.F., Frank, E., Kupfer, D.J., Manji, H.K., and Mallinger, A.G. (2000b). Concurrent measures of protein kinase C and phosphoinositides in lithium-treated bipolar patients and healthy individuals: A preliminary study. *Psychiatry Res*. 95(2), 109–118.

Soares, J.C., Dippold, C.S., Wells, K.F., Frank, E., Kupfer, D.J., and Mallinger, A.G. (2001). Increased platelet membrane phosphatidylinositol-4,5-bisphosphate in drug-free depressed bipolar patients. *Neurosci Lett*, 299, 150–152.

Sobczak, S., Riedel, W.J., Booij, I., Aan Het Rot, M., Deutz, N.E., and Honig, A. (2002). Cognition following acute tryptophan depletion: Difference between first-degree relatives of bipolar disorder patients and matched healthy control volunteers. *Psychol Med*, 32, 503–515.

Sofuoglu, S., Dogan, P., Kose, K., Esel, E., Basturk, M., Oguz, H., and Gonul, A.S. (1995). Changes in platelet monoamine oxidase and plasma dopamine-beta-hydroxylase activities in lithium-treated bipolar patients. *Psychiatry Res*, 59, 165–170.

Sohrabji, F., Miranda, R.C., and Toran-Allerand, C.D. (1994). Estrogen differentially regulates estrogen and nerve growth factor receptor mrnas in adult sensory neurons. *J Neurosci*, 14(2), 459–471.

Sokolski, K.N., and DeMet, E.M. (1999). Pupillary cholinergic sensitivity to pilocarpine increases in manic lithium responders. *Biol Psychiatry*, 45, 1580–1584.

Sokolski, K.N., and DeMet, E.M. (2000). Cholinergic sensitivity predicts severity of mania. *Psychiatry Res*, 95(3), 195–200.

Sonawalla, S.B., Renshaw, P.F., Moore, C.M., Alpert, J.E., Nierenberg, A.A., Rosenbaum, J.F., and Fava, M. (1999). Compounds containing cytosolic choline in the basal ganglia: A potential biological marker of true drug response to fluoxetine. *Am J Psychiatry*, 156, 1638–1640.

Song, L., and Jope, R.S. (1992). Chronic lithium treatment impairs phosphatidylinositol hydrolysis in membranes from rat brain regions. *J Neurochem*, 58, 2200–2206.

Sonino, N., and Fava, G.A. (2001). Psychiatric disorders associated with Cushing's syndrome. Epidemiology, pathophysiology and treatment. *CNS Drugs*, 15(5), 361–373.

Sorensen, P.S., Gjerris, A., and Hammer, M. (1985). Cerebrospinal fluid vasopressin in neurological and psychiatric disorders. *J Neurol Neurosurg Psychiatry*, 48, 50–57.

Soucek, K., Zvolsky, P., Krulik, R., Filip, V., Vinarova, E., and Dostal, T. (1974). The levels of lithium in serum and in red blood cells and its ratios in manic-depressive patients. *Act Nerv Super (Praha)*, 16(3), 193–194.

Souetre, E., Salvati, E., Pringuey, D., Krebs, B., Plasse, Y., and Darcourt, G. (1986). The circadian rhythm of plasma thyrotropin in depression and recovery. *Chronobiol Int*, 3, 197–205.

Souetre, E., Salvati, E., Wehr, T.A., Sack, D.A., Krebs, B., and Darcourt, G. (1988). Twenty-four-hour profiles of body temperature and plasma TSH in bipolar patients during depression and during remission and in normal control subjects. *Am J Psychiatry*, 145, 1133–1137.

Souza, F.G., Mander, A.J., Foggo, M., Dick, H., Shearing, C.H., and Goodwin, G.M. (1991). The effects of lithium discontinuation and the non-effect of oral inositol upon thyroid hormones and cortisol in patients with bipolar affective disorder. *J Affect Disord*, 22, 165–170.

Sparapani, M., Virgili, M., Ortali, F., and Contestabile, A. (1997). Effects of chronic lithium treatment on ornithine decarboxylase induction and excitotoxic neuropathology in the rat. *Brain Res*, 765, 164–168.

Sperling, R.I., Benincaso, A.I., Knoell, C.T., Larkin, J.K., Austen, K.F., and Robinson, D.R. (1993). Dietary omega-3 polyunsaturated fatty acids inhibit phosphoinositide formation and chemotaxis in neutrophils. *J Clin Invest*, 91, 651–660.

Spiegel, A. (1998). *G Proteins, Receptors, and Disease*. Totowa, NJ: Humana Press.

Spitz, R.A. (1946). Anaclitic depression: An inquiry into the genesis of psychiatric conditions in early childhood: II. *Psychoanal Study Child*, 2, 313–347.

Spleiss, O., van Calker, D., Scharer, L., Adamovic, K., Berger, M., and Gebicke-Haerter, P.J. (1998). Abnormal G protein alpha(s)–and alpha(i2)–subunit mRNA expression in bipolar affective disorder. *Mol Psychiatry*, 3, 512–520.

Sporn, J., and Sachs, G. (1997). The anticonvulsant lamotrigine in treatment-resistant manic-depressive illness. *J Clin Psychopharmacol*, 17, 185–189.

Sporn, J., Ghaemi, S.N., Sambur, M.R., Rankin, M.A., Recht, J., Sachs, G.S., Rosenbaum, J.F., and Fava, M. (2000). Pramipexole augmentation in the treatment of unipolar and bipolar depression: A retrospective chart review. *Ann Clin Psychiatry*, 12, 137–140.

Stambolic, V., Ruel, L., and Woodgett, J.R. (1996). Lithium inhibits glycogen synthase kinase-3 activity and mimics wingless signalling in intact cells. *Curr Biol.*, 6(12):1664–1668. Erratum in *Curr Biol* 1997 7(3), 196.

Stancer, H.C., and Persad, E. (1982). Treatment of intractable rapid-cycling manic-depressive disorder with levothyroxine. Clinical observations. *Arch Gen Psychiatry*, 39, 311–312.

Staner, L., Hilger, C., Hentges, F., Monreal, J., Hoffmann, A., Couturier, M., Le Bon, O., Stefos, G., Souery, D., and Mendlewicz, J. (1998). Association between novelty-seeking and the dopamine D3 receptor gene in bipolar patients: A preliminary report. *Am J Med Genet*, 81, 192–194.

Stanley, M., and Mann, J.J. (1983). Increased serotonin-2 binding sites in frontal cortex of suicide victims. *Lancet*, I, 214–216.

Stanley, M., Virgilio, J., and Gershon, S. (1982). Tritiated imipramine binding sites are decreased in the frontal cortex of suicides. *Science*, 216, 1337–1339.

Stanley, M., Mann, J.J., and Gershon, S. (1983). Alterations in pre- and postsynaptic serotonergic neurons in suicide victims. *Psychopharmacol Bull*, 19, 684–687.

Starkman, M.N., Giordani, B., Gebarski, S.S., Berent, S., Schork, M.A., and Schteingart, D.E. (1999). Decrease in cortisol reverses human hippocampal atrophy following treatment of Cushing's disease. *Biol Psychiatry*, 46(12), 1595–1602.

Staunton, D.A., Magistretti, P.J., Shoemaker, W.J., and Bloom, F.E. (1982a). Effects of chronic lithium treatment on dopamine receptors in the rat corpus striatum. I. Locomotor activity and behavioral supersensitivity. *Brain Res*, 232, 391–400.

Staunton, D.A., Magistretti, P.J., Shoemaker, W.J., Deyo, S.N., and Bloom, F.E. (1982b). Effects of chronic lithium treatment on dopamine receptors in the rat corpus striatum. II. No effect on denervation or neuroleptic-induced supersensitivity. *Brain Res*, 232, 401–412.

Steffens, D.C., and Krishnan, K.R. (1998). Structural neuroimaging and mood disorders: Recent findings, implications for classification, and future directions. *Biol Psychiatry*, 43, 705–712.

Steffens, D.C, Helms, M.J., Krishnan, K.R., and Burke, G.L. (1999). Cerebrovascular disease and depression symptoms in the cardiovascular health study. *Stroke*, 30, 2159–2166.

Stein, M.B., Chen, G., Potter, W.Z., and Manji, H.K. (1996). G-protein level quantification in platelets and leukocytes from patients with panic disorder. *Neuropsychopharmacology*, 15, 180–186.

Steketee, J.D. (1993). Injection of the protein kinase inhibitor H7 into the A10 dopamine region blocks the acute responses to cocaine: Behavioral and in vivo microdialysis studies. *Neuropharmacology*, 32, 1289–1297.

Steketee, J.D. (1994). Intra-A10 injection of H7 blocks the development of sensitization to cocaine. *Neuroreport*, 6, 69–72.

Steketee, J.D., and Kalivas, P.W. (1991). Sensitization to psychostimulants and stress after injection of pertussis toxin into the A10 dopamine region. *J Pharmacol Exp Ther*, 259, 916–924.

Steketee, J.D., Striplin, C.D., Murray, T.F., and Kalivas, P.W. (1991). Possible role for G-proteins in behavioral sensitization to cocaine. *Brain Res*, 545, 287–291.

Stenfors, C., Theodorsson, E., and Mathe, A.A. (1989). Effect of repeated electroconvulsive treatment on regional concentrations of tachykinins, neurotensin, vasoactive intestinal polypeptide, neuropeptide Y, and galanin in rat brain. *J Neurosci Res*, 24, 445–450.

Stengaard-Pedersen, K., and Schou, M. (1982). In vitro and in vivo inhibition by lithium of enkephalin binding to opiate receptors in rat brain. *Neuropharmacology*, 21, 817–823.

Steppuhn, K.G., and Turski, L. (1993). Modulation of the seizure threshold for excitatory amino acids in mice by antiepileptic drugs and chemoconvulsants. *J Pharmacol Exp Ther*, 265, 1063–1070.

Stewart, J., and Badiani, A. (1993). Tolerance and sensitization to the behavioral effects of drugs. *Behav Pharmacol*, 4(4), 289–312.

Stockmeier, C.A. (1997). Neurobiology of serotonin in depression and suicide. *Ann NY Acad Sci*, 836, 220–232.

Stockmeier, C.A. (2003). Involvement of serotonin in depression: Evidence from postmortem and imaging studies of serotonin receptors and the serotonin transporter. *J Psychiatr Res*, 37, 357–373.

Stockmeier, C.A., and Meltzer, H.Y. (1991). Beta-adrenergic receptor binding in frontal cortex of suicide victims. *Biol Psychiatry*, 29, 183–191.

Stockmeier, C.A., Dilley, G.E., Shapiro, L.A., Overholser, J.C., Thompson, P.A., and Meltzer, H.Y. (1996). Serotonin receptors in suicide victims with major depression. *Neuropsychopharmacology*, 16, 162–173.

Stockmeier, C.A., Dilley, G.E., Shapiro, L.A., Overholser, J.C., Thompson, P.A., and Meltzer, H.Y. (1997). Serotonin receptors in suicide victims with major depression. *Neuropsychopharmacology*, 16, 162–173.

Stockmeier, C.A., Shapiro, L.A., Dilley, G.E., Kolli, T.N., Friedman, L., and Rajkowska, G. (1998). Increase in serotonin-1A autoreceptors in the midbrain of suicide victims with major depression-postmortem evidence for decreased serotonin activity. *J Neurosci*, 18, 7394–7401.

Stockmeier, C.A., Mahajan, G.J., Konick, L.C., Overholser, J.C., Jurjus, G.J., Meltzer, H.Y., Uylings, H.B., Friedman, L., and Rajkowska, G. (2004). Cellular changes in the postmortem hippocampus in major depression. *Biol Psychiatry*, 56(9), 640–650.

Stokes, P.E., Pick, G.R., Stoll, P.M., and Nunn, W.D. (1975). Pituitary–adrenal function in depressed patients: Resistance to dexamethasone suppression. *J Psychiatr Res*, 12, 271–281.

Stokes, P.E., Frazer, A., and Casper, R. (1981). Unexpected neuroendocrine-transmitter relationships [proceedings]. *Psychopharmacol Bull*, 17, 72–75.

Stokes, P.E., Stoll, P.M., Koslow, S.H., Maas, J.W., Davis, J.M., Swann, A.C., and Robins, E. (1984). Pretreatment DST and hypothalamic–pituitary–adrenocortical function in depressed patients and comparison groups. A multicenter study. *Arch Gen Psychiatry*, 41, 257–267.

Stoll, A.L., Cohen, B.M., Snyder, M.B., and Hanin, I. (1991). Erythrocyte choline concentration in bipolar disorder: A predictor of clinical course and medication response. *Biol Psychiatry*, 29, 1171–1180.

Stoll, A.L., Renshaw, P.F., Sachs, G.S., Guimaraes, A.R., Miller, C., Cohen, B.M., Lafer, B., and Gonzalez, R.G. (1992). The human brain resonance of choline-containing compounds is similar in patients receiving lithium treatment and controls: An in vivo proton magnetic resonance spectroscopy study. *Biol Psychiatry*, 32, 944–949.

Stoll, A.L., Sachs, G.S., Cohen, B.M., Lafer, B., Christensen, J.D., and Renshaw, P.F. (1996). Choline in the treatment of rapid-cycling bipolar disorder: Clinical and neurochemical findings in lithium-treated patients. *Biol Psychiatry*, 40(5), 382–388.

Stork, C., and Renshaw, P.F. (2005). Mitochondrial dysfunction in bipolar disorder: Evidence from magnetic resonance spectroscopy research. *Mol Psychiatry*, 10(10), 900–919.

Strakowski, S.M., Wilson, D.R., Tohen, M., Woods, B.T., Douglass, A.W., and Stoll, A.L. (1993). Structural brain abnormalities in first-episode mania. *Biol Psychiatry*, 33, 602–609.

Strakowski, S.M., Adler, C.M., and DelBello, M.P. (2002). Volumetric MRI studies of mood disorders: Do they distinguish unipolar and bipolar disorder? *Bipolar Disord*, 4, 80–88.

Strandman, E., Wetterberg, L., Perris, C., and Ross, S.B. (1978). Serum dopamine-beta-hydroxylase in affective disorders. *Neuropsychobiology*, 4, 248–255.

Stratakis, C.A., Sarlis, N.J., Berrettini, W.H., Badner, J.A., Chrousos, G.P., Gershon, E.S., and Detera-Wadleigh, S.D. (1997). Lack of linkage between the corticotropin-releasing hormone (CRH) gene and bipolar affective disorder. *Mol Psychiatry*, 2, 483–485.

Strzyzewski, W., Rybakowski, J., Potok, E., and Zelechowska-Ruda, E. (1984). Erythrocyte cation transport in endogenous depression: Clinical and psychophysiological correlates. *Acta Psychiatr Scand*, 70, 248–253.

Styra, R., Joffe, R., and Singer, W. (1991). Hyperthyroxinemia in major affective disorders. *Acta Psychiatr Scand*, 83, 61–63.

Styron, W. (1990). *Darkness Visible: A Memoir of Madness*. New York: Random House.

Suhara, T., Nakayama, K., Inoue, O., Fukuda, H., Shimizu, M., Mori, A., and Tateno, Y. (1992). D1 dopamine receptor binding in mood disorders measured by positron emission tomography. *Psychopharmacology (Berl)*, 106, 14–18.

Sulser, F. (1978). Functional aspects of the norepinephrine receptor coupled adenylate cyclase system in the limbic forebrain and its modification by drugs which precipitate or alleviate depression: molecular approaches to an understanding of affective disorders. *Pharmakopsychiatr Neuropsychopharmakol*, 11, 43–52.

Sunahara, G.I., and Chiesa, A. (1992). Phorone (diisopropylidene acetone), a glutathione depletor, decreases rat glucocorticoid receptor binding in vivo. *Carcinogenesis*, 13(7), 1083–1089.

Sunahara, R.K., Guan, H.C., O'Dowd, B.F., Seeman, P., Laurier, L.G., Ng, G., George, S.R., Torchia, J., Van Tol, H.H., and Niznik, H.B. (1991). Cloning of the gene for a human dopamine D5 receptor with higher affinity for dopamine than D1. *Nature*, 350, 614–619.

Suomi, S.J. (1982). The development of social competence by rhesus monkeys. *Ann Ist Super Sanita*, 18, 193–202.

Suomi, S.J., Seaman, S.F., Lewis, J.K., DeLizio, R.D., and McKinney, W.T. Jr. (1978). Effects of imipramine treatment of separation-induced social disorders in rhesus monkeys. *Arch Gen Psychiatry*, 35, 321–325.

Suzuki, K., Kusumi, I., Sasaki, Y., and Koyama, T. (2001). Serotonin-induced platelet intracellular calcium mobilization in various psychiatric disorders: Is it specific to bipolar disorder? *J Affect Disord*, 64, 291–296.

Swann, A.C. (1984). Caloric intake and Na+-K+-ATPase: Differential regulation by alpha 1- and beta-noradrenergic receptors. *Am J Physiol*, 247(3 Pt. 2), R449–R455.

Swann, A.C. (1988). Norepinephrine and (Na+, K+)-ATPase: Evidence for stabilization by lithium or imipramine. *Neuropharmacology*, 27, 261–267.

Swann, A.C., Maas, J.W., Hattox, S.E., and Landis, H. (1980). Catecholamine metabolites in human plasma as indices of brain function: Effects of debrisoquin. *Life Sci*, 27, 1857–1862.

Swann, A.C., Secunda, S.K., Katz, M.M., Koslow, S.H., Maas, J.W., Chang, S., and Robins, E. (1986). Lithium treatment of mania: Clinical characteristics, specificity of symptom change, and outcome. *Psychiatry Res*, 18(2), 127–141.

Swann, A.C., Koslow, S.H., Katz, M.M., Maas, J.W., Javaid, J., Secunda, S.K., and Robins, E. (1987). Lithium carbonate treatment of mania. Cerebrospinal fluid and urinary monoamine metabolites and treatment outcome. *Arch Gen Psychiatry*, 44, 345–354.

Swann, A.C., Secunda, S.K., Stokes, P.E., Croughan, J., Davis, J.M., Koslow, S.H., and Maas, J.W. (1990). Stress, depression, and mania: Relationship between perceived role of stressful events and clinical and biochemical characteristics. *Acta Psychiatr Scand*, 81, 389–397.

Swann, A.C., Secunda, S.K., Koslow, S.H., Katz, M.M., Bowden, C.L., Maas, J.W., Davis, J.M., and Robins, E. (1991). Mania: Sympathoadrenal function and clinical state. *Psychiatry Res*, 37, 195–205.

Swann, A.C., Stokes, P.E., Casper, R., Secunda, S.K., Bowden, C.L., Berman, N., Katz, M.M., and Robins, E. (1992). Hypothalamic–pituitary–adrenocortical function in mixed and pure mania. *Acta Psychiatr Scand*, 85, 270–274.

Swann, A.C., Stokes, P.E., Secunda, S.K., Maas, J.W., Bowden, C.L., Berman, N., and Koslow, S.H. (1994). Depressive mania versus agitated depression: Biogenic amine and hypothalamic–pituitary–adrenocortical function. *Biol Psychiatry*, 35, 803–813.

Swann, A.C., Petty, F., Bowden, C.L., Dilsaver, S.C., Calabrese, J.R., and Morris, D.D. (1999). Mania: Gender, transmitter function, and response to treatment. *Psychiatry Res*, 88, 55–61.

Szabo, S., Gould, T.D., and Manji, H.K. (2003). Neurotransmitters, receptors, signal transduction pathways and second messengers. In C.B. Nemeroff and A.F. Schatzberg (Eds.), *American Psychiatric Textbook of Psychopharmacology* (pp. 3–52). Arlington, VA: American Psychiatric Publishing.

Szentistvanyi, I., and Janka, Z. (1979). Correlation between the lithium ratio and Na-dependent Li transport of red blood cells during lithium prophylaxis. *Biol Psychiatry*, 14, 973–977.

Szuba, M. P., Baxter, L.R. Jr., Fairbanks, L.A., Guze, B.H., and Schwartz, J.M. (1991). Effects of partial sleep deprivation on the diurnal variation of mood and motor activity in major depression. *Biol Psychiatry*, 30(8), 817–829.

Szuba, M.P., Baxter, L.R. Jr., Altshuler, L.L., Allen, E.M., Guze, B.H., Schwartz, J.M., and Liston, E.H. (1994). Lithium sustains the acute antidepressant effects of sleep deprivation: Preliminary findings from a controlled study. *Psychiatry Res*, 51, 283–295.

Szuba, M.P., Amsterdam, J.D., Fernando, A.T. III, Gary, K.A., Whybrow, P.C., and Winokur, A. (2005). Rapid antidepressant response after nocturnal TRH administration in patients with bipolar type I and bipolar type II major depression. *J Clin Psychopharmacol*, 25(4), 325–330.

Takashima, A., Yamaguchi, H., Noguchi, K., Michel, G., Ishiguro, K., Sato, K., Hoshino, T., Hoshi, M., and Imahori, K. (1995). Amyloid beta peptide induces cytoplasmic accumulation of amyloid protein precursor via tau protein kinase I/glycogen synthase kinase-3 beta in rat hippocampal neurons. *Neurosci Lett*, 198, 83–86.

Tan, C.H., Javors, M.A., Seleshi, E., Lowrimore, P.A., and Bowden, C.L. (1990). Effects of lithium on platelet ionic intracellular calcium concentration in patients with bipolar (manic-depressive) disorder and healthy controls. *Life Sci*, 46(16), 1175–1180.

Tan, C.H., Lee, H.S., Kua, E.H., and Peh, L.H. (1995). Resting and thrombin-stimulated cytosolic calcium in platelets of patients with alcoholic withdrawal, bipolar manic disorder and chronic schizophrenia. *Life Sci*, 56(21), 1817–1823.

Tandon, R., Channabasavanna, S.M., and Greden, J.F. (1988). CSF biochemical correlates of mixed affective states. *Acta Psychiatr Scand*, 78, 289–297.

Tanimoto, K., Maeda, K., and Terada, T. (1983). Inhibitory effect of lithium on neuroleptic and serotonin receptors in rat brain. *Brain Res*, 265, 148–151.

Tartaglia, N., Du, J., Tyler, W.J., Neale, E., Pozzo-Miller, L., and Lu, B. (2001). Protein synthesis-dependent and -independent regulation of hippocampal synapses by brain-derived neurotrophic factor. *J Biol Chem*, 276, 37585–37593.

Taylor, M.P., Reynolds, C.F. III, Frank, E., Cornes, C., Miller, M.D., Stack, J.A., Begley, A.E., Mazumdar, S., Dew, M.A., and Kupfer, D.J. (1999). Which elderly depressed patients remain well on maintenance interpersonal psychotherapy alone?: Report from the pittsburgh study of maintenance therapies in late-life depression. *Depress Anxiety*, 10(2), 55–60.

Terenius, L., and Wahlstrom, A. (1976). A method for site selectivity analysis applied to opiate receptors. *Eur J Pharmacol*, 40, 241–248.

Terenius, L., Wahlström, A., Lindström, L., and Widerlöv, E. (1976). Increased CSF levels of endorphins in chronic psychosis. *Neurosci Lett*, 3, 157–162.

Terenius, L., Wahlstrom, A., and Agren, H. (1977). Naloxone (Narcan) treatment in depression: Clinical observations and effects on CSF endorphins and monoamine metabolites. *Psychopharmacology (Berl)*, 54, 31–33.

Terry, J.B., Padzernik, T.L., and Nelson, S.R. (1990). Effect of LiCl pretreatment on cholinomimetic-induced seizures and seizure-induced brain edema in rats. *Neurosci Lett*, 114, 123–127.

Thakar, J.H., Lapierre, Y.D., and Waters, B.G. (1985). Erythrocyte membrane sodium-potassium and magnesium ATPase in primary affective disorder. *Biol Psychiatry*, 20, 734–740.

Thakore, J.H., O'Keane, V., and Dinan, T.G. (1996). d-fenfluramine-induced prolactin responses in mania: Evidence for serotonergic subsensitivity. *Am J Psychiatry*, 153, 1460–1463.

Thase, M.E., Mallinger, A.G., McKnight, D., and Himmelhoch, J.M. (1992). Treatment of imipramine-resistant recurrent depression: IV. A double-blind crossover study of tranylcypromine for anergic bipolar depression. *Am J Psychiatry*, 149, 195–198.

Thome, J., Sakai, N., Shin, K., Steffen, C., Zhang, Y.J., Impey, S., Storm, D., and Duman, R.S. (2000). cAMP response element–mediated gene transcription is upregulated by chronic antidepressant treatment. *J Neurosci*, 20, 4030–4036.

Thome, J., Pesold, B., Baader, M., Hu, M., Gewirtz, J.C., Duman, R.S., and Henn, F.A. (2001). Stress differentially regulates synaptophysin and synaptotagmin expression in hippocampus. *Biol Psychiatry*, 50, 809–812.

Thompson, P.M., Rosenberger, C., and Qualls, C. (1999). CSF SNAP-25 in schizophrenia and bipolar illness. A pilot study. *Neuropsychopharmacology*, 21, 717–722.

Tkachev, D., Mimmack, M.L., Ryan, M.M., Wayland, M., Freeman, T., Jones, P.B., Starkey, M., Webster, M.J., Yolken, R.H., and Bahn, S. (2003). Oligodendrocyte dysfunction in schizophrenia and bipolar disorder. *Lancet*, 362, 798–805.

Tollefson, G.D., Senogles, S.E., and Frey, W.H. II. (1982). Ionic regulation of antagonist binding to the human muscarinic cholinergic receptor of caudate nucleus. *J Psychiatr Res*, 17, 275–283.

Torok, T.L. (1989). Neurochemical transmission and the sodium-pump. *Prog Neurobiol*, 32(1), 11–76.

Traskman, L., Asberg, M., Bertilsson, L., and Sjostrand, L. (1981). Monoamine metabolites in CSF and suicidal behavior. *Arch Gen Psychiatry*, 38, 631–636.

Treiser, S., and Kellar, K.J. (1979). Lithium effects on adrenergic receptor supersensitivity in rat brain. *Eur J Pharmacol*, 58, 85–86.

Treiser, S., and Kellar, K.J. (1980). Lithium: Effects on serotonin receptors in rat brain. *Eur J Pharmacol*, 64, 183–185.

Treiser, S.L., Cascio, C.S., O'Donohue, T.L., Thoa, N.B., Jacobowitz, D.M., and Kellar, K.J. (1981). Lithium increases serotonin release and decreases serotonin receptors in the hippocampus. *Science*, 213, 1529–1531.

Tremolizzo, L., Doueiri, M.S., Dong, E., Grayson, D.R., Davis, J., Pinna, G., Tueting, P., Rodriguez-Menendez, V., Costa, E., and Guidotti, A. (2005). Valproate corrects the schizophrenia-like epigenetic behavioral modifications induced by methionine in mice. *Biol Psychiatry*, 57(5), 500–509.

Tricklebank, M.D., Singh, L., Jackson, A., and Oles, R.J. (1991). Evidence that a proconvulsant action of lithium is mediated by inhibition of myo-inositol phosphatase in mouse brain. *Brain Res*, 558, 145–148.

Trottier, E., Belzil, A., Stoltz, C., and Anderson, A. (1995). Localization of a phenobarbital-responsive element (PBRE) in the 5'-flanking region of the rat *CYP2B2* gene. *Gene*, 158(2), 263–268.

Tsai, G., and Coyle, J.T. (1995). N-acetylaspartate in neuropsychiatric disorders. *Prog Neurobiol*, 46, 531–540.

Tsankova, N.M., Berton, O., Renthal, W., Kumar, A., Neve, R.L., and Nestler, E.J. (2006). Sustained hippocampal chromatin regulation in a mouse model of depression and antidepressant action. *Nat Neurosci*, 9(4), 519–525.

Tudorache, B., and Diacicov, S. (1991). The effect of clonidine in the treatment of acute mania. *Rom J Neurol Psychiatry*, 29, 209–213.

Turktas, L., Gucuyener, K., and Ozden, A. (1997). Medication-induced psychotic reaction. *J Am Acad Child Adolesc Psychiatry*, 36(8), 1017–1018.

Turner, K.M., Burgoyne, R.D., and Morgan, A. (1999). Protein phosphorylation and the regulation of synaptic membrane traffic. *Trends Neurosci*, 22, 459–464.

Turski, L. (1990). The N-methyl-D-aspartate receptor complex. Various sites of regulation and clinical consequences. *Arzneimittelforschung*, 40, 511–514.

Tzschentke, T.M., and Schmidt, W.J. (1997). Interactions of MK-801 and GYKI 52466 with morphine and amphetamine in place preference conditioning and behavioural sensitization. *Behav Brain Res*, 84, 99–107.

Ueda, Y., and Willmore, L.J. (2000). Molecular regulation of glutamate and GABA transporter proteins by valproic acid in rat hippocampus during epileptogenesis. *Exp Brain Res*, 133, 334–339.

Uhde, T.W., Vittone, B.J., Siever, L.J., Kaye, W.H., and Post, R.M. (1986). Blunted growth hormone response to clonidine in panic disorder patients. *Biol Psychiatry*, 21, 1081–1085.

Ullian, E.M., Sapperstein, S.K., Christopherson, K.S., and Barres, B.A. (2001). Control of synapse number by glia. *Science*, 291, 657–661.

Uney, J.B., Marchbanks, R.M., and Marsh, A. (1985). The effect of lithium on choline transport in human erythrocytes. *J Neurol Neurosurg Psychiatry*, 48, 229–233.

Ur, E., Turner, T.H., Goodwin, T.J., Grossman, A., and Besser, G.M. (1992). Mania in association with hydrocortisone replacement for Addison's disease. *Postgrad Med J*, 68, 41–43.

Uranova, N., Orlovskaya, D., Vikhreva, O., Zimina, I., Kolomeets, N., Vostrikov, V., and Rachmanova, V. (2001). Electron microscopy of oligodendroglia in severe mental illness. *Brain Res Bull*, 55, 597–610.

Ushijama, I., Yamada, K., and Furukawa, T. (1986). Behavioral effects of lithium on presynaptic sites of catecholaminergic neurons in the mouse. *Arch Int Pharmachodyn*, 282, 58–67.

Vacheron-Trystram, M.N., Cheref, S., and Gauillard, J. (2002). A case report of mania precipitated by use of DHEA. *Encephale*, 28(6 Pt. 1), 563–566

Vaden, D.L., Ding, D., Peterson, B., and Greenberg, M.L. (2001). Lithium and valproate decrease inositol mass and increase expression of the yeast *INO1* and *INO2* genes for inositol biosynthesis. *J Biol Chem*, 276, 15466–15471.

Valberde, O., Tzavara, E., Hanoune, J., Roques, B.P., and Maldonado, R. (1996). Protein kinases in the rat nucleus accumbens are involved in the aversive component of opiate withdrawal. *Eur J Neurosci*, 8, 2671–2678.

Vallar, L., Muca, C., Magni, M., Albert, P., Bunzow, J., Meldolesi, J., and Civelli, O. (1990). Differential coupling of dopaminergic D2 receptors expressed in different cell types. Stimulation of phosphatidylinositol 4,5-bisphosphate hydrolysis in LtK-fibroblasts, hyperpolarization, and cytosolic-free Ca2+ concentration decrease in GH4C1 cells. *J Biol Chem*, 265, 10320–10326.

Valle, J., Ayuso-Gutierrez, J.L., and Abril, A. (1999). Evaluation of thyroid function in lithium-naive bipolar patients. *Eur Psychiatry*, 14(6), 341–345.

van Calker, D., and Belmaker, R.H. (2000). The high-affinity inositol transport system: Implications for the pathophysiology and treatment of bipolar disorder. *Bipolar Disord*, 2, 102–107.

van Calker, D., Steber, R., Klotz, K.N., and Greil, W. (1991). Carbamazepine distinguishes between adenosine receptors that mediate different second messenger responses. *Eur J Pharmacol*, 206, 285–290.

van Calker, D., Forstner, U., Bohus, M., Gebicke Harter, P., Hecht, H., Wark, H.J., and Berger, M. (1993). Increased sensitivity to agonist stimulation of the Ca2+ response in neutrophils of manic-depressive patients: Effect of lithium therapy. *Neuropsychobiology*, 27(3), 180–183.

van der Laan, J.W., de Boer, T., and Bruinvels, J. (1979). Di-n-propylacetate and GABA degradation. Preferential inhibition of succinic semialdehyde dehydrogenase and indirect inhibition of GABA-transaminase. *J Neurochem*, 32, 1769–1780.

Vanelle, J.M., Poirier, M.F., Benkelfat, C., Galinowski, A., Sechter, D., Suzini de Luca, H., and Loo, H. (1990). Diagnostic and therapeutic value of testing stimulation of thyroid-stimulating hormone by thyrotropin-releasing hormone in 100 depressed patients. *Acta Psychiatr Scand*, 81, 156–161.

Van Kammen, D.P., and Murphy, D.L. (1975). Attenuation of the euphoriant and activating effects of d- and l-amphetamine by lithium carbonate treatment. *Psychopharmacologia*, 44(3), 215–224.

Van Kammen, D.P., Docherty, J.P., Marder, S.R., Rosenblatt, J.E., and Bunney, W.E. Jr. (1985). Lithium attenuates the activation–euphoria but not the psychosis induced by d-amphetamine in schizophrenia. *Psychopharmacology (Berl)*, 87, 111–115.

Van Praag, H.M. (1982). Depression, suicide and the metabolism of serotonin in the brain. *J Affect Disord*, 4, 275–290.

Van Praag, H.M., and de Haan, S. (1979). Central serotonin metabolism and frequency of depression. *Psychiatry Res*, 1, 219–224.

Van Praag, H.M., and Korf, J. (1975). Central monoamine deficiency in depressions: Causative of secondary phenomenon? *Pharmakopsychiatr Neuropsychopharmakol*, 8, 322–326.

Van Praag, H., Christie, B.R., Sejnowski, T.J., and Gage, F.H. (1999). Running enhances neurogenesis, learning, and long-term potentiation in mice. *Proc Natl Acad Sci USA*, 96(23), 13427–13431.

Van Tits, L.J., Michel, M.C., Grosse-Wilde, H., Happel, M., Eigler, F.W., Soliman, A., and Brodde, O.E. (1990). Catecholamines increase lymphocyte beta 2-adrenergic receptors via a beta 2-adrenergic, spleen-dependent process. *Am J Physiol*, 258, E191–E202.

Vawter, M.P., Freed, W.J., and Kleinman, J.E. (2000). Neuropathology of bipolar disorder. *Biol Psychiatry*, 48(6), 486–504.

Vawter, M.P., Thatcher, L., Usen, N., Hyde, T.M., Kleinman, J.E., and Freed, W.J. (2002). Reduction of synapsin in the hippocampus of patients with bipolar disorder and schizophrenia. *Mol Psychiatry*, 7, 571–578.

Vecsei, L., and Widerlöv, E. (1988). Brain and CSF somatostatin concentrations in patients with psychiatric or neurological illness. An overview. *Acta Psychiatr Scand*, 78, 657–667.

Veith, R.C., Raskind, M.A., Barnes, R.F., Gumbrecht, G., Ritchie, J.L., and Halter, J.B. (1983). Tricyclic antidepressants and supine, standing, and exercise plasma norepinephrine levels. *Clin Pharmacol Ther*, 33, 763–769.

Veith, R.C., Halter, J.B., Murburg, M.M., et al. (1985). *Increased plasma NE appearance rate in dexamethasone resistant depression*. Fourth World Congress of Biological Psychiatry, Athens, Greece, October 13–17.

Veith, R.C., Barnes, R.F., Villacres, E., Murburg, M.M., Raskind, M.A., and Borson, S. (1988). Plasma catecholamines and norepinephrine kinetics in depression and panic disorder. In

R. Belmaker R (Ed.), *Catecholamines: Clinical Aspects* (pp. 197–202). New York: Alan R. Liss.

Veith, R.C., Lewis, N., Linares, O.A., Barnes, R.F., Raskind, M.A., Villacres, E.C., Murburg, M.M., Ashleigh, E.A., Castillo, S., and Peskind, E.R. (1994). Sympathetic nervous system activity in major depression. Basal and desipramine-induced alterations in plasma norepinephrine kinetics. *Arch Gen Psychiatry*, 51, 411–422.

Velayudhan, A., Sunitha, T.A., Balachander, S., Reddy, J.Y., and Khanna, S. (1999). A study of platelet serotonin receptor in mania. *Biol Psychiatry*, 45, 1059–1062.

Verbanck, P.M., Lotstra, F., Gilles, C., Linkowski, P., Mendlewicz, J., and Vanderhaeghen, J.J. (1984). Reduced cholecystokinin immunoreactivity in the cerebrospinal fluid of patients with psychiatric disorders. *Life Sci*, 34, 67–72.

Verimer, T., Goodale, D.B., Long, J.P., and Flynn, J.R. (1980). Lithium effects on haloperidol-induced pre- and postsynaptic dopamine receptor supersensitivity. *J Pharm Pharmacol*, 32, 665–666.

Virkkunen, M., De Jong, J., Bartko, J., and Linnoila, M. (1989). Psychobiological concomitants of history of suicide attempts among violent offenders and impulsive fire setters. *Arch Gen Psychiatry*, 46, 604–606.

Vogt, I.R., Shimron-Abarbanell, D., Neidt, H., Erdmann, J., Cichon, S., Schulze, T.G., Muller, D.J., Maier, W., Albus, M., Borrmann-Hassenbach, M., Knapp, M., Rietschel, M., Propping, P., and Nothen, M.M. (2000). Investigation of the human serotonin 6 [5-HT6] receptor gene in bipolar affective disorder and schizophrenia. *Am J Med Genet*, 96, 217–221.

Vollenweider, F.X., Maguire, R.P., Leenders, K.L., Mathys, K., and Angst, J. (1998). Effects of high amphetamine dose on mood and cerebral glucose metabolism in normal volunteers using positron emission tomography (PET). *Psychiatry Res*, 83(3), 149–162.

Volonte, C., and Rukenstein, A. (1993). Lithium chloride promotes short-term survival of PC12 cells after serum and NGF-deprivation. *Lithium*, 4, 211–219.

von Knorring, L., Oreland, L., Perris, C., and Runeberg, S. (1976). Lithium RBC/plasma ratio in subgroups of patients with affective disorders. *Neuropsychobiology*, 2(2-3), 74–80.

Vriend, J.P., and Alexiuk, N.A. (1996). Effects of valproate on amino acid and monoamine concentrations in striatum of audiogenic seizure-prone Balb/c mice. *Mol Chem Neuropathol*, 27, 307–324.

Vrontakis, M.E. (2002). Galanin: A biologically active peptide. *Curr Drug Targets CNS Neurol Disord*, 1(6), 531–541.

Wada, J.A., Osawa, T., Sato, M., Wake, A., Corcoran, M.E., and Troupin, A.S. (1976). Acute anticonvulsant effects of diphenylhydantoin, phenobarbital, and carbamazepine: A combined electroclinical and serum level study in amygdaloid kindled cats and baboons. *Epilepsia*, 17, 77–88.

Wada, K., Yamada, N., Suzuki, H., Lee, Y., and Kuroda, S. (2000). Recurrent cases of corticosteroid-induced mood disorder: Clinical characteristics and treatment. *J Clin Psychiatry*, 61(4), 261–267.

Wager-Smith, K., and Kay, S.A. (2000). Circadian rhythm genetics: From flies to mice to humans. *Nat Genet*, 26, 23–27.

Wahlestedt, C., Blendy, J.A., Kellar, K.J., Heilig, M., Widerlöv, E., and Ekman, R. (1990). Electroconvulsive shocks increase the concentration of neocortical and hippocampal neuropeptide Y (NPY)–like immunoreactivity in the rat. *Brain Res*, 507, 65–68.

Wakoh, H., and Hatotani, N. (1973). Endocrinological treatment of psychoses. In K. Lissák (Ed.), *Hormones and Brain Function* (pp. 491–498). New York: Plenum Press.

Waldman, I.D., Robinson, B.F., and Feigon, S.A. (1997). Linkage disequilibrium between the dopamine transporter gene (DAT1) and bipolar disorder: Extending the transmission disequilibrium test (TDT) to examine genetic heterogeneity. *Genet Epidemiol*, 14, 699–704.

Waldmeier, P.C., Baumann, P.A., Fehr, B., De Herdt, P., and Maitre, L. (1984). Carbamazepine decreases catecholamine turnover in the rat brain. *J Pharmacol Exp Ther*, 231, 166–172.

Wang, H.G., Rapp, U.R., and Reed, J.C. (1996). Bcl-2 targets the protein kinase Raf-1 to mitochondria. *Cell*, 87, 629–638.

Wang, H.Y., and Friedman, E. (1988). Chronic lithium: Desensitization of autoreceptors mediating serotonin release. *Psychopharmacology (Berl)*, 94, 312–314.

Wang, H.Y., and Friedman, E. (1996). Enhanced protein kinase C activity and translocation in bipolar affective disorder brains. *Biol Psychiatry*, 40, 568–575.

Wang, H.Y., and Friedman, E. (1999). Effects of lithium on receptor-mediated activation of G proteins in rat brain cortical membranes. *Neuropharmacology*, 38, 403–414.

Wang, H., and Friedman, E. (2001). Increased association of brain protein kinase C with the receptor for activated c kinase-1 (RACK1) in bipolar affective disorder. *Biol Psychiatry*, 50(5), 364–370.

Wang, H.Y., Markowitz, P., Levinson, D., Undie, A.S., and Friedman, E. (1999). Increased membrane-associated protein kinase C activity and translocation in blood platelets from bipolar affective disorder patients. *J Psychiatr Res*, 33, 171–179.

Wang, J.-F., Young, L.T., Li, P.P., and Warsh, J.J. (1997). Signal transduction abnormalities in bipolar disorder. In R.T. Joffe (Ed.), *Bipolar Disorder: Biological Models and Their Clinical Application* (pp. 41–79). New York: Dekker.

Wang, J.F., Asghari, V., Rockel, C., and Young, L.T. (1999). Cyclic AMP responsive element binding protein phosphorylation and DNA binding is decreased by chronic lithium but not valproate treatment of SH-SY5Y neuroblastoma cells. *Neuroscience*, 91, 771–776.

Wang, S.J., Huang, C.C., Hsu, K.S., Tsai, J.J., and Gean, P.W. (1996). Presynaptic inhibition of excitatory neurotransmission by lamotrigine in the rat amygdalar neurons. *Synapse*, 24, 248–255.

Warner-Schmidt, J.L., and Duman, R.S. (2006). Hippocampal neurogenesis: Opposing effects of stress and antidepressant treatment. *Hippocampus*, 16(3), 239–249.

Warsh, J., Young, L., and Li, P. (2000). Guanine nucleotide binding (G) proteindisturbances. In R. Belmaker (Ed.), *Bipolar Affective Disorder in Bipolar Medications: Mechanisms of Action* (pp. 299–329). Washington, DC: American Psychiatric Press.

Watanabe, Y., Gould, E., Daniels, D.C., Cameron, H., and McEwen, B.S. (1992). Tianeptine attenuates stress-induced morphological changes in the hippocampus. *Eur J Pharmacol*, 222, 157–162.

Watson, D.G., Watterson, J.M., and Lenox, R.H. (1998). Sodium valproate down-regulates the myristoylated alanine-rich C kinase substrate (MARCKS) in immortalized hippocampal cells: A property of protein kinase C–mediated mood stabilizers. *J Pharmacol Exp Ther*, 285(1), 307–316.

Watts, B.V., and Grady, T.A. (1997). Tramadol-induced mania. *Am J Psychiatry*, 154, 1624.

Weaver, I.C., Cervoni, N., Champagne, F.A., D'Alessio, A.C., Sharma, S., Seckl, J.R., Dymov, S., Szyf, M., and Meaney, M.J. (2004). Epigenetic programming by maternal behavior. *Nat Neurosci*, 7(8), 847–854.

Webster, E.L., Lewis, D.B., Torpy, D.J., Zachman, E.K., Rice, K.C., and Chrousos, G.P. (1996). In vivo and in vitro characterization of antalarmin, a nonpeptide corticotropin-releasing hormone (CRH) receptor antagonist: Suppression of pituitary ACTH release and peripheral inflammation. *Endocrinology*, 137(12), 5747–5750.

Webster, M.J., Knable, M.B., O'Grady, J., Orthmann, J., and Weickert, C.S. (1999). Decreased glucocorticoid receptor mRNA levels in individuals with depression, bipolar disorder and schizophrenia. *Schizophr Res*, 41, 111.

Webster, M.J., Knable, M.B., O'Grady, J., Orthmann, J., and Weickert, C.S. (2002). Regional specificity of brain glucocorticoid receptor mRNA alterations in subjects with schizophrenia and mood disorders. *Mol Psychiatry*, 7(9), 924, 985–994.

Weeke, A., and Weeke, J. (1978). Disturbed circadian variation of serum thyrotropin in patients with endogenous depression. *Acta Psychiatr Scand*, 57, 281–289.

Weeke, J. (1973). Circadian variation of the serum thyrotropin level in normal subjects. *Scand J Clin Lab Invest*, 31, 337–342.

Wehr, T.A. (1977). Phase and biorhythm studies of affective illness. In W.E. Bunney Jr. (Ed.), The switch process in manic-depressive psychosis. *Ann Intern Med*, 87, 319–335.

Wehr, T.A., and Goodwin, F.K. (1987). Can antidepressants cause mania and worsen the course of affective illness? *Am J Psychiatry*, 144, 1403–1411.

Wehr, T.A., Sack, D.A., and Rosenthal, N.E. (1987). Sleep reduction as a final common pathway in the genesis of mania. *Am J Psychiatry*, 144, 201–204.

Wehr, T.A., Sack, D.A., Rosenthal, N.E., and Cowdry, R.W. (1988). Rapid cycling affective disorder: Contributing factors and treatment responses in 51 patients. *Am J Psychiatry*, 145, 179–184.

Wei, H., Qin, Z.H., Senatorov, V.V., Wei, W., Wang, Y., Qian, Y., and Chuang, D.M. (2001). Lithium suppresses excitotoxicity-induced striatal lesions in a rat model of Huntington's disease. *Neuroscience*, 106(3), 603–612.

Wei, Q., Lu, X.Y., Liu, L., Schafer, G., Shieh, K.R., Burke, S., Robinson, T.E., Watson, S.J., Seasholtz, A.F., and Akil, H. (2004). Glucocorticoid receptor overexpression in forebrain: A mouse model of increased emotional lability. *Proc Natl Acad Sci USA*, 101(32), 11851–11856.

Weinberger, D.R., Egan, M.F., Bertolino, A., Callicott, J.H., Mattay, V.S., Lipska, B.K., Berman, K.F., and Goldberg, T.E. (2001). Prefrontal neurons and the genetics of schizophrenia. *Biol Psychiatry*, 50, 825–844.

Weiner, R.D., Krystal, A.D., Coffey, C.E., and Smith, P. (1992). The electrophysiology of ECT: Relevance to mechanism of action. *Clin Neuropharmacol*, 15(Suppl. 1, Pt. A), 671A–672A.

Weingartner, H., Gold, P., Ballenger, J.C., Smallberg, S.A., Summers, R., Rubinow, D.R., Post, R.M., and Goodwin, F.K. (1981). Effects of vasopressin on human memory functions. *Science*, 211, 601–603.

Weintraub, B. (1995). *Molecular Endocrinology: Basic Concepts and Clinical Correlations*. New York: Raven Press.

Weiss, S.R., and Post, R.M. (1994). Caveats in the use of the kindling model of affective disorders. *Toxicol Ind Health*, 10, 421–447.

Weiss, E.L., Bowers, M.B. Jr., and Mazure, C.M. (1999). Testosterone-patch-induced psychotic mania. *Am J Psychiatry*, 156, 969.

Weiss, J.M., and Kilts, C.D. (1998). Animal models of depression and schizophrenia. In A.F. Schatzerg and C.B. Nemeroff (Eds.), *Textbook of Psychopharmacology* (pp. 89–131). Washington, DC: American Psychiatric Press.

Weiss, J.M., Goodman, P., Ambrose, M.J., Webster, A., and Hoffman, L.J. (1984). Neurochemical basis of behavioral depression. In E. Katkin and S. Manuck (Eds.), *Advances in Behavioral Medicine* (pp. 233–276). Greenwich, CT: JAI Press.

Weiss, J.M., Bonsall, R.W., Demetrikopoulos, M.K., Emery, M.S., and West, C.H. (1998). Galanin: A significant role in depression? *Ann NY Acad Sci*, 863, 364–382.

Weiss, S.R., Post, R.M., Costello, M., Nutt, D.J., and Tandeciarz, S. (1990). Carbamazepine retards the development of cocaine-kindled seizures but not sensitization to cocaine-induced hyperactivity. *Neuropsychopharmacology*, 3, 273–281.

Weiss, S.R., Post, R.M., Sohn, E., Berger, A., and Lewis R. (1993). Cross-tolerance between carbamazepine and valproate on amygdala-kindled seizures. *Epilepsy Res*, 16(1), 37–44.

Weiss, S.R., Li, X.L., Rosen, J.B., Li, H., Heynen, T., and Post, R.M. (1995). Quenching: Inhibition of development and expression of amygdala kindled seizures with low frequency stimulation. *Neuroreport*, 6(16), 2171–2176.

Weissman, M.M., Leaf, P.J., Tischler, G.L., Blazer, D.G., Karno, M., Bruce, M.L., and Florio, L.P. (1988). Affective disorders in five United States communities. *Psychol Med*, 18, 141–153.

Weller, E.B., and Weller, R.A. (1988). Neuroendocrine changes in affectively ill children and adolescents. *Neurol Clin*, 6, 41–54.

Wellman, C.L. (2001). Dendritic reorganization in pyramidal neurons in medial prefrontal cortex after chronic corticosterone administration. *J Neurobiol*, 49, 245–253.

Weng, G., Bhalla, U.S., and Iyengar, R. (1999). Complexity in biological signaling systems. *Science*, 284, 92–96.

Wersinger, S.R., Ginns, E.I., O'Carroll, A.M., Lolait, S.J., and Young, W.S. III. (2002). Vasopressin v1b receptor knockout reduces aggressive behavior in male mice. *Mol Psychiatry*, 7(9), 975–984.

Werstiuk, E.S., Steiner, M., and Burns, T. (1990). Studies on leukocyte beta-adrenergic receptors in depression: A critical appraisal. *Life Sci*, 47(2), 85–105. Review. Erratum in: *Life Sci*, 47(21), 1979–1980.

Weston, P.G., and Howard, M.Q. (1922). The determination of Na, K, Ca, and Mg in the blood and spinal fluid of patients suffering from manic-depressive insanity. *Arch Neurol Psychiatry*, 8, 179–183.

Whalley, L.J., Christie, J.E., Bennie, J., Dick, H., Blackburn, I.M., Blackwood, D., Sanchez Watts, G., and Fink, G. (1985). Selective increase in plasma luteinising hormone concentrations in drug free young men with mania. *BMJ (Clin Res Ed)*, 290, 99–102.

Whalley, L.J., Kutcher, S., Blackwood, D.H., Bennie, J., Dick, H., and Fink, G. (1987). Increased plasma LH in manic-depressive illness: Evidence of a state-independent abnormality. *Br J Psychiatry*, 150, 682–684.

Whittle, S.R., and Turner, A.J. (1978). Effects of the anticonvulsant sodium valproate on gamma-aminobutyrate and aldehyde metabolism in ox brain. *J Neurochem*, 31, 1453–1459.

Whitworth, P., and Kendall, D.A. (1989). Effects of lithium on inositol phospholipid hydrolysis and inhibition of dopamine

D1 receptor-mediated cyclic AMP formation by carbachol in rat brain slices. *J Neurochem*, 53, 536–541.

Whybrow, P.C. (1994). The therapeutic use of triiodothyronine and high dose thyroxine in psychiatric disorder. *Acta Med Austriaca*, 21, 47–52.

Wiborg, O., Kruger, T., and Jakobsen, S.N. (1999). Region-selective effects of long-term lithium and carbamazepine administration on cyclic AMP levels in rat brain. *Pharmacol Toxicol*, 84(2), 88–93.

Widdowson, P.S., Ordway, G.A., and Halaris, A.E. (1992). Reduced neuropeptide Y concentrations in suicide brain. *J Neurochem*, 59, 73–80.

Widerlöv, E., Bissette, G., and Nemeroff, C.B. (1988a). Monoamine metabolites, corticotropin releasing factor and somatostatin as CSF markers in depressed patients. *J Affect Disord*, 14, 99–107.

Widerlöv, E., Lindstrom, L.H., Wahlestedt, C., and Ekman, R. (1988b). Neuropeptide Y and peptide YY as possible cerebrospinal fluid markers for major depression and schizophrenia, respectively. *J Psychiatr Res*, 22, 69–79.

Widner, B., Leblhuber, F., Walli, J., Tilz, G.P., Demel, U., and Fuchs, D. (1999). Degradation of tryptophan in neurodegenerative disorders. *Adv Exp Med Biol*, 467, 133–138.

Williams, D., Lee, T.D., Dinh, N., and Young, M.K. (2000). Oligosaccharide profiling: The facile detection of mono-, di- and oligosaccharides by electrospray orthogonal time-of-flight mass spectrometry using 3-aminophenylboronic acid derivatization. *Rapid Commun Mass Spectrom*, 14(16), 1530–1537.

Williams, J.A., and Sehgal, A. (2001). Molecular components of the circadian system in *Drosophila*. *Annu Rev Physiol*, 63, 729–755.

Williams, N., Layden, B.T., Suhy, J., Metreger, T., Foley, K., Abukhdeir, A.M., Borge, G., Crayton, J., Bryant, F.B., and Mota de Freitas, D. (2003). Testing competing path models linking the biochemical variables in red blood cells from li+-treated bipolar patients. *Bipolar Disord*, 5(5), 320–329.

Willner, P. (1983). Dopamine and depression: A review of recent evidence. I. Empirical studies. *Brain Res*, 287(3), 211–224.

Willner, P. (1984). The validity of animal models of depression. *Psychopharmacology*, 83, 1–16.

Willner, P. (1991). Animal models as simulations of depression. *Trends Pharmacol Sci*, 12, 131–136.

Willner, P. (1995). Animal models of depression: Validity and applications. In G. Serra (Ed.), *Depression and Mania: From Neurobiology to Treatment* (Vol. 49) (pp. 19–42). New York: Raven Press.

Witkin, J.M. (1993). Blockade of the locomotor stimulant effects of cocaine and methamphetamine by glutamate antagonists. *Life Sci*, 53(24), PL405–410.

Wolfe, N., Katz, D.I., Albert, M.L., Almozlino, A., Durso, R., Smith, M.C., and Volicer, L. (1990). Neuropsychological profile linked to low dopamine. In Alzheimer's disease, major depression, and Parkinson's disease. *J Neurol Neurosurg Psychiatry*, 53, 915–917.

Wolkowitz, O.M., and Reus, V.I. (1999). Treatment of depression with antiglucocorticoid drugs. *Psychosom Med*, 61(5), 698–711.

Wolkowitz, O.M., Reus, V.I., Weingartner, H., Thompson, K., Breier, A., Doran, A., Rubinow, D., and Pickar, D. (1990). Cognitive effects of corticosteroids. *Am J Psychiatry*, 147(10), 1297–1303.

Wolkowitz, O.M., Reus, V.I., Roberts, E., Manfredi, F., Chan, T., Raum, W.J., Ormiston, S., Johnson, R., Canick, J., Brizendine, L., and Weingartner, H. (1997). Dehydroepiandrosterone (DHEA) treatment of depression. *Biol Psychiatry*, 41(3), 311–318.

Wolkowitz, O.M., Reus, V.I., Keebler, A., Nelson, N., Friedland, M., Brizendine, L., and Roberts, E. (1999). Double-blind treatment of major depression with dehydroepiandrosterone. *Am J Psychiatry*, 156(4), 646–649.

Wong, M.L., Kling, M.A., Munson, P.J., Listwak, S., Licinio, J., Prolo, P., Karp, B., McCutcheon, I.E., Geracioti, T.D. Jr., DeBellis, M.D., Rice, K.C., Goldstein, D.S., Veldhuis, J.D., Chrousos, G.P., Oldfield, E.H., McCann, S.M., and Gold, P.W. (2000). Pronounced and sustained central hypernoradrenergic function in major depression with melancholic features: Relation to hypercortisolism and corticotropin-releasing hormone. *Proc Natl Acad Sci USA*, 97(1), 325–330.

Wood, A.J., Elphick, M., and Grahame-Smith, D.G. (1989). Effect of lithium and of other drugs used in the treatment of manic illness on the cation-transporting properties of Na+,K+-ATPase in mouse brain synaptosomes. *J Neurochem*, 52, 1042–1049.

Wood, K., and Coppen, A. (1983). Prophylactic lithium treatment of patients with affective disorders is associated with decreased platelet [3H]dihydroergocryptine binding. *J Affect Disord*, 5, 253–258.

Woodgett, J.R. (2001). Judging a protein by more than its name: GSK-3. *Sci STKE*, 2001, RE12.

Woodside, B., Zilli, C., and Fisman, S. (1989). Biologic markers and bipolar disease in children. *Can J Psychiatry*, 34, 128–131.

Wright, A.F., Crichton, D.N., Loudon, J.B., Morten, J.E., and Steel, C.M. (1984). Beta-adrenoceptor binding defects in cell lines from families with manic-depressive disorder. *Ann Hum Genet*, 48(Pt. 3), 201–214.

Wyatt, R.J., Portnoy, B., Kupfer, D.J., Snyder, F., and Engelman, K. (1971). Resting plasma catecholamine concentrations in patients with depression and anxiety. *Arch Gen Psychiatry*, 24, 65–70.

Xing, G.Q., Russell, S., Webster, M.J., and Post, R.M. (2004). Decreased expression of mineralocorticoid receptor mRNA in the prefrontal cortex in schizophrenia and bipolar disorder. *Int J Neuropsychopharmacol*, 7(2), 143–153.

Xu, J., Culman, J., Blume, A., Brecht, S., and Gohlke, P. (2003). Chronic treatment with a low dose of lithium protects the brain against ischemic injury by reducing apoptotic death. *Stroke*, 34(5), 1287–1292.

Yamawaki, S., Kagaya, A., Okamoto, Y., Shimizu, M., Nishida, A., and Uchitomi, Y. (1996). Enhanced calcium response to serotonin in platelets from patients with affective disorders. *J Psychiatry Neurosci*, 21, 321–324.

Yan, Q.S., Mishra, P.K., Burger, R.L., Bettendorf, A.F., Jobe, P.C., and Dailey, J.W. (1992). Evidence that carbamazepine and antiepilepsirine may produce a component of their anticonvulsant effects by activating serotonergic neurons in genetically epilepsy-prone rats. *J Pharmacol Exp Ther*, 261, 652–659.

Yang, J.C., and Cortopassi, G.A. (1998). Induction of the mitochondrial permeability transition causes release of the apoptogenic factor cytochrome c. *Free Radic Biol Med*, 24(4), 624–631.

Yatham, L.N. (1996). Prolactin and cortisol responses to fenfluramine challenge in mania. *Biol Psychiatry*, 39(4), 285–288.

Yatham, L.N., Zis, A.P., Lam, R.W., Tam, E., and Shiah, I.S. (1997). Sumatriptan-induced growth hormone release in patients with major depression, mania, and normal controls. *Neuropsychopharmacology*, 17, 258–263.

Yatham, L.N., Liddle, P.F., Shiah, I.S., Scarrow, G., Lam, R.W., Adam, M.J., Zis, A.P., and Ruth, T.J. (2000). Brain serotonin2 receptors in major depression: A positron emission tomography study. *Arch Gen Psychiatry*, 57, 850–858.

Yatham, L.N., Liddle, P.F., Shiah, I.S., Lam, R.W., Ngan, E., Scarrow, G., Imperial, M., Stoessl, J., Sossi, V., and Ruth, T.J. (2002). PET study of [¹⁸F]6-fluoro-L-dopa uptake in neuroleptic- and mood-stabilizer-naive first-episode nonpsychotic mania: Effects of treatment with divalproex sodium. *Am J Psychiatry*, 159, 768–774.

Yehuda, S., Carasso, R.L., and Mostofsky, D.I. (1994). Essential fatty acid preparation (SR-3) raises the seizure threshold in rats. *Eur J Pharmacol*, 254, 193–198.

Yildiz, A., Demopulos, C.M., Moore, C.M., Renshaw, P.F., and Sachs, G.S. (2001). Effect of lithium on phosphoinositide metabolism in human brain: A proton decoupled (31)P magnetic resonance spectroscopy study. *Biol Psychiatry*, 50, 3–7.

Yoon, I.S., Li, P.P., Siu, K.P., Kennedy, J.L., Cooke, R.G., Parikh, S.V., and Warsh, J.J. (2001). Altered *IMPA2* gene expression and calcium homeostasis in bipolar disorder. *Mol Psychiatry*, 6, 678–683.

Young, A.H. (2006) Antiglucocoticoid treatments for depression. *Aust N Z J Psychiatry*, 40(5), 402–405.

Young, A.H., Gallagher, P., Watson, S., Del-Estal, D., Owen, B.M., and Ferrier, I.N. (2004). Improvements in neurocognitive function and mood following adjunctive treatment with mifepristone (RU-486) in bipolar disorder. *Neuropsychopharmacology*, 29(8), 1538–1545.

Young, C.E., Arima, K., Xie, J., Hu, L., Beach, T.G., Falkai, P., and Honer, W.G. (1998). SNAP-25 deficit and hippocampal connectivity in schizophrenia. *Cereb Cortex*, 8(3), 261–268.

Young, E.A., Watson, S.J., Kotun, H., Haskett, R.J., Grunhaus, L., Murphy-Weinberg, V., Vale, W., Rivier, J., and Akil, H. (1990). Beta-lipotropin-beta-endorphin response to low-dose ovine corticotropin releasing factor in endogenous depression. *Arch Gen Psychiatry*, 47(5), 449–457.

Young, E.A., Lopez, J.F., Murphy-Weinberg, V., Watson, S.J., and Akil, H. (2003). Mineralocorticoid receptor function in major depression. *Arch Gen Psychiatry*, 60(1), 24–28.

Young, L.T., and Woods, C.M. (1996). Mood stabilizers have differential effects on endogenous ADP ribosylation in C6 glioma cells. *Eur J Pharmacol*, 309, 215–218.

Young, L.T., Li, P.P., Kish, S.J., Siu, K.P., Kamble, A, Hornykiewicz, O., and Warsh, J.J. (1993). Cerebral cortex Gs alpha protein levels and forskolin-stimulated cyclic AMP formation are increased in bipolar affective disorder. *J Neurochem*, 61, 890–898.

Young, L.T., Li, P.P., Kamble, A., Siu, K.P., and Warsh, J.J. (1994a). Mononuclear leukocyte levels of G proteins in depressed patients with bipolar disorder or major depressive disorder. *Am J Psychiatry*, 151(4), 594–596.

Young, L.T., Li, P.P., Kish, S.J., and Warsh, J.J. (1994b). Cerebral cortex beta-adrenoceptor binding in bipolar affective disorder. *J Affect Disord*, 30, 89–92.

Young, L.T., Warsh, J.J., Kish, S.J., Shannak, K., and Hornykeiwicz, O. (1994c). Reduced brain 5-HT and elevated NE turnover and metabolites in bipolar affective disorder. *Biol Psychiatry*, 35, 121–127.

Young, L.T., Wang, J.F., Woods, C.M., and Robb, J.C. (1999). Platelet protein kinase C alpha levels in drug-free and lithium-treated subjects with bipolar disorder. *Neuropsychobiology*, 40(2), 63–66.

Young, R.C., Moline, M., and Kleyman, F. (1997). Hormone replacement therapy and late-life mania. *Am J Geriatr Psychiatry*, 5, 179–181.

Yuan, P.X., Chen, G., Huang, L.D., and Manji, H.K. (1998). Lithium stimulates gene expression through the AP-1 transcription factor pathway. *Brain Res Mol Brain Res*, 58, 225–230.

Yuan, P.X., Huang, L.D., Jiang, Y.M., Gutkind, J.S., Manji, H.K., and Chen, G. (2001). The mood stabilizer valproic acid activates mitogen-activated protein kinases and promotes neurite growth. *J Biol Chem*, 276, 31674–31683.

Yuan, P.X., Gould, T.D., Gray, N.A., Bachmann, R.F., Schloesser, R.J., Lan, M., Du, J., Moore, G.J., and Manji, H.K. (2004). Neurotrophic signaling cascades are major long-term targets for lithium: Clinical implications. *Clin Neurosci Res*, 4, 137–153.

Yuan, P.X., Zhou, R., Farzad, N., Gould, T.D., Gray, N.A., Du, J., and Manji, H.K. (2005). Enhancing resilience to stress: The role of signaling cascades. In N. Steckler, J.M. Kalin, and H.M. Reul (Eds.), *Handbook on Stress, Immunology and Behaviour*. Amsterdam: Elsevier.

Zach, J., and Ackerman, S.H. (1988). Thyroid function, metabolic regulation, and depression. *Psychosom Med*, 50(5), 454–468.

Zachrisson, O., Mathe, A.A., Stenfors, C., and Lindefors, N. (1995). Limbic effects of repeated electroconvulsive stimulation on neuropeptide Y and somatostatin mRNA expression in the rat brain. *Brain Res Mol Brain Res*, 31, 71–85.

Zachrisson, O., Mathe, A.A., and Lindefors, N. (1996). Effects of chronic lithium and electroconvulsive stimuli on cholecystokinin mRNA expression in the rat brain. *Brain Res Mol Brain Res*, 43, 347–350.

Zanardi, R., Racagni, G., Smeraldi, E., and Perez, J. (1997). Differential effects of lithium on platelet protein phosphorylation in bipolar patients and healthy subjects. *Psychopharmacology (Berl)*, 129(1), 44–47.

Zanardi, R., Serretti, A., Rossini, D., Franchini, L., Cusin, C., Lattuada, E., Dotoli, D., and Smeraldi, E. (2001). Factors affecting fluvoxamine antidepressant activity: Influence of pindolol and 5-HTTLPR in delusional and nondelusional depression. *Biol Psychiatry*, 50, 323–330.

Zarate, C.A. Jr., and Quiroz, J.A. (2003). Combination treatment in bipolar disorder: A review of controlled trials. *Bipolar Disord*, 5(3), 217–225.

Zarate, C.A., Tohen, M., and Zarate, S.B. (1997). Thyroid function tests in first-episode bipolar disorder manic and mixed types. *Biol Psychiatry*, 42(4), 302–304.

Zarate, C.A. Jr., Quiroz J.A., Payne, J.L., and Manji, H.K. (2002). Modulators of the glutamatergic system: Implications for the development of improved therapeutics in mood disorders. *Psychopharmacol Bull*, 36, 35–83.

Zarate, C.A., Du, J., Quiroz, J., Gray, N.A., Denicoff, K.D., Singh, J., Charney, D.S., and Manji, H.K. (2003). Regulation of cellular plasticity cascades in the pathophysiology and treatment of mood disorder: Role of the glutamatergic system. *Ann N Y Acad Sci*, 1003, 273–291.

Zarate, C.A. Jr., Payne, J.L., Quiroz, J., Sporn, J., Denicoff, K.K., Luckenbaugh, D., Charney, D.S., and Manji, H.K. (2004a). An open-label trial of riluzole in patients with treatment-resistant major depression. *Am J Psychiatry*, 161(1), 171–174.

Zarate, C.A., Singh, J., Payne, J.L., Quiroz, J., Denicoff, K., Luckenbaugh, D.A., Charney, D.S., and Manji, H.K. (2004b). A double-blind, randomized, placebo-controlled pilot study examining the efficacy of pramipexole in bipolar II depression. *Biol Psychiatry*, 56, 54–60.

Zarate, C.A. Jr., Payne, J.L., Singh, J., Quiroz, J.A., Luckenbaugh, D.A., Denicoff, K.D., Charney, D.S., and Manji, H.K. (2004c). Pramipexole for bipolar II depression: A placebo-controlled proof of concept study. *Biol Psychiatry*, 56(1), 54–60.

Zarate, C.A., Quiroz, J.A., Singh, J., Denicoff, K., De Jesus, G., Luckenbaugh, D., Charney, D.S., and Manji, H.K. (2005). An open-label trial of the antiglutamatergic agent riluzole in treatment-resistant bipolar depression. *Biol Psychiatry*, 57, 430–432.

Zarate, C.A., Singh, J., Quiroz, J.A., DeJesus, G., Denicoff, K., Luckenbaugh, D.A., Manji, H.K., and Charney, D.S. (2006a). A double-blind, placebo-controlled study of memantine in the treatment of major depression. *Am J Psychiatry*, 163, 153–155.

Zarate, C.A. Jr., Singh, J., and Manji, H.K. (2006b). Cellular plasticity cascades: Targets for the development of novel therapeutics for bipolar disorder. *Biol Psychiatry*, 59(11), 1006–1020.

Zerahn, K. (1955). Studies on the active transport of lithium in the isolated frog skin. *Acta Physiol Scand*, 33, 347–358.

Zhang, L., Elmer, L.W., and Little, K.Y. (1998). Expression and regulation of the human dopamine transporter in a neuronal cell line. *Brain Res Mol Brain Res*, 59, 66–73.

Zhou, J.N., Riemersma, R.F., Unmehopa, U.A., Hoogendijk, W.J., van Heerikhuize, J.J., Hofman, M.A., and Swaab, D.F. (2001). Alterations in arginine vasopressin neurons in the suprachiasmatic nucleus in depression. *Arch Gen Psychiatry*, 58(7), 655–662.

Zhou, L., An, N., Jiang, W., Haydon, R., Cheng, H., Zhou, Q., Breyer, B., Feng, T., and He, T.C. (2002). Fluorescence-based functional assay for Wnt/beta-catenin signaling activity. *Biotechniques*, 33, 1126–1128, 1130, 1132 passim.

Zhou, R., Gray, N., Yuan, P., Li, X., Chen, J.S., Chen, G., Damschroder-Williams, P., Du, J., Zhang, L., and Manji, H.K. (2005). The anti-apoptotic, glucocorticoid receptor cochaperone protein BAG-1 is a long-term target for the actions of mood stabilizers. *J Neurosci*, 25, 4493–4502.

Zhu, G., Okada, M., Murakami, T., Kawata, Y., Kamata, A., and Kaneko, S. (2002). Interaction between carbamazepine, zonisamide and voltage-sensitive Ca2+ channel on acetylcholine release in rat frontal cortex. *Epilepsy Res*, 49, 49–60.

Zigova, T., Willing, A.E., Tedesco, E.M., Borlongan, C.V., Saporta, S., Snable, G.L., and Sanberg, P.R. (1999). Lithium chloride induces the expression of tyrosine hydroxylase in hNT neurons. *Exp Neurol*, 157, 251–258.

Zobel, A.W., Yassouridis, A., Frieboes, R.M., and Holsboer, F. (1999). Prediction of medium-term outcome by cortisol response to the combined dexamethasone-CRH test in patients with remitted depression. *Am J Psychiatry*, 156, 949–951.

Zobel, A.W., Nickel, T., Kunzel, H.E., Ackl, N., Sonntag, A., Ising, M., and Holsboer, F. (2000). Effects of the high-affinity corticotropin-releasing hormone receptor 1 antagonist R121919 in major depression: The first 20 patients treated. *J Psychiatr Res*, 34, 171–181.

Zohar, J., Bannet, J., Drummer, D., Fisch, R., Epstein, R.P., and Belmaker, R.H. (1983). The response of lymphocyte beta-adrenergic receptors to chronic propranolol treatment in depressed patients, schizophrenic patients, and normal controls. *Biol Psychiatry*, 18, 553–560.

Zohar, J., Drummer, D., Edelstein, E.D., Kaiser, N., Belmaker, R.H., and Nir, I. (1985). Effect of lysine vasopressin in depressed patients on mood and 24-hour rhythm of growth hormone, cortisol, melatonin and prolactin. *Psychoneuroendocrinology*, 10, 273–279.

Zubieta, J.K., Huguelet, P., Ohl, L.E., Koeppe, R.A., Kilbourn, M.R., Carr, J.M., Giordani, B.J., and Frey, K.A. (2000). High vesicular monoamine transporter binding in asymptomatic bipolar I disorder: Sex differences and cognitive correlates. *Am J Psychiatry*, 157, 1619–1628.

Zubieta, J.K., Huguelet, P., O'Neil, R.L., and Giordani, B.J. (2001). Cognitive function in euthymic bipolar I disorder. *Psychiatry Res*, 102, 9–20.

Zucker, M., Weizman, A., Harel, D., and Rehavi, M. (2001). Changes in vesicular monoamine transporter (VMAT2) and synaptophysin in rat substantia nigra and prefrontal cortex induced by psychotropic drugs. *Neuropsychobiology*, 44, 187–191.

CHAPTER 15

Abas, M.A., Sahakian, B.J., and Levy, R. (1990). Neuropsychological deficits and CT scan changes in elderly depressives. *Psychol Med*, 20(3), 507–520.

Abercrombie, H.C., Schaefer, S.M., Larson, C.L., Oakes, T.R., Lindgren, K.A., Holden, J.E., Perlman, S.B., Turski, P.A., Krahn, D.D., Benca, R.M., and Davidson, R.J. (1998). Metabolic rate in the right amygdala predicts negative affect in depressed patients. *Neuroreport*, 9(14), 3301–3307.

Abou-Saleh, M.T., Al Suhaili, A.R., Karim, L., Prais, V., and Hamdi, E. (1999). Single photon emission tomography with 99mTc-HMPAO in Arab patients with depression. *J Affect Disord*, 55(2-3), 115–123.

Adler, C.M., Holland, S.K., Schmithorst, V., Wilke, M., Weiss, K.L., Pan, H., and Strakowski, S.M. (2004). Abnormal frontal white matter tracts in bipolar disorder: A diffusion tensor imaging study. *Bipolar Disord*, 6(3), 197–203.

Adler, C.M., Levine, A.D., DelBello, M.P., and Strakowski, S.M. (2005). Changes in gray matter volume in patients with bipolar disorder. *Biol Psychiatry*, 58(2), 151–157.

Adler, C.M., Adams, J., DelBello, M.P., Holland, S.K., Schmithorst, V., Levine, A., Jarvis, K., and Strakowski, S.M. (2006). Evidence of white matter pathology in bipolar disorder adolescents experiencing their first episode of mania: A diffusion tensor imaging study. *Am J Psychiatry*, 163(2), 322–324.

Agam, G., and Shimon, H. (2000). Human evidence of the role of inositol in bipolar disorder and antibipolar treatment. In C.L. Bowden and R.H. Belmaker (Eds.), *Bipolar Medications: Mechanisms of Action* (pp. 31–45). Washington, DC: American Psychiatric Press.

Ahearn, E.P., Steffens, D.C., Cassidy, F., Van Meter, S.A., Provenzale, J.M., Seldin, M.F., Weisler, R.H., and Krishnan, K.R. (1998). Familial leukoencephalopathy in bipolar disorder. *Am J Psychiatry*, 155(11), 1605–1607.

Alexander, G.E., Crutcher, M.D., and DeLong, M.R. (1990). Basal ganglia–thalamocortical circuits: Parallel substrates for motor, oculomotor, prefrontal and limbic functions. *Prog Brain Res*, 85, 119–146.

Alexopoulos, G.S., Young, R.C., and Shindledecker, R.D. (1992). Brain computed tomography findings in geriatric depression and primary degenerative dementia. *Biol Psychiatry*, 31(6), 591–599.

Alexopoulos, G.S., Meyers, B.S., Young, R.C., Kakuma, T., Silbersweig, D., and Charlson, M. (1997). Clinically defined vascular depression. *Am J Psychiatry*, 154(4), 562–565.

Ali, S.O., Denicoff, K.D., Altshuler, L.L., Hauser, P., Li, X., Conrad, A.J., Mirsky, A.F., Smith-Jackson, E.E., and Post, R.M. (2000). A preliminary study of the relation of neuropsychological performance to neuroanatomic structures in bipolar disorder. *Neuropsychiatry Neuropsychol Behav Neurol*, 13(1), 20–28.

al-Mousawi, A.H., Evans, N., Ebmeier, K.P., Roeda, D., Chaloner, F., and Ashcroft, G.W. (1996). Limbic dysfunction in schizophrenia and mania. A study using ^{18}F-labelled fluorodeoxyglucose and positron emission tomography. *Br J Psychiatry*, 169(4), 509–516.

Altshuler, L.L., Devinsky, O., Post, R.M., and Theodore, W. (1990). Depression, anxiety, and temporal lobe epilepsy. Laterality of focus and symptoms. *Arch Neurol*, 47(3), 284–288.

Altshuler, L.L., Conrad, A., Hauser, P., Li, X.M., Guze, B.H., Denikoff, K., Tourtellotte, W., and Post, R. (1991). Reduction of temporal lobe volume in bipolar disorder: A preliminary report of magnetic resonance imaging [letter]. *Arch Gen Psychiatry*, 48(5), 482–483.

Altshuler, L.L., Curran, J.G., Hauser, P., Mintz, J., Denicoff, K., and Post, R. (1995). T$_2$ hyperintensities in bipolar disorder: Magnetic resonance imaging comparison and literature metaanalysis. *Am J Psychiatry*, 152(8), 1139–1144.

Altshuler, L.L., Bartzokis, G., Grieder, T., Curran, J., and Mintz, J. (1998). Amygdala enlargement in bipolar disorder and hippocampal reduction in schizophrenia: An MRI study demonstrating neuroanatomic specificity [letter]. *Arch Gen Psychiatry*, 55(7), 663–664.

Altshuler, L.L., Bartzokis, G., Grieder, T., Curran, J., Jimenez, T., Leight, K., Wilkins, J., Gerner, R., and Mintz, J. (2000). An MRI study of temporal lobe structures in men with bipolar disorder or schizophrenia. *Biol Psychiatry*, 48(2), 147–162.

Amaral, J.A., Lafer, B., et al. (2002). *A H-MRS study of the anterior cingulate gyrus in euthymic bipolar patients taking lithium.* 57th Annual Convention and Scientific Program of the Society of Biological Psychiatry, Philadelphia, PA, May 16–18.

Ames, D., Dolan, R., and Mann, A. (1990). The distinction between depression and dementia in the very old. *Int J Geriatr Psychiatry*, 5, 193–198.

Amsterdam, J.D. and Mozley, P.D. (1992). Temporal lobe asymmetry with iofetamine (IMP) SPECT imaging in patients with major depression. *J Affect Disord*, 24(1), 43–53.

Amsterdam, J.D., Mozley, P.D., et al. (1995). ^{123}I-iofetamine (IMP) SPECT brain imaging in depressed patients: Normalization of temporal lobe asymmetry during clinical recovery. *Depression*, 6(3), 273–283.

Andreasen, N.C., Swayze, V.W. II, Flaum, M., Alliger, R., and Cohen, G. (1990). Ventricular abnormalities in affective disorder: Clinical and demographic correlates. *Am J Psychiatry*, 147(7), 893–900.

Andreason, P.J., Altemus, M., Zametkin, A.J., King, A.C., Lucinio, J., and Cohen, R.M. (1992). Regional cerebral glucose metabolism in bulimia nervosa. *Am J Psychiatry*, 149(11), 1506–1513.

Andreason, P.J., Zametkin, A.J., Guo, A.C., Baldwin, P., and Cohen, R.M. (1994). Gender-related differences in regional cerebral glucose metabolism in normal volunteers. *Psychiatry Res*, 51(2), 175–183.

Anzalone, S.P., Pegues, M., et al. (2002). *Reduced hippocampal volumes in familial bipolar I disorder.* 57th Annual Convention and Scientific Program of the Society of Biological Psychiatry, Philadelphia, PA, May 16–18.

Ashtari, M., Greenwald, B.S., Kramer-Ginsberg, E., Hu, J., Wu, H., Patel, M., Aupperle, P., and Pollack, S. (1999). Hippocampal/amygdala volumes in geriatric depression. *Psychol Med*, 29(3), 629–638.

Auer, D.P., Putz, B., Kraft, E., Lipinski, B., Schill, J., and Holsboer, F. (2000). Reduced glutamate in the anterior cingulate cortex in depression: An in vivo proton magnetic resonance spectroscopy study. *Biol Psychiatry*, 47(4), 305–313.

Austin, M.P., Dougall, N., Ross, M., Murray, C., O'Carroll, R.E., Moffoot, A., Ebmeier, K.P., and Goodwin, G.M. (1992). Single photon emission tomography with ^{99m}Tc-exametazime in major depression and the pattern of brain activity underlying the psychotic/neurotic continuum. *J Affect Disord*, 26(1), 31–43.

Awata, S., Ito, H., Konno, M., Ono, S., Kawashima, R., Fukuda, H., and Sato, M. (1998). Regional cerebral blood flow abnormalities in late-life depression: Relation to refractoriness and chronification. *Psychiatry Clin Neurosci*, 52(1), 97–105.

Axelson, D.A., Doraiswamy, P.M., Boyko, O.B., Rodrigo Escalona, P., McDonald, W.M., Ritchie, J.C., Patterson, L.J., Ellinwood, E.H. Jr., Nemeroff, C.B., and Krishnan, K.R. (1992). In vivo assessment of pituitary volume with magnetic resonance imaging and systematic stereology: Relationship to dexamethasone suppression test results in patients. *Psychiatry Res*, 44(1), 63–70.

Axelson, D.A., Doraiswamy, P.M., McDonald, W.M., Boyko, O.B., Tupler, L.A., Patterson, L.J., Nemeroff, C.B., Ellinwood, E.H. Jr., and Krishnan, K.R. (1993). Hypercortisolemia and hippocampal changes in depression. *Psychiatry Res*, 47(2), 163–173.

Aylward, E.H., Roberts-Twille, J.V., Barta, P.E., Kumar, A.J., Harris, G.J., Geer, M., Peyser, C.E., and Pearlson, G.D. (1994). Basal ganglia volumes and white matter hyperintensities in patients with bipolar disorder. *Am J Psychiatry*, 151(5), 687–693.

Babb, S.M., Ke, Y., Lange, N., Kaufman, M.J., Renshaw, P.F., and Cohen, B.M. (2004). Oral choline increases choline metabolites in human brain. *Psychiatry Res*, 130(1), 1–9.

Baird, A.A., Gruber, S.A., Fein, D.A., Maas, L.C., Steingard, R.J., Renshaw, P.F., Cohen, B.M., and Yurgelun-Todd, D.A. (1999). Functional magnetic resonance imaging of facial affect recognition in children and adolescents. *J Am Acad Child Adolesc Psychiatry*, 38(2), 195–199.

Baker, S.C., Frith, C.D., and Dolan, R.J. (1997). The interaction between mood and cognitive function studied with PET. *Psychol Med*, 27(3), 565–578.

Baron, J.C., Lebrun-Grandie, P., Collard, P., Crouzel, C., Mestelan, G., and Bousser, M.G. (1982). Noninvasive measurement of blood flow, oxygen consumption, and glucose utilization in the same brain regions in man by positron emission tomography: Concise communication. *J Nucl Med*, 23(5), 391–399.

Baron, J.C., Rougemont, D., Soussaline, F., Bustany, P., Crouzel, C., Bousser, M.G., and Comar, D. (1984). Local interrelationships of cerebral oxygen consumption and glucose utilization in normal subjects and in ischemic stroke patients: A positron tomography study. *J Cereb Blood Flow Metab*, 4(2), 140–149.

Bauer, M., London, E.D., Rasgon, N., Berman, S.M., Frye, M.A., Altshuler, L.L., Mandelkern, M.A., Bramen, J., Voytek, B., Woods, R., Mazziotta, J.C., and Whybrow, P.C. (2005). Supraphysiological doses of levothyroxine alter regional cerebral metabolism and improve mood in bipolar depression. *Mol Psychiatry*, 10(5), 456–469.

Baumann, B., Bornschlegl, C., Krell, D., and Bogerts, B. (1997). Changes in CSF spaces differ in endogenous and neurotic depression. A planimetric CT scan study. *J Affect Disord*, 45(3), 179–188.

Baumann, B., Danos, P., Krell, D., Diekmann, S., Leschinger, A., Stauch, R., Wurthmann, C., Bernstein, H.G., and Bogerts, B. (1999). Reduced volume of limbic system–affiliated basal ganglia in mood disorders: Preliminary data from a postmortem study. *J Neuropsychiatry Clin Neurosci*, 11(1), 71–78.

Baxter, L.R., Jr., Phelps, M.E., Mazziotta, J.C., Schwartz, J.M., Gerner, R.H., Selin, C.E., and Sumida, R.M. (1985). Cerebral metabolic rates for glucose in mood disorders. Studies with positron emission tomography and fluorodeoxyglucose F 18. *Arch Gen Psychiatry*, 42(5), 441–447.

Baxter, L.R. Jr., Phelps, M.E., Mazziotta, J.C., Guze, B.H., Schwartz, J.M., and Selin, C.E. (1987a). Local cerebral glucose metabolic rates in obsessive-compulsive disorder. A comparison with rates in unipolar depression and in normal controls. *Arch Gen Psychiatry*, 44(3), 211–218.

Baxter, L.R., Mazziotta, J.C., Phelps, M.E., Selin, C.E., Guze, B.H., and Fairbanks, L. (1987b). Cerebral glucose metabolic rates in normal human females versus normal males. *Psychiatry Res*, 21(3), 237–245.

Baxter, L.R., Jr., Schwartz, J.M., Phelps, M.E., Mazziotta, J.C., Guze, B.H., Selin, C.E., Gerner, R.H., and Sumida, R.M. (1989). Reduction of prefrontal cortex glucose metabolism common to three types of depression. *Arch Gen Psychiatry*, 46(3), 243–250.

Beats, B., Levy, R., and Forstl, H. (1991). Ventricular enlargement and caudate hyperdensity in elderly depressives. *Biol Psychiatry*, 30(5), 452–458.

Beers, C.W. ([1908] 1980). *A Mind That Found Itself*. Pittsburgh: University of Pittsburgh Press.

Bell-McGinty, S., Butters, M.A., Meltzer, C.C., Greer, P.J., Reynolds, C.F. III, and Becker, J.T. (2002). Brain morphometric abnormalities in geriatric depression: Long-term neurobiological effects of illness duration. *Am J Psychiatry*, 159(8), 1424–1427.

Bench, C.J., Friston, K.J., Brown, R.G., Scott, L.C., Frackowiak, R.S., and Dolan, R.J. (1992). The anatomy of melancholia: Focal abnormalities of cerebral blood flow in major depression. *Psychol Med*, 22(3), 607–615.

Bench, C.J., Friston, K.J., Brown, R.G., Frackowiak, R.S., and Dolan, R.J. (1993). Regional cerebral blood flow in depression measured by positron emission tomography: The relationship with clinical dimensions. *Psychol Med*, 23(3), 579–590.

Bench, C.J., Frackowiak, R.S., and Dolan, R.J. (1995). Changes in regional cerebral blood flow on recovery from depression. *Psychol Med*, 25(2), 247–261.

Benes, F.M., Kwok, E.W., Vincent, S.L., and Todtenkopf, M.S. (1998). A reduction of nonpyramidal cells in sector CA2 of schizophrenics and manic depressives. *Biol Psychiatry*, 44(2), 88–97.

Berman, K.F., Doran, A.R., Pickar, D., and Weinberger, D.R. (1993). Is the mechanism of prefrontal hypofunction in depression the same as in schizophrenia? Regional cerebral blood flow during cognitive activation. *Br J Psychiatry*, 162, 183–192.

Berridge, M.J., Downes, C.P., and Hanley, M.R. (1989). Neural and developmental actions of lithium: A unifying hypothesis. *Cell*, 59(3), 411–419.

Bertolino, A., Frye, M., Callicott, J.H., Mattay, V.S., Rakow, R., Shelton-Repella, J., Post, R., and Weinberger, D.R. (2003). Neu-

ronal pathology in the hippocampal area of patients with bipolar disorder: A study with proton magnetic resonance spectroscopic imaging. *Biol Psychiatry*, 53(10), 906–913.

Besson, J.A., Henderson, J.G., Foreman, E.I., and Smith, F.W. (1987). An NMR study of lithium responding manic depressive patients. *Magn Reson Imaging*, 5(4), 273–277.

Beyer, J.L., Kuchibhatla, M., Payne, M.E., Moo-Young, M., Cassidy, F., Macfall, J., and Krishnan, K.R. (2004). Hippocampal volume measurement in older adults with bipolar disorder. *Am J Geriatr Psychiatry*, 12(6), 613–620.

Beyer, J.L., Taylor, W.D., MacFall, J.R., Kuchibhatia, M., Payne, M.E., Provenzale, J.M., Cassidy, F., and Krishnan, K.R. (2005). Cortical white matter microstructural abnormalities in bipolar disorder. *Neuropsychopharmacology*, 30(12), 2225–2229.

Biver, F., Goldman, S., Delvenne, V., Luxen, A., De Maertelaer, V., Hubain, P., Mendlewicz, J., and Lotstra, F. (1994). Frontal and parietal metabolic disturbances in unipolar depression. *Biol Psychiatry*, 36(6), 381–388.

Blair, R.J.R., Morris, J.S., Delvenne, V., Luxen, A., De Maertelaer, V., Hubain, P., Mendlewicz, J., and Lotstra, F. (1999). Dissociable neural responses to facial expressions of sadness and anger. *Brain*, 122(Pt. 5), 883–893.

Blumberg, H.P., Stern, E., Ricketts, S., Martinez, D., de Asis, J., White, T., Epstein, J., Isenberg, N., McBride, P.A., Kemperman, I., Emmerich, S., Dhawan, V., Eidelberg, D., Kocsis, J.H., and Silbersweig, D.A. (1999). Rostral and orbital prefrontal cortex dysfunction in the manic state of bipolar disorder. *Am J Psychiatry*, 156(12), 1986–1988.

Blumberg, H.P., Stern, E., Martinez, D., Ricketts, S., de Asis, J., White, T., Epstein, J., McBride, P.A., Eidelberg, D., Kocsis, J.H., and Silbersweig, D.A. (2000). Increased anterior cingulate and caudate activity in bipolar mania. *Biol Psychiatry*, 48(11), 1045–1052.

Blumberg, H.P., Martin, A., Kaufman, J., Leung, H.C., Skudlarski, P., Lacadie, C., Fulbright, R.K., Gore, J.C., Charney, D.S., Krystal, J.H., and Peterson, B.S. (2003a). Frontostriatal abnormalities in adolescents with bipolar disorder: Preliminary observations from functional MRI. *Am J Psychiatry*, 160(7), 1345–1347.

Blumberg, H.P., Leung, H.C., Skudlarski, P., Lacadie, C.M., Fredericks, C.A., Harris, B.C., Charney, D.S., Gore, J.C., Krystal, J.H., and Peterson, B.S. (2003b). A functional magnetic resonance imaging study of bipolar disorder: State- and trait-related dysfunction in ventral prefrontal cortices. *Arch Gen Psychiatry*, 60(6), 601–609.

Blumberg, H.P., Kaufman, J., Martin, A., Whiteman, R., Zhang, J.H., Gore, J.C., Charney, D.S., Krystal, J.H., and Peterson, B.S. (2003c). Amygdala and hippocampal volumes in adolescents and adults with bipolar disorder. *Arch Gen Psychiatry*, 60(12), 1201–1208.

Blumberg, H.P., Fredericks, C., Wang, F., Kalmar, J.H., Spencer, L., Papademetris, X., Pittman, B., Martin, A., Peterson, B.S., Fulbright, R.K., and Krystal, J.H. (2005). Preliminary evidence for persistent abnormalities in amygdale volumes in adolescents and young adults with bipolar disorder. *Bipolar Disord*, 7(6), 570–576.

Blumberg, H.P., Krystal, J.H., Bansal, R., Martin, A., Dziura, J., Durkin, K., Martin, L., Gerard, E., Charney, D.S., and Peterson, B.S. (2006). Age, rapid-cycling, and pharmacotherapy effects on ventral prefrontal cortex in bipolar disorder: A cross-sectional study. *Biol Psychiatry*, 59(7), 611–618.

Bocksberger, J.P., Young, R.C., et al. (1996). *Basal ganglia morphology in geriatric mania*. 50th Annual Meeting of the Society of Biological Psychiatry, New York, NY, May 1–5.

Bonne, O., Krausz, Y., Gorfine, M., Karger, H., Gelfin, Y., Shapira, B., Chisin, R., and Lerer, B. (1996a). Cerebral hypoperfusion in medication resistant, depressed patients assessed by Tc99m HMPAO SPECT. *J Affect Disord*, 41(3), 163–171.

Bonne, O., Krausz, Y., Shapira, B., Bocher, M., Karger, H., Gorfine, M., Chisin, R., and Lerer, B. (1996b). Increased cerebral blood flow in depressed patients responding to electroconvulsive therapy. *J Nucl Med*, 37(7), 1075–1080.

Boone, K.B., Miller, B.L., Lesser, I.M., Mehringer, C.M., Hill-Gutierrez, E., Goldberg, M.A., and Berman, N.G. (1992). Neuropsychological correlates of white-matter lesions in healthy elderly subjects. A threshold effect. *Arch Neurol*, 49(5), 549–554.

Botteron, K.N., Vannier, M.W., Geller, B., Todd, R.D., and Lee, B.C. (1995). Preliminary study of magnetic resonance imaging characteristics in 8- to 16-year-olds with mania. *J Am Acad Child Adolesc Psychiatry*, 34(6), 742–749.

Botteron, K.N., Raichle, M.E., et al. (1999). *An epidemiological twin study of prefrontal neuromorphometry in early onset depression*. 54th Annual Convention and Scientific Program of the Society of Biological Psychiatry, Washington, DC, May 13–15.

Botteron, K.N., Raichle, M.E., Drevets, W.C., Heath, A.C., and Todd, R.D. (2002). Volumetric reduction in left subgenual prefrontal cortex in early onset depression. *Biol Psychiatry*, 51(4), 342–344.

Bowley, M.P., Drevets, W.C., Ongur, D., and Price, J.L. (2002). Low glial numbers in the amygdala in major depressive disorder. *Biol Psychiatry*, 52(5), 404–412.

Brambilla, P., Harenski, K., Nicoletti, M., Mallinger, A.G., Frank, E., Kupfer, D.J., Keshavan, M.S., and Soares, J.C. (2001a). MRI study of posterior fossa structures and brain ventricles in bipolar patients. *J Psychiatr Res*, 35(6), 313–322.

Brambilla, P., Harenski, K., Nicoletti, M.A., Mallinger, A.G., Frank, E., Kupfer, D.J., Keshavan, M.S., and Soares, J.C. (2001b). Anatomical MRI study of basal ganglia in bipolar disorder patients. *Psychiatry Res*, 106(2), 65–80.

Brambilla, P., Nicoletti, M.A., Harenski, K., Sassi, R.B., Mallinger, A.G., Frank, E., Kupfer, D.J., Keshavan, M.S., and Soares, J.C. (2002). Anatomical MRI study of subgenual prefrontal cortex in bipolar and unipolar subjects. *Neuropsychopharmacology*, 27(5), 792–799.

Brambilla, P., Harenski, K., Nicoletti, M., Sassi, R.B., Mallinger, A.G., Frank, E., Kupfer, D.J., Keshavan, M.S., and Soares, J.C. (2003a). MRI investigation of temporal lobe structures in bipolar patients. *J Psychiatr Res*, 37(4), 287–295.

Brambilla, P., Nicoletti, M.A., Sassi, R.B., Mallinger, A.G., Frank, E., Kupfer, D.J., Keshavan, M.S., and Soares, J.C. (2003b). Magnetic resonance imaging study of corpus callosum abnormalities in patients with bipolar disorder. *Biol Psychiatry*, 54(11), 1294–1297.

Brambilla, P., Nicoletti, M., Sassi, R.B., Mallinger, A.G., Frank, E., Keshavan, M.S., Soares, J.C. (2004). Corpus callosum signal intensity in patients with bipolar and unipolar disorder. *J Neurol Neurosurg Psychiatry*, 75(2), 221–225.

Brambilla, P., Glahn, D.C., Balestrieri, M., and Soares, J.C. (2005). Magnetic resonance findings in bipolar disorder. *Psychiatr Clin North Am*, 28(2), 443–467.

Breiter, H.C., Etcoff, N.L., Whalen, P.J., Kennedy, W.A., Rauch, S.L., Buckner, R.L., Strauss, M.M., Hyman, S.E., and Rosen, B.R. (1996). Response and habituation of the human amygdala during visual processing of facial expression. *Neuron*, 17(5), 875–887.

Bremner, J.D., Innis, R.B., Salomon, R.M., Staib, L.H., Ng, C.K., Miller, H.L., Bronen, R.A., Krystal, J.H., Duncan, J., Rich, D., Price, L.H., Malison, R., Dey, H., Soufer, R., and Charney, D.S. (1997). Positron emission tomography measurement of cerebral metabolic correlates of tryptophan depletion–induced depressive relapse. *Arch Gen Psychiatry*, 54(4), 364–374.

Bremner, J.D., Narayan, M., Anderson, E.R., Staib, L.H., Miller, H.L., and Charney, D.S. (2000). Hippocampal volume reduction in major depression. *Am J Psychiatry*, 157(1), 115–118.

Bremner, J.D., Vythilingam, M., Vermetten, E., Nazeer, A., Adil, J., Khan, S., Staib, L.H., and Charney, D.S. (2002). Reduced volume of orbitofrontal cortex in major depression. *Biol Psychiatry*, 51(4), 273–279.

Bremner, J.D., Vythilingam, M., Ng, C.K., Vermetten, E., Nazeer, A., Oren, D.A., Berman, R.M., and Charney, D.S. (2003). Regional brain metabolic correlates of alpha-methylparatyrosine-induced depressive symptoms: Implications for the neural circuitry of depression. *JAMA*, 289(23), 3125–3134.

Bremner, J.D., Vythilingam, M., Vermetten, E., Vaccarino, V., and Charney, D.S. (2004). Deficits in hippocampal and anterior cingulate functioning during verbal declarative memory encoding in midlife major depression. *Am J Psychiatry*, 161(4), 637–645.

Broca, P. (1878). Anatomie comparée des circonvolutions cérébrales: Le grand lobe limbique et la scissure limbique dans la série des mammifères. [Anatomic considerations of cerebral convolutions: The great limbic lobe and limbic sulci in a series of mammals]. *Rev Anthropol*, 1(Ser. 2), 385–498.

Brody, A.L., Saxena, S., Mandelkern, M.A., Fairbanks, L.A., Ho, M.L., and Baxter, L.R. (2001a). Brain metabolic changes associated with symptom factor improvement in major depressive disorder. *Biol Psychiatry*, 50(3), 171–178.

Brody, A.L., Saxena, S., Stoessel, P., Gillies, L.A., Fairbanks, L.A., Alborzian, S., Phelps, M.E., Huang, S.C., Wu, H.M., Ho, M.L., Ho, M.K., Au, S.C., Maidment, K., and Baxter, L.R. Jr. (2001b). Regional brain metabolic changes in patients with major depression treated with either paroxetine or interpersonal therapy: Preliminary findings. *Arch Gen Psychiatry*, 58(7), 631–640.

Bromfield, E.B., Altshuler, L., Leiderman, D.B., Balish, M., Ketter, T.A., Devinsky, O., Post, R.M., and Theodore, W.H. (1992). Cerebral metabolism and depression in patients with complex partial seizures. *Arch Neurol*, 49(6), 617–623.

Brown, F.W., Lewine, R.J., Hudgins, P.A., and Risch, S.C. (1992). White matter hyperintensity signals in psychiatric and nonpsychiatric subjects. *Am J Psychiatry*, 149(5), 620–625.

Brühn, H., Stoppe, G., et al. (1993). *Quantitative proton MRS in vivo shows cerebral myo-inositol and cholines to be unchanged in manic-depressive patients treated with lithium* [abstract]. Proceedings of the Society of Magnetic Resonance in Medicine, New York, NY, August 14–20.

Bruno, S.D., Barker, G.J., Cercignani, M., Symms, M., and Ron, M.A. (2004). A study of bipolar disorder using magnetization transfer imaging and voxel-based morphometry. *Brain*, 127(Pt. 11), 2433–2440.

Buchsbaum, M.S., Cappelletti, J., Ball, R., Hazlett, E., King, A.C., Johnson, J., Wu, J., and DeLisi, L.E. (1984). Positron emission tomographic image measurement in schizophrenia and affective disorders. *Ann Neurol*, 15(Suppl.), S157–S165.

Buchsbaum, M.S., Wu, J., DeLisi, L.E., Holcomb, H., Kessler, R., Johnson, J., King, A.C., Hazlett, E., Langston, K., and Post, R.M. (1986). Frontal cortex and basal ganglia metabolic rates assessed by positron emission tomography with [^{18}F]2-deoxyglucose in affective illness. *J Affect Disord*, 10(2), 137–152.

Buchsbaum, M.S., Someya, T., and Bunney, W.E. (1997a). Neuroimaging bipolar illness with positron emission tomography and magnetic resonance imaging. *Psychiatr Ann*, 27(7), 489–495.

Buchsbaum, M.S., Wu, J., Siegel, B.V., Hackett, E., Trenary, M., Abel, L., and Reynolds, C. (1997b). Effect of sertraline on regional metabolic rate in patients with affective disorder. *Biol Psychiatry*, 41(1), 15–22.

Caetano, S.C., Sassi, R., Brambilla, P., Harenski, K., Nicoletti, M., Mallinger, A.G., Frank, E., Kupfer, D.J., Keshavan, M.S., and Soares, J.C. (2001). MRI study of thalamic volumes in bipolar and unipolar patients and healthy individuals. *Psychiatry Res*, 108(3), 161–168.

Caine, E.D., and Shoulson, I. (1983). Psychiatric syndromes in Huntington's disease. *Am J Psychiatry*, 140(6), 728–733.

Campbell, S., Marriott, M., Nahmias, C., and MacQueen, G.M. (2004). Lower hippocampal volume in patients suffering from depression: A meta-analysis. *Am J Psychiatry*, 161(4), 598–607.

Caparros-Lefebvre, D., Girard-Buttaz, I., Reboul, S., Lebert, F., Cabaret, M., Verier, A., Steinling, M., Pruvo, J.P., and Petit, H. (1996). Cognitive and psychiatric impairment in herpes simplex virus encephalitis suggest involvement of the amygdalo-frontal pathways. *J Neurol*, 243(3), 248–256.

Carson, A.J., MacHale, S., Allen, K., Lawrie, S.M., Dennis, M., House, A., and Sharpe, M. (2000). Depression after stroke and lesion location: A systematic review. *Lancet*, 356(9224), 122–126.

Castillo, M., Kwock, L., Courvoisie, H., and Hooper, S.R. (2000). Proton MR spectroscopy in children with bipolar affective disorder: Preliminary observations. *AJNR Am J Neuroradiol*, 21(5), 832–838.

Cecil, K.M., DelBello, M.P., Morey, R., and Strakowski, S.M. (2002). Frontal lobe differences in bipolar disorder as determined by proton MR spectroscopy. *Bipolar Disord*, 4(6), 357–365.

Cecil, K.M., DelBello, M.P., Sellars, M.C., and Strakowski, S.M. (2003). Proton magnetic resonance spectroscopy of the frontal lobe and cerebellar vermis in children with a mood disorder and a familial risk for bipolar disorders. *J Child Adolesc Psychopharmacol*, 13(4), 545–555.

Chakos, M.H., Lieberman, J.A., Bilder, R.M., Borenstein, M., Lerner, G., Bogerts, B., Wu, H., Kinon, B., and Ashtari, M. (1994). Increase in caudate nuclei volumes of first-episode schizophrenic patients taking antipsychotic drugs. *Am J Psychiatry*, 151(10), 1430–1436.

Chang, K.D., Blasey, C., Ketter, T.A., and Steiner, H. (2001). Family environment of children and adolescents with bipolar parents. *Bipolar Disord*, 3(2), 73–78.

Chang, K., Adleman, N.E., Dienes, K., Simeonova, D.I., Menon, V., and Reiss, A. (2004). Anomalous prefrontal–subcortical activation in familial pediatric bipolar disorder: A functional magnetic resonance imaging investigation. *Arch Gen Psychiatry*, 61(8), 781–792.

Charles, H.C., Lazeyras, F., Krishnan, K.R., Boyko, O.B., Patterson, L.J., Doraiswamy, P.M., and McDonald, W.M. (1994a). Proton spectroscopy of human brain: Effects of age and sex. *Prog Neuropsychopharmacol Biol Psychiatry*, 18(6), 995–1004.

Charles, H.C., Lazeyras, F., Krishnan, K.R., Boyko, O.B., Payne, M., and Moore, D. (1994b). Brain choline in depression: In vivo detection of potential pharmacodynamic effects of antidepressant therapy using hydrogen localized spectroscopy. *Prog Neuropsychopharmacol Biol Psychiatry*, 18(7), 1121–1127.

Chen, B.K., Sassi, R.. Axelson, D., Hatch, J.P., Sanches, M., Nicoletti, M., Brambilla, P., Keshavan, M.S., Ryan, N.D., Birmaher, B., and Soares, J.C. (2004). Cross-sectional study of abnormal amygdala development in adolescents and young adults with bipolar disorder. *Biol Psychiatry*, 56(6), 399–405.

Choi, S.J., Lim, K.O., et al. (2002). *Differential age-related decline in white matter integrity in late-life depression.* 57th Annual Convention and Scientific Program of the Society of Biological Psychiatry, Philadelphia, PA, May 16–18.

Chugani, H.T., Phelps, M.E., and Mazziotta, J.C. (1987). Positron emission tomography study of human brain functional development. *Ann Neurol*, 22(4), 487–497.

Churchill, C.M., Priolo, C.V., Nemeroff, C.B., Krishnan, K.R.R. (1991). Occult subcortical magnetic resonance findings in elderly depressives. *Int J Geriatr Psychiatry*, 6, 213–216.

Coffey, C.E., Hinkle, P.E., Weiner, R.D., Nemeroff, C.B., Krishnan, K.R., Varia, I., and Sullivan, D.C. (1987). Electroconvulsive therapy of depression in patients with white matter hyperintensity. *Biol Psychiatry*, 22(5), 629–636.

Coffey, C.E., Figiel, G.S., Djang, W.T., Cress, M., Saunders, W.B., and Weiner, R.D. (1988a). Leukoencephalopathy in elderly depressed patients referred for ECT. *Biol Psychiatry*, 24(2), 143–161.

Coffey, C.E., Figiel, G.S., Djang, W.T., Sullivan, D.C., Herfkens, R.J., and Weiner, R.D. (1988b). Effects of ECT on brain structure: A pilot prospective magnetic resonance imaging study. *Am J Psychiatry*, 145(6), 701–706.

Coffey, C.E., Figiel, G.S., Djang, W.T., Saunders, W.B., and Weiner, R.D. (1989). White matter hyperintensity on magnetic resonance imaging: Clinical and neuroanatomic correlates in the depressed elderly. *J Neuropsychiatry Clin Neurosci*, 1(2), 135–144.

Coffey, C.E., Figiel, G.S., Djang, W.T., and Weiner, R.D. (1990). Subcortical hyperintensity on magnetic resonance imaging: A comparison of normal and depressed elderly subjects. *Am J Psychiatry*, 147(2), 187–189.

Coffey, C.E., Weiner, R.D., Djang, W.T., Figiel, G.S., Soady, S.A., Patterson, L.J., Holt, P.D., Spritzer, C.E., and Wilkinson, W.E. (1991). Brain anatomic effects of electroconvulsive therapy. A prospective magnetic resonance imaging study. *Arch Gen Psychiatry*, 48(11), 1013–1021.

Coffey, C.E., Wilkinson, W.E., Parashos, I.A., Soady, S.A., Sullivan, R.J., Patterson, L.J., Figiel, G.S., Webb, M.C., Spritzer, C.E., and Djang, W.T. (1992). Quantitative cerebral anatomy of the aging human brain: A cross-sectional study using magnetic resonance imaging. *Neurology*, 42(3 Pt. 1), 527–536.

Coffey, C.E., Wilkinson, W.E., Weiner, R.D., Parashos, I.A., Djang, W.T., Webb, M.C., Figiel, G.S., and Spritzer, C.E. (1993a). Quantitative cerebral anatomy in depression. A controlled magnetic resonance imaging study. *Arch Gen Psychiatry*, 50(1), 7–16.

Coffey, C.E., Wilkinson, W.E., Weiner, R.D., Ritchie, J.C., and Aque, M. (1993b). The dexamethasone suppression test and quantitative cerebral anatomy in depression. *Biol Psychiatry*, 33(6), 442–449.

Coffey, C.E., Lucke, J.F., Saxton, J.A., Ratcliff, G., Unitas, L.J., Billig, B., and Bryan, R.N. (1998). Sex differences in brain aging:

A quantitative magnetic resonance imaging study. *Arch Neurol*, 55(2), 169–179.

Coffman, J.A., Bornstein, R.A., Olson, S.C., Schwarzkopf, S.B., and Nasrallah, H.A. (1990). Cognitive impairment and cerebral structure by MRI in bipolar disorder. *Biol Psychiatry*, 27(11), 1188–1196.

Cohen, R.M., Semple, W.E., Gross, M., Nordahl, T.E, King, A.C., Pickar, D., and Post, R.M. (1989). Evidence for common alterations in cerebral glucose metabolism in major affective disorders and schizophrenia. *Neuropsychopharmacology*, 2(4), 241–254.

Cohen, R.M., Gross, M., Nordahl, T.E., Semple, W.E., Oren, D.A., and Rosenthal N. (1992). Preliminary data on the metabolic brain pattern of patients with winter seasonal affective disorder. *Arch Gen Psychiatry*, 49(7), 545–552.

Cohen, B.M., Renshaw, P.F., Stoll, A.L., Wurtman, R.J., Yurgelun-Todd, D., and Babb, S.M. (1995). Decreased brain choline uptake in older adults. An in vivo proton magnetic resonance spectroscopy study. *JAMA*, 274(11), 902–907.

Colla, M., Meichel, K., et al. (2002). *Hippocampal volume reduction and hypercortisolemia in major depression*. 57th Annual Convention and Scientific Program of the Society of Biological Psychiatry, Philadelphia, PA, May 16–18.

Conca, A., Fritzsche, H., Peschina, W., Konig, P., Swoboda, E., Wiederin, H., and Haas, C. (2000). Preliminary findings of simultaneous 18F-FDG and 99mTc-HMPAO SPECT in patients with depressive disorders at rest: Differential correlates with ratings of anxiety. *Psychiatry Res*, 98(1), 43–54.

Connor, S.E., Ng, V., McDonald, C., Schulze, K., Morgan, K., Dazzan, P., and Murray, R.M. (2004). A study of hippocampal shape anomaly in schizophrenia and in families multiply affected by schizophrenia or bipolar disorder. *Neuroradiology*, 46(7), 523–534.

Constant, E.L., de Volder, A.G., Ivanoiu, A., Bol, A., Labar, D., Seghers, A., Cosnard, G., Melin, J., and Daumerie, C. (2001). Cerebral blood flow and glucose metabolism in hypothyroidism: A positron emission tomography study. *J Clin Endocrinol Metab*, 86(8), 3864–3870.

Coryell, W. (2005). Rapid cycling bipolar disorder: Clinical characteristics and treatment options. *CNS Drugs*, 19(7), 557–569.

Cowell, P.E., Turetsky, B.I., Gur, R.C., Grossman, R.I., Shtasel, D.L., and Gur, R.E. (1994). Sex differences in aging of the human frontal and temporal lobes. *J Neurosci*, 14(8), 4748–4755.

Curran, S.M., Murray, C.M., Van Beck, M., Dougall, N., O'Carroll, R.E., Austin, M.P., Ebmeier, K.P., and Goodwin, G.M. (1993). A single photon emission computerised tomography study of regional brain function in elderly patients with major depression and with Alzheimer-type dementia. *Br J Psychiatry*, 163, 155–165.

Curtis, V.A., Dixon, T.A., Morris, R.G., Bullmore, E.T., Brammer, M.J., Williams, S.C., Sharma, T., Murray, R.M., and McGuire, P.K. (2001). Differential frontal activation in schizophrenia and bipolar illness during verbal fluency. *J Affect Disord*, 66(2-3), 111–121.

Dager, S.R., Friedman, S.D., Parow, A., Demopulos, C., Stoll, A.L., Lyoo, I.K., Dunner, D.L., and Renshaw, P.F. (2004). Brain metabolic alterations in medication-free patients with bipolar disorder. *Arch Gen Psychiatry*, 61(5), 450–458.

Dahabra, S., Ashton, C.H., Bahrainian, M., Britton, P.G., Ferrier, I.N., McAllister, V.A., Marsh, V.R., and Moore, P.B. (1998). Structural and functional abnormalities in elderly patients clinically recovered from early- and late-onset depression. *Biol Psychiatry*, 44(1), 34–46.

Damasio, A.R., Grabowski, T.J., et al. (1998). Neural correlates of the experience of emotion [abstract 104.1]. *Soc Neurosci Abstr*, 24, 258.

Damasio, A.R., Grabowski, T.J., et al. (1999). *The contribution of subcortical nuclei to the processing of emotion and feeling* [abstract]. 5th International Conference on Functional Mapping of the Human Brain, Düsseldorf, Germany, June 22–26.

Davanzo, P., Thomas, M.A., Yue, K., Oshiro, T., Belin, T., Strober, M., and McCracken, J. (2001). Decreased anterior cingulate myo-inositol/creatine spectroscopy resonance with lithium treatment in children with bipolar disorder. *Neuropsychopharmacology*, 24(4), 359–369.

Davanzo, P., Yue, K., Thomas, M.A., Belin, T., Mintz, J., Venkatraman, T.N., Santoro, E., Barnett, S., and McCracken, J. (2003). Proton magnetic resonance spectroscopy of bipolar disorder versus intermittent explosive disorder in children and adolescents. *Am J Psychiatry*, 160(8), 1442–1452.

Davidson, R.J., Irwin, W., Anderle, M.J., and Kalin, N.H. (2003). The neural substrates of affective processing in depressed patients treated with venlafaxine. *Am J Psychiatry*, 160(1), 64–75.

Dean, B., Scarr, E., Pavey, G., and Copolov, D. (2003). Studies on serotonergic markers in the human hippocampus: Changes in subjects with bipolar disorder. *J Affect Disord*, 75(1), 65–69.

de Asis, J.M., Stern, E., Alexopoulos, G.S., Pan, H., Van Gorp, W., Blumberg, H., Kalayam, B., Eidelberg, D., Kiosses, D., and Silbersweig, D.A. (2001). Hippocampal and anterior cingulate activation deficits in patients with geriatric depression. *Am J Psychiatry*, 158(8), 1321–1323.

DeCarli, C., Murphy, D.G., Tranh, M., Grady, C.L., Haxby, J.V., Gillette, J.A., Salerno, J.A., Gonzales-Aviles, A., Horwitz, B., and Rapoport, S.I. (1995). The effect of white matter hyperintensity volume on brain structure, cognitive performance, and cerebral metabolism of glucose in 51 healthy adults. *Neurology*, 45(11), 2077–2084.

Dechent, P., Pouwels, P.J., and Frahm J. (1999a). Neither short-term nor long-term administration of oral choline alters metabolite concentrations in human brain. *Biol Psychiatry*, 46(3), 406–411.

Dechent, P., Pouwels, P.J., Wilken, B., Hanefeld, F., and Frahm, J. (1999b). Increase of total creatine in human brain after oral supplementation of creatine-monohydrate. *Am J Physiol*, 277(3 Pt. 2), R698–R704.

de Groot, J.C., de Leeuw, F.E., Oudkerk, M., Hofman, A., Jolles, J., and Breteler, M.M. (2000). Cerebral white matter lesions and depressive symptoms in elderly adults. *Arch Gen Psychiatry*, 57(11), 1071–1076.

Deicken, R.F., Reus, V.I., Manfredi, L., and Wolkowitz, O.M. (1991). MRI deep white matter hyperintensity in a psychiatric population. *Biol Psychiatry*, 29(9), 918–922.

Deicken, R.F., Calabrese, G., Merrin, E.L., Fein, G., and Weiner, M.W. (1995a). Basal ganglia phosphorous metabolism in chronic schizophrenia. *Am J Psychiatry*, 152(1), 126–129.

Deicken, R.F., Fein, G., and Weiner, M.W. (1995b). Abnormal frontal lobe phosphorous metabolism in bipolar disorder. *Am J Psychiatry*, 152(6), 915–918.

Deicken, R.F., Eliaz, Y., Feiwell, R., and Schuff, N. (2001). Increased thalamic N-acetylaspartate in male patients with familial bipolar I disorder. *Psychiatry Res*, 106(1), 35–45.

Deicken, R.F., Pegues, M.P., Anzalone, S., Feiwell, R., and Soher, B. (2003a). Lower concentration of hippocampal N-acetylaspartate in familial bipolar I disorder. *Am J Psychiatry*, 160(5), 873–882.

Deicken, R.F., Pegues, M.P., Anzalone, S., Feiwell, R., and Soher, B. (2003b). Lower concentration of hippocampal N-acetylaspartate in familial bipolar I disorder. *Am J Psychiatry*, 160(5), 873–882.

DelBello, M.P., Strakowski, S.M., Zimmerman, M.E., Hawkins, J.M., and Sax, K.W. (1999). MRI analysis of the cerebellum in bipolar disorder: A pilot study. *Neuropsychopharmacology*, 21(1), 63–68.

DelBello, M.P., Zimmerman, M.E., Mills, N.P., Getz, G.E., and Strakowski, S.M. (2004). Magnetic resonance imaging analysis of amygdala and other subcortical brain regions in adolescents with bipolar disorder. *Bipolar Disord*, 6(1), 43–52.

de Leon, M.J., Ferris, S.H., George, A.E., Christman, D.R., Fowler, J.S., Gentes, C., Reisberg, B., Gee, B., Emmerich, M., Yonekura, Y., Brodie, J., Kricheff, I.I., and Wolf, A.P. (1983). Positron emission tomographic studies of aging and Alzheimer disease. *AJNR Am J Neuroradiol*, 4(3), 568–571.

de Leon, M.J., George, A.E., Tomanelli, J., Christman, D., Kluger, A., Miller, J., Ferris, S.H., Fowler, J., Brodie, J.D., and van Gelder, P. (1987). Positron emission tomography studies of normal aging: A replication of PET III and 18-FDG using PET VI and 11-CDG. *Neurobiol Aging*, 8(4), 319–323.

Delvenne, V., Goldman, S., Biver, F., De Maertalaer, V., Wikler, D., Damhaut, P., and Lotstra, F. (1997a). Brain hypometabolism of glucose in low-weight depressed patients and in anorectic patients: A consequence of starvation? *J Affect Disord*, 44(1), 69–77.

Delvenne, V., Goldman, S., De Maertelaer, V., Wikler, D., Damhaut, P., and Lotstra, F. (1997b). Brain glucose metabolism in anorexia nervosa and affective disorders: Influence of weight loss or depressive symptomatology. *Psychiatry Res*, 74(2), 83–92.

Demopulos, C.D., Renshaw, P.F., et al. (1996). *Rapid cycling tended to be associated with low choline in the basal ganglia.* 149th Annual Meeting of the American Psychiatric Association, New York, NY, May 4–9.

Demopulos, C.M., Renshaw, P.F., et al. (1997). *Chronic choline administration does not increase brain choline:creatine.* 150th Annual Meeting of the American Psychiatric Association, San Diego, CA, May 17–22.

Devous, M.D., Husain, M., et al. (2002). *Effects of VNS on regional cerebral blood flow in depressed subjects.* 57th Annual Convention and Scientific Program of the Society of Biological Psychiatry, Philadelphia, PA, May 16–18.

Dewan, M.J., Haldipur, C.V., Lane, E., Donnelly, M.P., Boucher, M., and Major, L.F. (1987). Normal cerebral asymmetry in bipolar patients. *Biol Psychiatry*, 22(9), 1058–1066.

Dewan, M.J., Haldipur, C.V., Boucher, M., and Major, L.F. (1988a). Is CT ventriculomegaly related to hypercortisolemia? *Acta Psychiatr Scand*, 77(2), 230–231.

Dewan, M.J., Haldipur, C.V., Boucher, M.F., Ramachandran, T., and Major, L.F. (1988b). Bipolar affective disorder. II. EEG, neuropsychological, and clinical correlates of CT abnormality. *Acta Psychiatr Scand*, 77(6), 677–682.

Dewan, M.J., Haldipur, C.V., Lane, E.E., Ispahani, A., Boucher, M.F., and Major, L.F. (1988c). Bipolar affective disorder. I. Comprehensive quantitative computed tomography. *Acta Psychiatr Scand*, 77(6), 670–676.

Dickstein, D.P., Garvey, M., Pradella, A.G., Greenstein, D.K., Sharp, W.S., Castellanos, F.X., Pine, D.S., and Leibenluft, E.

(2005). Neurologic examination abnormalities in children with bipolar disorder or attention-deficit/hyperactivity disorder. *Biol Psychiatry*, 58(7), 517–524.

Dieckmann, N.F., Wang, P.W., et al. (2002). *Decreased left frontal lobe gray matter in men with bipolar I disorder.* 155th Annual Meeting of the American Psychiatric Association, Philadelphia, PA, May 18–23.

Direkze, M., Bayliss, S.G., and Cutting, J.C. (1971). Primary tumours of the frontal lobe. *Br J Clin Pract*, 25(5), 207–213.

Dolan, R.J., Calloway, S.P., and Mann, A.H. (1985). Cerebral ventricular size in depressed subjects. *Psychol Med*, 15(4), 873–878.

Dolan, R.J., Calloway, S.P., Thacker, P.F., and Mann, A.H. (1986). The cerebral cortical appearance in depressed subjects. *Psychol Med*, 16(4), 775–779.

Dolan, R.J., Bench, C.J., Brown, R.G., Scott, L.C., Friston, K.J., and Frackowiak, R.S. (1992). Regional cerebral blood flow abnormalities in depressed patients with cognitive impairment. *J Neurol Neurosurg Psychiatry*, 55(9), 768–773.

Dolan, R.J., Bench, C.J., Brown, R.G., Scott, L.C., and Frackowiak, R.S. (1994). Neuropsychological dysfunction in depression: The relationship to regional cerebral blood flow. *Psychol Med*, 24(4), 849–857.

Doris, A., Belton, E., Ebmeier, K.P., Glabus, M.F., and Marshall, I. (2004). Reduction of cingulate gray matter density in poor outcome bipolar illness. *Psychiatry Res*, 130(2), 153–159.

Drevets, W.C. (1999). Prefrontal cortical–amygdalar metabolism in major depression. *Ann NY Acad Sci*, 877, 614–637.

Drevets, W.C. (2000). Neuroimaging studies of mood disorders. *Biol Psychiatry*, 48(8), 813–829.

Drevets, W.C. (2001). Neuroimaging and neuropathological studies of depression: Implications for the cognitive-emotional features of mood disorders. *Curr Opin Neurobiol*, 11(2), 240–249.

Drevets, W.C., and Raichle, M.E. (1992). Neuroanatomical circuits in depression: Implications for treatment mechanisms. *Psychopharmacol Bull*, 28(3), 261–274.

Drevets, W.C., Videen, T.O., Price, J.L., Preskorn, S.H., Carmichael, S.T., and Raichle, M.E. (1992). A functional anatomical study of unipolar depression. *J Neurosci*, 12(9), 3628–3641.

Drevets, W.C., Price, J.L., Videen, T.O., and Todd, R.D. (1995). Metabolic abnormalities in the subgenual prefrontal cortex and ventral striatum in mood disorders. *Soc Neurosci Abstr*, 21(1), 260.

Drevets, W.C., Price, J.L., Simpson, J.R. Jr., Todd, R.D., Reich, T., Vannier, M., and Raichle, M.E. (1997). Subgenual prefrontal cortex abnormalities in mood disorders. *Nature*, 386(6627), 824–827.

Drevets, W.C., Gautier, C., Lowry, T., Bogers, W., and Greer, P. (2001). Abnormal hemodynamic responses to facially expressed emotion in major depression. *Soc Neurosci Abstr*, 31.

Drevets, W.C., Bogers, W., and Raichle, M.E. (2002a). Functional anatomical correlates of antidepressant drug treatment assessed using PET measures of regional glucose metabolism. *Eur J Neuropharmacol*, 12(6), 527–544.

Drevets, W.C., Price, J.L., Bardgett, M.E., Reich, T., Todd, R.D., and Raichle, M.E. (2002b). Glucose metabolism in the amygdala in depression: Relationship to diagnostic subtype and plasma cortisol levels. *Pharmacol Biochem Behav*, 71(3), 431–447.

Drevets, W.C., Thase, M., et al. (2002c). *Glucose metabolic correlates of depression severity and antidepressant treatment response.* 57th Annual Convention and Scientific Program of the Society of Biological Psychiatry, Philadelphia, PA, May 16–18.

Drevets, W.C., Thase, M. et al. (2002d). Antidepressant drug effects on regional glucose metabolism in major depression. *Soc Neurosci Abstr*, 32.

Drevets, W.C., Gadde, K., and Krishnan, R. (2006). Neuroimaging studies of mood disorders. In D.S. Charney and E.J. Nestler (Eds.), *The Neurobiological Foundation of Mental Illness* (Second Edition) (pp. 461–490). New York: Oxford University Press.

Dunn, R.T., Willis, M.W., Benson, B.E., Repella, J.D., Kimbrell, T.A., Ketter, T.A., Speer, A.M., Osuch, E.A., and Post, R.M. (2005). Preliminary findings of uncoupling of flow and metabolism in unipolar compared with bipolar affective illness and normal controls. *Psychiatry Res*, 140(2), 181–198.

Dupont, R.M., Jernigan, T.L., Gillin, J.C., Butters, N., Delis, D.C., and Hesselink, J.R. (1987). Subcortical signal hyperintensities in bipolar patients detected by MRI [letter]. *Psychiatry Res*, 21(4), 357–358.

Dupont, R.M., Jernigan, T.L., Butters, N., Delis, D., Hesselink, J.R., Heindel, W., and Gillin, J.C. (1990). Subcortical abnormalities detected in bipolar affective disorder using magnetic resonance imaging. Clinical and neuropsychological significance. *Arch Gen Psychiatry*, 47(1), 55–59.

Dupont, R.M., Butters, N., Schafer, K., Wilson, T., Hesselink, J., and Gillin, J.C. (1995a). Diagnostic specificity of focal white matter abnormalities in bipolar and unipolar mood disorder. *Biol Psychiatry*, 38(7), 482–486.

Dupont, R.M., Jernigan, T.L., Heindel, W., Butters, N., Shafer, K., Wilson, T., Hesselink, J., and Gillin, J.C. (1995b). Magnetic resonance imaging and mood disorders. Localization of white matter and other subcortical abnormalities. *Arch Gen Psychiatry*, 52(9), 747–755.

Ebert, D., Feistel, H., and Barocka, A. (1991). Effects of sleep deprivation on the limbic system and the frontal lobes in affective disorders: A study with Tc-99m-HMPAO SPECT. *Psychiatry Res*, 40(4), 247–251.

Ebert, D., Feistel, H., Barocka, A., Kaschka, W., and Mokrusch, T. (1993). A test–retest study of cerebral blood flow during somatosensory stimulation in depressed patients with schizophrenia and major depression. *Eur Arch Psychiatry Clin Neurosci*, 242(4), 250–254.

Ebert, D., Feistel, H., Barocka, A., and Kaschka, W. (1994). Increased limbic blood flow and total sleep deprivation in major depression with melancholia. *Psychiatry Res*, 55(2), 101–109.

Ebmeier, K.P., Glabus, M.F., Prentice, N., Ryman, A., and Goodwin, G.M. (1998). A voxel-based analysis of cerebral perfusion in dementia and depression of old age. *Neuroimage*, 7(3), 199–208.

Edmonstone, Y., Austin, M.P., Prentice, N., Dougall, N., Freeman, C.P., Ebmeier, K.P., and Goodwin, G.M. (1994). Uptake of ^{99m}Tc-exametazime shown by single photon emission computerized tomography in obsessive-compulsive disorder compared with major depression and normal controls. *Acta Psychiatr Scand*, 90(4), 298–303.

Elizagarate, E., Cortes, J., Gonzalez Pinto, A., Gutierrez, M., Alonso, I., Alcorta, P., Ramirez, M., de Heredia, J.L., Figuerido, J.L. (2001). Study of the influence of electroconvulsive therapy on the regional cerebral blood flow by HMPAO-SPECT. *J Affect Disord*, 65(1), 55–59.

Elkis, H., Friedman, L., Wise, A., Meltzer, H.Y. (1995). Meta-analyses of studies of ventricular enlargement and cortical sulcal prominence in mood disorders. Comparisons with controls or patients with schizophrenia. *Arch Gen Psychiatry*, 52(9), 735–746.

Elliott, R., Baker, S.C., Rogers, R.D., O'Leary, D.A., Paykel, E.S., Frith, C.D., Dolan, R.J., and Sahakian, B.J. (1997). Prefrontal dysfunction in depressed patients performing a complex planning task: A study using positron emission tomography. *Psychol Med*, 27(4), 931–942.

Elliott, R., Sahakian, B.J., Michael, A., Paykel, E.S., and Dolan, R.J. (1998). Abnormal neural response to feedback on planning and guessing tasks in patients with unipolar depression. *Psychol Med*, 28(3), 559–571.

Ende, G., Braus, D.F., Walter, S., Weber-Fahr, W., and Henn, F.A. (2000a). The hippocampus in patients treated with electroconvulsive therapy: A proton magnetic resonance spectroscopic imaging study. *Arch Gen Psychiatry*, 57(10), 937–943.

Ende, G., Braus, D.F., Walter, S., Weber-Fahr, W., Soher, B., Maudsley, A.A., and Henn, F.A. (2000b). Effects of age, medication, and illness duration on the N-acetyl aspartate signal of the anterior cingulate region in schizophrenia. *Schizophr Res*, 41(3), 389–395.

Epperson, C.N., Haga, K., Mason, G.F., Sellers, E., Gueorguieva, R., Zhang, W., Weiss, E., Rothman, D.L., and Krystal, J.H. (2002). Cortical gamma-aminobutyric acid levels across the menstrual cycle in healthy women and those with premenstrual dysphoric disorder: A proton magnetic resonance spectroscopy study. *Arch Gen Psychiatry*, 59(9), 851–858.

Ernst, M., Zametkin, A.J., Phillips, R.L., and Cohen, R.M. (1998). Age-related changes in brain glucose metabolism in adults with attention-deficit/hyperactivity disorder and control subjects. *J Neuropsychiatry Clin Neurosci*, 10(2), 168–177.

Escalona, P.R., Early, B., McDonald, W.M., and Doraiswamy, P.M. (1993). Reduction of cerebellar volume in major depression: A controlled MRI study. *Depression*, 1, 156–158.

Farchione, T.R., Moore, G.J., and Rosenberg, D.R. (2002). Proton magnetic resonance spectroscopic imaging in pediatric major depression. *Biol Psychiatry*, 52(2), 86–92.

Federoff, J.P., Starkstein, S.E., Forrester, A.W., Geisler, F.H., Jorge, R.E., Arndt, S.V., and Robinson, R.G. (1992). Depression in patients with acute traumatic brain injury. *Am J Psychiatry*, 149(7), 918–923.

Felber, S.R., Pycha, R., Hummer, M., Aichner, F.T., and Fleischhacker, W.W. (1993). Localized proton and phosphorus magnetic resonance spectroscopy following electroconvulsive therapy. *Biol Psychiatry*, 33(8-9), 651–654.

Figiel, G.S., Coffey, C.E., and Weiner, R.D. (1989a). Brain magnetic resonance imaging in elderly depressed patients receiving electroconvulsive therapy. *Convulsive Ther*, 5(1), 26–34.

Figiel, G.S., Krishnan, K.R., Breitner, J.C., and Nemeroff, C.B. (1989b). Radiologic correlates of antidepressant-induced delirium: The possible significance of basal-ganglia lesions. *J Neuropsychiatry Clin Neurosci*, 1(2), 188–190.

Figiel, G.S., Coffey, C.E., Djang, W.T., Hoffman, G. Jr., and Doraiswamy, P.M. (1990a). Brain magnetic resonance imaging findings in ECT-induced delirium. *J Neuropsychiatry Clin Neurosci*, 2(1), 53–58.

Figiel, G.S., Krishnan, K.R., and Doraiswamy, P.M. (1990b). Subcortical structural changes in ECT-induced delirium. *J Geriatr Psychiatry Neurol*, 3(3), 172–176.

Figiel, G.S., Krishnan, K.R., Doraiswamy, P.M., Rao, V.P., Nemeroff, C.B., and Boyko, O.B. (1991a). Subcortical hyperintensities on brain magnetic resonance imaging: A comparison between late age onset and early onset elderly depressed subjects. *Neurobiol Aging*, 12(3), 245–247.

Figiel, G.S., Krishnan, K.R., Rao, V.P., Doraiswamy, M., Ellinwood, E.H. Jr., Nemeroff, C.B., Evans, D., and Boyko, O. (1991b). Subcortical hyperintensities on brain magnetic resonance imaging: A comparison of normal and bipolar subjects. *J Neuropsychiatry Clin Neurosci*, 3(1), 18–22.

Folstein, S.E. and Folstein, M.F. (1983). Psychiatric features of Huntington's disease: Recent approaches and findings. *Psychiatr Dev*, 1(2), 193–205.

Fox, P.T. and Raichle, M.E. (1986). Focal physiological uncoupling of cerebral blood flow and oxidative metabolism during somatosensory stimulation in human subjects. *Proc Natl Acad Sci USA*, 83(4), 1140–1144.

Frazier, J.A., Chiu, S., Breeze, J.L., Makris, N., Lange, N., Kennedy, D.N., Herbert, M.R., Bent, E.K., Koneru, V.K., Dieterich, M.E., Hodge, S.M., Rauch, S.L., Grant, P.E., Cohen, B.M., Seidman, L.J., Caviness, V.S., and Biederman, J. (2005). Structural brain magnetic resonance imaging of limbic and thalamic volumes in pediatric bipolar disorder. *Am J Psychiatry*, 162(7), 1256–1265.

Frey, R., Metzler, D., Fischer, P., Heiden, A., Scharfetter, J., Moser, E., and Kasper, S. (1998). Myo-inositol in depressive and healthy subjects determined by frontal 1H-magnetic resonance spectroscopy at 1.5 tesla. *J Psychiatr Res*, 32(6), 411–420.

Friedman, S.D., Dager, S.R., Parow, A., Hirashima, F., Demopulos, C., Stoll, A.L., Lyoo, I.K., Dunner, D.L., and Renshaw, P.F. (2004). Lithium and valproic acid treatment effects on brain chemistry in bipolar disorder. *Biol Psychiatry*, 56(5), 340–348.

Frodl, T., Meisenzahl, E., Zetzsche, T., Bottlender, R., Born, C., Groll, C., Jager, M., Leinsinger, G., Hahn, K., and Moller, H.J. (2002a). Enlargement of the amygdala in patients with a first episode of major depression. *Biol Psychiatry*, 51(9), 708–714.

Frodl, T., Meisenzahl, E.M., Zetzsche, T., Born, C., Groll, C., Jager, M., Leinsinger, G., Bottlender, R., Hahn, K., and Moller, H.J. (2002b). Hippocampal changes in patients with a first episode of major depression. *Am J Psychiatry*, 159(7), 1112–1118.

Frodl, T., Meisenzahl, E.M., Zetzsche, T., Born, C., Jager, M., Groll, C., Bottlender, R., Leinsinger, G., and Moller, H.J. (2003). Larger amygdala volumes in first depressive episode as compared to recurrent major depression and healthy control subjects. *Biol Psychiatry*, 53(4), 338–344.

Frodl, T., Meisenzahl, E.M., Zetzsche, T., Hohne, T., Banac, S., Schorr, C., Jager, M., Leinsinger, G., Bottlender, R., Reiser, M., and Moller, H.J. (2004). Hippocampal and amygdala changes in patients with major depressive disorder and healthy controls during a 1-year follow-up. *J Clin Psychiatry*, 65(4), 492–499.

Frye, M.A., Bertolino, A., et al. (2000). *A ¹H-MRSI hippocampal study in bipolar patients with a history of alcohol abuse*. 55th Annual Convention and Scientific Program of the Society of Biological Psychiatry, Chicago, IL, May 11–13.

Frye, M.A., Yue, K., et al. (2001). *Decreased basal ganglia n-acetyl-aspartate in mania*. 40th Annual Meeting of the American College of Neuropsychopharmacology, Waikaloa, Hawaii, December 9–13.

Fujikawa, T., Yamawaki, S., and Touhouda, Y. (1993). Incidence of silent cerebral infarction in patients with major depression. *Stroke*, 24(11), 1631–1634.

Fujikawa, T., Yamawaki, S., and Touhouda, Y. (1995). Silent cerebral infarctions in patients with late-onset mania. *Stroke*, 26(6), 946–949.

Fujikawa, T., Yokota, N., Muraoka, M., and Yamawaki, S. (1996). Response of patients with major depression and silent cerebral infarction to antidepressant drug therapy, with emphasis on central nervous system adverse reactions. *Stroke*, 27(11), 2040–2042.

Fujikawa, T., Yanai, I., and Yamawaki, S. (1997). Psychosocial stressors in patients with major depression and silent cerebral infarction. *Stroke*, 28(6), 1123–1125.

Galynker, I.I., Cai, J., Ongseng, F., Finestone, H., Dutta, E., and Serseni, D. (1998). Hypofrontality and negative symptoms in major depressive disorder. *J Nucl Med*, 39(4), 608–612.

Gemar, M.C., Kapur, S., Segal, Z.V., Brown, G.M., and Houle, S. (1996). Effects of self-generated sad mood on regional cerebral activity: A PET study in normal subjects. *Depression*, 4(2), 81–88.

George, M.S., Ketter, T.A., Gill, D.S., Haxby, J.V., Ungerleider, L.G., Herscovitch, P., and Post, R.M. (1993). Brain regions involved in recognizing facial emotion or identity: An oxygen-15 PET study. *J Neuropsychiatry Clin Neurosci*, 5(4), 384–394.

George, M.S., Kellner, C.H., Bernstein, H., and Goust, J.M. (1994). A magnetic resonance imaging investigation into mood disorders in multiple sclerosis. *J Nerv Ment Dis*, 182(7), 410–412.

George, M.S., Ketter, T.A., Parekh, P.I., Herscovitch, P., and Post, R.M. (1995a). Brain activity during transient sadness and happiness in healthy women. *Am J Psychiatry*, 152(3), 341–351.

George, M.S., Kimbrell, T., et al. (1995b). *Actively depressed subjects have difficulty inducing, and blunted limbic rCBF during, transient sadness*. 148th Annual Meeting of the American Psychiatric Association, Miami, FL, May 20–25.

George, M.S., Wassermann, E.M., Williams, W.A., Callahan, A., Ketter, T.A., Basser, P., Hallett, M., and Post, R.M. (1995c). Daily repetitive transcranial magnetic stimulation (rTMS) improves mood in depression. *Neuroreport*, 6(14), 1853–1856.

George, M.S., Ketter, T.A., Parekh, P.I., Herscovitch, P., and Post, R.M. (1996). Gender differences in regional cerebral blood flow during transient self-induced sadness or happiness. *Biol Psychiatry*, 40(9), 859–871.

George, M.S., Ketter, T.A. Parekh, P.I., and Gill, D.S. (1997a). Depressed subjects have decreased rCBF activation during facial emotion recognition. *CNS Spectrums*, 2(10), 45–55.

George, M.S., Ketter, T.A., Parekh, P.I., Rosinsky, N., Ring, H.A., Pazzaglia, P.J., Marangell, L.B., Callahan, A.M., and Post, R.M. (1997b). Blunted left cingulate activation in mood disorder subjects during a response interference task (the Stroop). *J Neuropsychiatry Clin Neurosci*, 9(1), 55–63.

Giedd, J.N., Blumenthal, J., Jeffries, N.O., Castellanos, F.X., Liu, H., Zijdenbos, A., Paus, T., Evans, A.C., and Rapoport, J.L. (1999). Brain development during childhood and adolescence: A longitudinal MRI study. *Nat Neurosci*, 2(10), 861–863.

Ginsberg, M.D., Chang, J.Y., Kelley, R.E., Yoshii, F., Barker, W.W., Ingenito, G., and Boothe, T.E. (1988). Increases in both cerebral glucose utilization and blood flow during execution of a somatosensory task. *Ann Neurol*, 23(2), 152–160.

Gonzalez, R.G., Guimaraes, A.R., Sachs, G.S., Rosenbaum, J.F., Garwood, M., and Renshaw, P.F. (1993). Measurement of human brain lithium in vivo by MR spectroscopy. *AJNR Am J Neuroradiol*, 14(5), 1027–1037.

Goodwin, G.M., Austin, M.P., Dougall, N., Ross, M., Murray, C., O'Carroll, R.E., Moffoot, A., Prentice, N., and Ebmeier, K.P. (1993). State changes in brain activity shown by the uptake of ⁹⁹ᵐTc-exametazime with single photon emission tomography in major depression before and after treatment. *J Affect Disord*, 29(4), 243–253.

Goodwin, G.M., Cavanagh, J.T., Glabus, M.F., Kehoe, R.F., O'Carroll, R.E., and Ebmeier, K.P. (1997). Uptake of ^{99m}Tc-exametazime shown by single photon emission computed tomography before and after lithium withdrawal in bipolar patients: Associations with mania. *Br J Psychiatry*, 170, 426–430.

Goyer, P.F., Schulz, P.M., Semple, W.E., Gross, M., Nordahl, T.E., King, A.C., Wehr, T.A., and Cohen, R.M. (1992). Cerebral glucose metabolism in patients with summer seasonal affective disorder. *Neuropsychopharmacology*, 7(3), 233–240.

Grachev, I.D. and Apkarian, A.V. (2000). Chemical heterogeneity of the living human brain: A proton MR spectroscopy study on the effects of sex, age, and brain region. *Neuroimage*, 11(5 Pt. 1), 554–563.

Grachev, I.D., and Apkarian, A.V. (2001). Aging alters regional multichemical profile of the human brain: An in vivo 1H-MRS study of young versus middle-aged subjects. *J Neurochem*, 76(2), 582–593.

Grasso, M.G., Pantano, P., Ricci, M., Intiso, D.F., Pace, A., Padovani, A., Orzi, F., Pozzilli, C., and Lenzi, G.L. (1994). Mesial temporal cortex hypoperfusion is associated with depression in subcortical stroke. *Stroke*, 25(5), 980–985.

Greenwald, B.S., Kramer-Ginsberg, E., Krishnan, R.R., Ashtari, M., Aupperle, P.M., and Patel, M. (1996). MRI signal hyperintensities in geriatric depression. *Am J Psychiatry*, 153(9), 1212–1215.

Greenwald, B.S., Kramer-Ginsberg, E., Bogerts, B., Ashtari, M., Aupperle, P., Wu, H., Allen, L., Zeman, D., and Patel, M. (1997). Qualitative magnetic resonance imaging findings in geriatric depression. Possible link between later-onset depression and Alzheimer's disease? *Psychol Med*, 27(2), 421–431.

Greenwald, B.S., Kramer-Ginsberg, E., Krishnan, K.R., Ashtari, M., Auerbach, C., and Patel, M. (1998). Neuroanatomic localization of magnetic resonance imaging signal hyperintensities in geriatric depression. *Stroke*, 29(3), 613–617.

Grodd, W., Schneider, F., Klose, U., and Nagele, T. (1995). Functional magnetic resonance tomography of psychological functions exemplified by experimentally induced emotions. *Radiologe*, 35(4), 283–289.

Gruber, S., Frey, R., Mlynarik, V., Stadlbauer, A., Heiden, A., Kasper, S., Kemp, G.J., and Moser, E. (2003). Quantification of metabolic differences in the frontal brain of depressive patients and controls obtained by 1H-MRS at 3 Tesla. *Invest Radiol*, 38(7), 403–408.

Gur, R.E., Skolnick, B.E., Gur, R.C., Caroff, S., Rieger, W., Obrist, W.D., Younkin, D., and Reivich, M. (1984). Brain function in psychiatric disorders. II. Regional cerebral blood flow in medicated unipolar depressives. *Arch Gen Psychiatry*, 41(7), 695–699.

Gur, R.C., Mozley, L.H., Mozley, P.D., Resnick, S.M., Karp, J.S., Alavi, A., Arnold, S.E., and Gur, R.E. (1995). Sex differences in regional cerebral glucose metabolism during a resting state. *Science*, 267(5197), 528–531.

Guze, B.H., and Szuba, M.P. (1992). Leukoencephalopathy and major depression: A preliminary report. *Psychiatry Res*, 45(3), 169–175.

Gyulai, L., Bolinger, L., Leigh, J.S. Jr., Barlow, C., and Chance, B. (1984). Phosphorylethanolamine: The major constituent of the phosphomonoester peak observed by 31P-NMR on developing dog brain. *FEBS Lett*, 178(1), 137–142.

Gyulai, L., Wicklund, S.W., Greenstein, R., Bauer, M.S., Ciccione, P., Whybrow, P.C., Zimmerman, J., Kovachich, G., and Alves, W. (1991). Measurement of tissue lithium concentration by lithium magnetic resonance spectroscopy in patients with bipolar disorder. *Biol Psychiatry*, 29(12), 1161–1170.

Gyulai, L., Alavi, A., Broich, K., Reilley, J., Ball, W.B., and Whybrow, P.C. (1997). I-123 iofetamine single-photon computed emission tomography in rapid cycling bipolar disorder: A clinical study. *Biol Psychiatry*, 41(2), 152–161.

Hagman, J.O., Buchsbaum, M.S., Wu, J.C., Rao, S.J., Reynolds, C.A., and Blinder, B.J. (1990). Comparison of regional brain metabolism in bulimia nervosa and affective disorder assessed with positron emission tomography. *J Affect Disord*, 19(3), 153–162.

Hallcher, L.M., and Sherman, W.R. (1980). The effects of lithium ion and other agents on the activity of myo-inositol-1-phosphatase from bovine brain. *J Biol Chem*, 255(22), 10896–10901.

Hallett, M., Dubinsky, R.M., Zeffiro, T., and Bierner, S.M. (1994). Comparison of glucose metabolism and cerebral blood flow during cortical motor activation. *J Neuroimaging*, 4(1), 1–5.

Hamakawa, H., Kato, T., Murashita, J., and Kato, N. (1998). Quantitative proton magnetic resonance spectroscopy of the basal ganglia in patients with affective disorders. *Eur Arch Psychiatry Clin Neurosci*, 248(1), 53–58.

Hamakawa, H., Kato, T., Shioiri, T., Inubushi, T., and Kato, N. (1999). Quantitative proton magnetic resonance spectroscopy of the bilateral frontal lobes in patients with bipolar disorder. *Psychol Med*, 29(3), 639–644.

Hamidi, M., Drevets, W.C., and Price, J.L. (2004). Glial reduction in amygdala in major depressive disorder is due to oligodendrocytes. *Biol Psychiatry*, 55(6), 563–569.

Harvey, I., Persaud, R., Ron, M.A., Baker, G., and Murray, R.M. (1994). Volumetric MRI measurements in bipolars compared with schizophrenics and healthy controls. *Psychol Med*, 24(3), 689–699.

Hauser, P., Altshuler, L.L., Berrettini, W., Dauphinais, I.D., Gelernter, J., and Post, R.M. (1989a). Temporal lobe measurement in primary affective disorder by magnetic resonance imaging. *J Neuropsychiatry Clin Neurosci*, 1(2), 128–134.

Hauser, P., Dauphinais, I.D., Berrettini, W., DeLisi, L.E., Gelernter, J., and Post, R.M. (1989b). Corpus callosum dimensions measured by magnetic resonance imaging in bipolar affective disorder and schizophrenia. *Biol Psychiatry*, 26(7), 659–668.

Hauser, P., Matochik, J., Altshuler, L.L., Denicoff, K.D., Conrad, A., Li, X., and Post, R.M. (2000). MRI-based measurements of temporal lobe and ventricular structures in patients with bipolar I and bipolar II disorders. *J Affect Disord*, 60(1), 25–32.

Heath, R.G., Franklin, D.E., Walker, C.F., and Keating, J.W. Jr. (1982). Cerebellar vermal atrophy in psychiatric patients. *Biol Psychiatry*, 17(5), 569–583.

Hedges, L.V., and Olkin, I. (1985). *Statistical Methods for Meta-analysis*. Orlando, FL: National Academy Press.

Henry, M.E., Schmidt, M.E., Matochik, J.A., Stoddard, E.P., and Potter, W.Z. (2001). The effects of ECT on brain glucose: A pilot FDG PET study. *J ECT*, 17(1), 33–40.

Hickie, I., Scott, E., Mitchell, P., Wilhelm, K., Austin, M.P., and Bennett, B. (1995). Subcortical hyperintensities on magnetic resonance imaging: Clinical correlates and prognostic significance in patients with severe depression. *Biol Psychiatry*, 37(3), 151–160.

Hickie, I., Scott, E., Wilhelm, K., and Brodaty, H. (1997). Subcortical hyperintensities on magnetic resonance imaging in patients with severe depression: A longitudinal evaluation. *Biol Psychiatry*, 42(5), 367–374.

Hirayasu, Y., Shenton, M.E., Salisbury, D.F., Kwon, J.S., Wible, C.G., Fischer, I.A., Yurgelun-Todd, D., Zarate, C., Kikinis, R., Jolesz, F.A., and McCarley, R.W. (1999). Subgenual cingulate cortex volume in first-episode psychosis. *Am J Psychiatry*, 156(7), 1091–1093.

Hirono, N., Mori, E., Ishii, K., Ikejiri, Y., Imamura, T., Shimomura, T., Hashimoto, M., Yamashita, H., and Sasaki, M. (1998). Frontal lobe hypometabolism and depression in Alzheimer's disease. *Neurology*, 50(2), 380–383.

Ho, A.P., Gillin, J.C., Buchsbaum, M.S., Wu, J.C., Abel, L., and Bunney, W.E. Jr. (1996). Brain glucose metabolism during non-rapid eye movement sleep in major depression. A positron emission tomography study. *Arch Gen Psychiatry*, 53(7), 645–652.

Hoge, E.A., Friedman, L., and Schulz, S.C. (1999). Meta-analysis of brain size in bipolar disorder. *Schizophr Res*, 37(2), 177–181.

Holthoff, V.A., Beuthien-Baumann, B., Pietrzyk, U., Pinkert, J., Oehme, L., Franke, W.G., and Bach, O. (1999). Changes in regional cerebral perfusion in depression: SPECT monitoring of response to treatment. *Nervenarzt*, 70(7), 620–626.

Honer, W.G., Hurwitz, T., Li, D.K., Palmer, M., and Paty, D.W. (1987). Temporal lobe involvement in multiple sclerosis patients with psychiatric disorders. *Arch Neurol*, 44(2), 187–190.

Horn, S. (1974). Some psychological factors in Parkinsonism. *J Neurol Neurosurg Psychiatry*, 37(1), 27–31.

Hornig, M., Mozley, P.D., and Amsterdam, J.D. (1997). HMPAO SPECT brain imaging in treatment-resistant depression. *Prog Neuropsychopharmacol Biol Psychiatry*, 21(7), 1097–1114.

Horska, A., Kaufmann, W.E., Brant, L.J., Naidu, S., Harris, J.C., and Barker, P.B. (2002). In vivo quantitative proton MRSI study of brain development from childhood to adolescence. *J Magn Reson Imaging*, 15(2), 137–143.

Howard, R.J., Beats, B., et al. (1993). White matter changes in late onset depression: A magnetic resonance imaging study [letter]. *Int J Geriat Psychiatry*, 8, 183–185.

Howard, R., Cox, T., Almeida, O., Mullen, R., Graves, P., Reveley, A., and Levy, R. (1995). White matter signal hyperintensities in the brains of patients with late paraphrenia and the normal, community-living elderly. *Biol Psychiatry*, 38(2), 86–91.

Hsieh, M.H., McQuoid, D.R., Levy, R.M., Payne, M.E., MacFall, J.R., and Steffens, D.C. (2002). Hippocampal volume and antidepressant response in geriatric depression. *Int J Geriatr Psychiatry*, 17(6), 519–525.

Hurwitz, T.A., Clark, C., Murphy, E., Klonoff, H., Martin, W.R., and Pate, B.D. (1990). Regional cerebral glucose metabolism in major depressive disorder. *Can J Psychiatry*, 35(8), 684–688.

Husain, M.M., McDonald, W.M., Doraiswamy, P.M., Figiel, G.S., Na, C., Escalona, P.R., Boyko, O.B., Nemeroff, C.B., and Krishnan, K.R. (1991). A magnetic resonance imaging study of putamen nuclei in major depression. *Psychiatry Res*, 40(2), 95–99.

Iacono, W.G., Smith, G.N., Moreau, M., Beiser, M., Fleming, J.A., Lin, T.Y., and Flak, B. (1988). Ventricular and sulcal size at the onset of psychosis. *Am J Psychiatry*, 145(7), 820–824.

Iidaka, T., Nakajima, T., Kawamoto, K., Fukuda, H., Suzuki, Y., Maehara, T., and Shiraishi, H. (1996). Signal hyperintensities on brain magnetic resonance imaging in elderly depressed patients. *Eur Neurol*, 36(5), 293–299.

Iidaka, T., Nakajima, T., Suzuki, Y., Okazaki, A., Maehara, T., and Shiraishi, H. (1997). Quantitative regional cerebral flow measured by Tc-99M HMPAO SPECT in mood disorder. *Psychiatry Res*, 68(2-3), 143–154.

Irwin, W., Davidson, R.J., Lowe, M.J., Mock, B.J., Sorenson, J.A., and Turski, P.A. (1996). Human amygdala activation detected with echo-planar functional magnetic resonance imaging. *Neuroreport*, 7(11), 1765–1769.

Ito, H., Kawashima, R., Awata, S., Ono, S., Sato, K., Goto, R., Koyama, M., Sato, M., and Fukuda, H. (1996). Hypoperfusion in the limbic system and prefrontal cortex in depression: SPECT with anatomic standardization technique. *J Nucl Med*, 37(3), 410–414.

Jacoby, R.J., and Levy, R. (1980). Computed tomography in the elderly. 3. Affective disorder. *Br J Psychiatry*, 136, 270–275.

Jacoby, R.J., Levy, R., and Bird, J.M. (1981). Computed tomography and the outcome of affective disorder: A follow-up study of elderly patients. *Br J Psychiatry*, 139, 288–292.

Janowsky, D.S., el-Yousef, M.K., Davis, J.M, and Sekerke, H.J. (1972). A cholinergic-adrenergic hypothesis of mania and depression. *Lancet*, 2(778), 632–635.

Janssen, J., Hulshoff Pol, H.E., Lampe, I.K., Schnack, H.G., de Leeuw, F.E., Kahn, R.S., and Heeren, T.J. (2004). Hippocampal changes and white matter lesions in early-onset depression. *Biol Psychiatry*, 56(11), 825–831.

Jenkins, M., Malloy, P., Salloway, S., Cohen, R., Rogg, J., Tung, G., Kohn, R., Westlake, R., Johnson, E.G., and Richardson, E. (1998). Memory processes in depressed geriatric patients with and without subcortical hyperintensities on MRI. *J Neuroimaging*, 8(1), 20–26.

Jensen, H.V., Plenge, P., Stensgaard, A., Mellerup, E.T., Thomsen, C., Aggernaes, H., and Henriksen, O. (1996). Twelve-hour brain lithium concentration in lithium maintenance treatment of manic-depressive disorder: Daily versus alternate-day dosing schedule. *Psychopharmacology (Berl)*, 124(3), 275–278.

Jernigan, T.L., Press, G.A., and Hesselink, J.R. (1990). Methods for measuring brain morphologic features on magnetic resonance images: Validation and normal aging. *Arch Neurol*, 47(1), 27–32.

Jernigan, T.L., Archibald, S.L., Berhow, M.T., Sowell, E.R., Foster, D.S., and Hesselink, J.R. (1991). Cerebral structure on MRI, Part I: Localization of age-related changes. *Biol Psychiatry*, 29(1), 55–67.

Jeste, D.V., Lohr, J.B., and Goodwin, F.K. (1988). Neuroanatomical studies of major affective disorders. A review and suggestions for further research. *Br J Psychiatry*, 153, 444–459.

Johnstone, E.C., Owens, D.G., Crow, T.J., Colter, N., Lawton, C.A., Jagoe, R., and Kreel, L. (1986). Hypothyroidism as a correlate of lateral ventricular enlargement in manic-depressive and neurotic illness. *Br J Psychiatry*, 148, 317–321.

Johnstone, E.C., Owens, D.G., Crow, T.J., Frith, C.D., Alexandropolis, K., Bydder, G., and Colter, N. (1989). Temporal lobe structure as determined by nuclear magnetic resonance in schizophrenia and bipolar affective disorder. *J Neurol Neurosurg Psychiatry*, 52(6), 736–741.

Jorge, R.E., Robinson, R.G., Starkstein, S.E., Arndt, S.V., Forrester, A.W., and Geisler, F.H. (1993). Secondary mania following traumatic brain injury. *Am J Psychiatry*, 150(6), 916–921.

Jung, R.E., Yeo, R.A., Love, T.M., Petropoulos, H., Sibbitt, W.L. Jr., and Brooks, W.M. (2002). Biochemical markers of mood: A proton magnetic resonance spectroscopy study of normal human brain. *Biol Psychiatry*, 51(3), 224–229.

Kanakaratnam, G., and Direkze, M. (1976). Aspects of primary tumours of the frontal lobe. *Br J Clin Pract*, 30(11–12), 220–221.

Kanaya, T., and Yonekawa, M. (1990). Regional cerebral blood flow in depression. *Jpn J Psychiatry Neurol*, 44(3), 571–576.

Kato, T., Shioiri, T., Takahashi, S., and Inubushi, T. (1991). Measurement of brain phosphoinositide metabolism in bipolar patients using in vivo ^{31}P-MRS. *J Affect Disord*, 22(4), 185–190.

Kato, T., Takahashi, S., and Inubushi, T. (1992a). Brain lithium concentration by ^{7}Li- and ^{1}H-magnetic resonance spectroscopy in bipolar disorder. *Psychiatry Res*, 45(1), 53–63.

Kato, T., Takahashi, S., Shioiri, T., and Inubushi T. (1992b). Brain phosphorous metabolism in depressive disorders detected by phosphorus-31 magnetic resonance spectroscopy. *J Affect Disord*, 26(4), 223–230.

Kato, T., Shioiri, T., Inubushi, T., and Takahashi, S. (1993a). Brain lithium concentrations measured with lithium-7 magnetic resonance spectroscopy in patients with affective disorders: Relationship to erythrocyte and serum concentrations. *Biol Psychiatry*, 33(3), 147–152.

Kato, T., Takahashi, S., Shioiri, T., and Inubushi, T. (1993b). Alterations in brain phosphorous metabolism in bipolar disorder detected by in vivo ^{31}P and ^{7}Li magnetic resonance spectroscopy. *J Affect Disord*, 27(1), 53–59.

Kato, T., Inubushi, T., and Takahashi, S. (1994a). Relationship of lithium concentrations in the brain measured by lithium-7 magnetic resonance spectroscopy to treatment response in mania. *J Clin Psychopharmacol*, 14(5), 330–335.

Kato, T., Shioiri, T., Murashita, J., Hamakawa, H., Inubushi, T., and Takahashi, S. (1994b). Phosphorus-31 magnetic resonance spectroscopy and ventricular enlargement in bipolar disorder. *Psychiatry Res*, 55(1), 41–50.

Kato, T., Takahashi, S., Shioiri, T., Murashita, J., Hamakawa, H., and Inubushi, T. (1994c). Reduction of brain phosphocreatine in bipolar II disorder detected by phosphorus-31 magnetic resonance spectroscopy. *J Affect Disord*, 31(2), 125–133.

Kato, T., Shioiri, T., Murashita, J., Hamakawa, H., Inubushi, T., and Takahashi, S. (1995a). Lateralized abnormality of high-energy phosphate and bilateral reduction of phosphomonoester measured by phosphorus-31 magnetic resonance spectroscopy of the frontal lobes in schizophrenia. *Psychiatry Res*, 61(3), 151–160.

Kato, T., Shioiri, T., Murashita, J., Hamakawa, H., Takahashi, Y., Inubushi, T., and Takahashi, S. (1995b). Lateralized abnormality of high energy phosphate metabolism in the frontal lobes of patients with bipolar disorder detected by phase-encoded ^{31}P-MRS. *Psychol Med*, 25(3), 557–566.

Kato, T., Fujii, K., Shioiri, T., Inubushi, T., and Takahashi, S. (1996a). Lithium side effects in relation to brain lithium concentration measured by lithium-7 magnetic resonance spectroscopy. *Prog Neuropsychopharmacol Biol Psychiatry*, 20(1), 87–97.

Kato, T., Hamakawa, H., Shioiri, T., Murashita, J., Takahashi, Y., Takahashi, S., and Inubushi, T. (1996b). Choline-containing compounds detected by proton magnetic resonance spectroscopy in the basal ganglia in bipolar disorder. *J Psychiatry Neurosci*, 21(4), 248–254.

Kato, T., Murashita, J., Kamiya, A., Shioiri, T., Kato, N., and Inubushi, T. (1998). Decreased brain intracellular pH measured by 31P-MRS in bipolar disorder: A confirmation in drug-free patients and correlation with white matter hyperintensity. *Eur Arch Psychiatry Clin Neurosci*, 248(6), 301–306.

Kaufman, M.J., Henry, M.E., Frederick, B.D., Hennen, J., Villafuerte, R.A., Stoddard, E.P., Schmidt, M.E., Cohen, B.M., and Renshaw, P.F. (2003). Selective serotonin reuptake inhibitor discontinuation syndrome is associated with a rostral anterior cingulate choline metabolite decrease: A proton magnetic resonance spectroscopic imaging study. *Biol Psychiatry*, 54(5), 534–553.

Kaur, S., Sassi, R.B., Axelson, D., Nicoletti, M., Brambilla, P., Monkul, E.S., Hatch, J.P., Keshavan, M.S., Ryan, N., Birmaher, B., and Soares, J.C. (2005). Cingulate cortex anatomical abnormalities in children and adolescents with bipolar disorder. *Am J Psychiatry*, 162(9), 1637–1643.

Kegeles, L.S., Malone, K.M., Slifstein, M., Ellis, S.P., Xanthopoulos, E., Keilp, J.G., Campbell, C., Oquendo, M., Van Heertum, R.L., and Mann, J.J. (2003). Response of cortical metabolic deficits to serotonergic challenge in familial mood disorders. *Am J Psychiatry*, 160(1), 76–82.

Kellner, C.H., Rubinow, D.R., Gold, P.W., and Post, R.M. (1983). Relationship of cortisol hypersecretion to brain CT scan alterations in depressed patients. *Psychiatry Res*, 8(3), 191–197.

Kellner, C.H., Rubinow, D.R., and Post, R.M. (1986). Cerebral ventricular size and cognitive impairment in depression. *J Affect Disord*, 10(3), 215–219.

Kemmerer, M., Nasrallah, H.A., et al. (1994). *Increased hippocampal volume in bipolar disorder* [abstract]. 49th Annual Meeting of the Society of Biological Psychiatry, Philadelphia, PA, May 18–22.

Kennedy, S.H., Evans, K.R., Kruger, S., Mayberg, H.S., Meyer, J.H., McCann, S., Arifuzzman, A.I., Houle, S., and Vaccarino, F.J. (2001). Changes in regional brain glucose metabolism measured with positron emission tomography after paroxetine treatment of major depression. *Am J Psychiatry*, 158(6), 899–905.

Keshavan, M.S., Pettegrew, J.W., et al. (1992). Membrane phospholipids and lithium response in schizophrenia: A ^{31}P-MRS study. Abstract VIII.B.1. *Schizophr Res*, 6, 134.

Ketter, T.A., and Drevets, W.C. (2002). Neuroimaging studies of bipolar depression: Functional neuropathology, treatment effects, and predictors of clinical response. *Clin Neurosci Res*, 2(3-4), 182–192.

Ketter, T.A., and Wang, P.W. (2002). Predictors of treatment response in bipolar disorders: Evidence from clinical and brain imaging studies. *J Clin Psychiatry*, 63(Suppl. 3), 21–25.

Ketter, T.A., and Wang, P.W. (2003). The emerging differential roles of GABAergic and antiglutamatergic agents in bipolar disorders. *J Clin Psychiatry*, 64(Suppl. 3), 15–20.

Ketter, T.A., Andreason, P.J., et al. (1993). *Blunted CBF response to procaine in mood disorders*. 146th Annual Meeting of the American Psychiatric Association, San Francisco, CA, May 22–27.

Ketter, T.A., Andreason, P.J., George, M.S., Lee, C., Gill, D.S., Parekh, P.I., Willis, M.W., Herscovitch, P., and Post, R.M. (1996a). Anterior paralimbic mediation of procaine-induced emotional and psychosensory experiences. *Arch Gen Psychiatry*, 53(1)59–69.

Ketter, T.A., George, M.S., Kimbrell, T.A., and Benson, B.E. (1996b). Functional brain imaging, limbic function, and affective disorders. *Neuroscientist*, 2(1), 55–65.

Ketter, T.A., Winsberg, M.E., et al. (1997). *Amygdalar metabolism decreases with thirty minute self-induction of depressed mood by recalling sad memories*. 36th Annual Meeting of the American College of Neuropsychopharmacology, Waikoloa, HI, December 8–12.

Ketter, T.A., Kimbrell, T.A., George, M.S., Willis, M.W., Benson, B.E., Danielson, A., Frye, M.A., Herscovitch, P., and Post, R.M. (1999). Baseline cerebral hypermetabolism associated with carbamazepine response, and hypometabolism with nimodipine response in mood disorders. *Biol Psychiatry*, 46(10), 1364–1374.

Ketter, T.A., Wang, P.W., et al. (2000). *Baseline hypofrontality and divalproex response in bipolar disorders*. 55th Annual Convention and Scientific Program of the Society of Biological Psychiatry, Chicago, IL, May 11–13.

Ketter, T.A., Kimbrell, T.A., George, M.S., Dunn, R.T., Speer, A.M., Benson, B.E., Willis, M.W., Danielson, A., Frye, M.A., Herscovitch, P., and Post, R.M. (2001). Effects of mood and subtype on cerebral glucose metabolism in treatment-refractory bipolar disorders. *Biol Psychiatry*, 49(2), 97–109.

Ketter, T.A., Wang, P.W., et al. (2002). Brain anatomic circuits and the pathophysiology of affective disorders. In J.C. Soares (Ed.), *Brain Imaging in Affective Disorders* (pp. 79–118). New York: Marcel Dekker.

Ketter, T.A., Wang, P.W., Becker, O.V., Nowakowska, C., and Yang, Y. (2003). The diverse roles of anticonvulsants in bipolar disorders. *Ann Clin Psychiatry*, 15(2), 95–108.

Ketter, T.A., Wang, P.W., Becker, O.V., Nowakowska, C., and Yang, Y. (2004). Psychotic bipolar disorders: Dimensionally similar to or categorically different from schizophrenia? *J Psychiatry Res*, 38(1), 47–61.

Kimbrell, T.A., Little, J.T., Dunn, R.T., Frye, M.A., Greenberg, B.D., Wassermann, E.M., Repella, J.D., Danielson, A.L., Willis, M.W., Benson, B.E., Speer, A.M., Osuch, E., George, M.S., and Post, R.M. (1999). Frequency dependence of antidepressant response to left prefrontal repetitive transcranial magnetic stimulation (rTMS) as a function of baseline cerebral glucose metabolism. *Biol Psychiatry*, 46(12), 1603–1613.

Kimbrell, T.A., Ketter, T.A., George, M.S., Little, J.T., Benson, B.E., Willis, M.W., Herscovitch, P., and Post, R.M. (2002). Regional cerebral glucose utilization in patients with a range of severities of unipolar depression. *Biol Psychiatry*, 51(3), 237–252.

Kishimoto, H., Takazu, O., Ohno, S., Yamaguchi, T., Fujita, H., Kuwahara, H., Ishii, T., Matsushita, M., Yokoi, S., and Iio, M. (1987). ^{11}C-glucose metabolism in manic and depressed patients. *Psychiatry Res*, 22(1), 81–88.

Kling, A.S., Metter, E.J., Riege, W.H., and Kuhl, D.E. (1986). Comparison of PET measurement of local brain glucose metabolism and CAT measurement of brain atrophy in chronic schizophrenia and depression. *Am J Psychiatry*, 143(2), 175–180.

Kolbeinsson, H., Arnaldsson, O.S., Petursson, H., and Skulason, S. (1986). Computed tomographic scans in ECT-patients. *Acta Psychiatr Scand*, 73(1), 28–32.

Komoroski, R.A., Newton, J.E., Walker, E., Cardwell, D., Jagannathan, N.R., Ramaprasad, S., and Sprigg, J. (1990). In vivo NMR spectroscopy of lithium-7 in humans. *Magn Reson Med*, 15(3), 347–356.

Komoroski, R.A., Newton, J.E., Sprigg, J.R., Cardwell, D., Mohanakrishnan, P., and Karson, C.N. (1993). In vivo ^{7}Li nuclear magnetic resonance study of lithium pharmacokinetics and chemical shift imaging in psychiatric patients. *Psychiatry Res*, 50(2), 67–76.

Kowatch, R.A., Devous, M.D. Sr., Harvey, D.C., Mayes, T.L., Trivedi, M.H., Emslie, G.J., and Weinberg, W.A. (1999). A SPECT HMPAO study of regional cerebral blood flow in depressed adolescents and normal controls. *Prog Neuropsychopharmacol Biol Psychiatry*, 23(4), 643–656.

Krabbendam, L., Honig, A., Wiersma, J., Vuurman, E.F., Hofman, P.A., Derix, M.M., Nolen, W.A., and Jolles, J. (2000). Cognitive dysfunctions and white matter lesions in patients with bipolar disorder in remission. *Acta Psychiatr Scand*, 101(4), 274–280.

Kramer-Ginsberg, E., Greenwald, B.S., Krishnan, K.R., Christiansen, B., Hu, J., Ashtari, M., Patel, M., and Pollack, S. (1999). Neuropsychological functioning and MRI signal hyperintensities in geriatric depression. *Am J Psychiatry*, 156(3), 438–444.

Krishnan, K.R. (1993). Neuroanatomic substrates of depression in the elderly. *J Geriatr Psychiatry Neurol*, 6(1), 39–58.

Krishnan, K.R., Goli, V., Ellinwood, E.H., France, R.D., Blazer, D.G., and Nemeroff, C.B. (1988). Leukoencephalopathy in patients diagnosed as major depressive. *Biol Psychiatry*, 23(5), 519–522.

Krishnan, K.R., Doraiswamy, P.M., Lurie, S.N., Figiel, G.S., Husain, M.M., Boyko, O.B., Ellinwood, E.H. Jr., and Nemeroff, C.B. (1991). Pituitary size in depression. *J Clin Endocrinol Metab*, 72(2), 256–259.

Krishnan, K.R., McDonald, W.M., Escalona, P.R., Doraiswamy, P.M., Na, C., Husain, M.M., Figiel, G.S., Boyko, O.B., Ellinwood, E.H., and Nemeroff, C.B. (1992). Magnetic resonance imaging of the caudate nuclei in depression. Preliminary observations. *Arch Gen Psychiatry*, 49(7), 553–557.

Krishnan, K.R., McDonald, W.M., Doraiswamy, P.M., Tupler, L.A., Husain, M., Boyko, O.B., Figiel, G.S., and Ellinwood, E.H. Jr. (1993). Neuroanatomical substrates of depression in the elderly. *Eur Arch Psychiatry Clin Neurosci*, 243(1), 41–46.

Krishnan, K.R., Hays, J.C., and Blazer, D.G. (1997). MRI-defined vascular depression. *Am J Psychiatry*, 154(4), 497–501.

Kronhaus, D.M., Lawrence, N.S., Williams, A.M., Frangou, S., Brammer, M.J., Williams, S.C.R., Andrew, C.M., and Phillips, M.L. (2006). Stroop performance in bipolar disorder: Further evidence for abnormalities in the ventral prefrontal cortex. *Bipolar Disord*, 8, 28–39.

Krüger, S., Seminowicz, D., Goldapple, K., Kennedy, S.H., and Mayberg, H.S. (2003). State and trait influences on mood regulation in bipolar disorder: Blood flow differences with an acute mood challenge. *Biol Psychiatry*, 54(11), 1274–1283.

Krüger, S., Braunig, P., and Grunze, H. (2006). Official guidelines for the treatment of acute mania. *Psychiatr Prax*, 33(Suppl. 1), S2–S6.

Kuhl, D.E., Metter, E.J., Riege, W.H., and Phelps, M.E. (1982). Effects of human aging on patterns of local cerebral glucose utilization determined by the [18F]fluorodeoxyglucose method. *J Cereb Blood Flow Metab*, 2(2), 163–71.

Kuhl, D.E., Metter, E.J., et al. (1985). Patterns of cerebral glucose utilization in depression, multiple infarct dementia, and Alzheimer's disease. In L. Sokoloff (Ed.), *Brain Imaging and Brain Function* (pp. 211–226). New York: Raven Press.

Kumar, A., Mozley, D., et al. (1991). Semiquantitative I-123 IMP SPECT studies in late onset depression before and after treatment. *Int J Geriatr Psychiatry*, 6, 775–777.

Kumar, A., Newberg, A., Alavi, A., Berlin, J., Smith, R., and Reivich, M. (1993). Regional cerebral glucose metabolism in late-life depression and Alzheimer disease: A preliminary positron emission tomography study. *Proc Natl Acad Sci USA*, 90(15), 7019–7023.

Kumar, A., Miller, D.S., et al. (1996). *Focal anatomic substrates in late-life depression*. 149th Annual Meeting of the American Psychiatric Association, New York, NY, May 4–9.

Kumar, A., Schweizer, E., Jin, Z., Miller, D., Bilker, W., Swan, L.L., and Gottlieb, G. (1997). Neuroanatomical substrates of late-life minor depression. A quantitative magnetic resonance imaging study. *Arch Neurol*, 54(5), 613–617.

Kumar, A., Jin, Z., Bilker, W., Udupa, J., and Gottlieb, G. (1998). Late-onset minor and major depression: Early evidence for common neuroanatomical substrates detected by using MRI. *Proc Natl Acad Sci USA*, 95(13), 7654–7658.

Kumar, A., Bilker, W., Jin, Z., Udupa, J., and Gottlieb, G. (1999). Age of onset of depression and quantitative neuroanatomic measures: Absence of specific correlates. *Psychiatry Res*, 91(2), 101–110.

Kumar, A., Bilker, W., Jin, Z., and Udupa, J. (2000). Atrophy and high intensity lesions: Complementary neurobiological mechanisms in late-life major depression. *Neuropsychopharmacology*, 22(3), 264–274.

Kushner, M., Tobin, M., Alavi, A., Chawluk, J., Rosen, M., Fazekas, F., Alavi, J., and Reivich, M. (1987). Cerebellar glucose consumption in normal and pathologic states using fluorine-FDG and PET. *J Nucl Med*, 28(11), 1667–1670.

Kushnir, T., Itzchak, Y., Valevski, A., Lask, M., Modai, I., and Navon, G. (1993). Relaxation times and concentrations of ^{7}Li in the brain of patients receiving lithium therapy. *NMR Biomed*, 6(1), 39–42.

Kusumakar, V., MacMaster, F.P., Gates, L., Sparkes, S.J., and Khan, S.C. (2001). Left medial temporal cytosolic choline in early onset depression. *Can J Psychiatry*, 46(10), 959–964.

Kwon, A.H., Rogers, L.J., et al. (2002). *Reduced thalamic volumes in recurrent, familial major depressive disorder*. 57th Annual Convention and Scientific Program of the Society of Biological Psychiatry, Philadelphia, PA, May 16–18.

Lacerda, A.L., Nicoletti, M.A., Brambilla, P., Sassi, R.B., Mallinger, A.G., Frank, E., Kupfer, D.J., Keshavan, M.S., and Soares, J.C. (2003). Anatomical MRI study of basal ganglia in major depressive disorder. *Psychiatry Res*, 124(3), 129–140.

Lacerda, A.L., Keshavan, M.S., Hardan, A.Y., Yorbik, O., Brambilla, P., Sassi, R.B., Nicoletti, M., Mallinger, A.G., Frank, E., Kupfer, D.J., and Soares, J.C. (2004). Anatomic evaluation of the orbitofrontal cortex in major depressive disorder. *Biol Psychiatry*, 55(4), 353–358.

Lafer, B., Renshaw, P.F., et al. (1994). *Proton MRS of the basal ganglia in bipolar disorder*. 49th Annual Meeting of the Society of Biological Psychiatry, Philadelphia, PA, May 18–22.

Lai, T., Payne, M.E., Byrum, C.E., Steffens, D.C., and Krishnan, K.R. (2000). Reduction of orbital frontal cortex volume in geriatric depression. *Biol Psychiatry*, 48(10), 971–975.

Lammers, C.S., Doraiswamy, P.M., et al. (1991). MRI of corpus callosum and septum pellucidum in depression [letter]. *Biol Psychiatry*, 29(3), 300–301.

Lane, R.D., Reiman, E.M., Ahern, G.L., Schwartz, G.E., and Davidson, R.J. (1997). Neuroanatomical correlates of happiness, sadness, and disgust. *Am J Psychiatry*, 154(7), 926–933.

Lange, C., and Irle, E. (2004). Enlarged amygdala volume and reduced hippocampal volume in young women with major depression. *Psychol Med*, 34(6), 1059–1064.

Lauer, C.J., Wiegand, M., and Krieg, J.C. (1992). All-night electroencephalographic sleep and cranial computed tomography in depression. A study of unipolar and bipolar patients. *Eur Arch Psychiatry Clin Neurosci*, 242(2-3), 59–68.

Lavretsky, H., Kurbanyan, K., Ballmaier, M., Mintz, J., Toga, A., and Kumar, A. (2004). Sex differences in brain structure in geriatric depression. *Am J Geriatr Psychiatry*, 12(6), 653–657.

Lawrence, N.S., Williams, A.M., Surguladze, S., Giampietro, V., Brammer, M.J., Andrew, C., Frangou, S., Ecker, C., and Phillips, M.L. (2004). Subcortical and ventral prefrontal cortical neural responses to facial expressions distinguish patients with bipolar disorder and major depression. *Biol Psychiatry*, 55(6), 578–587.

Lebrun-Grandie, P., Baron, J.C., Soussaline, F., Loch'h, C., Sastre, J., and Bousser, M.G. (1983). Coupling between regional blood flow and oxygen utilization in the normal human brain. A study with positron tomography and oxygen 15. *Arch Neurol*, 40(4), 230–236.

Lennox, B.R., Park, S.B., Jones, P.B., and Morris, P.G. (1999). Spatial and temporal mapping of neural activity associated with auditory hallucinations [letter]. *Lancet*, 353(9153), 644.

Lenze, E.J., and Sheline, Y.I. (1999). Absence of striatal volume differences between depressed subjects with no comorbid medical illness and matched comparison subjects. *Am J Psychiatry*, 156(12), 1989–1991.

Lenze, E., Cross, D., McKeel, D., Neuman, R.J., and Sheline, Y.I. (1999). White matter hyperintensities and gray matter lesions in physically healthy depressed subjects. *Am J Psychiatry*, 156(10), 1602–1607.

Lesser, I.M., Miller, B.L., Boone, K.B., Hill-Gutierrez, E., Mehringer, C.M., Wong, K., and Mena, I. (1991). Brain injury and cognitive function in late-onset psychotic depression. *J Neuropsychiatry Clin Neurosci*, 3, 33–40.

Lesser, I.M., Mena, I., Boone, K.B., Miller, B.L., Mehringer, C.M., and Wohl, M. (1994). Reduction of cerebral blood flow in older depressed patients. *Arch Gen Psychiatry*, 51(9), 677–686.

Lesser, I.M., Boone, K.B., Mehringer, C.M., Wohl, M.A., Miller, B.L., and Berman, N.G. (1996). Cognition and white matter hyperintensities in older depressed patients. *Am J Psychiatry*, 153(10), 1280–1287.

Levine, J., Barak, Y., Gonzalves, M., Szor, H., Elizur, A., Kofman, O., and Belmaker, R.H. (1995). Double-blind, controlled trial of inositol treatment of depression. *Am J Psychiatry*, 152(5), 792–794.

Lewine, R.R., Risch, S.C., Risby, E., Stipetic, M., Jewart, R.D., Eccard, M., Caudle, J., and Pollard, W. (1991). Lateral ventricle–brain ratio and balance between CSF HVA and 5-HIAA in schizophrenia. *Am J Psychiatry*, 148(9), 1189–1194.

Lewine, R.R., Hudgins, P., Brown, F., Caudle, J., and Risch, S.C. (1995). Differences in qualitative brain morphology findings in schizophrenia, major depression, bipolar disorder, and normal volunteers. *Schizophr Res*, 15(3), 253–259.

Lim, K.O., Rosenbloom, M.J., Faustman, W.O., Sullivan, E.V., and Pfefferbaum, A. (1999). Cortical gray matter deficit in patients with bipolar disorder. *Schizophr Res*, 40(3), 219–227.

Liotti, M., Mayberg, H.S., Brannan, S.K., McGinnis, S., Jerabek, P., and Fox, P.T. (2000). Differential limbic—cortical correlates of sadness and anxiety in healthy subjects: Implications for affective disorders. *Biol Psychiatry*, 48(1), 30–42.

Liotti, M., Mayberg, H.S., McGinnis, S., Brannan, S.L., and Jerabek, P. (2002). Unmasking disease-specific cerebral blood flow abnormalities: Mood challenge in patients with remitted unipolar depression. *Am J Psychiatry*, 159(11), 1830–1840.

Lippmann, S., Manshadi, M., Baldwin, H., Drasin, G., Rice, J., and Alrajeh, S. (1982). Cerebellar vermis dimensions on computerized tomographic scans of schizophrenic and bipolar patients. *Am J Psychiatry*, 139(5), 667–668.

Lippmann, S., Manshadi, M., Baldwin, H., Drasin, G., Wagemaker, H., Rice, J., and Alrajeh, S. (1985). Cerebral CAT scan imaging in schizophrenic and bipolar patients. *J Ky Med Assoc*, 83(1), 13–15.

Lisanby, S.H., McDonald, W.M., Massey, E.W., Doraiswamy, P.M., Rozear, M., Boyko, O.B., Krishnan, K.R., and Nemeroff, C. (1993). Diminished subcortical nuclei volumes in Parkinson's disease by MR imaging. *J Neural Transm Suppl*, 40, 13–21.

Little, J.T., Ketter, T.A., Kimbrell, T.A., Danielson, A., Benson, B., Willis, M.W., and Post, R.M. (1996). Venlafaxine or bupropion responders but not nonresponders show baseline prefrontal and paralimbic hypometabolism compared with controls. *Psychopharmacol Bull*, 32(4), 629–635.

Little, J.T., Ketter, T.A., Kimbrell, T.A., Dunn, R.T., Benson, B.E., Willis, M.W., Luckenbaugh, D.A., and Post, R.M. (2005). Bupropion and venlafaxine responders differ in pretreatment regional cerebral metabolism in unipolar depression. *Biol Psychiatry*, 57(3), 220–228.

Lloyd, A.J., Ferrier, I.N., Barber, R., Gholkar, A., Young, A.H., and O'Brien, J.T. (2004). Hippocampal volume change in depression: Late- and early-onset illness compared. *Br J Psychiatry*, 184, 488–495.

Lochhead, R.A., Parsey, R.V., Oquendo, M.A., and Mann, J.J. (2004). Regional brain gray matter volume differences in patients with bipolar disorder as assessed by optimized voxel-based morphometry. *Biol Psychiatry*, 55(12), 1154–1162.

Loeber, R.T., Sherwood, A.R., Renshaw, P.F., Cohen, B.M., and Yurgelun-Todd, D.A. (1999). Differences in cerebellar blood volume in schizophrenia and bipolar disorder. *Schizophr Res*, 37(1), 81–89.

Loeber, R.T., Gruber, S.A., Cohen, B.M., Renshaw, P.F., Sherwood, A.R., and Yurgelun-Todd, D.A. (2002). Cerebellar blood volume in bipolar patients correlates with medication. *Biol Psychiatry*, 51(5), 370–376.

Lopez-Larson, M.P., DelBello, M.P., Zimmerman, M.E., Schwiers, M.L., and Strakowski, S.M. (2002). Regional prefrontal gray and white matter abnormalities in bipolar disorder. *Biol Psychiatry*, 52(2), 93–100.

Losfescu, D.V., Renshaw, P.F. et al. (2002). *Brain MRI white matter hyperintensities correlate with improved treatment outcome in depression*. 57th Annual Convention and Scientific Program of the Society of Biological Psychiatry, Philadelphia, PA, May 16–18.

Luchins, D.J., Lewine, R.R., and Meltzer, H.Y. (1984). Lateral ventricular size, psychopathology, and medication response in the psychoses. *Biol Psychiatry*, 19(1), 29–44.

Lyoo, I.K., Demopulos, C.M., Hirashima, F., Ahn, K.H., and Renshaw, P.F. (2003). Oral choline decreases brain purine levels in lithium-treated subjects with rapid-cycling bipolar disorder: A double-blind trial using proton and lithium magnetic resonance spectroscopy. *Bipolar Disord*, 5(4), 300–306.

Lyoo, I.K., Kim, M.J., Stoll, A.L., Demopulos, C.M., Parow, A.M., Dager, S.R., Friedman, S.D., Dunner, D.L., and Renshaw, P.F. (2004). Frontal lobe gray matter density decreases in bipolar I disorder. *Biol Psychiatry*, 55(6), 648–651.

Lyoo, I.K., Sung, Y.H., Dager, S.R., Friedman, S.D., Lee, J.Y., Kim, S.J., Kim, N., Dunner, D.L., and Renshaw, P.F. (2006). Regional cerebral cortical thinning in bipolar disorder. *Bipolar Disord*, 8(1), 65–74.

MacFall, J.R., Payne, M.E., Provenzale, J.E., and Krishnan, K.R. (2001). Medial orbital frontal lesions in late-onset depression. *Biol Psychiatry*, 49(9), 803–806.

MacHale, S.M., Lawrie, S.M., Cavanagh, J.T., Glabus, M.F., Murray, C.L., Goodwin, G.M., and Ebmeier, K.P. (2000). Cerebral perfusion in chronic fatigue syndrome and depression. *Br J Psychiatry*, 176, 550–556.

MacLean, P.D. (1952). Some psychiatric implications of physiological studies on the frontotemporal portion of limbic system (visceral brain). *Electroencephalogr Clin Neurophysiol*, 4, 407–418.

MacMaster, F.P., and Kusumakar, V. (2004a). MRI study of the pituitary gland in adolescent depression. *J Psychiatr Res*, 38(3), 231–236.

MacMaster, F.P., and Kusumakar, V. (2004b). Hippocampal volume in early-onset depression. *BMC Med*, 2, 2.

MacQueen, G.M., Campbell, S., McEwen, B.S., Macdonald, K., Amano, S., Joffe, R.T., Nahmias, C., and Young, L.T. (2003). Course of illness, hippocampal function, and hippocampal volume in major depression. *Proc Natl Acad Sci USA*, 100(3), 1387–1392.

Maes, M., Dierckx, R., Meltzer, H.Y., Ingels, M., Schotte, C., Vandewoude, M., Calabrese, J., and Cosyns, P. (1993). Regional cerebral blood flow in unipolar depression measured with Tc-^{99m}-HMPAO single photon emission computed tomography: Negative findings. *Psychiatry Res*, 50(2), 77–88.

Malberg, J.E. (2004). Implications of adult hippocampal neurogenesis in antidepressant action. *J Psychiatry Neurosci*, 29(3), 196–205.

Malhi, G.S., Lagopoulos, J., Sachdev, P., Mitchell, P.B., Ivanovski, B., and Parker, G.B. (2004). Cognitive generation of affect in hypomania: An fMRI study. *Bipolar Disord*, 6(4), 271–285.

Malhi, G.S., Lagopoulos, J., Sachdev, P.S., Ivanovski, B., and Shnier, R. (2005). An emotional stroop functional MRI study of euthymic bipolar disorder. *Bipolar Disord*, 7(Suppl. 5), 58–69.

Manji, H.K., and Lenox, R.H. (2000). Signaling: Cellular insights into the pathophysiology of bipolar disorder. *Biol Psychiatry*, 48(6), 518–530.

Manji, H.K., Drevets, W.C., and Charney, D.S. (2001). The cellular neurobiology of depression. *Nat Med*, 7(5), 541–547.

Mann, J.J., Malone, K.M., Diehl, D.J., Perel, J., Cooper, T.B., and Mintun, M.A. (1996). Demonstration in vivo of reduced serotonin responsivity in the brain of untreated depressed patients. *Am J Psychiatry*, 153(2), 174–182.

Marangell, L.B., Ketter, T.A., George, M.S., Pazzaglia, P.J., Callahan, A.M., Parekh, P., Andreason, P.J., Horwitz, B., Herscovitch, P., and Post, R.M. (1997). Inverse relationship of peripheral thyrotropin-stimulating hormone levels to brain activity in mood disorders. *Am J Psychiatry*, 154(2), 224–230.

Martinot, J.L., Hardy, P., Feline, A., Huret, J.D., Mazoyer, B., Attar-Levy, D., Pappata, S., and Syrota, A. (1990). Left prefrontal glucose hypometabolism in the depressed state: A confirmation. *Am J Psychiatry*, 147(10), 1313–1317.

Mason, G.F., Sanacora, G., et al. (2000). *Cortical GABA reduced in unipolar but not bipolar depression*. 55th Annual Convention and Scientific Program of the Society of Biological Psychiatry, Chicago, IL, May 11–13.

Matsuo, K., Kato, T., Fukuda, M., and Kato, N. (2000). Alteration of hemoglobin oxygenation in the frontal region in elderly depressed patients as measured by near-infrared spectroscopy. *J Neuropsychiatry Clin Neurosci*, 12(4), 465–471.

Matsuo, K., Kato, N., and Kato, T. (2002). Decreased cerebral haemodynamic response to cognitive and physiological tasks in mood disorders as shown by near-infrared spectroscopy. *Psychol Med*, 32(6), 1029–1037.

Mayberg, H.S. (1994). Frontal lobe dysfunction in secondary depression. *J Neuropsychiatry Clin Neurosci*, 6(4), 428–442.

Mayberg, H.S. (1997). Limbic-cortical dysregulation: A proposed model of depression. *J Neuropsychiatry Clin Neurosci*, 9(3), 471–481.

Mayberg, H.S., Starkstein, S.E., Sadzot, B., Preziosi, T., Andrezejewski, P.L., Dannals, R.F., Wagner, H.N. Jr., and Robinson, R.G. (1990). Selective hypometabolism in the inferior frontal lobe in depressed patients with Parkinson's disease. *Ann Neurol*, 28(1), 57–64.

Mayberg, H.S., Starkstein, S.E., and Morris, P.L. (1991). Remote cortical hypometabolism following focal basal ganglia injury: Relationship to secondary changes in mood. Abstract 540S. *Neurology*, 41(Suppl. 1), 266.

Mayberg, H.S., Starkstein, S.E., Peyser, C.E., Brandt, J., Dannals, R.F., and Folstein, S.E. (1992). Paralimbic frontal lobe hypometabolism in depression associated with Huntington's disease. *Neurology*, 42(9), 1791–1797.

Mayberg, H.S., Lewis, P.J., Regenold, W., and Wagner, H.N. Jr. (1994). Paralimbic hypoperfusion in unipolar depression. *J Nucl Med*, 35(6), 929–934.

Mayberg, H.S., Brannan, S.K., Mahurin, R.K., Jerabek, P.A., Brickman, J.S., Tekell, J.L., Silva, J.A., McGinnis, S., Glass, T.G., Martin, C.C., and Fox, P.T. (1997). Cingulate function in depression: A potential predictor of treatment response. *Neuroreport*, 8(4), 1057–1061.

Mayberg, H.S., Liotti, M., Brannan, S.K., McGinnis, S., Mahurin, R.K., Jerabek, P.A., Silva, J.A., Tekell, J.L., Martin, C.C., Lancaster, J.L., and Fox, P.T. (1999). Reciprocal limbic–cortical function and negative mood: Converging PET findings in depression and normal sadness. *Am J Psychiatry*, 156(5), 675–682.

Mayberg, H.S., Brannan, S.K., Tekell, J.L., Silva, J.A., Mahurin, R.K., McGinnis, S., and Jerabek, P.A. (2000). Regional metabolic effects of fluoxetine in major depression: Serial changes and relationship to clinical response. *Biol Psychiatry*, 48(8), 830–843.

Mayberg, H.S., Silva, J.A., Brannan, S.K., Tekell, J.L., Mahurin, R.K., McGinnis, S., and Jerabek, P.A. (2002). The functional neuroanatomy of the placebo effect. *Am J Psychiatry*, 159(5), 728–737.

McDonald, C., Bullmore, E., Sham, P., Chitnis, X., Suckling, J., MacCabe, J., Walshe, M., and Murray, R.M. (2005). Regional volume deviations of brain structure in schizophrenia and psychotic bipolar disorder: Computational morphometry study. *Br J Psychiatry*, 186, 369–377.

McDonald, W.M., Krishnan, K.R., Doraiswamy, P.M., and Blazer, D.G. (1991). Occurrence of subcortical hyperintensities in elderly subjects with mania. *Psychiatry Res*, 40(4), 211–220.

McDonald, W.M., Tupler, L.A., Marsteller, F.A., Figiel, G.S., DiSouza, S., Nemeroff, C.B., and Krishnan, K.R. (1999). Hyperintense lesions on magnetic resonance images in bipolar disorder. *Biol Psychiatry*, 45(8), 965–971.

McDonald, C., Zanelli, J., Rabe-Hesketh, S., Ellison-Wright, I., Sham, P., Kalidindi, S., Murray, R.M., and Kennedy, N. (2004). Meta-analysis of magnetic resonance imaging brain morphometry studies in bipolar disorder. *Biol Psychiatry*, 56(6), 411–417.

McIntosh, A.M., Job, D.E., Moorhead, T.W., Harrison, L.K., Forrester, K., Lawrie, S.M., and Johnstone, E.C. (2004).

Voxel-based morphometry of patients with schizophrenia or bipolar disorder and their unaffected relatives. *Biol Psychiatry*, 56(8), 544–552.

McIntosh, A.M., Job, D.E., Moorhead, T.W., Harrison, L.K., Lawrie, S.M., and Johnstone, E.C. (2005). White matter density in patients with schizophrenia, bipolar disorder and their unaffected relatives. *Biol Psychiatry*, 58(3), 254–257.

Mendez, M.F., Adams, N.L., and Lewandowski, K.S. (1989). Neurobehavioral changes associated with caudate lesions. *Neurology*, 39, 349–354.

Mervaala, E., Fohr, J., Kononen, M., Valkonen-Korhonen, M., Vainio, P., Partanen, K., Partanen, J., Tiihonen, J., Viinamaki, H., Karjalainen, A.K., and Lehtonen, J. (2000). Quantitative MRI of the hippocampus and amygdala in severe depression. *Psychol Med*, 30(1), 117–125.

Mervaala, E., Kononen, M., Fohr, J., Husso-Saastamoinen, M., Valkonen-Korhonen, M., Kuikka, J.T., Viinamaki, H., Tammi, A.K., Tiihonen, J., Partanen, J., and Lehtonen, J. (2001). SPECT and neuropsychological performance in severe depression treated with ECT. *J Affect Disord*, 66(1), 47–58.

Michael, N., Erfurth, A., Ohrmann, P., Arolt, V., Heindel, W., and Pfleiderer, B. (2003a). Metabolic changes within the left dorsolateral prefrontal cortex occurring with electroconvulsive therapy in patients with treatment-resistant unipolar depression. *Psychol Med*, 33(7), 1277–1284.

Michael, N., Erfurth, A., Ohrmann, P., Gossling, M., Arolt, V., Heindel, W., and Pfleiderer, B. (2003b). Acute mania is accompanied by elevated glutamate/glutamine levels within the left dorsolateral prefrontal cortex. *Psychopharmacology*, 168(3), 344–346.

Migliorelli, R., Starkstein, S.E., Teson, A., de Quiros, G., Vazquez, S., Leiguarda, R., and Robinson, R.G. (1993). SPECT findings in patients with primary mania. *J Neuropsychiatry Clin Neurosci*, 5(4), 379–383.

Miller, D.S., Kumar, A., et al. (1994). MRI high-intensity signals in depression and Alzheimer's disease. *Am J Geriatr Psychiatry*, 2(4), 332–337.

Mindham, R.H. (1970). Psychiatric symptoms in Parkinsonism. *J Neurol Neurosurg Psychiatry*, 33(2), 188–191.

Mitterschiffthaler, M.T., Kumari, V., Malhi, G.S., Brown, R.G., Giampietro, V.P., Brammer, M.J., Suckling, J., Poon, L., Simmons, A., Andrew, C., and Sharma, T. (2003). Neural response to pleasant stimuli in anhedonia: An fMRI study. *Neuroreport*, 14(2), 177–182.

Miura, S.A., Schapiro, M.B., Grady, C.L., Kumar, A., Salerno, J.A., Kozachuk, W.E., Wagner, E., Rapoport, S.I., and Horwitz, B. (1990). Effect of gender on glucose utilization rates in healthy humans: A positron emission tomography study. *J Neurosci Res*, 27(4), 500–504.

Moeller, J.R., Ishikawa, T., Dhawan, V., Spetsieris, P., Mandel, F., Alexander, G.E., Grady, C., Pietrini, P., and Eidelberg, D. (1996). The metabolic topography of normal aging. *J Cereb Blood Flow Metab*, 16(3), 385–398.

Moller, A., Wiedemann, G., Rohde, U., Backmund, H., and Sonntag, A. (1994). Correlates of cognitive impairment and depressive mood disorder in multiple sclerosis. *Acta Psychiatr Scand*, 89(2), 117–121.

Moore, C.M., Christensen, J.D., Lafer, B., Fava, M., and Renshaw, P.F. (1997). Lower levels of nucleoside triphosphate in the basal ganglia of depressed subjects: A phosphorous-31 magnetic resonance spectroscopy study. *Am J Psychiatry*, 154(1), 116–118.

Moore, C.M., Breeze, J.L., Kukes, T.J., Rose, S.L., Dager, S.R., Cohen, B.M., and Renshaw, P.F. (1999). Effects of myo-inositol ingestion on human brain myo-inositol levels: A proton magnetic resonance spectroscopic imaging study. *Biol Psychiatry*, 45(9), 1197–1202.

Moore, C.M., Breeze, J.L., Gruber, S.A., Babb, S.M., Frederick, B.B., Villafuerte, R.A., Stoll, A.L., Hennen, J,. Yurgelun-Todd, D.A., Cohen, B.M., and Renshaw, P.F. (2000). Choline, myo-inositol and mood in bipolar disorder: A proton magnetic resonance spectroscopic imaging study of the anterior cingulate cortex. *Bipolar Disord*, 2(3 Pt. 2), 207–216.

Moore, C.M., Demopulos, C.M., Henry, M.E., Steingard, R.J., Zamvil, L., Katic, A., Breeze, J.L., Moore, J.C., Cohen, B.M., and Renshaw, P.F. (2002). Brain-to-serum lithium ratio and age: An in vivo magnetic resonance spectroscopy study. *Am J Psychiatry*, 159(7), 1240–1242.

Moore, G.J., Bebchuk, J.M., Parrish, J.K., Faulk, M.W., Arfken, C.L., Strahl-Bevacqua, J., and Manji, H.K. (1999). Temporal dissociation between lithium-induced changes in frontal lobe myo-inositol and clinical response in manic-depressive illness. *Am J Psychiatry*, 156(12), 1902–1908.

Moore, G.J., Bebchuk, J.M., Hasanat, K., Chen, G., Seraji-Bozorgzad, N., Wilds, I.B., Faulk, M.W., Koch, S., Glitz, D.A., Jolkovsky, L., and Manji, H.K. (2000a). Lithium increases N-acetyl-aspartate in the human brain: In vivo evidence in support of bcl-2's neurotrophic effects? *Biol Psychiatry*, 48(1), 1–8.

Moore, G.J., Bebchuk, J.M., Wilds, I.B., Chen, G., and Manji, H.K. (2000b). Lithium-induced increase in human brain grey matter. *Lancet*, 356(9237), 1241–1242.

Moore, P.B., Shepherd, D.J., Eccleston, D., Macmillan, I.C., Goswami, U., McAllister, V.L., and Ferrier, I.N. (2001). Cerebral white matter lesions in bipolar affective disorder: Relationship to outcome. *Br J Psychiatry*, 178, 172–176.

Morris, J.S., Frith, C.D., Perrett, D.I., Rowland, D., Young, A.W., Calder, A.J., and Dolan, R.J. (1996). A differential neural response in the human amygdala to fearful and happy facial expressions. *Nature*, 383(6603), 812–815.

Morris, J.S., Friston, K.J., Buchel, C., Frith, C.D., Young, A.W., Calder, A.J., and Dolan, R.J. (1998a). A neuromodulatory role for the human amygdala in processing emotional facial expressions. *Brain*, 121(Pt. 1), 47–57.

Morris, J.S., Ohman, A., and Dolan, R.J. (1998b). Conscious and unconscious emotional learning in the human amygdala. *Nature*, 393(6684), 467–470.

Mozley, P.D., Hornig-Rohan, M., Woda, A.M., Kim, H.J., Alavi, A., Payer, F., and Amsterdam, J.D. (1996). Cerebral HMPAO SPECT in patients with major depression and healthy volunteers. *Prog Neuropsychopharmacol Biol Psychiatry*, 20(3), 443–458.

Mukherjee, S., Schnur, D.B., Lo, E.S., Sackeim, H.A., and Cooper, T.B. (1993). Post-dexamethasone cortisol levels and computerized tomographic findings in manic patients. *Acta Psychiatr Scand*, 88(3), 145–148.

Murashita, J., Kato, T., Shioiri, T., Inubushi, T., and Kato, N. (2000). Altered brain energy metabolism in lithium-resistant bipolar disorder detected by photic stimulated 31P-MR spectroscopy. *Psychol Med*, 30(1), 107–115.

Murata, T., Kimura, H., Omori, M., Kado, H., Kosaka, H., Iidaka, T., Itoh, H., and Wada, Y. (2001). MRI white matter hyperintensities, (1)H-MR spectroscopy and cognitive function in geriatric depression: A comparison of early- and late-onset cases. *Int J Geriatr Psychiatry*, 16(12), 1129–1135.

Murphy, D.G., DeCarli, C., Schapiro, M.B., Rapoport, S.I., and Horwitz, B. (1992). Age-related differences in volumes of subcortical nuclei, brain matter, and cerebrospinal fluid in healthy men as measured with magnetic resonance imaging. *Arch Neurol*, 49(8), 839–845.

Murphy, D.G., Murphy, D.M., Abbas, M., Palazidou, E., Binnie, C., Arendt, J., Campos Costa, D., and Checkley, S.A. (1993). Seasonal affective disorder: Response to light as measured by electroencephalogram, melatonin suppression, and cerebral blood flow. *Br J Psychiatry*, 163, 327–331, 335–337.

Murphy, D.G., DeCarli, C., McIntosh, A.R., Daly, E., Mentis, M.J., Pietrini, P., Szczepanik, J., Schapiro, M.B., Grady, C.L., Horwitz, B., and Rapoport, S.I. (1996). Sex differences in human brain morphometry and metabolism: An in vivo quantitative magnetic resonance imaging and positron emission tomography study on the effect of aging. *Arch Gen Psychiatry*, 53(7), 585–594.

Nasrallah, H.A., Jacoby, C.G., and McCalley-Whitters, M. (1981). Cerebellar atrophy in schizophrenia and mania [letter]. *Lancet*, 1(8229), 1102.

Nasrallah, H.A., McCalley-Whitters, M., and Jacoby, C.G. (1982a). Cerebral ventricular enlargement in young manic males: A controlled CT study. *J Affect Disord*, 4(1), 15–19.

Nasrallah, H.A., McCalley-Whitters, M., and Jacoby, C.G. (1982b). Cortical atrophy in schizophrenia and mania: A comparative CT study. *J Clin Psychiatry*, 43(11), 439–441.

Nasrallah, H.A., McCalley-Whitters, M., and Pfohl, B. (1984). Clinical significance of large cerebral ventricles in manic males. *Psychiatry Res*, 13(2), 151–156.

Navarro, V., Gasto, C., Lomena, F., Mateos, J.J., and Marcos, T. (2001). Frontal cerebral perfusion dysfunction in elderly late-onset major depression assessed by [99M]TC-HMPAO SPECT. *Neuroimage*, 14(1 Pt. 1), 202–205.

Nebes, R.D., Vora, I.J., Meltzer, C.C., Fukui, M.B., Williams, R.L., Kamboh, M.I., Saxton, J., Houck, P.R., DeKosky, S.T., and Reynolds, C.F. III. (2001). Relationship of deep white matter hyperintensities and apolipoprotein E genotype to depressive symptoms in older adults without clinical depression. *Am J Psychiatry*, 158(6), 878–884.

Nobler, M.S., Sackeim, H.A., Prohovnik, I., Moeller, J.R., Mukherjee, S., Schnur, D.B., Prudic, J., and Devanand, D.P. (1994). Regional cerebral blood flow in mood disorders, III. Treatment and clinical response. *Arch Gen Psychiatry*, 51(11), 884–897.

Nobler, M.S., Roose, S.P., Prohovnik, I., Moeller, J.R., Louie, J., Van Heertum, R.L., and Sackeim, H.A. (2000). Regional cerebral blood flow in mood disorders V: Effects of antidepressant medication in late-life depression. *Am J Geriatr Psychiatry*, 8(4), 289–296.

Nofzinger, E.A., Nichols, T.E., Meltzer, C.C., Price, J., Steppe, D.A., Miewald, J.M., Kupfer, D.J., and Moore, R.Y. (1999). Changes in forebrain function from waking to REM sleep in depression: Preliminary analyses of [18F]FDG PET studies. *Psychiatry Res*, 91(2), 59–78.

Nofzinger, E.A., Berman, S., Fasiczka, A., Miewald, J.M., Meltzer, C.C., Price, J.C., Sembrat, R.C., Wood, A., and Thase, M.E. (2001). Effects of bupropion SR on anterior paralimbic function during waking and REM sleep in depression: Preliminary findings using [18F]-FDG PET. *Psychiatry Res*, 106(2), 95–111.

Noga, J.T., Vladar, K., and Torrey, E.F. (2001). A volumetric magnetic resonance imaging study of monozygotic twins discordant for bipolar disorder. *Psychiatry Res*, 106(1), 25–34.

Nudmamud, S., Reynolds, L.M., and Reynolds, G.P. (2003). N-acetylaspartate and N-acetylaspartylglutamate deficits in superior temporal cortex in schizophrenia and bipolar disorder: A postmortem study. *Biol Psychiatry*, 53(12), 1138–1141.

Nugent, A.C., Milham, M.P., Bain, E.E., Mah, L., Cannon, D.M., Marrett, S., Zarate, C.A., Pine, D.S., Price, J.L., and Drevets, W.C. (2006). Cortical abnormalities in bipolar disorder investigated with MRI and voxel-based morphometry. *Neuroimage*, 30(2), 485–497.

O'Brien, J., Desmond, P., Ames, D., Schweitzer, I., Harrigan, S., and Tress, B. (1996). A magnetic resonance imaging study of white matter lesions in depression and Alzheimer's disease. *Br J Psychiatry*, 168(4), 477–485.

O'Connell, R.A., Van Heertum, R.L., Billick, S.B., Holt, A.R., Gonzalez, A., Notardonato, H., Luck, D., and King, L.N. (1989). Single photon emission computed tomography (SPECT) with [^{123}I]IMP in the differential diagnosis of psychiatric disorders. *J Neuropsychiatry Clin Neurosci*, 1(2), 145–153.

O'Connell, R.A., Van Heertum, R.L., Luck, D., Yudd, A.P., Cueva, J.E., Billick, S.B., Cordon, D.J., Gersh, R.J., and Masdeu, J.C. (1995). Single-photon emission computed tomography of the brain in acute mania and schizophrenia. *J Neuroimaging*, 5(2), 101–104.

Ohaeri, J.U., Adeyinka, A.O., Enyidah, S.N., and Osuntokun, B.O. (1995). Schizophrenic and manic brains in Nigerians. Computerised tomography findings. *Br J Psychiatry*, 166(4), 496–500.

Ohara, K., Isoda, H., Suzuki, Y., Takehara, Y., Ochiai, M., Takeda, H., Igarashi, Y., and Ohara, K. (1998). Proton magnetic resonance spectroscopy of the lenticular nuclei in bipolar I affective disorder. *Psychiatry Res*, 84(2-3), 55–60.

Öngür, D., Drevets, W.C., and Price, J.L. (1998). Glial reduction in the subgenual prefrontal cortex in mood disorders. *Proc Natl Acad Sci USA*, 95(22), 13290–13295.

Osuch, E.A., Ketter, T.A., Kimbrell, T.A., George, M.S., Benson, B.E., Willis, M.W., Herscovitch, P., and Post, R.M. (2000). Regional cerebral metabolism associated with anxiety symptoms in affective disorder patients. *Biol Psychiatry*, 48(10), 1020–1023.

Pande, A.C., Grunhaus, L.J., Aisen, A.M., and Haskett, R.F. (1990). A preliminary magnetic resonance imaging study of ECT-treated depressed patients. *Biol Psychiatry*, 27(1), 102–104.

Pantel, J., Schroder, J., Essig, M., Popp, D., Dech, H., Knopp, M.V., Schad, L.R., Eysenbach, K., Backenstrass, M., and Friedlinger, M. (1997). Quantitative magnetic resonance imaging in geriatric depression and primary degenerative dementia. *J Affect Disord*, 42(1), 69–83.

Pantel, J., Schroder, J., Essig, M., Schad, L.R., Popp, D., Eysenbach, K., Jauss, M., and Knopp, M.V. (1998). Volumetric brain findings in late depression. A study with quantified magnetic resonance tomography. *Nervenarzt*, 69(11), 968–974.

Papez, J.W. (1937). A proposed mechanism of emotion. *Arch Neurol Psychiatry*, 38, 725–743.

Parashos, I.A., Tupler, L.A., Blitchington, T., and Krishnan, K.R. (1998). Magnetic-resonance morphometry in patients with major depression. *Psychiatry Res*, 84(1), 7–15.

Pardo, J.V., Pardo, P.J., and Raichle, M.E. (1993). Neural correlates of self-induced dysphoria. *Am J Psychiatry*, 150(5), 713–719.

Pascual-Leone, A., and Pallardó, F. (1996). *Beneficial effects of repetitive transcranial magnetic stimulation (rTMS) in depression are associated with normalization of prefrontal hypometabolism.* 8th Congress of the Association of European Psychiatrists, London, England, July 7–12.

Passe, T.J., Rajagopalan, P., Tupler, L.A., Byrum, C.E., MacFall, J.R., and Krishnan, K.R. (1997). Age and sex effects on brain morphology. *Prog Neuropsychopharmacol Biol Psychiatry*, 21(8), 1231–1237.

Pearlson, G.D., and Veroff, A.E. (1981). Computerised tomographic scan changes in manic-depressive illness [letter]. *Lancet*, 2(8244), 470.

Pearlson, G.D., Garbacz, D.J., Breakey, W.R., Ahn, H.S., and DePaulo, J.R. (1984a). Lateral ventricular enlargement associated with persistent unemployment and negative symptoms in both schizophrenia and bipolar disorder. *Psychiatry Res*, 12(1), 1–9.

Pearlson, G.D., Garbacz, D.J., Tompkins, R.H., Ahn, H.S., Gutterman, D.F., Veroff, A.E., and DePaulo, J.R. (1984b). Clinical correlates of lateral ventricular enlargement in bipolar affective disorder. *Am J Psychiatry*, 141(2), 253–256.

Pearlson, G.D., Rabins, P.V., Kim, W.S., Speedie, L.J., Moberg, P.J., Burns, A., and Bascom, M.J. (1989). Structural brain CT changes and cognitive deficits in elderly depressives with and without reversible dementia ('pseudodementia'). *Psychol Med*, 19(3), 573–584.

Pearlson, G.D., Barta, P.E., Powers, R.E., Menon, R.R., Richards, S.S., Aylward, E.H., Federman, E.B., Chase, G.A., Petty, R.G., and Tien, A.Y. (1997). Ziskind-Somerfeld Research Award 1996. Medial and superior temporal gyral volumes and cerebral asymmetry in schizophrenia versus bipolar disorder. *Biol Psychiatry*, 41(1), 1–14.

Persaud, R., Russow, H., Harvey, I., Lewis, S.W., Ron, M., Murray, R.M., and du Boulay, G. (1997). Focal signal hyperintensities in schizophrenia. *Schizophr Res*, 27(1), 55–64.

Petit-Taboue, M.C., Landeau, B., Desson, J.F., Desgranges, B., and Baron, J.C. (1998). Effects of healthy aging on the regional cerebral metabolic rate of glucose assessed with statistical parametric mapping. *Neuroimage*, 7(3), 176–184.

Pettegrew, J.W., Keshavan, M.S., Panchalingam, K., Strychor, S., Kaplan, D.B., Tretta, M.G., and Allen, M. (1991). Alterations in brain high-energy phosphate and membrane phospholipid metabolism in first-episode, drug-naive schizophrenics. A pilot study of the dorsal prefrontal cortex by in vivo phosphorus 31 nuclear magnetic resonance spectroscopy. *Arch Gen Psychiatry*, 48(6), 563–568.

Petty, F., Rush, A.J., Davis, J.M., Calabrese, J.R., Kimmel, S.E., Kramer, G.L., Small, J.G., Miller, M.J., Swann, A.E., Orsulak, P.J., Blake, M.E., and Bowden, C.L. (1996). Plasma GABA predicts acute response to divalproex in mania. *Biol Psychiatry*, 39, 278–284.

Pfefferbaum, A., Mathalon, D.H., Sullivan, E.V., Rawles, J.M., Zipursky, R.B., and Lim, K.O. (1994). A quantitative magnetic resonance imaging study of changes in brain morphology from infancy to late adulthood. *Arch Neurol*, 51(9), 874–887.

Pfleiderer, B., Michael, N., Erfurth, A., Ohrmann, P., Hohmann, U., Wolgast, M., Fiebich, M., Arolt, V., and Heindel, W. (2003). Effective electroconvulsive therapy reverses glutamate/glutamine deficit in the left anterior cingulum of unipolar depressed patients. *Psychiatry Res*, 122(3), 185–192.

Phillips, M.L., Young, A.W., Senior, C., Brammer, M., Andrew, C., Calder, A.J., Bullmore, E.T., Perrett, D.I., Rowland, D., Williams, S.C., Gray, J.A., and David, A.S. (1997). A specific neural substrate for perceiving facial expressions of disgust. *Nature*, 389(6650), 495–498.

Phillips, M.L., Young, A.W., Scott, S.K., Calder, A.J., Andrew, C., Giampietro, V., Williams, S.C., Bullmore, E.T., Brammer, M., and Gray, J.A. (1998). Neural responses to facial and vocal expressions of fear and disgust. *Proc R Soc Lond B Biol Sci*, 265(1408), 1809–1817.

Philpot, M.P., Banerjee, S., Needham-Bennett, H., Costa, D.C., and Ell, P.J. (1993). ^{99m}Tc-HMPAO single photon emission tomography in late life depression: A pilot study of regional cerebral blood flow at rest and during a verbal fluency task. *J Affect Disord*, 28(4), 233–240.

Pillai, J.J., Friedman, L., Stuve, T.A., Trinidad, S., Jesberger, J.A., Lewin, J.S., Findling, R.L., Swales, T.P., and Schulz, S.C. (2002). Increased presence of white matter hyperintensities in adolescent patients with bipolar disorder. *Psychiatry Res*, 114(1), 51–56.

Pillay, S.S., Yurgelun-Todd, D.A., Bonello, C.M., Lafer, B., Fava, M., and Renshaw, P.F. (1997). A quantitative magnetic resonance imaging study of cerebral and cerebellar gray matter volume in primary unipolar major depression: Relationship to treatment response and clinical severity. *Biol Psychiatry*, 42, 79–84.

Pillay, S.S., Renshaw, P.F., Bonello, C.M., Lafer, B.C., Fava, M., and Yurgelun-Todd, D. (1998). A quantitative magnetic resonance imaging study of caudate and lenticular nucleus gray matter volume in primary unipolar major depression: Relationship to treatment response and clinical severity. *Psychiatry Res*, 84(2-3), 61–74.

Pizzagalli, D.A., Oakes, T.R., Fox, A.S., Chung, M.K., Larson, C.L., Abercrombie, H.C., Schaefer, S.M., Benca, R.M., and Davidson, R.J. (2004). Functional but not structural subgenual prefrontal cortex abnormalities in melancholia. *Mol Psychiatry*, 9(4), 325, 393–405.

Plenge, P., Stensgaard, A., Jensen, H.V., Thomsen, C., Mellerup, E.T., and Henriksen, O. (1994). 24-hour lithium concentration in human brain studied by Li-7 magnetic resonance spectroscopy. *Biol Psychiatry*, 36(8), 511–516.

Posener, J.A., Wang, L., Price, J.L., Gado, M.H., Province, M.A., Miller, M.I., Babb, C.M., and Csernansky, J.G. (2003). High-dimensional mapping of the hippocampus in depression. *Am J Psychiatry*, 160(1), 83–89.

Post, R.M., DeLisi, L.E., Holcomb, H.H., Uhde, T.W., Cohen, R., and Buchsbaum, M.S. (1987). Glucose utilization in the temporal cortex of affectively ill patients: Positron emission tomography. *Biol Psychiatry*, 22(5), 545–553.

Pouwels, P.J., and Frahm, J. (1998). Regional metabolite concentrations in human brain as determined by quantitative localized proton MRS. *Magn Reson Med*, 39(1), 53–60.

Pujol, J., Cardoner, N., Benlloch, L., Urretavizcaya, M., Deus, J., Losilla, J.M., Capdevila, A., and Vallejo, J. (2002). CSF spaces of the Sylvian fissure region in severe melancholic depression. *Neuroimage*, 15, 103–106.

Rabins, P.V., Pearlson, G.D., Aylward, E., Kumar, A.J., and Dowell, K. (1991). Cortical magnetic resonance imaging changes in elderly inpatients with major depression. *Am J Psychiatry*, 148(5), 617–620.

Raichle, M.E., Grubb, R.L. Jr., Gado, M.H., Eichling, J.O., and Ter-Pogossian, M.M. (1976). Correlation between regional cerebral blood flow and oxidative metabolism. In vivo studies in man. *Arch Neurol*, 33(8), 523–526.

Raichle, M.E., Taylor, J.R., et al. (1985). Brain circulation and metabolism in depression. In T. Greitz, D.H. Ingvar, and L. Widen (Eds.), *The Metabolism of the Human Brain Studied with Positron Emission Tomography* (pp. 453–456). New York: Raven Press.

Rajkowska, G. (1997). *Quantitative histopathology of prefrontal cortex in affective disorders*. 36th Annual Meeting of the American College of Neuropsychopharmacology, Waikoloa, HI, December 8–12.

Rao, V.P., Krishnan, K.R., Goli, V., Saunders, W.B., Ellinwood, E.H. Jr., Blazer, D.G., and Nemeroff, C.B. (1989). Neuroanatomical changes and hypothalamo–pituitary–adrenal axis abnormalities. *Biol Psychiatry*, 26(7), 729–732.

Rasgon, N.L., Thomas, M.A., Guze, B.H., Fairbanks, L.A., Yue, K., Curran, J.G., and Rapkin, A.J. (2001). Menstrual cycle–related brain metabolite changes using 1H magnetic resonance spectroscopy in premenopausal women: A pilot study. *Psychiatry Res*, 106(1), 47–57.

Raz, S. (1993). Structural cerebral pathology in schizophrenia: Regional or diffuse? *J Abnorm Psychol*, 102(3), 445–452.

Raz, S., and Raz, N. (1990). Structural brain abnormalities in the major psychoses: A quantitative review of the evidence from computerized imaging. *Psychol Bull*, 108(1), 93–108.

Reiman, E.M., Armstrong, S.M., Matt, K.S., and Mattox, J.H. (1996). The application of positron emission tomography to the study of the normal menstrual cycle. *Hum Reprod*, 11(12), 2799–2805.

Reischies, F.M., Hedde, J.P., and Drochner, R. (1989). Clinical correlates of cerebral blood flow in depression. *Psychiatry Res*, 29(3), 323–326.

Renshaw, P.F., and Wicklund, S. (1988). In vivo measurement of lithium in humans by nuclear magnetic resonance spectroscopy. *Biol Psychiatry*, 23(5), 465–475.

Renshaw, P.F., Johnson, K.A., et al. (1992). *New onset depression in patients with AIDS dementia complex (ADC) is associated with frontal lobe perfusion defects on HMPAO-SPECT scan*. 31st Annual Meeting of the American College of Neuropsychopharmacology, San Juan, Puerto Rico, December 14–18.

Renshaw, P.F., Yurgelun-Todd, D.A., Tohen, M., Gruber, S., and Cohen, B.M. (1995). Temporal lobe proton magnetic resonance spectroscopy of patients with first-episode psychosis. *Am J Psychiatry*, 152(3), 444–446.

Renshaw, P.F., Stoll, A.L., et al. (1996). *A choline deficit hypothesis for the progression of bipolar disorder with age*. 35th Annual Meeting of the American College of Neuropsychopharmacology, San Juan, Puerto Rico, December 9–13.

Renshaw, P.F., Lafer, B., Babb, S.M., Fava, M., Stoll, A.L., Christensen, J.D., Moore, C.M., Yurgelun-Todd, D.A., Bonello, C.M., Pillay, S.S., Rothschild, A.J., Nierenberg, A.A., Rosenbaum, J.F., and Cohen, B.M. (1997). Basal ganglia choline levels in depression and response to fluoxetine treatment: An in vivo proton magnetic resonance study. *Biol Psychiatry*, 41(8), 837–843.

Rieder, R.O., Mann, L.S., Weinberger, D.R., van Kammen, D.P., and Post, R.M. (1983). Computed tomographic scans in patients with schizophrenia, schizoaffective, and bipolar affective disorder. *Arch Gen Psychiatry*, 40(7), 735–739.

Riedl, U., Barocka, A., Kolem, H., Demling, J., Kaschka, W.P., Schelp, R., Stemmler, M., and Ebert, D. (1997). Duration of lithium treatment and brain lithium concentration in patients with unipolar and schizoaffective disorder: A study with magnetic resonance spectroscopy. *Biol Psychiatry*, 41(8), 844–850.

Ring, H.A., Bench, C.J., Trimble, M.R., Brooks, D.J., Frackowiak, R.S., and Dolan, R.J. (1994). Depression in Parkinson's disease. A positron emission study. *Br J Psychiatry*, 165(3), 333–339.

Risch, S.C., Lewine, R.J., Kalin, N.H., Jewart, R.D., Risby, E.D., Caudle, J.M., Stipetic, M., Turner, J., Eccard, M.B., and Pollard, W.E. (1992). Limbic–hypothalamic–pituitary–adrenal axis activity and ventricular-to-brain ratio studies in affective illness and schizophrenia. *Neuropsychopharmacology*, 6(2), 95–100.

Rosenberg, D.R., Paulson, L.D., et al. (2000). *Brain chemistry in pediatric depression*. 55th Annual Convention and Scientific Program of the Society of Biological Psychiatry, Chicago, IL, May 11–13.

Rossi, A., Stratta, P., Petruzzi, C., De Donatis, M., Nistico, R., and Casacchia, M. (1987). A computerised tomographic study in DSM-III affective disorders. *J Affect Disord*, 12(3), 259–262.

Rossi, A., Stratta, P., di Michele, V., Bolino, F., Nistico, R., de Leonardis, R., Sabatini, M.D., and Casacchia, M. (1989). A computerized tomographic study in patients with depressive disorder: A comparison with schizophrenic patients and controls. *Acta Psychiatr Belg*, 89(1-2), 56–61.

Rothschild, A.J., Benes, F., Hebben, N., Woods, B., Luciana, M., Bakanas, E., Samson, J.A., and Schatzberg, A.F. (1989). Relationships between brain CT scan findings and cortisol in psychotic and nonpsychotic depressed patients. *Biol Psychiatry*, 26(6), 565–575.

Roy, P.D., Zipursky, R.B., Saint-Cyr, J.A., Bury, A., Langevin, R., and Seeman, M.V. (1998). Temporal horn enlargement is present in schizophrenia and bipolar disorder. *Biol Psychiatry*, 44(6), 418–422.

Roy-Byrne, P.P., Post, R.M., Kellner, C.H., Joffe, R.T., and Uhde, T.W. (1988). Ventricular-brain ratio and life course of illness in patients with affective disorder. *Psychiatry Res*, 23(3), 277–284.

Rubin, E., Sackeim, H.A., Prohovnik, I., Moeller, J.R., Schnur, D.B., and Mukherjee, S. (1995). Regional cerebral blood flow in mood disorders: IV. Comparison of mania and depression. *Psychiatry Res*, 61(1), 1–10.

Rusch, B.D., Abercrombie, H.C., Oakes, T.R., Schaefer, S.M., and Davidson, R.J. (2001). Hippocampal morphometry in depressed patients and control subjects: Relations to anxiety symptoms. *Biol Psychiatry*, 50(12), 960–964.

Rush, A.J., Schlessor, M.A., Stokely, E., and Bonte, F.R. (1982). Cerebral blood flow in depression and mania. *Psychopharmacol Bull*, 18, 6–8.

Sachs, G.S., Renshaw, P.F., Lafer, B., Stoll, A.L., Guimaraes, A.R., Rosenbaum, J.F., and Gonzalez, R.G. (1995). Variability of brain lithium levels during maintenance treatment: A magnetic resonance spectroscopy study. *Biol Psychiatry*, 38(7), 422–428.

Sackeim, H.A. (1996). *Physiological perturbations in late-life depression: Implications for neuronal circuitry and effects of treatment*. 35th Annual Meeting of the American College of Neuropsychopharmacology, San Juan, Puerto Rico, December 9–13.

Sackeim, H.A., Prohovnik, I., Moeller, J.R., Brown, R.P., Apter, S., Prudic, J., Devanand, D.P., and Mukherjee, S. (1990). Regional cerebral blood flow in mood disorders. I. Comparison of major depressives and normal controls at rest. *Arch Gen Psychiatry*, 47(1), 60–70.

Sackeim, H.A., Prohovnik, I., Moeller, J.R., Mayeux, R., Stern, Y., and Devanand, D.P. (1993). Regional cerebral blood flow in mood disorders. II. Comparison of major depression and Alzheimer's disease. *J Nucl Med*, 34(7), 1090–1101.

Salloway, S., Malloy, P., Kohn, R., Gillard, E., Duffy, J., Rogg, J., Tung, G., Richardson, E., Thomas, C., and Westlake, R. (1996). MRI and neuropsychological differences in early- and late-life-onset geriatric depression. *Neurology*, 46(6), 1567–1574.

Salmon, E., Maquet, P., Sadzot, B., Degueldre, C., Lemaire, C., and Franck, G. (1991). Decrease of frontal metabolism demonstrated by positron emission tomography in a population of healthy elderly volunteers. *Acta Neurol Belg*, 91(5), 288–295.

Sanacora, G., Mason, G.F., Rothman, D.L., Behar, K.L., Hyder, F., Petroff, O.A., Berman, R.M., Charney, D.S., and Krystal, J.H. (1999). Reduced cortical gamma-aminobutyric acid levels in depressed patients determined by proton magnetic resonance spectroscopy. *Arch Gen Psychiatry*, 56(11), 1043–1047.

Sanacora, G., Mason, G.F., Rothman, D.L., and Krystal, J.H. (2002). Increased occipital cortex GABA concentrations in depressed patients after therapy with selective serotonin reuptake inhibitors. *Am J Psychiatry*, 159(4), 663–665.

Sanacora, G., Mason, G.F., Rothman, D.L., Hyder, F., Ciarcia, J.J., Ostroff, R.B., Berman, R.M., and Krystal, J.H. (2003). Increased cortical GABA concentrations in depressed patients receiving ECT. *Am J Psychiatry*, 160(3), 577–579.

Sanches, M., Sassi, R.B., Axelson, D., Nicoletti, M., Brambilla, P., Hatch, J.P., Keshavan, M.S., Ryan, N.D., Birmaher, B., and Soares, J.C. (2005). Subgenual prefrontal cortex of child and adolescent bipolar patients: A morphometric magnetic resonance imaging study. *Psychiatry Res*, 138(1), 43–49.

Sappey-Marinier, D., Calabrese, G., Hetherington, H.P., Fisher, S.N., Deicken, R., Van Dyke, C., Fein, G., and Weiner, M.W. (1992a). Proton magnetic resonance spectroscopy of human brain: Applications to normal white matter, chronic infarction, and MRI white matter signal hyperintensities. *Magn Reson Med*, 26(2), 313–327.

Sappey-Marinier, D., Deicken, R.F., Fein, G., Calabrese, G., Hubesch, B., Van Dyke, C., Dillon, W.P., Davenport, L., Meyerhoff, D.J., and Weiner, M.W. (1992b). Alterations in brain phosphorus metabolite concentrations associated with areas of high signal intensity in white matter at MR imaging. *Radiology*, 183(1), 247–256.

Sassi, R.B., Nicoletti, M., Brambilla, P., Harenski, K., Mallinger, A.G., Frank, E., Kupfer, D.J., Keshavan, M.S., and Soares, J.C. (2001). Decreased pituitary volume in patients with bipolar disorder. *Biol Psychiatry*, 50(4), 271–280.

Sassi, R.B., Brambilla, P., et al. (2002a). *Lithium influences the volume of the cingulate cortex in bipolar mood disorder patients*. 57th Annual Convention and Scientific Program of the Society of Biological Psychiatry, Philadelphia, PA, May 16–18.

Sassi, R.B., Nicoletti, M., Brambilla, P., Mallinger, A.G., Frank, E., Kupfer, D.J., Keshavan, M.S., and Soares, J.C. (2002b). Increased gray matter volume in lithium-treated bipolar disorder patients. *Neurosci Lett*, 329(2), 243–245.

Sassi, R.B., Brambilla, P., Nicoletti, M., Mallinger, A.G., Frank, E., Kupfer, D.J., Keshavan, M.S., and Soares, J.C. (2003). White matter hyperintensities in bipolar and unipolar patients with relatively mild-to-moderate illness severity. *J Affect Disord*, 77(3), 237–245.

Sassi, R.B., Brambilla, P., Hatch, J.P., Nicoletti, M.A., Mallinger, A.G., Frank, E., Kupfer, D.J., Keshavan, M.S., and Soares, J.C. (2004). Reduced left anterior cingulate volumes in untreated bipolar patients. *Biol Psychiatry*, 56(7), 467–475.

Sassi, R.B., Stanley, J.A., Axelson, D., Brambilla, P., Nicoletti, M.A., Keshavan, M.S., Ramos, R.T., Ryan, N., Birmaher, B., and Soares, J.C. (2005). Reduced NAA levels in the dorsolateral prefrontal cortex of young bipolar patients. *Am J Psychiatry*, 162(11), 2109–2115.

Sax, K.W., Strakowski, S.M., Zimmerman, M.E., DelBello, M.P., Keck, P.E. Jr., and Hawkins, J.M. (1999). Frontosubcortical neuroanatomy and the continuous performance test in mania. *Am J Psychiatry*, 156(1), 139–141.

Saxena, S., Brody, A.L., Ho, M.L., Alborzian, S., Ho, M.K., Maidment, K.M., Huang, S.C., Wu, H.M., Au, S.C., and Baxter, L.R. Jr. (2001). Cerebral metabolism in major depression and obsessive-compulsive disorder occurring separately and concurrently. *Biol Psychiatry*, 50(3), 159–170.

Scarr, E., Pavey, G., Sundram, S., MacKinnon, A., and Dean, B. (2003). Decreased hippocampal NMDA, but not kainite or AMPA receptors in bipolar disorder. *Bipolar Disord*, 5(4), 257–264.

Schlaepfer, T.E., Harris, G.J., Tien, A.Y., Peng, L.W., Lee, S., Federman, E.B., Chase, G.A., Barta, P.E., and Pearlson, G.D. (1994). Decreased regional cortical gray matter volume in schizophrenia. *Am J Psychiatry*, 151(6), 842–848.

Schlageter, N.L., Horwitz, B., Creasey, H., Carson, R., Duara, R., Berg, G.W., and Rapoport, S.I. (1987). Relation of measured brain glucose utilisation and cerebral atrophy in man. *J Neurol Neurosurg Psychiatry*, 50(6), 779–785.

Schlegel, S., and Kretzschmar, V. (1987). Computed tomography in affective disorders. Part I: ventricular and sulcal measurements. *Biol Psychiatry*, 22(1), 4–14.

Schlegel, S., Aldenhoff, J.B., Eissner, D., Lindner, P., and Nickel, O. (1989a). Regional cerebral blood flow in depression: Associations with psychopathology. *J Affect Disord*, 17(3), 211–218.

Schlegel, S., Frommberger, U., and Buller, R. (1989b). Computerized tomography (CT) in affective disorders: Relationship with psychopathology. *Psychiatry Res*, 29(3), 271–272.

Schlegel, S., von Bardeleben, U., Wiedemann, K., Frommberger, U., and Holsboer, F. (1989c). Computerized brain tomography measures compared with spontaneous and suppressed plasma cortisol levels in major depression. *Psychoneuroendocrinology*, 14(3), 209–216.

Schneider, F., Gur, R.E., Mozley, L.H., Smith, R.J., Mozley, P.D., Censits, D.M., Alavi, A., and Gur, R.C. (1995). Mood effects on limbic blood flow correlate with emotional self-rating: A PET study with oxygen-15 labeled water. *Psychiatry Res*, 61(4), 265–283.

Schneider, F., Grodd, W., Weiss, U., Klose, U., Mayer, K.R., Nagele, T., and Gur, R.C. (1997). Functional MRI reveals left amygdala activation during emotion. *Psychiatry Res*, 76(2-3), 75–82.

Schneider, F., Weiss, U., Kessler, C., Salloum, J.B., Posse, S., Grodd, W., and Muller-Gartner, H.W. (1998). Differential amygdala activation in schizophrenia during sadness. *Schizophr Res*, 34(3), 133–142.

Schneider, F., Hatbel, U., Kessler, C., Salloum, J.B., and Posse, S. (2000). Gender differences in regional cerebral activity during sadness. *Hum Brain Mapping*, 9(4), 226–238.

Schwartz, J.M., Baxter, L.R. Jr., Mazziotta, J.C., Gerner, R.H., and Phelps, M.E. (1987). The differential diagnosis of depression. Relevance of positron emission tomography studies of cerebral glucose metabolism to the bipolar–unipolar dichotomy. *JAMA*, 258(10), 1368–1374.

Schwartz, P.J., Loe, J.A., Bash, C.N., Bove, K., Turner, E.H., Frank, J.A., Wehr, T.A., and Rosenthal, N.E. (1997). Seasonality and pituitary volume. *Psychiatry Res*, 74(3), 151–157.

Scott, A.I., Dougall, N., Ross, M., O'Carroll, R.E., Riddle, W., Ebmeier, K.P., and Goodwin, G.M. (1994). Short-term effects of electroconvulsive treatment on the uptake of [99mTc]-exametazime into brain in major depression shown with single photon emission tomography. *J Affect Disord*, 30(1), 27–34.

Scott, M.L., Golden, C.J., Ruedrich, S.L., and Bishop, R.J. (1983). Ventricular enlargement in major depression. *Psychiatry Res*, 8(2), 91–93.

Shah, P.J., Ebmeier, K.P., Glabus, M.F., and Goodwin, G.M. (1998). Cortical grey matter reductions associated with treatment-resistant chronic unipolar depression. Controlled magnetic resonance imaging study. *Br J Psychiatry*, 172, 527–532.

Shah, S.A., Doraiswamy, P.M., Husain, M.M., Escalona, P.R., Na, C., Figiel, G.S., Patterson, L.J., Ellinwood, E.H. Jr., McDonald, W.M., and Boyko, O.B. (1992). Posterior fossa abnormalities in major depression: A controlled magnetic resonance imaging study. *Acta Psychiatr Scand*, 85(6), 474–479.

Sharma, R., Venkatasubramanian, P.N., Barany, M., and Davis, J.M. (1992). Proton magnetic resonance spectroscopy of the brain in schizophrenic and affective patients. *Schizophr Res*, 8(1), 43–49.

Sharma, V., Menon, R., Carr, T.J., Densmore, M., Mazmanian, D., and Williamson, P.C. (2003). An MRI study of subgenual prefrontal cortex in patients with familial and non-familial bipolar I disorder. *J Affect Disord*, 77(2), 167–171.

Sheline, Y.I., Wang, P.W., Gado, M.H., Csernansky, J.G., and Vannier, M.W. (1996). Hippocampal atrophy in recurrent major depression. *Proc Natl Acad Sci USA*, 93(9), 3908–3913.

Sheline, Y.I., Sanghavi, M., Mintun, M.A., and Gado, M.H. (1999). Depression duration but not age predicts hippocampal volume loss in medically healthy women with recurrent major depression. *J Neurosci*, 19(12), 5034–5043.

Sheline, Y.I., Barch, D.M., Barany, M., and Davis, J.M. (2001). Increased amygdala response to masked emotional faces in depressed subjects resolves with antidepressant treatment: An fMRI study. *Biol Psychiatry*, 50(9), 651–658.

Sheline, Y.I., Gado, M.H., and Kraemer, H.C. (2003). Untreated depression and hippocampal volume loss. *Am J Psychiatry*, 160(8), 1516–1518.

Shenton, M.E., Wible, C.G., and McCarley, R.W. (1997). A review of magnetic resonance imaging studies of brain abnormalities in schizophrenia. In K.R.R. Krishnan and P.M. Doriaswamy (Eds.), *Brain Imaging in Clinical Psychiatry* (pp. 297–380). New York: Marcel Dekker.

Shima, S., Shikano, T., Kitamura, T., Masuda, Y., Tsukumo, T., Kanba, S., and Asai, M. (1984). Depression and ventricular enlargement. *Acta Psychiatr Scand*, 70(3), 275–277.

Shiraishi, H., Koizumi, J., Hori, M., Terashima, Y., Suzuki, T., Saito, K., Mizukami, K., Tanaka, Y., and Yamaguchi, N. (1992). A computerized tomographic study in patients with delusional and non-delusional depression. *Jpn J Psychiatry Neurol*, 46(1), 99–105.

Silfverskiöld, P., and Risberg, J. (1989). Regional cerebral blood flow in depression and mania. *Arch Gen Psychiatry*, 46(3), 253–259.

Silverstone, P.H., Hanstock, C.C., Fabian, J., Staab, R., and Allen, P.S. (1996). Chronic lithium does not alter human myo-inositol or phosphomonoester concentrations as measured by 1H and 31P MRS. *Biol Psychiatry*, 40(4), 235–246.

Silverstone, P.H., Rotzinger, S., Pukhovsky, A., and Hanstock, C.C. (1999). Effects of lithium and amphetamine on inositol metabolism in the human brain as measured by 1H and 31P MRS. *Biol Psychiatry*, 46(12), 1634–1641.

Silverstone, P.H., Wu, R.H., O'Donnell, T., Ulrich, M., Asghar, S.J., and Hanstock, C.C. (2002). Chronic treatment with both lithium and sodium valproate may normalize phosphoinositol cycle activity in bipolar patients. *Hum Psychopharmacol*, 17(7), 321–327.

Silverstone, P.H., Wu, R.H., O'Donnell, T., Ulrich, M., Asghar, S.J., and Hanstock, C.C. (2003). Chronic treatment with lithium, but not sodium valproate, increases cortical N-acetyl-aspartate concentrations in euthymic bipolar patients. *Int Clin Psychopharmacol*, 18(2), 73–79.

Silverstone, P.H., Asghar, S.J., O'Donnell, T., Ulrich, M., and Hanstock, C.C. (2004). Lithium and valproate protect against dextro-amphetamine induced brain choline concentration changes in bipolar disorder patients. *World J Biol Psychiatry*, 5(1), 38–44.

Silverstone, T., McPherson, H., Li, Q., and Doyle, T. (2003). Deep white matter hyperintensities in patients with bipolar depression, unipolar depression and age-matched control subjects. *Bipolar Disord*, 5(1), 53–57.

Simpson, S., Baldwin, R.C., Jackson, A., and Burns, A.S. (1998). Is subcortical disease associated with a poor response to antidepressants? Neurological, neuropsychological and neuroradiological findings in late-life depression. *Psychol Med*, 28(5), 1015–1026.

Simpson, S.W., Baldwin, R.C., Burns, A., and Jackson, A. (2001). Regional cerebral volume measurements in late-life depression: Relationship to clinical correlates, neuropsychological impairment and response to treatment. *Int J Geriatr Psychiatry*, 16(5), 469–476.

Smith, E.A., Russell, A., Lorch, E., Banerjee, S.P., Rose, M., Ivey, J., Bhandari, R., Moore, G.J., and Rosenberg, D.R. (2003). Increased medial thalamic choline found in pediatric patients with obsessive-compulsive disorder versus major depression or healthy control subjects: A magnetic resonance spectroscopy study. *Biol Psychiatry*, 54(12), 1399–1405.

Smith, K.A., Morris, J.S., Friston, K.J., Cowen, P.J., and Dolan, R.J. (1999). Brain mechanisms associated with depressive relapse and associated cognitive impairment following acute tryptophan depletion. *Br J Psychiatry*, 174, 525–529.

Soares, J.C., Boada, F., et al. (1999). *NAA and choline measurements in the anterior cingulate of bipolar disorder patients.* 54th Annual Convention and Scientific Program of the Society of Biological Psychiatry, Washington, DC, May 13–15.

Soares, J.C., Boada, F., Spencer, S., Mallinger, A.G., Dippold, C.S., Wells, K.F., Frank, E., Keshavan, M.S., Gershon, S., and Kupfer, D.J. (2001). Brain lithium concentrations in bipolar disorder patients: Preliminary (7)Li magnetic resonance studies at 3 T. *Biol Psychiatry*, 49(5), 437–443.

Sonawalla, S.B., Renshaw, P.F., Moore, C.M., Alpert, J.E., Nierenberg, A.A., Rosenbaum, J.F., and Fava, M. (1999). Compounds containing cytosolic choline in the basal ganglia: A potential biological marker of true drug response to fluoxetine. *Am J Psychiatry*, 156(10), 1638–1640.

Speer, A.M., Upadhyaya, V.H., et al. (1997). *New windows into bipolar illness: Serial perfusion MRI scanning in rapid-cycling bipolar patients.* 150th Annual Meeting of the American Psychiatric Association, San Diego, CA, May 17–22.

Sprengelmeyer, R., Rausch, M., Eysel, U.T., and Przuntek, H. (1998). Neural structures associated with recognition of facial expressions of basic emotions. *Proc R Soc Lond B Biol Sci*, 265(1409), 1927–1931.

Standish-Barry, H.M., Hale, A.S., Honig, A., Bouras, N., Bridges, P.K., and Bartlett, J.R. (1985). Ventricular size, the dexamethasone suppression test and outcome of severe endogenous depression following psychosurgery. *Acta Psychiatr Scand*, 72(2), 166–171.

Starkstein, S.E., and Robinson, R.G. (1989). Affective disorders and cerebrovascular disease. *Br J Psychiatry*, 154, 170–182.

Starkstein, S.E., Mayberg, H.S., Berthier, M.L., Fedoroff, P., Price, T.R., Dannals, R.F., Wagner, H.N., Leiguarda, R., and Robinson, R.G. (1990). Mania after brain injury: Neuroradiological and metabolic findings. *Ann Neurol*, 7(6), 652–659.

Steffens, D.C., and Krishnan, K.R. (1998). Structural neuroimaging and mood disorders: Recent findings, implications for classification, and future directions. *Biol Psychiatry*, 43(10), 705–712.

Steffens, D.C., Byrum, C.E., McQuoid, D.R., Greenberg, D.L., Payne, M.E., Blitchington, T.F., MacFall, J.R., and Krishnan, K.R. (2000). Hippocampal volume in geriatric depression. *Biol Psychiatry*, 48(4), 301–309.

Steingard, R.J., Yurgelun-Todd, D.A., Hennen, J., Moore, J.C., Moore, C.M., Vakili, K., Young, A.D., Katic, A., Beardslee, W.R., and Renshaw, P.F. (2000). Increased orbitofrontal cortex levels of choline in depressed adolescents as detected by in vivo proton magnetic resonance spectroscopy. *Biol Psychiatry*, 48(11), 1053–1061.

Steingard, R.J., Renshaw, P.F., Hennen, J., Lenox, M., Cintron, C.B., Young, A.D., Connor, D.F., Au, T.H., and Yurgelun-Todd, D.A. (2002). Smaller frontal lobe white matter volumes in depressed adolescents. *Biol Psychiatry*, 52(5), 413–417.

Stern, R.A., and Bachmann, D.L. (1991). Depressive symptoms following stroke. *Am J Psychiatry*, 148, 351–356.

Stoll, A.L., Renshaw, P.F., Sachs, G.S., Guimaraes, A.R., Miller, C., Cohen, B.M., Lafer, B., and Gonzalez, R.G. (1992). The human brain resonance of choline-containing compounds is similar in patients receiving lithium treatment and controls: An in vivo proton magnetic resonance spectroscopy study. *Biol Psychiatry*, 32(10), 944–949.

Stoll, A.L., Renshaw, P.F., De Micheli, E., Wurtman, R., Pillay, S.S., and Cohen, B.M. (1995). Choline ingestion increases the resonance of choline-containing compounds in human brain: An in vivo proton magnetic resonance study. *Biol Psychiatry*, 37(3), 170–174.

Stoll, A.L., Sachs, G.S., Cohen, B.M., Lafer, B., Christensen, J.D., and Renshaw, P.F. (1996). Choline in the treatment of rapid-cycling bipolar disorder: Clinical and neurochemical findings in lithium-treated patients. *Biol Psychiatry*, 40(5), 382–388.

Strakowski, S.M., Wilson, D.R., Tohen, M., Woods, B.T., Douglass, A.W., and Stoll, A.L. (1993a). Structural brain abnormalities in first-episode mania. *Biol Psychiatry*, 33(8-9), 602–609.

Strakowski, S.M., Woods, B.T., Tohen, M., Wilson, D.R., Douglass, A.W., and Stoll, A.L. (1993b). MRI subcortical signal hyperintensities in mania at first hospitalization. *Biol Psychiatry*, 33(3), 204–206.

Strakowski, S.M., DelBello, M.P., Sax, K.W., Zimmerman, M.E., Shear, P.K., Hawkins, J.M., and Larson, E.R. (1999). Brain magnetic resonance imaging of structural abnormalities in bipolar disorder. *Arch Gen Psychiatry*, 56(3), 254–260.

Strakowski, S.M., DelBello, M.P., Zimmerman, M.E., Getz, G.E., Mills, N.P., Ret, J., Shear, P., and Adler, C.M. (2002). Ventricular and periventricular structural volumes in first- versus multiple-episode bipolar disorder. *Am J Psychiatry*, 159(11), 1841–1847.

Strasser, H.C., Honeycutt, N.A., et al. (2002). *Amygdala volumes in psychotic versus nonpsychotic bipolar disorder and schizophrenia.* 57th Annual Convention and Scientific Program of the Society of Biological Psychiatry, Philadelphia, PA, May 16–18.

Swayze, V.W. II, Andreasen, N.C., Alliger, R.J., Ehrhardt, J.C., and Yuh, W.T. (1990). Structural brain abnormalities in bipolar affective disorder. Ventricular enlargement and focal signal hyperintensities. *Arch Gen Psychiatry*, 47(11), 1054–1059.

Swayze, V.W. II, Andreasen, N.C., Alliger, R.J., Yuh, W.T., and Ehrhardt, J.C. (1992). Subcortical and temporal structures in affective disorder and schizophrenia: A magnetic resonance imaging study. *Biol Psychiatry*, 31(3), 221–240.

Tan, J., Bluml, S., Hoang, T., Dubowitz, D., Mevenkamp, G., and Ross, B. (1998). Lack of effect of oral choline supplement on the concentrations of choline metabolites in human brain. *Magn Reson Med*, 39(6), 1005–1010.

Tanaka, Y., Hazama, H., Fukuhara, T., and Tsutsuim T. (1982). Computerized tomography of the brain in manic-depressive patients: A controlled study. *Folia Psychiatr Neurol Jpn*, 36, 137–143.

Targum, S.D., Rosen, L.N., DeLisi, L.E., Weinberger, D.R., and Citrin, C.M. (1983). Cerebral ventricular size in major depressive disorder: Association with delusional symptoms. *Biol Psychiatry*, 18(3), 329–336.

Taylor, W.D., Payne, M.E., Krishnan, K.R., Wagner, H.R., Provenzale, J.M., Steffens, D.C., and MacFall, J.R. (2001). Evidence of white matter tract disruption in MRI hyperintensities. *Biol Psychiatry*, 50(3), 179–183.

Taylor, W.D., Steffens, D.C., MacFall, J.R., McQuoid, D.R., Payne, M.E., Provenzale, J.M., and Krishnan, K.R. (2003). White matter hyperintensity progression and late-life depression outcomes. *Arch Gen Psychiatry*, 60(11), 1090–1096.

Taylor, W.D., MacFall, J.R., Payne, M.E., McQuoid, D.R., Provenzale, J.M., Steffens, D.C., and Krishman, K.R. (2004). Late-life depression and microstructural abnormalities in dorsolateral prefrontal cortex white matter. *Am J Psychiatry*, 161(7), 1293–1296.

Teneback, C.C., Nahas, Z., Speer, A.M., Molloy, M., Stallings, L.E., Spicer, K.M., Risch, S.C., and George, M.S. (1999). Changes in prefrontal cortex and paralimbic activity in depression following two weeks of daily left prefrontal TMS. *J Neuropsychiatry Clin Neurosci*, 11(4), 426–435.

Thomas, K.M., Drevets, W.C., Whalen, P.J., Eccard, C.H., Dahl, R.E., Ryan, N.D., and Casey, B.J. (2001). Amygdala response to facial expressions in children and adults. *Biol Psychiatry*, 49(4), 309–316.

Thomas, P., Vaiva, G., Samaille, E., Maron, M., Alaix, C., Steinling, M., and Goudemand, M. (1993). Cerebral blood flow in major depression and dysthymia. *J Affect Disord*, 29(4), 235–242.

Trivedi, M.H., Blackburn, T., et al. (1995). *Effects of amphetamine in major depressive disorder using functional MRI.* 50th Annual Meeting of the Society of Biological Psychiatry, Miami, FL, May 17–20.

Tsai, L., Nasrallah, H.A., and Jacoby, C.G. (1983). Hemispheric asymmetries on computed tomographic scans in schizophrenia and mania. *Arch Gen Psychiatry*, 39, 1286–1289.

Tutus, A., Kibar, M., Sofuoglu, S., Basturk, M., and Gonul, A.S. (1998a). A technetium-^{99m} hexamethylpropylene amine oxime brain single-photon emission tomography study in adolescent patients with major depressive disorder. *Eur J Nucl Med*, 25(6), 601–606.

Tutus, A., Simsek, A., Sofuoglu, S., Nardali, M., Kugu, N., Karaaslan, F., and Gonul, A.S. (1998b). Changes in regional cerebral blood flow demonstrated by single photon emission computed tomography in depressive disorders: Comparison of unipolar vs. bipolar subtypes. *Psychiatry Res*, 83(3), 169–177.

Upadhyaya, A.K., Abou-Saleh, M.T., Wilson, K., Grime, S.J., and Critchley, M. (1990). A study of depression in old age using single-photon emission computerised tomography. *Br J Psychiatry Suppl*, 157(Suppl. 9), 76–81.

Vakili, K., Pillay, S.S., Lafer, B., Fava, M., Renshaw, P.F., Bonello-Cintron, C.M., and Yurgelun-Todd, D.A. (2000). Hippocampal volume in primary unipolar major depression: A magnetic resonance imaging study. *Biol Psychiatry*, 47(12), 1087–1090.

Van den Bossche, B., Maes, M., Brussaard, C., Schotte, C., Cosyns, P., De Moor, J., and De Schepper, A. (1991). Computed tomography of the brain in unipolar depression. *J Affect Disord*, 21(1), 67–74.

Vasile, R.G., Schwartz, R.B., Garada, B., Holman, B.L., Alpert, M., Davidson, P.B., and Schildkraut, J.J. (1996). Focal cerebral perfusion defects demonstrated by ^{99m}Tc-hexamethylpropyleneamine oxime SPECT in elderly depressed patients. *Psychiatry Res*, 67(1), 59–70.

Vasile, R.G., Sachs, G., Anderson, J.L., Lafer, B., Matthews, E., and Hill, T. (1997). Changes in regional cerebral blood flow following light treatment for seasonal affective disorder: Responders versus nonresponders. *Biol Psychiatry*, 42(11), 1000–1005.

Velakoulis, D., Pantelis, C., McGorry, P.D., Dudgeon, P., Brewer, W., Cook, M., Desmond, P., Bridle, N., Tierney, P., Murrie, V., Singh, B., and Copolov, D. (1999). Hippocampal volume in first-episode psychoses and chronic schizophrenia: A high-resolution magnetic resonance imaging study. *Arch Gen Psychiatry*, 56(2), 133–141.

Videbech, P. (1997). MRI findings in patients with affective disorder: A meta-analysis. *Acta Psychiatr Scand*, 96(3), 157–168.

Videbech, P., and Ravnkilde, B. (2004). Hippocampal volume and depression: A meta-analysis of MRI studies. *Am J Psychiatry*, 161(11), 1957–1966.

Videbech, P., Ravnkilde, B., Pedersen, A.R., Egander, A., Landbo, B., Rasmussen, N.A., Andersen, F., Stodkilde-Jorgensen, H., Gjedde, A., and Rosenberg, R. (2001). The Danish PET/depression project: PET findings in patients with major depression. *Psychol Med*, 31(7), 1147–1158.

Videbech, P., Ravnkilde, B., Pedersen, T.H., Hartvig, H., Egander, A., Clemmensen, K., Rasmussen, N.A., Andersen, F., Gjedde, A., and Rosenberg, R. (2002). The Danish PET/depression project: Clinical symptoms and cerebral blood flow. A regions-of-interest analysis. *Acta Psychiatr Scand*, 106(1), 35–44.

Vita, A., Sacchetti, E., and Cazzullo, C.L. (1988). A CT follow-up study of cerebral ventricular size in schizophrenia and major affective disorder. *Schizophr Res*, 1, 165–166.

Volk, S.A., Kaendler, S.H., Hertel, A., Maul, F.D., Manoocheri, R., Weber, R., Georgi, K., Pflug, B., and Hor, G. (1997). Can response to partial sleep deprivation in depressed patients be predicted by regional changes of cerebral blood flow? *Psychiatry Res*, 75, 67–74.

Volkow, N.D., Fowler, J.S., et al. (1991). *Abnormal dopamine brain activity in cocaine abusers.* 30th Annual Meeting of the American College of Neuropsychopharmacology, San Juan, Puerto Rico, December 9–13.

Volkow, N.D., Wang, G.J., Fowler, J.S., Hitzemann, R., Pappas, N., Pascani, K., and Wong, C. (1997). Gender differences in cerebellar metabolism: Test–retest reproducibility. *Am J Psychiatry*, 154(1), 119–121.

Volz, H.P., Rzanny, R., Riehemann, S., May, S., Hegewald, H., Preussler, B., Hubner, G., Kaiser, W.A., and Sauer, H. (1998). 31P magnetic resonance spectroscopy in the frontal lobe of major depressed patients. *Eur Arch Psychiatry Clin Neurosci*, 248(6), 289–295.

von Gunten, A., Fox, N.C., Cipolotti, L., and Ron, M.A. (2000). A volumetric study of hippocampus and amygdala in depressed patients with subjective memory problems. *J Neuropsychiatry Clin Neurosci*, 12(4), 493–498.

Vythilingam, M., Heim, C., Newport, J., Miller, A.H., Anderson, E., Bronen, R., Brummer, M., Staib, L., Vermetten, E., Charney, D.S., Nemeroff, C.B., and Bremner, J.D. (2002). Childhood trauma associated with smaller hippocampal volume in women with major depression. *Am J Psychiatry*, 159(12), 2072–2080.

Vythilingam, M., Charles, H.C., Tupler, L.A., Blitchington, T., Kelly, L., and Krishnan, K.R. (2003). Focal and lateralized subcortical abnormalities in unipolar major depressive disorder: An automated multivoxel proton magnetic resonance spectroscopy study. *Biol Psychiatry*, 54(7), 744–750.

Wang, G.J., Volkow, N.D., et al. (1994). Intersubject variability of brain glucose metabolic measurements in young normal males. *J Nucl Med*, 35(9), 1457–1466.

Wang, P.W., Dieckmann, N., et al. (2002). *3 Tesla ¹H-magnetic resonance spectroscopic measurements of prefrontal cortical gamma-aminobutyric acid (GABA) levels in bipolar disorder patients and healthy volunteers*. 57th Annual Convention and Scientific Program of the Society of Biological Psychiatry, Philadelphia, PA, May 16–18.

Ward, K.E., Friedman, L., Wise, A., and Schulz, S.C. (1996). Meta-analysis of brain and cranial size in schizophrenia. *Schizophr Res*, 22(3), 197–213.

Watanabe, A., Kato, N., and Kato, T. (2002). Effects of creatine on mental fatigue and cerebral hemoglobin oxygenation. *Neurosci Res*, 42(4), 279–285.

Weinberger, D.R., DeLisi, L.E., Perman, G.P., Targum, S., and Wyatt, R.J. (1982). Computed tomography in schizophreniform disorder and other acute psychiatric disorders. *Arch Gen Psychiatry*, 39(7), 778–783.

Whalen, P.J., Rauch, S.L., Etcoff, N.L., McInerney, S.C., Lee, M.B., and Jenike, M.A. (1998). Masked presentations of emotional facial expressions modulate amygdala activity without explicit knowledge. *J Neurosci*, 18(1), 411–418.

Wilke, M., Kowatch, R.A., DelBello, M.P., Mills, N.P., and Holland, S.K. (2004). Voxel-based morphometry in adolescents with bipolar disorder: First results. *Psychiatry Res*, 131(1), 57–69.

Willis, M.W., Ketter, T.A., Kimbrell, T.A., George, M.S., Herscovitch, P., Danielson, A.L., Benson, B.E., and Post, R.M. (2002). Age, sex and laterality effects on cerebral glucose metabolism in healthy adults. *Psychiatry Res*, 114(1), 23–37.

Wilson, J., Kupfer, D.J., et al. (2002). *Ventral striatal metabolism is increased in depression, and decreases with treatment*. 57th Annual Convention and Scientific Program of the Society of Biological Psychiatry, Philadelphia, PA, May 16–18.

Winsberg, M.E., Sachs, N., Tate, D.L., Adalsteinsson, E., Spielman, D., and Ketter, T.A. (2000). Decreased dorsolateral prefrontal *N*-acetyl aspartate in bipolar disorder. *Biol Psychiatry*, 47(6), 475–481.

Woods, B.T., Yurgelun-Todd, D., Benes, F.M., Frankenburg, F.R., Pope, H.G. Jr., and McSparren, J. (1990). Progressive ventricular enlargement in schizophrenia: Comparison to bipolar affective disorder and correlation with clinical course. *Biol Psychiatry*, 27(3), 341–352.

Woods, B.T., Brennan, S., Yurgelun-Todd, D., Young, T., and Panzarino, P. (1995a). MRI abnormalities in major psychiatric disorders: An exploratory comparative study. *J Neuropsychiatry Clin Neurosci*, 7(1), 49–53.

Woods, B.T., Yurgelun-Todd, D., Mikulis, D., and Pillay, S.S. (1995b). Age-related MRI abnormalities in bipolar illness: A clinical study. *Biol Psychiatry*, 38(12), 846–847.

Wu, J.C., Gillin, J.C., Buchsbaum, M.S., Hershey, T., Johnson, J.C., and Bunney, W.E. Jr. (1992). Effect of sleep deprivation on brain metabolism of depressed patients. *Am J Psychiatry*, 149(4), 538–543.

Wu, J.C., Buchsbaum, M.S., Johnson, J.C., Hershey, T.G., Wagner, E.A., Teng, C., and Lottenberg, S. (1993). Magnetic resonance and positron emission tomography imaging of the corpus callosum: Size, shape and metabolic rate in unipolar depression. *J Affect Disord*, 28(1), 15–25.

Wu, J., Buchsbaum, M.S., Gillin, J.C., Tang, C., Cadwell, S., Wiegand, M., Najafi, A., Klein, E., Hazen, K., Bunney, W.E. Jr., Fallon, J.H., and Keator, D. (1999). Prediction of antidepressant effects of sleep deprivation by metabolic rates in the ventral anterior cingulate and medial prefrontal cortex. *Am J Psychiatry*, 156(8), 1149–1158.

Wu, R.H., O'Donnell, T., Ulrich, M., Asghar, S.J., Hanstock, C.C., and Silverstone, P.H. (2004). Brain choline concentrations may not be altered in euthymic bipolar disorder patients chronically treated with either lithium or sodium valproate. *Ann Gen Hosp Psychiatry*, 3(1), 13.

Wurthmann, C., Bogerts, B., and Falkai, P. (1995). Brain morphology assessed by computed tomography in patients with geriatric depression, patients with degenerative dementia, and normal control subjects. *Psychiatry Res*, 61(2), 103–111.

Yates, W.R., Jacoby, C.G., and Andreasen, N.C. (1987). Cerebellar atrophy in schizophrenia and affective disorder. *Am J Psychiatry*, 144(4), 465–467.

Yazici, K.M., Kapucu, O., Erbas, B., Varoglu, E., Gulec, C., and Bekdik, C.F. (1992). Assessment of changes in regional cerebral blood flow in patients with major depression using the ⁹⁹ᵐTc-HMPAO single photon emission tomography method. *Eur J Nucl Med*, 19(12), 1038–1043.

Yildiz, A., Demopulos, C.M., Moore, C.M., Renshaw, P.F., and Sachs, G.S. (2001a). Effect of lithium on phosphoinositide metabolism in human brain: A proton decoupled (31)P magnetic resonance spectroscopy study. *Biol Psychiatry*, 50(1), 3–7.

Yildiz, A., Sachs, G.S., Dorer, D.J., and Renshaw, P.F. (2001b). 31P Nuclear magnetic resonance spectroscopy findings in bipolar illness: A meta-analysis. *Psychiatry Res*, 106(3), 181–191.

Yoshii, F., Barker, W.W., Chang, J.Y., Loewenstein, D., Apicella, A., Smith, D., Boothe, T., Ginsberg, M.D., Pascal, S., and Duara, R. (1988). Sensitivity of cerebral glucose metabolism to age, gender, brain volume, brain atrophy, and cerebrovascular risk factors. *J Cereb Blood Flow Metab*, 8(5), 654–661.

Young, R.C., Nambudiri, D., et al. (1988). *Ventricular-brain ratio and response to nortriptyline in geriatric depression* [abstract]. 43rd Annual Meeting of the Society of Biological Psychiatry.

Young, R.C., Bocksberger, J.P., et al. (1996). *Putamen volume and age at onset in geriatric mania*. 149th Annual Meeting of the American Psychiatric Association, New York, NY, May 4–9.

Yurgelun-Todd, D.A., Gruber, S.A., Kanayama, G., Killgore, W.D., Baird, A.A., and Young, A.D. (2000). fMRI during affect discrimination in bipolar affective disorder. *Bipolar Disord*, 2(3 Pt. 2), 237–248.

Zipursky, R.B., Seeman, M.V., Bury, A., Langevin, R., Wortzman, G., and Katz, R. (1997). Deficits in gray matter volume are present in schizophrenia but not bipolar disorder. *Schizophr Res*, 26(2-3), 85–92.

Zubenko, G.S., Sullivan, P., Nelson, J.P., Belle, S.H., Huff, F.J., and Wolf, G.L. (1990). Brain imaging abnormalities in mental disorders of late life. *Arch Neurol*, 47(10), 1107–1111.

CHAPTER 16

Abe, M., Herzog, E.D., and Block, G.D. (2000). Lithium lengthens the circadian period of individual suprachiasmatic nucleus neurons. *Neuroreport*, 11(14), 3261–3264.

Achermann, P., and Borbely, A.A. (1998). Coherence analysis of the human sleep electroencephalogram. *Neuroscience*, 85(4), 1195–1208.

Aeschbach, D., and Borbely, A.A. (1993). All-night dynamics of the human sleep EEG. *J Sleep Res*, 2(2), 70–81.

Aeschbach, D., Matthews, J.R., Postolache, T.T., Jackson, M.A., Giesen, H.A., and Wehr, T.A. (1999). Two circadian rhythms in the human electroencephalogram during wakefulness. *Am J Physiol*, 277(6 Pt. 2), R1771–R1779.

Aeschbach, D., Postolache, T. T., Sher, L., Matthews, J.R., Jackson, M.A., and Wehr, T.A. (2001a). Evidence from the waking electroencephalogram that short sleepers live under higher homeostatic sleep pressure than long sleepers. *Neuroscience*, 102(3), 493–502.

Aeschbach, D., Sher, L., Postolache, T.T., Matthews, J.R., Jackson, M.A., and Wehr, T.A. (2001b). A longer biological night in long sleepers than in short sleepers. *Sleep*, 24(Suppl.), 8.

Aeschbach, D., Sher, L., Postolache, T.T., Matthews, J.R., Jackson, M.A., and Wehr, T.A. (2003). A longer biological night in long sleepers than in short sleepers. *J Clin Endocrinol Metab*, 88(1), 26–30.

Albert, R., Merz, A., Schubert, J., and Ebert, D. (1998). Sleep deprivation and subsequent sleep phase advance stabilizes the positive effect of sleep deprivation in depressive episodes. *Nervenarzt*, 69(1), 66–69.

Allada, R., Emery, P., Takahashi, J. S., and Rosbash, M. (2001). Stopping time: The genetics of fly and mouse circadian clocks. *Annu Rev Neurosci*, 24, 1091–1119.

Allen, G., Rappe, J., Earnest, D. J., and Cassone, V. M. (2001). Oscillating on borrowed time: Diffusible signals from immortalized suprachiasmatic nucleus cells regulate circadian rhythmicity in cultured fibroblasts. *J Neurosci*, 21(20), 7937–7943.

Amzica, F., and Steriade, M. (1998). Electrophysiological correlates of sleep delta waves. *Electroencephalogr Clin Neurophysiol*, 107(2), 69–83.

Anand, A., Charney, D.S., Delgado, P.L., McDougle, C.J., Heninger, G.R., and Price, L.H. (1994). Neuroendocrine and behavioral responses to intravenous m-chlorophenylpiperazine (mCPP) in depressed patients and healthy comparison subjects. *Am J Psychiatry*, 151(11), 1626–1630.

Anderson, J.L., Vasile, R.G., Mooney, J.J., Bloomingdale, K.L., Samson, J.A., and Schildkraut, J.J. (1992). Changes in norepi-nephrine output following light therapy for fall/winter seasonal depression. *Biol Psychiatry*, 32(8), 700–704.

Anderson, J.L., Rosen, L.N., Mendelson, W.B., Jacobsen, F.M., Skwerer, R.G., Joseph-Vanderpool, J.R., Duncan, C.C., Wehr, T.A., and Rosenthal, N.E. (1994). Sleep in fall/winter seasonal affective disorder: Effects of light and changing seasons. *J Psychosom Res*, 38(4), 323–337.

Arbisi, P.A., Depue, R.A., Spoont, M.R., Leon, A., and Ainsworth, B. (1989). Thermoregulatory response to thermal challenge in seasonal affective disorder: A preliminary report. *Psychiatry Res*, 28(3), 323–334.

Arbisi, P.A., Depue, R.A., Krauss, S., Spoont, M.R., Leon, A., Ainsworth, B., and Muir, R. (1994). Heat-loss response to a thermal challenge in seasonal affective disorder. *Psychiatry Res*, 52(2), 199–214.

Archer, S.N., Robilliard, D.L., Skene, D.J., Smits, M., Williams, A., Arendt, J., and von Schantz, M. (2003). A length polymorphism in the circadian clock gene Per3 is linked to delayed sleep phase syndrome and extreme diurnal preference. *Sleep*, 26(4), 413–415.

Asada, H., Fukuda, Y., Tsunoda, S., Yamaguchi, M., and Tonoike, M. (1999). Frontal midline theta rhythms reflect alternative activation of prefrontal cortex and anterior cingulate cortex in humans. *Neurosci Lett*, 274(1), 29–32.

Aschoff, J.C. (1981a). History and clinical symptoms of brain tumors. *Aktuelle Probl Chir Orthop*, 18, 15–19.

Aschoff, J.C. (1981c). Free running and entrained circadian rhythms. In J. Aschoff (Ed.), *Handbook of Behavorial Neurobiology, Vol. 4 Biological Rhythms* (pp. 81–93). New York: Plenum Press.

Aschoff, J.C., and Wever, R. (1980). On reproducibility of circadian rhythms in man [in German]. *Klin Wochenschr*, 58(7), 323–335.

Aschoff, J.C., and Wever, R. (1981). The circadian system as discussed in psychiatric research. In T.A. Wehr and F.K. Goodwin (Eds.), *Circadian Rhythms in Psychiatry* (pp. 311–331). Pacific Grove, CA: The Boxwood Press.

Aschoff, U. (1981b). Scotopic and photopic parts of light and dark vibrations in the electrooculograph. *Dev Ophthalmol*, 4, 149–166.

Ashman, S.B., Monk, T.H., Kupfer, D.J., Clark, C.H., Myers, F.S., Frank, E., and Leibenluft, E. (1999). Relationship between social rhythms and mood in patients with rapid cycling bipolar disorder. *Psychiatry Res*, 86(1), 1–8.

Asikainen, M., Toppila, J., Alanko, L., Ward, D.J., Stenberg, D., and Porkka-Heiskanen, T. (1997). Sleep deprivation increases brain serotonin turnover in the rat. *Neuroreport*, 8(7), 1577–1582.

Avery, D.H., Bolte, M.A., Dager, S.R., Wilson, L.G., Weyer, M., Cox, G.B., and Dunner, D.L. (1993). Dawn simulation treatment of winter depression: A controlled study. *Am J Psychiatry*, 150(1), 113–117.

Avery, D.H., Bolte, M.A., and Ries, R. (1998). Dawn simulation treatment of abstinent alcoholics with winter depression. *J Clin Psychiatry*, 59(1), 36–42; quiz 43–34.

Baastrup, P.C., and Schou, M. (1967). Lithium as a prophylactic agent: Its effect agains recurrent depression and manic-depressive psychosis. *Arch Gen Psychiatry*, 16, 162–172.

Baillarger, J. (1854). Note sur un genre de folie dont les accés sont caractérisés par deux périodes régulières, l'une de depression et l'autre d'excitation. *Gazette Hebdomadaire de Medecine et Chirurgie*, 132, 263–265.

Barbini, B., Bertelli, S., Colombo, C., and Smeraldi, E. (1996). Sleep loss, a possible factor in augmenting manic episode. *Psychiatry Res*, 65(2), 121–125.

Barbini, B., Colombo, C., Benedetti, F., Campori, E., Bellodi, L., and Smeraldi, E. (1998). The unipolar–bipolar dichotomy and the response to sleep deprivation. *Psychiatry Res*, 79(1), 43–50.

Barinaga, M. (2002). Circadian clock. How the brain's clock gets daily enlightenment. *Science*, 295(5557), 955–957.

Bauer, M., Grof, P., Rasgon, N., Bschor, T., Glenn, T., and Whybrow, P.C. (2006). Temporal relation between sleep and mood in patients with bipolar disorder. *Bipolar Disord*, 8(2), 160–167.

Beersma, D.G. (1990). Do winter depressives experience summer nights in winter? *Arch Gen Psychiatry*, 47(9), 879–880.

Benca, R.M., Obermeyer, W.H., Thisted, R.A., and Gillin, J.C. (1992). Sleep and psychiatric disorders. A meta-analysis. *Arch Gen Psychiatry*, 49(8), 651–668, discussion 669–670.

Benedetti, F., Barbini, B., Campori, E., Colombo, C., and Smeraldi, E. (1996). Dopamine agonist amineptine prevents the antidepressant effect of sleep deprivation. *Psychiatry Res*, 65(3), 179–184.

Benedetti, F., Barbini, B., Lucca, A., Campori, E., Colombo, C., and Smeraldi, E. (1997). Sleep deprivation hastens the antidepressant action of fluoxetine. *Eur Arch Psychiatry Clin Neurosci*, 247(2), 100–103.

Benedetti, F., Colombo, C., Barbini, B., Campori, E., and Smeraldi, E. (1999a). Ongoing lithium treatment prevents relapse after total sleep deprivation. *J Clin Psychopharmacol*, 19(3), 240–245.

Benedetti, F., Serretti, A., Colombo, C., Campori, E., Barbini, B., di Bella, D., and Smeraldi, E. (1999b). Influence of a functional polymorphism within the promoter of the serotonin transporter gene on the effects of total sleep deprivation in bipolar depression. *Am J Psychiatry*, 156(9), 1450–1452.

Benedetti, F., Barbini, B., Campori, E., Fulgosi, M.C., Pontiggia, A., and Colombo, C. (2001a). Sleep phase advance and lithium to sustain the antidepressant effect of total sleep deprivation in bipolar depression: New findings supporting the internal coincidence model? *J Psychiatr Res*, 35(6), 323–329.

Benedetti, F., Campori, E., Barbini, B., Fulgosi, M.C., and Colombo, C. (2001b). Dopaminergic augmentation of sleep deprivation effects in bipolar depression. *Psychiatry Res*, 104(3), 239–246.

Benna, C., Scannapieco, P., Piccin, A., Sandrelli, F., Zordan, M., Rosato, E., Kyriacou, C.P., Valle, G., and Costa, R. (2000). A second *timeless* gene in *Drosophila* shares greater sequence similarity with mammalian *tim*. *Curr Biol*, 10(14), R512–R513.

Berger, M., Riemann, D., Hochli, D., and Spiegel, R. (1989). The cholinergic rapid eye movement sleep induction test with RS-86. State or trait marker of depression? *Arch Gen Psychiatry*, 46(5), 421–428.

Berger, M., Vollmann, J., Hohagen, F., Konig, A., Lohner, H., Voderholzer, U., and Riemann, D. (1997). Sleep deprivation combined with consecutive sleep phase advance as a fast-acting therapy in depression: An open pilot trial in medicated and unmedicated patients. *Am J Psychiatry*, 154(6), 870–872.

Berger, P.A., Watson, S.J., Akil, H., and Barchas, J.D. (1986). Investigating opioid peptides in schizophrenia and depression. *Res Publ Assoc Res Nerv Ment Dis*, 64, 309–333.

Berson, D.M., Dunn, F.A., and Takao, M. (2002). Phototransduction by retinal ganglion cells that set the circadian clock. *Science*, 295(5557), 1070–1073.

Blacker, C.V., Thomas, J.M., and Thompson, C. (1997). Seasonality prevalence and incidence of depressive disorder in a general practice sample: Identifying differences in timing by caseness. *J Affect Disord*, 43(1), 41–52.

Blacker, D., Faraone, S.V., Rosen, A.E., Guroff, J.J., Adams, P., Weissman, M.M., and Gershon, E.S. (1996). Unipolar relatives in bipolar pedigrees: A search for elusive indicators of underlying bipolarity. *Am J Med Genet*, 67(5), 445–454.

Blazer, D.G., Kessler, R.C., and Swartz, M.S. (1998). Epidemiology of recurrent major and minor depression with a seasonal pattern. The National Comorbidity Survey. *Br J Psychiatry*, 172, 164–167.

Blehar, M.C., and Lewy, A.J. (1990). Seasonal mood disorders: Consensus and controversy. *Psychopharmacol Bull*, 26(4), 465–494.

Booker, J.M., and Hellekson, C.J. (1992). Prevalence of seasonal affective disorder in Alaska. *Am J Psychiatry*, 149(9), 1176–1182.

Borbely, A. (1982). A two process model of sleep regulation. *Hum Neurobiol*, 1(3), 195–204.

Borbely, A.A., and Wirz-Justice, A. (1982). Sleep, sleep deprivation and depression. A hypothesis derived from a model of sleep regulation. *Hum Neurobiol*, 1(3), 205–210.

Borbely, A.A., Steigrad, P., and Tobler, I. (1980). Effect of sleep deprivation on brain serotonin in the rat. *Behav Brain Res*, 1(2), 205–210.

Borbely, A.A., Achermann, P., Trachsel, L., and Tobler, I. (1989). Sleep initiation and initial sleep intensity: Interactions of homeostatic and circadian mechanisms. *J Biol Rhythms*, 4(2), 149–160.

Bouhuys, A.L., van den Burg, W., and van den Hoofdakker, R.H. (1995). The relationship between tiredness prior to sleep deprivation and the antidepressant response to sleep deprivation in depression. *Biol Psychiatry*, 37(7), 457–461.

Braun, A.R., Balkin, T.J., Wesenten, N.J., Carson, R.E., Varga, M., Baldwin, P., Selbie, S., Belenky, G., and Herscovitch, P. (1997). Regional cerebral blood flow throughout the sleep–wake cycle. An H$_2$(15)O PET study. *Brain*, 120 (Pt. 7), 1173–1197.

Bremner, J.D., Innis, R.B., Salomon, R.M., Staib, L.H., Ng, C.K., Miller, H.L., Bronen, R.A., Krystal, J.H., Duncan, J., Rich, D., Price, L.H., Malison, R., Dey, H., Soufer, R., and Charney, D.S. (1997). Positron emission tomography measurement of cerebral metabolic correlates of tryptophan depletion–induced depressive relapse. *Arch Gen Psychiatry*, 54(4), 364–374.

Breslau, N., Roth, T., Rosenthal, L., and Andreski, P. (1996). Sleep disturbance and psychiatric disorders: A longitudinal epidemiological study of young adults. *Biol Psychiatry*, 39(6), 411–418.

Brewerton, T.D., Berrettini, W.H., Nurnberger, J.I. Jr, and Linnoila, M. (1988). Analysis of seasonal fluctuations of CSF monoamine metabolites and neuropeptides in normal controls: Findings with 5HIAA and HVA. *Psychiatry Res*, 23(3), 257–265.

Brown, L.F., Reynolds, C.F. III, Monk, T.H., Prigerson, H.G., Dew, M.A., Houck, P.R., Mazumdar, S., Buysse, D.J., Hoch, C.C., and Kupfer, D.J. (1996). Social rhythm stability following late-life spousal bereavement: Associations with depression and sleep impairment. *Psychiatry Res*, 62(2), 161–169.

Brown, R.P., Sweeney, J., Loutsch, E., Kocsis, J., and Frances, A. (1984). Involutional melancholia revisited. *Am J Psychiatry*, 141(1), 24–28.

Brunner, D.P., Krauchi, K., Dijk, D.J., Leonhardt, G., Haug, H.J., and Wirz-Justice, A. (1996). Sleep electroencephalogram in seasonal affective disorder and in control women: Effects of midday light treatment and sleep deprivation. *Biol Psychiatry*, 40(6), 485–496.

Buchsbaum, M.S., Hazlett, E.A., Wu, J., and Bunney, W.E. Jr. (2001). Positron emission tomography with deoxyglucose-F18 imaging of sleep. *Neuropsychopharmacology*, 25(5 Suppl.), S50–S56.

Bunney, W.E., and Bunney, B.G. (2000). Molecular clock genes in man and lower animals: Possible implications for circadian abnormalities in depression. *Neuropsychopharmacology*, 22(4), 335–345.

Bunney, W.E., Jr., Murphy, D.L., Goodwin, F.K., and Borge, G.F. (1972a). The "switch process" in manic-depressive illness. I. A systematic study of sequential behavioral changes. *Arch Gen Psychiatry*, 27(3), 295–302.

Bunney, W.E., Jr., Goodwin, F.K., Murphy, D.L., House, K.M., and Gordon, E.K. (1972b). The "switch process" in manic-depressive illness. II. Relationship to catecholamines, REM sleep, and drugs. *Arch Gen Psychiatry*, 27(3), 304–309.

Burgess, H.J., Fogg, L.F., Young, M.A., and Eastman, C.I. (2004). Bright light therapy for winter depression—Is phase advancing beneficial? *Chronobiol Int*, 21(4-5), 759–775.

Burton, R. ([1621] 2001). *The Anatomy of Melancholy*. New York: New York Review of Books.

Buysse, D.J., Frank, E., Lowe, K.K., Cherry, C.R., and Kupfer, D.J. (1997). Electroencephalographic sleep correlates of episode and vulnerability to recurrence in depression. *Biol Psychiatry*, 41(4), 406–418.

Campbell, S.S., and Murphy, P.J. (1998). Extraocular circadian phototransduction in humans. *Science*, 279(5349), 396–399.

Campbell, S.S., Dawson, D., and Zulley, J. (1993). When the human circadian system is caught napping: Evidence for endogenous rhythms close to 24 hours. *Sleep*, 16(7), 638–640.

Cantor, C.H., Hickey, P.A., and De Leo, D. (2000). Seasonal variation in suicide in a predominantly Caucasian tropical/subtropical region of Australia. *Psychopathology*, 33(6), 303–306.

Carlsson, A., Svennerholm, L., and Winblad, B. (1980). Seasonal and circadian monoamine variations in human brains examined post mortem. *Acta Psychiatr Scand Suppl*, 280, 75–85.

Carney, P.A., Fitzgerald, C.T., and Monaghan, C.E. (1988). Influence of climate on the prevalence of mania. *Br J Psychiatry*, 152, 820–823.

Cartwright, R.D. (1983). Rapid eye movement sleep characteristics during and after mood-disturbing events. *Arch Gen Psychiatry*, 40(2), 197–201.

Cassidy, F., and Carroll, B.J. (2002). Seasonal variation of mixed and pure episodes of bipolar disorder. *J Affect Disord*, 68(1), 25–31.

Chang, P.P., Ford, D.E., Mead, L.A., Cooper-Patrick, L., and Klag, M.J. (1997). Insomnia in young men and subsequent depression. The Johns Hopkins Precursors Study. *Am J Epidemiol*, 146(2), 105–114.

Chapman, J., Arlazoroff, A., Goldfarb, L.G., Cervenakova, L., Neufeld, M.Y., Werber, E., Herbert, M., Brown, P., Gajdusek, D.C., and Korczyn, A.D. (1996). Fatal insomnia in a case of familial Creutzfeldt-Jakob disease with the codon 200(Lys) mutation. *Neurology*, 46(3), 758–761.

Chen, D., Buchanan, G.F., Ding, J.M., Hannibal, J., and Gillette, M.U. (1999). Pituitary adenylyl cyclase–activating peptide: A pivotal modulator of glutamatergic regulation of the suprachiasmatic circadian clock. *Proc Natl Acad Sci USA*, 96(23), 13468–13473.

Chouvet, G., Mouret, J., Coindet, J., Siffre, M., and Jouvet, M. (1974). Periodicite bicircadienne due cycle veille-sommeil dans de conditions hors du temps: Etude polygraphique. *Electroencephalogr Clin Neurophysiol*, 37, 367–380.

Cohen, P., and Frame, S. (2001). The renaissance of GSK3. *Nat Rev Mol Cell Biol*, 2(10), 769–776.

Colombo, C., Benedetti, F., Barbini, B., Campori, E., and Smeraldi, E. (1999). Rate of switch from depression into mania after therapeutic sleep deprivation in bipolar depression. *Psychiatry Res*, 86(3), 267–270.

Colombo, C., Lucca, A., Benedetti, F., Barbini, B., Campori, E., and Smeraldi, E. (2000). Total sleep deprivation combined with lithium and light therapy in the treatment of bipolar depression: Replication of main effects and interaction. *Psychiatry Res*, 95(1), 43–53.

Cummings, M.A., Berga, S.L., Cummings, K.L., Kripke, D.F., Haviland, M.G., Golshan, S., and Gillin, J.C. (1989). Light suppression of melatonin in unipolar depressed patients. *Psychiatry Res*, 27(3), 351–355.

Czeisler, C.A., Shanahan, T.L., Klerman, E.B., Martens, H., Brotman, D.J., Emens, J.S., Klein, T., and Rizzo, J.F. III. (1995). Suppression of melatonin secretion in some blind patients by exposure to bright light. *N Engl J Med*, 332(1), 6–11.

Czeisler, C.A., Duffy, J.F., Shanahan, T.L., Brown, E.N., Mitchell, J.F., Rimmer, D.W., Ronda, J.M., Silva, E.J., Allan, J.S., Emens, J.S., Dijk, D.J., and Kronauer, R.E. (1999). Stability, precision, and near-24-hour period of the human circadian pacemaker. *Science*, 284(5423), 2177–2181.

Dahl, K., Avery, D.H., Lewy, A.J., Savage, M.V., Brengelmann, G.L., Larsen, L.H., Vitiello, M.V., and Prinz, P.N. (1993). Dim light melatonin onset and circadian temperature during a constant routine in hypersomnic winter depression. *Acta Psychiatr Scand*, 88(1), 60–66.

Davis, C., and Levitan, R.D. (2005). Seasonality and seasonal affective disorder (SAD): An evolutionary viewpoint tied to energy conservation and reproductive cycles. *J Affect Disord*, 87(1), 3–10.

Demet, E.M., Chicz-Demet, A., Fallon, J.H., and Sokolski, K.N. (1999). Sleep deprivation therapy in depressive illness and Parkinson's disease. *Prog Neuropsychopharmacol Biol Psychiatry*, 23(5), 753–784.

Dement, W., and Kleitman, N. (1957). Cyclic variations in EEG during sleep and their relation to eye movements, body motility, and dreaming. *Electroencephalogr Clin Neurophysiol*, 9, 673–690.

Depue, R.A., Arbisi, P., Spoont, M.R., Krauss, S., Leon, A., and Ainsworth, B. (1989). Seasonal and mood independence of low basal prolactin secretion in premenopausal women with seasonal affective disorder. *Am J Psychiatry*, 146(8), 989–995.

Depue, R.A., Arbisi, P., Krauss, S., Iacono, W.G., Leon, A., Muir, R., and Allen, J. (1990). Seasonal independence of low prolactin concentration and high spontaneous eye blink rates in unipolar and bipolar II seasonal affective disorder. *Arch Gen Psychiatry*, 47(4), 356–364.

Detre, T., Himmelhoch, J., Swartzburg, M., Anderson, C.M., Byck, R., and Kupfer, D.J. (1972). Hypersomnia and manic-depressive disease. *Am J Psychiatry*, 128(10), 1303–1305.

Devinsky, O., Morrell, M.J., and Vogt, B.A. (1995). Contributions of anterior cingulate cortex to behaviour. *Brain*, 118(Pt. 1), 279–306.

Dietzel, D.P., and Ciullo, J.V. (1996). Spontaneous pneumothorax after shoulder arthroscopy: A report of four cases. *Arthroscopy*, 12(1), 99–102.

Dijk, D.J., Duffy, J.F., and Czeisler, C.A. (1992). Circadian and sleep/wake dependent aspects of subjective alertness and cognitive performance. *J Sleep Res*, 1(2), 112–117.

Dijk, D.J., Duffy, J.F., and Czeisler, C.A. (2000). Contribution of circadian physiology and sleep homeostasis to age-related changes in human sleep. *Chronobiol Int*, 17(3), 285–311.

Ding, J.M., Faiman, L.E., Hurst, W.J., Kuriashkina, L.R., and Gillette, M.U. (1997). Resetting the biological clock: mediation of nocturnal CREB phosphorylation via light, glutamate, and nitric oxide. *J Neurosci*, 17(2), 667–675.

Ding, J.M., Buchanan, G.F., Tischkau, S.A., Chen, D., Kuriashkina, L., Faiman, L.E., Alster, J.M., McPherson, P.S., Campbell, K.P., and Gillette, M.U. (1998). A neuronal ryanodine receptor mediates light-induced phase delays of the circadian clock. *Nature*, 394(6691), 381–384.

Drevets, W.C. (1999). Prefrontal cortical–amygdalar metabolism in major depression. *Ann NY Acad Sci*, 877, 614–637.

Drevets, W.C., Price, J.L., Simpson, J.R. Jr., Todd, R.D., Reich, T., Vannier, M., and Raichle, M.E. (1997). Subgenual prefrontal cortex abnormalities in mood disorders. *Nature*, 386(6627), 824–827.

Duffy, J.F., Dijk, D.J., Klerman, E.B., and Czeisler, C.A. (1998). Later endogenous circadian temperature nadir relative to an earlier wake time in older people. *Am J Physiol*, 275(5 Pt. 2), R1478–R1487.

Duffy, J.F., Zeitzer, J.M., Rimmer, D.W., Klerman, E.B., Dijk, D.J., and Czeisler, C.A. (2002). Peak of circadian melatonin rhythm occurs later within the sleep of older subjects. *Am J Physiol Endocrinol Metab*, 282(2), E297–E303.

Duncan, W.C., Jr. (1996). Circadian rhythms and the pharmacology of affective illness. *Pharmacol Ther*, 71(3), 253–312.

Duncan, W.C., Jr., Gillin, J.C., Post, R.M., Gerner, R.H., and Wehr, T.A. (1980). Relationship between EEG sleep patterns and clinical improvement in depressed patients treated with sleep deprivation. *Biol Psychiatry*, 15(6), 879–889.

Eagles, J.M. (1994). The relationship between mood and daily hours of sunlight in rapid cycling bipolar illness. *Biol Psychiatry*, 36(6), 422–424.

Eagles, J.M., Mercer, G., Boshier, A.J., and Jamieson, F. (1996). Seasonal affective disorder among psychiatric nurses in Aberdeen. *J Affect Disord*, 37(2–3), 129–135.

Earnest, D.J., Liang, F.Q., Ratcliff, M., and Cassone, V.M. (1999). Immortal time: Circadian clock properties of rat suprachiasmatic cell lines. *Science*, 283(5402), 693–695.

Eastman, C.I., Gallo, L.C., Lahmeyer, H.W., and Fogg, L.F. (1993). The circadian rhythm of temperature during light treatment for winter depression. *Biol Psychiatry*, 34(4), 210–220.

Eastman, C., Young, M.A., Fogg, L.F., Liu, L., and Meaden. (1998). Bright light treatment of winter depression. *Arch Gen Psychiatry*, 55, 883–889.

Eastwood, M.R., and Peter, A.M. (1988). Epidemiology and seasonal affective disorder. *Psychol Med*, 18(4), 799–806.

Ebert, D., and Berger, M. (1998). Neurobiological similarities in antidepressant sleep deprivation and psychostimulant use: A psychostimulant theory of antidepressant sleep deprivation. *Psychopharmacology (Berl)*, 140(1), 1–10.

Ebert, D., Feistel, H., and Barocka, A. (1991). Effects of sleep deprivation on the limbic system and the frontal lobes in affective disorders: A study with tc-^{99m}-HMPAO SPECT. *Psychiatry Res*, 40(4), 247–251.

Ebert, D., Feistel, H., Kaschka, W., Barocka, A., and Pirner, A. (1994). Single photon emission computerized tomography assessment of cerebral dopamine D2 receptor blockade in depression before and after sleep deprivation—Preliminary results. *Biol Psychiatry*, 35(11), 880–885.

Ebisawa, T., Uchiyama, M., Kajimura, N., Mishima, K., Kamei, Y., Katoh, M., Watanabe, T., Sekimoto, M., Shibui, K., Kim, K., Kudo, Y., Ozeki, Y., Sugishita, M., Toyoshima, R., Inoue, Y., Yamada, N., Nagase, T., Ozaki, N., Ohara, O., Ishida, N., Okawa, M., Takahashi, K., and Yamauchi, T. (2001). Association of structural polymorphisms in the human period3 gene with delayed sleep phase syndrome. *EMBO Rep*, 2(4), 342–346.

Ehlers, C.L., Frank, E., and Kupfer, D.J. (1988). Social zeitgebers and biological rhythms: A unified approach to understanding the etiology of depression. *Arch Gen Psychiatry*, 45, 948–952.

Enoch, M.A., Goldman, D., Barnett, R., Sher, L., Mazzanti, C.M., and Rosenthal, N.E. (1999). Association between seasonal affective disorder and the 5-HT2A promoter polymorphism, −1438G/A. *Mol Psychiatry*, 4(1), 89–92.

Falret, J. (1890). La folie circulaire ou folie a formes alternes. In *Etudes Cliniques sur les Maladies Mentales et Nerveuses*. Paris: Librairie JB Bailliere et Fils.

Feldman-Naim, S., Turner, E.H., and Leibenluft, E. (1997). Diurnal variation in the direction of mood switches in patients with rapid-cycling bipolar disorder. *J Clin Psychiatry*, 58(2), 79–84.

Fernstrom, J.D., and Wurtman, R.J. (1971). Brain serotonin content: Increase following ingestion of carbohydrate diet. *Science*, 174, 1023–1025.

Field, M.D., Maywood, E.S., O'Brien, J.A., Weaver, D.R., Reppert, S.M., and Hastings, M.H. (2000). Analysis of clock proteins in mouse SCN demonstrates phylogenetic divergence of the circadian clockwork and resetting mechanisms. *Neuron*, 25(2), 437–447.

Foster, F.G., Kupfer, D.J., Coble, P., and McPartland, R.J. (1976). Rapid eye movement sleep density. An objective indicator in severe medical-depressive syndromes. *Arch Gen Psychiatry*, 33(9), 1119–1123.

Frank, E., Hlastala, S., Ritenour, A., Houck, P., Tu, X.M., Monk, T.H., Mallinger, A.G., and Kupfer, D.J. (1997). Inducing lifestyle regularity in recovering bipolar disorder patients: Results from the maintenance therapies in bipolar disorder protocol. *Biol Psychiatry*, 41(12), 1165–1173.

Frank, E., Swartz, H.A., and Kupfer, D.J. (2000). Interpersonal and social rhythm therapy: Managing the chaos of bipolar disorder. *Biol Psychiatry*, 48(6), 593–604.

Franken, P., Malafosse, A., and Tafti, M. (1999). Genetic determinants of sleep regulation in inbred mice. *Sleep*, 22(2), 155–169.

Friston, K.J., Sharpley, A.L., Solomon, R.A., and Cowen, P.J. (1989). Lithium increases slow wave sleep: Possible mediation by brain 5-HT2 receptors? *Psychopharmacology (Berl)*, 98(1), 139–140.

Fritzsche, M., Heller, R., Hill, H., and Kick, H. (2001). Sleep deprivation as a predictor of response to light therapy in major depression. *J Affect Disord*, 62(3), 207–215.

Gann, H., Riemann, D., Hohagen, F., Strauss, L.G., Dressing, H., Muller, W.E., and Berger, M. (1993). 48-hour rapid cycling: Results of psychopathometric, polysomnographic, PET imaging and neuro-endocrine longitudinal investigations in a single case. *J Affect Disord*, 28(2), 133–140.

Garcia-Borreguero, D., Jacobsen, F.M., Murphy, D.L., Joseph-Vanderpool, J.R., Chiara, A., and Rosenthal, N.E. (1995). Hormonal responses to the administration of m-chlorophenylpiperazine in patients with seasonal affective disorder and controls. *Biol Psychiatry*, 37(10), 740–749.

Gardner, J.P., Fornal, C.A., and Jacobs, B.L. (1997). Effects of sleep deprivation on serotonergic neuronal activity in the dorsal raphe nucleus of the freely moving cat. *Neuropsychopharmacology*, 17(2), 72–81.

Georgi, F. (1947). Psychophysische Korrelationen: III. Psychiatrische Probleme im Lichte der Rhythmusforschung. *Schweiz Med Wochenschr*, 49, 1276–1280.

Gerner, R.H., Post, R.M., Gillin, J.C., and Bunney, W.E. Jr. (1979). Biological and behavioral effects of one night's sleep deprivation in depressed patients and normals. *J Psychiatr Res*, 15(1), 21–40.

Ghadirian, A.M., Murphy, B.E., and Gendron, M.J. (1998). Efficacy of light versus tryptophan therapy in seasonal affective disorder. *J Affect Disord*, 50(1), 23–27.

Giles, D.E., Jarrett, R.B., Roffwarg, H.P., and Rush, A.J. (1987a). Reduced rapid eye movement latency. A predictor of recurrence in depression. *Neuropsychopharmacology*, 1(1), 33–39.

Giles, D.E., Roffwarg, H.P., and Rush, A.J. (1987b). REM latency concordance in depressed family members. *Biol Psychiatry*, 22(7), 910–914.

Giles, D.E., Biggs, M.M., Rush, A.J., and Roffwarg, H.P. (1988). Risk factors in families of unipolar depression. I. Psychiatric illness and reduced REM latency. *J Affect Disord*, 14(1), 51–59.

Giles, D.E., Jarrett, R.B., Biggs, M.M., Guzick, D.S., and Rush, A.J. (1989). Clinical predictors of recurrence in depression. *Am J Psychiatry*, 146, 764–767.

Gillin, J.C. (1983). The sleep therapies of depression. *Prog Neuropsychopharmacol Biol Psychiatry*, 7(2–3), 351–364.

Gillin, J.C., Wyatt, R.J., Fram, D., and Snyder, F. (1978). The relationship between changes in REM sleep and clinical improvement in depressed patients treated with amitriptyline. *Psychopharmacology (Berl)*, 59(3), 267–272.

Gillin, J.C., Duncan, W., Pettigrew, K.D., Frankel, B.L., and Snyder, F. (1979a). Successful separation of depressed, normal, and insomniac subjects by EEG sleep data. *Arch Gen Psychiatry*, 36(1), 85–90.

Gillin, J.C., Sitaram, N., and Duncan, W.C. (1979b). Muscarinic supersensitivity: A possible model for the sleep disturbance of primary depression? *Psychiatry Res*, 1(1), 17–22.

Gillin, J.C., Sitaram, N., and Mendelson, W.B. (1982). Acetylcholine, sleep, and depression. *Hum Neurobiol*, 1(3), 211–219.

Goldman, B.D. (2001). Mammalian photoperiodic system: Formal properties and neuroendocrine mechanisms of photoperiodic time measurement. *J Biol Rhythms*, 16(4), 283–301.

Goldman, B.D., and Eliott, J.A. (1988). Photoperiodism and seasonality in hamsters. Role of the pineal gland. In M.H. Stetson (Ed.), *Processing of Environmental Information in Vertebrates*. New York: Springer-Verlag.

Gooley, J.J., Lu, J., Chou, T.C., Scammell, T.E., and Saper, C.B. (2001). Melanopsin in cells of origin of the retinohypothalamic tract. *Nat Neurosci*, 4(12), 1165.

Gorman, M.R., and Zucker, I. (1997). Pattern of change in melatonin duration determines testicular responses in siberian hamsters, *Phodopus sungorus*. *Biol Reprod*, 56(3), 668–673.

Gould, T., and Manji, H. (2002a). Signaling networks in the pathophysiology and treatment of mood disorders. *J Psychosom Res*, 53(2), 687.

Gould, T.D., and Manji, H.K. (2002b). The Wnt signaling pathway in bipolar disorder. *Neuroscientist*, 8, 187–201.

Gresham, S.C., Agnew, H.W., and Williams. R.L. (1965). The sleep of depressed patients: An EEG and eye movement study. *Arch Gen Psychiatry*, 13, 503–507.

Griesinger, W. (1867). *Mental Pathology and Therapeutics*. Translated by C.L. Robertson and J. Rutherford. London: New Sydenhem Society.

Grunhaus, L., Shipley, J.E., Eiser, A., Pande, A.C., Tandon, R., Krahn, D.D., Demitrack, M.A., Remen, A., Hirschmann, S., Greden, J.F. (1997). Sleep-onset rapid eye movement after electroconvulsive therapy is more frequent in patients who respond less well to electroconvulsive therapy. *Biol Psychiatry*, 42(3), 191–200.

Guillemette, J., Hebert, M., Paquet, J., and Dumont, M. (1998). Natural bright light exposure in the summer and winter in subjects with and without complaints of seasonal mood variations. *Biol Psychiatry*, 44(7), 622–628.

Hakkarainen, R., Johansson, C., Kieseppa, T., Partonen, T., Koskenvuo, M., Kaprio, J., and Lonnqvist, J. (2003). Seasonal changes, sleep length and circadian preference among twins with bipolar disorder. *BMC Psychiatry*, 3, 6.

Halberg, G. (1968). Physiologic considerations underlying rhythmometry, with special reference to emotional illness. In J. DeAjuriaguerra (Ed.), *Cycles Biologiques et Psychiatrie* (pp. 73–126). Symposium Bel-Air III. Geneva: Masson et Cie.

Hallam, K.T., Olver, J.S., and Norman, T.R. (2005). Effect of sodium valproate on nocturnal melatonin sensitivity to light in healthy volunteers. *Neuropsychopharmacology*, 30(7), 1400–1404.

Hamada, T., Yamanouchi, S., Watanabe, A., Shibata, S., and Watanabe, S. (1999). Involvement of glutamate release in substance P–induced phase delays of suprachiasmatic neuron activity rhythm in vitro. *Brain Res*, 836(1–2), 190–193.

Han, L., Wang, K., Cheng, Y., Du, Z., Rosenthal, N.E., and Primeau, F. (2000a). Summer and winter patterns of seasonality in Chinese college students: A replication. *Compr Psychiatry*, 41(1), 57–62.

Han, L., Wang, K., Cheng, Y., Du, Z., and Rosenthal, N.E. (2000b). Seasonal variations in mood and behavior in Chinese medical students. *Am J Psychiatry*, 157, 133–135.

Hannibal, J., Hindersson, P., Knudsen, S.M., Georg, B., and Fahrenkrug, J. (2002). The photopigment melanopsin is exclusively present in pituitary adenylate cyclase–activating polypeptide-containing retinal ganglion cells of the retinohypothalamic tract. *J Neurosci*, 22(1), RC191.

Harding, G.F., Alford, C.A., and Powell, T.E. (1985). The effect of sodium valproate on sleep, reaction times, and visual evoked potential in normal subjects. *Epilepsia*, 26(6), 597–601.

Harvey, A.G., Schmidt, D.A., Scarna, A., Semier, C.N., and Goodwin, G.M. (2005). Sleep-related functioning in euthymic patients with bipolar disorder, patients with insomnia, and subjects without sleep problems. *Am J Psychiatry*, 162(1), 50–57.

Hattar, S., Liao, H.W., Takao, M., Berson, D.M., and Yau, K.W. (2002). Melanopsin-containing retinal ganglion cells: Architecture, projections, and intrinsic photosensitivity. *Science*, 295(5557), 1065–1070.

Hauri, P., Chernik, D., Hawkins, D., and Mendels, J. (1974). Sleep of depressed patients in remission. *Arch Gen Psychiatry*, 31(3), 386–391.

Healy, D., and Waterhouse, J.M. (1995). The circadian system and the therapeutics of the affective disorders. *Pharmacol Ther*, 65(2), 241–263.

Hebert, M., Dumont, M., and Lachapelle, P. (2002). Electrophysiological evidence suggesting a seasonal modulation of retinal sensitivity in subsyndromal winter depression. *J Affect Disord*, 68(2–3), 191–202.

Herzog, E.D., and Schwartz, W.J. (2002). Invited review: A neural clockwork for encoding circadian time. *J Appl Physiol*, 92(1), 401–408.

Herzog, E.D., Takahashi, J.S., and Block, G.D. (1998). Clock controls circadian period in isolated suprachiasmatic nucleus neurons. *Nat Neurosci*, 1(8), 708–713.

Hobson, J.A., and Steriade, M. (1986). Neuronal basis of behavioral state control. In V.B. Mountcastle, F. Blum, S.R. Geiger (Eds.), *Handbook of Physiology: A Critical, Comprehensive Presentation of Physiological Knowledge and Concepts* (Vol. IV, Section 1, The Nervous System) (pp. 701–823). Bethesda, MD: American Physiological Society.

Huber, R., Deboer, T., and Tobler, I. (2000). Effects of sleep deprivation on sleep and sleep EEG in three mouse strains: Empirical data and simulations. *Brain Res*, 857(1–2), 8–19.

Hudson, J.I., Lipinski, J.F., Frankenburg, F.R., Grochocinski, V.J., and Kupfer, D.J. (1988). Electroencephalographic sleep in mania. *Arch Gen Psychiatry*, 45(3), 267–273.

Hudson, J.I., Lipinski, J.F., Keck, P.E. Jr., Aizley, H.G., Lukas, S.E., Rothschild, A.J., Waternaux, C.M., and Kupfer, D.J. (1992). Polysomnographic characteristics of young manic patients. Comparison with unipolar depressed patients and normal control subjects. *Arch Gen Psychiatry*, 49(5), 378–383.

Hunt, N., Sayer, H., and Silverstone, T. (1992). Season and manic relapse. *Acta Psychiatr Scand*, 85(2), 123–126.

Illnerova, H., and Vanecek, J. (1982). Two-oscillator structure of the pacemaker controlling the circadian-rhythm of N-acetyltransferase in the rat pineal-gland. *J Comp Physiol*, 145(4), 539–548.

Ishii, R., Shinosaki, K., Ukai, S., Inouye, T., Ishihara, T., Yoshimine, T., Hirabuki, N., Asada, H., Kihara, T., Robinson, S.E., and Takeda, M. (1999). Medial prefrontal cortex generates frontal midline theta rhythm. *Neuroreport*, 10(4), 675–679.

Jac, M., Kiss, A., Sumova, A., Illnerova, H., and Jezova, D. (2000a). Daily profiles of arginine vasopressin mRNA in the suprachiasmatic, supraoptic and paraventricular nuclei of the rat hypothalamus under various photoperiods. *Brain Res*, 887(2), 472–476.

Jac, M., Sumova, A., and Illnerova, H. (2000b). c-Fos rhythm in subdivisions of the rat suprachiasmatic nucleus under artificial and natural photoperiods. *Am J Physiol Regul Integr Comp Physiol*, 279(6), R2270–R2276.

Jacobsen, F.M., Mueller, E.A., Rosenthal, N.E., Rogers, S., Hill, J.L., and Murphy, D.L. (1994). Behavioral responses to intravenous meta-chlorophenylpiperazine in patients with seasonal affective disorder and control subjects before and after phototherapy. *Psychiatry Res*, 52(2), 181–197.

Jang, K.L., Lam, R.W., Livesley, W.J., and Vernon, P.A. (1997a). Gender differences in the heritability of seasonal mood change. *Psychiatry Res*, 70(3), 145–154.

Jang, K.L., Lam, R.W., Livesley, W.J., and Vernon, P.A. (1997b). The relationship between seasonal mood change and personality: More apparent than real? *Acta Psychiatr Scand*, 95(6), 539–543.

Janowsky, D.S., el-Yousef, M.K., Davis, J.M., and Sekerke, H.J. (1972). A cholinergic–adrenergic hypothesis of mania and depression. *Lancet*, 2(7778), 632–635.

Johnsson, A., Pflug, B., Engelmann, W., and Klemke, W. (1979). Effect of lithium carbonate on circadian periodicity in humans. *Pharmakopsychiatr Neuropsychopharmakol*, 12(6), 423–425.

Johnsson, A., Engelmann, W., Pflug, B., and Klemke, W. (1980). Influence of lithium ions on human circadian rhythms. *Z Naturforsch [C]*, 35(5–6), 503–507.

Johnsson, A., Engelmann, W., Pflug, B., and Klemke, W. (1983). Period lengthening of human circadian rhythms by lithium carbonate, a prophylactic for depressive disorders. *Int J Chronobiol*, 8(3), 129–147.

Jones, C.R., Campbell, S.S., Zone, S.E., Cooper, F., DeSano, A., Murphy, P.J., Jones, B., Czajkowski, L., and Ptacek, L.J. (1999). Familial advanced sleep-phase syndrome: A short-period circadian rhythm variant in humans. *Nat Med*, 5(9), 1062–1065.

Jones, P.M., and Berney, T.P. (1987). Early onset rapid cycling bipolar affective disorder. *J Child Psychol Psychiatry*, 28, 731–738.

Jones, S.H., Hare, D.J., and Evershed, K. (2005). Actigraphic assessment of circadian activity and sleep patterns in bipolar disorder. *Bipolar Disord*, 7(2), 176–186.

Joseph-Vanderpool, J.R., Jacobsen, F.M., Murphy, D.L., Hill, J.L., and Rosenthal, N.E. (1993). Seasonal variation in behavioral responses to m-CPP in patients with seasonal affective disorder and controls. *Biol Psychiatry*, 33(7), 496–504.

Kafka, M.S., Marangos, P.J., and Moore, R.Y. (1985). Suprachiasmatic nucleus ablation abolishes circadian rhythms in rat brain neurotransmitter receptors. *Brain Res*, 327(1-2), 344–347.

Kalsbeek, A., van Heerikhuize, J.J., Wortel, J., and Buijs, R.M. (1996). A diurnal rhythm of stimulatory input to the hypothalamo-pituitary-adrenal system as revealed by timed intrahypothalamic administration of the vasopressin V1 antagonist. *J Neurosci*, 16(17), 5555–5565.

Kasper, S., Rogers, S.L., Yancey, A., Schulz, P.M., Skwerer, R.G., and Rosenthal, N.E. (1989a). Phototherapy in individuals with and without subsyndromal seasonal affective disorder. *Arch Gen Psychiatry*, 46(9), 837–844.

Kasper, S., Wehr, T.A., Bartko, J.J., Gaist, P.A., and Rosenthal, N.E. (1989b). Epidemiological findings of seasonal changes in mood and behavior. A telephone survey of Montgomery County, Maryland. *Arch Gen Psychiatry*, 46(9), 823–833.

Kavaliers, M., and Ralph, C.L. (1981). Encephalic photoreceptor involvement in the entrainment and control of circadian activity of young American alligators. *Physiol Behav*, 26(3), 413–418.

Klemfuss, H. (1992). Rhythms and the pharmacology of lithium. *Pharmacol Ther*, 56(1), 53–78.

Klemfuss, H., and Kripke, D.F. (1995). Antimanic drugs stabilize hamster circadian rhythms. *Psychiatry Res*, 57(3), 215–222.

Knowles, J.B., Cairns, J., MacLean, A.W., Delva, N., Prowse, A., Waldron, J., and Letemendia, F.J. (1986). The sleep of remitted bipolar depressives: Comparison with sex and age-matched controls. *Can J Psychiatry*, 31(4), 295–298.

Kraepelin, E. (1921). *Manic-Depressive Insanity and Paranoia*. Edinburgh: E & S Livingstone.

Kripke, D.F. (1983). Phase-advance theories for affective illness. In T.A. Wehr and F.K. Goodwin (Eds.), *Circadian Rhythms in Psychiatry* (pp. 41–69). Pacific Grove, CA: Boxwood Press.

Kripke, D.F. (1995). Mortality risk of major depression. *Am J Psychiatry*, 152(6), 962.

Kripke, D.F. (1998). Light treatment for nonseasonal depression: Speed, efficacy, and combined treatment. *J Affect Disord*, 49(2), 109–117.

Kripke, D.F., Mullaney, D.J., Atkinson, M.L., and Wolf, S. (1978). Circadian rhythms disorders in manic depressives. *Biol Psychiatry*, 13, 335–351.

Kripke, D.F., Ancoli-Israel, S., Klauber, M.R., Wingard, D.L., Mason, W.J., and Mullaney, D.J. (1997). Prevalence of sleep-disordered breathing in ages 40–64 years: A population-based survey. *Sleep*, 20(1), 65–76.

Kripke, D.F., Garfinkel, L., Wingard, D.L., Klauber, M.R., and Marler, M.R. (2002). Mortality associated with sleep duration and insomnia. *Arch Gen Psychiatry*, 59(2), 131–136.

Kuhs, H., and Tölle, R. (1991). Sleep deprivation therapy. *Biol Psychiatry*, 29(11), 1129–1148.

Kukopulos, A., and Reginaldi, D. (1973). Does lithium prevent depressions by suppressing manias? *Int Pharmacopsychiatry*, 8(3), 152–158.

Kupfer, D.J. (1976). REM latency: A psychobiologic marker for primary depressive disease. *Biol Psychiatry*, 11(2), 159–174.

Kupfer, D.J., and Foster, F.G. (1972). Interval between onset of sleep and rapid-eye-movement sleep as an indicator of depression. *Lancet*, 2(7779), 684–686.

Kupfer, D.J., Wyatt, R.J., Greenspan, K., Scott, J., and Snyder, F. (1970). Lithium carbonate and sleep in affective illness. *Arch Gen Psychiatry*, 23(1), 35–40.

Kupfer, D.J., Foster, F.G., Reich, L., Thompson, S.K., and Weiss, B. (1976). EEG sleep changes as predictors in depression. *Am J Psychiatry*, 133(6), 622–626.

Kupfer, D.J., Spiker, D.G., Coble, P.A., and Shaw, D.H. (1978). Electroencephalographic sleep recordings and depression in the elderly. *J Am Geriatr Soc*, 26(2), 53–57.

Kupfer, D.J., Spiker, D.G., Coble, P.A., Neil, J.F., Ulrich, R., and Shaw, D.H. (1981). Sleep and treatment prediction in endogenous depression. *Am J Psychiatry*, 138(4), 429–434.

Kupfer, D.J., Ehlers, C.L., Frank, E., Grochocinski, V.J., McEachran, A.B., and Buhari, A. (1994). Persistent effects of antidepressants: EEG sleep studies in depressed patients during maintenance treatment. *Biol Psychiatry*, 35(10), 781–793.

Kusumi, I., Koyama, T., and Yamashita, I. (1994). Serotonin-induced platelet intracellular calcium mobilization in depressed patients. *Psychopharmacology (Berl)*, 113(3–4), 322–327.

Lam, R.W., and Levitan, R.D. (1996). *Tryptophan Augmentation of Light Therapy in Patients with Seasonal Affective Disorder* (Vol. 8). Bethesda, MD: Society for Light Treatment and Biological Rhythms.

Lam, R.W., and Levitan, R.D. (2000). Pathophysiology of seasonal affective disorder: A review. *J Psychiatry Neurosci*, 25(5), 469–480.

Lam, R.V., and Levitt, A.J. (1999). *Canadian Consensus Guidelines for the Treatment of Seasonal Affective Disorder*. Vancouver, WA: Clinical & Academic Publishing.

Lam, R.W., Berkowitz, A.L., Berga, S.L., Clark, C.M., Kripke, D.F., and Gillin, J.C. (1990). Melatonin suppression in bipolar and unipolar mood disorders. *Psychiatry Res*, 33(2), 129–134.

Lam, R.W., Beattie, C.W., Buchanan, A., and Mador, J.A. (1992a). Electroretinography in seasonal affective disorder. *Psychiatry Res*, 43(1), 55–63.

Lam, R.W., Buchanan, A., Mador, J.A., Corral, M.R., and Remick, R.A. (1992b). The effects of ultraviolet-A wavelengths in light therapy for seasonal depression. *J Affect Disord*, 24(4), 237–243.

Lam, R.W., Beattie, C., Mador, J.A., Corral, M.R., Buchanan, A., and Zis, A.P. (1993). *The Effects of Light Therapy on Retinal Electrophysiologic Tests in Winter Depression*. Bethesda, MD: Society for Light Treatment and Biological Rhythms.

Lam, R.W., Gorman, C.P., Michalon, M., Steiner, M., Levitt, A.J., Corral, M.R., Watson, G.D., Morehouse, R.L., Tam, W., and Joffe, R.T. (1995). Multicenter, placebo-controlled study of fluoxetine in seasonal affective disorder. *Am J Psychiatry*, 152(12), 1765–1770.

Lam, R.W., Zis, A.P., Grewal, A., Delgado, P.L., Charney, D.S., and Krystal, J.H. (1996). Effects of rapid tryptophan depletion in patients with seasonal affective disorder in remission after light therapy. *Arch Gen Psychiatry*, 53(1), 41–44.

Lam, R.W., Levitan, R.D., Tam, E.M., Yatham, L.N., Lamoureux, S., and Zis, A.P. (1997). L-tryptophan augmentation of light therapy in patients with seasonal affective disorder. *Can J Psychiatry*, 42(3), 303–306.

Lam, R.W., Bowering, T.A., Tam, E.M., Grewal, A., Yatham, L.N., Shiah, I.S., and Zis, A.P. (2000). Effects of rapid tryptophan depletion in patients with seasonal affective disorder in natural summer remission. *Psychol Med*, 30(1), 79–87.

Lam, R.W., Lee, S.K., Tam, E.M., Grewal, A., and Yatham, L.N. (2001a). An open trial of light therapy for women with seasonal affective disorder and comorbid bulimia nervosa. *J Clin Psychiatry*, 62(3), 164–168.

Lam, R.W., Tam, E.M., Grewal, A., and Yatham, L.N. (2001b). Effects of alpha-methyl-para-tyrosine-induced catecholamine depletion in patients with seasonal affective disorder in summer remission. *Neuropsychopharmacology*, 25(Suppl. 5), S97–S101.

Lam, R.W., Tam, E.M., Yatham, L.N., Shiah, I.S., and Zis, A.P. (2001c). Seasonal depression: The dual vulnerability hypothesis revisited. *J Affect Disord*, 63(1–3), 123–132.

Lambert, G.W., Reid, C., Kaye, D.M., Jennings, G.L., and Esler, M.D. (2002). Effect of sunlight and season on serotonin turnover in the brain. *Lancet*, 360(9348), 1840–1842.

Larkin, J.E., Freeman, D.A., and Zucker, I. (2001). Low ambient temperature accelerates short-day responses in Siberian hamsters by altering responsiveness to melatonin. *J Biol Rhythms*, 16(1), 76–86.

Leibenluft, E., and Wehr, T.A. (1992). Is sleep deprivation useful in the treatment of depression? *Am J Psychiatry*, 149(2), 159–168.

Leibenluft, E., Turner, E.H., Feldman-Naim, S., Schwartz, P.J., Wehr, T.A., and Rosenthal, N.E. (1995). Light therapy in patients with rapid cycling bipolar disorder: Preliminary results. *Psychopharmacol Bull*, 31(4), 705–710.

Leibenluft, E., Albert, P.S., Rosenthal, N.E., and Wehr, T.A. (1996a). Relationship between sleep and mood in patients with rapid-cycling bipolar disorder. *Psychiatry Res*, 63(2–3), 161–168.

Leibenluft, E., Feldman-Naim, S., Turner, E.H., Schwartz, P.J., and Wehr, T.A. (1996b). Salivary and plasma measures of dim light melatonin onset (DLMO) in patients with rapid cycling bipolar disorder. *Biol Psychiatry*, 40(8), 731–735.

Lenox, R.H., Gould, T.D., and Manji, H.K. (2002). Endophenotypes in bipolar disorder. *Am J Med Genet*, 114(4), 391–406.

Leonhardt, G., Wirz-Justice, A., Krauchi, K., Graw, P., Wunder, D., and Haug, H. J. (1994). Long-term follow-up of depression in seasonal affective disorder. *Compr Psychiatry*, 35(6), 457–464.

Leu, S.J., Shiah, I.S., Yatham, L.N., Cheu, Y.M., and Lam, R.W. (2001). Immune-inflammatory markers in patients with seasonal affective disorder: Effects of light therapy. *J Affect Disord*, 63(1–3), 27–34.

Levitan, R.D., Kaplan, A.S., Brown, G.M., Vaccarino, F.J., Kennedy, S.H., Levitt, A.J., and Joffe, R.T. (1998). Hormonal and subjective responses to intravenous m-chlorophenylpiperazine in women with seasonal affective disorder. *Arch Gen Psychiatry*, 55(3), 244–249.

Levitan, R.D., Jain, U.R., and Katzman, M.A. (1999a). Seasonal affective symptoms in adults with residual attention-deficit hyperactivity disorder. *Compr Psychiatry*, 40(4), 261–267.

Levitan, R.D., Masellis, M., Kennedy, J.L., Kennedy, S.H., Kaplan, A.S., and Vaccario, F.J. (1999b). Polymorphism in serotonin genes in seasonal affective disorder and bulimia. *Biol Psychiatry*, 43(Suppl. 8), 271.

Levitt, A.J., Boyle, M.H., Joffe, R.T., and Baumal, Z. (2000). Estimated prevalence of the seasonal subtype of major depression in a Canadian community sample. *Can J Psychiatry*, 45(7), 650–654.

Lewis, P.R., and Lobban, M.C. (1957). Dissociation of diurnal rhythms in human subjects living in abnormal time routines. *Q J Exp Physiol Cognate Med Sci*, 42, 371–386.

Lewy, A.J., and Sack, R.L. (1988). The phase-shift hypothesis of seasonal affective disorder. *Am J Psychiatry*, 145(8), 1041–1043.

Lewy, A.J., and Sack, R.L. (1989). The dim light melatonin onset as a marker for circadian phase position. *Chronobiol Int*, 6(1), 93–102.

Lewy, A.J., Wehr, T.A., Goodwin, F.K., Newsome, D.A., and Markey, S.P. (1980). Light suppresses melatonin secretion in humans. *Science*, 210(4475), 1267–1269.

Lewy, A.J., Wehr, T.A., Goodwin, F.K., Newsome, D.A., and Rosenthal, N.E. (1981). Manic-depressive patients may be supersensitive to light. *Lancet*, 1(8216), 383–384.

Lewy, A.J., Kern, H.A., Rosenthal, N.E., and Wehr, T.A. (1982). Bright artificial light treatment of a manic-depressive patient with a seasonal mood cycle. *Am J Psychiatry*, 139, 1496–1498.

Lewy, A.J., Sack, R.L., and Singer, C.M. (1985). Immediate and delayed effects of bright light on human melatonin production: Shifting "dawn" and "dusk" shifts the dim light melatonin onset (DLMO). *Ann NY Acad Sci*, 453, 253–259.

Lewy, A.J., Nurnberger, J.I., Wehr, T.A., Pack, D., Becker, L.E., Powell, R.-L., and Newsome, D.A. (1985a). Supersensitivity to light: Possible trait marker for manic-depressive illness. *Am J Psychiatry*, 142, 725–727.

Lewy, A.J., Sack, R.L., Miller, L.S., and Hoban, T.M. (1987a). Antidepressant and circadian phase-shifting effects of light. *Science*, 235(4786), 352–354.

Lewy, A.J., Sack, R.L., Singer, C.M., and White, D.M. (1987b). The phase shift hypothesis for bright light's therapeutic mechanism of action: Theoretical considerations and experimental evidence. *Psychopharmacol Bull*, 23(3), 349–353.

Lewy, A.J., Bauer, V.K., Cutler, N.L., Sack, R.L., Ahmed, S., Thomas, K.H., Blood, M.L., and Jackson, J.M. (1998). Morning vs. evening light treatment of patients with winter depression. *Arch Gen Psychiatry*, 55(10), 890–896.

Lewy, A.J., Emens, J., Sack, R.L., Hasler, B.P., and Bernert, R.A. (2003). Zeitgeber hierarchy in humans: Resetting the circadian phase positions of blind people using melatonin. *Chronobiol Int*, 20(5), 837–852.

Lewy, A.J., Emens, J., Jackman, A., and Yuhas, K. (2006). Circadian uses of melatonin in humans. *Chronobiol Int*, 23(1–2), 403–412.

Linkowski, P., Mendlewicz, J., LeClercq, R., Brasseur, M., Hubain, P., Golstein, J., Copinschi, G., and Van Cauter, E. (1985a). The 24-hour profile of adrenocorticotropin and cortisol in major depressive illness. *J Clin Endocrinol Metab*, 61, 429–438.

Linkowski, P., Van Cauter, E., Leclercq, R., Desmedt, D., Brasseur, M., Golstein, J., Copinschi, G., and Mendlewicz, J. (1985b). ACTH, cortisol and growth hormone 24-hour profiles in major depressive illness. *Acta Psychiatr Belg*, 85(5), 615–623.

Linkowski, P., Kerkhofs, M., Rielaert, C., and Mendlewicz, J. (1986). Sleep during mania in manic-depressive males. *Eur Arch Psychiatry Neurol Sci*, 235(6), 339–341.

Linkowski, P., Kerkhofs, M., Van Onderbergen, A., Hubain, P., Copinschi, G., L'Hermite-Baleriaux, M., Leclercq, R., Brasseur, M., Mendlewicz, J., and Van Cauter, E. (1994). The 24-hour profiles of cortisol, prolactin, and growth hormone secretion in mania. *Arch Gen Psychiatry*, 51(8), 616–624.

Liu, C., and Reppert, S.M. (2000). GABA synchronizes clock cells within the suprachiasmatic circadian clock. *Neuron*, 25(1), 123–128.

Liu, C., Weaver, D.R., Jin, X., Shearman, L.P., Pieschl, R.L., Gribkoff, V.K., and Reppert, S.M. (1997a). Molecular dissection of two distinct actions of melatonin on the suprachiasmatic circadian clock. *Neuron*, 19(1), 91–102.

Liu, C., Weaver, D.R., Strogatz, S.H., and Reppert, S.M. (1997b). Cellular construction of a circadian clock: Period determination in the suprachiasmatic nuclei. *Cell*, 91(6), 855–860.

Lobban, M.C., Tredre, B., Elithorn, A., and Bridges, P. (1963). Diurnal rhythms of electrolyte excretion in depressive illness. *Nature*, 199, 667–669.

Lockley, S.W., Skene, D.J., Thapan, K., English, J., Ribeiro, D., Haimov, I., Hampton, S., Middleton, B., von Schantz, M., and Arendt, J. (1998). Extraocular light exposure does not suppress plasma melatonin in humans. *J Clin Endocrinol Metab*, 83(9), 3369–3372.

Loo, H., Hale, A., and D'Haenen, H. (2002). Determination of the dose of agomelatine, a melatoninergic agonist and selective 5-HT(2c) antagonist, in the treatment of major depressive disorder: A placebo-controlled dose range study. *Int Clin Psychopharmacol*, 17(5), 239–247.

Low, K.G., and Feissner, J.M. (1998). Seasonal affective disorder in college students: Prevalence and latitude. *J Am Coll Health*, 47(3), 135–137.

Lowrey, P.L., Shimomura, K., Antoch, M.P., Yamazaki, S., Zemenides, P.D., Ralph, M.R., Menaker, M., and Takahashi, J.S. (2000). Positional syntenic cloning and functional characterization of the mammalian circadian mutation *tau*. *Science*, 288(5465), 483–492.

Madden, P.A., Heath, A.C., Rosenthal, N.E., and Martin, N.G. (1996). Seasonal changes in mood and behavior. The role of genetic factors. *Arch Gen Psychiatry*, 53(1), 47–55.

Magnusson, A. (2000). An overview of epidemiological studies on seasonal affective disorder. *Acta Psychiatr Scand*, 101(3), 176–184.

Magnusson, A., and Axelsson, J. (1993). The prevalence of seasonal affective disorder is low among descendants of Icelandic emigrants in Canada. *Arch Gen Psychiatry*, 50(12), 947–951.

Magnusson, A., and Stefansson, J.G. (1993). Prevalence of seasonal affective disorder in Iceland. *Arch Gen Psychiatry*, 50(12), 941–946.

Malkoff-Schwartz, S., Frank, E., Anderson, B., Sherrill, J. T., Siegel, L., Patterson, D., and Kupfer, D.J. (1998). Stressful life events and social rhythm disruption in the onset of manic and depressive bipolar episodes: A preliminary investigation. *Arch Gen Psychiatry*, 55(8), 702–707.

Malpaux, B., Daveau, A., Maurice-Mandon, F., Duarte, G., and Chemineau, P. (1998). Evidence that melatonin acts in the pre-mammillary hypothalamic area to control reproduction in the ewe: Presence of binding sites and stimulation of luteinizing hormone secretion by in situ microimplant delivery. *Endocrinology*, 139(4), 1508–1516.

Maquet, P., Peters, J., Aerts, J., Delfiore, G., Degueldre, C., Luxen, A., and Franck, G. (1996). Functional neuroanatomy of human rapid-eye-movement sleep and dreaming. *Nature*, 383(6596), 163–166.

Martinek, S., Inonog, S., Manoukian, A.S., and Young, M.W. (2001). A role for the segment polarity gene *shaggy/GSK-3* in the *Drosophila* circadian clock. *Cell*, 105(6), 769–779.

Mayberg, H.S., Brannan, S.K., Mahurin, R.K., Jerabek, P.A., Brickman, J.S., Tekell, J.L., Silva, J.A., McGinnis, S., Glass, T.G., Martin, C.C., and Fox, P.T. (1997). Cingulate function in depression: A potential predictor of treatment response. *Neuroreport*, 8(4), 1057–1061.

McGrath, R.E., Buckwald, B., and Resnick, E.V. (1990). The effect of L-tryptophan on seasonal affective disorder. *J Clin Psychiatry*, 51(4), 162–163.

Mendels, J., and Chernik, D.A. (1973). The effect of lithium carbonate on the sleep of depressed patients. *Int Pharmacopsychiatry*, 8(3), 184–192.

Mendelson, W.B., and Basile, A.S. (2001). The hypnotic actions of the fatty acid amide, oleamide. *Neuropsychopharmacology*, 25(Suppl. 5), S36–S39.

Mendelson, W.B., Gillin, J.C., and Wyatt, R.J. (1997). *Human Sleep and Its Disorders.* New York: Plenum Press.

Meyer, T.D., and Maier, S. (2006). Is there evidence for social rhythm instability in people at risk for affective disorders? *Psychiatry Res*, 141(1), 103–114.

Middleton, B., Arendt, J., and Stone, B.M. (1996). Human circadian rhythms in constant dim light (8 lux) with knowledge of clock time. *J Sleep Res*, 5(2), 69–76.

Millar, A., Espie, C.A., and Scott, J. (2004). The sleep of remitted bipolar outpatients: A controlled naturalistic study using actigraphy. *J Affect Disord*, 80(2-3), 145–153.

Mistlberger, R.E., and Holmes, M.M. (2000). Behavioral feedback regulation of circadian rhythm phase angle in light–dark entrained mice. *Am J Physiol Regul Integr Comp Physiol*, 279(3), R813–R821.

Mizukawa, R., Ishiguro, S., Takada, H., Kishimoto, A., Ogura, C., and Hazama, H. (1991). Long-term observation of a manic-depressive patient with rapid cycles. *Biol Psychiatry*, 29(7), 671–678.

Modell, J.G., Rosenthal, N.E., Harriett, A.E., Krishen, A., Asgharian, A., Foster, V.J., Metz, A., Rockett, C.B., and Wightman, D.S. (2005). Seasonal affective disorder and its prevention by anticipatory treatment with bupropion XL. *Biol Psychiatry*, 58(8), 658–667.

Molin, J., Mellerup, E., Bolwig, T., Scheike, T., and Dam, H. (1996). The influence of climate on development of winter depression. *J Affect Disord*, 37(2-3), 151–155.

Monk, T.H., Flaherty, J.F., Frank, E., Hoskinson, K., and Kupfer, D.J. (1990). The Social Rhythm Metric. An instrument to quantify the daily rhythms of life. *J Nerv Ment Dis*, 178(2), 120–126.

Monk, T.H., Buysse, D.J., Reynolds, C.F. III, Jarrett, D.B., and Kupfer, D.J. (1992). Rhythmic vs. homeostatic influences on mood, activation, and performance in young and old men. *J Gerontol*, 47(4), P221–227.

Montgomery, S.A., Kennedy, S.H., Burrows, G.D., Lejoyeux, M., and Hindmarch, I. (2004). Absence of discontinuation symptoms with agomelatine and occurrence of discontinuation symptoms with paroxetine: A randomized, double-blind, placebo-controlled discontinuation study. *Int Clin Psychopharmacol*, 19(5), 271–280.

Moore, R.Y. (1996a). Entrainment pathways and the functional organization of the circadian system. *Prog Brain Res*, 111, 103–119.

Moore, R.Y. (1996b). Neural control of the pineal gland. *Behav Brain Res*, 73(1–2), 125–130.

Morgan, P.J., Messager, S., Webster, C., Barrett, P., and Ross, A. (1999). How does the melatonin receptor decode a photoperiodic signal in the pars tuberalis? *Adv Exp Med Biol*, 460, 165–174.

Morin, L.P. (1999). Serotonin and the regulation of mammalian circadian rhythmicity. *Ann Med*, 31(1), 12–33.

Morken, G., Lilleeng, S., and Linaker, O.M. (2002). Seasonal variation in suicides and in admissions to hospital for mania and depression. *J Affect Disord*, 69(1–3), 39–45.

Morrissey, S.A., Raggatt, P.T., James, B., and Rogers, J. (1996). Seasonal affective disorder: Some epidemiological findings from a tropical climate. *Aust N Z J Psychiatry*, 30(5), 579–586.

Moscovitch, A., Blashko, C., Wiseman, R., Goldberg, M., and Martindale, J. (1995). *A double-blind, placebo-controlled study of sertaline in patients with seasonal affective disorder.* New Research Abstracts. American Psychiatric Association Annual Meeting.

Mrosovsky, N. (1988). Phase response curves for social entrainment. *J Comp Physiol [A]*, 162, 35–46.

Mrosovsky, N., Salmon, P.A., and Vrang, N. (1998). Revolutionary science: An improved running wheel for hamsters. *Chronobiol Int*, 15(2), 147–158.

Mrugala, M., Zlomanczuk, P., Jagota, A., and Schwartz, W.J. (2000). Rhythmic multiunit neural activity in slices of hamster suprachiasmatic nucleus reflect prior photoperiod. *Am J Physiol Regul Integr Comp Physiol*, 278(4), R987–R994.

Murase, S., Murase, S., Kitabatake, M., Yamauchi, T., and Mathe, A.A. (1995). Seasonal mood variation among Japanese residents of Stockholm. *Acta Psychiatr Scand*, 92(1), 51–55.

Murray, G., Michalak, E.E., Levitt, A.J., Levitan, R.D., Enns, M.W., Morehouse, R., and Lam, R.W. (2006). O sweet spot where art thou? Light treatment of seasonal affective disorder and the circadian time of sleep. *J Affect Disord*, 90(2-3), 227–231.

Myers, D.H., and Davies, P. (1978). The seasonal incidence of mania and its relationship to climatic variables. *Psychol Med*, 8, 433–440.

Nagayama, H., Hasama, N., Tsuchiyama, K., Yamada, K., Ihara, J., and Yanagisawa, T. (1992). Circadian temperature and sleep–wake rhythms in depression. *Jpn J Psychiatry Neurol*, 46(1), 244–245.

Nelson, R.J. (1990). Photoperiodic responsiveness in house mice. *Physiol Behav*, 48, 403–408.

Nelson, R.J. (2004). Seasonal immune function and sickness responses. *Trends Immunol*, 25(4), 187–192.

Nelson, R.J., and Zucker, I. (1981). Photoperiodic control of reproduction in olfactory-bulbectomized rats. *Neuroendocrinology*, 32, 266–271.

Nelson, R.J., Demas, G.E., Klein, S.L., and Kriegsfeld, L.J. (2002). *Seasonal Patterns of Stress, Immune Function and Disease.* New York: Cambridge University Press.

Neumeister, A., Goessler, R., Lucht, M., Kapitany, T., Bamas, C., and Kasper, S. (1996). Bright light therapy stabilizes the antidepressant effect of partial sleep deprivation. *Biol Psychiatry*, 39(1), 16–21.

Neumeister, A., Praschak-Rieder, N., Besselmann, B., Rao, M.L., Gluck, J., and Kasper, S. (1997). Effects of tryptophan depletion on drug-free patients with seasonal affective disorder during a stable response to bright light therapy. *Arch Gen Psychiatry*, 54(2), 133–138.

Neumeister, A., Praschak-Rieder, N., Hesselmann, B., Vitouch, O., Rauh, M., Barocka, A., and Kasper, S. (1998a). Effects of tryptophan depletion in fully remitted patients with seasonal affective disorder during summer. *Psychol Med*, 28(2), 257–264.

Neumeister, A., Praschak-Rieder, N., Hesselmann, B., Vitouch, O., Rauh, M., Barocka, A., Tauscher, J., and Kasper, S. (1998b). Effects of tryptophan depletion in drug-free depressed patients who responded to total sleep deprivation. *Arch Gen Psychiatry*, 55(2), 167–172.

Neumeister, A., Turner, E.H., Matthews, J.R., Postolache, T.T., Barnett, R.L., Rauh, M., Vetticad, R.G., Kasper, S., and Rosenthal, N.E. (1998c). Effects of tryptophan depletion vs. catecholamine depletion in patients with seasonal affective disorder in remission with light therapy. *Arch Gen Psychiatry*, 55(6), 524–530.

Neumeister, A., Konstantinidis, A., Praschak-Rieder, N., Willeit, M., Hilger, E., Stastny, J., and Kasper, S. (2001). Monoaminergic function in the pathogenesis of seasonal affective disorder. *Int J Neuropsychopharmacol*, 4(4), 409–420.

Nievergelt, C.M., Kripke, D.F., Remick, R.A., Sadovnick, A.D., McElroy, S.L., Keck, P.E. Jr., and Kelsoe, J.R. (2005). Examination of the clock gene cryptochrome 1 in bipolar disorder: Mutational analysis and absence of evidence for linkage or association. *Psychiatr Genet*, 15(1), 45–52.

Nofzinger, E.A., Reynolds, C.F. III, Thase, M.E., Frank, E., Jennings, J.R., Fasiczka, A.L., Sullivan, L.R., and Kupfer, D.J. (1995). REM sleep enhancement by bupropion in depressed men. *Am J Psychiatry*, 152(2), 274–276.

Nofzinger, E.A., Mintun, M.A., Wiseman, M., Kupfer, D.J., and Moore, R.Y. (1997). Forebrain activation in REM sleep: An FDG PET study. *Brain Res*, 770(1–2), 192–201.

Nofzinger, E.A., Price, J.C., Meltzer, C.C., Buysse, D.J., Villemagne, V.L., Miewald, J.M., Sembrat, R.C., Steppe, D.A., and Kupfer, D.J. (2000). Towards a neurobiology of dysfunctional arousal in depression: The relationship between beta EEG power and regional cerebral glucose metabolism during NREM sleep. *Psychiatry Res*, 98(2), 71–91.

Norden, M.J., and Avery, D.H. (1993). A controlled study of dawn simulation in subsyndromal winter depression. *Acta Psychiatr Scand*, 88(1), 67–71.

Nurnberger, J.I. Jr., Berrettini, W., Tamarkin, L., Hamovit, J., Norton, J., and Gershon, E. (1988). Supersensitivity to melatonin suppression by light in young people at high risk for affective disorder. A preliminary report. *Neuropsychopharmacology*, 1(3), 217–223.

Nurnberger, J. Jr., Berrettini, W., Mendelson, W., Sack, D., and Gershon, E.S. (1989). Measuring cholinergic sensitivity: I. Arecoline effects in bipolar patients. *Biol Psychiatry*, 25(5), 610–617.

Nurnberger, J.I. Jr., Adkins, S., Lahiri, D.K., Mayeda, A., Hu, K., Lewy, A., Miller, A., Bowman, E.S., Miller, M.J., Rau, L., Smiley, C., and Davis-Singh, D. (2000). Melatonin suppression by light in euthymic bipolar and unipolar patients. *Arch Gen Psychiatry*, 57(6), 572–579.

Okawa, M., Shirakawa, S., Uchiyama, M., Oguri, M., Kohsaka, M., Mishima, K., Sakamoto, K., Inoue, H., Kamei, K., and

Takahashi, K. (1996). Seasonal variation of mood and behaviour in a healthy middle-aged population in Japan. *Acta Psychiatr Scand*, 94(4), 211–216.

Oren, D.A., Moul, D.E., Schwartz, P.J., Brown, C., Yamada, E.M., and Rosenthal, N.E. (1994a). Exposure to ambient light in patients with winter seasonal affective disorder. *Am J Psychiatry*, 151(4), 591–593.

Oren, D.A., Moul, D.E., Schwartz, P.J., Wehr, T.A., and Rosenthal, N.E. (1994b). A controlled trial of levodopa plus carbidopa in the treatment of winter seasonal affective disorder: A test of the dopamine hypothesis. *J Clin Psychopharmacol*, 14(3), 196–200.

Oren, D.A., Schulkin, J., and Rosenthal, N.E. (1994c). 1,25 $(OH)_2$ vitamin D_3 levels in seasonal affective disorder: Effects of light. *Psychopharmacology (Berl)*, 116(4), 515–516.

Oren, D.A., Levendosky, A.A., Kasper, S., Duncan, C.C., and Rosenthal, N.E. (1996). Circadian profiles of cortisol, prolactin, and thyrotropin in seasonal affective disorder. *Biol Psychiatry*, 39(3), 157–170.

O'Rourke, D.A., Wurtman, J.J., Brzezinski, A., Nader, T.A., and Chew, B. (1987). Serotonin implicated in etiology of seasonal affective disorder. *Psychopharmacol Bull*, 23(3), 358–359.

Ostenfeld, I. (1986). Abstinence from night sleep as a treatment for endogenous depressions. The earliest observations in a Danish mental hospital (1954) and an analysis of the causal mechanism. *Dan Med Bull*, 33(1), 45–49.

Ozaki, N., Rosenthal, N.E., Moul, D.E., Schwartz, P.J., and Oren, D.A. (1993). Effects of phototherapy on electrooculographic ratio in winter seasonal affective disorder. *Psychiatry Res*, 49(2), 99–107.

Ozaki, N., Ono, Y., Ito, A., and Rosenthal, N.E. (1995a). Prevalence of seasonal difficulties in mood and behavior among Japanese civil servants. *Am J Psychiatry*, 152(8), 1225–1227.

Ozaki, N., Rosenthal, N.E., Myers, F., Schwartz, P.J., and Oren, D.A. (1995b). Effects of season on electro-oculographic ratio in winter seasonal affective disorder. *Psychiatry Res*, 59(1-2), 151–155.

Palmai, G., and Blackwell, B. (1965). The diurnal pattern of salivary flow in normal and depressed patients. *Br J Psychiatry*, 111, 334–338.

Papoušek, M. (1975). Chronobiologische Aspekte der Zyklothymie. *Fortschritte der Neurologie, Psychatrie und Ihrer Grenzgebiete*, 43, 381–440.

Partinen, M., Kaprio, J., Koskenvuo, M., Putkonen, P., and Langinvainio, H. (1983). Genetic and environmental determination of human sleep. *Sleep*, 6(3), 179–185.

Partonen, T., and Lonnqvist, J. (1993). Effects of light on mood. *Ann Med*, 25(4), 301–302.

Partonen, T., and Lonnqvist, J. (1996). Seasonal variation in bipolar disorder. *Br J Psychiatry*, 169(5), 641–646.

Partonen, T., Appelberg, B., and Partinen, M. (1993a). Effects of light treatment on sleep structure in seasonal affective disorder. *Eur Arch Psychiatry Clin Neurosci*, 242(5), 310–313.

Partonen, T., Partinen, M., and Lonnqvist, J. (1993b). Frequencies of seasonal major depressive symptoms at high latitudes. *Eur Arch Psychiatry Clin Neurosci*, 243(3–4), 189–192.

Payne, J.L., Quiroz, J.A., Zarate, C.A. Jr., and Manji, H.K. (2002). Timing is everything: Does the robust upregulation of noradrenergically regulated plasticity genes underlie the rapid antidepressant effects of sleep deprivation? *Biol Psychiatry*, 52(10), 921–926.

Peck, D.F. (1990). Climatic variables and admissions for mania: A reanalysis. *J Affect Disord*, 20(4), 249–250.

Penn, J.S., and Williams, T.P. (1986). Photostasis: Regulation of daily photon-catch by rat retinas in response to various cyclic illuminances. *Exp Eye Res*, 43(6), 915–928.

Pereira, D.S., Tufik, S., Louzada, F.M., Benedito-Silva, A.A., Lopez, A.R., Lemos, N.A., Korczak, A.L., D'Almeida, V., and Pedrazzoli, M. (2005). Association of the length of polymorphism in the human *per3* gene with the delayed sleep-phase syndrome: Does latitude have an influence upon it? *Sleep*, 28(1), 29–32.

Perlman, C.A., Johnson, S.L., and Mellman, T.A. (2006). The prospective impact of sleep duration on depression and mania. *Bipolar Disord*, 8(3), 271–274.

Petridou, E., Papadopoulos, F.C., Frangakis, C.E., Skalkidou, A., and Trichopoulos, D. (2002). A role of sunshine in the triggering of suicide. *Epidemiology*, 13(1), 106–109.

Pfaffenberger, B., Hardt, I., Huhnerfuss, H., Konig, W.A., Rimkus, G., Glausch, A., Schurig, V., and Hahn, J. (1994). Enantioselective degradation of alpha-hexachlorocyclohexane and cyclodiene insecticides in roe-deer liver samples from different regions of Germany. *Chemosphere*, 29(7), 1543–1554.

Pflug, B., and Tölle, R. (1971). Disturbance of the 24-hour rhythm in endogenous depression and the treatment of endogenous depression by sleep deprivation. *Int Pharmacopsychiatry*, 6, 187–196.

Pflug, B., Erikson, R., and Johnsson, A. (1976). Depression and daily temperature: A long-term study. *Acta Psychiatr Scand*, 54, 254–266.

Pflug, B., Johnsson, A., and Ekse, A.T. (1981). Manic-depressive states and daily temperature. *Acta Psychiatr Scand*, 63, 277–289.

Pflug, B., Johnsson, A., and Martin, W. (1983). Alterations in the circadian temperature rhythms in depressed patients. In T.A. Weher and F.K. Goodwin (Eds.), *Circadian Rhythms in Psychiatry* (pp. 71–76). Pacific Grove, CA: Boxwood Press.

Phiel, C.J., and Klein, P.S. (2001). Molecular targets of lithium action. *Annu Rev Pharmacol Toxicol*, 41, 789–813.

Pittendrigh, C.S., and Daan, S. (1976). A functional analysis of circadian pacemakers in nocturnal rodents. V. Pacemaker structure: A clock for all seasons. *J Comp Physiol*, 106, 333–355.

Pizzagalli, D., Pascual-Marqui, R.D., Nitschke, J.B., Oakes, T.R., Larson, C.L., Abercrombie, H.C., Schaefer, S.M., Koger, J.V., Benca, R.M., and Davidson, R.J. (2001). Anterior cingulate activity as a predictor of degree of treatment response in major depression: Evidence from brain electrical tomography analysis. *Am J Psychiatry*, 158(3), 405–415.

Placidi, F., Diomedi, M., Scalise, A., Marciani, M. G., Romigi, A., and Gigli, G.L. (2000a). Effect of anticonvulsants on nocturnal sleep in epilepsy. *Neurology*, 54(5 Suppl. 1), S25–S32.

Placidi, F., Marciani, M.G., Diomedi, M., Scalise, A., Pauri, F., Giacomini, P., and Gigli, G.L. (2000b). Effects of lamotrigine on nocturnal sleep, daytime somnolence and cognitive functions in focal epilepsy. *Acta Neurol Scand*, 102(2), 81–86.

Placidi, F., Scalise, A., Marciani, M.G., Romigi, A., Diomedi, M., and Gigli, G.L. (2000c). Effect of antiepileptic drugs on sleep. *Clin Neurophysiol*, 111(Suppl. 2), S115–S119.

Plyte, S.E., Hughes, K., Nikolakaki, E., Pulverer, B.J., and Woodgett, J.R. (1992). Glycogen synthase kinase-3: Functions in oncogenesis and development. *Biochim Biophys Acta*, 1114(2–3), 147–162.

Postolache, T.T., and Oren, D.A. (2005). Circadian phase shifting, alerting, and antidepressant effects of bright light treatment. *Clin Sports Med*, 24(2), 381–413, xii.

Postolache, T.T., Hardin, T.A., Myers, F.S., Turner, E.H., Yi, L.Y., Barnett, R.L., Matthews, J.R., and Rosenthal, N.E. (1998). Greater improvement in summer than with light treatment in winter in patients with seasonal affective disorder. *Am J Psychiatry*, 155(11), 1614–1616.

Postolache, T.T., Benson, B.E., Guzman, A., Mathews, J.R., Turner, E.H., Wehr, T.A., Rosenthal, N.E., and Drevets, W.C. (2002a). Acute effects of light treatment on cerebral blood flow in healthy subjects. *Chronobiol Int*, 19, 984–985.

Postolache, T.T., Benson, B.E., Guzman, A., Mathews, J.R., Turner, E.H., Wehr, T.A., Rosenthal, N.E., and Drevets, W.C. (2002b). *Acute effects of light treatment on cerebral blood flow in healthy subjects and patients with seasonal affective disorder.* Symposium on Healthy Lighting. Eindhoven, The Netherlands: Light & Health Research Foundation.

Postolache, T.T., Matthews, J.R., Turner, E.H., Benson, B.E., Guzman, A., Rosenthal, N.E., and Drevets, W.C. (2002c). Cerebral blood flow in depressed individuals with sad as compared to matched controls. *Chronobiol Int*, 19(5), 986.

Postolache, T.T., Wehr, T.A., Doty, R.L., Sher, L., Turner, E.H., Bartko, J.J., and Rosenthal, N.E. (2002d). Patients with seasonal affective disorder have lower odor detection thresholds than control subjects. *Arch Gen Psychiatry*, 59(12), 1119–1122.

Postolache, T.T., Komarow, H.D., Stiller, J.W., and Tonelli, L.H. (2005a). Allergy, depression, and suicide. *Directions in Psychiatry*, 25(6), 59–70.

Postolache, T.T., Stiller, J.W., Herrell, R., Goldstein, M.A., Shreeram, S.S., Zebrak, R., Thrower, C.M., Volkov, J., No, M.J., Volkov, I., Rohan, K.J., Redditt, J., Parmar, M., Mohyuddin, F., Olsen, C., Moca, M., Tonelli, L.H., Merikangas, K., and Komarow, H.D. (2005b). Tree pollen peaks are associated with increased nonviolent suicide in women. *Mol Psychiatry*, 10, 232–238.

Provencio, I., Jiang, G., De Grip, W.J., Hayes, W.P., and Rollag, M.D. (1998). Melanopsin: An opsin in melanophores, brain, and eye. *Proc Natl Acad Sci USA*, 95(1), 340–345.

Provencio, I., Rodriguez, I.R., Jiang, G., Hayes, W.P., Moreira, E.F., and Rollag, M.D. (2000). A novel human opsin in the inner retina. *J Neurosci*, 20(2), 600–605.

Provencio, I., Rollag, M.D., and Castrucci, A.M. (2002). Photoreceptive net in the mammalian retina. *Nature*, 415(6871), 493.

Puchalski, W., and Lynch, G.R. (1986). Evidence for differences in the circadian organization of hamsters exposed to short day photoperiod. *J Comp Physiol [A]*, 159(1), 7–11.

Rasanen, M., Lehtinen, J.C., Niinikoski, H., Keskinen, S., Ruottinen, S., Salminen, M., Ronnemaa, T., Viikari, J., and Simell, O. (2002a). Dietary patterns and nutrient intakes of 7-year-old children taking part in an atherosclerosis prevention project in Finland. *J Am Diet Assoc*, 102(4), 518–524.

Rasanen, P., Hakko, H., Jokelainen, J., and Tiihonen, J. (2002b). Seasonal variation in specific methods of suicide: A national register study of 20,234 Finnish people. *J Affect Disord*, 71(1–3), 51–59.

Rasanen, T.L., Alhonen, L., Sinervirta, R., Keinanen, T., Herzig, K.H., Suppola, S., Khomutov, A.R., Vepsalainen, J., and Janne, J. (2002c). A polyamine analogue prevents acute pancreatitis and restores early liver regeneration in transgenic rats with activated polyamine catabolism. *J Biol Chem*, 277(42), 39867–39872.

Reinink, E., Bouhuys, N., Wirz-Justice, A., and van den Hoofdakker, R. (1990). Prediction of the antidepressant response to total sleep deprivation by diurnal variation of mood. *Psychiatry Res*, 32(2), 113–124.

Reinink, E., Bouhuys, A.L., Gordijn, M.C., and Van Den Hoof-dakker, R.H. (1993). Prediction of the antidepressant response to total sleep deprivation of depressed patients: Longitudinal versus single day assessment of diurnal mood variation. *Biol Psychiatry*, 34(7), 471–481.

Reme, C., Terman, M., and Wirz-Justice, A. (1990). Are deficient retinal photoreceptor renewal mechanisms involved in the pathogenesis of winter depression? *Arch Gen Psychiatry*, 47(9), 878–879.

Reppert, S.M., and Weaver, D.R. (2000). Comparing clockworks: Mouse versus fly. *J Biol Rhythms*, 15(5), 357–364.

Reppert, S.M., and Weaver, D.R.. (2001). Molecular analysis of mammalian circadian rhythms. *Annu Rev Physiol*, 63, 647–676.

Reynolds, C.F. III, Buysse, D.J., Brunner, D.P., Begley, A.E., Dew, M.A., Hoch, C.C., Hall, M., Houck, P.R., Mazumdar, S., Perel, J.M., and Kupfer, D.J. (1997). Maintenance nortriptyline effects on electroencephalographic sleep in elderly patients with recurrent major depression: Double-blind, placebo- and plasma-level-controlled evaluation. *Biol Psychiatry*, 42(7), 560–567.

Riemann, D., and Berger, M. (1989). EEG sleep in depression and in remission and the REM sleep response to the cholinergic agonist RS 86. *Neuropsychopharmacology*, 2(2), 145–152.

Riemann, D., and Berger, M. (1990). The effects of total sleep deprivation and subsequent treatment with clomipramine on depressive symptoms and sleep electroencephalography in patients with a major depressive disorder. *Acta Psychiatr Scand*, 81(1), 24–31.

Riemann, D., Wiegand, M., and Berger, M. (1991). Are there predictors for sleep deprivation response in depressed patients? *Biol Psychiatry*, 29(7), 707–710.

Riemann, D., Hohagen, F., Konig, A., Schwarz, B., Gomille, J., Voderholzer, U., and Berger, M. (1996). Advanced vs. normal sleep timing: Effects on depressed mood after response to sleep deprivation in patients with a major depressive disorder. *J Affect Disord*, 37(2–3), 121–128.

Riemann, D., Konig, A., Hohagen, F., Kiemen, A., Voderholzer, U., Backhaus, J., Bunz, J., Wesiack, B., Hermle, L., and Berger, M. (1999). How to preserve the antidepressive effect of sleep deprivation: A comparison of sleep phase advance and sleep phase delay. *Eur Arch Psychiatry Clin Neurosci*, 249(5), 231–237.

Riemann, D., Berger, M., and Voderholzer, U. (2001). Sleep and depression—results from psychobiological studies: An overview. *Biol Psychol*, 57(1-3), 67–103.

Rosenthal, N.E., Sack, D.A., Gillin, J.C., Lewy, A.J., Goodwin, F.K., Davenport, Y., Mueller, P.S., Newsome, D.A., and Wehr, T.A. (1984). Seasonal affective disorder. A description of the syndrome and preliminary findings with light therapy. *Arch Gen Psychiatry*, 41(1), 72–80.

Rosenthal, N.E., Sack, D.A., Carpenter, C.J., Parry, B.L., Mendelson, W.B., and Wehr, T.A. (1985). Antidepressant effects of light in seasonal affective disorder. *Am J Psychiatry*, 142(2), 163–170.

Rosenthal, N.E., Jacobsen, F.M., Sack, D.A., Arendt, J., James, S.P., Parry, B.L., and Wehr, T.A. (1988). Atenolol in seasonal affective disorder: A test of the melatonin hypothesis. *Am J Psychiatry*, 145(1), 52–56.

Rosenthal, N.E., Genhart, M.J., Caballero, B., Jacobsen, F.M., Skwerer, R.G., Coursey, R.D., Rogers, S., and Spring, B.J. (1989). Psychobiological effects of carbohydrate- and protein-rich meals in patients with seasonal affective disorder and normal controls. *Biol Psychiatry*, 25(8), 1029–1040.

Rosenthal, N.E., Levendosky, A.A., Skwerer, R.G., Joseph-Vanderpool, J.R., Kelly, K.A., Hardin, T., Kasper, S., Della-Bella, P., and Wehr, T.A. (1990). Effects of light treatment on core body temperature in seasonal affective disorder. *Biol Psychiatry*, 27(1), 39–50.

Rosenthal, N.E., Mazzanti, C.M., Barnett, R.L., Hardin, T.A., Turner, E.H., Lam, G.K., Ozaki, N., and Goldman, D. (1998). Role of serotonin transporter promoter repeat length polymorphism (5-HTTLPR) in seasonality and seasonal affective disorder. *Mol Psychiatry*, 3(2), 175–177.

Rudorfer, M.V., Skwerer, R.G., and Rosenthal, N.E. (1993). Biogenic amines in seasonal affective disorder: Effects of light therapy. *Psychiatry Res*, 46(1), 19–28.

Ruger, M., Gordijn, M.C., Beersma, D.G., de Vries, B., and Daan, S. (2003). Acute and phase-shifting effects of ocular and extraocular light in human circadian physiology. *J Biol Rhythms*, 18(5), 409–419.

Rush, A.J., Erman, M.K., Giles, D.E., Schlesser, M.A., Carpenter, G., Vasavada, N., and Roffwarg, H.P. (1986). Polysomnographic findings in recently drug-free and clinically remitted depressed patients. *Arch Gen Psychiatry*, 43(9), 878–884.

Saanjarvi, S., Lauerma, H., Helenius, S., and Saanlehto, S. (1997). Seasonal affective disorder common in Finland. *Biol Psychiatry*, 42, 255S.

Sack, D.A., Nurnberger, J., Rosenthal, N.E., Ashburn, E., and Wehr, T.A. (1985). Potentiation of antidepressant medications by phase advance of the sleep–wake cycle. *Am J Psychiatry*, 142(5), 606–608.

Sack, D.A., Duncan, W., Rosenthal, N.E., Mendelson, W.E., and Wehr, T.A. (1988). The timing and duration of sleep in partial sleep deprivation therapy of depression. *Acta Psychiatr Scand*, 77, 219–224.

Sack, R.L., Lewy, A.J., Wite, D.M., Singer, C.M., Fireman, M.J., and Vandiver, R. (1990). Morning vs. evening light treatment for winter depression. Evidence that therapeutic effects of light mediated by circadian phase shift. *Arch Gen Psychiatry*, 47, 343–351.

Saper, C.B., Chou, T.C., and Scammell, T.E. (2001). The sleep switch: Hypothalamic control of sleep and wakefulness. *Trends Neurosci*, 24, 726–731.

Sato, T., Bottlender, R., Sievers, M., and Moller, H.J. (2006). Distinct seasonality of depressive episodes differentiates unipolar depressive patients with and without depressive mixed states. *J Affect Disord*, 90(1), 1–5.

Schilgen, B., and Tölle, R. (1980). Partial sleep deprivation as therapy for depression. *Arch Gen Psychiatry*, 37, 267–271.

Schilling, A., and Perret, M. (1993). Removal of the olfactory bulbs modifies the gonadal responses of photoperiod in the lesser mouse lemur (microcebus murinus). *Biol Reprod*, 49, 58–65.

Schlager, D.S. (1994). Early-morning administration of short-acting beta blockers for treatment of winter depression. *Am J Psychiatry*, 151(9), 1383–1385.

Schreiber, W., Lauer, C.J., Krumrey, K., Holsboer, F., and Krieg, J.C. (1992). Cholinergic REM sleep induction test in subjects at high risk for psychiatric disorders. *Biol Psychiatry*, 32(1), 79–90.

Schremser, J.L., and Williams, T.P. (1995a). Rod outer segment (ROS) renewal as a mechanism for adaptation to a new intensity environment. I. Rhodopsin levels and ROS length. *Exp Eye Res*, 61(1), 17–23.

Schremser, J.L., and Williams, T.P. (1995b). Rod outer segment (ROS) renewal as a mechanism for adaptation to a new intensity environment. II. Rhodopsin synthesis and packing density. *Exp Eye Res*, 61(1), 25–32.

Schulz, H., and Lund, R. (1983). Sleep onset REM episodes are associated with circadian parameters of body temperature: A study in depressed patients and normal controls. *Biol Psychiatry*, 18, 1411–1426.

Schulz, H., and Lund, R. (1985). On the origin of early REM episodes in the sleep of depressed patients: A comparison of three hypotheses. *Psychiatry Res*, 16(1), 65–77.

Schulz, H., Lund, R., Cording, C., and Dirlich, G. (1979). Bimodal distribution of REM sleep latencies in depression. *Biol Psychiatry*, 14(4), 595–600.

Schwartz, P.J., Murphy, D.L., Wehr, T.A., Garcia-Borreguero, D., Oren, D.A., Moul, D.E., Ozaki, N., Snelbaker, A.J., and Rosenthal, N.E. (1997). Effects of meta-chlorophenylpiperazine infusions in patients with seasonal affective disorder and healthy control subjects. Diurnal responses and nocturnal regulatory mechanisms. *Arch Gen Psychiatry*, 54(4), 375–385.

Schwartz, P.J., Rosenthal, N.E., Kajimura, N., Han, L., Turner, E.H., Bender, C., and Wehr, T.A. (2000). Ultradian oscillations in cranial thermoregulation and electroencephalographic slow-wave activity during sleep are abnormal in humans with annual winter depression. *Brain Res*, 866(1–2), 152–167.

Schwartz, P.J., Rosenthal, N.E., and Wehr, T.A. (2001a). Band-specific electroencephalogram and brain cooling abnormalities during NREM sleep in patients with winter depression. *Biol Psychiatry*, 50(8), 627–632.

Schwartz, W.J., de la Iglesia, H.O., Zlomanczuk, P., and Illnerova, H. (2001b). Encoding le quattro stagioni within the mammalian brain: Photoperiodic orchestration through the suprachiasmatic nucleus. *J Biol Rhythms*, 16(4), 302–311.

Sharpley, A.L., Walsh, A.E., and Cowen, P.J. (1992). Nefazodone—a novel antidepressant—may increase REM sleep. *Biol Psychiatry*, 31(10), 1070–1073.

Shearman, L.P., Jin, X., Lee, C., Reppert, S.M., and Weaver, D.R. (2000a). Targeted disruption of the *mPer3* gene: Subtle effects on circadian clock function. *Mol Cell Biol*, 20(17), 6269–6275.

Shearman, L.P., Sriram, S., Weaver, D.R., Maywood, E.S., Chaves, I., Zheng, B., Kume, K., Lee, C.C., van der Horst, G.T., Hastings, M.H., and Reppert, S.M. (2000b). Interacting molecular loops in the mammalian circadian clock. *Science*, 288(5468), 1013–1019.

Shen, H., Watanabe, M., Tomasiewicz, H., Rutishauser, U., Magnuson, T., and Glass, J.D. (1997). Role of neural cell adhesion molecule and polysialic acid in mouse circadian clock function. *J Neurosci*, 17(13), 5221–5229.

Sher, L., Matthews, J.R., Turner, E.H., Postolache, T.T., Katz, K.S., and Rosenthal, N.E. (2001). Early response to light therapy partially predicts long-term antidepressant effects in patients with seasonal affective disorder. *J Psychiatry Neurosci*, 26(4), 336–338.

Shin, K., Schaffer, A., Levitt, A.J., and Boyle, M.H. (2005). Seasonality in a community sample of bipolar, unipolar and control subjects. *J Affect Disord*, 86(1), 19–25.

Siegel, J.M., and Rogawski, M.A. (1988). A function for REM sleep: Regulation of noradrenergic receptor sensitivity. *Brain Res*, 472(3), 213–233.

Siffre, M. (1975). Six months alone in a cave. *Natl Geographic*, 147, 426–435.

Silverstone, T., Romans, S., Hunt, N., and McPherson, H. (1995). Is there a seasonal pattern of relapse in bipolar affective disorders? A dual northern and southern hemisphere cohort study. *Br J Psychiatry*, 167(1), 58–60.

Sitaram, N., Wyatt, R.J., Dawson, S., and Gillin, J.C. (1976). REM sleep induction by physostigmine infusion during sleep. *Science*, 191(4233), 1281–1283.

Sitaram, N., Gillin, J.G., and Bunney, W.E. Jr. (1978a). Circadian variation in the time of "switch" of a patient with 48-hour manic-depressive cycles. *Biol Psychiatry*, 13(5), 567–574.

Sitaram, N., Moore, A.M., and Gillin, J.C. (1978b). Experimental acceleration and slowing of REM sleep ultradian rhythm by cholinergic agonist and antagonist. *Nature*, 274(5670), 490–492.

Sitaram, N., Nurnberger, J.I. Jr., Gershon, E.S., and Gillin, J.C. (1980). Faster cholinergic REM sleep induction in euthymic patients with primary affective illness. *Science*, 208(4440), 200–202.

Sitaram, N., Nurnberger, J.I. Jr., Gershon, E.S., and Gillin, J.C. (1982). Cholinergic regulation of mood and REM sleep: Potential model and marker of vulnerability to affective disorder. *Am J Psychiatry*, 139(5), 571–576.

Skene, D.J., Lockley, S.W., Thapan, K., and Arendt, J. (1999). Effects of light on human circadian rhythms. *Reprod Nutr Dev*, 39(3), 295–304.

Skwerer, R.G., Jacobsen, F.M., Duncan, C.C., Kelly, K.A., Sack, D.A., Tamarkin, L., Gaist, P.A., Kasper, S., and Rosenthal, N.E. (1988). Neurobiology of seasonal affective disorder and phototherapy. *J Biol Rhythms*, 3(2), 135–154.

Slater, E. (1938). Zur Periodic des manische-depressiven Irreseins. *Z Neurol Psychiatrie*, 162, 794–801.

Smeraldi, E., Benedetti, F., Barbini, B., Campori, E., and Colombo, C. (1999). Sustained antidepressant effect of sleep deprivation combined with pindolol in bipolar depression. A placebo-controlled trial. *Neuropsychopharmacology*, 20(4), 380–385.

Smith, G.S., Reynolds, C.F. III, Pollock, B., Derbyshire, S., Nofzinger, E., Dew, M.A., Houck, P.R., Milko, D., Meltzer, C.C., and Kupfer, D.J. (1999). Cerebral glucose metabolic response to combined total sleep deprivation and antidepressant treatment in geriatric depression. *Am J Psychiatry*, 156(5), 683–689.

Souêtre, E. (1990). Sleep disorders related to anxiety. *Presse Med*, 19(40), 1839–1841.

Souêtre, E., Pringuey, D., Salvati, E., and Robert, P. (1985). Rythmes circadiens de la température centrale et de la cortisolémie dans les dépressions endogènes. *L'Encéphale*, 11, 185–198.

Souêtre, E., Salvati, E., Wehr, T.A., Sack, D.A., Krebs, B., and Darcourt, G. (1988). Twenty-four-hour profiles of body temperature and plasma TSH in bipolar patients during depression and during remission and in normal control subjects. *Am J Psychiatry*, 145(9), 1133–1137.

Souêtre, E., Salvati, E., Belugou, J.L., Pringuey, D., Candito, M., Krebs, B., Ardisson, J.L., and Darcourt, G. (1989). Circadian rhythms in depression and recovery: Evidence for blunted amplitude as the main chronobiological abnormality. *Psychiatry Res*, 28(3), 263–278.

Spiegel, K., Leproult, R., and Van Cauter, E. (1999). Impact of sleep debt on metabolic and endocrine function. *Lancet*, 354(9188), 1435–1439.

Steiger, A., von Bardeleben, U., Herth, T., and Holsboer, F. (1989). Sleep EEG and nocturnal secretion of cortisol and growth hormone in male patients with endogenous depression before treatment and after recovery. *J Affect Disord*, 16(2-3), 189–195.

Steiger, A., Gerken, A., Benkert, O., and Holsboer, F. (1993a). Differential effects of the enantiomers R(−) and S(+) oxaprotiline on major endogenous depression, the sleep EEG and neuroendocrine secretion: Studies on depressed patients and normal controls. *Eur Neuropsychopharmacol*, 3(2), 117–126.

Steiger, A., Trachsel, L., Guldner, J., Hemmeter, U., Rothe, B., Rupprecht, R., Vedder, H., and Holsboer, F. (1993b). Neurosteroid pregnenolone induces sleep-EEG changes in man compatible with inverse agonistic GABAA-receptor modulation. *Brain Res*, 615(2), 267–274.

Steiger, A., von Bardeleben, U., Guldner, J., Lauer, C., Rothe, B., and Holsboer, F. (1993c). The sleep EEG and nocturnal hormonal secretion studies on changes during the course of depression and on effects of CNS-active drugs. *Prog Neuropsychopharmacol Biol Psychiatry*, 17(1), 125–137.

Stephan, F.K. (1983). Circadian rhythm dissociation induced by periodic feeding in rats with suprachiasmatic lesions. *Behav Brain Res*, 7(1), 81–98.

Steriade, M. (1994). Sleep oscillations and their blockage by activating systems. *J Psychiatry Neurosci*, 19(5), 354–358.

Swade, C., and Coppen, A. (1980). Seasonal variations in biochemical factors related to depressive illness. *J Affect Disord*, 2(4), 249–255.

Tafti, M., Chollet, D., Valatx, J.L., and Franken, P. (1999). Quantitative trait loci approach to the genetics of sleep in recombinant inbred mice. *J Sleep Res*, 8(Suppl. 1), 37–43.

Takano, A., Uchiyama, M., Kajimura, N., Mishima, K., Inoue, Y., Kamei, Y., Kitajima, T., Shibui, K., Katoh, M., Watanabe, T., Hashimotodani, Y., Nakajima, T., Ozeki, Y., Hori, T., Yamada, N., Toyoshima, R., Ozaki, N., Okawa, M., Nagai, K., Takahashi, K., Isojima, Y., Yamauchi, T., and Ebisawa, T. (2004). A missense variation in human casein kinase I epsilon gene that induces functional alteration and shows an inverse association with circadian rhythm sleep disorders. *Neuropsychopharmacology*, 29(10), 1901–1909.

Takei, N., O'Callaghan, E., Sham, P., Glover, G., Tamura, A., and Murray, R. (1992). Seasonality of admissions in the psychoses: Effect of diagnosis, sex, and age at onset. *Br J Psychiatry*, 161, 506–511.

Terman, J.S., and Terman, M. (1999). Photopic and scotopic light detection in patients with seasonal affective disorder and control subjects. *Biol Psychiatry*, 46(12), 1642–1648.

Terman, J.S., Terman, M., Lo, E.S., and Cooper, T.B. (2001). Circadian time of morning light administration and therapeutic response in winter depression. *Arch Gen Psychiatry*, 58(1), 69–75.

Terman, M., Boticelli, S.R., and Link, B.G., et al. (1989a). Seasonal symptom patters in New York: Patients and population. In C. Thomson, and T. Silverstone (Eds.), *Seasonal Affective Disorder* (pp. 77–95). London: CNS Publishers.

Terman, M., Terman J.-S., Quitkin, F., McGrath, P., Stewart, J., and Rafferty, B. (1989b). Light treatment for seasonal affective disorder: A review of efficacy. *Neuropsychopharmacology*, 2, 1–22.

Terman, M., Terman, J.S., and Ross, D.C. (1998). A controlled study of timed bright light and negative air ionization for treatment of winter depression. *Arch Gen Psychiatry*, 55, 875–882.

Thase, M.E., Himmelhoch, J.M., Mallinger, A.G., Jarrett, D.B., and Kupfer, D.J. (1989). Sleep EEG and DST findings in anergic bipolar depression. *Am J Psychiatry*, 146(3), 329–333.

Thase, M.E., Kupfer, D.J., Buysse, D.J., Frank, E., Simons, A.D., McEachran, A.B., Rashid, K.F., and Grochocinski, V.J. (1995). Electroencephalographic sleep profiles in single-episode and recurrent unipolar forms of major depression: I. Comparison during acute depressive states. *Biol Psychiatry*, 38(8), 506–515.

Thase, M.E., Fasiczka, A.L., Berman, S.R., Simons, A.D., and Reynolds, C.F. III. (1998). Electroencephalographic sleep profiles before and after cognitive behavior therapy of depression. *Arch Gen Psychiatry*, 55(2), 138–144.

Thomson, C., Rodin, I., and Birtwhistle, J. (1999). Light therapy for seasonal and nonseasonal affective disorder: A Cochrane meta-analysis, 11.

Thorell, L.H., Kjellman, B., Arned, M., Lindwall-Sundel, K., Walinder, J., and Wetterberg, L. (1999). Light treatment of seasonal affective disorder in combination with citalopram or placebo with 1-year follow-up. *Int Clin Psychopharmacol*, 14(Suppl. 2), S7–S11.

Toh, K.L., Jones, C.R., He, Y., Eide, E.J., Hinz, W.A., Virshup, D.M., Ptacek, L.J., and Fu, Y.H. (2001). An hPer2 phosphorylation site mutation in familial advanced sleep phase syndrome. *Science*, 291(5506), 1040–1043.

Tonelli, L.H., and Postolache, T.T. (2006). *Behavioral, cellular, and molecular responses in the brain induced by allergy to tree pollen.* Presented at the Neuroscience Meeting, Atlanta, GA.

Tonelli, L.H., Rujescu, D., Stiller, J.W., Giegling, I., Schneider, B., Maurer, K., Bratzke, H.J., Schnabel, A., and Postolache, T.T. (2006). Gender-specific cytokine gene expression in the brain of suicide victims. *Biol Psychiatry*, 59, 245S–246S.

Toth, L.A. (2001). Identifying genetic influences on sleep: An approach to discovering the mechanisms of sleep regulation. *Behav Genet*, 31(1), 39–46.

Totterdell, P., Reynolds, S., Parkinson, B., and Briner, R.B. (1994). Associations of sleep with everyday mood, minor symptoms and social interaction experience. *Sleep*, 17(5), 466–475.

Tsai, S.Y., Yang, Y.Y., Kuo, C.J., Chen, C.C., and Leu, S.J. (2001). Effects of symptomatic severity on elevation of plasma soluble interleukin-2 receptor in bipolar mania. *J Affect Disord*, 64(2–3), 185–193.

Tsujimoto, T., Yamada, N., Shimoda, K., Hanada, K., and Takahashi, S. (1990). Circadian rhythms in depression. Part II: Circadian rhythms in inpatients with various mental disorders. *J Affect Disord*, 18(3), 199–210.

Tsuno, N., Besset, A., and Ritchie, K. (1977). Sleep and depression. *J Clin Psychiatry*, 66(10), 1254–1269.

Van Cauter, E., and Turek, F.W. (1986). Depression: A disorder of timekeeping? *Perspect Biol Med*, 29(4), 510–519.

Van Den Burg, W., Beersma, D.G., Bouhuys, A.L., and Van Den Hoofdakker, R.H. (1992). Self-rated arousal concurrent with the antidepressant response to total sleep deprivation of patients with a major depressive disorder: A disinhibition hypothesis. *J Sleep Res*, 1(4), 211–222.

van den Hoofdakker, R.H. (1997). Total sleep deprivation: Clinical and theoretical aspects. In. A.V. Honig, and H.M. Praag (Eds.), *Depression: Neurobiological, Psychopathological and Therapeutic Advances* (pp. 564–589). Chichester, England: John Wiley & Sons,

van den Hoofdakker, R.H., and Beersma, D.G. (1985). On the explanation of short REM latencies in depression. *Psychiatry Res*, 16(2), 155–163.

van der Horst, G.T., Muijtjens, M., Kobayashi, K., Takano, R., Kanno, S., Takao, M., de Wit, J., Verkerk, A., Eker, A.P., van

Leenen, D., Buijs, R., Bootsma, D., Hoeijmakers, J.H., and Yasui, A. (1999). Mammalian Cry1 and Cry2 are essential for maintenance of circadian rhythms. *Nature*, 398(6728), 627–630.

van Houwelingen, C.A., and Beersma, D.G. (2001a). Seasonal changes in 24-h patterns of suicide rates: A study on train suicides in The Netherlands. *J Affect Disord*, 66(2–3), 215–223.

van Houwelingen, C.A., and Beersma, D.G. (2001b). Seasonal variation in suicides: Hidden not vanished. *Br J Psychiatry*, 178, 380.

Van Sweden, B. (1986). Disturbed vigilance in mania. *Biol Psychiatry*, 21(3), 311–313.

Vitaterna, M.H., King, D.P., Chang, A.M., Kornhauser, J.M., Lowrey, P.L., McDonald, J.D., Dove, W.F., Pinto, L.H., Turek, F.W., and Takahashi, J.S. (1994). Mutagenesis and mapping of a mouse gene, *Clock*, essential for circadian behavior. *Science*, 264(5159), 719–725.

Vitaterna, M.H., Selby, C.P., Todo, T., Niwa, H., Thompson, C., Fruechte, E.M., Hitomi, K., Thresher, R.J., Ishikawa, T., Miyazaki, J., Takahashi, J.S., and Sancar, A. (1999). Differential regulation of mammalian period genes and circadian rhythmicity by cryptochromes 1 and 2. *Proc Natl Acad Sci USA*, 96(21), 12114–12119.

Vogel, G.W., Vogel, F., McAbee, R.S., and Thurmond, A.J. (1980). Improvement of depression by REM sleep deprivation. New findings and a theory. *Arch Gen Psychiatry*, 37(3), 247–253.

Volk, S.A., Kaendler, S.H., Hertel, A., Maul, F.D., Manoocheri, R., Weber, R., Georgi, K., Pflug, B., and Hor, G. (1997). Can response to partial sleep deprivation in depressed patients be predicted by regional changes of cerebral blood flow? *Psychiatry Res*, 75(2), 67–74.

Vollmann, J., and Berger, M. (1993). Sleep deprivation with consecutive sleep-phase advance therapy in patients with major depression: A pilot study. *Biol Psychiatry*, 33(1), 54–57.

Vollrath, M., Wicki, W., and Angst, J. (1989). The Zurich study. VIII. Insomnia: Association with depression, anxiety, somatic syndromes, and course of insomnia. *Eur Arch Psychiatry Neurol Sci*, 239(2), 113–124.

von Economo, C. (1930). Sleep as a problem of localization. *J Nerv Ment*, 71, 249–259.

von Zerssen, D., Barthelmes, H., Dirlich, G., Doerr, P., Emrich, H.M., von Lindern, L., Lund, R., and Pirke, K.M. (1985). Circadian rhythms in endogenous depression. *Psychiatry Res*, 16(1), 51–63.

Wacker, H.R., Krauchi, K., Wirz-Justice, A., and Battegay, R. (1992). *"Seasonality" is correlated with affective and not with anxiety disorders.* 4th Annual Meeting on Light Treatment and Biological Rhythms, Bethesda, MD.

Wagner, S., Castel, M., Gainer, H., and Yarom, Y. (1997). GABA in the mammalian suprachiasmatic nucleus and its role in diurnal rhythmicity. *Nature*, 387(6633), 598–603.

Webb, W.B., and Campbell, S.S. (1983). Relationships in sleep characteristics of identical and fraternal twins. *Arch Gen Psychiatry*, 40(10), 1093–1095.

Wehr, T.A. (1989). Sleep loss: A preventable cause of mania and other excited states. *J Clin Psychiatry*, 50(Suppl.), 8–16, discussion 45–7.

Wehr, T.A. (1990). Manipulations of sleep and phototherapy: Nonpharmacological alternatives in the treatment of depression. *Clin Neuropharmacol*, 13(Suppl. 1), S54–S65.

Wehr, T.A. (1991a). The durations of human melatonin secretion and sleep respond to changes in daylength (photoperiod). *J Clin Endocrinol Metab*, 73(6), 1276–1280.

Wehr, T.A. (1991b). Sleep-loss as a possible mediator of diverse causes of mania. *Br J Psychiatry*, 159, 576–578.

Wehr, T.A. (1992a). A brain-warming function for REM sleep. *Neurosci Biobehav Rev*, 16(3), 379–397.

Wehr, T.A. (1992b). Improvement of depression and triggering of mania by sleep deprivation. *JAMA*, 267(4), 548–551.

Wehr, T.A. (1992c). In short photoperiods, human sleep is biphasic. *J Sleep Res*, 1(2), 103–107.

Wehr, T.A. (1996). A "clock for all seasons" in the human brain. *Prog Brain Res*, 111, 321–342.

Wehr, T.A. (2001). Photoperiodism in humans and other primates: Evidence and implications. *J Biol Rhythms*, 16, 348–364.

Wehr, T.A., and Goodwin, F.K. (Eds.). (1981). *Stress, Circadian Rhythms and Affective Disorders. Stress and Coping. Unit I: Psychophysiology.* Philadelphia: SmithKline Corporation.

Wehr, T.A., and Goodwin, F.K. (1983a). *Circadian Rhythms in Psychiatry.* Pacific Grove, CA: Boxwood Press.

Wehr, T.A., and Goodwin, F.K. (1983b). Introduction. In T.A. Wehr and F.K. Goodwin (Eds.), *Circadian Rhythms in Psychiatry* (pp. 1–15). Pacific Grove, CA: Boxwood Press.

Wehr, T.A., and Goodwin, F.K. (1983c). Biological rhythms in manic-depressive illness. In T.A. Wehr and F.K. Goodwin (Eds.), *Circadian Rhythms in Psychiatry* (pp. 129–184). Pacific Grove, CA: Boxwood Press.

Wehr, T.A., and Rosenthal, N.E. (1989). Seasonality and affective illness. *Am J Psychiatry*, 146(7), 829–839.

Wehr, T.A., and Sack, D.A. (1988). The relevance of sleep research to affective illness. In W.P. Koella, F. Obál, H. Schulz, and P. Visser, *Sleep '86* (pp. 207–211). New York: Gustav Fischer Verlag.

Wehr, T.A., and Wirz-Justice, A. (1981). Internal coincidence model for sleep deprivation and depression. In W.P. Koella (Ed.), *Sleep 80* (pp. 26–33). Basel: Karger.

Wehr, T.A., and Wirz-Justice, A. (1982). Circadian rhythm mechanisms in affective illness and in antidepressant drug action. *Pharmacopsychiatria*, 15(1), 31–39.

Wehr, T.A., Wirz-Justice, A., Goodwin, F.K., Duncan, W., and Gillin, J.C. (1979). Phase advance of the circadian sleep–wake cycle as an antidepressant. *Science*, 206(4419), 710–713.

Wehr, T.A., Goodwin, F.K., Wirz-Justice, A., Breitmaier, J., and Craig, C. (1982). 48-hour sleep–wake cycles in manic-depressive illness: Naturalistic observations and sleep deprivation experiments. *Arch Gen Psychiatry*, 39(5), 559–565.

Wehr, T.A., Rosenthal, N.E., Sack, D.A., and Gillin, J.C. (1985a). Antidepressant effects of sleep deprivation in bright and dim light. *Acta Psychiatr Scand*, 72, 161–165.

Wehr, T.A., Sack, D.A., Duncan, W.C., Mendelson, W.B., Rosenthal, N.E., Gillin, J.C., and Goodwin, F.K. (1985b). Sleep and circadian rhythms in affective patients isolated from external time cues. *Psychiatry Res*, 15(4), 327–339.

Wehr, T.A., Jacobsen, F.M., Sack, D.A., Arendt, J., Tamarkin, L., and Rosenthal, N.E. (1986). Phototherapy of seasonal affective disorder. Time of day and suppression of melatonin are not critical for antidepressant effects. *Arch Gen Psychiatry*, 43(9), 870–875.

Wehr, T.A., Sack, D.A., and Rosenthal, N.E. (1987). Sleep reduction as a final common pathway in the genesis of mania. *Am J Psychiatry*, 144(2), 201–204.

Wehr, T.A., Giesen, H.A., Schulz, P.M., Anderson, J.L., Joseph-Vanderpool, J.R., Kelly, K., Kasper, S., and Rosenthal, N.E. (1991). Contrasts between symptoms of summer depression and winter depression. *J Affect Disord*, 23(4), 173–183.

Wehr, T.A., Moul, D.E., Barbato, G., Giesen, H.A., Seidel, J.A., Barker, C., and Bender, C. (1993). Conservation of photoperiod-responsive mechanisms in humans. *Am J Physiol*, 265(4 Pt. 2), R846–R857.

Wehr, T.A., Giesen, H.A., Moul, D.E., Turner, E.H., and Schwartz, P.J. (1995). Suppression of men's responses to seasonal changes in day length by modern artificial lighting. *Am J Physiol*, 269(1 Pt. 2), R173–R178.

Wehr, T.A., Turner, E.H., Shimada, J.M., Lowe, C.H., Barker, C., and Leibenluft, E. (1998). Treatment of rapidly cycling bipolar patient by using extended bed rest and darkness to stabilize the timing and duration of sleep. *Biol Psychiatry*, 43(11), 822–828.

Wehr, T.A., Aeschbach, D., and Duncan, W.C. Jr. (2001a). Evidence for a biological dawn and dusk in the human circadian timing system. *J Physiol*, 535(Pt. 3), 937–951.

Wehr, T.A., Duncan, W.C. Jr., Sher, L., Aeschbach, D., Schwartz, P.J., Turner, E.H., Postolache, T.T., and Rosenthal, N.E. (2001b). A circadian signal of change of season in patients with seasonal affective disorder. *Arch Gen Psychiatry*, 58(12), 1108–1114.

Weissman, M.M., Greenwald, S., Nino-Murcia, G., and Dement, W.C. (1997). The morbidity of insomnia uncomplicated by psychiatric disorders. *Gen Hosp Psychiatry*, 19(4), 245–250.

Weitzman, E.D. (1982). Chronobiology of man. Sleep, temperature and neuroendocrine rhythms. *Hum Neurobiol*, 1(3), 173–183.

Welsh, D.K., and Moore-Ede, M.C. (1990). Lithium lengthens circadian period in a diurnal primate, *Saimiri sciureus. Biol Psychiatry*, 28(2), 117–126.

Welsh, D.K., Logothetis, D.E., Meister, M., and Reppert, S.M. (1995). Individual neurons dissociated from rat suprachiasmatic nucleus express independently phased circadian firing rhythms. *Neuron*, 14(4), 697–706.

Wever, R.A. (1979). *The Circadian System of Man: Results of Experiments under Temporal Isolation*. New York: Springer-Verlag.

Wever, R.A. (1980). Phase shifts of human circadian rhythms due to shifts of artificial zeitgebers. *Chronobiologia*, 7, 303–327.

Wever, R.A. (1983). Fractional desynchronization of human circadian rhythms. A method for evaluating entrainment limits and functional interdependencies. *Pflugers Arch*, 396(2), 128–137.

Wiegand, M., Berger, M., Zulley, J., Lauer, C., and von Zerssen, D. (1987). The influence of daytime naps on the therapeutic effect of sleep deprivation. *Biol Psychiatry*, 22(3), 389–392.

Wiegand, M., Riemann, D., Schreiber, W., Lauer, C.J., and Berger, M. (1993). Effect of morning and afternoon naps on mood after total sleep deprivation in patients with major depression. *Biol Psychiatry*, 33(6), 467–476.

Wilamowska, A., Pawlikowski, M., Klencki, M., and Kunert-Radek, J. (1992). Food restriction enhances melatonin effects on the pituitary-gonadal axis in female rats. *J Pineal Res*, 13(1), 1–5.

Williams, R.J., and Schmidt, G.G. (1993). Frequency of seasonal affective disorder among individuals seeking treatment at a northern Canadian mental health center. *Psychiatry Res*, 46(1), 41–45.

Winton, F., Corn, T., Huson, L.W., Franey, C., Arendt, J., and Checkley, S.A. (1989). Effects of light treatment upon mood and melatonin in patients with seasonal affective disorder. *Psychol Med*, 19(3), 585–590.

Wirz-Justice, A., and Richter, R. (1979). Seasonality in biochemical determinations: A source of variance and a clue to the temporal incidence of affective illness. *Psychiatry Res*, 1(1), 53–60.

Wirz-Justice, A., and Van den Hoofdakker, R.H. (1999). Sleep deprivation in depression: What do we know, where do we go? *Biol Psychiatry*, 46(4), 445–453.

Wirz-Justice, A., Pühringer, W., and Hole, G. (1979). Response to sleep deprivation as a predictor of therapeutic results with antidepressant drugs. *Am J Psychiatry*, 136, 1222–1223.

Wirz-Justice, A., Graw, P., Krauchi, K., Gisin, B., Jochum, A., Arendt, J., Fisch, H.U., Buddeberg, C., and Poldinger, W. (1993a). Light therapy in seasonal affective disorder is independent of time of day or circadian phase. *Arch Gen Psychiatry*, 50(12), 929–937.

Wirz-Justice, A., Graw, P., and Pecker, S. (1993b). The seasonal pattern questionnaire (SPAQ): Some comments. *Bull Soc Light Treat Biol Rhythms*, 5, 257–287.

Wirz-Justice, A., Graw, P., Roosli, H., Glauser, G., and Fleischhauer, J. (1999a). An open trial of light therapy in hospitalised major depression. *J Affect Disord*, 52(1–3), 291–292.

Wirz-Justice, A., Krauchi, K., Graw, P., Schulman, J., and Wirz, H. (1999b). *Seasonality in Switzerland: An epidemiological survey*. 4th Annual Meeting on Light Treatment and Biological Rhythms, Bethesda, MD.

Wirz-Justice, A., Quinto, C., Cajochen, C., Werth, E., and Hock, C. (1999c). A rapid-cycling bipolar patient treated with long nights, bedrest, and light. *Biol Psychiatry*, 45(8), 1075–1077.

Wirz-Justice, A., Benedetti, F., Berger, M., Lam, R.W., Martiny, K., Terman, M., and Wu, J.C. (2005). Chronotherapeutics (light and wake therapy) in affective disorders. *Psychol Med*, 35(7), 939–944.

Woodgett, J.R. (2001). Judging a protein by more than its name: GSK-3. *Sci STKE*, 2001(100), RE12.

Wu, J.C., and Bunney, W.E. (1990). The biological basis of an antidepressant response to sleep deprivation and relapse: Review and hypothesis. *Am J Psychiatry*, 147(1), 14–21.

Wu, J.C., Gillin, J.C., Buchsbaum, M.S., Hershey, T., Johnson, J.C., and Bunney, W.E. Jr. (1992). Effect of sleep deprivation on brain metabolism of depressed patients. *Am J Psychiatry*, 149(4), 538–543.

Wu, J., Buchsbaum, M.S., Gillin, J.C., Tang, C., Cadwell, S., Wiegand, M., Najafi, A., Klein, E., Hazen, K., Bunney, W.E. Jr., Fallon, J.H., and Keator, D. (1999). Prediction of antidepressant effects of sleep deprivation by metabolic rates in the ventral anterior cingulate and medial prefrontal cortex. *Am J Psychiatry*, 156(8), 1149–1158.

Wu, J.C., Buchsbaum, M., and Bunney, W.E. Jr. (2001). Clinical neurochemical implications of sleep deprivation's effects on the anterior cingulate of depressed responders. *Neuropsychopharmacology*, 25(Suppl. 5), S74–S78.

Yamada, N., Martin-Iverson, M.T., Daimon, K., Tsujimoto, T., and Takahashi, S. (1995). Clinical and chronobiological effects of light therapy on nonseasonal affective disorders. *Biol Psychiatry*, 37(12), 866–873.

Yamazaki, S., Goto, M., and Menaker, M. (1999). No evidence for extraocular photoreceptors in the circadian system of the Syrian hamster. *J Biol Rhythms*, 14(3), 197–201.

Yang, J.D., Elphick, M., Sharpley, A.L., and Cowen, P.J. (1989). Effects of carbamazepine on sleep in healthy volunteers. *Biol Psychiatry*, 26(3), 324–328.

Young, M.A., Watel, L.G., Lahmeyer, H.W., and Eastman, C.I. (1991). The temporal onset of individual symptoms in winter depression: Differentiating underlying mechanisms. *J Affect Disord*, 22(4), 191–197.

Young, M.A., Meaden, P.M., Fogg, L.F., Cherin, E.A., and East-man, C.I. (1997). Which environmental variables are related to the onset of seasonal affective disorder? *J Abnorm Psychol*, 106(4), 554–562.

Zheng, B., Larkin, D.W., Albrecht, U., Sun, Z.S., Sage, M., Eichele, G., Lee, C.C., and Bradley, A. (1999). The *mPer2* gene encodes a functional component of the mammalian circadian clock. *Nature*, 400(6740), 169–173.

Zis, A.P., and Goodwin, F.K. (1979). Major affective disorder as a recurrent illness: A critical review. *Arch Gen Psychiatry*, 36, 835–839.

Zylka, M.J., Shearman, L.P., Levine, J.D., Jin, X., Weaver, D.R., and Reppert, S.M. (1998a). Molecular analysis of mammalian *timeless*. *Neuron*, 21(5), 1115–1122.

Zylka, M.J., Shearman, L.P., Weaver, D.R., and Reppert, S.M. (1998b). Three period homologs in mammals: Differential light responses in the suprachiasmatic circadian clock and os-cillating transcripts outside of brain. *Neuron*, 20(6), 1103–1110.

CHAPTER 17

Abou-Saleh, M.T., and Coppen, A. (1986). Who responds to pro-phylactic lithium? *J Affect Disord*, 10, 115–125.

Almy, G.L., and Taylor, M.A. (1973). Lithium retention in mania. *Arch Gen Psychiatry*, 29, 232–234.

Altshuler, L., Suppes, T., Black, D., Nolen, W.A., Keck, P.E. Jr., Frye, M.A., McElroy, S., Kupka, R., Grunze, H., Walden, J., Leverich, G., Denicoff, K., Luckenbaugh, D., and Post, R. (2003). Impact of antidepressant discontinuation after acute bipolar depression remission on rates of depressive relapse at 1-year follow-up. *Am J Psychiatry*, 160(7), 1252–1262.

Baldessarini, R.J., Tondo, L., Hennen, J., and Floris, G. (1999). La-tency and episodes before treatment: Response to lithium main-tenance in bipolar I and II disorder. *Bipolar Disord*, 2, 91–97.

Baldessarini, R.J., Tondo, L., Floris, G., and Hennen, J. (2000). Ef-fects of rapid cycling on response to lithium maintenance treatment in 360 bipolar I and II disorder patients. *J Affect Disord*, 61(1-2), 13–22.

Baldessarini, R.J., Pompili, M., and Tondo, L. (2006). Suicidal risk in antidepressant drug trials. *Arch Gen Psychiatry*, 63(3), 246–248.

Bauer, M.S., Kirk, G.F., Gavin, C., and Williford, W.O. (2001). Determinants of functional outcome and healthcare costs in bipolar disorder: A high-intensity follow-up study. *J Affect Disord*, 65, 231–241.

Bauer, M., Grof, P., and Müller-Oerlinghausen, B. (Eds.) (2002). *Lithium in Neuropsychiatry: The Comprehensive Guide*. Abington, England: Informa UK.

Bauer, M.S., McBride, L., Williford, W.O., Glick, H., Kinosian, B., Altshuler, L., Beresford, T., Kilbourne, A.M., Sajatovic, M., and Cooperative Studies Program 430 Study Team. (2006a). Collaborative care for bipolar disorder: Part I. Intervention and implementation in a randomized effectiveness trial. *Psy-chiatr Serv*, 57(7), 927–936.

Bauer, M.S., McBride, L., Williford, W.O., Glick, H., Kinosian, B., Altshuler, L., Beresford, T., Kilbourne, A.M., Sajatovic, M., and Cooperative Studies Program 430 Study Team. (2006b). Collaborative care for bipolar disorder: Part II. Impact on clinical outcome, function, and costs. *Psychiatr Serv*, 57(7), 937–945.

Begley, C.E., Annegers, J.F., Swann, A.C., Lewis, C., Coan, S., Schnapp, W.B., and Bryant-Comstock, L. (2001). The lifetime cost of bipolar disorder in the U.S.: An estimate for new cases in 1998. *Pharmacoeconomics*, 19(5 Pt. 1), 483–495.

Benson, K., and Hartz, A.J. (2000). A comparison of observational studies and randomized, controlled trials. *N Engl J Med*, 342, 1878–1886.

Blanco, C., Lajc, G., Olfson, M., Marcus, S.C., and Pincus, H.A. (2002). Trends in the treatment of bipolar disorder by out-patient psychiatrists. *Am J Psychiatry*, 159, 1005–1010.

Bowden, C.L., Brugger, A.M., Swann, A.C., Calabrese, J.R., Jani-cak, P.G., Petty, F., Dilsaver, S.C., Davis, J.M., Rush, A.J., Small, J.G., for the Depakote Mania Study Group. (1994). Efficacy of divalproex vs. lithium and placebo in the treatment of mania. The Depakote Mania Study Group. *JAMA*, 271(12), 918–924.

Calabrese, J.R., and Rapport, D.J. (1999). Mood stabilizers and the evolution of maintenance study designs in bipolar I disor-der. *J Clin Psychiatry*, 60 (Suppl. 5), 5–13.

Calabrese, R.J., Hirschfeld, R.M.A., Reed, M., Davies, M.A., Frye, M.A., Keck, P.E., Lewis, L., McElroy, S.L., McNulty, J.P., and Wagner, K.D. (2003). Impact of bipolar disorder on a U.S. community sample. *J Clin Psychiatry*, 64, 425–432.

Chisholm, D., van Ommeren, M., Ayuso-Mateos, J.L., and Sax-ena, S. (2005). Cost-effectiveness of clinical interventions for reducing the global burden of bipolar disorder. *Br J Psychia-try*, 187, 559–567.

Coate, M. (1964). *Beyond all Reason*. London: Constable & Co.

Conus, P., Cotton, S., Abdel-Baki, A., Lambert, M., Berk, M., and McGorry, P.D. (2006). Symptomatic and functional outcome 12 months after a first episode of psychotic mania: Barriers to recovery in a catchment area sample. *Bipolar Disorders*, 8, 221–231.

Cooper, T.B., and Simpson, G.M. (1976). The 24-hour lithium level as a prognosticator of dosage requirements: A 2-year follow-up study. *Am J Psychiatry*, 133(4), 440–443.

Coryell, W., Scheftner, W., Keller, M., Endicott, J., Maser, J., and Klerman, G.L. (1993). The enduring psychosocial consequen-ces of mania and depression. *Am J Psychiatry*, 150(5), 720–727.

Dardennes, R., Thuile, J., Friedman, S., and Guelfi, J.D. (2006). The costs of bipolar disorder. *Encephale*, 32(1 Pt. 1), 18–25.

Dion, G., Tohen, M., Anthony, W., and Waternaux, C. (1988). Symp-toms and functioning of patients with bipolar disorder six months after hospitalization. *Hosp Commun Psychiatry*, 39, 652–657.

Ellenor, G.L., and Dishman, B.R. (1995). Pharmaceutical care role model in psychiatry—pharmacist prescribing. *Hosp Pharm*, 30(5), 377–378.

Fava, G.A., Molnar, G., Block, B., Lee, J.S., and Pereni, G.I. (1984). The lithium loading dose method in a clinical setting. *Am J Psychiatry*, 141, 812–813.

Fenn, H.H., Robinson, D., Luby, V., Dangel, C., Buxton, E., Beattie, M., Kraemer, H., and Yesavage, J.A. (1996). Trends in pharma-cotherapy of schizoaffective and bipolar affective disorders: A 5-year naturalistic study. *Am J Psychiatry*, 153(5), 711–713.

Fountoulakis, K.N., Vieta, E., Sanchez-Moreno, J., Kaprinis, S.G., Goikolea, J.M., and Kaprinis, G.S. (2005). Treatment guide-lines for bipolar disorder: A critical review. *J Affect Disord*, 86(1), 1–10.

Frances, A., Docherty, J.P., and Kahn, D.A. (1996). The Expert Consensus Guideline Series: Treatment of bipolar disorder. *J Clin Psychiatry*.

Franchini, L., Zanardi, R., Smeraldi, E., and Gasperini, M. (1999). Early onset of lithium prophylaxis as a predictor of good long-term outcome. *Eur Arch Psychiatry Clin Neurosci, 249,* 227–230.

Frangou, S., Raymont, V., and Bettany, D. (2002). The Maudsley bipolar disorder project: A survey of psychotropic prescribing patterns in bipolar I disorder. *Bipolar Disord, 4,* 378–385.

Gardner, H.H., Kleinman, N.L., Brook, R.A., Rajagopalan, K., Brizee, T.J., and Smeeding, J.E. (2006). The economic impact of bipolar disorder in an employed population from an employer perspective. *J Clin Psychiatry, 67*(8), 1209–1218.

Gelenberg, A.J., Kane, J.M., Keller, M.B., Lavori, P., Rosenbaum, J.F., Cole, K., and Lavelle, J. (1989). Comparison of standard and low serum levels of lithium for maintenance treatment of bipolar disorder. *N Engl J Med, 321,* 1489–1493.

Ghaemi, N., Sachs, G.S., and Goodwin, F.K. (2000). What is to be done? Controversies in the diagnosis and treatment of manic-depressive illness. *World J Biol Psychiatry, 1*(2), 65–74.

Ghaemi, S.N., Ko, J.Y., and Goodwin, F.K. (2002). "Cade's disease" and beyond: Misdiagnosis, antidepressant use, and a proposed definition for bipolar spectrum disorder. *Can J Psychiatry, 47*(2), 125–134.

Ghaemi, S.N., Hsu, D.J., Thase, M.E., Wisniewski, S.R., Nierenberg, A.A., Miyahara, S., and Sachs, G. (2006). Pharmacological treatment patterns at study entry for the first 500 STEP-BD participants. *Psychiatr Serv, 57*(5), 660–665.

Gillberg, I.C., Hellgren, L., and Gillberg, C. (1993). Psychotic disorders diagnosed in adolescence. Outcome at age 30 years. *J Child Psychol Psychiatry, 34*(7), 1173–1185.

Giroux, R. (Ed.) (1967). *Robert Lowell: Collected Prose.* New York: Farrar, Straus, Giroux.

Gitlin, M.J., Swendsen, J., Heller, T.L., and Hammen, C. (1995). Relapse and impairment in bipolar disorder. *Am J Psychiatry, 152*(11), 1635–1640.

Goldberg, J.F., and Ernst, C.L. (2002). Features associated with the delayed initiation of mood stabilizers at illness onset in bipolar disorder. *J Clin Psychiatry, 63*(11), 985–991.

Goodwin, F.K. (1999). Anticonvulsant therapy and suicide risk in affective disorders. *J Clin Psychiatry, 60* (Suppl. 2), 89–93.

Goodwin, F.K. (2003). Impact of formularies of clinical innovation. *J Clin Psychiatry, 64*(Suppl. 17), 11–14.

Goodwin, F.K., and Goldstein, M.A. (2003). Optimizing lithium treatment in bipolar disorder: A review of the literature and clinical recommendations. *J Psychiatr Pract, 9*(5), 333–343.

Goodwin, F.K., Murphy, D.L., and Bunney, W.E. Jr. (1969). Lithium carbonate treatment in depression and mania: A longitudinal double-blind study. *Arch Gen Psychiatry, 21,* 486–496.

Goodwin, F.K., Fireman, B., Simon, G.E., Hunkeler, E.M., Lee, J., and Revicki, D. (2003). Suicide risk in bipolar disorder during treatment with lithium and divalproex. *JAMA, 290*(11), 1467–1473.

Goodwin, G.M. (2003). Evidence-based guidelines for treating bipolar disorder: Recommendations from the British Association for Psychopharmacology. *J Psychopharmacol, 17,* 149–173.

Goodwin, G.M., and Young, A.H. (2003). The British Association for Psychopharmacology guidelines for treatment of bipolar disorder: A summary. *J Psychopharmacol, 17*(4 Suppl.), 3–6.

Gray, G. (2002). Evidence-based medicine: An introduction for psychiatrists. *J Psychiatr Pract, 8,* 5–13.

Greenspan, K., Green, R., and Durrell, J. (1968). Retention and distribution patterns of lithium, a pharmacological tool in studying the pathophysiology of manic-depressive psychosis. *Am J Psychiatry, 125,* 512–519.

Griffith, J.L., and Griffith, M.E. (2002). *Engaging the Sacred in Psychotherapy: How to Talk with People about Their Spiritual Lives.* New York: Guilford Press.

Grunze, H., Kasper, S., Goodwin, G., Bowden, C.L., Baldwin, D., Licht, R.W., Vieta, E., Möller, H.-J., and WFSBP Task Force on Treatment Guidelines for Bipolar Disorders. (2002). The World Federation of Societies of Biological Psychiatry (WFSBP) Guidelines for the Biological Treatment of Bipolar Disorders. Part I: Treatment of bipolar depression. *World J Psychiatry, 3,* 115–124.

Grunze, H., Kasper, S., Goodwin, G., Bowden, C.L., Baldwin, D., Licht, R.W., Vieta, E., Möller, H.-J., and WFSBP Task Force on Treatment Guidelines for Bipolar Disorders. (2003). The World Federation of Societies of Biological Psychiatry (WFSBP) Guidelines for the Biological Treatment of Bipolar Disorders. Part II: Treatment of mania. *World J Psychiatry, 4,* 5–13.

Grunze, H., Kasper, S., Goodwin, G., Bowden, C.L., Möller, H.-J., and WFSBP Task Force on Treatment Guidelines for Bipolar Disorders. (2004). The World Federation of Societies of Biological Psychiatry (WFSBP) Guidelines for the Biological Treatment of Bipolar Disorders. Part III: Maintenance treatment. *World J Psychiatry, 5,* 120–135.

Heres, S., Davis, J., Maino, K., Jetzinger, E., Kissling, W., and Leucht, S. (2006). Why olanzapine beats risperidone, risperidone beats quetiapine, and quetiapine beats olanzapine: An exploratory analysis of head-to-head comparison studies of second-generation antipsychotics. *Am J Psychiatry, 163*(2), 185–194.

Himmelhoch, J.M. (2003). On the usefulness of clinical case studies. *Bipolar Disord, 5,* 69–71.

Hirschfeld, R.M.A., Bowden, C.L., Gitlin, M.J., Keck, P.E., Perlis, R.H., and Suppes, T. (2002). Practice guideline for the treatment of patients with bipolar disorder (revision). *Am J Psychiatry, 159*(Suppl.), 1–50.

Hirschfeld, R.M.A., Calabrese, J.R., Weissman, M.M., Reed, M., Davies, M.A., Frye, M.A., Keck, P.E. Jr., Lewis, L., McElroy, S.L., McNulty, J.P., and Wagner, K.D. (2003). Screening for bipolar disorder in the community. *J Clin Psychiatry, 64,* 53–59.

Hunkeler, E.M., Westphal, J.R., and Williams, M. (1995). Developing a system for automated monitoring of psychiatric outpatients: A first step to improve quality. *HMO Pract, 9*(4), 162–167.

Jackson, A., Cavanagh, J., and Scott, J. (2003). A systematic review of manic and depressive prodromes. *J Affect Disord, 74*(3), 209–217.

Jaffe, S.L., and Yager, J. (1999). A pilot study of a district branch-based educational intervention: Awareness and reactions. *Acad Psychiatry, 23,* 9–13.

Josephson, A., and Peteet, J. (Eds.). (2004). *Handbook of Spirituality and Worldview in Clinical Practice.* Arlington, VA: American Psychiatric Publishing.

Judd, L.L., Akiskal, H.S., Schettler, P.J., Endicott, J., Leon, A.C., Solomon, D.A., Coryell, W., Maser, J.D., and Keller, M.B. (2005). Psychosocial disability in the course of bipolar I and II disorders: A prospective, comparative, longitudinal study. *Arch Gen Psychiatry, 62*(12), 1322–1330.

Keck, P.E., Strakowski, S.M., Hawkins, J.M., Dunayevich, E., Tugrul, K.C., Bennett, J.A., and McElroy, S.L. (2001). A pilot study of rapid lithium administration in the treatment of acute mania. *Bipolar Disord*, 4(4), 68–72.

Keck, P.E., Perlis, R.H., Otto, M.W., Carpenter, D., Ross, R., and Docherty, J.P. (2004). The Expert Consensus Guideline Series: Treatment of bipolar disorder 2004. *Postgrad Med Special Report*, 1, 120.

Kessler, R.C., Akiskal, H.S., Ames, M., Birnbaum, H., Greenberg, M.A., Jin, R., Merikangas, K.R., Simon, G.E., and Wang, P.S. (2006). Prevalence and effects of mood disorders on work performance in a nationally representative sample of U.S. workers. *Am J Psychiatry*, 163(9), 1561–1569.

Ketter, T.A., Frye, M.A., Cora-Locatelli, G., Kimbrell, T.A., and Post, R.M. (1999). Metabolism and excretion of mood stabilizers and new anticonvulsants. *Cell Mol Neurobiol*, 19(4), 511–532.

Kleinman, L., Lowin, A., Flood, E., Gandhi, G., Edgell, E., and Revicki, D. (2003). Costs of bipolar disorder. *Pharmacoeconomics*, 21(9), 601–622.

Kuhn, R. (1957). Über die Behandlung depressiver Zustände mit einem Iminodibenzylderivat (G 22355). [Treatment of depressive states with an iminodibenzyl derivative (G 22355)]. *Schweiz Med Wochenschrift*, 87, 1135–1140.

Kukopulos, A., Minnai, G., and Müller-Oerlinghausen, B. (1985). The influence of mania and depression on the pharmacokinetics of lithium: A longitudinal single-case study. *J Affect Disord*, 8, 159–166.

Levine, J., Chengappa, K.N.R., Brar, J.S., Gershon, S., Yablonsky, E., Stapf, D., and Kupfer, D.J. (2000). Psychotropic drug prescription patterns among patients with bipolar I disorder. *Bipolar Disord*, 2, 120–130.

Li, J., McCombs, J.S., and Stimmel, G.L. (2002). Cost of treating bipolar disorder in the California Medicaid (Medi-Cal) program. *J Affect Disord*, 71(1–3), 131–139.

Licht, R.W. (2002). Limits of the applicability and generalizability of drug trials in mania. *Bipolar Disord*, 4(Suppl. 1), 66–68.

Licht, R.W., Vestergaard, P., Kessing, L.V., Larsen, J.K., Thomsen, P.H., and Danish Psychiatric Association, and the Child and Adolescent Psychiatric Association in Denmark. (2003). Psychopharmacological treatment with lithium and antiepileptic drugs: Suggested guidelines from the Danish Psychiatric Association and the Child and Adolescent Psychiatric Association in Denmark. *Acta Psychiatr Scand*, 108(Suppl. 419), 1–22.

Lieberman, D.Z., Saggese, J.M., and Goodwin, F.K. (2006). Different views on the use of lithium across continents. In M. Bauer, P. Goff, and B. Muller-Oerlinghausen (Eds.), *Lithium and Neuropsychiatry: The Comprehensive Guide*. London: Taylor & Francis.

Lim, P.Z., Tunis, S.L., Edell, W.S., Jensik, S.E., and Tohen, M. (2001). Medication prescribing patterns for patients with bipolar I disorder in hospital settings: Adherence to published practice guidelines. *Bipolar Disord*, 3, 154–173.

Lish, J.D., Dime-Meenan, S., Whybrow, P.C., Price, R.A., and Hirschfeld, R.M. (1994). The National Depressive and Manic-Depressive Association (DMDA) survey of bipolar members. *J Affect Disord*, 31, 281–294.

Lloyd, A.J., Harrison, C.L., Ferrier, I.N., and Young, A.H. (2003). The pharmacological treatment of bipolar affective disorder: Practice is improving but could still be better. *J Psychopharmacol*, 17(2), 230–233.

Matza, L.S., Rajagopalan, K.S., Thompson, C.L., and de Lissovoy, G. (2005). Misdiagnosed patients with bipolar disorder:

Comorbidities, treatment patterns, and direct treatment costs. *J Clin Psychiatry*, 66(11), 1432–1440.

McElroy, S.L., Frye, M., Denicoff, K., Altshuler, L., Nolen, W., Kupka, R., Suppes, T., Keck, P.E. Jr., Leverich, G.S., Kmetz, G.F., and Post, R.M. (1998). Olanzapine in treatment-resistant bipolar disorder. *J Affect Disord*, 49(2), 119–122.

McIntyre, R.S., Konarski, J.Z., Soczynska, J.K., Wilkins, K., Panjwani, G., Bouffard, B., Bottas, A., and Kennedy, S.H. (2006). Medical comorbidity in bipolar disorder: Implications for functional outcomes and health service utilization. *Psychiatr Serv*, 57(8), 1140–1144.

Murray, C.J., and Lopez, A.D. (1996). Evidence-based health policy: Lessons from the global burden of disease study. *Science*, 274(5288), 740–743.

O'Connell, R.A., Mayo, J.A., and Flatow, L., Cuthbertson, B., and O'Brien, B.E. (1991). Outcome of bipolar disorder on long-term treatment with lithium. *Br J Psychiatry*, 159, 123–129.

Perlis, R.H. (2005). The role of pharmacologic treatment guidelines for bipolar disorder. *J Clin Psychiatry*, 66(Suppl. 3), 37–47.

Perlis, R.H., Ostacher, M.J., Patel, J.K., Marangell, L.B., Zhang, H., Wisniewski, S.R., Ketter, T.A., Miklowitz, D.J., Otto, M.W., Gyulai, L., Reilly-Harrington, N.A., Nierenberg, A.A., Sachs, G.S., and Thase, M.E. (2006). Predictors of recurrence in bipolar disorder: Primary outcomes from the Systematic Treatment Enhancement Program for Bipolar Disorder (STEP-BD). *Am J Psychiatry*, 163(2), 217–224.

Perry, A., Tarrier, N., Morriss, R., McCarthy, E., and Limb, K. (1999). Randomised controlled trial of efficacy of teaching patients with bipolar disorder to identify early symptoms of relapse and obtain treatment. *BMJ*, 318(7177), 149–153.

Perry, P.J., Alexander, B., Prince, R.A., and Dunner, F.J. (1984). Prospective evaluation of two lithium maintenance dose schedules. *J Clin Psychopharmacol*, 4, 242–246.

Post, R.M. (2005). The impact of bipolar depression. *J Clin Psychiatry*, 66(Suppl. 5), 5–10.

Post, R.M., and Luckenbaugh, D.A. (2003). Unique design issues in clinical trials of patients with bipolar affective disorder. *J Psychiatr Res*, 37(1), 61–73.

Prien, R.F., Caffey, E.M. Jr., and Klett, J. (1974). Factors associated with treatment success in lithium carbonate prophylaxis: Report of the Veterans Administration and National Institute of Mental Health Collaborative Study Group. *Arch Gen Psychiatry*, 31, 189–192.

Pugh, C.B., and Garnett, W.R. (1991). Current issues in the treatment of epilepsy. *Clin Pharmacol*, 10(5), 335–358.

Reinares, M., Vieta, E., Colom, F., Martinez-Aran, A., Torrent, C., Comes, M., Goikolea, J.M., Benabarre, A., Daban, C., and Sanchez-Moreno, J. (2006). What really matters to bipolar patients' caregivers: Sources of family burden. *J Affect Disord*, 94(1-3), 157–163.

Rush, A.J., Post, R.M., Nolen, W.A., Keck, P.E. Jr., Suppes, T., Altshuler, L., and McElroy, S.L. (2000). Methodological issues in developing new acute treatments for patients with bipolar illness. *Biol Psychiatry*, 48(6), 615–624.

Schaffer, A., Cairney, J., Cheung, A.H., Veldhuizen, S., and Levitt, A.J. (2006). Use of treatment services and pharmacotherapy for bipolar disorder in a general population-based mental health survey. *J Clin Psychiatry*, 67(3), 386–393.

Serry, M. (1969). The lithium excretion test I: Clinical application and interpretation. *Aust NZ J Psychiatry*, 3, 390–394.

Simon, G.E., and Unutzer, J. (1999). Health care utilization and costs among patients treated for bipolar disorder in an insured population. *Psychiatr Serv,* 50(10), 1303–1308.

Simon, G.E., Ludman, E.J., Unutzer, J., Bauer, M.S., Operskalski, B., and Rutter, C. (2005). Randomized trial of a population-based care program for people with bipolar disorder. *Psychol Med,* 35(1), 13–24.

Simon, G.E., Ludman, E.J., Bauer, M.S., Unutzer, J., and Operskalski, B. (2006). Long-term effectiveness and cost of a systematic care program for bipolar disorder. *Arch Gen Psychiatry,* 63(5), 500–508.

Soldani, F., Ghaemi, S.N., and Baldessarini, R.J. (2005). Research reports on treatments for bipolar disorder: Preliminary assessment of methodological quality. *Acta Psychiatr Scand,* 112(1), 72–74.

Spiker, D.G., and Pugh, D.D. (1976). Combining tricyclic and monoamine oxidase inhibitor antidepressants. *Arch Gen Psychiatry,* 33, 828–830.

Strakowski, S.M., Sax, K.W., McElroy, S.L., Keck, P.E., Hawkins, J.M., and West, S.A. (1998). Course of psychiatric and substance abuse syndromes co-occurring with bipolar disorder after a first psychiatric hospitalization. *J Clin Psychiatry,* 59(9), 465–471.

Strakowski, S.M., DelBello, M.P., Fleck, D.E., and Arndt, S. (2000). The impact of substance abuse on the course of bipolar disorder. *Biol Psychiatry,* 48(6), 477–485.

Suppes, T., Dennehy, E.B., Hirschfeld, R.M., Altshuler, L.L., Bowden, C.L., Calabrese, J.R., Crismon, M.L., Ketter, T.A., Sachs, G.S., and Swann, A.C. (2005). The Texas implementation of medication algorithms: Update to the algorithms for treatment of bipolar I disorder. *J Clin Psychiatry,* 66(7), 870–886.

Swann, A.C., Bowden, C.L., Calabrese, J.R., Dilsaver, S.C., and Morris, D.D. (1999). Differential effect of number of previous episodes of affective disorder on response to lithium or divalproex in acute mania. *Am J Psychiatry,* 156(8), 1264–1266.

Tohen, M., Waternaux, C.M., and Tsuang, M.T. (1990). Outcome in mania. A 4-year prospective follow-up of 75 patients utilizing survival analysis. *Arch Gen Psychiatry,* 47(12), 1106–1111.

Tohen, M., Tsuang, M.T., and Goodwin, D.C. (1992). Prediction of outcome in mania by mood-congruent or mood-incongruent psychotic features. *Am J Psychiatry,* 149(11), 1580–1584.

Tohen, M., Hennen, J., Zarate, C.M., Jr., Baldessarini, R.J., Strakowski, S.M., Stoll, A.L., Faedda, G.L., Suppes, T., Gebre-Medhin, P., and Cohen, B.M. (2000). Two-year syndromal and functional recovery in 219 cases of first-episode major affective disorder with psychotic features. *Am J Psychiatry,* 157(2), 220–228.

Tohen, M., Baker, R.W., Altshuler, L.L., Zarate, C.A., Suppes, T., Ketter, T.A., Milton, D.R., Risser, R., Gilmore, J.A., Breier, A., and Tollefson, G.A. (2002). Olanzapine versus divalproex in the treatment of acute mania. *Am J Psychiatry,* 159(6), 1011–1017.

Tohen, M., Calabrese, J.R., Sachs, G.S., Banov, M.D., Detke, H.C., Risser, R., Baker, R.W., Chou, J.C., and Bowden, C.L. (2006). Randomized, placebo-controlled trial of olanzapine as maintenance therapy in patients with bipolar I disorder responding to acute treatment with olanzapine. *Am J Psychiatry,* 163(2), 247–256.

Vestergaard, P. (2004). Guidelines for maintenance treatment of bipolar disorder: Are there discrepancies between European and North American recommendations? *Bipolar Disord,* 6(6), 519–522.

Vestergaard, P., and Schou, M. (1987). Does long-term lithium treatment induce diabetes mellitus? *Neuropsychobiology,* 17, 130–132.

Vieta, E., and Carne, X. (2005). The use of placebo in clinical trials on bipolar disorder: A new approach for an old debate. *Psychother Psychosom,* 74(1), 10–16.

Wang, P.S., Lane, M., Olfson, M., Pincus, H.A., Wells, K.B., and Kessler, R.C. (2005). Twelve-month use of mental health services in the United States. *Arch Gen Psychiatry,* 62, 629–640.

Wightman, W.P.D. (1971). *The Emergency of Scientific Medicine.* Edinburgh: Oliver & Boyd.

Winokur, G., Coryell, W., Keller, M., Endicott, J., and Akiskal, H. (1993). A prospective follow-up of patients with bipolar and primary unipolar affective disorder. *Arch Gen Psychiatry,* 50, 457–465.

Wyatt, R.J., and Henter, I. (1995). An economic evaluation of manic-depressive illness—1991. *Soc Psychiatry Psychiatr Epidemiol,* 30(5), 213–219.

Yatham, L.N., Kennedy, S.H., O'Donovan, C., Parikh, S., MacQueen, G., McIntyre, R., Sharma, V., Silverstone, P., Alda, M., Baruch, P., Beaulieu, S., Daigneault, A., Milev, R., Young, L.T., Ravindran, A., Schaffer, A., Connolly, M., and Gorman, C.P. (2005). Canadian Network for Mood and Anxiety Treatments (CANMAT) guidelines for the management of patients with bipolar disorder: Consensus and controversies. *Bipolar Disord,* 7(Suppl. 3), 5–69.

Zajecka, J.M., Weisler, R., Sachs, G., Swann, A.C., Wozniak, P., and Sommerville, K.W. (2002). A comparison of the efficacy, safety, and tolerability of divalproex sodium and olanzapine in the treatment of bipolar disorder. *J Clin Psychiatry,* 63(12), 1148–1155.

Ziegler, V.E., Wylie, L.T., and Biggs, J.T. (1978). Intrapatient variability of serial steady-state plasma tricyclic antidepressant concentrations. *J Pharm Sci,* 67(4), 554–555.

Chapter 18

Abbott Laboratories. (2005). *Abbott's Depakote® ER (Divalproex Sodium Extended-Release Tablets) approved for acute mania or mixed episodes associated with bipolar disorder.* Available: http://abbott.com/news/press_release.cfm?id=1034 [January 27, 2006].

Altshuler, L.L., Keck, P.E. Jr., McElroy, S.L., Suppes, T., Brown, E.S., Denicoff, K., Frye, M., Gitlin, M., Hwang, S., Goodman, R., Leverich, G., Nolen, W., Kupka, R., and Post, R. (1999). Gabapentin in the acute treatment of refractory bipolar disorder. *Bipolar Disord,* 1(1), 61–65.

Amann, B., and Grunze, H. (2005). Neurochemical underpinnings in bipolar disorder and epilepsy. *Epilepsia,* 46(Suppl. 4), 26–30.

Anand, A., Oren, D.A., Berman, R.M., Cappiello, A., and Charney, D.S. (1999). Lamotrigine treatment of lithium failure outpatient mania: A double-blind placebo-controlled trial. *Bipolar Disord,* S1(1), 23.

Aronson, T.A., Shukla, S., and Hirschowitz, J. (1989). Clonazepam treatment of five lithium-refractory patients with bipolar disorder. *Am J Psychiatry,* 146(1), 77–80.

Baker, R.W., Goldberg, J.F., Tohen, M., Milton, D.R., Stauffer, V.L., and Schuh, L.M. (2002). The impact of response to previous mood stabilizer therapy on response to olanzapine versus placebo for acute mania. *Bipolar Disord,* 4(1), 43–49.

Baker, R.W., Milton, D.R., Stauffer, V.L., Gelenberg, A., and To-hen, M. (2003a). Placebo-controlled trials do not find association of olanzapine with exacerbation of bipolar mania. *J Affect Disord*, 73(1-2), 147–153.

Baker, R.W., Tohen, M., Fawcett, J., Risser, R.C., Schuh, L.M., Brown, E., Stauffer, V.L., Shao, L., and Tollefson, G.D. (2003b). Acute dysphoric mania: Treatment response to olanzapine compared to placebo. *J Clin Psychopharmacol*, 23(2), 132–137.

Baker, R.W., Brown, E., Akiskal, H.S., Calabrese, J.R., Ketter, T.A., Schuh, L.M., Trzepacz, P.T., Watkin, J.G., and Tohen, M. (2004). Efficacy of olanzapine combined with valproate or lithium in the treatment of dysphoric mania. *Br J Psychiatry*, 185, 472–478.

Baldessarini, R.J., Tondo, L., Floris, G., and Hennen, J. (2000). Effects of rapid cycling on response to lithium maintenance treatment in 360 bipolar I and II disorder patients. *J Affect Disord*, 61(1-2), 13–22.

Baldessarini, R.J., Hennen, J., Wilson, M., Calabrese, J., Chengappa, R., Keck, P.E. Jr., McElroy, S.L., Sachs, G., Vieta, E., Welge, J.A., Yatham, L.N., Zarate, C.A. Jr., Baker, R.W., and Tohen, M. (2003). Olanzapine versus placebo in acute mania: Treatment responses in subgroups. *J Clin Psychopharmacol*, 23(4), 370–376.

Ballenger, J.C., and Post, R.M. (1980). Carbamazepine in manic-depressive illness: A new treatment. *Am J Psychiatry*, 137(7), 782–790.

Barbini, B., Scherillo, P., Benedetti, F., Crespi, G., Colombo, C., and Smeraldi, E. (1997). Response to clozapine in acute mania is more rapid than that of chlorpromazine. *Int Clin Psychopharmacol*, 12(2), 109–112.

Barton, B.M., and Gitlin, M.J. (1987). Verapamil in treatment-resistant mania: An open trial. *J Clin Psychopharmacol*, 7(2), 101–103.

Benabarre, A., Vieta, E., Colom, F., Martinez, A., Reinares, M., and Corbella, B. (2001). Treatment of mixed mania with risperidone and mood stabilizers. *Can J Psychiatry*, 46(9), 866–867.

Benazzi, F. (1998). Mania associated with donepezil. *Int J Geriatr Psychiatry*, 13(11), 814–815.

Benedetti, A., Lattanzi, L., Pini, S., Musetti, L., Dell'Osso, L., and Cassano, G.B. (2004). Oxcarbazepine as add-on treatment in patients with bipolar manic, mixed or depressive episode. *J Affect Disord*, 79(1-3), 273–277.

Bennett, J., Goldman, W.T., and Suppes, T. (1997). Gabapentin for treatment of bipolar and schizoaffective disorders. *J Clin Psychopharmacol*, 17(2), 141–142.

Berigan, T.R. (2002). Zonisamide treatment of bipolar disorder: A case report. *Can J Psychiatry*, 47(9), 887.

Berk, M., Ichim, L., and Brook, S. (1999). Olanzapine compared to lithium in mania: A double-blind randomized controlled trial. *Int Clin Psychopharmacol*, 14(6), 339–343.

Bersani, G. (2004). Levetiracetam in bipolar spectrum disorders: First evidence of efficacy in an open add-on study. *Hum Psycholpharmacol*, 19, 355–356.

Black, D.W., Winokur, G., and Nasrallah, A. (1987). Treatment of mania: A naturalistic study of electroconvulsive therapy versus lithium in 438 patients. *J Clin Psychiatry*, 48, 132–139.

Bowden, C.L. (1995). Predictors of response to divalproex and lithium. *J Clin Psychiatry*, 56(Suppl. 3), 25–30.

Bowden, C.L., Brugger, A.M., Swann, A.C., Calabrese, J.R., Janicak, P.G., Petty, F., Dilsaver, S.C., Davis, J.M., Rush, A.J., Small, J.G., Garza-Treviño, E.S., Risch, S.C., Goodnick, P.J., and Morris, D.D. (1994). Efficacy of divalproex vs. lithium and placebo in the treatment of mania. The Depakote Mania Study Group. *JAMA*, 271(12), 918–924.

Bowden, C.L., Janicak, P.G., Orsulak, P., Swann, A.C., Davis, J.M., Calabrese, J.R., Goodnick, P., Small, J.G., Rush, A.J., Kimmel, S.E., Risch, S.C., and Morris, D.D. (1996). Relation of serum valproate concentration to response in mania. *Am J Psychiatry*, 153(6), 765–770.

Bowden, C.L., Calabrese, J.R., McElroy, S.L., Rhodes, L.J., Keck, P.E. Jr., Cookson, J., Anderson, J., Bolden-Watson, C., Ascher, J., Monaghan, E., and Zhou, J. (1999). The efficacy of lamotrigine in rapid cycling and non-rapid cycling patients with bipolar disorder. *Biol Psychiatry*, 45(8), 953–958.

Bowden, C.L., Grunze, H., Mullen, J., Brecher, M., Paulsson, B., Jones, M., Vagero, M., and Svensson, K. (2005). A randomized, double-blind, placebo-controlled efficacy and safety study of quetiapine or lithium as monotherapy for mania in bipolar disorder. *J Clin Psychiatry*, 66(1), 111–121.

Bowden, C.L., Calabrese, J.R., Wallin, B.A., Swann, A.C., McElroy, S.L., Risch, S.C., and Hirschfeld, M.A. (1995). Illness characteristics of patients in clinical drug studies of mania. *Psychopharmacol Bull*, 31(1), 103–109.

Bowden, C.L., Swann, A.C., Calabrese, J.R., Rubenfaer, L.M., Wozniak, P.J., Collins, M.A., Abi-Saab, W., Saltarelli, M., for the Depakote ER Mania Study Group. (2006). A randomized, placebo-controlled, multicenter study of divalproex sodium extended release in the treatment of acute mania. *J Clin Psychiatry*, 67(10), 1501–1510.

Bozikas, V.P., Petrikis, P., Kourtis, A., Youlis, P., and Karavatos, A. (2002). Treatment of acute mania with topiramate in hospitalized patients. *Prog Neuropsychopharmacol Biol Psychiatry*, 26(6), 1203–1206.

Bradwejn, J., Shriqui, C., Koszycki, D., and Meterissian, G. (1990). Double-blind comparison of the effects of clonazepam and lorazepam in acute mania. *J Clin Psychopharmacol*, 10(6), 403–408.

Braunig, P., and Kruger, S. (2003). Levetiracetam in the treatment of rapid cycling bipolar disorder. *J Psychopharmacol*, 17, 239–241.

Brook, S., Lucey, J.V., and Gunn, K.P. (2000). Intramuscular ziprasidone compared with intramuscular haloperidol in the treatment of acute psychosis. Ziprasidone I.M. Study Group. *J Clin Psychiatry*, 61(12), 933–941.

Burt, T., Sachs, G.S., and Demopulos, C. (1999). Donepezil in treatment-resistant bipolar disorder. *Biol Psychiatry*, 45(8), 959–964.

Cabras, P.L., Hardoy, M.J., Hardoy, M.C., and Carta, M.G. (1999). Clinical experience with gabapentin in patients with bipolar or schizoaffective disorder: Results of an open-label study. *J Clin Psychiatry*, 60(4), 245–248.

Calabrese, J.R., and Delucchi, G.A. (1990). Spectrum of efficacy of valproate in 55 patients with rapid-cycling bipolar disorder. *Am J Psychiatry*, 147(4), 431–434.

Calabrese, J.R., Markovitz, P.J., Kimmel, S.E., and Wagner, S.C. (1992). Spectrum of efficacy of valproate in 78 rapid-cycling bipolar patients. *J Clin Psychopharmacol*, 12(Suppl. 1), 53S–56S.

Calabrese, J.R., Kimmel, S.E., Woyshville, M.J., Rapport, D.J., Faust, C.J., Thompson, P.A., and Meltzer, H.Y. (1996). Clozapine for treatment-refractory mania. *Am J Psychiatry*, 153(6), 759–764.

Calabrese, J.R., Bowden, C.L., McElroy, S.L., Cookson, J., Andersen, J., Keck, P.E. Jr., Rhodes, L., Bolden-Watson, C., Zhou, J., and Ascher, J.A. (1999). Spectrum of activity of lamotrigine in treatment-refractory bipolar disorder. *Am J Psychiatry*, 156(7), 1019–1023.

Calabrese, J.R., Suppes, T., Bowden, C.L., Sachs, G.S., Swann, A.C., McElroy, S.L., Kusumakar, V., Ascher, J.A., Earl, N.L., Greene, P.L., and Monaghan, E.T. (2000). A double-blind, placebo-controlled, prophylaxis study of lamotrigine in rapid-cycling bipolar disorder. Lamictal 614 Study Group. *J Clin Psychiatry*, 61(11), 841–850.

Calabrese, J.R., Keck, P.E. Jr., McElroy, S.L., and Shelton, M.D. (2001). A pilot study of topiramate as monotherapy in the treatment of acute mania. *J Clin Psychopharmacol*, 21(3), 340–342.

Calabrese, J.R., Shelton, M.D., Rapport, D.J., Youngstrom, E.A., Jackson, K., Bilali, S., Ganocy, S.J., and Findling, R.L. (2005). A 20-month, double-blind, maintenance trial of lithium versus divalproex in rapid-cycling bipolar disorder. *Am J Psychiatry*, 162(11), 2152–2161.

Chase, P.B., and Biros, M.H. (2002). A retrospective review of the use and safety of droperidol in a large, high-risk, inner-city emergency department patient population. *Acad Emerg Med*, 9(12), 1402–1410.

Chen, S.T., Altshuler, L.L., Melnyk, K.A., Erhart, S.M., Miller, E., and Mintz, J. (1999). Efficacy of lithium vs. valproate in the treatment of mania in the elderly: A retrospective study. *J Clin Psychiatry*, 60(3), 181–186.

Chengappa, K.N., Rathore, D., Levine, J., Atzert, R., Solai, L., Parepally, H., Levin, H., Moffa, N., Delaney, J., and Brar, J.S. (1999). Topiramate as add-on treatment for patients with bipolar mania. *Bipolar Disord*, 1(1), 42–53.

Chengappa, K.N., Baker, R.W., Shao, L., Yatham, L.N., Tohen, M., Gershon, S., and Kupfer, D.J. (2003). Rates of response, euthymia and remission in two placebo-controlled olanzapine trials for bipolar mania. *Bipolar Disord*, 5(1), 1–5.

Chengappa, K.N.R., Schwarzman, L.K., Hulihan, J.F., Xiang, J., and Rosenthal, N.R., for the Clinical Affairs Product Support Study-168 Investigators. (2006). Adjunctive topiramate therapy in patients receiving a mood stabilizer for bipolar disorder: A randomized, placebo-controlled trial. *J Clin Psychiatry*, 67, 1698–1706.

Chisholm, K.A., Dennehy, E.B., and Suppes, T. (2001). *Clinical responses to quetiapine add-on for the treatment of refractory bipolar disorder*. 8th International Conference on Bipolar Disorder, Pittsburgh, PA.

Chou, J.C., Zito, J.M., Vitrai, J., Craig, T.J., Allingham, B.H., and Czobor, P. (1996). Neuroleptics in acute mania: A pharmacoepidemiologic study. *Ann Pharmacother*, 30(12), 1396–1398.

Chou, J.C., Czobor, P., Charles, O., Tuma, I., Winsberg, B., Allen, M.H., Trujillo, M., and Volavka, J. (1999). Acute mania: Haloperidol dose and augmentation with lithium or lorazepam. *J Clin Psychopharmacol*, 19(6), 500–505.

Chouinard, G., Young, S.N., and Annable, L. (1983). Antimanic effect of clonazepam. *Biol Psychiatry*, 18(4), 451–466.

Chouinard, G., Annable, L., Turnier, L., Holobow, N., and Szkrumelak, N. (1993). A double-blind randomized clinical trial of rapid tranquilization with I.M. clonazepam and I.M. haloperidol in agitated psychotic patients with manic symptoms. *Can J Psychiatry*, 38(Suppl. 4), S114–S121.

Ciapparelli, A., Dell'Osso, L., Tundo, A., Pini, S., Chiavacci, M.C., Di Sacco, I., and Cassano, G.B. (2001). Electroconvulsive therapy in medication-nonresponsive patients with mixed mania and bipolar depression. *J Clin Psychiatry*, 62(7), 552–555.

Cipriani, A., Rendell, J.M., and Geddes, J.R. (2006). Haloperidol alone or in combination for acute mania. *Cochrane Database Syst Rev*, 19, 3:CD004362.

Curtin, F., and Schultz, P. (2004). Clonazepam and larazepam in acute mania: A Bayesian meta-analysis. *J Affect Disord*, 78, 201–208.

Dalkilic, A., Diaz, E., Baker, C.B., Pearsall, H.R., and Woods, S.W. (2000). Effects of divalproex versus lithium on length of hospital stay among patients with bipolar disorder. *Psychiatr Serv*, 51(9), 1184–1186.

Dam, M. (1994). Practical aspects of oxcarbazepine treatment. *Epilepsia*, 35(Suppl. 3), S23–S25.

Daniel, D.G., Zimbroff, D.L., Swift, R.H., and Harrigan, E.P. (2004). The tolerability of intramuscular ziprasidone and haloperidol treatment and the transition to oral therapy. *Int Clin Psychopharmacol*, 19(1), 9–15.

Dean, C.E. (2000). Prasterone (DHEA) and mania. *Ann Pharmacother*, 34(12), 1419–1422.

DelBello, M.P., Findling, R.L., Kushner, S., Wang, D., Olson, W.H., Capece, J.A., Fazzio, L., and Rosenthal, N.R. (2005). A pilot controlled trial of topiramate for mania in children and adolescents with bipolar disorder. *J Am Acad Child Adolesc Psychiatry*, 44(6), 539–547.

Denicoff, K.D., Smith-Jackson, E.E., Disney, E.R., Ali, S.O., Leverich, G.S., and Post, R.M. (1997). Comparative prophylactic efficacy of lithium, carbamazepine, and the combination in bipolar disorder. *J Clin Psychiatry*, 58(11), 470–478.

Desai, N.G., Gangahar, B.N., Channabasavanna, S.M., and Shetty, K.T. (1987). Carbamazepine hastens therapeutic action of lithium in mania. *Proceedings of the International Conference on New Directions in Affective Disorders*, 97.

Dose, M., Emrich, H.M., Cording-Tommel, C., and von Zerssen, D. (1986). Use of calcium antagonists in mania. *Psychoneuroendocrinology*, 11(2), 241–243.

Dubovsky, S.L., Franks, R.D., Allen, S., and Murphy, J. (1986). Calcium antagonists in mania: A double-blind study of verapamil. *Psychiatry Res*, 18(4), 309–320.

Dunayevich, E., and Strakowski, S.M. (2000). Quetiapine for treatment-resistant mania. *Am J Psychiatry*, 157(8), 1341.

Dunner, D.L. (2000). Optimizing lithium treatment. *J Clin Psychiatry*, 61(Suppl. 9), 76–81.

Dunner, D.L., and Fieve, R.R. (1974). Clinical factors in lithium carbonate prophylaxis failure. *Arch Gen Psychiatry*, (2), 229–233.

Dwight, M.M., Keck, P.E. Jr., Stanton, S.P., Strakowski, S.M., and McElroy, S.L. (1994). Antidepressant activity and mania associated with risperidone treatment of schizoaffective disorder. *Lancet*, 344(8921), 554–555.

Eden Evins, A., Demopulos, C., Nierenberg, A., Culhane, M.A., Eisner, L., and Sachs, G. (2006). A double-blind, placebo-controlled trial of adjunctive donepezil in treatment-resistant mania. *Bipolar Disord*, 8(1), 75–80.

Edwards, R., Stephenson, U., and Flewett, T. (1991). Clonazepam in acute mania: A double-blind trial. *Aust N Z J Psychiatry*, 25(2), 238–242.

Emilien, G., Maloteaux, J.M., Seghers, A., and Charles, G. (1996). Lithium compared to valproic acid and carbamazepine in the treatment of mania: A statistical meta-analysis. *Eur Neuropsychopharmacol*, 6(3), 245–252.

Emrich, H.M. (1990). Studies with oxcarbazepine in acute mania. *Int Clin Psychopharmacol*, 5(Suppl.), 83–88.

Emrich, H.M., Dose, M., and von Zerssen, D. (1985). The use of sodium valproate, carbamazepine and oxcarbazepine in patients with affective disorders. *J Affect Disord*, 8(3), 243–250.

Erfurth, A., Kammerer, C., Grunze, H., Normann, C., and Walden. J. (1998). An open label study of gabapentin in the treatment of acute mania. *J Psychiatr Res*, 32(5), 261–264.

Fink, M. (1999). Delirious mania. *Bipolar Disord*, 1(1), 54–60.

Fink, M., (2006). ECT in therapy-resistant mania: Does it have a place? *Bipolar Disord*, 8(3), 307–309.

Freeman, T.W., Clothier, J.L., Pazzaglia, P., Lesem, M.D., and Swann, A.C. (1992). A double-blind comparison of valproate and lithium in the treatment of acute mania. *Am J Psychiatry*, 149(1), 108–111.

Frye, M.A., Altshuler, L.L., Szuba, M.P., Finch, N.N., and Mintz, J. (1996). The relationship between antimanic agent for treatment of classic or dysphoric mania and length of hospital stay. *J Clin Psychiatry*, 57(1), 17–21.

Frye, M.A., Ketter, T.A., Kimbrell, T.A., Dunn, R.T., Speer, A.M., Osuch, E.A., Luckenbaugh, D.A., Cora-Ocatelli, G., Leverich, G.S., and Post, R.M. (2000). A placebo-controlled study of lamotrigine and gabapentin monotherapy in refractory mood disorders. *J Clin Psychopharmacol*, 20(6), 607–612.

Garfinkel, P.E., Stancer, H.C., and Persad, E. (1980). A comparison of haloperidol, lithium carbonate and their combination in the treatment of mania. *J Affect Disord*, 2(4), 279–288.

Garza-Trevino, E.S., Overall, J.E., and Hollister, L.E. (1992). Verapamil versus lithium in acute mania. *Am J Psychiatry*, 149(1), 121–122.

Ghaemi, S.N., and Goodwin, F.K. (2001). Gabapentin treatment of the non-refractory bipolar spectrum: An open case series. *J Affect Disord*, 65(2), 167–171.

Ghaemi, S.N., and Katzow, J.J. (1999). The use of quetiapine for treatment-resistant bipolar disorder: A case series. *Ann Clin Psychiatry*, 11(3), 137–140.

Ghaemi, S.N., and Sachs, G.S. (1997). Long-term risperidone treatment in bipolar disorder: 6-month follow up. *Int Clin Psychopharmacol*, 12(6), 333–338.

Ghaemi, S.N., Katzow, J.J., Desai, S.P., and Goodwin, F.K. (1998). Gabapentin treatment of mood disorders: A preliminary study. *J Clin Psychiatry*, 59(8), 426–429.

Giannini, A.J., Houser, W.L. Jr., Loiselle, R.H., Giannini, M.C., and Price, W.A. (1984). Antimanic effects of verapamil. *Am J Psychiatry*, 141(12), 1602–1603.

Goldberg, J.F., and Burdick, K.E. (2002). Levetiracetam for acute mania. *Am J Psychiatry*, 159(1), 148.

Gonzalez-Pinto, Lalaguna, B., Mosquera, F., Perez de Heredia, J.L., Gutierrez, M., Ezcurra, J., Gilaberte, I., and Tohen, M. (2001). Use of olanzapine in dysphoric mania. *J Affect Disord*, 66(2–3), 247–253.

Goodnick, P.J., and Meltzer, H.Y. (1984). Treatment of schizoaffective disorders. *Schizophr Bull*, 10, 30–48.

Goodwin, F.K., and Ebert, M. (1973). Lithium in mania: Clinical trials and controlled trials. In S. Gershon and B. Shopsin (Eds.), *Lithium: Its Role in Psychiatric Research* (pp. 237–252). New York: Plenum Press.

Goodwin, F.K., Murphy, D.L., and Bunney, W.E. Jr. (1969). Lithium-carbonate treatment in depression and mania. A longitudinal double-blind study. *Arch Gen Psychiatry*, 21(4), 486–496.

Gouliaev, G., Licht, R.W., Vestergaard, P., Merinder, L., Lund, H., and Bjerre, L. (1996). Treatment of manic episodes: Zuclopenthixol and clonazepam versus lithium and clonazepam. *Acta Psychiatr Scand*, 93(2), 119–124.

Green, A.I., Tohen, M., Patel, J.K., Banov, M., DuRand, C., Berman, I., Chang, H., Zarate, C., Jr., Posener, J., Lee, H., Dawson, R., Richards, C., Cole, J.O., and Schatzberg, A.F. (2000). Clozapine in the treatment of refractory psychotic mania. *Am J Psychiatry*, 157(6), 982–986.

Grisaru, N., Chudakov, B., Yaroslavsky, Y., and Belmaker, R.H. (1998). Transcranial magnetic stimulation in mania: A controlled study. *Am J Psychiatry*, 155(11), 1608–1610.

Grunze, H.C., Erfurth, A., Amann, B., Giupponi, G., Kammerer, C., and Walden, J. (1999a). Intravenous valproate loading in acutely manic and depressed bipolar I patients. *J Clin Psychopharmacol*, 19(4), 303–309.

Grunze, H.C., Erfurth, A., Marcuse, A., Amann, B., Normann, C., and Walden, J. (1999b). Tiagabine appears not to be efficacious in the treatment of acute mania. *J Clin Psychiatry*, 60(11), 759–762.

Grunze, H.C., Normann, C., Langosch, J., Schaefer, M., Amann, B., Sterr, A., Schloesser, S., Kleindienst, N., and Walden, J. (2001). Antimanic efficacy of topiramate in 11 patients in an open trial with an on-off-on design. *J Clin Psychiatry*, 62(6), 464–468.

Grunze, H.C., Kasper, S., Goodwin, G., Bowden, C., Baldwin, D., Licht, R.W., Vieta, E., Moller, H.J., and WFSBP Task Force on Treatment Guidelines for Bipolar Disorders. (2003). The World Federation of Societies of Biological Psychiatry (WFSBP) guidelines for the biological treatment of bipolar disorders, Part II: Treatment of mania. *World J Biol Psychiatry*, 4(1), 5–13.

Guille, C., Sachs, G.S., and Ghaemi, S.N. (2000). A naturalistic comparison of clozapine, risperidone, and olanzapine in the treatment of bipolar disorder. *J Clin Psychiatry*, 61(9), 638–642.

Hamilton, I. (1982). *Robert Lowell: A Biography*. New York: Random House.

Harada, T., and Otsuki, S. (1986). Antimanic effect of zotepine. *Clin Ther*, 8(4), 406–414.

Hatzimanolis, J., Lykouras, L., Oulis, P., and Christodoulou, G.N. (1999). Gabapentin as monotherapy in the treatment of acute mania. *Eur Neuropsychopharmacol*, 9(3), 257–258.

Heiden, A., Frey, R., Presslich, O., Blasbichler, T., Smetana, R., and Kasper, S. (1999). Treatment of severe mania with intravenous magnesium sulphate as a supplementary therapy. *Psychiatry Res*, 89, 239–246.

Hellewell, J.S. (2002). Oxcarbazepine (Trileptal) in the treatment of bipolar disorders: A review of efficacy and tolerability. *J Affect Disord*, 72(Suppl.), S23–S34.

Hillert, A., Maier, W., Wetzel, H., and Benkert, O. (1992). Risperidone in the treatment of disorders with a combined psychotic and depressive syndrome: A functional approach. *Pharmacopsychiatry*, 25(5), 213–217.

Hirschfeld, R.M., Allen, M.H., McEvoy, J.P., Keck, P.E. Jr., and Russell, J.M. (1999). Safety and tolerability of oral loading divalproex sodium in acutely manic bipolar patients. *J Clin Psychiatry*, 60(12), 815–818.

Hirschfeld, R.M., Baker, J.D., Wozniak, P., Tracy, K., and Sommerville, K.W. (2003). The safety and early efficacy of oral-loaded divalproex versus standard-titration divalproex, lithium, olanzapine, and placebo in the treatment of acute mania associated with bipolar disorder. *J Clin Psychiatry*, 64(7), 841–846.

Hirschfeld, R.M., Keck, P.E. Jr., Kramer, M., Karcher, K., Canuso, C., Eerdekens, M., and Grossman, F. (2004). Rapid antimanic effect of risperidone monotherapy: A 3-week multicenter, double-blind, placebo-controlled trial. *Am J Psychiatry*, 161(6), 1057–1065.

Hummel, B., Walden, J., Stampfer, R., Dittmann, S., Amann, B., Sterr, A., Schaefer, M., Frye, M.A., and Grunze, H. (2002). Acute antimanic efficacy and safety of oxcarbazepine in an open trial with an on-off-on design. *Bipolar Disord*, 4(6), 412–417.

Ichim, L., Berk, M., and Brook, S. (2000). Lamotrigine compared with lithium in mania: A double-blind randomized controlled trial. *Ann Clin Psychiatry*, 12(1), 5–10.

Isometsa, E.T., Henriksson, M.M., Aro, H.M., and Lonnqvist, J.K. (1994). Suicide in bipolar disorder in Finland. *Am J Psychiatry*, 151(7), 1020–1024.

Janicak, P.G., Sharma, R.P., Pandey, G., and Davis, J.M. (1998). Verapamil for the treatment of acute mania: A double-blind, placebo-controlled trial. *Am J Psychiatry*, 155(7), 972–973.

Jochum, T., Bar, K.J., and Sauer, H. (2002). Topiramate induced manic episode. *J Neurol Neurosurg Psychiatry*, 73(2), 208–209.

Juckel, G., Hegerl, U., Mavrogiorgou, P., Gallinat, J., Mager, T., Tigges, P., Dresel, S., Schroter, A., Stotz, G., Meller, I., Greil, W., and Moller, H.J. (2000). Clinical and biological findings in a case with 48-hour bipolar ultrarapid cycling before and during valproate treatment. *J Clin Psychiatry*, 61(8), 585–593.

Kanba, S., Yagi, G., Kamijima, K., Suzuki, T., Tajima, O., Otaki, J., Arata, E., Koshikawa, H., Nibuya, M., Kinoshita, N., and Asai, M. (1994). The first open study of zonisamide, a novel anticonvulsant, shows efficacy in mania. *Prog Neuropsychopharmacol Biol Psychiatry*, 18(4), 707–715.

Keck, P.E. Jr. (2005). Bipolar depression: A new role for atypical antipsychotics? *Bipolar Disord*, 7(Suppl. 4), 34–40.

Keck, P.E. Jr., Wilson, D.R., Strakowski, S.M., McElroy, S.L., Kizer, D.L., Balistreri, T.M., Holtman, H.M., and DePriest, M. (1995). Clinical predictors of acute risperidone response in schizophrenia, schizoaffective disorder, and psychotic mood disorders. *J Clin Psychiatry*, 56(10), 466–470.

Keck, P.E. Jr., Nabulsi, A.A., Taylor, J.L., Henke, C.J., Chmiel, J.J., Stanton, S.P., and Bennett, J.A. (1996). A pharmacoeconomic model of divalproex vs. lithium in the acute and prophylactic treatment of bipolar I disorder. *J Clin Psychiatry*, 57(5), 213–222.

Keck, P.E. Jr., Reeves, K.R., and Harrigan, E.P. (2001). Ziprasidone in the short-term treatment of patients with schizoaffective disorder: Results from two double-blind, placebo-controlled, multicenter studies. *J Clin Psychopharmacol*, 21(1), 27–35.

Keck, P.E. Jr., Marcus, R., Tourkodimitris, S., Ali, M., Liebeskind, A., Saha, A., Ingenito, G., and Aripiprazole Study Group. (2003a). A placebo-controlled, double-blind study of the efficacy and safety of aripiprazole in patients with acute bipolar mania. *Am J Psychiatry*, 160(9), 1651–1658.

Keck, P.E. Jr., Versiani, M., Potkin, S., West, S.A., Giller, E., Ice, K., and Ziprasidone in Mania Study Group. (2003b). Ziprasidone in the treatment of acute bipolar mania: A three-week, placebo-controlled, double-blind, randomized trial. *Am J Psychiatry*, 160(4), 741.

Ketter, T.A. (2005). *Advances in Treatment of Bipolar Disorder* (Review of Psychiatry). Arlington, VA: American Psychiatric Association.

Ketter, T.A., Kalali, A.H., Weisler, R.H., and SPD417 Study Group. (2004). A 6-month, multicenter, open-label evaluation of beaded, extended-release carbamazepine capsule monotherapy

in bipolar disorder patients with manic or mixed episodes. *J Clin Psychiatry*, 65(5), 668–673.

Khanna, S., Vieta, E., Lyons, B., Grossman, F., Eerdekens, M., and Kramer, M. (2005). Risperidone in the treatment of acute bipolar mania: A double-blind, placebo-controlled study of 290 patients. *Br J Psychiatry*, 187, 229–234.

Kinrys, G. (2000). Hypomania associated with omega3 fatty acids. *Arch Gen Psychiatry*, 57(7), 715–716.

Kushner, S.F., Khan, A., Lane, R., and Olson, W.H. (2006). Topiramate monotherapy in the management of acute mania: Results of four double-blind placebo-controlled trials. *Bipolar Disord*, 8(1), 15–27.

Lambert, P.A., Cavaz, G., Borselli, S., and Carrel, S. (1966). Action neuro-psychotrope d'un nouvel anti-épileptique: Le dépamide. *Ann Med Psychol*, 1, 707–710.

Lenox, R.H., Newhouse, P.A., Creelman, W.L., and Whitaker, T.M. (1992). Adjunctive treatment of manic agitation with lorazepam versus haloperidol: A double-blind study. *J Clin Psychiatry*, 53(2), 47–52.

Lerer, B., Moore, N., Meyendorff, E., Cho, S.R., and Gershon, S. (1987). Carbamazepine versus lithium in mania: A double-blind study. *J Clin Psychiatry*, 48(3), 89–93.

Lessig, M.C., Shapira, N.A., and Murphy, T.K. (2001). Topiramate for reversing atypical antipsychotic weight gain. *J Am Acad Child Adolesc Psychiatry*, 40(12), 1364.

Letmaier, M., Schreinzer, D., Wolf, R., and Kasper, S. (2001). Topiramate as a mood stabilizer. *Int Clin Psychopharmacol*, 16(5), 295–298.

Letmaier, M., Schreinzer, D., Thierry, N., Wolf, R., and Kasper, S. (2004). Drug therapy of acute manias: A retrospective data analysis of inpatients from 1997 to 1999. *Nervenarzt*, 75(3), 249–257.

Letmaier, M., Schreinzer, D., Reinfried, L., Glauninger, G., Thierry, N., Kapitany, T., and Kasper, S. (2006). Typical neuroleptics vs. atypical antipsychotics in the treatment of acute mania in a natural setting. *Int J Neuropsychopharmacol*, 9(5), 529–537.

Levy, N.A., and Janicak, P.G. (2000). Calcium channel antagonists for the treatment of bipolar disorder. *Bipolar Disord*, 2, 108–119.

Licht, R.W., Gouliaev, G., Vestergaard, P., and Frydenberg, M. (1997). Generalisability of results from randomised drug trials: A trial on antimanic treatment. *Br J Psychiatry*, 170, 264–267.

Maggs, R. (1963). Treatment of manic illness with lithium carbonate. *Br J Psychiatry*, 109, 56–65.

Manji, H.K., and Chen, G. (2002). PKC, MAP kinases and the bcl-2 family of proteins as long-term targets for mood stabilizers. *Mol Psychiatry*, 7(Suppl. 1), S46–S56.

Marcotte, D. (1998). Use of topiramate, a new anti-epileptic as a mood stabilizer. *J Affect Disord*, 50(2), 245–251.

Margolese, H.C., Beauclair, L., Szkrumelak, N., and Chouinard, G. (2003). Hypomania induced by adjunctive lamotrigine. *Am J Psychiatry*, 160(1), 183–188.

McElroy, S.L., and Keck, P.E. Jr. (2000). Pharmacologic agents for the treatment of acute bipolar mania. *Biol Psychiatry*, 48(6), 539–557.

McElroy, S.L., Keck, P.E. Jr., Pope, H.G. Jr., and Hudson, J.I. (1988). Valproate in the treatment of rapid-cycling bipolar disorder. *J Clin Psychopharmacol*, 8(4), 275–279.

McElroy, S.L., Keck, P.E. Jr., Pope, H.G. Jr., Hudson, J.I., Faedda, G.L., and Swann, A.C. (1992) Clinical and research implications of the diagnosis of dysphoric or mixed mania or hypomania. *Am J Psychiatry*, 149(12), 1633–1644.

McElroy, S.L., Keck, P.E., Stanton, S.P., Tugrul, K.C., Bennett, J.A., and Strakowski, S.M. (1996). A randomized comparison of divalproex oral loading versus haloperidol in the initial treatment of acute psychotic mania. *J Clin Psychiatry*, 57(4), 142–146.

McElroy, S.L., Soutullo, C.A., Keck, P.E. Jr., and Kmetz, G.F. (1997). A pilot trial of adjunctive gabapentin in the treatment of bipolar disorder. *Ann Clin Psychiatry*, 9(2), 99–103.

McElroy, S.L., Suppes, T., Keck, P.E., Frye, M.A., Denicoff, K.D., Altshuler, L.L., Brown, E.S., Nolen, W.A., Kupka, R.W., Rochussen, J., Leverich, G.S., and Post, R.M. (2000). Open-label adjunctive topiramate in the treatment of bipolar disorders. *Biol Psychiatry*, 47(12), 1025–1033.

McElroy, S.L., Suppes, T., Keck, P.E. Jr., Black, D., Frye, M.A., Altshuler, L.L., Nolen, W.A., Kupka, R.W., Leverich, G.S., Walden, J., Grunze, H., and Post, R.M. (2005). Open-label adjunctive zonisamide in the treatment of bipolar disorders: A prospective trial. *J Clin Psychiatry*, 66(5), 617–624.

McIntyre, R.S., Brecher, M., Paulsson, B., Huizar, K., and Mullen, J. (2005). Quetiapine or haloperidol as monotherapy for bipolar mania: A 12-week, double-blind, randomised, parallel-group, placebo-controlled trial. *Eur Neuropsychopharmacol*, 15(5), 573–585.

Meehan, K., Zhang, F., David, S., Tohen, M., Janicak, P., Small, J., Koch, M., Rizk, R., Walker, D., Tran, P., and Breier, A. (2001). A double-blind, randomized comparison of the efficacy and safety of intramuscular injections of olanzapine, lorazepam, or placebo in treating acutely agitated patients diagnosed with bipolar mania. *J Clin Psychopharmacol*, 21(4), 389–397.

Michael, N., and Erfurth, A. (2004). Treatment of bipolar mania with right prefrontal rapid transcranial magnetic stimulation. *J Affect Disord*, 78, 253–257.

Miller, D.S., Yatham, L.N., and Lam, R.W. (2001). Comparative efficacy of typical and atypical antipsychotics as add-on therapy to mood stabilizers in the treatment of mania. *J Clin Psychiatry*, 62(12), 9750–9980.

Milstein, V., Small, J.G., Klapper, M.H., Small, I.F., Miller, M.J., and Kellams, J.J. (1987). Uni- versus bilateral ECT in the treatment of mania. *Convuls Ther*, 3(1), 1–9.

Mishory, A., Yaroslavsky, Y., Bersudsky, Y., and Belmaker, R.H. (2000). Phenytoin as an antimanic anticonvulsant: A controlled study. *Am J Psychiatry*, 157(3), 463–465.

Modell, J.G., Lenox, R.H., and Weiner, S. (1985). Inpatient clinical trial of lorazepam for the management of manic agitation. *J Clin Psychopharmacol*, 5(2), 109–113.

Mukherjee, S., Sackeim, H.A., and Schnur, D.B. (1994). Electroconvulsive therapy of acute manic episodes: A review of 50 years' experience. *Am J Psychiatry*, 151(2), 169–176.

Muller, P., and Heipertz, R. (1977). Treatment of manic psychosis with clozapine [in German]. *Fortschr Neurol Psychiatr Grenzgeb*, 45(7), 420–424.

Muller-Oerlinghausen, B., Retzow, A., Henn, F.A., Giedke, H., and Walden, J. (2000). Valproate as an adjunct to neuroleptic medication for the treatment of acute episodes of mania: A prospective, randomized, double-blind, placebo-controlled, multicenter study. European Valproate Mania Study Group. *J Clin Psychopharmacol*, 20(2), 195–203.

Nierenberg, A.A., Burt, T., Matthews, J., and Weiss, A.P. (1999). Mania associated with St. John's Wort. *Biol Psychiatry*, 46(12), 1707–1708.

Normann, C., Langosch, J., Schaerer, L.O., Grunze, H., and Walden, J. (1999). Treatment of acute mania with topiramate. *Am J Psychiatry*, 156(12), 2014.

Okuma, T., Inanaga, K., Otsuki, S., Sarai, K., Takahashi, R., Hazama, H., Mori, A., and Watanabe, S. (1981). A preliminary double-blind study on the efficacy of carbamazepine in prophylaxis of manic-depressive illness. *Psychopharmacology (Berl)*, 73(1), 95–96.

Okuma, T., Yamashita, I., Takahashi, R., Itoh, H., Otsuki, S., Watanabe, S., Sarai, K., Hazama, H., and Inanaga, K. (1990). Comparison of the antimanic efficacy of carbamazepine and lithium carbonate by double-blind controlled study. *Pharmacopsychiatry*, 23(3), 143–150.

Pande, A.C., Crockatt, J.G., Janney, C.A., Werth, J.L., and Tsaroucha, G. (2000). Gabapentin in bipolar disorder: A placebo-controlled trial of adjunctive therapy. Gabapentin Bipolar Disorder Study Group. *Bipolar Disord*, 2 (3 Pt. 2), 249–255.

Pascual-Leone, A., and Catala, M.D. (1996). Lateralized effect of rapid-rate transcranial magnetic stimulation on the prefrontal contex on mood. *Neurology*, 46, 499–502.

Pazzaglia, P.J., Post, R.M., Ketter, T.A., Callahan, A.M., Marangell, L.B., Frye, M.A., George, M.S., Kimbrell, T.A., Leverich, G.S., Cora-Locatelli, G., and Luckenbaugh, D. (1998). Nimodipine monotherapy and carbamazepine augmentation in patients with refractory recurrent affective illness. *J Clin Psychopharmacol*, 18(5), 404–413.

Pecuch, P.W., and Erfurth, A. (2001). Topiramate in the treatment of acute mania. *J Clin Psychopharmacol*, 21(2), 243–244.

Perlis, R.H., Baker, R.W., Zarate, C.A. Jr., Brown, E.B., Schuh, L.M., Jamal, H.H., and Tohen, M. (2006a). Olanzapine versus risperidone in the treatment of manic or mixed states in bipolar disorder: A randomized, double-blind trial. *J Clin Psychiatry*, 67, 1747–1753.

Perlis, R.H., Welge, J.A., Vornik, L.A., Hirschfeld, R.M., and Keck, P.E. Jr. (2006b). Atypical antipsychotics in the treatment of mania: A meta-analysis of randomized, placebo-controlled trials. *J Clin Psychiatry*, 67(4), 509–516.

Perugi, G., Toni, C., Ruffolo, G., Sartini, S., Simonini, E., and Akiskal, H. (1999). Clinical experience using adjunctive gabapentin in treatment-resistant bipolar mixed states. *Pharmacopsychiatry*, 32(4), 136–141.

Peuskens, J., Moller, H.J., and Puech, A. (2002). Amisulpride improves depressive symptoms in acute exacerbations of schizophrenia: Comparison with haloperidol and risperidone. *Eur Neuropsychopharmacol*, 12(4), 305–310.

Phrolov, K., Applebaum, J., Levine, J., Miodovnick, H., and Belmaker, R.H. (2004). Single-dose intravenous valproate in acute mania. *J Clin Psychiatry*, 65(1), 68–70.

Pope, H.G., Jr., McElroy, S.L., Keck, P.E., and Hudson, J.I. (1991). Valproate in the treatment of acute mania. A placebo-controlled study. *Arch Gen Psychiatry*, 48(1), 62–68.

Post, R.M., Uhde, T.W., and Kramlinger, K.G. (1986a). Carbamazepine treatment of mania: Clinical and biochemical aspects. *Clin Neuropharmacol*, 9, 547–549.

Post, R.M., Uhde, T.W., Roy-Byrne, P.P., and Joffe, R.T. (1986b). Antidepressant effects of carbamazepine. *Am J Psychiatry*, 143(1), 29–34.

Post, R.M., Uhde, T.W., Roy-Byrne, P.P., and Joffe, R.T. (1987). Correlates of antimanic response to carbamazepine. *Psychiatry Research*, 21(1), 71–83.

Post, R.M., Frye, M.A., Denicoff, K.D., Leverich, G.S., Dunn, R.T., Osuch, E.A., Speer, A.M., Obrocea, G., and Jajodia, K. (2000). Emerging trends in the treatment of rapid cycling bipolar disorder: A selected review. *Bipolar Disord*, 2(4), 305–315.

Potkin, S.G., Keck, P.E. Jr., Segal, S., Ice, K., and English, P. (2005). Ziprasidone in acute bipolar mania: A 21-day randomized, double-blind, placebo-controlled replication trial. *J Clin Psychopharmacol*, 25(4), 301–310.

Powers, P., Sachs, G.S., Kushner, S.F., Wang, D., Olson, W., Capece, J., Fazzio, L., and Rosenthal, N. (2004). Topiramate in adults with acute bipolar I mania: Pooled results. In 157th Annual Meeting of the American Psychiatric Association. New York, NY: American Psychiatric Association.

Prien, R.F., and Caffey, E.M. Jr. (1976). Relationship between dosage and response to lithium prophylaxis in recurrent depression. *Am J Psychiatry*, 133(5), 567–570.

Prien, R.F., Caffey, E.M. Jr., and Klett, C.J. (1972). Comparison of lithium carbonate and chlorpromazine in the treatment of mania. Report of the Veterans Administration and National Institute of Mental Health Collaborative Study Group. *Arch Gen Psychiatry*, 26(2), 146–153.

Rifkin, A., Doddi, S., Karajgi, B., Borenstein, M., and Munne, R. (1994). Dosage of haloperidol for mania. *Br J Psychiatry*, 165, 113–116.

Rucci, P., Frank, E., Kostelnik, B., Fagiolini, A., Mallinger, A.G., Swartz, H.A., Thase, M.E., Siegel, L., Wilson, D., and Kupfer, D.J. (2002). Suicide attempts in patients with bipolar I disorder during acute and maintenance phases of intensive treatment with pharmacotherapy and adjunctive psychotherapy. *Am J Psychiatry*, 159(7), 1160–1164.

Rudorfer, M.V., Linnoila, M., and Potter, W.Z. (1987). Combined lithium and electroconvulsive therapy: Pharmacokinetic and pharmacodynamic interactions. *Convuls Ther*, 3(1), 40–45.

Sachs, G.S., Printz, D.J., Kahn, D.A., Carpenter, D., and Docherty, J.P. (2000). The expert consensus guideline series: Medication treatment of bipolar disorder 2000. *Postgrad Med*, Spec. No. 1–104.

Sachs, G.S., Grossman, F., Ghaemi, S.N., Okamoto, A., and Bowden, C.L. (2002). Combination of a mood stabilizer with risperidone or haloperidol for treatment of acute mania: A double-blind, placebo-controlled comparison of efficacy and safety. *Am J Psychiatry*, 159(7), 1146–1154.

Sachs, G., Chengappa, K.N., Suppes, T., Mullen, J.A., Brecher, M., Devine, N.A., and Sweitzer, D.E. (2004). Quetiapine with lithium or divalproex for the treatment of bipolar mania: A randomized, double-blind, placebo-controlled study. *Bipolar Disord*, 6(3), 213–223.

Sajatovic, M., Brescan, D.W., Perez, D.E., DiGiovanni, S.K., Hattab, H., Ray, J.B., and Bingham, C.R. (2001). Quetiapine alone and added to a mood stabilizer for serious mood disorders. *J Clin Psychiatry*, 62(9), 728–732.

Sanger, T.M., Tohen, M., Vieta, E., Dunner, D.L., Bowden, C.L., Calabrese, J.R., Feldman, P.D., Jacobs, T.G., and Breier, A. (2003). Olanzapine in the acute treatment of bipolar I disorder with a history of rapid cycling. *J Affect Disord*, 73(1–2), 155–161.

Schaffer, A., and Levitt, A.J. (2005). Double-blind, placebo-controlled pilot study of mexiletine for acute mania or hypomania. *J Clin Psychopharmacol*, 25(5), 507–508.

Schaffer, L.C., Schaffer, C.B., and Howe, J. (2002). An open case series on the utility of tiagabine as an augmentation in refractory bipolar outpatients. *J Affect Disord*, 71(1-3), 259–263.

Schatzberg, A.F., and Nemeroff, C.B. (Eds.). (1998). *The American Psychiatric Publishing Textbook of Psychopharmacology* (2nd Edition). Arlington, VA: American Psychiatric Association.

Schou, M., Juel-Nielsen, N, Strömgren, E., and Voldby, H. (1954). The treatment of manic psychoses by the administration of lithium salts. *J Neurol Neurosurg Psychiatry*, 17, 250–260.

Segal, J., Berk, M., and Brook, S. (1998). Risperidone compared with both lithium and haloperidol in mania: A double-blind randomized controlled trial. *Clin Neuropharmacol*, 21(3), 176–180.

Shaldubina, A., Stahl, Z., Furszpan, M., Regenold, W.T., Shapiro, J., Belmaker, R.H., and Bersudsky, Y. (2006). Inositol deficiency diet and lithium effects. *Bipolar Disord*, 8(2), 152–159.

Shi, L., Namjoshi, M.A., Zhang, F., Gandhi, G., Edgell, E.T., Tohen, M., Breier, A., and Haro, J.M. (2002). Olanzapine versus haloperidol in the treatment of acute mania: Clinical outcomes, health-related quality of life and work status. *Int Clin Psychopharmacol*, 17(5), 227–237.

Shopsin, B., Gershon, S., Thompson, H., and Collins, P. (1975). Psychoactive drugs in mania. A controlled comparison of lithium carbonate, chlorpromazine, and haloperidol. *Arch Gen Psychiatry*, 32(1), 34–42.

Short, C., and Cooke, L. (1995). Hypomania induced by gabapentin. *Br J Psychiatry*, 166(5), 679–680.

Small, J.G., Klapper, M.H., Kellams, J.J., Miller, M.J., Milstein, V., Sharpley, P.H., and Small, I.F. (1988). Electroconvulsive treatment compared with lithium in the management of manic states. *Arch Gen Psychiatry*, 45(8), 727–732.

Small, J.G., Klapper, M.H., Milstein, V., Kellams, J.J., Miller, M.J., Marhenke, J.D., and Small, I.F. (1991). Carbamazepine compared with lithium in the treatment of mania. *Arch Gen Psychiatry*, 48(10), 915–921.

Small, J.G., Klapper, M.H., Marhenke, J.D., Milstein, V., Woodham, G.C., and Kellams, J.J. (1995). Lithium combined with carbamazepine or haloperidol in the treatment of mania. *Psychopharmacol Bull*, 31(2), 265–272.

Smulevich, A.B., Khanna, S., Eerdekens, M., Karcher, K., Kramer, M., and Grossman, F. (2005). Acute and continuation risperidone monotherapy in bipolar mania: A 3-week placebo-controlled trial followed by a 9-week double-blind trial of risperidone and haloperidol. *Eur Neuropsychopharmacol*, 15(1), 75–84.

Sokolski, K.N., Green, C., Maris, D.E., and DeMet, E.M. (1999). Gabapentin as an adjunct to standard mood stabilizers in outpatients with mixed bipolar symptomatology. *Ann Clin Psychiatry*, 11(4), 217–222.

Stanton, S.P., Keck, P.E. Jr., and McElroy, S.L. (1997). Treatment of acute mania with gabapentin. *Am J Psychiatry*, 154(2), 287.

Stokes, P.E., Shamoian, C.A., Stoll, P.M., and Patton, M.J. (1971). Efficacy of lithium as acute treatment of manic-depressive illness. *Lancet*, 1(7713), 1319–1325.

Suppes, T., McElroy, S.L., Gilbert, J., Dessain, E.C., and Cole, J.O. (1992). Clozapine in the treatment of dysphoric mania. *Biol Psychiatry*, 32(3), 270–280.

Suppes, T., Webb, A., Paul, B., Carmody, T., Kraemer, H., and Rush, A.J. (1999). Clinical outcome in a randomized 1-year trial of clozapine versus treatment as usual for patients with treatment-resistant illness and a history of mania. *Am J Psychiatry*, 156(8), 1164–1169.

Suppes, T., Chisholm, K.A., Dhavale, D., Frye, M.A., Altshuler, L.L., McElroy, S.L., Keck, P.E., Nolen, W.A., Kupka, R., Denicoff, K.D., Leverich, G.S., Rush, A.J., and Post, R.M. (2002).

Tiagabine in treatment refractory bipolar disorder: A clinical case series. *Bipolar Disord*, 4(5), 283–289.

Swann, A.C., Bowden, C.L., Morris, D., Calabrese, J.R., Petty, F., Small, J., Dilsaver, S.C., and Davis, J.M. (1997). Depression during mania. Treatment response to lithium or divalproex. *Arch Gen Psychiatry*, 54(1), 37–42.

Swann, A.C., Bowden, C.L., Calabrese, J.R., Dilsaver, S.C., and Morris, D.D. (1999). Differential effect of number of previous episodes of affective disorder on response to lithium or divalproex in acute mania. *Am J Psychiatry*, 156(8), 1264.

Swann, A.C., Bowden, C.L., Calabrese, J.R., Dilsaver, S.C., and Morris, D.D. (2002). Pattern of response to divalproex, lithium, or placebo in four naturalistic subtypes of mania. *Neuropsychopharmacology*, 26(4), 530–536.

Tohen, M., Castillo, J., Pope, H.G. Jr., and Herbstein, J. (1994). Concomitant use of valproate and carbamazepine in bipolar and schizoaffective disorders. *J Clin Psychopharmacol*, 14(1), 67–70.

Tohen, M., Zarate, C.A. Jr., Centorrino, F., Hegarty, J.I., Froeschl, M., and Zarate, S.B. (1996). Risperidone in the treatment of mania. *J Clin Psychiatry*, 57(6), 249–253.

Tohen, M., Sanger, T.M., McElroy, S.L., Tollefson, G.D., Chengappa, K.N., Daniel, D.G., Petty, F., Centorrino, F., Wang, R., Grundy, S.L., Greaney, M.G., Jacobs, T.G., David, S.R., and Toma, V. (1999). Olanzapine versus placebo in the treatment of acute mania. Olanzapine HGEH Study Group. *Am J Psychiatry*, 156(5), 702–709.

Tohen, M., Jacobs, T.G., Grundy, S.L., McElroy, S.L., Banov, M.C., Janicak, P.G., Sanger, T., Risser, R., Zhang, F., Toma, V., Francis, J., Tollefson, G.D., and Breier, A. (2000). Efficacy of olanzapine in acute bipolar mania: A double-blind, placebo-controlled study. The Olanzipine HGGW Study Group. *Arch Gen Psychiatry*, 57(9), 841–849.

Tohen, M., Zhang, F., Taylor, C.C., Burns, P., Zarate, C., Sanger, T., and Tollefson, G. (2001). A meta-analysis of the use of typical antipsychotic agents in bipolar disorder. *J Affect Disord*, 65(1), 85–93.

Tohen, M., Baker, R.W., Altshuler, L.L., Zarate, C.A., Suppes, T., Ketter, T.A., Milton, D.R., Risser, R., Gilmore, J.A., Breier, A., and Tollefson, G.D. (2002). Olanzapine versus divalproex sodium for the treatment of acute mania. *Am J Psychiatry*, 159(6), 1011–1017.

Tohen, M., Ketter, T.A., Zarate, C.A., Suppes, T., Frye, M., Altshuler, L., Zajecka, J., Schuh, L.M., Risser, R.C., Brown, E., and Baker, R.W. (2003a). Olanzapine versus divalproex sodium for the treatment of acute mania and maintenance of remission: A 47-week study. *Am J Psychiatry*, 160(7), 1263–1271.

Tohen, M., Goldberg, J.F., Gonzalez-Pinto, Arrillaga, A.M., Azorin, J.M., Vieta, E., Hardy-Bayle, M.C., Lawson, W.B., Emsley, R.A., Zhang, F., Baker, R.W., Risser, R.C., Namjoshi, M.A., Evans, A.R., and Breier, A. (2003b). A 12-week, double-blind comparison of olanzapine vs. haloperidol in the treatment of acute mania. *Arch Gen Psychiatry*, 60(12), 1218–1226.

Tohen, M., Chengappa, K.N., Suppes, T., Baker, R.W., Zarate, C.A., Bowden, C.L., Sachs, G.S., Kupfer, D.J., Ghaemi, S.N., Feldman, P.D., Risser, R.C., Evans, A.R., and Calabrese, J.R. (2004). Relapse prevention in bipolar I disorder: 18-month comparison of olanzapine plus mood stabiliser vs. mood stabiliser alone. *Br J Psychiatry*, 184, 337–345.

Vieta, E., Gasto, C., Colom, F., Reinares, M., Martinez-Aran, A., Benabarre, A., and Akiskal, H.S. (2001). Role of risperidone in bipolar II: An open 6-month study. *J Affect Disord*, 67(1–3), 213–219.

Vieta, E., Brugue, E., Goikolea, J.M., Sanchez-Moreno, J., Reinares, M., Comes, M., Colom, F., Martinez-Aran, A., Benabarre, A., and Torrent, C. (2003). *Risperidone monotherapy in acute bipolar mania*. Poster, Meeting of the American College of Neuropsychopharmacology, Puerto Rico, 222.

Vieta, E., Bourin, M., Sanchez, R., Marcus, R., Stock, E., McQuade, R., Carson, W., Abou-Gharbia, N., Swanink, R., Iwamoto, T., and Aripoprazole Study Group. (2005). Effectiveness of aripiprazole vs. haloperidol in acute bipolar mania: Double-blind, randomised, comparative 12-week trial. *Br J Psychiatry*, 187, 235–242.

Walton, S.A., Berk, M., and Brook, S. (1996). Superiority of lithium over verapamil in mania: A randomized, controlled, single-blind trial. *J Clin Psychiatry*, 57(11), 543–546.

Weisler, R.H., Kalali, A.H., Ketter, T.A., and SPD417 Study Group. (2004). A multicenter, randomized, double-blind, placebo-controlled trial of extended-release carbamazepine capsules as monotherapy for bipolar disorder patients with manic or mixed episodes. *J Clin Psychiatry*, 65(4), 478–484.

Weisler, R.H., Keck, P.E. Jr., Swann, A.C., Cutler, A.J., Ketter, T.A., Kalali, A.H., and SPD417 Study Group. (2005). Extended-release carbamazepine capsules as monotherapy for acute mania in bipolar disorder: A multicenter, randomized, double-blind, placebo-controlled trial. *J Clin Psychiatry*, 66(3), 323–330.

Winokur, G., and Kadrmas, A. (1989). A polyepisodic course in bipolar illness: Possible clinical relationships. *Compr Psychiatry*, 30(2), 121–127.

Winokur, G., Coryell, W., Keller, M., and Scheftner, W.A. (1990). Relationship of electroconvulsive therapy to course in affective illness: A collaborative study. *Eur Arch Psychiatry Clin Neurosci*, 240(1), 54–59.

Yatham, L.N., Grossman, F., Augustyns, I., Vieta, E., and Ravindran, A. (2003). Mood stabilisers plus risperidone or placebo in the treatment of acute mania. International, double-blind, randomised controlled trial. *Br J Psychiatry*, 182, 141–147.

Yatham, L.N., Binder, C., Kusumakar, V., and Riccardelli, R. (2004). Risperidone plus lithium versus risperidone plus valproate in acute and continuation treatment of mania. *Int Clin Psychopharmacol*, 19(2), 103–109.

Zajecka, J.M., Weisler, R., Sachs, G., Swann, A.C., Wozniak, P., and Sommerville, K.W. (2002). A comparison of the efficacy, safety, and tolerability of divalproex sodium and olanzapine in the treatment of bipolar disorder. *J Clin Psychiatry*, 63(12), 1148–1155.

Zarate, C.A. Jr., Tohen, M., and Baldessarini, R.J. (1995). Clozapine in severe mood disorders. *J Clin Psychiatry*, 56(9), 411–417.

Zarate, C.A. Jr., Tohen, M., and Baraibar, G. (1997). Combined valproate or carbamazepine and electroconvulsive therapy. *Ann Clin Psychiatry*, 9(1), 19–25.

Zarate, C.A. Jr., Rothschild, A., Fletcher, K.E., Madrid, A., and Zapatel, J. (2000). Clinical predictors of acute response with quetiapine in psychotic mood disorders. *J Clin Psychiatry*, 61(3), 185–189.

CHAPTER 19

Abraham, G., Milev, R., and Stuart Lawson, J. (2006). T3 augmentation of SSRI resistant depression. *J Affect Disord*, 91(2-3), 211–215.

Abrams, R. (Ed.). (1997). *Electroconvulsive Therapy* (third edition). New York: Oxford University Press.

Ahokas, A., Aito, M., and Rimon, R. (2000). Positive treatment effect of estradiol in postpartum psychosis: A pilot study. *J Clin Psychiatry*, 61(3), 166–169.

Ahokas, A., Kaukoranta, J., Wahlbeck, K., and Aito, M. (2001). Estrogen deficiency in severe postpartum depression: Successful treatment with sublingual physiologic 17 beta-estradiol: A preliminary study. *J Clin Psychiatry*, 62(5), 332–336.

Akiskal, H.S. (1995). Switching from "unipolar" to bipolar II: An 11-year prospective study of clinical and temperamental predictors in 559 patients. *Arch Gen Psychiatry*, 52, 114–123.

Akiskal, H.S., Maser, J.D., Zeller, P.J., Endicott, J., Coryell, W., Keller, M., Warshaw, M., Clayton, P., and Goodwin, F. (1995). Switching from 'unipolar' to bipolar II. An 11-year prospective study of clinical and temperamental predictors in 559 patients. *Arch Gen Psychiatry*, 52(2), 114–123.

Akiskal, H.S., Hantouche, E.G., Allilaire, J.F., Sechter, D., Bourgeois, M.L., Azorin, J.M., Chatenet-Duchene, L., and Lancrenon, S. (2003). Validating antidepressant-associated hypomania (bipolar III): A systematic comparison with spontaneous hypomania (bipolar II). *J Affect Disord*, 73(1-2), 65–74.

Alpert, J.E., Papakostas, G., Mischoulon, D., Worthington, J.J. III, Petersen, T., Mahal, Y., Burns, A., Bottiglieri, T., Nierenberg, A.A., and Fava, M. (2004). S-Adenosyl-L-methionine (SAMe) as an adjunct for resistant major depressive disorder: An open trial following partial or nonresponse to selective serotonin reuptake inhibitors or venlafaxine. *J Clin Psychopharmacol*, 24(6), 661–664.

Altshuler, L.L., Post, R.M., Leverich, G.S., Mikalauskas, K., Rosoff, A., and Ackerman, L. (1995). Antidepressant-induced mania and cycle acceleration: A controversy revisited. *Am J Psychiatry*, 152(8), 1130–1138.

Altshuler, L.L., Keck, P.E. Jr., McElroy, S.L., Suppes, T., Brown, E.S., Denicoff, K., Frye, M., Gitlin, M., Hwang, S., Goodman, R., Leverich, G., Nolen, W., Kupka, R., and Post, R. (1999). Gabapentin in the acute treatment of refractory bipolar disorder. *Bipolar Disord*, 1(1), 61–65.

Altshuler, L., Kiriakos, L., Calcagno, J., Goodman, R., Gitlin, M., Frye, M., and Mintz, J. (2001a). The impact of antidepressant discontinuation versus antidepressant continuation on 1-year risk for relapse of bipolar depression: A retrospective chart review. *J Clin Psychiatry*, 62(8), 612–616.

Altshuler, L.L., Bauer, M., Frye, M.A., Gitlin, M.J., Mintz, J., Szuba, M.P., Leight, K.L., and Whybrow, P.C. (2001b). Does thyroid supplementation accelerate tricyclic antidepressant response? A review and meta-analysis of the literature. *Am J Psychiatry*, 158(10), 1617–1622.

Altshuler, L., Suppes, T., Black, D., Nolen, W.A., Keck, P.E. Jr., Frye, M.A., McElroy, S., Kupka, R., Grunze, H., Walden, J., Leverich, G., Denicoff, K., Luckenbaugh, D., and Post, R. (2003). Impact of antidepressant discontinuation after acute bipolar depression remission on rates of depressive relapse at 1-year follow-up. *Am J Psychiatry*, 160(7), 1252–1262.

Altshuler, L.L., Suppes, T., Black, D.O., Nolen, W.A., Leverich, G., Keck, P.E., Frye, M.A., Kupka, R., McElroy, S.L., Grunze, H., Kitchen, C.M., and Post, R. (2006). Lower switch rate in depressed patients with bipolar II than bipolar I disorder treated adjunctively with second-generation antidepressants. *Am J Psychiatry*, 163(2), 313–315.

American Psychiatric Association. (2002). Practice guidelines for the treatment of patients with bipolar depression (revision). *Am J Psychiatry*, 159(Suppl. 4), 1–50.

Amsterdam, J. (1998). Efficacy and safety of venlafaxine in the treatment of bipolar II major depressive episode. *J Clin Psychopharmacol*, 18(5), 414–417.

Amsterdam, J.D., and Garcia-Espana, F. (2000). Venlafaxine monotherapy in women with bipolar II and unipolar major depression. *J Affect Disord*, 59(3), 225–229.

Amsterdam, J.D., Garcia-Espana, F., Fawcett, J., Quitkin, F.M., Reimherr, F.W., Rosenbaum, J.F., Schweizer, E., and Beasley, C. (1998). Efficacy and safety of fluoxetine in treating bipolar II major depressive episode. *J Clin Psychopharmacol*, 18(6), 435–440.

Anand, A., Bukhari, L., Jennings, S.A., Lee, C., Kamat, M., Shekhar, A., Nurnberger, J.I. Jr., and Lightfoot, J. (2005). A preliminary open-label study of zonisamide treatment for bipolar depression in 10 patients. *J Clin Psychiatry*, 66(2), 195–198.

Angst, J. (1985). Switch from depression to mania: A record study over decades between 1920 and 1982. *Psychopathology*, 18(2-3), 140–154.

Angst, J., Angst, K., Baruffol, I., and Meinherz-Surbeck, R. (1992). ECT-induced and drug-induced hypomania. *Convuls Ther*, 8(3), 179–185.

Arieli, A., and Lepkifker, E. (1981). The antidepressant effect of lithium. *Curr Dev Psychopharmacol*, 6, 165–190.

Arnold, O.H., and Kryspin-Exner, K. (1965). Zur Frage der Beeinflussung des Verlaufes des manisch-depressiven Krankheitsgeschehens durch Antidepressiva. [The problem of control of manic-depressive processes by antidepressants]. *Wien Med Wochenschr*, 115, 929–934.

Aronson, R., Offman, H.J., Joffe, R.T., and Naylor, C.D. (1996). Triiodothyronine augmentation in the treatment of refractory depression. A meta-analysis. *Arch Gen Psychiatry*, 53(9), 842–848.

Artaud, A. (1965). *Artaud Anthology*. Edited by J. Hirschman. San Francisco: City Lights Press.

Aubry, J.M., Simon, A.E., and Bertschy, G. (2000). Possible induction of mania and hypomania by olanzapine or risperidone: A critical review of reported cases. *J Clin Psychiatry*, 61(9), 649–655.

Austin, M.P., Souza, F.G., and Goodwin, G.M. (1991). Lithium augmentation in antidepressant-resistant patients. A quantitative analysis. *Br J Psychiatry*, 159, 510–514.

Baastrup, P.C., and Schou, M. (1967). Lithium as a prophylactic agent. Its effect against recurrent depressions and manic-depressive psychosis. *Arch Gen Psychiatry*, 16(2), 162–172.

Baastrup, P.C., Poulsen, J.C., Schou, M., Thomsen, K., and Amdisen, A. (1970). Prophylactic lithium: Double-blind discontinuation in manic-depressive and recurrent-depressive disorders. *Lancet*, 2(7668), 326–330.

Baker, R.W., Milton, D.R., Stauffer, V.L., Gelenberg, A., and Tohen, M. (2003). Placebo-controlled trials do not find association of olanzapine with exacerbation of bipolar mania. *J Affect Disord*, 73(1-2), 147–153.

Baldassano, C.F., Sachs, G., and Stoll, A.L. (1995). Paroxetine for bipolar depression: Outcome in patients failing prior to antidepressant trials. *Depression*, 3182–3186.

Baldassano, C.F., Ghaemi, S.N., Chang, A., Lyman, A., and Lipari, M. (2004). Acute treatment of bipolar depression with adjunctive zonisamide: A retrospective chart review. *Bipolar Disord*, 6(5), 432–434.

Baldessarini, R.J., Tondo, L., Hennen, J., and Viguera, A.C. (2002). Is lithium still worth using? An update of selected recent research. *Harv Rev Psychiatry*, 10(2), 59–75.

Baldessarini, R.J., Pompili, M., and Tondo, L. (2006). Suicide in bipolar disorder: Risks and management. *CNS Spectr*, 11(6), 465–471.

Balon, R., Mufti, R., and Arfken, C.L. (1999). A survey of prescribing practices for monoamine oxidase inhibitors. *Psychiatr Serv*, 50(7), 945–947.

Barbini, B., Colombo, C., Benedetti, F., Campori, E., Bellodi, L., and Smeraldi, E. (1998). The unipolar–bipolar dichotomy and the response to sleep deprivation. *Psychiatry Res*, 79(1), 43–50.

Baron, M., Gershon, E.S., Rudy, V., Jonas, W.Z., and Buchsbaum, M. (1975). Lithium carbonate response in depression. Prediction by unipolar/bipolar illness, average-evoked response, catechol-O-methyl transferase, and family history. *Arch Gen Psychiatry*, 32(9), 1107–1111.

Bauer, M., and Döpfmer, S. (1999). Lithium augmentation in treatment-resistant depression: Meta-analysis of placebo-controlled studies. *J Clin Psychopharmacol*, 19(5), 427–434.

Bauer, M., and Döpfmer, S. (2000). Lithium augmentation in treatment-resistant depression: Meta-analysis of placebo-controlled studies. *J Clin.Psychopharmacol*, 20(2), 287.

Bauer, M.D., Hellweg, R., Graf, K.J., and Baumgartner, A. (1998). Treatment of refractory depression with high-dose thyroxine. *Neuropsychopharmacology*, 18(6), 444–455.

Bauer, M., Heinz, A., and Whybrow, P.C. (2002). Thyroid hormones, serotonin and mood: Of synergy and significance in the adult brain. *Mol Psychiatry*, 7(2), 140–156.

Bauer, M., London, E.D., Silverman, D.H., Rasgon, N., Kirchheiner, J., and Whybrow, P.C. (2003). Thyroid, brain and mood modulation in affective disorder: Insights from molecular research and functional brain imaging. *Pharmacopsychiatry*, 36(Suppl. 3), S215–S221.

Bauer, M., Rasgon, N., Grof, P., Altshuler, L., Gyulai, L., Lapp, M., Glenn, T., and Whybrow, P.C. (2005). Mood changes related to antidepressants: A longitudinal study of patients with bipolar disorder in a naturalistic setting. *Psychiatry Res*, 133(1), 73–80.

Bauer, M., Grof, P., and Muller-Oelingausen, B. (2006). The acute antidepressive effects of lithium: From monotherapy to augmentation therapy in major depression. In *Lithium in Neuropsychiatry: The Comprehensive Guide*. London: Taylor & Francis Book Ltd.

Bauer, M.S., and Whybrow, P.C. (1986). The effect of changing thyroid function on cyclic affective illness in a human subject. *Am J Psychiatry*, 142(5), 633–636.

Bauer, M.S., and Whybrow, P.C. (1990). Rapid cycling bipolar affective disorder. II. Treatment of refractory rapid cycling with high-dose levothyroxine: A preliminary study. *Arch Gen Psychiatry*, 47(5), 435–440.

Baumann, P., Nil, R., Souche, A., Montaldi, S., Baettig, D., Lambert, S., Uehlinger, C., Kasas, A., Amey, M., and Jonzier-Perey, M. (1996). A double-blind, placebo-controlled study of citalopram with and without lithium in the treatment of therapy-resistant depressive patients: A clinical, pharmacokinetic, and pharmacogenetic investigation. *J Clin Psychopharmacol*, 16(4), 307–314.

Benazzi, F. (1997). Antidepressant-associated hypomania in outpatient depression: A 203-case study in private practice. *J Affect Disord*, 46(1), 73–77.

Benazzi, F. (2001). Prevalence and clinical correlates of residual depressive symptoms in bipolar II disorder. *Psychother Psychosom*, 70(5), 232–238.

Benedetti, F., Barbini, B., Campori, E., Colombo, C., and Smeraldi, E. (1996). Dopamine agonist amineptine prevents the antidepressant effect of sleep deprivation. *Psychiatry Res*, 65(3), 179–184.

Benedetti, F., Colombo, C., Barbini, B., Campori, E., and Smeraldi, E. (1999). Ongoing lithium treatment prevents relapse after total sleep deprivation. *J Clin Psychopharmacol*, 19(3), 240–245.

Benedetti, F., Barbini, B., Campori, E., Fulgosi, M.C., Pontiggia, A., and Colombo, C. (2001a). Sleep phase advance and lithium to sustain the antidepressant effect of total sleep deprivation in bipolar depression: New findings supporting the internal coincidence model? *J Psychiatr Res*, 35(6), 323–329.

Benedetti, F., Campori, E., Barbini, B., Fulgosi, M.C., and Colombo, C. (2001b). Dopaminergic augmentation of sleep deprivation effects in bipolar depression. *Psychiatry Res*, 104(3), 239–246.

Benedetti, F., Colombo, C., Serretti, A., Lorenzi, C., Pontiggia, A., Barbini, B., and Smeraldi. E. (2003). Antidepressant effects of light therapy combined with sleep deprivation are influenced by a functional polymorphism within the promoter of the serotonin transporter gene. *Biol Psychiatry*, 154(7), 687–692.

Benedetti, F., Barbini, B., Fulgosi, M.C., Colombo, C., Dallaspezia, S., Pontiggia, A., and Smeraldi, E. (2005). Combined total sleep deprivation and light therapy in the treatment of drug-resistant bipolar depression: Acute response and long-term remission rates. *J Clin Psychiatry*, 66(12), 1535–1540.

Berger, M., Vollmann, J., Hohagen, F., Konig, A., Lohner, H., Voderholzer, U., and Riemann, D. (1997). Sleep deprivation combined with consecutive sleep phase advance as a fast-acting therapy in depression: An open pilot trial in medicated and unmedicated patients. *Am J Psychiatry*, 154(6), 870–872.

Berv, D., Klugman, J., Rosenquist, K.J., Hsu, D.J., and Ghaemi, S.N. (2002). *Oxcarbazepine treatment of refractory bipolar depression* [abstract]. 15th Congress of the European College of Neuropsychopharmacology, Barcelona, Spain.

Berzewski, H., Van Moffaert, M., and Gagiano, C.A. (1997). Efficacy and tolerability of reboxetine compared with imipramine in a double-blind study in patients suffering from major depressive offsodes. *Eur Neuropsychopharmacol*, 7(Suppl. 1), S37–S47.

Bhagwagar, Z., and Goodwin, G.M. (2002). The role of lithium in the treatment of bipolar depression. *Clin Neurosci Res*, 2(3-4), 222–227.

Black, D.W., Winokur, G., and Nasrallah, A. (1986). ECT in unipolar and bipolar disorders: A naturalistic evaluation of 460 patients. *Convuls Ther*, 2(4), 231–237.

Blanco, C., Laje, G., Olfson, M., Marcus, S.C., and Pincus, H.A. (2002). Trends in the treatment of bipolar disorder by outpatient psychiatrists. *Am J Psychiatry*, 159(6), 1005–1010.

Bodkin, J.A., and Amsterdam, J.D. (2002). Transdermal selegiline in major depression: A double-blind, placebo-controlled, parallel-group study in outpatients. *Am J Psychiatry*, 159(11), 1869–1875.

Boerlin, H.L., Gitlin, M.J., Zoellner, L.A., and Hammen, C.L. (1998). Bipolar depression and antidepressant-induced mania: A naturalistic study. *J Clin Psychiatry*, 59(7), 374–379.

Bottlender, R., Rudolf, D., Strauss, A., and Moller, H.J. (1998). Antidepressant-associated maniform states in acute treatment of patient with bipolar I depression. *Eur Arch Psychiatry Clin Neurosci*, 248, 296–300.

Bouckoms, A., and Mangini, L. (1993). Pergolide: An antidepressant adjuvant for mood disorders? *Psychopharmacol Bull*, 29(2), 207–211.

Bowden, C.L. (2001). Clinical correlates of therapeutic response in bipolar disorder. *J Affect Disord*, 67(1-3), 257–265.

Bowden, C.L., Brugger, A.M., Swann, A.C., Calabrese, J.R., Janicak, P.G., Petty, F., Dilsaver, S.C., Davis, J.M., Rush, A.J., and Small, J.G. (1994). Efficacy of divalproex vs. lithium and placebo in the treatment of mania. The Depakote Mania Study Group. *JAMA*, 271(12), 918–924.

Bowden, C.L., Calabrese, J.R., Sachs, G., Yatham, L.N., Asghar, S.A., Hompland, M., Montgomery, P., Earl, N., Smoot, T.M., DeVeaugh-Geiss, J., and Lamictal 606 Study Group. (2003). A placebo-controlled 18-month trial of lamotrigine and lithium maintenance treatment in recently manic or hypomanic patients with bipolar I disorder. *Arch Gen Psychiatry*, 60(4), 392–400.

Bowden, C.L., Collins, M.A., McElroy, S.L., Calabrese, J.R., Swann, A.C., Weisler, R.H., and Wozniak, P.J. (2005). Relationship of mania symptomatology to maintenance treatment response with divalproex, lithium, or placebo. *Neuropsychopharmacology*, 30(10), 1932–1939.

Bressa, G.M. (1994). S-adenosyl-l-methionine (SAMe) as antidepressant: Meta-analysis of clinical studies. *Acta Neurol Scand Suppl*, 154, 7–14.

Brown, E.S., Bobadilla, L., and Rush, A.J. (2001). Ketoconazole in bipolar patients with depressive symptoms: A case series and literature review. *Bipolar Disord*, 3(1), 23–29.

Bruijn, J.A., Moleman, P., Mulder, P.G., and van den Broek, W.W. (1998). Comparison of 2 treatment strategies for depressed inpatients: Imipramine and lithium addition or mirtazapine and lithium addition. *J Clin Psychiatry*, 59(12), 657–663.

Burt, T., Lisanby, S.H., and Sackeim, H.A. (2002). Neuropsychiatric applications of transcranial magnetic stimulation: A meta-analysis. *Int J Neuropsychopharmacol*, 5(1), 73–103.

Cade, J.F. (2000). Lithium salts in the treatment of psychotic excitement. 1949. *Bull World Health Organ*, 78(4), 518–520.

Calabrese J. (2005). One-year outcome with antidepressant treatment of bipolar depression: Is the glass half empty or half full? *Acta Psychiatr Scand*, 112(2), 85–87.

Calabrese, J.R., Bowden, C.L., McElroy, S.L., Cookson, J., Andersen, J., Keck, P.E. Jr., Rhodes, L., Bolden-Watson, C., Zhou, J., and Ascher, J.A. (1999a). Spectrum of activity of lamotrigine in treatment-refractory bipolar disorder. *Am J Psychiatry*, 156(7), 1019–1023.

Calabrese, J.R., Bowden, C.L., Sachs, G.S., Ascher, J.A., Monaghan, E., and Rudd, G.D. (1999b). A double-blind placebo-controlled study of lamotrigine monotherapy in outpatients with bipolar I depression. Lamictal 602 Study Group. *J Clin Psychiatry*, 60(2), 79–88.

Calabrese, J.R., Bowden, C.L., Sachs, G., Yatham, L.N., Behnke, K., Mehtonen, O.P., Montgomery, P., Ascher, J., Paska, W., Earl, N., DeVeaugh-Geiss, J., and Lamictal 605 Study Group. (2003). A placebo-controlled 18-month trial of lamotrigine and lithium maintenance treatment in recently depressed patients with bipolar I disorder. *J Clin Psychiatry*, 64(9), 1013–1024.

Calabrese, J.R., Keck, P.E. Jr., Macfadden, W., Minkwitz, M., Ketter, T.A., Weisler, R.G., Cutler, A.J., McCoy, R., Wilson, E., Mullen, J., and the Bolder Study Group. (2005). A randomized,

double-blind, placebo-controlled trial of quetiapine in the treatment of bipolar I or II depression. *Am J Psychiatry*, 162(7), 1351–1360.

Carlson, P.J., Merlock, M.C., and Suppes, T. (2004). Adjunctive stimulant use in patients with bipolar disorder: Treatment of residual depression and sedation. *Bipolar Disord*, 6(5), 416–420.

Chengappa, K.N., Levine, J., Gershon, S., Mallinger, A.G., Hardan, A., Vagnucci, A., Pollock, B., Luther, J., Buttenfield, J., Verfaille, S., and Kupfer, D.J. (2000). Inositol as an add-on treatment for bipolar depression. *Bipolar Disord*, 21(1), 47–55.

Cohn, J.B., Collins, G., Ashbrook, E., and Wernicke, J.F. (1989). A comparison of fluoxetine imipramine and placebo in patients with bipolar depressive disorder. *Int Clin Psychopharmacol*, 4(4), 313–322.

Cole, D.P., Thase, M.E., Mallinger, A.G., Soares, J.C., Luther, J.F., Kupfer, D.J., and Frank, E. (2002). Slower treatment response in bipolar depression predicted by lower pretreatment thyroid function. *Am J Psychiatry*, 159(1), 116–121.

Colombo, C., Benedetti, F., Barbini, B., Campori, E., and Smeraldi, E. (1999). Rate of switch from depression into mania after therapeutic sleep deprivation in bipolar depression. *Psychiatry Res*, 86(3), 267–270.

Colombo, C., Lucca, A., Benedetti, F., Barbini, B., Campori, E., and Smeraldi, E. (2000). Total sleep deprivation combined with lithium and light therapy in the treatment of bipolar depression: Replication of main effects and interaction. *Psychiatry Res*, 95(1), 43–53.

Corya, S.A., Perlis, R.H., Keck, P.E. Jr., Lin, D.Y., Case, M.G., Williamson, D.J., and Tohen, M.F. (2006). A 24-week open-label extension study of olanzapine-fluoxetine combination and olanzapine monotherapy in the treatment of bipolar depression. *J Clin Psychiatry*, 67(5), 798–806.

Coryell, W., Endicott, J., and Keller, M. (1992). Rapidly cycling affective disorder. Demographics, diagnosis, family history, and course. *Arch Gen Psychiatry*, 49(2), 126–131.

Coryell, W., Endicott, J., Maser, J.D., Keller, M.B., Leon, A.C., and Akiskal, H.S. (1995). Long-term stability of polarity distinctions in the affective disorders. *Am J Psychiatry*, 152, 385–390.

Coryell, W., Winokur, G., Solomon, D., Shea, T., Leon, A., and Keller, M. (1997). Lithium and recurrence in a long-term follow-up of bipolar affective disorder. *Psychol Med*, 27(2), 281–189.

Coupland, N.J., Ogilvic, C.J., Hegadoren, K.M., Seres, P., Hanstock, C.C., and Allen, P.S. (2005). Decreased prefrontal myo-inositol in major depressive disorder. *Biol Psychiatry*, 57(12), 1526–1534.

Crane, G.E. (1956). The psychiatric side effects of iproniazid. *Am J Psychiatry*, 112, 494–501.

Daly, J.J., Prudic, J., Devanand, D.P., Nobler, M.S., Lisanby, S.H., Peyser, S., Roose, S.P., and Sackeim, H.A. (2001). ECT in bipolar and unipolar depression: Differences in speed of response. *Bipolar Disord*, 3(2), 95–104.

Daskalakis, Z.J., Christensen, B.K., Fitzgerald, P.B., and Chen, R. (2002). Transcranial magnetic stimulation: A new investigational and treatment tool in psychiatry. *J Neuropsychiatry*, 14(4), 406–415.

Davidson, J.R., Abraham, K., Connor, K.M., and McLeod, M.N. (2003). Effectiveness of chromium in atypical depression: A placebo-controlled trial. *Biol Psychiatry*, 53(3), 261–264.

Davis, J.M., Janicak, P.G., and Hogan, D.M. (1999). Mood stabilizers in the prevention of recurrent affective disorders: A meta-analysis. *Acta Psychiatr Scand*, 100(6), 406–417.

Davis, L.L., Kabel, D., Patel, D., Choate, A.D., Foslien-Nash, C., Gurguis, G.N., Kramer, G.L., and Petty, F. (1996). Valproate as an antidepressant in major depressive disorder. *Psychopharmacol Bull*, 32(4), 647–652.

Davis, L.L., Bartolucci, A., and Petty, F. (2005). Divalproex in the treatment of bipolar depression: A placebo-controlled study. *J Affect Disord*, 85(3), 259–266.

Dean, C.E. (2000). Prasterone (DHEA) and mania. *Ann Pharmacother*, 34(12), 1419–1422.

DeBattista, C., Lembke, A., Solvason, H.B., Ghebremichael, R., and Poirier, J. (2004). A prospective trial of modafinil as an adjunctive treatment of major depression. *J Clin Psychopharmacol*, 24(1), 87–90.

DelBello, M.P., Schwiers, M.L., Rosenberg, H.L., and Strakowski, S.M. (2002). A double-blind, randomized, placebo-controlled study of quetiapine as adjunctive treatment for adolescent mania. *J Am Acad Child Adolesc Psychiatry*, 41(10), 1216–1223.

Delle Chiaie, R., Pancheri, P., and Scapicchio, P. (2002). Efficacy and tolerability of oral and intramuscular S-adenosyl-L-methionine 1,4-butanedisulfonate (SAMe) in the treatment of major depression: Comparison with imipramine in 2 multicenter studies. *Am J Clin Nutr*, 76(5), 1172S–1176S.

De Montigny, C., Grunberg, F., Mayer, A., and Deschenes, J.P. (1981). Lithium induces rapid relief of depression in tricyclic antidepressant drug non-responders. *Br J Psychiatry*, 138, 252–256.

Desai, A.K., and Grossberg, G.T. (2003). Herbals and botanicals in geriatric psychiatry. *Am J Geriatr Psychiatry*, 11(5), 498–506.

Detke, M.J., Lu, Y., Goldstein, D.J., McNamara, R.K., and Demitrack, M.A. (2002). Duloxetine 60 mg once daily dosing versus placebo in the acute treatment of major depression. *J Psychiatr Res*, 36(6), 383–390.

Dilsaver, S.C., Swann, S.C., Chen, Y.W., Shoaib, A., Joe, B., Krajewski, K.J., Gruber, N., and Tsai, Y. (1996). Treatment of bipolar depression with carbamazepine: Results of an open study. *Biol Psychiatry*, 40(9), 935–937.

Djousse, L., Pankow, J.S., Eckfeldt, J.H., Folsom, A.R., Hopkins, P.N., Province, M.A., Hong, Y., and Ellison, R.C. (2001). Relation between dietary linolenic acid and coronary artery disease in the National Heart, Lung, and Blood Institute Family Heart Study. *Am J Clin Nutr*, 74(5), 612–661.

Dolberg, O.T., Dannon, P.N., Schreiber, S., and Grunhaus, L. (2002). Transcranial magnetic stimulation in patients with bipolar depression: A double-blind, controlled study. *Bipolar Disord*, 4(Suppl. 1), 94–95.

Dube, S., Corya, S.A., and Andersen, S.W. (2002). Olanzapine-fluoxetine combination for treatment of psychotic depression. *Eur Psychiatry*, 17(Suppl. 1), 130.

Dunn, R.T., Gilmer, W., and Fleck, J. (2006). *Divalproex monotherapy for acute bipolar depression: A double-blind, randomized placebo-controlled trial.* Presented at the 159th Annual Meeting of the American Psychiatric Association, Toronto, Canada, May 20–25.

Eastman, C.I., Young, M.A., Fogg, L.F., Liu, L., and Meaden, P.M. (1998). Bright light treatment of winter depression: A placebo-controlled trial. *Arch Gen Psychiatry*, 55(10), 883–889.

Eden Evins, A., Demopulos, C., Yovel, I., Culhane, M., Ogutha, J., Grandin, L.D., Nierenberg, A.A., and Sachs, G.S. (2006). Inositol augmentation of lithium or valproate for bipolar depression. *Bipolar Disord*, 8 (2), 168–174.

El-Mallakh, R.S. (1999). Rapid fade of antidepressant effect of nefazodone in bipolar depression. *J Clin Psychiatry*, 60, 559.

El-Mallakh, R.S. (2000). An open study of methylphenidate in bipolar depression. *Bipolar Disord*, 2(1), 56–59.

Erfurth, A., Michael, N., Stadtland, C., and Arolt, V. (2002). Bupropion as add-on strategy in difficult-to-treat bipolar depressive patients. *Neuropsychobiology*, 45(Suppl. 1), 33–36.

Ernst, C.L., and Goldberg, J.F. (2002). The reproductive safety profile of mood stabilizers, atypical antipsychotics, and broad-spectrum psychotropics. *J Clin Psychiatry*, 63(Suppl. 4), 42–55.

Faedda, G.L., Tondo, L., Teicher, M.H., Baldessarini, R.J., Gelbard, H.A., and Floris, G.F. (1993). Seasonal mood disorders. Patterns of seasonal recurrence in mania and depression. *Arch Gen Psychiatry*, 50(1), 17–23.

Fagiolini, A., Kupfer, D.J., Scott, J., Swartz, H.A., Cook, D., Novick, D.M., and Frank E. (2006). Hypothyroidism in patients with bipolar I disorder treated primarily with lithium. *Epidemiol Psychiatr Soc*, 15(2), 123–127.

Fava, M. (2000). Management of nonresponse and intolerance: Switching strategies. *J Clin Psychiatry*, 61(Suppl. 2), 10–12.

Fava, M., Rosenbaum, J.F., McGrath, P.J., Stewart, J.W., Amsterdam, J.D., and Quitkin, F.M. (1994). Lithium and tricyclic augmentation of fluoxetine treatment for resistant major depression: A double-blind, controlled study. *Am J Psychiatry*, 151(9), 1372–1374.

Fava, M., Thase, M.E., and DeBattista, C. (2005). A multicenter, placebo-controlled study of modafinil augmentation in partial responders to selective serotonin reuptake inhibitors with persistent fatigue and sleepiness. *J Clin Psychiatry*, 66(1), 85–93.

Fieve, R.R., Platman, S.R., and Plutchik, R.R. (1968). The use of lithium on affective disorders. I: Acute endogenous depression. *Am J Psychiatry*, 125, 487–491.

Fink, M. (2001). Convulsive therapy: A review of the first 55 years. *J Affect Disord*, 63(1-3), 1–15.

Fogelson, D.L., Bystritsky, A., and Pasnau, R. (1992). Bupropion in the treatment of bipolar disorders: The same old story? *J Clin Psychiatry*, 53(12), 443–446.

Frangou, S., and Lewis, M. (2002). The Maudsley Bipolar Disorder Project: A double-blind, randomized, placebo controlled trial of Ethyl-EPA as an adjunct treatment of depression in bipolar disorder. *Bipolar Disord*, 4, 123.

Frangou, S., Lewis, M., and McCrone, P. (2006). Efficacy of ethyl-eicosapentaenoic acid in bipolar depression: Randomised double-blind placebo-controlled study. *Br J Psychiatry*, 188, 46–50.

Frankenburg, F.R., and Zanarini, M.C. (2002). Divalproex sodium treatment of women with borderline personality disorder and bipolar II disorder: A double-blind placebo-controlled pilot study. *J Clin Psychiatry*, 63(5), 442–446.

Frankle, W.G., Perlis, R.H., Deckersbach, T., Grandin, L.D., Gray, S.M., Sachs, G.S., and Nierenberg, A.A. (2002). Bipolar depression: Relationship between episode length and antidepressant treatment. *Psychol Med*, 32(8), 1417–1423.

Freeman, M.P., Hibbeln, J.R., Wisner, K.L., Davis, J.M., Mischoulon, D., Peet, M., Keck, P.E., Jr., Marangell, L.B., Richardson, A.J., Lake, J., and Stoll, A.L. (2006). Omega-3 fatty acids: Evidence basis for treatment and future research in psychiatry. *J Clin Psychiatry*, 67, 1954–1967.

Frye, M.A., Denicoff, K.D., Bryan, A.L., Smith-Jackson, E.E., Ali, S.O., Luckenbaugh, D., Leverich, G.S., and Post, R.M. (1999). Association between lower serum free T4 and greater mood instability and depression in lithium-maintained bipolar patients. *Am J Psychiatry*, 156(12), 1909–1914.

Frye, M., Ketter, T.A., Kimbrell, T.A., Dunn, R.T., Speer, A.M., Osuch, E.A., Luckenbaugh, D.A., Cora-Ocatelli, G., Leverich, G.S., and Post, R.M. (2000). A placebo-controlled sudy of lamotrigine and gabapentin monotherapy in refractory mood disorders. *J Clin Psychopharmacol*, 20(6), 607–612.

Frye, M.A., Calabrese, J.R., Reed, M.L., Wagner, K.D., Lewis, L., McNulty, J., and Hirschfeld, R.M. (2005). Use of health care services among persons who screen positive for bipolar disorder. *Psychiatr Serv*, 56(12), 1529–1533.

Frye, M.A., Yatham, L.N., Calabrese, J.R., Bowden, C.L., Ketter, T.A., Suppes, T., Adams, B.E., and Thompson, T.R. (2006). Incidence and time course of subsyndromal symptoms in patients with bipolar I disorder: An evaluation of 2 placebo-controlled trials. *J Clin Psychiatry*, 67(11), 1721–1728.

Gao, K., and Calabrese, J.R. (2005). New treatment studies for bipolar depression. *Bipolar Disord*, 7(Suppl. 5), 13–23.

Gelenberg, A.J., Kane, J.M., Keller, M.B., Lavori, P., Rosenbaum, J.F., Cole, K., and Lavelle, J. (1989). Comparison of standard and low serum levels of lithium for maintenance treatment of bipolar disorder. *N Engl J Med*, 321(22), 1489–1493.

Geller, B., Zimerman, B., Williams, M., Bolhofner, K., and Craney, J.L. (2001). Bipolar disorder at prospective follow-up of adults who had prepubertal major depressive disorder. *Am J Psychiatry*, 158(1), 125–127.

George, M.S., Sackeim, H.A., Rush, A.J., Marangell, L.B., Nahas, Z., Husain, M.M., Lisanby, S., Burt, T., Goldman, J., and Ballenger, J.C. (2000). Vagus nerve stimulation: A new tool for brain research and therapy. *Biol Psychiatry*, 47(4), 287–295.

George, M.S., Rush, A.J., Marangell, L.B., Sackeim, H.A., Brannan, S.K., Davis, S.M., Howland, R., Kling, M.A., Moreno, F., Rittberg, B., Dunner, D., Schwartz, T., Carpenter, L., Burke, M., Ninan, P., and Goodnick, P. (2005). A one-year comparison of vagus nerve stimulation with treatment as usual for treatment-resistant depression. *Biol Psychiatry*, 58(5), 364–373.

Ghaemi, S.N., and Goodwin, F.K. (2001a). Gabapentin treatment of the non-refractory bipolar spectrum: An open case series. *J Affect Disord*, 65, 167–171.

Ghaemi, S.N., and Goodwin, F.K. (2001b). Long-term naturalistic treatment of depressive symptoms in bipolar illness with divalproex vs. lithium in the setting of minimal antidepressant use. *J Affect Disord*, 65(3), 281–287.

Ghaemi, S.N., and Goodwin, F.K. (2005). Antidepressants for bipolar depression. *Am J Psychiatry*, 162(8), 1545–1546.

Ghaemi, S.N., and Hsu, D.J. (2005). Evidence-based treatment of bipolar disorder. In D.J. Stein, B. Lerer, and S. Stahl (Eds.), *Evidence-Based Psychopharmacology* (pp. 22–55). Cambridge, UK: Cambridge University Press.

Ghaemi, S.N., Katzow, J.J., Desai, S.P., and Goodwin, F.K. (1998). Gabapentin treatment of mood disorders: A preliminary study. *J Clin Psychiatry*, 59(8), 426–429.

Ghaemi, S.N., Boiman, E.E., and Goodwin, F.K. (2000). Diagnosing bipolar disorder and the effect of antidepressants: A naturalistic study. *J Clin Psychiatry*, 61(10), 804–808.

Ghaemi, S.N., Lenox, M.S., and Baldessarini, R.J. (2001). Effectiveness and safety of long-term antidepressant treatment in bipolar disorder. *J Clin Psychiatry*, 62, 565–569.

Ghaemi, S., Ko, J.Y., and Katzow, J.J. (2002). Oxcarbazepine treatment of refractory bipolar disorder: A retrospective chart review. *Bipolar Disord*, (1), 70–74.

Ghaemi, S.N., Berv, D.A., Klugman, J., Rosenquist, K.J., and Hsu, D.J. (2003a). Oxcarbazepine treatment of bipolar disorder. *J Clin Psychiatry*, 64(8), 943–945.

Ghaemi, S.N., Soldani, F., and Hsu, D. (2003b). Evidenced-based pharmacotherpy of bipolar disorder. *Int J Neuropsychopharmacol*, 6(3), 303–308.

Ghaemi, S.N., Hsu, D.J., Soldani, F., and Goodwin, F.K. (2003c). Antidepressants in bipolar disorder: The case for caution. *Bipolar Disord*, (6), 421–433.

Ghaemi, S.N., Rosenquist, K.J., Ko, J.Y., Baldassano, C.F., Kontos, N.J., and Baldessarini, R.J. (2004). Antidepressant treatment in bipolar versus unipolar depression. *Am J Psychiatry*, 161(1), 163–165.

Ghaemi, S.N., Hsu, D.J., Thase, M.E., Wisniewski, S.R., Nierenberg, A.A., Miyahara, S., and Sachs, G. (2006). Pharmacological treatment patterns at study entry for the first 500 STEP-BD participants. *Psychiatr Serv*, 57(5), 660–665.

Giedke, H., Klingberg, S., Schwarzler, F., and Schweinsberg, M. (2003). Direct comparison of total sleep deprivation and late partial sleep deprivation in the treatment of major depression. *J Affect Disord*, 85–93.

Gijsman, H.J., Geddes, J.R., Rendell, J.M., Nolen, W.A., and Goodwin, G.M. (2004). Antidepressants for bipolar depression: A systematic review of randomized, controlled trials. *Am J Psychiatry*, 161(9), 1537–1547.

Gjessing, R. (1938). Disturbances of somatic functions in catatonia with periodic course, and their compensation. *J Mental Sci*, 84, 608–621.

Goldberg, J.F., and Truman, C.J. (2003). Antidepressant-induced mania: An overview of current controversies. *Bipolar Disord*, 5, 407–420.

Goldberg, J.F., and Whiteside, J.E. (2002). The association between substance abuse and antidepressant-induced mania in bipolar disorder: A preliminary study. *J Clin Psychiatry*, 63(9), 791–795.

Goldberg, J.F., Singer, T.M., and Garno, J.L. (2001). Suicidality and substance abuse in affective disorders. *J Clin Psychiatry*, 62(Suppl. 25), 35–43.

Goldberg, J.F., Burdick, K.E., and Endick, C.J. (2004). Preliminary randomized, double-blind, placebo-controlled trial of pramipexole added to mood stabilizers for treatment-resistant bipolar depression. *Am J Psychiatry*, 161(3), 564–566.

Goldberg, J.F., and Nassir Ghaemi, S. (2005). Benefits and limitations of antidepressants and traditional mood stabilizers for treatment of bipolar depression. *Bipolar Disord*, 7(Suppl. 5), 3–12.

Golden, R.N., Gaynes, B.N., Ekstrom, R.D., Hamer, R.M., Jacobsen, F.M., Suppes, T., Wisner, K.L., and Nemeroff, C.B. (2005). The efficacy of light therapy in the treatment of mood disorders: A review and meta-analysis of the evidence. *Am J Psychiatry*, 162(4), 656–662.

Goldstein, D.J., Mallinckrodt, C., Lu, Y., and Demitrack, M.A. (2002). Duloxetine in the treatment of major depressive disorder: A double-blind clinical trial. *J Clin Psychiatry*, 63(3), 225–231.

Gonzalez-Pinto, A., Lalaguna, B., Mosquera, F., Perez de Heredia, J.L., Gutierrez, M., Ezcurra, J., Gilaberte, I., and Tohen, M. (2001). Use of olanzapine in dysphoric mania. *J Affect Disord*, 66(2–3), 247–253.

Goodwin, F.K., Murphy, D.L., and Bunney, W.F. Jr. (1969). Lithium carbonate treatment in depression and mania: A longitudinal double blind study. *Arch Gen Psychiatry*, 21, 486–496.

Goodwin, F.K., Murphy, D.L., Dunner, D.L., and Bunney, W.E. (1972). Lithium response in unipolar vs. bipolar depression. *Am J Psychiaty*, 129, 44–47.

Goodwin, F.K., Prange, A.J. Jr., Post, R.M., Muscettola, G., and Lipton, M.A. (1982). Potentiation of antidepressant effects by L-triiodothyronine in tricyclic nonresponders. *Am J Psychiatry*, 139, 34–38.

Goodwin, G.M., Bowden, C.L., Calabrese, J.R., Grunze, H., Kasper, S., White, R., Greene, P., and Leadbetter, R. (2004). A pooled analysis of 2 placebo-controlled 18-month trials of lamotrigine and lithium maintenance in bipolar I disorder. *J Clin Psychiatry*, 65(3), 432–441.

Goren, J.L., and Levin, J.M. (2000). Mania with bupropion: A dose-related phenomenon? *Ann Pharmacother*, 34(5), 619–621.

Grunebaum, M.F., Ellis, S.P., Li, S., Oquendo, M.A., and Mann, J.J. (2004). Antidepressants and suicide risk in the United States, 1985–1999. *J Clin Psychiatry*, 65(11), 1456–1462.

Grunhaus, L., Schreiber, S., Dolberg, O.T., Hirshman, S., and Dannon, P.N. (2002). Response to ECT in major depression: Are there differences between unipolar and bipolar depression? *Bipolar Disord*, 4(Suppl. 1), 91–93.

Grunze, H., Kasper, S., Goodwin, G., Bowden, C., Baldwin, D., Licht, R., Vieta, E., Moller, H.J., and World Federation of Societies of Biological Psychiatry Task Force on Treatment Guidelines for Bipolar Disorders. (2002). World Federation of Societies of Biological Psychiatry (WFSBP) guidelines for biological treatment of bipolar disorders. Part I: Treatment of bipolar depression. *World J Biol Psychiatry*, 3(3), 115–124.

Hantouche, E.G., Akiskal, H.S., Lancrenon, S., Allilaire, J.F., Sechter, D., Azorin, J.M., Bourgeois, M., Fraud, J.P., and Chatenet-Duchene, L. (1998). Systematic clinical methodology for validating bipolar-II disorder: Data in mid-stream from a French national multi-site study (EPIDEP). *J Affect Disord*, 50(2-3), 163–173.

Hantouche, E.G., Akiskal, H.S., Lancrenon, S., and Chatenet-Duchene, L. (2005). Mood stabilizer augmentation in apparently "unipolar" MDD: Predictors of response in the naturalistic French national EPIDEP study. *J Affect Disord*, 84(2-3), 243–249.

Henderson, L., Yue, Q.Y., Bergquist, C., Gerden, B., and Arlett, P. (2002). St. John's wort (*Hypericum perforatum*): Drug interactions and clinical outcomes. *Br J Clin Pharmacol*, 54(4), 349–356.

Hendrick, V., Altshuler, L.L., and Szuba, M.P. (1994). Is there a role for neuroleptics in bipolar depression? *J Clin Psychiatry*, 55(12), 533–535.

Henry, C., and Demotes-Mainard, J. (2003). Avoiding drug-induced switching in patients with bipolar depression. *Drug Safety*, 26(5), 337–351.

Henry, C., Sorbara, F., Lacoste, J., Gindre, C., and Leboyer, M. (2001). Antidepressant-induced mania in bipolar patients: Identification of risk factors. *J Clin Psychiatry*, 62(4), 249–255.

Hibbeln, J.R. (2002). Seafood consumption, the DHA content of mothers' milk and prevalence rates of postpartum depression: A cross-national, ecological analysis. *J Affect Disord*, 69(1-3), 15–29.

Hibbeln, J.R., Umhau, J.C., Linnoila, M., George, D.T., Ragan, P.W., Shoaf, S.E., Vaughan, M.R., Rawlings, R., and Salem, N. (1998). A replication study of violent and nonviolent subjects: CSF metabolites of serotonin and dopamine are predicted by plasma essential fatty acids. *Biol Psychiatry*, 44, 243–249.

Himmelhoch, J.M., Thase, M.E., Mallinger, A.G., and Houck, P. (1991). Tranylcypromine versus imipramine in anergic bipolar depression. *Am J Psychiatry*, 148(7), 910–916.

Hirschfeld, R.M., Fochtmann, L.J., and McIntyre, J.S. (2005). Antidepressants for bipolar depression. *Am J Psychiatry*, 162(8), 1546–1547.

Hirschfeld, R.M., Weisler, R.H., Raines, S.R., Macfadden, W. for the BOLDER Study Group. (2006). Quetiapine in the treatment of anxiety in patients with bipolar I or II depression: A secondary analysis from a randomized, double-blind, placebo-controlled study. *J Clin Psychiatry*, 67(3), 355–362.

Hlastala, S.A., Frank, E., Mallinger, A.G., Thase, M.E., Ritenour, A.M., and Kupfer, D.J. (1997). Bipolar depression: An underestimated treatment challenge. *Depress Anxiety*, 5(2), 73–83.

Hoencamp, E., Haffmans, J., Dijken, W.A., and Huijbrechts, I.P. (2000). Lithium augmentation of venlafaxine: An open-label trial. *J Clin Psychopharmacol*, 20(5), 538–543.

Holsboer, F. (2001). Prospects for antidepressant drug discovery. *Biol Psychol*, 57(1-3), 47–65.

Holtzheimer, P.E. III, Russo, J., and Avery, D.H. (2001). A meta-analysis of repetitive transcranial magnetic stimulation in the treatment of depression. *Psychopharmacol Bull*, 35(4), 149–169.

Hussain, M.Z., and Chaudhry, Z. (1999). Treatment of bipolar depression with topiramate. *Eur Neuropsychopharmacol*, 9(Suppl. 5), S222.

Hypericum Depression Trial Study Group. (2002). Effect of *Hypericum perforatum* (St. John's wort) in major depressive disorder: A randomized controlled trial. *JAMA*, 287(14), 1807–1814.

Isometsa, E.T., Henriksson, M.M., Aro, H.M., and Lonnqvist, J.K. (1994). Suicide in bipolar disorder in Finland. *Am J Psychiatry*, 151(7), 1020–1024.

Jackson, A., Cavanagh, J., and Scott, J. (2003). A systematic review of manic and depressive prodromes. *J Affect Disord*, 74(3), 209–217.

Janicak, P.G., Davis, J.M., Gibbons, R.D., Ericksen, S., Chang, S., and Gallagher, P. (1985). Efficacy of ECT: A meta-analysis. *Am J Psychiatry*, 142(3), 297–302.

Joffe, R.T. (1988). Triiodothyronine potentiation of the antidepressant effect of phenelzine. *J Clin Psychiatry*, 49, 409–410.

Joffe, R.T. (1992). Triiodothyronine potentiation of fluoxetine in depressed patients. *Can J Psychiatry*, 37(1), 48–50.

Joffe, R.T. (1998). The use of thyroid supplements to augment antidepressant medication. *J Clin Psychiatry*, 59(Suppl. 5), 26–29.

Joffe, R.T., Singer, W., Levitt, A.J., and MacDonald, C. (1993). A placebo-controlled comparison of lithium and triiodothyronine augmentation of tricyclic antidepressants in unipolar refractory depression. *Arch Gen Psychiatry*, 50(5), 387–393.

Joffe, R.T., MacQueen, G.M., Marriott, M., Robb, J., Begin, H., and Young, L.T. (2002). Induction of mania and cycle acceleration in bipolar disorder: Effect of different classes of antidepressant. *Acta Psychiatr Scand*, 105(6), 427–430.

Joffe, R.T., MacQueen, G.M., Marriott, M., and Young, L.T. (2005). One-year outcome with antidepressant—treatment of bipolar depression. *Acta Psychiatr Scand*, 112(2), 105–109.

Johnson, G. (1974). Antidepressant effect of lithium. *Compr Psychiatry*, 15(1), 43–47.

Judd, L.L., Schettler, P.J., Akiskal, H.S., Maser, J., Coryell, W., Solomon, D., Endicott, J., and Keller, M. (2003). Long-term symptomatic status of bipolar I vs. bipolar II disorders. *Int J Neuropsychopharmacol*, 6(2), 127–137.

Kanba, S., Yagi, G., Kamijima, K., Suzuki, T., Tajima, O., Otaki, J., Arata, E., Koshikawa, H., Nibuya, M., and Kinoshita, N. (1994). The first open study of zonisamide, a novel anticonvulsant, shows efficacy in mania. *Prog Neuropsychopharmacol Biol Psychiatry*, 18(4), 707–715.

Kaplan, B.J., Simpson, J.S., Ferre, R.C., Gorman, C.P., McMullen, D.M., and Crawford, S.G. (2001). Effective mood stabilization with a chelated mineral supplement: An open-label trial in bipolar disorder. *J Clin Psychiatry*, 62(12), 936–944.

Kasper, S., and Dienel, A. (2002). Cluster analysis of symptoms during antidepressant treatment with Hypericum extract in mildly to moderately depressed out-patients. A meta-analysis of data from three randomized, placebo-controlled trials. *Psychopharmacology (Berl)*, 164(3), 301–308.

Katona, C.L., Abou-Saleh, M.T., Harrison, D.A., Nairac, B.A., Edwards, D.R., Lock, T., Burns, R.A., and Robertson, M.M. (1995). Placebo-controlled trial of lithium augmentation of fluoxetine and lofepramine. *Br J Psychiatry*, 166(1), 80–86.

Kaufman, K.R. (1998). Adjunctive tiagabine treatment of psychiatric disorders: Three cases. *Ann Clin Psychiatry*, 10(4), 181–184.

Keck, P.E., Mintz, J., McElroy, S., Freeman, M., Suppes, T., Frye, M., Altshuler, L., Kupka, R., Nolen, W., Leverich, G., Denicoff, D., Grunze, H., Duan, N., and Post, R. (2006). Double-blind, randomized, placebo-controlled trials of ethyl-eicosapentanoate in the treatment of bipolar depression and rapid cycling bipolar disorder. *Biol Psychiatry*, 60(9), 1020–1022.

Keitner, G.I., Solomon, D.A., Ryan, C.E., Miller, I.W., Mallinger, A., Kupfer, D.J., and Frank, E. (1996). Prodromal and residual symptoms in bipolar I disorder. *Compr Psychiatry*, 37(5), 362–367.

Kennedy, S.H. (1997). Continuation and maintenance treatments in major depression: The neglected role of monoamine oxidase inhibitors. *J Psychiatry Neurosci*, 22(2), 127–131.

Khan, A.U. (1981). A comparison of the therapeutic and cardiovascular effects of a single nightly dose of Prothiaden (dothiepin, dosulepin) and Lentizol (sustained-release amitriptyline) in depressed elderly patients. *J Int Med Res*, 9(2), 108–112.

Kielholz, P., Terzani, S., and Poldinger, W. (1979). The long-term treatment of periodical and cyclic depressions with flupenthixol decanoate. *Int Pharmacopsychiatry*, 14(6), 305–309.

Klein, E., Kreinin, I., Chistyakov, A., Koren, D., Mecz, L., Marmur, S., Ben-Shachar, D., and Feinsod, M. (1999). Therapeutic efficacy of right prefrontal slow repetitive transcranial magnetic stimulation in major depression: A double-blind controlled study. *Arch Gen Psychiatry*, 56(4), 315–320.

Kline, M.D., and Jaggers, E.D. (1999). Mania onset while using dehydroepiandrosterone. *Am J Psychiatry*, 156(6), 971.

Klufas, A., and Thompson, D. (2001). Topiramate-induced depression. *Am J Psychiatry*, 158(10), 1736.

Koukopoulos, A., Reginaldi, D., Laddomada, P., Floris, G., Serra, G., and Tondo, L. (1980). Course of the manic-depressive cycle and changes caused by treatment. *Pharmakopsychiatr Neuropsychopharmakol*, 13(4), 156–167.

Koukopoulos, A., Faedda, G., Proietti, R., D'Amico, S., de Pisa, E., and Simonetto, C. (1992). Mixed depressive syndrome. *Encephale*, 18(1), 19–21.

Kovacs, M. (1996). Presentation and course of major depressive disorder during childhood and later years of the life span. *J Am Acad Child Adolesc Psychiatry*, 35(6), 705–715.

Krahl, S.E., Senanayake, S.S., Pekary, A.E., and Sattin, A. (2004). Vagus nerve stimulation (VNS) is effective in a rat model of antidepressant action. *J Psychiatr Res*, 38(3), 237–240.

Kripke, D.F. (1998). Light treatment for nonseasonal depression: Speed, efficacy, and combined treatment. *J Affect Disord*, 49(2), 109–117.

Kuhn, R. (1958). The treatment of depressive states with G22355 (imipramine hydrochloride). *Am J Psychiatry*, 115, 459–464.

Kupfer, D.J., and Spiker, D.G. (1981). Refractory depression: Prediction of non-response by clinical indicators. *J Clin Psychiatry*, 42(8), 307–312.

Kupfer, D.J., Chengappa, K.N., Gelenberg, A.J., Hirschfeld, R.M., Goldberg, J.F., Sachs, G.S., Grochocinski, V.J., Houck, P.R., and Kolar, A.B. (2001). Citalopram as adjunctive therapy in bipolar depression. *J Clin Psychiatry*, 62(12), 985–990.

Kusumakar, V., and Yatham, L.N. (1997). An open study of lamotrigine in refractory bipolar depression. *Psychiatry Res*, 72(2), 145–148.

Lake, C.R., Tenglin, R., Chernow, B., and Holloway, H.C. (1983). Psychomotor stimulant-induced mania in a genetically predisposed patient: A review of the literature and report of a case. *J Clin Psychopharmacol*, 3(2), 97–100.

Lecrubier, Y., Boyer, P., Turjanski, S., and Rein, W. (1997). Amisulpride versus imipramine and placebo in dysthymia and major depression. Amisulpride Study Group. *J Affect Disord*, 43(2), 95–103.

Levine, J., Barak, Y., Gonzalves, M., Szor, I.I., Elizur, A., Kofman, O., and Belmaker, R.H. (1995). Double-blind, controlled trial of inositol treatment of depression. *Am J Psychiatry*, 152(5), 792–794.

Lewis, J.L., and Winokur, G. (1982). The induction of mania: A natural history study with controls. *Arch Gen Psychiatry*, 39, 303–306.

Lewy, A.J., Bauer, V.K., Cutler, N.L., Sack, R.L., Ahmed, S., Thomas, K.H., Blood, M.L., and Jackson, J.M. (1998). Morning vs. evening light treatment of patients with winter depression. *Arch Gen Psychiatry*, 55(10), 890–896.

Lieber, C.S., and Packer, L. (2002). S-adenosylmethionine: Molecular, biological, and clinical aspects: An introduction. *Am J Clin Nutr*, 76(5), 1148S–1150S.

Linder, J., Fyro, B., Pettersson, U., and Werner, S. (1989). Acute antidepressant effect of lithium is associated with fluctuation of calcium and magnesium in plasma. A double-blind study on the antidepressant effect of lithium and clomipramine. *Acta Psychiatr Scand*, 80(1), 27–36.

Lipinski, J.F., Cohen, B.M., Frankenburg, F., Tohen, M., Waternaux, C., Altesman, R., Jones, B., and Harris, P. (1984). Open trial of S-adenosylmethionine for treatment of depression. *Am J Psychiatry*, 141(3), 448–450.

Lisanby, S.H., Schlaepfer, T.E., Fisch, H.U., and Sackeim, H.A. (2001a). Magnetic seizure therapy of major depression. *Arch Gen Psychiatry*, 58(3), 303–305.

Lisanby, S.H., Gutman, D., Luber, B., Schroeder, C., and Sackeim, H.A. (2001b). Sham TMS: Intracerebral measurement of the induced electrical field and the induction of motor-evoked potentials. *Biol Psychiatry*, 49(5), 460–463.

MacQueen, G.M., and Trevor Young, L. (2001). Bipolar II disorder: Symptoms, course, and response to treatment. *Psychiatr Serv*, 52(3), 358–361.

MacQueen, G.M., Trevor Young, L., Marriott, M., Robb, J., Begin, H., and Joffe, R.T. (2002). Previous mood state predicts response and switch rates in patients with bipolar depression. *Acta Psychiatr Scand*, 105(6), 414–418.

Malison, R.T., Anand, A., Pelton, G.H., Kirwin, P., Carpenter, L., McDougle, C.J., Heninger, G.R., and Price, L.H. (1999). Limited efficacy of ketoconazole in treatment-refractory major depression. *J Clin Psychopharmacol*, 19(5), 466–470.

Manji, H., Moore, G., and Chen, G. (2001). Bipolar disorder: Leads from the molecular and cellular mechanisms of action of mood stabilizers. *Br J Psychiatry*, 178(41), 107s–119s.

Manwani, S., Pardo, T.B., and Ghaemi, S.N. (2004). *Bipolar disorder, substance-abuse, and antidepressant-induced mania* [abstract]. 157th Annual Meeting of the American Psychiatric Association, New York City, NY.

Manwani, S.G., Pardo, T.B., Albanese, M.J., Zablotsky, B., Goodwin, F.K., Ghaemi, S.N. (2006). Substance use disorder and other predictors of antidepressant-induced mania: A retrospective chart review. *J Clin Psychiatry*, 67(9), 1341–1345.

Marangell, L.B. (2004). The importance of subsyndromal symptoms in bipolar disorder. *J Clin Psychiatry*, 65(Suppl. 10), 24–27.

Marangell, L.B., Rush, A.J., George, M.S., Sackeim, H.A., Johnson, C.R., Husain, M.M., Nahas, Z., and Lisanby, S.H. (2002). Vagus nerve stimulation (VNS) for major depressive episodes: One-year outcomes. *Biol Psychiatry*, 51(4), 280–287.

Marangell, L.B., Martinez, J.M., Zboyan, H.A., Kertz, B., Kim, H.F., and Puryear, L.J. (2003). A double-blind, placebo-controlled study of the omega-3 fatty acid docosahexaenoic acid in the treatment of major depression. *Am J Psychiatry*, 160(5), 996–998.

Marcotte, D. (1998). Use of topiramate, a new anti-epileptic as a mood stabilzer. *J Affect Disord*, 50, 245–251.

McAskill, R., Mir, S., and Taylor, D. (1998). Pindolol augmentation of antidepressant therapy. *Br J Psychiatry*, 173, 203–208.

McElroy, S.L., and Keck, P.E. Jr. (1993). Treatment guidelines for valproate in bipolar and schizoaffective disorders. *Can J Psychiatry*, 38(3 Suppl. 2), S62–S66.

McElroy, S.L., Suppes, T., Keck, P.E. Jr., Black, D., Frye, M.A., Altshuler, L.L., Nolen, W.A., Kupka, R.W., Leverich, G.S., Walden, J., Grunze, H., and Post, R.M. (2005). Open-label adjunctive zonisamide in the treatment of bipolar disorders: A prospective trial. *J Clin Psychiatry*, 66(5), 617–624.

McIntyre, R.S., Mancini, D.A., McCann, S., Srinivasan, J., Sagman, D., and Kennedy, S.H. (2002). Topiramate versus bupropion SR when added to mood stabilizer therapy for the depressive phase of bipolar disorder: A preliminary single-blind study. *Bipolar Disord*, 4, 207–213.

McLeod, M.N., and Golden, R.N. (2000). Chromium treatment of depression. *Int J Neuropsychopharmacol*, 3(4), 311–314.

McQuade, R., and Young, A.H. (2000). Future therapeutic targets in mood disorders: The glucocorticoid receptor. *Br J Psychiatry*, 177, 390–395.

Mendels, J., Sedcunda, S.K., and Dyson, W.L. (1972). A controlled study of the antidepressant effects of lithium carbonate. *Arch Gen Psychiatry*, 26, 154–157.

Menza, M.A., Kaufman, K.R., and Castellanos, A. (2000). Modafinil augmentation of antidepressant treatment in depression. *J Clin Psychiatry*, 61(5), 378–381.

Miller, L.J. (1994). Use of electroconvulsive therapy during pregnancy. *Hosp Community Psychiatry*, 45(5), 444–450.

Mischoulon, D., and Fava, M. (2000). Docosahexanoic acid and omega-3 fatty acids in depression. *Psychiatr Clin North Am*, 23(4), 785–794.

Moller, H.J., and Grunze, H. (2000). Have some guidelines for the treatment of acute bipolar depression gone too far in the restriction of antidepressants? *Eur Arch Psychiatry Clin Neurosci*, 250(2), 57–68.

Moller, H.J., Bottlender, R., Grunze, H., Strauss, A., and Wittmann, J. (2001). Are antidepressants less effective in the acute treatment of bipolar I compared to unipolar depression? *J Affect Disord*, 67(1–3), 141–146.

Montgomery, S.A., and Asberg, M. (1979). A new depression scale designed to be sensitive to change. *Br J Psychiatry*, 134, 382–389.

Moustgaard, G. (2000). Treatment-refractory depression successfully treated with the combination of mirtazapine and lithium. *J Clin Psychopharmacol*, 20(2), 268.

Mundo, E., Walker, M., Cate, T., Macciardi, F., and Kennedy, J.L. (2001). The role of serotonin transporter protein gene in antidepressant-induced mania in bipolar disorder: Preliminary findings. *Arch Gen Psychiatry*, 58, 539–544.

Mundo, E., Cattaneo, E., Russo, M., and Altamura, A.C. (2006). Clinical variables related to antidepressant-induced mania in bipolar disorder. *J Affect Disord*, 92(2–3), 227–230.

Nahas, Z., Kozel, F.A., Li, X., Anderson, B., and George, M.S. (2003). Left prefrontal transcranial magnetic stimulation (TMS) treatment of depression in bipolar affective disorder: A pilot study of acute safety and efficacy. *Bipolar Disord*, 5(1), 40–47.

Nahas, Z., Marangell, L.B., Husain, M.M., Rush, A.J., Sackeim, H.A., Lisanby, S.H., Martinez, J.M., and George, M.S. (2005). Two-year outcome of vagus nerve stimulation (VNS) for treatment of major depressive episodes. *J Clin Psychiatry*, 66(9), 1097–1104.

Nasr, S., Wendt, B., and Steiner, K. (2006). Absence of mood switch with and tolerance to modafinil: A replication study from a large private practice. *J Affect Disord*, 95(1-3), 111–114.

Nemeroff, C.B., Evans, D.L., Gyulai, L., Sachs, G.S., Bowden, C.L., Gergel, I.P., Oakes, R., and Pitts, C.D. (2001). Double-blind, placebo-controlled comparison of imipramine and paroxetine in the treatment of bipolar depression. *Am J Psychiatry*, 158(6), 906–912.

Nemeroff, C.B., Schatzberg, A.F., Goldstein, D.J., Detke, M.J., Mallinckrodt, C., Lu, Y., and Tran, P.V. (2002). Duloxetine for the treatment of major depressive disorder. *Psychopharmacol Bull*, 36(4), 106–132.

Nemets, B., Stahl, Z., and Belmaker, R.H. (2002). Addition of omega-3 fatty acid to maintenance medication treatment for recurrent unipolar depressive disorder. *Am J Psychiatry*, 159(3), 477–479.

Nierenberg, A.A., Burt, T., Matthews, J., and Weiss, A.P. (1999). Mania associated with St. John's wort. *Biol Psychiatry*, 46(12), 1707–1708.

Nierenberg, A.A., Trivedi, M.H., Fava, M., Biggs, M.M., Shores-Wilson, K., Wisniewski, S.R., Balasubramani, G.K., and Rush, A.J. (2006). Family history of mood disorder and characteristics of major depressive disorder: A STAR(*)D (sequenced treatment alternatives to relieve depression) study. *J Psychiatr Res*, 41(3-4), 214–221.

Normann, C., Hummel, B., Scharer, L.O., Horn, M., Grunze, H., and Walden, J. (2002). Lamotrigine as adjunct to paroxetine in acute depression: A placebo-controlled, double-blind study. *J Clin Psychiatry*, 63(4), 337–344.

Noyes, R. Jr., Dempsey, G.M., Blum, A., and Cavanaugh, G.L. (1974). Lithium treatment of depression. *Compr Psychiatry*, 15, 187–193.

Obrocea, G.V., Dunn, R.M., Frye, M.A., Ketter, T.A., Luckenbaugh, D.A., Leverich, G.S., Speer, A.M., Osuch, E.A., Jajodia, K., and Post, R.M. (2002). Clinical predictors of response to lamotrigine and gabapentin monotherapy in refractory affective disorders. *Biol Psychiatry*, 51(3), 253–260.

Osher, Y., Bersudsky, Y., and Belmaker, R.H. (2005). Omega-3 eicosapentaenoic acid in bipolar depression: Report of a small open-label study. *J Clin Psychiatry*, 66(6), 726–729.

Osser, D.N., Najarian, D.M., and Dufresne, R.L. (1999). Olanzapine increases weight and serum triglyceride levels. *J Clin Psychiatry*, 60(11), 767–770.

Parker, G., Gibson, N.A., Brotchie, H., Heruc, G., Rees, A.M., and Hadzi-Pavlovic, D. (2006). Omega-3 fatty acids and mood disorders. *Am J Psychiatry*, 163(6), 969–978.

Peet, M. (1994). Induction of mania with selective serotonin reuptake inhibitors and tricyclic antidepressants. *Br J Psychiatry*, 164(4), 549–550.

Peet, M. (2004). Nutrition and schizophrenia: Beyond omega-3 fatty acids. *Prostaglandins Leukot Essent Fatty Acids*, 70(4), 417–422.

Peet, M., and Horrobin, D.F. (2002). A dose-ranging study of the effects of ethyl-eicosapentaenoate in patients with ongoing depression despite apparently adequete treatment with standard drugs. *Arch Gen Psychiatry*, 59(10), 913–919.

Penland, H.R., and Ostroff, R.B. (2006). Combined use of lamotrigine and electroconvulsive therapy in bipolar depression: A case series. *J ECT*, 22(2), 142–147.

Perlis, R.H., Brown, E., Baker, R.W., and Nierenberg, A.A. (2006). Clinical features of bipolar depression versus major depressive disorder in large multicenter trials. *Am J Psychiatry*, 163(2), 225–231.

Perugi, G., Toni, C., Ruffolo, G., Frare, F., and Akiskal, H. (2001). Adjunctive dopamine agonists in treatment-resistant bipolar II depression: An open case series. *Pharmacopsychiatry*, 34(4), 137–141.

Physicians' Desk Reference. (2006). *2006 Physicians' Desk Reference (PDR): Your Complete Print and Electronic Drug Information Solution*. Montvale, NJ: Thomson Healthcare.

Post, R.M., Uhde, T.W., Roy-Byrne, P.P., and Joffe, R.T. (1986). Antidepressant effects of carbamazepine. *Am J Psychiatry*, 143(1), 29–34.

Post, R.M., Ketter, T.A., Denicoff, K., Pazzaglia, P.J., Leverich, G.S., Marangell, L.B., Callahan, A.M., George, M.S., and Frye, M.A. (1996). The place of anticonvulsant therapy in bipolar illness. *Psychopharmacology*, 128(2), 115–129.

Post, R.M., Leverich, G.S., Nolen, W.A., Kupka, R.W., Altshuler, L.L., Frye, M.A., Suppes, T., McElroy, S., Keck, P., Grunze, H., Walden, J., and Stanley Foundation Bipolar Network. (2003). A re-evaluation of the role of antidepressants in the treatment of bipolar depression: Data from the Stanley Foundation Bipolar Network. *Bipolar Disord*, 5(6), 396–406.

Post, R.M., Altshuler, L.L., Leverich, G.S., Frye, M.A., Nolen, W.A., Kupka, R.W., Suppes, T., McElroy, S., Keck, P.E. Jr., Denicoff, K.D., Grunze, H., Walden, J., Kitchen, C.M., and Mintz, J. (2006). Mood switch in bipolar depression: Comparison of adjunctive venlafaxine, bupropion, and sertraline. *Br J Psychiatry*, 189, 124–131.

Price, L.H., Charney, D.S., and Heninger, G.R. (1985). Efficacy of lithium-tranylcypromine treatment in refractory depression. *Am J Psychiatry*, 142(5), 619–623.

Prien, R.F. (1984). NIMH report. Five-center study clarifies use of lithium, imipramine for recurrent affective disorders. *Hosp Community Psychiatry*, 35(11), 1097–1098.

Prien, R.F., Kupfer, D.J., Mansky, P.A., Small, J.G., Tuason, V.B., Voss, C.B., and Johnson, W.E. (1984). Drug therapy in the prevention of recurrences in unipolar and bipolar affective diorders: A report of the NIMH Collaborative Study Group comparing lithium carbonate, imipramine, and a lithium carbonate-imipramine combination. *Arch Gen Psychiatry*, 41, 1096–1104.

Prien, R.F., Himmelhoch, J.M., and Kupfer, D.J. (1988). Treatment of mixed mania. *J Affect Disord*, 15, 9–15.

Quitkin, F.M., Kane, J., Rifkin, A., Ramos-Lorenzi, J.R., and Nayak, D.V. (1981). Prophylactic lithium carbonate with and without imipramine for bipolar 1 patients. A double-blind study. *Arch Gen Psychiatry*, 38(8), 902–907.

Rachid, F., Bertschy, G., Bondolfi, G., and Aubry, J.M. (2004). Possible induction of mania or hypomania by atypical antipsychotics: An updated review of reported cases. *J Clin Psychiatry*, 65(11), 1537–1545.

Ranjan, S., and Chandra, P.S. (2005). Modafinil-induced irritability and aggression: A report of 2 bipolar patients. *J Clin Psychopharmacol*, 25(6), 628–629.

Rao, A.V., and Nammalvar, N. (1977). The course and outcome in depressive illness: A follow-up study of 122 cases in Madurai, India. *Br J Psychiatry*, 130, 392–396.

Raskin, S., Teitelbaum, A., Zislin, J., and Durst, R. (2006). Adjunctive lamotrigine as a possible mania inducer in bipolar patients, *Am J Psychiatry*, 163(1), 159–160.

Riemann, D., Voderholzer, U., and Berger, M. (2002). Sleep and sleep–wake manipulations in bipolar depression. *Neuropsychobiology*, 45(Suppl. 1), 7–12.

Rocca, P., Fonzo, V., Ravizza, L., Rocca, G., Scotta, M., Zanalda, E., and Bogetto, F. (2002). A comparison of paroxetine and amisulpride in the treatment of dysthymic disorder. *J Affect Disord*, 70(3), 313–317.

Rohan, M., Parow, A., Stoll, A.L., Demopulos, C., Friedman, S., Dager, S., Hennen, J., Cohen, B.M., and Renshaw, P.F. (2004). Low-field magnetic stimulation in bipolar depression using an MRI-based stimulator. *Am J Psychiatry*, 161(1), 93–98.

Rosenthal, N.E., Sack, D.A., Gillin, J.C., Lewy, A.J., Goodwin, F.K., Davenport, Y., Mueller, P.S., Newsome, D.A., and Wehr, T.A. (1984). Seasonal affective disorder. A description of the syndrome and preliminary findings with light therapy. *Arch Gen Psychiatry*, 41(1), 72–80.

Rozans, M., Dreisbach, A., Lertora, J.J., and Kahn, M.J. (2002). Palliative uses of methylphenidate in patients with cancer: A review. *J Clin Oncol*, 20(1), 335–339.

Rudas, S., Schmitz, M., Pichler, P., and Baumgartner, A. (1999). Treatment of refractory chronic depression and dysthymia with high-dose thyroxine. *Biol Psychiatry*, 45(2), 229–233.

Rush, A.J., George, M.S., Sackeim, H.A., Marangell, L.B., Husain, M.M., Giller, C., Nahas, Z., Haines, S., Simpson, R.K. Jr., and Goodman, R. (2000). Vagus nerve stimulation (VNS) for treatment-resistant depressions: A multicenter study. *Biol Psychiatry*, 47(4), 276–286.

Rush, A.J., Marangell, L.B., Sackeim, H.A., George, M.S., Brannan, S.K., Davis, S.M., Howland, R., Kling, M.A., Rittberg,

B.R., Burke, W.J., Rapaport, M.H., Zajecka, J., Nierenberg, A.A., Husain, M.M., Ginsberg, D., and Cooke, R.G. (2005). Vagus nerve stimulation for treatment-resistant depression: A randomized, controlled acute phase trial. *Biol Psychiatry*, 58(5), 347–354.

Rybakowski, J.K., Suwalska, A., Lojko, D., Rymaszewska, J., and Kiejna, A. (2005). Bipolar mood disorder among Polish psychiatric outpatients treated for major depression. *J Affect Disord*, 84(2-3), 141–147.

Sachs, G. (2004). Strategies for improving treatment of bipolar disorder: Intergration of measurement and management. *Acta Psychiatr Scand*, 422(Suppl.), 7–17.

Sachs, G. (2005). *Advances in the treatment of acute bipolar depression. Advances in the treatment of bipolar disorders.* Washington, DC: American Psychiatric Association.

Sachs, G.S., Thase, M.E., Otto, M.W., Bauer, M., Miklowitz, D., Wisniewski, S.R., Lavori, P., Lebowitz, B., Rudorfer, M., Frank, E., Nierenberg, A.A., Fava, M., Bowden, C., Ketter, T., Marangell, L., Calabrese, J., Kupfer, D., and Rosenbaum, J.F. (1994). A double-blind trial of bupropion versus desipramine for bipolar depression. *J Clin Psychiatry*, 55(9), 391–393.

Sachs, G.S., Printz, D.J., Kahn, D.A., Carpenter, D., and Docherty, J.P. (2000). The expert consensus guideline series: Medication treatment of bipolar disorder 2000. *Postgrad Med*, 1–104.

Sachs, G.S., Altshuler, L.L., and Ketter, T.A. (2001). *Divalproex versus placebo for the treatment of bipolar depression* [abstract]. Annual Meeting of the American College of Neuropsychopharmacology, Puerto Rico.

Sachs, G.S., Thase, M.E., Otto, M.W., Bauer, M., Miklowitz, D., Wisniewski, S.R., Lavori, P., Lebowitz, B., Rudorfer, M., Frank, E., Nierenberg, A.A., Fava, M., Bowden, C., Ketter, T., Marangell, L., Calabrese, J., Kupfer, D., and Rosenbaum, J.F. (2003). Rationale, design, and methods of the systematic treatment enhancement program for bipolar disorder (STEP-BD). *Biol Psychiatry*, 53(11), 1028–1042.

Sachs, G., Chengappa, K.N., Suppes, T., Mullen, J.A., Brecher, M., Devine, N.A., and Sweitzer, D.E. (2004). Quetiapine with lithium or divalproex for the treatment of bipolar mania: A randomized, double-blind, placebo-controlled study. *Bipolar Disord*, 6(3), 213–223.

Sackeim, H.A., Rush, A.J., George, M.S., Marangell, L.B., Husain, M.M., Nahas, Z., Johnson, C.R., Seidman, S., Giller, C., Haines, S., Simpson, R.K. Jr., and Goodman, R.R. (2001). Vagus nerve stimulation (VNS) for treatment-resistant depression: Efficacy, side effects, and predictors of outcome. *Neuropsychopharmacology*, 25(5), 713–728.

Sajatovic, M., Brescan, D.W., Perez, D.E., DiGiovanni, S.K., Hattab, H., Ray, J.B., and Bingham, C.R. (2001). Quetiapine alone and added to a mood stabilizer for serious mood disorders. *J Clin Psychiatry*, 62(9), 728–732.

Sajatovic, M., Mullen, J.A., and Sweitzer, D.E. (2002). Efficacy of quetiapine and risperidone against depressive symptoms in outpatients with psychosis. *J Clin Psychiatry*, 63(12), 1156–1163.

Salzman, C., Wong, E., and Wright, B. (2002). Drug and ECT treatment of depression in the elderly, 1996–2001: A literature review. *Biol Psychiatry*, 52(3), 265.

Satel, S.L., and Nelson, J.C. (1989). Stimulants in the treatment of depression: A critical overview. *J Clin Psychiatry*, 50(7), 241–249.

Sato, T., Bottlender, R., Sievers, M., Schroter, A., Kleindienst, N., and Moller, H.J. (2004). Evaluating the inter-episode stability of depressive mixed states. *J Affect Disord*, 81(2), 103–113.

Schaffer, A., Zuker, P., and Levitt, A. (2006). Randomized, double-blind pilot trial comparing lamotrigene versus citalopram for the treatment of bipolar depression. *J Affect Disord*, 96, 95–99.

Schatzberg, A.F. (2000). Clinical efficacy of reboxetine in major depression. *J Clin Psychiatry*, 61(Suppl. 10), 31–38.

Schlatter, F.J., Soutullo, C.A., and Cervera-Enguix, S. (2001). First break of mania associated with topiramate treatment. *J Clin Psychopharmacol*, 21(4), 464–466.

Schweiger, U., Deuschle, M., Weber, B., Korner, A., Lammers, C.H., Schmider, J., Gotthardt, U., and Heuser, I. (1999). Testosterone, gonadotropin, and cortisol secretion in male patients with major depression. *Psychosom Med*, 61(3), 292–296.

Seidman, S.N., and Rabkin, J.G. (1998). Testosterone replacement therapy for hypogonadal men with SSRI-refractory depression. *J Affect Disord*, 48(2-3), 157–161.

Serby, M. (2001). Manic reactions to ECT. *Am J Geriatr Psychiatry*, 9(2), 180.

Serretti, A., Artioli, P., Zanardi, R., and Rossini, D. (2003). Clinical features of antidepressant associated manic and hypomanic switches in bipolar disorder. *Progr Neuropsychopharmacol Biol Psychiatry*, 27, 751–757.

Shapira, B., Oppenheim, G., Zohar, J., Segal, M., Malach, D., and Belmaker, R.H. (1985). Lack of efficacy of estrogen supplementation to imipramine in resistant female depressives. *Biol Psychiatry*, 20(5), 576–579.

Sharma, B., Khan, M., and Smith, A. (2005). A closer look at treatment resistant depression: Is it due to a bipolar diathesis? *J Affect Disord*, 84(2-3), 251–257.

Shelton, R.C., Keller, M.B., Gelenberg, A., Dunner, D.L., Hirschfeld, R., Thase, M.E., Russell, J., Lydiard, R.B., Crits-Cristoph, P., Gallop, R., Todd, L., Hellerstein, D., Goodnick, P., Keitner, G., Stahl, S.M., and Halbreich, U. (2001). Effectiveness of St. John's wort in major depression: A randomized controlled trial, *JAMA*, 285(15), 1978–1986.

Shergill, S.S., and Katona, C.L. (1997). Pharmacological choices after one antidepressant fails: A survey of UK psychiatrists. *J Affect Disord*, 43(1), 19–25.

Shimon, H., Agam, G., Belmaker, R.H., Hyde, T.M., and Kleinman, J.E. (1997). Reduced frontal cortex inositol levels in postmortem brain of suicide victims and patients with bipolar disorder. *Am J Psychiatry*, 154(8), 1148–1150.

Silverstone, T. (2001). Moclobemide vs. imipramine in bipolar depression: A multicentre double-blind clinical trial. *Acta Psychiatr Scand*, 104(2), 104–109.

Simpson, S.G., and DePaulo, J.R. (1991). Fluoxetine treatment of bipolar II depression. *J Clin Psychopharmacol*, 11(1), 52–54.

Smeraldi, E. (1998). Amisulpride versus fluoxetine in patients with dysthymia or major depression in partial remission: A double-blind, comparative study. *J Affect Disord*, 48(1), 47–56.

Smeraldi, E., Benedetti, F., Barbini, B., Campori, E., and Colombo, C. (1999). Sustained antidepressant effect of sleep deprivation combined with pindolol in bipolar depression. A placebo-controlled trial. *Neuropsychopharmacology*, 20(4), 380–385.

Smeraldi, E., Benedetti, F., Barbini, B., Campori, E., and Colombo, C. (2003). Sustained antidepressant effect of sleep deprivation combined with pindolol in bipolar depression: A placebo controlled trial. *Neuropsychopharmacology*, 20(4), 380–383.

Soares, C.N., Almeida, O.P., Joffe, H., and Cohen, L.S. (2001). Efficacy of estradiol for the treatment of depressive disorders in perimenopausal women: A double-blind, randomized, placebo-controlled trial. *Arch Gen Psychiatry*, (6), 529–534.

Sporn, J., and Sachs, G. (1997). The anticonvulsant lamotrigine in treatment-resistant manic-depressive illness. *J Clin Psychopharmacol*, 17(3), 185–189.

Sporn, J., Ghaemi, S.N., Sambur, M.R., Rankin, M.A., Recht, J., Sachs, G.S., Rosenbaum, J.F., and Fava, M. (2000). Pramipexole augmentation in the treatment of unipolar and bipolar depression: A retrospective chart review. *Ann Clin Psychiatry*, 12(3), 137–140.

Stokes, P.E., Shamoian, C.A., Stoll, P.M., and Patton, M.J. (1971). Efficacy of lithium as acute treatment of manic-depressive illness. *Lancet*, 1, 1319–1325.

Stoll, A.L., Mayer, P.V., Kolbrener, M., Goldstein, E., Suplit, B., Lucier, J., Cohen, B.M., and Tohen, M. (1994). Antidepressant-associated mania: A controlled comparison with spontaneous mania. *Am J Psychiatry*, 151(11), 1642–1650.

Stoll, A.L., Pillay, S.S., Diamond, L., Workum, S.B., and Cole, J.O. (1996). Methylphenidate augmentation of serotonin selective reuptake inhibitors: A case series. *J Clin Psychiatry*, 57(2), 72–76.

Stoll, A.L., Severus, W.E., Freeman, M.P., Rueter, S., Zboyan, H.A., Diamond, E., Cress, K.K., and Marangell, L.B. (1999). Omega 3 fatty acids in bipolar disorder: A preliminary double-blind, placebo-controlled trial. *Arch Gen Psychiatry*, 56(5), 407–412.

Su, K.P., Huang, S.Y., Chiu, C.C., and Shen, W.W. (2003). Omega-3 fatty acids in major depressive disorder. A preliminary double-blind, placebo-controlled trial. *Eur Neuropsychopharmacol*, 13(4), 267–271.

Suppes, T., Brown, E.S., McElroy, S.L., Keck, P.E. Jr., Nolen, W., Kupka, R., Frye, M., Denicoff, K.D., Altshuler, L., Leverich, G.S., and Post, R.M. (1999). Lamotrigine for the treatment of bipolar disorder: A clinical case series. *J Affect Disord*, 53(1), 95–98.

Suppes, T., McElroy, S.L., Keck, P.E., Altshuler, L., Frye, M.A., Grunze, H., Leverich, G.S., Nolen, W.A., Chisholm, K., Dennehy, E.B., and Post, R.M. (2004). Use of quetiapine in bipolar disorder: A case series with prospective evaluation. *Int Clin Psychopharmacol*, 19(3), 173–174.

Suppes, T., Mintz, J., McElroy, S.L., Altshuler, L.L., Kupka, R.W., Frye, M.A., Keck, P.E. Jr., Nolen, W.A., Leverich, G.S., Grunze, H., Rush, A.J., and Post, R.M. (2005). Mixed hypomania in 908 patients with bipolar disorder evaluated prospectively in the Stanley Foundation Bipolar Treatment Network: A sex-specific phenomenon. *Arch Gen Psychiatry*, 62(10), 1089–1096.

Szuba, M.P., Baxter, L.R. Jr., Altshuler, L.L., Allen, E.M., Guze, B.H., Schwartz, J.M., and Liston, E.H. (1994). Lithium sustains the acute antidepressant effects of sleep deprivation: Preliminary findings from a controlled study. *Psychiatry Res*, 51(3), 283–295.

Tamada, R.S., Issler, C.K., Amaral, J.A., Sachs, G.S., and Lafer, B. (2004). Treatment emergent affective switch: A controlled study. *Bipolar Disord*, 6(4), 333–337.

Taylor, D.M., and McAskill, R. (2000). Atypical antipsychotics and weight gain—a systematic review. *Acta Psychiatr Scand*, 101(6), 416–432.

Terman, M., and Terman, J.S. (1999). Bright light therapy: Side effects and benefits across the symptom spectrum. *J Clin Psychiatry*, 60(11), 799–808.

Terman, M., Terman, J.S., Quitkin, F.M., McGrath, P.J., Stewart, J.W., and Rafferty, B. (1989). Light therapy for seasonal affective disorder. A review of efficacy. *Neuropsychopharmacology*, 2(1), 1–22.

Terman, M., Terman, J.S., and Ross, D.C. (1998). A controlled trial of timed bright light and negative air ionization for treatment of winter depression. *Arch Gen Psychiatry*, 55(10), 875–882.

Tevar, R., Jho, D.H., Babcock, T., Helton, W.S., and Espat, N.J. (2002). Omega-3 fatty acid supplementation reduces tumor growth and vascular endothelial growth factor expression in a model of progressive non-metastasizing malignancy. *JPEN J Parenter Enteral Nutr*, 26(5), 285–289.

Thase, M.E. (2002). What role do atypical antipsychotic drugs have in treatment-resistant depression? *J Clin Psychiatry*, 63(2), 95–103.

Thase, M.E., Mallinger, A.G., McKnight, D., and Himmelhoch, J.M. (1992). Treatment of imipramine-resistant recurrent depression, IV: A double-blind crossover study of tranylcypromine for anergic bipolar depression. *Am J Psychiatry*, 149(2), 195–198.

Thase, M.E., Blomgren, S.L., Birkett, M.A., Apter, J.T., and Tepner, R.G. (1997). Fluoxetine treatment of patients with major depressive disorder who failed initial treatment with sertraline. *J Clin Psychiatry*, 58(1), 16–21.

Thase, M.E., Entsuah, A.R., and Rudolph, R.L. (2001). Remission rates during treatment with venlafaxine or selective serotonin reuptake inhibitors. *Br J Psychiatry*, 178, 234–241.

Thase, M.E., Bhargava, M., and Sachs, G.S. (2003). Treatment of bipolar depression: Current status, continued challenges, and the STEP-BD approach. *Psychiatr Clin North Am*, 26(2), 495–518.

Till, E., and Vuckovic, S. (1970). Uber den Einfluss der thymoleptischen Behandlung auf den Verlauf endogener Depressionen. *Int Pharmacopsychiatry*, 4, 210–219.

Tohen, M., Risser, R.C., Baker, R.W., Evans, A.R., Tollefson, G., and Breier, A. (2002). *Olanzapine in the treatment of bipolar depression*. Poster presented at 155th Annual Meeting. Philadelphia: American Psychiatric Association.

Tohen, M., Vieta, E., Calabrese, J., Ketter, T.A., Sachs, G., Bowden, C., Mitchell, P.B., Centorrino, F., Risser, R., Baker, R.W., Evans, A.R., Beymer, K., Dube, S., Tollefson, G.D., and Breier, A. (2003a). Efficacy of olanzapine and olanzapine-fluoxetine combination in the treatment of bipolar I depression. *Arch Gen Psychiatry*, 61(2), 176.

Tohen, M., Zarate, C.A. Jr., Hennen, J., Khalsa, H.M., Strakowski, S.M., Gebre-Medhin, P., Salvatore, P., and Baldessarini, R.J. (2003b). The McLean-Harvard First-Episode Mania Study: Prediction of recovery and first recurrence. *Am J Psychiatry*, 160(12), 2099–2107.

Trivedi, M.H., Rush, A.J., Wisniewski, S.R., Nierenberg, A.A., Warden, D., Ritz, L., Norquist, G., Howland, R.H., Lebowitz, B., McGrath, P.J., Shores-Wilson, K., Biggs, M.M., Balasubramani, G.K., and Fava, M., for the STAR*D Study Team. (2006). Evaluation of outcomes with citalopram for depression using measurement-based care in STAR*D: Implications for clinical practice. *Am J Psychiatry*, 163(1), 28–40.

Tuuainen, A., Kripke, D.F., and Endo, T. (2004). Light therapy for non-seasonal depression. *Cochrane Database Syst Rev*, (2), CD004050.

UK ECT Review Group. (2003). Efficacy and safety of electroconvulsive therapy in depressive disorders: A systematic review and meta-analysis. *Lancet*, 361(9360), 799–808.

Versiani, M., Mehilane, L., Gaszner, P., and Arnaud-Castiglioni, R. (1999). Reboxetine, a unique selective NRI, prevents relapse and recurrence in long-term treatment of major depressive disorder. *J Clin Psychiatry*, 60(6), 400–406.

Vieta, E., Colom, F., Martinez-Aran, A., Reinares, M., Benabarre, A., Corbella, B., and Gasto, C. (2001). Reboxetine-induced hypomania. *J Clin Psychiatry*, 62(8), 655–656.

Vieta, E., Martinez-Aran, A., Goikolea, J.M., Torrent, C., Colom, F., Benabarre, A., and Reinares, M. (2002). A randomized trial comparing paroxetine and venlafaxine in the treatment of bipolar depressed patients taking mood stabilizers. *J Clin Psychiatry*, 63(6), 508–512.

Visser, H., and Van der Mast, R. (2005). Bipolar disorder, antidepressants, and induction of hypomania or mania: A systemic review. *World J Biol Psychiatry*, 6, 231–241.

Wagner, G.J., and Rabkin, R. (2000). Effects of dextroamphetamine on depression and fatigue in men with HIV: A double-blind, placebo-controlled trial. *J Clin Psychiatry*, 61(6), 436–440.

Waldmeier, P.C. (1993). Newer aspects of the reversible inhibitor of MAOA and serotonin reuptake, brofaromine. *Prog Neuropsychopharmacol Biol Psychiatry*, 17(2), 183–198.

Walker, S.E., Shulman, K.I., Tailor, S.A., and Gardner, D. (1996). Tyramine content of previously restricted foods in monoamine oxidase inhibitor diets. *J Clin Psychopharmacol*, 16(5), 383–388.

Walter, G., Lyndon, B., and Kubb, R. (1998). Lithium augmentation of venlafaxine in adolescent major depression. *Aust NZ J Psychiatry*, 32(3), 457–459.

Watanabe, S., Ishino, H., and Otsuki, S. (1975). Double-blind comparison of lithium carbonate and imipramine in treatment of depression. *Arch Gen Psychiatry*, 32(5), 659–668.

Wehr, T., and Goodwin, F.K. (1979a). Tricyclics modulate frequency of mood cycles. *Chronobiologia*, 6(4), 377–385.

Wehr, T., and Goodwin, F.K. (1979b). Rapid cycling in manic-depressives induced by tricyclic antidepressants. *Arch Gen Psychiatry*, 36(5), 555–559.

Wehr, T.A., Goodwin, F.K., Wirz-Justice, A., Breitmaier, J., and Craig, C. (1982). 48-hour sleep–wake cycles in manic-depressive illness: Naturalistic observations and sleep deprivation experiments. *Arch Gen Psychiatry*, 39(5), 559–565.

Wehr, T.A., Sacks, D.A., Rosenthal, N.E., and Cowdry, R.W. (1988). Rapid cycling affective disorder: Contributing factors and treatment responses in 51 patients. *Am J Psychiatry*, 145(2), 179–184.

Whybrow, P.C. (1994). The therapeutic use of triiodothyronine and high-dose thyroxine in psychiatric disorder. *Acta Med Austriaca*, 21(2), 47–52.

Wiegand, M., Riemann, D., Schreiber, W., Lauer, C.J., and Berger, M. (1993). Effect of morning and afternoon naps on mood after total sleep deprivation in patients with major depression. *Biol Psychiatry*, 33(6), 467–476.

Williamson, D., Brown, E., Perlis, R.H., Ahl, J., Baker, R.W., and Tohen, M. (2006). Clinical relevance of depressive symptom improvement in bipolar I depressed patients. *J Affect Disord*, 92(2-3), 261–266.

Winsberg, M.E., DeGolia, S.G., Strong, C.M., and Ketter, T.A. (2001). Divalproex therapy in medication-naive and mood-stabilizer-naive bipolar II depression. *J Affect Disord*, 67(1-3), 207–212.

Wirshing, D.A., Spellberg, B.J., Erhart, S.M., Marder, S.R., and Wirshing, W.C. (1998). Novel antipsychotics and new-onset diabetes. *Biol Psychiatry*, 44(8), 778–783.

Wirz-Justice, A., and van den Hoofdakker, R.H. (1999). Sleep deprivation in depression: What do we know, where do we go? *Biol.Psychiatry*, 46(4), 445–453.

Wolkowitz, O.M., and Reus, V.I. (1999). Treatment of depression with antiglucocorticoid drugs. *Psychosom Med*, 61(5), 698–711.

Wolkowitz, O.M., Reus, V.I., Chan, T., Manfredi, F., Raum, W., Johnson, R., and Canick, J. (1999a). Antiglucocorticoid treatment of depression: Double-blind ketoconazole. *Biol Psychiatry*, 45(8), 1070–1074.

Wolkowitz, O.M., Reus, V.I., Keebler, A., Nelson, N., Friedland, M., Brizendine, L., and Roberts, E. (1999b). Double-blind treatment of major depression with dehydroepiandrosterone. *Am J Psychiatry*, 156(4), 646–649.

Wong, A.H., Smith, M., and Boon, H.S. (1998a). Herbal remedies in psychiatric practice. *Arch Gen Psychiatry*, 55(11), 1033–1044.

Wong, A.H., Smith, M., and Boon, H.S. (1998b). Herbal remedies in psychiatric practice. *Arch Gen Psychiatry*, 55(11), 1033–1044.

Wong, E.H., Sonders, M.S., Amara, S.G., Tinholt, P.M., Piercey, M.F., Hoffmann, W.P., Hyslop, D.K., Franklin, S., Porsolt, R.D., Bonsignori, A., Carfagna, N., and McArthur, R.A. (2000). Reboxetine: A pharmacologically potent, selective, and specific norepinephrine reuptake inhibitor. *Biol Psychiatry*, 47(9), 818–829.

Worrall, E.P., Moody, J.P., Peet, M., Dick, P., Smith, A., Chambers, C., Adams, M., and Naylor, G.J. (1979). Controlled studies of the acute antidepressant effects of lithium. *Br J Psychiatry*, 135, 255–262.

Wu, J.C., and Bunney, W.E. (1990). The biological basis of an antidepressant response to sleep deprivation and relapse: Review and hypothesis. *Am J Psychiatry*, 147(1), 14–21.

Yatham, L.N., Calabrese, J.R., and Kusumakar, V. (2003). Bipolar depression: Criteria for treatment selection, definition of refractoriness, and treatment options. *Bipolar Disord*, 5(2), 85–97.

Yildiz, A., and Sachs, G.S. (2003). Do antidepressants induce rapid cycling? A gender-specific association. *J Clin Psychiatry*, 64(7), 814–818.

Young, A.H., Gallagher, P., and Porter, R.J. (2002). Elevation of the cortisol-dehydroepiandrosterone ratio in drug-free depressed patients. *Am J Psychiatry*, 159(7), 1237–1239.

Young, E.A., and Korszun, A. (2002). The hypothalamic-pituitary-gonadal axis in mood disorders. *Endocrinol Metab Clin North Am*, 31(1), 63–78.

Young, L., Robb, J.C., Patelis-Siotis, I., MacDonald, C., and Joffe, R.T. (1997). Acute treatment of bipolar depression with gabapentin. *Biol Psychiatry*, 42(9), 851–853.

Young, L.T., Joffe, R.T., Robb, J.C., MacQueen, G.M., Marriott M., and Patelis-Siotis, I. (2000). Double-blind comparison of addition of a second mood stabilizer versus an antidepressant to an initial mood stabilizer for treatment of patients with bipolar depression. *Am J Psychiatry*, 1, 124–126.

Zabara, J. (1988). Neuroinhibition of xylazine induced emesis. *Pharmacol Toxicol*, 63(2), 70–74.

Zanarini, M.C., and Frankenburg, F.R. (2003). Omega-3 fatty acid treatment of women with borderline personality disorder: A double-blind, placebo-controlled pilot study. *Am J Psychiatry*, 160(1), 167–169.

Zarate, C.A. Jr., Rothschild, A., Fletcher, K.E., Madrid, A., and Zapatel, J. (2000). Clinical predictors of acute response with quetiapine in psychotic mood disorders. *J Clin Psychiatry*, 61(3), 185–189.

Zarate, C.A. Jr., Payne, J.L., Singh, J., Quiroz, J.A., Luckenbaugh, D.A., Denicoff, K.D., Charney, D.S., and Manji, H.K. (2004). Pramipexole for bipolar II depression: A placebo-controlled proof of concept study. *Biol Psychiatry*, 56(1), 54–60.

Zarate, C.A. Jr., Quiroz, J.A., Singh, J.B., Denicoff, K.D., De Jesus, G., Luckenbaugh, D.A., Charney, D.S., and Manji, H.K. (2005). An open-label trial of the glutamate-modulating agent riluzole in combination with lithium for the treatment of bipolar depression. *Biol Psychiatry*, 57(4), 430–432.

Zornberg, G.L., and Pope, H.G. Jr. (1993). Treatment of depression in bipolar disorder: New directions for research. *J Clin Psychopharmacol*, 13(6), 397–408.

Zwil, A.S., Bowring, M.A., Price, T.R., Goetz, K.L., Greenbarg, J.B., and Kane-Wanger, G. (1990). Prospective electroconvulsive therapy in the presence of intracranial tumor. *Convuls Ther*, 6(4), 299–307.

CHAPTER 20

Aagaard, J., and Vestergaard, P. (1990). Predictors of outcome in prophylactic lithium treatment: A 2-year prospective study. *J Affect Disord*, 18(4), 259–266.

Abrams, R. (1990). ECT as prophylactic treatment for bipolar disorder. *Am J Psychiatry*, 147(3), 373–374.

Ahlfors, U.G. Baastrup, P.C., Dencker, S.J., Elgen, K., Lingjaerde, O., Pedersen, V., Schou, M., and Aaskoven, O. (1981). Flupenthixol decanoate in recurrent manic-depressive illness: A comparison with lithium. *Acta Psychiatr Scand*, 64(3), 226–237.

Ahmed, Z., and Anderson, I.M. (2001). Treatment of bipolar affective disorder in clinical practice. *J Psychopharmacol*, 15(1), 55–57.

Ahrens, B., Grof, P., Moller, H.J., Muller-Oerlinghausen, B., and Wolf, T. (1995). Extended survival of patients on long-term lithium treatment. *Can J Psychiatry*, 241–246.

Akiskal, H. 2000. Mood disorders. In M.H. Beers, R. Berkow (Eds.), *The Merck Manual of Diagnosis and Therapy* (17th edition). Rahway, NJ: Merck Research Laboratories.

Allan, S.J., Kavanagh, G.M., Herd, R.M., and Savin, J.A. (2004). The effect of inositol supplements on the psoriasis of patients taking lithium: A randomized, placebo-controlled trial. *Br J Dermatol*, 150(5), 966–969.

Allen, M.H., Hirschfeld, R.M., Wozniak, P.J., Baker, J.D., and Bowden, C.L. (2006). Linear relationship of valproate serum concentration to response and optimal serum levels for acute mania. *Am J Psychiatry*, 163(2), 272–275.

Allison, D.B. (2001). Antipsychotic-induced weight gain: A review of the literature. *J Clin Psychiatry*, 62(Suppl. 7), 22–31.

Altshuler, L.L., Cohen, L., Szuba, M.P., Burt, V.K., Gitlin, M., and Mintz, J. (1996). Pharmacologic management of psychiatric illness during pregnancy: Dilemmas and guidelines. *Am J Psychiatry*, 153(5), 592–606.

Altshuler, L.L., Keck, P.E. Jr., McElroy, S.L., Suppes, T., Brown, E.S., Denicoff, K., Frye, M., Gitlin, M., Hwang, S., Goodman, R., Leverich, G., Nolen, W., Kupka, R., and Post, R. (1999). Gabapentin in the acute treatment of refractory bipolar disorder. *Bipolar Disord*, 1(1), 61–65.

American Psychiatric Association. (2002). Practice guideline for the treatment of patients with bipolar disorder (revision). *Am J Psychiatry*, 159(Suppl. 4), 1–50.

Amsterdam, J.D., Garcia-Espana, F., Fawcett, J., Quitkin, F.M., Reimherr, F.W., Rosenbaum, J.F., Schweizer, E., and Beasley, C. (1998). Efficacy and safety of fluoxetine in treating bipolar II major depressive episode. *J Clin Psychopharmacol*, 18(6), 435–440.

Andrade, C., and Kurinji, S. (2002). Continuation and maintenance ECT: A review of recent research. *J ECT*, 18(3), 149–158.

Angst, J., Weis, P., Grof, P., Baastrup, P.C., and Schou, M. (1970). Lithium prophylaxis in recurrent affective disorders. *Br J Psychiatry*, 116, 604–614.

Appleby, L., Mortensen, P.B., Faragher, E.B. (1998). Suicide and other causes of mortality after post-partum psychiatric admission. *Br J Psychiatry*, 173, 209–211.

Atmaca, M. (2002). Weight gain and serum leptin levels in patients on lithium treatment. *Neuropsychobiology*, 46(2), 67–69.

Austin, M.P. (1992). Puerperal affective psychosis: Is there a case for lithium prophylaxis? *Br J Psychiatry*, 161, 692–694.

Baastrup, P.C., and Schou, M. (1967). Lithium as a prophylactic agent: Its effect against recurrent depressions and manic-depressive psychosis. *Arch Gen Psychiatry*, 16(2), 162–172.

Baastrup, P.C., Poulsen, J.C., Schou, M., Thomsen, K., and Amdisen, A. (1970). Prophylactic lithium: Double blind discontinuation in manic-depressive and recurrent-depressive disorders. *Lancet*, 2(7668), 326–330.

Baethge C., Smolka, M.N., Gruschka, P., Berghofer, A., Schlattmann, P., Bauer, M., Altshuler, L., Grof, P., and Muller-Oerlinghausen, B. (2003). Does prophylaxis-delay in bipolar disorder influence outcome? Results for a long-term study of 147 patients. *Acta Psychiatr Scand*, 107, 260–267.

Baethge, C., Baldessarini, R.J., Mathiske-Schmidt, K., Hennen, J., Berghofer, A., Muller-Oerlinghausen, B. (2005). Long-term combination therapy versus monotherapy with lithium and carbamazepine in 46 bipolar I patients. *J Clin Psychiatry*, 66(2), 174–182.

Baldessarini, R.J. (1988). A summary of current knowledge of tardive dyskinesia. *Encephale*, 14, 263–268.

Baldessarini, R.J., and Tondo, L. (2000). Does lithium treatment still work? Evidence of stable responses over three decades. *Arch Gen Psychiatry*, 57(2), 187–190.

Baldessarini, R.J., Tondo, L., Faedda, G., Floris, G., Suppes, T., and Rudas, N. (1996). Effects of the rate of discontinuing lithium maintenance treatment in bipolar disorders. *J Clin Psychiatry*, 57, 441–448.

Baldessarini, R.J., Tondo, L., Floris, G., and Rudas, N. (1997). Reduced morbidity after gradually discontinuing lithium in bipolar I and II disorders: A replication study. *Am J Psychiatry*, 154, 551–553.

Baldessarini, R.J., Tondo, L., Hennen, J., and Floris, G. (1999a). Latency and episodes before treatment: Response to lithium maintenance in bipolar I and II disorders. *Bipolar Disord*, 1(2), 91–97.

Baldessarini, R.J., Tondo, L., and Viguera, A.C. (1999b). Discontinuing lithium maintenance treatment in bipolar disorders: Risks and implications. *Bipolar Disord*, 1(1), 17–24.

Baldessarini, R.J., Tondo, L., Floris, G., and Hennen, J. (2000). Effects of rapid cycling on response to lithium maintenance treatment in 360 bipolar I and II disorder patients. *J Affect Disord*, 61(1-2), 13–22.

Baldessarini, R.J., Tondo, L., Hennen, J., and Viguera, A.C. (2002). Is lithium still worth using? An update of selected recent research. *Harv Rev Psychiatry*, 10(2), 59–75.

Baldessarini, R.J., Tondo, L., and Hennen, J. (2003). Treatment-latency and previous episodes: Relationships to pretreatment morbidity and response to maintenance treatment in bipolar I and II disorders. *Bipolar Disord*, 5(3), 169–179.

Baldessarini, R.J., Pompili, M., and Tondo, L. (2006). Suicidal risk in antidepressant drug trials. *Arch Gen Psychiatry*, 63(3), 246–248.

Ballenger, J.C., and Post, R.M. (1978). Therapeutic effects of carbamazepine in affective illness: A preliminary report. *Commun Psychopharmacol*, 2, 159–175.

Ballenger, J.C., and Post, R.M. (1980). Carbamazepine in manic-depressive illness: A new treatment. *Am J Psychiatry*, 137(7), 782–790.

Banov, M.D., Zarate, C.A. Jr., Tohen, M., Scialabba, D., Wines, J.D. Jr., Kolbrener, M., Kim, J.W., and Cole, J.O. (1994). Clozapine therapy in refractory affective disorders: Polarity predicts response in long-term follow-up. *J Clin Psychiatry*, 55(7), 295–300.

Baptista, T., Lacruz, A., de Mendoza, S., Guillen, M.M., Burguera, J.L., de Burguera, M., and Hernandez, L. (2000). Endocrine effects of lithium carbonate in healthy premenopausal women: Relationship with body weight regulation. *Prog Neuropsychopharmacol Biol Psychiatry*, 24(1), 1–16.

Baptista, T., Kin, N.M., Beaulieu, S., and de Baptista, E.A. (2002). Obesity and related metabolic abnormalities during antipsychotic drug administration: Mechanisms, management and research perspectives. *Pharmacopsychiatry*, 35(6), 205–219.

Barton, C.D. Jr., Dufer, D., Monderer, R., Cohen, M.J., Fuller, H.J., Clark, M.R., and DePaulo, J.R. Jr. (1993). Mood variability in normal subjects on lithium. *Biol Psychiatry*, 34(12), 878–884.

Bauer, J., Jarre, A., Klingmuller, D., and Elger, C.E. (2000). Polycystic ovary syndrome in patients with focal epilepsy: A study in 93 women. *Epilepsy Res*, 41(2), 163–167.

Bauer, M.S., and Mitchner, L. (2004). What is a "mood stabilizer"? An evidence-based response. *Am J Psychiatry*, 161(1), 3–18.

Bauer, M.S., and Whybrow, P.C. (1990). Rapid cycling bipolar affective disorder: II. Treatment of refractory rapid cycling with high-dose levothyroxine: A preliminary study. *Arch Gen Psychiatry*, 47(5), 435–440.

Bauer, M., and Whybrow, P.C. (2001). Thyroid hormones, neural tissue, and mood modulation. *World J Biol Psychiatry*, 2, 59–69.

Bauer, M., Berghofer, A., Bschor, T., Baumgartner, A., Kiesslinger, U., Hellweg, R., Adli, M., Baethge, C., and Muller-Oerlinghausen, B. (2002). Supraphysiological doses of L-thyroxine in the maintenance treatment of prophylaxis-resistant affective disorders. *Neuropsychopharmacology*, 27(4), 620–628.

Baumgartner, A. (2000). Thyroxine and the treatment of affective disorders: An overview of the results of basic and clinical research. *Int J Neuropsychopharmacol*, 3(2), 149–165.

Bech, P. (2006). The full story of lithium: A tribute to Mogens Schou (1918–2005). *Psychother Psychosom* 75(5), 265–269.

Berghofer, A., Kossmann, B., and Muller-Oerlinghausen, B. (1996). Course of illness and pattern of recurrences in patients with affective disorders during long-term lithium prophylaxis: A retrospective analysis over 15 years. *Acta Psychiatr Scand*, 93(5), 349–354.

Bendz, H., Aurell, M., and Lanke, J. (2001). A historical cohort study of kidney damage in long-term lithium patients: Continued surveillance needed. *Eur Psychiatry*, 16(4), 199–206.

Birt, J. (2003). Management of weight gain associated with antipsychotics. *Ann Clin Psychiatry*, 15(1), 49–58.

Blackwell, B., and Shepherd, M. (1968). Prophylactic lithium: Another therapeutic myth? *Lancet*, 968–971.

Bocchetta, A., Chillotti, C., Severino, G., Ardau, R., and Del Zompo, M. (1997). Carbamazepine augmentation in lithium-refractory bipolar patients: A prospective study on long-term prophlyactic effectiveness. *J Clin Psychopharmacol*, 17(2), 92–96.

Bocchetta, A., Mossa, P., Velluzzi, F., Mariotti, S., Zompo, M.D., and Loviselli, A. (2001). Ten-year follow-up of thyroid function in lithium patients. *J Clin Psychopharmacol*, 21(6), 594–598.

Bollini, P., Pampallona, S., Orza, M.J., Adams, M.E., and Chalmers, T.C. (1994). Antipsychotic drugs: Is more worse? A meta-analysis of the published randomized control trials. *Psychol Med*, 24(2), 307–316.

Bonari, L., Pinto, N., Ahn, E., Einarson, A., Steiner, M., and Koren, G. (2004). Perinatal risks of untreated depression during pregnancy. *Can J Psychiatry*, 49(11), 726–735.

Bowden, C.L. (1998). Key treatment studies of lithium in manic-depressive illness: Efficacy and side effects. *J Clin Psychiatry*, 59(Suppl. 6), 13–19; discussion 20.

Bowden, C.L., Brugger, A.M., Swann, A.C., Calabrese, J.R., Janicak, P.G., Petty, F., Dilsaver, S.C., Davis, J.M., Rush, A.J., and Small, J.G. (1994). Efficacy of divalproex vs lithium and placebo in the treatment of mania. The Depakote Mania Study Group. *JAMA*, 271(12), 918–924.

Bowden, C.L., Calabrese, J.R., McElroy, S.L., Rhodes, L.J., Keck, P.E. Jr., Cookson, J., Anderson, J., Bolden-Watson. C., Ascher, J., Monaghan, E., and Zhou, J. (1999). The efficacy of lamotrigine in rapid cycling and non-rapid cycling patients with bipolar disorder. *Biol Psychiatry*, 45(8), 953–958.

Bowden, C.L., Calabrese, J.R., McElroy, S.L., Gyulai, L., Wassef, A., Petty, F., Pope, H.G. Jr., Chou, J.C., Keck, P.E. Jr., Rhodes, L.J., Swann, A.C., Hirschfeld, R.M., and Wozniak, P.J. (2000a). A randomized, placebo-controlled 12-month trial of divalproex and lithium in treatment of outpatients with bipolar I disorder. Divalproex Maintenance Study Group. *Arch Gen Psychiatry*, 57(5), 481–489.

Bowden, C.L., Lecrubier, Y., Bauer, M., Goodwin, G., Greil, W., Sachs, G., and von Knorring, L. (2000b). Maintenance therapies for classic and other forms of bipolar disorder. *J Affect Disord*, 59(Suppl. 1), S57–S67.

Bowden, C.L., Calabrese, J.R., Sachs, G., Yatham, L.N., Asghar, S.A., Hompland, M., Montgomery, P., Earl, N., Smoot, T.M., DeVeaugh-Geiss, J., and Lamictal 606 Study Group. (2003a). A placebo-controlled 18-month trial of lamotrigine and lithium maintenance treatment in recently manic or hypomanic patients with bipolar I disorder. *Arch Gen Psychiatry*, 60(4), 392.

Bowden, C.L., Calabrese, J.R., Sachs, G., Yatham, L.N., Asghar, S.A., Hompland, M., Montgomery, P., Earl, N., Smoot, T.M., DeVeaugh-Geiss, J., for Lamictal 606 Study Group. (2003b). A placebo-controlled 18-month trial of lamotrigine and lithium maintenance treatment in recently manic or hypomanic patients with bipolar I disorder. *Arch Gen Psychiatry*, 60(4), 392–400.

Bowden, C.L., Myers, J.E., Grossman, F., and Xie, Y. (2004). Risperidone in combination with mood stabilizers: A 10-week continuation phase study in bipolar I disorder. *J Clin Psychiatry*, 65(5), 707–714.

Bowden, C.L., Collins, M.A., McElroy, S.L., Calabrese, J.R., Swann, A.C., Weisler, R.H. (2005). Relationship of mania symptomatology to maintenance treatment response with divalproex, lithium, or placebo. *Neuropsychopharmacology*, 30(10), 1932–1939.

Bowden, C.L., Calabrese, J.R., Ketter, T.A., Sachs, G.S., White, R.L., and Thompson, T.R. (2006). Impact of lamotrigine and lithium on weight in obese and nonobese patients with bipolar I disorder. *Am J Psychiatry*, 163(7), 1199–1201.

Bowden, R.C., Grof, P., and Grof, E. (1991). Less frequent lithium administration and lower urine volume. *Am J Psychiatry*, 148(2), 189–192.

Burt, T., Sachs, G.S., and Demopulos, C. (1999). Donepezil in treatment-resistant bipolar disorder. *Biol Psychiatry*, 45(8), 959–964.

Byrne, S.E., and Rothschild, A.J. (1998). Loss of antidepressant efficacy during maintenance therapy: Possible mechanisms and treatments. *J Clin Psychiatry*, 59(6), 279–288.

Cade, J.F.J. (1949). Lithium salts in the treatment of psychotic excitement. *Med J Aust*, 36, 349–352.

Calabrese, J.R., and Delucchi, G.A. (1990). Spectrum of efficacy of valproate in 55 patients with rapid-cycling bipolar disorder. *Am J Psychiatry*, 147(4), 431–434.

Calabrese, J.R., and Rapport, D.J. (1999). Mood stabilizers and the evolution of maintenance study designs in bipolar I disorder. *J Clin Psychiatry*, 60(Suppl. 5), 5–13; discussion 14–15.

Calabrese, J.R., Rapport, D.J., Kimmel, S.E., Reece, B., and Woyshville, M.J. (1993). Rapid cycling bipolar disorder and its treatment with valproate. *Can J Psychiatry*, 38(3 Suppl. 2), S57–S61.

Calabrese, J.R., Bowden, C.L., McElroy, S.L., Cookson, J., Andersen, J., Keck, P.E. Jr., Rhodes, L., Bolden-Watson, C., Zhou, J., and Ascher, J.A. (1999a). Spectrum of activity of lamotrigine in treatment-refractory bipolar disorder. *Am J Psychiatry*, 156(7), 1019–1023.

Calabrese, J.R., Bowden, C.L., Sachs, G.S., Ascher, J.A., Monaghan, E., and Rudd, G.D. (1999b). A double-blind placebo-controlled study of lamotrigine monotherapy in outpatients with bipolar I depression. Lamictal 602 Study Group. *J Clin Psychiatry*, 60(2), 79–88.

Calabrese, J.R., Suppes, T., Bowden, C.L., Sachs, G.S., Swann, A.C., McElroy, S.L., Kusumakar, V., Ascher, J.A., Earl, N.L., Greene, P.L., and Monaghan, E.T. (2000). A double-blind, placebo-controlled, prophylaxis study of lamotrigine in rapid-cycling bipolar disorder. Lamictal 614 Study Group. *J Clin Psychiatry*, 61(11), 841–850.

Calabrese, J.R., Shelton, M.D., Rapport, D.J., Kujawa, M., Kimmel, S.E., and Caban, S. (2001). Current research on rapid cycling bipolar disorder and its treatment. *J Affect Disord*, 67(1–3), 241–255.

Calabrese, J.R., Sullivan, J.R., Bowden, C.L., Suppes, T., Goldberg, J.F., Sachs, G.S., Shelton, M.D., Goodwin, F.K., Frye, M.A., and Kusumakar, V. (2002). Rash in multicenter trials of lamotrigine in mood disorders: Clinical relevance and management. *J Clin Psychiatry*, 63(11), 1012–1019.

Calabrese, J.R., Bowden, C.L., Sachs, G., Yatham, L.N., Behnke, K., Mehtonen, O.P., Montgomery, P., Ascher, J., Paska, W., Earl, N., DeVeaugh-Geiss, J., and Lamictal 605 Study Group. (2003). A placebo-controlled 18-month trial of lamotrigine and lithium maintenance treatment in recently depressed patients with bipolar I disorder. *J Clin Psychiatry*, 64(9), 1013–1024.

Calabrese, J.R., Shelton, M.D., Rapport, D.J., Youngstrom, E.A., Jackson, K., Bilali, S., Ganocy, S.J., and Findling, R.L. (2005). A 20-month, double-blind, maintenance trial of lithium versus divalproex in rapid-cycling bipolar disorder. *Am J Psychiatry*, 162(11), 2152–2161.

Calabrese, J.R., Goldberg, J.F., Ketter, T.A., Suppes, T., Frye, M., White, R., DeVeaugh-Geiss, A., and Thompson, T.R. (2006). Recurrence in bipolar I disorder: A post hoc analysis excluding relapses in two double-blind maintenance studies. *Biol Psychiatry*, 59(11), 1061–1064.

Calil, H.M., Zwicker, A.P., and Klepacz, S. (1990). The effects of lithium carbonate on healthy volunteers: Mood stabilization? *Biol Psychiatry*, 27(7), 711–722.

Carta, M.G. Hardoy, M.C., Grunze, H., and Carpiniello, B. (2002). The use of tiagabine in affective disorders. *Pharmacopsychiatry*, 35(1), 33–34.

Cavanagh, J., Smyth, R., and Goodwin, G.M. (2004). Relapse into mania or depression following lithium discontinuation: A 7-year follow-up. *Acta Psychiatr Scand*, 109(2), 91–95.

Champion, L.M., Nem, J.Y., Culver, J.L., Wong, P.W., Marsh, W.K., Bonner, J.C., and Ketter, T.C. (2006). *Effectiveness of lamotrigine in a clinical setting*. APA New Research Poster. Presented at American Psychiatric Association Meeting, Toronto, Canada.

Chang, J.S., Ha, K-S., Lee, K.Y., Kim, Y.S., and Ahn, Y.M. (2006). The effects of long-term clozapine add-on therapy on the rehospitalization rate and the mood polarity patterns in bipolar disorders. *J Clin Psychiatry*, 67(3), 461–467.

Chaudron, L.H., and Jefferson, J.W. (2000). Mood stabilizers during breastfeeding: A review. *J Clin Psychiatry*, 61(2), 79–90.

Chaudron, L.H., and Pies, R.W. (2003). The relationship between postpartum psychosis and bipolar disorder: A review. *J Clin Psychiatry*, 64(11), 1284–1292.

Chen, S.T., Altshuler, L.L., Melnyk, K.A., Erhart, S.M., Miller, E., and Mintz, J. (1999). Efficacy of lithium vs. valproate in the treatment of mania in the elderly: A retrospective study. *J Clin Psychiatry*, 60(3), 181–186.

Chengappa, K.N., Chalasani, L., Brar, J.S., Parepally, H., Houck, P., and Levine, J. (2002). Changes in body weight and body mass index among psychiatric patients receiving lithium, valproate, or topiramate: An open-label, nonrandomized chart review. *Clin Ther*, 24(10), 1576–1584.

Ciapparelli, A., Dell'Osso, L., Pini, S., Chiavacci, M.C., Fenzi, M., and Cassano, G.B. (2000). Clozapine for treatment-refractory schizophrenia, schizoaffective disorder, and psychotic bipolar disorder: A 24-month naturalistic study. *J Clin Psychiatry*, 61(5), 329–334.

Cohen, L.S., Friedman, J.M., Jefferson, J.W., Johnson, E.M., and Weiner, M.L. (1994). A reevaluation of risk of in utero exposure to lithium. *JAMA*, 271(2), 146–150.

Cole, D.P., Thase, M.E., Mallinger, A.G., Soares, J.C., Luther, J.F., Kupfer, D.J., and Frank, E. (2002). Slower treatment response in bipolar depression predicted by lower pretreatment thyroid function. *Am J Psychiatry*, 159(1), 116–121.

Conney, J., and Kaston, B. (1999). Pharmacoeconomic and health outcome comparison of lithium and divalproex in a VA geriatric nursing home population: Influence of drug-related morbidity on total cost of treatment. *Am J Manag Care*, 5(2), 197–204.

Coppen, A., Noguera, R., Bailey, J., Burns, B.H., Swani, M.S., Hare, E.H., Gardner, R., and Maggs, R. (1971). Prophylactic lithium in affective disorders: Controlled trial. *Lancet*, 2(7719), 275–279.

Coppen, A., Peet, M., Bailey, J., Noguera, R., Burns, B.H., Swani, M.S., Maggs, R., and Gardner, R. (1973). Double-blind and open prospective studies on lithium prophylaxis in affective disorders. *Psychiatr Neurol Neurochir*, 76(6), 501–510.

Correll, C.U., Frederickson, A.M., Kane, J.M., and Manu, P. (2006). Metabolic syndrome and the risk of coronary disease in 367 patients treated with second-generation antipsychotic drugs. *J Clin Psychiatry*, 67(4), 575–583.

Coryell, W., Winokur, G., Solomon, D., Shea, T., Leon, A., and Keller, M. (1997). Lithium and recurrence in a long-term follow-up of bipolar affective disorder. *Psychol Med*, 27(2), 281–289.

Coryell, W., Solomon, D., Leon, A.C., Akiskal, H.S., Keller, M.B., Scheftner, W.A., and Mueller, T. (1998). Lithium discontinuation and subsequent effectiveness. *Am J Psychiatry*, 155(7), 895.

Coxhead, N., Silverstone, T., and Cookson, J. (1992). Carbamazepine versus lithium in the prophylaxis of bipolar affective disorder. *Acta Psychiatr Scand*, 85(2), 114–118.

Crawford, P. (2002). Interactions between antiepileptic drugs and hormonal contraception. *CNS Drugs*, 16(4), 263–272.

Cundall, R.L., Brooks, P.W., and Murray, L.G. (1972). A controlled evaluation of lithium prophylaxis in affective disorders. *Psychol Med*, 2(3), 308–311.

Cunnington, M., and Tennis, P. (2005). Lamotrigine and the risk of malformations in pregnancy. *Neurology*, 64(6), 955–960.

Davis, J.M., Janicak, P.G., and Hogan, D.M. (1999). Mood stabilizers in the prevention of recurrent affective disorders: A meta-analysis. *Acta Psychiatr Scand*, 100(6), 406–417.

Dean, C., Williams, R.J., and Brockington, I.F. (1989). Is puerperal psychosis the same as bipolar manic-depressive disorder? A family study. *Psychol Med*, 19(3), 637–647.

de Camargo, O.A., and Bode, H. (1999). Agranulocytosis associated with lamotrigine. *BMJ*, 318(7192), 1179.

Denicoff, K.D., Smith-Jackson, E.E., Bryan, A.L., Ali, S.O., and Post, R.M. (1997a). Valproate prophylaxis in a prospective clinical trial of refractory bipolar disorder. *Am J Psychiatry*, 154(10), 1456–1458.

Denicoff, K.D., Smith-Jackson, E.E., Disney, E.R., Ali, S.O., Leverich, G.S., and Post, R.M. (1997b). Comparative prophylactic efficacy of lithium, carbamazepine, and the combination in bipolar disorder. *J Clin Psychiatry*, 58(11), 470–478.

DePaulo, J.R. Jr., Folstein, M.F., and Correa, E.I. (1982). The course of delirium due to lithium intoxication. *J Clin Psychiatry*, 43(11), 447–449.

Deshauer, D., Fergusson, D., Duffy, A., Albuquerque, J., and Grof, P. (2005). Re-evaluation of randomized control trials of lithium monotherapy: A cohort effect. *Bipolar Disord*, 7(4), 382–387.

Dettling, M., and Anghelescu, I.G. (2006). Antipsychotic drugs and schizophrenia. *N Engl J Med*, 354(3), 298–300.

Dickson, W.E., and Kendell, R.E. (1986). Does maintenance lithium therapy prevent recurrences of mania under ordinary clinical conditions? *Psychol Med*, 16(3), 521–530.

Duffy, A., Alda, M., Kutcher, S., Cavazzoni, P., Robertson, C., Grof, E., and Grof, P. (2002). A prospective study of the offspring of bipolar parents responsive and nonresponsive to lithium treatment. *J Clin Psychiatry*, 63(12), 1171–1178.

Dunner, D.L., and Fieve, R.R. (1974). Clinical factors in lithium carbonate prophylaxis failure. *Arch Gen Psychiatry*, 30(2), 229–233.

Dunner, D.L., Dwyer, T., and Fieve, R.R. (1976). Depressive symptoms in patients with unipolar and bipolar affective disorder. *Compr Psychiatry*, 17(3), 447–451.

Dunner, D.L., Patrick, V., and Fieve, R.R. (1977). Rapid cycling manic depressive patients. *Compr Psychiatry*, 18(6), 561–566.

Eberhard-Gran, M., Eskild, A., and Opjordsmoen, S. (2005). Treating mood disorders during pregnancy: Safety considerations. *Drug Saf*, 28(8), 695–706.

Ernst, C.L., and Goldberg, J.F. (2002). The reproductive safety profile of mood stabilizers, atypical antipsychotics, and broad-spectrum psychotropics. *J Clin Psychiatry*, 63(Suppl. 4), 42–55.

Esparon, J., Kolloori, J., Naylor, G.J., McHarg, A.M., Smith, A.H., and Hopwood, S.E. (1986). Comparison of the prophylactic action of flupenthixol with placebo in lithium treated manic-depressive patients. *Br J Psychiatry*, 148, 723–725.

Eyer, F., Pfab, R., Felgenhauer, N., Lutz, J., Heemann, U., Steimer, W., Zondler, S., Fichtl, B., and Zilker, T. (2006). Lithium poisoning: pharmacokinetics and clearance during different therapeutic measures. *J Clin Psychopharmacol*, 26(3), 325–330.

Faedda, G.L., Tondo, L., Baldessarini, R.J., Suppes, T., and Tohen, M. (1993). Outcome after rapid vs. gradual discontinuation of lithium treatment in bipolar mood disorders. *Arch Gen Psychiatry*, 50, 448–455.

Fagiolini, A., Frank, E., Houck, P.R., Mallinger, A.G., Swartz, H.A., Buysse, D.J., Ombao, H., and Kupfer, D.J. (2002). Prevalence of obesity and weight change during treatment in patients with bipolar I disorder. *J Clin Psychiatry*, 63(6), 528–533.

Fagiolini, A., Frank, E., Scott, J.A., Turkin, S., and Kupfer, D.J. (2005). Metabolic syndrome in bipolar disorder: Findings from the Bipolar Disorder Center for Pennsylvanians. *Bipolar Disord*, 7(5), 424–430.

Fava, G.A. (2003). Can long-term treatment with antidepressant drugs worsen the course of depression? *J Clin Psychiatry*, 64(2), 123–133.

Fieve, R.R., Kumbaraci, T., and Dunner, D.L. (1976). Lithium prophylaxis of depression in bipolar I, bipolar II, and unipolar patients. *Am J Psychiatry*, 133(8), 925–929.

Folstein, M.F., DePaulo, J.R. Jr., and Trepp, K. (1982). Unusual mood stability in patients taking lithium. *Br J Psychiatry*, 140, 188–191.

Forty, L., Jones, L., Macgregor, S., Caesar, S., Cooper, C., Hough, A., Dean, L., Dave, S., Farmer, A., McGuffin, P., Brewster, S., Craddock, N., and Jones, I. (2006). Familiality of postpartum depression in unipolar disorder: Results of a family study. *Am J Psychiatry*, 163(9), 1549–1553.

Frangou, S., Raymont, V., and Bettany, D. (2002). The Maudsley bipolar disorder project: A survey of psychotropic prescribing patterns in bipolar I disorder. *Bipolar Disord*, 4(6), 378–385.

Frank, E., Kupfer, D.J., Wagner, E.F., McEachran, A.B., and Cornes, C. (1991). Efficacy of interpersonal psychotherapy as a maintenance treatment of recurrent depression: Contributing factors. *Arch Gen Psychiatry*, 48(12), 1053–1059.

Frankenburg, F.R., and Zanarini, M.C. (2002). Divalproex sodium treatment of women with borderline personality disorder and bipolar II disorder: A double-blind placebo-controlled pilot study. *J Clin Psychiatry*, 63(5), 442–446.

Freeman, M.P., and Stoll, A.L. (1998). Mood stabilizer combinations: A review of safety and efficacy. *Am J Psychiatry*, 155(1), 12–21.

Frye, M.A., Denicoff, K.D., Bryan, A.L., Smith-Jackson, E.E., Ali, S.O., Luckenbaugh, D., Leverich, G.S., and Post, R.M. (1999).

Association between lower serum free T4 and greater mood instability and depression in lithium-maintained bipolar patients. *Am J Psychiatry*, 156(12), 1909–1914.

Frye, M., Ketter, T.A., Kimbrell, T.A., Dunn, R.T., Speer, A.M., Osuch, E.A., Luckenbaugh, D.A., Cora-Ocatelli, G., Leverich, G.S., and Post, R.M. (2000). A placebo-controlled study of lamotrigine and gabapentin monotherapy in refractory mood disorders. *J Clin Psychopharmacol*, 20(6), 607–612.

Garza-Trevino, E.S., Overall, J.E., and Hollister, L.E. (1992). Verapamil versus lithium in acute mania. *Am J Psychiatry*, 149(1), 121–122.

Geddes, J.R., Rendell, J.M., and Goodwin, G. (2002). BALANCE: A large simple trial of maintenance treatment for bipolar disorder. *World Psychiatry*, 1(1), 48–51.

Geddes, J.R., Burgess, S., Hawton, K., Jamison, K., and Goodwin, G.M. (2004). Long-term lithium therapy for bipolar disorder: Systematic review and meta-analysis of randomized controlled trials. *Am J Psychiatry*, 161(2), 217–222.

Gelenberg, A.J., Kane, J.M., Keller, M.B., Lavori, P., Rosenbaum, J.F., Cole, K., and Lavelle, J. (1989). Comparison of standard and low serum levels of lithium for maintenance treatment of bipolar disorder. *N Engl J Med*, 321(22), 1489–1493.

Gentile, S. (2004). Clinical utilization of atypical antipsychotics in pregnancy and lactation. *Ann Pharmacother*, 38(7–8), 1265–1271.

Gentile, S. (2006). Prophylactic treatment of bipolar disorder in pregnancy and breastfeeding: Focus on emerging mood stabilizers. *Bipolar Disord*, 8(3), 207–220.

Ghaemi, S.N. (2001). On defining "mood stabilizer." *Bipolar Disord*, 3(3), 154–158.

Ghaemi, S.N., and Goodwin, F.K. (2001). Long-term naturalistic treatment of depressive symptoms in bipolar illness with divalproex vs. lithium in the setting of minimal antidepressant use. *J Affect Disord*, 65(3), 281–287.

Ghaemi, S.N., and Goodwin, F.K. (2005). Antidepressants for bipolar depression. *Am J Psychiatry*, 162(8), 1545–1546.

Ghaemi, S.N., and Sachs, G.S. (1997). Long-term risperidone treatment in bipolar disorder: 6-Month follow up. *Int Clin Psychopharmacol*, 12(6), 333–338.

Ghaemi, S.N., Boiman, E.E., and Goodwin, F.K. (2000). Diagnosing bipolar disorder and the effect of antidepressants: A naturalistic study. *J Clin Psychiatry*, 804–808.

Ghaemi, S.N., Lenox, M.S., and Baldessarini, R.J. (2001a). Effectiveness and safety of long-term antidepressant treatment in bipolar disorder. *J Clin Psychiatry*, 62(7), 565–569.

Ghaemi, S.N., Manwani, S.G., Katzow, J.J., Ko, J.Y., and Goodwin, F.K. (2001b). Topiramate treatment of bipolar spectrum disorders: A retrospective chart review. *Ann Clin Psychiatry*, 13(4), 185–189.

Ghaemi, S.N., Ko, J.Y., and Katzow, J.J. (2002). Oxcarbazepine treatment of refractory bipolar disorder: A retrospective chart review. *Bipolar Disord*, 4, 70–74.

Ghaemi, S.N., Hsu, D.J., Rosenquist, K.J., Pardo, T.B., and Goodwin, F.K. (2000). Extrapyramidal side effects with atypical neuroleptics in bipolar disorder. *Prog Neuropsychopharmacol Biol Psychiatry*, 30(2), 209–213.

Gitlin, M. (1999). Lithium and the kidney: An updated review. *Drug Saf*, 20(3), 231–243.

Glazer, W.M., Sonnenberg, J.G., Reinstein, M.J., and Akers, R.F. (2004). A novel, point-of-care test for lithium levels: Description and reliability. *J Clin Psychiatry*, 65(5), 652–655.

Goldberg, J.F., Garno, J.L., Leon, A.C., Kocsis, J.H., and Portera, L. (1998). Rapid titration of mood stabilizers predicts remission from mixed or pure mania in bipolar patients. *J Clin Psychiatry*, 59(4), 151–158.

Goodnick, P.J. (1993). Verapamil prophylaxis in pregnant women with bipolar disorder. *Am J Psychiatry*, 150(10), 1560.

Goodwin, F.K. (1989). The biology of recurrence: New directions for the pharmacologic bridge. *J Clin Psychiatry*, 50(Suppl.), 40–44; discussion 45–47.

Goodwin, F.K. (2003). Rationale for using lithium in combination with other mood stabilizers in the management of bipolar disorder. *J Clin Psychiatry*, 64(Suppl. 5), 18–24.

Goodwin, F.K., and Goldstein, M. (2003). Optimizing lithium treatment in bipolar disorder: A review of the literature and clinical recommendations. *J Psychiatr Pract*, 9(5), 1–11.

Goodwin, F.K., and Jamison, K.R. (1990). *Manic-Depressive Illness*. New York: Oxford University Press.

Goodwin, G.M. (1994). Recurrence of mania after lithium withdrawal: Implications for the use of lithium in the treatment of bipolar affective disorder. *Br J Psychiatry*, 164(2), 149–152.

Goodwin, G.M., and Geddes, J.R. (2003). Latest maintenance data on lithium in bipolar disorder. *Eur Neuropsychopharmacol*, 13(Suppl. 2), S51–S55.

Goodwin, G.M., Cavanagh, J.T., Glabus, M.F., Kehoe, R.F., O'Carroll, R.E., and Ebmeier, K.P. (1997). Uptake of ^{99m}Tc-exametazime shown by single photon emission computed tomography before and after lithium withdrawal in bipolar patients: Associations with mania. *Br J Psychiatry*, 170, 426–430.

Goodwin, G.M., Bowden, C.L., Calabrese, J.R., Grunze, H., Kasper, S., White, R., Greene, P., and Leadbetter, R. (2004). A pooled analysis of 2 placebo-controlled 18-month trials of lamotrigine and lithium maintenance in bipolar I disorder. *J Clin Psychiatry*, 65(3), 432–441.

Graham, K.A., Gu, H., Lieberman, J.A., Harp, J.B., and Perkins, D.O. (2005). Double-blind, placebo-controlled investigation of amantadine for weight loss in subjects who gained weight with olanzapine. *Am J Psychiatry*, 162(9), 1744–1746.

Greil, W., and Kleindienst, N. (1999). Lithium versus carbamazepine in the maintenance treatment of bipolar II disorder and bipolar disorder not otherwise specified. *Int Clin Psychopharmacol*, 14(5), 283–285.

Greil, W., Ludwig-Mayerhofer, W., Erazo, N., Engel, R.R., Czernik, A., Giedke, H., Muller-Oerlinghausen, B., Osterheider, M., Rudolf, G.A., Sauer, H., Tegeler, J., and Wetterling, T. (1997). Lithium vs. carbamazepine in the maintenance treatment of schizoaffective disorder: A randomised study. *Eur Arch Psychiatry Clin Neurosci*, 247(1), 42–50.

Grof, P., and Alda, M. (2000). Discrepancies in the efficacy of lithium. *Arch Gen Psychiatry*, 57(2), 191.

Grof, P., Cakulis, P., and Dostal, T. (1970). Lithium dropouts: A follow-up study of patients who discontinued prophylactic treatment. *Int Pharmacopsychiatry*, 5, 162–169.

Grof, P., Alda, M., Grof, E., Zvolsky, P., and Walsh, M. (1994). Lithium response and genetics of affective disorders. *J Affect Disord*, 32(2), 85–95.

Grof, P., Robbins, W., Alda, M., Berghoefer, A., Vojtechovsky, M., Nilsson, A. (2000). Protective effect of pregnancy in women with lithium-responsive bipolar disorder. *J Affect Disord*, 61(1–2), 31–39.

Gruenwald J., The Medical Economics Team, and PDR Physicians Desk Reference Team (Eds.). (2004). *PDR for Herbal Medicines* (3rd edition). Montvale, NJ: Thompson PDR.

Grunze, H., Erfurth, A., Marcuse, A., Amann, B., Normann, C., and Walden, J. (1999). Tiagabine appears not to be efficacious in the treatment of acute mania. *J Clin Psychiatry*, 60(11), 759–762.

Grunze, H., Kasper, S., Goodwin, G., Bowden, C., Baldwin, D., Licht, R. (2002). World Federation of Societies of Biological Psychiatry (WFSBP) guidelines for biological treatment of bipolar disorders. Part I: Treatment of bipolar depression. *World J Biol Psychiatry*, 3(3), 115–124.

Grunze, H., Kasper, S., Goodwin, G., Bowden, C., Moller, H.J., WFSBP Task Force on Treatment Guidelines for Bipolar Disorders. (2004). The World Federation of Societies of Biological Psychiatry (WFSBP) guidelines for the biological treatment of bipolar disorders, part III: Maintenance treatment. *World J Biol Psychiatry*, 5(3), 120–135.

Guo, J.J., Keck, P.E., Corey-Lisle, P.K., Li, H., Jiang, D., Jang, R., and L'italien, G.J. (2006). Risk of diabetes mellitus associated with atypical antipsychotic use among patients with bipolar disorder: A retrospective, population-based, case-control study. *J Clin Psychiatry*, 67(7), 1055–1061.

Gyulai, L., Bowden, C.L., McElroy, S.L., Calabrese, J.R., Petty, F., Swann, A.C., Chou, J.C., Wassef, A., Risch, C.S., Hirschfeld, R.M., Nemeroff, C.B., Keck, P.E. Jr., Evans, D.L., and Wozniak, P.J. (2003). Maintenance efficacy of divalproex in the prevention of bipolar depression. *Neuropsychopharmacology*, 28(7), 1374–1382.

Harrow, M., Goldberg, J.F., Grossman, L.S., and Meltzer, H.Y. (1990). Outcome in manic disorders: A naturalistic follow-up study. *Arch Gen Psychiatry*, 47(7), 665–671.

Hartong, E.G., Moleman, P., Hoogduin, C.A., Broekman, T.G., Nolen, W.A., and LitCar Group. (2003). Prophylactic efficacy of lithium versus carbamazepine in treatment-naive bipolar patients. *J Clin Psychiatry*, 64(2), 144–151.

Henderson, D.C., Cagliero, E., Gray, C., Nasrallah, R.A., Hayden, D.L., Schoenfeld, D.A., and Goff, D.C. (2000). Clozapine, diabetes mellitus, weight gain, and lipid abnormalities: A five-year naturalistic study. *Am J Psychiatry*, 157(6), 975–981.

Hendrick, V., Altshuler, L., and Whybrow, P. (1998). Psychoneuroendocrinology of mood disorders: The hypothalamic-pituitary-thyroid axis. *Psychiatr Clin North Am*, 21(2), 277–292.

Holinger, P.C., and Wolpert, E.A. (1979). A ten year follow-up of lithium use. *IMJ Ill Med J*, 156(2), 99–104.

Hopkins, H.S., and Gelenberg, A.J. (2000). Serum lithium levels and the outcome of maintenance therapy of bipolar disorder. *Bipolar Disord*, 3(5), 174–179.

Isaksson, A., Ottosson, J.O., and Perris, C. (1969). Methologische aspekte der Forschung über prophylaktische Behandlung bei affektiven Psychosen. In H. Hippius and H. Selbach (Eds.), *Das Depressive Syndrom* (pp. 561–574). Munich: Urban and Schwarzenberg.

Isojarvi, J.I., Laatikainen, T.J., Pakarinen, A.J., Juntunen, K.T., and Myllyla, V.V. (1993). Polycystic ovaries and hyperandrogenism in women taking valproate for epilepsy. *N Engl J Med*, 329(19), 1383–1388.

Jacobsen, F.M., and Comas-Diaz, L. (1999). Donepezil for psychotropic-induced memory loss. *J Clin Psychiatry*, 60(10), 698–704.

Jacobson, S.J., Jones, K., Johnson, K., Ceolin, L., Kaur, P., Sahn, D., Donnenfeld, A.E., Rieder, M., Santelli, R., Smythe, J. (1992). Prospective multicentre study of pregnancy outcome after lithium exposure during first trimester. *Lancet*, 339(8792), 530–533.

Jamison, K.R., Gerner, R.H., and Goodwin, F.K. (1979). Patient and physician attitudes toward lithium: Relationship to compliance. *Arch Gen Psychiatry*, 36(Spec. No. 8), 866–869.

Joffe, H., Hall, J.E., Cohen, L.S., Taylor, A.E., and Baldessarini, R.J. (2003). A putative relationship between valproic acid and polycystic ovarian syndrome: Implications for treatment of women with seizure and bipolar disorders. *Harv Rev Psychiatry*, 11(2), 99–108.

Joffe, H., Cohen, L.S., Suppes, T., McLaughlin, W.L., Lavori, P., and Adams, J.M. (2006). Valproate is associated with new-onset oligoamenorrhea with hyperandrogenism in women with bipolar disorder. *Biol Psychiatry*, 59(11), 1078–1086.

Johnston, A.M., and Eagles, J.M. (1999). Lithium-associated clinical hypothyroidism: Prevalence and risk factors. *Br J Psychiatry*, 175, 336–339.

Jones, I., and Craddock, N. (2001). Familiality of the puerperal trigger in bipolar disorder: Results of a family study. *Am J Psychiatry*, 158(6), 913–917.

Jones, I., and Craddock, N. (2005). Bipolar disorder and childbirth: The importance of recognising risk. *Br J Psychiatry*, 186, 453–454.

Judd, L.L., Akiskal, H.S., Schettler, P.J., Endicott, J., Leon, A.C., and Solomon, D.A. (2005). Psychosocial disability in the course of bipolar I and II disorders: A prospective, comparative, longitudinal study. *Arch Gen Psychiatry*, 62(12), 1322–1330.

Kahn, D.A., Sachs, G.S., Printz, D.J., Carpenter, D., Docherty, J.P., and Ross, R. (2000). Medication treatment of bipolar disorder 2000: A summary of the expert consensus guidelines. *J Psychiatr Pract*, 6(4), 197–211.

Kallen, A.J. (1994). Maternal carbamazepine and infant spina bifida. *Reprod Toxicol*, 8(3), 203–205.

Kallner, G., Lindelius, R., Petterson, U., Stockman, O., and Tham, A. (2000). Mortality in 497 patients with affective disorders attending a lithium clinic or after having left it. *Pharmacopsychiatry*, 33(1), 8–13.

Kane, J.M., Quitkin, R.A., Ramos-Lorenzi, J.R., Nayak, D.D., and Howard, A. (1982). Lithium carbonate and imipramine in the prophylaxis of unipolar and bipolar II illness: A prospective, placebo-controlled comparison. *Arch Gen Psychiatry*, 39, 1065–1069.

Kanner, A.M., and Frey, M. (2000). Adding valproate to lamotrigine: A study of their pharmacokinetic interaction. *Neurology*, 55(4), 588–591.

Kaplan, B.J., Simpson, J.S., Ferre, R.C., Gorman, C.P., McMullen, D.M., and Crawford, S.G. (2001). Effective mood stabilization with a chelated mineral supplement: An open-label trial in bipolar disorder. *J Clin Psychiatry*, 62(12), 936–944.

Kaplan, B.J., Fisher, J.E., Crawford, S.G., Field, C.J., and Kolb, B. (2004). Improved mood and behavior during treatment with a mineral-vitamin supplement: A open-label case series of children. *J Child Adolesc Psychopharmacol*, 14(1), 115–122.

Keck, P.E. Jr., and McElroy, S.L. (2003). Redefining mood stabilization. *J Affect Disord*, 73(1–2), 163–169.

Keck, P.E., McElroy, S.L., Strakowski, S.M., Balistreri, T.M., Kizer, D.I., and West, S.A. (1996). Factors associated with maintenance antipsychotic treatment of patients with bipolar disorder. *J Clin Psychiatry*, 57(4), 147–151.

Keck, P.E. Jr., Mendlwicz, J., Calabrese, J.R., Fawcett, J., Suppes, T., Vestergaard, P.A., and Carbonell, C. (2000). A review of randomized, controlled clinical trials in acute mania. *J Affect Disord*, 59(Suppl. 1), S31–S37.

Keck, P.E. Jr., Calabrese, J.R., McQuade, R.D., Carson, W.H., Carlson, B.X., Rollin, L.M., Marcus, R.N., Sanchez, R., and Aripiprazole Study Group. (2006). A randomized, double-blind, placebo-controlled 26-week trial of aripiprazole in recently manic patients with bipolar I disorder. *J Clin Psychiatry*, 67(4), 626–637.

Keller, M.B., Lavori, P.W., Mueller, T.I., Endicott, J., Coryell, W., Hirschfeld, R.M., and Shea, T. (1992). Time to recovery, chronicity, and levels of psychopathology in major depression: A 5-year prospective follow-up of 431 subjects. *Arch Gen Psychiatry*, 49(10), 809–816.

Keller, M.B., Lavori, P.W., Coryell, W., Endicott, J., and Mueller, T.I. (1993). Bipolar I: A five-year prospective follow-up. *J Nerv Ment Dis*, 181(4), 238–245.

Ketter, T.A., and Calabrese, J.R. (2002). Stabilization of mood from below versus above baseline in bipolar disorder: A new nomenclature. *J Clin Psychiatry*, 63(2), 146–151.

Ketter, T.A., Wang, P.W., Chandler, R.A., Alarcon, A.M., Becker, O.V., Nowakowska, C., O'Keeffe, C.M., and Schumacher, M.R. (2005). Dermatology precautions and slower titration yield low incidence of lamotrigine treatment-emergent rash. *J Clin Psychiatry*, 66(5), 642–645.

Ketter, T.A., Houston, J.P., Adams, D.H., Risser, R.C., Meyers, A.L., Williamson, D.J., and Tohen, M. (2006). Differential efficacy of olanzapine and lithium in preventing manic or mixed recurrence in patients with bipolar I disorder based on number of previous manic or mixed episodes. *J Clin Psychiatry*, 67(1), 95–101.

King, J.R., and Hullin, R.P. (1983). Withdrawal symptoms from lithium: Four case reports and a questionnaire study. *Br J Psychiatry*, 143, 30–35.

Kirov, G., Tredget, J., John R., Owen, M.J., and Lazarus, J.H. (2005). A cross-sectional and a prospective study of thyroid disorders in lithium-treated patients. *J Affect Disord*, 87(2-3), 313–317.

Kishimoto, A. (1992). The treatment of affective disorder with carbamazepine: Prophylactic synergism of lithium and carbamazepine combination. *Prog Neuropsychopharmacol Biol Psychiatry*, 16(4), 483–493.

Kishimoto, A., Ogura, C., Hazama, H., and Inoue, K. (1983). Long-term prophylactic effects of carbamazepine in affective disorder. *Br J Psychiatry*, 143, 327–331.

Kleindienst, N., and Greil, W. (2002). Inter-episodic morbidity and drop-out under carbamazepine and lithium in the maintenance treatment of bipolar disorder. *Psychol Med*, 32(3), 493–501.

Kleindienst, N., Greil, W., Ruger, B., and Moller, H.J. (1999). The prophylactic efficacy of lithium—transient or persistent? *Eur Arch Psychiatry Clin Neurosci*, 249(3), 144–149.

Kleindienst, N., Engel, R., and Greil, W. (2005). Which clinical factors predict response to prophylactic lithium? A systematic review for bipolar disorders. *Bipolar Disord*, 7(5), 404–417.

Kleiner, J., Altshuler, L., Hendrick, V., and Hershman, J.M. (1999). Lithium-induced subclinical hypothyroidism: Review of the literature and guidelines for treatment. *J Clin Psychiatry*, 60(4), 249–255.

Knoll, J., Stegman, K., and Suppes, T. (1998). Clinical experience using gabapentin adjunctively in patients with a history of mania or hypomania. *J Affect Disord*, 49(3), 229–233.

Kukopulos, A., Reginaldi, D., Laddomada, P., Floris, G., Serra, G., and Tondo, L. (1980). Course of the manic-depressive cycle and changes caused by treatment. *Pharmakopsychiatr Neuropsychopharmakol*, 13(4), 156–167.

Kupka, R.W., Nolen, W.A., Post, R.M., McElroy, S.L., Altshuler, L.L., Denicoff, K.D., Frye, M.A., Keck, P.E. Jr., Leverich, G.S., Rush, A.J., Suppes, T., Pollio, C., Drexhage, H.A. (2002). High rate of autoimmune thyroiditis in bipolar disorder: Lack of association with lithium exposure. *Biol Psychiatry*, 51(4), 305–311.

Kupka, R.W., Luckenbaugh, D.A., Post, R.M., Leverich, G.S., and Nolen, W.A. (2003). Rapid and non-rapid cycling bipolar disorder: A meta-analysis of clinical studies. *J Clin Psychiatry*, 64(12), 1483–1494.

Kusalic, M. (1992). Grade II and grade III hypothyroidism in rapid-cycling bipolar patients. *Neuropsychobiology*, 25(4), 177–181.

Lambert, P.A., Borselli, S., Marcou, G., Bouchardy, M., and Cabrol, G. (1971). Long-term thymoregulative action of Depamide in manic-depressive psychoses. *Ann Med Psychol (Paris)*, 2(3), 442–448.

Laurell, B., and Ottosson, J.O. (1968). Prophylactic lithium? *Lancet*, 2(7580), 1245–1246.

Lepkifker, E., Sverdlik, A., Iancu, I., Ziv, R., Segev, S., and Kotler, M. (2004). Renal insufficiency in long-term lithium treatment. *J Clin Psychiatry*, 65(6), 850–856.

Leucht, S., Wahlbeck, K., Hamann, J., and Kissling, W. (2003). New generation antipsychotics versus low-potency conventional antipsychotics: A systematic review and meta-analysis. *Lancet*, 361(9369), 1581–1589.

Levy, E., Margolese, H.C., and Chouinard, G. (2002). Topiramate produced weight loss following olanzapine-induced weight gain in schizophrenia. *J Clin Psychiatry*, 63(11), 1045.

Licht, R.W., Vestergaard, P., Rasmussen, N.A., Jepsen, K., Brodersen, A., and Hansen, P.E. (2001). A lithium clinic for bipolar patients: 2-Year outcome of the first 148 patients. *Acta Psychiatr Scand*, 104(5), 387–390.

Lieberman, D.Z., and Goodwin, F.K. (2004). Separate and concomitant use of lamotrigine, lithium, and divalproex in bipolar disorders. *Curr Psychiatry Rep*, 6(6), 459–465.

Lipkovich, I., Citrome, L., Perlis, R., Deberdt, W., Houston, J.P., Ahl, J., and Hardy, T. (2006). Early predictors of substantial weight gain in bipolar patients treated with olanzapine. *J Clin Psychopharmacol*, 26(3), 316–320.

Littlejohn, R., Leslie, F., and Cookson, J. (1994). Depot antipsychotics in the prophylaxis of bipolar affective disorder. *Br J Psychiatry*, 165(6), 827–829.

Luby, E.D., and Singareddy, R.K. (2003). Long-term therapy with lithium in a private practice clinic: A naturalistic study. *Bipolar Disord*, 5(1), 62–68.

Luznat, R.M., Murphy, D.P., and Nunn, C.M.H. (1988). Carbamazepine vs. lithium treatment and prophylaxis of mania. *Br J Psychiatry*, 153, 198–204.

Lydon, E., and El-Mallakh, R.S. (2006). Naturalistic long-term use of methylphenidate in bipolar disorder. *J Clin Psychopharmacol*, 26(5), 516–518.

Macritchie, K.A., Geddes, J.R., Scott, J., Haslam, D.R., and Goodwin, G.M. (2001). Valproic acid, valproate and divalproex in the maintenance treatment of bipolar disorder. *Cochrane Database Syst Rev*, (3):CD003196.

Macritchie, K.A.N., Geddes, J.R., Scott, J., Haslam, D.R.S., and Goodwin, G.M. (2002). Valproic acid, valproate and divalproex in the maintenance treatment of bipolar disorder. *Cochrane Database Syst Rev*, (3), CD003196.

Maj, M., Starace, F., Nolfe, G., and Kemali, D. (1986). Minimum plasma lithium levels required for effective prophylaxis in DSM III bipolar disorder: A prospective study. *Pharmacopsychiatry*, 19, 420–423.

Maj, M., Pirozzi, R., and Magliano, L. (1995). Nonresponse to re-instituted lithium prophylaxis in previously responsive bipolar patients: prevalence and predictors. *Am J Psychiatry*, 152(12), 1810–1811.

Maj, M., Pirozzi, R., and Magliano, L. (1996). Late non-response to lithium prophylaxis in bipolar patients: Prevalence and predictors. *J Affect Disord*, 39(1), 39–42.

Maj, M., Pirozzi, R., Magliano, L., and Bartoli, L. (1998). Long-term outcome of lithium prophylaxis in bipolar disorder: A 5-year prospective study of 402 patients at a lithium clinic. *Am J Psychiatry*, 155(1), 30–35.

Maj, M., Pirozzi, R., Bartoli, L., and Magliano, L. (2002). Long-term outcome of lithium prophylaxis in bipolar disorder with mood-incongruent psychotic features: A prospective study. *J Affect Disord*, 71(1–3), 195–198.

Malone, K., Papagni, K., Ramini, S., and Keltner, N.L. (2004). Antidepressants, antipsychotics, benzodiazepines, and the breast-feeding dyad. *Perspect Psychiatr Care*, 40(2), 73–85.

Marcotte, D. (1998). Use of topiramate, a new anti-epileptic as a mood stabilizer. *J Affect Disord*, 50(2–3), 245–251.

Markar, H.R., and Mander, A.J. (1989). Efficacy of lithium prophylaxis in clinical practice. *Br J Psychiatry*, 155, 496–500.

Markowitz, G.S., Radhakrishnan, J., Kambham, N., Valeri, A.M., Hines, W.H., D'Agati, V.D. (2000). Lithium nephrotoxicity: A progressive combined glomerular and tubulointerstitial nephropathy. *J Am Soc Nephrol*, 11(8), 1439–1448.

McElroy, S.L., Suppes, T., Keck, P.E., Frye, M.A., Denicoff, K.D., Altshuler, L.L., Brown, E.S., Nolen, W.A., Kupka, R.W., Rochussen, J., Leverich, G.S., and Post, R.M. (2000). Open-label adjunctive topiramate in the treatment of bipolar disorders. *Biol Psychiatry*, 47(12), 1025–1033.

McIntyre, R.S., Girgla, S., Binder, C., Riccardelli, R., and Kennedy, S.H. (2002). *Efficacy of topiramate as adjunctive therapy to mood stabilizers in patients with bipolar I or II disorder.* Poster presented at the Meeting of the American College of Neurosychopharmacology, Puerto Rico.

McIntyre, R.S., Mancini, D.A., McCann, S., Srinivasan, J., and Kennedy, S.H. (2003). Valproate, bipolar disorder and polycystic ovarian syndrome. *Bipolar Disord*, 5(1), 28–35.

McKenna, K., Koren, G., Tetelbaum, M., Wilton, L., Shakir, S., Diav-Citrin, O., Levinson, A., Zipursky, R.B., and Einarson, A. (2005). Pregnancy outcome of women using atypical antipsychotic drugs: A prospective comparative study. *J Clin Psychiatry*, 66(4), 444–449; quiz 546.

McQuade, R.D., Stock, E., Marcus, R., Jody, D., Gharbia, N.A., Vanveggel, S., Archibald, D., Carson, W.H. (2004). A comparison of weight change during treatment with olanzapine or aripiprazole: Results from a randomized, double-blind study. *J Clin Psychiatry*, 65(Suppl. 18), 47–56.

Melia, P.I. (1970). Prophylactic lithium: A double-blind trial in recurrent affective disorders. *Br J Psychiatry*, 115, 621–624.

Miller, A.L., Bowden, C.L., and Plewes, J. (1985). Lithium and impairment of renal concentrating ability. *J Affect Disord*, 9(2), 115–119.

Mishory, A., Winokur, M., and Bersudsky, Y. (2003). Prophylactic effect of phenytoin in bipolar disorder: A controlled study. *Bipolar Disord*, 5, 464–467.

Mockenhaupt, M., Messenheimer, J., Tennis, P., and Schlingmann, J. (2005). Risk of Stevens-Johnson syndrome and toxic epidermal necrolysis in new users of antiepileptics. *Neurology*, 64, 1134–1138.

Moretti, M.E., Koren, G., Verjee, Z., and Ito, S. (2003). Monitoring lithium in breast milk: An individualized approach for breast-feeding mothers. *Ther Drug Monit*, 25(3), 364–366.

Movig, K.L., Leufkens, H.G., Belitser, S.V., Lenderink, A.W., and Egberts, A.C. (2002). Selective serotonin reuptake inhibitor-induced urinary incontinence. *Pharmacoepidemiol Drug Saf*, 11(4), 271–279.

Movig, K.L., Baumgarten, R., Leufkens, H.G., van Laarhoven, J.H., and Egberts, A.C. (2003). Risk factors for the development of lithium-induced polyuria. *Br J Psychiatry*, 182, 319–323.

Munoz, R. (2002). *Oxcarbazepine for the treatment of bipolar disorder.* Poster presented to the Meeting of the American Psychiatric Association, Philadelphia, PA.

Murray, M., Hopwood S., Balfour, D.J.K., Ogston, S., and Hewick, D.S. (1983). The influence of age on lithium efficacy and side effects in out-patients. *Pscychol Med*, 13, 53–60.

Narendran, R., Young, C.M., Valenti, A.M., Pristach, C.A., Pato, M.T., and Grace, J.J. (2001). Olanzapine therapy in treatment-resistant psychotic mood disorders: A long-term follow-up study. *J Clin Psychiatry*, 62(7), 509–516.

Nascimento, A.L., Appolinario, J.C., Segenreich, D., Cavalcanti, M.T., and Brasil, M.A. (2006). Maintenance electroconvulsive therapy for recurrent refractory mania. *Bipolar Disord*, 8(3), 301–303.

Nasr, S., and Caspar, M. (2002). *Oxcarbazepine for the treatment of bipolar disorder.* Poster presented to the Meeting of the American Psychiatric Association, Philadelphia, PA.

Nemeroff, C.B. (2003). Advancing the treatment of mood and anxiety disorders: The first 10 years' experience with paroxetine. *Psychopharmacol Bull*, 37(Suppl. 1), 6–7.

Newcomer, J.W. (2006). Medical risk in patients with bipolar disorder and schizophrenia. *J Clin Psychiatry*, 67(Suppl. 9), 25–30.

Newcomer, J.W., Haupt, D.W., Fucetola, R., Melson, A.K., Schweiger, J.A., Cooper, B.P., and Selke, G. (2002). Abnormalities in glucose regulation during antipsychotic treatment of schizophrenia. *Arch Gen Psychiatry*, 59(4), 337–345.

Newport, D.J., Viguera, A.C., Beach, A.J., Ritchie, J.C., Cohen, L.S., and Stowe, Z.N. (2005). Lithium placental passage and obstetrical outcome: Implications for clinical management during late pregnancy. *Am J Psychiatry*, 162(11), 2162–2170.

Noack, C.H., and Trautner, E.M. (1951). The lithium treatment of maniacal psychosis. *Med J Aust*, 2(7), 219–222.

Nonacs, R., and Cohen, L.S. (2003). Assessment and treatment of depression during pregnancy: An update. *Psychiatr Clin North Am*, 26, 547–562.

Nulman, I., Rovet, J., Stewart, D.E., Wolpin, J., Pace-Asciak, P., Shuhaiber, S., and Koren, G. (2002). Child development following exposure to tricyclic antidepressants or fluoxetine throughout fetal life: A prospective, controlled study. *Am J Psychiatry*, 159(11), 1889–1895.

O'Donovan, C., Kusumakar, V., Graves, G.R., and Bird, D.C. (2002). Menstrual abnormalities and polycystic ovary syndrome in women taking valproate for bipolar mood disorder. *J Clin Psychiatry*, 63(4), 322–330.

Okuma, T. (1993). Effects of carbamazepine and lithium on affective disorders. *Neuropsychobiology*, 27(3), 138–145.

Okuma, T., Kishimoto, A., Inoue, K., Matsumoto, H., and Ogura, A. (1973). Anti-manic and prophylactic effects of carbamazepine (Tegretol) on manic depressive psychosis: A preliminary report. *Folia Psychiatr Neurol Jpn*, 27(4), 283–297.

Okuma, T., Koga, I., and Uchida, Y. (1976). Sensitivity to chlorpromazine effects on brain function of schizophrenics and normals: A preliminary report. *Psychopharmacology (Berl)*, 51(1), 101–105.

Okuma, T., Inanaga, K., Otsuki, S., Sarai, K., Takahashi, R., Hazama, H., Mori, A., and Watanabe, S. (1981). A preliminary double-blind study on the efficacy of carbamazepine in prophylaxis of manic-depressive illness. *Psychopharmacology (Berl)*, 73(1), 95–96.

Pande, A.C., Crockatt, J.G., Janney, C.A., Werth, J.L., and Tsaroucha, G. (2000). Gabapentin in bipolar disorder: A placebo-controlled trial of adjunctive therapy. Gabapentin Bipolar Disorder Study Group. *Bipolar Disord*, 2 (3 Pt. 2), 249–255.

Parker, G., Tully, L., Olley, A., and Hadzi-Pavlovic, D. (2006). SSRIs as mood stabilizers for bipolar II disorder? A proof of concept study. *J Affect Disord*, 92(2-3), 205–214.

Passmore, M.J., Garnham, J., Duffy, A., MacDougall, M., Munro, A., Slaney, C., Teehan, A., and Alda, M. (2003). Phenotypic spectra of bipolar disorder in responders to lithium versus lamotrigine. *Bipolar Disord*, 5(2), 110–114.

Pazzaglia, P.J., Post, R.M., Ketter, T.A., George, M.S., and Marangell, L.B. (1993). Preliminary controlled trial of nimodipine in ultra-rapid cycling affective dysregulation. *Psychiatry Res*, 49(3), 257–272.

Pazzaglia, P.J., Post, R.M., Ketter, T.A., Callahan, A.M., Marangell, L.B., Frye, M.A., George, M.S., Kimbrell, T.A., Leverich, G.S., Cora-Locatelli, G., and Luckenbaugh, D. (1998). Nimodipine monotherapy and carbamazepine augmentation in patients with refractory recurrent affective illness. *J Clin Psychopharmacol*, 18(5), 404–413.

Perlis, R.H., Sachs, G.S., Lafer, B., Otto, M.W., Faraone, S.V., Kane, J.M., and Rosenbaum, J.F. (2002). Effect of abrupt change from standard to low serum levels of lithium: A reanalysis of double-blind lithium maintenance data. *Am J Psychiatry*, 159(7), 1155.

Perlis, R.H., Ostacher, M.J., Patel, J.K., Marangell, L.B., Zhang, H., Wisniewski, S.R., Ketter, T.A., Miklowitz, D.J., Otto, M.W., Gyulai, L., Reilly-Harrington, N.A., Nierenberg, A.A., Sachs, G.S., and Thase, M.E. (2006). Predictors of recurrence in bipolar disorder: Primary outcomes from the Systematic Treatment Enhancement Program for Bipolar Disorder (STEP-BD). *Am J Psychiatry*, 163(2), 217–224.

Perselow, E.D., Dunner, D.L., Fieve, R.R., and Lautin A. (1980). Lithium carbonate and weight gain. *J Affect Disord*, 2, 303–310.

Petrides, G., Dhossche, D., Fink, M., and Francis, A. (1994). Continuation ECT: Relapse prevention in affective disorders. *Convuls Ther*, 10(3), 189–194.

Pies, R. (2000). Free drug fraction versus free drug concentration. *J Clin Psychiatry*, 61(6), 449.

Placidi, G.F., Lenzi, A., Lazzerini, F., Cassano, G.B., and Akiskal, H.S. (1986). The comparative efficacy and safety of carbamazepine versus lithium: A randomized, double blind three year trial in 83 patients. *J Clin Psychiatry*, 47, 490–494.

Plenge, P., Mellerup, E.T., and Bolwig, T.G. (1982). Lithium treatment: Does the kidney prefer one daily dose instead of two? *Acta Psychiatr Scand*, 66, 121–128.

Poole, A.J., James, H.D., and Hughes, W.C. (1978). Treatment experiences in the lithium clinic at St. Thomas Hospital. *J R Soc Med*, 71(12), 890–894.

Popper, C.W. (2001). Do vitamins or minerals (apart from lithium) have mood stabilizing effects? *J Clin Psychiatry*, 62(12), 933–935.

Post, R.M., Uhde, T.W., Roy-Byrne, P.P., and Joffe, R.T. (1986). Antidepressant effects of carbamazepine. *Am J Psychiatry*, 143(1), 29–34.

Post, R.M., Uhde, T.W., Roy-Byrne, P.P., and Joffe, R.T. (1987). Correlates of antimanic response to carbamazepine. *Psychiatry Res*, 21(1), 71–83.

Post, R.M., Leverich, G.S., Altshuler, L., and Mikalauskas, K. (1992). Lithium-discontinuation-induced refractoriness: Preliminary observations. *Am J Psychiatry*, 149(12), 1727–1729.

Post, R.M., Altshuler, L.L., Frye, M.A., Suppes, T., Rush, A.J., Keck, P.E. Jr., McElroy, S.L., Denicoff, K.D., Leverich, G.S., Kupka, R., and Nolen, W.A. (2001). Rate of switch in bipolar patients prospectively treated with second-generation antidepressants as augmentation to mood stabilizers. *Bipolar Disord*, 3(5), 259–265.

Presne, C., Fakhouri, F., Noel, L.H., Stengel, B., Even, C., Kreis, H., Mignon, F., and Grunfeld, J.P. (2003). Lithium-induced nephropathy: Rate of progression and prognostic factors. *Kidney Int*, 64(2), 585–592.

Prien, R.F., Caffey, E.M. Jr., and Klett, C.J. (1973a). Prophylactic efficacy of lithium carbonate in manic-depressive illness: Report of the Veterans Administration and National Institute of Mental Health collaborative study group. *Arch Gen Psychiatry*, 28(3), 337–341.

Prien, R.F., Klett, C.J., and Caffey, E.M. Jr. (1973b). Lithium carbonate and imipramine in prevention of affective episodes: A comparison in recurrent affective illness. *Arch Gen Psychiatry*, 29(3), 420–425.

Prien, R.F., Klett, C.J., and Caffey, E.M. Jr. (1974). Lithium prophylaxis in recurrent affective illness. *Am J Psychiatry*, 131(2), 198–203.

Prien, R.F., Kupfer, D.J., Mansky, P.A., Small, J.G., Tuason, V.B., Voss, C.B., and Johnson, W.E. (1984). Drug therapy in the prevention of recurrences in unipolar and bipolar affective disorders: Report of NIMH Collaborative study group comparing lithium carbonate, imipramine, and a lithium carbonate-imipramine combination. *Arch Gen Psychiatry*, 41, 1096–1104.

Quitkin, F.M., Kane, J.M., Rifkin, A., Ramos-Lorenzi, J.R., Saraf, K., Howard, A., and Klein, D.F. (1981). Lithium and imipramine in the prophylaxis of unipolar and bipolar II depression: A prospective, placebo-controlled comparison [proceedings]. *Psychopharmacol Bull*, 17(1), 142–144.

Revicki, D.A., Hirschfeld, R.M., Ahearn, E.P., Weisler, R.H., Palmer, C., and Keck, P.E. Jr. (2005). Effectiveness and medical costs of divalproex versus lithium in the treatment of bipolar disorder: Results of a naturalistic clinical trial. *J Affect Disord*, 86(2-3), 183–193.

Rhodes, L.J. (2000). Maintenance ECT replaced with lamotrigine. *Am J Psychiatry*, 157(12), 2058.

Rybakowski, J., Chlopocka-Wozniak, M., Kapelski, Z., and Strzyzewski, W. (1980). The relative prophylactic efficacy of lithium against manic and depressive recurrences in bipolar patients. *Int Pharmacopsychiatry*, 15(2), 86–90.

Rzany, B., Correia, O., Kelly, J.P., Naldi, L., Auquier, A., and Stern, R. (1999). Risk of Stevens-Johnson syndrome and toxic epidermal necrolysis during first weeks of antiepileptic therapy: A case-control study. Study Group of the International Case Control Study on Severe Cutaneous Adverse Reactions. *Lancet*, (353), 2190–2194.

Sachs, G.S. (1996). Bipolar mood disorder: practical strategies for acute and maintenance phase treatment. *J Clin Psychopharmacol*, 16(2 Suppl. 1), 32S–47S.

Sachs, G.S., Lafer, B., Stoll, A.L., Banov, M., Thibault, A.B., Tohen, M., and Rosenbaum, J.F. (1994). A double-blind trial of bupropion versus desipramine for bipolar depression. *J Clin Psychiatry*, 55(9), 391–393.

Sachs, G., Bowden, C., Calabrese, J.R., Ketter, T., Thompson, T., White, R., and Bentley, B. (2006). Effects of lamotrigine and lithium on body weight during maintenance treatment of bipolar I disorder. *Bipolar Disord*, 8(2), 175–181.

Sajatovic, M., Gyulai, L., Calabrese, J.R., Thompson, T.R., Wilson, B.G., White, R., and Evoniuk, G. (2005). Maintenance treatment outcomes in older patients with bipolar I disorder. *Am J Geriatr Psychiatry*, 13(4), 305–311.

Sanger, T.M., Grundy, S.L., Gibson, P.J., Namjoshi, M.A., Greaney, M.G., and Tohen, M.F. (2001). Long-term olanzapine therapy in the treatment of bipolar I disorder: An open-label continuation phase study. *J Clin Psychiatry*, 62(4), 273–281.

Sashidharan, S.P., and McGuire, R.J. (1983). Recurrence of affective illness after withdrawal of long-term lithium treatment. *Acta Psychiatr Scand*, 68, 126–133.

Schaffer, L.C., and Schaffer, C.B. (1999). Tiagabine and the treatment of refractory bipolar disorder. *Am J Psychiatry*, 156(12), 2014–2015.

Schaffer, L.C., Schaffer, C.B., and Howe, J. (2002). An open case series on the utility of tiagabine as an augmentation in refractory bipolar outpatients. *J Affect Disord*, 71(1-3), 259–263.

Schou, M. (1963). Normothymics, "mood-normalizer." *Br J Psychiatry*, 109, 803–809.

Schou, M. (1968). Lithium in psychiatric therapy and prophylaxis. *J Psychiatr Res*, 6(1), 67–95.

Schou, M. (2001). Lithium treatment at 52. *J Affect Disord*, 67(1-3), 21–32.

Schou, M., Juel-Nielsen, N., Stromgren, E., and Voldby, H. (1954). The treatment of manic psychoses by the administration of lithium salts. *J Neurochem*, 17(4), 250–260.

Schou, M., Amdisen, A., Eskjer, J.S., and Olsen, T. (1968). Occurrence of goitre during lithium treatment. *BMJ*, 3, 710–713.

Schou, M., Baastrup, P.C., Grof, P., Weis, P., and Angst, J. (1970). Pharmacological and clinical problems of lithium prophylaxis. *Br J Psychiatry*, 116(535), 615–619.

Schrauwen, E., and Ghaemi, S.N. (2006). Galantamine treatment of cognitive impairment in bipolar disorder: Four cases. *Bipolar Disord*, 8(2), 196–199.

Schumann, C., Lenz, G., Berghofer, A., and Muller-Oerlinghausen, B. (1999). Non-adherence with long-term prophylaxis: A 6-year naturalistic follow-up study of affectively ill patients. *Psychiatry Res*, 89(3), 247–257.

Severus, W.E., Grunze, H., Kleindienst, N., Frangou, S., and Moeller, H.J. (2005). Is the prophylactic antidepressant efficacy

of lithium in bipolar I disorder dependent on study design and lithium level? *J Clin Psychopharmacol*, 25(5), 457–462.

Sharma, V., Smith, A., and Mazmanian, D. (2006). Olanzapine in the prevention of postpartum psychosis and mood episodes in bipolar disorder. *Bipolar Disord*, 8(4), 400–404.

Shulman, K.I., Sykora, K., Gill, S., Mamdani, M., Bronskill, S., Wodchis, W.P., Anderson, G., and Rochon, P. (2005). Incidence of delirium in older adults newly prescribed lithium or valproate: A population-based cohort study. *J Clin Psychiatry*, 66(4), 424–427.

Sienaert, P., and Peuskens, J. (2006). Electroconvulsive therapy: An effective therapy of medication-resistant bipolar disorder. *Bipolar Disord*, 8(3), 304–306.

Silverstone, T., McPherson, H., Hunt, N., and Romans, S. (1998). How effective is lithium in the prevention of relapse in bipolar disorder? A prospective naturalistic follow-up study. *Aust NZ J Psychiatry*, 32(1), 61–66.

Sobotka, J.L., Alexander, B., and Cook, B.L. (1990). A review of carbamazepine's hematologic reactions and monitoring recommendations. *DICP*, 24(12), 1214–1219.

Solomon, D.A., Ryan, C.E., Keitner, G.I., Miller, I.W., Shea, M.T., Kazim, A., and Keller, M.B. (1997). A pilot study of lithium carbonate plus divalproex sodium for the continuation and maintenance treatment of patients with bipolar I disorder. *J Clin Psychiatry*, 58(3), 95–99.

Solomon, D.A., Leon, A.C., Mueller, T.I., Coryell, W., Teres, J.J., Posternak, M.A., Judd, L.L., Endicott, J., and Keller, M.B. (2005). Tachyphylaxis in unipolar major depressive disorder. *J Clin Psychiatry*, 66(3), 283–290.

Solvason, H.B. (2000). Agranulocytosis associated with lamotrigine. *Am J Psychiatry*, 157(10), 1704.

Souza, F.G., Mander, A.J., and Goodwin, G.M. (1990). The efficacy of lithium in prophylaxis of unipolar depression: Evidence from its discontinuation. *Br J Psychiatry*, 157, 718–722.

Spinelli, M.G. (2004). Maternal infanticide associated with mental illness: Prevention and promise of saved lives. *Am J Psychiatry*, 161(9), 1548–1557.

Sporn, J., and Sachs, G. (1997). The anticonvulsant lamotrigine in treatment-resistant manic-depressive illness. *J Clin Psychopharmacol*, 17(3), 185–189.

Stallone, F., Shelley, E., Mendlewicz, J., and Fieve, R.R. (1973). The use of lithium in affective disorders: 3. A double-blind study of prophylaxis in bipolar illness. *Am J Psychiatry*, 130(9), 1006–1010.

Steckler, T.L. (1994). Lithium- and carbamazepine-associated sinus node dysfunction: Nine-year experience in a psychiatric hospital. *J Clin Psychopharmacol*, 14(5), 336–339.

Stewart, D.E. (2000). Antidepressant drugs during pregnancy and lactation. *Int Clin Psychopharmacol*, 15(Suppl. 3), S19–S24.

Stewart, D.E., Klompenhouwer, J.L., Kendell, R.E., and van Hulst, A.M. (1991). Prophylactic lithium in puerperal psychosis: The experience of three centres. *Br J Psychiatry*, 158, 393–397.

Suppes, T., and Dennehy, E.B. (2002). Evidence-based long-term treatment of bipolar II disorder. *J Clin Psychiatry*, 63(Suppl. 10), 29–33.

Suppes, T., Baldessarini, R.J., Faedda, G.L., and Tohen, M. (1991). Risk of recurrence following discontinuation of lithium treatment in bipolar disorder. *Arch Gen Psychiatry*, 48(12), 1082–1088.

Suppes, T., Brown, E.S., McElroy, S.L., Keck, P.E. Jr., Nolen, W., Kupka, R., Frye, M., Denicoff, K.D., Altshuler, L., Leverich,

G.S., and Post, R.M. (1999a). Lamotrigine for the treatment of bipolar disorder: A clinical case series. *J Affect Disord*, 53(1), 95–98.

Suppes, T., Webb, A., Paul, B., Carmody, T., Kraemer, H., and Rush, A.J. (1999b). Clinical outcome in a randomized 1-year trial of clozapine versus treatment as usual for patients with treatment-resistant illness and a history of mania. *Am J Psychiatry*, 156(8), 1164–1169.

Suppes, T., Ozcan, M.E., and Carmody, T. (2004). Response to clozapine of rapid cycling versus non-cycling patients with a history of mania. *Bipolar Disord*, 6(4), 329–332.

Suppes, T., Brown, E., Schuh, L.M., Baker, R.W., and Tohen, M. (2005). Rapid versus non-rapid cycling as a predictor of response to olanzapine and divalproex sodium for bipolar mania and maintenance of remission: Post hoc analyses of 47-week data. *J Affect Disord*, 89(1–3), 69–77.

Swann, A.C., Bowden, C.L., Calabrese, J.R., Dilsaver, S.C., and Morris, D.D. (1999). Differential effect of number of previous episodes of affective disorder on response to lithium or divalproex in acute mania. *Am J Psychiatry*, 156(8), 1264–1266.

Swann, A.C., Bowden, C.L., Calabrese, J.R., Dilsaver, S.C., and Morris, D.D. (2000). Mania: Differential effects of previous depressive and manic episodes on response to treatment. *Acta Psychiatr Scand*, 101(6), 444–451.

Thisted, E., and Ebbesen, F. (1993). Malformations, withdrawal manifestations, and hypoglycaemia after exposure to valproate in utero. *Arch Dis Child*, 69(Spec. No. 3), 288–291.

Tohen, M., Castillo, J., Baldessarini, R.J., Zarate, C. Jr., and Kando, J.C. (1995). Blood dyscrasias with carbamazepine and valproate: A pharmacoepidemiological study of 2,228 patients at risk. *Am J Psychiatry*, 152(3), 413–418.

Tohen, M., Bowden, C., Greil, W., Jacobs, T.G., Baker, R.W., Evans, A.R., and Cassano, G. (2002). *Olanzapine in relapse prevention of bipolar disorder*. Poster presented to the Meeting of the American College of Neurosychopharmacology, Puerto Rico.

Tohen, M., Ketter, T.A., Zarate, C.A., Suppes, T., Frye, M., Altshuler, L., Zajecka, J., Schuh, L.M., Risser, R.C., Brown, E., and Baker, R.W. (2003). Olanzapine versus divalproex sodium for the treatment of acute mania and maintenance of remission: A 47-week study. *Am J Psychiatry*, 160(7), 1263–1271.

Tohen, M., Chengappa, K.N., Suppes, T., Baker, R.W., Zarate, C.A., Bowden, C.L., Sachs, G.S., Kupfer, D.J., Ghaemi, S.N., Feldman, P.D., Risser, R.C., Evans, A.R., and Calabrese, J.R. (2004). Relapse prevention in bipolar I disorder: 18-Month comparison of olanzapine plus mood stabilizer v. mood stabilizer alone. *Br J Psychiatry*, 184, 337–345.

Tohen, M., Calabrese, J.R., Sachs, G.S., Banov, M.D., Detke, H.C., Risser, R., Baker, R.W., Chou, J.C., and Bowden, C.L. (2006). Randomized, placebo-controlled trial of olanzapine as maintenance therapy in patients with bipolar I disorder responding to acute treatment with olanzapine. *Am J Psychiatry*, 163(2), 247–256.

Tondo, L., Baldessarini, R.J., Floris, G., and Rudas, N. (1997). Effectiveness of restarting lithium treatment after its discontinuation in bipolar I and bipolar II disorders. *Am J Psychiatry*, 154(4), 548–550.

Tondo, L., Baldessarini, R.J., Hennen, J., and Floris, G. (1998). Lithium maintenance treatment of depression and mania in bipolar I and bipolar II disorders. *Am J Psychiatry*, 155(5), 638–645.

Tondo, L., Baldessarini, R.J., and Floris, G. (2001). Long-term clinical effectiveness of lithium maintenance treatment in types I and II bipolar disorders. *Br J Psychiatry*, 41, S184–S190.

Tondo, L., Hennen, J., and Baldessarini, R.J. (2003). Rapid-cycling bipolar disorder: Effects of long term treatments. *Acta Psychiatr Scand*, 108, 4–14.

Trivedi, M.H., Rush, A.J., Wisniewski, S.R., Nierenberg, A.A., Warden, D., Ritz, L., Norquist, G., Howland, R.H., Lebowitz, B., McGrath, P.J., Shores-Wilson, K., Biggs, M.M., Balasubramani, G.K., Fava, M., and STAR*D Study Team. (2006). Evaluation of outcomes with citalopram for depression using measurement-based care in STAR*D: Implications for clinical practice. *Am J Psychiatry*, 163(1), 28–40.

Tsankov, N., Angelova, I., and Kazandjieva, J. (2000). Drug-induced psoriasis: Recognition and management. *Am J Clin Dermatol*, 1(3), 159–165.

Vaidya, N.A., Mahableshwarkar, A.R., and Shahid, R. (2003). Continuation and maintenance ECT in treatment-resistant bipolar disorder. *J ECT*, 19(1), 10–16.

Van Gerpen, M.W., Johnson, J.E., and Winstead, D.K. (1999). Mania in the geriatric patient population: A review of the literature. *Am J Geriatr Psychiatry*, 7(3), 188–202.

Vanelle, J.M., Loo, H., Galinowski, A., de Carvalho, W., Bourdel, M.C., Brochier, P., Bouvet, O., Brochier, T., and Olie, J.P. (1994). Maintenance ECT in intractable manic-depressive disorders. *Convuls Ther*, 10(3), 195–205.

Vestergaard, P. (2004). Guidelines for maintenance treatment of bipolar disorder: Are there discrepancies between European and North American recommendations? *Bipolar Disord*, 6(6), 519–522.

Vestergaard, P., and Schou, M. (1987). Does long-term lithium treatment induce diabetes mellitus? *Neuropsychobiology*, 17(3), 130–132.

Vestergaard, P., Licht, R.W., Brodersen, A., Rasmussen, N.A., Christensen, H., Arngrim, T., Gronvall, B., Kristensen, E., and Poulstrup, I. (1998). Outcome of lithium prophylaxis: A prospective follow-up of affective disorder patients assigned to high and low serum lithium levels. *Acta Psychiatr Scand*, 98(4), 310–315.

Vieta, E., Goikolea, J.M., Corbella, B., Benabarre, A., Reinares, M., Martinez, G., Fernandez, A., Colom, F., Martinez-Aran, A., Torrent, C., and Group for the Study of Risperidone in Affective Disorders (GSRAD). (2001a). Risperidone safety and efficacy in the treatment of bipolar and schizoaffective disorders: Results from a 6-month, multicenter, open study. *J Clin Psychiatry*, 62(10), 818–825.

Vieta, E., Reinares, M., Corbella, B., Benabarre, A., Gilaberte, I., Colom, F., Martinez-Aran, A., Gasto, C., and Tohen, M. (2001b). Olanzapine as long-term adjunctive therapy in treatment-resistant bipolar disorder. *J Clin Psychopharmacol*, 21(5), 469–473.

Vieta, E., Torrent, C., Garcia-Ribas, G., Gilabert, A., Garcia-Pares, G., Rodriguez, A., Cadevall, J., Garcia-Castrillon, J., Lusilla, P., and Arrufat, F. (2002). Use of topiramate in treatment-resistant bipolar spectrum disorders *J Clin Psychopharmacol*, 22(4), 431–435.

Vieta, E., Sanchez-Moreno, J., Goikolea, J.M., Torrent, C., Benabarre, A., Colom, F., Martinez, A., Reinares, M., Comes, M., and Corbella, B. (2003). Adjunctive topiramate in bipolar I disorder. *World J Biol Psychiatry*, 4(4), 172–176.

Vieta, E., Sanchez-Moreno, J., Goikolea, J. M., Colom, F., Martinez-Aran, A., Benabarre, A., Corbella, B., Torrent, C.,

Comes, M., Reinares, M., and Brugue, E. (2004). Effects on weight and outcome of long-term olanzapine-topiramate combination treatment in bipolar disorder. *J Clin Psychopharmacol*, 24(4), 374–378.

Vieta, E., Goikolea, J.M., Martinez-Aran, A., Comes, M., Verger, K., Masramon, X., Sanchez-Moreno, J., and Colom, F. (2006). A double-blind, randomized, placebo-controlled, prophylaxis study of adjunctive gabapentin for bipolar disorder. *J Clin Psychiatry*, 67(3), 473–477.

Viguera, A.C., Nonacs, R., Cohen, L.S., Tondo, L., Murray, A., and Baldessarini, R.J. (2000). Risk of recurrence of bipolar disorder in pregnant and nonpregnant women after discontinuing lithium maintenance. *Am J Psychiatry*, 157(2), 179–184.

Viguera, A.C., Cohen, L.S., Baldessarini, R.J., and Nonacs, R. (2002). Managing bipolar disorder during pregnancy: Weighing the risks and benefits. *Can J Psychiatry*, 47(5), 426–436.

Walden, J., Hesslinger, B., van Calker, D., and Berger, M. (1996). Addition of lamotrigine to valproate may enhance efficacy in the treatment of bipolar affective disorder. *Pharmacopsychiatry*, 29(5), 193–195.

Walden, J., Schaerer, L., Schloesser, S., and Grunze, H. (2000). An open longitudinal study of patients with bipolar rapid cycling treated with lithium or lamotrigine for mood stabilization. *Bipolar Disord*, 2(4), 336–339.

Warner, J.P. (2000). Evidence-based psychopharmacology: 3. Assessing evidence of harm: What are the teratogenic effects of lithium carbonate? *J Psychopharmacol*, 14(1), 77–80.

Watkins, S.E., Callender, K., Thomas, D.R., Tidmarsh, S.F., and Shaw, D.M. (1987). The effect of carbamazepine and lithium on remission from affective illness. *Br J Psychiatry*, 150, 180–182.

Wehr, T.A., and Goodwin, F.K. (1979). Rapid cycling in manic-depressives induced by tricyclic antidepressants. *Arch Gen Psychiatry*, 36(5), 555–559.

Wehr, T.A., Sack, D.A., Rosenthal, N.E., and Cowdry, R.W. (1988). Rapid cycling affective disorder: Contributing factors and treatment responses in 51 patients. *Am J Psychiatry*, 145(2), 179–184.

Wehr, T.A., Turner, E.H., Shimada, J.M., Lowe, C.H., Barker, C., and Leibenluft, E. (1998). Treatment of rapidly cycling bipolar patient by using extended bed rest and darkness to stabilize the timing and duration of sleep. *Biol Psychiatry*, 43(11), 822–828.

Whitwell, J.R. (1936). *Historical Notes on Psychiatry: Early Times—End of 16th Century*. London: H.K. Lewis & Co.

Wisner, K.L., Peindl, K.S., Perel, J.M., Hanusa, B.H., Piontek, C.M., and Baab, S. (2002). Verapamil treatment for women with bipolar disorder. *Biol Psychiatry*, 51(9), 745–752.

Wisner, K.L., Hanusa, B.H., Peindl, K.S., and Perel, J.M. (2004). Prevention of postpartum episodes in women with bipolar disorder. *Biol Psychiatry*, 56(8), 592–596.

Wong, I.C., Mawer, G.E., and Sander, J.W. (1999). Factors influencing the incidence of lamotrigine-related skin rash. *Ann Pharmacother*, 33(10), 1037–1042.

Yonkers, K.A., Wisner, K.L., Stowe, Z., Leibenluft, E., Cohen, L., Miller, L., Manber, R., Viguera, A., Suppes, T., and Altshuler, L. (2004). Management of bipolar disorder during pregnancy and the postpartum period. *Am J Psychiatry*, 161(4), 608–620.

Young, A., Geddes, J., Macritchie, K., Rao, S., and Vasudev, A. (2006). Tiagabine in the maintenance treatment of bipolar disorders. *Cochrane Database Syst Rev*, 19(3), CD005173.

Zarate, C.A. Jr., and Quiroz, J.A. (2003). Combination treatment in bipolar disorder: A review of controlled trials. *Bipolar Disord*, 5(3), 217–225.

Zarate, C.A. Jr., Tohen, M., and Baldessarini, R.J. (1995). Clozapine in severe mood disorders. *J Clin Psychiatry*, 56(9), 411–417.

CHAPTER 21

Aagaard, J., and Vestergaard, P. (1990). Predictors of outcome in prophylactic lithium treatment: A 2-year prospective study. *J Affect Disord*, 18, 259–266.

Abou-Saleh, M.T., and Coppen, A. (1983). Subjective side-effects of amitriptyline and lithium in affective disorders. *Br J Psychiatry*, 142, 391–397.

Adams, J., and Scott, J. (2000). Predicting medication adherence in severe mental disorders. *Acta Psychiatr Scand*, 101(2), 119–124.

Amador, X.F., Flaum, M., Andreasen, N.C., Strauss, D.H., Yale, S.A., Clark, S.C., and Gorman, J.M. (1994). Awareness of illness in schizophrenia, schizoaffective and mood disorders. *Arch Gen Psychiatry*, 51, 826–836.

Angst, J., Weis, P., Grof, P., Baastrup, P.C., and Schou, M. (1970). Lithium prophylaxis in recurrent affective disorders. *Br J Psychiatry*, 116, 604–614.

Ball, J.R., Mitchell, P.B., Corry, J.C., Skillecorn, A., Smith, M., and Malhi, G.S. (2006). A randomized controlled trial of cognitive therapy for bipolar disorder: Focus on long-term change. *J Clin Psychiatry*, 67, 277–286.

Bech, P. (1981). Rating scales for affective disorders: Their validity and consistency. *Acta Psychiatr Scand*, 295, 1–101.

Bech P., Vendsborg, P.B., and Rafaelsen, O.J. (1976). Lithium maintenance treatment of manic-melancholic patients: Its role in the daily routine. *Acta Psychiatr Scand*, 53, 70–81.

Becker, M.H., and Maiman, L.A. (1980). Strategies for enhancing compliance. *J Community Health*, 6, 113–135.

Blackwell, B. (1973). Patient adherence. *N Engl J Med*, 289, 249–252.

Blackwell, B. (1976). Treatment adherence. *Br J Psychiatry*, 129, 513–531.

Blackwell, B. (1980, January). *Why don't patients take their medicines?* Paper presented at the annual meeting of the American Association for the Advancement of Science, Toronto, Canada.

Blackwell, B. (1982). Treatment adherence. In J.H. Greist, J.W. Jefferson, and R.L. Spitzer (Eds.), *Treatment of Mental Disorders* (pp. 501–516). New York: Oxford University Press.

Bonin, J.P. (1999). Psychosocial determinants of lithium compliance in patients with bipolar disorder. *Can J Nurs Res*, 31, 24–40.

Bowskill, R., Clatworthy, J., Parham, R., Rank, T., and Horner, R. (2006). Patient dissatisfaction with information provided about medicines prescribed for bipolar disorder. *J Affect Disord*, Dec. 14 [epub ahead of print].

Boyd, J.R., Covington, T.R., Stanaszek, W.F., and Coussons, R.T. (1974a). Drug defaulting: Part I. Determinants of adherence. *Am J Hosp Pharm*, 31, 362–367.

Boyd, J.R., Covington, T.R., Stanaszek, W.F., and Coussons, R.T. (1974b). Drug defaulting: Part II. Analysis of non-adherence patterns. *Am J Hosp Pharm*, 31, 485–491.

Brookmeyer, R., Johnson, E., and Bollinger, R. (2003). Modeling the optimum duration of antibiotic prophylaxis in an anthrax outbreak. *Proc Natl Acad Sci USA*, 100(17), 10129–10132.

Cade, J.F.J. (1978). Past, present and future. In F.N. Johnson, and S. Johnson (Eds.), *Lithium in Medical Practice* (pp. 5–16). Baltimore: University Park Press.

Cassidy, F., Ahearn, E., and Carroll, B.J. (2001). A prospective study of inter-episode consistency of manic and mixed subtypes of bipolar disorder. *J Affect Disord*, 67(1-3), 181–185.

Clarkin, J.F., Carpenter, D., Hull, J., Wilner, P., and Glick, I. (1998). Effects of psychoeducational intervention for married patients with bipolar disorder and their spouses. *Psychiatr Serv*, 49(4), 531–533.

Cochran, S.D. (1982). *Strategies for Preventing Lithium Non-Adherence in Bipolar Affective Illness*. Unpublished doctoral dissertation, University of California, Los Angeles, CA.

Cochran, S.D. (1984). Preventing medical noncompliance in the outpatient treatment of bipolar affective disorders. *J Consult Clin Psychol*, 52, 873–878.

Cochran, S.D., and Gitlin, M.J. (1988). Attitudinal correlates of lithium adherence in bipolar affective disorders. *J Nerv Ment Dis*, 176, 457–464.

Colom, F., and Vieta, E. (2002). Treatment adherence in bipolar patients. *Clin Approaches Bipolar Disord*, 1, 49–56.

Colom, F., Vieta, E., Martínez-Arán, A., Reinares, M., Benabarre, A., and Gasto, C. (2000). Clinical factors associated with treatment noncompliance in euthymic bipolar patients. *J Clin Psychiatry*, 61, 549–555.

Colom, F., Vieta, E., Martínez-Arán, A., Reinares, M., Goikolea, J.M., Benabarre, A., Torrent, C., Comes, M., Corbella, B., Parramon, G., and Corominas, J. (2003). A randomized trial on the efficacy of group psychoeducation in the prophylaxis in bipolar patients whose disease is in remission. *Arch Gen Psychiatry*, 60, 402–407.

Connelly, C.E., Davenport, Y.B., and Nurnberger, J.I. (1982). Adherence to treatment regimen in a lithium carbonate clinic. *Arch Gen Psychiatry*, 39, 585–588.

Dailey, L.F., Townsend, S.W., Dysken, M.W., and Kuskowski, M.A. (2005). Recidivism in medication-noncompliant serious juvenile offenders with bipolar disorder. *J Clin Psychiatry*, 66, 477–484.

Danion, J.M., Neunreuther, C., Krieger-Finance, F., Imbs, J.L., and Singer, L. (1987). Compliance with long-term lithium treatment in major affective disorders. *Pharmacopsychiatry*, 20, 230–231.

Day, J.C., Bertall, R.P., Roberts, C., Randall, F., Rogers, A., Cattell, D., Healy D., Rae, P., and Power, C. (2005). Attitudes toward antipsychotic medication: The impact of clinical variables and relationships with health professionals. *Arch Gen Psychiatry*, 62, 717–724.

Dell'Osso, L., Pini, S., Tundo, A., Sarno, N., Musetti, L., and Cassano, G.B. (2000). Clinical characteristics of mania, mixed mania, and bipolar depression with psychotic features. *Compr Psychiatry*, 41(4), 242–247.

Dell'Osso, L., Pini, S., Cassano, G.B., Mastrocinque, C., Seckinger, R.A., Saettoni, M., Papasogli, A., Yale, S.A., and Amador, X.F. (2002). Insight into illness in patients with mania, mixed mania, bipolar depression and major depression with psychotic features. *Bipolar Disord*, 4(5), 315–322.

DiMatteo, M.R. (2004). Variations in patients' adherence to medical recommendations: A quantitative review of 50 years of research. *Med Care*, 42(3), 200–209.

Docherty, J.P., and Fiester, S.J. (1985). The therapeutic alliance and compliance with psychopharmacology. In R.E. Hales and A.J. Frances (Eds.), *American Psychiatric Association Annual Review, Vol. 4* (pp. 607–632). Washington, DC: American Psychiatric Press.

Dolder, C., Lacro, J., Dunn, L., and Jeste, D. (2002). Antipsychotic medication adherence: Is there a difference between typical and atypical agents? *Am J Psychiatry*, 159, 103–108.

Fennig, S., Bromet, E.G., Jandorf, L., Schwartz, J., Lavelle, J., and Ram, R. (1995). Eliciting psychotic symptoms using a semistructured interview. *J Nerv Ment Dis*, 181, 20–26.

Fenton, W.S., Blyer, C.R., and Heinssen, R.K. (1997). Determinants of medication adherence in schizophrenia: Empirical and clinical findings. *Schizophrenia Bull*, 23, 637–651.

Fitzgerald, R.G. (1972). Mania as a message: Treatment with family therapy and lithium carbonate. *Am J Psychotherapy*, 26, 547–553.

Frank, E., Prien, R.F., Kupfer, D.J., and Alberts, L. (1985). Implications of nonadherence on research in affective disorders. *Psychopharmacol Bull*, 21, 37–42.

Frank, J.D., and Frank, J.B. (1991). *Persuasion and Healing: A Comparative Study of Psychotherapy*, 3rd ed. Baltimore: Johns Hopkins University Press.

Ghaemi, S.N. (1997). Insight and psychiatric disorder: A review of the literature, with a focus on its clinical relevance for bipolar disorder. *Psychiatr Ann*, 27, 782–790.

Ghaemi, S.N., Stoll, A.L., and Pope, H.G. Jr. (1995). Lack of insight in bipolar disorder: The acute manic episode. *J Nerv Ment Dis*, 183(7), 464–467.

Gianfrancesco, F.D., Rajagopalan, K., Sajatovic M., Wang, R.H. (2006). Treatment adherence among patients with bipolar or manic disorder taking atypical and typical antipsychotics. *J Clin Psychiatry*, 67(2), 222–232.

Gitlin, M.J., and Jamison, K.R. (1984). Lithium clinics: Theory and practice. *Hosp Community Psychiatry*, 35(4), 363–368.

Gitlin, M.J., Cochran, S.D., and Jamison, K.R. (1989). Maintenance lithium treatment: Side effects and adherence. *J Clin Psychiatry*, 50, 127–131.

Glazer, W.M., Sonnenberg, J.G., Reinstein, M.J., and Akers, R.F. (2004). A novel, point-of-case test for lithium levels: Description and reliability. *J Clin Psychiatry*, 65, 652–656.

Goldberg, J.F., Harrow, M., and Leon, A.C. (1996). Lithium treatment of bipolar affective disorders under naturalistic followup conditions. *Psychopharmacol Bull*, 32, 47–54.

Gonzalez-Pinto, A., Mosquera, F., Alonso, M., Lopez, P., Ramirez, F., Vieta, E., and Baldessarini, R.J. (2006). Suicidal risk in bipolar I disorder patients and adolescence to long-term lithium treatment. *Bipolar Disord*, 8, 618–624.

Greenhouse, W.J., Meyer, B., and Johnson, S.L. (2000). Coping and medication adherence in bipolar disorder. *J Affect Disord*, 59, 237–241.

Grof, P., Cakulis, P., and Dostal, T. (1970). Lithium dropouts: A follow-up study of patients who discontinued prophylactic treatment. *Int Pharmacopsychiatry*, 5, 162–169.

Harvey, N.S., and Peet, M. (1991). Lithium maintenance: 2. Effects of personality and attitude on health information acquisition and compliance. *Br J Psychiatry*, 158, 200–204.

Haynes, R.B., Taylor, D.W., and Sackett, D.L. (Eds.). (1979). *Compliance in Health Care*. Baltimore: The Johns Hopkins University Press.

Haynes, R.B., McDonald, H., Garg, A.X., and Montague, P. (2002). Interventions for helping patients to follow prescriptions for medications. *Cochrane Database Syst Rev*, (2):CD000011.

Horne, R., Clatworthy, J., Parham, R., Rank, T., Bowskill, R. (2006). Medication prescribed for bipolar disorder: The role of patients' treatment perceptions in predicting nonadherence. *J Affect Disord*, 915, 566.

Jamison, K.R. (1995). *An Unquiet Mind: A Memoir of Moods and Madness*. New York: Alfred A. Knopf.

Jamison, K.R., Gerner, R.H., and Goodwin, F.K. (1979). Patient and physician attitudes toward lithium: Relationship to adherence. *Arch Gen Psychiatry*, 36, 866–869.

Johnson, R.E., and McFarland, B.H. (1996). Lithium use and discontinuation in a health maintenance organization. *Am J Psychiatry*, 153, 993–1000.

Johnson, S., Winett, C., Miller, I., Bauer, M., Solomon, D., Keitner, G., and Ryan, C. (1998). Life events, medications and bipolar-I disorder. *J Bipolar Disord*, 1, 37–39.

Keck, P.E., McElroy, S.L., Strakowski, S.M., Bourne, M.L., and West, S.A. (1997). Compliance with maintenance treatment in bipolar disorder. *Psychopharmacol Bull*, 33, 87–91.

Keck, P.E., McElroy, S.L., Strakowski, S.M., West, S.A., Sax, K.W., Hawkins, J.M., Bourne, M.L., and Haggard, P. (1998). 12-month outcome of patients with bipolar disorder following hospitalization for a manic or mixed episode. *Am J Psychiatry*, 155, 646–652.

Kerry, J. (1978). Recent developments in patient management. In F.N. Johnson and S. Johnson (Eds.), *Lithium in Medical Practice* (pp. 337–353). Baltimore: University Park Press.

Kleindienst, N., and Greil, W. (2004). Are illness concepts a powerful predictor of adherence to prophylactic treatment in bipolar disorder? *J Clin Psychiatry*, 65, 966–974.

Kucera-Bozarth, K., Beck, N.C., and Lyss, L. (1982). Compliance with lithium regimens. *J Psychosoc Nurs Ment Health Serv*, 20, 11–15.

Kulhara, P., Basu, D., Matoo, S.K., Sharan, P., and Chopra, R. (1999). Lithium prophylaxis of recurrent bipolar affective disorder: Long-term outcome and its psychosocial correlates. *J Affect Disord*, 54, 87–96.

Lam, D., Bright, J., Jones, S., Hayward, P., Schuck, N., Chisholm, D., and Sham, P. (2000). Cognitive therapy for bipolar illness: A pilot study of relapse prevention. *Cognitive Ther Res*, 24, 503–520.

Lam, D.H., Watkins, E.R., Hayward, P., Bright, J., Wright, K., Kerr, N., Parr-Davis, G., and Sham, P. (2003). A randomized controlled study of cognitive therapy for relapse prevention for bipolar affective disorder: Outcome of the first year. *Arch Gen Psychiatry*, 60, 145–152.

Lam, D.H., Hayward, P., Watkins, E.R., Wright, K., and Sham, P. (2005). Relapse prevention in patients with bipolar disorder: Cognitive therapy outcome after 2 years. *Am J Psychiatry*, 162, 324–329.

Lenzi, A., Lazzerini, F., Placidi, G.F., Cassano, G.B., and Akiskal, H.S. (1989). Predictors of adherence with lithium and carbamazepine regimens in the long-term treatment of recurrent mood and related psychotic disorders. *Pharmacopsychiatry*, 22, 34–37.

Maarbjerg, K., Aagaard, J., and Vestergaard, P. (1988). Adherence to lithium prophylaxis: I. Clinical predictors and patient's reasons for non adherence. *Pharmacopsychiatry*, 21, 121–125.

Marken, P.A., Stanislac, W.S., Lacombe, S., Pierce, C., Hornstra, R., and Sommi, R.W. (1992). Profile of a sample of subjects admitted to an acute care psychiatric facility with manic symptoms. *Psychopharmacol Bull*, 28, 201–205.

Mazullo, J.M., and Lasagna, L. (1972). Take thou . . . But is your patient really taking what you prescribed? *Drug Ther*, 2, 11–15.

McDonald, H.P., Garg, A.X., and Haynes, R.B. (2002). Interventions to enhance patient adherence to medication prescriptions: Scientific review. *JAMA*, 288, 2868–2879.

Michalakeas, A., Skoutas, C., Charalambous, A., Peristeris, A., Marinos, V., and Keramari, E. (1994). Insight in schizophrenia and mood disorders and its relation to psychopathology. *Acta Psychiatr Scand*, 90, 46–49.

Miklowitz, D.J. (1992). Longitudinal outcome and medication nonadherence among manic patients with and without mood-incongruent psychotic features. *J Nerv Ment Di*, 180, 703–711.

Miklowitz, D.J., Simoneau, T.L., George, E.L., Richards, J.A., Kalbag, A., Sachs-Ericsson, N., and Suddath, R. (2000). Family-focused treatment of bipolar disorder: 1-Year effects of a psychoeducational program in conjunction with pharmacotherapy. *Biol Psychiatry*, 48(6), 582–592.

Miklowitz, D.J., Richard, J.A., George, E.L., Frank, E., Suddath, R.L., Powell, K.B., and Sacher, J.A. (2003). Integrated family and individual therapy for bipolar disorder: Results of a treatment development study. *J Clin Psychiatry*, 64, 182–191.

Morselli, P.L., Elgie, R., GAMIAN-Europe. (2003). GAMIAN-Europe/BEAM Survey I-global analysis of a patient questionnaire circulated to 3450 members of 12 European advocacy groups operating in the field of mood disorders. *Bipolar Disord* 5, 265–278.

Mukherjee, S., Rosen, A.M., and Skukla, S. (1993). Acceptance by patients of maintenance lithium treatment. *Lithium*, 2, 63–69.

Osterberg, L., and Blaschke, T. (2005). Adherence to medication. *N Engl J Med*, 353, 487–497.

Pallanti, S., Quercioli, L., Pazzagli, A., Rossi, A., Dell'Osso, L., Pini, S., Cassano, G.B. (1999). Awareness of illness and subjective experience of cognitive complaints in patients with bipolar I and bipolar II disorder. *Am J Psychiatry*, 156(7), 1094–1096.

Pampallona, S., Bollini, P., Tibaldi, G., Kupelnick, B., and Munizza, C. (2002). Patient adherence in the treatment of depression. *Br J Psychiatry*, 180, 104–109.

Peralta, V., and Cuetsa, M.J. (1998). Lack of insight in mood disorders. *J Affect Disord*, 49, 55–58.

Perkins, D.O., Johnson, J.L., Hamer, R.M., Zipursky, R.B., Keefe, R.S., Centorrhino, F., Green, A.I., Glick, I.B., Kahn, R.S., Sharma, T., Tohen, M., McEvoy, J.P., Weiden, P.J., and Lieberman, J.A. (2006). Predictors of antipsychotic medication adherence in patients recovering from a first psychotic episode. *Schizophr Res*, 83, 53–63.

Perlick, D.A., Rosenheck, R.A., Clarkin, J.F., Maciejewski, P.K., Sirey, J., Struening, E., and Link, B.G. (2004a). Impact of family burden and affective response on clinical outcome among patients with bipolar disorder. *Psychiatr Serv*, 55, 1029–1035.

Perlick, D.A., Rosenheck, R.A., Kaczynski, R., and Kozma, L. (2004b). Medication non-adherence in bipolar disorder: A patient-centered review of research findings. *Clin Approaches Bipolar Disord* 3, 56–64.

Perry, A., Tarrier, N., Morriss, R., McCarthy, E., and Limb, K. (1999). Randomised controlled trial of efficacy of teaching patients with bipolar disorder to identify early symptoms of relapse and obtain treatment. *BMJ*, 318(7177), 149–153.

Pini, S., Cassano, G.B., Dell'Osso, L., and Amador, X.F. (2001). Insight into illness in schizophrenia, schizoaffective disorder, and mood disorders with psychotic features. *Am J Psychiatry*, 158(1), 122–125.

Polatin, P., and Fieve, R.R. (1971). Patient rejection of lithium carbonate prophylaxis. *JAMA,* 218, 864–866.

Pope, M., and Scott, J. (2003). Do clinicians understand why individuals stop taking lithium? *J Affect Disord,* 74, 287–291.

Sajatovic, M., Davies, M., and Hrouda, D.R. (2004). Enhancement of treatment adherence among patients with bipolar disorder. *Psychiatr Serv,* 55, 264–269.

Sajatovic, M., Bauer, M.S., Kilbourne, A.M., Vertrees, J.E., and Williford, W. (2006a). Self-reported medication treatment adherence among veterans with bipolar disorder. *Psychiatr Serv,* 57, 56–62.

Sajatovic, M., Valenstein, M., Blow, F.C., Ganoczy, D., and Ignacio, R.V. (2006b). Treatment adherence with antipsychotic medications in bipolar disorder. *Bipolar Disord,* 8, 232–241.

Schou, M. (1997). The combat of non-adherence during prophylactic lithium treatment. *Acta Psychiatr Scand,* 95, 361–363.

Schou, M., and Baastrup, P.C. (1973). Personal and social implications of lithium maintenance treatment. In T.A. Ban, J.R. Boissier, G.H. Gessa, H. Heimann, L. Hollister, H.E. Lehmann, I. Munkvad, H. Steinberg, F. Sulser, A Sundwall, and O. Vinar (Eds.), *Psychopharmacology, Sexual Disorders and Drug Abuse* (pp. 65–68). Amsterdam and London: North-Holland Publishing Co.

Schou, M., Baastrup, P. C., Grof, P., Weis, P., and Angst, J. (1970). Pharmacological and clinical problems of lithium prophylaxis. *Br J Psychiatry,* 116, 615–619.

Schumann, C., Lenz, G., Berghofer, A., and Muller-Oerlinghausen, B. (1999). Non-adherence with long-term prophylaxis: A 6-year naturalistic follow-up study of affectively ill patients. *Psychiatry Res,* 89, 247–257.

Scott, J., and Pope, M. (2002a). Nonadherence with mood stabilizers: Prevalence and predictors. *J Clin Psychiatry,* 63, 384–390.

Scott, J., and Pope, M. (2002b). Self-reported adherence to treatment with mood stabilizers, plasma levels, and psychiatric hospitalization. *Am J Psychiatry,* 159, 1927–1929.

Scott, J., Paykel, E., Morriss, R., Bentall, R., Kinderman, P., Johnson, T., Abbott, R., and Hayhurst, H. (2006). Cognitive-behavioural therapy for severe and recurrent bipolar disorders: Randomised controlled trial. *Br J Psychiatry,* 188, 313–320.

Shakir, S.A., Volkmar, F.R., Bacon, S., and Pfefferbaum, A. (1979). Group psychotherapy as an adjunct to lithium maintenance. *Am J Psychiatry,* 136, 455–456.

Silverstone, T., McPherson, H., Hunt, N., and Romans, S. (1998). How effective is lithium in the prevention of relapse in bipolar disorder? A prospective naturalistic follow-up study. *Aust NZ J Psychiatry,* 32, 61–66.

Slavney, P.R. (2005). *Psychotherapy: An Introduction for Psychiatry Residents and Other Mental Health Trainees.* Baltimore: Johns Hopkins University Press.

Stratigos, K., Peselowe, L., Sobel, M., Fieve, R., and Laje, G. (2002, October). *Non-Adherence with Long-Term Mood Stabilizers in Patients with Bipolar Disorder.* Poster presented at the Institute on Psychiatric Services Meeting, Chicago, IL.

Suppes, T., Baldessarini, R.J., Faedda, G.L., and Tohen, M. (1991). Risk of recurrence following discontinuation of lithium treatment in bipolar disorder. *Arch Gen Psychiatry,* 48, 1082–1088.

Svarstad, B.L., Shireman, T., and Sweeney, J.K. (2001). Using drug claims data to assess the relationship of medication adherence with hospitalization costs. *Psychiatr Serv,* 52, 805–811.

Tohen, M., Chengappa, K.N., Suppes, T., Baker, R.W., Zarate, C.A., Bowden, C.L., Sachs, G.S., Kupfer, D.J., Ghaemi, S.N.,

Feldman, P.D., Risser, R.C., Evans, A.R., and Calabrese, J.R. (2004). Relapse prevention in bipolar I disorder: 18-Month comparison of olanzapine plus mood stabilizer vs. mood stabilizer alone. *Br J Psychiatry,* 184, 337–345.

Tsai, S.M., Chen, C., Kuo, C., Lee, J., Lee, H., and Strakowski, S.M. (2001). 15-year outcome of treated bipolar disorder. *J Affect Disord,* 63(1-3), 215–220.

van Gent, E.M., and Zwart, F.M. (1991). Psychoeducation of partners of bipolar-manic patients. *J Affect Disord,* 21(1), 15–18.

Van Putten, T. (1975). Why do patients with manic-depressive illness stop their lithium? *Compr Psychiatry,* 16, 179–183.

Van Putten, T., and Jamison, K.R. (1980). Rejecting of lithium maintenance therapy by the patient. In Johnson, F.N. (ed.), *Handbook of Lithium Therapy* (pp. 103–108). Lancaster, England: NTP Press.

Vestergaard, P., and Amdisen, A. (1983). Patient attitudes toward lithium. *Acta Psychiatr Scand,* 67, 8–12.

Weiss, R.D., Greenfield, S.F., Najavits, L.M., Soto, J.A., Wyner, D., Tohen, M., and Griffin, M.L. (1998). Medication adherence among patients with bipolar disorder and substance use disorder. *J Clin Psychiatry,* 59, 172–174.

Weiss, R.D., Kolodziej, M.E., Najavits, L.M., Greenfield, S.F., and Fucito, L.M. (2000). Utilization of psychosocial treatments by patients diagnosed with bipolar disorder and substance dependence. *Am J Addict,* 9(4), 314–320.

World Health Organization. (2003). *Adherence to Long-Term Therapies: Evidence for Action.* Geneva: World Health Organization.

Yen, C.-F., Chen, C.-S., Yeh, M.-L., Yang, S.-J., Ke, J.-H., and Yen, J.-Y. (2003). Changes of insight in manic episodes and influencing factors. *Compr Psychiatry,* 44, 404–408.

Yen, C.-F., Chen, C.-S., Yeh, M.-L., Ker, J.-H., Yang, S.-J., and Yen, J.-Y. (2004). Correlates of insight among patients with bipolar I disorder in remission. *J Affect Dis,* 78, 57–60.

Young, J.L., Spitz, R.T., Hillbrand, M., and Daneri, G. (1999). Medication adherence failure in schizophrenia: A forensic review of rates, reasons, treatments, and prospects. *J Am Acad Psychiatry Law,* 27, 426–444.

Chapter 22

Abraham, K. (1911). Notes on the psycho-analytical investigation and treatment of manic-depressive insanity and allied conditions. In *Selected Papers of Karl Abraham, M.D.* (pp. 137–156). Translated by D. Bryan and A. Strachey. London: Hogarth Press.

Abraham, K. (1927). Notes on the psycho-analytical investigation and treatment of manic-depressive insanity and allied conditions, 1911. In D. Bryan and A. Strachey (Eds.), *Selected Papers of Karl Abraham, M.D.* (pp. 137–156). London: Hogarth Press.

Aleman, A., Agrawal, N., Morgan, K.D., and David, A.S. (2006). Insight in psychosis and neuropsychological function: Meta-analysis. *Br J Psychiatry,* 189, 204–212.

Alloy, L.B., Reilly-Harrington, N., Fresco, D.M., Whitehouse, W.G., and Zechmeister, J.S. (1999). Cognitive styles and life events in subsyndromal unipolar and bipolar disorders: Stability and prospective prediction of depressive and hypomanic mood swings. *J Cogn Psychotherapy,* 13, 21–40.

American Psychiatric Association (APA). (2002). Practice guideline for the treatment of patients with bipolar disorder. *Am J Psychiatry,* 159(Suppl.), 4–50.

Anonymous. (1984). Manic depressive illness. *Lancet,* 2(8414), 1268.

Anthony, E.J. (1975). The influence of a manic-depressive environment on the developing child. In E.J. Anthony and T. Benedek (Eds.), *Depression and Human Existence* (pp. 279–315). Boston: Little, Brown.

Baastrup, P.C., and Schou, M. (1967). Lithium as a prophylactic agent: Its effect against recurrent depression and manic-depressive psychosis. *Arch Gen Psychiatry,* 16, 162–172.

Basco, M.R., and Rush, A.J. (1996). *Cognitive Behavioral Therapy for Bipolar Disorder.* New York: The Guilford Press.

Bauer, M.S., Crits-Christoph, P., Ball, W.A., Dewees, E., McAllister, T., Alahi, P., Cacciola, J., and Whybrow, P.C. (1991). Independent assessment of manic and depressive symptoms by self-rating: Scale characteristics and implications for the study of mania. *Arch Gen Psychiatry,* 48, 807–812.

Beck, A.T., Rush, A.J., Shaw, B.F., and Emery, G. (1979). *Cognitive Therapy of Depression.* New York: The Guilford Press.

Benson, R. (1976). Psychological stress as a cause of lithium prophylaxis failure: A report of three cases. *Dis Nerv Syst,* 37(12), 699–700.

Berk, M., Berk, L., and Castle, D. (2004). A collaborative approach to the treatment alliance in bipolar disorder. *Bipolar Disord,* 6, 504–518.

Callahan, A.M., and Bauer, M.S. (1999). Psychosocial interventions for bipolar disorder. *Psychtr Clin North Am,* 22, 675–688.

Cassidy, F., Murry, E., Forest, K., and Carroll, B.J. (1998). Signs and symptoms of mania in pure and mixed episodes. *J Affect Disord,* 50(2-3), 187–201.

Cassidy, F., McEvoy, J.P., Yang, Y.K., and Wilson, W.H. (2001). Insight is greater in mixed than in pure manic episodes of bipolar I disorder. *J Nerv Ment Dis,* 189(6), 398–399.

Clarkin, J.F., Carpenter, D., Hull, J., Wilner, P., and Glick, I. (1998). Effects of psychoeducational intervention for married patients with bipolar disorder and their spouses. *Psychiatr Serv,* 49, 531–533.

Cochran, S.D. (1984). Preventing medical nonadherence in the outpatient treatment of bipolar affective disorders. *J Consult Clin Psychol,* 52, 873–878.

Cohen, M.B., Baker, G., Cohen, R.A., Fromm-Reichmann, F., and Weighert, E.V. (1954). An intensive study of twelve cases of manic-depressive psychosis. *Psychiatry,* 17, 103–137.

Colom, F., and Vieta, E. (2006). The pivotal note of psychoeducation with long-term treatment of bipolar disorder. In H.S. Akiskal and M. Tohen (Eds.), *Bipolar Psychopharmacotherapy: Caring for the Patient* (pp. 333–345). New York: John Wiley & Sons.

Colom, F., Vieta, E., Martinez-Avan, A., Reinares, M., Goikolea, J.M., Benabarre, A., Torrent, C., Comes, M., Corbella, B., Parramon, G., and Corominas, J. (2003a). A randomized trial on the efficacy of group psychoeducation in the prophylaxis of recurrences in remitted bipolar patients. *Arch Gen Psychiatry,* 60, 402–407.

Colom, F., Vieta, E., Reinares, M., Martinez-Aran, A., Torrent, C., Goikolea, J.M., and Gasto, C. (2003b). Psychoeducation efficacy in bipolar disorders beyond compliance enhancement. *J Clin Psychiatry,* 64, 1101–1105.

Colom, F., Vieta, E., Sánchez-Moreno, J., Martinez-Arán, A., Reinares, M., Goikolea, J.M., and Scott, J. (2005). Stabilizing the stabilizer: Group psychoeducation enhances the stability of serum lithium levels. *Bipolar Disord,* 7(Suppl. 5), 32–36.

Coryell, W., Scheftner, W., Keller, M., Endicott, J., Maser, J., and Klerman, G.L. (1993). The enduring psychosocial consequences of mania and depression. *Am J Psychiatry,* 150, 720–727.

Culver, J.L., Nam, J.Y., Ullal, A., Wang, P.W., Marsh, W., and Ketter, T.A. (2006). *Finding a silver lining: Benefit-finding in bipolar disorder.* Poster presented at the annual meeting of the American Psychiatric Association, Toronto, Canada.

Custance, J. (1952). *Wisdom, Madness, and Folly: The Philosophy of a Lunatic.* New York: Farrar, Strauss, & Cudahy.

Davenport, Y.B., Aldland, M.L., Gold, P.W., and Goodwin, F.K. (1979). Manic-depressive illness: Psychodynamic features of multigenerational families. *Am J Orthopsychiatry,* 49, 24–35.

de Andrés, R.D., Aillon, N., Bardiot, M.C., Bourgeois, P., Mertel, S., Nerfin, F., Romailler, G., Gex-Fabry, M., and Aubry, J.M. (2006). Impact of the life goals group therapy program for bipolar patients: an open study. *J Affect Disord,* 93, 253–257.

Dell'Osso, L., Pini, S., Tundo, A., Sarno, N., Musetti, L., and Cassano, G.B. (2000). Clinical characteristics of mania, mixed mania, and bipolar depression with psychotic features. *Conpr Psychiatry,* 41(4), 242–247.

Dell'Osso, L., Pini, S., Cassano, G.B., Mastrocinque, C., Seckinger, R.A., Saettoni, M., Papasogli, A., Yale, S.A., and Amador, X.F. (2002). Insight into illness in patients with mania, mixed mania, bipolar depression and major depression with psychotic features. *Bipol Disord,* 4(5), 315–322.

Denicoff, K.D., Smith-Jackson, E.E., Disney, E.R., Suddath, R.L., Leverich, G.S., and Post, R.M. (1997). Preliminary evidence of the reliability and validity of the prospective life-chart methodology (LCM-p). *J Psychiatr Res,* 31, 593–603.

Depression and Bipolar Support Alliance (DBSA). http://www.dbsalliance.org/site/PageServer?pagename=home&printer_friendly=1.

Depression and Bipolar Support Alliance (DBSA). http://www.dsballiance.org/site/PageServer?pagename=empower_advance_advancedirectives2. Page created 5/8/2006.

Ehlers, C.L., Frank, E., and Kupfer, D.J. (1988). Social zeitgebers and biological rhythms: A unified approach to understanding the etiology of depression. *Arch Gen Psychiatry,* 45, 948–952.

Endler, A.T., and Gabi, F. (1982). The role of drug level determination in therapy control [in German]. *Med Lab (Stuttg),* 35(5), 133–136.

English, O.S. (1949). Observations of trends in manic-depressive psychosis. *Psychiatry,* 12, 125–133.

Fallon, I.R.H., Boyd, J.L., and McGill, C.W. (1984). *Family Care of Schizophrenia.* New York: The Guilford Press.

Frank, E., Kupfer, D.J., Ehlers, C.L., Monk, T.H., and Cornes, C. (1994). Interpersonal and social rhythm therapy for bipolar disorder: Integrating interpersonal and behavior approaches. *The Behavior Therapist,* 17, 143–149.

Frank, E., Kupfer, D.J., and Siegel, L.R. (1995). Alliance not adherence: A philosophy of outpatient care. *J Clin Psychiatry,* 56(Suppl.), 11–16.

Frank, E., Swartz, H.A., Mallinger, A.G., Thase, M.E., Weaver, E.V., and Kupfer, D.J. (1999). Adjunctive psychotherapy for bipolar disorder: Effects of changing treatment modality. *J Abnorm Psychol,* 108, 579–587.

Frank, E., Swartz, H.A., and Kupfer, D.J. (2000). Interpersonal and social rhythm therapy: Managing the chaos of bipolar disorder. *Biol Psychiatry,* 48, 593–604.

Frank, E., Kupfer, D.J., Thase, M.E., Mallinger, A.G., Swartz, H.A., Faglioni, A.M., Grochocinski, V., Houck, P., Scott, J.,

Thompson, W., and Monk, T. (2005). Two-year outcomes for interpersonal and social rhythm therapy in individuals with bipolar IV. *Arch Gen Psychiatry*, 62, 996–1004.

Frank, J.D. (1961). *Persuasion and Healing*. New York: Oxford University Press.

Fristad, M.A., Teare, M., Weller, E.B., Weller, R.A., and Salmon, P. (1998). Study III: Development and concurrent validity of the Children's Interview for Psychiatric Syndromes–parent version (P-ChIPS). *J Child Adolesc Psychopharmacol*, 8(4), 221–226.

Fristad, M.A., Goldberg-Arnold, J.S., and Gavazzi, S.M. (2002). Multifamily psychoeducation groups (MFPG) for families of children with bipolar disorder. *Bipolar Disord*, 4(4), 254–262.

Fromm-Reichman, F. (1949). Intensive psychotherapy of manic-depressives: A preliminary report. *Confina Neurologica*, 9, 158–165.

Ghaemi, S.N., Stoll, A.L., and Pope H.R. (1995). Lack of insight in bipolar disorder. The acute manic episode. *J Nerv Ment Dis*, 183(7), 464–467.

Gitlin, M.J., Cochran, S.D., and Jamison, K.R. (1989). Maintenance lithium treatment: Side effects and compliance. *J Clin Psychiatry*, 50(4), 127–131.

Goldberg, J.F., and Harrow, M. (1999). Poor-outcome bipolar disorders. In J.F. Goldberg and M. Harrow (Eds.), *Bipolar Disorders: Clinical Course and Outcome* (pp. 1–19). Washington, DC: American Psychiatric Press.

Goldberg, J.F., Harrow, M., and Grossman, L.S. (1995). Course and outcome in bipolar affective disorder: A longitudinal follow-up study. *Am J Psychiatry*, 152, 379–384.

Goodale, L.C., and Lewis, L. (1999). The effects of support group participation on treatment adherence. In J.C. Soares, S. Gershon (Eds.), Bipolar Disorders. Poster presented at the Third International Conference on Bipolar Disorder, Pittsburgh, PA, June 17–19. *Int J Psychiatry Neurosci*, 1(Suppl. 1), 32.

Goodwin, G. (2002). Hypomania: What's in a name? *Br J Psychiatry*, 181, 94–95.

Graves, A. (1942). *The Eclipse of a Mind*. New York: The Medical Journal Press.

Greene, J. (2001). Benchmarking. Guidelines on kids. *Hosp Health Netw*, 75(7), 26, 28.

Greenson, R.R. (1967). *The Technique and Practice of Psychoanalysis*. New York: International Universities Press.

Haas, G.L., Glick, I.D., Clarkin, J.F., Spencer, J.H., Lewis, A.B., Peyser, J., DeMane, N., Good-Ellis, M., Harris, E., and Lestelle, V. (1988). Inpatient family intervention: A randomized clinical trial: II: Results at hospital discharge. *Arch Gen Psychiatry*, 45, 217–224.

Hamilton, I. (1982). *Robert Lowell: A Biography*. New York: Random House.

Hibbs, E.D., Clarke, G., Hechtman, L., Abikoff, H.B., Greenhill, L.L., and Jensen, P.S. (1997). Manual development for the treatment of child and adolescent disorders. *Psychopharmacol Bull*, 33, 619–629.

Highet, N., Thompson, M., and McNair, B. (2005). Identifying depression in a family member: The carers' experience. *J Affect Disord*, 87, 25–33.

Hirschfeld-Becker, D.R., Gould, R.A., Reilly-Harrington, N., Morabito, C., Cosgrove, V., Guille, C., Fredman, S., and Sachs, G. (1998). *Short-Term Adjunctive Cognitive-Behavioral Group Therapy for Bipolar Disorder: Preliminary Results from a Controlled Trial*. Poster presented at the 32nd Annual Convention of the Association for the Advancement of Behavior Therapy, Washington, DC, November 5–8.

Hollon, S.D., Kendall, P.C., and Lamry, A. (1986). Specificity of depressogenic cognitions in clinical depression. *J Abnorm Psychol*, 95, 52–59.

Honig, A., Hofman, A., Rozendaal, N., and Dingemans, P. (1997). Psycho-education in bipolar disorder: Effect on expressed emotion. *Psychiatry Res*, 72(1), 17–22.

Jackson, A., Cavanagh, J., and Scott, J. (2003). A systematic review of manic and depressive prodromes. *J Affect Disord*, 74, 209–217.

Jamison, K.R. (1991). Manic-depressive illness: The overlooked need for psychotherapy. In B.D. Beitman and G. Klerman (Eds.), *Integrating Pharmacotherapy and Psychotherapy* (pp. 409–420). Washington, DC: American Psychiatric Press.

Jamison, K.R. (1995). *An Unquiet Mind: A Memoir of Moods and Madness*. New York: Alfred A. Knopf.

Jamison, K.R. (2004). *Exuberance: The Passion for Life*. New York: Alfred A. Knopf.

Jamison, K.R. (2006). The many stigmas of mental illness. *Lancet*, 367(9520), 1396–1397.

Jamison, K.R., and Goodwin, F.K. (1983). Psychotherapeutic treatment of manic-depressive patients on lithium. In M. Greenhill and A. Gralnick (Eds.), *The Interrelationship of Psychopharmacology and Psychotherapy* (pp. 53–74). New York: Macmillan.

Jamison, K.R., Gerner, R.H., and Goodwin, F.K. (1979). Patient and physician attitudes toward lithium: Relationship to adherence. *Arch Gen Psychiatry*, 36, 866–869.

Jamison, K.R., Gerner, R.H., Hammen, C., and Padesky, C. (1980). Clouds and silver linings: Positive experiences associated with primary affective disorders. *Am J Psychiatry*, 137, 198–202.

Janowsky, D.S., Leff, M., and Epstein, R.S. (1970). Playing the manic game: Interpersonal maneuvers of the acutely manic patient. *Arch Gen Psychiatry*, 22, 252–261.

Jones, I., Scourfield, J., McCandless, F., and Craddock, N. (2002). Attitudes towards future testing for bipolar disorder susceptibility genes: A preliminary investigation. *J Affect Disord*, 71, 189–193.

Jones, L., Scott, J., Hague, S., Gordon-Smith, K., Heron, J., Caesar, S., Cooper, C., Forty, L., Hyde, S., Lyon, L., Greening, J., Sham, P., Farmer, A., McGuffin, P., Jones, I., and Craddock, N. (2005). Cognitive style in bipolar disorder. *Br J Psychiatry*, 187, 431–437.

Joshi, K.G. (2003). Psychiatric advance directives. *J Psychiatr Prac*, 9, 303–306.

Keck, P.E. Jr., McElroy, S.L., Strakowski, S.M., Bourne, M.L., and West, S.A. (1997). Adherence with maintenance treatment in bipolar disorder. *Psychopharmacol Bull*, 33, 87–91.

Keck, P.E. Jr., McElroy, S.L., and Strakowski, S.M. (1998). Anticonvulsants and antipsychotics in the treatment of bipolar disorder. *J Clin Psychiatry*, 59(Suppl. 6), 74–81.

Kim, E.Y., and Miklowitz, D.J. (2004). Expressed emotion as a predictor of outcome among bipolar patients undergoing family therapy. *J Affect Disord*, 82, 343–352.

Klerman, G.L., Weissman, M.M., Rounsaville, B.J., and Chevron, E.S. (1984). *Interpersonal Psychotherapy of Depression*. New York: Basic Books.

Kraepelin, E. (1904). *Lectures on Clinical Psychiatry*. London: Ballière, Tindall & Cox.

Lam, D.H. (2006). What can we conclude from studies on psychotherapy in bipolar disorder? Invited commentary on . . . Cognitive-behavioral therapy for severe and recurrent bipolar disorders. *Br J Psychiatry*, 188, 321–322.

Lam, D.H., and Wong, G. (1997). Prodromes, coping strategies, insight and social functioning in bipolar affective disorder. *Psychol Med*, 27, 1091–1100.

Lam, D.H., Bright, J., Jones, S., Hayward, P., Schuck, N., Chisholm, D., and Sham, P. (2000). Cognitive therapy of bipolar illness: A pilot study. *Cogn Ther Res*, 24, 503–520.

Lam, D.H., Watkins, E.R., Hayward, P., Bright, J., Wright, K., Kerr, N., Parr-Davis, G., and Sham P. (2003). A randomized controlled study of cognitive therapy for relapse prevention for bipolar affective disorder: Outcome of the first year. *Arch Gen Psychiatry*, 60(2), 145–152.

Lam, D.H., McCrone, P., Wright, K., and Kerr, N. (2005a). Cost-effectiveness of relapse-prevention cognitive therapy for bipolar disorder: 30-month study. *Br J Psychiatry*, 186, 500–506.

Lam, D.H., Hayward, P., Watkins, E.R., Wright, K., and Sham, P. (2005b). Relapse prevention in patients with bipolar disorder: Cognitive therapy outcome after 2 years. *Am J Psychiatry*, 162, 324–329.

Leverich, G.S., and Post, R.M. (1993). *The NIMH Life Chart Manual for Recurrent Affective Illness: The LCM*. Bethesda, MD: Monograph.

Lish, J.D., Dime-Meenan, S., Whybrow, P.C., Price, R.A., and Hirschfeld, R.M.A. (1994). The National Depressive and Manic-depressive Association (DMDA) survey of bipolar members. *J Affect Disord*, 31, 281–294.

Logan, J. (1976). *Josh: My Up and Down, In and Out Life*. New York: Delacorte Press.

Lowell, R. (1959). Home after three months away. In *Life Studies*. New York: Farrar, Strauss, and Cudahy.

Lowell, R. (1977). Since 1939. In *Day by Day*. New York: Farrar, Straus & Giroux.

Marlatt, G.A., and Gordon, J.R. (1985). *Relapse Prevention*. New York: The Guilford Press.

McAlpin, R.N., Goodnick, P.J. (1998). Psychotherapy, in mania: Clinical and research perspectives (pp. 363–381). P.J. Goodnick (Ed.). Washington, DC: American Psychiatric Press.

Miklowitz, D.J., and Goldstein, M.J. (1990). Behavioral family treatment for patients with bipolar affective disorder. *Behav Modif*, 14, 457–489.

Miklowitz, D.J., and Goldstein, M.J. (1997). *Bipolar Disorder: A Family Focused Treatment Approach*. New York: The Guilford Press.

Miklowitz, D.J., Frank, E., and George, E.L. (1996). New psychosocial treatments for the outpatient management of bipolar disorder. *Psychopharm Bull*, 32, 613–621.

Miklowitz, D.J., Simoneau, T.L., George, E.L., Richards, J.A., Kalbag, A., Sachs-Ericsson, N., and Suddath, R. (2000). Family-focused treatment of bipolar disorder: One-year effects of a psychoeducational program in conjunction with pharmacotherapy. *Biol Psychiatry*, 48, 582–592.

Miklowitz, D.J., George, E.L., Axelson, D.A., Kim, E.Y., Birmaher, B., Schneck, C., Beresford, C., Craighead, W.E., and Brent, D.A. (2004). Family-focused treatment for adolescents with bipolar disorder. *J Affect Disord*, 825, S113–S128.

Miklowitz, D.J., Wisniewski, S.R., Miyahara, S., Otto, M.W., and Sachs, G.S. (2005). Perceived criticism from family members as a predictor of the one-year course of bipolar disorder. *Psychiatry Res*, 136, 101–111.

Miklowitz, D.J., Otto, M.W., Wisniewski, S.R., Araga, M., Frank, E., Reilly-Harrington, N.A., Lembke, A., and Sachs, G.S. (2006). Psychotherapy, symptom outcomes, and role functioning over one year among patients with bipolar disorder. *Psychiatr Serv*, 57, 959–969.

Miller, I.W., Keitner, G.I., Bishop, D.S., and Ryan, C.I. (1991). *Families of Bipolar Patients: Dysfunction, Course of Illness, and Pilot Treatment Study*. Presented at the annual meeting of the Association for Advancement of Behavior Therapy, New York.

Miller, I.W., Solomon, D.A., Ryan, C.E., and Keitner, G.I. (2004). Does adjunctive family therapy enhance recovery from bipolar I mood episodes? *J Affect Disord*, 82(3), 431–436.

Molnar, G., Feeney, M.G., and Fava, G.A. (1988). Duration and symptoms of bipolar prodromes. *Am J Psychiatry*, 145, 1576–1578.

Monk, T.H., Kupfer, D.J., Frank, E., and Ritenour, A.M. (1991). The Social Rhythm Metric (SRM): Measuring daily social rhythms over 12 weeks. *Psychiatry Res*, 36, 195–207.

Pallanti, S., Quercioli, L., Pazzagli, A., Rossi, A., Dell'Osso, L., Pini, S., and Cassano, G.B. (1999). Awareness of illness and subjective experience of cognitive complaints in patients with bipolar I and bipolar II disorder. *Am J Psychiatry*, 156(7), 1094–1096.

Pavuluri, M.N., Naylor, M., and Janicak, P. (2002). Recognition and treatment of pediatric bipolar disorder. *Contemp Psychiatry*, 1, 1–10.

Pavuluri, M.N., Graczyk, P.A., Henry, D.B., Carbray, J.A., Heidenreich, J., and Miklowitz, D.J. (2004). Child- and family-focused cognitive-behavioral therapy for pediatric bipolar disorder: Development and preliminary results. *J Am Acad Child Adolesc Psychiatry*, 43, 528–537.

Peet, M., and Harvey, N.S. (1991). Lithium maintenance: 1. A standard education programme for patients. *Br J Psychiatry*, 158, 197–200.

Peralta, V., and Cuesta, M.J. (1998). Lack of insight in mood disorders. *J Affect Disord*, 49(1), 55–58.

Perlick, D.A., Rosenheck, R.A., Clarkin, J.F., Maciejewski, P.K., Sirey, J., Struening, E., and Link, B.G. (2004). Impact of family burden and affective response on clinical outcome among patients with bipolar disorder. *Psychiatr Serv*, 55(9), 1029–1035.

Perry, A., Tarrier, N., Morriss, R., McCarthy, E., and Limb, K. (1999). Randomised controlled trial of efficacy of teaching patients with bipolar disorder to identify early symptoms of relapse and obtain treatment. *BMJ*, 318, 149–153.

Pini, S., Cassano, G.B., Dell'Osso, L., and Amador, X.F. (2001). Insight into illness in schizophrenia, schizoaffective disorder, and mood disorders with psychotic features. *Am J Psychiatry*, 158(1), 122–125.

Post, R.M., Rubinow, D.R., and Ballenger, J.C. (1986). Conditioning and sensitization in the longitudinal course of affective illness. *Br J Psychiatry*, 149, 191–201.

Prien, R.F., and Potter, W.Z. (1990). *Report from the NIMH Workshop on the Treatment of Bipolar Disorder*. Rockville, MD: NIMH Division of Clinical Research.

Rado, S. (1928). The problem of melancholia. *Int J Psychoanal*, 9, 420–438.

Rea, M., Tompson, M., Miklowitz, D., Goldstein, M., Hwang, S., and Mintz, J. (2003). Family-focused treatment versus individual treatment for bipolar disorder: Results of a randomized clinical trial. *J Consult Clin Psychol, 71,* 482–492.

Reiss, E. (1910). *Konstitutionelle Verstimmung und manisch-depressives Irresein: Klinische Untersuchungen über den Zusammenhang von Veranlagung und Psychose.* Berlin: J. Springer.

Rosenfeld, H. (1963). Notes on the psychopathology and psychoanalytic treatment of depressive and manic depressive patients. In H. Azima and B.C. Glueck (Eds.), *Psychiatric Research Report 17* (pp. 73–83). Washington, DC: American Psychiatric Association.

Roy, C.K., and Williams, P. (2005). Barriers to the effective management of bipolar disorder: A survey of psychiatrists based on the UK and USA. *Bipolar Disord, 7*(Suppl. 1), 38–42.

Schou, M. (1980). Social and psychological implications of lithium therapy. In F.N. Johnson (Ed.), *Handbook of Lithium Therapy* (pp. 378–381). Baltimore: University Park Press.

Schou, M., and Baastrup, P.C. (1973). Personal and social implications of lithium maintenance treatment. In T.A. Ban, J.R. Boissier, G.J. Gessa, H. Heimann, L. Hollister, H.E. Lehmann, I. Munkvad, H. Steinberg, F. Sulser, A. Sundwall, and O. Vinar (Eds.), *Psychopharmacology, Sexual Disorders and Drug Abuse.* Amsterdam and London: North-Holland Publishing Company.

Scott, J. (1996). Cognitive therapy of affective disorders: A review. *J Affect Disord, 37,* 1–11.

Scott, J., and Gutierrez, M.J. (2004). The current status of psychological treatments in bipolar disorders: A systematic review of relapse prevention. *Bipolar Disord, 6,* 498–503.

Scott, J., and Pope, M. (2003). Cognitive styles in individuals with bipolar disorders. *Psychol Med, 33,* 1082–1088.

Scott, J., Stanton, B., Garland A., and Ferrier, I.N. (2000). Cognitive vulnerability in patients with bipolar disorder. *Psychol Med, 30,* 467–472.

Scott, J., Garland, A., and Moorhead, S. (2001). A pilot study of cognitive therapy in bipolar disorder. *Psychol Med, 31*(3), 459–467.

Simon, G.E., Ludman, E.J., Unützer, J., Bauer, M.S., Operskalski, B., and Rutter, C. (2005). Randomized trial of a population-based care program for people with bipolar disorder. *Psychol Med, 35,* 13–24.

Slavney, P.R. (2005). *Psychotherapy: An Introduction for Psychiatry Residents and Other Mental Health Trainees.* Baltimore: Johns Hopkins University Press.

Smith, J.A., and Tarrier, N. (1992). Prodromal symptoms in manic depressive psychosis. *Soc Psychiatry Psychiatr Epidemiol, 27,* 245–248.

Smith, L.B., Sapers, B., Reus, V.I., and Freimer, N.B. (1996). Attitudes towards bipolar disorder and predictive genetic testing among patients and providers. *J Med Genet, 33,* 544–559.

Squillace, K., Post, R.M., Savard, R., and Erwin-Gorman, M. (1984). Life charting of the longitudinal course of recurrent affective illness. In: R.M. Post, J.C. Ballenger (Eds.), *Neurobiology of Mood Disorders* (pp. 38–59). Baltimore: Williams & Wilkins.

Srebnik, D.S., Rutherford, L.T., Peto, T., Russo, J., Zick, E., Jaffe, C., and Holtzheimer, P. (2005). The content and clinical utility of psychiatric advance directives. *Psychiatr Serv, 56,* 592–598.

Suppes, T., Swann, A.C., Dennehy, E.B., Habermacher, E.D., Mason, M., Crismon, M.L., Toprac, M.G., Rush, A.J., Shon, S.P., and Altshuler, K.Z, (2001). Texas Medication Algorithm Project: Development and feasability testing of a treatment algorithm for patients with bipolar disorder. *J Clin Psychiatry, 62,* 439–447.

Suppes, T., Dennehy, E.B., Swann, A.C., Bowden, C.L., Calabrese, J.R., Hirschfeld, R.M., Keck, P.E., Sachs, G.S., Crismon, M.L., Toprac, M.G., Shon, S.P., Texas Consensus Conference Panel on Medication Treatment of Bipolar Disorder. (2002). Report of the Texas Consensus Conference Panel on medication treatment of bipolar disorder 2000. *J Clin Psychiatry, 63*(4), 288–299.

Swanson, J.W., Swartz, M.S., Elbogen, E.G., Van Dorn, R.A., Ferron, J., Wagner, H.R., McCauley, B.J., and Kim, M. (2006). Facilitated psychiatric advance directives: A randomized trial of an intervention to foster advance treatment planning among persons with severe mental illness. *Am J Psychiatry, 163,* 1943–1951.

Szmukler, G.I., and Bloch, S. (1997). Family involvement in the care of people with psychoses: An ethical argument. *Br J Psychiatry, 171,* 401–405.

Toprac, M.G., Hopkins, C., Conner, T., Rush, A.J., Crismon, M.L., Dees, M., Rowe, V., and Shon, S.P. (1998). *Texas Medication Algorithm Project (TMAP) Patient Education Plan Guidebook.* Austin, TX: Texas Department of Mental Health and Mental Retardation (TDMHMR).

Toprac, M.G., Rush, J.A., Conner, T.M., Crismon, M.L., Dees, M., Hopkins, C., Rowe, V., and Shon, S.P. (2000). The Texas Medication Algorithm Project Patient and Family Education Program: A consumer-guided initiative. *J Clin Psychiatry, 61,* 477–486.

Trippitelli, C.L., Jamison, K.R., Folstein, M.F., Bartko, J.J., and DePaulo, J.R. (1998). Pilot study on patients' and spouses' attitudes toward potential genetic testing for bipolar disorder. *Am J Psychiatry, 155,* 899–904.

van Gent, E.M., and Zwart, F.M. (1991). Psychoeducation of partners of bipolar-manic patients. *J Affect Disord, 21*(1), 15–18.

Varga, M., Magnusson, A., Flekkøy, K., Rønnerg, U., and Opjordsmoen, S. (2006). Insight, symptoms and neurocognition in bipolar I patients. *J Affect Disord, 91,* 1–9.

Vasile, R.G., Samson, J.A., Bemporad, J., Bloomingdale, K.L., Creasey, D., Fenton, B.T., Gudeman, J.E., and Schildkraut, J.J. (1987). A biopsychosocial approach to treating patients with affective disorders. *Am J Psychiatry, 144,* 341–344.

Verdeli, H. (2004, October). *Modifying IPT for Prevention for Symptomatic Offspring of Bipolar Parents.* Presented at the Symposium, "New Developments in IPT with Adolescents" (L. Mufson Chair). Washington, DC: American Academy of Child and Adolescent Psychiatry.

Wehr, T.A., and Goodwin, F.K. (1987). Can antidepressants cause mania and worsen the course of affective illness? *Am J Psychiatry, 144,* 1403–1411.

Wehr, T.A., Sach, D.A., and Rosenthal, N.E. (1987a). Sleep reduction as a final common pathway in the genesis of mania. *Am J Psychiatry, 144,* 201–204.

Wehr, T.A., Sach, D.A., and Rosenthal, N.E. (1987b). Seasonal affective disorder with summer depression and winter hypomania. *Am J Psychiatry, 144,* 1602–1603.

Weiss, R.D., Griffin, M.L., Greenfield, S.F., Najavits, L.M., Wyner, D., Soto, J.A., and Hennen, J.A. (2000). Group therapy for patients with bipolar disorder and substance dependence: Results of a pilot study. *J Clin Psychiatry, 61,* 361–365.

Weissman, M.M., Markowitz, J.C., and Klerman, G.L. (2000). *Comprehensive Guide to Interpersonal Psychotherapy.* New York: Basic Books.

Wilson, S. (1976). *What Shall We Wear to This Party? The Man in the Gray Flannel Suit: Twenty Years Before and After*. New York: Arbor House.

Wodehouse, P.G. (1975). *The Code of the Woosters*. New York: Random House.

Yen, C.F., Chen, C.S., Yeh, M.L., Yang, S.J., Ke, J.H., and Yen, J.Y. (2003). Changes of insight in manic episodes and influencing factors. *Compr Psychiatry*, 44(5), 404–408.

Zaretsky, A.E., Zindel, V.S., and Gemar, M. (1999). Cognitive therapy for bipolar depression: A pilot study. *Can J Psychiatry*, 44, 491–494.

CHAPTER 23

Akiskal, H.S., Downs, J., Jordan, P., Watson, S., Daugherty, D., and Pruitt, D.B. (1985). Affective disorders in referred children and younger siblings of manic depressives. *Arch Gen Psychiatry*, 42, 996–1004.

Allison, D.B., Mentore, J.L., Heo, M., Chandler, L.P., Cappelleri, J.C., Infante, M.C., and Weiden, P.J. (1999). Antipsychotic-induced weight gain: A comprehensive research synthesis. *Am J Psychiatry*, 156(11), 1686–1696.

Altshuler, L., Suppes, T., Black, D., Nolen, W.A., Keck, P.E. Jr., Frye, M.A., McElroy, S., Kupka, R., Grunze, H., Walden, J., Leverich, G., Denicoff, K., Luckenbaugh, D., and Post, R. (2003). Impact of antidepressant discontinuation after acute bipolar depression remission on rates of depressive relapse at 1-year follow-up. *Am J Psychiatry*, 160(7), 1252–1262.

Aman, M.G., Singh, N.N., Stewart, A.W., and Field, C.J. (1985). The aberrant behavior checklist: A behavior rating scale for the assessment of treatment effects. *Am J Ment Defic*, 89(5), 485–491.

Aman, M.G., Tasse, M.J., Rojahn, J., and Hammer, D. (1996). The Nisonger CBRF: A child behavior rating form for children with developmental disabilities. *Res Dev Disabil*, 17(1), 41–57.

Aman, M.G., De Smedt, G., Derivan, A., Lyons, B., Findling, R.L., and Risperidone Disruptive Behavior Study Group. (2002). Double-blind, placebo-controlled study of risperidone for the treatment of disruptive behaviors in children with subaverage intelligence. *Am J Psychiatry*, 159(8), 1337–1346.

American Diabetes Association. (2004). Consensus Development Conference on Antipsychotic Drugs and Obesity and Diabetes. http://www.diabetes.org/for=media/2004=press=releases/jan=27-04.jsp.

Annell, A.L. (1969). Lithium in the treatment of children and adolescents. *Acta Psychiatr Scand Suppl*, 207, 19.

Anthony, E.J., and Scott, P. (1960). Manic-depressive psychosis in childhood. *J Child Psychol Psychiatry*, 1, 53–72.

Baldessarini, R.J., Tondo, L., and Viguera, A.C. (1999). Discontinuing lithium maintenance treatment in bipolar disorders: Risks and implications. *Bipolar Disord*, 1(1), 17–24.

Barnett, M.S. (2004). Ziprasidone monotherapy in pediatric bipolar disorder. *J Child Adolesc Psychopharmacol*, 14(3), 471–477.

Barzman, D.H., DelBello, M.P., Kowatch, R.A., Gernert, B., Fleck, D.E., Pathak, S., Rappaport, K., Delgado, S.V., Campbell, P., and Strakowski, S.M. (2004). The effectiveness and tolerability of aripiprazole for pediatric bipolar disorders: A retrospective chart review. *J Child Adolesc Psychopharmacol*, 14(4), 593–600.

Barzman, D.H., Adler, C.M., DelBello, M.P., Stanford, K.E., Kowatch, R.A., and Strakowski, S.M. (2006). Quetiapine efficacy in bipolar adolescents with depressive symptoms. *New Research Abstract*, May 22, 2006. American Psychiatric Association.

Baumer, F.M., Howe, M., Gallelli, K., Simeonova, D.I., Hallmayer, J., and Chang, K.D. (2006). A pilot study of antidepressant-induced mania in pediatric bipolar disorder: Characteristics, risk factors, and the serotonin transporter gene. *Biol Psychiatry*, 60(9), 1005–1012.

Biederman, J., Wozniak, J., Kiely, K., Ablon, S., Faraone, S., Mick, E., Mundy, E., and Kraus, I. (1995). CBCL Clinical Scales discriminate prepubertal children with structured-interview-derived diagnosis of mania from those with ADHD. *J Am Acad Child Adolesc Psychiatry*, 34, 133–140.

Biederman, J., Faraone, S., Mick, E., Wozniak, J., Chen, L., Ouellette, C., Marrs, A., Moore, P., Garcia, J., Mennin, D., and Lelon, E. (1996). Attention-deficit hyperactivity disorder and juvenile mania: An overlooked comorbidity? *J Am Acad Child Adolesc Psychiatry*, 35(8), 997–1008.

Biederman, J., Klein, R.G., Pine, D.S., and Klein, D.F. (1998). Resolved: Mania is mistaken for ADHD in prepubertal children. *J Am Acad Child Adolesc Psychiatry*, 37(10), 1091–1096; discussion 1096–1099.

Biederman, J., Mick, E., Spencer, T.J., Wilens, T.E., and Faraone, S.V. (2000a). Therapeutic dilemmas in the pharmacotherapy of bipolar depression in the young. *J Child Adolesc Psychopharmacol*, 10(3), 185–192.

Biederman, J., Faraone, S.V., Wozniak, J., and Monuteaux, M.C. (2000b). Parsing the associations between bipolar, conduct, and substance use disorders: A familial risk analysis. *Biol Psychiatry*, 48, 1037–1044.

Biederman, J., Mick, E., Wozniak, J., Aleardi, M., Spencer, T., and Faraone, S.V. (2005a). An open-label trial of risperidone in children and adolescents with bipolar disorder. *J Child Adolesc Psychopharmacol*, 15(2), 311–317.

Biederman, J., McDonnell, M.A., Wozniak, J., Spencer, T., Aleardi, M., Falzone, R., Mick, E. (2005b). Aripiprazole in the treatment of pediatric bipolar disorder: A systematic chart review. *CNS Spectr*, 10(2), 141–148.

Buitelaar, J.K., van der Gaag, R.J., Cohen-Kettenis, P., and Melman, C.T. (2001). A randomized controlled trial of risperidone in the treatment of aggression in hospitalized adolescents with subaverage cognitive abilities. *J Clin Psychiatry*, 62(4), 239–248.

Calabrese, J.R., Shelton, M.D., Rapport, D.J., Youngstrom, E.A., Jackson, K., Bilali, S., Ganocy. S.J., and Findling, R.L. (2005). A 20-month, double-blind, maintenance trial of lithium versus divalproex in rapid-cycling bipolar disorder. *Am J Psychiatry*, 162(11), 2152–2161.

Campbell, M., Fish, B., Korein, J., Shapiro, T., Collins, P., and Koh, C. (1972). Lithium and chlorpromazine: A controlled crossover study of hyperactive severely disturbed young children. *J Autism Child Schizophr*, 2(3), 234–263.

Campbell, M., Small, A.M., Green, W.H., Jennings, S.J., Perry, R., Bennett, W.G., and Anderson, L. (1984). Behavioral efficacy of haloperidol and lithium carbonate: A comparison in hospitalized aggressive children with conduct disorder. *Arch Gen Psychiatry*, 41(7), 650–656.

Campbell, M., Adams, P.B., Small, A.M., Kafantaris, V., Silva, R.R., Shell, J., Perry, R., and Overall, J.E. (1995). Lithium in hospitalized aggressive children with conduct disorder: A double-blind and placebo-controlled study. *J Am Acad Child Adolesc Psychiatry*, 34(4), 445–453.

Carandang, C.G., Maxwell, D.J., Robbins, D.R., and Oesterheld, J.R. (2003). Lamotrigine in adolescent mood disorders. *J Am Acad Child Adolesc Psychiatry*, 42(7), 750–751.

Carlson, G.A. (2005a). Early onset bipolar disorder: Clinical and research considerations. *J Clin Child Adolesc Psychol*, 34(2), 333–343.

Carlson, G.A. (2005b). Medication-induced activation in children and adolescents. *Psychiatr Times*, Vol. XXII, issue 10.

Carlson, G.A., and Kelly, K.L. (1998). Manic symptoms in psychiatrically hospitalized children: What do they mean? *J Affect Disord*, 51(2), 123–135.

Carlson, G.A., and Kelly, K.L. (2003). Stimulant rebound: How common is it and what does it mean? *J Child Adolesc Psychopharmacol*, 13(2), 137–142.

Carlson, G.A., and Meyer, S.E. (2006). Phenomenology and diagnosis of bipolar disorder in children, adolescents, and adults: Complexities and developmental issues. *Dev Psychopathol*, 18, 939–969.

Carlson, G.A., and Mick, E. (2003). Drug-induced disinhibition in psychiatrically hospitalized children. *J Child Adolesc Psychopharmacol*, 13, 153–164.

Carlson, G.A., and Strober, M. (1978). Affective disorder in adolescence: Issues in misdiagnosis. *J Clin Psychiatry*, 39, 59–66.

Carlson, G.A., Rapport, M.D., Pataki, C., and Kelly, K.K. (1992a). Lithium in hospitalized children at 4 and 8 weeks: Mood, behavior and cognitive effects. *J Child Psychol Psychiatry*, 33, 411–425.

Carlson, G.A., Rapport, M.D., Pataki, C., and Kelly, K.K. (1992b). The effects of methylphenidate and lithium on attention and activity level. *Am Acad Child Adolesc Psychiatry*, 31, 262–270.

Carlson, G.A., Loney, J., Salisbury, H., and Volpe, R.J. (1998). Young referred boys with DICA-P manic symptoms versus two comparison groups. *J Affect Disord*, 51, 113–121.

Carlson, G.A., Bromet, E.J., and Lavelle, J. (1999). Medication treatment in adolescents versus adults with psychotic mania. *J Child Adolesc Psychopharmacol*, 9, 221–231.

Carlson, G.A., Loney, J., Salisbury, H., Kramer, J.R., and Arthur, C. (2000). Stimulant treatment in young boys with symptoms suggesting childhood mania: A report from a longitudinal study. *J Child Adolesc Psychopharmacol*, 10, 175–184.

Carlson, G.A., Bromet, E.J., Driessens, C., Mojtabai, R., and Schwartz, J.E. (2002). Age at onset, childhood psychopathology, and 2-year outcome in psychotic bipolar disorder. *Am J Psychiatry*, 159, 307–309.

Carlson, G.A., Jensen, P.S., Findling, R.L., Meyer, R.E., Calabrese, J., DelBello, M.P., Emslie, G., Flynn, L., Goodwin, F., Hellander, M., Kowatch, R., Kusumakar, B., Laughren, T., Leibenluft, E., McCracken, J., Nottelmann, E., Pine, D., Sachs, G., Shaffer, D., Simar, R., Strober, M., Weller, E.B., Wozniak, J., and Youngstrom, E.A. (2003). Methodological issues and controversies in clinical trials with child and adolescent patients with bipolar disorder: Report of a consensus conference. *J Child Adolesc Psychopharmacol*, 13(1), 13–27.

Carlson, G.A., Finch, S., Kang, S., Ye, Q., and Bromet, E. (in press). Conversion from depression to mania in 1st admission patients with psychotic bipolar disorder. *J Affect Disord*.

Casey, D.E. (2004). Dyslipidemia and atypical antipsychotic drugs. *J Clin Psychiatry*, 65(Suppl. 18), 27–35.

Chang, K.D., and Ketter, T.A. (2000). Mood stabilizer augmentation with olanzapine in acutely manic children. *J Child Adolesc Psychopharmacol*, 10(1), 45–49.

Chang, K.D., Dienes, K., Blasey, C., Adleman, N., Ketter, T., and Steiner, H. (2003). Divalproex monotherapy in the treatment of bipolar offspring with mood and behavioral disorders and at least mild affective symptoms. *J Clin Psychiatry*, 64(8), 936–942.

Chang, K., Saxena, K., and Howe M. (2006). An open-label study of lamotrigine adjunct or monotherapy for the treatment of adolescents with bipolar depression. *J Am Acad Child Adolesc Psychiatry*, 45(3), 298–304.

Cheung, A.H., Emslie, G.J., and Mayes, T.L. (2005). Review of the efficacy and safety of antidepressants in youth depression. *J Child Psychol Psychiatry*, 46(7), 735–754.

Correll, C.U., and Carlson, H.E.C. (2006). Endocrine and metabolic adverse effects of psychotropic medications in children and adolescents. *J Am Acad Child Adolesc Psychiatry*, 45(7), 771–791.

Correll, C.U., Parikh, U.H., Mughal, T., Olshanskiy, V., Moroff, M., Pleak, R.R., Foley, C., Shah, M., Gutkovich, Z., Kane, J.M., and Malhotra, A.K. (2005). Body composition changes associated with second-generation antipsychotics. *Biol Psychiatry*, 57(Suppl. 8), 36.

Craney, J., and Geller, B. (2003). Clinical implications of antidepressant and stimulant use on switching from depression to mania in children. *J Child Adolesc Psychopharmacol*, 13(2), 201–204.

Craven, C., and Murphy, M. (2000) Carbamazepine treatment of bipolar disorder in an adolescent with cerebral palsy. *J Am Acad Child Adolesc Psychiatry*, 39(6), 680–681.

Davanzo, P.A., Krah, N., Kleiner, J., and McCracken, J. (1999). Nimodipine treatment of an adolescent with ultradian cycling bipolar affective illness. *J Child Adolesc Psychopharmacol*, 9(1), 51–61.

DelBello, M.P., Soutullo, C.A., Hendricks, W., Niemeier, R.T., McElroy, S.L., and Strakowski, S.M. (2001). Prior stimulant treatment in adolescents with bipolar disorder: Association with age at onset. *Bipolar Disord*, 3(2), 53–57.

DelBello, M.P., Schwiers, M.L., Rosenberg, H.L., and Strakowski, S.M. (2002). A double-blind, randomized, placebo-controlled study of quetiapine as adjunctive treatment for adolescent mania. *J Am Acad Child Adolesc Psychiatry*, 41(10), 1216–1223.

DelBello, M.P., Carlson, G.A., Tohen, M., Bromet, E.J., Schwiers, M., and Strakowski, S.M. (2003). Rates and predictors of developing a manic or hypomanic episode 1 to 2 years following a first hospitalization for major depression with psychotic features. *J Child Adolesc Psychopharmacol*, 13, 173–186.

DelBello, M.P., Findling, R.L., Kushner, S., Wang, D., Olson, W.H., Capece, J.A., Fazzio, L., and Rosenthal, N.R. (2005). A pilot controlled trial of topiramate for mania in children and adolescents with bipolar disorder. *J Am Acad Child Adolesc Psychiatry*, 44(6), 539–547.

DelBello, M.P., Kowatch, R.A., Adler, C.M., Stanford, K.E., Welge, J.A., Barzman, D.H., Nelson, E., and Strakowski, S.M. (2006). A double-blind randomized pilot study comparing quetiapine and divalproex for adolescent mania. *J Am Acad Child Adolesc Psychiatry*, 45(3), 305–313.

DeLong, G.R. (1978). Lithium carbonate treatment of select behavior disorders in children suggesting manic depressive illness. *J Pediatr*, 93, 689–694.

DeLong, G.R., and Aldershof, A.L. (1987). Long-term experience with lithium treatment in childhood: Correlation with clinical diagnosis. *Am Acad Child Adolesc Psychiatry*, 26, 389–394.

Deltito, A.J., Levitan, J., Damore, J., Hajal, F., and Zambenedetti, M. (1998). Naturalistic experience with the use of divalproex sodium on an in-patient unit for adolescent psychiatric patients. *Acta Psychiatr Scand*, 97, 236–240.

Donovan, S.J., Stewart, J.W., Nunes, E.V., Quitkin, F.M., Parides, M., Daniel, W., Susser, E., and Klein, D.F. (2000). Divalproex treatment for youth with explosive temper and mood lability: A double-blind, placebo-controlled crossover design. *Am J Psychiatry*, 157(5), 818–820.

Duffy, A., Alda, M., Kutcher, S., Fusee, C., and Grof, P. (1998). Psychiatric symptoms and syndromes among adolescent children of parents with lithium-responsive or lithium-nonresponsive bipolar disorder. *Am J Psychiatry*, 155(3), 431–433.

Dyson, W.L., and Barcai, A. (1970). Treatment of children of lithium-responding parents. *Curr Ther Res Clin Exp*, 12(5), 286–290.

Egeland, J.A., Hostetter, A.M., Pauls, D.L., and Sussex, J.N. (2000). Prodromal symptoms before onset of manic-depressive disorder suggested by first hospital admission histories. *J Am Acad Child Adolesc Psychiatry*, 39(10), 1245–1252.

Egeland, J.A., Shaw, J.A., Endicott, J., Pauls, D.L., Allen, C.R., Hostetter, A.M., and Sussex, J.N. (2003). Prospective study of prodromal features for bipolarity in well Amish children. *J Am Acad Child Adolesc Psychiatry*, 42(7), 786–796.

Endicott, J., and Spitzer, R.L. (1978). A diagnostic interview: The Schedule for Affective Disorders and Schizophrenia. *Arch Gen Psychiatry*, 35(7), 837–844.

Faedda, G.L., Baldessarini, R.J., Glovinsky, I.P., and Austin, N.B. (2004). Treatment-emergent mania in pediatric bipolar disorder: A retrospective case review. *J Affect Disord*, 82(1), 149–158.

Faraone, S.V., Biederman, J., Wozniak, J., Mundy, E., Mennin, D., and O'Donnell, D. (1997). Is comorbidity a marker for juvenile-onset mania? *J Am Acad Child Adolesc Psychiatry*, 36, 1046–1055.

Findling, R.L., and McNamara, N.K. (2004). Atypical antipsychotics in the treatment of children and adolescents: Clinical applications. *J Clin Psychiatry*, 65(Suppl. 6), 30–44.

Findling, R.L., McNamara, N.K., Branicky, L.A., Schluchter, M.D., Lemon, E., and Blumer, J.L. (2000). A double-blind pilot study of risperidone in the treatment of conduct disorder. *J Am Acad Child Adolesc Psychiatry*, 39(4), 509–516.

Findling, R.L., Gracious, B.L., McNamara, N.K., Youngstrom, E.A., Demeter, C.A., Branicky, L.A., and Calabrese, J.R. (2001). Rapid, continuous cycling and psychiatric co-morbidity in pediatric bipolar I disorder. *Bipolar Disord*, 3(4), 202–210.

Findling, R.L., McNamara, N.K., Gracious, B.L., Youngstrom, E.A., Stansbrey, R.J., Reed, M.D., Demeter, C.A., Branicky, L.A., Fisher, K.E., and Calabrese, J.R. (2003). Combination lithium and divalproex sodium in pediatric bipolarity. *J Am Acad Child Adolesc Psychiatry*, 42(8), 895–901.

Findling, R.L., McNamara, N.K., Youngstrom, E.A., Stansbrey, R., Gracious, B.L., Reed, M.D., and Calabrese, J.R. (2005). Double-blind 18-month trial of lithium versus divalproex maintenance treatment in pediatric bipolar disorder. *J Am Acad Child Adolesc Psychiatry*, 44(5), 409–417.

Frazier, J.A., Meyer, M.C., Biederman, J., Wozniak, J., Wilens, T.E., Spencer, T.J., Kim, G.S., and Shapiro, S. (1999). Risperidone treatment for juvenile bipolar disorder: A retrospective chart review. *J Am Acad Child Adolesc Psychiatry*, 38(8), 960–965.

Frazier, J.A., Biederman, J., Tohen, M., Feldman, P.D., Jacobs, T.G., Toma, V., Rater, M.A., Tarazi, R.A., Kim, G.S., Garfield, S.B., Sohma, M., Gonzalez-Heydrich, J., Risser, R.C., and Nowlin, Z.M. (2001). A prospective open-label treatment trial of olanzapine monotherapy in children and adolescents with bipolar disorder. *J Child Adolesc Psychopharmacol*, 11(3), 239–250.

Fristad, M.A., Cummins, J., Verducci, J.S., Teare, M., Weller, E.B., and Weller, R.A. (1998). Study IV: Concurrent validity of the DSM-IV revised Children's Interview for Psychiatric Syndromes (ChIPS). *J Child Adolesc Psychopharmacol*, 8(4), 227–236.

Fristad, M.A., Goldberg-Arnold, J.S., Gavazzi, S.M. (2002). Multifamily psychoeducation groups (MFPG) for families of children with bipolar disorder. *Bipolar Disord*, 4(4), 254–262.

Fristad, M.A., Gavazzi, S.M., and Mackinaw-Koons, B. (2003). Family psychoeducation: An adjunctive intervention for children with bipolar disorder. *Biol Psychiatry*, 53(11), 1000–1008.

Fuchs, D.C. (1994). Clozapine treatment of bipolar disorder in a young adolescent. *J Am Acad Child Adolesc Psychiatry*, 33(9), 1299–1302.

Galanter, C.A., Carlson, G.A., Jensen, P.S., Greenhill, L., Davies, M., Li, W., Chuang, S.Z., Glen Elliott, G.R., Arnold, L.E., March, J.S., Hechtman, L., Pelham, W.E., and Swanson, J.M. (2003). Response to methylphenidate in children with ADHD and manic symptoms in the MTA titration trial. *J Child Adolesc Psychopharmacol*, 13, 123–137.

Geller, B., Cooper, T.B., Sun, K., Zimerman, B., Frazier, J., Williams, M., and Heath, J. (1998a). Double-blind and placebo-controlled study of lithium for adolescent bipolar disorders with secondary substance dependency. *J Am Acad Child Adolesc Psychiatry*, 37(2), 171–178.

Geller, B., Zimerman, B., Williams, M., Bolhofner, K., and Craney, J.L. (2001). Bipolar disorder at prospective follow-up of adults who had prepubertal major depressive disorder. *Am J Psychiatry*, 158(1), 125–127.

Geller, B., Zimerman, B., Williams, M., DelBello, M.P., Frazier, J., and Beringer, L. (2002). Phenomenology of prepubertal and early adolescent bipolar disorder: Examples of elated mood, grandiose behaviors, decreased need for sleep, racing thoughts and hypersexuality. *J Child Adolesc Psychopharmacol*, 12(1), 3–9.

Geller, B., Tillman, R., Craney, J.L., and Bolhofner, K. (2004). Four-year prospective outcome and natural history of mania in children with a prepubertal and early adolescent bipolar disorder phenotype. *Arch Gen Psychiatry*, 61(5), 459–467.

Ghaemi, S.N., Hsu, D.J., Soldani, F., and Goodwin, F.K. (2003). Antidepressants in bipolar disorder: The case for caution. *Bipolar Disord*, 5(6), 421–433.

Ghaziuddin, N., Kutcher, S.P., Knapp, P., and American Academy of Child and Adolescent Psychiatry Work Group on Quality Issues. (2004). Summary of the practice parameter for the use of electroconvulsive therapy with adolescents. *J Am Acad Child Adolesc Psychiatry*, 43(1), 119–122.

Gijsman, H.J., Geddes, J.R., Rendell, J.M., Nolen, W.A., and Goodwin, G.M. (2004). Antidepressants for bipolar depression: A systematic review of randomized, controlled trials. *Am J Psychiatry*, 161(9), 1537–1547.

Glovinsky, I. (2002). A brief history of childhood-onset bipolar disorder through 1980. *Child Adolesc Psychiatr Clin North Am*, 11(3), 443–460.

Gracious, B.L., Findling, R.L., Seman, C., Youngstrom, E.A., Demeter, C.A., and Calabrese, J.R. (2004). Elevated thyrotropin in bipolar youths prescribed both lithium and divalproex sodium. *J Am Acad Child Adolesc Psychiatry*, 43(2), 215–220.

Gram, L.F., and Rafaelsen, O.J. (1972). Lithium treatment of psychotic children and adolescents: A controlled clinical trial. *Acta Psychiatr Scand*, 48(3), 253.

Greene, R.W., and Ablon, J.S. (2005). *Treating Explosive Kids: The Collaborative Problem-Solving Approach.* New York: Guilford Press.

Greene, R.W., Ablon, J.S., and Goring, J.C. (2003). A transactional model of oppositional behavior: Underpinnings of the collaborative problem solving approach. *J Psychosom Res*, 55(1), 67–75.

Greenhill, L.L., Rieder, R.O., Wender, P.H., Buchsbaum, M., and Zhan, T.P. (1973). Lithium carbonate in the treatment of hyperactive children. *Arch Gen Psychiatry*, 28(5), 636.

Harrington, R., and Myatt, T. (2003). Is preadolescent mania the same condition as adult mania? A British perspective. *Biol Psychiatry*, 53, 961–969.

Hazell, P., O'Connell, D., Heathcote, D., and Henry, D. (2002). Tricyclic drugs for depression in children and adolescents. *Cochrane Database Syst Rev*, 2, CD002317.

Hazell, P.L., Carr, V., Lewin, T.J., and Sly, K. (2003). Manic symptoms in young males with ADHD predict functioning but not diagnosis after 6 years. *J Am Acad Child Adolesc Psychiatry*, 42(5), 552–560.

Hill, M.A., Courvoisie, H., Dawkins, K., Nofal, P., and Thomas, B. (1997). ECT for the treatment of intractable mania in two prepubertal male children. *Convuls Ther*, 13(2), 74–82.

Hsu, L.K.G., and Starzynski, J.M. (1986). Mania in adolescence. *J Clin Psychiatry*, 47(12), 596–599.

Humphrey, L.L. (1982). Children's and teachers' perspectives on children's self-control: The development of two rating scales. *J Consult Clin Psychol*, 50(5), 624–633.

Joffe, R.T., MacQueen, G.M., Marriott, M., and Young, L.T. (2005). One-year outcome with antidepressant treatment of bipolar depression. *Acta Psychiatr Scand*, 112(2), 105–109.

Johnson, S.L., Winett, C.A., Meyer, B., Greenhouse, W.J., and Miller, I. (1999). Social support and the course of bipolar disorder. *J Abnorm Psychol*, 108(4), 558–566.

Kafantaris, V., Coletti, D.J., Dicker, R., Padula, G., and Pollack, S. (1998). Are childhood psychiatric histories of bipolar adolescents associated with family history, psychosis, and response to lithium treatment? *J Affect Disord*, 51, 153–164.

Kafantaris, V., Coletti, D.J., Dicker, R., Padula, G., and Kane, J.M. (2001). Adjunctive antipsychotic treatment of adolescents with bipolar psychosis. *J Am Acad Child Adolesc Psychiatry*, 40(12), 1448–1456.

Kafantaris, V., Coletti, D.J., Dicker, R., Padula, G., and Kane, J.M. (2003). Lithium treatment of acute mania in adolescents: A large open trial. *J Am Acad Child Adolesc Psychiatry*, 42(9), 1038–1045.

Kafantaris, V., Coletti, D.J., Dicker, R., Padula, G., Pleak, R.R., and Alvir, J.M. (2004). Lithium treatment of acute mania in adolescents: A placebo-controlled discontinuation study. *J Am Acad Child Adolesc Psychiatry*, 43(8), 984–993.

Kant, R., Chalansani, R., Chengappa, K.N., and Dieringer, M.F. (2004). The off-label use of clozapine in adolescents with bipolar disorder, intermittent explosive disorder, or posttraumatic stress disorder. *J Child Adolesc Psychopharmacol*, 14(1), 57–63.

Kastner, T., and Friedman D.L. (1992). Verapamil and valproic acid treatment of prolonged mania. *J Am Acad Child Adolesc Psychiatry*, 31(2), 271–275.

Kowatch, R.A., Suppes, T., Carmody, T.J., Bucci, J.P., Hume, J.H., Kromelis, M., Emslie, G.J., Weinberg, A., and Rush, A.J. (2000). Effect size of lithium, divalproex sodium, and carbamazepine in children and adolescents with bipolar disorder. *J Am Acad Child Adolesc Psychiatry*, 39(6), 713–720.

Kowatch, R.A., Sethuraman, G., Hume, J.H., Kromelis, M., and Weinberg, W.A. (2003). Combination pharmacotherapy in children and adolescents with bipolar disorder. *Biol Psychiatry*, 53(11), 978–984.

Kowatch, R.A., Fristad, M., Birmaher, B., Wagner, K.D., and Findling, R. (2005). Treatment guidelines for children and adolescents with bipolar disorder. *J Am Acad Child Adolesc Psychiatry*, 44(3), 213–235.

Kusumakar, V., and Yatham, L.N. (1997). An open study of lamotrigine in refractory bipolar depression. *Psychiatry Res*, 72, 145–148.

Lapalme, M., Hodgins, S., and LaRoche, C. (1997). Children of parents with bipolar disorder: A metaanalysis of risk for mental disorders. *Can J Psychiatry*, 42(6), 623–631.

Leibenluft, E., Blair, R.J., Charney, D.S., and Pine, D.S. (2003). Irritability in pediatric mania and other childhood psychopathology. *Ann N Y Acad Sci*, 1008, 201–218.

Lewinsohn, P.M., Klein, D.N., and Seeley, J.R. (2000). Bipolar disorder during adolescence and young adulthood in a community sample. *Bipolar Disord*, 2(3 Pt. 2), 281–293.

Maj, M., Pirozzi, R., Magliano, L., and Bartoli, L. (2002). The prognostic significance of "switching" in patients with bipolar disorder: A 10-year prospective follow-up study. *Am J Psychiatry*, 159(10), 1711–1717. Erratum in *Am J Psychiatry*, 159(12), 2132.

Malone, R.P., Delaney, M.A., Luebbert, J.F., Cater, J., and Campbell, M. (2000). A double-blind placebo-controlled study of lithium in hospitalized aggressive children and adolescents with conduct disorder. *Arch Gen Psychiatry*, 57(7), 649–654.

Mannuzza, S., Klein, R.G., Bessler, A., Malloy, P., and LaPadula, M. (1998). Adult psychiatric status of hyperactive boys grown up. *Am J Psychiatry*, 155(4), 493–498.

Martin, A., Young, C., Leckman, J.F., Mukonoweshuro, C., Rosenheck, R., and Leslie, D. (2004). Age effects on antidepressant-induced manic conversion. *Arch Pediatr Adolesc Med*, 158(8), 773–780.

Masi, G., Mucci, M., and Millepiedi, S. (2002). Clozapine in adolescent inpatients with acute mania. *J Child Adolesc Psychopharmacol*, 12(2), 93–99.

McClellan, J. (2005). Commentary: Treatment guidelines for child and adolescent bipolar disorder. *J Am Acad Child Adolesc Psychiatry*, 44(3), 236–239.

McClellan, J., and Werry, J. (1997). Practice parameters for the assessment and treatment of children and adolescents with bipolar disorder. American Academy of Child and Adolescent Psychiatry. *J Am Acad Child Adolesc Psychiatry*, 36(10 Suppl.), 157S–176S.

McConville, B.J., Arvanitis, L.A., Thyrum, P.T., Yeh, C., Wilkinson, L.A., Chaney, R.O., Foster, K.D., Sorter, M.T., Friedman, L.M., Brown, K.L., and Heubi, J.E. (2000). Pharmacokinetics, tolerability, and clinical effectiveness of quetiapine fumarate: An open-label trial in adolescents with psychotic disorders. *J Clin Psychiatry*, 61(4), 252–260.

McCracken, J.T., McGough, J., Shah, B., Cronin, P., Hong, D., Aman, M.G., Arnold, L.E., Lindsay, R., Nash, P., Hollway, J., McDougle, C.J., Posey, D., Swiezy, N., Kohn, A., Scahill, L.,

Martin, A., Koenig, K., Volkmar, F., Carroll, D., Lancor, A., Tierney, E., Ghuman, J., Gonzalez, N.M., Grados, M., Vitiello, B., Ritz, L., Davies, M., Robinson, J., McMahon, D., and Research Units on Pediatric Psychopharmacology Autism Network. (2002). Risperidone in children with autism and serious behavioral problems. *N Engl J Med*, 347(5), 314–321.

McKnew, D.H., Cytryn, L., Buchsbaum, M.S., Hamovit, J., Lamour, M., Rapoport, J.L., and Gershon, E.S. (1981). Lithium in children of lithium-responding parents. *Psychiatry Res*, 4(2), 171–180.

Meyer, S.E., Carlson, G.A., Wiggs, E.A., Martinez, P.E., Ronsaville, D.S., Klimes-Dougan, B., Gold, P.W., and Radke-Yarrow, M. (2004). A prospective study of the association among impaired executive functioning, childhood attentional problems, and the development of bipolar disorder. *Dev Psychopathol*, 16(2), 461–476.

Mick, E., Biederman, J., Pandina, G., and Faraone, S.V. (2003). A preliminary meta-analysis of the child behavior checklist in pediatric bipolar disorder. *Biol Psychiatry*, 53(11), 1021–1027.

Miklowitz, D.J., Simoneau, T.L., George, E.L., Richards, J.A., Kalbag, A., Sachs-Ericsson, N., and Suddath, R. (2000). Family-focused treatment of bipolar disorder: 1-Year effects of a psychoeducational program in conjunction with pharmacotherapy. *Biol Psychiatry*, 48(6), 582–592.

Miklowitz, D.J., George, E.L., Axelson, D.A., Kim, E.Y., Birmaher, B., Schneck, C., Beresford, C., Craighead, W.E., and Brent, D.A. (2004). Family-focused treatment for adolescents with bipolar disorder. *J Affect Disord*, 82(Suppl. 1), S113–S128.

Papatheodorou, G., Kutcher, S.P., Katic, M., and Szalai, J.P. (1995). The efficacy and safety of divalproex sodium in the treatment of acute mania in adolescents and young adults: An open clinical trial. *J Clin Psychopharmacol*, 15, 110–116.

Pappadopulos, E., Macintyre, J.C. II, Crismon, M.L., Findling, R.L., Malone, R.P., Derivan, A., Schooler, N., Sikich, L., Greenhill, L., Schur, S.B., Felton, C.J., Kranzler, H., Rube, D.M., Sverd, J., Finnerty, M., Ketner, S., Siennick, S.E., and Jensen, P.S. (2003). Treatment Recommendations for the Use of Antipsychotics for Aggressive Youth (TRAAY): Part II. *J Am Acad Child Adolesc Psychiatry*, 42(2), 145–161.

Patel, N.C., DelBello, M.P., Bryan, H.S., Adler, C.M., Kowatch, R.A., Stanford, K., Strakowski, S.M. (2006). Open-label lithium for the treatment of adolescents with bipolar depression. *J Am Acad Child Adolesc Psychiatry*, 45(3), 289–297.

Pavuluri, M.N., Graczyk, P.A., Henry, D.B., Carbray, J.A., Heidenreich, J., and Miklowitz, D.J. (2004a). Child- and family-focused cognitive-behavioral therapy for pediatric bipolar disorder: Development and preliminary results. *J Am Acad Child Adolesc Psychiatry*, 43(5), 528–537.

Pavuluri, M.N., Henry, D.B., Carbray, J.A., Sampson, G., Naylor, M.W., and Janicak, P.G. (2004b). Open-label prospective trial of risperidone in combination with lithium or divalproex sodium in pediatric mania. *J Affect Disord*, 82(Suppl. 1), S103–S111.

Pavuluri, M.N., Henry, D.B., Carbray, J.A., Naylor, M.W., and Janicak, P.G. (2005). Divalproex sodium for pediatric mixed mania: A 6-month prospective trial. *Bipolar Disord*, 7(3), 266–273.

Post, R.M., and Kowatch, R.A. (2006). The health care crisis of childhood-onset bipolar illness: Some recommendations for its amelioration. *J Clin Psychiatry*, 67(1), 115–125.

Post, R.M., Leverich, G.S., Fergus, E., Miller, R., and Luckenbaugh, D. (2002). Parental attitudes towards early intervention in children at high risk for affective disorders. *J Affect Disord*, 70(2), 117–124.

Post, R.M., Leverich, G.S., Nolen, W.A., Kupka, R.W., Altshuler, L.L., Frye, M.A., Suppes, T., McElroy, S., Keck, P., Grunze, H., and Walden, J. (2003). A re-evaluation of the role of antidepressants in the treatment of bipolar depression: Data from the Stanley Foundation Bipolar Network. *Bipolar Disord*, 5(6), 396–406.

Poznanski, E.O., Israel, M.G., and Grossman, J. (1984). Hypomania in a four-year-old. *J Am Acad Child Psychiatry*, 23, 105–110.

Reinblatt, S.P., and Walkup, J.T. (2005). Psychopharmacologic treatment of pediatric anxiety disorders. *Child Adolesc Psychiatr Clin North Am*, 14(4), 877–908.

Rey, J.M., and Walter, G. (1997). Half a century of ECT use in young people. *Am J Psychiatry*, 154(5), 595–602.

Robertson, J.M., and Tanguay, P.E. (1997). Case study: The use of melatonin in a boy with refractory bipolar disorder. *J Am Acad Child Adolesc Psychiatry*, 36(6), 822–825.

Russell, P.S., Tharyan, P., Arun Kumar, K., and Cherian, A. (2002). Electro convulsive therapy in a pre-pubertal child with severe depression. *J Postgrad Med*, 48(4), 290–291.

Schaller, J.L., and Behar, D. (1999). Quetiapine for refractory mania in a child. *J Am Acad Child Adolesc Psychiatry*, 38(5), 498–499.

Scheffer, R.E., Kowatch, R.A., Carmody, T., and Rush, A.J. (2005). Randomized, placebo-controlled trial of mixed amphetamine salts for symptoms of comorbid ADHD in pediatric bipolar disorder after mood stabilization with divalproex sodium. *Am J Psychiatry*, 162(1), 58–64.

Schreier, H.A. (1982). Mania responsive to lecithin in a 13-year-old girl. *Am J Psychiatry*, 139(1), 108–110.

Schur, S.B., Sikich, L., Findling, R.L., Malone, R.P., Crismon, M.L., Derivan, A., Macintyre, J.C. II, Pappadopulos, E., Greenhill, L., Schooler, N., Van Orden, K., and Jensen, P.S. (2003). Treatment Recommendations for the Use of Antipsychotics for Aggressive Youth (TRAAY). Part I: A review. *J Am Acad Child Adolesc Psychiatry*, 42(2), 132–144.

Shaffer, D., Gould, M.S., Brasic, J., Ambrosini, P., Fisher, P., Bird, H., and Aluwahlia, S. (1983). A Children's Global Assessment Scale (CGAS). *Arch Gen Psychiatry*, 40(11), 1228–1231.

Shaw, J.A., Egeland, J.A., Endicott, J., Allen, C.R., and Hostetter, A.M. (2005). A 10-year prospective study of prodromal patterns for bipolar disorder among Amish youth. *J Am Acad Child Adolesc Psychiatry*, 44(11), 1104–1111.

Silva, R.R., Campbell, M., Golden, R.R., Small, A.M., Pataki, C.S., and Rosenberg, C.R. (1992). Side effects associated with lithium and placebo administration in aggressive children. *Psychopharmacol Bull*, 28(3), 319–326.

Snyder, R., Turgay, A., Aman, M., Binder, C., Fisman, S., Carroll, A., and Risperidone Conduct Study Group. (2002). Effects of risperidone on conduct and disruptive behavior disorders in children with subaverage IQs. *J Am Acad Child Adolesc Psychiatry*, 41(9), 1026–1036.

Soutullo, C.A., Casuto, L.S., and Keck, P.E. Jr. (1998). Gabapentin in the treatment of adolescent mania: A case report. *J Child Adolesc Psychopharmacol*, 8, 81–85.

Soutullo, C.A., Sorter, M.T., Foster, K.D., McElroy, S.L., and Keck, P.E. (1999). Olanzapine in the treatment of adolescent acute mania: A report of seven cases. *J Affect Disord*, 53(3), 279–283.

Soutullo, C.A., DelBello, M.P., Ochsner, J.E., McElroy, S.L., Taylor, S.A., Strakowski, S.M., Keck, P.E. Jr. (2002). Severity of bipolarity in hospitalized manic adolescents with history of stimulant or antidepressant treatment. *J Affect Disord*, 70(3), 323–327.

Steiner, H., Petersen, M.L., Saxena, K., Ford, S., and Matthews, Z. (2003). Divalproex sodium for the treatment of conduct disorder: A randomized controlled clinical trial. *J Clin Psychiatry*, 64(10), 1183–1191.

Strakowski, S.M., DelBello, M.P., Kowatch, R., Whitsel, R., and Adler, C. (2006). A single-blind prospective study of quetiapine for the treatment of mood disorders in adolescents who are at high risk for developing bipolar disorder. *New Research Abstract*, May 22, 2006. American Psychiatric Association.

Strober, M., and Carlson, G. (1982). Bipolar illness in adolescents with major depression: Clinical, genetic, and psychopharmacologic predictors in a three- to four-year prospective follow-up investigation. *Arch Gen Psychiatry*, 39(5), 549–555.

Strober, M., Morrell, W., Burroughs, J., Lampert, C., Danforth, H., and Freeman, R. (1988). A family study of bipolar I disorder in adolescence: Early onset of symptoms linked to increased familial loading and lithium resistance. *J Affect Disord*, 15(3), 255–268.

Strober, M., Morrell, W., Lampert, C., and Burroughs, J. (1990). Relapse following discontinuation of lithium maintenance therapy in adolescents with bipolar I illness: A naturalistic study. *Am J Psychiatry*, 147, 457–461.

Strober, M., DeAntonio, M., Schmidt-Lackner, S., Freeman, R., Lampert, C., and Diamond, J. (1998). Early childhood attention deficit hyperactivity disorder predicts poorer response to acute lithium therapy in adolescent mania. *J Affect Disord*, 51, 145–151.

Suppes, T., Baldessarini, R.J., and Faedda, G.L. (1991). Risk of recurrence following discontinuation of lithium in bipolar disorder. *Arch Gen Psychiatry*, 48, 1082–1088.

Taieb, O., Flament, M.F., Chevret, S., Jeammet, P., Allilaire, J.F., Mazet, P., and Cohen, D. (2002). Clinical relevance of electroconvulsive therapy (ECT) in adolescents with severe mood disorder: Evidence from a follow-up study. *Eur Psychiatry*, 17(4), 206–212.

Tillman, R., Geller, B., Craney, J.L., Bolhofner, K., Williams, M., Zimerman, B., Frazier, J., and Beringer, L. (2003). Temperament and character factors in a prepubertal and early adolescent bipolar disorder phenotype compared to attention deficit hyperactive and normal controls. *J Child Adolesc Psychopharmacol*, 13(4), 531–543.

Tohen, M., Kryzhanovskay, L., Carlson, G., DelBello, M., Wozniak, J., Kowatch, R., Wagner, K., Findling, R., Lin, D., Robertson-Plouch, C., Xu, W., Huang, X., Dittman, R., and Biederman, J. (2006). Olanzapine in the treatment of acute mania in adolescents with bipolar I disorder: A 3-week randomized double-blind placebo-controlled study. *New Research Abstract*, May 22, 2006. American Psychiatric Association.

Towbin, K.E., Pradella, A., Gorrindo, T., Pine, D.S., and Leibenluft, E. (2005). Autism spectrum traits in children with mood and anxiety disorders. *J Child Adolesc Psychopharmacol*, 15(3), 452–464.

Tuke, D.H. (1892). *A Dictionary of Psychological Medicine*. Philadelphia: P. Blaikston, Son & Co.

Turgay, A., Binder, C., Snyder, R., and Fisman, S. (2002). Long-term safety and efficacy of risperidone for the treatment of disruptive behavior disorders in children with subaverage IQs. *Pediatrics*, 110(3), e34.

U.S. Food and Drug Administration (FDA). (2004). T.A. Hammad (Ed.), *Relationship between Psychotropic Drugs and Pediatric Suicidality: Review and Evaluation of Clinical Data*. Available: http://www.fda.gov/ohrms/dockets/ac/04/briefing/2004–4065b1-10-TAB08-Hammads-Review.pdf [November 2004].

Varanka, T.M., Weller, R.A., and Weller, E.B. (1988). Fristad, M.A. (Ed.), Lithium treatment of manic episodes with psychotic features in prepubertal children. *Am J Psychiatry*, 145(12), 1557–1559.

Wagner, K.D., Weller, E.B., Carlson, G.A., Sachs, G., Biederman, J., Frazier, J.A., Wozniak, P., Tracy, K., Weller, R.A., and Bowden, C. (2002). An open-label trial of divalproex in children and adolescents with bipolar disorder. *J Am Acad Child Adolesc Psychiatry*, 41(10), 1224–1230.

Wagner, K.D., Jonas, J., Findling, R.L., Ventura, D., and Saikali, K. (2006a). A double-blind, randomized, placebo-controlled trial of escitalopram in the treatment of pediatric depression. *J Am Acad Child Adolesc Psychiatry*, 45(3), 280–288.

Wagner, K.D., Kowatch, R.A., Emslie, G.J., Findling, R.L., Wilens, T.E., McCague, K., D'Souza, J., Wamil, A., Lehman, R.B., Berv, D., and Linden, D. (2006b). A double-blind, randomized, placebo-controlled trial of oxcarbazepine in the treatment of bipolar disorder in children and adolescents. *Am J Psychiatry*, 163(7), 1179–1186.

Walter, G., and Rey, J.M. (2003). Has the practice and outcome of ECT in adolescents changed? Findings from a whole-population study. *J ECT*, 19(2), 84–87.

Walter, G., Rey, J.M., and Mitchell, P.B. (1999). Practitioner review: Electroconvulsive therapy in adolescents. *J Child Psychol Psychiatry*, 40(3), 325–334.

Weissman, M.M., Wolk, S., Goldstein, R.B., Moreau, D., Adams, P., Greenwald, S., Klier, C.M., Ryan, N.D., Dahl, R.E., and Wickramaratne, P. (1999a). Depressed adolescents grown up. *JAMA*, 281(18), 1707–1713.

West, S.A., Keck, P.E., Jr., McElroy, S.L., Strakowski, S.M., Minnery, K.L., McConville, B.J., and Sorter, M.T. (1994). Open trial of valproate in the treatment of adolescent mania. *J Child Adolesc Psychopharmacol*, 4, 263–267.

Woolston, J.L. (1999). Case study: Carbamazepine treatment of juvenile-onset bipolar disorder. *J Am Acad Child Adolesc Psychiatry*, 38(3), 335–338.

Wudarsky, M., Nicolson, R., Hamburger, S.D., Spechler, L., Gochman, P., Bedwell, J., Lenane, M.C., and Rapoport, J.L. (1999). Elevated prolactin in pediatric patients on typical and atypical antipsychotics. *J Child Adolesc Psychopharmacol*, 9(4), 239–245.

Youngerman, J., and Canino, I.A. (1978). Lithium carbonate use in children and adolescents. A survey of the literature. *Arch Gen Psychiatry*, 35(2), 216–224.

Youngstrom, E.A., Findling, R.L., Calabrese, J.R., Gracious, B.L., Demeter, C., Bedoya, D.D., and Price, M. (2004). Comparing diagnostic accuracy of six potential screening instruments for bipolar disorder in youths aged 5 to 17 years. *J Am Acad Child Adolesc Psychiatry*, 43(7), 847–858.

CHAPTER 24

Ahrens, B., Grof, P., Moller, H.J., Muller-Oerlinghausen, B., and Wolf, T. (1995). Extended survival of patients on long-term lithium treatment. *Can J Psychiatry*, 40, 241–246.

Alevizos, B., Lykouras, L., Zervas, I.M., and Christodoulou, G.N. (2002). Risperidone-induced obsessive-compulsive symptoms: A series of six cases. *J Clin Psychopharmacol*, 22(5), 461–467.

Anderson, J.W., Greenway, F.L., Fujioka, K., Gadde, K.M., McKenney, J., and O'Neil, P.M. (2002). Bupropion SR enhances weight loss: A 48-week double-blind, placebo-controlled trial. *Obes Res*, 10, 633–641.

Appolinario, J.C., Bacaltchuk, J., Sichieri, R., Claudino, A.M., Godoy-Matos, A., Morgan, C., Zanella, M.T., and Coutinho, W. (2003). A randomized, double-blind, placebo-controlled study of sibutramine in the treatment of binge-eating disorder. *Arch Gen Psychiatry*, 60, 1109–1116.

Aronson, R., Offman, H.J., Joffe, R.T., and Naylor, C.D. (1996). Triiodothyronine augmentation in the treatment of refractory depression: A meta-analysis. *Arch Gen Psychiatry*, 53, 842–848.

Ballenger, J.C., Davidson, J.R., Lecrubier, Y., Nutt, D.J., Marshall, R.D., Nemeroff, C.B., Shalev, A.Y., and Yehuda, R. (2004). Consensus statement update on posttraumatic stress disorder from the international consensus group on depression and anxiety. *J Clin Psychiatry*, 65(Suppl. 1), 55–62.

Barbarich, N.C., McConaha, C.W., Gaskill, J., La Via, M., Frank, G.K., Achenbach, S., Plotnicov, K.H., and Kaye, W.H. (2004). An open trial of olanzapine in anorexia nervosa. *J Clin Psychiatry*, 65, 1480–1482.

Bauer, M.S., and Whybrow, P.C. (1990). Rapid cycling bipolar affective disorder: II. Treatment of refractory rapid cycling with high-dose levothyroxine: A preliminary study. *Arch Gen Psychiatry*, 47, 435–440.

Bauer, M.S., Berghofer, A., Bschor, T., Baumgartner, A., Kiesslinger, U., Hellweg, R., Adli, M., Baethge, C., and Muller-Oerlinghausen, B. (2002). Supraphysiological doses of L-thyroxine in the maintenance treatment of prophylaxis-resistant affective disorders. *Neuropsychopharmacology*, 27, 620–628.

Bellack, A.S., Bennett, M.E., Gearon, J.S., Brown, C.H., and Yang, Y. (2006). A randomized clinical trial of a new behavioral treatment for drug abuse in people with severe and persistent mental illness. *Arch Gen Psychiatry*, 63, 426–432.

Berton, F., Francesconi, W.G., Madamba, S.G., Zieglgansberger, W., and Siggins, G.R. (1998). Acamprosate enhances *N*-methyl-D-aspartate receptor-mediated neurotransmission but inhibits presynaptic GABA(B) receptors in nucleus accumbens neurons. *Alcohol Clin Exp Res*, 22, 183–191.

Bjorkqvist, S.E., Isohanni, M., Makela, R., and Malinen, L. (1976). Ambulant treatment of alcohol withdrawal symptoms with carbamazepine: A formal multicentre double-blind comparison with placebo. *Acta Psychiatr Scand*, 53, 333–342.

Brady, K.T., Sonne, S.C., Anton, R., and Ballenger, J.C. (1995). Valproate in the treatment of acute bipolar affective episodes complicated by substance abuse: A pilot study. *J Clin Psychiatry*, 56(3), 118–121.

Brady, K.T., Sonne, S.C., Malcolm, R.J., Randall, C.L., Dansky, B.S., Simpson, K., Roberts, J.S., and Brondino, M. (2002). Carbamazepine in the treatment of cocaine dependence: Subtyping by affective disorder. *Exp Clin Psychopharmacol*, 10, 276–285.

Bray, G.A., Hollander, P., Klein, S., Kushner, R., Levy, B., Fitchet, M., and Perry, B.H. (2003). A 6-month randomized, placebo-controlled, dose-ranging trial of topiramate for weight loss in obesity. *Obes Res*, 11, 722–733.

Brown, E.S. (2006). Management of comorbid bipolar disorder and substance abuse. *J Clin Psychiatry*, 67(8), e05.

Brown, E.S., Nejtek, V.A., Perantie, D.C., and Bobadilla, L. (2002). Quetiapine in bipolar disorder and cocaine dependence. *Bipolar Disord*, 4(6), 406–411.

Brown, E.S., Nejtek, V.A., Perantie, D.C., Orsulak, P.J., and Bobadilla, L. (2003). Lamotrigine in patients with bipolar disorder and cocaine dependence. *J Clin Psychiatry*, 64(2), 197–201.

Brown, E.S., Beard, L., Dobbs, L., and Rush, A.J. (2006). Naltrexone in patients with bipolar disorder and alcohol dependence. *Depress Anxiety*, 23(8), 492–495.

Brown, J., Kranzler, H.R., and Del Boca, F.K. (1992). Self-reports by alcohol and drug abuse inpatients: Factors affecting reliability and validity. *Br J Addict*, 87, 1013–1024.

Calabrese, J.R., Shelton, M.D., Bowden, C.L., Rapport, D.J., Suppes, T., Shirley, E.R., Kimmel, S.E., and Caban, S.J. (2001). Bipolar rapid cycling: Focus on depression as its hallmark. *J Clin Psychiatry*, 62(Suppl. 14), 34–41.

Chick, J., Anton, R., Checinski, K., Croop, R., Drummond, D.C., Farmer, R., Labriola, D., Marshall, J., Moncrieff, J., Morgan, M.Y., Peters, T., and Ritson, B. (2000). A multicentre, randomized, double-blind, placebo-controlled trial of naltrexone in the treatment of alcohol dependence or abuse. *Alcohol Alcohol*, 35, 587–593.

Denys, D., de Geus, F., van Meger, H.J., and Westenberg, H.G. (2004). A double blind, randomized, placebo controlled trial of quetiapine addition in patients with obsessive-compulsive disorder refractory to serotonin reuptake inhibitors. *J Clin Psychiatry*, 1040–1048.

Drake, R.E., Xie, H., McHugo, G.J., and Shumway, M. (2004). Three-year outcomes of long-term patients with co-occurring bipolar and substance use disorders. *Biol Psychiatry*, 56(10), 749–756.

Driessen, M., Veltrup, C., Wetterling, T., John, U., and Dilling, H. (1998). Axis I and Axis II comorbidity in alcohol dependence and the two types of alcoholism. *Alcohol Clin Exp Res*, 22, 77–86.

Driessen, M., Meier, S., Hill, A., Wetterling, T., Lange, W., and Junghanns, K. (2001). The course of anxiety, depression and drinking behaviours after completed detoxification in alcoholics with and without comorbid anxiety and depressive disorders. *Alcohol Alcohol*, 36, 249–255.

Dymek, M.P., le Grange, D., Neven, K., and Alverdy, J. (2001). Quality of life and psychosocial adjustment in patients after Roux-en-Y gastric bypass: A brief report. *Obes Surg*, 11, 32–39.

Estroff, T.W., Dackis, C.A., Gold, M.S., and Pottash, A.L. (1985). Drug abuse and bipolar disorders. *Int J Psychiatry Med*, 15, 37–40.

Famularo, R., Stone, K., and Popper, C. (1985). Preadolescent alcohol abuse and dependence. *Am J Psychiatry*, 142, 1187–1189.

Feltner, D.E., Crockatt, J.G., Dubovsky, S.J., Cohn, C.K., Shrivastava, R.K., Targum, S.D., Liu-Dumaw, M., Carter, C.M., and Pande, A.C. (2003). A randomized, double-blind, placebo-controlled, fixed-dose, multicenter study of pregabalin in patients with generalized anxiety disorder. *J Clin Psychopharmacol*, 23(3), 240–249.

Fesler, F.A. (1991). Valproate in combat-related posttraumatic stress disorder. *J Clin Psychiatry*, 52, 361–364.

Foa, E.B., Zoellner, L.A., Feeny, N.C., Hembree, E.A., and Alvarez-Conrad, J. (2002). Does imaginal exposure exacerbate PTSD symptoms? *J Consult Clin Psychol*, 70, 1022–1028.

Forster, P.L., Schoenfeld, F.B., Marmar, C.R., and Lang, A.J. (1995). Lithium for irritability in post-traumatic stress disorder. *J Trauma Stress*, 8, 143–149.

Friedman, M.A., Schwartz, M.B., and Brownell, K.D. (1998). Differential relation of psychological functioning with the history and experience of weight cycling. *J Consult Clin Psychol*, 66, 646–650.

Gadde, K.M., Parker, C.B., Maner, L.G., Wagner, H.R. II, Logue, E.J., Drezner, M.K., and Krishnan, K.R. (2001). Bupropion for weight loss: An investigation of efficacy and tolerability in overweight and obese women. *Obes Res*, 9(9), 544–551.

Gadde, K.M., Francisy, D.M., Wagner, H.R. II, and Krishnan, K.R. (2003). Zonisamide for weight loss in obese adults: A randomized controlled trial. *JAMA*, 289, 1820–1825.

Gawin, F.H., and Kleber, H.D. (1984). Cocaine abuse treatment: Open pilot trial with deipramine and lithium carbonate. *Arch Gen Psychiatry*, 41, 903–909.

Geller, B., Cooper, T.B., Sun, K., Zimerman, B., Frazier, J., Williams, M., and Heath, J. (1998). Double-blind and placebo-controlled study of lithium for adolescent bipolar disorders with secondary substance dependency. *J Am Acad Child Adolesc Psychiatry*, 37(2), 171–178.

Goldberg, J.F., and Whiteside, J.E. (2002). The association between substance abuse and antidepressant-induced mania in bipolar disorder: A preliminary study. *J Clin Psychiatry*, 63, 791–795.

Goldberg, J.F., Garno, J.L., Leon, A.C., Kocsis, J.H., and Portera, L. (1999). A history of substance abuse complicates remission from acute mania in bipolar disorder. *J Clin Psychiatry*, 60, 733–740.

Goodman, W.K., and Charney, D.S. (1987). A case of alprazolam, but not lorazepam, inducing manic symptoms. *J Clin Psychiatry*, 48, 117–118.

Goodwin, F.K., Prange, A.J. Jr., Post, R.M., Muscettola, G., and Lipton, M.A. (1982). Potentiation of antidepressant effects by L-triiodothyronine in tricyclic nonresponders. *Am J Psychiatry*, 139, 34–38.

Gross, H.A., Ebert, M.H., Faden, V.B., Goldberg, S.C., Nee, L.E., and Kaye, W.H. (1981). A double-blind controlled trial of lithium carbonate primary anorexia nervosa. *J Clin Psychopharmacol*, 1, 376–381.

Haffenden, J. (1982). *The Life of John Berryman*. Boston: Routledge & Kegan Paul.

Hamner, M., Deitsch, S., Brodrick, P., Ulmer, H., and Lorberbaum, J. (2003). Quetiapine treatment in patients with post-traumatic stress disorder: An open trial of adjunctive therapy. *J Clin Psychopharmacol*, 23, 15–20.

Henderson, D.C., Cagliero, E., Copeland, P.M., Borba, C.P., Evins, E., Hayden, D., Weber, M.T., Anderson, E.J., Allison, D.B., Daley, T.B., Schoenfeld, D., and Goff D.C. (2005). Glucose metabolism in patients with schizophrenia treated with atypical antipsychotic agents: A frequently sampled intravenous glucose tolerance test and minimal model analysis. *Arch Gen Psychiatry*, 62, 19–28.

Hertzberg, M.A., Butterfield, M.I., Feldman, M.E., Beckham, J.C., Sutherland, S.M., Connor, K.M., and Davidson, J.R. (1999). A preliminary study of lamotrigine for the treatment of post-traumatic stress disorder. *Biol Psychiatry*, 45, 1226–1229.

Hirschfeld, R.M., Weisler, R.H., Raines, S.R., Macfadden, W., and the BOLDER Study Group. (2006). Quetiapine in the treatment of anxiety in patients with bipolar I or II depression: A secondary analysis from a randomized, double-blind, placebo-controlled study. *J Clin Psychiatry*, 67(3), 355–362.

Hollander, E., Kaplan, A., and Stahl, S.M. (2003). A double-blind, placebo-controlled trial of clonazepam in obsessive-compulsive disorder. *World J Biol Psychiatry*, 4, 30–34.

Hollister, L.E., Johnson, K., Boukhabza, D., and Gillespie, H.K. (1981). Aversive effects of naltrexone in subjects not dependent on opiates. *Drug Alcohol Depend*, 8, 37–41.

Hoopes, S.P., Reimherr, F.W., Hedges, D.W., Rosenthal, N.R., Kamin, M., Karim, R., Capece, J.A., and Karvois, D. (2003). Treatment of bulimia nervosa with topiramate in a randomized, double-blind, placebo-controlled trial: Part 1. Improvement in binge and purge measures. *J Clin Psychiatry*, 64, 1335–1341.

Hsu, L.K., Clement, L., Santhouse, R., and Ju, E.S. (1991). Treatment of bulimia nervosa with lithium carbonate: A controlled study. *J Nerv Ment Dis*, 179, 351–355.

Hutterfield, M., Becker, M., and Conner, K. (2001). Olanzapine in the treatment of post-traumatic stress disorder: A pilot study. *Int Clin Psychopharmacol*, 16, 197–203.

Jain, A.K., Kaplan, R.A., Gadde, K.M., Wadden, T.A., Allison, D.B., Brewer, E.R., Leadbetter, R.A., Richard, N., Haight, B., Jamerson, B.D., Buaron, K.S., and Metz, A. (2002). Bupropion SR vs. placebo for weight loss in obese patients with depressive symptoms. *Obes Res*, 10(10), 1049–1056.

Johnson, B.A., Ait-Daoud, N., Bowden, C.L., DiClemente, C.C., Roache, J.D., Lawson, K., Javors, M.A., and Ma, J.Z. (2003). Oral topiramate for treatment of alcohol dependence: A randomised controlled trial. *Lancet*, 361, 1677–1685.

Kanba, S., Yagi, G., Kamijima, K., Suzuki, T., Tajima, O., Otaki, J., Arata, E., Koshikawa, H., Nibuya, M., and Kinoshita, N. (1994). The first open study of zonisamide, a novel anticonvulsant, shows efficacy in mania. *Prog Neuropsychopharmacol Biol Psychiatry*, 18, 707–715.

Keck, P.E., Jr., McElroy, S.L., and Friedman, L.M. (1992). Valproate and carbamazepine in the treatment of panic and posttraumatic stress disorders, withdrawal states, and behavioral dyscontrol syndromes. *J Clin Psychopharmacol*, 12, 36S–41S.

Keck, P.E., Jr., Taylor, V.E., Tugrul, K.C., McElroy, S.L., and Bennett, J.A. (1993). Valproate treatment of panic disorder and lactate-induced panic attacks. *Biol Psychiatry*, 33, 542–546.

Latt, N.C., Jurd, S., Houseman, J., and Wutzke, S.E. (2002). Naltrexone in alcohol dependence: A randomised controlled trial of effectiveness in a standard clinical setting. *Med J Aust*, 176, 530–534.

Leibow, D. (1983). L-thyroxine for rapid-cycling bipolar illness. *Am J Psychiatry*, 140, 1255.

Lensi, P., Cassano, G.B., Correddu, G., Ravagli, S., Kunovac, J.L., and Akiskal, H.S. (1996). Obsessive-compulsive disorder: Familial-developmental history, symptomatology, comorbidity and course with special reference to gender-related differences. *Br J Psychiatry*, 169, 101–107.

Leverich, G.S., Altshuler, L.L., Frye, M.A., Suppes, T., McElroy, S.L., Keck, P.E. Jr., Kupka, R.W., Denicoff, K.D., Nolen, W.A., Grunze, H., Martinez, M.I., and Post, R.M. (2006). Risk of switch in mood polarity to hypomania or mania in patients with bipolar depression during acute and continuation trials of venlafaxine, sertraline, and bupropion as adjuncts to mood stabilizers. *Am J Psychiatry*, 163(2), 232–239.

Levin, F.R., and Hennessy, G. (2004). Bipolar disorder and substance abuse. *Biol Psychiatry*, 56, 738–748.

Longo, L.P., Campbell, T., and Hubatch, S. (2002). Divalproex sodium (Depakote) for alcohol withdrawal and relapse prevention. *J Addict Dis*, 21, 55–64.

Magura, S., Laudet, A.B., Mahmood, D., Rosenblum, A., and Knight, E. (2002). Adherence to medication regimens and participation in dual-focus self-help groups. *Psychiatr Serv*, 53, 310–316.

Malcolm, R., Ballenger, J.C., Sturgis, E.T., and Anton, R. (1989). Double-blind controlled trial comparing carbamazepine to oxazepam treatment of alcohol withdrawal. *Am J Psychiatry*, 146, 617–621.

Malcolm, R., Myrick, H., and Roberts., J. (2002). The effects of carbamazepine and lorazepam on single versus multitude previous alcohol withdrawals in an outpatient randomized trial. *J Gen Intern Med*, 17, 349–355.

McDougle, C.J., Price, L.H., Goodman, W.K., Charney, D.S., and Heninger, G.R. (1991). A controlled trial of lithium augmentation in fluvoxamine-refractory obsessive-compulsive disorder: Lack of efficacy. *J Clin Psychopharmacol*, 11(3), 175–184.

McDougle, C.J., Epperson, C., Peltion, G., Wasylink, S., and Price, L. (2000). A double blind placebo controlled study of risperidone addition in serotonin reuptake inhibitor-refractory obsessive compulsive disorder. *Arch Gen Psychiatry*, 57, 794–801.

McElroy, S.L., Arnold, L.M., Shapira, N.A., Keck, P.E. Jr., Rosenthal, N.R., Karim, M.R., Kamin, M., and Hudson, J.I. (2003). Topiramate in the treatment of binge eating disorder associated with obesity: A randomized, placebo-controlled trial. *Am J Psychiatry*, 160, 255–261.

McElroy, S.L., Kotwal, R., Hudson, J.I., Nelson, E.B., and Keck, P.E. (2004). Zonisamide in the treatment of binge-eating disorder: An open-label, prospective trial. *J Clin Psychiatry*, 65, 50–56.

Monnelly, E., Ciraulo, D., Knapp, C., and Keane, T. (2003). Low-dose risperidone as adjunctive therapy for irritable aggression in post-traumatic stress disorder. *J Clin Psychopharmacol*, 23, 193–196.

Montgomery, S.A., Tobias, K., Zornberg, G.L., Kasper, S., and Pande, A.C. (2006). Efficacy and safety of pregabalin in the treatment of generalized anxiety disorder: A 6-week, multicenter, randomized, double-blind, placebo-controlled comparison of pregabalin and venlafaxine. *J Clin Psychiatry*, 67(5), 771–782.

Morrison, J.R. (1975). The family histories of manic-depressive patients with and without alcoholism. *J Nerv Ment Dis*, 160, 227–229.

Mueller, T.I., Stout, R.L., Rudden, S., Brown, R.A., Gordon, A., Solomon, D.A., and Recupero, P.R. (1997). A double-blind, placebo-controlled pilot study of carbamazepine for the treatment of alcohol dependence. *Alcohol Clin Exp Res*, 21, 86–92.

Muller-Oerlinghausen, B., Wolf, T., Ahrens, B., Glaenz, T., Schou, M., Grof, E., Grof, P., Lenz, G., Simhandl, C., Thau, K., Vestergaard, P., and Wolf, R. (1996). Mortality of patients who dropped out from regular lithium prophylaxis: A collaborative study by the International Group for the Study of Lithium-treated Patients (IGSLI). *Acta Psychiatr Scand*, 94, 344–347.

Najavits, L.M., Weiss, R.D., Shaw, S.R., and Muenz, L.R. (1998). "Seeking safety": Outcome of a new cognitive-behavioral psychotherapy for women with posttraumatic stress disorder and substance dependence. *J Trauma Stress*, 11, 437–456.

Nunes, E.V., McGrath, P.J., Wager, S., and Quitkin, F.M. (1990). Lithium treatment for cocaine abusers with bipolar spectrum disorders. *Am J Psychiatry*, 147(5), 655–657.

Nuzzo, V., Lupoli, G., Esposito Del Puente, A., Rampone, E., Carpinelli, A., Del Puente, A.E., and Oriente, P. (1998). Bone mineral density in premenopausal women receiving levothyroxine suppressive therapy. *Gynecol Endocrinol*, 12, 333–337.

Ogborne, A.C., and Glaser, F.B. (1985). Evaluating Alcoholics Anonymous. In T.E. Bratter (Ed.), *Alcoholism and Substance Abuse* (pp. 176–192). New York: Free Press.

Olson, G.A., Olson, R.D., and Kastin, A.J. (1996). Endogenous opiates: 1995. *Peptides*, 17, 1421–1466.

Pande, A.C., Davidson, J.R., Jefferson, J.W., Janney, C.A., Katzelnick, D.J., Weisler, R.H., Greist, J.H., and Sutherland, S.M. (1999). Treatment of social phobia with gabapentin: A placebo-controlled study. *J Clin Psychopharmacol*, 19(4), 341–348.

Pande, A.C., Pollack, M.H., Crockatt, J., Greiner, M., Chouinard, G., Lydiard, R.B., Taylor, C.B., Dager, S.R., and Shiovitz, T. (2000). Placebo-controlled study of gabapentin treatment of panic disorder. *J Clin Psychopharmacol*, 20, 467–471.

Pande, A.C., Crockatt, J.G., Feltner, D.E., Janney, C.A., Smith, W.T., Weisler, R., Londborg, P.D., Bielski, R.J., Zimbroff, D.L., Davidson, J.R., and Liu-Dumaw, M. (2003). Pregabalin in generalized anxiety disorder: A placebo-controlled trial. *Am J Psychiatry*, 160(3), 533–540.

Perugi, G., Akiskal, H.S., Pfanner, C., Presta, S., Gemignani, A., Milanfranchi, A., Lensi, P., Ravagli, S., and Cassano, G.B. (1997). The clinical impact of bipolar and unipolar affective comorbidity on obsessive-compulsive disorder. *J Affect Disord*, 46, 15–23.

Perugi, G., Toni, C., Frare, F., Travierso, M.C., Hantouche, E., and Akiskal, H.S. (2002). Obsessive-compulsive-bipolar comorbidity: A systematic exploration of clinical features and treatment outcome. *J Clin Psychiatry*, 63, 1129–1134.

Pigott, T.A., Pato, M.T., L'Heureux, F., Hill, J.L., Grover, G.N., Bernstein, S.E., and Murphy, D.L. (1991). A controlled comparison of adjuvant lithium carbonate or thyroid hormone in clomipramine-treated patients with obsessive-compulsive disorder. *J Clin Psychopharmacol*, 11(4), 242–248.

Pohl, R.B., Feltner, D.E., Fieve, R.R., and Pande, A.C. (2005). Efficacy of pregabalin in the treatment of generalized anxiety disorder: Double-blind, placebo-controlled comparison of BID versus TID dosing. *J Clin Psychopharmacol*, 25(2), 151–158.

Post, R.M., Kramlinger, K.G., Joffe, R.T., Roy-Byrne, P.P., Rosoff, A., Frye, M.A., and Huggins, T. (1997). Rapid cycling bipolar affective disorder: Lack of relation to hypothyroidism. *Psychiatry Res*, 72, 1–7.

Powers, P.S., Santana, C.A., and Bannon, Y.S. (2002). Olanzapine in the treatment of anorexia nervosa: An open label trial. *Int J Eat Disord*, 32, 146–154.

Prange, A.J., Jr., Wilson, I.C., Rabon, A.M., and Lipton, M.A. (1969). Enhancement of imipramine antidepressant activity by thyroid hormone. *Am J Psychiatry*, 126, 457–469.

Reinhold, R.B. (1994). Late results of gastric bypass surgery for morbid obesity. *J Am Coll Nutr*, 13, 326–331.

Rickels, K., Pollack, M.H., Feltner, D.E., Lydiard, R.B., Zimbroff, D.L., Bielski, R.J., Tobias, K., Brock, J.D., Zornberg, G.L., and Pande, A.C. (2005). Pregabalin for treatment of generalized anxiety disorder: A 4-week, multicenter, double-blind, placebo-controlled trial of pregabalin and alprazolam. *Arch Gen Psychiatry*, 62(9), 1022–1030.

Rubio G., Lopez-Munoz. F., and Alamo, C. (2006). Effects of lamotrigine in patients with bipolar disorder and alcohol dependence. *Bipolar Disord*, 8, 289–293.

Rychtarik, R.G., Connors, G.J., Dermen, K.H., and Stasiewicz, P.R. (2000). Alcoholics Anonymous and the use of medications to prevent relapse: An anonymous survey of member attitudes. *J Stud Alcohol*, 61, 134–138.

Salloum, I.M., Cornelius, J.R., Daley, D.C., Kirisci, L., Himmel-hoch, J.M., and Thase, M.E. (2005). Efficacy of valproate maintenance in patients with bipolar disorder and alcoholism: A double-blind placebo-controlled study. *Arch Gen Psychiatry*, 62, 37–45.

Sass, H., Soyka, M., Mann, K., and Zieglgansberger, W. (1996). Relapse prevention by acamprosate: Results from a placebo-controlled study on alcohol dependence. *Arch Gen Psychiatry*, 53, 673–680.

Saxena, S., Wang, D., Bystritsky, A., and Baxter, L.R. Jr. (1996). Risperidone augmentation of SRI treatment for refractory obsessive-compulsive disorder. *J Clin Psychiatry*, 57(7), 303–306.

Schuckit, M. (1983). Alcoholic patients with secondary depression. *Am J Psychiatry*, 140, 711–714.

Shapira, N.A., Ward, H.E., Mandoki, M., Murphy, T.K., Yang, M.C., Blier, P., and Goodman, W.K. (2004). A double-blind, placebo-controlled trial of olanzapine addition in fluoxetine-refractory obsessive-compulsive disorder. *Biol Psychiatry*, 55, 553–555.

Solyom, L., DiNicola, V.F., Phil, M., Sookman, D., and Luchins, D. (1985). Is there an obsessive psychosis? Aetiological and prognostic factors of an atypical form of obsessive-compulsive neurosis. *Can J Psychiatry*, 30(5), 372–380.

Sonne, S.C., and Brady, K.T. (2000). Naltrexone for individuals with comorbid bipolar disorder and alcohol dependence. *J Clin Psychopharmacol*, 20, 114–115.

Stancer, H.C., and Persad, E. (1982). Treatment of intractable rapid-cycling manic-depressive disorder with levothyroxine: Clinical observations. *Arch Gen Psychiatry*, 39, 311–312.

Strakowski, S.M., Sax, K.W., McElroy, S.L., Keck, P.E. Jr., Hawkins, J.M., and West, S.A. (1998). Course of psychiatric and substance abuse syndromes co-occurring with bipolar disorder after a first psychiatric hospitalization. *J Clin Psychiatry*, 59(9), 465–471.

Swartz, H.A., Pilkonis, P.A., Frank, E., Proietti, J.M., and Scott, J. (2005). Acute treatment outcomes in patients with bipolar I disorder and comorbid borderline personality disorder receiving medication and psychotherapy. *Bipolar Disord*, 7(2), 192–197.

Tarrier, N., Pilgrim, H., Sommerfield, C., Faragher, B., Reynolds, M., Graham, E., and Barrowclough, C. (1999a). A randomized trial of cognitive therapy and imaginal exposure in the treatment of chronic posttraumatic stress disorder. *J Consult Clin Psychol*, 67, 13–18.

Tarrier, N., Sommerfield, C., Pilgrim, H., and Humphreys, L. (1999b). Cognitive therapy or imaginal exposure in the treatment of post-traumatic stress disorder: Twelve-month follow-up. *Br J Psychiatry*, 175, 571–575.

Taylor, C.B., Youngblood, M.E., Catellier, D., Veith, R.C., Carney, R.M., Burg, M.M., Kaufmann, P.G., Shuster, J., Mellman, T., Blumenthal, J.A., Krishnan, R., Jaffe, A.S., and ENRICHD Investigators (2005). Effects of antidepressant medication on morbidity and mortality in depressed patients after myocardial infarction. *Arch Gen Psychiatry*, 62, 792–798.

Tiihonen, J., Lönnqvist, J., Wahlbeck, K., Klaukka, T., Tanskanen, A., and Haukka, J. (2006). Antidepressants and the risk of suicide, attempted suicide, and overall mortality in a nationwide cohort. *Arch Gen Psychiatry*, 63, 1368–1367.

Tonigan, J.S., Toscova, R., and Miller, W.R. (1996). Meta-analysis of the literature on Alcoholics Anonymous: Sample and study characteristics moderate findings. *J Stud Alcohol*, 57, 65–72.

Uhde, T.W., Stein, M.B., and Post, R.M. (1988). Lack of efficacy of carbamazepine in the treatment of panic disorder. *Am J Psychiatry*, 145, 1104–1109.

Vaillant, G.E. (1978). Alcoholism and drug dependence. In A.M. Nicholi (Ed.), *The Harvard Guide to Modern Psychiatry* (pp. 567–577). Cambridge, MA: Belknap Press.

Vulink, N.C., Denys, D., and Westenberg, H.G. (2005). Bupropion for patients with obsessive-compulsive disorder: An open-label, fixed-dose study. *J Clin Psychiatry*, 66, 228–230.

Weiss, R.D., Greenfield, S.F., Najavits, L.M., Soto, J.A., Wyner, D., Tohen, M., and Griffin, M.L. (1998). Medication compliance among patients with bipolar disorder and substance use disorder. *J Clin Psychiatry*, 59, 172–174.

Weiss, R.D., Najavits, L.M., and Greenfield, S.F. (1999). A relapse prevention group for patients with bipolar and substance use disorders. *J Subst Abuse Treat*, 16, 47–54.

Weiss, R.D., Kolodziej, M.E., Najavits, L.M., Greenfield, S.F., and Fucito, L.M. (2000). Utilization of psychosocial treatments by patients diagnosed with bipolar disorder and substance dependence. *Am J Addict*, 9, 314–320.

Weiss, R.D., Griffin, M.L., Kolodziej, M.E., Greenfield, S.F., Najavits, L.M., Daley, D.C., Doreau, H.R., and Hennen, J.A. (2007). A randomized trial of integrated group therapy versus group drug counseling for patients with bipolar disorder and substance dependence. *Am J Psychiatry*, 164, 100–107.

Whitworth, A.B., Fischer, F., Lesch, O.M., Nimmerrichter, A., Oberbauer, H., Platz, T., Potgieter, A., Walter, H., and Fleischhacker, W.W. (1996). Comparison of acamprosate and placebo in long-term treatment of alcohol dependence. *Lancet*, 347, 1438–1442.

Wilner, K.D., Anziano, R.J., Johnson, A.C., Miceli, J.J., Fricke, J.R., and Titus, C.K. (2002). The anxiolytic effect of the novel antipsychotic ziprasidone compared with diazepam in subjects anxious before dental surgery. *J Clin Psychopharmacol*, 22, 206–210.

Chapter 25

Advisory Committee to U.S. Food and Drug Administration. (2004). Center for Drug Evaluation and Research, Psychopharmacologic Drugs Advisory Committee with the Pediatric Subcommittee of the Anti-Infective Drugs Advisory Committee. *February 2 Transcript*. Available: http://www.fda.gov/ohrms/dockets/ac/04/transcripts/4006t1.htm (accessed September 19, 2006).

Akiskal, H.S., Benazzi, F., Perugi, G., and Rihmer, Z. (2005). Agitated "unipolar" depression re-conceptualized as a depressive mixed state: Implications for the antidepressant-suicide controversy. *J Affect Disord*, 85(3), 245–258.

Allen, M.H., and Currier, G.W. (2004). Use of restraints and pharmacotherapy in academic psychiatric emergency services. *Gen Hosp Psychiatry*, 26, 42–49.

American Psychiatric Association. (2003). Practice guidelines for the assessment and treatment of patients with suicidal behaviors. *Am J Psychiatry,* 117 pp. Available at: http://www.psych.org/psych_pract/treatg/pg/pg_suicidalbehaviors.pdf.

Angst, F., Stassen, H.H., Clayton, P.J., and Angst, J. (2002). Mortality of patients with mood disorders: Follow-up over 34–38 years. *J Affect Disord,* 68(2), 167–181.

Angst, J., Angst, F., Gerber-Werder, R., and Gamma, A. (2005b). Suicide in 406 mood-disorder patients with and without long-term medication: A 40 to 44 years' follow-up. *Arch Suicide Res,* 9(3), 279–300.

Appleby, L., Shaw, J., Amos, T., McDonnell, R., Harris, C., McCann, K., Kiernan, K., Davies, S., Bickley, H., and Parsons, R. (1999). Suicide within 12 months of contact with mental health services: National clinical survey. *BMJ,* 318(7193), 1235–1239.

Baldessarini, R.J., and Goodwin, F.K. (2003). *Psychiatric treatments versus suicidal risk.* Submitted to ACNP Task Force on Treatment Effects and Suicide, by invitation.

Baldessarini, R.J., and Goodwin, F.K. (2005). Citizens Petition to the United States Food and Drug Administration: Lithium and Suicide Prevention.

Baldessarini, R.J., and Jamison, K. (1999). Effects of medical interventions on suicidal behavior. *J Clin Psychiatry,* 60(Suppl. 2), 117–122.

Baldessarini, R.J., Tondo, L., and Hennen, J. (1999). Effects of lithium treatment and its discontinuation on suicidal behavior in bipolar manic-depressive disorder. *J Clin Psychiatry,* 60(Suppl. 2), 77–84.

Baldessarini, R.J., Tondo, L., and Hennen, J. (2001). Treating the suicidal patient with bipolar disorder: Reducing suicide risk with lithium. *Ann N Y Acad Sci,* 932:24–38; discussion 39–43.

Baldessarini, R.J., Tondo, L., and Hennen, J. (2003). Lithium treatment and suicide risk in major affective disorders: Update and new findings. *J Clin Psychiatry,* 64(Suppl. 5), 44–52.

Baldessarini, R.J., Pompili, M., and Tondo, L. (2006a). Suicide in bipolar disorder: Risks and management. *CNS Spectr,* 11(6), 465–471.

Baldessarini, R.J., Tondo, L., Davis, P., Pompili, M., Goodwin, F.K., and Hennen, J. (2006b). Decreased risks of suicides and suicide attempts during long-term lithium treatment: A meta-analytic review. *Bipolar Disord,* 8, 625–639.

Barraclough, B., Bunch, J., Nelson, B., and Sainsbury, P. (1974). A hundred cases of suicide: Clinical aspects. *Br J Psychiatry,* 125, 355–373.

Battaglia, J. (2005). Pharmacologic management of acute agitation. *Drugs,* 65, 1207–1222.

Bauer, M.S., Wisniewski, S.R., Marangell, L.B., Chessick, C.A., Allen, M.H., Dennehy, E.B., Miklowitz, D.J., Thase, M.E., and Sachs, G.S. (2006). Are antidepressants associated with new-onset suicidality in bipolar disorder? A prospective study of participants in the Systematic Treatment Enhancement Program for Bipolar Disorder (STEP-BD). *J Clin Psychiatry,* 67, 48–55.

Bradvik, L., and Berglund, M. (2000). Treatment and suicide in severe depression: A case-control study of antidepressant therapy at last contact before suicide. *J ECT,* 16(4), 399–408.

Brent, D.A., Moritz, G., Bridge, J., Perper, J., and Canobbio, R. (1996). Long-term impact of exposure to suicide: A three-year controlled follow-up. *J Am Acad Child Adolesc Psychiatry,* 35(5), 646–653.

Brodersen, A., Licht, R.W., Vestergaard, P., Olesen, A.V., and Morensen, P.B. (2000). Sixteen-year mortality in patients with affective disorder commenced on lithium. *Br J Psychiatry,* 176, 429–433.

Brown, G.K., Ten Have, T., Henriques, G.R., Xie, S.X., Hollander, J.E., and Beck, A.T. (2005). Cognitive therapy for the prevention of suicide attempts: A randomized controlled trial. *JAMA,* 294, 563–570.

Bruce, M.L., Ten Have, T.R., Reynolds, C.F. III, Katz, I.I., Schulberg, H.C., Mulsant, B.H., Brown, G.K., McAvay, G.J., Pearson, J.L., and Alexopoulos, G.S. (2004). Reducing suicidal ideation and depressive symptoms in depressed older primary care patients: A randomized controlled trial. *JAMA,* 291(9), 1081–1091.

Busch, K.A., Fawcett, J., and Jacobs, D.G. (2003). Clinical correlates of inpatient suicide. *J Clin Psychiatry,* 64(1), 14–19.

Cassem, N.H. (1978). Treating the person confronting death. In A.M. Nicholi (Ed.), *Harvard Guide to Modern Psychiatry* (pp. 579–606). Cambridge, MA: Belknap Press of Harvard University Press.

Cerel, J., Fristad, M.A., Weller, E.B., and Weller, R.A. (1999). Suicide-bereaved children and adolescents: A controlled longitudinal examination. *J Am Acad Child Adolesc Psychiatry,* 38(6), 672–679.

Chemtob, C.M., Hamada, R.S., Bauer, G., Kinney, B., and Torigoe, R.Y. (1988a). Patients' suicides: Frequency and impact on psychiatrists. *Am J Psychiatry,* 145(2), 224–228.

Chemtob, C.M., Hamada, R.S., Bauer, G., Torigoe, R.Y., and Kinney, B. (1988b). Patients' suicides: Frequency and impact on psychologists. *Prof Psychol,* 19, 416–420.

Ciapparelli, A., Dell'Osso, L., Pini, S., Chiavacci, M.C., Fenzi, M., and Cassano, G.B. (2000). Clozapine for treatment-refractory schizophrenia, schizoaffective disorder, and psychotic bipolar disorder: A 24-month naturalistic study. *J Clin Psychiatry,* 61(5), 329–334.

Cipriani, A., Wilder, H., Hawton, K., and Geddes, J.R. (2005). Lithium in the prevention of suicidal behavior and all-cause mortality in patients with mood disorders: A systematic review of randomized trials. *Am J Psychiatry,* 162(10), 1805–1819.

Coate, M. (1964). *Beyond All Reason.* London: Constable & Co.

Coppen, A., Standish-Barry, H., Bailey, J., Houston, G., Silicocks, P., and Hermon, C. (1990). Long-term lithium and mortality. *Lancet,* 335, 1347.

Coppen, A., Standish-Barry, H., Bailey, J., Houston, G., Silicocks, P., and Hermon, C. (1991). Does lithium reduce the mortality of recurrent mood disorders? *J Affect Disord,* 23, 1–7.

Coryell, W. (1988). Panic disorder and mortality. *Psychiatr Clin North Am,* 11(2), 433–440.

Dixon, J.F., and Hokin, L.E. (1998). Lithium acutely inhibits and chronically up-regulates and stabilizes glutamate uptake by presynaptic nerve endings in mouse cerebral cortex. *Proc Natl Acad Sci USA,* 95(14), 8363–8368.

Dubicka, B., Hadley, S., and Roberts, C. (2006). Suicidal behavior in youths with depression treated with new-generation antidepressants. *Br J Psychiatry,* 189, 393–398.

Duke University. (2005). *Duke University program on psychiatric advance directives.* Available: http://pad.duhs.duke.edu/index.html [accessed September 19, 2006].

Emslie, G.J., Heiligenstein, J.H., Wagner, K.D., Hoog, S.L., Ernest, D.E., Brown, E., Nilsson, M., and Jacobson, J.G. (2002). Fluoxetine for acute treatment of depression in children and adolescents: A placebo-controlled randomized clinical trial. *J Am Acad Child Adolesc Psychiatr,* 41, 1205–1215.

Faedda, G., Tondo, L., Baldessarini, R.J., Suppes, T., and Tohen, M. (1993). Outcome after rapid vs. gradual discontinuation of lithium treatment in bipolar mood disorders. *Arch Gen Psychiatry,* 50, 448–455.

Fawcett, J., and Barkin, R.L. (1998). Review of the results from clinical studies on the efficacy, safety and tolerability of mirtazapine for the treatment of patients with major depression. *J Affect Disord,* 51(3), 267–285.

Fawcett, J., Scheftner, W., Clark, D., Hedeker, D., Gibbons, R., and Coryell, W. (1987). Clinical predictors of suicide in patients with major affective disorders: A controlled prospective study. *Am J Psychiatry,* 144(1), 35–40.

Fawcett, J., Scheftner, W.A., Fogg, L., Clark, D.C., Young, M.A., Hedeker, D., and Gibbons, R. (1990). Time-related predictors of suicide in major affective disorder. *Am J Psychiatry,* 147(9), 1189–1194.

Fergusson, D., Doucette, S., Glass, K.C., Shapiro, S., Healy, D., Hebert, P., and Hutton, B. (2005). Association between suicide attempts and selective serotonin in reuptake inhibitors: Systematic review of randomized controlled trials. *BMJ,* 330, 396.

Fieve, R.R. (1975). The lithium clinic: A new model for the delivery of psychiatric services. *Am J Psychiatry,* 132, 1018–1022.

Gibbons, R.D., Hur, K., Bhaumik, D.K., and Mann, J.J. (2005). The relationship between antidepressant medication use and rate of suicide. *Arch Gen Psychiatry,* 62(2), 165–172.

Gibbons, R.D., Hur, K., Bhaumik, D.K., and Mann, J.J. (2006). The relationship between antidepressant prescription rates and rate yearly adolescent suicide. *Am J Psychiatry,* 163, 1898–1904.

Gitlin, M.J. (1999). A psychiatrist's reaction to a patient's suicide. *Am J Psychiatry,* 156(10), 1630–1634.

Gitlin, M.J., and Jamison, K.R. (1984). Lithium clinics: Theory and practice. *Hosp Community Psychiatry,* 35, 363–368.

Glazer, W.M. (1997). Olanzapine and the new generation of antipsychotic agents: Patterns of use. *J Clin Psychiatry,* 58(Suppl. 10), 18–21.

Goldstein, R.B., Black, D.W., Nasrallah, A., and Winokur, G. (1991). The prediction of suicide: Sensitivity, specificity and predictive value of a multivariate model applied to suicide among 1906 patients with affective disorders. *Arch Gen Psychiatry,* 48(5), 418–422.

Goodwin, F.K., and Jamison, K.R. (1984). The natural course of manic-depressive illness. In R.M. Post and J.C. Ballenger (Eds.), *Neurobiology of Mood Disorders* (pp. 20–37). Baltimore: Williams & Wilkins.

Goodwin, F.K., Fireman, B., Simon, G.E., Hunkeler, E.M., Lee, J., and Revicki, D. (2003). Suicide risk in bipolar disorder during treatment with lithium and divalproex. *JAMA,* 290(11), 1467–1473.

Grunebaum, M.F., Oquendo, M.A., Burke, A.K., Ellis, S.P., Echavarria, G., Brodsky, B.S., Malone, K.M., and Mann, J.J. (2003). Clinical impact of a 2-week psychotropic medication washout in unipolar depressed inpatients. *J Affect Disord,* 75(3), 291–296.

Hankoff, L.D. (1982). Suicide and attempted suicide. In E.S. Paykel (Ed.), *Handbook of Affective Disorders* (pp. 416–428). New York: Guildford Press.

Hartigan, G.P. (1959). *Experiences with Treatment with Lithium Salts.* Paper read to the Southeastern branch of the Royal Medicopsychological Society, London, UK.

Hawton, K., and Catalan, J. (1982). *Attempted Suicide: A Practical Guide to Its Nature and Management.* New York: Oxford University Press.

Hawton, K., Arensman, E., Townsend, E., Bremner, S., Feldman, E., Goldney, R., Gunnell, D., Hazell, P., van Heeringen, K., House, A., Owens, D., Sakinofsky, I., and Traskman-Bendz, L. (1998). Deliberate self harm: Systematic review of efficacy of psychosocial and pharmacological treatments in preventing repetition. *BMJ,* 317(7156), 441–447.

Hawton, K., Townsend, E., Arensman, E., Gunnell, D., Hazell, P., House, A., and van Heeringen, K. (2000). Psychosocial versus pharmacological treatments for deliberate self harm. *Cochrane Database Syst Rev,* (2), CD001764.

Hendin, H., Lipschitz, A., Maltsberger, J.T., Haas, A.P., and Wynecoop, S. (2000). Therapists' reactions to patients' suicides. *Am J Psychiatry,* 157(12), 2022–2027.

Hendin, H., Haas, A.P., Maltsberger, J.T., Szanto, K., and Rabinowicz, H. (2004). Factors contributing to therapists' distress after the suicide of a patient. *Am J Psychiatry,* 161(8), 1442–1446.

Hepp, U., Wittmann, L., Schnyder, U., and Michel, K. (2004). Psychological and psychosocial interventions after attempted suicide: An overview of treatment studies. *Crisis,* 25(3), 108–117.

Institute of Medicine (IOM). (2002). *Reducing Suicide: A National Imperative.* Washington, DC: National Academy Press.

Isacsson, G. (2000). Suicide prevention: A medical breakthrough? *Acta Psychiatr Scand,* 102(2), 113–117.

Isacsson, G., Redfors, I., Wasserman, D., and Bergman, U. (1994). Choice of antidepressants: Questionnaire survey of psychiatrists and general practitioners in two areas of Sweden. *BMJ,* 309(6968), 1546–1549.

Isacsson, G., Holmgren, P., Druid, H., and Bergman, U. (1997). The utilization of antidepressants—A key issue in the prevention of suicide: An analysis of 5281 suicides in Sweden during the period 1992–1994. *Acta Psychiatr Scand,* 96(2), 94–100.

Isometsa, E.T., Henriksson, M.M., Aro, H.M., Heikkinen, M.E., Kuoppasalmi, K.I., and Lonnqvist, J.K. (1994). Suicide in major depression. *Am J Psychiatry,* 151(4), 530–536.

Isometsa, E.T., Heikkinen, M.E., Marttunen, M.J., Henriksson, M.M., Aro, H.M., and Lonnqvist, J.K. (1995). The last appointment before suicide: Is suicide intent communicated? *Am J Psychiatry,* 152(6), 919–922.

Jacobs, D.G., Baldessarini, R.J., Conwell, Y., Fawcett, J., Horton, L., Meltzer, H., Pfeffer, C.R., and Simon, R.L. (2003). *Practice Guideline for the Assessment and Treatment of Patients with Suicide Behaviors.* Available: http://www.psych.org/psych_pract/treatg/quick_ref_guide/Suibehavs_QRG.pdf (accessed September 19, 2006).

Jamison, K.R. (1995). *An Unquiet Mind.* New York: Knopf.

Jamison, K.R. (1999). *Night Falls Fast: Understanding Suicide.* New York: Random House.

Khan, A., Shad, M.U., and Preskorn, S.H. (2000). Lack of sertraline efficacy probably due to an interaction with carbamazepine. *J Clin Psychiatry,* 61(7), 526–527.

Khan, A., Khan, S., Kolts, R., and Brown, W.A. (2003). Suicide rates in clinical trials of SSRIs, other antidepressants, and placebo: Analysis of FDA reports. *Am J Psychiatry,* 160(4), 790–792.

Kessing, L.V., Sondergard, L., Kvist, K., and Andersen, P.K. (2005). Suicide risk in patients treated with lithium. *Arch Gen Psychiatry,* 62(8), 860–866.

King, R.A., Riddle, M.A., Chappell, P.B., Hardin, M.T., and Anderson, G.M. (1991). Emergence of self-destructive phenomena in children and adolescents during fluoxetine treatment. *J Am Acad Child Adolesc Psychiatry*, 30(2), 179–186.

Knox, K.L., Litts, D.A., Talcott, G.W., Feig, J.C., and Caine, E.D. (2003). Risk of suicide and related adverse outcomes after exposure to a suicide prevention programme in the U.S. Air Force: Cohort study. *BMJ*, 327(7428), 1376.

Knox, K.L., Conwell, Y., and Caine, E.D. (2004). If suicide is a public health problem, what are we doing to prevent it? *Am J Public Health*, 94(1), 37–45.

Leon, A.C. (2005). Fluoxetine plus cognitive behavioural therapy improves symptoms of major depressive disorder in adolescents. *Evid Based Ment Health*, 8, 10.

Londborg, P.D., Smith, W.T., Glaudin, V., and Painter, J.R. (2000). Short-term cotherapy with clonazepam and fluoxetine: Anxiety, sleep disturbance and core symptoms of depression. *J Affect Disord*, 61(1–2), 73–79.

Ludwig, J., and Marcotte, D.E. (2005). Anti-depressants, suicide, and drug regulation. *J Policy Anal Manage*, 24, 249–272.

Luoma, J.B., Martin, C.E., and Pearson, J.L. (2002). Contact with mental health and primary care providers before suicide: A review of the evidence. *Am J Psychiatry*, 159(6), 909–916.

MacKinnon, D.R., and Farberow, N.L. (1976). An assessment of the utility of suicide prediction. *Suicide Life Threat Behav*, 6(2), 86–91.

Malone, K.M., Oquendo, M.A., Haas, G.L., Ellis, S.P., Li, S., and Mann, J.J. (2000). Protective factors against suicidal acts in major depression: Reasons for living. *Am J Psychiatry*, 157(7), 1084–1088.

Marco, C.A., and Vaughan, J. (2005). Emergency management of agitation in schizophrenia. *Am J Emerg Med*, 23, 767–776.

Marder, S.R., (2006). A review of agitation in mental illness: Treatment guidelines and current therapies. *J Clin Psychiatry*, 67(Suppl. 10), 13–21.

McElroy, S.L., Kotwal, R., Kaneria, R., and Keck, P.E. (2006). Antidepressants and suicidal behavior in bipolar disorder. *Bipolar Disord*, 8, 596–617.

Meltzer, H.Y., and Okayli, G. (1995). Reduction of suicidality during clozapine treatment of neuroleptic-resistant schizophrenia: Impact on risk-benefit assessment. *Am J Psychiatry*, 152(2), 183–190.

Meltzer, H.Y., Alphs, L., Green, A.I., Altamura, A.C., Anand, R., Bertoldi, A., Bourgeois, M., Chouinard, G., Islam, M.Z., Kane, J., Krishnan, R., Lindenmayer, J.P., Potkin, S., and International Suicide Prevention Trial Study Group. (2003). Clozapine treatment for suicidality in schizophrenia: International Suicide Prevention Trial (InterSePT). *Arch Gen Psychiatry*, 60(1), 82–91.

Middlebrook, D.W. (1991). *Anne Sexton: A Biography* (p. 36). Boston: Houghton Mifflin.

Miklowitz, D.J., and Taylor, D.O. (2006). Family-focused treatment of the suicidal bipolar patient. *Bipolar Disord*, 8, 640–651.

Modestin, J., Pian, D.D., and Agarwall, P. (2005). Clozapine diminishes suicidal behavior: A retrospective evaluation of clinical record. *J Clin Psychiatry*, 66, 534–538.

Motto, J.A. (1975). The recognition and management of the suicidal patient. In F.F. Flach and S.C. Draghi (Eds.), *The Nature and Treatment of Depression* (pp. 229–254). New York: John Wiley & Sons.

Muller-Oerlinghausen, B., Muser-Causemann, B., and Volk, J. (1992a). Suicides and parasuicides in a high-risk patient group on and off lithium long-term medication. *J Affect Disord*, 25, 261–269.

Muller-Oerlinghausen, B., Berghofer, A., and Ahrens, B. (2003). The antisuicidal and mortality-reducing effect of lithium prophylaxis: Consequences for guidelines in clinical psychiatry. *Can J Psychiatry*, 48(7), 433–439.

Murphy, G.E. (1975). The physician's responsibility for suicide: II. Errors of omission. *Ann Intern Med*, 82(3), 305–309.

Murphy, G.E., Simons, A.D., Wetzel, R.D., and Lustman, P.J. (1984). Cognitive therapy and pharmacotherapy: Singly and together in the treatment of depression. *Arch Gen Psychiatry*, 41, 33–41.

Norton, B., and Whalley, L.J. (1984). Mortality of a lithium-treated population. *Br J Psychiatry*, 145, 277–282.

Nutt, D.J. (1999). Care of depressed patients with anxiety symptoms. *J Clin Psychiatry*, 60(Suppl. 17), 23–27; discussion, 46–48.

Olfson, M., Shaffer, D., Marcus, S.C., and Greenberg, T. (2003). Relationship between antidepressant medication treatment and suicide in adolescents. *Arch Gen Psychiatry*, 60(10), 978–982.

Olfson, M., Marcus, S.C., and Shaffer, D. (2006). Antidepressant drug therapy and suicide in severely depressed children and adults. *Arch Gen Psychiatry*, 63, 865–872.

Oquendo, M.A., Malone, K.M., Ellis, S.P., Sackeim, H.A., and Mann, J.J. (1999). Inadequacy of antidepressant treatment for patients with major depression who are at risk for suicidal behavior. *Am J Psychiatry*, 156(2), 190–194.

Oquendo, M.A., Galfalvy, H., Russo, S., Ellis, S.P., Grunebaum, M.F., Burke, A., and Mann, J.J. (2004). Prospective study of clinical predictors of suicidal acts after a major depressive episode in patients with major depressive disorder or bipolar disorder. *Am J Psychiatry*, 161(8), 1433–1441.

Osman, A., Gutierrez, P.M., Muehlenkamp, J.J., Dix-Richardson, F., Barrios, F.X., and Kopper, B.A. (2004). Suicide Resilience Inventory-25: Development and preliminary psychometric properties. *Psychol Rep*, 94(3 Pt. 2), 1349–1360.

Pirraglia, P.A., Stafford, R.S., and Singer, D.E. (2003). Trends in prescribing of selective serotonin reuptake inhibitors and other newer antidepressant agents in adult primary care. *Prim Care Companion J Clin Psychiatry*, 5(4), 153–157.

Pokorny, A.D. (1983). Prediction of suicide in psychiatric patients: Reports of a prospective study. *Arch Gen Psychiatry*, 40(3), 249–257.

Pokorny, L.J. (1991). A summary measure of client level of functioning: Progress and challenges for use within mental health agencies. *J Ment Health Adm*, 18(2), 80–87.

Prudic, J., and Sackeim, H.A. (1999). Electroconvulsive therapy and suicide risk. *J Clin Psychiatry*, 60(Suppl. 2), 104–110; discussion, 111–116.

Reid, W.H., Mason, M., and Hogan, T. (1998). Suicide prevention effects associated with clozapine therapy in schizophrenia and schizoaffective disorder. *Psychiatr Serv*, 49(8), 1029–1033.

Rihmer, Z. (2004). Decreasing national suicide rates—fact or fiction? *World J Biol Psychiatry*, 5, 55–56.

Rihmer, Z., Rutz, W., and Pihlgren, H. (1995). Depression and suicide on Gotland. An intensive study of all suicides before and after a depression-training programme. *J Affect Disord*, 35, 147–152.

Robins, E., Murphy, G.E., Wilkinson, R.H., Gassner, S., and Kayes, J. (1959). Some clinical considerations in the prevention of suicide based on a study of 134 successful suicides. *Am J Public Health*, 49, 888–899.

Robins, L.N., Helzer, J.E., Croughan, J., and Ratcliff, K.S. (1981). National Institute of Mental Health Diagnostic Interview Schedule: Its history, characteristics, and validity. *Arch Gen Psychiatry*, 38, 381–389.

Roose, S.P., Glassman, A.H., Walsh, B.T., Woodring, S., and Vital-Herne, J. (1983). Depression, delusions, and suicide. *Am J Psychiatry*, 140, 1159–1162.

Rothschild, A.J., and Locke, C.A. (1991). Reexposure to fluoxetine after serious suicide attempts by three patients: The role of akathisia. *J Clin Psychiatry*, 52(12), 491–493.

Roy, A. (1982). Risk factors for suicide in psychiatric patients. *Arch Gen Psychiatry*, 39, 1089–1095.

Rucci, P., Frank, E., Kostelnik, B., Fagiolini, A., Mallinger, A.G., Swartz, H.A., Thase, M.E., Siegel, L., Wilson, D., and Kupfer, D.J. (2002). Suicide attempts in patients with bipolar I disorder during acute and maintenance phases of intensive treatment with pharmacotherapy and adjunctive psychotherapy. *Am J Psychiatry*, 159(7), 1160–1164.

Rush, B. (1812). *Medical Inquiries and Observations upon the Diseases of the Mind*. Philadelphia: Kimber and Richardson.

Sachs, G.S. (2006). A review of agitation in mental illness: Burden of illness and underlying pathology. *J Clin Psychiatry*, 67(Suppl. 10), 5–12.

Schatzberg, A.F. (1998). Noradrenergic versus serotonergic antidepressants: Predictors of treatment response. *J Clin Psychiatry*, 59(Suppl. 14), 15–18.

Sernyak, M.J., Desai, R., Stolar, M., and Rosenheck, R. (2001). Impact of clozapine on completed suicide. *Am J Psychiatry*, 158(6), 931–937.

Sharma, V. (1999). Retrospective controlled study of inpatient ECT: Does it prevent suicide? *J Affect Disord*, 56(2–3), 183–187.

Sharma, V. (2001). Loss of response to antidepressants and subsequent refractoriness: Diagnostic issues in a retrospective case series. *J Affect Disord*, 64(1), 99–106.

Sheard, M.H. (1975). Effect of lithium on human aggression. *Nature*, 230, 113–114.

Shi, L., Thieband, P., and McCombs, J.S. (2004). The impact of unrecognized bipolar disorders for patients treated with depression with antidepressants in the fee-for-services California Medicaid (Medi-Cal) programme. *J Affect Disord*, 82, 373–383.

Simon, G.E., Savarino, J., Operskalski, B., and Wang, P.S. (2006). Suicide risk during antidepressant treatment. *Am J Psychiatry*, 163, 41–47.

Smith, W.T., Londborg, P.D., Glaudin, V., and Painter, J.R. (2002). Summit research: Is extended clonazepam cotherapy of fluoxetine effective for outpatients with major depression? *J Affect Disord*, 70(3), 251–259.

Soomro, G.M. (2004). Deliberate self harm. *Clin Evid*, (12), 1348–1360.

Storosum, J.G., Elferink, A.J., van Zwieten, B.J., van Strik, R., Hoogendijk, W.J., and Broekmans, A.W. (2002). Amisulpride: Is there a treatment for negative symptoms in schizophrenia patients? *Schizophr Bull*, 28(2), 193–201.

Teicher, M.H., Glod, C.A., and Cole, J.O. (1990). Emergence of intense suicidal preoccupation during fluoxetine treatment. *Am J Psychiatry*, 147(2), 207–210.

Teicher, M.H., Glod, C.A., and Cole, J.O. (1993). Antidepressant drugs and the emergence of suicidal tendencies. *Drug Saf*, 8(3), 186–212.

Tiihonen, J., Lönnqvist, J., Wahlbeck, K., Klaukka, T., Tanskanen, A., and Haukka, J. (2006). Antidepressants and the risk of suicide, attempted suicide, and overall mortality in a nationwide cohort. *Arch Gen Psychiatry*, 63, 1358–1367.

Tondo, L., and Baldessarini, R.J. (2000). Reduced suicide risk during lithium maintenance treatment. *J Clin Psychiatry*, 61(Suppl. 9), 97–104.

Tran, P.V., Dellva, M.A., Tollefson, G.D., Wentley, A.L., and Beasley, C.M. (1998). Oral olanzapine versus oral haloperidol in the maintenance treatment of schizophrenia and related psychoses. *Br J Psychiatry*, 172, 499–505.

Treiser, S.L., Cascio, C.S., O'Donohue, T.L., Thoa, N.B., Jacobowitz, D.M., and Kellar, K.J. (1981). Lithium increases serotonin release and decreases serotonin receptors in the hippocampus. *Science*, 213, 1529–1531.

U.S. Food and Drug Administration (FDA). (2004). T.A. Hammad (Ed.), *Relationship between Psychotropic Drugs and Pediatric Suicidality: Review and Evaluation of Clinical Data*. Available: http://www.fda.gov/ohrms/dockets/ac/04/briefing/2004-4065b1-10-TAB08-Hammads-Review.pdf (accessed September 19, 2006).

U.S. Public Health Service. (1999). *The Surgeon General's Call to Action to Prevent Suicide*. Washington, DC: Department of Health and Human Services.

Vestergaard, P., and Aagaard, J. (1991). Five-year mortality in lithium-treated manic-depressive patients. *J Affect Disord*, 21, 33–38.

Wagner, K.D., Robb, A.S., Findling, R.L., Jin, J., Gutierrez, M.M., and Heydorn, W.E. (2004). A randomized, placebo-controlled trial of citalopram for the treatment of major depression in children and adolescents. *Am J Psychiatry*, 161, 1079–1083.

Walker, A.M., Lanza, L.L., Arellano, F., and Rothman, K.J. (1997). Mortality in current and former users of clozapine. *Epidemiology*, 8(6), 671–677.

Weeke, A. (1979). Causes of death in manic-depressives. In M. Schou and E. Strömgren (Eds.), *Origin, Prevention and Treatment of Affective Disorders* (pp. 289–299). London: Academic Press.

West, L.J. (1975). Integrative psychotherapy of depressive illness. In F.F. Flach and S.C. Draghi (Eds.), *The Nature and Treatment of Depression*. New York: John Wiley & Sons.

Winokur, G., Clayton, P.J., and Reich, T. (1969). *Manic Depressive Illness*. St. Louis: CV Mosby.

Wolf, T., Muller-Oerlinghausen, B., Ahrens, B., Grof, P., Schou, M., Feiber, W., Grof, E., Lenz, G., Nilsson, A., Simhandl, C., Thau, K., Vestergaard, P., and Wolf, R. (1996). How to interpret findings on mortality of long-term lithium treated manic-depressive patients? Critique of different methodological approaches. *J Affect Disord*, 39, 127–132.

Yerevanian, B.I., Koek, R.J., and Mintz, J. (2003). Lithium, anticonvulsants and suicidal behavior in bipolar disorder. *J Affect Disord*, 73, 223–228.

Zito, J.M., Safer, D.J., dosReis, S., Gardner, J.F., Magder, L., Soeken, K., Boles, M., Lynch, F., and Riddle, M.A. (2003). Psychotropic practice patterns for youth: A 10-year perspective. *Arch Pediatr Adolesc Med*, 157(1), 17–25.

Index

Note: Page numbers followed by the letter b refer to boxes, those followed by f refer to figures, and those followed by t refer to tables.